FUNDAMENTALS

PERSPECTIVES ON THE ART AND SCIENCE OF CANADIAN NURSING

FUNDAMENTALS

PERSPECTIVES ON THE ART AND SCIENCE OF CANADIAN NURSING

DAVID GREGORY, RN, PhD
Dean, Faculty of Nursing
University of Regina
Regina, Saskatchewan

CHRISTY RAYMOND-SENIUK, RN, BScN, MEd, PhD (candidate)
Instructor, Faculty of Health and Community Studies
MacEwan University
Edmonton, Alberta

LINDA PATRICK, RN, PhD
Dean, Faculty of Nursing
University of Windsor
Windsor, Ontario

TRACEY STEPHEN, BScN, MN, RN
Faculty Lecturer, Faculty of Nursing
University of Alberta
Edmonton, Alberta

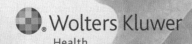
Wolters Kluwer
Health

Philadelphia • Baltimore • New York • London
Buenos Aires • Hong Kong • Sydney • Tokyo

Acquisitions Editor: Sherry Dickinson
Product Development Editor: Annette Ferran
Development Editor: Barbara Price
Editorial Assistant: Dan Reilly
Production Project Manager: Joan Sinclair
Design Coordinator: Joan Wendt
Illustration Coordinator: Jennifer Clements
Marketing Manager: Dean Karampelas
Manufacturing Coordinator: Karin Duffield
Prepress Vendor: Absolute Service, Inc.

9 8 7 6 5 4 3 2

Printed in China

Library of Congress Cataloging-in-Publication Data

Fundamentals (Gregory)
  Fundamentals : perspectives on the art and science of Canadian nursing / [edited by] David Gregory, Christy Raymond-Seniuk, Linda Patrick, Tracey C. Stephen.
    p. ; cm.
  Perspectives on the art and science of Canadian nursing
  Includes bibliographical references and index.
  ISBN 978-1-60547-090-0 (alk. paper)
  I. Gregory, David Michael, 1958- editor. II. Raymond-Seniuk, Christy, editor. III. Patrick, Linda, editor. IV. Stephen, Tracey C., editor. V. Title. VI. Title: Perspectives on the art and science of Canadian nursing.
  [DNLM: 1. Nursing Process—Canada. 2. Education, Nursing—Canada. 3. Nurses—psychology—Canada. 4. Nursing—Canada. WY 100 DC2]
  RT81.C23
  610.73071'171—dc23
                                                                            2014007100

Care has been taken to confirm the accuracy of the information presented and to describe generally accepted practices. However, the authors, editors, and publisher are not responsible for errors or omissions or for any consequences from application of the information in this book and make no warranty, expressed or implied, with respect to the currency, completeness, or accuracy of the contents of the publication. Application of this information in a particular situation remains the professional responsibility of the practitioner; the clinical treatments described and recommended may not be considered absolute and universal recommendations.

The authors, editors, and publisher have exerted every effort to ensure that drug selection and dosage set forth in this text are in accordance with the current recommendations and practice at the time of publication. However, in view of ongoing research, changes in government regulations, and the constant flow of information relating to drug therapy and drug reactions, the reader is urged to check the package insert for each drug for any change in indications and dosage and for added warnings and precautions. This is particularly important when the recommended agent is a new or infrequently employed drug.

Some drugs and medical devices presented in this publication have Food and Drug Administration (FDA) clearance for limited use in restricted research settings. It is the responsibility of the health care provider to ascertain the FDA status of each drug or device planned for use in his or her clinical practice.

Contributors

Susan E. Anthony, RN, PhD
Assistant Professor, Arthur Labatt Family School of
    Nursing
Western University
London, Ontario

Velna Clarke Arnault, RN, MN
Aboriginal Nursing Student Advisor, Nursing
Saskatchewan Institute of Applied Arts and Sciences
Buffalo Narrows, Saskatchewan

Sherry Arvidson, RN, MN
Instructor, Faculty of Nursing
University of Regina
Regina, Saskatchewan

Karen Scott Barss, RPN, BHSc, MA
Faculty, Saskatchewan Collaborative Bachelor of Science in
    Nursing
Saskatchewan Institute of Applied Science and Technology
Undergraduate Adjunct Professor, University of Regina
Saskatoon, Saskatchewan

E. Joyce Black, RN, EdD
Senior Education Consultant, Registration, Inquiry
    and Discipline
College of Registered Nurses of British Columbia
Vancouver, British Columbia

Judy A. K. Bornais, RN, MSc, CDE
Experiential Learning Specialist, Faculty of Nursing
University of Windsor
Windsor, Ontario

Elizabeth Borycki, RN, PhD
Associate Professor, School of Health Information Science
University of Victoria
Victoria, British Columbia

Joan Bray, RN, BN, MEd
Holistic Nurse Educator and Clinical Consultant, Raven
    Brae Services Ltd.
Staff Nurse, Interior Health Authority
Home and Community Care
Cranbrook, British Columbia

Annette J. Browne, PhD, RN
Professor, School of Nursing
University of British Columbia
Vancouver, British Columbia

Seanna Chesney-Chauvet, RN, MN
Faculty Lecturer, Faculty of Nursing
University of Alberta
Edmonton, Alberta

Andrea Chute, RN, BN, MN
Instructor, Faculty of Health and Community Studies
MacEwan University
Edmonton, Alberta

Donna K. Ciliska, RN, PhD
Professor, School of Nursing
McMaster University
Hamilton, Ontario

Roni L. Clubb, RN, MScN
Faculty, Practical Nursing Program
Saskatchewan Institute of Applied Science and Technology
Regina, Saskatchewan

Laurie Clune, RN, BA, BScN, MEd, PhD
Associate Dean, Graduate Programs and Research
Faculty of Nursing
University of Regina
Regina, Saskatchewan

Catherine Cotter, RN, BScN
Nursing Practice Advisor, Policy, Practice and Quality Assurance
College of Registered Nurses of British Columbia
Vancouver, British Columbia

Betty Cragg, RN, EdD
Professor Emeritus, School of Nursing
University of Ottawa
Ottawa, Ontario

Michelle L. Cullen, BN
Nursing Practice Instructor, Faculty of Nursing
University of Calgary
Registered Nurse, Child and Adolescent Mental Health
South Health Campus
Calgary, Alberta

William Diehl-Jones, RN, PhD
Associate Professor, Faculty of Health Disciplines
Athabasca University
Athabasca, Alberta

Elizabeth L. Domm, RN, PhD
Assistant Professor, Faculty of Nursing
University of Regina
Regina, Saskatchewan

Glenn Donnelly, RN, ENC,BScN MN, PhD
Associate Professor, Faculty of Nursing
University of Regina
Regina, Saskatchewan

Kathryn A. Edmunds, RN, PhD(c)
Adjunct Assistant Professor, Faculty of Nursing
University of Windsor
Windsor, Ontario

Colette Foisy-Doll
Faculty of Nursing, Professional Resource Faculty,
    Clinical Simulation Centre
MacEwan University
Edmonton, Alberta

Debbie Fraser, MN, RNC-NIC
Associate Professor, Faculty of Health Disciplines
Athabasca University
Athabasca, Alberta
Advanced Practice Nurse, Neonatal Intensive Care Unit
St. Boniface Hospital
Winnipeg, Manitoba

Michelle Freeman, PhD, RN, CPPS
Assistant Professor, Faculty of Nursing
University of Windsor
Windsor, Ontario

Noreen Cavan Frisch, PhD, RN, FAAN
Professor and Director, School of Nursing
University of Victoria
Victoria, British Columbia

David Gregory, RN, PhD
Dean, Faculty of Nursing
University of Regina
Regina, Saskatchewan

Melanie J. Hamilton, MN, BN, RN
NESA BN Programs Faculty, Theory Course Coordinator
NESA BN Program
Lethbridge College
Lethbridge, Alberta

B. Nicole Harder, RN, PhD
Assistant Professor, Faculty of Nursing
University of Manitoba
Winnipeg, Manitoba

Jean N. Harrowing, RN, BSc, MN, PhD
Associate Professor, Faculty of Health Sciences
University of Lethbridge
Lethbridge, Alberta

Joy L. Johnson, PhD, RN, FCAHS
Professor, School of Nursing
University of British Columbia
Vancouver, British Columbia

Peter Kellett, BN, MN, RN
Nursing Instructor III, Faculty of Health Sciences
University of Lethbridge
Lethbridge, Alberta

Kelly N. Kilgour, RN, MScN, CHPCN(c), PhD (candidate)
Professor, School of Nursing, Faculty of Health
    Sciences
University of Ottawa
Ottawa, Ontario

Sarah Kostiuk, BScN, RN, MN, EdD(c)
Faculty, Saskatchewan Collaborative Bachelor of Science
    in Nursing
Saskatchewan Institute of Applied Science and
    Technology
Regina, Saskatchewan

Mary Anne Krahn, RN, BScN, MScN
Collaborative Bachelor of Science in Nursing Program
    and Year Two Coordinator, School of Nursing
Faculty of Health Sciences, Human Services and
    Nursing
Fanshawe College
Adjunct Faculty, Western University
London, Ontario

How Lee, RN, MN
Faculty Lecturer, Faculty of Nursing
University of Alberta
Edmonton, Alberta

Sarah Lopez, RN, BScN, MScN (Student)
Clinical Instructor, Faculty of Nursing
University of Windsor
Registered Nurse, Family Birthing Centre
Windsor Regional Hospital
Windsor, Ontario

Marie Sherry McDonald, RN, BScN, MPS
Undergraduate Adjunct Professor, Saskatchewan
    Collaborative Bachelor of Science in Nursing
Saskatchewan Institute of Applied Science and Technology
Saskatoon, Saskatchewan

Amanda McEwen, RN, BScN, BSc (Honours Biology), MScN
(Student)
Clinical Instructor, Faculty of Nursing
University of Windsor
Windsor, Ontario

Pertice Moffitt, RN, BScN, MN, PhD
Manager, Health Research Programs, Aurora Research
    Institute
Aurora College, BAS Service 9700
Yellowknife, Northwest Territories

Nadine Moniz, RN, BScN, MN
Faculty Lecturer, Faculty of Nursing
University of Alberta
Edmonton, Alberta

Elaine Mordoch, RN, BN, MN, PhD
Assistant Professor, Faculty of Nursing
University of Manitoba
Winnipeg, Manitoba

Natasha L. Hubbard Murdoch, PhD(c), MN, CMSN(C), RN
Faculty, Saskatchewan Collaborative Bachelor of Science in
    Nursing
Saskatchewan Institute of Applied Science and Technology
Saskatoon, Saskatchewan

Sarah Painter, BN, RN
Registered Nurse, Emergency Department
Saint Boniface General Hospital
Winnipeg, Manitoba

Michèle Parent, RN, BN, MSc, PhD
Adjunct Professor, School of Nursing
Master of Science in Nursing Program
Laurentian University
Sudbury, Ontario

Barbara L. Paterson, RN, PhD
Adjunct Professor, School of Nursing
Thompson Rivers University
Kamloops, British Columbia

Linda Patrick, RN, PhD
Dean, Faculty of Nursing
University of Windsor
Windsor, Ontario

Bernadette M. Pauly, RN, PhD
Associate Professor, School of Nursing
Scientist, Centre for Addictions Research of British Columbia
University of Victoria
Victoria, British Columbia

Em M. Pijl-Zieber, BScN, MEd, RN, PhD (candidate)
Nursing Instructor, Faculty of Health Sciences
University of Lethbridge
Lethbridge, Alberta

Joanne Profetto-McGrath, PhD, MEd, BScN, BA (Psych), RN
Professor and Vice Dean, Faculty of Nursing
University of Alberta
Edmonton, Alberta

Bonnie Raisbeck, RN, BScN, MN
Faculty Member, Nursing Division
Saskatchewan Institute of Applied Science and Technology
Regina, Saskatchewan

Christy Raymond-Seniuk, RN, BScN, MEd, PhD (candidate)
Instructor, Faculty of Health and Community Studies
MacEwan University
Edmonton, Alberta

Sandra Regan, RN, PhD
Assistant Professor, Arthur Labatt Family School of Nursing
Western University
London, Ontario

Debbie Rickeard, RN, MSN
Experiential Learning Specialist, Faculty of Nursing
University of Windsor
Staff Nurse, Cardiac Care Unit
Windsor Regional Hospital - Ouellette Campus
Windsor, Ontario

Elizabeth C. Robertson, BA, LLB
Legal Counsel (Retired), Alberta Law Reform Institute
Law Centre
University of Alberta
Edmonton, Alberta

Kathleen S. Rodger, RN, BSN, MN, CMSN (C)
Faculty, Saskatchewan Collaborative Bachelor of Science in
    Nursing
Saskatchewan Institute of Applied Science and Technology
University of Regina
Regina, Saskatchewan

Kathryn Rousseau, BA, MScN, RN
Professor, School of Nursing
St. Clair College
Windsor, Ontario

Joan Samuels-Dennis, RN, BScN, MSc, PhD
Assistant Professor, School of Nursing
York University
Toronto, Ontario

Lynn Sheridan, BScN, MHSc, MDDE
Faculty Member, Saskatchewan Collaboration Bachelor
    Science Nursing, Simulation Learning Centre,
    Occupational Health and Safety Practitioner Program
Saskatchewan Institute Applied Science Technology
Saskatoon, Saskatchewan

Julie Stanton, BScN, MSc, RN
Faculty Lecturer, Faculty of Nursing
University of Alberta
Edmonton, Alberta

Tracey Stephen, BScN, MN, RN
Faculty Lecturer, Faculty of Nursing
University of Alberta
Edmonton, Alberta

Claire Tellier, MN, RN
Faculty Lecturer, Faculty of Nursing
University of Alberta
Edmonton, Alberta

Colleen Varcoe, RN, PhD
Professor, School of Nursing
University of British Columbia
Vancouver, British Columbia

Michael J. Villeneuve, RN, MSc
Lecturer, Lawrence S. Bloomberg Faculty of Nursing
University of Toronto
Toronto, Ontario

Joan I. J. Wagner, RN, PhD
Assistant Professor, Faculty of Nursing
University of Regina
Regina, Saskatchewan

P. Susan Wagner
Professor Emeritus, College of Nursing
University of Saskatchewan
Saskatoon, Saskatchewan

Nancy Walton, BScN, RN, PhD
Director, e-Learning
Associate Professor, Daphne Cockwell School of Nursing
Ryerson University
Toronto, Ontario

Fjola Hart Wasekeesikaw, RN, MN
Executive Director
Aboriginal Nurses Association of Canada
Ottawa, Ontario

Christine Wellington, RD, MS, BSc
Adjunct Assistant Professor, Department of Family
    Medicine
Sessional Instructor, Family Medicine
Faculty of Nursing
Schulich School of Medicine and Dentistry
University of Windsor
Windsor, Ontario

Leanne J. Wyrostok, MN, BN, RN
Senior Instructor (Emeritus), Faculty of Nursing
University of Calgary
Calgary, Alberta

Lynne E. Young, PhD, RN
Professor, School of Nursing
University of Victoria
Victoria, British Columbia

*For a list of the contributors to the Student and Instructor
Resources accompanying this book, please visit* the**Point**.

Reviewers

Anna Boyechko
North Island College
Vancouver Island, British Columbia

Dianne Brown, RN, BScN, MN, GDID
Coordinator, Curriculum Development and
    Quality Assurance
Educator & Instructional Designer
Department of Nursing
Red River College
Winnepeg, Manitoba

Elaine Bush-Simmons
Fleming College
Peterborough, Ontario

Shari Cherney
George Brown College
Toronto, Ontario

Sharon Chin, RN, MHScN, CPMHN(c)
Professor of Nursing
Nipissing University
Collaborative Bachelor of Science in Nursing Program
Canadore College
North Bay, Ontario

Vlad Chiriac
Paramedic Program
Durham College
Oshawa, Ontario

Judith Findlay, RN, BScN, MEd
Nursing Instructor
John Abbott College
Sainte-Anne-de-Bellevue, Quebec

Karen Fletcher, RN, MN, CON(C)
Instructor II, Faculty of Nursing
University of Manitoba
Winnipeg, Manitoba

Katherine Fukuyama, RN, BSN, MEd, EdD
Department Head, Bachelor of Science in Nursing Program
Vancouver Community College
Vancouver, British Columbia

Joanne Gullison, RN, BScN
Instructor, Practical Nurse and Personal Support Worker
    Programs
New Brunswick Community College
Fredericton, New Brunswick

Judy Hainstock, RN, BScN, MN
Coordinator, LPN Program (retired)
Kingstec Campus, Nova Scotia Community College
Kentville, Nova Scotia

*For a list of the reviewers of the Test Generator accompanying
this book, please visit* thePoint.

Preface

Nursing is a dynamic profession that is all-at-once rewarding and challenging. Nurses enact many complex roles and responsibilities in the provision of care. Their work ultimately fosters a greater level of health for all. Nursing students are also an important and influential part of nursing, illuminating the vital importance of curiosity, commitment, and courage along lifelong learning paths. Nurse educators inspire learners and journey with them. And thus, a great responsibility in the formation of what it is to "be a nurse" is shared between the teacher and the learner. And it is in this educator–learner relationship that the possibility of transformation is realized. We offer this textbook in support of and to honor nurses, educators, scholars, and students whose professional and personal lives intersect with an extraordinary profession: nursing.

When we first conceptualized this textbook, we thought it should be, foremost, a learner-centered resource that spoke to, and with, each individual about the adventure and excitement of nursing practice. We viewed learners as individuals in various stages of their careers, including students experiencing their first exposure to nursing through our textbook as well as experienced nurses looking to refresh their knowledge about the foundations of care. We committed to the creation of a Canadian textbook that represented nursing perspectives from all parts of Canada; such perspectives embody the richness of nursing in such a diverse, unique, and vast country.

Fundamentals: Perspectives on the Art and Science of Canadian Nursing is a fully Canadian, newly developed textbook that explores the multifaceted role of the nurse along a lifelong learning journey. All of the content in this textbook has been developed by talented Canadian students, nurses, scholars, and educators who share a passion for representing the realities of Canadian nursing and nursing education. The voice used by all of the contributors in this textbook speaks to the uniqueness of Canadian nursing. It is an authentic voice, encouraging students to discover the art and science of a profession.

Fundamentals: Perspectives on the Art and Science of Canadian Nursing is uniquely organized. We have categorized the chapters into clusters that represent processes of a learning continuum in nursing, represented by the five units of Knowing, Thinking, Being, Interacting, and Understanding. We have purposefully scaffolded the content in the five units; each chapter builds on previous chapters in the textbook to promote an integrated understanding of nursing fundamentals.

- **Knowing:** The authors of the chapters in the "Knowing" unit offer important information and provide foundational knowledge on which nursing practice is built. The content in this unit offers key insights into the unique historical and present context of nursing in Canada today.
- **Thinking:** Authors of the chapters in the "Thinking" unit offer content unique to current nursing practice. These are chapters that provide specific foundational and highly applicable knowledge for nursing practice. The chapters will cause students to pause and "think" about nursing and their future place in the profession. Whereas the chapters in the initial "Knowing" unit provide the broad foundation on which nursing as a health profession exists, these chapters are focused on specific foundational issues.
- **Being:** The authors of chapters in the "Being" unit address more broad integrative skills, assessments, and knowledge that nurses incorporate into their daily practice while in a variety of roles and settings. This unit includes specific skill-related chapters.
- **Interacting:** Authors of chapters in the "Interacting" unit introduce content that builds on the "Being" chapters (i.e., from more broad-based skills, we move into the realm of more complex and detailed interventions that require concurrent application of the knowledge from the previous unit). Furthermore, authors emphasize the relational aspect of nursing whereby students are encouraged to apply Knowing, Thinking, and Being all at once. This unit also focuses on how the nurse interacts with others in the health-care setting.
- **Understanding:** Finally, in our last unit, "Understanding," authors present a series of unique contextual and compelling chapters, which provide insight into the current place nursing occupies while also looking ahead to where nurses can take the profession. This is the unit where authors share their expertise on the "reality" of nursing practice in Canada today and the unique challenges that go along with this practice. Although grounding the previous units in the reality of Canada today, these chapters also provide a forward-looking perspective, acknowledging the diversity and dynamic nature of nursing and the populations for which we, as nurses, provide care.

*J*onathan is a second-year nursing student starting his first medical-surgical clinical placement. He reads the course outline and wonders what it will be like giving medications. Jonathan is worried about the difficulty of this skill and wonders how he might learn the steps necessary to master this skill.

We have also included exciting features in each chapter that emphasize important content, perspectives, and thinking skills.

Case Study

Each chapter introduces and follows a nursing student or patient, presented in a "Case Study," (shown above) whose case exemplifies the information and issues covered in the chapter. The Case Study helps bring theoretical concepts into the real world, illustrating what it might be like to be a nursing student or nurse caring for a real patient with real human attributes, conditions, and needs.

Think Boxes

The "Think" box feature facilitates critical thinking skills and gives learners opportunities to take what they know and apply it to different situations. The goal of the "Think" box is to stimulate the reader to think "outside the box" and explore different perspectives. These boxes appear in most chapters, as appropriate, and pose important questions to guide critical inquiry into the identified issue or practice. Because thinking critically is an important feature of the nursing role, Think boxes bring important content to life and help with application and prioritization of knowledge.

 Think *Implications of Food Intolerances on Medication Administration*

Patient allergies and intolerances of food can cause catastrophic events post administration. These allergies should be well documented before medication administration. The most frequently experienced allergies in food such as peanuts, shellfish, soy, eggs, nuts, and dyes as well as intolerances to such items as gluten, lactose, and soy can be experienced with medication administration as many contain these very items. Although there are no concrete guidelines to ensuring that patients do not have certain allergies or intolerances to medications prior to their administration, it is important for the practitioner to know the food allergies and intolerances that the patient has in order to question whether the medications are appropriate for that individual. As well, it is important to know which medications pose an allergy or intolerance risk in order to better screen patients for potentially serious reactions. Although many parents of small children and adults know food items to which they are allergic, many do not often mention the intolerances they have to certain foods or ingredients. Asking patients about allergies as well as intolerances will elicit more useful information than just questioning about allergies alone.

"Through the Eyes" Features

Given the diverse realities found in Canadian nursing, a key innovative feature we use in this text is the emphasis on multiple perspectives. The varying viewpoints represented in this feature include those of students, nurses, and patients, highlighting the critical understanding of varying perceptions on different issues. "Through the eyes of a student" validates the need to appreciate and honor the student perspective, one which embodies learning, curiosity, and courage. This perspective also affirms nurses as "lifelong learners" in the nursing profession and emphasizes the importance of reflective nursing practice. "Through the eyes of a nurse" showcases the experience and professional growth apparent among expert nurses. This feature often addresses how a nurse thinks and deals with challenges of nursing practice in a variety of settings. We round out this feature by looking "Through the eyes of a patient." This patient-centered features emphasizes the important viewpoint of the patient and/or patient's family in care interactions or during caring interventions. This feature reminds us that the patient has a unique perception of our care. These personal accounts demonstrate how effective nursing care can make a difference in the lives of patients and their families.

Through the eyes of a nurse

I am always nervous on Day 1 when students are giving medications for the first time. I think that there is so much stress in the medication room; this tension doesn't really help a student learn. The students who spend most of their time copying and memorizing the drug book and not really thinking about their patients and why they need the medication are often the most nervous. It is really important that students are prepared and understand the rationale for the medications they are administering as well as basic information about how they work and possible side effects. Learning medications takes time, and nursing instructors have the ability and capacity to really foster calmness in a student.

(personal reflection of a nurse)

Research

Where possible, the "Research" feature is used to illuminate cutting-edge and/or pertinent Canadian research that directly affects health-care practice today. This feature focuses on an important aspect of health care or nursing education that impacts nursing practice. Authors address the specific nursing implications of Canadian research studies they feature to promote the application of research into nursing care and foster, in part, the development of evidence-informed practice.

RESEARCH
MEDICATION RECONCILIATION

Adverse events in medication administration can result in serious consequences for both the patient and health-care provider. Understanding medication prescription and administration practices, policies, and procedures

Nursing Skills

This feature is not evident in every chapter but is used mainly in the skill-related chapters. To outline each of the included skills, knowledge in this feature is organized using five main headings.

1. Reviewing Pertinent Information
2. Preparing for (the skill)
3. The name of the actual skill (e.g., in the medication chapter, the heading reads "Administering the Medication")
4. Engaging in Evaluation
5. Documenting Effectively

This feature (shown below) includes effectively placed pictures to help support learner-friendly application of the chapter information.

At the end of every chapter, valuable resources are listed to assist the reader in further application of the text content. These features include the following:

- **Critical Thinking Case Scenarios.** These present real-life situations encouraging the reader to think critically and focus on pertinent material.

- **Multiple-Choice Questions.** Questions that emphasize critical material are also included at the end of each chapter. These questions have been developed to help learners explore their understanding of the knowledge covered in the chapter. The answers to these questions are provided as an Instructor Resource on **thePoint**.
- **Suggested Lab Activities.** These activities (based on chapter content) consist of ideas for encouraging active learning in a skills lab, class room, or small group setting.
- **References and Suggested Readings.** Important information sources are included in the reference section of each chapter. In this section, authors have included references used to write each chapter, along with suggested readings, which are helpful for learners to explore the topic further.

The constellation of multiple features in this textbook makes it a valuable learning tool. More specifically, we offer a unique organization of content that focuses on a purposeful learning continuum, a student-engaged voice and writing style that will speak to various learners, and the inclusion of quality features aimed at making application and understanding of the material rewarding and fun. The additional emphasis on Canadian realities and diverse issues that directly impact nursing care in Canada enhances this textbook's ability to represent cross-Canadian perspectives on important foundational issues in nursing. We hope readers enjoy their journey through this textbook as much as we have enjoyed facilitating its creation.

Resources for Instructors and Students

Instructors and students can visit **thePoint** at http://thepoint .lww.com/Gregory1e for resources to support teaching and learning. For instructors, available tools to assist you with teaching your course include the following:

- An Image Bank, which lets you use the photographs and illustrations from this textbook in your lecture slides, class handouts, or as you see fit in your course

SKILL 22.1	Administering Oral Medications
Reviewing Pertinent Information	
Step	**Rationale**
Review the medication(s) ordered from the medication record or patient chart.	Important to know why the patient is receiving the medication, if the medication is appropriate for the patient's situation, and actual appropriateness of the dose and route ordered
Review patient allergies to medications and food products.	Some food products are found in medications and can cause an allergic reaction as well as medication allergic reaction to the active medicinal ingredient.
Review the applicable pharmacological principles of the medication including the onset and duration of action.	Knowing the pharmacological mechanism of action can aid in monitoring for therapeutic and adverse effects of the medication. This information is also useful when teaching your patient the expected outcome(s) of the medication.
Review pertinent lab results pertaining to the medication indication for your patient.	Lab and diagnostic results offer more information into why the patient is receiving the medication and if the medication is having a therapeutic or adverse effect.

- Answers to the end-of-chapter multiple-choice questions in the book, which you can release to your students to help them in their studies, or use to assess their responses to the questions
- A robust Test Generator of NCLEX-style questions, written by a subject matter expert and professional test question writer, lets you put together exclusive new tests to help you in assessing your students' understanding of the material.
- You also have access to the resources provided for students.

For students, available study aids and additional learning opportunities include the following:

- Watch & Learn and Practice & Learn videos, which demonstrate key nursing skills and practices
- Concepts in Action animations, which visually illustrate some of the more complex concepts of the medical science behind nursing care
- Journal articles on recent research studies relevant to the chapter content
- Web resources selected by the chapter authors to give you access to a wider body of information
- Assorted readings and resources of interest for select chapters

Acknowledgments

We would like to acknowledge the many individuals who are responsible for making this textbook a reality. From conceptualization to publication, we would like to thank our families, students, colleagues, contributors, reviewers, and the publication team from Wolters Kluwer Health, Lippincott Williams & Wilkins. This textbook would not have been possible without their support, dedication, and belief in its existence.

We have had the pleasure of working with many individuals throughout this process, including Barry Wight and Corey Wolfe, who originally planted the seed which led to the germination of a Canadian fundamentals textbook. We are grateful to the publication team and those who supported it, including Annette Ferran, Jean Findley, Barbara Price, and Harold Medina, making miracles happen amidst all the challenges that face a new textbook.

The students were truly the impetus that led us to consider the possibility of such a textbook. Thank you for providing us with your treasured gifts of learning.

To our contributors, your patience and perseverance are remarkable, along with your ability to share your knowledge and passion for nursing.

—david Gregory
—Christy Raymond-Seniuk
—Linda Patrick
—Tracey C. Stephen

The book is there for inspiration and as a foundation, the fundamentals on which to build.
Thomas Keller

NANDA-I content in this book is from Nursing Diagnoses – Definitions and Classifications, 2012–2014. Copyright 2012, 1994–2012 by NANDA International. Used by arrangement with John Wiley and Sons Limited.

Contents

unit three

Being   339

chapter 19

chapter 20

chapter 21

chapter 41

Nursing as Lifelong Learning 1093

one

Knowing

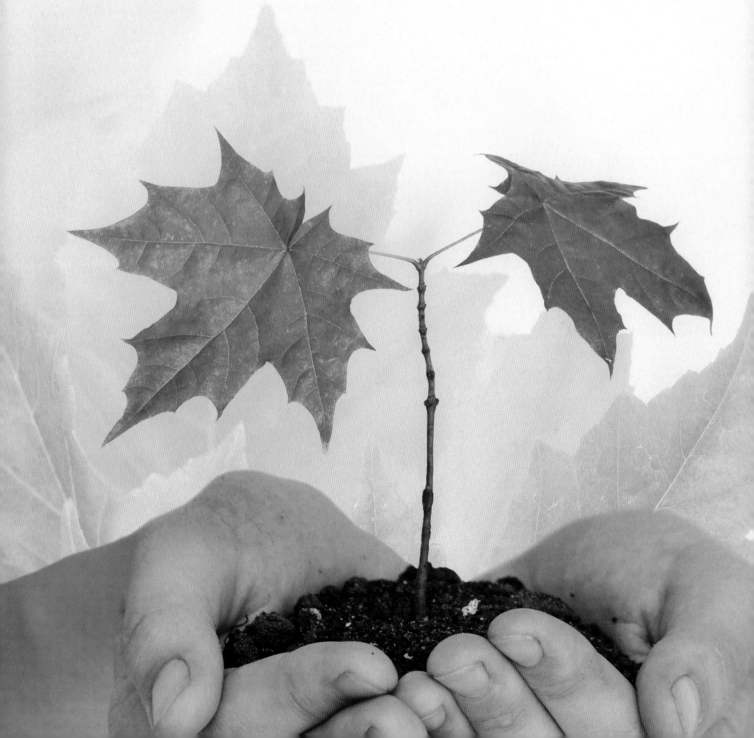

An Introduction to Canadian Nursing

DAVID GREGORY, CHRISTY RAYMOND-SENIUK,
LINDA PATRICK, AND TRACEY STEPHEN

Mike and Britney are first-year nursing students. They sat beside each other during their mandatory program orientation during the first week of September. Mike wonders if nursing is the right career choice. He has never heard of men as nurses. He was relieved to see some other fellows at the orientation session. Britney's mother is a nurse. Her mother was not very encouraging of her to enter nursing. However, Britney is convinced that nursing is right for her. After the orientation, they meet for a coffee to talk about nursing and their program. They both have their fundamentals textbook with them. Mike wants to learn more about men in nursing. Britney wants to know more about the realities of nursing in Canada and why her mother was hesitant to recommend that she consider nursing as a career.

CHAPTER OBJECTIVES

By the end of this chapter, you will be able to:

1. Identify the social forces that are serving as agents of change for nursing education and practice.
2. Discuss the relevancy of nursing history with respect to contemporary nursing.
3. Identify some of the early nursing leaders and their respective contributions to the nursing profession.
4. Discern how societal perceptions of women, historical and current, influence the public's perception of nurses and the nursing profession.
5. Describe some of the issues faced by men and other minorities in nursing.
6. Articulate dimensions of the art and the science of nursing.
7. Reflect on the nurse–patient relationship and the complexity that characterizes it.

Put the patient in the best condition for nature to act upon him.

—NIGHTINGALE, 1860/1969, p. 133

Caring is the most common criterion of humanness. . . . No discipline is seen to be so directly and intimately involved in caring needs and behaviours as nursing. . . . Nursing is (in essence) the professionalization of caring.

—ROACH, 1992, p. 11

Both the healthcare system and nursing are at a crossroad. Nursing can and should become a major player in turning the healthcare system around. Nurses can do so by providing the vision, creating the direction and leading the way. As the healthcare system transforms itself, nursing faces a choice. It can wait to see how things unfold and how nurses will fit into the new system once it takes shape; or, nursing can lead the way. The profession can do so by setting forth a new vision rooted in nursing values of holism and restoring the centrality of the nurse-person relationship as expressed through a strengths-based approach.

—GOTTLIEB, GOTTLIEB, AND SHAMIAN, 2012, p. 47

The Changing Face of Health Care and Nursing in Canada

Florence Nightingale, considered the founder of modern-day nursing, precipitated a revolution in the education and practice of nursing. Sister Simone Roach, a recipient of the Order of Canada, enacted major reform in nursing through her work on ethics and her theory of caring. She oversaw the development of the first ever Canadian code of ethics for Canadian nurses. Dr. Laurie Gottlieb, editor-in-chief of the *Canadian Journal of Nursing Research*, and Dr. Judith Shamian, former president of the Canadian Nurses Association and the second Canadian president of the International Council of Nursing, observed that our Canadian health-care system and nursing are at a crossroads.

Expert nurses from across Canada have collectively written this textbook to offer the essential knowledge and skills that will assist you as you start your nursing journey. In addition to fundamentals, we want you to learn about the realities of nursing; this includes an honest account of Canadian nursing. You will be introduced to the domains of practice that includes education, clinical, research, and policy/administration.

Transforming Nursing Education

That the health-care system needs to change is a reality in Canada. Accompanying the urgency to transform the Canadian health-care system is the clarion call by nurse leaders and educators from across the globe for revolution in registered nurse (RN) education and practice in Canada. Commissioned by the Canadian Nurses Association, the National Expert Commission's call to action recommends a 9-point action plan (Canadian Nurses Association, 2012). One of the recommendations concerns the need to prepare service providers (including RNs) differently, with new topics, teaching methods, science, and research to match the transformation of the Canadian health-care system. In response to Commission's report, a think tank was held at the Dalhousie University School of Nursing (MacMillan, 2013), finding there is a need to transform undergraduate nursing education, with particular attention paid to curriculum and pedagogy, generalist and specialist education, interprofessional education, and safety and quality (MacMillan, 2013). "Just as pressing . . . is the need to give renewed focus to the *fundamentals of care* in undergraduate nursing education and in the transition to practice" (MacMillan, 2013, p. 11). Both reports are clear: There is a need for change.

This fundamentals text presents the realities of Canadian nursing. You are entering nursing education at a time of significant change. You will not only learn the fundamentals of nursing care but also learn about teaching, pedagogy, generalist and specialist education, interprofessional education, patient and cultural safety, and the ethical foundations of quality nursing practice. You will come to experience first-hand how the Canadian Association of Schools of Nursing (CASN), the Canadian Nurses Association, the Canadian Council of Registered Nurses Regulators, and schools and faculties of nursing are transforming the education of RNs.

There are many good things about being a nurse and the nursing profession. No other health profession touches the lives of patients, clients, families, and communities globally like nursing, and none is more trusted by members of society. A recent Gallup Poll reveals that nurses have the highest honesty and ethical standards rating among 22 professions (Newport, 2012). You should know that nursing consistently outranks physicians, pharmacists, police officers, firefighters, and minister in terms of public trust. Despite such trust accorded to the profession by society, there are also disputes, difficulties, and disappointments within the profession and in relation to the health-care system. We come back to these issues later in this chapter and reflect on them throughout the book.

Developing a Foundation

To develop a foundational understanding of Canadian nursing, you will need to learn a brief history of the profession; about the sociocultural, environmental, and political contexts

in which nursing takes place; and the extraordinary changes that have occurred in nursing since the advent of the millennium. You will come to understand and recognize the many factors that impact nurses and nursing in the 21st century. You will encounter more detailed accounts of these and other issues and trends in Canadian nursing in Years 3 and 4 of your nursing program. The same social, economic, and political events that have shaped Canada's unique experience and position in the global community have also influenced nursing. In turn, nursing has evolved alongside these national and global events, adapting to the changing needs of individuals, families, and communities with responsiveness and relevance. Nurses and nursing were participants from the colonization of the New World, to the sexual revolution, to severe acute respiratory syndrome (SARS), and the influenza A (H1N1) influenza outbreaks.

Our role as nurses, as clinicians, as agents, and as advocates of social change has developed over time. Over the last 100 years, nurses have transformed from being apprentice-like extensions of the physician's role to being independent, collaborative, and vital professionals with unique roles and responsibilities.

Why Consider Nursing?

Each of us has our own reason why we want to become a nurse. People enter nursing because they encountered a nurse during the care of a family member, relative, or friend and were inspired to consider nursing. For some students, a mother or father (aunt, uncle, brother, sister) was a nurse, so becoming a nurse was second nature to them. For others, it is simply a reasonable employment opportunity. Nursing unions across Canada have worked diligently to increase the pay and benefits associated with nursing. In terms of financial recompense (salary) and benefits, nursing has become a viable career option for many more men and women. However, most people become nurses, regardless of influences, out of a sense of concern and caring for people. They want to make a difference in the lives of others.

Through the eyes of a student

I decided to become a registered nurse because I wanted to help people. I want to make a different in their lives. I'm the first nurse in the family, and I'm very excited about the possibility of nursing as a career. *(personal reflection of a student)*

Nursing Across the Lifespan

Nurses are present at all life transitions, from birth to death, and by promoting the health of women even before they conceive, nurses work to improve the health of future generations. Nurses accompany patients who live with diseases or conditions, both chronic and acute, helping them to live as fully as possible despite their ailments. Nurses are there in the care of dying. Nurses are there promoting the health and well-being of clients, families, groups, and communities. Nurses come to know fully the human condition. Through encounters with patients and clients, they are empathic witnesses to joy and sorrow, life and death, and the frailty and resilience of the human body and spirit. Nurses are also present with patients and clients as highly educated, knowledgeable, ethical, and skilled care providers.

A Career in Nursing

There are astounding possibilities found within this remarkable and dynamic profession. It is just a matter of discovering where your talents, skills, and abilities are best applied. Over time and through the course of your nursing program, you will be exposed to many clinical practice settings, and you will discover an area of nursing practice that resonates with you.

Through the eyes of a student

I remember thinking that I had to be absolutely certain about where I was first employed in nursing. We were all thinking that this was a career decision. In the end, it wasn't, although I really did struggle with this decision. I talked with my professors, my clinical instructors, and with many of the staff nurses. In the end, I opted to begin my nursing career in gerontology. I've always enjoyed working with the elderly. There are lots of opportunities for me within this area of nursing. You know what? Just do the kind of nursing that speaks to you—that you really enjoy. Go for it!
(personal reflection of a student)

Your entry-level preparation (your degree, BN or BScN, and your professional credentials, e.g., RN) and ongoing occasions for further education (continuing competency, continuing education, certificates, master's and doctoral degrees) create unique and intersecting career opportunities and paths in practice, education, research, and administration. Some of these opportunities are highlighted in Table 1.1.

A Brief History of Nursing

Reflecting on the past will provide you with a greater understanding of how the nursing profession has evolved. Knowing where we have been may also help us to decide where we would like to go in the future. In Canadian history, nurses played key roles in immigration and settlement, contributing to the foundation of health care in Canada.

Early History

Prior to the arrival of nursing in New France, the religious orders (e.g., the Jesuits and others) provided rudimentary health and nursing care (Waldram, Herring, & Young, 1995). These religious were men, and it was difficult for them to provide medical care to women (e.g., labour and delivery). Furthermore, as the number of indigenous people and settlers requiring care increased, so did the need for nursing care. Female religious orders in France were asked to come and minister to the sick. Consequently, nursing played an integral role in the colonization of the New World.

Spreading Christianity

Two key goals of the colonization of the New World from Europe were to spread Christian values and try to convert Aboriginals to Christianity while ensuring that the settlements were safe and healthy for new settlers and those living on the land (Ross-Kerr & Wood, 2010). This same mandate applied to many nurses arriving in the New World (Ross-Kerr & Wood, 2010).

Colonialism is Canada's dark stain on its historical fabric. Colonialism, the policies, laws, and systems associated with controlling people or geographic areas, has been characterized by multiple losses: the loss of culture, knowledge, traditions, a way of life, the role of the family and community; the loss of spirituality and health; and so on. The impact of colonization (aspects of which have lasted into the 21st century) and the trauma it caused is still being felt by the Aboriginal peoples of Canada. Please see Chapter 39 ("Aboriginal Peoples and Nursing") for a more detailed account of colonization and the suffering it precipitated.

Early Settlers

The immigration of settlers to early Canada was replete with hardships and challenges. Crossing the Atlantic from Europe was like heading into the great unknown; it was a risky journey. Immigrating and settling involved risking one's life (Bates, Dodd, & Rousseau, 2005). Life was brutal and often short. As the new immigrants traveled and settled, colonization spread, and so did the diseases and ailments they carried, such as cholera, typhus, and smallpox (Ross-Kerr & Wood, 2010). Most often, these epidemics decimated the Aboriginal peoples (causing a demographic catastrophe) because they had little resistance to them. Trade centres were points of contact between Aboriginal peoples and Europeans and often became the places for disease outbreaks and the diffusion of epidemics along trading routes to the hinterland.

Early Nursing Leaders in Canada

As the demand for nursing care increased, many lay women responded. A few key figures such as Marie Rollet Hébert, Jeanne Mance, and Marguerite d'Youville were instrumental in the establishment of nursing as a healing and helping vocation

TABLE 1.1	Where Can I Work in Nursing? What Can I Do?
Area of Nursing Practice	
Hospital—staff nurse	Maternal-child care, labour and delivery, pediatrics, and the care of children
	Operating room
	Care of people living with mental illness
	Intensive care units
	Emergency department
	Medical/surgical units
Oncology	Cancer nursing care
Palliative and hospice care	Care of the dying and their families and friends
Instructor/Professor	Working with students in classroom or clinical settings
Gerontology	Nursing care of elderly persons
Street links	Working with the homeless and street people
Telehealth	Nursing care through multimedia
Community health	Working with aggregates, families, and communities
Communicable disease control	Preventing and treating diseases such as tuberculosis
Aboriginal nursing	Working with Canada's Aboriginal People, including outpost nursing (nursing stations)
Nursing home/Long-term care	
Self-employed	
Community health centre/Agency	
Private nursing agency	
Home care agency	
Nursing station	
Educational institution	
Administration/Management	
Inventor/Researcher/Scientist	
Colleges and Associations of Nursing	
Nursing unions	
Rehabilitation/Convalescent centre	
Clinical nurse specialist	
Mental health centre	
Primary health care	
Nurse practitioner	
Business/Industry	
School nurse	

This is not an exhaustive list of possibilities. It illustrates where you might find your place within the nursing profession.

in Canada (Bates et al., 2005; Ross-Kerr & MacPhail, 1996; Ross-Kerr & Wood, 2010).

Long before Nightingale ushered in the era of modern nursing in Britain, French nursing sisters were practicing a comprehensive type of nursing care in the New World. Marie Rollet Hébert, Jeanne Mance, and Marguerite d'Youville each took risks and challenged conventional ideas and doctrines. By taking on the tough and often patronizing (and arrogant) stance of the colonists and their leaders, they promoted equality of care and fairness in the treatment of all.

Marie Rollet Hébert

Marie Rollet Hébert (1588–1649) arrived in New France in 1617. Louis, her husband, was to serve as the apothecary of Québec. The couple and their three children built the second stone house at The Habitation (Québec City). Madame Hébert was a layperson who assisted her physician husband to care for the early settlers in New France (Fig. 1.1). Madame Hébert was the first European women to live in

New France. She confronted the notion that the Aboriginal peoples were in need of saving in terms of their physical or spiritual lives (Brown, 1966; Ross-Kerr & Wood, 2010). Instead, she sought their advice on remedies and cures in treating the ill (Ross-Kerr & Wood, 2010). Madame Hébert was committed to educating Aboriginal children, instructing them in the Christian faith; she is commonly referred to as Canada's first teacher. She also was a godmother to many Aboriginal children whose families converted to the Catholic faith. She took in orphans and young Aboriginal girls who were taught by the Jesuits. Madame Hébert died in May 1649 at the age of 61 years after living in New France for some 30 years. Although it was common for physicians' wives to help with care of the ill, her concern for and treatment of the Aboriginal peoples was noteworthy.

Jeanne Mance

Jeanne Mance (1606–1673), originally a socialite in France, felt a call to help in New France, establishing a hospital soon after her arrival in 1642 (Fig. 1.2). Few detailed

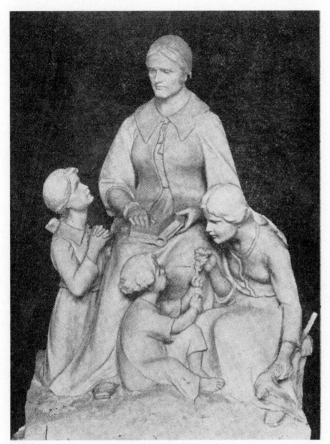

Figure 1.1 Marie Rollet Hébert, who arrived in New France in 1617. (Source: Library and Archive Canada.)

accounts and historical documents about Madame Mance exist; however, scholars agree that she was not only one of the first lay nurses in North America but that she also had considerable skill and expertise in medicine and surgery and in the provision of nursing care (Bates et al., 2005).

Many consider Jeanne Mance to be the founder of the Hôtel Dieu de Ville Marie in Montréal and through this role, one of the founders of the City of Montréal (Gibbon & Mathewson, 1947). Madame Mance lived in New France for more than 30 years. The Religious Hospitallers of Saint Joseph, founded in France and dedicated to the care of the sick, joined Jeanne Mance in Montréal in 1659, where members of the congregation still carry on the work she began. The Hotel-Dieu continues as one of Montréal's great hospitals. Since 1971, the Canadian Nurses Association has honoured a nurse at its biennial convention and annual meeting with the Jeanne Mance Award. Nurse nominees have made a significant contribution to the health of Canadians.

Marguerite d'Youville

Marguerite d'Youville (1701–1771), a widow, changed the way that nursing was practiced in Canada by moving nursing care out of the cloistered and sheltered Christian sanctuaries and into the community (Fig. 1.3). d'Youville founded Les Soeurs Grises (the Grey Nuns), considered the first group of visiting nurses in Canada, providing quality nursing care to all without consideration of race or social class to justify provision of care (Gibbon & Mathewson, 1947; Ross-Kerr & Wood, 2010). In 1749, the Montréal authorities, recognizing d'Youville's goodwill and talents,

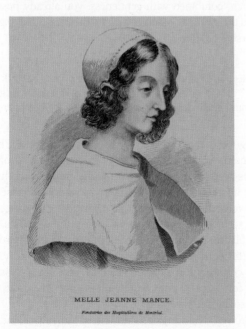

MELLE JEANNE MANCE.
Fondatrice des Hospitalières de Montréal

Figure 1.2 Jeanne Mance. (Source: Library and Archive Canada.)

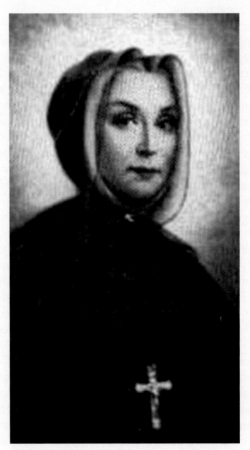

Figure 1.3 Marguerite d'Youville.

asked her to take over the management of the faltering general hospital. King Louis XV confirmed the appointment. d'Youville opened the hospital not only to the settlers but also to Aboriginal peoples and to people suffering from epilepsy, the mentally ill, people living with leprosy, the blind, the victims of contagious diseases, foundlings (abandoned babies), and the aged.

Other women joined d'Youville, giving up their homes, possessions, and social favours to care for; and offer refuge to the poor, the disadvantaged, and the ill. The gradual shift of care into the communities anticipated the movement on a broader scale in Canada, setting the stage for such prominent groups such as the Victoria Order of Nurses established in 1897. Marguerite d'Youville was canonized in 1990 by Pope John Paul II. She is the first native-born Canadian to be elevated to sainthood by the Roman Catholic Church.

The Impact of Florence Nightingale

Alongside groundbreaking discoveries such as the microscope and anesthesia came an increasing willingness to turn to the modern methods of care for illness or injury. Health care moved from the domain of religion and the church to root itself in the foundations of empirical science (as it was understood at the time). With the changing relevance of the church came a new consideration and respect for medical science and nursing.

The work and theories of Florence Nightingale began moving into the collective consciousness of hospitals and nursing education, providing a new image of nursing as a respectable vocation for young women (Mansell, 2004). Nightingale, as befits the era, held a view of nursing as fundamentally women's work, best practiced under the supervision and guidance of (male) physicians. Nurses trained and practiced in hospital-based nursing schools, removing them from the community. This seclusion provided an opportunity to develop a culture and skills unique from medicine and paved the way for a distinct professional nursing to evolve (Bates et al., 2005).

Nightingale (Fig. 1.4) played an important global role in the evolution of nursing. She characterized nursing as a vocation for those women with a higher moral calling, closely linked to pious values. The good nurse displayed the attributes of sobriety, loyalty, altruism, and self-sacrifice, all deeply rooted in Christianity and the virtues (Ross-Kerr & Wood, 2003). These qualities were readily embraced by a rapidly evolving Victorian society, often torn between the new liberal view and the changing position of the church in society and morality. The public opinion of nurses improved and their position as a necessary part of the provision of health care began to be widely accepted. There was an increased willingness to recognize hospitals as the venue for treatment of illness and disease, although they remained the domains of physicians with nurses as trusted and subservient assistants.

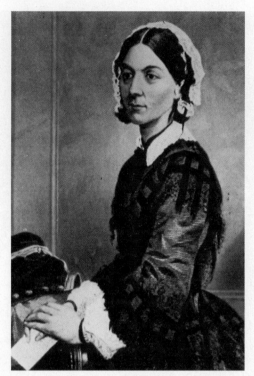

Figure 1.4 Florence Nightingale.

The Role and Character of Victorian Women

If you were applying to work as a nurse toward the turn of the 20th century, the job qualifications and prerequisites listed in *Ambulance Lectures on Home Nursing and Hygiene*, a British handbook published in 1885, would look like this:

> To be a competent nurse, a slight knowledge of anatomy, physiology, and surgery is necessary . . . delicacy of touch, combined with gentleness, you already possess, and these are the qualities that are most essential to good nursing (p. 1).

Think Would you have met the job criteria to work as a nurse in 1895, including a slight knowledge of anatomy, and a delicacy of touch, combined with gentleness?

A good home, basic education, and a solid Christian character were requisites for entering the profession. Nurses were to bring a sense of the moral and the good to the hospital wards. Christian character and closeness to God were character traits that the ideal nurse needed in order to face the challenges in caring for the ill as well as to fulfill the responsibility of being the "moral barometer" of 19th century health care. Such demands and expectations countered the perception of nursing as disdained work for women who were not proper (meaning obediently socialized) women.

Through Nightingale's influence, nursing came to be viewed less as the labour of unskilled women and wives and more as a desirable vocation for proper young women to pursue. Although this movement was a positive step forward on one hand, through an acknowledgment of the scientific basis for many nursing actions, it also contributed to an image of the nurse as a proper and virtuous young woman, with characteristics that might include "wifely obedience to the physician, motherly devotion to the patient, and a firm mistress-servant disciples to those below her" (Mansell, 2004, p. 35).

The contemporary reader should understand that what we now see as the misguided treatment of women and nurses was a reflection of how society treated and valued women and their work.

> The formidable Miss Nightingale imposed on her nurses a regime similar to that of nuns in holy orders. They had to be devout, chaste, good women.
>
> Thus was born the "tyranny of niceness" that made nursing, like motherhood, a universal source of admiration. But like motherhood, it did not always involve a lot of economic support.
>
> With chastity came poverty and obedience. Nightingale's legacy lives on in the form of economic disadvantage and often poor conditions for nurses throughout the world. (Kirby, 2002, para. 2–4)

However, the flaws and faults within the early legacy of nursing are not exclusively a consequence of Florence Nightingale and her contemporaries' vision of women (and men) in nursing but the lasting influence of patriarchal constraints on women's roles.

Men in Nursing

Nightingale believed there was no place in nursing for men, except where physical strength might be required. During the Victorian era, this was not an unreasonable or unexpected stance. The presence of men in nursing, however, has not greatly increased; despite 130 years of modern nursing, men held only 6.6% of positions in the RN workforce as of 2011 (Canadian Institute for Health Information [CIHI], 2013).

The First Nursing Schools in Canada

Early nursing schools, based on the Nightingale model, were established in hospitals in Montréal, Hamilton, and St. Catharines (Mansell, 1996). Dr. Theophilus Mack established the first official training school for nurses in Canada at Mack's General and Marine Hospital in St. Catharines, Ontario (McPherson, 1996). Named the *Mack Training School for Nurses*, it offered a 2-year program based on practical nursing experience in the hospital. The school's infamous motto was, "I see and am silent," indicative of the attitudes toward

(and plight of) Victorian-era women. The first graduating class in 1878 was composed of six nurses. The St. Catharines Marine and General Hospital employed nurses trained in the Nightingale tradition who passed along the educational approach and values, as well as knowledge, to those in training. These nurses, after graduation, moved on to positions in other hospitals in cities across Canada and made up part of the growing number of trained nurses working in and establishing nursing programs in places such as Winnipeg, Montréal, Victoria, and Toronto. These early graduates were instrumental in establishing some of the first nursing educational programs in Canada.

The Organization of Canadian Nursing Begins

At the turn of the 20th century, most nursing education was provided by male physicians, who also dictated the ideal virtues of the female nurse. Yet women were moving into leadership roles. Women such as Mary Agnes Snively took on roles of supervision and education of nurses in training. When Snively assumed the position of lady superintendent of the Toronto General Hospital's School of Nursing (1884–1910), she observed the deplorable conditions in which students were required to work, and she strove to make improvements and changes to nursing education. She was responsible for the formation in 1908 of the Canadian National Association of Trained Nurses, a burgeoning professional group that proposed a cohesive group of professionals that eventually became the Canadian Nurses Association (CNA) in 1924. In doing so, there was clear recognition that the nursing profession held promise and potential of its own. Ms. Snively also cofounded the International Council of Nurses. The International Council of Nurses (ICN) was established in 1899, reflecting the similar reform and evolution of nursing as a unique profession that was happening across the globe. In 1909, Canada joined the ICN. The first precursor to the modern nursing journal, *The Canadian Nurse*, Canada's oldest peer-reviewed academic journal, had already been in publication for 4 years. The ICN currently advances nursing and health worldwide.

Nurses in the 20th Century

The demand for nurses increased with more and busier hospitals. Nursing students took on an apprentice role, working long hours during their training to fill the growing need for skilled nurses. Days were lengthy and the work strenuous, with poor compensation and challenging working conditions. The First World War served to accentuate the growing need for trained and skilled nurses. The workforce of nurses, estimated at approximately 300 at the outset of the new century, grew to 20,000 by the First World War (Bates et al., 2005). See Box 1.1, the Nursing Sisters' Memorial, which is located in the Hall of Honour in the centre block on Parliament Hill.

BOX 1.1   Nursing Sisters' Memorial

The Nursing Sisters' Memorial is located in the Hall of Honour in the centre block on Parliament Hill. Mr. G. W. Hill, R.C.A., of Montréal, sculpted this work in Italy, using marble from the Carrara quarries. The completed panel was mounted in the Hall of Honour during the summer of 1926.

In the Programme of the Unveiling Ceremony of the Canadian Nurses' Memorial, the artist interprets the sculptured panel: *"The design for the sculptured panel embraces the history of the nurses of Canada from the earliest days to the First World War. The right-hand side of the base represents the contribution made by the religious sisters who came to Canada from France during l'ancien régime, and depicts a sister nursing a sick Indian child while an Iroquois warrior looks on suspiciously. To the left, a group of two nursing sisters in uniform tending a wounded soldier symbolizes the courage and self-sacrifice of the Canadian nurses who served in the war. In the centre stands the draped figure of 'Humanity' with outstretched arms. In her left hand she holds the caduceus, the emblem of healing; with the other hand, she indicates the courage and devotion of nurses through the ages. In the background, 'History' holds the book of records containing the deeds of heroism and sacrifice of Canadian nurses through almost three centuries of faithful service."*

More than eight hundred nurses from across Canada had assembled in Ottawa that week, for the 13th general meeting of the CNA. The President of the Association, Miss Jean Brown, presented the memorial to the acting Prime Minister, Sir Henry Drayton, during a ceremony in front of the Centre Bloc. Sir Drayton accepted the memorial in the name of the people of Canada.

Veterans Affairs Canada. (2014). *The Nursing Sisters' Memorial*. Retrieved from https://www.veterans.gc.ca/eng/memorials/memcan/memnurse

War Years

The early 20th century was dominated by two World Wars. Nurses operated on the front lines in both wars, furthering the image of the profession as one of self-sacrifice and heroism. Although there are varying reports of the numbers, 2,000 to 3,000 nurses enlisted, and 50 active duty nurses were killed (including 14 nurses who died with the sinking of the Canadian hospital ship, the Llandovery Castle) in the First World War (Bates et al., 2005; Mansell, 1996; Ross-Kerr & MacPhail, 1996; Ross-Kerr & Wood, 2003).

Nurses in the military assumed an active part in the highly specialized provision of modern care on the front lines (McPherson, 1996). The profession quickly progressed from a religious vocation to a widely publicized profession of specialization, skill, and bravery. The Royal Canadian Army Medical Corps maintained a registry of nurses who actively served in situations of conflict (Ross-Kerr & MacPhail, 1996). Read more about one extraordinary nurse, Helen Kathleen Mussallem (Fig. 1.5 and Box 1.2), who contributed greatly to the profession during this period.

War meant an increased demand for expertise in nurses; enlisted female nurses were rewarded with officer status. Male nurses in the military did not fare as well. Male RNs were not permitted to hold officer status in the Nursing Division of the Canadian military. Prior to 1967, only female nurses were permitted to join the Nursing Division. A 25-year struggle by the Registered Nurses' Association of Ontario (RNAO), its Male Nurses Committee (MNC), and the CNA was required to change this discriminatory policy. The struggle for equality on behalf of Canadian male nurses was successfully resolved because of the united stand taken by the MNC, the RNAO, and the CNA (Care, Gregory, English, & Venkatesh, 1996).

With the end of the First World War came the advent of the Roaring Twenties. Postwar, nurses were moving toward enhancing their professional image; yet during this time, nurses were also moving toward deprofessionalization and a shift back to the role of compliant and acquiescent handmaiden to the physician (Ross-Kerr & Wood, 2003, p. 68).

The deprofessionalization of nursing arose primarily out of the kinds of conditions that existed in many hospital-based nursing schools. Nurses who trained in the hospitals were used as cheap labour, working under appallingly bad conditions; low pay, high workload and responsibility; and

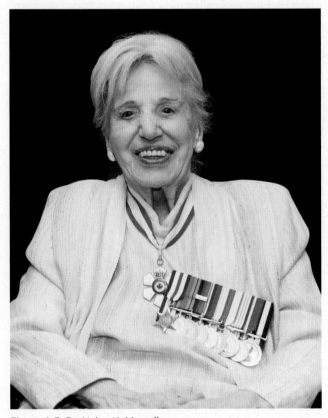

Figure 1.5 Dr. Helen K. Mussallem.

BOX 1.2 Helen Kathleen Mussallem

Helen Kathleen Mussallem was born in Prince Rupert (BC), into a Lebanese family. Dr. Mussallem, Canada's most decorated nurse leader, began her career as a staff nurse at the Vancouver General Hospital. She served overseas during World War II as a lieutenant in the Royal Canadian Army Medical Corps—serving as an operating room nurse in battlefield hospitals in England, France, and The Netherlands. A graduate of Columbia University's Teacher's College, she was an instructor, then director of education, at the Victoria General Hospital School of Nursing. She was the first Canadian nurse to earn a doctoral degree from Columbia University, New York, in 1962.

Dr. Mussallem served as executive director of the CNA, 1963–1981. She advised international organizations such as the ICN and the World Health Organization (WHO), and was the first non-governmental representative on a Canadian Government delegation at the World Health Assembly (1977). In 1981, she received the highest award of the International Committee of the Red Cross, the Florence Nightingale Medal. The National CNA Nursing Library was renamed the Helen K. Mussallem Library in her honour that same year. She was made an officer in the Order of Canada in 1969 and was promoted within the Order to Companion in 1992. Dr. Mussallem held honorary doctorates from UBC and for other universities. The School of Nursing at UBC established a fund in her name, supporting nursing students to attend international conferences.

In 2006, Her Excellency, the Right Honourable Michaëlle Jean, governor general of Canada, appointed Dr. Mussallem Capilano herald extraordinary within the Canadian Heraldic Authority.

Dr. Mussallem died in Ottawa at the age of 97 on 9 November 2012.

Sources: Historica Canada. (n.d.). *Helen Kathleen Mussallem.* Retrieved from http://www.thecanadianencyclopedia.com/en/article/helen-kathleen-mussallem; UBC Nursing News. (2012). UBC Nursing honours Dr. Helen Mussallem. Retrieved from http://www.nursing.ubc.ca/News/NewsItem.aspx?id=197

Nursing Education for Men

In 1939 as World War II was taking shape in Europe, there were four all-male schools of nursing in the United States of America. The last of these (Alexian Brothers School) closed in 1972 as nursing education moved from diploma programs to the university setting (Tranbarger, 2006).

Through the eyes of a student

I wasn't sure that nursing was for me. I mean, as a male, I was a visible minority in my program. I had never experienced that kind of status before. My classmates were really good, and I always felt accepted by them. My teachers and clinical instructors were great. I never had any problems. One of my professors was male, and that made a big difference for me. And the patients! They were great and responded well to me. I found labour and delivery difficult, but my clinical instructor helped me to provide professional care.

(personal reflection of a student)

In 1961, only 25 out of 170 schools of nursing in Canada accepted male applicants (Evans, 2004). At present, men are eligible to apply to all nursing programs in Canada.

Our intent is to whet your appetite for nursing history by covering 100 years in a few pages, giving you an idea of how far we have come. If you want more information about nursing history, read more (see "References and Suggested Readings" at the end of this chapter) and visit websites; for example, the Nursing History Research Unit at the University of Ottawa, the Canadian Nursing History Collection, and the Nursing History Digitization Project (Nursing Education in Nova Scotia).

exploitive long shifts with few lectures or educational activities (McPherson, 1996; Ross-Kerr & Wood, 2003). This phenomenon devalued and diminished the nurse as a professional, furthering the view of nursing as unskilled labour that required little education. The atrocities of the Second World War spurred a cultural shift; a natural reaction to one of the darkest eras in modern history. Societal trends turned to conservative values, embracing the hearth and home and the values of stable nuclear family life. America embraced the values of home and family, where women were encouraged to marry, stay at home, and care for children, tending to the home and taking on domestic responsibilities as their primary role. Nursing was heralded as a respected career choice; however, it was also viewed as an extension of the conservative female role—maternal, nurturing, and reactive (Ross-Kerr & Wood, 2003). Women who embraced the career of a nurse were certainly esteemed, but not more so than those women who epitomized the reputable married woman—at home, with children.

The Development of Nursing Education in Canada

Changes in the practice of nursing resulted in parallel changes in the education of nurses. Nursing education gradually shifted from physicians-as-teachers and the apprenticeship model, to institutional training as hospital-based schools of nursing developed across the country. Almost every hospital, whether in an urban or rural setting and whether small or large, had a school of nursing; for example, the Ninette Sanatorium (Ninette, Manitoba) and the Galt School of Nursing (Lethbridge, Alberta). These, and hundreds of other small schools of nursing, are now long closed. See Figure 1.6 for a picture of nurses from Lethbridge. In 1909, there were approximately 70 hospital-based schools of nursing across Canada (Mussallem, 1965), a model of nursing education that remained prominent until the 1970s.

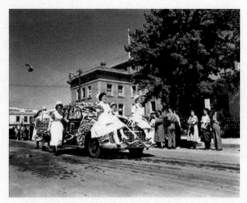

Figure 1.6 Galt School of Nursing car with student and RNs riding on the hood. (Source: Archives of Manitoba.)

University-Based Nursing Education

The first university program in Canada was established in 1919 at the University of British Columbia (UBC) through a school of nursing created within the Faculty of Applied Science (Pringle, Green, & Johnson, 2004). University programs emphasized the theoretical aspects of nursing. Students studied at the university for a year and then moved into the hospitals for hands-on training experiences. Nurses would engage in this dynamic (university practice; theory followed by practice) over several years before earning their degrees. The Canadian Red Cross Society funded one-year university certificate programs in public health for graduate nurses at Dalhousie, McGill, Toronto, Western Ontario, Alberta and UBC in 1920. It was the University of Toronto that developed the integrated theory/practice model on which most nursing education in Canada is based today (Canadian Nurses Association [CNA], 2006b, p. 25).

Nursing Education Leadership: University of Manitoba

In Manitoba, Dr. Margaret Elder Hart provided leadership for the advancement of nursing education at the University of

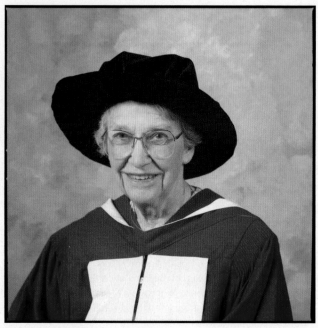

Figure 1.7 Dr. Margaret Elder Hart.

Manitoba. She served as director of the School of Nursing for 24 years (1948–1972). Furthermore, she was one of several graduates from Columbia University who would have a significant impact on the nursing education landscape in Canada for years to come (Fig. 1.7 and Box 1.3). Dr. Hart's tenure as director was succeeded by Dr. Helen Preston Glass. Dr. Glass played an important role in establishing the Master of Nursing program in the then School of Nursing as well as creating the Manitoba Nursing Research Institute. Dr. Glass also served as president of the CNA and influenced the wording and scope of the Canada Health Act in 1984 such that RNs were added to the Act. In addition to being an officer of the Order of Canada and member of the Order of Manitoba, Dr. Glass was inducted in the Teacher's College Nursing Hall of Fame

---

BOX 1.3   Margaret Elder Hart

Margaret Elder Hart graduated in 1930 from the Winnipeg General Hospital School of Nursing. She obtained her B.Sc., M.A., Ed.D., and LL.D. degrees from Teachers College, Columbia University. Upon completion of her studies, Dr. Hart returned to Manitoba. Her pioneer work in Public Health Nursing had a significant impact in the Province of Manitoba; she also developed nursing programs in public health and administration.

Dr. Hart served as director of the School of Nursing from 1948 until her retirement in 1972. During the 1960s, she submitted the School's first proposal for a Master of Nursing program. Dr. Hart was active in the provincial nursing association. She served as a charter member and honorary member (1972) of the Canadian Association of University Schools of Nursing (now CASN, the Canadian Association of Schools of Nursing; see http://www.casn

.ca/en/), a founding member of the National League for Nursing, and a fellow of both the American Public Health Association, and the Royal Society of Health.

Dr. Hart was the recipient of several notable awards and honours including: the Manitoba Medal, Canada Centennial medal, and the Manitoba Association of Registered Nurses Award for Excellence in Nursing Education (1986). In memory of Dr. Hart, the Faculty of Nursing established the Margaret Elder Hart Distinguished Lecture Series in 1991. Dr. Hart was awarded an honourary Doctor of Laws Degree by the University of Manitoba during the Faculty's 50th Anniversary Year.

The Dr. Margaret Elder Hart Heritage Room, Faculty of Nursing University of Manitoba, bears her name in recognition of her contribution to nursing education and her lifelong interest in nursing history.

University of Manitoba Faculty of Nursing. (n.d.). *Manitoba nurse: Margaret Elder Hart*. Retrieved from http:// umanitoba.ca/faculties/nursing/info/hart.html

at Columbia University, New York. You can access Dr. Glass's inventory of her papers at the University of Manitoba: http://umanitoba.ca/libraries/units/archives/collections/complete_holdings/ead/html/glass.shtml.

Collaborative Nursing Programs

Throughout the 1970s and 1980s, the nonuniversity diploma programs eventually moved from hospital schools of nursing to community colleges. From about the mid-1980s onward, collaborative partnerships and programs were established between the colleges and universities. The outcome was collaborative or joint baccalaureate degree programs in nursing, where both the college and university participated in the education of RNs. Several program partners have evolved and are now offering their own baccalaureate programs; for example, Mount Royal College (Alberta), Red River College (Manitoba), and several of the university colleges in British Columbia. The most recent collaborative nursing program (the Saskatchewan Collaborative Bachelor of Science in Nursing [SCBScN]) is offered through a partnership between the University of Regina and the Saskatchewan Institute of Applied Science and Technology (SIAST). Canada's newest faculty of nursing (University of Regina) was established in 2010, in part, to support the SCBScN program.

Baccalaureate Nursing Degree

Nursing has long advocated for the baccalaureate degree as entry to the profession. That is, to become a nurse (RN), a university education is required. Establishing this education standard has taken many, many years. Although the baccalaureate degree is the desired standard throughout Canada, there are some jurisdictions that still offer a nursing diploma or combination of diploma-baccalaureate programming. For example, in Québec, there are diploma programs, as well as baccalaureate partnerships between Collège d'enseignement général et professionnel (CEGEP). However, the Ordre des infirmières et des infirmiers du Québec voted to lobby the Québec government to require baccalaureate degrees as the entry to practice. Despite this lobby, the government has halted any further progress requiring the baccalaureate degree as entry to practice in Québec. Of the 270,724 RNs employed in nursing in Canada in 2011, 57.3% (155,110) had achieved a diploma as their highest education level. There were 104,932 (38.8%) RNs with baccalaureate degrees. A small percentage of RNs (3.9%) held master's and/or doctorates.

Graduate Nursing Education

RNs throughout Canada have access to higher education opportunities such as master's and doctoral (PhD) programs. RNs recognize the need for master's and PhD programs in order to advance the knowledge base of the profession. The first master's program in nursing was established in 1959 at the University of Western Ontario. It took 40 years before graduate education became readily available to baccalaureate-educated nurses in Canada. It would be another 30 years before doctoral nursing education was established at the University of Alberta in 1991. There are now at least 15 nursing PhD programs in Canada (Canadian Association of Schools of Nursing [CASN], 2010).

Advanced Practice Nursing

In Canada, nurses who undertake further study, typically at the graduate or master's level, can become advanced practice nurses. In its national framework for advanced nursing practice, the CNA defines this practitioner as follows:

> Advanced nursing practice is an umbrella term describing an advanced level of clinical nursing practice that maximizes the use of graduate educational preparation, in-depth nursing knowledge and expertise in meeting the health needs of individuals, families, groups, communities and populations. It involves analyzing and synthesizing knowledge; understanding, interpreting and applying nursing theory and research; and developing and advancing nursing knowledge and the profession as a whole. (CNA, 2008b, p. ii)

Advanced nursing practice includes clinical nurse specialists (CNSs) and nurse practitioners (NPs). Both NPs and CNSs require graduate-level education, in-depth nursing knowledge, and clinical expertise. These nurses address health needs at the individual, family, community, and population levels. "The distinctions between the CNS and NP roles are in their history, education, regulated authority, reporting structures, and emphasis on domains of practice" (Winnipeg Regional Health Authority, 2012). The Winnipeg Regional Health Authority's (WRHA) document outlining the differences in the practice of NPs and CNSs is very helpful to understand these different roles. NP programs focus on clinical skills and primary care services. NPs are licensed to practice on an extended practice registry maintained by the nursing regulatory body. Such registries acknowledge that NPs have the authority to perform activities beyond the scope of RN practice. This includes independently prescribing medications, ordering and managing the results of screening and diagnostic tests, and performing minor surgical and invasive procedures. In contrast, the CNS functions within the full scope of an RN and does not require additional regulatory authority (Winnipeg Regional Health Authority [WRHA], 2012, p. 4). The CNS engages in at least three domains influencing direct and indirect care activities: collaboration, scholarship, and empowerment. In the CNS role, RNs consult, collaborate, and build coalitions within and external to nursing and at all levels of the health-care system—all with the goal to foster quality patient care.

Social Forces Affecting Nursing

Never doubt that a small group of thoughtful, committed citizens can change the world; indeed, it's the only thing that ever has.

—Margaret Mead

By the mid-1960s, there were other forces that contributed to a changing image not only of nurses but also of women in general. In many contexts and environments, every day, citizens and noteworthy heroes were challenging the status quo by raising attention to issues such as the protection of the civil rights and liberties of those most oppressed. Those active in the African American Civil Rights Movements (1955–1968) and the Women's Rights Movement opened the doors to discussions of equality, fairness and justice for all. The Civil Rights Movement, while calling attention to the oppression of non-Whites in much of America, also provided momentum for those concerned about the oppression of all individuals because of their gender, sexuality, choices, or social class. Out of this rapidly changing time came new views of rights and liberties. Women were deemed to be in control of their sexuality and their reproductive rights. This was furthered through the availability of the oral contraceptive and the acceptance of the changing role of women in society, both in and out of the home. There are many sources for history of the Women's Rights Movement in Canada, including the Canadian Human Rights Commission.

Alongside this empowerment came a less positive view of women as sexual objects, reflected in some of the media depictions of nurses from that era. Television shows such as M*A*S*H portrayed the nurse as a sexual object for the pleasure of men, often physicians (Ross-Kerr & Wood, 2003). Although many women in society were making strides forward, they were also being viewed as sex objects. This paved the way for careers and roles that women adopted while at the same time objectifying them.

An Ongoing Challenge for the Profession

Why do we examine the roles and perceptions of women to get a sense of the public view of nurses? Nursing has been traditionally viewed as a feminized profession, strongly linked to notions of traditional female roles and virtues. As women's work, nursing has been accorded the characteristics that many have historically thought of as being feminine, including care, nurturing, and tenderness (McLaughlin, Muldoon, & Moutray, 2010). This view is changing but remains largely in the public consciousness. Nursing also remains one of the most sexualized professions (Fig. 1.8). The Ontario Nurses' Association (ONA) has initiated a campaign against the MTV reality show, Scrubbing In. The cast comprises young, hard-partying, buxom nurses in California. The ONA president observes, "The nurses portrayed in the show [are presented] as sexual objects, exploit negative stereotypes and diminish the

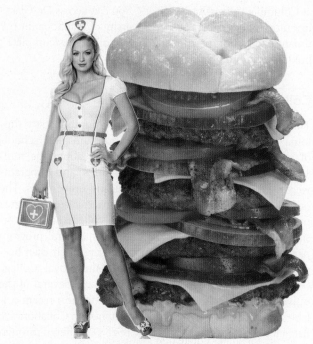

Figure 1.8 "Sexy Nurse" from Heart Attack Grill®.

fact that we are knowledgeable health care professionals who make the difference between life and death for patients every day." (Krashinsky, 2013).

Think Go to the website for a restaurant called Heart Attack Grill®. Waitresses dressed in nurse's uniforms serve a mostly male clientele ultra-high caloric foods ("triple bypass" burgers, "flat-liner" fries) and alcoholic beverages. Note that several of the waitresses are wearing caps, although the nurses' cap disappeared from the nursing landscape beginning in the 1970s. It is not by chance that the wait staff consists of sexualized nurses, an image that plays into contemporary male sexual fantasies. Recently, spanking nurse videos were added to the website. Male customers who do not finish their meals don patient gowns and are publicly spanked and humiliated by a nurse-waitress.

The Tempe, Arizona-based restaurant advertises, "The young servers in the small burger joint sport sexed-up nurse outfits (fishnet stockings, revealing tops, super short skirts, etc.) and cooks wear surgical scrubs." The management offers the following disclaimer:

The use of the word "Nurse" above is only intended as a parody. None of the women pictured on our website actually have any medical training, nor do they attempt to provide any real medical services. It should be made clear that the Heart Attack Grill® and its employees do NOT offer any therapeutic treatments (aside from laughter) whatsoever.

The Arizona State Board of Nursing expressed its concern about the representation of the wait staff as nurses but has not pursued litigation.

Do nursing uniforms (outfits?) really include fishnet stockings, revealing tops, and super short skirts? What do you think of this image of nurses?

Stereotypes of Male Nurses

Men in nursing are not immune from stereotypes. For example, male nurses are often stereotyped as effeminate or homosexual because nursing is viewed by most societies as women's work. The character Jack McFarland on the television situation comedy *Will & Grace* was a nursing student for several episodes. Male nursing was parodied in several episodes of the television comedy *Scrubs* by having an effeminate, but clearly gay, male nurse named Paul Flaurs (*flowers*). A male nurse was also the basis for humour in the film *Meet the Parents*.

The Evolving Public Image of Nurses

Much of the image of nursing rests with the present and future generations of nurses and nursing students. Some steps that nursing students can take to help change the public image of nursing include critical viewing of images of nurses, "monitoring the media" (Kalisch & Kalisch, 1987, p. 187), speaking out in an articulate and organized way against images that present an inaccurate portrayal of nurses and nursing, and promoting an improved image through one's own practice.

Strong, autonomous, intelligent, and compassionate nurses are more prevalent today in media representations, with organizations such as the CNA monitoring the media for nursing images, both negative and positive. Moreover, the CNA is also making strides by promoting an image of nursing that is professional and progressive, moving away from attention to gender and focusing instead on educational qualifications, evidence-based quality care practice, and research involvement.

Thus, there is a move away from the notion and public image of nursing as based solely on the concept of care. Of course, nurses care, but the concept of *care* is a vague, ill-defined term, highly associated with the female gender and often set in contrast to knowledge, science, and power. Caring is not a domain reserved solely for women, and it is not a naturally occurring default for women. Nurses exercise best practices where patient care is based on knowledge, evidence including research, and clinical experience. There is greater awareness of the nursing profession as a career for men and women that requires a high level of postsecondary education, application of specialized knowledge, and a keen understanding of health and illness. Public awareness, not only of the altruism and bravery of individual nurses in situations such as the SARS outbreak of 2003, has led to increased respect, a more positive, progressive public image of nurses. Coinciding with this increased recognition of the importance and unique contribution of the role, the profession remains vigilant for negative and stereotypical portrayal of nurses in the public domain.

Nurses Agitate for Change

In more than one way, nurses cannot and must not see and remain silent. People's lives are at stake when nurses do not speak up. For example, it was the power of nurses that launched the Winnipeg Inquest. The Inquest examined the deaths of 12 children who had undergone cardiac surgery in 1994 at the Winnipeg Health Sciences Centre.

> The deaths and the events that led to them were "a tragic example of health care system design flaws and system failure . . . a high-profile example of the need for action in Canada on systems and patient safety." Justice Murray Sinclair, who oversaw the three-year inquest, wrote in his report that of the 12 children who died in the cardiac paediatric surgical unit at the Winnipeg Health Sciences Centre, at least five deaths were preventable, another four might have been prevented and only one death was not preventable (Sinclair 2001). (Dick, Weisbrod, Gregory, Dyck, & Neudorf, 2006, p. 35)

The RNs who provided expert care for these children spoke up, repeatedly and at some risk, to bring this terrible situation to light. Their persistence and their courage ostensibly launched the patient safety movement in Canada.

Nurses in Research, Administration, and Policy

Thus far, you have read about nursing, its historical roots, and the domains of practice that include clinical, education, and research. Recently, a fifth pillar, policy, has been added to the domains in which nurses are active.

> A very small cadre of nurses also worked in formal policy roles, but only in the last decade has that fifth pillar of nursing practice expanded significantly. As nurses moved into the four domains, they created an extensive network of professional, union and regulatory associations based on their regulated categories, work areas (such as management or education), service setting (operating rooms or community health) disease categories (such as spinal cord injury or diabetes) and other interests (e.g., nursing history and cultural affiliation). (CNA, 2006b, p. 21)

To practice contemporary nursing, nurses are increasingly relying on both a scientific basis and a human science basis for their work, with valid research and scholarly activities, and a unique body of nursing knowledge essential to health and health care. We've discussed education and clinical nursing; let's look briefly at the three remaining pillars: research, administration, and policy.

Nursing Research

Research and evaluation have always been important aspects of nursing practice. Research in nursing can have two meanings. A broad definition of research could encompass any gathering of data, information, and facts for the advancement of knowledge. This involves reading research and would include your search among nursing journals or web sources for current articles on best practices. Original or scientific research involves conducting research, a process used to collect and analyze information to increase our understanding or knowledge on a specific topic or issue. The process is composed of three steps: posing the question, collecting data, and a presentation of the results (or answer). Your ability to learn about research, how to read it, and to determine whether it has any implications for practice is important to professional nursing.

Nursing research in Canada did not evolve with the same profile or speed as clinical practice. Clinical and research operated in separate spheres, even if the research was focused on clinical nursing. For many years, research was seen as reserved for academics, an activity focused on universities and their graduate programs, and led by people with doctoral degrees, rather than an integral part of the practice of all nurses. Some sense of this separation still exists today, but "clearly research is a fundamental concept that now underpins all undergraduate RN . . . degree programs, and it is an essential component of all modern clinical environments" (CNA, 2006b, p. 26). Knowledge translation and/or knowledge uptake (the application of research evidence to nursing practice) has gained not only momentum but also a centrality as increasingly nurses become knowledge workers. See for example the journal *Evidence-Based Nursing*. There are also some excellent websites that address nursing research in Canada; for example, the Canadian Association for Nursing Research and the Canadian Journal of Nursing Research. Nursing research in Canada is discussed further in Chapter 12.

Nursing Administration

At one time, there were head nurses on nursing units. These administrators were typically seasoned nurses with considerable clinical skill and experience. Although the head nurse model had its roots in the hierarchies of the military and religious traditions, these nurses were vital to the practice of nursing. "In the early days nurses controlled how care was organized and head nurses especially wielded significant power over patient care, nurses and even physicians, depending on the setting" (CNA, 2006b, p. 27). During the 1990s, a significant change occurred. Fiscally driven (the intent was to reduce costs) hospitals and community-based programs across Canada moved to a generic management model where leadership was provided to multiprofessional teams. The leaders of these teams were not necessarily nurses. Nursing's influence on (and some would suggest power in) patient care was greatly reduced and more than 5,500 nurse managers were deleted from their head nurse positions (CNA, 2006b). As Villeneuve and MacDonald observe,

> It also meant an end to the best features of the old head nurse role: the coaching, mentoring, teaching and support that many head nurses had offered to nurses,

families and organizations. Directors of nursing became program managers and in some cases professional nurse leaders who were not part of the senior decision-making team. (CNA, 2006b, p. 27)

Vibrant and effective nurse leaders, managers, and union representatives are vital to improving the working conditions for nurses in the field and a critical focus to retain nurses currently in the health-care system and for attracting newcomers to the profession. The empowering behaviours of nurse leaders can be pivotal to how nurses not only react to their work environment but their satisfaction in their work (Laschinger, Almost, & Tuer-Hodes, 2003). Recently, a lot of research is being done about the quality of nurses' work life. For example, see the following Internet resources: the Academy of Canadian Executive Nurses (ACEN), Nursing Leadership (the Canadian Journal of Nursing Leadership), and the Nursing Health Services Research Unit.

Nursing Policy

Nurses have a long history of developing policy in all areas of the profession (practice, education, research, and the policy sector itself). Development and implementation of policies that are in the best interest of the nursing profession fall to

- regulatory bodies (e.g., the College of Registered Nurses of Nova Scotia, the Association of New Brunswick Licensed Practical Nurses, College of Registered Psychiatric Nurses of Manitoba),
- professional associations (e.g., CNA, RNAO),
- nursing unions (e.g., United Nurses of Alberta, Federation des infirmières et infirmiers du Québec, Canadian Federation of Nurses Unions [CFNU]), and
- the academy (e.g., CASN).

Most provinces and territories have nurses in senior policy positions to provide advice and leadership regarding the profession within their jurisdictions. The federal government of Canada has had a senior or chief nurse since 1953. The federal government created the Office of Nursing Policy (ONP) in 1999 to strengthen the focus on nursing policy issues within Health Canada. The ONP advises Health Canada on policy issues and programs, contributes to the development of health policy and programs, and networks with the nursing community in developing advice to the minister of health. Recently, the ONP has focused on the supply and mix of nurses (human resource management) in Canada and the quality of workplaces for nurses.

> We frequently hear that nurses love nursing. However, the toll of health reform has overshadowed many of the positive aspects of nursing practice. The office is committed to rekindling nurses' enthusiasm and passion for their profession, by promoting efforts to increase job satisfaction and decrease burnout,

stimulate innovative care-delivery models, and mobilize rewards and recognition for outstanding practice. (Health Canada, Office of Nursing Policy, 2009).

For more information, visit the ONP website.

Trends in 21st Century Nursing

In Canada, new concerns and issues have come to the attention of the public, such as the rights of same gender couples; access to health care for new immigrants; quality of life and health care for First Nations, Inuit and Métis peoples; appropriateness of new technologies; the state of the public health system; and our preparedness for the unforeseen. These are only a few of the current broader health care–related concerns of all Canadians.

Nontraditional nurses, those who have not been represented in great numbers within nursing, are writing new narratives of nursing history. These nurses with legitimate histories often remain unknown within the profession, among them men, black nurses, Aboriginal nurses (Box 1.4), immigrant and new Canadian nurses, Filipino nurses, Asian nurses, and Indo-Canadian nurses.

In Canada, there is a multiplicity of nursing identities and experiences. As a result, no one narrative, story, or account can speak for all. Think of all the unwritten and emergent histories in nursing that are happening today. Such histories will address the diverse demographics of nurses and patients, the changing focus on the importance of the environment and our health, the emergence of new health challenges in the modern world, the changing emphasis on costs and priorities, and in the context of globalization. These are all trends having a direct and indirect effect on the daily and overarching experience of nurses in today's world.

The Context of Canadian Nursing

There are significant shifts and changes taking place in Canadian society that are having an impact on nursing education and practice. The future of nursing is being shaped by this constellation of change, influenced by factors in demographics, economics, science and technology, family structures, and social and cultural issues. As a nursing student, you will encounter these changes first hand.

The Importance of the Social Determinants of Health

What makes Canadians healthy? We know that it is not simply a matter of having more nurses, physicians, and health-care providers, or more hospitals and expensive technology. Since the 1970s, the WHO has helped us understand that what contributes to health (and good health) must be viewed holistically (Box 1.5). Canada has also contributed to the understanding of the social determinants of health and how they shape the health of people. In 1974, the Department of Health and Welfare published *A New Perspective on the Health of Canadians*, acknowledging that the health-care system was only one of several factors that contributed to health. This notion was revolutionary for its time.

This vision was developed and shared with the world in 1978 through the "The Declaration of Alma-Ata" (http://www.euro.who.int/AboutWHO/Policy/20010827_1). The Declaration provided the foundation for "primary health care" and

---

BOX 1.4 Jean Cuthand Goodwill

Jean Cuthand Goodwill, was born on Little Pine First Nation in Saskatchewan. She lived with tuberculosis as a child and spent several years at the TB sanatorium in Prince Albert, Saskatchewan. She completed her nursing diploma from the Holy Family Hospital in Prince Albert in 1954. She was the first Aboriginal person to finish a nursing program in Saskatchewan.

She was executive director of the Indian-Métis Friendship Centre in Winnipeg, head of the Department of Indian Health Studies at the Saskatchewan Indian Federated College of the University of Regina, a member of the Board of Directors for the Canadian Public Health Association and founding member of the Aboriginal Women's Association of Canada, to name but a few. She was also a founding member of the Aboriginal Nurses Association of Canada, where she served as president for 7 years.

Goodwill wrote four books, including a profile of Indian and Inuit nurses of Canada, and a biography of her father, John Tootoosis, a Cree leader from Poundmaker First Nation in Saskatchewan.

Jean Goodwill devoted herself to politics but was committed to improving the living conditions of Aboriginal people. In 1978, she became a nursing consultant for the Medical Services Branch and an advisor to Assistant Deputy Minister D. Lyall Black at Aboriginal Affairs. Two years later, she became the first Aboriginal woman in the federal public service to be appointed to the position of special advisor to the minister of National Health and Welfare, Monique Bégin.

Dr. Goodwill received numerous distinctions throughout her career. In 1981, she received the Jean Goodwill Award, created in her honour by the Manitoba Indian Nurses Association. Queen's University gave her an Honourary Doctorate of Law in 1986. In 1992, she was named an Officer of the Order of Canada in recognition of her achievements. Then, in 1994, she won a national excellence award from the National Aboriginal Achievement Foundation. In 2000, three years after her death, Goodwill was named recipient of the Ron Draper Health Promotion Award, bestowed by the Canadian Public Health Association. The award recognizes those who have made a significant contribution to health promotion.

Sources: Indspire. (n.d.). *Ms. Jean Cuthand Goodwill*. Retrieved from https://indspire.ca/laureates/jean-cuthand-goodwill; Library and Archives Canada. (n.d.). *Jean Goodwill*. Retrieved from http://www.collectionscanada.gc.ca/femmes/030001-1406-e.html; Aboriginal Multi-Media Society. (n.d.). *Jean Goodwill—Footprints*. Retrieved from http://www.ammsa.com/content/jean-goodwill-footprints

BOX 1.5   Social Determinants of Health

- Income and income distribution
- Education
- Unemployment and job security
- Employment and working conditions
- Early childhood development
- Food insecurity
- Housing
- Social exclusion
- Social safety network
- Health services
- Aboriginal status
- Gender
- Race
- Disability

Source: Mikkonen, J., & Raphael, D. (2010). *Social determinants of health: The Canadian facts.* Toronto, ON: York University School of Health Policy and Management.

"health for all by 2000." In 1986, Canada hosted an international meeting that developed and adopted the First International Charter on Health Promotion (the Ottawa Charter). The authors of the charter highlighted the need for health promotion actions through healthy public policy, supportive environments, community action, development of personal skills, and the reorientation of health-care services.

The Canadian population experiences alterations in health, and these differ according to gender, region, education, and income. The major health issues concerning Canadians, cancer, heart disease, mental health issues, AIDS, asthma, obesity, and diabetes, are influenced by social, economic, and cultural factors. Chronic conditions (e.g., diabetes) are on the rise, and the percentage of Canadians who report that they have two or more chronic conditions has increased from 26% in 2007 to 31% in 2010 (Health Council of Canada, 2013). Physical inactivity, smoking, and obesity (lifestyle factors) greatly influence health status and the prevention and management of chronic diseases (Health Council of Canada, 2013). You can read more on the social determinants of health in Chapter 8.

An Aging Population

The aging population is growing, and the greater prevalence of age-related illnesses and specific concerns are causing a shift in priorities and the allocation of resources in health care. The number of seniors aged 65 years and older increased 14.1% between 2006 and 2011 to nearly 5 million. This rate of growth was higher than that of children aged 14 years and younger (0.5%) and people aged 15 to 64 years (5.7%) (Statistics Canada, 2012). Not only is there a significantly aging general population but also an aging nursing workforce. In 2011, regulated nurses aged 50 years or older represented more than 40% of the RN workforce (CIHI, 2011). With higher numbers of nurses retiring en masse, the workforce will lose a group of nurses and mentors with a wealth of experience. The number of RNs approaching retirement continued to increase: In 2011, 11.9% of RNs were age 60 years or older,

and 0.8% (2,180) were older than age 70 years. A larger proportion of RNs older than age 60 years (58.1%) were working on a part-time or casual basis (CIHI, 2011).

Chronic Disease

Chronic diseases, such as heart disease, stroke, cancer, respiratory diseases, and diabetes, are estimated to cause 36 million deaths around the world each year (World Health Organization [WHO], 2005). In Canada, 3 out of 5 people older than the age of 25 years live with one of these diseases; 4 out of 5 are at risk (Public Health Agency of Canada [PHAC], 2013b). The Public Health Agency of Canada (PHAC) has developed the "Preventing Chronic Disease Strategic Plan," which serves as an integrated strategy to foster healthy living and prevent chronic disease (PHAC, 2013a). There are five pillars supporting the plan:

- Tracking trends and filling data gaps;
- Healthy weights: A priority for preventing chronic disease;
- Targeting specific diseases;
- Putting evidence into action; and
- Supporting our workforce.

Although Canadians are by most indicators among the healthiest people in the world, rising rates of obesity, diabetes, cardiovascular disease, cancer and chronic obstructive pulmonary disease have major implications for the country, the health-care system, and the education of nurses and their practice.

Stress and Mental Health Issues

Stress and mental health issues have vaulted to the top of the list for health-related concerns; 20% of Canadians will suffer mental illness at some time (Health Canada, 2002a; Mental Health Commission of Canada, 2012). Most Canadians are affected by mental illness, either directly or indirectly, through family, friends, or colleagues. Yet, a stigma remains attached to this range of diseases that is a barrier to correct diagnosis and treatment as well as to the acceptance and support of people with mental illness within the community. Although most mental illnesses begin during adolescence and young adulthood, people of all ages, cultures, educational, and income levels experience mental illnesses.

Mental illness can have a serious impact on a person's ability to function effectively over a long period of time. Along with the profound costs to livelihood, the economic costs of mental illness are also enormous to society. Most people with mental illness can be helped through health professionals and community-based services, whereas some may need hospitalization to stabilize their symptoms. The PHAC has some excellent information regarding mental health promotion, mental health problems and disorders, and mental health services.

Poverty

In Canada and worldwide, the gap between the rich and the poor is widening. The claim that 90% of the world's health care is used by 10% of the population is no longer considered to be merely rhetoric but an accurate reflection of the precarious and deleterious condition of many of the world's peoples. As the world becomes more accessible through television and the Internet, so does our knowledge of the strife and challenges of those who are exploited by poverty and this widening gap. Many are moving beyond being witnesses and are actively involved in global health-care reform and sustainability of systems at both policy and grassroots levels. Even in our own country, poverty and deprivation are evident. In 2012, a record of 882,000 Canadians used food banks each month, the highest level of food bank usage ever (Canada Without Poverty, 2013). Homelessness in Canada has grown in complexity and size in recent years. The demographic profile of those who are homeless is also changing. At one time, most homeless were men. Although men remain the majority, women and children represent the fastest growing subgroup of the homeless population. The notion of the social safety net that is the philosophical foundation of Canada's social system is changing with increased need for assistance and a lack of sustainable and relevant social assistance programs.

Family Patterns

What constitutes a family is changing in Canada. Traditional notions of family are being challenged and expanded. As nurses, we provide care not only for individual patients but also for people within dynamic contexts and complex family situations. Our view of a patient is a snapshot from his or her life. By recognizing and acknowledging individuals within their unique family context, our nursing care becomes that much more dynamic, relevant, and sustainable.

Where We Live and How We Work

The daily life of Canadians is changing. Urban sprawl, commuting, and long work hours—these trends are having an effect on the health of Canadians and their families. New technologies have allowed us to be connected to work at all times, which again has a notable effect on the health of families and the way that their time is spent together. Children are more involved in technology at an earlier stage. The shift from the park to the video console as a locus of play and socialization is beginning to give rise to new concerns for the health and well-being of the younger generations. Inactivity and obesity are a growing problem in Canadian society.

New Canadians and the Changing Nation

As a nation, our growth is increasingly dependent on immigration of new Canadians. As Canada becomes more ethno-culturally diverse, the needs, priorities, and traditions of individuals and groups are increasingly unique and varied. New concerns and stress related to immigration, separation of families, settlement, and isolation all contribute to health-care needs. Nursing education (and practice) must expand understanding of the real limitations and challenges associated with the concepts of culture and cultural competence and look more closely at the concept of cultural safety (Ramsden, 1993; Smye, Josewski, & Kendall, 2010). Each of us bears culture; it is not simply the exotica of the other. Fundamentally, cultural safety is about power over another; for example, in a nursing care situation, or with

respect to Canadian federal policy (The Indian Act). Cultural safety can open up space in the nurse–patient relationship to understand the realities and complexities of racism, prejudice, and discrimination. See Chapter 13 on cultural safety.

First Nations, Inuit and Métis Peoples

Of increasing concern are the health, education, and well-being of Canada's founding peoples. Deplorable conditions related to basic health needs such as clean water, adequate housing, and affordable healthy food exist in some communities (reserves) in our own country. Quality education, opportunities and outreach for adolescents at risk, and health-care systems that address the unique needs of these communities remain elusive. Although we look outward at conditions of extreme poverty and deprivation in other countries in the world, the reality is that these kinds of conditions exist in Canada. Nursing's commitment to our Aboriginal peoples is validated, in part, by actions to increase the number of First Nations, Inuit and Métis, nursing students in Canada. See also the Aboriginal Nurses Association of Canada.

Disease Patterns

With increased access to global travel, new patterns of immigration and settlement, and a weak but improving global public health system, new patterns of illness and disease are emerging. Moreover, older diseases are reoccurring. Although cheap effective interventions such as the oral polio vaccine often exist, there are also political barriers or competing priorities for health-care dollars that impede efforts to introduce and deliver proposed safe and effective solutions. Polio has resurfaced in Africa; and diseases of poverty, such as tuberculosis and malnutrition, are on the rise again in Canadian cities and on Indian reserves. AIDS continues to devastate families and communities worldwide. "In some African countries an entire generation of young adults has been virtually wiped out. Child-led families have become commonplace in many of these nations" (CNA, 2006b, p. 18). The WHO and countries across the globe are anxiously anticipating a flu pandemic (e.g., the H1N1 flu of 2009) and strengthening and supporting the weak infrastructures of public health systems. As immigration and settlement patterns evolve, so do the evolutionary patterns of global epidemics and pandemics.

Health-Care Systems

New models of practice are being implemented across all health-care disciplines. Emergence of trends such as evidence-informed practice, interprofessional and collaborative education, patient safety, and continuous quality improvement affect not only the overarching practice of nursing but also the day-to-day experiences of nurses in various contexts. Changing priorities and foci within the health-care system have shifted the public's attention. In Canada, the degree of privatization of the system, sustainability and accountability, definitions of health-care reform, priorities for limited health-care dollars, and perceived inequities in access to and quality of health care are all key issues that are currently foremost in the minds of many Canadians. Differences between provinces in the provision of health care have sparked ongoing debates about the responsibility and appropriateness of governments administrating the health-care system—one founded on the principle of egalitarianism, embedded in the Canada Health Act, and considered alongside our Canadian Charter of Rights and Freedoms.

The Nursing Shortage: A Cyclic and Ongoing Issue

Perhaps of all the factors affecting nursing (education and practice) in the future, the nursing shortage will have direct consequences for graduates over the next decade. The CFNU observes that there is an insufficient supply of nurses required to sustain the workforce. There is a significant disparity in terms of shortages from one part of the country to another (Canadian Charter of Rights and Freedoms [CFNU], 2012). For example, the situation in northern, rural, and remote areas and in Aboriginal communities is especially serious. The CNA predicts a shortfall of 60,000 full-time equivalent nurses by 2022 (CNA, 2009).

Many health human resource planners have warned that Canada, like the rest of the industrialized world, is facing a nursing shortage. Nearly one-third of RNs in the workforce are aged 50 years or older and will soon reach the typical retirement age of 65 years. Research also indicates that an increasing proportion of RNs are retiring early, many by age 56 years. For the first time in recent history, the workforce spans four generations (veterans, baby boomers, generation X, and generation Y). This presents significant challenges and opportunities for health human resource planners. Different strategies may be required to entice and motivate the members of each generation. Regardless, the coming waves of retiring nurses will have an impact on how nurses are educated (the four-year degree will likely be only one of several options to completing a university education, i.e., accelerated programs such as the second-degree or post-degree option will be needed). Of course, whatever options are available, graduates of these programs will need to meet the competencies expected of newly graduated or novice nurses. In addition, the practice context will likely undergo changes; for example, ideal mix of nurses given their respective competencies and the need to hold on to our most seasoned and experienced nurses pre- and post-retirement.

The Environment

The contamination of our environment, the phenomenon of global warming, and other environmental challenges have the potential to affect the health of Canadians. The impact of the environment on health was readily felt during the latter half of the 20th century. For example, in Canada, *Escherichia coli* (*E. coli*) in the drinking water in Walkerton, Ontario, claimed six lives and sent over 2,000 people to the hospital in May 2000 (CNA, 2006b). The Intergovernmental Panel on Climate Change (IPCC) is predicting significant climate change at an alarming rate (Intergovernmental Panel on Climate Change [IPCC], 2007). The IPCC consists of scientists from the World Meteorological Organization and the United Nations Environment Programme. Temperature increases are forecast for Canada over the next 100 years. Water sources, rising sea levels, increasingly volatile weather patterns and storms, floods, and droughts are consequences of environmental changes related to alterations in the climate.

The Art and Science of Nursing

The purpose of this textbook is to provide nursing students with the foundations of nursing. Each chapter serves to progressively ground you in nursing as you complete your education journey to novice nurse status. To engage in nursing is to embrace ways of knowing. Although published many years ago, Barbara Carper's work remains relevant and important to contemporary Canadian nursing (Carper, 1978). She proposed four fundamental ways of knowing (empirical, personal, ethical, and aesthetic) that constitute nursing.

As a nurse, you make use of factual knowledge from science (empirical knowledge). You require understanding that is based in basic and applied science as well as the human sciences. Clinical decision-making and clinical judgment draw on consummate assessment skills and a kind of knowing that discerns changes in a patient's condition over time. Empirical knowing means bringing general knowledge to bear on the patient, and the particular knowledge of assessment findings from the patient to general knowledge with the goal of providing appropriate and effective nursing care.

Your personal knowing—revealed through reflection and reflective practice—concerns self-understanding, empathy, and compassion. Nursing will foster a profound self-awareness as you engage in relational practice with others. Authentic knowing reveals one's feelings, prejudices, biases, and understanding of power in the patient encounter. In this aspect of knowledge, you encounter the "Other" as an empathic witness to suffering and as an empathetic, compassionate nurse.

Ethical knowing is core to nursing practice. This is a matter of knowing what is right and just—and what ought to be done in a patient care situation. It is reasoning about what is right and wrong. Although the Code of Ethics of the CNA (2008c) serves as a moral compass for nursing, it is in those moments of profound patient vulnerability where you will make decisions and engage in behaviours rooted in the ethical, both with respect to intent and to action.

And finally, there is the aesthetics of nursing. This is an awareness of nursing in the moment of caring. It is enacting the wholeness of nursing care with patients and clients. For nurses, clinical epiphanies are revealed in the aesthetics of nursing. Suddenly, and all-at-once, a profound understanding of a patient care situation is realized; it is in this moment that space and time become suspended and the unity of being with the "Other" (patient) becomes known. The privilege and the power in nursing, in this relational connection, is revealed.

Enacting the art and science of nursing requires, in part, knowledge from each of these four knowledge domains. The possibility of wholistic nursing care also becomes a reality through these four ways of knowing. Communication, grounded in understanding and connection with patients, will enable you to offer a kind of nursing that is respectful of patients, families, and communities. Core to nursing practice is the nurse–patient relationship.

The nurse–patient relationship is always professional and therapeutic. It is characterized by the following components (College of Nurses of Ontario, 2006; College of Registered Nurses of British Columbia [CRNBC], n.d.):

- *Trust* is core to the nurse–patient relationship given the vulnerability of patients (clients). A loss of trust in this relationship is profoundly significant, and it may be very difficult, if not impossible, to reestablish it.
- *Respect* recognizes the inherent dignity, worth, and uniqueness of every individual regardless of socioeconomic status, gender, ethno-cultural heritage, sexuality, age, personal attributes, and the nature of the health problem.
- *Professional intimacy* is often present in the nature of care provided by nurses. This can be related to physical activities (e.g., bathing), other kinds of care, and conversations that create closeness between the nurse and the patient. "Professional intimacy can also involve psychological, spiritual and social elements . . ." (CRNBC, n.d., p. 5).
- *Empathy* is the nurse's expression of understanding that validates and resonates the meaning of the health-care experience for the client. In this textbook, the "Through the Eyes

of a Patient" feature is not only instructive about the need for empathy in the nurse–patient relationship but reveals the importance of listening to and really hearing patients.
- *Power* is always present in the nurse–patient relationship. The nurse can potentially exercise more power in this relationship than the patient (e.g., the nurse has specialized knowledge, access to privileged information, influence in the health-care system). When a nurse enacts power over a patient in a non-caring manner, he or she then places a patient at risk for harm (see Chapter 13 on cultural safety). The patient is a partner in this caring relationship and every effort should be taken to involve the patient as such.

At this point in your education journey, and for most nursing students in their first year of nursing, the art and science of nursing remains something theoretical. As soon as you enter in the practice landscape, something amazing will occur; the possibility and reality of the nurse–patient relationship. It is through this relationship that the art and science of nursing will become real to you.

After a long talk and some leafing through their fundamentals text, Mike and Britney agree that, although they are both feeling a bit nervous, they are excited to begin their nursing program.

REFERENCES AND SUGGESTED READINGS

Bates, C., Dodd, D., & Rousseau, N. (2005). *On all frontiers: Four centuries of Canadian nursing.* Ottawa, ON: University of Ottawa Press.

Brown, G. (1966). *Dictionary of Canadian biography: 1000 to 1700* (Vol. 1). Toronto, ON: University of Toronto Press.

Canada Without Poverty. (2013). *Just the facts.* Retrieved from http://www.cwp-csp.ca/poverty/just-the-facts/

Canadian Association of Schools of Nursing. (2010). *CASN 2010 Environmental scan on doctoral programs.* Ottawa, ON: Author.

Canadian Federation of Nurses Unions. (2012a). *The nursing workforce.* Retrieved from http://www.nursesunions.ca/publications/factsheets

Canadian Federation of Nurses Unions. (2012b). *The nursing workforce: Canadian federation of nurses unions backgrounder.* Ottawa, ON: Author.

Canadian Health Services Research Foundation. (2005). *A systematic approach to maximizing nursing scopes of practice.* Ottawa, ON: Author.

Canadian Institute for Health Information. (2004). *Improving the health of Canadians.* Ottawa, ON: Author.

Canadian Institute for Health Information. (2011). *Regulated nurses: Canadian trends, 2007 to 2011.* Ottawa, ON: Author. Retrieved from http://secure.cihi.ca/cihiweb/dispPage.jsp?cw_page=PG_1710_E&cw_topic=1710&cw_rel=AR_2529_E

Canadian Institute for Health Information. (2013). *Regulated nurses, 2012—Summary report.* Ottawa, ON: Author. Retrieved from https://secure.cihi.ca/free_products/RegulatedNurses2012Summary_EN.pdf

Canadian Nurses Association. (2002). *Advanced nursing practice: Position statement.* Retrieved from http://www.cna-aiic.ca/en/advocacy/policy-support-tools/cna-position-statements

Canadian Nurses Association. (2006a). *Joint position statement. Practice environments: Maximizing client, nurse and system outcomes.* Retrieved from http://www.cna-/~/media/cna/page%20content/pdf%20en/2013/07/26/10/40/ps88-practice-environments-e.pdf

Canadian Nurses Association. (2006b). *Toward 2020: Visions for nursing.* Ottawa, ON: Author.

Canadian Nurses Association. (2008a). *Advanced nursing practice: A national framework.* Retrieved from http://www2.cna-aiic.ca/CNA/documents/pdf/publications/ANP_National_Framework_e.pdf

Canadian Nurses Association. (2008b). *Code of ethics for registered nurses* (2008 centennial edition). Retrieved from http://www.cna-aiic.ca/~/media/cna/page%20content/pdf%20fr/2013/09/05/18/05/code_of_ethics_2008_e.pdf

Canadian Nurses Association. (2009). *Tested solutions for eliminating Canada's nursing shortage.* Retrieved from http://www2.cna-aiic.ca/cna/documents/pdf/publications/RN_Highlights_e.pdf

Canadian Nurses Association. (2010). *Taking action on nurse fatigue* [Position statement]. Ottawa, ON: Author.

Canadian Nurses Association. (2012). *A nursing call to action.* Ottawa, ON: National Expert Commission.

Care, D., Gregory, D., English, J., & Venkatesh, P. (1996). A struggle for equality: Resistance to commissioning of male nurses in the military, 1952-1967. *Canadian Journal of Nursing Research, 28*(1), 103–117.

Carper, B. (1978). Fundamental patterns of knowing in nursing. *Advances in Nursing Science, 1*(1), 13–24.

Cho, J., Laschinger, H., & Wong, C. (2006). Workplace empowerment, work engagement and organizational commitment of new graduate nurses. *Nursing Research, 19*, 43–60.

College & Association of Registered Nurses of Alberta. (2008). *Nursing practice standards.* Edmonton, AB: Author.

College of Nurses of Ontario. (2006). *Therapeutic nurse-client relationship.* Toronto, ON: Author. Retrieved from http://www.cno.org/en/learn-about-standards-guidelines/educational-tools/learning-modules/therapeutic-nurse-client-relationship/

College of Registered Nurses of British Columbia. (n.d.). *Nurse-client relationships.* Vancouver, BC: Author. Retrieved from https://

www.crnbc.ca/Standards/Lists/StandardResources/406Nurse
ClientRelationships.pdf

Dick, D., Weisbrod, L., Gregory, D., Dyck, N., & Neudorf, K. (2006). Case study: On the leading edge of new curricula concepts: Systems and safety in nursing education. *Canadian Journal of Nursing Leadership, 19*(3), 34–42.

Evans, J. (2004). Men nurses: An historical perspective. *Journal of Advanced Nursing, 47*(3), 321–328.

Gibbon, J. M., & Mathewson, M. S. (1947). *Three centuries of Canadian nursing.* Toronto, ON: MacMillan.

Gottlieb, L., Gottlieb, B., & Shamian, J. (2012). Principles of strengths-based nursing leadership for strengths-based nursing care: A new paradigm for nursing and healthcare for the 21st century. *Nursing Leadership, 25*(2), 38–50.

Health Canada. (2002a). *Mental health—Mental illness.* Ottawa, ON: Author.

Health Canada. (2002b). *Our health, our future: Creating quality workplaces for Canadian nurses.* Ottawa, ON: Advisory Committee on Health Human Resources.

Health Canada, Office of Nursing Policy. (2009). *Quality of workplace settings.* Retrieved from http://www.hc-sc.gc.ca/ahc-asc/branch-dirgen/spb-dgps/onp-bpsi/issues-enjeux-eng.php

Health Council of Canada. (2013). *Better health, better care, better value for all: Refocusing health care reform in Canada.* Retrieved from http://healthcouncilcanada.ca/content_bh.php?mnu=2&mnu1=48&mnu2=30&mnu3=53

Intergovernmental Panel on Climate Change. (2007). *Fourth assessment report: Climate change 2007.* Geneva, Switzerland: Author.

Kalisch, P., & Kalisch, B. (1982). Anatomy of the image of the nurse: Dissonant and ideal models. In C. Williams (Ed.), *Image-making in nursing: Papers of the 1982 scientific session* (pp. 3–23). Washington, DC: American Academy of Nursing.

Kalisch, P., & Kalisch, B. (1987). *The changing image of the nurse.* Toronto, ON: Addison Wesley.

Kirby, M. (2002). *How the tyranny of niceness handicaps nurses.* Retrieved from http://www.theage.com.au/articles/2002/06/13/1023864323033.html

Krashinsky, S. (2013, October 21). Ontario nurses campaign to stop MTV reality show. *The Globe and Mail.* Retrieved from http://www.theglobeandmail.com/report-on-business/industry-news/marketing/nurses-campaign-to-stop-mtv-%adreality-show/article14967822/

Laschinger, H. K. S., Almost, J., & Tuer-Hodes, D. (2003). Workplace empowerment as a predictor of nurse burnout in restructured healthcare settings. *Longwoods Review, 1*(3), 2–11.

MacMillan, K. (Ed.). (2013). *Proceedings of a think tank on the future of undergraduate nursing education in Canada.* Halifax, NS: Dalhousie University School of Nursing.

Mansell, D. (1996). *The history of nursing in Canada: Spiritual vocation to secular profession* (Doctoral dissertation). University of Calgary, NN12790, Calgary, AB.

Mansell, D. J. (2004). *Forging the future: A history of nursing in Canada.* Ann Arbor, MI: Thomas Press.

McLaughlin, K., Muldoon, R., & Moutray, M. (2010). Gender, gender roles and completion of nursing education: A longitudinal study. *Nurse Education Today, 30*(4), 303–307.

McPherson, K. (1996). *Bedside matters: The transformation of Canadian nursing, 1900-1990.* Toronto, ON: Oxford University Press.

Med-Emerg, Inc. (2006). *Building the future: An integrated strategy for nursing human resources in Canada. Phase II: Final report.* Ottawa, ON: The Nursing Sector Study Corporation.

Mental Health Commission of Canada. (2012). *The mental health strategy for Canada.* Retrieved from http://www.mentalhealthcommission.ca/English/Pages/Strategy.aspx?routetoken=51c004116981247ad9c2ed27c81875e7&terminitial=41

Mussallem, H. K. (1965). *Nursing education in Canada.* Ottawa, ON: Queen's Printer.

Newport, F. (2012). *Congress retains low honesty rating. Nurses have highest honesty rating; car salespeople, lowest.* Retrieved from http://www.gallup.com/poll/159035/congress-retains-low-honesty-rating.aspx

Nightingale, F. (1969). *Notes on nursing.* New York, NY: Dover. (Original work published 1860).

Nurses Association of New Brunswick. (1996). *Position statement: Scope of nursing practice.* Fredericton, NB: Author.

Osborn, S. (1885). *Ambulance lectures on home nursing and hygiene.* London, United Kingdom: H. K. Lewis. Retrieved from http://books.google.ca/books?hl=en&lr=&id=gAkFAAAAQAAJ&oi=fnd&pg=PA1&dq=Ambulance+Work+and+Nursing,+1885&ots=vg7nqEnaar&sig=gCIOj_uOuHN9QVGLP7OiaPK6VxA#v=snippet&q=graceful%20carriage&f=false

Pringle, D., Green, L., & Johnson, S. (2004). *Nursing education in Canada: Historical review and current capacity.* Ottawa, ON: The Nursing Sector Study Corporation. Retrieved from http://umanitoba.ca/faculties/nursing/info/hart.html

Public Health Agency of Canada. (2013a). *Preventing chronic disease strategic plan 2013-2016.* Retrieved from http://www.phac-aspc.gc.ca/cd-mc/diabetes-diabete/strategy_plan-plan_strategique-eng.php

Public Health Agency of Canada. (2013b). *Risk factor atlas.* Retrieved from http://www.phac-aspc.gc.ca/cd-mc/atlas/index-eng.php

Ramsden, I. (1993). Kawa Whakaruruhau: Cultural safety in nursing education in Aotearoa (New Zealand). *Nursing Praxis, 8*(3), 4–10.

Roach, S. (1992). *The human act of caring* (Rev. ed.). Ottawa, ON: Canadian Hospital Association Press.

Roach, S. M. (2002). *Caring, the human mode of being: A blueprint for the health professions* (2nd ed.). Ottawa, ON: Canadian Hospital Association Press.

Rosen, R. (2001). Filipino nurses in Canada. *Canadian Women's Health Network, 4*(3), 13.

Ross-Kerr, J. C., & MacPhail, J. (1996). *Concepts in Canadian nursing.* St. Louis, MO: Mosby.

Ross-Kerr, J. C., & Wood, M. (2003). *Canadian nursing: Issues and perspectives.* Toronto, ON: Mosby.

Ross-Kerr, J. C., & Wood, M. (2010). *Canadian nursing: Issues and perspectives.* Toronto, ON: Elsevier.

Royal College of Nursing. (2003). *Defining nursing: def. Nursing is . . . .* London, United Kingdom: Author.

Sinclair, M. (2001). Findings and recommendations. In *The Report of the Manitoba Pediatric Cardiac Surgery Inquest: An Inquiry into Twelve Deaths at the Winnipeg Health Sciences Centre in 1994* (pp. 465–501). Retrieved from http://www.pediatriccardiacinquest.mb.ca/

Smith, P., Fritschi, L., Reid, A., & Mustard, C. (2013). The relationship between shift work and body mass index among Canadian nurses. *Applied Nursing Research, 26*(1), 24–31.

Statistics Canada. (2012). *The Canadian population in 2011: Age and sex* (Catalogue no. 98-311-X2011001). Ottawa, ON: Author.

Syme, V., Josewski, V., & Kendall, E. (2010). *Cultural safety: An overview.* Retrieved from http://e4e701.mediainsights.net.au/files/e4e/docs/CulturalSafety.pdf

Tranbarger, R. (2006). American schools of nursing for men. In C. O'Lynn & R. Tranbarger (Eds.), *Men in nursing: History, challenges, and opportunities* (pp. 43–66). New York, NY: Springer Publishing.

Waldram, J., Herring, A., & Young, K. (1995). *Aboriginal health in Canada.* Toronto, ON: University of Toronto Press.

Winnipeg Regional Health Authority. (2012). *A guide for successful integration of a clinical nurse specialist.* Winnipeg, MB: Author.

World Health Organization. (1986). *Ottawa charter for health promotion.* Retrieved from http://www.who.int/healthpromotion/conferences/previous/ottawa/en/

World Health Organization. (2005). *Preventing chronic diseases: A vital investment.* Geneva, Switzerland: Author.

Health Care in Canada and Issues of Health-Care Reform

SUSAN E. ANTHONY AND MARY ANNE KRAHN

Louis is a first-generation Canadian who lives at home while studying nursing at university. He lives in a multigenerational family. His parents and grandparents moved together from Mexico to Canada a few months before Louis was born. He has a younger brother who has severe cerebral palsy. Louis's father was an engineer in Mexico but drives a taxi in Canada. His mother was a psychologist in Mexico but now is employed as a housekeeper at a local hotel. Louis's mother and grandparents speak little English. His grandparents do not have a family doctor or a primary care nurse practitioner; they do have health cards but have not sought out or needed medical care since arriving in Canada. Louis's grandmother has just experienced a dizzy spell during which she nearly blacked out. Louis's parents have asked him to accompany his grandmother to the urgent care centre for several reasons: They cannot get time off work; he is a nursing student so he understands the health-care system, and he can interpret for his grandmother. Louis wonders if an urgent care centre is the correct point/type of care for his grandmother and is concerned that she will have a long wait time before being seen.

CHAPTER OBJECTIVES

By the end of this chapter, you will be able to:

1. Demonstrate appreciation for the evolution of Canada's health-care system, including jurisdictional matters and provincial versus federal involvement.
2. Describe the culture and process of current Canadian health care and distinguish between private and publicly funded health care.
3. Recognize the implications of the Canada Health Act for the health and wellness of Canadian citizens and health professionals.
4. Explain the concept of Canadian health-care reform and give examples of the role of health-care reform to the health and well-being of Canadians.
5. Comprehend contemporary past and present Canadian health and health-care structures as a platform for understanding future health-care needs.
6. Identify the relevance of the Canadian health-care system to your professional nursing education and practice knowledge.

KEY TERMS

Canada Health Act (CHA) Act setting out the criteria, conditions, and national standards for insured health-care services the provinces and territories must meet to receive federal funding from the Canada Health and Social Transfer (CHST). The act was passed into law in 1984, replacing earlier legislation: the Hospital Insurance and Diagnostic Services Act (1957) and the Medical Care Act (1968).

Determinants of Health Also referred to as the *social determinants of health*, the elements at biologic, psycho-emotional, social, environmental, individual, and societal levels that can affect the health and well-being of all humans. These elements include income and social status, social support networks, education, employment, working conditions, physical environment, social environments, biologic and genetic endowment, physical health practices and coping skills, healthy child development, health services, gender, and culture.

Health-Care Reform General term referring to changes made by government through the creation of health policy that influences the delivery of health care.

Health Professional A broad expression that refers to practitioners within the health system; typically refers to licensed and regulated health professions, including nursing, medicine, physical and occupational therapy, speech language pathology and audiology, respiratory therapy, pharmacy, and dietetics, among others.

(continued on page 24)

Point of Care Term used to refer to the level or place at which a person receives health care.

Primary Health Care "Refers to an approach to health and a spectrum of services beyond the traditional health care system. It includes all services that play a part in health, such as income, housing, education, and environment. Primary care is the element within primary health care that focuses on health care services, including health promotion, illness and injury prevention, and the diagnosis and treatment of illness and injury" (Health Canada, 2012a, para. 1).

Public Administration Within the context of the Canadian health system, refers to planning, organizing, directing, coordinating, and controlling the publicly funded, not-for-profit health-care system, including policies, programs, and other matters related to the health of Canadians, by all levels of governments elected by public citizenry who, in turn, bear some responsibility for determining the health policies and programs of these governments.

Secondary Health Care The level of care when Canadians have been referred by a primary care provider to specialized care at a hospital or some other facility; usually involves diagnosis and treatment of health challenges of varying complexities by specialists. Additionally, secondary care may result in referral to a tertiary level of care.

Socialized Medicine Refers to Canada's publicly funded universal health insurance system designed to ensure that all residents have reasonable access to medically necessary hospital and physician services. Unofficially, socialized medicine may be referred to as *medicare*.

Tertiary Health Care Specialized consultative care involving specialized supports and resources that is usually referred from primary or secondary health-care providers and includes diagnosis and treatment of disease and disability in sophisticated large research and teaching hospitals. Specialized intensive care units, advanced diagnostic support services, and highly specialized personnel are characteristic of tertiary health-care services.

The Canadian Health-Care System

By building healthy public policy, creating supportive environments, and strengthening communities across the provinces and territories, Canadians can work collaboratively to improve the health-care system and to promote its future sustainability. The Canadian constitution outlines the organization of Canada's health-care system, including how health-care responsibilities are divided between the federal, provincial, and territorial governments. According to Health Canada (2009), administration of publicly funded health care is the responsibility of Canada's 10 provinces and three territories, outlined in the Canada Health Act (CHA).

Importance for Nurses

It is important for us to understand our Canadian health-care system in the broad context because this information contributes to our knowledge-based practice. For example, in the opening scenario, Louis's nursing program likely included classes on the Canadian health-care system. For Louis's safe and competent professional practice, it is important for him to know about and understand the Canadian health-care system because it is the professional context in which he practices. Within his personal context, this same information about the Canadian health-care system helps him provide informed support to his grandmother and family, including anticipatory guidance regarding an appropriate type and level of available care as well as patient health-care rights. What information about the Canadian health-care system is important to Louis's grandmother as she seeks health care in a culture different from her culture of origin? How is an understanding of the history, evolution, and reform in Canadian health care important to Louis as a beginning health professional and advocate for his grandmother?

Context of Concepts

The Canadian health-care system is composed of all of the health services provided by health professionals to eligible residents, ensuring that they have reasonable access to medically necessary insured services on a prepaid basis without direct charges (Health Canada, 2006a). Canada as a nation is the broad context for health services not only for patients but also for professional nursing practice and education. Social, cultural, and physical dimensions of our country impact the complexity, diversity, and richness of health services delivery as well as nursing practice and education. The term *context* refers to the surroundings, circumstances, environment, background, setting (*Oxford English Dictionary*, 2006), and interconnected events that help determine, specify, or clarify the meaning of an event. In nursing, the concept of context takes into consideration factors that influence patient care and may include historic, social, cultural, physical, economic, and global dimensions.

As a beginning practitioner, what is important for you to know about health care in Canada and the Canadian health-care system? According to Storch (2010), within a Canadian health-care context, a large percentage of Canadians younger than 60 years of age have not experienced living without full coverage of medical and hospital care expenses. To understand our current Canadian health-care system and context as well as health-care reform for the future, it is useful to revisit where we have been.

Health Care in Canada: The Historic Context

Romanow (2002, p. xix) stated that "Canadians are the shareholders of the public health care system. They own it and are the sole reason the health care system exists." For many years, our publicly funded health-care system, also termed as *medicare*, has been a source of Canadian pride. Our current health-care system has evolved to provide the comprehensive, accessible, and universal health services that Canadians currently enjoy. Even before confederation in 1867, Canadians struggled to build a health-care system responsive to social, economic, and technological change (Thompson, 2010). The effort has continued post confederation, with the creation of landmark laws and documents outlining jurisdiction for health care and the process of health services delivery. For example, the British North America (BNA) Act of 1867 that created the Dominion of Canada from Ontario, Quebec, New Brunswick, and Nova Scotia set out terms and provisions for federal and provincial responsibilities for health care. This early document set a precedent for organization and management of the health of Canadians.

Approaches to Health Care in Canada

The organization and management of Canadian health care and approaches to health care are interdependent. Historically, approaches to health care in Canada have been categorized as medical, behavioural, and socioenvironmental.

Medical Approach to Health Care in Canada

Throughout the 20th century, a medical approach to health was predominant. This approach equated health problems with physiological risk factors that conveyed disease. Health problems were pathologized, which means that the focus of health care was on curing diseases and health problems. Medical intervention for restoration of health was emphasized. Health care was reactive and did not incorporate proactive approaches for disease prevention and health promotion. Consequently, with a medical approach to health care, many Canadians needed health-care procedures that were largely performed by physicians, with heavy reliance on in-hospital patient care. Until the 1960s, payment for health care came directly out of the pockets of Canadians. Understandably, during this era, not all Canadians could afford routine or lifesaving procedures.

In 1947, the Saskatchewan government, led by leader Tommy Douglas, introduced the first provincial hospital insurance program. A serious health challenge plagued Mr. Douglas in his youth, an experience that had a profound influence on his life and prompted him to champion the introduction of **socialized medicine**, or publicly funded insurance-based health coverage (Box 2.1). Mr. Douglas is

reported saying, "I came to believe that health services ought not to have a price tag on them, and that people should be able to get whatever health services they required irrespective of their individual capacity to pay" (Waiser, 2006, p. 4). Mr. Douglas, the illustrious and influential former Premier of Saskatchewan, features prominently in the history of Canada as the father of socialized medicine.

Using a medical approach to health, how would Louis's grandmother's dizzy spell be understood? Would the dizzy spell be pathologized and attributed to a disease process for which she has physiological risk factors? Might the primary focus of her care be looking for disease that caused the dizzy spells rather than developing a holistic health assessment inclusive of psycho-emotional, nutritional, and stress assessment that might reveal others causes? Because she has not sought any type of health care in Canada, is there a potential for her care to be reactive, excluding discussion about disease prevention and health promotion? Using a medical approach to understand and treat Louis's grandmother's dizzy spell, how reliant is she on physicians and in-hospital patient care? The answers to these questions help us understand the medical approach to health and health care and allow us to see that this approach does not meet completely the current holistic health-care needs of Canadians.

Behavioural Approach to Health Care in Canada

In the 1970s, a shift away from a medical model approach to health care gave way to a behavioural perspective. During this time, Canada led the way in expanding understanding health, prompted by concern over the meager increase in individual health outcomes relative to the increased funding spent on health care. A report entitled *A New Perspective on the Health of Canadians* (Lalonde, 1974/1981), commonly called the Lalonde Report, promoted individual responsibility for health, shifting the emphasis away from seeing health problems solely as physiological risk factors that conveyed disease. A refocused perspective of health that looked at causal influences beyond risk factors predominant in the medical approach was a groundbreaking shift in thinking about health and well-being of Canadians and the structure of health services needed to support them. The behavioural approach de-emphasized medical intervention for restoration of health by proposing the integration of the relatively new concepts of health promotion and disease prevention into the medical approach. It was at this time that the Canadian public was first introduced in the Lalonde Report to health field concepts that are now known as **determinants of health**; for example, biology, lifestyle, environment, and health-care organizations, or access to care. Canadians' awareness of the complexity of health and what it meant to be healthy (i.e., not just governmental and physician-determined events such as immunization) was raised. If it was true that health was within individual control, then it was thought that poor health could

---

> ### BOX 2.1 Tommy Douglas's Early Experience With Health Care
>
> At the age of 10 years, Tommy Douglas was hospitalized due to a bone infection, osteomyelitis, suffered 4 years earlier. His knee required several operations—none of which were successful. Without the money to pay for a specialist, his parents were told that the only option was to amputate their son's leg before the infection spread to the rest of his body. But before that could happen, a visiting surgeon offered to operate on Douglas for free, as long as his students were allowed to attend. The surgery saved Douglas's leg—quite possibly his life—and would serve as his inspiration for his dream of universally accessible medical care.
>
> Source: *Making Medicare Work: The History of Healthcare in Canada 1914–2007* (2010). Retrieved from http://www.civilization.ca/cmc/exhibitions/hist/medicare/medic-3g03e.shtml

be related to lack of knowledge. If lifestyle was a major factor contributing to health, then providing education could improve health by decreasing risk factors within individual control. The Lalonde Report and subsequent theories spawned several educational initiatives, including the introduction of Canada's Food Guide. Although the individual responsibility approach to health seems realistic now, 40 years ago, this approach was criticized for implying that individuals were not taking responsibility for healthy choices and were therefore to blame for their poor health. During this time, health behaviour changes were made primarily by well-educated and well-employed Canadians. The behavioural approach fell out of favour because it neglected to recognize socioeconomic, sociocultural, environmental, and geographic barriers to making healthy lifestyle choices. Critics of the behavioural approach to health believed that individuals could not be separated from their context. As a result, Lalonde's original health field concepts have been expanded to include social context and the relationship between personal health and social physical environments.

The Epp Report

Two additional landmark reports from 1986 have informed approaches to Canadian health and health care. These reports are Achieving Health for All: A Framework for Health Promotion (Epp, 1986), commonly called the Epp Report, and the Ottawa Charter for Health Promotion (Canadian Public Health Association, Health and Welfare Canada, & World Health Organization, 1986). The First International Conference on Health Promotion was hosted in Ottawa by Canada in 1986. The then Canadian Minister of Health and Welfare and an author, the Hon. Jake Epp, first shared his report at the conference, during which he outlined health promotion initiatives that later became Canada's blueprint to meet the World Health Organization's 1978 mandate of Health for All by the Year 2000 (World Health Organization [WHO], 1978) (Box 2.2).

The Ottawa Charter was created and signed by delegates representing 38 countries who shared a common belief in health equity. The charter incorporated socioenvironmental criteria to health promotion, expanding on Lalonde's (1974/1981) four health field concepts but renaming them health prerequisites. Since then, the Ottawa Charter has been used globally as a template for health promotion (Box 2.3).

Using a behavioural approach to health, how would Louis's grandmother's dizzy spell be understood? Although this approach would shift the emphasis away from seeing her dizzy spell solely as a result of physiological risk factors and an indicator of disease, she has not sought any type of health care since arriving in Canada, making it difficult to know about her understanding of health, health promotion, and disease prevention. Within a behavioural approach that focuses on individual responsibility for health, would Louis's grandmother feel blamed for not seeking health care since

BOX 2.2 Achieving Health for All: A Framework for Health Promotion (The Epp Report)

The Epp Report (Epp, 1986) followed the contributions of the Lalonde Report (Lalonde, 1974/1981) in which health was conceptualized as a function of more than the advancement of medicine and stressed the important contribution to health of lifestyle, nutrition, and physical environment. Through the government's 1980s initiatives to modify individual behaviour, the concept of health promotion was born. Responding to changes in thought beyond the government, the Epp Report broadened health promotion from the emphasis on lifestyle to include environmental determinants. It introduced the idea of healthy public policy as a health promotion intervention that went beyond what could be done by the government alone. Epp maintained that health promotion initiatives needed support from all levels of government, local groups, and employers to promote success and change over time. The key health promotion challenges stressed by the Epp Report were (1) assessing the health status of disadvantaged groups and reducing inequities (e.g., shorter life expectancies, higher prevalence of disability, and poorer health than average Canadians), (2) detecting and managing chronic disease, (3) identifying diseases that were preventable and focusing on prevention, and (4) enhancing people's abilities to cope. To overcome these challenges, suggested health promotion strategies included self-care, mutual aid (i.e., people helping each other), and creation of health environments. The legacy of the Epp Report includes fostering public participation in implementing health promotion programs, strengthening community health services, and coordinating health public policy to achieve health for all Canadians.

Source: Epp, J. (1986). *Achieving health for all: A framework for health promotion*. Ottawa, ON: Health Canada.

coming to Canada? Does a behavioural approach to health consider the cultural context of health and health care and the influence of both on the experience of a new immigrant? Does a behavioural approach support culture as a determinant of health and the provision of culturally safe (Browne, Smye, & Varcoe, 2005) health care? Additionally, how does a behavioural approach to health consider the role and impact of family as context for care? Information about and insight to the responses to these questions may be revealed in an exploration of a socioenvironmental approach to health.

The Socioenvironmental Approach to Health Care in Canada

The introduction of health fields, or social determinants of health (WHO, 2011), led the way for a socioenvironmental approach to health. The socioenvironmental approach builds on the behavioural perspective that humans' purposeful/chosen interaction with biology, lifestyles, environment, and health-care organizations, or access to care, is a legitimate factor in determining health and health outcomes. The socioenvironmental approach combines previous approaches with an exploration of possible other

Ottawa Charter for Health Promotion

The Ottawa Charter for Health Promotion is a landmark Canadian document that expanded on Lalonde's (1974/1981) work with "health fields." Health fields became "health prerequisites" that included peace, shelter, education, food, a stable ecosystem, income/employment, sustainable resources, and social justice and equity. The Ottawa Charter stressed the importance of a collaborative approach to explore and manage health issues, maintaining that many factors outside of health care are integral to the improvement of individual and population health. This document includes the following five strategies that have served as a health promotion framework for countries around the world.

1. Build public health promotion policies at all levels of government.
2. Create and maintain supportive physical, social, cultural, spiritual, and economic environments.
3. Strengthen community action to achieve better health via priority setting and responsible decision-making inclusive of diligent assessment, planning, and implementation.
4. Develop personal skills to enable preparation for all life stages, including illness and injury.
5. Redefine and/or reorient health services to better meet the individual and community health needs.

Source: Canadian Public Health Association, Health and Welfare Canada, & World Health Organization. (1986). *Ottawa Charter for Health Promotion.* Retrieved from http://www.who.int/hpr/NPH/docs/ottawa_charter_hp.pdf

contributors to health beyond those impacting the individual. For example, the social context as a contributor to health refers to family and community environment (e.g., social support network, housing and education, social status) in which we live and interact and the resultant impact on our knowledge development and way of being. Our environmental context refers to the collective impact on health and health outcomes related to human-built environments (Natural Resources Canada, 2010), encompassing growth in energy use (e.g., expansion of nuclear wind and electric power) and communication/entertainment technology (i.e., worldwide connectivity and sedentary activity), the reliance on car transportation (i.e., increased air pollution and decreased exercise), or food availability (e.g., convenience and fast foods). Combined social and environmental contexts inform a socioenvironmental approach to health. This perspective asks how individuals, groups, and communities can realize their aspirations and satisfy their health, health care, and other needs and at the same time cope with (or change) the socioenvironment to benefit health and health outcomes. This approach includes the perspective that health is self-defined. A sense of health may be present even in the company of a medical diagnosis (e.g., diabetes). Using a socioenvironmental approach to health, health resources (e.g., nurse practitioners, physiotherapists, centres for a broad range of health care) should be comprehensive, available, and accessible to all. Yet, we must question how a

socioenvironmental perspective considers cultural components of health (e.g., Aboriginal health care) and changing demographics, such as the emergence of a large cohort of aging baby boomers; as well as geography and the impact of rural/urban locations on the health of Canadians; and the needs of Canada's growing immigrant population, to name a few factors that are known to impact health and health behaviour (Romanow, 2002).

For Louis as a first-generation Canadian tasked with helping his grandmother manage her health challenge, what is the meaning of a socioenvironmental approach to health care? Is this approach appropriate in providing holistic care for his grandmother? What elements of care might be missing? How might a socioenvironmental approach to health be changed to incorporate Louis's grandmother's holistic health-care needs? Your suggestions are integral in creating a platform for health-care reform, discussed later in this chapter.

Summary of Historical Context

Since confederation, the changes in approach to Canadian health care and the health-care system occurred in response to the needs of Canadians and how they live their lives across all socioeconomic, sociocultural, and socioenvironmental sectors. Simultaneously, socially, economically, and technologically prompted growth was supported by health-care legislation. However, the path of change has not always been smooth. The differences between provinces in the provision of health care have sparked ongoing debates about the responsibility and appropriateness of governments administrating the health-care system. As an example, consider the Canadian Health Care System, founded on the principle of egalitarianism embedded in the CHA alongside the complexity of the Canadian Charter of Rights and Freedoms. Integral components of the ongoing discussion about what health care and health human resource framework best suits the holistic health-care needs of Canadians are where and how people live their lives, including their views and responses to health and illness, and the kind of treatment they expect.

Reflecting on the case of Louis's grandmother, what approach to health care is evident in the family and health-care system's management of her care? How does the CHA support her health-care needs? Information and insight into the answers to these questions may be revealed in the following discussion of contemporary context of health care in Canada.

1984 Canada Health Act

By 1971, under the CHA, all Canadians were guaranteed access to essential medical services, regardless of employment, income, or health (Kraker, 2001). During the early 1970s, with health-care costs rising, many physicians decided to charge patients privately rather than receive payment through provincial/territorial health plans. To bill privately for health care was antithetical to the intent of the CHA, which was to "protect, promote and restore the physical and mental well-being of Canada and to facilitate reasonable access to health services without financial or other barriers" (Health Canada, 2010).

In order to uphold the principles of medicare, the Hospital Insurance and Diagnostic Services Act of 1957 (Turner, 1958) and the Medical Care Act of 1966 (Thompson, 2010) were replaced by the **Canada Health Act (CHA)**, possibly the most important landmark legislation in support of Canadian health care (Health Canada, 2010). Today, the CHA is the federal legislation that governs Canada's publicly funded, not-for-profit health-care system. This Act was first passed in 1984 and includes a condition that provinces/territories that allow private and extra billing within their respective plans would be denied federal financial support. At the same time, physicians who had opted out of the insurance plan were forbidden to charge patients beyond the scheduled fee-for-service set for the province/territory (Department of Justice, 2011).

A history of Canada's socialized medicine program, or medicare, entitled *Making Medicare: The History of Health Care in Canada, 1914-2007*, can be found at the Canadian Museum of Civilization website.

The Organization of Health Care in Canada: The Contemporary Context

The federal government provides national leadership and oversight for health care in Canada. The federal ministry responsible for the health of Canadians is Health Canada, which is "committed to improving the lives of all of Canada's people and to making this country's population among the healthiest in the world as measured by longevity, lifestyle and effective use of the public health care system" (Health Canada, 2011a). Although the provinces and territories have authority for health care, Health Canada ensures that they are compliant with the CHA and can impose penalties (such as withholding funding) on those provinces and territories that do not comply. Health Canada is responsible for transferring federal dollars to the provinces and territories to fund health care.

Five Pillars of the Canadian Health-Care System

The CHA of 1984 continues to define the five principles, also called pillars, of Canada's socialized medicine, or medicare program. These pillars ensure that all eligible residents of Canada have reasonable access to insured health services on a prepaid basis without direct charges at the point of care for such services.

Public Administration

Public administration is the first pillar of Canada's health-care system. Each provincial and territorial health insurance plan must be administered and operated on a not-for-profit basis by a public authority. The public authority is accountable to its respective provincial or territorial government for decisions regarding benefits and levels of service, and its records are publicly audited (Parliament of Canada, 2005). To meet CHA requirements, provincial and territorial ministries or departments of health oversee health plans. At local levels, health service plans are delivered through regional health authorities (RHAs; Thompson, 2010).

Comprehensiveness

The health-care insurance plan of a province or territory must cover all insured services provided by hospitals, physicians, or dentists (e.g., dental services that require surgery in a hospital setting) and where the law of the province permits, select services provided by other health-care practitioners for eligible people (Parliament of Canada, 2005). Services available under the insurance plan must be available to all provincial or territorial residents with equal opportunity. Comprehensiveness of health services (e.g., coverage for components of home care, chiropractic care, or pharmacy care) may vary across provinces and territories as determined by their respective governments (Thompson, 2010). For information about uninsured health services, consult provincial and territorial ministries of health.

Universality

Universality in public health means all insured residents of a province or territory are entitled to the insured health services provided by their respective provincial or territorial health insurance plan on uniform terms and conditions (Parliament of Canada, 2005). To become insured and therefore entitled to receive health services, all residents must register with their respective government. For persons new to Canada (e.g., landed immigrants, returning Canadians) following the application process, there may be a waiting period before becoming eligible to receive insured health services. However, by law, this waiting period must not exceed 3 months. The CHA orders 100% coverage of insured costs, in contrast to the earlier Medical Care Act of 1967 that required only 95% coverage (Thompson, 2010).

Portability

Portability in public health means that residents moving from one province or territory to another continue to be covered for insured health services by their home jurisdiction during any waiting period (not longer than 3 months) before coverage is transferred to their new jurisdiction. During any temporary absence from a home province or territory, or from Canada, insured health services coverage continues for a prescribed period of time set by each province and territory. However, the intent of the portability criterion is not to entitle persons to seek health services outside their home province. Rather, it is intended to provide seamless coverage in the event of an emergency or urgent need during the temporary absence (e.g., business, education, vacation) (Parliament of Canada, 2005; Thompson, 2010). Provincial and territorial websites for ministries of health offer information about the specific details of health-care coverage in each respective jurisdiction.

Accessibility

Accessibility protects all insured people of Canada's provinces and territories from extra charges for health care or from discrimination. They are guaranteed reasonable access to insured hospital, medical, and surgical-dental care on uniform terms and conditions without discrimination on the basis of age, health status, or financial circumstances (Parliament of Canada, 2005). The term *reasonable access* means access to services when and where they are available, as they are available. For example, an insured person must be granted access to a service in another jurisdiction (i.e., at the closest location) if the health-care service is required but is not available in their home territory or province (Thompson, 2010).

Organization of Canada's Health System

As mentioned previously, Canada's health system is governed by federal, provincial, and territorial governments. This means that Health Canada, in accordance with the CHA (2009), outlines the principles of health care for Canadians. Thus, the provinces and territories must follow these principles to manage and provide health care for their residents under the authority of provincial and territorial ministries of health.

Health Canada is headed by the minister of health, who is an elected member of parliament appointed to the position by the prime minister of Canada. The current minister of health is Leona Aglukkaq. Because the minister of health is responsible for promoting, preserving, and improving the health of the people of Canada, the minister oversees health-related laws and regulations and works collaboratively with the provinces and territories on health system issues. Included in the minister of health's portfolio, which has over 12,000 employees with an annual budget of more than $3.8 billion, are the Public Health Agency of Canada, the Canadian Institutes of Health and Research, the Hazardous Materials Information Review Commission, the Patented Medicine Prices Review Board, and Assisted Human Reproduction Canada (Health Canada, 2009). The minister is responsible for preparing an annual report including how the provinces have met the conditions of the CHA. This report is presented in parliament and is a public document (Health Canada, 2013). In 2009 to 2010, the most prominent concerns with respect to compliance with the CHA remained the practice at private clinics of extra billing and queue jumping for medically necessary health services at private clinics. Health Canada has made these concerns known to the provinces that allow these charges.

Administration of Health Canada

The administrative structure of Health Canada includes the deputy minister of health and associate deputy ministers, all of whom are appointed from the civil service. They are not elected members of parliament; rather, they are considered apolitical (Thompson, 2010). The deputy minister can assume some of the duties of the minister of health if the minister is unavailable.

Health Canada also is a service provider. This means that Health Canada is responsible for providing health care for serving members of the Royal Canadian Mounted Police and the military; Inuit, Innu, and First Nations Canadians living on reserves; eligible veterans; refugee claimants; and inmates in federal penitentiaries. Health Canada also provides primary health-care services in remote and isolated areas of Canada when provincial and territorial services are not available (Health Canada, 2011b).

Branches of Health Canada

Health Canada is organized into branches and agencies to fulfill its roles and mission (Box 2.4). In addition to the roles of overseeing laws and regulations, upholding the pillars of medicare, and providing service, this ministry is a funder of health programs and research and provides information essential to maintaining health care and safety of Canadians (Health Canada, 2011b).

BOX 2.4 Health Canada: Branches and Agencies

Ministers and Officers
- Minister of Health
- Deputy Minister
- Associate Deputy Minister
- Chief Public Health Officer

Branches, Offices and Bureaus
- Audit and Accountability Bureau
- Chief Financial Officer Branch
- Corporate Services Branch
- Departmental Secretariat
- First Nations & Inuit Health Branch
- Health Products & Food Branch
- Healthy Environments & Consumer Safety Branch
- Legal Services
- Pest Management Regulatory Agency
- Communications and Public Affairs Branch
- Regions and Programs Branch
- Strategic Policy Branch

Agencies
- Assisted Human Reproduction Canada
- Canadian Institutes of Health Research
- Hazardous Materials Information Review Commission
- Patented Medicines Prices Review Board
- Public Health Agency of Canada

Source: http://www.hc-sc.gc.ca/ahc-asc/branch-dirgen/index-eng.php

The Strategic Policy Branch of Health Canada is of particular interest to nurses. This branch "strive[s] to develop effective policy responses to a range of priority, emerging, and cross-cutting issues that impact the health of Canadians" (Health Canada, 2011c). For example, the Office of Nursing Policy was created in 1999 to advise Health Canada on policy issues and programs and recommendations regarding the nursing workforce to better meet the health-care needs of Canadians (Thompson, 2010).

Through the Strategic Policy Branch, Health Canada also plays an important role in global health by collaborating with international health agencies and governments. This is another way that Health Canada protects the health of Canadians and shares health information with the global community. The International Affairs Directorate "initiates, coordinates and monitors departmental policies, strategies and activities in the international field. It provides advice on the department's strategic approach to international affairs, ensures the department's international activities are internally coherent and consistent with government-wide policies and recommends departmental representation at international meetings" (Health Canada, 2007). This directorate coordinates Canada's representation in international organizations such as WHO.

Separate Provincial and Territorial Plans

Although the CHA outlines the principles and responsibilities of medicare, each province and territory is responsible for managing and providing primary, secondary, and tertiary health care for its citizens. This means there are 13 separate health-care insurance programs across Canada to cover hospital care and medically necessary procedures for eligible residents. Each province and territory determines the services covered; therefore, this varies across the country. For example, because Canada does not have a national vaccination strategy, having 14 different immunization schedules across the country means that the influenza vaccine is free for all residents in some provinces, and in others, only to those in high-risk groups (Picard, 2010). Canada also lacks a national pharmacare plan for prescription drugs. According to Gagnon and Hébert (2010), if Canada were to develop a national plan for prescription drugs that respected provincial health jurisdictions, savings of up to $10.7 billion could be realized while giving all Canadians equal access to affordable prescription drugs.

Like the federal government, each province and territory has a ministry responsible for health care with various branches. Similar to the federal minister, the provincial ministers responsible for health care are appointed by the premier, and the deputy ministers are civil servants. Where there are gaps in funding, provinces and territories finance health-care services through various means (depending on the context of the province or territory), such as health-care premiums, payroll taxes, or through general revenues (Thompson, 2010). Third-party insurance or private health insurance such as that provided by employee benefit plans offset much of the cost of health-care services not provided by the provinces and territories.

Health-care costs in Canada are consuming a growing proportion of the federal, provincial, and territorial budgets—a trend which experts warn is unsustainable. According to the Fraser Institute, government spending on health care has grown faster than provincial revenues. In Quebec and Ontario, health-care spending currently consumes half of total revenues. Saskatchewan, Alberta, British Columbia, and New Brunswick will spend half of their total revenues by 2017. By 2028, Manitoba and Prince Edward Island will join the other provinces in health-care spending levels (Skinner & Rovere, 2011).

Reorganization of Health Systems

In order to make the health system more responsive and accountable to the public and to streamline decision-making in a more cost-effective manner, every province and territory has undertaken regionalization of health systems. In order to engage the community, RHAs have formed, made up of citizens, with the mandate to "identify the health needs of its area, to prioritize and develop plans to address these, and to ensure that funds are allocated and services delivered accordingly" (Chessie, 2009, p. 706). The intent of RHAs is to decentralize decision-making and streamline services. RHAs oversee long-term care; residential and acute care services; and, in some regions, public and mental health, addiction, and health promotion programs, reporting financial statements and performance indicators to their respective provincial or territorial ministries of health (Thompson, 2010, p. 155). For example, Local Health Integration Networks (LHINs) are RHAs that have been developed across Ontario to make decisions at the community level about health needs for constituents. Their goal is to integrate health services in order to provide the best and most appropriate care in the right setting. To achieve this goal, LHINs are responsible for funding and managing a wide range of health services and service providers (Government of Ontario, 2014), including hospitals, Community Care Access Centres (CCAC), mental health and addiction agencies, and community support services, among others.

Points of Care

According to the CHA criteria of accessibility, all insured Canadians have the right to access care. This criterion is well implemented within Canada's regionalized health system, and Canadians can access health care in various settings, or at various **points of care**. These points of care can be described using broad categories, including public health units, offices and clinics, health-care institutions, and private homes. Descriptive details about points of care are included in Table 2.1. Each point of care is designed to meet the current and future needs of Canadians.

Point of Care	Examples	Type of Care	Health Professional
Public health	Public health unit clinics	Primary	Physicians, nurses
	Public health unit website	Primary	Information dedicated to public health generated by government, physicians, nurses, and other health professionals
	Public health unit phone lines	Primary	Nurses
Office	Family doctor	Primary	Family doctor, nurse practitioner, family therapist
	Physician specialist	Secondary	Physician specialist (e.g., cardiology, orthopedic surgeon)
	Naturopathic specialist	Primary, secondary	Naturopathic health provider
Clinic	Community rehabilitation specialist	Primary	Family doctor, nurse practitioner, rehabilitation specialist, social worker, family therapist
Institution	Community hospital	Secondary	Physician specialists, nurses, nurse practitioners, other health specialists may include but not limited to OT, PT, SLP, pastoral care, social work, psychologists, respiratory therapists
	Acute care hospital	Tertiary, quaternary	
	Long-term care centre	Primary, secondary	
	Hospice, palliative care centre	Primary, secondary	
Phone	Telehealth	Primary	Nurses
Home	Palliative care, for example	Primary, secondary, tertiary	Physicians, nurses, and others

TABLE 2.1 Canadian Health System Points of Care

OT, occupational therapist; PT, physical therapist; SLP, speech-language pathologist.

Louis's grandmother is using the urgent care centre for care. Because the emergency room is her first point of contact with the health system, she will receive the primary level of health care. If she requires the services of a physician specialist, she will experience secondary level of care services. If Louis's grandmother requires care in an institution, she may be admitted to a secondary care or community-based hospital, where specialist and nursing care is available. If her health needs are more acute, requiring a different type of specialist care, she may be admitted to a health-care institution for tertiary or quaternary level of care by various **health professionals**, often involving specialized technology. The Canadian health system is organized according to complexity and type of care required and is framed as levels including primary, secondary, tertiary, and quaternary care.

Primary Health Care

"**Primary health care** refers to an approach to health and a spectrum of services beyond the traditional health care system. It includes all services that play a part in health, such as income, housing, education, and environment. Primary care is the element within primary health care that focuses on health care services, including health promotion, illness and injury prevention, and the diagnosis and treatment of illness and injury" (Health Canada, 2012a, para. 1). At this first level of care, supports and services to promote the health and well-being of Canadians include direct provision of care from health professionals (e.g., nurses, nurse practitioners, doctors, physiotherapists, occupational therapists, speech language pathologists, chiropractors, psychologists, and other regulated

health providers) as well as direct links to diagnostic and hospital services (Health Canada, 2006a). Increasingly, primary health-care services are provided by an interprofessional team composed of health- and social-care (e.g., social work) professionals best suited to caring for individuals' needs. Additionally, primary health care refers to coordination of care services to promote continuity of care across the health system so that Canadians requiring more specialized care can move easily from primary to the next level of care if health challenges are best addressed in-hospital or by a physician specialist (e.g., cardiologist or neurologist) (Health Canada, 2006a).

The variety and arrangement of primary health services and their respective models of administration and funding vary across the provinces and territories in order to meet the needs of Canadians within their personal and geographic contexts. Generally, primary health-care services may include health promotion, prevention and treatment of common diseases and injuries, basic emergency services, primary mental health care, palliative and end-of-life care, well-baby care and healthy child development, primary maternity care, rehabilitation services, and referral specialist and in-hospital care. Primary health care is integral to the health of Canadians. To uphold this health-care responsibility, an emphasis on primary health-care reform is active and described later in this text.

Louis has taken his grandmother to an urgent care centre for care. How does this type of care fit with what you know about primary care? Is the urgent care centre the most appropriate place for her to receive primary care? What primary health-care options are available to Louis, his family, and other Canadians facing similar health challenges?

Secondary Health Care

Secondary care usually involves diagnosis and treatment of health challenges of varying complexities by specialists (e.g., surgeon, psychiatrist, or ophthalmologist) (Ontario Ministry of Health and Long-Term Care, 2009). For **secondary health care**, Canadians are referred by a primary care provider to specialized care at a hospital (e.g., community-based general hospital), at a long-term care facility, or in the community (Health Canada, 2005). Importantly, primary care providers work with specialists to provide diagnostic and treatment services. Care by specialists may be short term, with care being resumed by primary care providers. Additionally, secondary care may involve/result in referral to a tertiary level of care (Thompson, 2010).

Whom are the health system criteria that need to be met to support a referral to secondary care for Louis's grandmother? Using your nursing knowledge, what is the likelihood that Louis's grandmother is in need of a referral to secondary care? What would her secondary health care look like?

Tertiary and Quaternary Health Care

Tertiary health care is specialized consultative care involving dedicated supports and resources usually based on a referral from primary or secondary health-care providers. This highly technical level of health care includes diagnosis and treatment of disease and disability in sophisticated large research and teaching hospitals. Specialized intensive care units, advanced diagnostic support services, and highly trained personnel are characteristic of tertiary health-care services. Specialist care from an interprofessional team may include acute, rehabilitative, or palliative care. Similar to secondary levels of care, referral is required, and once tertiary health care is no longer required, the primary provider resumes provision of care. Commonly, tertiary and quaternary health care is provided at academic health science centres, also called teaching hospitals, which have an affiliation with universities with health profession schools, often including medicine and nursing. Teaching hospitals are involved in education, research, and patient care, providing complex or specialized care for their communities, districts, and regions (Ontario Ministry of Health and Long-Term Care, 2009). Although both tertiary and quaternary levels provide extremely specialized care, quaternary care is distinguished by the difference in type and availability of specialized care provided. With highly complex subspecialty services, the providers may act as provincial, national, and international resources (e.g., Hospital for Sick Children) (Ontario Ministry of Health and Long-Term Care, 2009).

Nurses and Canadian Health Care: The Professional Context

Currently, baccalaureate degree as entry to registered nurse (RN) practice is required by all provinces and territories, except Quebec (Canadian Nurses Association [CNA], 2009).

At the Ordre des infirmières et infirmiers du Québec annual meeting, the baccalaureate degree as entry to practice was endorsed by the membership (Ordre des infirmières et infirmiers du Québec [OIIQ], 2012). In addition to RN practice, other nursing roles across the country include registered practical nurse (RPN) (e.g., RPN in Ontario), licensed practical nurse (LPN), and registered psychiatric nurse (RPN) (CNA, 2010). Educational programs leading to a baccalaureate nursing degree have expanded beyond the historic 4-year program to include compressed time frame (or fast-track) 2-year programs for students in possession of a degree and the requisite adjunct nursing courses (e.g., anatomy, pharmacology, research methods). Other baccalaureate programs are tailored specifically for internationally educated or foreign nursing graduates, with programs to bridge LPN and registered practical and psychiatric nurses to baccalaureate degrees. There are post-RN programs for diploma-prepared nurses educated in the era prior to the baccalaureate entry to practice mandate who wish to obtain a nursing degree. A list of nurse education programs in Canada can be found on the Canadian Nurses Association (CNA) website.

Scopes of practice for RNs and RPNs differ and are outlined clearly by provincial and territorial licensing bodies (e.g., College of Nurses of Ontario [CNO]). These provincial and territorial regulatory bodies have developed and agreed on RN entry to practice competencies (CNA, 2010) that can also be found on the CNA website. The Canadian Registered Nurse Exam (CRNE) is the national RN licensing exam for all eligible nursing graduates across the country, except Quebec. In 2015, the national RN licensing exam will be changing to the National Council Licensure Examination (NCLEX), and consideration by the province of Quebec to have their nursing graduates write the NCLEX is ongoing at the time of writing this chapter. You can read more about the NCLEX in Chapter 7. A core requirement for eligibility is successful graduation from an accredited nursing program. Because responsibility for health-care education is a provincial and territorial jurisdiction, each jurisdiction determines its own baccalaureate program goals and success criteria. Program accreditation follows a framework established by the Canadian Association of Schools of Nursing (CASN). In general, nursing education and practice in Canada is governed by *Standards of Practice* established by provincial and territorial regulatory bodies yet adheres to a *Codes of Ethics* established by the CNA (2008). Nursing programs strive to develop relevant and responsive curricula. In view of the challenge of human health resources and national nursing shortage (Thompson, 2010), the implications for nursing education and practice today include graduating significant numbers of nurses and the retention of an experienced workforce to serve as valued mentors to novice practitioners. Historically, nurses are trusted and respected health professionals, yet the current Canadian health context challenges nurses to address seemingly irresolvable and recurring issues in health-care delivery, education, and practice with diminishing resources and insufficient support (McIntyre & McDonald, 2010).

Nursing in Practice

Nursing is an academic and practice profession that continues to evolve in response to the changing landscape of Canadian health and health services. Health promotion is the focus of RNs across all provinces and territories, yet increasingly, there are "incongruities between what nurses are prepared to do educationally and philosophically and the expectations encountered in practice" (McDonald & McIntyre, 2010, p. 284). The nature of nurses' work and workplaces and the significance of both are impacted by the broader context of Canadian's health, Canadian health services, and Canadian **health-care reform**. What is the role of nursing in today's health-care environment and what is the changing face of nursing are questions that need to be addressed by nurses for nurses. However, what is certain is that nurses work with people throughout the life continuum in multiple contexts across wellness and illness situations. Currently and following traditional patterns, most nurses practice in hospitals, with community-based and long-term care as the next most common practice areas (CNA & Canadian Association of Schools of Nursing [CASN], 2010; McDonald & McIntyre, 2010). Within the shifting context of Canadian health care, not only are scopes of nursing practice changing but also locations where nurses work and the nature of the workplace are changing accordingly. For example, with current health-care reform and structures among many provinces and territories, the role of the primary care nurse practitioner is gaining recognition as an appropriate first point of care for a growing population of Canadians (Thompson, 2010), a first point of care often made by choice. Changing scopes of practice and the nature of nurses' work are evolving to meet the shifting needs of Canada's diverse population.

Health-Care Reform: The Changing Context of Canadian Health Care

For decades, Canadians have enjoyed the benefits of a health-care system that upholds the principles and values outlined in the CHA of 1984 (i.e., health as a public good). Since the inception of the CHA over a quarter of a century ago, changes in medicine have occurred alongside changes in Canadian society. For example, the baby boom population has changed population demographics as this large age cohort approaches retirement and experiences the changes of aging. Despite the fact that this cohort is aging, many enjoy good health and are actively involved in second careers, community activities, and sports. The health needs of this cohort are different from those of earlier generations, making new demands on the health-care system. Health ecology is changing, and the advent of superbugs is upon us. At the same time, the prevalence of chronic health challenges exists across all age sectors, and increased acuity in secondary, tertiary, and quaternary health institutions has risen. Further changes to Canadian health care include decentralization of mental health care and advances in health-care technology

and pharmacology (e.g., pharmacogenomics). Challenges with health human resources and concern about access to health care for rural populations (Romanow, 2002) continue to be present. Perhaps due to these changes in Canadian society and in the health sector, issues about privatization of health care are resurfacing (Irvine, Ferguson, & Cackett, 2005). Uppermost in the minds of many Canadians is concern about our publicly funded health-care system and whether or not it can continue to meet the expanding and changing needs of the Canadian public. Canadian health-care spending is growing (Thompson, 2010), raising questions about the sustainability of our single-payer medicare system. Is one model for the entire country relevant in this era?

Health-Care Reform

The answers to these and other questions are being explored, and the concept of health-care reform has become prominent over the last decade as funding restraints have imposed the need for change (Rankin, 2003). *Health-care reform* is a general term that refers to discussion about, changes to, and creation of health policy (i.e., by government) that affects health-care delivery. Health-care reform might address issues related to the relative lack of emphasis on health promotion and disease prevention, lack of continuity among providers and institutions, health system access problems (e.g., lack of care in rural and remote areas or after-hours services in urban centres), and quality of work life for health providers (Health Canada, 2006a).

In 2001, Mr. Roy Romanow, QC, was commissioned by the prime minister to review and explore Canada's health-care system and to make recommendations to enhance its quality and sustainability. To understand the situation and to collect data, Romanow consulted Canadians. The outcome of this large consultative process is documented in *Building on Values: The Future of Health Care in Canada* (Romanow, 2002), including 47 recommendations that "serve as a roadmap for a collective journey by Canadians to reform and renew their health care system" (p. xxiii). The full Romanow report can be found as a media link in Web Resources on **thePoint**.

Since the work of the Romanow commission, other important gatherings have aimed to explore and review the future of Canadian health care. For example, the first ministers (Canadian heads of government including the prime minister and the provincial and territorial premiers) have met numerous times to identify and work on health-care issues across the provinces and territories. These reforms are a work in progress and first ministers continue to meet periodically. Of prime significance to the health of Canada's population is an agreement among first ministers, entitled the Kelowna Accord (Government of Canada: Justice Laws Website, 2013), in which the government attaches specific significance to the health of Canada's Aboriginal population (Box 2.5).

Health-care reform applies to all levels of health care, including primary, secondary, tertiary, and quaternary care.

BOX 2.5   Kelowna Accord

The Kelowna Accord is a series of agreements between the government of Canada, first ministers of the provinces, territorial leaders, and the leaders of five national Aboriginal organizations in Canada. The purpose of the Accord was to improve the education, employment, and living conditions for Aboriginal peoples through governmental funding and other programs. Background consultation with stakeholder groups, including those listed, informed the November 2005 First Ministers' Meeting in Kelowna, British Columbia and resulted in a paper entitled *First Ministers and National Aboriginal Leaders Strengthening Relationships and Closing the Gap*, or Kelowna Accord as named by the media. Aboriginal leaders considered the Accord a step forward because it involved a process of cooperation and consultation that brought all parties to the table. Changes in Canada's governing political party since the creation of the Kelowna Accord in 2005 resulted in changes in perspective on funding, expenditure, and process, although commitment to intent of the document and the targets set out at the First Ministers' Meeting in Kelowna were supported. Concerns have been raised by Aboriginal leaders about the value of the Accord in eliminating gaps between Aboriginal and non-Aboriginal Canadians that exist in the areas of education, skills development, health care, housing, and access to clean water and employment, as provided for in the Kelowna Accord. The Kelowna Accord Implementation Act received final government assent on June 18, 2008 (Government of Canada: Justice Laws Website 2013).

However, as the first point of contact and the foundation of the health-care system, primary health-care reform has been of particular focus (Health Council of Canada, 2005).

Primary Health-Care Reform

The ways in which primary health-care services are organized and delivered have been the focus of much discussion and debate (Health Council of Canada, 2005; Romanow, 2002). As a result, several key changes have been recommended for primary health-care reform. First, we have seen a shift from individual health provider (e.g., physician) to teams of health providers (e.g., physician, nurses/nurse practitioners, and other health professionals as partners) who can provide comprehensive services that can result in better health, improved access to services, more efficient use of resources, and better satisfaction for both patients and providers (Health Canada, 2006b). The focus of health teams is health promotion and improving management of chronic health challenges. The advent of telephone advice (i.e., telehealth) can support primary health-care services after hours. The goals of these primary care reforms are to reduce the need for costly emergency room visits, to prevent unnecessary repetition of personal health information and diagnostic tests, and to promote greater collaboration. Changes to primary health care are ongoing as the provinces and territories implement their own plans for care reform suited to the specific needs of their respective jurisdictions. Time-limited (i.e., from 2000 to 2006) federal funding for primary health-care reform was provided directly to these jurisdictions to support transitional costs associated with introducing new approaches to care delivery, to support sustainability, and to promote a lasting impact on the health-care system (Health Canada, 2006b). At the same time, successful adoption of primary health reform and effective delivery of primary care is reliant on an adequate supply of human resources (the health workforce, e.g., nurses, physiotherapists, doctors), appropriate and up-to-date information technology (e.g., electronic health records [EHR]), changes to infrastructure and governance to support collaborative team-based care, and a move to a culture of accountability inclusive of personal feedback performance measurement and quality improvement (Health Canada, 2006b).

Secondary Health-Care Reform

Over the last decade, significant reform has occurred in the hospital sector. For example, hospitals are being restructured, business models are being imposed on health institution management, and transition to electronic rather than text-based records is growing (Rankin, 2003). At the same time, pressures exist to alter hospital structures to accommodate changing patterns of care from an institutional to a community-based model. This type of reform is aimed at providing the best care in the most client-appropriate environment while managing health care more efficiently. Following the business model, context also focuses on effectiveness and efficiency in secondary care. For example, because funding for Canadian hospitals is a global, provincially provided budget, some challenges to cost efficiency include decreasing wait times, upgrading technology and equipment, and providing adequate health human resources (e.g., nurses).

Health-care reform also involves changes to the supportive infrastructure for health services (e.g., pharmaceuticals). In 2003, the First Ministers' Accord on Health Care Renewal outlined a 10-year plan, starting in 2004, for health-care reforms including improved wait times, pharmaceuticals management, EHR, and teletriage. A document released by the Health Council of Canada (2011), entitled *Progress Report 2011: Health Care Renewal in Canada*, describes progress achieved to date among these areas of reform and other health-care innovations since 2003.

What Lies Ahead for Canadian Health Care: The Future Context

Canadians value and support their publicly funded, provincially administered, single-payer health-care system (Romanow, 2002; White & Nanan, 2009). The health-care system aims to protect, promote, and restore physical and mental well-being and to facilitate reasonable access to health services without financial barrier (Health Canada, 2010). In support of this aim, our understanding of health has grown over the last few decades to include many determinants such as gender and sex, employment, income inequality and poverty, education and literacy, social status and power, stress, food security, and environments among others (CNA, 2005; WHO, 2011). Toward this end, health-care interests are focused heavily on health promotion and illness prevention over illness treatment (Thompson, 2010). As a result of this shift, Canadians seeking health care will continue to have access to health promotion and primary and secondary illness prevention programs. Experiencing a health change no longer means an obligatory visit to a physician or a hospital.

It has been almost 40 years since the landmark work of the Lalonde Report (Lalonde, 1974/1981) and over 25 years that Canadians have enjoyed the legacy of the Epp Report (Epp, 1986) and the Ottawa Charter (Canadian Public Health Association et al., 1986). The vision for reducing health inequities through development of a framework in which governmental and individual attention intersected deliberately has triggered significant and sustained health promotion work, health policy development, and health research that continues today. A positive future of health care for Canadians focused on health promotion and illness prevention can hold health-care costs down and improve quality of life in the long term (Health Canada, 2012b). Meeting the health-care challenges of tomorrow means continuous assessment and review of current health-care frameworks and services, supporting health and health systems research (Collins & Hayes, 2007), and fostering partnerships with practice partners and researchers across the country and the world (Health Canada, 2012b).

Critical Thinking Exercises

1. Considering the diversity among Canadians, what is the relevance of the CHA in today's society?
2. In the opening case study, we learn that Mexico is Louis's grandparents' and parents' country and culture of origin. How does the CHA take culture into consideration?
3. Approaches to health care in Canada have been categorized as medical, behavioural, and socioenvironmental. How relevant is context to Canadians' health experience generally and to Louis and his family specifically?
4. The Ottawa Charter recognizes prerequisites for health, including food, shelter, justice, and income among others. How is the Ottawa Charter a template for health promotion? What health-promoting activities could be recommended for Louis's grandmother?

5. How do the CHA and the current model of health care contribute to the health of all Canadians, including Inuit, Innu, First Nations Canadians, and Canadians living in rural and northern jurisdictions?

Multiple-Choice Questions

1. Which pillars of the CHA provide for Louis's grandmother to receive care?
   a. Public administration, comprehensiveness, universality, portability
   b. Comprehensiveness, universality, portability, accessibility
   c. Universality, portability, accessibility, public administration
   d. Public administration, comprehensiveness, universality, accessibility

2. Health Canada fulfills all of the following roles except:
   a. Regulating of hospitals
   b. Providing information essential to maintaining health care and safety of Canadians
   c. Overseeing health and health-related laws and regulations
   d. Providing health care to Inuit, Innu, and First Nations Canadians living on reserves; eligible veterans; refugee claimants; and inmates in federal penitentiaries

3. What is the responsibility of the provinces and territories in health care?
   a. Administration of publicly funded system outlined in the CHA
   b. Administration of publicly funded system outlined by each regional health authority
   c. Administration of privately funded system as outlined in the CHA
   d. Administration of privately funded system outlined by each regional health authority

4. The Canadian health system is organized according to complexity and type of care required and is framed as levels, including primary, secondary, tertiary, and quaternary care. To what level of care did Louis accompany his grandmother?
   a. Primary
   b. Secondary
   c. Tertiary
   d. Quaternary

5. If Louis's grandmother is referred to a specialist for further investigation of her dizziness, what levels of care might she receive?
   a. Primary, secondary, and tertiary
   b. Primary, tertiary, and quaternary

c. Secondary, tertiary, and quaternary

d. Primary, secondary, and quaternary

6. In contemporary nursing practice, how do regulatory bodies promote safe and competent patient care?

   a. By adhering to international regulations

   b. By adhering to hospital-specific standards

   c. By adhering to provincial and territorial guidelines

   d. By adhering to national nursing competencies for entry to practice

7. Our understanding of health has grown over the last few decades such that the determinants of health established originally by the legislation of the 1980s have changed. Which of the following can be considered determinants of health in contemporary Canadian society?

   a. Siblings, family size, social life

   b. Gender, sex, stress

   c. Hobbies, political opinion, culture

   d. Family composition, social life, amount of paid vacation

REFERENCES AND SUGGESTED READINGS

Baris, E. (1998). Reforming health care in Canada: Current issues. *Salud Pública de México, 40*(3), 276–280.

Browne, A. J., Smye, V. L., & Varcoe, C. (2005). The relevance of postcolonial theoretical perspectives to research in Aboriginal health. *Canadian Journal of Nursing Research, 37*(4), 16–37.

Canadian Nurses Association. (2005). *Social determinants of health and nursing: A summary of the issues.* Ottawa, ON: Author.

Canadian Nurses Association. (2008). *Code of ethics for registered nurses: 2008 centennial edition.* Ottawa, ON: Author.

Canadian Nurses Association. (2009). *Registered nurses and baccalaureate education.* Ottawa, Canada: CNA Public Policy Department.

Canadian Nurses Association. (2010). *Canadian Registered Nurse Examination competencies June 2010-May 2015. Professional practice.* Retrieved from http://www.cna-aiic.ca/CNA/nursing/rnexam/competencies/default_e.aspx

Canadian Nurses Association. (2011). *Canadian Registered Nurse Examination: CRNE exam development.* Retrieved from http://www2.cna-aiic.ca/CNA/nursing/rnexam/history/default_e.aspx

Canadian Nurses Association, & Canadian Association of Schools of Nursing. (2010). *Nursing education in Canada statistics 2008-2009: Registered nurse workforce, Canadian production: Potential new supply.* Ottawa, ON: Author.

Canadian Public Health Association, Health and Welfare Canada, & World Health Organization. (1986). *Ottawa Charter for Health Promotion.* Retrieved from http://www.who.int/hpr/NPH/docs/ottawa_charter_hp.pdf

Chessie, K. (2009). Health system regionalization in Canada's provincial and territorial health systems: Do citizen governance boards represent, engage, and empower? *International Journal of Health Services, 39*(4), 705–724. doi: 10.2190/HS.34.4.g

Collins, P. A., & Hayes, M. V. (2007). Twenty years since Ottawa and Epp: Researchers' reflections on challenges, gains and future prospects for reducing health inequities in Canada. *Health Promotion International, 22*(4), 337–345. doi: 10.1093/heapro/dam031

Deber, R. B. (2003). Health care reform: Lessons from Canada. *American Journal of Public Health, 93*(1), 20–24.

Department of Justice. (2011). *Canada Health Act.* Retrieved from http://laws-lois.justice.gc.ca/eng/acts/C-6/

Epp, J. (1986). *Achieving health for all: A framework for health promotion.* Ottawa, ON: Health Canada.

Gagnon, M-A., & Hébert, G. (2010). *The economic case for universal pharmacare. Costs and benefits of publicly funded drug coverage for all Canadians.* Retrieved from http://www.theglobeandmail.com/life/health/new-health/andre-picard/why-is-there-no-national-vaccination-strategy/article1830159/

Government of Canada: Justice Laws Website. (2013). *Kelowna Accord Implementation Act.* Retrieved from http://laws.justice.gc.ca/eng/acts/K-0.65/page-1.html

Government of Ontario. (2014). *Ontario's local health integration networks: What are LHINs?* Retrieved from http://www.lhins.on.ca/aboutlhin.aspx

Health Canada. (2005). *Canada's health care system.* Ottawa, ON: Author.

Health Canada. (2006a). *Overview of the Canadian health care system.* Retrieved from http://www.hc-sc.gc.ca/hcs-sss/delivery-prestation/fptcollab/2003accord/fs-if_hcs-sds-eng.php

Health Canada. (2006b). *Primary health care.* Retrieved from http://www.hc-sc.gc.ca/hcs-sss/prim/about-apropos-eng.php#a4

Health Canada. (2007). *International Affairs Directorate.* Retrieved from http://www.hc-sc.gc.ca/ahc-asc/branch-dirgen/spb-dgps/iad-dai/index-eng.php

Health Canada. (2009). *Health care system.* Ottawa, ON: Author.

Health Canada. (2010). *Canada Health Act.* Retrieved from http://www.hc-sc.gc.ca/hcs-sss/medi-assur/cha-lcs/index-eng.php

Health Canada. (2011a). *About Health Canada.* Ottawa, ON: Author. Retrieved from http://www.hc-sc.gc.ca/ahc-asc/index-eng.php

Health Canada. (2011b). *About Health Canada: About mission, values, activities.* Retrieved from http://hc-sc.gc.ca/ahc-asc/activit/about-apropos/index-eng.php

Health Canada. (2011c). *Strategic policy branch.* Retrieved from http://www.hc-sc.gc.ca/ahc-asc/branch-dirgen/spb-dgps/index-eng.php

Health Canada. (2012a). *About primary health care.* Retrieved from http://www.hc-sc.gc.ca/hcs-sss/prim/about-apropos-eng.php

Health Canada. (2012b). *What is Health Canada's goal?* Retrieved from http://www.hc-sc.gc.ca/ahc-asc/index-eng.php

Health Canada. (2013). *Canada Health Act annual reports.* Retrieved from http://www.hc-sc.gc.ca/hcs-sss/pubs/cha-lcs/index-eng.php

Health Council of Canada. (2005). *Primary health care. A background paper to health care renewal in Canada: Accelerating change.* Toronto, ON: Author.

Health Council of Canada. (2011). *Progress report 2011: Health care renewal in Canada.* Retrieved from http://healthcouncilcanada.ca/en/index.php?page=shop.product_details&flypage=shop.flypage&product_id=137&category_id=14&manufacturer_id=0&option=com_virtuemart&Itemid=170

Irvine, B., Ferguson, S., & Cackett, B. (2005). *Background briefing: The Canadian health care system.* Retrieved from http://www.civitas.org.uk/pdf/Canada.pdf

Kraker, D. (2001). The Canadian cure. *In Motion Magazine.* Retrieved from http://www.inmotionmagazine.com/hcare/canadahc.html

Lalonde, M. (1981). *A new perspective on the health of Canadians.* Ottawa, ON: Government of Canada. (Original work published 1974)

Madore, O. (2005). *The Canada Health Act: Overview and options* (Library of Parliament No. 94-4E). Retrieved from http://www.parl.gc.ca/Content/LOP/ResearchPublications/944-e.pdf

McDonald, C., & McIntyre, M. (2010). Issues arising from the nature of nurses' work and workplaces. In M. McIntyre & C. McDonald (Eds.), *Realities of Canadian nursing: Professional, practice, and power issues* (3rd ed., pp. 283–315). Philadelphia, PA: Lippincott Williams & Wilkins.

McIntyre, M., & McDonald, C. (2010). Nursing issues: A call to political action. In M. McIntyre & C. McDonald (Eds.), *Realities of Canadian nursing: Professional, practice, and power issues* (3rd ed., pp. 3–16). Philadelphia, PA: Lippincott Williams & Wilkins.

Ministry of Health and Long-Term Care. (2002). *Local Health Integration Networks*. Toronto, ON: Author.

Natural Resources Canada. (2010). *Moving forward on energy efficiency in Canada: A foundation for action*. Ottawa, ON: Author. Retrieved from http://www.nrcan.gc.ca/com/resoress/publications/cemcme/buibat-eng.php?PHPSESSID=6b5e298bd24500ce56ae64181c59b47f

Ontario Ministry of Health and Long-Term Care. (2009). *Access to quality health care in rural and northern Ontario*. Retrieved http://www.health.gov.on.ca/english/public/pub/ministry_reports/rural/ruralca.html

Ordre des infirmières et infirmiers du Québec. (2012). *Rehaussement de la formation pour les infirmières de la relève*. Retrieved from http://www.oiiq.org/salle-de-presse/espace-oiiq/rehaussement-de-la-formation-pour-les-infirmieres-de-la-releve

Oxford English Dictionary. (2006). Oxford, United Kingdom: Oxford University Press.

Parliament of Canada. (2005). *The Canada Health Act: Overview and options*. Retrieved from http://www.parl.gc.ca/Content/LOP/ResearchPublications/944-e.htm#1criteriatxt

Picard, A. (2010). *Why is there no national vaccination strategy?* Retrieved from http://www.theglobeandmail.com/life/health/new-health/andre-picard/why-is-there-no-national-vaccination-strategy/article1830159/

Randall, G. E., & Williams, A. P. (2009). Health-care reform and the dimensions of professional autonomy. *Canadian Public Administration, 52*(1), 51–69.

Rankin, J. M. (2003). 'Patient satisfaction': Knowledge for ruling hospital reform—An institutional ethnography. *Nursing Inquiry, 10*(1), 57–65.

Raphael, D. (2003). Addressing the social determinants of health in Canada: Bridging the gap between research findings and public policy. *Policy Options*. Retrieved from http://www.irpp.org/po/archive/mar03/raphael.pdf

Romanow, R. J. (2002). *Building our values: The future of health care in Canada—Final report*. Ottawa, ON: Commission on the Future of Health Care in Canada.

Ryan-Nicholls, K. D. (2004). Impact of health reform on registered psychiatric nursing practice. *Journal of Psychiatric and Mental Health Nursing, 11*(6), 644–653.

Shannon, V., & French, S. (2005). The impact of the re-engineered world of health-care in Canada on nursing patient outcomes. *Nursing Inquiry, 12*(3), 231–239.

Skinner, B. J., & Rovere, M. (2011, April 19). Without some privatization, medicare will collapse. *National Post*. Retrieved from http://fullcomment.nationalpost.com/2011/04/19/brett-j-skinner-and-mark-rovere-without-some-privatization-medicare-will-collapse/

Storch, J. L. (2010). Canadian healthcare system. In M. McIntyre & C. McDonald (Eds.), *Realities of Canadian nursing: Professional, practice, and power issues* (3rd ed., pp. 34–55). Philadelphia, PA: Lippincott Williams & Wilkins.

Thompson, V. D. (2010). *Health and health care delivery in Canada*. Toronto, ON: Mosby/Elsevier.

Thorpe, K., & Loo, R. (2003). Balancing professional and personal satisfaction of nurse managers: Current and future perspectives in a changing health care system. *Journal of Nursing Management, 11*(5), 321–330.

Turner, J. G. (1958). The Hospital Insurance and Diagnostic Services Act: Its impact on hospital administration. *Canadian Medical Association Journal, 78*(10), 768–770.

Villeneuve, M. J. (2010). Looking back, moving forward: Taking nursing toward 2020. In M. McIntyre & C. McDonald (Eds.), *Realities of Canadian nursing: Professional, practice, and power issues* (3rd ed., pp. 470–481). Philadelphia, PA: Lippincott Williams & Wilkins.

Waiser, B. (2006). *The Canadians. Tommy Douglas*. Markham, ON: Fitzhenry & Whiteside.

White, F., & Nanan, D. (2009). A conversation on health in Canada: Revisiting universality and the centrality of primary care. *Journal of Ambulatory Care Management, 32*(2), 141–149.

World Health Organization. (1978). *Declaration of Alma-Alta*. Retrieved from http://www.who.int/social_determinants/tools/multimedia/alma_ata/en/index.html

World Health Organization. (2011). *Social determinants of health*. Retrieved from http://www.who.int/social_determinants/en/

Complementary and Alternative Medicine: Health and Healing for Patients and Nurses

PERTICE MOFFITT

Morgan is a third-year nursing student working in a maternity unit of a rural hospital in Northern Canada. After learning that her assignment is observation and support of a labouring woman, Morgan thinks about the many ways she can prepare herself in this supportive role. She considers the importance of centering, but what exactly does this mean? She also researches alternative approaches to dealing with the pain of labour. She wonders which supportive modalities will best meet the needs of her patients.

CHAPTER OBJECTIVES

By the end of this chapter, you will be able to:

1. Explain the concepts important to healing from a complementary and alternative medicine perspective.
2. Reflect on the importance of self-care for healing and practice.
3. Describe and differentiate complementary and alternative modalities and consider the application of these modalities within health care.
4. Explore ways in which integrative healing supports and enables health and healing for yourself and your patients.
5. Discuss the role of the nurse in assisting patients with the use of complementary and alternative modalities.

KEY TERMS

Aboriginal Healer   A person known to his or her community as a spiritual leader and guide to well-being who practices traditional approaches based on cultural beliefs and medicines. Although colonialism disrupted the use of traditional healing methods, Aboriginal healers have reclaimed their practices and through ceremony and protocols are providing direction and care to their communities.

Acupressure   A technique of traditional Chinese medicine where digital pressure is applied to points on the body to produce therapeutic effects on organs of the body and to relieve nausea and pain. Acupressure is sometimes combined with massage to enhance relaxation.

Allopathic Medicine   The practice of conventional Western medicine, which is biologically based to treat symptoms of diseases or parts of the body. Symptoms are isolated and treated rather than addressing the wholeness of the person.

Alternative Medicine   The term used to consider medical and health practices that are alternative to the Western biomedical model of health care.

Art Therapy   A means of expressing emotions and feelings in an artistic manner, such as drawing, sculpting, painting, dancing, and other ways of nonverbally expressing ourselves to enhance healing, self-awareness, and well-being.

Ayurveda   One of the world's oldest Hindu health-care systems; it originated in India. It is a holistic practice that addresses all aspects of mind, body, and spirit. Ayurveda focuses on maintaining the body's

balance and preventing illness by focusing on good health. Along with teaching and practicing a healthy lifestyle, herbal medicines and oils are prescribed.

Biofeedback   A measure of the body's physiological responses; for example, heart rate, blood pressure, skin temperature, sweat gland activity and so on, to promote greater self-awareness and enhance health through an understanding of how the body is reacting.

Complementary Medicine   A broad range of therapies/modalities that are considered complementary to conventional Western medicine. Some of these therapies have been highlighted in this chapter; for example, psychotherapy, art therapy, music therapy, massage therapy, and so on.

Five Elements   Within traditional Chinese medicine, the five elements are wood, fire, earth, metal, and water and are used to classify all phenomena.

Holistic Care   Care involving consideration of the complexity, interrelationship, and connectedness of the patient's entire system. Holism is a theoretical premise that whole entities exist as a unique system (as one) and are more than only the sum of their parts.

Homeopathy (Homeopathic Medicine)   A type of alternative medicine that is based on an understanding that health can be restored from certain diseases by introducing small amounts of the substance that caused the disease into individuals that are experiencing the illness. Homeopathic remedies are made from natural substances and geared to each individual's unique requirements.

Hypnosis One of the many techniques of psychotherapy where an altered state of consciousness is created through the use of words, instructions, and sometimes instruments. Hypnosis is used to treat illness, for smoking cessation, and to induce relaxation.

Imagery The use of images for healing. One example often used to relieve pain is guided imagery.

Integrative Healing A term that has grown out of the integrative health-care movement, which combines complementary and alternative medicine with conventional medicine based on a biomedical model. *Integrative* is used rather than *integration* to denote that the work between complementary and alternative medicine and conventional health care is an active process without an endpoint. Healing is holistic and dynamic and is a process of becoming and self-transformation.

Massage Therapy The manipulation of the soft tissue of the body to relieve muscle tension and pain and promote relaxation and health. Massage therapists use their hands to rub, stroke, knead and push on various parts of the body with the aid of lotions, oils, and such items as hot stones.

Meditation A self-care discipline that involves focused and controlled breathing to clear the mind and relax the body. Meditation is a therapy that originated from Ayurvedic medicine.

Meridians In traditional Chinese medicine, the energy pathways of the body that move and store qi.

Music Therapy The use of music as an intervention or tool to promote healing, memory, and relaxation and to alleviate pain. Music is effective alone or when combined with other therapies and has a personal and diverse application.

Naturopathy (Naturopathic Medicine) Natural medicine that can heal and maintain the body through healthy lifestyle and natural plant substances. Exercise, good nutrition, fresh air, massage, and other natural healing practices are all considered part of naturopathic medicine.

Prayer A personal act whereby God, the Creator, or a spiritual guide is addressed with an intention of request, confession, plea, petition, praise, and/or thanks regarding a personal need, event, or condition.

Prayers may be silent or spoken aloud. They may be individual or with a group. Prayer is a source of personal strength and spirituality.

Psychotherapy A group of therapies that involve a relationship and interaction with a therapist to guide an individual through practices that address emotions, feelings, psychological issues, and subconscious emotional issues.

Qi A traditional Chinese medicine term, the life energy that each person is born with and that is acquired from air, food, and water.

Reiki A Japanese technique that promotes health and well-being by transferring life-force energy from a Reiki master to the patient through a laying on of hands and energy shift. As well, like many other complementary and alternative medicines, Reiki is a philosophy of life that evokes harmony with all living creatures.

Therapeutic Touch A healing modality that was brought into nursing primarily by Dr. Dolores Krieger. It is a technique whereby hands are used a slight distance from the patient's body to assess, treat, and evaluate the exchange of energy. Therapeutic touch boosts the immune system and promotes healing.

Traditional Aboriginal Medicine An alternative medicine that involves the traditional and holistic (mind, body, spirit, and emotions) health and healing practices of Aboriginal (First Nations, Inuit, and Métis) healers in Canada. Healing practices include, for example, ceremonies, drumming, sweat lodge, plant, and animal treatments through the work of a shaman or healer.

Traditional Chinese Medicine Often abbreviated as TCM, includes traditional practices that originated in China and are being used throughout the world.

Yin and Yang Terms used within traditional Chinese medicine to describe opposing forces within the body that are interconnected and complement each other to maintain the body's equilibrium of qi, the life force.

Yoga A lifestyle practice that originated from Ayurvedic medicine and includes such things as meditation, postures, and controlled breathing to promote and maintain well-being. *Yama* and *niyama* are the negative and positive aspects of behaviour that guide yoga.

Nursing as a discipline embraces many knowledge systems that theoretically and conceptually form the basis of practice. As students, you are practitioners of complementary and alternative medicine (CAM), and in this introductory chapter, you are developing an understanding of how CAM is used by your patients. As well, you will encounter nurses and other health-care professionals who have received certification and advanced education to provide CAM. Nurses are particularly interested in **integrative healing**; that is, healing that considers holistic care of the patient that is meaningful to the patient and his or her family and which is provided by a nurse who is grounded, healthy, competent, and whole. Nursing knowledge stems from many sources. The biomedical knowledge of Western medicine, known as **allopathic medicine**, has formed many of our present-day nursing practices, but this is only one perspective on health and healing. **Alternative medicine** involves knowledge that stems from worldviews, some of which are as old as humankind. These ways of knowing about health and healing stem from non-Western philosophies and include traditional Aboriginal knowledge, Chinese medicine, Ayurveda, and homeopathic and naturopathic medicine. **Complementary medicine** includes mind-body therapies (psychotherapy,

art therapy, music therapy, imagery, hypnosis, meditation, and yoga), touch therapies (massage therapy, acupressure, reflexology), energy therapies (biofeedback, healing touch, magnet therapy, neurofeedback, polarity, Reiki, prayer, and therapeutic touch), and plant therapies (herbal medicine).

CAM is considered a complement to conventional medicines (biomedical) and/or as an alternative to conventional medicine. CAM has influenced our present-day nursing practice and the everyday lives of our patients. In 1999, the Fraser Institute (a conservative think-tank) conducted a national survey about CAM use in Canada, which was followed in 2006 by a second survey to investigate the prevalence, costs, and patterns of CAM use in Canada. Fifty-four percent of Canadians used at least one form of alternative therapy; the most commonly used were massage, prayer, chiropractic care, relaxation techniques, and herbal therapies (Esmail, 2007). Data from the 1999 survey provided a baseline to which the 2006 data collected could be compared. Some of the findings suggest that little has changed in access to a physician's office, clinic, or health centre for medical care from 1997 (88%) to 2006 (88%) (Esmail, 2007). From 73% of Canadians using some CAM in 1997 to 74% in 2006 reflects a slight increase. The change was not significant, but the percentage of users is impressive. CAM is not considered a part of the essential service of Canada's publicly funded health care, so often, the cost of CAM is paid by the individual. Some private health insurance plans may cover the cost of CAM therapies.

Whole Person Systems

There are certain concepts that are common to all of the complementary and alternative therapies (Box 3.1). These concepts are interrelated and include healing, holistic care, self-care, mindfulness, multiple realities, lived experience and storytelling, and spirituality. These concepts developed from a knowledge system that grew from indigenous people's experiences with living in close interaction with the land and plants and animals that live there. Healing is central to living life in a healthy way. The biomedical model views healing as a way of becoming well again, but many of the alternative healing

systems incorporate healing as a way of life. When we consider health and healing holistically, developing and growing is all about healing. The healer provides holistic care that is focused on the whole person and the environment in which he lives. Self-care for the healer, and for nurses as healers, is essential. To be fully present for a patient, you must be mindful of your personal health and your role in caring for another human. Furthermore, people's knowledge, beliefs, and values warrant respect, inclusion, and engagement in the healing process. The stories of our patients are precious and central to the care we give them. Together, we create new stories that inform experiences of health and healing that we reflect on and learn from.

Aboriginal Medicine

Traditional Aboriginal medicine, from the Aboriginal people of our country, is described as healing based on knowledge that involves a holistic approach through

---

BOX 3.1 Integrative Healing Concepts

Healing
Healing is "the act or process of curing or of restoring to health, the process of getting well" (Merriam-Webster, Inc., 1993). Healing also involves a journey of self-discovery, fulfillment, and enlightenment. It is active work through the self, and with the help of others, to achieve a balance of body, mind, spirit, emotion, and environment. This healing work is reparative, restorative, and transformative and creates a deep level of understanding and meaning in a person's life and living. Perkins (2003) describes healing as rendered through love. Love is a powerful energy source that has potential to open our human "being" to a greater potential.

Holistic Care
Holistic care is focused on the whole person, concerned with mind, body, spirit, emotion, and environment (Dossey & Keegan, 2009). Caring of this nature places the patient at the centre. Care providers (nurses and other health-care team members) work with the patient to support his or her choices, growth, health, and healing. In a concept analysis of holistic nursing practice for pediatric nursing, Tjale and Bruce (2007) describe two dimensions: "whole person" and "mind-body-spirit." Recognition of the person as a spiritual being with beliefs and values that extend to the family, community, and country is central to holistic caring.

Self-Care
Self-care is essential for nurses in their roles as caregivers. Nurses routinely practice many of the modalities presented in this chapter in their daily lives in part in order to maintain a healthy presence with their patient(s). The goal of self-care is to seek out activities and practices that heighten self-awareness and fulfillment. As individuals, we engage in emotional, physical, and spiritual actions that nourish our inner spirit, mind, and body. Thus, self-care gives meaning, purpose, and understanding that transcends the self.

Mindfulness
Mindfulness is one way that we grow and become whole. Mindfulness, "the art of conscious living" (Dossey & Keegan, 2009, p. 722),

is the self-awareness of both the internal and external environment that occurs in the moment to create a personal healing intention (Kabat-Zinn, 2003; Schmidt, 2004). Schmidt (2004) describes mindfulness qualities as nonjudging, accepting, nonattachment, openness of mind, nonstriving (taking your lead from the patient), gentleness, and kindness. As has been demonstrated through the health program called mindfulness, stress reduction mindfulness can be learned (Carmody & Baer, 2008).

Multiple Realities
Nurses recognize that there are multiple realities or truths that inform the lives of the patients in our care. Through the realization that there are many perspectives (or personal truths or perceptions of reality), we are able to open our hearts and practices to healing modalities that have developed from many knowledge systems.

Lived Experience and Storytelling
Nursing as a relational and experiential profession recognizes that telling, reflecting, and interpreting lived experience is integral to our development as individuals and as nurses. We share and learn from each other through narratives that capture the moments of living that we are experiencing. Hearing each other's stories is essential to health and healing modalities. Our stories help us to experience the whole event again and unravel what lies beneath in order to act on new insights.

Spirituality
Spirituality is a dimension of self, of connection to others, and to a higher being that creates meaning, purpose of life, and living. *Spirituality* is a term used to capture "the essence of being human" (Miner-Williams, 2006, p. 817). The attributes of spirituality are meaning, value, transcendence, connecting, and becoming (Martsolf & Mickley, 1998). An alleviation of suffering occurs through engaging in spiritual practices or acts of love, joy, hope, peacefulness, forgiveness, and comfort (Coyle, 2002; Miner-Williams, 2006; Tanyi, 2002, 2006).

interaction with the entire universe, the interrelationship of all living things, and meaningfully lived encounters (Royal Commission on Aboriginal Peoples [RCAP], 1996). The National Aboriginal Health Organization (2008) provided case studies as illustrations of the integration of traditional knowledge into conventional health-care systems. In brief, the three exemplars included the Inuulitsivik Health Centre in Puvirnituq, Nunavik, where traditional midwifery has returned birthing to the community; the First Nations Health Program at the Whitehorse General Hospital, where an elders working group developed a program that includes services of a traditional healer and the use of traditional medicines; and the Métis Addictions Council of Saskatchewan, where traditional approaches such as cleansing ceremonies and sweat lodge ceremonies are available.

The Medicine Wheel and the Circle

Aboriginal people recognize the importance of ceremony to healing. McCabe (2008) describes Aboriginal mind, body, emotions, and spirit dialogue as occurring through the medicine wheel, burning tobacco, sweat lodge, and storytelling. The medicine wheel is structured on four directions, demonstrating the interconnectedness of mind, body, emotion, and spirit (Fig. 3.1). The medicine wheel encompasses a philosophy for living and healing through ceremony and through the teachings that guide the development of inner self dialogue.

The medicine wheel has also been used as a conceptual guide for research (Hart-Wasekeesikaw, 1996; Lavallee, 2008, 2009; Waldram, 2008). Hart-Wasekeesikaw (1996) interviewed 46 Aboriginal people from Anishinaabe communities in Manitoba to learn about their experience of cancer. The participants used terms to describe their cancer such as "the stranger" and "manitoch," which in Ojibwa translates to

cancer-as-worm. The participants went to Indian medicine healers as well as conventional health professionals. An important aspect of Ojibwa care when they were hospitalized was the gathering of friends, family, and community members at their bedside.

What can we learn from studies like this? One of the most important contributions to nursing is the help we get from understanding the cultural beliefs and values central to care. We learn about the importance of the extended family. We need to make room for the gathering of families in our facilities. We need to access local **Aboriginal healers** and implement their recommended supportive measures; for example, the use of Indian medicine tea. Elders should be consulted to organize talking circles and support groups in home communities.

In some nursing programs, opportunities are provided for students to learn from elders in a land experience. A land experience encompasses more than the physical setting but includes a way of life (beliefs and practices) that evolved over many generations from a sacredness, spirituality, understanding of the metaphysical creation, and existence of mankind. Through a land experience, students and faculty learn about Aboriginal life and culture. This enhances cultural knowledge of local people and leads to respect and understanding. These experiences include engaging in traditional practices such as pulling in the fish nets or other activities such as plucking ducks, smoking meat and fish, beading, and listening to stories.

Although not all Aboriginal people in Canada use the medicine wheel, the underlying principle of the circle is relevant to many. All aspects of living are considered in the circle: the four directions—north, east, south, and west; the seasons—winter, spring, summer, and fall; the stages of life—infant, child, adult, and elder, and so on. The concept of the circle is relevant to all aspects of living a life. The circle is also a principle in teaching and learning. Sharing circles involve participants sitting together and sharing stories with one another in a respectful and cyclical manner and with the underlying principle that each person in the circle is equal.

Another way to see the symbolism and sacredness of the circle is to visit an Aboriginal community and participate in a drum dance (Fig. 3.2). This also is conducted in a circle and accompanied by the drum. An integral part of healing through drumming, prayer songs, and songs of celebration are shared. Drumming has also been used to revitalize culture and identity through such activities as drum making and hand drumming (Goudreau, Weber-Pillwax, Cote-Meek, Madill, & Wilson, 2008).

The sweat lodge involves ceremony in a special place to enhance inner dialogue and self-awareness. The sweat lodge is located on land that is determined to be a place of healing. People sit in a circle within the lodge with hot stones at the centre of the structure. An elder leads the session through prayers, assisted by a helper to prepare the stones. People make prayers regarding issues current in their lives. Following the sweat, the participants share a meal.

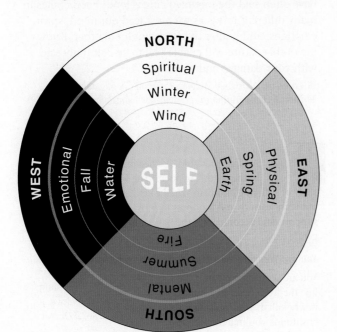

Figure 3.1 Medicine wheel.

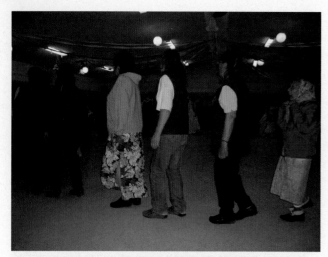

Figure 3.2 Drum dance. (Reproduced with permission from Moffitt, P. [2008]. *Keep myself well: Perinatal health beliefs and health promotion practices of pregnant Tlicho women* [Doctoral dissertation]. Retrieved from http://amicus.collectionscanada .gc.ca/aaweb-bin/aamain/itemdisp?sessionKey=999999999_142 &l=0&d=2&v=0&lvl=1&itm=34492030)

Making offerings of tobacco to the land is another sacred ritual that strengthens and restores identity and spirit. For Dene people in Northern Canada, *feeding the fire* is a unique ceremony where tobacco and/or food are offered into the fire, which is at the centre of the circle. The drummers warm their drums over this fire before beginning to play and singing a prayer song. All of these functions demonstrate the interconnection of the philosophy of the circle.

Traditional Dene Medicine

Two separate projects in the Northwest Territories have described the traditional medicinal use of plants and animals by specific peoples, the Tlicho and the Gwich'in (Andre & Fehr, 2001; Ryan & Johnson, 1994). The Ryan and Johnson (1994) study described the traditional medicine system of the Dene, documented in a carefully catalogued database. This preserves the information they obtained through participatory action research with the elders. The authors advise that the teaching of Dene medicine remains with the elders' verbal traditions to convey all the ritualistic and spiritual requirements. Dene medicine continues to be practiced today, as an adjunct to Western medicine or by itself at the request of an individual in need of healing (Ryan & Johnson, 1994).

Ryan and Johnson (1994) reported that Dene medicine is based on well-being, which is described as "balance between the individual, the group, the human, animal and spiritual worlds" (p. 36). Within the Dene, there were individuals with special knowledge of healing, those with medicine or *ink'on*, but if someone were ill, the group would collectively assist in the individual's return to health by collecting the medicine, gift giving, and providing support. They explain the existence of traditional Dene medicine as "rooted in their understanding of the spiritual world and the ecological natural world" (Ryan & Johnson, 1994, p. 18). The use of specific plants, roots and

berries, along with animals, fish, and birds in healing are outlined. There are specific rituals that must be performed when collecting the plants so essential to survival on the land.

Spiritual Leaders

Spiritual healers are people with a special gift (Helm, 1994, 2000; Ryan & Johnson, 1994). These healers acquired their spiritual power through a Spring ritual when they were most receptive to receiving the energy of the spirit. Dreaming was a part of the process of receiving the special gift.

In traditional practice as in nursing, establishing a relationship of trust and rapport is significant to healing. There is mutuality and reciprocity between patient and healer as they undertake the journey together. Healing occurs through the Creator. The medicine power comes from the Creator and gives the healer special skills, such as the ability to see and predict the future, to read the mind, and to mend the body (Blondin, 1990). Healers are intuitive, perceptive, and observant. Through touch, the healer identifies the problem, and through ceremony, the healing occurs. Ceremony affects all four spheres of the human being: the body, the mind, the spirit, and the heart.

Through the eyes of a nurse

I have found in my practice as Aboriginal Wellness Coordinator that it is most important for health-care providers to come from a place of awareness and understanding of historical and present power relations with all patients and themselves as health-care providers. This is the crux of cultural safety. Holistic health care requires us to understand our collective history and the collective implications of Treaty (the treaty that was made between the government and First Nations people). The elders have often said the first medicine is food. Food comes in many different forms as we must feed our mind, spirit, emotions, and bodies to be present for another. Knowing of this nature will enable you to be culturally safe with your patients and coworkers.

(S. Lockhart, Aboriginal Wellness Program Coordinator, Stanton Territorial Health Authority, personal communication, June 9, 2009)

Think An interpretation of a healing journey is illuminated in the following poem. The words unfold to tell a story of suffering and pain. The healer listens carefully, reaches out with warmth and kindness to provide positive intent and support, and accompanies the patient in an empowering and gentle way.

You are Wearing Your Hurt Like the Fresh Heart of a Buffalo

You are wearing your hurt
like the fresh heart of a buffalo
newly killed. Your pulsing hurt
enshrouds you in a thick robe
of dark shadows and shades.

Your hurt speaks to me clearly
through a muted voice with
vibrations not easily detected
by the unlistening ear

but

I hear you.
I hear and I see you.
I feel your body's desire to fold, curl, and nestle;
to find a path through the thick skin of pain
encasing your heart;
to find solace in some other place-
a place you call "norm".

I feel your spine begin to strengthen
as the timbre of who you are
leans into this fierce wind,
this crouching evil,
this cunning misery in your life.

The love tip-toes toward you,
Reluctant to intrude,
unsure of how to approach,
desirous of offering to shelter you
in a rabbit-skin robe; to sing out for you
your sorrows and strengths, to honour your protests and pain,
to walk beside you towards salvation and peace.

You raise an invisible hand to halt my approach.

I pause
I watch
Silently, I step aside.

Still, I see your wounds.
I hear your unspoken sorrow.

My heart slips quietly over
to stand near yours.
Here I remain,
the unwavering witness
to your stark journey.

(Copied with permission from Aline La Flamme, Métis grandmother and healer, June 12, 2009.)

Read over the poem. Describe the relationship between the healer and the patient. What is her approach? What relational skills can you identify? What metaphors are used and what is the significance for the Aboriginal healer?

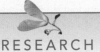

RESEARCH

SPIRITUAL HEALING IN CANCER PATIENTS

Study
In this qualitative study conducted in Manitoba, the researcher examined narratives of 47 cancer patients, with 10% or less chance of survival at 5 years, before and after their care by an Aboriginal healer. Panels of medical students, graduate students, health-care providers, and patients reviewed and rated the narratives for themes. The explanatory themes identified included

present-centeredness, forgiveness of others, release of the past, process orientation, humour, life meaning and dignity, faith and hope, refusal to accept death, plausible explanation, supportive community, quantum change, and spiritual change. Comparison was made between exceptional survivors and nonsurvivors using these themes. Meaning and dignity and faith and hope were dimensions shared by all of the patients with cancer being cared for by the Aboriginal healer. The researcher named the treatment by the Aboriginal healer as "spiritual healing" (p. 502).

Nursing Implications
We can provide preliminary evidence and hope to our patients that positive states of mind can lengthen survival. As well, ceremonies provided by Aboriginal healers can prompt a change that enables healing. Faith and trust in both the healer and the method of healing increases survivorship.

Mehl-Madrona, L. (2008). Narratives of exceptional survivors who work with Aboriginal healers. Journal of Alternative and Complementary Medicine, 14(5), 497–504.

Traditional Chinese Medicine

Traditional Chinese medicine, an ancient system of health care, centers on beliefs about the body's state of unbalance in terms of qi, yin and yang, five elements, and meridians (Kong, Tan, Goh, & Chia, 2004). **Qi** (pronounced *chee*) is the life energy that each person is born with and that is acquired from air, food, and water. **Yin and yang** are opposing forces within the body that are interconnected and complement each other to maintain the body's equilibrium of qi, the life force. The **five elements**—wood, fire, earth, metal, and water—are used to classify all phenomena. Healers providing care apply these five elements to the physiology and pathology of the human body. The **meridians** are the energy pathways of the body that move and store qi. Healing modalities that have originated from this philosophy are therapies designed to restore balance.

Qigong (pronounced *chee-gung*) is an ancient Chinese technique that has become popular in North America (McCaffrey & Fowler, 2003). Qigong involves training of the body, breath, voice, and mind. Qigong includes disciplined work every day, repeatedly completing exercises with a certified Qigong teacher. T'ai Chi is one component of Qigong.

Ayurveda

Ayurveda is a Sanskrit word defined as the science of life and longevity. Ayurveda is an ancient Indian science that considers *prakratti*, a person's natural constitution identified through assessment of the body, mind, and emotional well-being. The focus of Ayurvedic medicine is on having a healthy body and mind to cope with life's everyday stresses.

The prakratti is composed of *Tridosha*, the three elements of diagnosis and therapeutics. According to Joshi (2004),

Tridosha is the term used for *vata* (energy of movement), *pitta* (energy of digestions and metabolism), and *kapha* (energy of lubrication and structure). A person's constitution is a unique combination of vata, pitta, and kapha. It is important for Tridosha to be balanced. When there is an imbalance, disease or disorder is present. Ayurveda medicine emphasizes diet, lifestyle, and herbal tonics to boost the immune system.

Through the eyes of a patient

When I learned I had high cholesterol, it was a wake-up call. My physician offered me pills. He was treating the cholesterol, a tiny bit of me. I thought of the impact that high cholesterol has on me and my life. I wanted to be healthy and to live a healthy lifestyle. This is what drew me to Ayurvedics. Ayurvedics is all about living a natural life based on wellness. The worldview of Ayurvedics originates in Hinduism, the oldest living tradition that encompasses all facets of life. In fact, it is a way of life. I met with an Ayurvedic physician to learn about my *dosha*. His approach to me was holistic. By that I mean that he didn't just examine me and take my blood, he questioned me about my entire life. He then diagnosed my dosha as pitta. He gave me a booklet that included a diet plan—what I could eat daily, weekly, and what I could never eat. He advised an exercise program of yoga and walking and prescribed herbs. I followed this advice explicitly, and my cholesterol level became normal. When I returned to my Western family doctor, he was astounded and thought my case should be written up.

(*A. Veylan, personal communication, July 20, 2009*)

Ayurveda and yoga overlap in teachings from Indian science, both working to keep the body and mind balanced. Yoga includes *pranayama* or breathing exercises, *asanas* or postures, and meditation. Through diagnosis of dosha (body type), Ayurvedic treatment along with a yoga regime can be planned to meet an individual need. Yoga is presented in further detail in a following section.

Homeopathic Medicine

Homeopathy is a system of medicine developed in Germany in the 1800s by Samuel Hahemann. Homeopathy treats the whole person by matching remedies to the individual. These remedies are put through a repetitive diluting process. The advantages of homeopathy are that the remedies are not habit-forming; can be used intermittently; have no side effects; reportedly provide improved sleep, energy, and self-esteem; and are inexpensive. A nurse, nurse practitioner, physician, pharmacist, and others can all become homeopaths through a certification process (Lennihan, 2004). A homeopath provides an in-depth intake assessment that includes

a detailed interview to learn about the patient's complaints, ailments, and experiences of health and illness.

All homeopathic medicines must be licensed before being sold in Canada (Health Canada, 2007). The Natural Health Products Directorate has assessed and approved all products and provided regulation for natural health products since 2004. Some of the more commonly known remedies are in response to common health problems such as migraine headaches, allergies, and asthma. The remedies are related to each patient's symptoms; for example, there are various treatments for headache. Belladonna is used for headaches that manifest as right-sided and throbbing; *Bryonia alba* is prescribed for headaches that pulsate near the left eye; and *Cimicifuga* is recommended for headache associated with menstruation (Shalts, 2005).

Naturopathic Medicine

Naturopathy is a system of medicine based on the belief that healing is integral to living organisms and that healing involves a restoration to equilibrium that can be done by self-healing and/or with the help of others. The principles foundational to naturopathy are the healing force of nature and restoring health by treating the whole person. Refer to Box 3.2 for the guiding principles of naturopathic doctors. The patient learns the importance of self-care from the naturopath. Within naturopathic medicine, self-care is an important lifestyle practice to prevent illness (Dunne et al., 2005). The naturopathic doctor provides a thorough assessment by

---

BOX 3.2   Principles of Naturopathic Medicine

Naturopathic doctors are guided by six fundamental healing principles:

1. **First, to do no harm**, by using methods and medicines that minimize the risk of harmful side effects.
2. **To treat the causes of disease**, by identifying and removing the underlying causes of illness, rather than suppressing symptoms.
3. **To teach the principles of healthy living and preventative medicine**, by sharing knowledge with patients and encouraging individual responsibility for health.
4. **To heal the whole person through individualized treatment**, by understanding the unique physical, mental, emotional, genetic, environmental and social factors that contribute to illness, and customizing treatment protocols to the patient.
5. **To emphasize prevention**, by partnering with the patient to assess risk factors and recommend appropriate naturopathic interventions to maintain health and prevent illness.
6. **To support the healing power of the body**, by recognizing and removing obstacles to the body's inherent self-healing process.

Source: Canadian College of Naturopathic Medicine. (n.d.). *Principles of naturopathic medicine*. Retrieved from http://www.ccnm.edu/?q=about_ccnm/principles_naturopathic_medicine

conducting a physical examination, blood and stool laboratory tests, and a complete individual and family history. The detailed history includes such things as diet, exercise, lifestyle, stressors, and environmental context (where the patient works and lives). This thorough examination and history allows the naturopath to treat the patient holistically by offering treatments not only attentive to physical symptomology but also to social and spiritual lifestyle. For example, treatments may include nutritional counseling, herbal medicine, acupuncture, hydrotherapy, spiritual development, lifestyle counseling, and other treatments that are aimed at holistically improving health.

Naturopathic doctors take a 4-year degree program and must pass a Naturopathic Physicians Licensing Exam to become licensed in Canada. Currently, there is a process for licensure in five Canadian jurisdictions (Alberta, British Columbia, Manitoba, Ontario, and Nova Scotia).

Mind-Body Therapies

Many of the following mind-body therapies are creative activities that trigger positive responses in the internal and external environment. The mind works within a directed consciousness to transform the body to a healing place. Directed consciousness is the purposeful exercise of allowing the mind to fixate or focus so that a situational awareness is created of self and the environment.

Psychotherapy

Although **psychotherapy** is a more broadly defined modality, some practices can be used as complementary of alternative health interventions. There are many techniques used in psychotherapy to promote healing. Methods such as **hypnosis** create an altered state of consciousness that not only improves self-empowerment but also creates a state where suggestions by the therapist are more acceptable and useable to the patient. Relaxation therapy is often used, and some therapists recommend a prescribed set of actions that are followed as a repetitive and exact protocol and in that respect become what is considered "ritual." The ritual therapy model includes five steps: centering, assessment, gathering energy, directing energy, and gratitude and closure (Cole, 2003).

Stone (2008) refers to the helping relationship of the psychoanalyst as wounded healing. Within the relationship, love through compassion is the energy that is shared between the patient and therapist. There is a shared suffering that facilitates the healing process and leaves both the patient and therapist feeling better.

Biofeedback

Biofeedback is patient-guided treatment that alerts the patient to biologic cues (such as pulse rate, respirations, temperature, and muscle tension). Biofeedback has been used by various practitioners and for various purposes. In some hospitals, physical therapists use biofeedback to assist stroke patients to regain movement following paralysis, and in some health clinics, psychologists have used biofeedback to help anxious people to relax. With this feedback, the patient uses techniques to manipulate the biologic response. Biofeedback uses technology to display the body's response to stress and the energy fields and pathways of the body. Nurses can use objective biofeedback data to teach the patient by showing the measured improvements they made with interventions or treatments; for example, with muscle tone. In one study, nurses worked with postpartum women to help them recover muscle tone in the pelvic floor after having a baby (Day & Goad, 2010). By using a probe that provides electrical stimulation to the pelvic floor muscles, the muscles contract and become stronger. The patient is given a visual of the way the muscle is responding to treatment, and this visual aspect maintains the motivation to continue with treatment. The technique of biofeedback is through the use of sensors attached to the body, a monitor or screen that displays the body's response, and personal intent to focus deliberately on that part of the body or body response. The feedback through the technique is what makes it so powerful, in that the patient is able to see how he or she is enabling the mind and body connection. Biofeedback is a growing scientific field, as evidenced in the numerous studies published in an international and interdisciplinary journal entitled *Applied Psychophysiology and Biofeedback*.

Art Therapy

Art therapy is especially suited for people who have difficulty verbally expressing feelings and emotions. Self-expression through writing, sculpting, music, and dance are all ways of improving and enhancing healing. Art therapy is an example of self-expression that leads to aesthetic knowing. Aesthetic knowing is another way of making sense of experience through an awareness or understanding that comes from sensing, feeling, and thinking while being fully present in the moment. This ability to be present in the moment requires an intentional focus in where you are right now and maximizing that moment with positive attention. By reflecting in this creative manner, healing is taken to a new height and the joy of recognition of inner meaning and understanding provides new insights that enable health. Art therapy has been used for cancer patients as a way of expressing their experiences (Ponto et al., 2003).

Sometimes, in nursing education, art therapy is used in the classroom to assist in the reflective process. One example is the creation of a self-mandala (Fig. 3.3). *Mandala*, a Sanskrit word translated to mean circle, represents wholeness and is used to seek spiritual renewal. Through a personal mandala, you as a nursing student can explore inner meanings and thoughts that will provide personal insight.

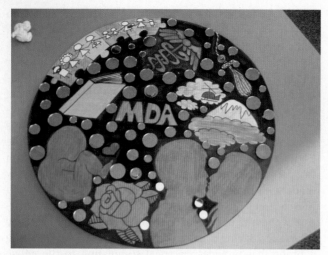

Figure 3.3 Mandala.

This self-enlightenment helps you to achieve wellness and highlight important connections. The creation of a mandala allows you to consider who you are and how you are situated in the world around you. Therefore, you realize important connections and interrelationships and become open to further possibilities and change. The mandala is a symbol that represents you. It can be made from any material you choose. With the mandala, you explore who you are, what you value, what you believe in, and what or who has influenced your growth as a human being. Some artists create mandalas to use in meditation to assist with finding focus and inner peace (Tenzin-Dolma, 2008).

Art therapy is effective for people of all ages. Through creative expression, healing occurs. For this reason, art therapy is introduced in a wide range of settings. For example, people experiencing recovery from addictions undertake painting, drawing, and sculpting, which offer positive outlets for emotion and feelings. The painting or the drawing can also elicit a story or be used to facilitate dialogue that enhances reflection that leads to growth and healing. Hospitalized children are often encouraged to use drawings to portray their experiences.

A personal story may help with this point. My son was hospitalized for osteomyelitis when he was 8 years old. During his hospitalization, he required surgery and had packing in his leg. When the packing was to be removed, the resident provided a brief explanation and began the procedure. My son screamed loudly and upset everyone in attendance. He was terrified. By working with the play therapist and completing a drawing, he was able to talk about the incident. We learned that he thought the doctor was pulling the bone out of his leg. Although this was retrospective, the art and dialogue with the play therapist provided an opportunity to talk about his fears. This story illustrates the knowledge that can be generated with art therapy and also illuminates the importance of communicating to children in words they understand.

In Canada, many art therapists belong to the Canadian Art Therapy Association, which was launched in 1977 by Dr. Martin Fisher as a nonprofit organization. Along with the national association, there are three provincial associations in Ontario, British Columbia, and Quebec. Art therapists complete both undergraduate and graduate studies and publish in a national journal. These sources describe art therapy as beneficial to people of all ages. Art therapy promotes health and healing in many settings (individual, counseling, rehabilitative, treatment centres, elder care centres, correctional institutes, schools, and hospitals).

Music Therapy

Music therapy is more than an effective healing technique for patients in all stages of life, from newborns to the elderly. Music therapy is a program of study led by recognized professionals, as described by the Canadian Association for Music Therapists that was founded in 1974. There is substantial research that supports the positive effect of music therapy on quality of life and well-being (O'Callaghan, 2009), described in a relatively new journal in the Sage collection called *Music and Medicine*. Music therapy, facilitated by a music therapist, involves a comprehensive assessment of the individual patient and family to develop interventions tailored to their beliefs and practices. There are various techniques that assist in alleviating suffering of various chronic illnesses.

Music therapy has been used extensively in palliative care. For example, the therapist engages with the patient and family to enable the expression of the patient's unique life history and story through guided reflection. Individual life stories can be produced in a DVD as a narrative or in a song with lyrics created by the patient, and this process can assist the patient to a new understanding and meaning of her life. The DVD also becomes a tool of remembrance for the family. As well, patients express pain relief when they listen to various music that provides distraction from the physical pain caused by disease. This can be simply an auditory intervention or can include guided imagery (walking through a forest or on an ocean front). For many years, nurses have been singing informally as they go about their work, bringing a smile to many of their patients but not realizing that research supports their singing as best practice. Music is a cognitive stimulant that soothes and calms patients, reduces anxiety and pain, and restores emotional balance (Stuckley & Nobel, 2010). In some hospitals, formal music therapy programs have been created. Listening to music brings relief to patients with cancer, using compositions that are creative, open, and interpretive. Music is so personal and versatile that it is beneficial for a diversity of people.

Music is also combined with techniques such as progressive relaxation and deep breathing to promote relaxation. Progressive relaxation is a technique that instructs the patient to tense and relax successive muscle groups; for example, starting at the toes and working up the body. Simply say, "Tighten your toes, now relax your toes," then proceed to the lower leg, and repeat the exercise, and so on, up the entire body. Ask the patient to notice the difference between the muscle when it is tense and the muscle when it is relaxed. Progression relaxation can be taught quickly, conducted through the use of audiotapes or by providing simple instructions in a calm voice and quiet controlled environment. Soft music in the background further facilitates the relaxation process. Researchers report that progressive relaxation combined with music resulted in behavioural and self-reported positive effects (Scheufele, 2000).

Through the eyes of a student

When I was a first-year student, I was coming to know my patient with dementia and learned that the staff had trouble bathing her because of her agitation. I learned that she loved music and loved to sing. One of the recreational therapists said one of her favorite songs was "I'm Forever Blowing Bubbles." I thought music and singing might help with the bath. I prepared for practice by looking up the words of the song on the Internet and memorizing them. The next day, while I gave my patient a bath in the century tub, I sang to her and she sang with me. She relaxed on hearing the song, and her bathing became an enjoyable experience.

(L. Westman, personal communication, June 8, 2009)

Imagery

Imagery in health care is used at all levels to improve health outcomes. At the corporate level, imagery is used in positive health messaging for health promotion and advocacy and as artwork strategically placed in hospitals and health centres to foster positive patient experiences. As a research method, imagery has been used to trigger stories. Photovoice is an example of a community-based participatory research method that uses photographs and stories to promote health and healing (Moffitt & Vollman, 2004).

Imagery or visualization, at the personal level, is an everyday technique that is not only often used for relaxation but is also used by athletes to enhance performance. Imagery can be self-guided or guided by a professional. Most modes of imagery are visual (seeing) but can also be auditory (hearing) and kinesthetic (feeling). Some people use a particular painting or photograph to focus and help with visualization, whereas other people may use music to create a relaxed environment while imagining an experience. When you are practicing self-guided imagery, you think about a goal that you have been hoping to reach and imagine that experience. In other words, you visualize yourself performing a skill at peak performance. By performing self-guided imagery, athletes have found that their performance improves; they have increased energy and motivation along with more confidence and positive thinking.

Imagery and visualization can be used in a similar fashion to improve health outcomes. Imagery is a versatile and safe method to heal the body and spirit through both mental rehearsal as performed by athletes and by visualizing images through self-imagining or guided by the words of a facilitator. This guided method is often used to take the mind to another place to ease the suffering caused by pain. Kingwatsiaq and Pii (2003) use this technique within a healing team working with community residential school survivors. Residential school survivors include Aboriginal people who were taken from their homes to be assimilated in mainstream North American culture in the Canadian residential school system. There has been an intergenerational legacy of trauma related to the physical, emotional, and sexual abuse experienced by students in residential schools. Because of these atrocities, the Aboriginal Healing Foundation was created and spearheads community-based healing efforts. For further information, visit the Aboriginal Healing Foundation website.

Through the eyes of a patient

I closed my eyes and sat very still on the cushion on the floor listening to the voice of Miya. I breathed in and deeply listened to her words. She took me on a healing journey. I envisioned happy people, birds singing, and heard the rippling brook. As a calmness and peace became my reality, I unloaded my burdens and suffering to a blue boat that was readily available in my imaginings. I sent my pain out to sea. Then through the guiding words, I visited a white boat and came to see all that was beautiful in my heart and soul. I let go of the burden and pain that I have carried so long. I took in all that was beautiful about myself, and I loved me for who I am. I felt immense joy and release.

(personal reflection, cancer patient)

Meditation

The mind is constantly on the move. **Meditation** is a technique to slow the mind in order to remove the psychological stress that comes from rushing and unbidden thoughts and unwarranted conclusions. A goal of meditation is to intentionally focus, so thinking is slowed and deliberate. Calming the mind helps us to find the core of our inner wisdom and resource. Inner peace and positive feelings of joy, happiness, and hope are spiritual benefits of meditation. Ott (2004) describes two types of meditation as concentrative and mindfulness meditation. Concentrative meditation focuses on creating one-pointed thinking by focusing on an image, message, or object and ridding the mind of straying thinking. Mindfulness meditation requires the practitioner be present in the moment.

There are three underlying principles of meditation. First, focus on one thing at a time; second, as thoughts wonder, slowly bring back the focus; and third, try to ignore distractions, thoughts, and sensations while focusing. Furthermore in yoga, active meditation occurs while doing asana and pranayama. Posture and breathing assist in the focus required to meditate.

There are many ways to meditate. Walking meditation is an intentional focus on the feel of your body while you walk. This focus provides calm and relaxation. You can experience body meditation in a similar way by finding a quiet space and focusing on all parts of your body deliberately. You can also use a mantra or verse to meditate. For examples, visit the Blue Mountain Center of Meditation online and review many passages that can be used for meditation. All forms of meditation yield greater benefits when practiced regularly.

Yoga

Yoga is a healing modality for the body, mind, and soul. Nurses themselves are advised to practice yoga to strengthen the musculoskeletal system and develop body awareness, inner self-attention, and self-efficacy (Kollack, 2009). The asana or posture practiced in yoga accelerates muscle activity, which in turn increases pulse rate, breathing rate, and muscle oxygenation. It takes concentration to maintain yoga postures, and with repetition and time, muscle strength is enhanced and stress is eased. Yoga practice improves posture and, combined with breathing, recognition of muscle tension is learned. As you learn to recognize muscle tension and relaxation, self-awareness grows.

The yoga most people are familiar with, called Hatha yoga, was introduced in India during the 15th century. This form of health and physical exercise became popular in the West during the second half of the 20th century. Yoga involves exercise and movement to strengthen and tone the muscles of the body (Fig. 3.4). It is based on asanas (postures) and pranayama (breathing techniques). As a person moves through various positions, breathing is controlled to heighten awareness. The deliberate practice of postures and breathing uses *prana* or life force that circulates through energy pathways in the body. When we are in good health, prana flows freely through the body. In this way, yoga is more than an exercise regime. It is a facet of living that will promote lifelong health.

There are different types of yoga. For example, Zen yoga (empty mind), which is considered to be breathing and moving with the whole body, has been reported to be good medicine for surgical patients (Bottalini, 2008). When yoga is included in preoperative teaching, health outcomes include evidence that controlled movements restore and repair and that established deep breathing calms and energizes. However, depending on the teacher, the style of yoga, and the health/flexibility of the patient, it is possible to experience soft tissue injuries from yoga. While using the breathing yoga, pranayama is relatively harmless at the beginning stages, safely progressing to more advanced practice requires the guidance of a knowledgeable teacher.

Touch Therapies

Touch therapies involve manual touch to promote healing. Touch provides an exchange of energy that acts to relax, soothe, and comfort. Although many people are open to touch therapies, there is considerable intimacy with touch, and there are differing cultural norms and attitudes about what is acceptable. For this reason, you should talk with your patients about their views and beliefs about touch. They most likely will tell you their past experiences, what they have found most and least helpful, and what their preferences are.

Massage Therapy

Massage therapy is an ancient healing modality that involves therapeutic manipulation of the soft tissues of the body by various hand movements, including rubbing, kneading, pressing, and rolling. Massage therapists include both regulated and unregulated workers in Canada. Most jurisdictions of Canada have developed standards of practice for registered massage therapists (RMTs), but only three provinces have legislation to regulate RMTs (British Columbia, Ontario, and Newfoundland). Although nurses are educated in the importance of touch and ways to provide touch to comfort patients, entry-level curriculum provides an introduction to many therapies but not to certification in massage. Many nurses in various specialties take continuing education courses and programs to advance this aspect of their practice.

The benefits of massage have been documented through physiological responses such as reduced heart rate, blood pressure, and respiratory rate and reduced anxiety and stress through an elicitation of the relaxation response. Some palliative care nurses find that massage is a tool that expresses compassion and empathy when words are not enough (Buckley, 2002; Mackey, 1998).

Touch is an essential component to nursing practice. Although therapeutic massage is not the same as, for example, a back rub to promote sleep and relieve tension, it is a comfort measure that has been an effective intervention and part of nurses' practice (Fig. 3.5). You may be thinking, "Okay, but I have never given another person a back rub or massage of any kind." With a friend, practice different types of touch and have him tell you what feels good and what irritates. Some suggestions are as follows: Place your hands on either side of the spine at the lower back, and with firm pressure, go from the base of the spine to the shoulders. Rotate your hands across the shoulders, providing even compression, and move back

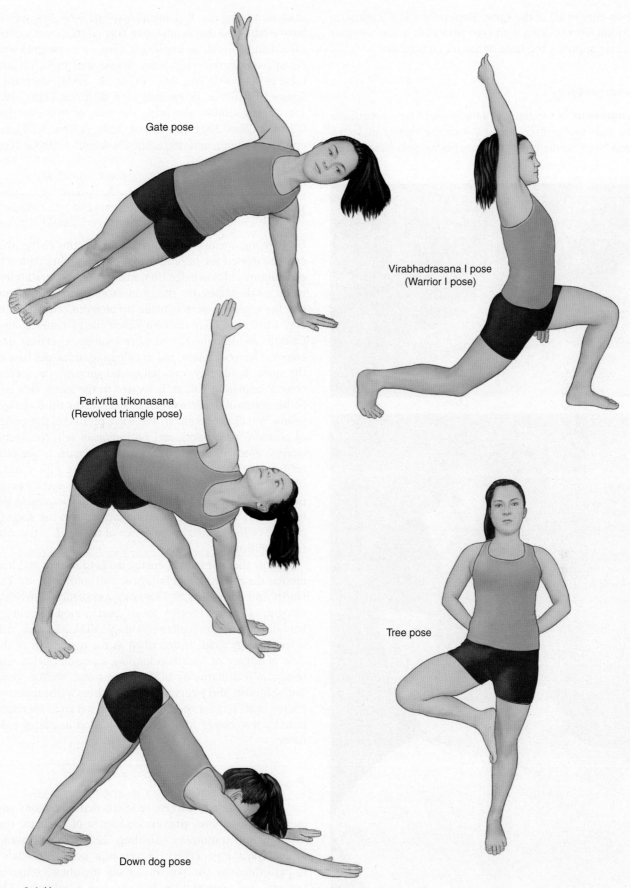

Gate pose

Virabhadrasana I pose
(Warrior I pose)

Parivrtta trikonasana
(Revolved triangle pose)

Tree pose

Down dog pose

Figure 3.4 Yoga.

down either side of the spine. Repeat for a full 5 minutes, periodically checking with your patient to assess whether you are applying too little or too much pressure.

Acupressure

Acupressure is a technique of traditional Chinese medicine that uses touch (firm pressure with the fingers or something blunt) to the body's pressure points, sometimes called

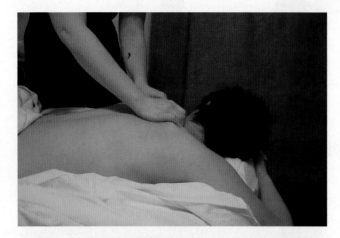

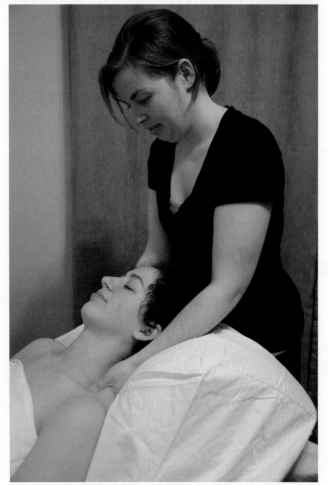

Figure 3.5 **Massage therapist providing back and neck massage.**

acupuncture points, and meridians (Fig. 3.6). Researchers have established that acupressure is effective in many clinical situations, such as improving dyspnea in patients with chronic obstructive pulmonary disease and bronchiectasis (Maa et al., 2007; Wu, Wu, Lin, & Lin, 2004), decreasing agitated behaviour in patients with dementia (Yang, Wu, Lin, & Lin, 2007), alleviating the pain of dysmenorrhea (Chen & Chen, 2004; Jun, Chang, Kang, & Kim, 2007) and childbirth labour, and decreasing the length of labour (Lee, Chang, & Kang, 2004).

Energy Therapies

Every living organism has energy, and it is this energy that can be targeted for healing. Based on the accumulation of generations of knowledge from many countries, traditional medicine describes this energy in various ways. For example, the chakra system is made up of seven centres of energy within the body through which energy patterns flow. Chakras are described by number, location, character, and colour. The first chakra, red in colour, found at the base of the spine, holds physical vitality and survival; the second chakra, orange in colour, is located in the sacral area and is the centre of desire and sexual energy; the third chakra, yellow in colour, found in the solar plexus, is the centre of creation, perception, and projection of self; the fourth chakra, green in colour, located in the heart, is the centre for love, compassion, and empathy; the fifth chakra, blue, is found in the pit of the throat and is the energy for communication; the sixth chakra, indigo, located in the forehead, is responsible for visualization; and the seventh chakra, violet, located at the crown of the head, is the centre for spirituality.

Energy therapies target energy fields to restore and harmonize the physical, psychological, and spiritual body. The North American Nursing Diagnosis Association (NANDA) recognizes energy therapy as an intervention for energy field disturbance or depletion. This NANDA diagnosis, disturbed energy field, is described as the disruption of the flow of energy or aura surrounding a person's being that results in a disharmony of the body, mind, and/or spirit. The diagnosis and interventions to address a disruption in energy fields require specialized instruction and supervised practice that comes from formal education in energy field theory.

Prayer

For many people of diverse religious denominations and cultural distinctions, **prayer** is a source of strength, restoration, and tranquility (Ameling, 2000; Narayanasamy & Narayanasamy, 2008). Prayer as a healing modality is performed by the patient, family members, religious leaders, and community friends and neighbors. The power of prayer is believed to increase with the number

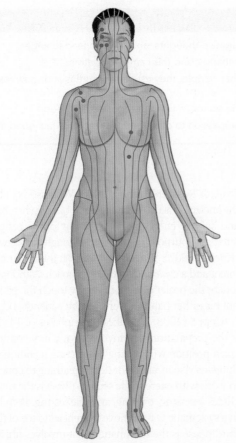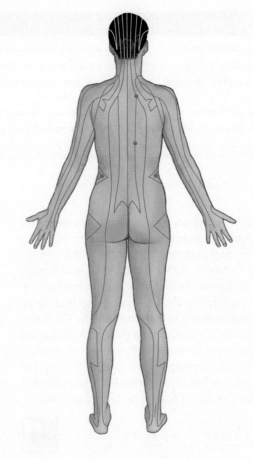

Figure 3.6 Pressure points and meridians.

of people who pray for and with the patient. Prayer is a form of connection with the sacred and divine, through communication with God or the Creator. There are different kinds of prayer based on need or intention; for example, praying for self and others, meditative praying, inner healing prayers, listening prayers, praying for worship, praying for thanks, and praying for confession (Tan, 2007). According to the national survey conducted by the Fraser Institute, 50% of respondents had total confidence in their provider using spiritual or religious healing modalities, and 56% of Canadians used prayer for wellness in the 12 months prior to the 2006 survey (Esmail, 2007). One example is the trust and respect that is given to an elder conducting a Sundance ceremony and the collective healing that occurs through praying and dancing to the Creator and ancestors.

Nurses are particularly concerned with providing spiritual care to their patients. Whether they have the skills and abilities to address these needs themselves is a philosophical debate (Hussey, 2009). However, NANDA has identified Spiritual Distress as a nursing diagnosis. The intervention is to provide spiritual support with the rationale to facilitate a sense of inner peace. The nurse can facilitate spiritual comfort through listening and then incorporating resources into the patient's care.

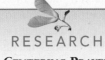

RESEARCH
CENTERING PRAYER

Study
In this descriptive study conducted in the United States, the researchers investigated the use of centering prayer with 10 chemotherapy patients diagnosed with recurrent ovarian cancer to find out if centering prayer is useful in influencing well-being and quality of life. Most participants found centering prayer beneficial. The instrument used to measure emotional well-being, anxiety, depression, and faith demonstrated improvement.

Nursing Implications
Centering prayer is a useful intervention to incorporate into our care of patients with recurrent ovarian cancer. The authors also identify the centering prayer process in four easy steps that nursing students could learn and practice in nursing labs.

Johnson, M. E., Dose, A. M., Pipe, T. B., Petersen, W. O., Huschka, M., Gallenberg, M. M., . . . Frost, M. H. (2009). Centering prayer for women receiving chemotherapy for recurrent ovarian cancer: A pilot study. Oncology Nursing Forum, 36(4), 421–428.

TABLE 3.1	The Five Spiritual Principles of Reiki
1. Just for today, do not worry.	When we worry, we create negative thoughts, and this can lead to anger.
2. Just for today, do not anger.	When we are angry, we are unhappy, and this can lead to stress.
3. Honour your parents, teachers, and elders.	When we show respect to other people, they usually mirror this and show respect to us.
4. Earn your living honestly.	By doing this, we feel safe and secure in that our reputation is good.
5. Give gratitude to every living thing.	Live by kindness and show compassion to others; this will make us feel good and positive.

From Bourne, L. (2009). The art of Reiki and its uses in general. *Practice Nursing, 20,* 11–14.

Reiki

Reiki (pronounced *ray-key*) is a Japanese healing method used by health-care professionals from many disciplines, including nursing, medicine, and occupational therapy (Bossi, Ott, & DeCristofaro, 2008; Bourne, 2009; Swann, 2008), and settings and practices with patients with various health challenges. A Reiki healer uses his or her hands to channel energy from his or her body to the chakra system in the patient's body. The healer uses movements across the chakras from the head to the toe. As the healer proceeds down the body, negative energy is removed and replaced with positive energy. The five spiritual principles of Reiki are summarized in Table 3.1. To learn Reiki, you will need to study with a Reiki master through an accredited program.

Through the eyes of a nurse

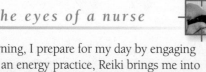

*E*ach morning, I prepare for my day by engaging in self-Reiki. As an energy practice, Reiki brings me into greater alignment with my spiritual self, grounding and centering me and reminding me of my commitment to my human/spiritual journey. In doing so, I feel more prepared to face the challenges that might arise, and to be open to the unexpected blessings that often surface in my encounters with others. Such self-care has been essential in the cultivation of the consciousness required for "being" as a component of effective relational practice. It has been essential for allowing me to begin to grow into responsiveness and out of reactiveness. It nurtures me and helps me to remain objective. . . . I also receive Reiki from others as a routine and engage in it in response to challenging situations. By doing so, my ability to process and integrate the lessons of a given situation are expedited.

(D. Newman-Fuhr, personal communication, June 8, 2009)

Therapeutic Touch and Healing Touch

Therapeutic touch (TT) and healing touch (HT) are similar healing modalities. TT (also known as noncontact therapeutic touch [NCTT]) was initiated in 1972 and is used throughout the world to decrease anxiety by increasing the relaxation response, accelerating wound healing, decreasing pain, and stimulating the immunological system (Coppa, 2008; Daley, 1997; Eschiti, 2007; Kerr, Wasserman, & Moore, 2007; Moore,

Ting, & Rossiter-Thorton, 2008; Wilkinson et al., 2002). TT is the ancient practice of laying on of hands whereby healers assess and balance energy fields by caring for the patient from a centered and purposeful state and through a process of handwork (Krieger, 2002). When providing TT, the healer must have good intent and a clear and focused approach. Although referred to as touch, the healer does not actually touch the patient during TT, but his or her hands hover over the patient's body/energy field.

Coppa (2008) describes three phases of TT. The first phase is the preparation that involves lying in a comfortable and relaxed position while using a centering technique through such things as visualizations or deep breathing to concentrate the self to work with energy. The second phase is the treatment that includes assessing, treating, and reassessing. Both hands are used in a systematic way to move from head to toe of the patient. The third phase is the termination that involves finishing when the energy field feels intact; the practitioner then disengages.

Through the eyes of a nurse

*I*n my mind, as a nurse, I would set my intention for healing with the highest good of the patient and then I would trust that is happening. I need to be grounded, centered, and focused within myself. Also, I need to be connected to my divine source. So then, for example, after I have taken an IV out, I set my connection, ground myself and put my hands over the site, and trust that healing is taking place.

(C. Landry, RN, personal communication, June 5, 2009)

Through the eyes of a patient

I was diagnosed with multiple myeloma and attended several sessions based on energetic healing. In the beginning, I used deep breathing exercises. I cleared my mind, letting go of invading thoughts, and focused on my simple mantra, "I will survive." I breathed in and out deeply focusing on each in and out breath. I visualized the air filling my lungs and then emptying out. I felt my body relax. After practicing this exercise for many days, I could call it up when I was dealing with specific issues, like a treatment event or my fear during a test.

(patient living with multiple myeloma)

Morgan, the third-year student you met at the beginning of the chapter, met a registered nurse (RN) on the maternity unit who was a Reiki master. Morgan had an opportunity to chat with her about the patients she saw in her practice as a Reiki master. The RN described several Reiki sessions with an oncology patient who was experiencing a great deal of pain. The energy that was transferred from the Reiki practitioner to the patient reduced the pain by restoring balance to pain receptors. Morgan was asked to write a paper on therapeutic touch. Through that process, she realized CAM practitioners certified or licensed in their practices quite often operate outside of the health-care system. She learned how to access the classes to become a therapeutic touch practitioner.

SUMMARY

Throughout this chapter, you have learned about some of the most recognized CAM modalities. You have been given real examples from the practice of nurses and the experiences of patients. Examples of research that identifies the effectiveness of CAM for health and healing have been included. The chapter offers a basis for how you could use these therapies within your nursing practice. Alternative medicine and worldviews reveal a wealth of cultural perspectives and approaches that provide supportive and compassionate care.

Critical Thinking Case Scenarios

▶ Mary is a 55-year-old Dene woman admitted to the medicine unit for hypertension. Mary tells you that she has not been able to sleep for the past 2 days in the hospital because spirits are visiting her. She is concerned that the room has not been cleansed. You are confused by what Mary is requesting. You know that the room had a terminal clean by housekeeping, and the staff tell you that occasionally, an Aboriginal healer comes to the unit to perform a cleansing ceremony. How will you respond to Mary? What will you do? Where can you go to for resources? How will you learn about the cleansing ceremony?

▶ Clara is a 40-year-old Métis woman who visits you while you are working in the community health centre. She has a leg ulcer that for the past 2 weeks she has been treating with her own dressing of caribou skin and spruce gum. The ulcer is healing beautifully. Clara is here for advice. She asks you if she should continue to use her medicine or if she should have something different. How will you respond to her? What will you do? What are the healing properties of spruce gum? What resources are available to you?

▶ Sam is a 55-year-old businessman scheduled for exploratory abdominal surgery with a preliminary diagnosis of cancer of the bowel. You admit Sam to the surgical floor. He is anxious. You notice that he is wringing his hands while talking with you and that his speech is rapid. He verbalizes that he is scared about what is going to happen to him. He has never had surgery before. He is worried about the loss of time from work, and he is especially concerned about his wife and children and the unpredictable future that he is now facing. You ask Sam what he does to relax. He says he watches television, and occasionally, he rides his bike. He enjoys classical music. You know the benefits of relaxation for surgical patients. Your job is to develop a teaching plan for Sam. Which of the mind-body therapies will you include? What is your rationale for the selection of this therapy?

Multiple-Choice Questions

1. Alternative medicine is considered as an alternative to Western medicine. How would you describe Aboriginal medicine?
   a. Traditional knowledge that addresses mind, body, emotions, and spirit using various ceremonies
   b. Remedies of plants and animals from the land to treat specific symptoms
   c. A system of healing that was used many years ago but has been proven to be ineffective
   d. A type of medicine that focuses on natural products

2. Mindfulness is an important attribute for the nurse as healer because it is a way of:
   a. Centering prior to providing care
   b. Developing new knowledge
   c. Being present for the patient
   d. Showing what you know

3. Self-care is a vital tool for nurses who use complementary modalities because:
   a. A healthy healer delivers positive energy to the patient.
   b. A deliberate approach is needed for a specific ailment.
   c. Stress and tension create chaos in the workplace.
   d. To be a nurse, you must be fit.

4. Therapeutic touch is an energy modality that nurses perform by:
   a. Taking vital signs, massaging the body, and covering with a warm blanket
   b. Assessing the energy field, performing a treatment, and concluding the treatment
   c. Assessing the pathways, applying pressure to each of the chakras, and concluding the treatment
   d. Warming the hands, rubbing from head to toe, and concluding the treatment

5. Joe tells you his anxiety is reduced when people pray with him. He asks you if you will pray with him before he goes for surgery. Your best response would be:
   a. "I do not believe that prayer will do anything for you."
   b. "The administration forbid me from praying with patients."
   c. "Is there a special prayer you would like or will I use one of my own?"
   d. "Yes, what do you find most helpful?"

6. Sarah is visibly anxious. She is to go for an magnetic resonance imaging (MRI). She has confirmed that massage helps her to relax. Massage works by:
   a. Encouraging patients to rest in bed
   b. Manipulating the soft tissues with the hands
   c. Alleviating muscle pain and tension by applying various techniques with the hands
   d. Rubbing oil into the skin

Suggested Lab Activities

● Visit and interview an Aboriginal elder to learn about traditional knowledge and health. Consider questions such as, "What are cultural beliefs and practices about birth and death?" "How would a community member access an Aboriginal healer?" and "How can cultural practices be honoured in health care?"

● Visit a clinical herbalist and discuss the use of plants for various common illnesses; for example, "What plant could you use to boost your immune system?" and "Are there plants that can be used to help with symptoms of menstruation and menopause?"

● Visit a meditation website, for example, http://www.how-to-meditate.org, and practice meditation. You may also like to consider exploring how this makes you feel. By recognizing pleasant and unpleasant feelings, we may learn how to change our feelings through focused meditation. See if you can train your mind to go to a positive state and thus reduce your stress and bring you a peaceful feeling.

References and Suggested Readings

Adams, J., & Tovey, P. (Eds.). (2008). *Complementary and alternative medicine in nursing and midwifery. Towards a critical social science.* New York, NY: Routledge.

Ameling, A. (2000). Prayer: An ancient healing practice becomes new again. *Holistic Nursing Practice, 14*(3), 40–48.

Andre, A., & Fehr, A. (2001). *Gwich'in ethnobotany: Plants used by the Gwich'in for food, medicine, shelter and tools.* Tsiigehtchic, Northwest Territories: Gwich'in Social and Cultural Institute and Aurora Research Institute.

Blondin, G. (1990). *When the world was new: Stories of the Sahtu Dene.* Yellowknife, NT: Outcrop.

Bossi, L. M., Ott, M., & DeCristofaro, S. (2008). Reiki as a clinical intervention on oncology nursing practice. *Clinical Journal of Oncology Nursing, 12*(3), 489–494.

Bottalini, C. (2008). Zen Yoga: Good medicine for surgical patients. *RN, 71*(7), 20–22.

Bourne, L. (2009). The art of Reiki and its uses in general. *Practice Nursing, 20,* 11–14.

Buckley, J. (2002). Massage and aromatherapy massage: Nursing art and science. *International Journal of Palliative Nursing, 8*(6), 276–280.

Carmody, J., & Baer, R. A. (2008). Relationships between mindfulness practice and levels of mindfulness, medical and psychological symptoms and well-being in a mindfulness-based stress reduction program. *Journal of Behavioral Medicine, 31,* 23–33.

Chen, H., & Chen, C. (2004). Effects of acupressure at the sanyinjiao point on primary dysmenorrhoea. *Journal of Advanced Nursing, 48*(4), 380–387.

Cole, V. L. (2003). Healing principles: A model for the use of ritual in psychotherapy. *Counseling & Values, 47*(3), 344–346.

Coppa, D. (2008). The internal process of therapeutic touch. *Journal of Holistic Nursing, 26*(1), 17–24.

Coyle, J. (2002). Spirituality and health: Towards a framework for exploring the relationship between spirituality and health. *Journal of Advanced Nursing, 37*(6), 589–597.

Daley, B. (1997). Therapeutic touch, nursing practice and contemporary wound healing research. *Journal of Advanced Nursing, 25,* 1123–1132.

Day, J., & Goad, K. (2010). Recovery of the pelvic floor after pregnancy and childbirth. *British Journal of Midwifery, 18,* 51–53.

Dossey, B., & Keegan, L. (2009). *Holistic nursing: A handbook for practice* (5th ed.). Mississauga, ON: Jones and Bartlett.

Dunne, N., Benda, W., Kim, L., Mittman, P., Barrett, R., Snider, P., & Pizzomo, J. (2005). Naturopathic medicine: What can patients expect? *Journal of Family Practice, 54*(12), 1067–1072.

Eschiti, V. S. (2007). Healing touch: A low-tech intervention in high-tech settings. *Critical Care Nursing, 26*(1), 9–14.

Esmail, N. (2007). *Complementary and alternative medicine in Canada: Trends in use and public attitudes, 1997–2006.* Vancouver, BC: Fraser Institute. Retrieved from http://www.fraserinstitute.org/commerce.web/product_files/ComplementaryAlternativeMedicine.pdf

Goudreau, G., Weber-Pillwax, C., Cote-Meek, S., Madill, H., & Wilson, S. (2008). Hand-drumming: Health-promoting experiences of Aboriginal women from a Northern Ontario urban community. *Journal of Aboriginal Health.* Retrieved from http://www.naho.ca/english/journal/jah04_01/10HandDrumming_72-83.pdf

Hart-Wasekeesikaw, F. (1996). *First Nations peoples' perspectives and experiences with cancer* (Unpublished master's thesis). University of Manitoba, Winnipeg, MB.

Health Canada. (2007). *Evidence for homeopathic medicines.* Ottawa, ON: National Health Products Directorate.

Helm, J. (1994). *Prophecy and power among the Dogrib Indians.* Lincoln, NE: University of Nebraska Press.

Helm, J. (2000). *The people of Denendeh: Ethnohistory of the Indian's of Canada's Northwest Territories.* Montreal, QC: McGill-Queen's University Press.

Hussey, T. (2009). Nursing and spirituality. *Philosophy, 18,* 71–80.

Joshi, R. R. (2004). A biostatistical approach to Ayurveda: Quantifying the Tridosha. *The Journal of Alternative and Complementary Medicine, 10*(5), 879–889.

Jun, E. M., Chang, S., Kang, D. H., & Kim, S. (2007). Effects of acupressure on dysmenorrhea and skin temperature changes in college students: A non-randomized controlled trial. *International Journal of Nursing Studies, 44*(6), 973–981.

Kabat-Zinn, J. (2003). Mindfulness-based interventions in context: Past, present, and future. *Clinical Psychology, Science and Practice, 10*(2), 144–156.

Kerr, C. E., Wasserman, R. H., & Moore, C. I. (2007). Cortical dynamics as a therapeutic mechanism for touch healing. *Journal of Alternative and Complementary Medicine, 13*(1), 59–66.

Kingwatsiaq, N., & Pii, K. (2003). Healing the body and the soul through visualization: A technique used by the Community Healing Team of Cape Dorset, Nunavut. *Arctic Anthropology, 40*(2), 90–92.

Kollack, I. (2009). *Yoga for nurses.* New York, NY: Springer Publishing.

Kong, J., Tan, K., Goh, N., & Chia, L. (2004). Traditional Chinese medicine. *Asia Pacific Biotech News, 8*(23), 1244–1251.

Krieger, D. (2002). *Therapeutic touch as transpersonal healing.* New York, NY: Lantern Books.

Lavallee, L. F. (2008). Balancing the medicine wheel through physical activity. *Journal of Aboriginal Health.* Retrieved from http://www.naho.ca/english/journal/jah04_01/09MedicineWheel_64-71.pdf

Lavallee, L. F. (2009). Practical application of an Indigenous research framework and two qualitative Indigenous research methods: Sharing circles and Anishnaabe symbol-based reflection. *International Journal of Qualitative Methods, 8*(1), 21–40. Retrieved from http://creativecommons.org/licences/by/2.0

Lee, M. K., Chang, S. B., & Kang, D. H. (2004). Effects of SP6 acupressure on labour pain and length of delivery time in women during labour. *Journal of Alternative and Complementary Medicine, 10*(6), 959–965.

Lennihan, B. (2004). Homeopathy: Natural mind-body healing. *Journal of Psychosocial Nursing and Mental Health Services, 42*(7), 30–40.

Maa, S. H., Tsou, T. S., Wang, K. Y., Wang, C. H., Lin, H. C., & Huang, Y. H. (2007). Self-administered acupressure reduces the symptoms that limit daily activities in bronchiectasis patients: Pilot study findings. *Journal of Clinical Nursing, 16,* 794–804.

Mackey, S. (1998). Massage as a nursing intervention: Using reflection to achieve change in practice. *Contemporary Nurse, 7*(1), 18–23.

Martsolf, D. S., & Mickley, J. R. (1998). The concept of spirituality in nursing theories: Differing world-views and extent of focus. *Journal of Advanced Nursing, 27,* 294–303.

McCabe, G. (2008). Mind, body, emotions and spirit: Reaching to the ancestors for healing. *Counselling Psychology Quarterly, 21*(2), 143–152.

McCaffrey, R., & Fowler, N. L. (2003). Qigong practice: A pathway to health and healing. *Holistic Nursing Practice, 17*(2), 110–116.

Merriam-Webster, Inc. (1993). *Webster's Third New International Dictionary of the English Language Unabridged.* Springfield, MA: Author.

Miner-Williams, D. (2006). Putting a puzzle together: Making spirituality meaningful for nursing using an evolving theoretical framework. *Journal of Clinical Nursing, 15,* 811–821.

Moffitt, P., & Vollman, A. (2004). Photovoice: Picturing the health of Aboriginal women in a remote northern community. *Canadian Journal of Nursing Research, 36*(4), 189–201.

Moore, T., Ting, B., & Rossiter-Thornton, M. (2008). A pilot study of the experience of participating in a therapeutic touch practice group. *Journal of Holistic Nursing, 26*(3), 161–168.

Narayanasamy, A., & Narayanasamy, M. (2008). The healing power of prayer and its implications for nursing. *British Journal of Nursing, 17*(6), 394–398.

National Aboriginal Health Organization. (2008). *An overview of traditional knowledge and medicine and public health in Canada.* Ottawa, ON: Author.

O'Callaghan, C. (2009). Objectivist and constructivist music therapy in oncology and palliative care: An overview and reflection. *Music and Medicine, 1*(1), 41–60.

Ott, M. J. (2004). Mindfulness meditation: A path of transformation and healing. *Journal of Psychosocial Nursing and Mental Health Services, 42*(7), 22–29.

Perkins, J. B. (2003). Healing through spirit: The experience of the eternal in the everyday. *Visions, 11*(1), 29–42.

Ponto, J. A., Frost, M. H., Thompson, R., Allers, T., Reed-Will, T., Zahasky, K., . . . Hartmann, L. C. (2003). Stories of breast cancer through art. *Oncology Nursing Forum, 30*(6), 1007–1013.

Royal Commission on Aboriginal Peoples. (1996). *Report of the Royal Commission on Aboriginal Peoples.* Ottawa, ON: Author.

Ryan, J., & Johnson, M. (1994). *Traditional Dene medicine, Part one and part two, Lac La Martre, NWT.* Hay River, NT: Dene Cultural Institute.

Scheufele, P. M. (2000). Effects of progressive relaxation and classical music on measurements of attention, relaxation and stress responses. *Journal of Behavioral Medicine, 23*(2), 207–228.

Schmidt, S. (2004). Mindfulness and healing intention: Concepts, practice, and research evaluation. *Journal of Alternative and Complementary Medicine, 10,* S7–S14.

Shalts, E. (2005). *Easy homeopathy: The 7 essential remedies you need for common illness and first aid.* New York, NY: McGraw-Hill.

Stone, D. (2008). Wounded healing: Exploring the circle of compassion in the helping relationship. *The Humanistic Psychologist, 36,* 45–51.

Stuckley, H. L., & Nobel, J. (2010). The connection between art, healing, and public health: A review of the literature. *American Journal of Public Health, 100,* 254–263. doi:10.2105/AJPH.2008.156497

Swann, J. (2008). An introduction to Reiki as an alternative therapy in care homes. *Nursing & Residential Care, 11*(1), 31–34.

Tan, S. (2007). Use of prayer and scripture in cognitive-behavioral therapy. *Journal of Psychology and Christianity, 26*(2), 101–111.

Tanyi, R. A. (2002). Towards clarification of the meaning of spirituality: Nursing theory and concept development or analysis. *Journal of Advanced Nursing, 39*(5), 500–509.

Tanyi, R. A. (2006). Spirituality and family nursing: Spiritual assessment and interventions for families. *Journal of Advanced Nursing, 53*(3), 287–294.

Tenzin-Dolma, L. (2008). *Healing mandalas.* London, United Kingdom: Duncan Baird.

Tjale, A. A., & Bruce, J. (2007). A concept analysis of holistic nursing care in paediatric nursing. *Curationis, 30*(4), 45–52.

Waldram, J. B. (Ed.). (2008). *Aboriginal healing in Canada: Studies in therapeutic meaning and practice.* Ottawa, ON: Aboriginal Healing Foundation.

Wilkinson, D. S., Knox, P. L., Chatman, J. E., Johnson, T. L., Barbour, N., Myles, Y., & Reel, A. (2002). The clinical effectiveness of healing touch. *Journal of Alternative and Complementary Medicine, 8*(1), 33–47.

Wu, H. S., Wu, S. C., Lin, J. G., & Lin, L. C. (2004). Effectiveness of acupressure in improving dyspnoea in chronic obstructive pulmonary disease. *Journal of Advanced Nursing, 43*(3), 252–259.

Yang, M. H., Wu, S. C., Lin, J. G., & Lin, L. C. (2007). The efficacy of acupressure for decreasing agitated behavior in dementia: A pilot study. *Journal of Clinical Nursing, 16,* 308–315.

Nursing as a Regulated Profession: Standards of Practice

E. JOYCE BLACK, SANDRA REGAN, AND CATHERINE COTTER

Jas is a first-year nursing student in a baccalaureate education program in Eastern Canada. He and other first-year students are starting to learn about nursing as a regulated profession and its standards of practice. He understands that the standards of practice are set by another organization, not by his nursing program. He wonders: Who sets these standards? Why do I have to follow these standards, and what do they mean for me as a student?

CHAPTER OBJECTIVES

By the end of this chapter, you will be able to:

1. Describe the purpose of professional regulation and self-regulation.
2. Identify the ways regulatory bodies influence what you need to learn by the time you graduate to be eligible for registration.
3. Differentiate between the professional behaviours expected of a professional registered nurse and a student nurse.
4. Compare and contrast the mandates of two or more provincial/territorial nursing regulatory bodies.
5. Explain the significance of fitness to practice and the strategies you will use as a student to ensure your fitness to practice.
6. Discuss the privileges with the related responsibilities and accountabilities that nurses must demonstrate to practice safely, competently, and ethically.
7. Describe what you learn in your nursing education program that will enable you to become a self-regulating professional nurse and meet the continuing competence or quality assurance requirements for registration.

KEY TERMS

Accountability   Nurses have the obligation to answer for the professional, ethical, and legal responsibilities of their activities and duties.

Competencies   The knowledge, abilities, skills, attitudes, and clinical judgment required to provide competent, safe, and ethical patient care.

Continuing Competence   The ongoing ability of a registered nurse to integrate and apply the knowledge, skills, judgment, and personal attributes required to practice safely and ethically in a designated role and setting.

Duty to Provide Care   Nurses have a legal and ethical duty to provide safe, ethical, and competent care.

Duty to Report   Nurses or others who observe practice in nurses or other health professionals who place patients at risk have an obligation to report significant concerns about an individual to their regulatory body.

Fitness to Practice   All the qualities and capabilities of an individual relevant to his or her capability to practice as a nurse, including, but not limited to, freedom from any cognitive, physical, psychological, or emotional condition or a dependence on alcohol or drugs, that impair his or her ability to practice nursing.

Professional Presence   Nurses act with confidence, integrity, optimism, passion, and empathy in accordance with professional standards, guidelines, and code of ethics. Professional presence includes reflective practice, verbal and nonverbal communications, and the ability to articulate a positive role and professional image.

Public Interest   The common good or benefit that applies to a broad group of people, such as patients or the public for which nurses provide care.

Quality Assurance   Programs developed by regulatory bodies to help nurses to maintain and improve their competence from year to year.

Regulation   Rules established to govern behaviour of people or groups.

Regulatory Body   A nonprofit organization with the legal authority to establish, monitor, and enforce standards of practice within a professional group for the purposes of public protection. In Canada, the authority of regulatory bodies comes from legislation enacted by the provincial and territorial governments.

Scope of Practice   Activities that nurses are educated and legally authorized to perform.

Self-regulation   Self-regulation recognizes that a profession is in the best position to determine standards for education and practice and to ensure that standards are met. Self-regulation means that the government has granted a professional group, such as registered nurses, the privilege and responsibility to regulate themselves. In essence, society contracts with the registered nursing profession to regulate its own members in order to protect the public from harm that could be caused by registered nurses in the course of their practice.

Standard   An authoritative statement that describes the required behaviour of every nurse and is used to evaluate individual performance.

Standards of Practice   All types of standards about nursing practice to which nurses are held accountable.

Use of Title   Criteria defined in legislation that set out who can use the title *nurse*.

Professional Regulation

What comes to mind when you hear the terms *regulation* and *self-regulation*? If you are thinking about human pathophysiology, you might think about the complex systems that help regulate body functions. Of course, the terms *regulation* and *self-regulation* will have different meanings when we discuss them within the context of the profession of nursing.

This chapter introduces you to how regulatory bodies protect the public interest through standards and what it means to be a member of the regulated profession of nursing.

What Is Professional Regulation?

Regulation and *self-regulation* are terms that are sometimes used interchangeably. Although related, they are defined separately and used to mean specific things. In the broadest sense, **regulation** is simply establishing and enforcing rules to govern behaviour of people or groups. Regulations exist for how drugs are approved or how food is inspected. Regulations are in place to govern professional groups from accountants to engineers to health professionals. In all these cases, regulations safeguard the public in some way. **Self-regulation** recognizes that a profession is in the bet position to determine standards for education an practice and to ensure that standards are met" (Canadian Nurses Association, 2007, p. 1). With the privilege to self-regulate comes the expectation that not only will the profession define standards but that it will also monitor and enforce these standards. This occurs in two broad ways. First, an organization called a **regulatory body** sets up processes for this monitoring and enforcement, and second, each individual nurse monitors and enforces standards. Nursing is one of these self-regulating professions.

What Does It Mean to Regulate in the Public Interest?

Not every profession is granted the authority to self-regulate. The government and the public place a great deal of trust in nurses self-regulating in a way that protects the public and ensures the public interest is upheld.

Public interest refers to how a profession enacts its obligations to ensure the welfare of society; in nursing, this means the provision of safe, competent, and ethical patient care for all people. To ensure this, the government, as steward of the public interest, sets out expectations in the form of legislation for professions. When we talk about regulating nurses in the public interest, it means we place the interests of the public above interests of the profession or individual nurses. The benefit to the public is the assurance that a registered nurse is providing safe, competent, and ethical care to the public. The College of Registered Nurses of Manitoba states, "Self-regulation means that the government has granted a professional group, such as registered nurses, the privilege and responsibility to regulate themselves". In essence, society contracts with the registered nursing profession to regulate its own members in order to protect the public from harm that could be caused by registered nurses in the course of their practice. When there is a conflict between public interest and professional self-interest, regulatory bodies such as the College of Registered Nurses of Manitoba are expected to support the public interest" (College of Registered Nurses of Manitoba, 2011, p. 1). This relationship between the nursing profession and society (the public) is a type of social contract where professional rights and responsibilities are set as well as expectations for public accountability. This relationship might contrast with the mandate of a union or professional association; for example, where the primary interest is first its membership, then the public or other interest. Unions safeguard the interests of nurses through collective agreements for the socioeconomic benefits of nurses. This does not mean that they are not concerned about the public interest but rather that the interests of their members are a dominant consideration. For regulatory bodies, the first priority is always with public interest before individual or professional interest. This is a challenging idea because in our society, there are often competing priorities between public interest and professional or individual rights. Some of the competing interests that arise in nursing will be discussed later in this chapter in the section on professional obligations.

The concept of trust is an important one in professional self-regulation. Public opinion polls consistently identify nursing as one of the most trusted professions. Society places a higher standard of accountability and responsibility on those whom we entrust with the well-being of the public. Nurses take this trust very seriously. One way the profession maintains that trust is ensuring nurses practice safely, competently, and ethically. When challenges arise and nursing practice is not safe, competent, or ethical, regulatory bodies intervene, placing the interests of the public ahead of the interests of the individual nurse.

What Is a Regulatory Body?

In self-regulation, who actually regulates and how do they do this? Health professional regulation in Canada is a provincial/territorial matter. Provincial/territorial governments, through legislation, establish regulatory bodies. A regulatory body is given authority, through legislation, to set out standards, among other duties it must perform, to ensure that the public is protected.

Some provinces/territories have a health professions legislation, called an *act*, which sets out the framework for how regulatory bodies operate, specifying their duties and obligations. This legislation is often very broad and applicable to several health professions such as physicians, pharmacists, and others. In some provinces/territories, each profession has its own legislation or act (e.g., rather than a broad Health Professions Act, they may have a specific Nurses Act). Along with the act, government sets out regulations that are specific to a given profession. The regulation is often where you will find the definition of the profession (what nursing is), who can call themselves a nurse and under what conditions they can do so (use of title and title protection), and what nurses can and cannot do (scope of practice). Nursing regulatory bodies have authority to regulate individual nurses, not the organizations in which they work. These organizations and health-care facilities such as hospitals operate under different regulations and have different processes, such as licensing and accreditation. For more information on nursing regulation, refer to Box 4.1.

How Are Regulatory Bodies Organized?

The health profession does not self-regulate on its own; it involves the public in various ways. One important way is through the appointment by government of public representatives who sit on the board or council that governs a regulatory body. As part of the governance of a regulatory body, it will have a board of directors or council made up of members of the profession and representatives of the public. The public representatives are usually appointed by the government and have an important decision-making role in a

BOX 4.1   More on Nursing Regulation

Regulation of health professionals has a long history in Canada. Nurses, along with physicians and pharmacists, are among the oldest regulated professions. Of course, 100 years ago, regulation looked quite different from today! Regulation has changed over time, adapting to changing expectations of government and the public. This is another way that we regulate in the public interest—by ensuring that we remain responsive to public concerns regarding health professionals. If you would like to understand more about the history of nursing regulation and the specific activities of a regulatory body, we encourage you to read the following reference:

Brunke, L. (2010). Canadian provincial and territorial professional associations and colleges. In M. McIntyre & C. McDonald (Eds.), *Realities of Canadian nursing: Professional, practice, and power issues* (3rd ed., pp. 147–165). Philadelphia, PA: Lippincott Williams & Wilkins.

regulatory body. They are expected to represent the public interest to assist the regulatory body in self-regulation and ensure that the public interest is included when setting standards and policies that govern the practice of that profession.

There are different ways that nursing regulatory bodies are organized. In some provinces/territories, the college (another name for a regulatory organization, not to be confused with an educational institution) and association functions are combined (such as with the College and Association of Registered Nurses of Alberta). In other provinces, the organizations are called *associations*, but actually combine regulatory and association functions as well (such as the Registered Nurses Association of Northwest Territories and Nunavut). In Ontario, there is a separate college and association: The College of Nurses of Ontario regulates nurses, and the Registered Nurses Association of Ontario is the professional association for nurses. What is the name of the regulatory body in your province/territory? Refer to Table 4.1 for a list of regulatory bodies by province. How does that fit with the descriptions we have just discussed?

TABLE 4.1	Websites of Regulatory Bodies in Canada	
Province/Territory	**Regulatory Body**	**Website Address**
Alberta	College and Association of Registered Nurses of Alberta	http://www.nurses.ab.ca
British Columbia	College of Registered Nurses of British Columbia	http://www.crnbc.ca
Manitoba	College of Registered Nurses of Manitoba	http://www.crnm.mb.ca
New Brunswick	Nurses Association of New Brunswick	http://www.nanb.nb.ca
Newfoundland and Labrador	Association of Registered Nurses of Newfoundland and Labrador	http://www.arnnl.ca
Northwest Territories and Nunavut	Registered Nurses Association of the Northwest Territories and Nunavut	http://www.rnantnu.ca
Nova Scotia	College of Registered Nurses of Nova Scotia	http://www.crnns.ca
Ontario	College of Nurses of Ontario	http://www.cno.org
Prince Edward Island	Association of Registered Nurses of Prince Edward Island	http://www.arnpei.ca
Quebec	Ordre des infirmières et des infirmiers du Québec	http://www.oiiq.org
Saskatchewan	Saskatchewan Registered Nurses Association	http://www.srna.org
Yukon	Yukon Registered Nurses Association	http://www.yrna.ca

What Does a Regulatory Body Do?

There are several activities that a regulatory body undertakes to regulate the profession and protect the public. Many of these activities are set out explicitly in legislation. The regulatory body protects the public by being a gatekeeper, setting out requirements for those entering the profession and how they maintain their registration in the profession. In fact, in nursing, registration is mandatory to practice; it is illegal to call yourself a nurse or practice nursing without being registered with the provincial/territorial nursing regulatory body. Setting requirements for entering the profession, including the competencies that shape your education program, and annual requirements for maintaining registration are only some of the better known activities of a regulatory body. Regulatory bodies also ensure that nurses maintain their competence to practice and address concerns when a nurse practices in a manner that is unsafe, incompetent, or unethical. Providing supports to nurses to assist them to provide safe, ethical, and competent patient care is also an important part of what the regulatory body does.

What Is Nursing?

There are numerous definitions of *nursing*; however, each province/territory will set out a broad definition of nursing in legislation. This helps to differentiate nursing from other health professions. For example, in Ontario, the Nursing Act describes the practice of nursing as "the promotion of health and the assessment of, the provision of care for, and the treatment of health conditions by supportive, preventive, therapeutic, palliative and rehabilitative means in order to attain or maintain optimal function" (College of Nurses of Ontario, 2011, p. 1). In Manitoba, the Registered Nurses Act defines the practice of nursing as "the application of nursing knowledge, skill and judgment to promote, maintain and restore health, prevent illness and alleviate suffering, and includes, but is not limited to, (a) assessing health status; (b) planning, providing and evaluating treatment and nursing interventions; (c) counselling and teaching to enhance health and well-being; and (d) education, administration and research related to providing health services" (Manitoba Government, n.d.).

Has your nursing education program defined *nursing*? You might want to compare the legislation in your province/territory with that definition or other definitions you find in this and other textbooks.

When Can You Call Yourself a Nurse?

In most cases, the title *nurse* is protected by legislation. This means that only those who meet criteria defined in legislation can use the title; this is often called **use of title**. One of the most important reasons for limiting the use of *nurse* is to ensure that the public is protected. By ensuring that only those who meet specific criteria set out by the regulatory body call themselves nurses, the public can be assured that when someone calls himself or herself a nurse, he or she meets agreed-upon standards. In fact, one of the activities of the regulatory body is to investigate when someone uses the title *nurse* inappropriately.

Although students are not specifically mentioned in legislation, they are usually granted permission to use the title *student nurse* because the regulatory body has some oversight for nursing education programs. The public is protected because they are made aware of your learner status, and you have guidance from a registered nurse faculty member or preceptor when practicing with patients. Calling yourself a *student nurse* is a privilege and comes with responsibilities and accountability to use the title appropriately.

What Can a Nurse Do?

Scope of practice refers to those activities that nurses are educated and legally authorized to perform. The scope of practice is usually set out in legislation, and just like the definition of nursing, it is fairly broad. In some provinces, the scope of practice includes a list of activities. These activities have been identified as posing significant risk of harm to the public, and only certain health professions are permitted to perform these activities. Some of these activities include medication administration, insertion of instruments or tubes into the body, and administration of oxygen or blood products. Because the scope of nursing practice is broad, it only gives direction for what the profession as a whole is legally authorized to perform. The regulatory body will set out further boundaries for the legal scope of practice by taking into consideration the extent to which certain activities pose a significant risk of harm to the public; the education required, including whether additional education beyond the basic nursing education program is required; and the appropriateness of having nurses perform the activities.

Nurses need to know when they require an order from another regulated health professional such as a pharmacist, physician, or nurse practitioner to perform an activity; when they can perform activities without an order; or even whether they can perform certain activities at all. It is also important for nurses to know which regulated health professionals they can take orders from. An individual nurse would be required to practice within the boundaries of the scope of practice and only perform those activities for which he or she has the competence—the collective knowledge, skills, attitude, and judgment—and is authorized by legislation and the nursing regulatory body to perform. The scope of practice for an individual nurse is dependent on where he or she practices nursing, the needs of the patient, and the nurse's education and experience. Does this sound familiar to you? In your nursing program, you may have learned that you can only carry out those activities that you have learned in your studies, have been authorized to perform by a nursing faculty member, and are consistent with the organization policies—both in your education program and in the health-care facility. These are similar boundaries that registered nurses comply with when they practice within the scope of practice.

National and International Perspectives on Nursing Regulation

The Canadian Nurses Association (CNA) is the national professional association of registered nurses. As an association and a national organization, it does not regulate nurses. It does, however, work with provincial/territorial nursing regulatory bodies on areas where a collaborative approach might fit with the public interest.

The International Council of Nurses (ICN) is a federation of national nurses' associations representing nursing worldwide; CNA is a member of ICN. Like CNA, ICN does not directly regulate individual nurses, but ICN considers regulation one of its three pillars (along with professional practice and socioeconomic welfare). ICN provides a global forum for member countries to establish or reform nursing professional regulatory practices. If you wish to know more about CNA or ICN, you can go to their websites and read more about their work on health policy issues that are pertinent to regulation. This will be of particular importance if you are travelling to another country for a student placement or to work as a nurse. Box 4.2 has suggestions for accessing student resources on the websites of regulatory bodies.

Students and Regulation

Professionals are regulated. Students have not yet assumed the professional role. In Canada, with the exception of British Columbia, nursing regulatory bodies do not regulate students. In British Columbia, registration is mandatory for those students who choose to work as employed student nurses. Nursing students in British Columbia should check with the regulatory body regarding what aspects of regulation apply to them and under what conditions. In a recent report in the United Kingdom, the authors briefly discuss whether students in health professional education programs such as nursing and medicine should be regulated. They concluded that the need to regulate students is dependent

---

BOX 4.2   Accessing Student Resources on the Nursing Regulatory Website

Most nursing regulatory bodies have resources specifically for students. Go to the website for your provincial/territorial nursing regulatory body. What resources can you find specific to students? Tip: You might enter the search word *student* to more easily find these resources. If your provincial/territorial regulatory body does not have information, try another website. Are there ways for you to be involved in the regulatory body?

---

on the risk of harm to the public and will vary depending on the health profession (Secretary of State for Health, 2007). Even though most nursing students are not regulated in Canada, they are still expected to practice within their competence level as a student, to practice within the standards, and to practice within the policies of the education program in which they are enrolled. These standards are similar to what we would expect of a registered nurse. You are meeting these expectations as a student, whereas a registered nurse is meeting expectations as a professional.

Nursing as a Regulated Profession

What makes nursing a profession and not just an occupation? Sociologists and others commonly use a set of characteristics to define a profession (Chitty, 2007; Volti, 2008). Some of these characteristics include accountability, specialized body of knowledge, competent application of knowledge, code of ethics, service to the public, and self-regulation. These characteristics form the basis of the professional standards for Canadian nursing regulatory bodies.

Practitioner Accountability

Professional registered nurses are held accountable for the professional decisions we make and the nursing services we provide. That is, we are legally answerable for our practice to our patients, our employers, and our regulating body. However, there is also the collective accountability of the nursing profession that arises from self-regulation. Along with the privilege of regulating nursing practice comes the responsibility to do this effectively. The regulatory body is accountable to the public for the way in which it implements, monitors, and enforces regulatory activities such as registration of individual nurses and approval of nursing education programs.

A Specialized Body of Knowledge

Over the past few decades, much work has been done on the development of nursing theory, which helps us to clarify the unique nursing approach with patients and their needs. As well as contributing to the definition of what is and what is not nursing, this work assists others to see more clearly that nursing knowledge is unique to the profession and is complementary to that of the other health disciplines. Each nursing regulatory body has a legal definition of nursing which clarifies that registered nursing is different from another health profession such as medicine or physiotherapy and broadly describes the practice of registered nurses.

Competent Application of Knowledge

A major expectation of the public is that nurses will apply their nursing knowledge competently. The patient receiving nursing services is likely to be far more interested in our competence than in almost anything else about us. One of the hallmarks of being professional is the ability, as individuals, to recognize and act on our ongoing learning needs. As a student, you are learning about the boundaries of your competence; for example, what you can and cannot do when you are in your clinical placement and when you need to seek guidance from a registered nurse. Maintaining competence is a responsibility that never ends and demands our commitment to lifelong learning. You will learn more about lifelong learning in a later chapter in this book.

Code of Ethics

A profession's code of ethics is its public statement of values and acceptable professional conduct. The CNA has developed a code of ethics that has been adopted or adapted by most of the nursing regulatory bodies. The CNA code sets out the foundational "nursing values and ethical responsibilities." These are the ethical responsibilities for all nurses including students (as shown in Box 4.3). In addition, the CNA code sets out "ethical endeavours" which are broad statements regarding how nurses can make changes in systems and societies for the betterment of all. You will be learning more about ethics and the CNA code in a later chapter in this book.

A Tradition of Service to the Public

The public has come to expect that nurses, as professionals, will always see public service as an important role. It is this belief in public service—the commitment to do good—that drives nurses in their concern for individual patient rights and for the well-being of families, groups, entire communities, and populations. The idea of public service also provides the basis for working in cooperation with other health-care disciplines to serve our patients better.

Engaging in Self-Regulation

Just as individual nurses regulate themselves by maintaining their competence and fitness to practice, the nursing profession regulates its members collectively in order to protect the public from harm. Professional groups regulate themselves because few outside of their profession have their specialized body of knowledge. This knowledge is important to understand what constitutes appropriate and acceptable practice for the profession and evaluate the performance of individuals using bona fide standards of practice. The need for this specialized knowledge about nursing practice in order to inform decisions makes external regulation difficult. The inclusion of government-appointed public representatives to regulatory boards and councils means there is a balance between specialized professional knowledge and public input. It makes good sense for the public to have professionals regulate themselves as long as they do it using fair, transparent, unbiased, comprehensive, and timely processes to ensure the public interest is protected.

Jas had no idea that so much about what a nurse does is governed by legislation and is subject to self-regulation. He is curious about the nursing regulatory body that sets the standards in his province. He especially wants to find out more about how public representatives participate in the nursing regulatory body. He was pleased to learn that the regulatory body permits observers at the board meetings and decides to contact them to ask if he can attend a meeting.

Regulation and Nursing Education

Who decides what is included in a nursing program to ensure safe patient care? Regulatory bodies, educational institutions, and nursing faculty all play essential roles. One of the major ways regulatory bodies protect the public is through measures to determine that students learn to provide safe patient care by graduation. The regulatory bodies do this by setting the standards of practice and **competencies** to be demonstrated in order to be eligible for registration following graduation. The competencies encompass the knowledge, abilities, skills, attitudes, and clinical judgments required to provide competent, safe, and ethical patient care. Educational institutions and nursing faculty decide many other aspects of nursing education, especially the learning opportunities to demonstrate student use of the standards of practice and achievement of the competencies. Faculty decisions include how the competencies and standards of practice are placed in different nursing courses, what courses are required, how courses are structured and sequenced, what learning activities and practice experiences

---

| BOX 4.3 | Canadian Nurses Association Code of Ethics for Registered Nurses |

Primary Nursing Values

1. Providing safe, compassionate, competent and ethical care
   Nurses provide safe, compassionate, competent and ethical care.
2. Promoting health and well-being
   Nurses work with people to enable them to attain their highest possible level of health and well-being.
3. Promoting and respecting informed decision-making
   Nurses recognize, respect and promote a person's right to be informed and make decisions.
4. Preserving dignity
   Nurses recognize and respect the intrinsic worth of each person.
5. Maintaining privacy and confidentiality
   Nurses recognize the importance of privacy and confidentiality and safeguard personal, family and community information obtained in the context of a professional relationship.
6. Promoting justice
   Nurses uphold principles of justice by safeguarding human rights, equity and fairness and by promoting the public good.
7. Being accountable
   Nurses are accountable for their actions and answerable for their practice.

Source: Canadian Nurses Association. (2008). *Code of ethics for registered nurses* (2008 centennial edition). Retrieved from http://www.cna-aiic.ca/CNA/practice/ethics/code/default_e.aspx. © Canadian Nurses Association. Reprinted with permission. Further reproduction prohibited.

with patients are required at different stages of the program, evaluation to ensure safe care with patients, and the policies used to decide whether a student will pass or fail. Most regulatory bodies in Canada conduct regular reviews of nursing education programs to determine that all students will learn the standards of practice and competencies in order to be eligible to register to practice nursing after graduation.

Standards of Practice

The phrase *standards of practice* is the general language used to refer to all types of standards to which nurses are held accountable. A **standard** is an authoritative statement that describes the required behaviour of every nurse and is used to evaluate individual performance. The standards of practice usually fall in two or more categories. In addition to professional standards, there are often other types of standards such as those about the legislated scope of practice that stipulates what nurses can and cannot do and more specific practice standards or guidelines about certain topics. The professional standards referred in this chapter apply to all nurses throughout their career regardless of where they work or the different positions they hold. Hence, the professional standards may be considered global in their application.

Practice standards are different from professional standards because practice standards are normally short documents that describe standards for carrying out particular aspects of patient care that are essential to patient's physical and psychological safety. The most common are about medications, documentation of patient care on patient records or charts, and nurse–patient relationships. Some regulatory bodies have many additional practice standards, including ones for confidentiality and the privacy of patient information, patient consent to care, duty to provide care, and duty to report.

All of the standards of practice for nurses are set and kept up-to-date by regulatory bodies. They are revised regularly with input from nurses with different experiences and roles reviewing what needs to be changed based on new developments in practice. All nurses are expected to practice in accordance with whatever standards of practice are set by the province/territory where they are registered and work. If a question arises about whether a nurse is practicing safely, competently, and ethically, the standards of practice are applied to evaluate the facts of the situation. In other words, the regulatory bodies, on behalf of patients and the general public, hold nurse registrants accountable to the established standards of practice.

Many regulatory bodies provide information and guidance to help nurses meet the standards; for example, fact sheets or guidelines for meeting registration requirements. It is important to differentiate these resources from the standards of practice to which nurses are held accountable. For example, see the website for the College of Nurses of Ontario, *Complete Standards and Guidelines* (College of Nurses of Ontario, n.d.). If you are a student nurse outside Ontario, have a look at the website of your regulatory body to become familiar with the standards of practice you need to learn and find the resources that may be provided to help nurses meet them. You will likely find the same resources useful in your nursing course assignments.

You will not learn all of the standards of practice in the first nursing courses. However, you will be expected to learn all of them by the time you graduate. The faculty will decide how to evaluate your performance in relation to the standards of practice in different stages of your learning and in different ways throughout the program.

Where Can I Get the Competencies?

The list of competencies can be found through the website of the regulatory body in the province/territory in which you are studying. The respective council or board for each regulatory body approves the required competencies. National collaborative processes have enhanced the consistency of the entry-level registered competencies in most Canadian provinces/territories (Black et al., 2008). You will find that the participating regulatory bodies organize the competencies in a similar way using categories derived from professional standards of practice. The Ordre des infirmières et des infirmiers du Québec (2009) uses the concept of a mosaic to present the clinical competencies required for initial registration in Quebec.

The competencies publication will have some key statements about nursing education that are usually listed under a heading called "Assumptions." For example, all registered nurses in Canada must have a broad generalist nursing education before they are eligible for registration. Generalist means having the introductory knowledge and beginning skills necessary to practice safely with all age groups and genders of patients in various practice settings; for example, homes, community clinics, hospitals, schools, and residential care facilities. As a generalist, you need to learn to practice safely with patients who are in different states of health and illness. That is why some nursing courses deal with health promotion, prevention, and population health, and you will learn how to care for patients who have acute or chronic illnesses in other courses. You will also need to learn how to provide care for patients who require rehabilitative, palliative, or end-of-life care.

Knowledge-Based Practice

Knowledge-based practice is based on up-to-date knowledge and the latest research findings, not on myth, intuition, or how things have always been done. You need an extensive knowledge base from nursing and other disciplines to know the reasons behind what you are doing, know enough to decide what care patients want or need, and know how to talk therapeutically with patients while giving patient care. The nature, breadth, and depth of knowledge needed to practice safely are extensive. They include nursing knowledge and specialized knowledge about health and illness, the pathophysiology of diseases, pharmacology, microbiology, health promotion, health-care systems, and global health issues. Knowledge from the health sciences and the humanities is combined with nursing knowledge about how to care for patients. In addition, it does not end with knowing about individual patients. You need knowledge about how individuals interact in families, groups, and entire communities. Some of this knowledge is found in non-nursing courses taught by other disciplines; for example, sociology, psychology, and philosophy. The competencies are usually under a specialized body of knowledge section of knowledge-based practice. It will be interesting for you to compare the competencies with what you learn in the courses you are or will be taking. Notice what references are made to the competencies published by the regulatory body where you are studying. Different courses will help you gain the knowledge base you need to provide safe patient care. Often, certain competencies are introduced in the first nursing courses and built upon as you learn more in each nursing course until the end of your program.

Through the eyes of a student

I can't believe I have to take so many courses that are not nursing courses. I thought I would be able to care for patients right away. Working with patients is what I really want to learn about. The courses in human anatomy, physiology, pathophysiology, psychology, sociology, and English are tough. I don't have time for anything else. The nursing courses start with general topics, laboratory skills, and observation. We don't get to see patients for any length of time until later in the program. This doesn't make sense to me.

(personal reflection of Gordon, a first-year nursing student)

Through the eyes of a student

*N*ow that I am in the last year of the program, I can see how much I combine knowledge from other disciplines with nursing knowledge to care for patients. At first, I was sceptical about how useful the non-nursing courses would be. I really did not know the value of this knowledge until I used it in clinical, and one has to gain knowledge before using it, so I now see why the program was front-end loaded with non-nursing courses. I also did not know how to write papers well. The English course helped, and I also got help from the writing centre. Now, I do pretty well in my papers.

(personal reflection of Linda, a fourth-year nursing student)

Through the eyes of a nurse

I am always impressed by the breadth of knowledge the nursing students and new graduates have. They know how to look up everything and get the latest information. They bring a lot of good ideas and make us all think about how to provide the best patient care. This is a big positive for us. . . . The caveat is that students need to be careful to recognize the knowledge staff have from different sources, especially from many years of working with patients.

(personal reflection of Peggy, a nurse)

Using Your Knowledge to Care for Patients

Regulatory bodies require that you apply specialized knowledge from nursing and other disciplines during experiences where you learn to practice nursing directly with patients. You will begin to apply knowledge in nursing laboratories with simulated patients and other learning techniques in preparation for interacting directly with patients in hospitals and other settings. The regulatory body looks at the kind and length of the clinical experiences in the program when it is reviewed. The review looks for evidence that these learning opportunities are sufficient to achieve the required competencies. The competencies about using knowledge are commonly stated in a category called *competent application of knowledge*. Typically, this category has the highest number of competencies in the publication of the regulatory body because this is the crux of providing safe patient care. The other categories of competencies address professional responsibility and accountability, ethical practice, service to the public, and self-regulation, consistent with the characteristics of a profession. The competencies are specific to what you need to learn before entering the profession and could be considered the clinical practice indicators for the professional standards of practice. In Saskatchewan, the entry-level competencies are considered foundational and are presented in combination with the professional standards (Saskatchewan Registered Nurses Association, 2013). Later chapters cover topics relevant to the professional standards of practice; for example, ethics and lifelong learning.

Skills and Abilities to Achieve the Competencies

Nursing students need certain basic skills and abilities to meet the entry-level competencies required for registration. Some regulatory bodies have published these as a guide to the kinds of activities nursing students need to perform and the general demands of registered nurse education. The original publications were by the College of Registered Nurses of British Columbia (CRNBC, 2007a) and the College of Registered Nurses of Nova Scotia (2009a) and later adapted by other regulatory bodies. The skills and abilities fall into seven categories, as listed in Box 4.4.

BOX 4.4   Requisite Skills and Abilities to Attain Entry-Level Competencies

The following seven categories of requisite skills and abilities were developed by the College of Registered Nurses of British Columbia (CRNBC) and adopted by the College of Registered Nurses of Nova Scotia:

1. **Cognitive**
   * Remember information over a brief period of time.
   * Remember information from past experiences.
   * Problem-solve to develop professional judgment.
   * Reason to develop professional judgment.
   * Exercise critical inquiry skills to develop professional judgment.
   * Apply mathematical skills and abilities in order to:
     * add, subtract, multiply and divide
     * calculate ratios, percentages and apply algebraic equations.

   Examples: The student can make sense of complex knowledge; use knowledge and theory appropriately; use past experience to inform current decision making.

2. **Behavioural**
   * Manage own behaviour well enough to provide safe, competent and ethical patient care.
   * Engage with self and others to create a safe environment.
   * Respond appropriately in situations that are stressful or that involve conflict.
   * React appropriately to giving and receiving physical touch and working in close proximity with a full range of clients.
   * Fulfill responsibility as part of a team.
   * Manage time appropriately.

   Examples: The student remains calm in stressful situations; recognizes client priorities; and responds appropriately in conflict situations.

3. **Communication**
   * Speak and understand spoken English well enough to avoid mixing up words and meanings: includes the ability to understand complex medical and technical knowledge.
   * Write and understand written English well enough to avoid mixing up words and meanings.
   * Recognize own non-verbal signals and interpret those received from others while considering individual differences in expression and associated meaning.

   Examples: The student recognizes her/his own non-verbal behaviour; demonstrates awareness that each individual's behaviour has different meanings; listens appropriately to clients.

4. **Interpersonal**
   * Develop professional relationships and rapport with individuals and groups for the purpose of education, support and counselling.
   * Recognize the needs of clients and colleagues.
   * Recognize the importance of maintaining interpersonal boundaries.

   Examples: The student recognizes the importance of maintaining interpersonal boundaries with clients; supports clients to make healthy choices; recognizes the importance of client perspectives and feelings.

5. **Physical**
   Ability to perform each of the following requisites well enough to provide client care and participate in educational activities:
   * Stand and maintain balance.
   * Manual dexterity
   * Move within limited spaces.
   * Push and pull.
   * Perform repetitive movements.
   * Perform complex sequences of hand eye coordination.
   * Bend
   * Reach
   * Lift
   * Walk
   * Climb
   * Carry objects.

   Examples: The student can carry a case weighing 8 kg up a flight of stairs; give intramuscular injections; remove wound sutures.

6. **Sensory Perceptual**
   Ability to perceive with each of the following senses well enough to provide care and participate in educational activities:
   * Sight
   * Hearing
   * Touch

   Examples: The student can accurately assess blood pressure and pulse; read the small print on medication packages and bottles; and assess client colour.

7. **Environmental**
   Ability to function in the presence of each of the following commonly encountered and unavoidable environmental factors:
   * Noxious smells
   * Disease agents
   * Distractions
   * Noise
   * Chemicals
   * Unpredictable behaviour in others

   Examples: The student can recognize dangers in the client environment; tolerate disposing of body waste; and tolerate unpleasant odours.

Source: College of Registered Nurses of British Columbia. (2007). *Becoming a registered nurse in British Columbia: Requisite skills and abilities.* Retrieved from http://www.crnbc.ca/downloads/464.pdf; College of Registered Nurses of Nova Scotia. (2009). *Becoming a registered nurse in Nova Scotia: Requisite skills and abilities.* Retrieved from http://www.nursing.dal.ca/Files/CRNNSfinal.pdf

This information may be useful to those deciding whether a nursing career is a good fit with their aspirations and capabilities. As you progress in your nursing education program, the requisite skills and abilities may be useful if you need to discuss with faculty and others any particular learning supports or accommodation you may need to achieve the competencies. If you have any concerns about your capabilities at any time during your studies, take the initiative to disclose this to faculty or a student services support person, for example, student counsellor or disabilities service provider, within the educational institution. You will be required to provide evidence of your needs and negotiate in good faith to arrive at a reasonable plan that allows you to achieve the competencies and standards of practice. Although the legislation governing human rights issues related to student accommodation varies somewhat by province/territory, the principles and requirements in the landmark document published by the Alberta Human Rights Commission (2010) generally apply.

How Regulatory Bodies Review Nursing Education Programs

Although the review processes vary by province/territory, there are commonalities in most regulatory bodies. These commonalities include the requirement to undergo a review process on a regular basis; for example, at least once every 4 to 7 years. Reviews may be more frequent for the startup of new programs, for those making substantial changes, and for programs that need to make certain improvements. Each regulatory body has nursing education standards used to evaluate programs. The review process is a systematic evaluation to determine whether the provincial/territorial regulatory body will approve or recognize the nursing education program. This is done to establish the eligibility of program graduates to proceed in the registration process. Programs that are not approved by the regulatory body cannot assume that the graduates will be eligible for registration. Those nursing education programs approved or recognized by a regulatory body may be listed on the website of the regulatory body.

Some regulatory bodies use all or parts of the accreditation process conducted by the Canadian Association of Schools of Nursing (CASN, 2011) using its nursing education standards. Accreditation itself is a voluntary rather than a mandatory process. Exceptions to this exist where the legislation allows the regulatory organization to designate another body to approve programs (College of Nurses of Ontario [CNO]) or where regulatory bodies have established contractual agreements with CASN to conduct approval processes jointly (College of Registered Nurses of Nova Scotia and Association of Registered Nurses of Newfoundland and Labrador). The list of approved/recognized programs by each jurisdiction is the most important one in relation to your eligibility to become registered after graduation. The review process typically begins with the submission of a self-evaluation report by the nursing education program. The self-evaluation report provides evidence about the ways the nursing education standards are addressed. Evidence is submitted that a student will have learned and practiced in accordance with the required competencies and standards of practice. A committee of experts reviews the evidence, and two or three external reviewers visit the program (also called *site visitors*). The external reviewers are nurses with extensive experience in baccalaureate nursing education and/or with new graduates working in health-care facilities. For 2 or more days, the reviewers are present at the location(s) where the nursing education program is offered to verify and elaborate on evidence in the self-evaluation report. Among other things, the reviewers may talk with students in all years of the program, faculty, administrators, committees, nurses who work with students or graduates in health-care facilities, and graduates of the program. For example, see the *Nursing Education Program Approval Process* of the Saskatchewan Registered Nurses Association (2009b).

Broad statements about the purpose of program reviews usually include "for the purposes of registration" related to registration requirements. This means that graduates of nursing education programs approved or recognized by a regulatory body are eligible to proceed in the registration process. Once you are registered, you are able to practice legally and use the protected title, *registered nurse*. The administrative head of your nursing program, for example, the dean, director, chair, or department head, conveys to the regulatory body the names of graduates who have successfully completed the program. After you complete an application form, one of the first steps is to write and pass regulatory examinations. Toward the end of your program, you will naturally be more concerned about what regulatory examination you need to successfully complete. The regulatory bodies have information and exam preparation resources materials available online.

Interacting in a Responsible and Accountable Way

You interact with others all the time and have been doing so since birth. So what is the big deal about interacting as a professional nurse? The reasons include privileged professional relationships, patient rights, informed consent, and confidentiality issues. All of these reasons result in the need for nurses as professionals to act responsibly in accordance with standards of practice set by regulatory bodies to which nurses are held to account. **Accountability** is the obligation to answer for the professional, ethical, and legal responsibilities of one's activities and duties. Professional responsibility and accountability are so important that they usually form the overarching professional standards used by regulatory bodies and nurses in their practice. The entry-level competencies are those that students need to attain to meet the expectations about professional responsibility and accountability. Other chapters in this text are devoted to related topics because they pervade nursing practice and merit extensive discussion.

Be Taken Seriously

...urse, during all of your experiences with ...you have access to private, confidential informa-...on. You are privileged to know patients and provide care in very personal and emotionally sensitive situations. Because of this, you have a special professional relationship with patients and are expected to communicate according to established standards for nurse–patient relationships. The public trusts nurses will act responsibly and be accountable in all their interactions. That is why patients will disclose and discuss such personal experiences and feelings with you.

As a professional, you are held to a higher standard than you are in everyday social situations. These standards uphold the public trust that nurses:

1. Ensure the privacy and confidentiality of all patient information.
2. Answer for all of their actions when providing care.
3. Practice in the best interests of the public to provide patient care and protect the public from harm in all interactions.

Crossing the Line

When does the relationship you have with your patient cross the line from professional to nonprofessional or from a therapeutic to a social one? What are the consequences for the patient and for you when you cross over boundaries? These are questions that the nursing regulatory bodies address to develop practice standards and interpretative documents about appropriate nurse–patient relationships. Take a moment to reflect on the ways in which you automatically interact in social situations and what the norms are for your social relationships. For example, you may use blogs, cell phones, and Twitter to share what you did during the day, with most of the information centered on your own experiences, feelings, and needs.

You now need to learn about relating in a different way to establish, maintain, and terminate a professional, therapeutic relationship with patients. This aspect of safe nursing practice is so important that regulatory bodies often develop stand-alone documents about the requirements for a therapeutic relationship, including their boundaries and the consequences of their violation. Recent examples are the 2011 publications of the College and Association of Registered Nurses of Alberta (2011a) and the Nurses Association of New Brunswick (2011b). Your competence in developing therapeutic relationships with appropriate boundaries is so essential that related theory and practice are usually integrated or woven together with other topics, student assignments in different courses, and evaluations of your interactions with patients.

The Patient's Right to Know

Introducing yourself by your name and professional designation is a first step toward practicing in a responsible and accountable manner. It also initiates the development of a therapeutic relationship and begins to establish the boundaries for your relationship with patients. Patients have the right to know who is providing their care. This may seem simple, yet often, patients do not know the names or roles of their care providers. Sometimes, this is because of the number of different people involved. You may be surprised that patients also may not know because of the way people introduce themselves. You will have considerable practice in introducing yourself to patients and others to meet the entry-level competencies required by regulatory bodies. You are responsible for ensuring patients know who you are and what you will be doing. You are then also holding yourself accountable because patients can identify you and ask questions or express any concerns they may have about your care. Patients and the public have the right to complain about their care; if they do not know your name and role, patients are hampered in acting on this right.

Through the eyes of a patient

*T*he name of the student nurse here today is about the only one I know. The instructor was here too and made sure I did not mind having a student. I know how to get the instructor when I want to. I suppose everyone learns to let patients know who they are and not keep them in the dark. That sure is not what happens here most of the time. There are so many people around, and they all do different things. I cannot keep track of them all. . . . They are just faces coming and going. The nurses who stand out for me make sure I know who they are.

(personal reflection of Bruce, a patient)

Beyond Introductions to Informed Consent

Nurses have ethical and legal responsibilities to ensure patients give their consent to accept care based on their full understanding of what is being done. There are several kinds of informed consent; the most common one you will see is consent for care or treatment. Normally, patient consent for treatment including surgery is carried out by the most appropriate health professional. Health-care facilities and regulatory bodies often have guidelines or practice standards related to consent that must be followed; for example, the Nurses Association of New Brunswick (2011a). The same applies in cases of the patient's right to refuse treatment and to participate or not in a research study. Patients must also consent to the release of any of their health information, which is strictly confidential and private.

Jas wondered if his nursing education program had policies or professional conduct requirements for students practicing with patients. He found the policies on the school website and also in a nursing student handbook. There were a lot of guidelines and requirements about how students should introduce themselves, how they sign their name, and what title to use. Jas also found policies about the responsibilities of students in patient consent. Jas decided he would need to use this reference often. There are some things students cannot do and other things students have to do in certain ways. Jas concluded that the responsible and accountable thing to do is to learn these policies and those established by the nursing education program and act accordingly. He was able to see how the policies considered legal implications and standards of practice.

Confidentiality and Privacy of Information

You will have the privilege to access and the significant responsibility to safeguard confidential and private information about patients. Patients are the owners of any information about them, and you will be held to account for any breaches of confidentiality or inappropriate disclosure of their information. There are legal requirements and ethical obligations to uphold (CNA, 2011; Canadian Nurses Protective Society, 2008). Regulatory bodies may set out the requirements in standards that address specific provincial/territorial legislation (College and Association of Registered Nurses of Alberta, 2011b).

In the past, when written patient records and documents were the only ones readily available, the protection of patient information seemed easier. Now, with the use of quickly and widely distributed electronic information, it is very easy to make serious errors of judgment that may have legal consequences. That is why you need to stop and think twice if you tend to automatically share your experiences with your classmates, friends, and others. Patient information is shared only on a need-to-know basis; that is, by those health-care providers who need the information to plan, provide, and evaluate patient care. The privacy of health information is a national and international concern of nurses. For more information, read *Health Information: Protecting Patient Rights*; visit the website of the ICN (2008).

Text messaging and social networking websites, for example, Facebook, Twitter, YouTube, and others, present you with a host of ways to breach confidentiality and privacy of patient information without intending to do so. To avoid getting yourself into a serious situation, it is essential that you think through the appropriateness of your actions. Writing a simple e-mail to a friend about your patient is not acceptable; neither is talking about your patients outside the nursing and formal learning situation. Taking a photograph of a patient and sharing it without informed consent are inappropriate. If you use electronic social networks, ask yourself if you are presenting appropriate information. Is the information strictly your own personal information? Seriously consider the risks of making the information public and the possible consequences (Canadian Nurses Protective Society, 2010). The National Council of State Boards of Nursing (2012) publication includes scenarios where student and practicing nurses have become involved in disciplinary procedures for violations committed through inappropriate use of social media. In some cases, students have been expelled from nursing education programs.

If you are representing yourself as a professional in any way, you have the responsibility to ensure that your use of information is professional. Ask yourself if anyone else might possibly perceive your comments as derogatory of the profession or revealing a negative aspect of your own personal behaviour or views that might leave you open to allegations of professional misconduct. You will be held accountable for your actions, so it is a good idea to think about it and make sure you are acting appropriately. When in doubt, ask your nursing faculty. Before you graduate, you will be learning much more about this issue and how to present yourself as a professional.

Jas reflects on what he has been learning about confidentiality, privacy, and protecting patient information. Some of the students in his class have discussed setting up a blog to debrief their clinical experiences. He joins in the discussion and suggests that a standard on patient confidentiality from their regulatory body's website might provide more direction on whether this is appropriate. Another student finds information on patient confidentiality in their nursing program's student handbook. After much discussion, the students identified several concerns and decided that a blog could potentially violate patient confidentiality with possible legal consequences.

Professional Presence

What is the difference between being there in person and a professional presence? One of the common entry-level competencies you need to attain is to demonstrate a professional presence and model professional behaviour. **Professional presence** means acting with confidence, integrity, optimism, passion, and empathy in accordance with professional standards, guidelines, and codes of ethics. It includes reflective practice, verbal and nonverbal communications, and the ability to articulate a positive role and professional image (Association of Registered Nurses of Newfoundland and Labrador, 2013; College of Registered Nurses of Nova Scotia, 2013; Nurses Association of New Brunswick, 2013b). When you introduce yourself by name and professional designation or protected title, you contribute to a professional presence. Not only do you need to explain your role and responsibilities to patients, but you also need to do so with all others involved in providing patient care. You may even be able to be a leader in how you approach this.

Leadership Comes in All Sizes

You may ask how you can be a leader when you are still learning what to do and how to do things well. Leadership is not limited to formal or high-level roles. Leadership includes many attributes that you can demonstrate in significant, although seemingly small ways. These attributes, as stated in entry-level competencies, include self-awareness, commitment to individual growth, ethical values and beliefs, presence, reflection and foresight, advocacy, integrity, intellectual energy, being involved, being open to new ideas, having confidence in one's own capabilities, and a willingness to make an effort to guide and motivate others (Association of Registered Nurses of Newfoundland and Labrador, 2013; College of Registered Nurses of Nova Scotia, 2013; Nurses Association of New Brunswick, 2013b).

You may be surprised at how many learning opportunities you will have to develop leadership attributes while providing patient care and interacting with others. Situations will arise when you can display leadership by taking the initiative to meet patient needs and preferences for care, especially when this goes beyond taken-for-granted practices and usual routines. Many students demonstrate leadership by bringing new and emerging knowledge to patient care situations that may lead to quality improvement. In your early years as a student, you will need to discuss your assessments and plans first with nursing faculty to make sure they are well-reasoned, timely, framed in a respectful manner, and therefore likely to have positive results. As you near graduation, you will have opportunities to practice more complex leadership skills and use basic conflict resolution skills to transform situations of conflict into healthier interpersonal interactions.

Being: How to Be a Professional

As a nursing student, you are on your way to becoming a registered nurse, in the transition from student to professional. During your time in your education program, you will be learning about the expectations of a professional and provided with opportunities to understand these expectations. For example, as a student, you are still expected to meet the professional standards for practice. But you meet these standards as a student, which has a different, but no less important, level of expectation.

As you make the transition from student role to professional role, you will be provided with guidance by nursing faculty members and other registered nurses on how to approach professional issues such as the duty to report, the duty to provide care, and professional conduct.

Duty to Provide Care: Risk and Patient Care

Is there ever a time when you can refuse to give care? Yes, under certain conditions. To provide care for which you are not competent, educated, and authorized to perform is considered unsafe practice. The first condition depends on your self-assessed competence to provide the patient care required. Ask yourself if you have studied the theory and practiced the skill in a laboratory. Find out how the patient care required fits with the policies of your nursing education program regarding whether you can perform certain care

without nursing faculty being with you. Whenever in doubt, ask the nursing faculty responsible for the course.

Nurses have a legal and ethical duty to provide safe, ethical, and competent care. We call this a **duty to provide care**. Once a nurse has initiated patient care, that is, agreed to provide care to a patient or patients, he or she enters into another obligation, a duty to provide care. However, there may be situations where a nurse will have to withdraw or refuse care. Because of the nature of nursing practice, nurses accept that a certain amount of risk is inherent in provision of patient care. However, nurses are not expected to place themselves or remain in situations of unnecessary risk. In recent years, a great deal of the discussion about the nurse's duty to provide care has focused on pandemic planning. The College of Registered Nurses of Nova Scotia (2009b) has adapted an ethical values and decision-making framework for disaster and/or emergency. This framework applies concepts such as duty to provide care, protection of the public from harm, risk, and equity to assist nurses to make appropriate decisions regarding their duty to provide care during an emergency situation such as a pandemic.

In addition to pandemic or emergency situations, there are other situations where the nurse may have to consider withdrawing or refusing to provide care. In all cases, the nurse never abandons the patient(s) and is always expected to follow a process to communicate concerns to the appropriate authority such as the employer and ensure that the patient's care and safety is not compromised. The CRNBC (2012) lists four broad categories which may influence your duty to provide care: unreasonable burden, personal danger, individual competence, and conscientious objection. These are described in Box 4.5. Do you think expectations

BOX 4.5   Categories of Situations That May Influence Your Duty to Provide Care

1. Unreasonable burden—An unreasonable burden exists when your ability to provide safe care and meet standards of practice is compromised by unreasonable expectations, lack of resources, or ongoing threats to personal well-being.

2. Personal danger—While you are not entitled to abandon your clients, you are not obligated to place yourself in situations where care delivery would entail unreasonable danger to your personal safety. This includes situations involving violence, communicable diseases, and physical or sexual abuse.

3. Individual competence—You are expected to practice competently and to continually acquire new knowledge and skills in your areas of practice. You are not obligated, however, to provide care beyond your level of competence.

4. Conscientious objection—When a specific type of care conflicts with your moral or religious beliefs, you may arrange with your employer to refrain from providing the care. Personal biases or judgments against the client or the client's lifestyle, however, are not grounds for conscientious objection.

Source: College of Registered Nurses of British Columbia. (2012). *Duty to provide care*. Vancouver, BC: Author. Retrieved from http://www.crnbc.ca/downloads/398.pdf

are different for you in the student role versus the professional role?

Through the eyes of a nurse

I have been working a lot lately and am suffering from fatigue. Before I left work, they asked me to work an extra shift. I refused, although I worry about the patients who need care because I don't know if another registered nurse is available and able to work. I often wonder if I have done the right thing when I say no to overtime and whether I am fulfilling my professional obligations to provide care.

I know, though, that meeting my standards means that I have to look after myself to make sure I practice safely and do not make mistakes because I am fatigued. That means sometimes saying no to working extra. One of the things I have done is talk with the charge nurse about the impact of overtime on my well-being. I also brought in a resource from my regulatory body on working short-staffed so that my colleagues and I can try to sort out what other things we could do to minimize pressure to work overtime.

(personal reflection of Martin, a nurse)

The Duty to Report

Nurses, along with other health professionals, have long had an ethical **duty to report** unsafe, incompetent, or unethical practice. This means that nurses who observe practices by nurses or other health professionals that place patients at risk have an obligation to report significant concerns about an individual professional to their regulatory body. Although this has been an ethical duty, in recent years, many provinces/territories have made this a legal duty set out in legislation. This means that nurses (and other health professionals) have an obligation to report misconduct or incompetent behaviour. In fact, failure to report may place you in a position of professional misconduct. Why have governments placed this legal duty alongside the ethical duty for health professionals? In part, it is the continued evolution of regulation and self-regulation. We identify where we can improve our accountability to the public and implement mechanisms for maintaining their trust. The duty to report is one such mechanism.

Although we expect professionals to meet the duty to report, what is your obligation as a student in reporting misconduct or incompetent behaviour? One of the competencies expected of entry-level registered nurses is the reporting of "unsafe practice within the context of professional self-regulation" (Association of Registered Nurses of Newfoundland and Labrador, 2013; College of Registered Nurses of Nova Scotia, 2013; Nurses Association of New Brunswick, 2013b). One of the first steps you might take if you are concerned about someone's practice is to discuss this concern with a nursing faculty member. They should be able to help you understand the policies and processes for students who observe a practice issue, including whether to raise

the issue with the individual or the employer or to discuss it with the regulatory body. Not all situations or concerns will require that you report directly to the regulatory body. Part of the learning process is being able to reflect on concerns, discuss them with others, and begin to understand what issues require reporting to a higher authority. However, if you have concerns that are not addressed to your satisfaction, you may call your provincial/territorial nursing regulatory body for further advice. Because you are not yet a regulated member, you may choose to raise concerns as a member of the public. Most regulatory bodies have someone who deals with the public, and this information is posted on their websites.

Professional Conduct Review

Many educational institutions have a student code of conduct that sets out rules, obligations, and expectations for students in academic programs and may also address behavioural expectations in terms of civility, respect, and responsibilities as a student in a community of learning. Further, many nursing education programs have developed codes of conduct that detail specific expectations for nursing students. In many cases, these codes of conduct are a precursor to what will be expected of you as a professional nurse and often align with professional standards and codes of ethics.

Regulatory bodies working for the public interest typically want foremost to promote quality nursing practice and prevent poor practice. In a minority of cases, unsafe and unacceptable practice occurs, and disciplinary action is necessary to protect the public from harm. For this reason, regulatory bodies have the legal authority to intervene in cases of unsafe or unacceptable practice.

The commonly used processes for intervening are through receiving and investigating complaints, professional conduct review, and discipline. On the websites of regulatory bodies, you will note information about how the public, employers, other nurses, or health professionals may make a report about the practice of a nurse. Following due consideration of a report to determine if there is a reason to investigate further, most regulatory bodies proceed with a professional conduct review process (Yukon Registered Nurses Association, 2006). During this process, the nurse whose practice was deemed unsafe or unacceptable may have the opportunity to take part in developing the remedy to address the practice issues and the conditions for improvement. Various individualized remedies or disciplinary actions may be taken. Discipline by the regulatory body may range from requiring an individual to take additional education to suspension of registration to practice until there is evidence that certain improvements have been made, and in the most serious offenses, to complete rescinding of registration to practice.

Fit for Nursing Practice

One of the requirements to enter the profession of nursing is that you are fit to engage in the practice of nursing. What does being fit to practice mean? Although each regulatory body may define fitness to practice somewhat differently, there are a lot of commonalities. Here, we use **fitness to practice** to mean all the qualities and capabilities of an individual relevant to his or her capability to practice as a nurse, including freedom from any cognitive, physical, psychological, or emotional condition or a dependence on alcohol or drugs, that impair his or her ability to practice nursing (Association of Registered Nurses of Newfoundland and Labrador, 2008; College of Registered Nurses of Nova Scotia, 2013; Nurses Association of New Brunswick, 2013b). The CNA Code of Ethics (2008) addresses how nurses maintain their fitness to practice and actions to take when they become aware that they are not fit to practice.

The standards of practice set by regulatory bodies and the codes of ethics establish the expectation that it is the individual nurse's responsibility for maintaining fitness to practice. This is one of the essentials you need to learn about and practice in your self-assessments, reflections on your practice, and development of effective learning plans. All of these learning activities are aimed at helping you learn to self-regulate in order to consistently provide safe, competent, and ethical patient care.

Learning about and maintaining your fitness to practice begins early in your nursing studies. There are many conditions that might impair your fitness to practice. They may be short term, for example, acute illness or injury due to an accident; or they may be long term, for example, chronic illnesses or various sustained demands on your psychological and emotional health. A cognitive condition impacts a nurse's ability to think things through and make safe, evidence-informed, clinical decisions and give sound reasons for his or her actions. Impaired thinking or cognitive ability could result from a head injury following sports or vehicle accidents, prolonged sleep deprivation, side effects of medications/drugs, or severe emotional stress. A physical condition may prevent a nurse from providing certain kinds of care with patients, especially care that requires fine muscle movements, walking, lifting, and so on. Problematic substance use is a situation in which the use of a substance, for example, drugs of any kind, alcohol, or over-the-counter products, negatively impacts a nurse's ability to practice in a safe, competent, and ethical manner (College of Registered Nurses of Nova Scotia, 2008).

As a student, you have the right to request help and support or accommodation to overcome and work around any impairments you may have or develop during your studies. The supports would be designed to enable you to achieve the entry-level competencies and standards of practice. You also have a responsibility to seek out the help and support that you need to be successful. These responsibilities include disclosing the strengths and limitations you have, providing information from a medical or other expert about your capabilities, and engaging in good faith efforts to negotiate reasonable arrangements with the nursing education program so you can be successful. The same general principles apply when you need to request accommodation in an employment situation, although there will be differences in the demands or occupational requirements of your employment position than the role of a student learning to become a nurse.

Your nursing education program will have policies and procedures to follow related to your fitness to practice; for example, what you should do if you are ill and cannot attend class or clinical. Normally, policies address the responsibilities of students to be prepared to practice safely. When you practice nursing with patients in nursing courses, you will be required to prepare with the knowledge base and planning needed to provide safe, competent, and ethical care. If you are not prepared for clinical assignments or are not performing at the level expected in the course, policies usually allow for faculty or nurses in the practice setting to require that you leave. Should this happen, students may be able to improve their performance sufficiently through a learning plan or contract developed with nursing faculty. Otherwise, failure in a course and possibly in the program may result. Regulatory bodies look for such policies during nursing education program reviews and want to see evidence that policies support nursing faculty to fail students for safety reasons in the best interests of public protection. From the perspective of regulatory bodies, these kinds of policies and administrative supports for nursing faculty are necessary to ensure students who graduate and apply for registration are prepared to practice safely, competently, and ethically. This is another means by which the regulatory body meets its mandate to regulate in the public interest.

Through the eyes of a student

I feel overwhelmed, getting to all my classes and the labs. The nursing language is so different and soon we start clinical. I'm not feeling well, but I am really afraid that if I stay home, I will miss so much. On the other hand, if I go, how much will I retain, and what if I pass this bug to someone else? I don't know what to do about how I am feeling or who I can speak to.
(personal reflection of Caroline, a nursing student)

Students often feel overwhelmed by all the responsibilities of being a student. It is very hard work and stressful. The first step a student can take when experiencing these feelings is to talk with a faculty person in the program who has responsibility for students. They might have the title *student advisor* or *academic advisor*. If you are not sure, ask someone in your program who fills this role. Student advisors can help you identify the source of your stress and work with you to identify appropriate strategies to deal with the tensions.

Significance of Fitness to Practice

The demands in the profession of nursing require that nurses have the capacity to monitor and maintain their fitness to practice. "Nursing is a stressful profession. Caring for clients—individuals, families, groups, populations or entire communities—with multiple, complex and distressing problems can be overwhelming for even the most experienced practitioner" (CRNBC, 2008, p. 4). In response to the stressors that often impact negatively on fitness to practice, the regulatory bodies often develop resources to help nurses meet fitness to practice requirements. These resources may apply equally as well to your role as a student nurse. Some of the stressors that nurses encounter in their work include lack of staff, equipment, and resources, together with multiple demands and needs of patients. In addition, nurses do all this in a time of uncertainty, with many health system challenges and limited resources. This is sometimes referred to as *workplace adversity*, which is any negative, stressful, traumatic, or difficult situation or episode of hardship encountered in the occupational setting (Jackson, Firtko, & Edenborough, 2007). How an individual responds to these stressful situations can have an effect on his or her physical, emotional, psychological, and spiritual well-being and ultimately can affect his or her fitness to practice. Regulatory bodies offer supports for nurses in practice including resources or consultation with individual nurses to discuss issues and identify strategies to effectively manage stressors. For a specific example, the website for the Association of Registered Nurses of Prince Edward Island provides guidance on working extra hours, fitness to practice, and duty to provide care.

You must also keep in mind that situations arise when someone's fitness to practice requires you to report that individual to his or her regulatory body. This is a case where your duty to report unsafe practice is a requirement. See Box 4.6 for tips from faculty and students for maintaining fitness to practice.

BOX 4.6 Tips From Faculty and Students for Maintaining Fitness to Practice

If you make a mistake in clinical, own up to it right away.

Find a good mentor. If your school does not have this already, initiate the creation of a social club within your nursing program that facilitates learning from each other, from all levels and experience within the program.

Always think critically about everything, and always ask questions!

If you are struggling with a course/concept, ask for help right away. Don't wait until the last second before an exam or competency test.

When you have an issue or concern regarding the program, peers or instructors, talk to someone right away. Don't wait until the end of the semester.

It is strongly encouraged that you inform your classroom instructor when you are off ill. It is imperative to call your clinical instructor and the unit you are working on that you will be off ill. Moreover, it is best to support your call with an email to your instructor.

Source: Personal communication with Nursing Students and Faculty at Langara College, School of Nursing, Vancouver, BC.

Through the eyes of a nurse

I know that maintaining my own physical well-being contributes to my fitness to practice. I spoke to these new graduate registered nurses who offered the following advice for students.

Pamela says, "Walk everywhere! If you drive to school, park a few blocks away and walk. Take the stairs, not the elevator. Drink water. Get a good night's sleep, especially before clinical days. Try to maintain pre-nursing school regular activities like going to the gym, hiking, swimming, playing sports, etc. Exercise your soul, too; every once in a while, indulge yourself, but be careful in what you choose."

Kevin advised that another crucial way to maintain your fitness is to "eat right! Avoid the food that is bad for your body and consume more smart food, which can actually help you with your energy level and improve your memory."
(personal reflection of Cathy, a nurse)

Understanding the Requirements for Individual Self-Regulation

One of the essential things to learn before graduation is how to become self-regulating in your everyday work as an individual nurse. Earlier in this chapter, we discussed the authority given to an organization to set rules and principles for oversight of the profession in the public interest. We defined this as self-regulation. Self-regulation also refers to how you, as an individual, regulate your practice. Regulatory bodies establish the entry-level competencies about individual self-regulation that you need to achieve by the time you graduate. Because of their importance to safe practice and public protection, you will likely find these competencies listed by themselves in a category about self-regulation. Additionally, the professional standards of practice have a category about self-regulation to address requirements for self-assessment, fitness to practice, and meeting quality assurance requirements throughout your nursing career.

Individual self-regulation starts with you as a student by understanding yourself, your capabilities, and your learning needs. The main foundations of individual self-regulation you need to practice as a student are self-assessment and reflective practice; developing and evaluating your own learning plans; understanding and maintaining your fitness to practice, as discussed already; and ongoing learning to maintain and enhance your competence.

Why Is There So Much Emphasis on Self-Assessment?

The quick answer is that self-assessment of one's own competence is a cornerstone of safe practice and lies at the heart of self-regulation by individuals. Self-assessment may be called *self-evaluation* in your assignments and other evaluations in nursing courses. A student self-assessment is a part of the evaluation in courses where ability to provide direct patient care is evaluated. We use the term *self-assessment* here because this is typically the language used by regulatory bodies in the entry-level competencies and in the expectations of the quality assurance and continuing competence program in the province/territory where you will seek registration after graduation.

The ability to self-assess and fully understand your level of competence will develop over time through many learning activities, assignments, and evaluation methods throughout the program. Accurate self-assessment of your competence is essential to your ability to practice safely within the boundaries of your own competence as well as the legislated scope of nursing practice.

Reflecting on your practice goes hand in hand with self-assessment of your competence because self-reflection enables you to look back at your performance and feelings to identify what you did well and what you can improve as well as what things you need to learn about, practice, and plan to do next. Nursing students learn to reflect on their practice through assignments and during group discussions or seminars. Self-reflective writing about your experiences and what you have learned from them, often called *journal writing*, is a common assignment in nursing programs. Such assignments help you learn the competencies required for individual self-regulation. Your reflections add to the self-assessment of your competencies, that is, knowledge, skills, attitudes, and judgments, and form the basis of developing a learning plan, a usual requirement in clinical practice courses. You will read more on reflection in a later chapter of this book.

Learning Plans

The use of learning plans, developed by students working together with faculty and others, helps you learn one of the typical quality assurance/continuing competence requirements for nurses. You take your self-assessment to an action step when you develop a learning plan. Nursing programs usually provide students with information about what is needed in learning plans for specific courses and how students are expected to use their learning plans. Look at your course materials and student handbook to see if learning plans and learning contracts are mentioned. Note what the requirements are and what language is used. Part of a learning plan is to evaluate its effectiveness in order to develop future learning plans that enable you to maintain and advance your ability to consistently provide safe, competent, and ethical care with patients. Sometimes, learning contracts are used as well to ensure you are achieving the entry-level competencies and standards of practice. It will be important for you to find out what the main difference is between a learning plan and a learning contract or equivalent if different language is used.

Quality Assurance or Continuing Competence Requirements

Today, nothing stands still, especially the knowledge and skills required to practice nursing safely, competently, and ethically. This is why government legislation typically requires that regulatory bodies have a quality assurance and/or continuing competence program to ensure the continued competence of nurses to provide safe care.

Quality assurance and continuing competence are the broad terms for programs developed by regulatory bodies to help nurses maintain and improve their competence from year to year (College of Nurses of Ontario, 2009c). Although there are variations by province/territory, the commonalities of these programs include self-assessments; reflections on practice; using peer feedback; and developing, implementing, and evaluating personal learning plans. A requirement for practice hours is also common, which means a nurse must actively practice or work as a nurse for a certain amount of time over several years to be eligible to renew registration. When a nurse takes time off or chooses to discontinue a nursing career for several years (usually five or more), there is a requirement to obtain additional education to become qualified for registration again.

Many regulatory bodies develop assessment tools, checklists, and other resources to help nurses meet continuing competence requirements. For example, the CRNBC has an online tutorial that provides an overview of its continuing competence program and how to meet the requirements.

Continuing Competency

When you become a registered nurse, you will be required to engage in learning activities on a regular basis to keep your competencies up-to-date and demonstrate that you continue to meet the standards of practice and the expectations of the quality assurance programs specific to the provincial/territorial jurisdiction where you work. You will likely not be able to renew your registration to practice if you do not meet these expectations. **Continuing competence** means the ongoing ability of a registered nurse to integrate and apply the knowledge, skills, judgment, and personal attributes required to practice safely and ethically in a designated role and setting. Maintaining ongoing abilities involves a continual process linking the code of ethics, standards of practice, and lifelong learning. The registered nurse reflects on his or her practice on an ongoing basis and takes action to continually improve that practice (Association of Registered Nurses of Newfoundland and Labrador, 2009; Nurses Association of New Brunswick, 2013a).

Participating in Setting Standards and Regulation

The regulatory bodies develop and keep the standards of practice up-to-date by consulting with nurses in practice, education, research, and administration as well as other stakeholders, including employers and government. Often, the experiences and feedback of newly graduated nurses are sought out as one target group. This provides you with an opportunity to participate in professional regulation. This may be one of the ways you choose to learn new things, thereby maintaining and enhancing your competence.

You will have opportunities in your nursing education program to give feedback about and participate in quality improvement of the program. Completing course and instructor evaluation forms and being a member/student representative on program committees, for example, curriculum, program evaluation, or student affairs, are important ways to contribute your perspective and make sure that the voice of students is considered. Six to 12 months after you have graduated, you may receive a survey from the nursing education program or an invitation to provide feedback in a focus group about how well the program prepared you for nursing practice. Regulatory bodies look for evidence of feedback from graduates and their employers during nursing education program reviews. Regulatory bodies ask to see what you have to say about the program, looking back after you have worked for a while. The possibilities for participating are abundant as a student and during your nursing career. Think about how you want to contribute to make the standards of nursing practice and professional regulation the best it can be in the interests of the public. This will benefit you in return by helping you meet the continuing competence expectations.

Jas graduated from his nursing education program 2 years ago and became a registered nurse after successfully writing the nursing registration exam and meeting the other registration requirements set out by the provincial nursing regulatory body. He just got back from small group discussions about what changes are needed in the entry-level competencies. When he got the e-mail invitation from the regulatory body, he wasn't sure he would have anything to say but decided to volunteer anyway. What a great learning experience! He found it was exhilarating to meet nurses from different places and talk about what's happening where they work. It turns out he had lots to talk about too. He was able to remember and use what he learned about self-regulation in his education program. After working for a while, he had quite a few ideas about what competencies should be required for registration. Jas will be writing about this experience in his file of continuing competence evidence.

Critical Thinking Case Scenarios

▶ Susan is in a clinical placement where there is a lot of preparation and talk about pandemic planning. The staff anticipates that the upcoming flu season will be particularly challenging for the health-care system. Susan is uncertain about what her responsibilities are as a student in the planning process and what her responsibilities are during an actual pandemic. What do you know about competencies and standards of practice for nurses in pandemic planning? What are the expectations of the regulatory body where you are located? If you were asked, as a student, to participate in patient care during a pandemic, what factors would you expect to have to consider?

▶ I am a new graduate and have just completed my final night of four consecutive 12-hour shifts on a busy acute medical unit. Near the end of my shift, I was asked to do an overtime shift. I said no because I felt I would not be able to provide safe care being so mentally and physically exhausted. I haven't been sleeping well lately. I am afraid they will say I have to stay. If I say no, can I be reported and lose my license?

▶ Kelly, a second-year nursing student, is often late for class and her labs. She complains of feeling tired, and often, her group work isn't complete so she asks the rest of the group to help. Sometimes, she has to nap during breaks to keep going. Students in her group have tried to talk with Kelly because they are concerned about her. They suggest that Kelly speak to her instructor or a student counsellor. Kelly is worried about how she will be perceived by others if she seeks help. Kelly is really finding second year tough, trying to juggle school and work to pay her bills. She feels like she is running on empty with so much to do at school and at home. She knows that she has been late recently for her classes and labs, so this is beginning to affect her performance. She doesn't have the energy or time to get group work done. She feels bad about asking her classmates for help but does it to manage anyway. She knows she should not need to nap during any breaks and notices that others have more energy than she does. Kelly knows that she needs help to sort things out so she can pass her courses. Kelly remembers learning about fitness to practice in class and that it is her responsibility to maintain her fitness to practice. Kelly decides to talk with a nursing faculty advisor about how she can juggle things better or find a way to get more financial support so she does not have to work so much. What would you do in Kelly's place? What would you do if you were her classmate? What do you know about expectations of an entry-level nurse related to fitness to practice?

Multiple-Choice Questions

1. Professional self-regulation is:
   a. A physiological process in the human body
   b. A right of all professions
   c. A privilege granted to some professions
   d. A strategy to inform the public about professionals

2. Match these regulatory terms to the appropriate definition.
   a. Duty to report
   b. Fitness to practice
   c. Standard
   d. Continuing competence

   I. All the qualities and capabilities of an individual relevant to his or her capability to practice as a nurse, including, but not limited to, freedom from any cognitive, physical, psychological, or emotional condition or a dependence on alcohol or drugs, that impair his or her ability to practice nursing.

II. Nurses or others who observe practice in nurses or other health professionals who place patients at risk have an ethical and legal duty to report concerns to the appropriate person or organization including the regulatory body if appropriate.

III. An authoritative statement that describes the required behaviour of every nurse and is used to evaluate individual performance.

IV. The ongoing ability of a registered nurse to integrate and apply the knowledge, skills, judgment, and personal attributes required to practice safely and ethically in a designated role and setting.

3. The nursing regulatory bodies influence what you need to learn in your nursing education program by establishing which of the following?
   a. The structure and sequence of nursing and non-nursing courses
   b. The forms used to evaluate student performance with patients
   c. The entry-level competencies and standards of practice
   d. The policies for student grades and conduct

4. Nurses acknowledge their professional privileges when they do which of the following?
   a. Act responsibly and accountably in all their interactions.
   b. Write e-mails to their friends about patients for self-reflection.
   c. Talk with patients the same way they do with family members.
   d. Explain patient care plans only when patients ask questions.

5. Individual self-regulation and evidence of your continued competence are requirements for registration to practice. The typical requirements of continuing competence set by the regulatory bodies are:
   a. Written examinations every 3 years
   b. Learning plans based on self-assessment
   c. Learning plans developed by the nurse manager
   d. Certificates of short course completion

6. Student nurses are learning about regulation and the standards of practice. To what extent are students held accountable to practice in accordance with the standards of practice before they graduate?
   a. To the same extent as newly graduated registered nurses
   b. To the extent that students have been educated so far to practice competently

   c. To a limited extent and only when ethical and integrity issues arise
   d. To the full extent that the scope of nursing practice allows

7. Fitness to practice requirements are set through standards of practice and the CNA Code of Ethics. Who has the primary responsibility for assessing and maintaining a nurse's fitness to practice?
   a. The nurse manager who evaluates the performance of nursing staff
   b. The employer who develops policies and monitors the work environment
   c. The regulatory body that provides resources about fitness to practice
   d. The individual nurse who self-assesses and maintains his or her own fitness to practice

Suggested Lab Activities

● Go to the website of the regulatory body in your province/territory. What is the definition of nursing in your province/territory? Who can use the title *nurse* and under what conditions? What does the scope of practice for a registered nurse look like in your province/territory? What types of activities can registered nurses do, and what can't they do?

● Look at the websites of two or more regulatory bodies in Canada to locate their standards of practice. How do they differentiate different types of standards, or do they? Compare the similarities and differences you find in the standards used by the two provinces/territories. Do either of them have standards about how you are to be supervised as a nursing student while learning to provide patient care?

● When in a health-care facility, observe how different health-care providers introduce themselves. What is the variation? Determine whether the patients actually know who different people are and what they do. If a patient has a question for, or was dissatisfied with a particular person, how would the patient exercise his or her right to ask or complain? To do so, the patient would need to know the name and professional designation of the health-care provider. Think about how what you witness erodes or upholds patient rights. Think about how professionals may unintentionally absolve themselves of their accountabilities by how they introduce themselves.

● Have another look at the standards of practice from the website of your province/territory. What do the professional standards say about fitness to practice? Tip: Look for a category dealing with self-regulation. What other resources, if any, does the regulatory body have available about understanding and maintaining your fitness to practice? Now look at the policies of your nursing education program. What policies are related to the fitness to practice of nursing students? What overall direction do the policies give students who have fitness to practice issues?

● Examine the entry-level competencies established by the regulatory body where you are located and find the competencies about demonstrating continuing competence.

Compare them to the quality assurance/continuing competence requirements in the same regulatory body. Tip: This information may be a section by itself or may be found in registration or practice support. What assessment tools, checklists, or other resources, if any, are developed by the regulatory body to help nurses meet the quality assurance/ continuing competence requirements?

REFERENCES AND SUGGESTED READINGS

Alberta Human Rights Commission. (2010). *Duty to accommodate students with disabilities in post-secondary education institutions.* Retrieved from http://www.albertahumanrights.ab.ca/Bull_DutytoAccom_web.pdf

Association of Registered Nurses of Newfoundland and Labrador. (2009). *Continuing competence program. Framework: Strengthening and growing nursing practice.* Retrieved from http://www.arnnl.ca/documents/pages/CCP_Framework_09.pdf

Association of Registered Nurses of Newfoundland and Labrador. (2013). *Competencies in the Context of Entry Level Registered Nurse Practice 2013–2018.* Retrieved from http://www.arnnl.ca/documents/pages/Competencies_required_for_entry_level_RN_08_13.pdf

Association of Registered Nurses of Prince Edward Island. (2009). *Working extra hours: Fitness to practice/duty of care.* Retrieved from http://www.arnpei.ca/default.asp?mn=1.45

Black, J., Allen, D., Redfern, L., Muzio, L., Rushowick, B., Balaski, B., . . . Round, B. (2008). Competencies in the context of entry-level registered nurse practice: A collaborative project in Canada. *International Nursing Review, 55,* 171–178.

Canadian Association of Schools of Nursing. (2011). *Accreditation program information.* Retrieved from http://www.casn.ca/en/62.html

Canadian Nurses Association (2007). Understanding self-regulation. *Nursing Now: issues and Trends in Canadian Nursing, 21,* 1–5.

Canadian Nurses Association. (2008). *Code of ethics for registered nurses* (2008 centennial edition). Retrieved from http://www.cnaaiic.ca/CNA/practice/ethics/code/default_e.aspx

Canadian Nurses Association. (2011). *Fact sheet: Privacy of personal health information.* http://www.cnaaiic.ca/~/media/cna/page%20content/pdf%20fr/2013/09/09/22/50/fs28_privacy_personal_health_info_2011_e.pdf

Canadian Nurses Protective Society. (2008). Confidentiality of health information. *InfoLaw, 1*(2), 1–2.

Canadian Nurses Protective Society. (2012). Social media. *InfoLaw, 19*(3), 1–2.

Chitty, K. K. (2007). The professionalization of nursing. In K. K. Chitty & B. P. Black (Eds.), *Professional nursing: Concepts and challenges* (pp. 69–85). St. Louis, MO: Saunders.

College and Association of Registered Nurses of Alberta. (2007). *Documenting your continuing competence activities.* Retrieved from http://www.nurses.ab.ca/Carna/index.aspx?WebStructureID=2227

College and Association of Registered Nurses of Alberta. (2011a). *Professional boundaries for registered nurses: Guidelines for the nurse-client relationship.* Retrieved from https://www.nurses.ab.ca/Carna-Admin/Uploads/professional_boundaries_May_%202011.pdf

College and Association of Registered Nurses of Alberta. (2011b). *Privacy and management of health information: Standards for CARNA's regulated members.* http://www.nurses.ab.ca/Carna-Admin/Uploads/Privacy%20of%20Health%20Info.pdf

College of Nurses of Ontario. (n.d.). *Complete Standards and Guidelines.* Retrieved from http://www.cno.org/en/learn-about-standards-guidelines/standards-and-guidelines/

College of Nurses of Ontario. (2009). *Quality assurance reflective practice.* Retrieved from http://www.cno.org/Global/docs/qa/44008_fsRefprac.pdf

College of Nurses of Ontario. (2011). *Legislation and regulation: An introduction to the Nursing Act, 1991.* Retrieved from http://www.cno.org/Global/docs/prac/41064_fsNursingact.pdf

College of Registered Nurses of British Columbia. (2007). *Becoming a registered nurse in British Columbia: Requisite skills and abilities.* Retrieved from https://crnbc.ca/Standards/Lists/StandardResources/464requisiteskillsabilities.pdf

College of Registered Nurses of British Columbia. (2008). *Fitness to practice: The challenge to maintain physical, mental and emotional health.* Retrieved from http://www.crnbc.ca/downloads/329.pdf

College of Registered Nurses of British Columbia. (2012). *Duty to provide care.* Vancouver, BC: Author. Retrieved from http://www.crnbc.ca/downloads/398.pdf

College of Registered Nurses of Manitoba. (2011). *Self-regulation.* http://cms.tng-secure.com/file_download.php?fFile_id=165

College of Registered Nurses of Nova Scotia. (2008). *Problematic substance use in the workplace: A resource guide for registered nurses.* Retrieved from http://www.crnns.ca/documents/Problematic%20Substance%20Use%20Resource%20Guide.pdf

College of Registered Nurses of Nova Scotia. (2009a). *Becoming a registered nurse in Nova Scotia: Requisite skills and abilities.* Retrieved from http://www.nursing.dal.ca/Files/CRNNSfinal.pdf

College of Registered Nurses of Nova Scotia. (2009b). *Emergency preparedness plan (Version 1.6).* Retrieved from http://www.crnns.ca/documents/CRNNS%20Emergency%20Preparedness%20Plan%20with%20Appendices%20-%20V1.6.pdf

College of Registered Nurses of Nova Scotia. (2013). *Entry-level competencies for registered nurses in Nova Scotia.* Retrieved from http://www.crnns.ca/documents/Entry-LevelCompetenciesRNs.pdf

International Council of Nurses. (2008). *Health information: Protecting patient rights.* Retrieved from http://www.icn.ch/PS_E05_HealthInformation.pdf

Jackson, D., Firtko, A., & Edenborough, M. (2007). Personal resilience as a strategy for surviving and thriving in the face of workplace adversity: A literature review. *Journal of Advanced Nursing, 60*(1), 1–9.

Manitoba Government. (n.d.). *The Registered Nurses Act.* Retrieved from http://web2.gov.mb.ca/laws/statutes/ccsm/r040e.php

National Council of State Boards of Nursing. (2011). *White paper: A nurse's guide to the use of social media.* Chicago, IL: Author.

Nurses Association of New Brunswick (2011a). *Practice standard: Consent.* Retrieved from http://www.nanb.nb.ca/downloads/Practice%20Guideline%20Consent_E(3).pdf

Nurses Association of New Brunswick (2011b). *Practice standard: The therapeutic nurse-client relationship.* Retrieved from http://www.nanb.nb.ca/downloads/Practice%20Standard-Nurse-Client%20Relationship_E.pdf

Nurses Association of New Brunswick. (2013a). *Continuing competence program: Learning in action.* Retrieved from http://www.nanb.nb.ca/downloads/CCP%20Document_2014_%20FINAL_English.pdf

Nurses Association of New Brunswick. (2013b). *Entry-level competencies for registered nurses in New Brunswick*. Retrieved from http://www.nanb.nb.ca/downloads/Entry%20level%20Competencies%20May%202013-E.pdf

Ordre des infirmières et des infirmiers du Québec. (2009). *Mosaic of nurses' clinical competencies* (2nd ed.). Montreal, QC: Author.

Saskatchewan Registered Nurses Association. (2009a). *A SRNA discussion paper on hours of work, fatigue and patient safety*. Retrieved from http://www.srna.org/images/stories/pdfs/nurse_practitioner/documents/work_hours.pdf

Saskatchewan Registered Nurses Association. (2009b). *Nursing education program approval process*. Retrieved from http://www.srna.org/images/stories/pdfs/nurse_resources/Program_Approval_Nov_26.pdf

Saskatchewan Registered Nurses Association. (2013). *Standards and foundation competencies for the practice of registered nurses*. Retrieved from http://www.srna.org/images/stories/Nursing_Practice/Resources/Standards_and_Foundation_2013_06_10_Web.pdf

Secretary of State for Health. (2007). *Trust, assurance and safety—The regulation of health professionals in the 21st century*. London, United Kingdom: The Stationary Office. Retrieved from http://www.official-documents.gov.uk/document/cm70/7013/7013.pdf

Volti, R. (2008). *An introduction to the sociology of work and occupations*. Los Angeles, CA: Pine Forge Press.

Yukon Registered Nurses Association. (2006). *Professional conduct review complaints and discipline policy*. Whitehorse, YT: Author. Retrieved from http://www.yrna.ca/pdf/wp-content/uploads/PCRPolicy.pdf

Health Care and the Law in Canada

ELIZABETH C. ROBERTSON

Hélène is in the first year of her nursing program at a university in western Canada. She is very interested in current affairs and regularly reads several newspapers from across the country. Since beginning her nursing studies, she has noticed media reports of patients suing health professionals for medical negligence. This has frightened her, and she is worried that she might be involved in a lawsuit in the future. She wonders if there are any steps she can take in her nursing practice to minimize her risk of being sued for medical negligence. To protect herself and her patients, Hélène will need to learn about the legal concepts that govern nursing practice and understand some basics about the legal system in Canada.

CHAPTER OBJECTIVES

By the end of this chapter, you will be able to:

1. Demonstrate knowledge of the basic legal process and concepts involved in a medical negligence lawsuit.
2. Describe the structure of the Canadian legal system and the steps involved in bringing a lawsuit to court.
3. List the required elements for proof of negligence.
4. Define the legal standard of care.
5. Discuss examples of ways in which nurses have been found to be negligent.
6. Explain the nature of patient consent.
7. Name the steps a nurse can take to minimize risk and the legal protections of nurses in practice.

KEY TERMS

Approved Practice A defence that says a health professional has acted in accordance with the generally accepted practice at the time.

Civil Law A legal system based on a code that contains a comprehensive set of rules that are followed by judges in deciding court cases.

Common Law A legal system based on judge-made law where cases are decided following precedents.

Consent A patient must give consent before any medical intervention takes place. Consent must be voluntary, given by a patient with capacity, referable to the intervention, and informed. Consent may be either express or implied by the circumstances.

Error of Judgment An error may not be negligent if the health professional has acted with reasonable care, exercising the skills of a normal, prudent professional.

Informed Consent A patient must be given the necessary information to give an informed consent to a medical intervention. A patient must be informed of the material risks that a reasonable person in the position of the patient would want to know.

Negligence An action will be negligent in law where the defendant owes the plaintiff a duty of care, the defendant breached the

standard of care, the plaintiff suffered an injury or loss, and the defendant's conduct was the actual and legal cause of the plaintiff's injury or loss.

Precedent A principle or rule established by a prior court decision with similar fact situations that are used by judges to make decisions on subsequent cases.

Standard of Care The law requires a medical practitioner to exercise the care and skill that could reasonably be expected of a normal, prudent practitioner of the same experience and standing.

Statement of Claim A document used to initiate a lawsuit that sets out the alleged facts and the amount of compensation being asked for.

Statement of Defence A document that outlines the reasons why the court should not find the practitioner responsible.

Tort Law The area of law that enables a victim to get compensation from a wrongdoer, not including wrongs covered by contract or criminal law.

Vicarious Liability The employer is liable for the negligent acts of an employee and will be responsible for paying any damages awarded to the injured patient.

All nurses who practice in Canada need to have a basic understanding of the Canadian legal system because the law impacts the nurse in many aspects of practice. For example, the Canada Health Act (1985) and provincial law govern health-care delivery in Canada. Laws govern the regulation of the nursing profession and the employee–employer relationship.

You will recall that Hélène in the opening chapter scenario has noticed media reports of medical negligence lawsuits. She is worried that in the future, she might become a defendant in a lawsuit as a result of her nursing practice. The prospect of being involved in a lawsuit brought by an injured patient can cause great concern. This chapter introduces you to basic knowledge of the legal processes involved in a medical negligence lawsuit and the standard of care expected of nurses in the practice of their profession. This is knowledge that will enable you to take steps in your practice to minimize the risk of being sued for medical negligence.

Understanding the Canadian Legal System

The law in Canada is roughly divided into two areas: private law and public law. Private law focuses on the individual. It is concerned with relationships between people or things. For example, business disputes and divorces are governed by private law. In general, private law disputes are resolved through monetary payments. In contrast, public law refers to the relationships between government or society and individuals. Areas of law that fall within the category of public law are human rights, tax, criminal, and constitutional law.

Private law in Canada is governed by two different legal traditions: the **common law** and the **civil law**. The common law is the legal system adopted by all the provinces of Canada except Quebec. In Quebec, private law disputes are decided under civil law. Under both systems, the courts are required to apply the laws passed by the Parliament of Canada or provincial legislatures. Legislation takes precedence over any case law on the same subject.

In a common law system, judges develop the law by referring to the law as decided in previous cases (known as **precedents**). Sometimes, a judge will conclude that no precedents apply to a particular case, and this gives the common law the ability to evolve to meet new and novel situations. The law in Quebec is a civil law system based on Roman law, as is the French legal system. A civil law system is based on a code that contains a comprehensive set of rules that judges follow in deciding court cases. Medical negligence will be discussed in terms of the common law. However, many of the same principles apply to cases decided under the civil law.

The Canadian Court System

The structure of the court system is basically the same in all provinces. For private law disputes, there is a trial court for disputes involving claims for small amounts of compensation.

These courts are often called *small claims courts* and are often handled by the individuals involved without a lawyer. Above this is a superior court for all other trials and then a court of appeal. Provincially, the lower courts must follow the decisions of a higher court. These decisions are called *precedents*. Decisions from other provinces are not binding but can often be followed, especially when it is a decision from a higher court. Decisions made by the appeal courts of the provinces can be appealed to the Supreme Court of Canada. The Supreme Court of Canada decides cases involving issues of national importance or uncertain areas of law. All courts in Canada must follow the decisions of the Supreme Court (Keatings & Smith, 2010).

Anatomy of a Lawsuit

The basic steps involved in a lawsuit for medical professional negligence are discussed here. A patient who has been injured by an adverse event while being treated may decide to commence a lawsuit against some or all of the health professionals involved in the adverse event. If the treatment took place in hospital, the hospital is often sued as well. The patient, as the person initiating the lawsuit, is called the *plaintiff*. The people and/or organizations being sued are termed *defendants*.

A lawsuit is initiated by a document usually called a **statement of claim**. The statement of claim sets out the alleged facts and the amount of compensation being asked for. The defendants respond with a **statement of defence**, which outlines the reasons why the court should not find them responsible. *Discoveries* are usually the next major step. This involves exchanging all relevant documents and an examination of the parties by opposing lawyers. Following discoveries, *out-of-court settlement* discussions and/or mediation often take place, which in most cases result in an agreement to end the lawsuit. If a settlement cannot be reached, the case will proceed to trial to be decided by the court. A judge alone decides most medical negligence cases in Canada, not a jury (Canadian Nurses Protective Society, 2007a).

Tort Law

It is not easy to define the area of law comprised by **tort law**. It is the area of law that enables a victim to get compensation from a wrongdoer. However, it does not include wrongs covered by contract or criminal law. There are various kinds of torts. A tort may be either intentional or unintentional. Examples of intentional torts are battery, defamation, and false imprisonment. Negligent actions are unintentional torts. Most lawsuits against health professionals are actions for negligent conduct. Although this chapter focuses on negligence, brief descriptions of some of the intentional torts that may affect nursing practice are presented later.

Battery

Battery consists of intentionally touching someone without consent. The person need not have been injured. Thus, if consent is not obtained from a patient prior to medical treatment, the health professional may have committed a battery (Kerr & Ross-Kerr, 2003). However, a health professional who fails to provide informed consent will be liable for negligence only and not battery.

Defamation

A nurse may be sued for defamation of character. "A defamatory statement is any communication, oral or written, which would tend to lower the plaintiff's reputation in the estimation of right thinking people generally, or lead to the plaintiff being shunned or avoided" (Picard & Robertson, 2007, p. 438). This can arise in nursing practice in several ways. For example, untrue patient information may be given out that could be seen as defamatory in nature, or a nurse might write statements about a supervisor who is perceived as defamatory (Tapp, 1999).

False Imprisonment

A patient may bring a lawsuit based on the tort of false imprisonment in circumstances where a patient has been intentionally prevented from leaving a hospital. Patients are at liberty to leave hospital in the same way that they are able to refuse any medical treatment.

Proof of Negligence

There are four elements which must be proved before a **negligence** lawsuit will be successful. These elements are

"(a) the defendant must owe the plaintiff a duty of care;
(b) the defendant must breach the standard of care established by law;
(c) the plaintiff must suffer an injury or loss; and
(d) the defendant's conduct must have been the actual and legal cause of the plaintiff's injury." (Picard & Robertson, 2007, p. 212)

Duty of Care

The duty of care may arise from the nurse's employment, from the provision of patient care, or when a patient believes that the nurse will be providing services (Adlersberg, 2006, p. 25). As a rule, the existence of a duty of care toward the particular patient is self-evident and will not be an issue in the lawsuit.

Injury

The plaintiff must also have been injured as a result of the nurse's actions. The damage suffered by a plaintiff is most often a physical injury. The required presence of a measurable injury flows from the purpose of negligence law, which is to reinstate the plaintiff to his or her pre-accident position to the extent that an award of money is able to do so.

Causation

In addition, the plaintiff's injury must have been caused by the nurse's actions, both factually and legally. To prove the factual element of causation, scientific and technical evidence is presented to prove that the injury would not have happened but for the actions of the nurse. Proof of the legal element involves an inquiry by the court as to whether it was reasonably foreseeable that the nurse's actions would cause the plaintiff's injuries (Canadian Nurses Protective Society, 2004b).

Breach of Standard of Care

The last requirement, and the one which lies at the heart of every medical negligence action, is that the nurse must have contravened or failed to observe the required **standard of care**. The classic statement of the required standard of care is contained in the case of *Crits v. Sylvester* (1956):

> Every medical practitioner must bring to his task a reasonable degree of skill and knowledge and must exercise a reasonable degree of care. He is bound to exercise that degree of care and skill which could reasonably be expected of a normal, prudent practitioner of the same experience, standing, and if he holds himself out as a specialist, a higher degree of skill is required of him than of one who does not profess to be so qualified by special training and ability.

Standard of Care

The standard of care expected of a health professional by the law is a broad umbrella covering a wide area of expectations. The courts have outlined several specific duties and corresponding standards of care. For example, there is a duty to attend a patient, a duty to treat a patient, and a duty to refer a patient when appropriate. In general, the same legal principles apply to nurses as are applied to physicians.

The case of *Bauer (Litigation Guardian of) v. Seager* (Manitoba, 2000) outlined in Box 5.1 provides a good illustration of the required standard of care for nurses and contains a valuable discussion of the overarching principles. The case concerned an induced birth of a fetus in the breech position. The mother needed to be monitored carefully as there was a risk of cord compression. Before going on a break, one of the nursing team

---

BOX 5.1   *Bauer (Litigation Guardian of) v. Seager* and Standards of Care

Facts
- An infant was born with severe brain injuries as a result of hypoxia during labour.
- There was a lack of proper communication between the nurses that resulted in no one contacting the doctor for over 30 minutes.

What the Court Said
- A nurse "is bound to exercise that degree of skill and care which could reasonably be expected of a normal prudent practitioner of the same training."
- Nurses "have a duty to use [their] skills in making appropriate assessments of patients and to communicate accurately those assessments to physicians."

What the Court Held
- The nurses had been negligent and were responsible for the injuries suffered by the infant.

observed deep decelerations in the foetal heartbeat. She testified that she told the charge nurse to call the doctor; however, the charge nurse had no recollection of this. The doctor was actually notified approximately 30 minutes after the first problems with the fetus were noticed. By this time, it was too late to perform a caesarean section, and the foetal brain damage had already occurred. The court summarized the standard of care expected of nurses as follows:

> Nurses are professionals who possess special skills and knowledge and the same principles apply as in the case of doctors, residents and interns. They have a duty to use those skills in making appropriate assessments of patients and to communicate accurately those assessments to physicians. (Manitoba, 2000)

It is essential to remember that the standard is not a standard of perfection. The nurse is simply expected to perform her duties in the same way as another ordinary skilled nurse working in the same area would.

In Canadian hospitals, health professionals work as a team, and members must perform their roles by meeting the appropriate standard of care. Other members of the team must be able to rely on team members to carry out their duties.

> If staff obstetricians, for example, cannot rely upon staff obstetrical nurses to provide accurate assessments, given all of the constraints under which they are operating, I am satisfied our system would fail. . . . It is not for the obstetrical nurse to fully understand all of the subtleties that may be determined on a foetal heart strip, but it is the responsibility of that nurse to understand and report problems to someone else on the obstetrical team, problems such as severe and persistent variable decelerations. (*Granger [Litigation Guardian of] v. Ottawa General Hospital*, 1996)

In *Bauer (Litigation Guardian of) v. Seager*, the court found that the nurses had failed to meet the required standard of care because they had not made sure that the doctors had been notified when the problems with the fetus were first noticed. "Time is of the essence and it simply took too long for the nurses to alert the doctors as to the emergent status of this fetus" (*Bauer [Litigation Guardian of] v. Seager* [Manitoba, 2000]).

The court applied the principle that the standard of care expected of a nurse was that of the reasonable nurse in similar circumstances. This means that the nurses in this case were expected to perform their duties in the same manner as a prudent nurse working as part of an obstetrical team. The court determined the appropriate standard through expert evidence given in court by obstetrical nurses and obstetricians.

Inexperience and Specialized Training

Two important points must be emphasized in connection with the required standard of care. The first point is that a nurse's inexperience does not provide an excuse. A nurse fresh from her training is held to the same standard as the ordinary skilled nurse working in the particular area. The second point is that a specialist, such as a nurse practitioner, must perform at the higher level of skill and knowledge expected as a result of the expert training. Thus, the performance of the obstetrical nurse practitioner would be measured against the skills required of other obstetrical nurse practitioners (*Gemoto v. Calgary Regional Hospital Authority*, Alberta 2006).

Specific Duties

Gemoto v. Calgary Regional Hospital Authority (2006) is a recent case from Alberta that details the various duties expected of nurses. As outlined in Box 5.2, the case law has established that the nurse has many legal duties to fulfill in caring for his patients.

The *Gemoto* case involved the death as a result of a ruptured appendix of a seven and one-half month old boy at the Alberta Children's Hospital. He was treated both in the emergency room and subsequently in a ward. Both the nurses and physicians involved in the case were found to have been negligent. The emergency room nurses had failed to meet their obligations to properly care for the infant in several areas. First, they had failed to document the deteriorating condition of the infant. Second, they had failed to take his vital signs as required by hospital policy. Thirdly, they had failed to properly monitor and assess the patient, including failing to monitor the infant's hydration and urine output, failing to see the abdominal distension, and failing to address concerns raised by the parents. The ward nurse had been negligent as well. Although she had done a full assessment and had charted properly, she was a recent graduate and had been negligent in not appreciating the gravity of the infant's condition. The court stated that there was "no lower or separate standard for a beginner" (*Gemoto v. Calgary Regional Hospital Authority*, 2006).

Working With Physicians

In most situations, nurses play a subordinate role in relation to physicians in the sense that they routinely follow instructions from doctors and, in fact, are under a legal duty to do so. However, there are exceptional circumstances in

---

BOX 5.2   Specific Duties Expected of Nurses

- Assess patients.
- Maintain accurate records and notes.
- Review patient records.
- Follow hospital policy and inform physicians of changes in their patients' conditions.
- Ensure that drugs are properly administered.
- Seek guidance from physicians.
- Adhere to physicians' instructions, absent clear and obvious neglect or incompetence.
- Communicate both with the doctor and the charge nurse in a timely fashion.

Derived from the court's findings in *Gemoto v. Calgary Health Authority* (Alberta, 2006).

which a nurse will have a legal duty to either intervene in a physician's handling of a patient or summon the assistance of another physician.

In *Skeels Estate v. Iwashkiw* (Alberta, 2006), complications (shoulder dystocia) arose during the delivery of a baby. The physician conducting the delivery had difficulties handling the emergency situation and was emotionally distressed following the delivery. This resulted in his being unable to resuscitate the baby. After some minutes of failed resuscitation, the nursing team called for another physician. Throughout the delivery and resuscitation, the defendant physician had not asked that another physician be called although this was part of the standard protocol for treating shoulder dystocia.

The court found that the nurses could have summoned help both when they first recognized the emergency, and again when they knew the physician was emotionally distressed following the delivery. The court held the nurses had acted appropriately when they first recognized the emergency. At this point, the physician was still in charge, and it would have been difficult for the nurses to second-guess the doctor.

The court found that the nurses should have summoned help immediately after the delivery when it was clear that the physician was very distressed and unable to do his job. The nurses had been negligent in failing to do so. The court decided that there was "a positive duty to intervene when there is 'clear and obvious neglect or incompetence on the part of the physician'." Intervention is required in these exceptional circumstances.

Defences

There are several defences available to a nurse who has been accused of professional negligence. Two important defences are *approved practice* and excusable *error of judgment*.

Error of Judgment

The defence of **error of judgment** plays an important part in many cases. Medical treatment is a science and an art. Some decisions or actions will be taken which involve the exercise of professional judgment. If a health professional has acted with reasonable care, exercising the skills of a normal, prudent professional and has nevertheless made an error, the court may find that the error was not negligent (*Wilson v. Swanson*, 1956).

Approved Practice

The defence of **approved practice** involves providing the court with evidence that the conduct named in the legal complaint was in accordance with generally accepted practice at the time. In the words of the Supreme Court of Canada, "It is generally accepted that when a doctor acts in accordance with a recognized and respectable practice of the profession, he or she will not be found to be negligent." (*ter Neuzen v. Korn*, 1995)

This defence underlines the importance of acting in accordance with hospital policies and other protocols. Following these policies will often provide evidence that the standard of care was met (*Crouch [Guardian ad litem of] v. B.C. Women's Hospital & Health Centre*, 2001/2003; Hardingham, 2000).

Vicarious Liability

In many instances, negligent acts by a nurse will be held by the court to be the responsibility of his or her employer; for example, a physician or a hospital. This is termed **vicarious liability**, and it means that the employer is liable for the negligent acts of employees and will be responsible for paying any damages awarded to the injured patient. Vicarious liability only applies to acts done during the course of employment, although this is a flexible concept (Canadian Nurses Protective Society, 1998).

Consent

A patient must have given **consent** before any medical intervention, such as a diagnostic test or treatment, takes place (Fig. 5.1). A mentally competent individual has the right to refuse treatment even in a situation where the refusal may result in death. Consent may be either express or implied from the situation. An example of an express consent is a written consent. Consent can be implied, for example, in a situation when a patient holds out his arm to receive a vaccination although he has not said that he wishes to receive the vaccine

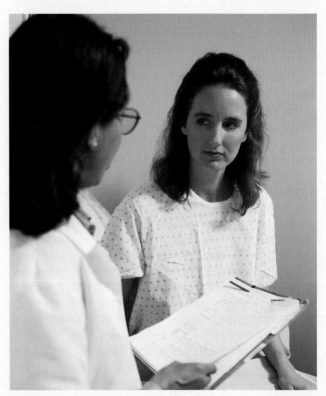

Figure 5.1 An appropriate environment should be provided when obtaining patient consent.

(Keatings & Smith, 2010, p. 162). A health professional who treats a patient without consent may be liable for the tort of battery if the patient decided to sue and won the case.

There are some exceptions to this rule. Most notably, in an emergency situation, a person may be unable to give consent due to injury, illness, or unconsciousness. In these circumstances, the person may be given necessary treatment to safeguard her health or life (Picard & Robertson, 2007, pp. 54–61). Under public health legislation, treatment of some conditions may be carried out without consent. In addition, in some provinces, there is legislation that allows testing for certain conditions without consent (Bailey, Caulfield, & Ries, 2008). Some provinces have passed laws dealing with consent to treatment (Keatings & Smith, 2010, pp. 171–183).

In nursing practice, consent is usually obtained by the physician. When carrying out invasive nursing treatments, it is good practice for a nurse to explain the procedure and obtain consent. This should be documented (Canadian Nurses Protective Society, 1994).

Elements of Consent

There are four elements of consent: It must be voluntarily, given by a person who has the mental capacity to do so, must be referable to the treatment and to the provider, and must be informed.

Voluntarily Given

For consent to be voluntary, the person must not have been overly influenced or coerced into giving the consent. Sometimes, a patient may be facing undue pressure from family or friends. A patient giving consent after receiving preoperative sedation is another example of a situation when it may be questionable whether the consent is voluntary.

Mental Competence

A person must be mentally competent to give consent. There are many reasons why a person's capacity to give consent may be affected (e.g., illness, dementia, psychiatric conditions). To give valid consent, an individual must be able to comprehend the character and results of the choices being made. If an individual is incapable of giving consent, some provinces have substitute consent legislation, and almost all provinces have legislation providing for proxy appointments and advance directives (Canadian Nurses Protective Society, 2004a).

In general, young children do not have the capacity to give consent, and parental consent must be obtained. In *Toews v. Weisner* (2001), a community health nurse gave an 11-year-old child a vaccination because the nurse thought the parents had given oral consent. The parents had not consented, and the court found the nurse's action was a battery.

For older children, some provinces have legislation governing when an older child may give consent. In other provinces, the situation is governed by the common law, and the child may give consent if he has the maturity to comprehend the treatment and the consequences of choosing or refusing consent (Kuz, 2006).

Referable to the Treatment and Provider

To be valid, consent must be referable to the treatment and the health professional providing the treatment. For example, a patient who consents to surgery done by a specific surgeon does not normally consent to the treatment being performed by a different surgeon. The same applies to categories of treatments; for example, consent to a caesarean section is not consent to a tubal ligation.

Informed

A failure to give **informed consent** is a frequent allegation in medical negligence lawsuits. The requirement that consent be informed is an outgrowth of the physician–patient relationship. The physician possesses extensive knowledge that the patient does not have. There is an inherent inequality in the relationship. The right of the patient to make his or her own health-care decisions mandates the requirement that the patient has been given the necessary information to make an informed decision.

What information must be given to a patient? The patient must be informed of the material risks that a reasonable person in the position of the patient would want to know. The patient must also be informed of the consequences of the risk (i.e., the type of injury that might occur if the risk materialized). Patients must also be informed if there are alternative treatments available. Any specific questions that the patient asks need to be answered.

It is important to be aware that the patient may withdraw consent at any time. A nurse may be faced with a situation where a patient wishes to withdraw consent. For example, a physician has obtained a patient's consent, and the patient changes the written consent form in the nurse's presence, making a change to the nature and/or scope of the treatment. In this situation, the nurse must inform the physician and may be found to have been negligent if she fails to do so (*Keane v. Craig*, 2000). In nursing practice, there are many steps that can be taken to ensure that consents are obtained in an appropriate environment, giving the patient sufficient time to reflect about the decision (Box 5.3).

BOX 5.3 Obtaining Informed Consent

- It is necessary to be aware of any cultural differences or difficulties with language that the patient may have which might affect his or her understanding of the discussion. It may be necessary to have an interpreter present.
- Everyone is different in the time it takes to understand information and make decisions.
- The consent discussion should take place in an appropriate environment, and the patient's privacy and comfort should be considered.
- It is often helpful to give the patient written material as well as an oral explanation.
- The patient may choose to have a family member or friend with him or her during the discussion.
- The nurse should listen carefully to the patient and ensure that the patient understands the information.

Source: Keatings, M., & Smith, O. (2010). *Ethical and legal issues in Canadian nursing* (3rd ed., pp. 161–162). Toronto, ON: Mosby.

Good Nursing Practice and Medical Negligence

Following good nursing practices on every shift, when documenting nursing care as well as when giving telephone advice, is an important step to minimize the risk of being involved in a lawsuit. It is also very important to be aware of the advice and services offered by your professional liability insurer.

Documentation

Complete and accurate documentation is one of the most important things a nurse can do to protect himself or herself in the event of a lawsuit (Fig. 5.2). Numerous cases have found nurses to be negligent as a result of inadequate documentation. The recent case of *Aristorenas v. Comcare Health Services* (2004) provides a good example of the consequences of inaccurate charting. A patient was discharged home with a wound infection after a caesarean section. Her physician monitored her and a team of home care nurses. Her infection deteriorated for a week. She was admitted to hospital where she was diagnosed with necrotizing fasciitis (called the *flesh-eating disease*), a life-threatening condition. The court found that the home care nurses had been negligent in several respects. There was no record that the patient's vital signs had been taken and documented. This is very important in tracking the progress of an infection. In addition, the court found the documenting of symptoms had been "sketchy and inconsistent." The lack of charting on the part of all members of the team made it difficult for other members of the team and the physician to accurately assess the deterioration in the patient's condition.

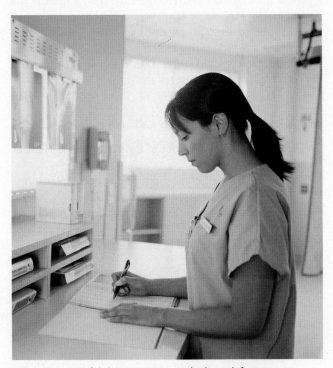

Figure 5.2 Careful documentation is the best defence.

In contrast, in *Ewert v. Marshall* (2009), the patient alleged there had been negligence in diagnosing appendicitis. He alleged that he had told the nurse and physician that he was suffering from severe pain in his lower right abdomen. The court found that the nurse had documented in accordance with accepted nursing practice, and the entries in the record had been made shortly after observing the patient. The records did not contain any evidence that the patient's symptoms had been ignored nor that he had told the nurse or physician that he had severe pain in his lower right abdomen. The records were a more accurate reflection of the patient's condition at the time than the patient's recollection. The court dismissed the patient's lawsuit, mainly on the basis of the evidence contained in the clinical records.

The previous cases illustrate the importance of proper documentation. Maintaining thorough, accurate, and timely records of a patient's condition may provide evidence of appropriate care. In this respect, it is important that entries are legible, accurate and clear, and entered on a regular and timely basis (Canadian Nurses Protective Society, 2007c; Wade, 2009).

Through the eyes of a nurse

*T*he unit that I work on is so busy that I often find it a struggle to do the most accurate and timely documentation. I have learned over the years to chart throughout the shift and not leave it all to the end of the day. In my career, I have also experienced improvements that have made documentation easier for nurses; for example, having documents closer to the point of care for recording vital signs and having electronic charting stations closer to patient rooms.

(personal reflection of a nurse)

Telephone Advice

The provision of telephone advice by nurses is becoming more frequent. Giving advice over the phone creates special challenges because the nurse cannot see the patient and may not even be talking with the patient. The nurse is legally responsible for the advice given. Extra care should be taken to make sure enough information is gathered from the patient. Accurate and complete documentation of all the details of the conversation is vital (Canadian Nurses Association, 2000; Canadian Nurses Protective Society, 2008).

Specific Practice Areas

Some areas of nursing practice result in more lawsuits than others. This is the case for nurses practicing in the areas of surgery and obstetrics. It is important for nurses practicing in these areas to be familiar with the types of errors that have resulted in frequent negligence claims and the steps that can be taken to minimize risks (Canadian Nurses Protective Society, 2002, 2007b).

The Role of the Canadian Nurses Protective Society and Other Insurers

Insurance coverage for professional liability is available as part of a nurse's membership in his professional association or college. In most provinces in Canada, the Canadian Nurses Protective Society provides this coverage. The Society provides information about potential legal issues, legal assistance, and payment of lawyers' fees and damages. It is important to be familiar with the services provided by your insurer and to contact your insurer if you suspect that you may be involved in a lawsuit or have been involved in any out-of-the-ordinary occurrence.

Hélène is feeling much better now that she has learned more about the legal concepts that govern nursing practice, and she is beginning to understand some basics about the legal system in Canada. She is feeling more confident about the steps a nurse can take to minimize risk and the legal protections of nurses in practice. Hélène also acknowledges that she will need to revisit health-care legal issues throughout her nursing career and stay informed in order to maintain good nursing practice and to protect herself and her patients from harm.

SUMMARY

This chapter has outlined medical negligence law with the aim of giving the student studying to be a registered nurse an understanding of the steps involved in a medical malpractice lawsuit and a knowledge of some of the actions that can be taken to avoid being involved in a lawsuit. Nurses must be aware of their legal duties in the day-to-day practice of their profession. A nurse must meet the standard of care expected of an ordinary skilled member of the profession working in the same area. The law expects nurses to properly document, follow hospital policies, properly administer drugs, be guided by physicians, and communicate with other team members. To minimize liability in a possible lawsuit, careful and thorough documentation is probably the most important practice a nurse can undertake.

Critical Thinking Case Scenarios

▶ You are a nurse on an overflow ward and have the care of a patient who has been transferred for observation overnight. The male patient presented with abdominal pain. The patient was admitted overnight for observation of a possible small bowel obstruction. The physician ordered morphine for pain as the patient reported pain on a scale of 8 out of 10. Between 11:00 pm and 4:00 pm, you went to attend to the patient on three occasions after the patient had requested the bathroom or more morphine. At 5:00 pm, the patient rang again and said that his pain was now 10 out of 10.

You conducted an assessment, taking vital signs and listening for bowel sounds, which appeared normal. You documented that the patient said the pain was 10 out of 10. In your view, the patient's pain wasn't as severe as he said it was, but you didn't note that on the chart, nor did you note the results of your other assessments. Because he continues to report pain, you gave the patient two more doses of morphine. At 7:00 pm, you documented that the patient had a temperature and was shivering and that you were having trouble getting a pulse. Out of an abundance of caution, you decided to call the doctor. On the phone, you told the doctor that the patient was still in pain despite the morphine. The doctor ordered an increase in the dosage and said that she would be at the hospital to see the patient in 10 minutes. Did your actions in this scenario meet the legally required standard of care expected of a nurse? If not, discuss the areas in which you might be held liable for professional negligence.

▶ You are an emergency room nurse. You receive a telephone call from a member of the public who asks what would happen if someone took four tablets of an antidepressant. You ask a physician standing nearby, and she tells you that four tablets are in the normal therapeutic range. The caller asks if the antidepressant could cause confusion or hallucinations. You tell the caller that if it did the person would sleep it off. Ten minutes later, the doctor decides to call back to get further information but is unable to do so because you didn't ask the caller for his name or phone number. Were your actions appropriate? If not, discuss in what respects your actions might result in a court finding that you were negligent.

▶ You are preparing to administer preoperative sedation to a patient undergoing elective surgery to repair a hernia. The patient is 19 years old. You are aware that the surgeon had talked to the patient and obtained a written consent form. The patient asks you if the surgery may affect his fertility in the future. How should you answer the patient's question? Do you think that you must tell the surgeon?

Multiple-Choice Questions

1. The court will judge a nurse in the performance of his or her duties by:
   a. Looking at whether he or she has a good explanation for why he or she acted as he or she did
   b. Considering whether his or her performance was perfect
   c. The conduct expected of the ordinary skilled nurse in similar circumstances
   d. His or her educational background

2. In Canada, courts make decisions by:
   a. Following the decisions made by the Supreme Court of Canada and other higher courts in the province
   b. Making the decision that the judge feels is the right decision

c. Looking only at the decisions made by the Supreme Court of Canada

d. Following the decisions made by courts in the United States

3. If a plaintiff is awarded damages by a court, the nurse defendant:

a. Never has to pay any money to the defendant himself

b. Must pay any monetary damages awarded to the plaintiff from his or her own money

c. Will not be responsible for paying the money himself or herself in many cases, as the hospital or his or her employer will be vicariously liable for the payment

d. Will not be responsible for paying the money himself or herself in almost all cases, as either the hospital, his or her employer, or his or her insurance will cover the payment

4. Consent from a patient must be:

a. Timely, detailed, and appropriate

b. Informed, timely, and referable

c. Voluntary

d. Voluntary, with capacity, referable, and informed

5. Proper documentation should:

a. Be complete, legible, and accurate

b. State personal opinions about patients or other staff

c. Contain the minimum of information to save time

d. Be legible so the notes are easy to read

6. The standard of care required of a nurse practitioner working in an emergency room will be measured by the standard expected of:

a. The ordinary skilled emergency room physician

b. The nurse working on any ward in the hospital

c. The ordinary skilled emergency room nurse practitioner

d. The newly graduated nurse

7. The nurse working with a treating physician has a legal duty to summon another physician:

a. In exceptional circumstances where there is clear or obvious neglect or incompetence on the part of the physician

b. When he or she remembers gossip about the competence of the treating physician

c. When he or she thinks the doctor is making a wrong diagnosis

d. When it appears that the physician is tired

8. To consent to treatment, a patient must be told:

a. The date and time when the treatment will take place

b. The information that a reasonable person in the position of the patient would want to know

c. The name of the treating physician

d. What public transit is available to get to the place where the treatment will take place

Suggested Lab Activities

● Break into small groups and discuss the principles involved in obtaining informed consent. When is it appropriate for nurses to be obtaining consents? Can you think of any situations that present particular challenges for nurses? Devise a role-play to be presented to the other groups in the class illustrating an informed consent scenario involving a nurse and patient. Following presentation of the role-play, discuss how the role-play illustrates a difficult situation for a nurse and discuss possible courses of action.

Break into small groups and prepare a poster presentation on one of the following topics:

Legal Duty of Care and the Nurse
Documentation, the Law, and the Nurse
Informed Consent and the Nurse

Invite two lawyers specializing in medical negligence law to speak to the lab class on the topic of the medical negligence lawsuit from the perspectives of both the plaintiff and the defendant. Your provincial or territorial law society or university law school may be able to provide suitable references.

REFERENCES AND SUGGESTED READINGS

Adlersberg, M. (2006). Duty to provide care. *Nursing BC, 38*(1), 25.

Aristorenas v. Comcare Health Services, O.J. No. 3647 (S.C.J.) (2004).

Bailey, T., Caulfield, T., & Ries, N. M. (2008). *Public health law and policy in Canada* (2nd ed.). Toronto, ON: LexisNexis.

Bauer (Litigation Guardian of) v. Seager, M.J. No. 356 (Q.B.) (2000).

Canada Health Act, R.S.C., 1985, c. C-6

Canadian Nurses Association. (2000). Telehealth: Great potential or risky terrain? *Nursing Now, 9,* 1–4.

Canadian Nurses Protective Society. (1994). Consent to treatment: The role of the nurse. *InfoLaw, 3*(2), 1.

Canadian Nurses Protective Society. (1998). Vicarious liability. *InfoLaw, 7*(1).

Canadian Nurses Protective Society. (2002). Obstetrical nursing. *InfoLaw, 11*(1).

Canadian Nurses Protective Society. (2004a). Consent for the incapable adult. *InfoLaw, 13*(3), 1–2.

Canadian Nurses Protective Society. (2004b). Negligence. *InfoLaw, 3*(1).

Canadian Nurses Protective Society. (2007a). Malpractice lawsuits. *InfoLaw, 7*(2).

Canadian Nurses Protective Society. (2007b). Operating room nursing. *InfoLaw, 16*(1).

Canadian Nurses Protective Society. (2007c). Quality documentation: Your best defence. *InfoLaw, 1*(1).

Canadian Nurses Protective Society. (2008). Telephone advice. *InfoLaw, 6*(1).

College of Nurses of Ontario. (2009). *Practice guideline: Telepractice.* Toronto, Canada: Author.

Crits v. Sylvester, 1 D.L.R. (2d) 502 at 508 (Ont. C.A.) (1956).

Croutch (Guardian ad litem of) v. B.C. Women's Hospital & Health Centre (2001) B.C.J. No. 1430 (S.C.), *aff'd,* B.C.J. No. 2029 (C.A.) (2003).

Ewert v. Marshall, B.C.J. No. 114 (S.C.) (2009).

Gall, G. L. (2004). *The Canadian legal system.* Scarborough, ON: Carswell.

Gemoto v. Calgary Regional Hospital Authority, A.J. No. 1278 (Q.B.) (2006).

Granger (Litigation Guardian of) v. Ottawa General Hospital, O.J. No. 2129 (Gen. Div.) (1996).

Hardingham, L. (2000). Meeting nursing practice standards. *Alberta RN,* 56(1).

Keane v. Craig, O.J. No. 2160 (S.C.) (2000).

Keatings, M., & Smith, O. (2010). The Canadian legal system. In M. Keatings & O. Smith (Eds.), *Ethical and legal issues in Canadian nursing* (pp. 87–119). Toronto, ON: Mosby.

Kerr, L. L., & Ross-Kerr, J. C. (2003). The practising nurse and the law. In J. C. Ross-Kerr & M. J. Wood (Eds.), *Canadian nursing: Issues and perspectives* (4th ed., pp.195–228). Toronto, ON: Mosby.

Kuz, K. M. (2006). Young teenagers providing their own surgical consents: An ethical-legal dilemma for perioperative Registered Nurses. *Canadian Operating Room Nursing Journal,* 24(2), 6–8, 10–11, 14–15.

Picard, E., & Robertson, G. (2007). *Legal liability of doctors and hospitals in Canada.* Toronto, ON: Carswell.

Poole Estate v. Mills Memorial Hospital, B.C.J. No. 635 (S.C.) (1994).

Skeels Estate v. Iwashkiw, A.J. No. 666 (Q.B.) (2006).

Tapp, A. (1999). Defamation actions. *The Canadian Nurse,* 95(3), 49–50.

ter Neuzen v. Korn, 10 W.W.R. 1 (S.C.C.) (1995).

Toews v. Weisner, B.C.J. No 30 (S.C.) (2001).

Wade, S. (2009). Documentation. *Nursing BC,* 41(3), 28–30.

Wilson v. Swanson, 5 D.L.R. (2d) 113 (S.C.C.) (1956).

Nursing Organizations: Nursing Leadership in Action

MICHAEL J. VILLENEUVE AND JOAN I. J. WAGNER

Katie is a senior nursing student completing her final semester of study in a four-year Bachelor of Science in Nursing (BScN) program in Ontario. She is in a preceptor placement in a local hospital on an acute care unit and is hoping to be hired in the same hospital following graduation in a few weeks. She loves the clinical area and patients but notices that there is a lot of fatigue among the nurses who are working consistently high levels of overtime. More worrying to her, she thinks their fatigue is contributing to errors in patient care. In doing some scanning, she finds that this problem is not uncommon and has been reported in other units across Canada caring for the same kinds of patients. Upset with the situation, for her final assignment, she drafts a letter to the Canadian Nurses Association (CNA), urging them to take action on this unsafe and unprofessional situation.

CHAPTER OBJECTIVES

By the end of this chapter, you will be able to:

1. Identify the roles of leadership, management, and mentorship for nurses.
2. Reflect on the roles of leadership, management, and mentorship for students.
3. Classify major leadership theories as relationally-focused or task-focused leadership styles.
4. Discuss how nurse leaders promote healthy work environments.
5. Envision how nurse leaders address health inequities.
6. Differentiate between the mandates, roles, and purposes of the national professional, regulatory, and union organizations for registered nurses.
7. Explain how membership in a national professional organization for nurses can benefit the individual nurse and the nursing profession.
8. Describe strategies that student nurses can engage in to learn more about the roles of the provincial regulatory bodies.

KEY TERMS

Accreditation A quality assurance process. In Canada, accreditation of undergraduate nursing programs is the role of the Canadian Association of Schools of Nursing (CASN).

Leadership The process of pursuing and influencing the thoughts, feelings, and behaviours of others regarding a course of action.

Licensed Practical Nurse The regulated category of licensed practical nurses in all Canadian jurisdictions including Ontario, where the category is titled *registered practical nurse*.

Management Directing and leading others to meet desired outcomes in the workplace through the effective and efficient use of resources. As a nurse in a management role, this may include planning and organizing the work of nurses on your unit, planning for adequate staffing, and managing the unit's financial resources.

Nursing Association/Organization A group of nurses who come together for a common purpose. This purpose may include political

action, advocacy, and professional development opportunities for its membership. In some associations, membership is voluntary and in other associations membership may be mandatory.

Registered Nurse The category of general nurses regulated in all Canadian jurisdictions.

Registered Psychiatric Nurse The category of psychiatric nurses that focus on mental and developmental health, regulated in Canada's four western provinces and Yukon.

Registration The formal entry point for graduates of approved educational programs in nursing into the profession of nursing in Canada. The regulatory bodies in each province require graduates to successfully pass a registration examination as part of the entry to practice requirements. Acceptance into the professional body also requires compliance with the regulations that govern the profession of nursing.

Nursing Leadership, Management, and Mentorship

A nursing leader can be any nurse who has the courage to fulfill a vision focused on achieving goals or outcomes related to the provision of quality health care. This courage to lead others comes from passion, not position. Farias (2009) speaks about the study of **leadership** as "the study of how men and women guide us through adversity, uncertainty, hardship, disruption, transformation, transition, recovery, new beginnings, and other significant challenges. It's also the study of how men and women, in times of constancy and complacency, actively seek to disturb the status quo and awaken new possibilities" (p. 13).

As a graduate nurse, you will be a leader in the provision of patient care. As the health-care provider who is with the patient around the clock in the hospital, or, alternatively, the provider who routinely supports and monitors the community patient within his or her home, you are designated as a patient or client advocate. Who better knows the needs of the patient? A knowledgeable nurse who is passionate about patient and client care provides crucial leadership to the health-care team and contributes to the optimal health and well-being of care recipients.

As a student leader, you also play a critical role in the provision of quality patient and client care. Who better than you, the student, to inform the educational processes that lead to the graduation of knowledgeable and professional nurses? For example, your feedback on courses, assignments, and clinical practices through the completion of course evaluations is essential for the continued improvement of nursing education. In addition, your leadership on committees where students gather side by side with faculty actively contributes to the nursing education processes. Your participation in various student association activities is vital to your professional growth as a nursing student and, eventually, as a graduate nurse. The collective voices of student associations play a powerful role in shaping the nursing educational environment.

Although leadership is not exclusive to **management** (officers, executive level professionals, and board members), leaders are frequently found in management positions; however, managers are not always leaders. Managers are appointed and given the authority to make all aspects of an organization run smoothly. Most often, visions are provided by the leaders but implemented by the managers. Management implementation of a vision often occurs through use of the five traditional management functions of planning, organization, commanding, coordinating, and controlling to achieve organizational objectives (MacLeod, 2012). Not everybody can be a manager, but anyone with vision and a passion to take action can be a leader.

You may ask yourself—"This all sounds wonderful, but how do I find the courage to be a leader?" Very few people are natural leaders. It is important that you look at the leaders around you. When you find a person with leadership traits that you truly admire, ask if he or she is willing to mentor you in the development of the leadership and management skills that you so admire. You will be surprised at his or her willingness to assist you. Mentoring is not a process of supervision and instruction; rather, it is a relational process of growth and development that requires the support and guidance of individuals with exemplary skills and abilities. Opportunities for formal and informal mentoring of staff are plentiful within most organizations—you just need to look for them.

Leadership Theories

Take a few minutes to research the phrase *leadership theory* on the Internet. You are sure to find many different leadership theories. These theories are grouped by some experts into three major categories, starting with the behavioural theories such as autocratic leadership, democratic leadership, and laissez-faire leadership from the 1930s; to assorted contingency and situational approaches; and, finally, to contemporary theories such as charismatic and transformational theories (Kelly & Crawford, 2008). As you look at the different theories, you will need to decide how to use them within your nursing practice. You are encouraged to take a critical look at Goleman's (1995) classic writings about emotional intelligence and use this knowledge to guide your choice of leadership theories. These writings suggest that we focus on the leader's relationship with followers, rather than on tasks. Later work by Goleman, Boyatzis, and McKee (2002) identifies four domains of emotional intelligence that help emotionally intelligent leaders to generate excitement, optimism, and passion among followers while also maintaining an atmosphere of cooperation and trust. Refer to the definitions of domains of emotional intelligence in Table 6.1.

TABLE 6.1	Definitions of Domains of Emotional Intelligence
Domain	**Definition**
Self-awareness	Leaders are aware of how their emotions affect themselves and their performance on the job.
Self-management	Leaders display self-control, transparency, and adaptability that are directed toward achievement.
Social awareness	Leaders display empathy and organizational awareness throughout their service to others.
Relational management	Leaders are change catalysts who manage conflict and encourage collaborative teamwork by inspiring, influencing, and developing others.

Source: Goleman, D., Boyatzis, R., & McKee, A. (2002). *The new leaders: Transforming the art of leadership into the science of results.* London, United Kingdom: Little, Brown.

You found multiple leadership theories during your Internet search, so now, how are you going to apply them to your nursing practice? Although it is important to familiarize yourself with the different approaches to leadership, you do not have to remember all the details of each theory to be a good leader. A simplified approach that identifies the organizational leadership as either relationally focused (emphasis on people and relationships to achieve the common goal) (Table 6.2) or task-focused (emphasis on tasks to be accomplished, or non-relationally focused) (Table 6.3) may help you along the path to understanding leadership theories. Many leaders match their leadership style with the characteristics of the situation, or in other words, use a contingency approach to leadership. Hibberd and Smith (2006) clarify this approach further stating, "The effectiveness of a leadership style is determined by the appropriateness of the style for the environment" (p. 378).

TABLE 6.2	Leadership Styles Classified as Relationally Focused
Leadership Style	**Description**
Transformational	Transformational leaders have four characteristics including idealized influence, inspirational motivation, intellectual stimulation, and idealized consideration. Transformational leaders are sensitive to the needs of others and change the organizational culture by realigning it with a new vision (Bass & Avolio, 1993).
Resonant	Relational energy is made evident by building relationships and managing emotion in the workplace (Cummings, 2004).
Individualized consideration	This leader is attentive to the needs of each staff member and supports individuals to reach their full potential (Avolio et al., 1999).
Servant	Robert Greenleaf proposed servant leadership as a way of life. The leader displays stresses service to others and recognizes that the role of organizations is to create people who can build a better tomorrow (Parris & Peachey, 2012).
Quantum	The leader is a change agent, anticipating change and communicating with others, guiding them to adapt and respond appropriately to prepare for the "unfolding reality." The leader is "a good signpost reader" (Porter-O'Grady & Malloch, 2011, p. 7)

Source: Cummings, G. G., MacGregor, T., Davey, M., Lee, H., Wong, C. A., Lo, E., . . . Stafford, E. (2010). Leadership styles and outcome patterns for the nursing workforce and work environment: A systematic review. *International Journal of Nursing Studies, 47*, 363–385.

TABLE 6.3	Leadership Styles Classified as Task-Focused
Leadership Style	**Description**
Management by exception	This leader focuses on appropriate completion of tasks to maintain current performance. Failure to adequately complete tasks requires correction (Avolio, Bass, & Jung, 1999).
Laissez-faire	Refers to leaders who are not concerned about organizational outcomes or follower behaviour. Leaders refuse to take responsibility to address important outcomes (Xirasager, 2008).
Transactional	These leaders tend to (1) clarify expected performance and provide rewards for good performance, (2) correct variations from the expected standard, and (3) work to prevent problems (Xirasager, 2008).
Dissonant	These leaders lack empathy, and tend to be negative, lacking emotional intelligence. Goleman et al. (2002) describes them as the "bosses people dread working for" (p. 30).
Passive avoidant	These leaders often avoid taking action, reacting with corrective action once problems have become serious (Avolio et al., 1999).
Instrumental	These behaviours are not values-based, rather they are focused on strategy and facilitation of work outcomes (Antonakis & Atwater, 2002).
Initiating structure	These leaders define individual's roles, focused on goal achievement and create clear communication channels (Judge, Piccolo, & Ilies, 2004).

Source: Cummings, G. G., MacGregor, T., Davey, M., Lee, H., Wong, C. A., Lo, E., . . . Stafford, E. (2010). Leadership styles and outcome patterns for the nursing workforce and work environment: A systematic review. *International Journal of Nursing Studies, 47*, 363–385.

Promoting Healthy Work Environments

We have introduced the characteristics of different types of leadership and how leadership style may vary according to the individual and/or the workplace environment, but we have not discussed how a nurse leader can support a healthy workplace. You will find that examination of the organization's vision, mission, and value statements provides you with a valuable picture of how each organization treats employees and patients or clients. These guiding statements reflect the values of the organization and provide the organizational community with a focus for the provision of health care (Hibberd & Smith, 2006). Therefore, as a nurse leader, your

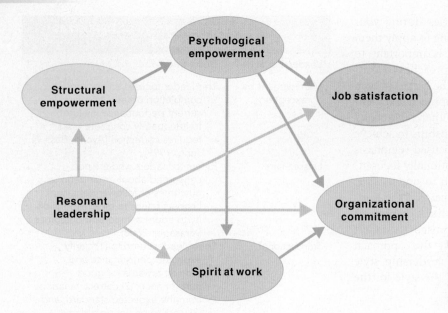

Figure 6.1   Relationships indicated in recent RN research (Wagner et al., 2010) between SAW (Kinjerski & Skrypnek), workplace empowerment theory (Laschinger, 2008, and resonant leadership (Cummings, 2004).

success will be measured according to the achievement of established goals or targets that are derived from the organization's vision, mission, and values.

Through the eyes of a nurse

We are in the process of computerizing all of our patient records. This new technology is requiring extra time and energy from us. Many RNs are staying overtime to complete their electronic charting. I am exhausted, and all I ever wanted to do was to get home to the kids; however, as a nurse leader, I felt that I needed to do something. So, last week I asked the unit manager if we could have an in-service on how to use the new system. She just didn't seem to be interested. This is so discouraging. What type of leadership is she providing?

(personal reflection of a nurse)

Understanding how to build healthy work environments that support health-care teams to deliver quality health services and, ultimately, achieve the organization's vision, mission, values, and goals is essential for your success as a leader (Pangman & Pangman, 2010). Canadian researcher, Dr. Heather Laschinger, brought a new perspective to workplace research when she studied Kanter's (1993, 1997) empowerment theory within the Canadian workplace (Havens & Laschinger, 1997). Her research and work are considered groundbreaking.

Research on workplace empowerment indicates a strong link between critical structural components and registered nurse (RN) positive work behaviours and attitudes, including increased job satisfaction and retention (Wagner et al., 2010). As a nurse leader, your attention to the four structural empowerment concepts: *support* from superiors, peers, and subordinates, which can take the form of

evaluations and informal comments; *information*, which refers to the knowledge and expertise required for the RN to work effectively; *resources*, which may refer to adequate staffing and appropriate equipment, supplies, and materials; and finally, the *opportunity* to learn and grow and experience a sense of challenge (Havens & Laschinger, 1997), will assist you to develop and maintain a healthy workplace (Fig. 6.1).

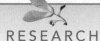

RESEARCH

RESONANT LEADERSHIP, WORKPLACE EMPOWERMENT AND SPIRIT AT WORK: IMPACT ON JOB SATISFACTION AND ORGANIZATIONAL COMMITMENT

Why should nurse leaders be interested in spirituality in the workplace? Spirit at work (SAW), with its four concepts of engaging work (individual's conviction that work is engaging), sense of community (feeling of trust and connectedness to coworkers), mystical experience (a feeling associated with energy and vitality), and spiritual connection (contributing to something larger than themselves) (Kinjerski & Skrypnek, 2004), provides nursing leaders with a wholistic measurement of the nurse work environment. Fostering spirituality in the workplace is proposed as a solution to the significant influences of nurse shortages, aging demographics, professional autonomy issues, restructuring, occupational health and safety issues (Jackson, Firtko, & Edenborough, 2007), and difficulties in professional and interprofessional relationships (Webber, 2009).

A theoretical model exploring the relationship between leadership, workplace empowerment, SAW, and workplace outcomes of job satisfaction and organizational commitment was tested using LISREL 8.80 and survey data from 148 randomly selected RNs from across the province of Alberta, Canada. The survey consisted of six questionnaires previously tested for reliability and a single open-ended question labeled "comments" at the end of the survey. This sample was representative of the provincial demographics, save for the significantly higher number of RNs in management and RNs with master or doctoral preparation within the survey data. The fit indices of the final model fit the observed data, or in other words, the proposed model described statistically significant relationships for this sample of RNs. This healthy workplace model indicates multiple significant relationships between concepts, with SAW receiving effects from resonant leadership, structural empowerment, and psychological empowerment while culminating in increased workplace commitment. The model shows that RNs experienced higher levels of SAW when they believed that they had a resonant leader and they felt empowered.

Recommendations coming out of the research included a suggestion that leaders ask RNs for their perceptions of SAW. Leaders can then tailor workplace changes to meet RNs needs. Management awareness of the relationship between workplace structures/processes and SAW can lead to health-promoting changes for both RN and patients alike. The model also indicates that select leadership actions optimize RN's perceptions of organizational commitment. Leaders are encouraged to use resonant leadership behaviours such as listen to staff feedback and act on staff concerns, focus on successes and potential, support and mentor teams and individuals, engage staff to work toward a shared vision, and promote RN autonomy. Managers had similar needs to staff, and they also required organizational and social support, information, and opportunities for education adequate resources within their workplace for job satisfaction to occur.

This study provides RNs and health-care leaders with information on which to base decisions related to evaluation and design of future workplaces. The research introduces SAW as a wholistic measure of the nurse's voice within the health-care setting. As nurses, we work to provide wholistic care to our patients; in turn, is it not appropriate that, as nurses, we practice within a healthy wholistic work environment?

Wagner, J., Cummings, G., Smith, D. L., Olson, J., & Warren, S. (2013). Resonant leadership, workplace empowerment and spirit at work: Impact on job satisfaction and organizational commitment for registered nurses. Canadian Journal of Nursing Research, 45(4), 1–16.

The Leader's Role in Addressing Health Inequities

In other chapters, you discovered that primary health care (PHC), with its focus on promoting health and preventing illness through interprofessional health-care teams, is regarded as the foundation for a health-care system that supports and promotes universal accessibility of essential health care to individuals and families across Canada and throughout the world (World Health Organization [WHO], 1978). Why do you think that experts describe PHC as supporting equitable access to health services by everybody, regardless of age, socioeconomic status, geographic location, or lifestyle (Cueto, 2004)? Nurses play an important role in PHC by providing leadership through interprofessional collaboration with health professionals, regulators, educators, and professional associations. Please read the CNA position statement on interprofessional collaboration (2011) for suggestions on how to work within a PHC team.

A growing awareness of the multiple factors or health determinants that influence the health of individuals within the larger population requires all sectors in society to collaborate on enhancing the health of the population as a whole. Because health-care systems do not exist in isolation from other social systems, it is important that, as nurses, we play a role in ensuring the presence of social policy that promotes equity for all (Starfield, 2011). Can you think of anybody better than a nurse to provide leadership in introducing and lobbying for promotion of the principles of population health throughout the global community? Who better than the nurse who stands beside the individual patient or client?

The Value and Purpose of Nursing Organizations

As you can see, nursing leaders do more than delegate, dictate, and direct others in clinical settings. Leadership involves helping others to reach for their highest potential.

Effective, modern nursing organizations represent a potentially important resource that can help shape a professional leadership orientation by nurses. There are many steps between presenting one's first paper at a chapter meeting of a regional nursing association and becoming a chief nurse, director of a home care company, or the minister of health. Our nursing organizations often serve as the testing ground for learning about political action and policy. They can help groom important practical skills such as honing public speaking, writing and publishing articles, and even teaching us how to behave as a member of a board of directors.

Nursing organizations and **nursing associations** bring nurses together for a common goal and purpose, which may include political action, advocacy, and professional development opportunities. At their best, nursing organizations and nursing associations nourish a long-term combination of social and professional interactions that can test, educate, support, motivate, and help sustain members over the course of a career. Among their many outcomes, effective organizations give focus to individual nurse leaders, leveraging their talents and influence to boost the leadership prestige and influence of the organization itself. Although nursing organizations and associations can groom, position, and boost individual nurse leaders, the most effective ones galvanize that energy to put a collective shine on themselves and on broader nursing profession leadership on any given set of issues.

History of Nursing Organizations in Canada

There are three regulated categories of nurses in Canada, totaling some 360,000 individuals. They can be found in clinical and management settings across the health system working with people who are sick, helping people to stay well, teaching in classrooms, conducting research, and developing public policy. **Registered nurses** are the category of general nurses, now increasingly baccalaureate-prepared in Canada and regulated in all Canadian jurisdictions. **Licensed practical nurses** are the category of nurses who hold a diploma in practical nursing and are regulated in all Canadian jurisdictions (including Ontario, where the category is *registered practical nurses*). **Registered psychiatric nurses** are the category of nurses that focus on mental and developmental health. They are regulated in Canada's four western provinces and the Yukon Territory. Canada's RNs (275,000), licensed or registered practical nurses (80,000), and registered psychiatric nurses (5,000) are spread across 6 time zones and 13 provinces and territories that make up the second largest nation on earth—and one of its least densely populated. Canadians are irregularly dispersed; for example, Nunavut alone is the size of Western Europe but is home to just 34,000. Some 80% of us live within about an hour's drive of the 6,400-km long border between Canada and the 48 lower U.S. states. If finding ways to come together to discuss (sometimes to discover) issues of common concern has been a major geopolitical challenge for nurses over the past century, then finding ways to modernize and move the profession forward has been an even bigger leadership hurdle.

Canada was just 26 years old when its first nursing association—the Society of Superintendents of Training Schools for Nurses of the United States and Canada—was established in 1893. That organization was the forerunner of today's CNA and Canadian Association of Schools of Nursing (CASN).

Society of Superintendents of Training Schools for Nurses

The Society of Superintendents of Training Schools for Nurses of the United States and Canada, established in 1893, was the first major nursing association in our country. Superintendents—the nursing school directors of their day—came together to tackle one of nursing's earliest serious challenges, and one that to some extent still haunts us. They realized that the vexing problem of multiple entry points into the nursing profession through widely varying kinds of education was coupling very early in nursing's history with the problem of defining just who could call themselves *nurses*. Remember, that organization predated nurse registration. These early nurse leaders understood that the public could be harmed—and the nursing profession tainted by association—when unqualified persons operated using the title *nurse*. Their organization (then called a *society*) represents our first attempt to talk about what nurses and nursing really mean, what the education should involve and where it should take place, and how we should designate the title *nurse*, so that the public has some assurance that it is dealing with a legitimately educated and tested professional. This first association was the mother of nursing regulation, advocacy and education in Canada and the United States.

Nursing Organizations Worldwide

Who in 1893 might have imagined that a few members under one association would explode to 360,000 Canadian nurses belonging to more than 100 national, provincial, and territorial associations and countless more nursing interest groups and local associations?

These numbers reflect just the major domestic nursing associations. To those, we must add all the other Canadian organizations to which nurses may belong (e.g., the Canadian Public Health Association) and then multiply the numbers by hundreds when we look at similar structures across other countries and myriad international structures such as the International Council of Nurses (ICN). One can quickly get lost in the vast number of organizations, their purposes and activities, and their relationship to nurses and nursing.

The Conundrum of Nursing Organizations

The tremendous proliferation of nursing organizations over the past century has served to develop and strengthen Canadian and international nursing. But for all the good that can come of them, there are many points of overlap, duplication of effort, gaps, strained funding, and sometimes a lack of effective impact. Further, because membership criteria keep some people out of groups, our efforts to come together can also push us apart. Having three regulated categories of nurses exacerbates the challenge. Many of these structures mirror Canada's perennial federal (or national), provincial, and territorial health system tussles. The political and policy challenges of a federated governance structure such as Canada's can play out in very similar ways among regulated professions such as nursing.

Why Have Nursing Organizations?

People come together in groups, clubs, and associations for all sorts of reasons—to share hobbies, solve problems in a systematic way, teach and learn, develop strategies to change something, and sometimes just to socialize with others around a common interest. Nursing's organizations exist for all these same reasons.

It is useful to take a step back and think about our nursing organizations. Why they were created? Do they work in the 21st century, and if so, how many of them are really needed?

At their best, organizations representing nurses or the profession can hone complex problems and concepts into punchy messages that capture the attention and imagination of the public, casting nurses as credible advocates and leaders. Among many benefits, they provide structure and forums for professional development, publication of research, and national discussion on issues of importance to nurses. For example, we might see nurse leaders speaking with the prime minister and federal minister of health during a meeting about the importance of strengthening the public health-care system. The existence of a credible, strong nursing association can help bring these sorts of expert voices together at one table in the interest of the public.

On the other hand, the existence of so many organizations may also blur the message of individual groups. Who really does speak for nursing? And where many claim to be the voice of nursing, whose messages carry weight and really bear attention? Too many poorly coordinated voices and messages can be as ineffective as none at all; they can even create a convenient excuse for some decision-makers to throw their hands up and choose to ignore nursing.

Professional Issues, Policy, Advocacy, and Regulation

The professional, public policy and advocacy sides of associations exist to represent nurses, advance the discipline and the profession, and advocate for health system policy changes. These are different mandates than those of unions; a discussion of unions appears later in this chapter. Historically, our national and provincial/territorial nursing associations held a mix of both professional and regulatory functions. Many are now moving away from those mixed mandates to having mostly (or only) a regulatory function. At the national level for RNs, CNA has always held a strong professional mandate and has been seeking ways to link with nurses in jurisdictions where the former professional association now has a solely regulatory function.

Special Cases

Ontario and British Columbia are different from their provincial counterparts; there are separate organizations for regulation and professional representation.

Ontario

Nurses must register with the College of Nurses of Ontario (the regulatory body) to practice, but the College is not a member of CNA. There are approximately 95,000 practicing RNs in Ontario, about 23,500 of whom are voluntary members of the Registered Nurses Association of Ontario (RNAO). There are also student members of RNAO. RNAO belongs to CNA, so its members are also part of CNA and ICN. Because the College of Nurses of Ontario is not a member of CNA, the 67,000+ RNs registered in Ontario who are not RNAO members also are not members of CNA or ICN.

British Columbia

There are approximately 36,000 practicing RNs registered with the College of Registered Nurses of British Columbia (the regulatory body), which withdrew from CNA in 2011. With the transition of professional representation to the Association of Registered Nurses of British Columbia, the College maintains universal fee collection and all members of the College remain members of CNA and, in turn, of ICN.

Categories of Nursing Associations and Organizations

Canada's myriad nursing organizations today can be categorized loosely around the traditional domains of nursing—that is to say, administration, clinical practice, education, policy and research. But the largest organizations, those focused on regulation and professional/advocacy issues, in some ways crosscut and impact all the domains of practice. The list rapidly starts to grow as we find many organizations existing at a national (or pan-Canadian) level as well as at provincial and territorial levels. To this mix of associations, we add unions, which also have national and provincial/territorial structures. And finally, some of these structures also exist for student nurses, licensed practical nurses, and registered psychiatric nurses.

Given this matrix of nursing roles and areas of interest, it is easy to imagine how the number of organizations very quickly grows to more than 100. Their names and purposes can be confusing to governments, the public, and even nurses ourselves. As we see in Table 6.4, there are nine overarching organizations that touch on nursing's traditional domains of practice; some have interests that relate to all the places nurses learn and practice. Box 6.1 lists the names of 39 more national organizations dedicated to specialty areas of nursing practice.

Let's take a look at the main national nursing organizations listed in Table 6.4. We briefly clarify their missions and objectives before we talk about what they mean to nursing, to the health-care system, and to your career.

The Canadian Nurses Association

CNA is Canada's oldest, continuous, pan-Canadian nursing organization. Established originally as the Canadian National Association of Trained Nurses in 1908, the name was modernized to CNA in 1924. Although nurses worldwide are familiar with the soaring career of Florence Nightingale, many Canadian nurses know little about Mary Agnes Snively, the founding president of CNA. She had such a giant influence on Canadian nursing that she is sometimes called the "mother of Canadian nursing." A founding member of ICN before CNA existed, Snively was the most influential figure in Canadian nursing in the first half of the 20th century.

TABLE 6.4	Major Pan-Canadian Registered Nurse Organizations by Domain of Nursing	
Domain of Nursing	Organizational Title	Year Founded
Administration	ACEN	1982
Culture	ANAC	Registered Nurses of Canadian Indian Ancestry, 1975; Indian and Inuit Nurses of Canada, 1983; Aboriginal Nurses Association of Canada, 1992
Education	CASN	Society of Superintendents of Training Schools for Nurses of the United States and Canada, 1893; CASN, 2002
	CNSA	Canadian University Nursing Students' Association, 1971; CNSA, 1992
Professional issues, health policy, and advocacy	CNA	Canadian National Association of Trained Nurses, 1908; CNA, 1924
Regulation: protecting the public	Canadian Council of Registered Nurse Regulators	2011
	CNA	Canadian National Association of Trained Nurses, 1908; CNA, 1924
Research and history	CANR	1986
	Canadian Association for the History of Nursing	1987
Unionization: representing nurses	CFNU	National Federation of Nurses Unions, 1981; CFNU, 1999

CNA is the "national professional voice of registered nurses . . . [advancing] the practice and profession of nursing to improve health outcomes and strengthen Canada's publicly funded, not-for-profit health system" (CNA, 2013a, "CNA's Goals," para. 2). To that end, the goals of CNA's external work are to

- Promote and enhance the role of RNs to strengthen nursing and the Canadian health system.
- Shape and advocate for healthy public policy provincially/territorially, nationally, and internationally.
- Advance nursing leadership for nursing and for health.
- Broadly engage nurses in advancing nursing and health.

Think In 2011, CNA launched the first National Expert Commission led by nurses. After commissioning three research syntheses, undertaking public polling, conducting background research, and consulting in person with Canadians across the country, commissioners release a 9-point action plan in June 2012. What is your school doing to respond to the Commission? Your employer? Your government?

BOX 6.1	Pan-Canadian Registered Nurses Organizations for Specialty Nurses and Clinical Practice

Canadian Association for Enterostomal Therapy
Canadian Association for International Nursing
Canadian Association for Parish Nursing Ministry
Canadian Association for Rural and Remote Nursing
Canadian Association of Advanced Practice Nurses
Canadian Association of Burn Nurses
Canadian Association of Critical Care Nurses
Canadian Association of Hepatology Nurses
Canadian Association of Medical and Surgical Nurses
Canadian Association of Neonatal Nurses
Canadian Association of Nephrology Nurses and Technologists
Canadian Association of Neuroscience Nurses
Canadian Association of Nurses in AIDS Care
Canadian Association of Nurses in Hemophilia Care
Canadian Association of Nurses in Oncology
Canadian Association of Perinatal and Women's Health Nurses
Canadian Association of Rehabilitation Nurses
Canadian Council of Cardiovascular Nurses
Canadian Family Practice Nurses Association
Canadian Federation of Mental Health Nurses

Canadian Gerontological Nurses Association
Canadian Holistic Nurses Association
Canadian Hospice Palliative Care Association Nurses Interest Group
Canadian Nurse Continence Advisors Association
Canadian Nurses Interested in Ethics
Canadian Nurses for the Health and the Environment
Canadian Nursing Informatics Association
Canadian Nursing Students' Association
Canadian Occupational Health Nurses Association, Inc.
Canadian Orthopaedic Nurses Association
Canadian Pain Society Special Interest Group Nursing Issues
Canadian Respiratory Health Professionals
Canadian Society of Gastroenterology Nurses and Associates
Community and Hospital Infection Control Association
Community Health Nurses of Canada
Forensic Nurses' Society of Canada
National Association of PeriAnesthesia Nurses of Canada
National Emergency Nurses' Affiliation Inc.
Operating Room Nurses Association of Canada

These goals reflect the complex mix of professional and regulatory activities that have shaped Canadian nursing for a century. CNA gave rise over the years to all our other modern nursing organizations, and it remains the only national association with the capacity and credibility to stand as the steward of professional Canadian nursing. CNA members automatically become members of ICN, where CNA sits for Canada on the Council of National Representatives.

Katie describes the clinical situation on her unit in a letter to the nursing policy department at CNA. She receives a helpful response, in which she is reminded that although CNA is deeply concerned about the issue and pleased Katie reported it, the national body has no authority when it comes to intervening in jurisdictional issues at the level of a province or territory and cannot become involved in a care delivery issue within an institution. Katie learns that she needs to tackle the problem on three fronts: by involving her union, her professional association, and most importantly, the regulatory body—in this case, the College of Nurses of Ontario.

The Canadian Federation of Nurses Unions: Representing Nurses

Stand-alone nurses unions are relatively new players on the scene, emerging only during the 1970s. Some of the functions of today's unions were previously embedded in the roles of organizations such as CNA. To some degree, they remain unique among unions, sometimes being accorded a special status because they represent only one category of worker: nurses. Differing from other unions, nurses' unions must conduct all negotiations, job actions, and resolution of grievances related to their members with a keen eye on the impacts of their decisions on human beings to whom nurses deliver services.

Labour relations and working conditions were early policy concerns for CNA and indeed remain an important part of its work today. But through the 20th century, CNA also took stands against the idea of unions and the right to strike—even implying in a 1970s version of its code of ethics that striking was unethical. The Canadian Federation of Nurses Unions (CFNU) now represents 136,000 nurses from eight provincial unions (Table 6.5) plus 25,000 student members of the Canadian Nursing Students' Association (CNSA) (CFNU, 2013) and is a respected leader in all national discussions of nursing practice. In tandem with its focus on the working condition of nurses, CFNU is a vigorous and effective national advocate for safe patient care, the public medicare system, and a broad range of other social justice issues. Although there certainly is some overlap across the organizations (e.g., in the area of research), with the founding of the national union organization and its focus on representing the working conditions concerns of nurses, CNA now focuses on professional representation, policy advocacy, and regulatory policy and does not involve itself in labour relations or negotiations.

Canadian Council of Registered Nurse Regulators

The Canadian Council of Registered Nurse Regulators (CCRNR) is a new organization that includes representatives of the "12 provincial/territorial bodies that regulate

TABLE 6.5	Unions for Registered Nurses	
Jurisdiction	Name	Year Founded
National	CFNU	The National Federation of Nurses Unions, 1981; CFNU, 1999
Alberta	United Nurses of Alberta	1977
British Columbia	British Columbia Nurses' Unions	1981
Manitoba	Manitoba Nurses' Union	Provincial Staff Nurses' Council, 1970; MB Organization of Nurses' Association, 1975; MB Nurses' Union, 1990
New Brunswick	New Brunswick Nurses Union	NB Association of RNs Provincial Collective Bargaining Council, 1968; the council becomes autonomous in 1971; NB Nurses Union, 1978
Newfoundland and Labrador	Newfoundland and Labrador Nurses' Union	Newfoundland and Labrador Nurses' Union, 1974
Nova Scotia	Nova Scotia Nurses' Union	1976
Ontario	Ontario Nurses' Association	1973
Prince Edward Island	Prince Edward Island Nurses' Union	Provincial Collective Bargaining Committee of the Association of Nurses of PE, 1974; PE Nurses' Union, 1987
Quebec	Fédération interprofessionnelle de la santé du Québec	Grew out of the United Nurses Union and United Nurses Federation
Saskatchewan	Saskatchewan Union of Nurses	1974

the practice of registered nurses" in Canada (CCRNR, 2013b, para. 1). It was established to "promote excellence in professional nursing regulation and serve as a national forum and voice regarding interprovincial/territorial, national and global regulatory matters for nursing regulation" (CCRNR, 2013a, para. 1).

For most of the past century, the national voice in regulatory policy came from CNA, which has a lengthy record in establishing or helping to develop standards for Canadian nursing education, testing, and regulation. CNA's letters patent state that one of its objects is "to promote profession-led regulation in the public interest" (CNA, 2013, p. v). This aspect of CNA's leadership is about protecting the public, which is the purpose of regulation, from trucking standards, to food safety, to knowing what it means when someone says, "I am a registered nurse," whether they are in Cape Breton, Windsor, or Yellowknife.

CNA is the original home of the Canadian Registered Nurse Examination, the written test all nurses must pass to use the title registered nurse and to practice in Canada.

However, after 2015 CNA's relationship to licensing will change in most jurisdictions. CCRNR has chosen to use the NCLEX-RN exam, administered by the National Council of State Boards of Nursing in the United States, as the examination all future nurses will have to pass in order to practice in Canada (Table 6.6).

Regulation

Regulation is sometimes an area of confusion for nurses. Each nurse who graduates from a nursing education program must be further tested through the provincial regulator where he or she wants to practice to show that he or she has the knowledge to meet a set of standards that grant him or her the privilege to use the title *registered nurse*. Those regulatory bodies, often called *colleges*, exist to protect the public, not to advocate for nurses. They simply establish, and then apply, standards of practice so that care will be of high quality and consistent across practice settings and borders. RNs must register to practice in each province and territory (Table 6.7), and as

TABLE 6.6	Regulatory and Professional Associations for Registered Nurses	
Jurisdiction	Name	Year Founded
National	CNA	Canadian National Association of Trained Nurses, 1908; CNA, 1924
	CCRNR	2011
Alberta	College and Association of Registered Nurses of Alberta	AB Association of Graduate Nurses, 1916; AB Association of RNs, 1921; College and Association of RNs, 2005
British Columbia	Association of Registered Nurses of British Columbia	Graduate Nurses Association of BC, 1912; RN Association of BC, 1918; College of RNs of BC, 2005; Association of RNs of BC, 2012
	College of Registered Nurses of British Columbia	2005
Manitoba	College of Registered Nurses of Manitoba	MB Association of Graduate Nurses, 1906; MB Association of RNs, 1913; College of RNs of MB, 2001
New Brunswick	Nurses Association of New Brunswick	NB Association of Graduate Nurses, 1916; NB Association of RNs, 1957; Nurses Association of NB, 1984
Newfoundland and Labrador	Association of Registered Nurses of Newfoundland and Labrador	Newfoundland Graduate Nurses Association, 1916; Association of RNs of NL, 1954
Northwest Territories and Nunavut	Registered Nurses Association of Northwest Territories and Nunavut	RN Association of NT, 1975; RN Association of NT and NU, 2004
Nova Scotia	College of Registered Nurses of Nova Scotia	Graduate Nurses Association of NS, 1910; RNs' Association of NS, 1926; College of RNs of NS, 2002
Ontario	College of Nurses of Ontario	1963
	Registered Nurses Association of Ontario	Graduate Nurses Association of ON, 1904; RNs Association of ON, 1927
Prince Edward Island	Association of Registered Nurses of Prince Edward Island	1911
Québec	L'Ordre des infirmières et infirmiers du Québec (OIIQ)/The Order of Nurses of Québec	l'Association des infirmières diplômées de la province de Québec/Association of Graduate Nurses of Québec, 1917; OIIQ/Order of Nurses of Québec, 1974
Saskatchewan	Saskatchewan Registered Nurses Association	1917
Yukon Territory	Yukon Registered Nurses Association	YT Nurses Society, 1982; YT RNs Association, 1992

TABLE 6.7	Regulatory and Professional Associations for Licensed Practical Nurses (LPNs)	
Jurisdiction	Name	Year Founded
National	Canadian Council for Practical Nurse Regulators	2004
Alberta	College of Licensed Practical Nurses of Alberta	AB Certified Nursing Aide Association, 1961; AB Association of Registered Nursing Assistants, 1978; College of LPNs of AB, 2003
British Columbia	College of Licensed Practical Nurses of British Columbia Licensed Practical Nurses Association of British Columbia	Council of LPNs of BC, 1991; College of LPNs of BC, 1996
Manitoba	College of Licensed Practical Nurses of Manitoba	MB Association of LPNs, 1945; College of LPNs of MB, 2001
New Brunswick	Association of New Brunswick Licensed Practical Nurses	Association of NB Registered Nursing Assistants, 1965; regulatory responsibilities added in 1977; Association of NB LPNs, 2002
Newfoundland and Labrador	College of Licensed Practical Nurses of Newfoundland and Labrador	1984
Northwest Territories	Registrar for Licensed Practical Nurses, Health and Social Services Government of the Northwest Territories	No professional association exists at the time of this writing.
Nova Scotia	College of Licensed Practical Nurses of Nova Scotia	Practical Nurses Licensing Board, 1957; LPNs Association of NS merged with the Board in 2001–2002; College of LPNs of NS, 2002
Nunavut	Nunavut Department of Human Resources/Health	No professional association exists at the time of this writing.
Ontario	College of Nurses of Ontario	1963
	Registered Practical Nurses Association of Ontario	ON Association of Registered Nursing Assistants, 1958; Registered Practical Nurses Association of ON, 1993
Prince Edward Island	Licensed Practical Nurses Association of Prince Edward Island Prince Edward Island Licensed Practical Nursing Registration Board	Association founded 1999
Quebec	Ordre des infirmières et infirmiers auxiliaires du Québec	Commission of LPN Schools founded 1951. Quebec Assoc of LPNs founded in 1960. The 2 merged in 1964.
Saskatchewan	Saskatchewan Association of Licensed Practical Nurses	Sask Nursing Assistants Assoc 1957 founded.
Yukon Territory	Registrar for Nursing Assistants, Justice Service Division, Yukon Government	No professional association exists at the time of this writing.

noted earlier, with the exception of Ontario, they then automatically become members of CNA and ICN.

Canadian Association of Schools of Nursing

Splitting off from the original group that included both Canada and the United States, the Canadian Society of Superintendents of Training Schools for Nurses was established in 1907. More correctly reflecting its real purpose (i.e., a focus on nursing education, not its superintendents), the organization's name was changed in 1917 to the Canadian Association of Nursing Education (CANE). The organization was merged into CNA in 1924 where a new department for nursing education was created. That structure remained in effect until 1942 when the Provisional Council of University Schools and the Departments of Nursing were created. The Council became the Canadian Association of University Schools of Nursing in 1971, and then CASN in 2002 when the organization admitted the original diploma schools (by then largely affiliated with university degree-granting programs.)

The CASN mission is to be "the national voice for nursing education, research, and scholarship" representing baccalaureate and graduate nursing programs in Canada. Its overarching objective is "to lead nursing education and nursing scholarship in the interest of healthier Canadians" (CASN, 2013, para. 1). The organization lists 92 schools of nursing as its members along with four regional affiliate members. A core part of CASN's business lies in the accreditation of Canada's nursing education programs, which it has led since 1987; a new accreditation program was established in 2005. **Accreditation** is a process that assures certain standards, outcomes, and quality are met in an education program, a health-care delivery setting, or a business. In many cases, accreditation is a voluntary process, but because of the perceived prestige of accreditation, many programs and businesses see it as essential to their success.

Canadian Nursing Students' Association

Canadian nursing students have their own national association—the Canadian Nursing Students' Association (CNSA). Welcoming RN, licensed practical nurse, and registered psychiatric nurse students as members, CNSA is still the only national nursing association integrating all three regulated categories. With some 25,000 members, CNSA represents the voice and "interests of nursing students to federal, provincial, and international governments and to other nursing and health care organizations" (CNSA, 2013, para. 2). Increasingly strategic over the years, CNSA is an affiliate member of CNA (where in 2008, it gained a nonvoting position on the board of directors) and an associate member of CFNU. As of 2013, CNSA is a full voting member of the CNA board of directors. It maintains a close relationship with CASN and serves as cochair of the New Health Professionals Network. Read more on CNSA in Chapter 7.

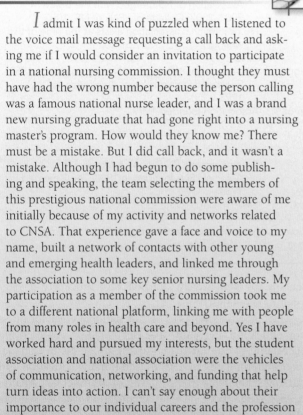

Through the eyes of a student

I admit I was kind of puzzled when I listened to the voice mail message requesting a call back and asking me if I would consider an invitation to participate in a national nursing commission. I thought they must have had the wrong number because the person calling was a famous national nurse leader, and I was a brand new nursing graduate that had gone right into a nursing master's program. How would they know me? There must be a mistake. But I did call back, and it wasn't a mistake. Although I had begun to do some publishing and speaking, the team selecting the members of this prestigious national commission were aware of me initially because of my activity and networks related to CNSA. That experience gave a face and voice to my name, built a network of contacts with other young and emerging health leaders, and linked me through the association to some key senior nursing leaders. My participation as a member of the commission took me to a different national platform, linking me with people from many roles in health care and beyond. Yes I have worked hard and pursued my interests, but the student association and national association were the vehicles of communication, networking, and funding that help turn ideas into action. I can't say enough about their importance to our individual careers and the profession at large.

(personal reflection of a nursing student)

Academy of Canadian Executive Nurses

The Academy of Canadian Executive Nurses (ACEN) was founded in 1982 to share support and information among senior nurse executives. To date, it is the only Canadian nursing organization dedicated to leadership development of executives and other senior leaders (e.g., deans, senior researchers) in settings where research is an important part of the organization's mandate. In 2013, ACEN broadened its mandate to include influencing health-care policy and aligning and advancing the national nursing practice, education, research, and leadership agendas. Membership is voluntary and members receive the quarterly *Canadian Journal of Nursing Leadership*. The Academy is an associate member of CNA.

Aboriginal Nurses Association of Canada

Originally called Registered Nurses of Canadian Indian Ancestry, today's Aboriginal Nurses Association of Canada (ANAC) was founded in 1975 "to improve the health of Aboriginal people, by supporting Aboriginal Nurses and by promoting the development and practice of Aboriginal Health Nursing" (Aboriginal Nurses Association of Canada [ANAC], 2013, para. 1). The organization has members across the country, strives to influence Aboriginal health and healing, and hosts an annual conference to share research and practice issues relevant to Aboriginal nurses, nursing, and health.

Canadian Association for Nursing Research

The Canadian Association for Nursing Research (CANR) was established in 1986 to "foster research-based nursing practice and practice-based nursing research" (Canadian Association for Nursing Research [CANR], 2013, para. 2). Among its stated objectives are to provide information about research, strengthen linkages between research and education, administration, and clinical practice and educate educating professionals and the public about the significance of the nursing research–practice partnership (CANR, 2013). Members receive the quarterly *Canadian Journal of Nursing Research*. Established in 1987, the Canadian Association for the History of Nursing promotes interest in the history of nursing and strives to develop scholarship in this domain of nursing. Both organizations hold associate member status in CNA.

After speaking with the CNA staff, Katie brings their response to the attention of her clinical instructor and the patient care manager. The patient care manager provides good advice, suggesting that because there has been no major safety incident, before getting the college of nurses involved, first look at what can be done to prevent one from happening. She calls together a meeting of the patient safety and quality officer in the hospital with several of the senior staff, and the students on the unit where Katie presents her concerns, actions, and findings to date. Katie is surprised to learn that the nurses who seemed silent on the issue were very concerned about it; they were just too tired fighting the issue to keep talking about it and had given up trying.

Specialty Nurses and Clinical Practice

Canada is home to 39 national organizations focused on specialty nurses and a wide range of areas of clinical practice (refer to Table 6.4). These are the closest of all groups to the nurse–patient interface. They tend to have strong mandates around focused clinical care issues or areas of practice. Generally, they provide education, advocacy, and support to the nurses who practice in these areas across Canada. Many are involved in developing specialty standards of care and also hold an interest advocacy related to their respective areas of human health. For example, the Canadian Council of Cardiovascular Nurses promotes "the health and well-being of Canadians through standards, research, education, health promotion, specialty certification, advocacy and strategic alliances" (Canadian Council of Cardiovascular Nurses, 2013, "CCCN's Mission," para. 1). Apart from its emphasis on nursing excellence, the Canadian Association of Nurses in AIDS Care promotes "the health, rights and dignity of persons affected by HIV/AIDS" (Canadian Association of Nurses in AIDS Care [CANAC], 2013, para. 1).

Other than CNA, CFNU, and CNSA, some of these groups are larger in membership than our other national associations. And mirroring other federated structures, many of them are associated with provincial and territorial specialty associations and chapters—another layer of nursing groups in the mix. A number of them are associated with international associations, conferences, and journals related to their respective specialties; the World Federation of Neuroscience Nurses, for example, claims 15 member organizations across 32 nations having some 5,000 members.

Currently, the specialty groups all maintain status as associate members of CNA (CNA, 2013c). Nineteen specialty groups offer certification examinations within the CNA program—an indicator "to patients, employers, the public and professional licensing bodies that [the nurse is] qualified, competent and current in a nursing specialty/area of nursing practice" (CNA, 2013b, para. 1). In a world of increasing specialization, an important function for many of the national associations now lies in the development of these specialty credentials.

Some of the organizational structures around registered nursing emerged in the history of Canada's other regulated categories of nurses. Nearly 80,000 in number (Canadian Institute for Health Information, 2013), Canada's licensed practical nurses (74,000+), and registered psychiatric nurses (5,100+) also have a matrix of regulatory, professional, union, and other organizations with which they are affiliated. We take a look here at the largest of these.

Licensed Practical Nurses

The Canadian Council for Practical Nurse Regulators (see Table 6.7) was established in 2004 to "provide leadership in practical nurse regulation" (Canadian Council for Practical Nurse Regulators [CCPNR], 2011, "Our Mission," para. 1) and "support excellence in practical nursing from a public policy perspective" (CCPNR, 2011, "Our Vision," para. 1). The Council's members include provincial regulators in Alberta, British Columbia, Manitoba, New Brunswick, Newfoundland and Labrador, Nova Scotia, Prince Edward Island, and Saskatchewan. Similar to the situation with RNs, licensed practical nurses in Quebec are not members of the national licensed practical nurse organization. The professional counterpart to the Council, established originally as the Canadian Practical Nurses Association in 1975, was dissolved during the past decade.

Registered Psychiatric Nurses

Canada's registered psychiatric nurses have regulatory, professional, union, and other needs just like the other categories of nurses and have created organizations to meet them (Table 6.8). At the national level, the Registered Psychiatric Nurses of Canada "provides a unified provincial, national and international voice for Canadian registered psychiatric nurses with a vision to provide quality mental health services for all Canadians" (Registered Psychiatric Nurses of Canada,

TABLE 6.8	Regulatory and Professional Associations for Registered Psychiatric Nurses (RPNs)	
Jurisdiction	Name	Year Founded
National	Registered Psychiatric Nurses of Canada	Canadian Council of Psychiatric Nurses, 1951; Psychiatric Nurses Association of Canada, 1960; RPNs of Canada, 2001
Alberta	College of Registered Psychiatric Nurses of Alberta	AB Psychiatric Nurses Association, 1950; Psychiatric Nurses Association of AB, 1963; Registered Psychiatric Nurses Association of AB, 1988; College of Registered Psychiatric Nurses of AB, 2005
British Columbia	College of Registered Psychiatric Nurses of British Columbia	Founded 1947 as the BC Psychiatric Nurses Association.
Manitoba	College of Registered Psychiatric Nurses of Manitoba	1960
Saskatchewan	Registered Psychiatric Nurses Association of Saskatchewan	Founded in 1948 as Sask Psychiatric Nurses Association
Yukon	Office of the Registrar of Registered Psychiatric Nurses, Consumer Services, Government of the Yukon	YT regulates RPNs through the four provincial regulators; no professional association as of this writing

2013, para. 1). Its member associations from Alberta, British Columbia, Manitoba, and Saskatchewan hold mixed regulatory and professional mandates, much as registered nursing associations have done through most of the past century. At one time, during the mid-1970s, the organization also had individual members in Nova Scotia, Ontario, and the Northwest Territories. In 1983, the association was reorganized so that the four western provincial associations became the members. Most recently, Yukon proclaimed legislation of registered psychiatric nurses in that territory.

Katie was referred by CNA to two important groups: the jurisdictional member of CNA in Ontario, RNAO, and the associated member nurses working in her clinical specialty. From RNAO, she learns about two different "best practice guidelines" that could apply to her clinical unit, and from the specialty nurses, she learns more about a whole group of nurses who are worried about the very same problem on their unit in Alberta. She also learns that a rigorous study of care of these patients is already underway in Arizona. Katie meets with the union representative for the unit—a senior nurse who is a long-standing member of the Ontario Nurses Association, the provincial jurisdictional member of CFNU. She is directed to the CFNU website, where Katie discovers a wealth of information about nursing working conditions, even finding some that apply to her specific kind of situation. She contacts the national office only to find out that CNA and CFNU are in the process of launching together a special national project focused on ramping up patient safety and quality in response to the National Expert Commission. The team is thinking ahead to finding test sites, and soon, Katie and her patient care manager are involved in discussions about whether the problem on their unit can be tested as part of a national demonstration project that weaves patients' safety with quality in nursing working conditions.

Complexities and Conflicts in Nursing: The World of Nursing Organizations

For better or worse, we have the nursing discipline and practice we see around us today because of the leadership of these organizations. Many of the things we think work well about nursing and its practice relate back in some way to the efforts of these groups, and they justifiably claim credit.

But just as we can point to links between nursing organizations and successes, some of the areas where we have concerns about nursing also link to the action—or inaction—of our nursing organizations. As noted earlier in this chapter, the number, style, membership, and funding of nursing organizations sometimes have had a constraining effect on the effectiveness of some of their initiatives. Sometimes, we simply have lagged too long in our responses, failed to step

out front in a leadership position, or been too averse to taking risks, clinging to the familiar even if not fully comfortable with it.

Still, long-standing troubles that dog nursing certainly cannot be placed fully at the feet of our nursing organizations. All sorts of dynamics are at play, sometimes many of them concurrently. For example, the best lobbying efforts and most compelling evidence can fall on deaf ears at the political level; the gender implications of nursing and the place of women in society should never be underestimated; and world events like the terrorist actions of September 11, 2001, the severe acute respiratory syndrome (SARS) and influenza A (H1N1) outbreaks, and the global economic upheaval beginning in late 2007 can quickly hijack attention away from even the most effective and best-planned strategies to influence policy. Nursing organizations and nurse leaders cannot be held to account for global events beyond their control.

Action and Strength From Crisis and Cutbacks: The Example of Canadian Nursing Association

The federal Office of Nursing Policy serves as an example of a success of the advocacy strategies of national-level groups such as CNA when they are functioning at their best. Nurses and nursing organizations had no influence over the dire warnings of groups such as the World Bank and International Monetary Fund in the early 1990s that led to federal decisions to rein in Canadian debts and deficits. And nurses were impacted along with many other public services in the tumultuous ensuing years wherein large chunks of funding were carved out of the health-care system. But having no influence on the World Bank does not mean that nursing organizations stood by in silence; they lobbied government agencies. But they did so in the context of an elected government that had made fairly clear its intentions to make major cuts.

Effective Nursing Lobbying Efforts

At the end of that fiscal crisis, Canada emerged with a robust economy, balanced and surplus budgets that were for a decade the envy of the world, and a banking system that withstood the economic recession of 2008–2010 that collapsed some other national economies. But getting there was very tough. Drastic cuts to health care began to play out in earnest by 1994 and 1995. However, some of the behind-the-scenes lobbying efforts of CNA were effective. Even as cuts were being made and budget deficits were successfully being reined in, plans were being formed for the ensuing phase of rebuilding. By the time of CNA's June 1998 convention, then federal minister of health, the Hon. Allan Rock, appeared before the audience to make his now-famous comment that health system cutbacks of the previous 5 years had been borne disproportionately on the backs of nurses. That kind of comment comes directly from a real understanding of the situation, arising from many hours of behind-the-scenes lobbying, meetings, letters, and quiet discussions by nursing organizations with political and policy staff.

Concurrent efforts were underway across the country with strong lobbies coming from groups such as RNAO, which had influenced the creation of Ontario's Nursing Task Force (1998), and first provincial chief nursing officer role, which was placed highly and effectively in the bureaucracy of Ontario's health ministry. Similar activities were taking place in most provinces and territories, with the result that by 2002, most provinces had some form of chief nursing officer role in place within the government—again, the result of effective nursing organization lobbying efforts.

At the 1998 CNA convention, the federal minister responded to the Quiet Crisis lobby in decisive ways. For example, he announced that a new federal Office of Nursing Policy would be created to position nurses more forcefully in the development of Canada's national nursing and health policy. In previous years, the federal principal nursing officer role did not have the status of a full office nor the resources to go with it. The role had been eliminated along with many other cuts in 1994. The resurrection of a nursing policy voice within Health Canada was an important signal to nursing organizations and the country's nurses. And to help strengthen the discipline itself, Minister Rock announced the creation of the 10-year, $25 million national nursing research fund.

National Nursing Strategy for Canada

Those efforts moved federal and provincial/territorial governments to generate the national Nursing Strategy for Canada (Advisory Committee on Health Human Resources, 2000), which gave rise to the Canadian Nursing Advisory Committee (2002), and they also funded the national nursing sector study (The Nursing Sector Study Corporation, 2006). For example, the federal government provided $8.9 million to CNA to lead the national project to establish and build the regulatory base for nurse practitioners—a seminal example of a mix of professional and regulatory policy functions working together at national and provincial/territorial levels to build a better health-care system. In fact, CNA would receive more than $30 million in funding in the decade 2000–2010 for an impressive roster of activities including its international policy and development programs.

Katie learns a bit more about nurse leaders because the CNA officer tells her about the body of work on safe, quality nursing practice settings by the federal Office of Nursing Policy in partnership with CNA over the past 12 years. Katie had never heard of the federal government chief nurse, and she finds now that work done by the office in tandem with nursing leaders nationally over a decade led to measurements of the quality of nursing working conditions being included among the indicators in the hospital accreditation program for the very place she is practicing.

In Partnership With Canadian Nursing Association

CNA's capacity and credibility began to attract important partnerships. Late in the decade, for example, ANAC asked CNA to partner in a project with CASN under Aboriginal leadership to strengthen cultural competency across Canadian nursing education. They did not come to CNA for funding but rather for its expertise and the credibility of its name.

Given that the national Nursing Research Fund of 1999 would come to its end in 2009, CNA took leadership of the effort to lobby for establishment of new funding beginning in 2007. CNA and the Canadian Nurses Foundation worked with national counterparts in what came to be called the "Consortium for Nursing Research and Innovation," including ACEN, CASN, and CANR. These sorts of efforts of nursing organizations are important to students because they include lobbying for scholarship and other funding for nursing education. However, severe funding challenges arose as a result of the global economic collapse of 2008–2009, and as yet, a new national nursing science fund has not been built.

Students in Nursing Organizations

Although all these organizations may seem quite distant to a nursing student, they are the forces that have shaped your education, the number of students sharing the classrooms around you, the clinical settings in which you test your knowledge, and the content of the examinations you will face until you escape into the world of professional nursing.

How Students Affect Change

Change often arises from the bottom up, despite the efforts of leaders to lead (or resist) it from the top down. And social movements often find their greatest energy among youth. Canada's nursing students are a political force to reckon with. Whether strategically or inadvertently, the courageous precedent set by CNSA when it included all categories of nurses among its members may have set the course for major shifts in the future. This is the first time, at the national level, where nurses in the three regulated groups share membership in one organization.

The decision of the students' association reflects language that became de rigueur during the 2000 decade—that is, a focus on teams, teamwork, and collaboration. This was not the first precedent set by students; in 1992, they were a decade ahead of their teachers in opening the old university nursing students' association to diploma students. And in the current decade, they are the first (and to date, only) group to truly integrate the principles of team functioning by integrating all students in programs leading to practice in one of the three regulated categories of nurses.

Implications for Students

Why does this matter to you as a student? In many other examples, the student world sometimes differs significantly from the world of work. Students who graduate from generalist programs are thrust into a world of work, where they are nearly always required to operate from the start in highly specialized clinical settings. For those who grow up in the increasingly integrated milieu and philosophy of CNSA during this decade, it may be an equally striking reality to graduate and find that nursing organizations and associations generally do not look and feel like student groups. The vast majority of our leading national and provincial associations remain starkly segregated by regulatory categories and roles. Even in the face of shrinking resources, they have not moved from using the language of teams and collaboration to actually turning it into action by reshaping the structures of organizations. Far from collapsing down the number of organizations or their structures over the past decade, new associations continue to emerge. The existing ones often do not sit on each other's boards, have not made their memberships more inclusive, and, in many ways, still compete for the attention of governments and decision-makers even within regulated categories.

These dynamics matter to nursing students: Our organizations shape the way all of us are licensed (or registered), our employment experiences, and the ways we deliver care—including what kind of care and with what team members. It is not overstating the case to say that in many ways, the behaviours of our organizations today will shape nursing careers through the coming decades.

Knowing these things, the question we must ask is how we want our organizations to look. How can we take hold of and sustain their best qualities while influencing them to let go of traditions that do not bring a modernizing, synergizing, quality-improving value to nurses, nursing, patients, and systems? What can you, as a student and soon a graduate, do to shape these organizations in ways that will better shape the kind of innovative and satisfying career you want to have in nursing?

Getting Involved

Creating change always means seeing a need and making a decision to get involved. First, although we all understand nursing as a series of caring services that we provide based on scientific knowledge, we also need to imagine nursing as a political act (Calnan, 2003). Although nursing may be expressed as a very intimate, one-on-one act of caring, the larger profession is a major political force for change in which we all have an obligation to act. This does not mean every nurse has to enter into political action in a formal way but rather to see himself or herself as an important actor in a movement much bigger than those important nursing services delivered at bedsides, in clinics, and in classrooms.

Think Join organizations representing people and topics you know, and where you can input and make a difference. But do more than that: It's just as important to join the ones that can teach you something new and help take you where you want to be in the future. If there is a leader you want to meet in any field, find out the organizations that person belongs to and go to one of their meetings, wedge yourself in through free offerings, and sit at the lunch table with the person you want to meet!

If we imagine our importance to the larger political action that nursing represents, then it's easy to imagine another important action you can take as a student: Join and participate in your student organization and other professional and advocacy organizations that welcome students. Many of them welcome students as members at a reduced (or even no) cost, and most of them offer reduced rates at their major meetings and conferences where you can start to build the support and professional networks that will introduce you to influential nurses and other leaders, enrich you personally, and help build your career. Many nursing organizations encourage and invite students to attend board meetings and annual general meetings as observers at no cost—these are terrific opportunities to start to expand your understanding of the breadth of activities going on and how associations are run and importantly, to meet and start to build networks of nurse leaders with whom you want to engage as a professional.

Look beyond nursing to other health and social organizations where your nursing voice may be linked with those of other professionals and the public. For example, at the time of writing of this chapter, Canada's Mental Health Commission has issued a call for members of a youth council—an opportunity for younger voices to merge into an effective and supported coalition. All such opportunities can fuel and inform your interest in political action and strategies to make change.

The Power of Membership

Linda Silas, president of CFNU, often speaks of the power of membership. As she words it, "information is power." The union constantly brings information and education to its members; the power of the union comes about when members are able to articulate its messages with credibility and passion (personal communication, January 8, 2010). Silas says, "you get out of it what you put into it." In the case of her union that can mean general education, negotiating skills, leadership training, and paid travel. Although she was talking specifically about her organization, the principles she outlines so well apply to any organization. Organizations must be seen as (and behave as) living things; they are not physical places, but they are people and members. They are sustained by our choice to join them. They carry out the activities we champion, condone, or merely tolerate. And they grow, change, and innovate when we participate in them, challenge them, help them, and work for them.

Strength in Numbers—But Weaknesses Too!

We have seen some examples of successes and challenges experienced by CNA and its partners. In some of these examples, it has been to the association's advantage to say it represents 149,000 nurses from 12 provinces and territories, and more than 40 associate and affiliate members; impressive numbers to be sure. But operations on a daily basis are a major challenge for many of those organizations.

Our federated structure, where health delivery and the regulation of health professions falls largely to provinces and territories, gave rise to its own roster of organizations—and here, challenges of disparities arise. In fact, disparity is in some ways a watchword when we think about the shape and population of our nation. The combined population of the four Atlantic provinces and all three territories (Statistics Canada, 2012), for example, is less than that of the Greater Toronto Area. The three northern territories combined support a population less dense than the city of Peterborough, Ontario. The size of nursing organizations and their membership vary widely across the country.

Complications of Funding

It is a very human response to create a group; humans often feel safer and supported when they come together. All those forces have given rise to the 100+ organizations mentioned in this chapter. But the reality is that very few of these organizations and associations have the membership, funding, and resources of the larger national groups such as CFNU or CNA or regulatory colleges in large provinces such as Ontario, British Columbia, or Alberta. Even at the national level, some groups have a few dozen paying members, and are run by volunteers, or a small paid staff, that can mean as little as one part-time person. Those realities do not augur well for success in their goals to influence the big game of national health system policy, to influence the public, or shape nursing practice. The challenges can be particularly hard on clinical specialty groups who rely solely on small numbers of working clinical nurses for their fiscal support and who may have little or no experience in the strange land of public policy.

Modernizing Organizational Structures

How long nurses can afford—or should attempt—to support this long list of organizations is unclear. With 360,000 nurses belonging to more than a hundred organizations, which among them is effective in meeting the visions and missions for which they were created? Whose messages are "right"? To which one(s) would you send an elected official in your city or province if they asked you for the latest information about some aspect of nursing or population health?

The motives of the nurses and leaders in all these groups are not an issue; they are all on a mission to make the world a better place for those coming after them. But, beyond minor tweaks, some of our organizational structures exist today pretty much as they did before there were cars and airplanes, telephones, and televisions. What must be on the table now is whether the time has come to have a very hard look at ourselves and our organizations. Is it time to make some tough decisions about whether nurses, patients, and systems might benefit by modernizing the structures we built to meet nursing's needs a century ago in favour of new ones that could streamline our ways of coming together and synergize our energies?

Future Directions for Nursing Organizations

We arrive in the present with a broad and solid base of nursing organizations representing nearly every possible facet of nursing's domains of practice spread across regulatory categories and across 14 national, provincial, and territorial jurisdictions. This remarkable legacy has been passed on to us by a century of leaders who built the profession we know today and who worked entire careers to shape its education, leadership, science base, and practice to make it relevant and safe. Our challenge is to take stock of the strengths of all these organizations and shape them so that they are able to take us efficiently in the directions we need nursing to go in this century.

Taking action in five areas could help instigate changes to take our nursing associations in stronger, more effective, and more sustainable directions going forward.

Streamlining

To overcome our geographic reality and federated structure, the vast numbers of Canadian nursing organizations need to be reshaped and streamlined to synergize the power of members currently spread sparsely in small nursing groups across the country. The sustainability of those organizations is uncertain, and their effectiveness could be better harnessed if coalesced into strategic coalitions. Imagine how much more effective a group of small organizations might be, even on a regional basis, if they came under one roof to share resources such as administrative staff, databases, and information technology while maintaining their own identities. Clearly, a leading-edge stance on the use of information and communication technologies to supplement or even supplant paper documents and large in-person meetings are essential in the modernization of our nursing associations.

Building Pan-Canadian Organizations

The distribution of membership within and across our major national associations must be addressed. For example, Quebec does not belong to the national professional associations of any of the categories of nursing. And of the nearly 262,000 Canadian RNs working in nursing, some 122,000 are not members of CNA nor are they members of ICN. Similar problems challenge licensed practical nurses and registered psychiatric nurses, where in both cases national membership leaves out major parts of the country.

Resolution of this problem is important to building truly pan-Canadian associations and may be triggered by CNSA's decision to admit all regulated categories as members. Perhaps, their integrated undergraduate experience in a national organization will equip them with the imagination and courage to help us resolve old hurts and geopolitical agendas to dream of a different future together.

Resetting Organizational Goals

Nursing organizations in every domain of practice must commit themselves to meeting the challenge of being an essential and active element in promoting and nourishing professional formation and leadership skills for individuals and translating that to effective policy leadership by the profession. They can do this by contributing to and then reinforcing skills provided in undergraduate and graduate programs; participating together to influence and support specialty training; and providing opportunities for nurses at all career stages to meet, talk, collaborate, support, and learn.

Active Roles in the National Agenda

Nursing organizations must be active participants in the health system transformation agenda. Regardless of mandate, our nursing organizations can and must show leadership and provide opportunities for members to take part meaningfully in transformations such as those recommended by the National Expert Commission (2012). And our organizations themselves must change too; they cannot stand still while the world around them is changing in direction and tone.

Focus on Multiprofessional Teams and Practice Settings

Transforming the health system; improving population health; and delivering safer, more effective health-care services demands that nurses be able to work effectively in multiprofessional teams and practice settings. Stand-alone nursing organizations can support these goals by (a) contributing to the formation of professional nursing knowledge sets and skills that build the profession-based confidence and skills of nurses to participate effectively in interprofessional teams and (b) providing interprofessional role modeling in some meeting and educational offerings (e.g., conferences).

Final Thoughts

Amelia Earhart said, "Create your future from your future, not your past." No less is demanded of nurse leaders and organizations today.

The roster of structures we built in the last century, many established before antibiotics were discovered, still serve us well in many ways. Yet, to be ever more relevant forces as we move ahead, we all need to think about the discipline and practice of nursing and about the leaders and organizations that will shape them. Some of the new ideas may seem radical. Organizational leaders have sometimes spoken out in informed and imaginative ways that did not always please their boards and irritated other players by being too provocative. Therein lies the difference between leadership in action and leader inaction. We need all our nursing organizations to muster similar courage, and students can help fuel that energy.

Early 21st Century Leaders

Past president of CNA, Dr. Judith Shamian, was elected the 27th president of ICN, serving 2013–2017. She is only the second Canadian to have ever held the post. Dr. Marlene Smadu, another former CNA president, was elected to a second, four-year term as an ICN vice president. So Canada is politically poised as never before to exert an impact on global health and nursing. And indeed, *impact* has been chosen by Shamian as the watchword of her presidency. She intends to steer the global nursing ship to impact (a) quality of nursing care and patients safety; (b) global health through nursing knowledge, voice, experience, and participation; (c) social determinants of health; and (d) the level of knowledge and skills we use to bring about better health and better nursing.

Modern nursing leaders and organizations must be technologically nimble and politically savvy. They must be well versed in and able to represent the realities of nurses' lives and practice today. But we don't want them just dreaming about those things. Whatever the domain of nursing, we need them to be thinking and acting forward—staying well ahead of the pack, studying the health-care needs of Canadians years down the line, imagining how nursing should be shaped to meet those needs, and then articulating ways to help us feel safe moving toward them. It is important for you, as a student, to engage in your own future by getting involved in shaping those organizations so that they are able to meet these daunting but exciting challenges.

In advancing her knowledge of the regulatory body, professional associations, her union, and specialty nursing groups, Katie also came to learn a great deal about the hospital where she is a student and hopes to launch her professional career. Important to her professional development, she came to know many of the players in various levels of leadership across the professions in that hospital. She knew that in a future situation, she could shortcut the amount of work she did by speaking earlier in the process to her union leader, the local chapter of specialty nurses in her clinical area, and the interprofessional practice council leader—because she quickly found that she was not alone in her concerns and was certainly not the first to notice them. But with her eyes being new on the situation, she was able to muster her team to tackle the problem again.

Critical Thinking Exercises

▶ A group of nurses on a rehabilitation unit has been getting a lot of positive feedback from patients and families about their model of care. They are encouraged by their clinical instructor to present what they are doing at a conference. They are excited by the idea, but none of them have ever done that. Where might they start?

▶ If the large numbers of nursing organizations in Canada are not fiscally sustainable, why not just combine them? For example, why do unions and professional bodies have to be separate? Couldn't we just collapse all these associations into one?

▶ David is a home care nurse who's becoming increasingly frustrated with the poor information and communication technology made available to him to do his job. What options does he have?

Multiple-Choice Questions

1. As a student nurse, it is your responsibility to complete your assignments to the best of your ability in a timely and accurate manner. Your responsibility is to learn and grow as a nurse, not to provide leadership in evaluation of the educational processes. True or false?

2. Match the following management styles with their definitions:

Leadership style	Description
1. Management by exception	A. The leader displays stresses service to others and recognizes that the role of organizations is to create people who can build a better tomorrow.
2. Laissez-faire	B. Leaders have four characteristics including idealized influence, inspirational motivation, intellectual stimulation, and idealized consideration. Transformational leaders are sensitive to the needs of others and change the organizational culture by realigning it with a new vision.
3. Transactional	C. Relational energy is made evident by building relationships and managing emotion in the workplace.
4. Servant	D. These leaders often avoid taking action, reacting with corrective action once problems have become serious.
5. Passive avoidant	E. This leader focuses on appropriate completion of tasks to maintain current performance. Failure to adequately complete tasks requires correction.
6. Transformational	F. Refers to leaders who are not concerned about organizational outcomes or follower behaviour. Leaders refuse to take responsibility to address important outcomes.
7. Resonant	G. These leaders tend to (1) clarify expected performance and provide rewards for good performance, (2) correct variations from the expected standard, and (3) work to prevent problems.

3. Match the following pan-Canadian organizations with their functions:

Organization	Function
I. ACEN	A. National voice of Canadian nursing students
II. CASN	B. Advances solutions to improve patient care, working conditions, and our public health-care system
III. CCRNR	C. National professional voice of RNs
IV. CFNU	D. National voice for nursing education, research, and scholarship
V. CNA	E. Aligning and advancing the national nursing practice, education, research, and leadership
VI. CNSA	F. National forum and voice regarding interprovincial/territorial, national and global regulatory matters for nursing regulation

4. RNs, licensed (or registered) practical nurses, and registered psychiatric nurses are licensed to practice in all Canadian provinces and territories. True or false?

5. RNs, licensed practical nurses, and registered psychiatric nurses may all belong to which of the following organizations?
   a. ACEN
   b. CASN
   c. CNA
   d. CNSA
   e. None of the above

6. Approximately how many RNs are registered to practice in Canada?
   a. 80,000
   b. 149,000
   c. 275,000
   d. 360,000

7. All members of CFNU have reciprocal membership in CNA. True or false?

8. Which of the following nursing organizations have primarily a *professional* mandate?
   a. CNA, College and Association of Registered Nurses of Alberta, and ACEN
   b. CASN, CNA, and ANAC
   c. Association of Registered Nurses of British Columbia, CNA, and RNAO
   d. CCRNR, CNA, and College of Registered Nurses of British Columbia

9. The federal Office of Nursing Policy was housed under which organization?
   a. Health Canada
   b. CFNU

c. The ministry of health in each province

d. CNA headquarters in Ottawa

10. Match the type of nursing organization with its purpose:

Type of Organization	Purpose
I. Clinical specialty	**A.** Represent nurses and their working conditions
II. Professional	**B.** Quality of practitioners and protection of the public
III. Regulatory	**C.** Education, advocacy, and support to clinical specialty nurses
IV. Union	**D.** Advance the practice and profession

11. Members of which of the following clinical organizations automatically become affiliate members of CNA?

a. Canadian Council of Cardiovascular Nurses, Association of Registered Nurses of British Columbia, and Canadian Gerontological Nurses Association

b. RNAO, Ontario Nurses Association, and Nurse Practitioners Association of Ontario

c. Canadian Federation of Mental Health Nurses, Registered Psychiatric Nurses of Canada, and Canadian Association of Nurse Counsellors

d. Canadian Association of Neuroscience Nurses, National Emergency Nurses' Affiliation, and Canadian Association of Burn Nurses

Suggested Lab Activities

● Point your browser to the website of CNA. What does CNA say about the move from its national RN examination (CRNE) to the American NCLEX-RN examination? Look at the website of the regulatory body (college) in your home province; what does it say about the change? Is there any statement about this issue on the website of the National Council of State Boards of Nursing in the United States?

• Do these various nursing leadership organizations adequately explain their position and the change?

• What does CNSA have to say about this change?

• What are some implications of this change for nursing students?

● Look up the websites of one or more clinical specialty organizations in areas of your clinical interest. What is their membership policy for nursing students? What benefits do they offer students who join the organization? With what other nursing (or other) organizations/associations are they affiliated?

● Nursing leadership skills must be learned. What are some options for leadership education after graduation that you are able to find online?

● Look up the website of the professional association in your home province. What options does it offer students for networking and leadership development?

REFERENCES AND SUGGESTED READINGS

Aboriginal Nurses Association of Canada. (2013). *Mission statement.* Retrieved from http://anac.on.ca/mission.php

Academy of Canadian Executive Nurses. (2013). *Objectives.* Retrieved from http://acen.ca/about/objectives/

Advisory Committee on Health Human Resources. (2000). *The nursing strategy for Canada.* Ottawa, ON: Health Canada. Retrieved from http://www.hc-sc.gc.ca/hcs-sss/pubs/nurs-infirm/2000-nurs-infirm-strateg/index-eng.php

American Heritage Stedman's Medical Dictionary. (2002.). *Definition: "organization."* Retrieved from http://dictionary.reference.com/browse/organization.

Antonakis, J., & Atwater, L. (2002). Leader distance: A review and proposed theory. *The Leadership Quarterly, 13*(6), 673–704.

Avolio, B. J., Bass, B. M., & Jung, D. I. (1999). Re-examining the components of transformational and transactional leadership using the multifactor leadership questionnaire. *Journal of Occupational and Organizational Psychology, 72*(4), 441–462.

Bass, B. M., & Avolio, B. J. (1993). Transformational leadership and organizational culture. *Public Administration Quarterly, 17*(1), 112–121.

Calnan, R. (2003). Message from the president. *The Canadian Nurse, 99*(9).

Canadian Association for Nursing Research. (2013). *Mission.* Retrieved from http://www.canr.ca/index.php

Canadian Association of Nurses in AIDS Care. (2013). *About us.* Retrieved from http://www.canac.org/English/index.html

Canadian Association of Schools of Nursing. (2013). *About CASN.* Retrieved from http://www.casn.ca/en/CASNACESIMission_20/

Canadian Council for Practical Nurse Regulators. (2011). *Mission, vision and values.* Retrieved from http://www.ccpnr.ca/mission visionvalues.html

Canadian Council of Cardiovascular Nurses. (2013). *Vision and mission.* Retrieved from http://www.cccn.ca/content.php?doc=90

Canadian Council of Registered Nurse Regulators. (2013a). *What We Do.* Retrieved from http://www.ccrnr.ca/index.htm

Canadian Council of Registered Nurse Regulators. (2013b). *Who We Are.* Retrieved from http://www.ccrnr.ca/index.htm

Canadian Federation of Nurses Unions. (2013). *Welcome.* Retrieved from http://cfnu.ca/

Canadian Institute for Health Information. (2013). *Regulated nurses: Canadian trends, 2007 to 2011. Updated February 2010.* Ottawa, ON: Author.

Canadian Nurses Association. (2011). *Position statement on interprofessional collaboration.* Retrieved from http://www.nurseone.ca/docs/NurseOne/CNAPrimaryCareToolkit/PS117_Interprofessional_Collaboration_2011_e.pdf

Canadian Nurses Association. (2013a). *About CNA.* Retrieved from http://www.cna-aiic.ca/en/about-cna/

Canadian Nurses Association. (2013b). *Benefits of certification.* Retrieved from http://www.nurseone.ca/Default.aspx?portlet=Static HtmlViewerPortlet&plang=1&ptnme=Specialty+Certification+What+Is+Certification

Canadian Nurses Association. (2013c). *Our members.* Retrieved from http://www.cna-aiic.ca/en/about-cna/our-members/

Canadian Nurses Association. (in press). *The Canadian Nurses Association 1908–2008: One hundred years of service.* Ottawa, ON: Author.

Canadian Nursing Advisory Committee. (2002). *Our health, our future: Final report of the Canadian Nursing Advisory Committee.* Ottawa, ON: Health Canada. Retrieved from http://www.hc-sc.gc.ca/hcs-sss/pubs/nurs-infirm/2002-cnac-cccsi-final/index-eng.php

Canadian Nursing Students' Association. (2013). *About us.* Retrieved from http://www.cnsa.ca/english/aboutus

Collins English Dictionary Complete & Unabridged 10th Edition. (2009). *Definition: "association."* Retrieved from http://dictionary.reference.com/browse/association

Cowden, T., Cummings, G., & Profetto-McGrath, J. (2011). Leadership practices and staff nurses' intent to stay: A systematic review. *Journal of Nursing Management, 19,* 461–477.

Cueto, M. (2004). The ORIGINS of primary health care and SELECTIVE primary health care. *American Journal of Public Health, 94*(11), 1864–1874.

Cummings, G. G. (2004). Investing relational energy: The hallmark of resonant leadership. *Canadian Journal of Nursing Leadership, 17*(4), 76–87.

Cummings, G. G., MacGregor, T., Davey, M., Lee, H., Wong, C. A., Lo, E., . . . Stafford, E. (2010). Leadership styles and outcome patterns for the nursing workforce and work environment: A systematic review. *International Journal of Nursing Studies, 47,* 363–385.

Farias, M. T. (2009). *Breathing fire: Unleashing the leader in you.* Mustang, OK: Tate Publishing & Enterprise.

Goleman, D. (1995). *Emotional intelligence: Why it can matter more than IQ.* New York, NY: Bantam Books.

Goleman, D., Boyatzis, R., & McKee, A. (2002). *The new leaders: Transforming the art of leadership into the science of results.* London, United Kingdom: Little, Brown.

Government of Canada. (2012). *Registered psychiatric nurse.* Retrieved from http://www.credentials.gc.ca/immigrants/fact-sheets/psychiatric.asp

Greenleaf, R. K. (1977). *Servant leadership: A journey into the nature of legitimate power and greatness.* New York, NY: Paulist Press.

Havens, D. S., & Laschinger, H. K. S. (1997). Creating the environment to support shared governance: Kanter's theory of power in organizations. *Journal of Shared Governance, 3*(1), 15–23.

Hibberd, J. M., & Smith, D. L. (2006). *Nursing leadership and management in Canada* (3rd ed.). Toronto, ON: Elsevier Canada.

Jackson, D., Firtko, A., & Edenborough, M. (2007). Personal resilience as a strategy for surviving and thriving in the face of workplace adversity: A literature review. *Journal of Advanced Nursing, 60*(1), 1–9.

Judge, T. A., Piccolo, R. F., & Ilies, R. (2004). The forgotten ones?: The validity of consideration and initiating structure in leadership research. *Journal of Applied Psychology, 89*(1), 36–51.

Kanter, R. (1993). *Men and women of the corporation* (2nd ed.). New York, NY: Basic Books.

Kanter, R. (1977). *Men and women of the corporation.* New York, NY: Basic Books.

Kelly, P., & Crawford, H. (2008). *Nursing leadership and management* (1st Canadian ed.). Toronto, ON: Nelson Education.

Kinjerski, V., & Skrypnek, B. (2004). Defining spirit at work: Finding common ground. *Journal of Organizational Change Management, 17,* 26–42.

Kinjerski, V., & Skrypnek, B. J. (2008). The promise of spirit at work. *Journal of Gerontological Nursing, 34*(10), 17–26.

Kouzes, J. M., & Posner, B. Z. (2013). The leadership challenge. How to make extraordinary things happen in organizations. *Choice Reviews Online, 50*(5), 50–2759. doi:10.5860/CHOICE.50-2759

Kouzes, J. M., & Posner, B. Z. (2007). *The leadership challenge* (4th ed.). San Francisco, CA: John Wiley & Sons.

Laschinger, H. K. S. (2008). Effect of empowerment on professional practice environments, work satisfaction, and patient care quality: Further testing of the Nursing Worklife Model. *Journal of Nursing Care Quality, 20*(2), 25–41. doi:10.1097/01.NCQ.0000318028.67910.6b

Laschinger, H. K. S., Finegan, J., Shamian, J., & Wilk, P. (2004). A longitudinal analysis of the impact of workplace empowerment on work satisfaction. *Journal of Organizational Behavior, 25,* 527–554.

Laschinger, H. K. S., Wong, E. A., Grau, A. I. L., Read, E. A., & Stam, L. M. P. (2011). The influence of leadership practices and empowerment on Canadian nurse manager outcomes. *Journal of Nursing Management, 20,* 877–888. doi:10.1111/j.1365-2834.2011.01307.x

MacLeod, L. (2012). A broader view of nursing leadership: Rethinking manager–leader functions. *Nurse Leader, 10*(3), 57–61.

National Expert Commission. (2012). *The health of our nation, the future of our health system. A nursing call to action.* Ottawa, ON: Canadian Nurses Association.

The Nursing Sector Study Corporation. (2006). *Building the future: An integrated strategy for nursing human resources in Canada.* Ottawa, ON: Author.

Pangman, C., & Pangman, V. C. (2010). *Nursing leadership from a Canadian perspective.* Philadelphia, PA: Lippincott Williams & Wilkins.

Parris, D. L., & Peachey, J. W. (2012). A systematic literature review of servant leadership for organizational contexts. *Journal of Business Ethics, 113,* 377–393.

Porter-O'Grady, T., & Malloch, K. (2011). *Quantum leadership* (3rd ed.). Mississauga, ON : Jones & Bartlett Learning.

Registered Psychiatric Nurses of Canada. (2013). *Welcome.* Retrieved from http://rpnc.ca

Royal College of Nursing. (2013). *Extraordinary general meeting (EGM).* London, United Kingdom: Author. Retrieved from http://www.rcn.org.uk/newsevents/egm

Starfield, B. (2011). Politics, primary healthcare and health: Was Virchow right? *Journal of Epidemiology and Community Health, 65,* 653–655.

Statistics Canada. (2012). *Population by year, by province and territory.* Retrieved from http://www.statcan.gc.ca/tables-tableaux/sum-som/l01/cst01/demo02a-eng.htm

Wagner, J. I. J., Cummings, G., Smith D. L., Olson, J., Anderson, L., & Warren, S. (2010). The relationship between structural empowerment and psychological empowerment for nurses: A systematic review. *Journal of Nursing Management, 18,* 448–462.

Wagner, J., Cummings, G., Smith, D. L., Olson, J., & Warren, S. (2013). Resonant leadership, workplace empowerment and spirit at work: Impact on job satisfaction and organizational commitment for registered nurses. *Canadian Journal of Nursing Research, 45*(4), 1–16.

Webber, C. (2009). *Between a rock and a hard place: When healthcare providers experience moral distress: Report on the world café exercise.* Edmonton, AB: Provincial Health Ethics Network.

World Conference on Social Determinants of Health (2011). Rio political declaration on social determinants of health. Found at http://www.who.int/sdhconference/declaration/en/

World Health Organization. (1978). *Alma-Ata 1978. Primary health care. Report of the International Conference on Primary Health Care, Alma-Ata, USSR, 6–12 September 1978.* Geneva, Switzerland: Author.

Xirasager, S. (2008). Transformational, transactional and laissez-faire leadership among physician executives. *Journal of Health Organization and Management, 22*(6), 599–613.

The Journey From Student to Graduate Nurse

LINDA PATRICK, MICHELLE FREEMAN, AND SARAH PAINTER

Jaswinder was looking forward to the first day of nursing school, but now that it had arrived, she was feeling very anxious. She did not sleep much the night before the first class, and she worried about what to bring and what to wear. Jaswinder reflected on the decision that she made to apply to nursing school and to move away from home to live in residence. It was very difficult to say goodbye to her parents and her younger brother but exciting at the same time. Making the decision to be a nurse was one of the most important decisions that she had made in her life so far. As she walked into the room to meet her teachers and her fellow students, she hoped that it was going to be the right decision for her.

CHAPTER OBJECTIVES

By the end of this chapter, you will be able to:

1. Differentiate between campus and external services that offer student support.
2. Use learning strategies to enhance your success in both theory and clinical.
3. Reflexively examine the theory of "transition shock" and the potential impact on new nursing graduates.
4. Explain the purpose of the licensing exam for Canadian registered nurses.
5. Identify who has the responsibility for developing and maintaining the exam after 2015.
6. Describe the four major Client Needs categories used to structure the NCLEX.
7. Critique resources to assist in preparing for entry to practice examinations.

KEY TERMS

Canadian Council of Registered Nurse Regulators (CCRNR) Representatives from Canada's 12 provincial/territorial bodies comprise the organization that regulates the practice of registered nurses (RNs) in Canada.

Canadian Nursing Students' Association (CNSA) A national voice for Canadian nursing students

Computerized Adaptive Testing (CAT) Computer technology that is being used by NCLEX to administer the examination that will be used to determine if a graduate nurse can become an RN in Canada after 2015.

Jurisprudence Exam In preparation for the transition to the NCLEX process in 2015, provinces are developing jurisprudence examinations. The purpose of the jurisprudence examination is to assess knowledge and comprehension of the laws, regulations, bylaws, practice standards, and guidelines that regulate the profession of nursing (College of Nurses of Ontario, 2013). Check to see if your province has one by contacting your provincial regulatory body.

OSCE The acronym for objective structured clinical examination. OSCE's are increasingly being use in nursing education to evaluate student learning; for example, health assessment skills.

Preceptor In nursing, refers to the one-on-one relationship that a senior level nursing student has with an RN in a clinical setting for an assigned period of time. The student is expected to achieve increasing independence, under the supervision of the assigned RN, in preparation for graduation.

Prioritizing An approach to decision-making and the ordering of tasks to ensure that the most critical or important tasks are completed first.

Problem-Based Learning (PBL) An approach used in some nursing schools to engage students in a process of discovery to solve a problem. It could be a clinical practice scenario that requires students to learn some new knowledge to solve the problem.

Time Management Skills Refer to personal skills of organization used to manage one's time effectively and complete tasks efficiently.

Getting Started on the Right Foot

This is a very unique chapter in a nursing fundamentals textbook and has been designed to explore your student experience from various perspectives, including current students and recent graduates. This chapter does not hold all the answers, but it generates ideas for thoughtful dialogue with other students, nurse educators, and nurses in clinical practice. The topics are intended to be supportive, even though some of the content may shock you; for example, bullying by other nurses. Shedding light on some of the hidden issues that nurses may experience is one strategy for improving the quality of the student learning experience and nurses' work. This is your chosen profession, and each day in practice should bring you professional and personal satisfaction. No one is saying that your days as a student or graduate nurse won't be challenging, but there should be moments of joy that empower you to want to make a difference for your patients and the next generation of nurses that will come after you.

This chapter is divided into sections that begin with your admission into nursing school and end with your graduation and successful registration as a nurse. The pages contain information on resources and articles that you may want to return to visit often as you transition from a beginning student nurse to graduate nurse. If you are reading this chapter as part of an assignment, you may want to read it from beginning to end. If you are skimming through this on your own time, then we suggest that you make this chapter work for you. You may choose to flip through it and skim for whatever catches your eye, as long as you know that it's here and that you can come back to it freely for support and guidance when the timing is right for you.

A Survival Guide to Nursing School

Across Canada, thousands of students enter college and university nursing programs each year with the same hopes and dreams of entering the nursing profession. You may have a parent, aunt, or neighbor who is a nurse and who mentored you in your choice for a career. However, it will soon become very clear to you that your experience is unique to you and will require motivation, organization, and strategies for success.

Nursing students were traditionally high school graduates entering postsecondary settings immediately following high school. Today, students may also enter nursing schools as adults seeking a second career, returning to school after other completed or partially completed degree or diploma programs, and after years of employment in a different field. Regardless of how you ended up enrolled in a nursing program, you are all beginning the same journey from the same starting line with the same or similar determination to be successful and the same or similar physical and emotional demands.

Students often begin their studies with worries that are in addition to the concerns associated with studying and getting good grades. Postsecondary education is expensive, so you may be planning to work to help pay for your tuition and living costs. If you have returned to school after working and you have a family, then your worries may include paying a mortgage, managing time to spend with your family, and finding time to do homework. Colleges and universities recognize this by providing student support services. Take a moment to search your school's website for information about support services offered on your campus. Table 7.1 provides some guidance about the most frequent services available on campuses to support student health and well-being.

Student Success Strategies

If you are feeling frightened and nervous, you are certainly not alone. Nursing school can make even the most confident person feel overwhelmed. The first thing that we need to get settled, right here and right now, is that this is a normal feeling. Most of your classmates would probably join you in saying, "I don't know if I am cut out for this." Even the ones that seem confident likely have some small part of them that feels nervous. Take a deep breath—don't panic. These feelings are normal and healthy, so long as you use them in a positive way.

Through the eyes of a student

*W*alking into my first day of clinical of my first year in nursing school, felt like walking into an already lost battle. I remember the first thing we did was sit and observe the shift change report, and I sat there trying to look like I had a clue what was going on. Throughout the day, I had many trips to the bathroom where I stood there staring in the mirror saying to myself, "You can do this!"

(personal reflection of Stephanie Painter, a nursing student)

Many first-year students often become so overwhelmed by workload and the stress that it creates that their life gets out of balance. An important aspect of doing well in school is to have a balanced and healthy life. Learning strategies that you can employ to achieve school-life balance will continue to be useful to manage your work-life balance as an employed nurse.

It is important to become skilled at managing your priorities so that you can harness your stress to enhance your performance but not allow it to consume your life. Look around at your peers; some of them are probably so panicked that they doubt they'll make it through the first month, let alone 4 years. You'll also find students that seem calm, cool, and collected. They are making the grade or excelling in their studies. So what's the difference? It's not that the calm ones

TABLE 7.1 Campus Student Support Services

Resource		Examples of Services
Academic calendar	The academic calendar is a guide to the courses, programs, admission requirements, and student services offered at your school. Most schools have their calendar available online with specific headings to identify key content.	In the academic calendar, you will find official information about fees, courses, programs, related policies and regulations, as well as general information about your school.
Academic advising services	Academic advisors are available to help you with course selection, program planning, and educational goal setting.	Academic advisors provide guidance for such things as choosing majors and minors, adding courses, dropping courses, and withdrawing from programs.
Career services	The career development office will help you to move from the academic setting to the workplace. The office may also have coordinators to assist you in choosing cooperative placements for work experience while still a student.	Internships/externships, resume building, preparation for job interviews
Accessibility services	Accessibility service counselors partner with students, faculty, and staff to coordinate and facilitate accommodations to support student development and success.	Services may include support for note taking, provision of extra time for exam writing or a quiet exam room.
Student learning services	Some schools have writing labs or offer peer tutoring programs. Workshops may be offered to help you develop your time management skills, test taking ability, note taking, textbook reading, and writing skills.	A focus on supporting your academic success through the skills development and learning support
New student orientation	Student orientation programs help you to transition to campus life and your college or university campus setting. Events are a mix of social activities and academic support.	Adjusting to campus life and the academic standards of postsecondary settings
Student counseling services	Counseling services provide crisis intervention; personal, career, and educational counseling; and various workshops. Some centres are now offering "puppy rooms" during high stress times such as final exams (see chapter for more information).	Services may be provided by psychologists, a clinical therapist, a registered nurse, or master's-level graduate students.
Student registration and records	The registrar's office serves as the heart of campus for academic information at your school. Services include credit, registration, fees, confirmation of enrolment, exam deferrals, student academic records, official transcripts, critical dates, and graduation.	All records—from fees due, scholarship fund balance, transcripts, etc.
Campus services	The services listed above are only a small sample of services and supports that may be available on your campus.	Go to your campus home page for links to student services at your school.

aren't also feeling the same pressure. It's usually that the calm students are controlling their stress and keeping the balance in their life. The students who are frazzled are usually so consumed by school, and the stress that it brings that they burn themselves out. It may be helpful to test your stress using the Canadian Mental Health Stress Meter; find it on the Canadian Mental Health website.

You will need to work hard at maintaining balance throughout school and the rest of your career. Keeping things in balance is difficult, and sometimes, you will find that you are missing the mark. That's okay—as long as you

can work to get back to your most healthy mental and physical space. Some survival tips for nursing school include strategies that will support you in your studies and also prepare you for nurses' work in practice. Over the course of the next few years, you will hear your teachers speak about "being organized" and **time management skills**. Nurses need to be skillful at both to be able to juggle the many demands on their time in practice settings. Thompson (2012a) identified three key strategies for nurses to use for managing their time, and two of them are applicable for nursing students. The three strategies for time management are (1) plan,

(2) anticipate, and (3) delegate (Thompson, 2012b, p. 18). Spend a little time each day deciding what you must do, what you should do, and what you could do. By organizing your tasks this way, you will be **prioritizing** (Thompson, 2012b). Adhering to this easy-to-remember process increases your sense of control and your chances of staying on top of your workload. How do you manage all of your schoolwork and keep life in balance? Let's break it down into manageable pieces, and then we'll look at each one and talk about some strategies that will help you to conquer them.

Your Life in the Balance

As a nursing student, it is critical that you claim a certain amount of personal time for yourself and protect it. This may not be something that you have had to think about before, but postsecondary education and studying for a profession are very different from being in high school. Each of you will choose to approach personal time in a way that is unique to meet your own needs. Some of you may have been involved in team sports or other similar activities while in high school. University and college campuses have both varsity and intramural sports and clubs for special interests. These activities are good for meeting new friends with similar interests and for continuing with activities that have brought you enjoyment. Attending university and college does not mean that you have to give up your special interests. Academic advisors in your school can provide direction about how to fit these activities into your nursing school schedule. Also, coaches for the varsity teams are often advocates for students on school teams to assist them to fit practices and games into class and clinical schedules. It is worth seeking advice if this is of interest to you.

Perhaps, you'll find that exercising relieves your stress or maybe hanging out with friends and family most helps you relax. Whatever you enjoy that makes you feel relaxed and comfortable will contribute to balancing your life. This precious period of time is meant to preserve your mental and physical health and well-being.

A word of caution about social activities is warranted here. Socializing with peers is a very important and special part of postsecondary education. You have lots in common including the need to share stories and experiences and enjoy breaks between studies. Remember to remain balanced and safe especially when socializing in public and consuming alcohol. Some students have learned the hard way that driving under the influence or being in the wrong place when a fight breaks out at a party can lead to an unsatisfactory police clearance. It is a good idea to know your school's policy and the implications of having a positive police clearance on your progression in a nursing program.

The reality of self-care practices when it comes to students is that we live in a world that does not always insist that we take care of ourselves first. The **Canadian Nursing Students' Association (CNSA)** believes that "nursing students have a responsibility to protect their own health, as well as the health of others" (Canadian Nursing Students' Association [CNSA], 2009, para. 1). However in their position statement, "Self-Care Practices Among Nursing Students," they note that nursing students often place self-care at the bottom of their list of responsibilities. The notion that you must be healthy to care for others is an important one. If you don't develop adequate self-care practices in nursing school, what do you think the chances are that you'll have them when you are a nurse? Neglecting self-care has major ramifications for more than just the individual nurse because fatigue can contribute to making errors that put your patients at risk.

Staying in Balance

General advice for staying in balance includes being well rested by maintaining a normal sleep schedule. Each of us has our own sleep pattern, but sleep deprivation is something we should strive to avoid. Health promotion advice usually includes telling us to eat a healthy and balanced diet that can sometimes be a challenge on campus. In recent years, food services on both college and university campuses have made an extra effort to include healthy choices including vegan and gluten-free options. Also, you may be able to expand your food choices to include ethnic dishes provided by food services on many campuses to meet the preferences of international students.

In addition to the earlier selections, you will also find the usual pizza, hamburgers, etc., so just try to balance your favorites with some healthy choices. Students often complain that they gain weight in postsecondary settings due to being less physically active. Monitor your alcohol consumption and make sure that it is in moderation. One last word of advice is to eat breakfast so that your mind is well fuelled for classes and clinical. It is true that you will be better prepared for new clinical experiences when you are not feeling faint from skipping breakfast.

Taking Care of Your Mental and Physical Health

If you are feeling overwhelmed or stressed, find someone to talk to. Friends that you trust or family are always an excellent place to turn. Professors may be able to assist you with problems related to deadlines and academic resources, but when things feel like they are getting out of control, you may want to visit your student health services. Student health services on campus are a good resource for health promotion activities, counseling for mental health concerns and clinics for when you are ill. Most of the clinics offer yearly flu shots and assistance to fill out the required health forms that you must complete for nursing school each year. More and more campuses are looking for creative ways to reduce student stress during exam times; see Box 7.1 to learn more about "puppy rooms."

Dalhousie University used "puppy rooms" to reduce student stress during the fall semester exam period in 2012 (Southey, 2012). The dogs are trained therapy dogs and a little past the puppy stage but provide considerable comfort to students who may be missing a favorite pet from home. The article reported that exams create considerable stress for students, and the dogs were able to reduce stress and anxiety because they have the potential to raise brain neurotransmitters through their unconditional love. So, a cuddle with a Labradoodle may be available on your campus, but if not, then speak to a representative on your student union to see about arranging one in the future.

To share your view about what universities and colleges should do to address student stress and mental health, visit http://www.theglobeandmail.com/news/national/education /tell-us-what-should-universities-do-to-address-student-stress -and-mental-health/article5912294/

How Will You Learn to Be a Nurse?

Lectures, exams, scholarly papers, skills lab, objective structured clinical examination or **OSCE** testing, clinical, . . . and the list goes on. Nursing school is unique because there are both theory and practical requirements for the program, regardless of what school you attend. It can be challenging to be expected to perform in all of these different ways, but it's important that you do. Nurses need to be accomplished in knowledge, skills performance, and in delivery of the written and spoken word. Nursing programs are designed to prepare you to be competent professionals. That's why you are evaluated in all kinds of different ways, to make sure that you are prepared to think critically and perform safely in the real world. Everything that you do, whether it's hard or easy, has a purpose in the big picture.

Lectures

Lectures are the cornerstone of your education. They guide your learning and help to prepare you for clinical practice. They are often delivered in a format that is complementary to the appropriate clinical section. Lots of students find this to be helpful, as you have weekly time slots dedicated to the theory that informs your practice. Of course, this would never replace the clinical preparation that you're required to do. However, it does help you along and gives you the big picture ideas that spending 6 (or 12) weeks on one or two clinical settings simply can't give you.

Let's say it's your first week of school, and you've attended all of your classes and met the teachers and the other students in the classes. The first thing you should do is read each courses syllabus. Mark down all of the important dates in your day planner, read the objectives, and start to get you head around how you will manage your time throughout the term. Laying down this kind of groundwork will go a long way in the grand scheme of things. The consequence of poor planning is that you feel like you're constantly scrambling to make the grade.

It is also important that you attend classes even if the lectures are not mandatory. Students who are engaged in their own learning and participate in discussions about difficult topics and ask questions are way ahead of the game with keeping up and maintaining balance. If you must miss a class, it is helpful to follow up with a classmate to see what you missed. Reading over the posted class PowerPoint slides will usually only provides you with the outline of the larger discussions that took place.

Exams

Exams or tests can be among the most stressful aspect of your education. Late night study sessions fueled by caffeine and panic is not balance, and it never will be. The cliché idea that this is what being a student is all about is as senseless as it is dated. It also works against you in the end. In the long run, you retain information much better when you are exposed to it repeatedly, over a greater period of time. The whole point of studying is to make yourself a better nurse, not do marginally better on one test in one course.

Preparation will go a long way to reducing stress and anxiety when we're talking exams. Well in advance of test dates, read your syllabus and figure out what you're responsible to review. Make a study plan where you spend 1 or more hours at a time, spread over numerous days. Book more time than you think you need rather than less and then being flexible with your personal limits. If you get too tired, take a break or call it quits until the next day. The beauty of this approach is that you are not going to end up being frazzled because you've planned for the human factor—the possibility that things might not go according to plan. For the actual study sessions, ensure that you have gone through the required readings and reviewed the notes. After you do a preliminary review of all testable material, take a look at the objectives listed in the syllabus. The objectives are the goals for the course. Typically, these items represent what the student should be taking away as knowledge. Objectives are a handy guide for choosing your focus, and because they should be in sequential order, they suggest approximately where in the text you will find the information.

After you write an exam—try to relax and avoid worrying about the outcome. This doesn't necessarily mean give up for the afternoon and leave campus but don't dwell on what you may or may not have done. Until you get your mark, don't waste your time comparing your answers with other people. Once you get your results, if you are pleased, then pat yourself on the back and move on. If you are disappointed, schedule a meeting with your professor to discuss where you might have gone wrong and how you can improve. Your professors are there to help; go to them with the attitude that you want to learn, try hard, and do better.

Try to keep a calm, level head when you're not achieving excellence. If you write a test or exam that doesn't go your way, use it as a lesson. Every student that you're in school with has had ups and downs. A poor student may become disgruntled and shut down after an exam that doesn't quite go as planned. A big thinker will look at the situation constructively, try earnestly to find the problem, and address it through action. That might mean getting a study group together, changing the way they study, or just studying more. When you are met with a challenge, rise to the occasion. One test or even one rough course will not define you as a nurse.

Think of how Jaswinder felt when she first started in Year 1 of the program. Compare this to how she may be feeling as she enters into Year 2 and the expectations for her academic and clinical performance become more demanding. Jaswinder is experiencing an additional source of stress because English is not her first language, and there all these writing rules for her course assignments. In Year 1, she could make a mistake once in a while, but this year marks are deducted for each mistake. What should she do?

Scholarly Papers

First of all, when assigned a paper, give yourself enough time, so make sure to write the due date into your planner. To write a good paper, you need to plan your approach to the topic and organize your time and materials. Research, note taking, and typing multiple drafts are all parts to fit in to the equation. Go to your syllabus or the assignment handout and review it thoroughly. Contact your instructor if you have any questions to be sure that you're clear about what he or she wants want to see from you. One last bit of advice is to seek out resources on your campus to strengthen writing skills. A workshop about writing or some tutoring can go a long way toward reducing your stress and increasing your success.

Through the eyes of a student

Ah . . . the scholarly paper! It truly is your best friend or perhaps your worst nightmare. After my time in university, I think for me it's a bit of both. I learned that there are a few things that you have to get in order before you can discover a *love of papers* that I bet you never thought you had.

(personal reflection of a graduate nursing student)

Nursing Labs

Each nursing school will use nursing labs in its own unique way to fit best with its curriculum and available resources (Fig. 7.1). You will be informed early in your program about the expectations for clinical lab experiences and practice opportunities outside of class at your school. Some schools

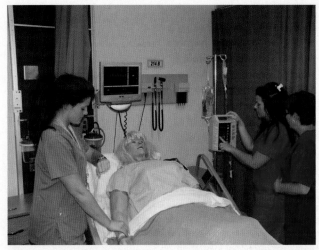

Figure 7.1 Nursing students in a nursing lab with a simulated adult patient.

have scheduled hours for practice, and some may have open hours that you can fit into your own personal schedule depending on your needs. It is important that you use your time wisely to prepare for clinical testing and clinical experiences. Explore all the resources available to you and find out if there is an expectation for small group work, **problem-based learning**, seminars, workshops, and independent lab practice with peer tutors or lab technologists. The more you know, the better your chances of success.

Clinical Practice

Students who enter nursing school come with the knowledge that they will have clinical practice experiences as part of their learning journey. Some students choose the school that they will attend based on the curriculum and where in the program the first clinical experiences are placed. Clinical for nursing students is offered across Canada in unique ways that fit with program design and also with opportunities determined by location, geography, available clinical placements, and competition with other students from, for example, medicine and practical nursing.

Traditional clinical experiences would include a clinical instructor assigned to a group of students placed in a setting for a semester. The agencies determine how large the clinical groups can be so the numbers vary. One teacher may also have to cover more than one unit in a hospital or more than one community agency to accommodate placement. In the early years of a program, the clinical instructor is usually close for student supervision. More nontraditional clinical experiences are being developed as the health-care setting moves to more community-based care and different roles for registered nurses (RNs) in practice evolve.

The final year of clinical may have a different model that includes **preceptors**. The preceptor or RN that you are assigned to for a semester or a predetermined period of time works closely with a faculty advisor to ensure that you are gradually progressing toward more independence in

Get to Know Your Preceptor

It is the relationship with a preceptor that determines new graduate confidence and competence. A positive relationship is critical for your success. Spend time getting to know your preceptor beyond the work environment. This can help to build a trusting and nurturing relationship that can transcend beyond orientation. Ask questions about family, pets, activities, and stories from when he/she was a new nurse. Take breaks together.

Take Charge of Your Learning

Let your preceptor know how you like to learn. Are you somebody with somebody talking you through it? Having this conversation up front can save you and your preceptor a lot of time and potential frustration.

Ask for Feedback

If you're not getting any feedback from your preceptor, ask. Make sure you ask for both positive and negative feedback. "What did I do really well today? What do I need to improve?" Tell your preceptor that you want to know when you are not doing something right. If all you hear are the things you do well, you limit your ability to grow as a professional.

Take Responsibility for Your Orientation if It's Not Working Well

Identify that the relationship isn't working. Within 2 weeks, you should have a good idea if you and your preceptor are a good fit. If not, don't suffer in silence. It's YOUR orientation. You only get one, and it can set the tone for your career as a professional nurse.

Overall, take an active role in the relationship. Don't assume that your preceptor should know the best way to teach you everything you need to know as a new nurse.

"What did I do really well today?" "What do you think I need to work on?" "The relationship I have with you is important to me. I'm not sure we are working well together and I'd like to talk about it."

Excerpt printed with Permission from Thompson, R. (2012b). *"Survive 1 thrive: A guide: Helping new nurses succeed."* Pittsburgh, PA: RT Connections, LLC.

preparation for graduation and professional practice. Myrick and Yonge (2005) described this approach to teaching-learning as a pairing that "intends to foster professional socialization, enhance learning, promote critical thinking, cultivate practical wisdom, and facilitate competence" (p. 3).

Students most often have an idea of where they would like to spend this senior-level experience in preparation for employment. Explore whether or not you can suggest a setting with a faculty advisor at your school. You may not get exactly what you ask for, but it may assist with your placement in a setting that matches your learning needs with your career goals (Box 7.2).

Jaswinder is now feeling more confident at the end of Year 3 and is looking forward to being a senior-level student in the final year of the program. She has heard about preceptors and is curious about how she is going to work independently with an RN instead of being in a clinical group with an instructor. What should she do to make this a good experience and prepare her for professional practice?

Through the eyes of a student

Preparation for every clinical day is crucial. Your instructor or preceptor will be evaluating you to ensure that you're ready to provide safe and effective patient care. The evaluation is defined by things as small as having a clean and pressed uniform, with all of your pre-clinical patient assignments ready. It also looks at things as large as if you understand what you are doing and are equipped to perform the assessments and skills at the expected level for where you are in your program. *(personal reflection of a student nurse)*

Patient Safety

All of the sections that we have discussed earlier come back to patient safety. Through preparation, organization, competent performance, and accountability, we create an environment where safety is the result. Doing well in clinical is the goal, but every single day that you go into the hospital, you must concern yourself with providing the safest care possible. Understand hospital policy for how to perform assisted lifts and transfer techniques. Learn how to help patients to be mobile and how to prevent falls. If you don't know how to do something or it is your first time, get your instructor or preceptor to help you. Some students think they will look unprepared or dependent if they asked for help. To the contrary, this demonstrates that you know your limits and are most concerned with making sure that patients are safe.

Be an Active Participant in Creating a Culture of Safety

If you feel that something unsafe is happening in clinical, speak up. Tell your instructor or preceptor that you are not comfortable. If this doesn't get the response that you need, follow the chain of command and take it to a person with higher authority. You can also be proactive and ask your school what they are doing to facilitate patient safety and protect their own students. In their position statement on patient safety, the CNSA describes approaches that encourage schools to improve the safety culture for students. This might include asking for supplemental clinical experiences with the replication of real-life crises using simulation technology to educate students on patient safety. Or perhaps lobbying for the faculty administration and clinical instructors to adopt the perspective that mistakes are an opportunity to learn and improve rather than a culture of blame. Whatever your approach, it is important that if you see a problem, you speak up on behalf of yourself, other students, and patients. The safety culture will not improve if we don't participate in the change.

It is important in your role as a student nurse that you ingrain safe practice in your work. Some of the safe practices that you will learn in your nursing program include effective hand hygiene to prevent infections, correctly identifying patients using two patient identifiers (such as full name and date of birth) before administering any treatment/medication, using independent double checks before administering high-risk medications, and effective communication and teamwork techniques. It is also important that you participate in reporting of both errors that you were involved in or discover. Every reported error is an opportunity to prevent a future error. Near misses should also be shared. A near miss (also called a *good catch*) is an error that was caught before it reached the patient. Near misses are free lessons and allow an institution to identify and address system problems which, if not addressed, can result in patient harm. As patient advocates, nursing students are encouraged to report near misses. To achieve safe care, it is also essential that patients and families are active participants in their care and accepted as members of the health-care team. They should also be encouraged and supported to speak up if they have any concerns.

Opportunities for Personal and Professional Development

The previous section described nursing school from the perspective of required activities that you must do to progress from entry to successful completion of the program. This section will introduce you to other opportunities that are voluntary but will add to your nursing school experience, build your leadership skills, and help to achieve the balance in your life that was referred to earlier. How much you do and when you do it are critical decisions that you must make based on your ability to balance these activities with other competing demands for your time.

Student Council

The student council can be a tremendous opportunity. Impressively, these groups have almost all been established by a few people like you that decided that there should be a voice for students at your school. Some of them are small, and some are large, but regardless of the size, there is a lot of good work happening at campuses all over the country. Student councils keep students in touch with what is happening with faculty in your city, province, and country. They allow you to meet new friends and participate in fundraising, professional development, and business activities. This is a great place to start, whether you are in first year or at the very end of your program.

Canadian Nursing Students' Association

With approximately 25,000 members, CNSA is the voice of nursing students in Canada. Since 1971, CNSA has represented the interests of nursing students to federal, provincial, and international governments and to other nursing and health-care organizations. They are an affiliate member of the Canadian Nurses Association (CNA) and an associate member of the Canadian Federation of Nurses Unions (CFNU). They also have a reciprocal relationship with the Canadian Association of Schools of Nursing (CASN). Through these relationships, members of the CNSA Board of Directors convey the student perspective by holding positions on the boards of directors of the cited organizations. It took a long time for the CNSA to establish themselves with each of these major groups but was worth the work. Canadian nurses value nursing student input, and the CNA, CFNU, and CASN have demonstrated this by ensuring that the CNSA is always involved. The CNSA also liaises with several other groups, including Registered Practical Nurses of Canada, Registered Psychiatric Nurses of Canada, Nursing the Future, the Canadian Association of Pharmacy Students and Interns, the Canadian Federation of Medical Students, the International Council of Nurses—Student Network, and various provincial organizations.

One benefit of membership of CNSA is their regional and national conferences that are held each year. At these conferences, the business of the organization is conducted. Using *Robert's Rules of Order*, important issues of concern are discussed by nursing student leaders, and the board of directors is given direction on how to proceed. In addition to hosting the business meetings of the association, the conferences represent a tremendous professional development opportunity for nursing students. Each January, approximately 600 nursing students converge to network and learn together at the CNSA National Conference. The conference is held by a member school and is completely student-run. Past highlights have included workshops on the Canadian Registered Nurse Examination; career development workshops; an interprofessional panel, featuring the CNSA Vice President, in addition to the Presidents of the Canadian Federation of Medical Students and the Canadian Association of Pharmacy Students and Interns; and an international panel, with invited guests from other nursing student organizations within the International Council of Nurses—Student Network. In past conferences, registrants have enjoyed presentations from representatives from Africa, Iceland, Poland, and the United States.

CNSA also provides all its members with access to the CNA's NurseONE database. This essential reference tool provides nursing students and nurses with access to clinical resources, journals, online Compendium of Pharmaceuticals and Specialties, and learning modules on several topics, such as the Code of Ethics. This resource normally comes at a high price but is included with CNSA membership fees.

CNSA is a nationally respected organization whose student leaders have gone on to work in a wide variety of sectors within nursing. The skills that students gain by getting involved in advocacy and professional development early in their nursing careers prove very beneficial in work as in life. Although it is a lot of work, CNSA leaders never regret their roles—and most couldn't imagine their lives without having been involved.

Professional Memberships

Students in nursing schools also have the opportunity to join professional organizations with student membership fees. Examples include nursing associations such as the RNs associations in your province and Sigma Theta Tau International (STTI) with headquarters in Indianapolis, Indiana, USA. STTI is an honour society with membership criteria and yearly dues. It was started by six nursing students in 1922 and has now grown worldwide (Sigma Theta Tau International [STTI], 2013). The best way to find out more about these opportunities is to visit the websites of each association or honour society. There will also be information available on your campus, especially if your school has an STTI chapter or your community has a local RNs association chapter.

Conferences

A good conference offers a wealth of enrichment. Although students can start attending events right from the beginning, third year is a good time to start looking for opportunities such as this. Conferences can be instrumental in developing your interests in nursing and the health-care field at large. The conferences included in the following sections are specific to being a student nurse and the student nurse journey. Speak to your faculty advisors about other conference opportunities, e.g., research conferences.

The Canadian Nursing Students National Conference
The CNSA holds several events throughout the year, and this can be a great way to be introduced to the world of conferences. The biggest event is the national conference that is hosted annually by a member school in different areas all over Canada. It has a rich schedule including free workshops, speaker sessions, and national assembly, which is the annual general meeting of the association. This is an opportunity to meet nursing students from across the country and will undoubtedly get you excited about what it means to be a Canadian nursing student. Many schools generously provide funding through your local student council for students to attend. For more information, contact your local council or student society and visit the website http://www.cnsa.ca.

There are also many local, regional, and national conference events that will be available. Look up the different groups online that interest you to find out if and when they hold their functions. The CNA and the CFNU host wonderful conferences that are enlightening and inspiring to attend. Provincial colleges and unions will have similar events that you may find a little easier to get to. Also, if you know that you are interested in a specific type of nursing, you might find it valuable to attend an event hosted by a specific group.

While you are in school, you might feel that it will be difficult to afford to attend conferences or are reluctant to be absent from the classroom or a clinical day. Many schools value this type of professional development and will be willing to provide funding for your attendance at the conference. As for the absenteeism, you may actually be able to have a conference day counted as a school or clinical day. As a professional nurse, you will be expected to attend functions such as this as continuing education and professional development. Many schools will uphold this standard and even encourage students to behave in a similar way. If you would like more information on the rationale for this or you require a tool to help you substantiate a request, the CNSA has a "Conference Time Equals Clinical Time" position statement that you may find helpful.

Nursing the Future Annual Conference
An annual conference located in Canada and organized by the Workplace Integration of New Nurses-Nursing the Future (WINN-NTF) organization. The leaders of WINN-NTF intend the annual conference to offer new graduates and all the nurse leaders who support them (teachers, preceptors, nurse managers, employers) an opportunity to come together to learn more about the challenges associated with being a new nurse entering practice.

This conference increases awareness for all participants of the needs of new nurses around preparation for practice, orientation, integration into workplace settings, and stabilization in new roles. Perhaps, more importantly, it provided participants with the most up-to-date research on transition issues and tangible strategies to take back to their workplaces. New graduate participants are provided with resources to assist them in building relationships and a support base that has proven to be extremely important during the transition period.

Committees

A committee is a small group that gathers to do specific work. This as a way to familiarize yourself with nursing issues as well as professional development. Many schools will have committees that require one or two students to take part. They might be concerned with program review or perhaps even student appeals. This experience will allow you to become comfortable in a meeting-type setting and take part in some interesting work.

On the local front, if you think that you are interested in getting involved with a committee, get in touch with your student council or a faculty member to see if there is anything available. Based on what information you get, you should look at your options and decide what is a good fit. There may even be a committee that doesn't have a student position but would be willing to have you sit in on the meetings just so that you can be exposed to the business. There are also many CNSA committees that are always looking for new members. They do work around global health, community and public health, diversity, and much more. For more information, check out http://www.cnsa.ca.

Volunteering

There are many volunteering opportunities that can get you involved early on. Volunteering is also a great activity to list on your resume to demonstrate that you take an interest in your profession. It would be impossible to list all of the ways that you might be able to locate a suitable position, but here are a few hints.

Hospitals in your city or town are always looking for people to help. This could include working at an information desk, delivering specimens to laboratories, spending time with patients, and much more. An added bonus is the fact that you can get familiar with the flow of the hospital. This is always a benefit if you still have clinical sections to complete. The more time that you spend in a hospital, the more comfortable you get and that is always an advantage to a student nurse.

Opportunities With Monetary Benefits

The ability to earn a little money while doing something that is contributing to your learning and professional development is a bonus. There are opportunities, but they may require a little effort to find out what they are and how you apply for them on your campus.

Research Assistant

Professors are engaged in research projects and hire research assistants even at the undergraduate level. These positions may be for a short period of time but often depending on the nature of the project may extend longer. You will be paid, and in addition, you will learn about the research process and contribute in a meaningful to the final outcome of a study. Specific tasks may include, but are not limited to, conducting a literature search, collecting data with the professor or a graduate student, and entering data into a computer data analysis program. This is a great opportunity to be mentored for future graduate studies.

Peer Tutor

Many schools have opportunities for senior nursing students to work in the clinical lab as tutors. As a peer tutor, you would support student learning for the basic nursing skills usually after hours when nursing students are coming to the lab setting for individual practice. An added benefit to helping someone else with his or her clinical skill development is that you get very good at your own.

Proctoring Exams and Marking Papers as a Teaching Assistant

This practice varies school to school, but you may be able to proctor or monitor exams. You will need to investigate if you would be allowed to monitor nursing exams, because in most schools, you would be paid to monitor exam writing in other faculties or departments. This is especially important so that you are not monitoring a nursing exam that you have not written yet but will write in the future. Marking papers may have the same restrictions. This means that if you are in the final year of your program, you would mark papers for a teacher who has first- or second-year students. Marking papers is one really good way to reinforce your skills at writing.

Other opportunities exist on campuses across Canada. There can be employment opportunities in the campus bookstore, the residence, and in the campus recreation services. Explore what is available on your campus by checking out your school's websites.

Dealing With Difficult Situations

Supportive learning environments and work environments are foremost on the minds of nursing leaders today. As a student, it might be difficult to "find your voice" when you feel that you have experienced negative behaviour directed toward you by another student, a teacher, or perhaps another nurse. In 2010, the World Health Organization (Srabstein & Leventhal, 2010) identified bullying as a global threat to nurses' health and well-being. Read more about bullying and nursing students in the Research Review box.

How Do I Know If I Am Being Bullied?

As a student, you may not be familiar with all the ways in which another person can undermine your self-confidence and damage your self-esteem, but if you are the victim, you may feel sad, unmotivated, and unsure of yourself, deliberately avoiding activities that used to make you happy. See the Research Review for more ways in which others could be undermining your success.

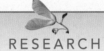

RESEARCH

REPORTING BEHAVIOURS OF NURSING STUDENTS WHO HAVE EXPERIENCED VERBAL ABUSE

It has been recognized internationally that nurses are vulnerable to verbal abuse in workplace settings, but the reporting of this abuse is not well documented. Student nurses may experience the same kind of abuse in their clinical placements in the form of verbal abuse from patients or bullying from staff. The purpose of this study was to explore the reporting behaviours of nursing students who had experienced verbal abuse while gaining clinical experience.

Study

The research method is survey or questionnaire with a convenience sample of 156 Year 3 nursing students in England.

Conclusion

Fifty-one students reported that they had experienced verbal abuse in their practicum settings, but only 62% of those who answered (32 students) said that they reported the abuse. Even more disturbing is that only 4 students formally documented the abuse in writing, so that there was a record. Students most frequently said that they did not report the abuse because it was embarrassing or that they felt sorry for the person who verbally abused them.

(continued on page 118)

REPORTING BEHAVIOURS OF NURSING STUDENTS WHO HAVE EXPERIENCED VERBAL ABUSE (CONTINUED)

Implications for Nursing Students
This study identified the need for a reporting system or process for nursing students to report abuse and the need to establish formal support services for students who experience abuse. The responsibility for the development of the reporting system and the support services rests with the educational institutions and health-care providers.

Ferns, T., & Meerabeau, E. (2009). Reporting behaviours of nursing students who have experienced verbal abuse. Journal of Advanced Nursing, 65(12), 2678–2688.

Successful transition of newly graduated nurses is also threatened by unhealthy work environments that do not recognize the stress that a new graduate nurse experience upon entering the workforce. Constructive relationships with co-workers in a respectful work environment ease transition. The courses that you take as a student nurse will enlighten you about the issues that nurses' experience and build your skills in communication, conflict management, and leadership. There are many articles about using your knowledge and skills as a nurse to have a positive influence on your future colleagues and workplaces.

Transition to Professional Practice

It may seem a little strange to be reading a chapter in an introduction to nursing textbook and see a title about moving into professional practice. The reality is that you are preparing for your career as a nurse from the day you apply to nursing school. This section contains information that is worth referring back to multiple times during your program. We will begin with career development and tips for moving into a nursing career that thrives.

Transition Theory

Adjusting to professional practice as a newly graduated nurse is a process that has been studied and written about in the literature. Although it is not within the scope of this chapter to review the entire journey, references and interesting websites are provided later. The most recent studies have focused on the milieu of the contemporary work environment: its increasing complexity being characterized by intensifying patient acuity and demanding workloads (Duchscher, 2008). New graduates struggle to "hit the ground running," due in part to limited practice experience and low self-confidence. Experienced nurses, who may have long forgotten the stresses and strains of this tumultuous transition, do not always appreciate the challenges faced by a generation of graduates who are entering our health-care system at much more dynamic and intense time. With fiscal restraints and resource cutbacks, nurses are called on to "do more with less." Not having lived through or had time to adjust to the tremendous changes in health-care workload and nursing workplace intensity over the last decade, new nurses are oftentimes inadvertently "thrown in at the deep end" by their more experienced nurse colleagues. Inadequately supported or mentored, some of these new professionals flounder, whereas others experiencing near-drowning experiences as they grow their sea-legs in a profession more an ocean than a stream. In recognition of this phenomenon, more schools of nursing are including the theory of Transition Shock and the Stages of Transition in their senior level courses. As a student preparing for graduation, having knowledge about the transition journey can both remove the mystery and empower the next phase of professional evolution. Figure 7.2 identifies the stages of Transition Shock theory.

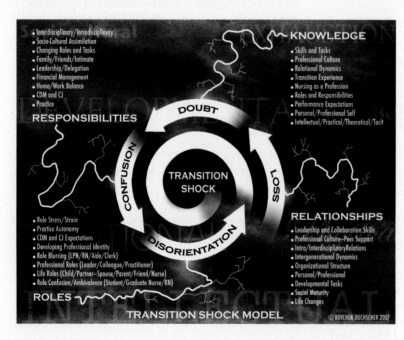

Figure 7.2 Diagram Transition Shock theory.

Career Development

An early start on developing your career is a critical component in moving toward success. This doesn't mean that you need to have a 10-year plan laid out, ensuring that you arrive to your anticipated goal on a fixed or rigid schedule. Leave yourself open to different things that might interest you. Crafting narrow plans for yourself might distract you from once-in-a-lifetime opportunities and make you feel unsuccessful if you don't stay on course.

As we mentioned earlier, prepare for your senior practicum, assess the practice areas that you are interested in. Inquire regarding the kind of support that a potential employer will give you in the way of continuing education and professional development. Assess for opportunities that would be present for advancement, should you decide this is the direction that you want to go. A preliminary look at other degree or diploma programs can assist you in achieving future goals, can clarify or inspire your interests, and show you how you might consider getting there.

Preparing for Registration

Preparation for graduation and the transition to professional practice actually begins on your first day of nursing school. Your learning is deliberately paced and begins with the more simple concepts and competencies and gradually moves from concrete facts to abstract thinking. No one will ever dispute that over the course of 4 years, you learn a massive amount of information. Application of this information is required in your professional practice and will be tested in the registration examinations that you write prior to entering practice as an RN in your province and Canada. Provinces are also developing **jurisprudence examinations** that students are expected to take prior to receiving their registration with the provincial regulatory bodies. The examinations were at varying stages of development across Canada at the time of this chapter being written. It is strongly recommended that you check with your own provincial regulatory body website or your academic advisor well in advance of your final year of nursing studies to prepare for the examination process.

It is impossible to study for an exam of this type in the last few months of school because the test questions are designed to measure your readiness to enter practice and to safely and effectively provide care to your patients. Organization will be helpful and reviewing each, and every time that you care for a patient in clinical will also help you to retain the knowledge required to pass an examination of this type.

The National Council Licensure Examination for Registered Nurses

The purpose of the RN licensing exam is to ensure that the individual has the entry-level competencies to provide safe and effective nursing care. Prior to 2015, the Canadian Registration Nursing Exam (CRNE), developed and maintained by the CNA, was the exam used nationally. In 2012, the **Canadian Council of Registered Nurse Regulators (CCRNR)** made the decision to adapt the National Council Licensure Examination (NCLEX) to replace the CRNE as the registration exam for RNs. The NCLEX provides a universal structure for defining nursing actions and competencies. It focuses on clients of all ages and in all settings. See Table 7.2 for links to more information on the CNA, CCRNR, and National Council of State Boards of Nursing (NCSBN).

How Is the National Council Licensure Examination Developed to Reflect the Knowledge Required by Entry-Level Nurses to Practice?

NCSBN (2013) conducts practice analyses to determine the level of competency that entry-level nurses must possess in order to provide safe and effective care and

TABLE 7.2	Nursing Organizations	
Organization	**Purpose**	**Website**
What is the CNA role in CRNE?	Prior to January 2015, the CNA developed and maintained the CRNE.	http://www.cna-aiic.ca/en/becoming-an-rn/rn-exam/
What is the CCRNR?	National organization formed in 2011 and is made up of representatives from Canada's 12 provincial/territorial bodies that regulate the practice of registered nurses	http://www.ccrnr.ca/
What is the NCSBN?	Not-for-profit organization whose purpose is to provide an organization through which boards of nursing act and counsel together on matters of common interest and concern affecting the public health, safety, and welfare, including the development of licensing examinations in nursing	https://www.ncsbn.org/index.htm

TABLE 7.3	Resources for Preparing for National Council Licensure Examination for Registered Nurses Examination	
Question	Guidance	Website for Information
How do I register and prepare for the exam?	Review NCLEX candidate bulletin prior to registering or taking the exam.	https://www.ncsbn.org/1213.htm
What is the NCLEX passing standard?	Information on process used to set passing standard and the current passing standard	https://www.ncsbn.org/2630.htm
Where can I get an example of the test plan and sample questions?	Test plan provides a concise summary of the content and scope of the examination and serve as a guide for preparation.	https://www.ncsbn.org/1287.htm
What is CAT?	Video and information explaining CAT	https://www.ncsbn.org/1216.htm
What if I have other questions?	NCLEX Frequently Asked Questions for Canadian Educators & Students	http://www.cno.org/Global/new/NCLEX/Canadia_NCLEX_FAQs_toPost.pdf

uses this information to construct a test plan. The items developed are based on all health-care settings in which entry-level RNs practice including acute/critical care, long-term/rehabilitation care, outpatient care, and community based/home care. The complete process used to develop the exam questions is explained on the NCSBN website (Table 7.3).

How Is the Exam Structured?

The exam uses a framework that is organized into four major categories of Client Needs. Two categories, Safe and Effective Care Environment and Physiological Integrity are divided into subcategories (Box 7.3).

What Is the Process for Taking the Exam?

The NCLEX is administered using **computerized adaptive testing (CAT)** (https://www.ncsbn.org/1216.htm). CAT allows the computer to choose items based on the individual's ability. Every time an item is answered, the computer re-estimates the individual's ability based on all the previous answers and the difficulty of those items.

BOX 7.3   Client Needs Exam Framework

1. Safe and Effective Care Environment
   Management of Care
   Safety and Infection Control
2. Health Promotion and Maintenance
3. Psychosocial Integrity
4. Physiological Integrity
   Basic Care and Comfort
   Pharmacological and Parenteral Therapies
   Reduction of Risk Potential
   Physiological Adaptation

Source: National Council of State Boards of Nursing. (2012). *NCLEX-RN® Examination. Test plan for the National Council Licensure Examination for Registered Nurses.* Retrieved from https://www.ncsbn.org/2013_NCLEX_RN_Test_Plan.pdf

---

Jaswinder is now preparing to write the NCLEX for entry to practice. She has been thinking about the exams every semester and feels confident about her ability but admits she is afraid of the unknown and wants to do well. It has been her dream for 4 years to reach graduation and become an RN. Jaswinder reflects on strategies for success that she has been using to study for exams as a student in her nursing program but wonders if there is anything else that she can do to prepare for national exams.

How Can I Prepare for This Exam?

You should review the regularly updated resources that are available on the NCSBN website (see Table 7.3). It provides guidance on what to do prior to taking the exam, what to do on exam day, and what to do after the exam. Also see Box 7.4 for some advice on preparing for exams from actual students.

SUMMARY

Graduation is just the beginning of the next chapter of your professional development. As you will see in the final chapter of this book, you are expected to continually develop and refresh your nursing skills and build on your knowledge from your first day of work to the day you retire or longer. I know many retired nurses who still do volunteer work, attend conferences and are valuable contributors as researchers, mentors, adjunct faculty, and the list goes on. This chapter has touched on some interesting topics and in reality has only just scratched the surface on the student journey from admission to graduation and entrance to professional practice. Celebrate the destination once you reach your goal but remember to enjoy the journey along the way. The memories and the friendships that you make in nursing school have been known to last a lifetime, and reunions are something that nursing graduates cherish and look forward to throughout their careers.

BOX 7.4 **Student Advice: Preparing for the National Council Licensure Examination for Registered Nurses Examination**

Note: The students below who are providing personal views about writing the NCLEX, voluntarily chose to write the NCLEX in addition to writing the CRNE prior to 2015. In 2015, the NCLEX is the required examination for registration in Canada, and the CRNE is no longer offered.

"Firstly, remember that the NCLEX is just another exam. You have survived through years of nursing school, and this is the finale to all those years of study. That being said, keep in mind that you have been studying for this exam for years. This is the mad dash to the finish line. So, when you get ready to study, I would recommend looking back at your nursing education and reviewing what is important. You know your anatomy and physiology; don't study what you already know. Use the time before the exam to supplement your existing knowledge with anything you feel is important. Do some research and see what the foci are of the exam and tailor your studying to optimize your time. What I did was focused on studying and learning test-taking techniques, specifically looking exactly what the NCLEX is asking you to answer and what means are best used to answer each question. For example, if a question asks for an intervention, being able to identify and eliminate non-intervention options can be difficult if you don't learn how to do it properly. A month prior to writing the NCLEX, I only did practice questions. Do a lot of practice questions! Not only does it help you study content, but it [also] gets you used to answering NCLEX style questions. After a few hundred, you will start to see specific patterns that make things much easier for your actual exam. So good luck and remember: Focus on what's important and practice lots of questions."—Conrad Lauko

"I bought a[n] NCLEX prep book and reviewed the content briefly, making sure to focus on the differences between Canada and the USA; for example, lab values. Since all the NCLEX prep books are formatted differently, make sure to browse around to find the one you like best. Mostly importantly, answer as many practice questions as you can. Since you don't know the style of the actual NCLEX questions, I found it beneficial to answer practice questions from different prep books."—Tomasina Malott

"When it comes to prepping for the NCLEX, first and foremost, give yourself enough time to thoroughly review all material. This is not a psychosocial exam to assess your personality; this exam is a test of one's knowledge base. I would recommend at least 6 weeks to review material—4 weeks as a solid overview where you can determine your strengths and weaknesses, followed by 2 weeks of focused review on areas where you feel you could improve. In addition to this, if you are having difficulty remembering a specific fact (e.g., specific ABG values), move on. It is best to have an understanding rather than to memorize facts; you will never see a repeat of a practice question in the NCLEX, as the exam is not assessing your ability to recall facts, but rather your understanding of concepts, pathways, and clinical judgement—how you put it all together."—Kyla Wortley

"The first step in preparing for the NCLEX is evaluating your current study skills and habits. Cramming may have worked in the past for previous nursing school exams, but cramming here will set you up for failure. You also need to acknowledge that trying to memorize 4 years of information in a very short period of time will get you nowhere. The NCLEX doesn't want to know what you've memorized; it wants to evaluate your knowledge base by having you apply critical thinking skills to scenarios. Plan out a study schedule and be reasonable. Two weeks will not be enough time to prepare, but waiting 3 or 4 months to write is just prolonging the inevitable. I found 6 weeks was a good time frame. I studied about 2–3 hours a day for those 6 weeks. It's not how long you study for—it's what you study that makes the difference. Divide and conquer—group subjects together and study. I did lab values and tests for a few days, cardiac for a few days, obstetrics and peds for a few days, and so on. However, the NCLEX wants to evaluate your general knowledge base in medical-surgical nursing because you're a novice. Do lots of practice questions. This really helps you get in the mindset of what to expect when you're actually writing and makes you feel more comfortable. Stop studying the day before. Do not cram! You'll amp up your stress levels and panic. Give yourself lots of time to get to the test center—the last thing you need to be worrying about is being late for the exam. And the most helpful thing to remember—try not to listen to the horror stories of other people's exam writing experiences. Easier said than done, but sometimes, it's just easier to plug your ears, ignore them, and worry about yourself and do your own thing! Have a little bit of confidence in yourself—you got this far, so you're doing something right!"—Victoria Ziraldo

Critical Thinking Case Scenarios

▶ Braden is a fourth-year student who is eagerly anticipating entry to practice. As such, he is starting to think more critically during his clinical shifts by synthesizing all components of his nursing education. On more than one occasion, he has witnessed or been involved in situations that he is uncertain if they had been handled ethically. As a student, describe some of the different types of situations that you could be involved in that would make you feel like Braden.

▶ The CNSA has been on Matthew's mind for some time. As a motivated yet fatigued third-year student, he wonders if he should even think about trying to get involved. In the spirit of good decision-making, he asks a few of his professors what they think about his wanting to get involved, to which he receives mixed reviews. Feeling hopeful and brave, he decides to get involved and work very hard to ensure that he can manage all of his responsibilities. How would you go about making the decision that Matthew has made?

Multiple-Choice Questions

1. An error that is caught before it happens is called a:
   a. Near miss
   b. Good save
   c. Stroke of luck
   d. Timely discovery

2. CNSA: The voice of nursing students in Canada has been in existence since:
   a. 2000
   b. 1971
   c. 1999
   d. 2005

3. Which of the following behaviours could be perceived as "bullying" behaviours?
   a. Eye rolling by a nurse at you or another nurse
   b. Having other nurses refuse to help you with patient care
   c. Being excluded by certain nurses from lunches or social events
   d. All of the above

4. CAT allows for:
   a. The computer to choose items based on the individual's ability
   b. The student to control the questions being asked
   c. The testing process to be shorter
   d. A longer wait time for the results

5. The jurisprudence examination is taken:
   a. Prior to receiving registration by your provincial regulatory body.
   b. At the beginning of your final year of nursing school.
   c. With the CRNE or the NCLEX.
   d. Annually, once you are an RN.

6. The exam uses a framework that is organized into four major categories. A Safe and Effective Care Environment is further divided into which two subcategories:
   a. Management of Care and Falls Prevention
   b. Falls Prevention and Safe Medication Administration
   c. Management of Care and Safety and Infection Control
   d. Safety and Infection Control and Safe Medication Administration

7. Transition Shock may involve the following:
   a. Denial, Confusion, Panic and Fear
   b. Denial, Confusion, Loss and Doubt
   c. Doubt, Disorientation, Loss and Confusion
   d. Doubt, Disorientation, Panic and Confusion

REFERENCES AND SUGGESTED READINGS

Canadian Council of Registered Nurse Regulators. (2013). *Who we are*. Retrieved from http://www.ccrnr.ca/

Canadian Mental Health Association. (2013). *Canadian mental health stress meter*. Retrieved from http://www.cmha.ca/mental_health/mental-health-meter/#.UmbcFRaRP8s/

Canadian Nurses Association. (2013). *RN exam*. Retrieved from http://www.cna-aiic.ca/en/becoming-an-rn/rn-exam/

Canadian Nursing Students' Association. (2009). *Patient safety*. Retrieved from http://www.cnsa.ca/english/publications/resolutions-and-position-statements/position-statements/self-care-practices-among-nursing-students

College of Nurses of Ontario. (2013). *Jurisprudence exam*. Retrieved from http://www.cno.org/become-a-nurse/about-registration/entry-to-practice-examinations/jurisprudence-examination/

Duchscher, J. B. (2008). A process of becoming: The stages of new nursing graduate professional role transition. *The Journal of Continuing Education in Nursing, 39*(10), 441–450.

Duchscher, J. B. (2012). *From surviving to thriving: Navigating the first year of professional nursing practice*. Saskatoon, SK: Saskatoon Fastprint.

Myrick, F., & Yonge, O. (2005). *Nursing preceptorship: Connecting practice & education*. Philadelphia, PA: Lippincott Williams & Wilkins.

National Council Licensure Examination for Registered Nurses. (n.d.). *Candidate bulletin & information*. Retrieved from https://www.ncsbn.org/1213.htm

National Council of State Boards of Nursing. (2013). *For the nursing community*. Retrieved https://www.ncsbn.org/index.htm

Sigma Theta Tau International Records. (1920–2007). Ruth Lilly Special Collections and Archives, IUPUI University Library, Indiana University Purdue University Indianapolis.

Southey, T. (2012, December 12). 'What did you just eat?' The lessons of a university minor in 'dog.' *The Globe and Mail*. Retrieved from http://www.theglobeandmail.com/commentary/columnists/what-did-you-just-eat-the-lessons-of-a-university-minor-in-dog/article6122173

Srabstein, J. C., & Leventhal, B. L. (2010). Prevention and bullying-related morbidity and mortality: A call for public health policies. *Bulletin of the World Health Organization, 88*, 403. doi:10.2471/BLT.10.077123

Thompson, R. (2012a). *"Do no harm" applies to nurses too! Strategies to protect and bully-proof yourself at work*. Pittsburgh, PA: inCredible Messages Press.

Thompson, R. (2012b). *"Survive + thrive: A guide: Helping new nurses succeed."* Pittsburgh, PA: RT Connections, LLC.

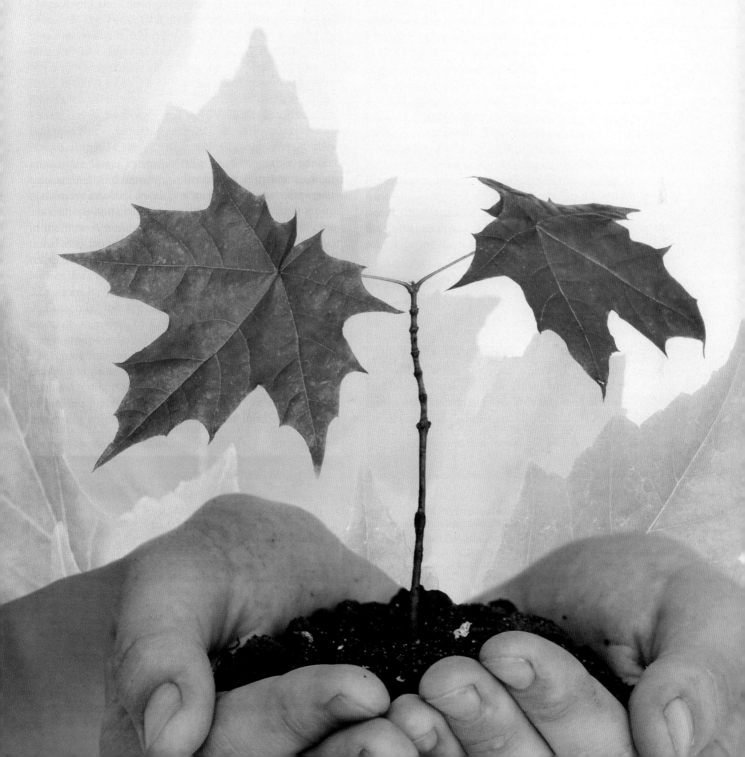

two
Thinking

Health, Wellness, and Illness

NATASHA L. HUBBARD MURDOCH

Katia is a first-year nursing student. She is from the Philippines. In her first nursing seminar, each student offers an introduction and tells a story of what brought them to nursing. Katia is quiet and waits until she is asked to share her story. Katia reveals that she enjoys "nursing" her grandmother who has been living with the family for 2 years following a stroke. She is thinking of writing her first nursing paper on what it means to be healthy following a stroke.

CHAPTER OBJECTIVES

By the end of this chapter, you will be able to:

1. Differentiate between health, wellness, and illness.
2. Compare types of knowing.
3. Describe the value of a health risk assessment tool.
4. Offer examples of each domain of wellness.
5. Describe wellness for specific patient populations.
6. Describe the roles of a nurse in promoting health.
7. Describe the Health Promotion Model.

KEY TERMS

Determinants Factors that impact health, such as income and social status, social support networks, education, working conditions, social environments, physical environments, personal health practices and coping skills, biology, gender, and culture.

Disease The physiological deviation from "normal," that is, therefore, objective or measurable.

Health A positive concept, beyond physical capabilities, emphasizes social and personal resources. Holistic understanding of health is central to the definition of health promotion. The Ottawa Charter emphasizes certain prerequisites for health, which include peace, adequate economic resources, food and shelter, and a stable ecosystem and sustainable resource use. These prerequisites highlight the inextricable links between social and economic conditions, the physical environment, individual lifestyles, and health. Although health is a positive, it is not the point to living; health is a resource for living well.

Health Promotion Health promotion is, in part, the promotion of healthy ideas and concepts in order to motivate individuals to adopt healthy behaviours. Health promotion is also the provision of information and/or education to families and communities encouraging family unity, community commitment, and spirituality, all of which make positive contributions to health.

Illness The subjective experience of living with a disease or condition and its accompanying symptoms.

Nursing Process A multistep framework used to create a plan of care, including assessment, nursing diagnosis, planning, interventions, and evaluation.

Objective Knowing Concrete, measurable knowledge; often easily defined as the "opposite of subjective."

Population Health Improving the determinants of health from the perspective of a nation.

Self-Change Behaviour An action the patient is willing to employ to meet health outcomes.

Self-Efficacy The judgment a person makes of his or her personal ability to organize and carry out a particular course of action.

Subjective Knowing Knowledge informed by perception, personal views, experience, or background.

Well-Being The presence of the highest possible quality of life, including such aspects as good living standards and education; robust health; a sustainable environment; vital communities with high levels of civic participation; and access to and participation in arts, culture, and recreation.

Wellness There is no universally accepted definition of wellness. Wellness is an evolving process of becoming aware of and making choices toward a fulfilling sense of individual life accomplishments. Dimensions of wellness include both physical and mental components. Wellness describes a multidimensional state of being involving the existence of positive health, exemplified by the individual's experience of life quality and his or her sense of well-being.

Beginning to Understand What We Know About Health

What does a healthy person look like? Is health the same as wellness? What causes a person to be ill? How does a nurse know when others are feeling well or ill? This chapter begins with thinking about the way nurses and patients perceive health, wellness, and illness. The roles of nursing require interacting with diverse patient populations and health-care professionals. In addition, the nurse's understanding of personal, provincial, national, and global motivations for health shapes how he or she interacts with patients.

When patients relay their stories about health, nurses gather knowledge that shapes a clinical picture. Knowing in nursing is a complex concept. Nurses gain or use knowledge through experience, with reflection, and to improve practice. It has been a topic of interest and research since the 1970s when Carper (1978) published her important work on fundamental patterns of knowing in nursing.

You will learn about patterns of knowing throughout this textbook. However, for the purpose of this chapter, the focus is on subjective and objective knowing. **Subjective knowing** is a way of thinking and feeling based on personal experiences and interactions with others or the environment (Bonis, 2009). Subjective knowing constantly changes with each new experience; we develop meanings about our experiences and how they affect us. This type of knowing is difficult to measure and may be interpreted differently between nurses. For example, a patient may report excruciating pain, but have no change in facial expression, whereas another patient may be crying and grimacing. **Objective knowing** is concrete, measurable, often easily defined and coined as the "opposite of subjective" (Venes, 2009). Therefore, we can seek the patient's subjective answer to such questions as, "Do you think you are healthy?" "What are your favourite foods?" We can also explore with the patient objective measures that inform us about his or her "health status" such as weight or height.

Nurses use both subjective and objective information to develop a plan of care with the patient. Both subjective and objective information are data. The more data or pieces of information, the more thorough a picture of the patient and his perception about being healthy or the measures that show health. Collecting data is part of the first step, assessment, in the **nursing process**, a multi-step framework used to create a plan of care. Nurses use patient data to make decisions about the most appropriate actions to support the patient. The data collected leads the nurse to nursing diagnoses and subsequently appropriate plans of care based on a continual evaluation of each action and decision in collaboration with the patient. The nursing process is discussed further in Chapter 10. For the moment, consider subjective and objective knowing as you read through the eyes of a nurse working with a patient who smokes cigarettes.

Health, Wellness, Illness, and Disease

The difficulty with concepts related to health and illness is that, despite all the research from numerous specialties and disciplines within and outside nursing, there is a little agreement regarding a singular definition. Our understanding of health, wellness, illness, and disease has evolved over time (and continues to evolve), and we are now able to understand it in ways that make sense to nurses.

What Is Health?

Historically, being healthy was an objective concept that meant stability and balance (Jensen & Allen, 1993a; Mackey, 2009); a "wholeness or completeness" (Jensen & Allen, 1993b, p. 220) that superseded wellness (Mackey, 2009). Even the word *healthy* means "being whole, sound or well" (Harper, 2001). But what does wholeness look like? How can we measure wholeness? Dr. Halbert Dunn was a biostatistician who developed a computer program to classify and collect medical information on patients (U.S. Census Bureau, 2012). We use those statistics to determine how healthy our communities are and find evidence for decisions we make in practice. Dr. Dunn's work is a foundation for health promotion, discussed later in this chapter. He described the differing states of being healthy: "Sometimes you are more well than at other times . . . you are fairly alive with the glow of good health—with wellness" (Dunn, 1961, p. 2). There is a close relationship between being healthy and being well, and either or both of those concepts are equated to well-being. As a result, the three terms are often used interchangeably; but healthiness, wellness, and well-being are distinctly different from each other.

The constitution of the World Health Organization (WHO, 1948, p. 1) has defined **health** as "a state of complete physical, mental, and social well-being and not merely the absence of disease or infirmity," a definition that has not changed since 1948. To reach full health, a person must have the capacity to "identify and to realize aspirations, to satisfy needs, and to change or cope with the environment" (World Health Organization [WHO], 1986, p. 1). Although good health is a positive, it is not the point of living; instead, health is a resource for living well.

What Is Wellness?

The WHO's new definition of **wellness** is the optimal state of health of individuals and groups. There are two focal concerns: the realization of the fullest potential of an individual physically, psychologically, socially, spiritually, and economically and the fulfillment of one's role expectations in the family, community, place of worship, workplace, and other settings (Smith, Tang, & Nutbeam, 2006).

Wellness is often characterized as a subjective experience (Jensen & Allen, 1993a). From a nursing perspective, wellness is a match between a person's reason for living, actions, and potential (Benner & Wrubel, 1989). Dunn (1961) stated, "Wellness is an integrated method of functioning which is oriented toward maximizing the potential of which the individual is capable" (p. 4). If health is considered an objective measure, then wellness is the person's subjective experience of being healthy.

What Is Disease and Illness?

Disease and illness are often seen in opposition to health and wellness (Jensen & Allen, 1993b). **Disease** is the physiological deviation from normal, which is objective or measurable. Disease "implies a focus on pathological processes that may or may not produce symptoms and that result in a patient's illness" (Association of Faculties of Medicine of Canada [AFMC], n.d., p. 1). Typically, diseases cause altered functioning (Jensen & Allen, 1993a). Being ill is frequently defined as synonymous with disease (Pugh, 2006). **Illness**, however, is the experience of living with a disease. It is subjective, depending on the personal experience of associated symptoms, suffering, or distress. The impact of this altered function is different for each individual and is noticeable as a difference in behaviour (Kiefer, 2008), a change in how the individual relates or acts in conversation (Paterson, 2001), or whether the individual can do the same tasks and live in the same environment as before the change in health (Breen, Green, Roarty, & Saggers, 2008; Freund, 2001).

Think *Whose Wellness?*

I worked with a patient who had been diagnosed with breast cancer. At the time she met me, she had completed her surgery. This was her first appointment at the clinic, and I gave her educational materials on the chemotherapy and radiation she was expected to have next. Because she was young, the chemotherapy was going to put her into premature menopause. In her household, she would not be considered a woman anymore if she did not have the potential to have children. If she were not a woman, her husband could end their marriage. The difficulty with cancer, the disease, is that it was not causing her any measurable symptoms. This woman experienced distress because of the potential impact on her relationship with her husband.

The best approach for me in this situation was to give her all the information possible about the next treatment steps and make another appointment where she could share her decision. In the meantime, I needed to find out more about her sociocultural situation, debrief with my colleagues, and be clear on my health values and her right to make an informed decision.
What is the definition of health for the nurse?
What is the definition of wellness for this woman?

What Do Canadians Think About Health?

Although the WHO defines health as "a state of complete physical, mental, or social well-being and not merely the absence of disease or infirmity" (WHO, 1948, p.1), what do Canadians think about health?

Perceptions of Health

A Health Canada report (2011) combining data on the health status of Canadians included 54 health and disease indicators and revealed that in general, life expectancy for men and women had increased, fewer teenagers smoked, and there was less incidence of breast and prostate cancer. Conversely, one third of Canadians were overweight, and over 15% were obese. The researchers asked Canadians whether they felt healthy, and overall Canadians rated their health at least very good.

Health Canada (2009) observes that when people consider how they perceive their own health, they think about their chances of having a "chronic disease, loss of ability to function, and ultimately, survival" (p. 44). This has interesting implications for the general health of Canadians. How do people actually judge their health (Singh-Manoux et al., 2006)? When Canadians are asked about "age, early life factors and measures of family history, sociodemographic variables, psychosocial factors, health behaviours, and measures of health and disease" (Singh-Manoux et al., 2006, p. 364), the response contrasts with Health Canada's (2009) report. Measures of health, such as the symptoms of illness, and psychosocial factors, such as emotions, are how people decide whether they are healthy, not how old they are, where they have lived, or where they grew up. Health is what is happening, in the moment, in the body, mind, and spirit.

Sometimes, people continue with poor health practices, such as smoking for example, because they perceive they are already healthy and well (Mackey, 2009; Paterson, 2001; Peterson, 1996). Nurses can listen to a patient's perceptions of health values and beliefs, work with the patient on what optimal health could be, and encourage him or her to consider wellness programs that would match his or her family and work lifestyle. Consider how having information about a patient's health values and beliefs might be of value to nurses. As a fourth-year baccalaureate nursing student, Serena writes about comparing the objective health perceptions written in a patient chart with her personal subjective experiences.

Through the eyes of a student

Definitions and perceptions are two completely different things. My definition of health may be completely different than what another person perceives health to be. An example of this is a person I knew all my life: someone who had polio as a child, was in a wheelchair, and on large doses of opiates for pain. His legs had complete muscle atrophy and were no bigger than just the bone covered in skin. He would regularly call me, excited that his weight was over 100 lb. (He was over 6 ft tall if he could have stood upright!) On first glance, would I have defined him as healthy? If I had not known this person and had just seen him on paper, probably not. Yet, he perceived himself to be healthy, and he lived to the highest optimum health he could. He was a writer, enjoyed the company of others and was quite social, was involved in the arts, and always told me never to let anything that any other person perceives define who you are and what you can do.

This person died a few years ago, but I will always remember not to let what is written in a chart define what I perceive as health for a patient. Until I have had a chance to talk to the patient, I keep an open mind.

(personal reflection of Serena, a student nurse)

Health Risk Assessments

Health risk assessments are one kind of resource available to nurses to help patients assess their health. This data provides a snapshot of the patient's knowledge about health, current behaviours, and areas of knowledge deficit based on past medical history, family history, and exposure to harmful substances (Fig. 8.1). After completing the assessment, the nurse and patient can discuss behaviours that are risky. The nurse should consider three components when working with a patient to determine health risks: psychological, scientific, and media-related factors (Mahon, 2006).

Psychologically, the patient's perception of risk may depend on how much control or fear is associated with the potential harm, such as the impact on quality of life. An example might be children exposed to secondhand smoke.

The patient may continue to expose his or her child to secondhand smoke if he or she does not view any harm arising from the smoke of just one cigarette an hour.

Scientifically, the statistical information may be difficult to comprehend or to place in context of the patient's life. He or she may simply reject the scientific evidence as unbelievable, untrustworthy, or not valuable. For example, knowing that exposure to the sun can cause skin cancer, will he or she wear sunscreen, hats, and sunglasses all the time? Finally, media-related factors affect understanding of risks. Health information has become readily available because of technology, but much of it may be inaccurate, not thorough, or sensationalized through reality television (TV).

There are numerous health risk assessment tools available. As a student, you will want to use an assessment that prompts questions and ensures thorough consideration of the patient. The important thing to remember is that completely filling in the tool is not the goal. Instead, use the tool to better understand the patient. A nonverbal reaction to a specific question may lead to a story about unhealthy behaviours (and therefore, provide you with an opportunity to teach about the risky behaviour and ways to reduce the associated harm). Alternatively, the patient may reveal his or her commitment and good habits or appropriate knowledge and use of resources, providing an opportunity for you to encourage and support positive health behaviours.

Humans have always been driven to optimize health, evolving from the earlier perceptions of the body as a machine (to be fixed) toward emphasis on patient self-responsibility (Grasser & Craft, 1984). Just because the patient knows the risks or has been provided education does not mean that he is motivated to change risk behaviours. The patient may be unwilling or unable to change (Grasser & Craft, 1984; V. D. Johnson, 2007). The sense of health and well-being is different between patients even if they have similar symptoms (Erickson, Stapleton, Erickson, Giannokopoulos, & Wilson, 2006). Thus, a patient's health values impact his or her tolerance of disease-related symptoms. Factors such as well-being, access to resources, the need for control, the ability to be flexible and adapt to situations, self-esteem, and competence in enacting health behaviours affect the patient's perception of how prone he or she is to health problems.

Think of how Katia felt at the beginning of the academic year: rested from her summer and having chosen a career path. Compare this to how she might feel at the end of the semester or term—with exams, full-time studies, and working part-time to meet rent payments. Although Katia is exhausted from the workload, she is more concerned about spending the break away from her family. Sometimes, Katia feels like she's going to burst from the stress, but she cannot seem to put her finger on what is bothering her more—physical tiredness or being close to tears all the time. She just does not feel well.

Demographics

Age _____   Occupation (in or outside?) _____

Gender _____   Type of residence _____

Ethnic background _____   Education achieved _____

Lifestyle behaviors

Activity   *Nutrition*

Physical x/week _____   Diet _____

Types _____   Meals and snacks / day _____

Hobbies _____   Junk foods _____

Drugs

Prescription			
Complementary			
Over-the-counter			
Vitamins			
Recreational			
Smoking			
Alcohol			
'Street drugs'			

Genetics

Anyone in family been for counseling?	
Birth anomalies	

Family History

Medical diagnosis	Member	Age at death	Mental illness diagnosis
	Mother		
	Father		
	Paternal grandmother		
	Paternal grandfather		
	Maternal grandmother		
	Maternal grandfather		
	Siblings		

Screening

Sunscreen	PAP smear
Long sleeved clothing	Rectal exam
Immunizations	BSE/TSE
Seatbelt/helmet	BP

Figure 8.1 Health risk assessment.

The need for patients to be independent, competent, and supported affects their motivation to make healthy choices (V. D. Johnson, 2007). If patients find that inspiration within themselves, that is, intrinsic motivation, they are "doing an activity because it is interesting or enjoyable and it provides satisfaction of the basic needs" (V. D. Johnson, 2007, p. 234). In contrast, extrinsic motivators, the driving forces from outside, are often perceived as controlling. For example, "deadlines, imposed goals, surveillance, threats, orders, and pressured evaluations," are not as effective in motivating behaviour change (V. D. Johnson, 2007, p. 234). A patient may choose to stay on a diet because he or she knows it helps him or her lose weight, whereas a diet is not so compelling if it is suggested by someone else (V. D. Johnson, 2007). Nurses can reflect on their own motivation to keep themselves healthy but also foster the intrinsic investment and responsibility toward wellness in others (Grasser & Craft, 1984; V. D. Johnson, 2007; Mahon, 2006). Think about a time when making a lifestyle change was a priority for you. Reflect on the internal, the feeling-good implications, in contrast to the external, or obligatory, factors that had an impact on your motivation.

Perceptions of Wellness

Wellness is the process of trying to reach optimal health. In that sense, wellness is "always ahead of the person, a state of being to strive towards, always in the future" (Mackey, 2009, p. 104). People usually do not think about wellness unless they are ill, and thus, it is often defined based on what it is not.

Wellness is subjective and therefore difficult to measure, yet numerous wellness assessment tools exist. Wellness is assessed through the emotional, intellectual, occupational, physical, sexual, spiritual, environmental, and social domains. Similar to health risk assessments, wellness assessments provide nurses opportunity to learn what patients think and feel about being healthy. There are three fundamental ideas behind wellness: (1) the domains are interrelated, (2) wellness seems to ebb and flow within and among domains, and (3) the patient is responsible for making choices toward reaching higher levels of wellness; the nurse cannot make choices for the patient.

Depending on how a patient accepts injury or disease, even an illness could be perceived as wellness (Jensen & Allen, 1994). For example, some people who become infected with HIV begin to live their lives in a positive way; that is, they perceive their infection as an opportunity not only for wellness but also for self-transformation (Mulkins, Morse, & Best, 2002). Similarly, a diagnosis of cancer can spur the patient and his or her family to live more fully.

There is no agreement about which domains should or should not be included in a wellness assessment (Canadian Nurses Association [CNA], 2010; Labonté, Muhajarine, Winquist et al., 2010; Roscoe, 2009; WHO, 1998). Examples of wellness assessments include the Life Assessment Questionnaire and the Wellness Index (see web resources at the**Point**).

Wellness Domains

Wellness tools measure the extent to which wellness domains are fulfilled; domains being a way to separate wellness into parts to be assessed (Mackey, 2009). The eight domains—emotional, intellectual, occupational, physical, sexual, spiritual, environmental, and social—are explored in the following sections.

Emotional Wellness

The emotional domain involves understanding feelings, managing or controlling those feelings when necessary, and being able to express feelings appropriately (Engel & Kieffer, 2008). A nursing student must think about where his or her clinical placements will take him. As one clinical group works on the oncology ward, new patients are met, and plans of care are developed. For each member of that clinical group, some feelings to process may include, "Is that what my friend will go through now that she's been diagnosed with cancer?" or "Being a nursing student feels different than when I visited my grandma in hospital." When patients are quite ill, the clinical group may talk about how it would feel to be the nursing student for someone who dies. One nursing student stated, "It is going to be hard for me to hold back tears." Think about how you would feel crying with a patient. Showing vulnerability takes strength. Care is required, however, to maintain the focus of the interaction on the patient. Nurses can build empathy and rapport by showing respect for a patient's situation and experience.

Through the eyes of a nurse

*W*hat I have found helpful working on oncology is ensuring I do two things to keep perspective on stories that can vary from saddening to satisfying. First, journaling, in a diary-like way, about the reality of being human and how emotional some stories make me feel. Then, debriefing with a nurse, or clinical instructor, who can provide explanations, relay similar experiences, or offer resources and evidence. These two steps separate the personal from the professional. This reflective process allows the nurse to plan appropriate care.

(personal reflection of Natasha, a nurse)

Through the eyes of a patient

I was diagnosed with adenocarcinoma of the rectum. At first, I wasn't sure who they were talking about because it couldn't have been me. It just wasn't part of my belief that I would come down with this. After the initial shock of being diagnosed, that's when the fear set in. It feels like disbelief, and then you're scared. All I can say for myself is that I had very little hope. I tried to play it down for my family's sake. I think too; it was denial on my part. I didn't want to believe that this was happening to me. You go through a lot of emotions; you go through the whole thing over and over again. Just because you deal with one emotion doesn't mean it doesn't come back again. My husband and I had talked about the ramifications of cancer and treatment. I knew what I was facing, but I didn't want my children to know. I thought I could prevent them from knowing how serious it was. After the fear was betrayal. I thought I had been betrayed. Cancer is your own body attacking you. It is your own cells that have gone rampant, and they are attacking your good cells. So, it's your body fighting against itself and making you die. All I could think of was, let's get this out of here, before it goes any further. I have to put my life on hold; I have to basically face my own death.

(*personal reflection of Penny, a patient*)

Intellectual Wellness

Conversely, in the intellectual domain, the advancement of knowledge and creative potential is a priority (Roscoe, 2009). Individuals search for stimulating activity and opportunities for critical thinking to ensure the growth of self. Paluck, Allerdings, Kealy, and Dorgan (2006) compared three age groups of women to understand their needs for wellness activities in a rural setting. The researchers stated that "older women were unique in their focus on keeping an 'active mind'" (Paluck et al., 2006, p. 113), which might include visiting, hobbies, or volunteering. Recent research in neuroscience has use playing brainteasers and memory games to increase attention and performance. What a great reason to buy that app, download a podcast, or register for an open course!

Occupational Wellness

The occupational domain, sometimes called the *vocational domain*, relates specifically to the value that individuals place on work, whether paid or volunteer (Roscoe, 2009). Optimal wellness in this domain is attained through being satisfied with providing service to others (Engel & Kieffer, 2008) by using personal skills to advance the community and society at large. This includes the attitude and desire to enjoy the benefits of both work and play. Stamm et al. (2009) interviewed people with rheumatoid arthritis to understand their experiences of being well in relation to employment. Because rheumatoid arthritis affects patients' roles as employees, they were challenged to find a new balance within their work worlds and home contexts. The researchers discovered that people considered the following: challenging versus relaxing occupations and activities, activities meaningful to the individual, and emphasizing self-care activities versus caring for others.

Katia thinks back to her family. Her father was the sole income earner and seemed pleased at how well his small business was doing. Because Katia has three brothers and two sisters and her grandmother required 24-hour care, Katia's mother was the "stay-at-home" parent. Katia reflects on her future role as a nurse and as the primary wage earner when she brings her family to Canada.

Physical Wellness

The physical domain encompasses activities directed at sustaining states of health including lifestyle choices (not smoking or using recreational drugs, consuming alcohol in moderation, and engaging in regular physical activity), maintaining a nutritious diet, and self-care (Engel & Kieffer, 2008). There are many facets to the decision to maintain physical health. Nurses perform warm-up exercises prior to their shifts for safe functioning when assisting patients to mobilize, which is a task in the occupational domain. However, choosing to consume more than a moderate amount of alcohol when around friends may be related to peer pressure in the social domain.

Nurse researchers in Saskatchewan surveyed high school students to determine how adolescents view wellness (Spurr, Bally, Ogenchuk, & Walker, 2012). The researchers stipulated at the start of the study that for adolescents to achieve holistic wellness, they must grow in four specific dimensions: physical, psychological, social, and spiritual. What is interesting about their study is the premise that there is an ideal state of wellness to be achieved. The researchers found an unexpected result; the domains "were not equally important" for the students (Spurr et al., 2012, p. 323) when compared to the researcher's ideal.

This finding is significant for nurses performing wellness assessments. First, the patient defines health, wellness, and well-being for himself or herself. Second, nurses need to understand physical well-being according to the developmental stage of the patient. Metabolism, strength, flexibility, and endurance might be different for an adolescent compared to an elder. Nurses can stress wellness through education and also by understanding the patient's viewpoint and pressures that exist. Look at Figure 8.2 and note the ages of the children and how similar they all look. Consider what you know of this age group: How do they feel about their bodies? What do they talk about with friends? What amount of physical activity is suggested for children in Canada?

Sexual Wellness

Sexuality is often not included in wellness assessments. Researchers lament that limited data exists about people's view of their sexuality, possibly because of our discomfort with asking or even answering questions about sex.

Sexual wellness is directly related to health. As health declines, so does sexual satisfaction (Hooghe, 2012). Consider physiological changes in functioning associated with a spinal cord injury or a stroke and how sexuality then ties to the physical domain. Linkages to the intellectual, emotional, and social domains are through the concepts that help define sexuality (Hucker, Mussap, & McCabe, 2010). Sexual identity comprises what preferences and values are chosen in relationships and how sexuality is expressed. Sexual self-efficacy, which is confidence in making appropriate healthy decisions, and sexual self-esteem, which is a sense of worth, positively influence views on wellness. Sexual satisfaction, which includes positive relationships, contributes to overall happiness with life (Hooghe, 2012).

Nurses can target support and education by respecting sexual identity, self-efficacy, and self-esteem. Traditionally, sexual education focuses on anatomy and physiology or the

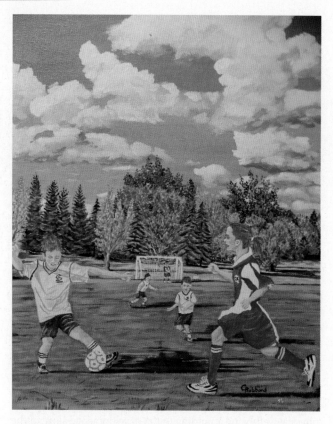

Figure 8.2 Children playing soccer. (Source: Hubbard, C. [2012]. Children Playing Soccer. Used with Permission.)

use of condoms. But consider education across the lifespan. Those between the ages of 30 and 50 years tend to feel less satisfied, but this may be because of work, responsibilities, and stress or increased commitments to children (Hooghe, 2012). Sexual satisfaction also increases with years of education, which may relate to education leading to better employment and better health. As people get older, sexuality declines; to be sexually well often is tied to having a partner. Think about how many older adults, 75 or 85 years or older, have someone to live with and to engage in sexual practices.

Also, consider how sociocultural environment affects expression of sexuality. A worldwide study of 27,500 respondents older than the age of 40 years wondered whether countries with a male-dominated culture would have a lower sexual well-being (Laumann et al., 2006). *Male-dominated* was defined as "emphasis[ing] the centrality of men in controlling the sexual conduct of women" (Laumann et al., 2006, p. 146) as compared to gender-equal regimes, which do not stress sex as a duty of marriage or procreation. Despite cultural variety, it was physical and mental health and positive relationships that determined sexual wellness.

Sexual wellness contributes to identity and personality; is affected by physical and intellectual domains; and has an impact on occupational experiences, emotions, and social relationships. Because of these links between mind, body, and quality relationships with others, sexuality is also tied to spirituality.

Spiritual Wellness

Assessing wellness in the spiritual domain requires a holistic view of the individual—the person as a mingling of mind, body, and spirit. The WHO (2002a) notes the need for impeccable assessment of physical, psychological, social, and spiritual needs. A variety of perspectives on spirituality exist. The humanistic perspective suggests that "persons have a soul or spirit (a spiritual dimension), that life is sacred, and that life has a higher purpose" (Delgado, 2007, p. 281). Other perspectives describe spiritual wellness as sustained through having a sense of meaning in life (Engel & Kieffer, 2008; Kiefer, 2008). Meaning and purpose in life evolve during the course of a lifetime. The relational perspective describes spirituality as having a relationship with nature, or relationships with the self, others, or a higher being (Fisher, Francis, & Johnson, 2000; McBrien, 2006). Fisher et al. (2000) gathered data on the perceptions of spiritual health from teachers and found that the components of spirituality include such things as being happy to be alive, being trusting and truthful with others, enjoying beauty and time to reflect, and having a relationship with God. However, the authors of the study point out that within the domain of spirituality, an individual will choose which aspects mean the most to her—not everyone will choose a conventional relationship with God. Fisher et al. (2000) state, "it is such individuals who enable us to see more clearly the unique qualities" (p. 135) that are incorporated in a spiritual assessment. The individual is the nurse's best source of information for whether optimal spiritual wellness is achieved.

In working toward meeting the spiritual needs of patients, challenges to providing support become apparent. One difficulty exists because the innate character of spirituality (Roscoe, 2009) makes it difficult to separate the spirit from other domains (Delgado, 2007) such as intellectual or emotional. This, in turn, necessitates assessing and planning patient-specific nursing care because each person involved, whether nurse, patient, family member, other health-care providers, and other professionals (e.g., clergy), has a unique perspective on spirituality. Other difficulties with providing spiritual care include lack of confidence among nurses, limited knowledge, lack of self-awareness (of one's own spirituality), lack of time, and an inappropriate environment (e.g., a four-bed ward in a hospital; Barss, 2012; Delgado, 2007).

In addition, differing orientations to spirituality exist; for example, the scientific, medical-model approach, versus a more ephemeral, inclusive, and relational approach (Chuengsatiansup, 2003). The Canadian Nurses Association (CNA) position statement was developed on spirituality in the context of suffering (CNA, 2010) and the WHO Quality of Life Spirituality, Religiousness and Personal Beliefs (QoL-SRPB) group developed a questionnaire for assessment based in concerns (WHO, 2002b). The work of both the CNA and the WHO was based in a medical approach that focused on health and quality of life in relation to illness and disability rather than to wellness and well-being. This scientific approach contrasts with the relational perspective in which spirituality is revealed through connection with something or someone else (Chuengsatiansup, 2003). Refer to Chapter 40, Spirituality and Nursing, for discussion of using a relational model to promote spiritual well-being for both the nurse and the patient (Barss, 2012).

However, despite the challenges, spirituality remains theoretically tied to nursing (Delgado, 2007). It follows then, that nurses may assist patients to deal with loss, suffering, or death; turmoil related to beliefs; or the opportunity to grow spiritually (Delgado, 2007) in relationships with the self, others, and/or a higher being (Fisher et al., 2000).

RESEARCH

THE MEANING OF HEALTH FOR LUTSEL K'E DENE FIRST NATION

The meaning of health among members of the Lutsel K'e Dene First Nation on Great Slave Lake in the Northwest Territories was explored as they were undergoing an environmental assessment prior to a diamond mine being built. The purpose of the study was to understand the meaning of health in order to be able to assess any health impact on the Dene people once the mine was functional.

Study
The research method is participatory action research using narratives from interviews and thematic analysis to develop a framework noting health indicators to be assessed. The community has then used the results to monitor their health.

Conclusions
The main definition of health is described as "the Dene way of life." The first theme, self-governance, meant "power and capacity to control and manage community affairs, lands, and resources" (p. 120). The second theme was healing for individuals, families, and the community. The third theme was cultural preservation, with narratives about land, traditions, language, and caribou harvesting. The authors suggest that a wellness orientation more closely aligns with the cultural perspective. The WHO definition of health, although widely cited, is not universally accepted.

Implications for Nursing Students
This particular research article provides a unique perspective on each domain of wellness from an individual and community perspective. For the purposes of a nursing environmental assessment, there is significance in the relationship of people to land and resources. This not only includes considering large-scale developments but also the significance of historical and traditionally spiritual landmarks as well as the effects of a change in diet from hunting to prepared foods.

Parlee, B., O'Neil, J., & Lutsel K'e Dene First Nation. (2007). "The Dene way of life": Perspectives on health from Canada's north. Journal of Canadian Studies, 41(3), 112–133.

Environmental Wellness

The context of the environmental domain includes the use of and need for natural resources (Roscoe, 2009). Assessment in this domain includes the impact of humans on the environment and vice versa. Numerous resources are available about the environmental health concerns that exist for patients based on the relationship between humans and the environment (Box 8.1; CNA, 2012; Health Canada (2010). For example, one universal concern is climate change, which is the result of pollution caused by human use of natural resources. Wider temperature ranges resulting in increased smog in large cities may lead to respiratory effects especially for the very young and the elderly because of their lower ability to adapt to temperature changes. Toxins in the drinking water or pollution in the air from factories may impact a community. The impact to the global community may lead to increasing disparities between modern and developing countries. As the more affluent countries increase their impact on the environment to sustain their comfortable way of life, people in the rest of the world are left with the environmental aftermath and none of the benefit. Nurses can direct attention "to the relationship between personal well-being, and broader issues such as the collective wellness of humanity and the planet" (Carlisle, Henderson, & Hanlon, 2009, p. 1559). Optimizing the environmental domain could be achieved through individuals taking responsibility by reducing their carbon footprint on the world.

Social Wellness

The social domain concerns the relationship of the individual to others or the environment (Roscoe, 2009). Aspects of this relationship include respect, cooperation, support, and communication skills. Roles, boundaries, cultural identity, and family context all impact on wellness. Canadian community vitality is conceptualized as social relationships, civic relationships, and economic partnerships including safety and support, which incorporate the values of trust, respect, altruism, and belonging (Scott, 2010). Canada's most recent assessment revealed that we value relationships and our relationships determine our well-being: Canadian well-being is improving.

Although the words *social* and *community* suggest face-to-face interactions, the advent of the Internet offers unique opportunities for the creation of virtual social supports and communities as well. A few years ago, TJ Sweeney wrote a

---

BOX 8.1	Environmental Health Issues in Nursing

Air quality
Contamination of country foods
Drinking and recreational water quality
Radiological effects
Electric and magnetic fields
Noise

Source: Health Canada (2010); with permission from the Minister of Health, 2014.

blog about quitting smoking. He wrote about the importance of social support to help quitters "escape" from an unhealthy behaviour. That specific blog no longer exists, but TJ graciously shared his thoughts about the ties of smoking to wellness for him, his new blog on tools for quitting smoking, and his current work on tobacco control (personal communication, TJ Sweeney, April 25, 2013). The following is his original blog post, and his current blog is listed in the web resources at the**Point**.

> The words illness and wellness hold an odd illustration for me. . . .
> Illness-Wellness
> **I**llness-**We**llness
> **I - We**
> By myself (as "I") I am not well. But as part of a "we" (a couple or community) I am well.
> My "I-ness" reveals my insecurities, flaws, and failures.
> My "We-ness" affords me assurance, shared strengths and experience.
> The difference between Illness and Wellness is the difference between I and We.

TJ wrote, "Together we can accomplish things that perhaps none of the I's in the room can accomplish." Therein lies the value of a wider view when working with a patient. The nurse's role in assessing this domain ranges from one-on-one interactions, to family and friends, to World Wide Web contacts. For example, a nursing student worked with a patient in a private hospital room because he was immunocompromised. Because of this forced isolation, the patient had limited contact with his family and friends, and the student decided to interview her patient to gain an understanding of what his life would be like outside this environment. After learning about his mom and siblings, the conversation led to the patient's hobbies, which included gaming and his connection with friends sometimes in person but often online. The student's plan was to get the patient a laptop and set up Internet access while the patient was in hospital, reconnecting this isolated patient with his community. This was an example of optimizing the social domain of wellness despite the physical domain being compromised.

Think *The Web of Wellness*

If you perform an Internet search for wellness, the results are wheels, continuums, balance scales, or collages. Even some of the resources suggested at the end of this chapter include questionnaires, which seem very objective and concrete. Wellness is subjective and fluid. Picture a spider web, malleable and intricate, yet having incredible tensile strength for the purpose it serves.

Choose eight different colours of yarn to represent each domain. Cut the length according to your level of happiness or confidence in that domain. Then tie your web together. Make sure you knot the ends to create a strong web. Think about the length of yarn in relation to its purpose in the web. Is the centre of the web and shorter strand the most important? Stronger? Or protected? What happens to your web if you pull one strand toward you? What visual relation does this have to wellness in your own life (like when a stressor pulls your last nerve!)?

Canadian Well-Being

The Canadian Index of Wellbeing provides information that Canadians can use to work toward well-being as a nation. The working definition of **well-being** is

> The presence of the highest possible quality of life in its full breadth of expression, focused on but not necessarily exclusive to: good living standards, robust health, a sustainable environment, vital communities, an educated populace, balanced time use, high levels of civic participation, and access to and participation in dynamic arts, culture and recreation. (Canadian Index of Wellbeing, 2012, p. 5)

The Institute reports the movement of the indicators of wellness, such as the rate of employment or how many hours children spend in physical activity, as well as the impact of one indicator on another, such as whether the number of people employed can also afford housing. What is the result of these effects on society? The purpose of each report is to highlight the interconnectedness of the domains of wellness in relation to Canadian values. From this knowledge, policies can be developed to improve living conditions for all members of society. "Disparities in health by social groups speak to the need for stronger policy and program emphasis on social justice and equity-oriented measures" (Labonté, Muhajarine, Winquist, et al., 2009, p. 93).

The Institute of Wellbeing is a Canadian initiative, prompted by a worldwide impetus toward understanding societal progress. Although wellness continues to be the highlight in the current health-care climate, programs remain directed at the specific health event that is being measured (e.g., blood pressure clinics, exercise for weight loss, and nutrition for diabetes). The possibility exists that advocating at a societal level will also address unique patient concerns for health and wellness.

Special Population Considerations

The individual uniquely defines wellness for himself. Within special populations, perspectives are further refined, especially related to disability and age.

Disability

Patients living with disability have a unique relationship with their bodies, themselves, and others. In a health context, disability is viewed from medical, disability, and social models. In the medical model, the health-care provider is considered powerful, and the patient is a victim, unable to function normally, at a psychological loss without the health-care provider (Breen et al., 2008). The disability model views the patient as the result of a tragedy to be adjusted to and overcome; oppressed because of inability (Breen et al. 2008; Freund, 2001). In contrast, the social model focuses on the limits that have been placed on the patient based on the space (environment, context) where the patient interacts. The significance of this viewpoint is that, although patients' "impairments might cause restrictions in activity, they are not the cause of the disability" (Breen et al., 2008, p. 174). The design or use of space can benefit or disadvantage a person with a disability, whereas others might see that disability as belonging to the patient (Freund, 2001). For example, a wheelchair can be viewed as confining or as a mode of transportation. When you are next working in long-term care, think about whether a wheelchair is a restraint or limiting device, or whether it is the source of an opportunity to take a walk outside. When you are next in a movie theater, think about the space. Compare seating for couples versus room for a family to sit together, with a wheelchair and stroller.

As members of our society get older, the normal effects of aging will result in a population that is, in effect, disabled (if we use current definitions; Freund, 2001). How spaces are designed in society is based on the needs of the widest range of people. Consider what a major shopping centre looks like and where the nearest elevators are or who can use the escalators. Three unique people—one with rheumatoid arthritis, one with dementia, and one with a spinal cord injury—each have "very different interests, desires, wishes and needs [yet] all three, because of their conditions, will most likely find themselves segregated and sequestered in either institutional or domestic space" (Freund, 2001, p. 690). A wellness model approach maintains the individuality of the patient, yet offers shared control by having the patient collaborate with his or her health-care team (Breen et al., 2008). An ergonomic keyboard might be available for arthritic joints, a locked ward may not be necessary for the person with dementia, and the patient with the spinal cord injury could see the occupational therapist about an electric wheelchair.

Older Adults

A worldwide picture of wellness for the older adult can be illustrated through the following perspectives from the United States, United Kingdom, and Canada. In the United States, a physician and nurse team developed a community-based program geared to reducing health-care costs for older adults who have multiple medical conditions or who are frail. The premise of the program was that members of this population "do not get better and they will not live longer, but they can live better" (Chess, Krentzman, & Charde, 2007, p. 36); and by extending the time they can continue to live in their own community, their quality of life will be better. This team planned to provide more care up front so less intense and costly care would be required later. The difficulty with this program is the lack of profitability for managed care organizations. However, the translation to the Canadian system would suggest a decrease in the need to access health care, an increase in satisfaction with health services, and increased perception of health.

A large study from the United Kingdom and Europe investigated the relation of physical activity to psychological well-being (Fox, Stathi, McKenna, & Davis, 2007). The researchers used questionnaires and interviews to compare low, moderate, and high levels of physical activity in relation to mental well-being. The researchers made two observations.

First, older people, "who move more often and spend less time sitting down, experience higher levels of self-rated mental health and well-being than those who are less active" (Fox et al., 2007, p. 600). Inversely, older adults with higher levels of mental well-being might be more inclined to move. The connection between the two domains (physical and intellectual) has implications for other domains because mobility is required to attend gatherings (social), volunteer for activities (occupational), connect with nature (Fig. 8.3) or participate in traditional practices (environmental and spiritual).

Student Wellness

A few nurses have reported the development of campus wellness programs that were designed with nursing students in mind but included students in other professions. Clemmens, Engler, and Chinn (2004) developed an Introduction to Health course. The authors viewed the student body as a microcosm of society and listed the common behaviours of young adults in college, including smoking, drinking, poor nutrition, and decreased emotional health (stress, fear of failure, relationship issues, and sexual safety). Comparably, Ewing, Ryan, and Zarco (2007) listed the top health issues that could impact progress through school, including stress, minor illnesses, sleep disturbance, a close significant other in trouble, and depression or anxiety.

The first steps for each program included creating participants' awareness through surveys or assessments of domains

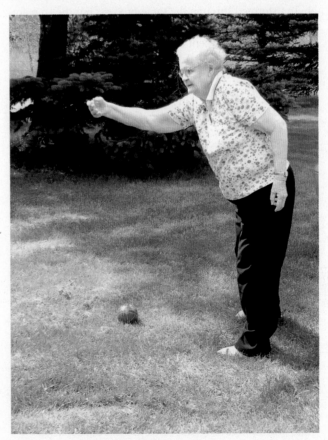

Figure 8.3 Older adult playing bocci ball.

including health risk assessments (Clemmens et al., 2004; Ewing et al., 2007). The intent of the programs was to promote students' recognition of factors that might influence health, policy and advocacy opportunities, components and partners in the health-care system, and options for wellness activities.

Students were required to complete assessment tools that advanced their learning of health and wellness, including *genograms* (schematics that are similar to a family tree but track other information such as medical history and life events), food menus, health risk assessment and wellness questionnaires, and development of health promotion activities for others. The researchers stated that as students examined the context of their own health, "they began to realize the importance of wellness as a starting point" (Clemmens et al., 2004, p. 317) with the ultimate benefits being good health through individual capacity, opportunity to teach and collaborate, and strong relationships (Ewing et al., 2007).

Health and Wellness: Putting It All Together

Understanding results from gaining knowledge about health, wellness, and illness and reflecting on personal values and beliefs that are reflected in the multiple domains (Bonis, 2009). Patients and nurses create meaning in going through the process of learning. "Both nurses and patients are transformed through the same process, but the transformation for each is unique to the individual" (Bonis, 2009, p. 1335); and the patient care provided must be modified to fit that uniqueness. Read Nancy's story about changing her perspectives on health.

Through the eyes of a nurse

I chose to become a nurse over 27 years ago because I wanted to care for others. I married and planned to start a family—the usual and expected course in life. When I went into labour with my first child, I anticipated the usual course of events for the birth. The usual did not happen. The doctor and the nurse asked for consent for a "do not resuscitate" order if our son stopped breathing. I froze. I was thinking, "I am usually the one asking this question, not the one having to answer."

We did take our son home 7 days later. I was so proud of how strong he was despite all the scenarios the doctor gave before his discharge; he could die, he could be severely mentally damaged, or he could be a year behind in school.

I really can't remember the exact moment that I started to appreciate what I had been given. I started to look at life differently. My perspective shifted as a whole new way of "knowing" appeared to me. I have learned many lessons from my son, who has surpassed all the expectations that the medical professionals set for him so many years ago. He is self-sufficient with his activities of daily living, surprising those who said he would "never walk and never talk." He graduated from high school (a year behind) and is now an accomplished songwriter.

A special son has made me a better person and a better nurse. So, the next time you are given the opportunity to work with someone who has a disability, look for what is special and ask yourself, "What can I learn from this experience? What unusual lessons might this unique person have for me?"

(personal reflection of Nancy, a nurse)

Promoting Health

The first part of this chapter put definitions to health and illness and broke apart wellness so that each domain could be understood separately. However, nurses see their patients as holistic or unified beings. Nurses help patients achieve wellness by assisting them to adopt healthy behaviours within the context of their lives. After assessing the wellness domains and asking about health values, the next step is understanding what factors may be strengths or barriers to achieving optimal health and wellness.

Determinants of Health

Factors that impact health are **determinants**. These include "income and social status, social support networks, education and literacy, employment/working conditions, social environments, physical environments, personal health practices and coping skills, healthy child development, biology and genetic endowment, health services, gender, and culture" (PHAC, 2010). Determinants can affect an individual patient, a family, a community, or a larger population.

Population Health

The concept of **population health** involves improving the determinants of health from the perspective of a nation. Data on health status, inequities between social and ethno-cultural groups, and emerging health issues are gathered and used to determine what health priorities exist for the nation (PHAC, 2012). Priorities are determined by analyzing what factors indicate health for the entire group.

The Senate Subcommittee on Population Health, which researched and witnessed the concerns related to the health and care of Canadians as compared to the rest of the world (Keon & Pépin, 2009), is a specifically Canadian example of addressing health factors. In considering the health services determinant, the senators realized that the health-care system (e.g., medical clinics, hospitals, public health offices) is only one way to keep people healthy. No matter how much funding the health-care system receives, there is no guarantee that health will improve. Therefore, health is determined outside the health-care system (e.g., at home, at work, at school, in the park).

An example from the determinant of socioeconomic status is that Canadians living in poverty have higher incidences of poor health. People with a low socioeconomic status are more likely to smoke longer and less likely to quit, which results in smoking-related diseases (Narcisse, Dedobbeleer, Contandriopoulos, & Ciampi, 2009). As well, women smoke more than men, leading to added concerns for children in the home. The Senate Subcommittee found that "Canada spends more money on health care to achieve worse results than the other countries surveyed" (Keon & Pépin, 2009, p. 15). Further, they report that "it is unacceptable for a wealthy country like ours to continue to tolerate such disparities in health" (Keon & Pépin, 2009, p. 42). To promote a healthy nation, the goals need to be matched with the health indicators (Table 8.1).

Health Promotion

Health promotion "is the process of enabling people to increase control over, and to improve their health" (WHO, 1986, p. 2). The goal is to optimize the human experience, especially well-being, health, and survival (McMichael & Butler, 2006) through building the strengths and skills of individuals, changing the conditions and determinants that impact health, and encouraging participation in the health of the community (WHO, 1998).

Health promotion action includes mobilizing communities and societies and advocating for the health and safety of others (WHO, 1998).

Health promotion is action; it is movement toward successful living (R. L. Johnson, 2005). All definitions, no matter the discipline, suggest direction, force, movement toward a positive, not necessarily disease to health or illness to wellness but including health to well-being. "Health promotion action takes place where people live, work, play and love—in communities" (Health Canada, 1997a, p. 32). As the largest group of health-care providers, nurses have a unique role in their ability to affect differing levels of governments and also affect the well-being of individual patients. Note the photo (Fig. 8.4) of nurses immunizing the community, affecting the health of each patient provided with a vaccine and education while implementing public safety.

Health promotion is a process that is relational; it is based on the relationship between a health-care provider and an individual, families, the community, or other professionals.

Health Promotion Model

Health professionals are always concerned about providing quality care to patients. Quality is achieved by applying research evidence to practice. In health promotion, a few nursing models exist that explain a patient's beliefs and values surrounding health. Through understanding patient attitudes toward healthy behaviours, a nurse can plan appropriate care. The Health Promotion Model (HPM) (Pender, Murdaugh, & Parsons, 2011) attempts

TABLE 8.1 Health Goals for Canada	
Health Goals for Canada	As a nation, we aspire to a Canada in which every person is as healthy as they can be—physically, mentally, emotionally, and spiritually.
Canada is a country where:	
Basic Needs (Social and Physical Environments)	Our children reach their full potential, growing up happy, healthy, confident, and secure.
	The air we breathe, the water we drink, the food we eat, and the places we live, work and play are safe and healthy—now and for generations to come.
Belonging and Engagement	Each and every person has dignity, a sense of belonging, and contributes to supportive families, friendships and diverse communities.
	We keep learning throughout our lives through formal and informal education, relationships with others, and the land.
	We participate in and influence the decisions that affect our personal and collective health and well-being.
	We work to make the world a healthy place for all people, through leadership, collaboration and knowledge.
Healthy Living	Every person receives the support and information they need to make healthy choices.
A System for Health	We work to prevent and are prepared to respond to threats to our health and safety through coordinated efforts across the country and around the world.
	A strong system for health and social well-being responds to disparities in health status and offers timely, appropriate care.

Rewritten from Public Health Agency of Canada. (2005). *Health Goals for Canada*. Retrieved from http://www.phac-aspc.gc.ca/hgc-osc/pdf/goals-e.pdf, with permission.

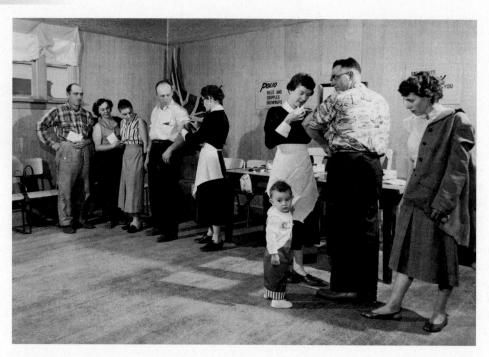

Figure 8.4 Public health nurses. (Source: Canadian Nurses Association and Library and Archives Canada. [1960]. *Two public health nurses are vaccinating adults at a polio clinic in Southey, SK.* Retrieved from http://collectionscanada.gc.ca/)

to explain and predict patient health behaviours. This model is significant to nursing for several reasons. First, the model is strongly grounded in nursing and therefore in the goal of nursing to assist others to achieve optimal health. Second, the model has been thoroughly researched and applied to differing patient populations and health conditions, proving that the model is a reliable and valid evidence-based tool for practice. Thirdly, for a nurse, almost every interaction with a patient involves educating about some aspect of promoting health. Think about the first few moments you spend with your patient at the beginning of your clinical. You might be asking how he slept and assessing what he ate for breakfast. Or you might be performing anthropomorphic measurements—those objective numbers that bring a human body to life—such as blood pressure, pulse, respiration, temperature, weight, height, body fat, and body mass index. Each one of these measurements provides a telltale sign that supports the nurse's subjective data collection about an individual's personal characteristics or health behaviours. The combination of subjective and objective data is the beginning of the path through the HPM.

The basic premise in using the HPM is that when the factors leading to health promotion are known, and then nurses can better understand a patient's behaviours and suggest interventions that could foster a healthy lifestyle (Pender et al., 2011). The model was developed in 1975, revised once, and incorporates nursing, behavioural, and social-cognitive concepts. Pender et al.'s (2011) definition of health is "the actualization of inherent and acquired human potential through goal-directed behavior, competent self-care, and satisfying relationships with others, while making adjustments as needed to maintain

structural integrity and harmony with the relevant environment" (p. 23). A caveat to be aware of is noting how the authors include wellness concepts within this definition, another example where wellness and health are used interchangeably.

Patients exhibit health behaviours depending on whether they are motivated to change (Pender et al., 2011). Negative motivation is action or behaviour to avoid illness or disease. For example, a patient stops smoking because she knows that smoking causes lung cancer. Smoking cessation is an example of primary prevention. Often, these primary interventions are aimed at protecting a person just in case, such as immunizations. Secondary prevention interventions are aimed at detecting a disease early; for example, recommending every woman over 50 years old have a mammogram every 2 years to detect breast cancer in an effort to treat the cancer early. Tertiary (third level) prevention interventions are aimed at restoring functioning or rehabilitating to potential. An example might be a patient learning to walk again after an acquired brain injury.

Avoidance of a negative perception of health is based on a medical model; the goal being to treat and limit the effects of a specific disease. Alternatively, a positive perception of health (quality of life, living longer, well-being) can be achieved with health promotion. Pender et al. (2011) agree that a multitude of factors have an effect on health outcomes, and therefore, the focus of health promotion is on health over a lifetime rather than on a specific disease process. For this reason, the concept of self-change is embedded in the HPM. A **self-change behaviour** is an action the patient is willing to take to meet health outcomes. Patients "have the power and skill to change health behaviors or modify health-related lifestyles" (Pender et al., 2011, p. 37). The design of an individual health promotion program makes use of the patient's strengths and incorporates individual beliefs about health and cultural values. The major components of the model are shown in Figure 8.5.

A key concept in the HPM is **self-efficacy**, which is the "judgment of personal capability to organize and carry out a particular course of action. Self-efficacy is not concerned with the skill one has but with judgments of what one can do with whatever skills one possesses" (Pender et al., 2011, p. 47). Health promotion emphasizes personal responsibility and motivation to use inherent strengths (e.g., having the willpower to quit smoking). Alternative models focus on preventing risks (e.g., wearing sunscreen to prevent skin cancer) and avoiding negative threats (e.g., wearing a helmet when riding a bicycle). The positive approach to well-being is exhibited in research about general healthy lifestyle behaviours within differing contexts. Examples include (a) occupational safety, such as hearing protection for construction workers (Ronis, Hong, & Lusk, 2006); (b) sociocultural context, such as learning from Chinese elders (Kwong & Kwan, 2007); or (c) behaviours, such as physical activity (Pender et al., 2011; Taymoori et al., 2008).

As with any model, judgment is required in choosing the best evidence to apply and the appropriate context for the patient. There are limitations to incorporating the HPM into nursing practice. As mentioned previously, the HPM uses the definitions of health and well-being interchangeably, so ensuring a thorough assessment of how your patient defines health is important. As well, understanding health promotion behaviours requires the patient to self-report. Like wellness measures and health risk assessments, self-reporting means the patient might choose to answer either with what they "should," what they "desire," or the "truth." Ensuring a trusting relationship and creating a rapport with the patient will shift the focus of the assessment from what the patient thinks you want to hear to his or her view of optimal health.

A nurse's purpose in meeting with a patient regarding health promotion behaviours must be reflective of the patient's current health. The priority may initially be to assist the patient to manage the current disease or illness and then to suggest health promotion possibilities. Pender et al. (2011) describe the role for nurses in promoting healthy behaviours. The nurse may raise consciousness, promote patient self-efficacy, support the patient in controlling the environment, and assist the patient to manage barriers to change. Take a look at Amanda's experience of her changing views toward health. As a first-year nursing student, she shares stories of the challenges overcome by herself, a family member going through treatment, and her elderly patients in first-year clinical. Think about how her approaches are encouraging a patient view of optimal health.

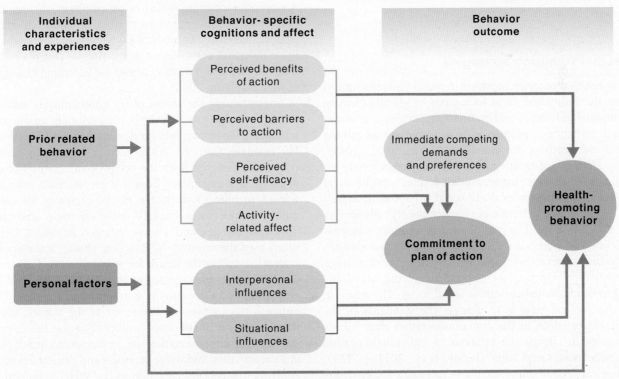

Figure 8.5 Health Promotion Model. (Redrawn from Pender, N. J., Murdaugh, C. L., & Parson, M. A. [2011]. *Health promotion in nursing practice* [6th ed.]. Upper Saddle River, NJ: Pearson Prentice Hall, with permission.)

Through the eyes of a student

*T*here have been a few experiences in my life that have redefined my definitions of health, illness, and wellness. The process of losing 70 lb changed my thoughts from "being healthy means you are skinny" to where I am now, having a healthy lifestyle (nutrition, exercise, relationships) is something that I crave.

What made me really question the concept of health was when my mom was diagnosed with cancer. I didn't perceive illness as having cancer and wellness as not having cancer but rather wellness as what she did to try and live happily and as healthy as possible while having cancer.

I compare that to when I was younger and thought the elderly couldn't do activities because they were lazy or didn't want to. Since I started working in a care home, I realize that elderly people can't do things because of physical changes. That doesn't mean that they aren't healthy, it just means that you need to look at being healthy from a different perspective.

What I wanted to show by writing about my experiences is that health, wellness, and illness are defined differently by different people and populations based on the experiences they have had in their lives. As a nursing student, I think it is important to really get to know my patients to better understand their unique definitions of wellness and illness.

(personal reflection of Amanda, a student nurse)

Health Promotion Strategies

Most health promotion literature in recent years has moved from the individual focus to societal or global. Coming to understand family and community perspectives about health and health promotion is as important as talking about the needs of the individual (Pender et al., 2011). "Any strategy for health promotion that focuses only on individual behavior change will fail without simultaneous efforts to alter the physical and social environment as well as the collective behavior of the community" (Pender et al., 2011, p. 338). The goal of societal wellness is to provide all members with a standard of living that ensures they can achieve their potential. Nurses can encourage participation, empowerment, problem solving, and leadership of individuals toward a social focus. The purpose of this societal view is to change "the standards of acceptable behavior in the community rather than by attempting to change the behavior of individuals against overwhelming social odds" (Pender et al., 2011, p. 339). Nurses and community members can work for environmental, policy, and economic change. The Ottawa Charter

lists actions for health promotion, including "build health public policy, create supportive environments, strengthen community actions, develop personal skills, and reorient health services" (WHO, 1986). These actions encompass numerous strategies nurses can share with patients and their communities.

Healthy public policy means action toward strengthening the health of communities and nations and "includes, but goes beyond, policies that support healthy personal behaviors (such as no-smoking or healthy diet policies) to include policies that address socioenvironmental risk conditions, such as poverty and working conditions" (Reutter & Williamson, 2000). Strategies include developing policy (such as no smoking on public grounds), advocating, and organizational change (WHO, 1986). Policy often determines the funding available for health promotion programs. As a result, there are provincial strategies based in the priorities of the people and culture. For example, Saskatchewan's focus is on Aboriginal well-being and "the Northern way," whereas many Atlantic Canada strategies focus on children and the workplace.

A socioecological approach is the strategy that underlies creating supportive environments (WHO, 1986). Nurses work toward respecting natural resources and understanding the patterns between work and leisure, those environmental contexts where we spend our time and which directly impact our health. For example, a nurse may encourage breast-feeding for a new mother, yet the new mom may refuse to breast-feed because of concern for contaminants in the local water supply and thereby the breast milk. A workplace example would be an employer offering and promoting wellness programs at work to reduce absenteeism because of illness, to decrease workplace injury, and to lower insurance costs. Rather than caring for patients with a focus on illness and disease, nurses are becoming managers of wellness (Bean, 2003).

Strengthening the action of the community is assisted through strategies such as supporting self-help groups and mobilizing the community for development (WHO, 1986). For example, Carriere (2008) reports on a 1-day health conference designed with the needs of vulnerable women in mind. The organizers from a street outreach program wanted to offer more than a needle exchange for community members who engaged in the sex trade, who used intravenous drugs, and who were largely homeless. Organizers used the acronym ACE (action, choice, and empowerment) to reflect the desire for women to build on their own strengths, take control of their own health, and be empowered by a community partnering for wellness. The outreach nurses assessed the needs of the women (from the perspective of the street, rather than the health-care providers), planned a conference, implemented health promotion activities, and wrote an article and designed posters applying this conceptualization to the WHO definition of health.

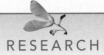

RESEARCH

STREET OUTREACH

The need for this study arose out of the awareness that the traditional outreach services were not meeting the needs of current patients. The nurses ascertained that health promotion strategies had expanded beyond needle exchange and were being provided to a growing group of patients. Because a larger number of men were being seen, the nurses were concerned that a focus on disparities for women were not being addressed.

Study

The research group was a team of Street Outreach nurses, upper level B.S. in Nursing students and public health nurses. The participants were 96 women living in Kamloops, BC.

A needs assessment was performed with questions related to determinants of health, access to health care, barriers to wellness, health needs, and interests. The results were used to plan day-to-day nursing activities, a 1-day health conference, and knowledge dissemination through posters depicting the influence of social determinants for two fictitious women; one meeting significant barriers to health.

Conclusions

The outcome of the programs and posters created by the outreach nurses was a paradigm shift in the assessment, development, and evaluation of nursing services for women from a time-consuming individual approach to a wellness partnership approach for the women, their families, and the community.

Implications for Nursing Students

Understanding the social determinants of health, patient's perspectives regarding their own health, and health promotion strategies for marginalized populations—including the contexts that create vulnerability—should inform how nurses engage patients and work with them in partnership. Acknowledgement, safety, and respect are important for any patient interaction and encourage empowerment, inclusivity, and decision-making. Communicating caring promotes positive nurse–patient relationships.

Carriere, G. L. (2008). Linking women to health and wellness: Street Outreach takes a population health approach. International Journal of Drug Policy, 19(3), 205–210. doi:10.1016/j.drugpo.2008.03.006

Another strategy is developing capacity and personal skills through activities such as health communication and health education (WHO, 1986). You might have already completed health communication promotion in your program. Tools developed under this strategy include posters about diseases or illnesses, pamphlets on prevention measures, or even wiki development about wellness opportunities. A neat assignment is developing and uploading a YouTube video on a health concern or a nursing theorist. Imagine how that health communication has now advanced from a poster delivered to your nursing peers to a worldwide audience! That is the power of health promotion.

Health education is the next step; "an activity that seeks to inform the individual on the nature and causes of health/illness and that individual's personal level of risk associated with their lifestyle-related behavior" (Whitehead, 2004, p. 313). Health education requires a relationship between the nurse and patient and includes motivating, changing, and influencing values, beliefs, and attitudes. This concurs with the WHO (1998) definition of health education as strategies to increase a patient's self-efficacy through literacy, knowledge, or life skills. Nurses can offer education activities which "are voluntary, create understanding, provide skills for rational choices and assist patients in clarifying their values as well as respect and contribute to the autonomy of the patient" (Whitehead, 2009, p. 870). Both of these strategies of communication and education assist with building the patient's personal capacity to better care for herself and her family (Health Canada, 1997). A nurse's role on a national scale, for example, might be to promote awareness of physical activity to decrease obesity in Canada. Yet the role in a developing region, such as some countries in Africa, might be to teach about the local foods that have higher calories for young pregnant mothers to increase the chance that their babies survive.

The final action is reorienting health services to achieve better health for all within a nation (WHO, 1986). Assessments of health services have previously been discussed, including the Canadian Index of Wellbeing and the Senate Subcommittee on Health Promotion review of the health of Canadians. Others engaged in strategies to attain a system change are Nurses for Medicare or the Canadian Alliance for Sustainable Health Care. In a recent summit on the Canadian health system (Hodgson, 2012), five key ideas emerged, including (1) changing the way patients access the health-care system; (2) using technology more appropriately; (3) increasing the accountability of health-care providers by compensating them based on patient outcomes, not the number of patients assessed; (4) enabling elders to stay in their homes and communities rather than be admitted to institutions; and (5) promoting health of Canadians to reduce chronic health conditions and the use of the health-care system. Health promotion continues to drive the Canadian health-care system.

SUMMARY

The first half of this chapter provided language on how to differentiate between health, wellness, and illness. By using tools such as health risk assessments or wellness domains, nurses combine objective and subjective data to gain a holistic view of the patient, including his or her beliefs about health. In developing a therapeutic relationship and coming to understand the patterns of health and wellness, the nurse and patient collaborate on a health promotion plan. The HPM (revised) is one such tool for encouraging self-efficacy and building patient capacity. These individual interactions filter to families and communities and signal the nurse's role in population health. By acknowledging the WHO (1986) actions toward health promotion globally, nurses implement strategies to change health systems through health communication policy development or community mobilization. Nurses should remember that "health promotion proceeds by small, incremental steps that only slowly result in major change, [therefore] health promotion can only be evaluated over a time frame spanning decades or even generations!" (Health Canada, 1997b, p. 25). Successful change may yet be measured by patient satisfaction with the health-care system.

Critical Thinking Case Scenarios

Eva

▶ I am 92 years old, and I am alone. I have outlived my husband of 50 years, my four children, and three siblings. I have worked hard all my life, taking care of the children, the dairy farm, and my husband, who had Alzheimer's disease. I do sometimes feel lonely, but I am happy living in the home I've been in all my life. I can see the ocean from this window, and when it's not foggy, the boats fill my imagination with the fishing I used to love so much. My grandchildren live far away but visited earlier this year. I love to watch mainlanders try oysters for the first time (giggles). The hardest part is getting motivated to move since there is no one to move for!

1. Develop one question to ask Eva from each wellness domain.
2. Which domain(s) may be out of balance? Explain.
3. What activities might you suggest as a nursing student working with Eva's Home Care nurse?

Laura

▶ Laura is 12 years old and attends public school. Her school is part of a provincial/territorial and national initiative to create healthy exercise habits for life. However, Laura thinks the activities are boring, no fun, and the attitude of the older kids in school brings down those who like to exercise. The purpose of the Healthy Bodies Active Minds (H-BAM!) program is to encourage breaks from sitting in desks all day. Laura calls it "exercising your body inside of your mind." She likes getting out of the classroom and thinks it's neat that the school is starting to advertise H-BAM! in the community: There are t-shirts, bulletin boards, and newsletter updates. You are the student nurse working in this Grade 6 classroom.

1. What assessments could you perform with this group of students to get a picture of health for children in Grade 6?
2. How could you evaluate whether this health promotion program is working?
3. How could H-BAM! be moved to the community? Which WHO (1986) action could you implement as a student in this setting?

Brian and Carlyle

▶ Brian is a teacher, father, husband, and Ironman participant. Ironman is a triathlon where the goal is to swim 3,800 m, bike 180 km, and run 42.2 km all in 1 day. Brian likes to train and spends 10 to 14 hours/week exercising. There is no goal to completing Ironman, just to finish. Brian is happy to be more active, to be eating better, and to have lost weight.

Carlyle is an Ironman competitor. He trains to meet a personal best time. He really enjoys training, exercising 20 to 24 hours/week with sessions that push his body to the outward limits. Carlyle realizes that rest is important to body healing but sometimes pushes when he knows he should rest.

1. What are the definitions of health, wellness, and illness for Brian and Carlyle?
2. Is there balance between domains when training for Ironman?

Multiple-Choice Questions

1. Which is an example of a health risk assessment?
   a. A family genogram
   b. Past medical history
   c. A general health survey
   d. Exposure to harmful substances

2. Thomas wants to compete in a local 5-km run. Which wellness domain does this represent?
   a. Physical
   b. Intellectual
   c. Occupational
   d. Environmental

3. What is the best example of a spiritual wellness intervention?
   a. Plan a walk to the hospital lobby.
   b. Test the patient with a mini-mental exam.
   c. Observe how much the patient ingested for breakfast.
   d. Sit with a young child until asleep on his first night in hospital.

4. Limits placed on a patient in the space where he or she lives and works is an example of which approach to disability?
   a. Social model
   b. Medical model
   c. Disability model
   d. Chronic illness model

5. Where does the concept of social support networks fit?
   a. Self-change behaviours
   b. Determinants of health
   c. Health education activities
   d. Health promotion behaviours

6. Mary chooses to quit drinking coffee when she studies because the caffeine is affecting her sleep. Twice this last week, she stayed up late to study and then slept through her morning class! Mary decides she will quit today. Mary's decision is an example of which concept in the revised HPM?
   a. Self-change behaviour
   b. Self-efficacy
   c. Self-assessment
   d. Self-concept

Suggested Lab Activities

Wellness Index

● Print off a copy of the full Wellness Index (see web resources at **thePoint**) and split it up in sections for pairs of students. Have each pair complete the section and note which statements reflect which domain. One of the concerns with filling out the index is that the individual knows the index is asking about healthy behaviour. Have a discussion about self-reporting questionnaires. Can they always be true measures of wellness if the expected answer is easy to guess?

Environmental Wellness

● The CNA website offers resources for nursing students to learn about environmental issues and the role of nurses. Watch the 3-minute video available at http://www2.cna-aiic.ca/CNA/pop-up/environment/principles/default_e.html and discuss the following: current impact of your lab group on the immediate environment, suggested opportunities to improve the environment, ways to overcome barriers, and methods for evaluating your effectiveness.

Canadian Index of Wellbeing

● With your knowledge of the working definition of well-being, engage in a discussion with your small group about what well-being *looks* like. Next, create a photovoice of well-being for your group based on photos group members have submitted and present that to your group. Consider that the Index is only one representation of a worldwide community. View the video at http://www.youtube.com/watch?v=sh6esxa2e3o and discuss your perceptions of your world compared to this perspective of the larger one.

Health Promotion or Health Education

● Download a copy of the article, "The Practice of Patient Education: The Theoretical Perspective," by Rebecca Syx (2008). Split into small groups and give each group one model/theory from the journal article. Describe and explain the components of the chosen model/theory in relation to the case study and whether the model/theory is a best fit. Do you agree that using a model/theory is most beneficial for patient care planning?

REFERENCES AND SUGGESTED READINGS

The Association of Faculties of Medicine of Canada. (n.d.). *Illness, sickness, and disease*. Retrieved from http://phprimer.afmc.ca/Part1-TheoryThinkingAboutHealth/Chapter1ConceptsOfHealthAndIllness/IllnessSicknessandDisease

Barss, K. S. (2012). T.R.U.S.T.: An affirming model for inclusive spiritual care. *Journal of Holistic Nursing, 30*(1), 24–34. doi:10.1177/0898010111418118

Bean, S. (2003). Making well-being a team effort. *Occupational Health, 55*(4), 22.

Benner, P., & Wrubel, J. (1989). *The primacy of caring: Stress and coping in health and illness*. Don Mills, ON: Addison-Wesley.

Bonis, S. A. (2009). Knowing in nursing: A concept analysis. *Journal of Advanced Nursing, 65*(6), 1328–1341. doi:10.1111/j.1365-2648.2008.04951.x

Breen, L. J., Green, M. J., Roarty, L., & Saggers, S. (2008). Toward embedding wellness approaches to health and disability in the policies and practices of allied health providers. *Journal of Allied Health, 37*(3), 173–179.

Canadian Index of Wellbeing. (2012). *How are Canadians really doing? The 2012 CIW report*. Waterloo, ON: Canadian Index of Wellbeing and University of Waterloo. Retrieved from https://uwaterloo.ca/canadian-index-wellbeing/sites/ca.canadian-index-wellbeing/files/uploads/files/CIW2012-HowAreCanadiansReallyDoing-23Oct2012_0.pdf

Canadian Nurses Association. (2010). *Position statement: Spirituality, health and nursing practice*. Ottawa, ON: Author.

Canadian Nurses Association. (2012). *Position statement: Nurses and environmental health*. Ottawa, ON: Author.

Carlisle, S., Henderson, G., & Hanlon, P. W. (2009). 'Wellbeing': A collateral casualty of modernity? *Social Science and Medicine, 69*(10), 1556–1560. doi:10.1016/j.socscimed.2009.08.029

Carper, B. (1978). Fundamental patterns of knowing in nursing. *Advances in Nursing Science, 1*(1), 13–23.

Carriere, G. L. (2008). Linking women to health and wellness: Street Outreach takes a population health approach. *International Journal of Drug Policy, 19*(3), 205–210. doi:10.1016/j.drugpo.2008.03.006

Chess, D., Krentzman, M., & Charde, J. (2007). Creating a wellness program/safety net for the medically complex and frail patient. *Journal of Ambulatory Care Management, 30*(1), 30–38.

Chuengsatiansup, K. (2003). Spirituality and health: An initial proposal to incorporate spiritual health in health impact assessment. *Environmental Impact Assessment Review, 23*, 3–15.

Clemmens, D., Engler, A., & Chinn, P. L. (2004). Learning and living health: College students' experiences with an introductory health course. *Journal of Nursing Education, 43*(7), 313–318.

Delgado, C. (2007). Meeting clients' spiritual needs. *Nursing Clinics of North America, 42*(2), 279–293. doi:10.1016/j.cnur.2007.03.002

Dunn, H. L. (1961). *High-level wellness*. Arlington, VA: Beatty Press.

Engel, R. J., & Kieffer, T. (2008). A comprehensive individual and organizational wellness assessment of older adults. *Seniors Housing & Care Journal, 16*(1), 83–95.

Erickson, D., Stapleton, F., Erickson, P., Giannokopoulos, E., & Wilson, C. (2006). The development and validation of the Health Proneness Questionnaire. *Journal of Clinical Psychology in Medical Settings, 13*(4), 415–423.

Ewing, B., Ryan, M., & Zarco, E. P. (2007). A campus wellness program: Accepting the challenge. *Journal of the New York State Nurses Association, 38*(1), 13–16.

Fisher, J. W., Francis, L. J., & Johnson, P. (2000). Assessing spiritual health via four domains of spiritual wellbeing: The SH4DI. *Pastoral Psychology, 49*(2), 133–145.

Fox, K., Stathi, A., McKenna, J., & Davis, M. G. (2007). Physical activity and mental wellbeing in older people participating in the Better Ageing Project. *European Journal of Applied Physiology, 100*(5), 591–602.

Freund, P. (2001). Bodies, disability and spaces: The social model and disabling spatial organisations. *Disability & Society, 16*(5), 689–706. doi:10.1080/09687590120070079

Grasser, C., & Craft, B. J. (1984). The patient's approach to wellness. *Nursing Clinics of North America, 19*(2), 207–218.

Harper, D. (2001). Health. In *Online etymology dictionary*. Retrieved from http://www.etymonline.com/index.php?term=health

Health Canada. (1997a). *Health promotion in Canada*: A case study. Ottawa, ON: Author.

Health Canada. (1997b). Health promotion in Canada: A case study. *Health Promotion International, 13*(1), 7–32.

Health Canada. (2009). *Healthy Canadians—A federal report on comparable health indicators 2008*. Retrieved from http://www.hc-sc.ca/hcs-sss/pubs/system-regime/index-eng.php

Health Canada. (2010). *Useful information for environmental assessments*. Retrieved from http://www.hc-sc.gc.ca/ewh-semt/alt_formats/hecs-sesc/pdf/pubs/eval/environ_assess-eval/environ_assess-eval-eng.pdf

Health Canada. (2011). *Healthy Canadians—A federal report on comparable health indicators 2010*. Retrieved from http://www.hc-sc.gc.ca/hcs-sss/pubs/system-regime/index-eng.php

Hodgson, G. (2012). *Five priorities for fixing the Canadian health care system*. Retrieved from http://www.conferenceboard.ca/economics/hot_eco_topics/default/12-11-06/five_priorities_for_fixing_the_canadian_health_care_system.aspx

Hooghe, M. (2012). Is sexual well-being part of subjective well-being? An empirical analysis of Belgian (Flemish) survey data using an extended well-being scale. *Journal of Sex Research, 49*(2–3), 264–273. doi:10.1080/00224499.2010.551791

Hucker, A., Mussap, A. J., & McCabe, M. M. (2010). Self-concept clarity and women's sexual well-being. *The Canadian Journal of Human Sexuality, 19*(3), 67–77.

Jensen, L., & Allen, M. (1993a). Insights from latent partition analysis into categories inherent in wellness-illness. *Journal of Advanced Nursing, 18*(7), 1118–1124. doi:10.1046/j.1365-2648.1993.18071118.x

Jensen, L., & Allen, M. (1993b). Wellness: The dialectic of illness. *Image: The Journal of Nursing Scholarship, 25*(3), 220–224. doi:10.1111/j.1547-5069.1993.tb00785.x

Jensen, L., & Allen, M. (1994). A synthesis of qualitative research on wellness-illness. *Qualitative Health Research, 4*(4), 349–369. doi:10.1177/104973239400400402

Johnson, R. L. (2005). Health promotion: A theoretical overview with an African American perspective comparison. *The Journal of Theory Construction & Testing, 9*(1), 6–10.

Johnson, V. D. (2007). Promoting behavior change: Making healthy choices in wellness and healing choices in illness—Use of self-determination theory in nursing practice. *Nursing Clinics of North America, 42*(2), 229–241. doi:10.1016/j.cnur.2007.02.003

Keon, W., & Pépin, L. (2009). *A healthy, productive Canada: A determinant of health approach. The Standing Senate Committee on Social Affairs, Science and Technology final report of Senate Subcommittee on Population Health*. Retrieved on from http://www.parl.gc.ca/content/sen/committee/402/popu/rep/rephealth1jun09-e.pdf

Kiefer, R. A. (2008). An integrative review of the concept of wellbeing. *Holistic Nursing Practice, 22*(5), 244–252.

Kwong, E. W., & Kwan, A. Y. (2007). Participation in health-promoting behaviour: Influences on community-dwelling older Chinese people. *Journal of Advanced Nursing, 57*(5), 522–534. doi:10.1111/j.1365-2648.2006.04132.x

Labonte, R., Muhajarine, N., Winquist, B., & Quail, J. (2010). *Healthy populations: A report of the Canadian Index of Wellbeing (CIW)*. Retrieved from https://uwaterloo.ca/canadian-index-wellbeing/sites/ca.canadian-index-wellbeing/files/uploads/files/HealthyPopulation_DomainReport.sflb_.pdf

Laumann, E. O., Paik, A., Glasser, D. B., Kang, J. H., Wang, T., Levinson, B., . . . Gingell, C. (2006). A cross-national study of subjective sexual well-being among older women and men: Findings from the Global Study of Sexual Attitudes and Behaviors. *Archives of Sexual Behaviour, 35*(2), 145–161. doi:10.1008/s10508-005-9005-3

Mackey, S. (2009). Towards an ontological theory of wellness: A discussion of conceptual foundations and implications for nursing. *Nursing Philosophy, 10*(2), 103–112. doi:10.1111/j.1466-769X.2008.00390.x

Mahon, S. M. (2006). What are the chances? Risk in the real world. *Clinical Journal of Oncology Nursing, 10*(1), 99–101, 107. doi:10.1188/06.CJON.99-101

McBrien, B. (2006). A concept analysis of spirituality. *British Journal of Nursing, 15*(1), 42–45.

McMichael, A. J., & Butler, C. D. (2006). Emerging health issues: The widening challenge for population health promotion. *Health Promotion International, 21*(S1), 15–24. doi:10.1093/heapro/dal047

Mitton, C., O'Neil, D., Simpson, L., Hoppins, Y., & Harcus, S. (2007). Nurse–physician collaborative partnership: A rural model for the chronically ill. *Canadian Journal of Rural Medicine, 12*(4), 208–216.

Mulkins, A., Morse, J., & Best, A. (2002). Complementary therapy use in HIV/AIDS. *Canadian Journal of Public Health, 93*(4), 308–312.

Narcisse, M. R., Dedobbeleer, N., Contandriopoulos, A. P., & Ciampi, A. (2009). Understanding the social patterning of smoking practices: A dynamic typology. *Sociology of Health & Illness, 31*(4), 583–601. doi:10.1111/j.1467-9566.2009.01159.x

Paluck, E. C., Allerdings, M., Kealy, K., & Dorgan, H. (2006). Health promotion needs of women living in rural areas: An exploratory study. *Canadian Journal of Rural Medicine, 11*(2), 111–116.

Paterson, B. L. (2001). The shifting perspectives model of chronic illness. *Journal of Nursing Scholarship, 33*(1), 21–26.

Pender, N. J., Murdaugh, C. L., & Parsons, M. A. (2011). *Health promotion in nursing practice* (6th ed.). Upper Saddle River, NJ: Pearson Prentice Hall.

Peterson, M. (1996). Health perception and behavior comparison between wellness program participants and non-participants. *Journal of Wellness Perspectives, 12*(3), 155.

Public Health Agency of Canada. (2012). *What is the population health approach?* Retrieved from http://www.phac-aspc.gc.ca/ph-sp/approach-approche/index-eng.php#What

Public Health Agency of Canada. (2010). *Environment health*. Retrieved from http://www.phac-aspc.gc.ca/hp-ps/dca-dea/stages-etapes/childhood-enfance/environnement-eng.php

Pugh, M. (Ed.). (2006). *Stedman's medical dictionary* (28th ed.). Retrieved from http://www.statref.com

Reutter, L., & Williamson, D. L. (2000). Advocating healthy public policy: Implications for baccalaureate nursing. *Journal of Nursing Education, 39*(1), 21–26.

Ronis, D. L., Hong, O., & Lusk, S. L. (2006). Comparison of the original and revised structures of the Health Promotion Model in predicting construction workers' use of hearing protection. *Research in Nursing & Health, 29*(1), 3–17.

Roscoe, L. J. (2009). Wellness: A review of theory and measurement for counselors. *Journal of Counseling & Development, 87*(2), 216–226.

Scott, K. (2010). *Community vitality: A report of the Canadian Index of Wellbeing.* Retrieved from https://uwaterloo.ca/canadian-index-wellbeing/sites/ca.canadian-index-wellbeing/files/uploads/files/CommunityVitality_DomainReport.sflb_.pdf

Singh-Manoux, A., Martikainen, P., Ferrie, J., Zins, M., Marmot, M., & Goldberg, M. (2006). What does self rated health measure? Results from the British Whitehall II and French Gazel cohort studies. *Journal of Epidemiology and Community Health, 60*(4), 364–372. doi:10.1136/jech.2005.039883

Smith, B. J., Tang, K. C., & Nutbeam, D. (2006). WHO health promotion glossary: New terms. *Health Promotion International, 21*(4), 340–345. doi:10.1093/heapro/dal033

Smith, K. R., & Ezzati, M. (2005). How environmental health risks change with development: The epidemiologic and environmental risk transitions revisited. *Annual Review of Environmental Resources, 30,* 291–333. doi:10.1146/annurev.energy.30.050504.144424

Spurr, S., Bally, J., Ogenchuk, M., & Walker, K. (2012). A framework for exploring adolescent wellness. *Pediatric Nursing, 38*(6), 320–326.

Stamm, T., Lovelock, L., Stew, G., Nell, V., Smolen, J., Machold, K., . . . Sadlo, G. (2009). I have a disease but I am not ill: A narrative study of occupational balance in people with rheumatoid arthritis. *OTJR: Occupation, Participation & Health, 29*(1), 32–39. doi:10.3928/15394492-20090101-05

Syx, R. L. (2008). The practice of patient education: The theoretical perspective. *Orthopedic Nursing, 27*(1), 50–54. doi:10.1097/01.NOR.0000310614.31168.6b

Taymoori, P., Niknami, S., Berry, T., Lubans, D., Ghofranipour, F., & Kazemnejad, A. (2008). A school-based randomized controlled trial to improve physical activity among Iranian high school girls. *International Journal of Behavioral Nutrition and Physical Activity, 5*(18). doi:10.1186/1479-5868-5-18

U.S. Census Bureau. (2012). *United States Census Bureau, Halbert L. Dunn.* Retrieved from http://www.census.gov/history/www/census_then_now/notable_alumni/halbert_l_dunn.html

Venes, D. (Ed.). (2009). *Taber's cyclopedic medical dictionary* (21st ed.). Retrieved from http://www.statref.com

Whitehead, D. (2004). Health promotion and health education: Advancing the concepts. *Journal of Advanced Nursing, 47*(3), 311–320. doi:10.1111/j.1365-2648.2004.03095.x

Whitehead, D. (2009). Reconciling the differences between health promotion in nursing and 'general' health promotion. *International Journal of Nursing Studies, 46*(6), 865–874. doi:10.1016/j.ijnurstu.2008.12.014

World Health Organization. (1948). *Constitution of the World Health Organization.* Retrieved from http://apps.who.int/gb/bd/PDF/bd47/EN/constitution-en.pdf

World Health Organization. (1986). *Ottawa charter for health promotion.* Ottawa, ON: World Health Organization, Health and Welfare Canada, and Canadian Public Health Association. Retrieved from http://www.phac-aspc.gc.ca/ph-sp/docs/charter-chartre/pdf/charter.pdf

World Health Organization. (2002a). *National cancer control programmes: Policies and managerial guidelines* (2nd ed.). Geneva, Switzerland: Author. Retrieved from http://www.who.int/cancer/publications/nccp2002/en/index.html

World Health Organization. (2002b). *WHOQOL-SRPB field-test instrument.* Geneva, Switzerland: Author. Retrieved from http://www.who.int/mental_health/media/en/622.pdf

chapter

9

Ethics and Integrity in Practice: Moral Dilemmas and Moral Issues

NANCY WALTON

Jason is a fourth-year nursing student doing his final clinical placement in a long-term care institution. During his time there, Jason has often cared for Emily, a 20-year-old woman with an acquired brain injury from a motorboat accident at age 16 years that left her paralyzed and unable to care for herself. She requires complete care and has been in the institution for nearly 4 years with frequent serious complications, including severe infections and painful bedsores. She must undergo burdensome and painful treatments and is completely ventilator-dependent. Before her injury, Emily was a serious athlete and a popular student with a close-knit group of friends. Emily's friends visit once or twice monthly, but their times together have become infrequent, as they have moved on to university. Her parents are busy caring for their elderly parents and her two younger siblings, one of whom has asthma. Family counselling has been ongoing but sporadic, and eventually, last month, Emily asked that it be discontinued.

Jason and Emily are close in age, and Emily has found she can confide in Jason easily. Most of the residents in the institution are elderly so she has few friends or people her age to talk to. Jason feels that Emily has become more withdrawn and quiet. She has also asked several times about his experiences with dying patients and what he has observed about the dying process.

Jason decides to address this in a straightforward way, asking if she is thinking about suicide. She smiles when he asks and tells Jason that she is relieved that someone "finally had the guts to ask me." She tells Jason that she fully understands her prognosis and considers her future to be a bleak one. She tells Jason that she has no desire to continue living in this way. She also informs him that she is at peace with her decision and feels hopeful for the first time in years. Her parents are aware of her desire to die, and they have expressed an understanding, although they find it hard to support such a decision. She reiterates to Jason her relief at being able to talk about this with him.

CHAPTER OBJECTIVES

By the end of this chapter, you will be able to:

1. Define ethics, morality, and ethical dilemma.
2. Identify values and beliefs we each hold and the sources of these values.
3. Demonstrate an understanding of the following concepts related to moral integrity: moral autonomy, steadfastness, and wholeness.
4. Differentiate between approaches to moral dilemmas found in nursing ethics, feminist ethics, and bioethics.
5. Apply basic ethical principles and theories to the examination of challenging clinical situations.
6. Explore issues of academic honesty and ethical dilemmas for nursing students.
7. Examine and analyze three specific ethical issues commonly encountered in nursing practice: patient autonomy, care at the end of life, and truth-telling.
8. Examine two ethical decision-making models and explore their effectiveness in helping to resolve ethical dilemmas.

KEY TERMS

Academic Integrity   Maintaining truth, soundness, and honesty in academic matters.

Advance Directives   Instructions, usually written, describing a person's explicit wishes for medical and health care should that person be unable to communicate these wishes in a time of illness.

Assisted Suicide   The act of killing oneself with the advice or help of another person.

Autonomy   The ability to govern oneself. In health care, this concept refers to the right of the individual to have control over decision-making concerning one's own life and health.

Beneficence   Acting in a way intended to promote the best interests of another person.

Bioethics   The branch of philosophy of inquiry that can involve a range of health-care professionals, activities, and issues.

Deontological Ethics   The ethical soundness or moral rightness of an action lies in our adherence to our duties. Our moral obligation involves knowing what our moral duties are and acting in accordance with those duties.

Ethical Dilemma   A situation involving values and beliefs in which we find that the clear course of action is not obvious and in which we find that there may be strong ethical reasons to support each possible alternative or option.

Ethical Theories   Systematic approaches to help us examine why some things might seem more wrong or more right when we are attempting to resolve ethical dilemmas.

Ethics   The branch of philosophy that helps us organize our thinking and reasoning about what we consider to be right and wrong, particularly in the social context.

Euthanasia   Causing the painless death of a person, with a goal to be merciful, in order to end or prevent suffering or pain.

Feminist Ethics   An approach to examining moral dilemmas that acknowledges gender and the social construction of gender as an important and influential factor in our view of the world.

Fiduciary Duty   A duty to protect the needs and the best interests of others and hold that responsibility above one's own needs or interests. A fiduciary relationship must be built on trust, disclosure, and care.

Justice   A broad concept that encompasses notions of fairness in the distribution of resources, benefits, and risks as well as fairness in procedures and processes.

Moral Autonomy   A state in which we feel responsibility and ownership for our chosen values and beliefs.

Moral Distress   Knowing the right thing to do but being constrained from doing it.

Moral Integrity   A virtue that relates to reliability, wholeness, an integration of character, and fidelity in adhering to moral norms that are sustained over time.

Moral Seamlessness   Our ability to integrate all the roles we have into one morally consistent person.

Morality   The beliefs and traditions we hold in how we conduct ourselves toward others.

Nonmaleficence   A guiding principle that requires that we avoid harming or acting with malice toward others.

Nursing Ethics   The examination of the norms, values, and principles in nursing practice.

Principlism   A widely used framework for solving real-world ethical dilemmas in health care, developed by Thomas Beauchamp and James Childress in 1979, involving four principles: autonomy, beneficence, nonmaleficence, and justice.

Quality of Life   One's overall well-being and satisfaction with the conditions under which one lives.

Steadfastness   Being true to our own values and beliefs even in the face of adversity.

Utilitarian Theory   An ethical theory in which the moral rightness or ethical soundness of an action is judged by how much good, satisfaction, or happiness it might produce.

Ethics and Morality: Values and Choices

Every day in our lives, we make judgments about what we consider to be right and wrong. Arguably, we all have ideas about what ethical behaviour or moral character involves, and we make decisions every day about what we should and should not do. The notions of what we consider to be right or wrong are based on the values and beliefs we hold. These values and beliefs are often instilled in us as children and evolve as we grow and become more morally autonomous adults. In our daily lives, we don't spend a lot of time explicitly stating what our values are. Instead, they are quietly reflected in the kinds of decisions we make, the actions we take, and the opinions we express to others. The following examples demonstrate that we often express our values and beliefs through the choices we make without consciously examining them first.

- If you are driving your car behind someone who is turning left illegally, you make a choice whether to honk to alert the driver to the fact that left turns are disallowed or simply wait and do nothing, although it means you'll be waiting longer at the intersection. You may feel justified in honking because it is more than simply an issue of your waiting; it involves someone doing something that is illegal.

- If you leave the grocery store and realize that the cashier did not charge you for the magazines at the bottom of your cart, you are faced with a choice. You can either return to the store and pay for the magazines or take them without paying. You may justify your choice to take the magazines without paying by telling yourself that the store charges too much for other items and, as a struggling student, you need the money more. Alternatively, you might feel that the right thing to do is return to the store and pay because you are opposed to stealing in any context.

- If you have 20 dollars to give to a charity, you'll likely give to the charity that provides help to a group or population you relate to most strongly or feel is the most deserving of help.

In each of these circumstances, you are expressing your values and beliefs through the choices you make without consciously examining them first. However, as nursing students and practicing nurses, we may find ourselves immersed in serious, complex personal situations that challenge our beliefs, thereby forcing us to explicitly examine and analyze the values and beliefs we hold.

Ethics and Morality

The terms *ethics* and *morality* are often used interchangeably, although depending on the field of study, they are quite different. Having an understanding of what each of these terms means to you and deciding then how they are related is the beginning of understanding what it means to be an ethical nurse.

Ethics is the critical, structured examination of how we should behave in the social context in particular (Burkhardt, Nathaniel, & Walton, 2013). It is a way of reflecting on and understanding norms, beliefs, and values alongside practices and issues that have a moral dimension. What do we mean by issues with a moral dimension? These are typically situations that we find most complex, often involving conflicting values and beliefs and usually very difficult to resolve easily or practically (Jameton, 1984; Oberle & Bouchal, 2009). Moral issues are those that we find ourselves in the midst of, often thinking that this should or should not happen, someone ought to make a particular decision or act with a specific intention, a person has a right to something or we must act according to a particular moral duty we have in this case.

Morality may refer to the beliefs and traditions we hold in how we conduct ourselves toward others. Often, our ideas about morality are realized in more action-oriented ways, as we tend to examine ethical or moral dilemmas and focus on what we think people ought to do or the choices that we feel they ought to make. The ideas we have about what ought to happen are how we express our morality; however, even these ideas and expressions may not always help us figure out what is the right thing to do in particular ethical dilemmas. Furthermore, our ideas about morality may be grounded in the values that have been instilled in us throughout our lives and those beliefs and values we explore and choose as our own as we grow. Because of this very individualized basis for our ideas about morality, we inevitably find disagreement on ethical and moral issues, even among rational, reasonable, and free-minded people.

What Are Ethical Dilemmas?

Differences in beliefs about what constitutes the morally correct thing to do underpin many of the **ethical dilemmas** we find both in our daily lives and in particular contexts, such as health care. Ethical dilemmas may be situations in which we find that the clear course of action is not obvious. There may be strong ethical reasons we can think of to support each position, and no one position or choice will please everyone involved (Beauchamp & Walters, 1999). We may feel that, when faced with an ethical dilemma, any of the two or more alternatives might be reasonable, plausible, or morally acceptable. It may be quite easy to understand how very reasonable people might disagree and also to understand the different viewpoints or perspectives of others. Yet, we might also feel, when faced with an ethical dilemma, that no one alternative will be completely perfect or without some kind of downside.

Where Do We Find Ethical Dilemmas?

Years ago, the most common likely ethical dilemmas involved trying to figure out what to do. With more choices, alternatives, interventions, and possibilities, the ethical dilemmas we face in health care today are much more complex. We must also consider that patients today are far more knowledgeable and have access to a virtual library of information and are able to make informed choices. Unlike many years ago when the physician tended to make decisions for the patient, we now find that patients are actively involved in decision-making about their care. For the most part, they are no longer passive recipients of care in a mostly patriarchal-type of health-care system. With the multitude of choices and alternatives for medical care along with the move toward ensuring patients can exercise autonomous, informed choices, nurses may find that their practice is much more complex and challenging, from both practical and ethical perspectives.

Many people imagine that most ethical dilemmas occur in an acute care setting, such as an intensive care unit (ICU) or an operating room, where dealing with life and death can be a daily, almost routine, occurrence. However, ethical dilemmas occur in all kinds of health-care contexts, not just critical care contexts. Nurses in public health and community care face ethical dilemmas all the time. Rural and remote nursing presents special ethical dilemmas that a nurse working in a busy downtown emergency room (ER) might not encounter. Nurse practitioners who work in family practice clinics or offices also face ethical issues that reflect the unique collaboration that is an inherent part of being a team member in such a context. We cannot claim that ethical dilemmas only occur in acute, emergent or urgent settings. Clearly, from the decision-makers in federal government offices to the triage nurse in a busy urban emergency department, all the way to the nurse at the bedside in a quiet rural hospice, health care is full of moral issues and ethical dilemmas.

Values and Beliefs

Values can be defined as our conception of what is good and what is most desirable. We seek to promote that which we value through our actions and behaviours (Heath, 2003). We hold many values and beliefs about the world, the way things happen, and the choices people make. These values and beliefs arise from various sources that influence us throughout our lives. As children, we lack moral autonomy, and for the most part, our parents and guardians make choices about what happens to us in our daily life and what we should value. Whether to go to church and what church to attend, how we will be educated, what kind of food we eat, what we wear, or what music we listen to—all these choices are made for us. Our parents act as our moral authorities. As we grow into adolescence, most young people find that they wish to explore alternative choices. In addition, through school, extracurricular activities, and peer groups, we are often exposed to a wider variety of differing values. What many adults refer to as teenage rebellion is really the normal developmental stage of challenging the values of our parents and guardians and beginning the process of figuring out what values fit us better as we develop new ideas about the world around us. It is at this time that we see young people rejecting the choices that have already been made for them in favour of exploration of alternative choices and values. This trying on of other values and beliefs for fit can be thought of as a kind of moral exploration and is a part of establishing our **moral autonomy**. Moral autonomy refers to a state in which we feel responsibility and ownership for our chosen values and beliefs. Being accountable and standing up for what we believe in makes us morally autonomous. Of course, we don't simply wake up 1 day as persons with moral autonomy. Becoming morally autonomous people is an iterative and ongoing process—one that takes patience, time, and, often, a significant amount of moral courage.

As we are faced with new ethical challenges and develop each of these four elements in our own roles as moral agents, we also develop our moral integrity. Clearly, this is an iterative process and one that requires a great deal of honest self-reflection along the journey.

Moral Integrity

Moral integrity can be thought of as a virtue that relates to reliability, wholeness, an integration of character, and fidelity in adhering to moral norms that are sustained over time. Inherent in moral integrity is the sense of trustworthiness and of consistency between our convictions and our actions (Burkhardt et al., 2013).

We can think of persons who we would consider to have moral integrity as those we would say have good moral character. These might be persons we would consider to be moral mentors; those whose advice we would seek out if we were faced with a difficult ethical decision. We can also think about moral integrity as an attribute of being whole, complete, or intact. People who we consider to have integrity in moral matters are those that we may notice are obviously committed to a clear set of values and beliefs. They maintain consistency by remaining true to the values that they explicitly embrace.

Moral Distress

Even the person we would think of as having the most moral integrity may find it difficult to maintain if he or she is pushed too hard or his or her values are pushed to their own limits (Yeo, Moorhouse, Khan, & Rodney, 2010). This can happen in any of the ethical dilemmas that we'll be talking about in this chapter. Our values can be pushed to a limit by being consistently disrespected, trivialized, ignored, or compromised. If we find that, for some reason, it is difficult or impossible to stay true to our convictions, we may then feel that our values have been pushed to a limit. This can lead to feelings of anger, resentment, despair, and powerlessness. Throughout the literature and in many working environments, nurses vocalize that they feel powerless to make changes or take actions that they feel are morally correct. This feeling of being unable to effect meaningful change in challenging ethical circumstances is known as **moral distress**. Simply stated, someone who knows the right thing to do but is unable to do it may experience moral distress (Jameton, 1993). This inability may stem from any number of sources, including (but not limited to) institutional constraints, real or perceived powerlessness, strong hierarchies, lack of ethical leadership, and lack of resources or access to resources. Moral distress can also result when ethical dilemmas are not acknowledged or are simply ignored; when communication between team members, patients, and families is ineffective; or when nurses feel alone or unsupported in dealing with difficult situations. Feelings of moral distress can result in serious negative consequences for nurses: feeling of anxiety, frustration and guilt, and dissatisfaction with nursing practice and performance. In turn, these kinds of feelings can lead to nurses vacating their positions, which can contribute to the already-standing problems of recruitment and retention in settings where there is a high level of moral distress (Jameton, 1993; Keatings & Smith, 2010).

Ethical Environments

Reducing feelings of moral distress comes as a result of creating ethical environments in places where we work. Ethical environments are those in which we feel supported in ethical approaches to nursing practice and patient care. These are practice environments in which we feel that we can actively and genuinely participate in decision-making about patient care and treatment. Finally, they are environments with strong ethical leaders and mentors, who encourage open discussion and collaborative approaches to decision-making in ethical dilemmas. An ethical environment is one in which we, as individual nurses, feel that meaningful change can happen and that we are not alone when dealing with problems that have a moral or ethical dimension.

It is within ethical environments that nurses find that they can maintain their moral integrity. They may find it easier to remain true to their values even in the face of adversity or disagreement if they feel supported and that they are not alone. It may help nurses to maintain moral integrity through shared values that are articulated through a professional code of ethics and supported in ethical environments. The Canadian Nurses Association (CNA) Code of Ethics for Registered Nurse (see Box 4.3) outlines seven values of professional nurses, which include providing safe, ethical, and compassionate care; the promotion of health and general well-being of our patients and populations; the promotion of informed decision-making facilitated by nurses; the preservation of dignity, maintaining confidentiality and respective privacy of our patients; promoting justice and rights of others in processes; and being accountable in all areas of our practice (Canadian Nurses Association [CNA], 2008).

Moral Autonomy

Being morally autonomous refers to being in a state in which we feel accountable and responsible for our chosen values and beliefs. It is through embracing our own values that we become more morally autonomous and develop our authentic self rather than simply being guided by those values that are imposed on us by others. Standing up for what we believe in helps to makes us more morally autonomous. But moral autonomy is only one part of moral integrity. In addition to moral autonomy, other parts of moral integrity include keeping our promises, being steadfast, and moral seamlessness (Yeo et al., 2010).

Keeping Our Promises

Keeping our promises is an important part of being a person with moral integrity. From the smallest promise to the most serious public oath we might take, making and keeping promises achieves two important outcomes. First, a willingness to actually make a promise to another person means that we are willing to put aside our own priorities to ensure something happens for someone else. The willingness to make a promise means we are also willing to take a personal risk and do our best to make sure something happens. If we manage to also keep the promises we make, those around us may see us as having integrity and trustworthiness. Trust is an important component of any relationship: patient–nurse, nurse–coworker, and student–professor. "Trust is a confident believe in and reliance upon the moral character and competence of another person. Trust entails a confidence that another will act with the right motives and in accordance with appropriate moral norms" (Beauchamp & Childress, 2012, p. 34).

Think back to the case of Jason and Emily, where we see the trust that Emily has in Jason that allowed her to open up about a difficult and controversial request, for assistance with dying. In this case, Emily's trust in Jason is absolutely necessary in order for her to make herself quite vulnerable by opening up about such a deeply personal, serious, and sensitive topic.

We trust that people will be predictable and consistent when choosing whether or not to follow moral norms. Trustworthiness can be demonstrated in the keeping of a promise. We make promises all the time, both implicitly and explicitly. By signing an employment contract, we promise that we will abide by the terms of employment. By getting married, two persons make explicit promises to each other while their closest friends and family act as witnesses. When we take a loan at a bank, we essentially promise to repay the loan abiding by the rules of the banking institution. These are all explicit promises: observable, clearly expressed, detailed, and, in most cases, precise. There are other kinds of promises that are less observable. When we make plans to meet a friend for dinner, we are making a promise to show up and be on time as much as we can and not leave our friend waiting alone in a restaurant. When a nurse assures a patient that he or she will return in 10 minutes with a pain medication and a cup of tea, that is a promise. If the same nurse assures the patient that he or she will check on the test ordered for tomorrow and forgets to do so, the patient may well feel as if a promise has been broken. Although these kinds of situations do not involve a specific oath or a verbal promise, the notion of a promise is implied, although perhaps not expressed out loud. These kinds of promises we can call implicit promises.

In the acceptance of either kind of promise, there is an assumption that the person who is making the promise is trustworthy. Making a promise to another person implies that we are willing to abide by social rules and that our moral norms include keeping our word to others.

Being Steadfast

Maintaining **steadfastness** is perhaps the most challenging part of being a person or a professional with moral integrity. Being steadfast means being true to our own values and beliefs even in the face of adversity. This is difficult in many situations, and sticking to our values is never done without some risk or courage. There are several reasons why we might find it hard to be steadfast in standing up for something we feel is right: a desire to be liked, a hesitance to challenge the status quo, fear of reprisal, fear of being isolated or socially shunned, lack of perceived power, and temptation to go along with others.

Consider these other examples of steadfastness:

- The nurse who questions the value of an ordered treatment that the patient states she does not want
- The nursing student who gently reminds the two senior nurses who are discussing a patient in the hospital elevator that the practice is unacceptable
- The professor who stands up for a student's rights when the university administration is not responsive
- The community nurse who stands up for a patient from a typically marginalized and underserved group who finds himself fighting the system
- The nurse who questions a family's plan to lie to a patient about her poor prognosis in order to keep the patient from losing hope and possibly becoming depressed

Moral Seamlessness

The last part of moral integrity is **moral seamlessness**. This refers to our ability to integrate all the roles we have into one morally consistent person. In addition to being nurses and nursing students, we are also sons, daughters, brothers, and sisters. Some of us are wives or husbands. Some of us are mothers or fathers. We may be caregivers for others. We may be students and also employees. In addition to our roles in a professional capacity, we may have roles in extracurricular activities at work or school. In each context, we find that our approach to moral problems or our expectations of how we should act may change. Caring and compassionate toward your patients, you may find that you are impatient and unfriendly with your coworkers. In another case, you may be very respectful to those who you mentor in your volunteer work at a homeless shelter but find that you are very hard on the new recruits on your unit. As a nurse working in a youth shelter, you may counsel your patients about the dangers of illicit drug use yet not worry about your close friends who use illicit drugs when you're around. Each of these cases highlights how difficult it can be to maintain a kind of moral seamlessness. It is a challenge to try to be the same kind of moral agent in every situation, context, or role. We might not agree with lying to patients, even with good intentions, but we may find ourselves lying to our friends and families. This kind of inconsistency can result in confusion and unease at best and, at worst, a kind of moral distress.

Ethics as Inquiry

Ethics is a complex topic, the study of the formalized system of rules. Topics such as bioethics, nursing, and feminist ethics (among others) fall under the topic of applied ethics. **Ethical theories** help us to answer the question, what should be done here? What is the *right* thing to do? Although they do not provide easy answers to difficult questions, these theories can help to focus on actions and the rationales behind actions.

Bioethics

Bioethics can be defined as the branch of philosophy of inquiry that can involve a range of health-care professionals, activities, and issues. Relatively new, bioethics has arisen in the mid to late 20th century in response to a plethora of emerging technologies in areas of health care, research, and the environment and the subsequent new choices that we may have as people living in this complex and rapidly changing world (Storch, Rodney, & Starzomski, 2013). Many people call this field of study *biomedical ethics* or *health-care ethics*, whereas others feel that these two terms refer more specifically to issues of health care and health research.

Global Trends in Health Care

Alongside the rise of bioethics, we see three distinct global trends in health care. First, there are rapidly evolving technological advances in the care of those who are ill as well as new frontiers in the enhancement and sustenance of human life. Second, historic advances in the reach of the media have occurred in the latter half of the 20th century. The power of the media to disseminate health information and, in turn, our ability to access a monumental amount of health information at the touch of a mouse click has had a significant change in all of our lives. Third, a change in the traditional patriarchal doctor–patient relationship has resonated throughout many health-care settings. As patients become more knowledgeable

not only about their own health care and their rights but also the obligations of their health-care providers, they have also become more empowered and in doing so, challenged the traditional "doctor knows best" model of health care and medicine. Modern health care is complex, and the associated legal rights and professional obligations are also highly complicated. Once we have even a basic understanding of this complexity, we can then see how all three of these trends both contribute to and help in resolving difficult issues in bioethics.

Nursing Ethics

Although bioethics highlights issues in modern medicine and can also address the perspectives and issues that arise in the practice of other health-care professionals, nursing is considered to be unique and highly diverse. **Nursing ethics** is defined as the examination of the norms, values, and principles in nursing practice (Yeo et al., 2010). The one key consideration in thinking about nursing ethics separately from bioethics is the focus nurses have on relationships. Nursing is seen as consistently existing within a relational context. Because of this, the moral aspect of nursing practice must be constantly and explicitly examined and discussed (Gastmans, Dierckx de Casterle, & Schotsmans, 1998).

Nurses work in various settings including the acute care hospital, the community, rural settings, ambulatory care or clinics, home care, and institutional settings such as schools or correctional facilities. They take on a range of responsibilities and duties including provision of direct patient care, management and administration, education and welfare, and public health and health promotion. Their work is independent, interdisciplinary or multidisciplinary, and may be carried out under the title of *registered nurse*, *licensed practical nurse*, *registered practical nurse*, *nurse clinician*, *clinical nurse specialist*, *nurse midwife*, or *nurse practitioner*. As nursing practice continues to change and grow, so do our obligations, as professionals, to reflect on and analyze the kinds of ethical challenges and issues that these changes might bring.

Feminist Ethics

The rise of **feminist ethics** is relevant to the discussion of nursing ethics. The realization that moral dilemmas necessarily involved human relationships means that in order to resolve such dilemmas, there is the necessity for an approach that encompasses an explicit awareness of power imbalances, assumptions, competing priorities, marginalization, and oppression. Scholars in feminist ethics approach moral dilemmas using a perspective that acknowledges how important and influential gender is in our socially constructed ideas about the way that the world works. Carol Gilligan, a feminist scholar, states that the differences in the experiences and relationships of men or women have an effect on our moral development and, in turn, how we approach moral dilemmas (Gilligan, 1982). In a world in which many of our social structures have traditionally been patriarchal, or male-dominated, the social experiences of men and women, in many ways, are quite different. From a historical perspective, females, as a gender, have often been oppressed, marginalized, and dominated within patriarchal social structures created for the benefits of males (Liaschenko & Peter, 2003; Sherwin, 1992). Although there are many different ways of thinking about moral dilemmas even just within the field of feminist ethics, there is a common underlying belief that the moral experiences of persons involve relationships and that these relationships occur within various social structures and contexts. These contextual relationships may involve power imbalances, strong hierarchies, assumptions and stereotypes, diverse moral beliefs, and political stances, all of which may be grounded in issues related to gender. To fail to consider these kinds of factors when examining moral dilemmas is to ignore the very real social structures in which moral dilemmas occur. Feminist ethicists aim to uncover nontraditional ways of approaching complicated moral dilemmas that prioritize the consideration of these contexts, social structures, and gender influences.

Although the notion of a patriarchal world is constantly being challenged and, in many ways, is antiquated, there are many resultant legacies that have an effect on the lives of many persons today. In the profession of nursing, we can see that issues of gender are highly relevant. Nursing has traditionally been seen as a female profession alongside medicine, which is traditionally viewed as a male profession. Much of the work of nursing has been feminized: viewed as less skilled and more intuitive and aligned with what are often assumed to be natural tendencies of females to be more caring and nurturing. This feminization of nursing work has, many times, resulted in a devaluing of nursing rather than an acknowledgement of the unique and necessary contribution that nursing practice makes in the provision of holistic health care.

Ethical Theories

Ethical theories are systematic approaches to help us examine why some things might seem more wrong or more right when we attempt to resolve ethical dilemmas. Theories can be used like straightforward tools to help us think through complex ethical challenges. Our discussion of ethical theories here will be an introduction. Keep in mind that ethical theories have been developed based on elaborately thoughtful and often prolific writings in philosophy. We will focus here on two specific types of ethical theories: the consequentialist (or teleological) theories and the deontological (or nonteleological) theories. We will also discuss principlism—a more modern and widely cited ethical theory.

Consequentialist Theories

Consequentialists put forth that the most important (the only) consideration in resolving ethical dilemmas are the consequences or outcomes. They posit that when trying to sort through ethical dilemmas, the most crucial moral obligation is to maximize the positive outcomes and minimize the negative outcomes (Thomas & Waluchow, 2002). In order to resolve an ethical dilemma using a consequentialist stance, knowledge of possible outcomes is required as is the ability to evaluate outcomes ahead of time. One problem with consequentialist theories is that it is sometimes difficult to reach consensus, even among reasonable persons, about what is a good or bad outcome or consequence. Many times, even reasonable persons might disagree about what constitutes a good outcome or a negative one. The most commonly discussed type of consequentialist theories is **utilitarian theories**.

Utilitarian Theories

Utilitarians assess the moral rightness of a possible action by how much good, satisfaction, or happiness it might produce. In looking at possible alternatives that might be considered when approaching an ethical dilemma, a utilitarian will choose the alternative that will produce the most good. There are three distinct steps in this utilitarian calculation. First, the outcomes of each possible alternative must be established. Then, the balance of good to bad outcomes for each alternative must be calculated or estimated. Finally, the alternative that appears to have the capacity to produce the greatest amount of good (happiness, satisfaction, pleasure) should be chosen (Yeo et al., 2010). It's not difficult to imagine problems or challenges presented by a utilitarian stance. Even very reasonable persons might disagree about what constitutes a good consequence or a negative one. A utilitarian perspective assumes that we have accurate predictive powers, which clearly we don't always have, and highly subjective and complex concepts such as happiness and satisfaction are very difficult to measure. On the other hand, utilitarianism is often seen as a straightforward, future-focused, and clear approach to complex ethical problems. In many areas of social policy, we see a utilitarian stance being used to resolve difficult priority-setting problems. Excessive security measures in airports and taxation are two examples of social policies that aim to produce the most good for the most persons involved. Public health measures such as quarantining sick persons during pandemics or vaccinating people against communicable diseases are both examples of utilitarian approaches; that is, doing the most good for the most people. If we look at the example of vaccination, we realize that there are possible negative outcomes related to vaccination; for example, rare negative side effects as well as the localized pain and discomfort of receiving a vaccination. However, if we look at what produces the most good for the most people—either vaccinating persons or not—we realize that the good of vaccinations far outweighs the bad.

Deontological Ethics

Where we consider utilitarian approaches to be future-focused, that is, looking toward the future consequences, **deontological ethics** tends to focus on what lies behind our chosen actions and states that our ideas about what it means to adhere to our duties should dictate the moral rightness of our actions in ethical dilemmas. According to deontologists, our moral obligation involves knowing what our moral duties are and acting in accordance with those duties (Yeo et al., 2010). Unlike consequentialists, deontologists do not consider possible outcomes or consequences of actions. Immanuel Kant (1724–1804) is probably the most well-known and often cited deontologist. According to Kant, an action is morally permissible if it can meet the categorical imperative, which gives no credence to outcomes or consequences. As Kant describes it, his concept of imperative compels us to choose an action that can be universalized to all other similar kinds of situations (Oberle & Bouchal, 2009). For example, if we are considering lying to a patient (even with very good intentions of trying to protect them from something hurtful or painful), we must imagine that in all similar kinds of situations, it can be morally acceptable to lie to patients. When we look at it that way, lying to a patient might be more difficult to justify as the morally acceptable alternative. If however, we can, in fact, see our action universalized; that is, the action that is morally correct and the one that we must take in accordance with our duty.

Application of Deontological Theory

Although adherence to duty is an important and relevant concept to nursing, deontological theories are difficult to use in real life. It's not always clear what our duties are. As nurses, we have several obligations: to our patients, to the institution that employs us, to our profession, to our colleagues, and to society. As compelling as our professional responsibilities are, we also have personal, familial, and social duties. Sometimes, these duties or our ideas about what these duties are may conflict.

When we have duties that conflict (and we often do), deontological theories provide little guidance to help us resolve these conflicts or prioritize duties. The fact that outcomes do matter is another objection that many have to the use of this set of theories to solve complex real-world ethical dilemmas. Even if we are very cognizant of our moral duties, to simply ignore consequences or outcomes seems unrealistic and impossible to support. What happens as a result of our actions is important. On the other hand, however, deontologists may make a similar claim of a consequentialist approach. To pay attention only to outcomes and ignore motivations, intentions, or duties that lie behind those actions is to fail to attend to something that most of us consider to be very important. The legal system considers both motive and intent as key concepts in deciding just how wrong an action is. We more easily forgive someone for a wrongdoing if we believe that he or she genuinely intended to do something good but his or her plans went awry. Alternatively, we punish someone more severely for a morally wrong action if wrongdoing was his or her clear intention. Neither of the two most popular ethical theories we've discussed deals effectively with all the important considerations of a real-world ethical dilemma. Although these two theories seem worlds apart, it is possible that a deontologist and a consequentialist might agree on what is the most morally right action in a situation.

When examined critically, the common ethical theories we have identified seem to omit one or more important considerations. To approach real-world ethical dilemmas as a deontologist or utilitarian would mean neglecting relevant aspects. To many who are entrenched in the ethical dilemmas of an ICU or a transplant team, deontology and utilitarianism provide very limited guidance to help tackle complex and captivating ethical dilemmas. In some ways, the problems of health care have always been approached in a much different way than philosophical problems. Whereas work in academic philosophy has been to examine, explore, and analyze ethical theories, in biomedicine, the focus has traditionally been on doing good for patients, avoiding harm, and advocating for the rights of individuals.

Principlism

Ethical values or principles have often been articulated within professional codes of ethics or codes of conduct; however, these have also been discipline-specific, traditionally narrow, and focused on the behaviour of the professional, which is not a particularly good fit with solving multidimensional ethical dilemmas. In an attempt to make academic philosophical principles more accessible to solve real-world ethical dilemmas in health care, an approach or framework called **principlism** was developed in 1979 by Thomas Beauchamp and James Childress (Beauchamp & Childress, 2012; Holm, 2002). Principlism quickly became widely popular in the burgeoning field of medical ethics (Holm, 2002). The framework continues to be taught across disciplines and is felt by many to be a highly accessible and realistic approach to complex ethical problems faced in health care today.

Principlism consists of four guiding principles that are intended to be the middle ground between high-level idealistic values based on moral theory and a lower everyday morality (Holm, 2002). They are principles to which health-care professionals should hold themselves accountable because they are drawn from traditional values found in professions such as medicine or nursing (Beauchamp & Childress, 2012). Principles are ideas that constitute goodness that can be held constant across various contexts, places, and times. This framework identifies four guiding principles in considering ethical issues: (a) respect for autonomy, (b) beneficence, (c) nonmaleficence, and (d) justice.

Four Guiding Principles

Autonomy refers the ability to govern oneself. In health-care ethics, this concept is overarching and refers to the right of the individual to have control over processes and decision-making concerning one's own life and health.

Health-care professionals are expected to apply **benefi-cence** in their practice, to be attentive to the best interests of others, and advocate for those interests. Whereas beneficence compels us to act in the best interests of others, **nonmaleficence** requires that we avoid harming or acting with malice toward others. **Justice** is a broad concept encompassing the notion of fairness in the distribution of resources, benefits, and risks as well as fairness in procedures and processes (Beauchamp & Childress, 2012; Beauchamp & DeGrazia, 2004).

We can see that although ethical theories answer what should be done in a situation and what is the right thing to do, they do not provide easy answers. Theories help to focus on actions and the rationales behind actions. What is important to remember is that the use of ethical theories is intended to be helpful in providing clear rationale for difficult decisions. Ethical theories are meant to help us focus on what is important and what values we are prioritizing as we attempt to resolve the ethical dilemmas that we are facing.

Ethics in Practice: Real-World Problems

There are many kinds of ethical dilemmas that you will be faced with, as a nursing student and, eventually, a nurse in practice. It would be beyond the scope of this chapter to touch on all the possible kinds of professional and academic issues that might arise in your career that will have ethical aspects. For now, we'll focus on four kinds of real-world ethical dilemmas that are relevant to you today and in the near future. First, we'll discuss ethical issues in academic settings. Then, we'll explore three common sources of ethical dilemmas in practice: patient autonomy and informed consent, truth-telling, and care at the end of life.

Student Ethics

Academic integrity is a term used to describe maintaining truth, soundness, and honesty in academic matters. It is, many times, viewed simply as a policy or a set of rules to which students and professors must adhere. However, it is and should be much more than that. As nursing students, we are evolving professionals on our way to becoming responsible for the most intimate and important of role: the skilled care of other people. In working toward embracing that professional role, you will be expected to conduct yourself in a way that reflects a particular set of values including honesty and accountability. As a nursing student, you are going to be expected to demonstrate responsibility, respect for others, and fair treatment of those around you.

Academic integrity includes a set of values (as noted, even in the face of adversity) that can include honesty, trust, fairness, respect, and responsibility (The Center for Academic Integrity, 1999). Interestingly, these are the same kinds of

values that will be expected of you in the role of a nurse. Intellectual and personal honesty, mutual trust, clear standards, opportunities for participation, personal accountability, and action in the face of wrongdoing are all values that are present in both discussions of academic integrity and those of professional integrity as well (Office of the Vice-Principal, Queen's University, n.d.).

Through the eyes of a student

*I*t is midterm, and I have a number of assignments due, all at once. Each one is really important, and I am finding it difficult to decide which one to prioritize. I'm far behind on two of the biggest assignments, both due tomorrow. Additionally, I'm on academic probation from last term, as I failed my pharmacology course. It's imperative that I achieve a good mark on both of the assignments in order to meet the requirements of my probationary contract with the university. I remember that, for the first assignment, I wrote another paper on the same topic 2 years ago in another course. I find it, "cut and paste" sections from my older paper into my new assignment, and finish my work very quickly. For the second assignment, which involves contributing to an online discussion, I have found a significant number of good lay sources on the Internet. I quickly cut and paste them into my discussion text, change a few words and add a couple of my own words. I figure that since they weren't scholarly sources, since I changed a few words, and this wasn't a scholarly paper after all, my actions were acceptable. Later that night, I begin to feel far less comfortable with my approach to both assignments. I'm really not sure who to talk to about this and I'm worried.

(personal reflection of a nursing student)

The tremendous pressure to succeed, both from within and from external sources, can lead to choices that might not be reflective of one's typical values. Students who value truth-telling and honesty have found themselves in precarious academic situations and made the choice to commit plagiarism or take short cuts that constitute academic dishonesty. For students in nonprofessional programs, this is a matter of academic integrity. For students in programs such as nursing or medicine, academic dishonesty can be seen even more seriously, keeping in mind that you are evolving professionals. You may well be held to higher standards in terms of conduct in your academic program. Choices you make in your academic life may be seen as reflective of the kind of professional you will eventually become. Taking short cuts, acting dishonestly, covering something up to avoid exposure of an error, cheating—these are all behaviours that we would not typically want to discover in the nurse who is providing patient care and it may be viewed as more seriously problematic for a nursing student.

Think Your closest friend and study partner, Hiro, is in a different section of the same nursing theory course, and his section meets 3 days after yours. Last semester, his father died, and he has been having a hard time dealing with his grief and keeping up with his studies. You know Hiro needs to maintain his good grades in order to maintain his scholarship—a scholarship that he now needs even more than ever without his dad around. You have just finished writing the midterm today and feel very good about the test. You have a high average in this class and understand the complex concepts well. Your friend approaches you after the midterm and says that he has been having trouble sleeping and studying and was hoping you could give him an idea of the questions and your answers so that he can focus his studying. How would this make you feel in this situation? What kinds of principles would guide your decision-making?

In this situation, you may be finding it difficult to assess just what is in Hiro's best interests. He needs help right now, but providing him with the information he has asked for makes you uncomfortable, and you know that while it will make him feel better in the short term, it won't help him in a meaningful way. If he doesn't learn this for himself, he won't be able to pass the course or move forward to other courses. The information is important in learning about providing patient care, and you know Hiro wants to be an accountable and responsible nurse. With beneficence guiding you, you feel that helping Hiro in some way will be in his best interests, but that providing the questions and answers outright will not be in his or your best interests or those of the patients who are in Hiro's care in his clinical placement. Based on this, a suggestion might be to take time to study with Hiro, teach him about the concepts you understand well, and help him to be as prepared as possible for the midterm.

Professional Ethics

In the following section, we explore four topics related to professional and nursing ethics: autonomy, informed consent, truth-telling, and end-of-life care. These are important topics to explore from a nursing perspective because nurses have unique roles and responsibilities related to these four topics.

Patient Autonomy and Informed Consent

Autonomy refers to our ability to make decisions about our own lives. In health care, autonomy is often seen as the prevailing principle; we respect the autonomous decisions of others, even if they are different than the decisions we would have made. Autonomy refers to our ability to make decisions about our own lives. Competent patients have the right to make decisions about their care, and in turn, health-care professionals must ensure that patients' autonomy, and their wishes are respected. This can present challenges in patient–clinician relationships. Many times, patients make choices that may not be what the nurse or the health-care team considers to be in their best interests.

Let's revisit our case from the beginning of the chapter. During their conversation, Emily asks Jason to advocate for her in her request to the medical team to discontinue the respirator. Jason replies that he feels this is assisted suicide and that it is illegal for him to help her and unethical, in his opinion, for him to advocate for her in this way. Although he tells her that he respects her autonomous decision, he can't possibly agree to it and can't see himself, in his role as a caregiver, helping "to kill" a patient, especially a young person. He also wonders aloud if perhaps her current depression is affecting her ability to be positive, and he suggests that perhaps he could be a better advocate for her by helping her find reasons to live. Emily nods and tells Jason she understands his reaction; however, she has thought a great deal about this. She is puzzled that, as a nursing student, he would respect her autonomous wishes in every other way but not the most important way. She also points out that the medical team have allowed other treatments and interventions to be discontinued at her request, so why should this be any different? She asks Jason, "Isn't this just like respecting my wishes in any other way? It's no different!"

In today's health-care settings, patients are faced with many choices: surgery or medicine, this physician or the one in another hospital, the standard of care or the new experimental procedure, and urgent surgery or wait and see. Patients have to make difficult decisions about their care and their future. Sometimes, they make a choice that is not seen as the obviously beneficial one. Patients who leave the hospital against medical advice or refuse a lifesaving therapy or prescribed medications may be seen by members of the health-care team to be making decisions that are not in the best interests of their health. However, we respect autonomy over other ethical principles and allow patients to make choices for themselves. We do have clear responsibilities, of course. From the most simple to the most complex decisions, patients must be allowed to make informed choices and must be provided with clear, relevant, and thorough information about their possible choices.

Through the eyes of a patient

It's been 3 years since I was diagnosed with stage 2 lung cancer. I've had chemotherapy and radiation and even one surgery. I've been in and out of hospital for treatment and monitoring; more doctor visits than I could have ever imagined. Despite all that, I've been able to travel, enjoy time with my kids and my grandchildren, and spend time at my cottage. At my last doctor's appointment, I was told that my lung cancer has gotten worse and that it's now stage 4. I'm feeling a lot less well than before, and I don't think I have the energy to keep fighting. I decided I'd like to learn more about palliative care, and

(continued on page 156)

Through the eyes of a patient (continued)

my doctor said that was probably an okay idea. I've talked a lot about it with my kids, with my oncologist, and with the oncology clinic nurse, Ray, who really helped me out. Ray just talked about all my options with me, let me talk about what I needed, and he tried to answer all my questions. He also helped me connect with the palliative care team that helps patients stay at home and be comfortable as long as they can. He really helped me make this difficult decision, and I feel good about it. I feel relaxed and at peace with this decision and happy that I can just stop fighting so hard.

(personal reflection of a patient)

Informed consent is probably the most widely discussed topic within the larger body of literature on patient autonomy. Respecting autonomy by ensuring the patients' rights to provide informed consent for care is a clear priority in health care, and many professional codes of ethics reflect this as a value. The CNA Code of Ethics for Registered Nurses in Canada includes, as one of the seven key values, the responsibility of the nurse to "promote and respect informed decision-making" (CNA, 2008, p. 11). Acting autonomously means not only having information about choices but also the freedom or ability to make a choice without constraint or interference. Informed consent, then, has two important aspects: the cognitive aspect and the volitional aspect (Appelbaum, Lidz, & Meisel, 2001). As patient advocates, nurses should ensure that patients have access to as much information as possible in order to make informed decisions. They should also ensure that the information provided is both relevant and appropriate for the patient's understanding and decision-making. A patient who does not speak English should have a translator present the information in the language that he or she can understand. Someone who has a developmental disability or a cognitive deficit may only be able to understand information when provided in simple small chunks. Literacy and reading comprehension are important factors for consideration if there is written material involved such as a consent form or information brochure. A patient who is competent but who may have short periods of transient delirium occasionally at night in the ICU should be provided with information at a time of day that allows him to focus and be as clearheaded as possible. All these considerations are relevant to the cognitive aspect of informed consent. In addition to confirming that the patient clearly understands the information provided—the choices and their risks, benefits, and alternatives—the nurse also ensures that the patient has the ability to make a voluntary choice and that he or she does not feel coerced, unduly influenced, or pressured to choose a particular course of action. This kind of pressure may not be obvious or intentional. It may simply be that the patient finds it difficult to question or refuse the prescribed option for fear of displeasing or angering health-care providers.

Informed consent for therapy and for research is an intrinsically complex notion. There are many debatable issues and gray areas within the topic of informed consent. For example, who is the most appropriate person to obtain consent? In the age of the Internet and seemingly limitless information, just how much information is required in order to be fully informed? What about persons with fluctuating or limited capacity? Are they competent to provide informed consent for themselves? Can children provide informed consent? What happens if a patient consents and then changes his mind?

In many cases, the health-care professional who is directly seeking the patients' informed consent for procedures, surgeries, research, or interventions is the physician, not the nurse. The physician who is responsible for carrying out the procedure is the one who obtains the patient's informed consent. The nurse has a role as a facilitator and an advocate in respecting patient autonomy. Nurses develop trusting relationships with patients and within these relationships can facilitate access to current, complete, and relevant information; create opportunities for patients to make informed choices; advocate for patients' decisions; and respect past decisions, sometimes as articulated through an advance directive or substitute decision-maker. As nurses are most often at the bedside, they must be attentive to the fact that consent is a dynamic notion, and there are times when patients change their minds. For example, a patient who has previously expressed consent for a surgical procedure may wake up afraid or hesitant, with additional questions that change their mind about consent until the questions are answered and their fears addressed. Although most interventions such as surgical procedures and invasive diagnostic tests require a formal, written consent process, nurses must use less formal ways of ensuring that patients' consent to the care they receive. All patients have the right to provide (or refuse) consent for any kind of touching, be it a bed bath, having vital signs taken, insertion of a catheter, a physical assessment, or a dressing change. In a court of law, any kind of touch that is done without the consent of another person could potentially be considered battery (Keatings & Smith, 2000), should a patient pursue a complaint. Thus, nurses must ensure that they have open and trusting channels of communication with their patients. Before initiating any kind of nursing action, the patient is provided the opportunity to express consent. Just like the patient who changes his or her mind about surgery, a patient who has agreed to allow the nurse to do a nonurgent dressing change may be in pain or fatigued and wish to postpone the dressing change until later. The nurse, in turn, must respect that decision and delay the dressing change until the patient provides consent.

Truth-Telling, Deception, and Withholding Knowledge

Trusting relationships are an important part of a nurse–patient relationship. Trusting others means that we tend to assume that people will be truthful and fair with us, and in turn, we will also act in an honest and fair manner. In everyday life, we may be less than truthful in many kinds of situations for many different reasons. You tell a friend that his or her haircut looks nice when you really feel it doesn't, or you may tell the phone company that you paid the overdue bill 2 days ago when you haven't paid it at all. We avoid truth-telling in some situations in order to avoid harming someone by hurting their feelings, to protect ourselves from harm, or to avoid unnecessary disputes or misunderstandings. People may be less than honest at times in an attempt to smooth things over or to avoid difficult emotional situations. However, the nature of the relationships in everyday life is quite different from the relationships we have in clinical settings with patients. Nurses and other health-care professionals have a **fiduciary duty** toward those for whom we care. Originally a legal term, a *fiduciary* is a person who has the responsibility to protect the needs and the best interests of others and holds that responsibility above his or her own needs or interests. Typically, a person who requires a fiduciary has little choice but to trust that person with his or her best interests. By upholding principles of beneficence and nonmaleficence, a fiduciary relationship is built on trust, disclosure, and care. Part of the responsibility of this kind of duty is the obligation to be truthful in communications with patients (Collis, 2006). In the CNA Code of Ethics for Registered Nurses (2008), honesty and truth-telling are referred to as ethical responsibilities in the discussions of two values: promoting justice and being accountable. Although nurses are not typically the members of the health-care team who are responsible for the provision of difficult news, diagnoses, or prognoses, they still have important roles in communicating with patients. Nurses in advance practice roles are communicating diagnoses and prognoses to patients in some cases. It is reasonable to say that we need to consider truth-telling a value in all situations, not just in communicating difficult or bad news to patients. In all kinds of relationships and communication, truthfulness should be a priority in order to protect the autonomy of the patient and prevent potential harm. Moreover, truthfulness is an intrinsic good and an expectation within a trusting relationship (Collis, 2006; Tuckett, 2004).

Deception is often justified by the intention to act out of nonmaleficence, to protect the patient from harm, or to avoid damaging the nurse–patient relationship (Hébert, Hoffmaster, Glass, & Singer, 1997). However, the literature clearly shows that patients prefer truthfulness, even if facing difficult or painful information (Tuckett, 2004). Truthfulness helps to reduce patients' potential mistrust, fear, resentment, and loss of faith in both individuals and the health-care system. By promoting truth-telling in all aspects of care and communication, the trust that is nurtured helps to strengthen the supportive nurse–patient relationship, which can be comforting and reassuring for the patient who is facing bad news. Meaningful communication; helping patients to access relevant and complete information; providing advice and counsel in a judicious and nonbiased way; educating patients about their health, their choices, and their rights; and finally, advocating for truth-telling in all modes of communication between patients and health-care professionals are all ways that nurses can contribute to an environment in which truthfulness is communicated as an intrinsic good.

The commonly cited expression coined by Francis Bacon in the 16th century, "knowledge is power" (Bacon, 1996), is relevant to this discussion. In health-care settings, the inherent power imbalances that are created by the possession of specialized knowledge can be overwhelming and intimidating to patients who can feel confused, resentful, deceived, or uninformed. By withholding knowledge or being dishonest with patients, we may further emphasize the negative consequences of these power imbalances. Nurses must realize that they are gatekeepers to information and knowledge, and their role involves a serious responsibility to provide care with integrity and honesty, alongside an overarching commitment to build and foster trusting relationships.

Care at the End of Life

There are many kinds of ethical issues that arise in care of patients who are dying. More than any other health-care professional, nurses are the ones who often provide total care and support throughout the dying process, across various settings. As part of this intense involvement, nurses are often a part of difficult conversations, heart-wrenching, decision-making processes, and direct care of patients at the end of life. In turn, nurses face ethical dilemmas in the provision of care and involvement in the lives of persons who are dying.

Historically, death and dying have been private and family processes, often occurring at home and without the assistive technologies that have become a common part of dying in today's health-care settings. The capacity of technology to help sustain life, prolong functioning, and delay the dying process has created new dilemmas and shifted the locus of control for matters of life and death to specialists in ICU.

Davis and Aroskar (1983) classify three types of ethical dilemmas in death and dying: those that involve interventions of modern medicine (e.g., resuscitation; prolonging life by artificial means; withdrawal of food, fluids, or assistive technology), interventions of people who might be close to the patient (e.g., determining futility, carrying out advance directives, hastening death), and interventions by the patient (e.g., suicide, requests for assistance with suicide, refusal of lifesaving interventions). Although certainly not exhaustive, this collection of ethical dilemmas covers key issues at the end of life, some of which we will touch on here.

Medical Interventions

Medical interventions at the end of life are highly involved and now almost an accepted part of dying. Common processes include cardiopulmonary resuscitation (CPR), ventilation, and medications to prolong life and improve functioning. In most hospital settings, respiratory or cardiac arrest results in rapid intervention (calling a code) to take over the functions of the heart and lungs, and by doing so, prevent a person's death. In many cases, CPR and full resuscitation measures prevent deaths and prolong life, which we deem intrinsically good. However, in some cases, resuscitation is arguably too invasive, too painful or only serving to sustain a life that has poor quality or lengthen an already difficult dying process (CNA, 1995). In cases like these, do not resuscitate (DNR) orders may be most appropriate and in the best interests of patients. When patients or family members feel that a DNR order may be desired, a frank and honest discussion with the health-care team is initiated. Typically, only physicians can write DNR orders for patients (which are also usually reviewed on an ongoing regular basis); however, it is imperative that the entire health-care team understands not only that the order is in place but also how that order intervenes in a sudden health crisis. Clarity about roles and responsibilities and opportunities for revisiting the DNR decision in an open discussion are both important considerations when establishing such an order. Additionally, nurses may be the health-care team members who are responsible for educating staff, families, and patients about what a DNR status means. Even after making such a difficult decision, many patients and family members have questions, worries, and concerns. Nursing team members maintain an open, approachable, and well-informed attitude around choices regarding resuscitation.

Quality of Life

Discussions about medical interventions at the end of life inevitably turn to values about **quality of life**. For many people, quality of life is a highly subjective and imprecise term, but it usually refers to one's overall well-being and satisfaction with the conditions under which one lives. Advancements in health care have been responsible for significant quality-of-life gains in recent years as we are living longer on average and in better health. Although not a widely embraced phrase, what we are actually talking about is "quality of death." Reasonable people might agree that at the end of our life, quality of life means retaining some control over the process and being as pain-free, peaceful, and comfortable as possible. Little is known about self-perceived quality of life near the end of life because such information is so difficult to collect and to interpret. The diversity of patient philosophical, cultural, religious, and spiritual beliefs will have an impact on individual perceptions about what quality of life means. In one study, patients at the end of life identified five domains that were important to them at the end of life: management of pain and unpleasant symptoms, sustaining life only when appropriate, having some degree of control, relieving burden on caregivers, and ensuring that relationships with families and loved ones were intact and even strengthened (Singer, Martin, & Kelner, 1999).

Advance Directives

At the end of life, patients may not be able to articulate their wishes or take part in a discussion about alternatives for their care. However, one way that they can make sure that their authentic wishes will be respected is to have them written down in the form of a living will. Living wills can outline a patient's specific wishes regarding how they are cared for at the end of life: whether or not CPR will be done, whether they wish to be treated in the event of a respiratory infection or organ failure, or whether they wish to have surgery and what kind of palliative care they would accept. A living will, more commonly referred to as an **advance directive**, achieves two specific goals: It allows for the authentic wishes of a competent person to be carried out when that person is no longer competent or able to speak for himself or herself. An advance directive essentially prolongs the autonomy of a person beyond the point of his or her ability to communicate his or her autonomous choices freely. Second, it requires the appointment of a substitute decision-maker (or a proxy) who can ensure that the wishes, as articulated in the advance directives, are carried out

as much as possible (Singer, Robertson, & Roy, 1996). Across Canada, advance directive documents look very different and use various terms to mean the same thing. In different provinces, living wills have different names and powers or are legal documents in most provinces and not in others. A living will is called a *representation agreement* in British Columbia, a *personal directive* in Alberta, a *health-care directive* in Manitoba, and a *power of attorney for personal care* in New Brunswick. Whereas Ontario refers to the appointed proxy as the *attorney for personal care*, a person in the same role in Quebec is called a *mandatory* and a *substitute decision-maker* in Newfoundland. It's clear that advance directives and legislation about how their contents can be enacted is confusing and highly variable between jurisdictions. In institutions and hospitals, there is often a certain amount of uncertainty over how to deal with advance directives. Furthermore, some family members may not understand how the advance directive affects care of their loved one. Fear, hesitation, lack of knowledge, and lack of understanding are all contributors to not following the wishes of an advance directive.

Facing Death

There may be situations in end-of-life care when the health-care team is approached to ease suffering or hasten death. These kinds of requests may be made explicitly by patients or loved ones, or they may be requested through more implicit means, such as gestures or actions; for example, refusing medications or interventions.

Euthanasia can be defined as causing the painless death of a person, with a goal to be merciful, in order to end or prevent suffering or pain. Euthanasia may be further categorized as voluntary, involuntary, or nonvoluntary, depending on the person's voiced or known wishes, competence, or awareness (Lavery, Dickens, Boyle, & Singer, 1997). There are also distinctions made between the kinds of interventions carried out to cause death. Cases where treatment is withheld or ceased and the patient then becomes more vulnerable to underlying processes that may cause death are usually referred to as passive euthanasia. In cases of active euthanasia, bodily processes necessary to sustain life are actively interfered with or stopped (Battin, 1994). Whereas some people feel that these are very different, others posit that there is no clear moral distinction between these classifications; stopping a ventilator required to sustain respiration and cardiac function may not be morally different from withholding antibiotics to treat an impending respiratory infection. The notion of passivity (allowing a body process such as infection or cancer to cause death without intervention) is somehow, to many people, more morally palatable than to actively cause death by an injection or by taking an action to stop something that is sustaining life, such as a feeding tube, a ventilator, or a cardiac assistive device. This debate is ongoing and reflects how different values have an effect on how we classify things as morally acceptable. **Assisted suicide** is defined as the act of killing oneself with the advice or help of another person. The other person may provide the means by which to commit suicide, the knowledge to carry out a suicide plan, or both. A person who seeks counsel on how much of a narcotic is necessary for an overdose or who seeks a prescription to explicitly stockpile for this purpose is an example of seeking assistance with suicide. Physician-assisted suicide implies that a doctor helps or counsels a patient who wishes to commit suicide. Assisted suicide is illegal in most places, including Canada, with notable exceptions being Belgium, Switzerland, the Netherlands, and the state of Oregon in the United States. In Canada, euthanasia and physician-assisted suicide are both illegal under the Criminal Code of Canada, regardless of the stated wishes of the person (Criminal Code of Canada, 1985, Part VIII). The issue remains a legal gray area in many countries where there is no law explicitly prohibiting physician-assisted suicide.

Nurses play several important roles for patients and families facing death. Not only are they the health-care providers who often are present for the entire dying process and the immediate time after death but also are often the persons who family members and patients themselves turn to with difficult questions and requests. Nurses are trained to care for persons in all stages and to facilitate reaching a level of optimal well-being in any state: health, illness, acutely injured, or dying. This implies that providing care for the dying patient is more than simply making them comfortable or ensuring that they are free of pain, although all are important roles. There are other equally significant responsibilities of the nurse caring for a dying patient, including protecting the patient's right to self-determination by advocating for the patient's wishes and involvement in decision-making. Nurses also provide accurate and up-to-date information, facilitating communication among patients, their families, and the health-care team, and respect the patient's right to refuse treatment while advocating for adequate resources and settings for end of life, such as a palliative care unit with an appropriate level of patient care (CNA, 2000).

Ethical Decision-Making Models

Ethical decisions are not made within a vacuum. We don't work in isolation nor are we ever asked to face difficult ethical dilemmas alone. Ethical dilemmas commonly involve relationships and are intrinsically convoluted by virtue of diverse values and multiple stakeholders, all with their own perspectives and interests. Although ethical theories may assist us in analysis and reasoning about cases, they may not adequately address the contextual nature of ethical dilemmas. Even within a health-care team made up of reasonable individuals with a common goal, ideas on ethical rightness and moral integrity can be quite different.

You might be wondering how anyone ever makes decisions when faced with ethical dilemmas. In light of the complexity of contexts and diversity of persons and values, how can we find an acceptable solution when faced with an ethical dilemma? Models for ethical decision-making will not point to the actual answer or solution, but they may serve to provide a framework for discussion and systematic analysis of ethical problems (Rodney, 1991; Storch et al., 2013). Boxes 9.1 and 9.2 present two ethical decision-making models for you to try on for size. Both models are presented here to show the similarities between them and demonstrate that ethical decision-making can be, to some degree, quite systematic. You'll notice differences between the two models, but many of the important steps are present in both models.

BOX 9.1 A Guide to Moral Decision-Making

1. **Recognize the moral dimension.** This first very important stage involves recognizing that you are, in fact, facing an issue that has moral or ethical significance. According to MacDonald, a key to recognizing moral significance is noting that there is a conflict of values.

2. **Decide who the relevant parties are and determine their relationships.** Once you have recognized that the issue is a morally significant issue, you need to determine who the key stakeholders are. Who has an interest in the outcome or processes? MacDonald advises us to be both careful and yet "imaginative and sympathetic" at this stage because at first glance, it may not always be obvious who is involved or who might be affected by decisions. Once you have determined who might in fact have a stake in the situation, it is important to figure out what kinds of relationships exist between the identified persons as well as with yourself. Once you can identify the kinds of relationships that exist, you can also identify what expectations or obligations will necessarily be involved.

3. **Figure out what values are involved.** At this stage, you need to think about the values that are at stake. What is the key question or dilemma? Is this a case of autonomy like Emily's case at the beginning of the chapter? Or is this an issue of justice or rights? Is there a risk of harm to anyone in this case?

4. **Weigh the benefits and burdens.** Benefits, according to MacDonald, can range from things that may have intrinsic or instrumental good to attempt to satisfy people's preferences or respect their wishes. On the other hand, burdens may involve costs, harms, or pain.

5. **Look for analogous cases.** Have you ever faced this kind of situation before? Do you know of other cases similar to this one? If so, think about what happened in those cases. Are the outcomes or processes relevant for consideration in this case?

6. **Discuss with relevant others.** Deliberation involving others is a valuable way to see the problem from various perspectives. Discussion and disclosure about cases, however, must be done with attention to maintaining confidentiality.

7. **Determine if the proposed decision is in accordance with legal and organizational rules.** At this point, once you have decided upon possible alternatives, you must note the context and location in which the ethical dilemma exists. In doing this, pay attention to policies or laws that might have an effect upon your decision.

8. **Reflect on your own level of comfort with this decision.** Once you've decided what the best course of action is, you should note your gut reaction. Can you live with this option? Would you be comfortable telling others about it? Living by it?

Adapted from MacDonald, C. (2002). *A guide to moral decision making*. Retrieved from http://www.ethicsweb.ca/guide/

BOX 9.2   An Ethical Decision-Making Model for Critical Care Nursing

1. **Gather background information.** This first stage is characterized by the collection of relevant information to help you define and describe the problem.
2. **Identify whether the problem is an ethical one.** Determine, through collecting as much information as possible, whether the problem is in fact an ethical one or whether it may instead be a practical, legal, or professional issue. There may certainly be overlap between these categories of issues, but it is most important at this point to determine whether the problem has an ethical dimension.
3. **Identify key stakeholders.** Identify the key players; that is, anyone who might be affected by this ethical issue. Relational

concepts such as responsibility, authority, professional roles, and conflicting duties may be relevant.
4. **Identify possible courses of action.** Identify possible options and consequences.
5. **Reconcile the facts of the case with relevant principles.** As you have already determined the relevant principles, you must now consider the outcomes along with these principles to make sure you haven't missed an important consideration.
6. **Resolution.** Try to achieve consensus among all those involved in resolving the issue, keeping in mind that there may be constraints such as professional obligations or legal restrictions that may affect realization of the chosen alternative.

Adapted from Rodney, P. (1991). Dealing with ethical problems: An ethical decision-making model for critical care nursing. *Canadian Critical Care Nursing Journal, 8*(1), 8–10.

When we revisit Emily's case using either of these ethical decision-making models, we find that we can think about the case in a more organized way to help move toward resolution. Assuming the role of Jason, let's use the MacDonald's (2002) *Guide to Moral Decision Making* to help guide our thinking about the ethical dilemma he is facing.

1. **Recognize the moral dimension.** It's clear that there is a moral dimension to Emily's case. Cases involving death and dying are often fraught with ethical issues. Emily is requesting assistance to die, and there are apparent conflicting values. A highly normative concept such as quality of life is relevant in this case.
2. **Decide who the relevant parties are and determine their relationships.** In this case, the key stakeholder is Emily and her family. Her close friends may also be affected to some degree by the outcome of the dilemma. The health-care team who will provide care to Emily needs to be considered because team members may well find it either rewarding or deeply troubling to care for Emily at this point. Certainly, Jason has identified that he has an emotional and professional stake in the outcome of the case. If we were to think about the allocation of scarce resources, we might also consider other patients as peripherally relevant as well. The demands of 24-hour care for Emily take human and financial resources away from other patients. In terms of relationships, the trusting relationship that Jason and Emily have formed has allowed Emily to speak her mind and to disclose her innermost wishes. The relationships that she currently maintains with others, such as her family and friends, seem tenuous. As this is the case, Jason is clearly in the role of confidante for Emily. She views him as an advocate and as someone who might be able to understand her position.
3. **Figure out what values are involved.** This following values or principles are apparent in this case: autonomy, beneficence, and nonmaleficence. Emily is a competent

and autonomous individual. However, she cannot carry out her wish to die without assistance. Some might question her competency in the face of depression, whereas others would argue this, claiming that her situational depression should not be a factor in deciding whether she is capable of making decisions. Jason feels that to assist someone with dying is to harm him or her. It is quite clear that Emily considers that acting in her best interests means respecting her wishes and providing assistance for her to die.
4. **Weigh the benefits and burdens.** Emily has thought a great deal about this desire. She states that she feels at peace for the first time. The burdens she carries are great: painful treatments, a bleak outlook, a life spent in a long-term care setting, few friends, and complete dependence on others for even the simplest needs. The benefits of respecting her wishes include promoting her dignity by allowing her to control the one and perhaps only thing she feels that she can still control: her own death. However, in respecting her wishes, burdens may be shifted to others. Her family, friends, and caregivers may experience feelings of guilt, sorrow, and grief. Yet even now, her parents are finding it difficult to cope with her condition, and to continue in this condition for many years to come means that the burden on Emily's parents would be great. Jason bears a burden as the one person to whom Emily has disclosed. Whether he chooses to approach the health-care team with her request and how he does so will have an effect on how the request is viewed by others. He bears the burden of conflicting values. He would like to act in Emily's best interests, but it isn't entirely clear what that means.
5. **Look for analogous cases.** Jason is a nursing student. Like many nursing students, the difficult ethical dilemmas that he may encounter during his training will likely be a series of firsts. Although he may have taken a course in ethics and has read a great deal on death and dying, this is probably the first time that he has been this directly involved in such a case.

6. **Discuss with relevant others.** Jason needs to discuss this with someone other than Emily. He can turn to his preceptor or his faculty advisor or a nurse he trusts. He might see who has been closely involved in Emily's care to include them in a discussion. As Emily and her family did see a counselor, it might be prudent to discuss this with him as well. Jason needs to discuss this case not only in order to effectively deliberate on a difficult choice but also to help sort out his own conflicting feelings and values. In this case, a mentor or trusted teacher might be someone whom Jason could approach while ensuring he maintains confidentiality in order to adhere to professional rules of conduct. Legal and institutional guidelines about disclosure of personal information dictate that Jason might only be able to talk about this case in hypothetical terms with persons outside of Emily's circle of care. For Emily's benefit and with her permission, Jason might think about expanding the discussion to other members of the health-care team.

7. **Determine if the proposed decision is in accordance with legal and organizational rules.** Assisting someone to end his or her life is considered illegal in Canada. The institution where Jason is doing his clinical placement may not have a policy in place that addresses euthanasia or assisted suicide directly, but it may well have policies around palliative care, withdrawal of treatment, and respect for the wishes of competent patients. Jason is not yet a fully licensed nurse, so he practices under the license of his preceptor who assumes responsibility for his actions. Although the only decision he currently has to make is whether or not to support Emily's request to advocate for her, the implications and possible outcomes from this initial step may result in professional issues for both Jason and his preceptor.

8. **Reflect on your own level of comfort with this decision.** Even after exploring Emily's case using this ethical decision-making model, we still find that the answer is not obvious. Jason needs to decide how he will proceed from here and what ethical principles will guide his actions. What would you do, if you were Jason, and why?

SUMMARY

Thinking about our professional practice from an ethical perspective is something we do all the time. Without knowing it, we are often reflecting on and demonstrating to others what values we hold by our actions, our words, and our deliberative choices. We will certainly encounter many situations in our practice when our values conflict with others, and the challenge is to work through these kinds of ethically challenging circumstances while maintaining our moral integrity and standing up for what we believe is the right thing to do. Being concretely steadfast in holding to our values is not always the absolute best course of action. Having moral integrity often means maintaining an open attitude to the diverse values and beliefs of others, and in doing so, viewing the world in a different way. We have much to learn from each other when faced with ethical dilemmas, and as nurses, that lifelong learning continues throughout our career with each new encounter. Many of the nursing practice situations we will come upon will have an ethical dimension to them. Learning to recognize that a practice problem or issue is an ethical one is the first step to being a nurse with moral integrity and a keen ethical awareness.

Critical Thinking Case Scenarios

Working on the street

▶ You are a nurse in a mental health outreach unit. The unit is in a storefront and provides support, services, and referral for those living with mental health issues in the community. You find that you often see the same patients time and time again, and many are transitioning from being institutionalized to living independently or semi-independently. Today, you are seeing Carter, a young patient with schizophrenia, who has been discharged from the hospital on medication but who has not been showing up to his halfway house at night. When you ask him about this, Carter says that the halfway house is noisy, frightening, and lacking in privacy. The house makes him feel very nervous. He also discloses to you that along with the nervousness, he is having terrible side effects from his medication and feels that it is in his best interest to stop taking it now that he has been discharged. You explain to Carter that if he stops taking his medication, he may risk the symptoms of schizophrenia returning. You are also aware that winter is only a few weeks away and living on the street in this area of town means facing bad weather and very real threats to safety. You offer several concrete suggestions for him to deal with his specific side effects and offer to make him an appointment with the clinic physician the next day. Carter refuses your help and leaves the clinic but says he'll come by the clinic soon. As you watch him leave, you are at once very nervous for him but realize he has the right to make his own decision. However, you are still uncomfortable with this. Why? What ethical principles are in conflict in this situation? What should you do, if anything?

Steadfastness

▶ You are a third-year nursing student, with a placement in a long-term care setting, working with a preceptor, Kathy. You are working your first night shift. On rounds at 2 AM, you find Mrs. Wong disoriented and yelling. She is waking up other residents. You know that speaking to her in Cantonese can easily reorient Mrs. Wong, and you also know that the nursing supervisor working tonight is fluent in Cantonese. You suggest calling the supervisor, but Kathy tells you not to, and she instead speaks loudly and harshly to Mrs. Wong, saying, "That's enough! Stop making so much noise! You'll wake others up! Stop!" Mrs. Wong becomes quieter but still appears confused and begins to cry. Kathy says to you, "Oh, don't worry, she's fine. At least she'll be quiet now. She'll go back to sleep and won't remember this tomorrow. This is what you do on nights, kid! You're learning." You feel uncomfortable with this, especially as the patient is still crying, and you felt that there were several alternatives to calm her that could have easily been done. Why do you think you are uncomfortable despite Kathy's reassurance? What would you do?

Conflicting duties

▶ It is the end of a busy shift, and you are almost ready to go home. The manager approaches you and tells you that you have a professional obligation to stay longer and provide coverage for a critically ill patient because two nurses from the next shift are quite late and have not yet arrived. You fully understand that patient care is a priority; however, as a single father, you are also aware that your babysitter is waiting at home for you anxiously with your young son who has been ill. You are torn between two important and yet competing or conflicting duties, and at this moment, you are unclear which duty should override. What factors do you need to consider in this situation? What decision do you think you would end up making? What broader implications does this situation have?

What's the right thing to do and why?

▶ You are a licensed practical nurse in a busy ER. Today has been a hectic day, and the ER staff has been faced with difficult challenges and patients and barely any time to debrief. When you go for your lunch break, you overhear your ER colleagues at the next table in the full cafeteria talking animatedly and in great detail about a particularly difficult case this morning. They are making jokes about the overbearing family and the patient. They see you and call you over to join the discussion. You face a difficult choice. Should you join the discussion with your colleagues, risking your own moral integrity and knowing that the group could be easily overheard by anyone? Or should you tell your colleagues that you wish to join them but not to discuss the patient and the family because you clearly have a professional obligation not to do so? Use what you've learned about the various theories of ethics in thinking about this dilemma. What are the possible outcomes, negative and positive, of your decision?

Multiple-Choice Questions

1. Which of the following best describes an ethical dilemma?
   a. A situation involving conflicting or overlapping professional roles
   b. A situation in which there are conflicting values and beliefs
   c. Any clinical situation that involves informed consent
   d. A situation that highlights cultural or gender differences

2. Mr. Lindon, a married father of two, is a competent 36-year-old man who is refusing to have an intravenous (IV) line started and also refusing antibiotic therapy for endocarditis, a fatal infection. What should the nurse realize?
   a. Mr. Lindon is legally and ethically bound to make the right choice by accepting treatment.
   b. The nurse must start the IV and administer the lifesaving treatment to Mr. Lindon.
   c. Refusal can be overruled because Mr. Lindon has a potentially fatal infection.
   d. Mr. Lindon is within his legal rights to refuse treatment.

3. Which of the following statements best describes moral distress?
   a. When there is uncertainty about moral principles in a given situation
   b. When there are professional practice requirements that are difficult to abide by
   c. When a person knows the right thing to do but cannot carry out that action
   d. When a person's autonomous choice is not accepted by others

4. Which of the following is the best example of steadfastness?
   a. The nursing student who hands all his assignments in completed and on time
   b. The nursing educator who ensures that her class is well prepared for the exam
   c. The nursing student who takes a patients' concerns with care to his preceptor
   d. The nurse who makes sure that all colleagues sign the narcotic sheet properly

5. Which of the following is a global trend in health care that has important ethical implications?
   a. The effect and power of the media has decreased over time.
   b. The traditional hierarchal model of the doctor–patient relationship persists.
   c. The use of technology in health care is prevalent and continues to increase.
   d. The legal rights of patients are well aligned with the health-care professionals' obligations.

6. Which of the following best describes the major difference between deontological and consequentialist ethical theories?
   a. Deontologists focus on duties to guide ethical action, whereas consequentialists look to outcomes.

b. Deontologists believe that the most ethical action is that which aligns with individual values while consequentialists emphasize collective values.

c. Deontologists state that we should act in a way that maximizes good, whereas consequentialists focus on maximizing utility.

d. Deontologists would state that one should never lie, whereas consequentialists would claim that lying is always permissible.

7. Which of the following best describes the responsibility of nurses in terms of informed consent?

a. Nurses must act as witnesses to patients' signatures on consent forms.

b. Nurses should explain detailed surgical procedures to patients.

c. Nurses should seek written consent for all patient care activities, including dressing changes and injections.

d. Nurses should provide patients with the chance to express consent for patient care.

REFERENCES AND SUGGESTED READINGS

Appelbaum, P. S., Lidz, C. W., & Meisel, A. (2001). *Informed consent: Legal theory and clinical practice* (2nd ed.). New York, NY: Oxford University Press.

Bacon, F. (1996). *Meditations sacrae and human philosophy*. Whitefish, MO: Kessinger.

Battin, M. (1994). *The least worst death: Essays in bioethics on the end of life*. New York, NY: Oxford Press.

Beauchamp, T. L., & Childress, J. (2012). *Principles of biomedical ethics* (7th ed.). New York, NY: Oxford University Press.

Beauchamp, T. L. & DeGrazia, D. (2004). Principles and principlism. In G. Khushf (Ed.), *Handbook of bioethics* (pp. 55–74). Dordrecht, The Netherlands: Kluwer Academic.

Beauchamp, T. L., & Walters, L. (1999). *Contemporary issues in bioethics* (5th ed.). Belmont, CA: Wadsworth.

Berg, J. W., Applebaum, P. S., Lidz, C. W., & Parker, L. (2001). *Informed consent: Legal theory and clinical practice*. New York, NY: Oxford University Press.

Burkhardt, M. A., Nathaniel, A. K., & Walton, N. (2013). *Ethics and issues in contemporary nursing* (2nd Canadian ed.). Toronto, ON: Nelson.

Canadian Nurses Association. (1995). *Joint statement on resuscitation interventions*. Ottawa, ON: Author.

Canadian Nurses Association. (2000). *Position statement: End-of-life issues*. Ottawa, ON: Author.

Canadian Nurses Association. (2008). *Code of ethics for registered nurses* (2008 centennial edition). Ottawa, ON: Author.

Collis, S. P. (2006). The importance of truth-telling in health care. *Nursing Standard, 20*(17), 41–45.

Criminal Code of Canada (R.S.C., 1985, c. C-46). Retrieved from http://laws.justic.gc.ca.en/C-46/

Davis, A. J., & Aroskar, M. A. (1983). *Ethical dilemmas and nursing practice*. Norwalk, CT: Appleton.

Gastmans, C., Dierckx de Casterle, B., & Schotsmans, P. (1998). Nursing considered as moral practice: A philosophical-ethical interpretation of nursing. *Kennedy Institute of Ethics Journal, 8*(1), 43–69.

Gilligan, C. (1982). *In a different voice*. Cambridge, MA: Harvard University Press.

Heath, J. (2003). *The myth of shared values in Canada*. Ottawa, ON: Government of Canada.

Hébert, P. C., Hoffmaster, B., Glass, K. C., & Singer, P. A. (1997). Bioethics for clinicians: 7. Truth-telling. *Canadian Medical Association Journal, 156*(2), 225–228.

Holm, S. (2002). Book review: Principles of biomedical ethics (5th ed.). *Journal of Medical Ethics, 28*, 332.

Jameton, A. (1984). *Nursing practice: The ethical issues*. New Jersey, NY: Prentice Hall.

Jameton, A. (1993). Dilemmas of moral distress: Moral responsibility and nursing practice. *AWHONN Clinical Issues in Perinatal Women's Health Nursing, 4*(4), 542–551.

Keatings, M., & Smith, O. B. (2010). *Ethical and legal issues in Canadian nursing* (3rd ed.). Toronto, ON: Elsevier.

Lavery, J. V., Dickens, B. M., Boyle, J. M., & Singer, P. A. (1997). Bioethics for clinicians: 11. Euthanasia and assisted suicide. *Canadian Medical Association Journal, 156*(10), 1405–1408.

Liaschenko, J., & Peter, E. (2003). Feminist ethics. In V. Tschudin (Ed.), *Approaches to ethics: Nursing beyond boundaries* (pp. 33–44). New York, NY: Butterworth.

MacDonald, C. (2002). *A guide to moral decision making*. Retrieved from http://www.ethicsweb.ca/guide/

Oberle, K., & Bouchal, S. R. (2009). *Ethics in Canadian nursing practice: Navigating the journey*. Toronto, ON: Pearson.

Office of the Vice-Principal, Queen's University. (n.d.). *Academic integrity*. Kingston, ON: Queen's University. Retrieved from http://www.queensu.ca/academicintegrity/index.html.

Rodney, P. (1991). Dealing with ethical problems: An ethical decision-making model for critical care nursing. *Canadian Critical Care Nursing Journal, 8*(1), 8–10.

Sherwin, S. (1992). *No longer patient: Feminist ethics and health care*. Philadelphia, PA: Temple University Press.

Singer, P. A., Robertson, G., & Roy, D. J. (1996). Bioethics for clinicians: Advance care planning. *Canadian Medical Association Journal, 155*, 1689–1692.

Singer, P. A. (2002). *University of Toronto Joint Centre for Bioethics: Living will*. Toronto, ON: University of Toronto. Retrieved from http://www.jointcentreforbioethics.ca/tools/livingwill.shtml

Singer, P. A., & Bowman, K. (2002). Quality care at the end of life. *British Medical Journal, 324*, 1291–1292.

Singer, P. A., Martin, D. K., & Kelner, M. (1999). Quality end-of-life care: Patients' perspectives. *Journal of the American Medical Association, 281*(2), 163–168.

Storch, J., Rodney, P., & Starzomski. R. (2013). *Toward a moral horizon: Nursing ethics for leadership and practice* (2nd ed.). Toronto, ON: Pearson.

The Center for Academic Integrity. (1999). *The fundamental values of academic integrity*. Des Plaines, IL: Oakton Community College. Retrieved from http://www.academicintegrity.org/fundamental_values_project/index.php

Thomas, J., & Waluchow, W. (2002). *Well and good: A case study approach to bioethics* (3rd ed.). Peterborough, ON: Broadview Press.

Tuckett, A. G. (2004). Truth-telling in clinical practice and the arguments for and against: A review of the literature. *Nursing Ethics, 11*(5), 500–513.

Yeo, M., Moorhouse, A., Khan, P., & Rodney, P. (2010). *Concepts and cases in nursing ethics* (3rd ed.). Peterborough, ON: Broadview Press.

The Nursing Process in the 21st Century

MICHELLE L. CULLEN AND P. SUSAN WAGNER

Tanja is a third year nursing student. This is her second clinical shift on a medical unit. She has been assigned to care for Amarina. Amarina is 23 years old and was diagnosed with Crohn disease and rheumatoid arthritis when she was 7 years of age. Amarina lives at home with her parents and has an older sister in good health who is attending university. Until recently, Amarina has independently cared for her colostomy and her nutritional needs and has been responsible for her medication. However, over the last 2 months, Amarina has lost a significant amount of weight (13.6 kg) and has had to supplement her nutrition through a G-tube. Amarina is also aware that she will need another surgery within the next few months to remove the rest of her colon. Her mother is very concerned about her daughter's weight loss and unwillingness to participate in her own care. After hearing her mother's concerns, Amarina's medical doctor hospitalized her because she was not following the care plan at home, not following her medication regime, and continuing to lose weight.

CHAPTER OBJECTIVES

By the end of this chapter, you will be able to:

1. Identify the five steps of the nursing process and describe how they are interrelated.
2. Describe how each step in the nursing process contributes to patient-centered care.
3. Identify the resources used to gather information.
4. Formulate appropriate nursing diagnoses.
5. Develop a comprehensive nursing care plan.
6. Identify factors affecting patient care priorities.
7. Compare and contrast the effectiveness of interventions planned by the health-care team to those interventions that include the patient in such planning.
8. Evaluate patient care outcomes as they relate to the treatment goals and list potential changes that may be required to increase the effectiveness of the care provided.

KEY TERMS

Assessment A systematic and ongoing process of gathering, organizing, validating, and documenting data related to the patient's health status through inquiry, collaboration, and using various resources.

Clarification Seeks more information to confirm your understanding.

Closed-Ended Questions Specific questions that are used to limit the scope of the response or to focus on a specific area of interest.

Diagnosis Involves analyzing data, identifying health problems and risks, as well as strengths, and formulating diagnostic statements.

Ecomap A pictorial depiction of how a person values his or her attachments to people or activities.

Evaluation To review and measure whether the care goals were met, to identify if there were any unintended outcomes, and to determine if any changes to the plan are required in order to accomplish any unmet goals.

Genogram A pictorial representation of the patient's family and health patterns.

Implementation An intentional effort to achieve the goals related to the patient's health status.

Interpreting Understanding the clinical significance of how the assessment data fits together to inform clinical decisions regarding patient care.

Interventions Planned nursing actions taken to address patient or family needs, working toward previously established collaborative goals for patient or family outcomes.

Leading Questions Questions that suggest a direction for the conversation.

Neutral Questions Questions that provide an opportunity for the patient to respond according to his or her own perceptions.

Nonverbal Communication Includes a person's facial expressions, gestures, posture, and attentiveness.

Nursing Diagnosis A clinical judgment that identifies a patient's response to actual or potential health problems.

Nursing Interventions Classification (NIC) An internationally recognized list of nursing actions with standardized labels and descriptions.

Nursing Judgment The process nurses use to critically evaluate and interpret patient data and then make informed decisions about their patient's care.

Nursing Outcomes Classification (NOC) An internationally recognized list of the results of nursing care with standardized labels and descriptions.

Nursing Process A systematic and rational method of planning and providing patient care organized around a series of phases that facilitates evidence-informed, and ethical nursing practice.

Objective Data The information collected from examining the patient and from the patient's chart and medical records that is measurable and evaluated against a standard which is considered the norm.

Open-Ended Questions Questions without a yes or no answer that encourage patients to provide additional information about their situation.

Paraphrasing Interprets the patient's words.

Planning The steps taken by the patient, nurse, and interprofessional team to formulate goals, identify timelines, and coordinate resources.

Prioritizing Using nursing knowledge and experience to determine which patient needs are most important and what care will be given at a particular time.

Restatement Repeats the patient's words.

Subjective Data The information collected during an interview or conversation from listening to the experiences of the patient or a family member.

Synthesis Combining assessment data, nursing knowledge, and clinical experience to determine the provision of care.

Taxonomy A codified way of categorizing and classifying information.

Verbal Communication Includes what is said and the tone and rhythm of a person's voice.

Overview of the Nursing Process

If you were the nursing student caring for Amarina, you may have felt overwhelmed by the complexity of her situation, or you may have been afraid you did not have enough knowledge or experience to provide her with excellent care. A nurse would provide comprehensive care for Amarina's complex health needs using the **nursing process**, a systematic and rational method of planning and providing patient care organized around a series of phases that facilitates evidence-informed, and ethical practice (Huckabay, 2009).

In this chapter, you will explore how nurses use the nursing process along with evidence-informed practice and excellent problem-solving skills to provide safe, competent, ethical, and holistic patient care through nursing interventions. The nursing process assists nurses to provide quality care by applying a systematic process that fosters critical thinking and optimizes patient care outcomes (Table 10.1).

Five Phases of the Nursing Process

This chapter discusses the five basic steps of the nursing process: assessment, nursing diagnosis, planning, implementation, and evaluation (Fig. 10.1).

With practice and experience, it will take progressively less time to collect and interpret data, identify significant clinical changes, and provide appropriate interventions (Fig. 10.2A).

The nurse will also be able to provide a comprehensive evaluation of patient outcomes, drawing conclusions about the status of the problem and whether patient care can be ended or additional care needs to be provided. As part of ongoing professional accountability, the nurse evaluates the quality of patient care.

The Nurse's Experience

In addition, nurses use the nursing process to provide multiple aspects of care simultaneously. Figure 10.2B illustrates how additional aspects of care can be identified throughout the nursing process.

It is nurses' breadth and depth of experience, including critical reasoning and problem-solving skills, that enables them to apply the nursing process seemingly without effort and all at once. Some nurses may refer to this rapid decision-making as *intuition*; however, there is clinical evidence to support their knowledge and clinical reasoning. This complex and holistic process ensures that comprehensive patient and family care is provided wherever nursing is practiced.

Assessment

As a nurse, you will use knowledge and your assessment skills to gather information or data from multiple sources. The goal is to gather sufficient information that results in a comprehensive understanding of the patient's situation. **Assessment** is the phase of the nursing process where we collect, organize, validate, and document data.

Assessment is the first step, the beginning of providing patient-centered care, and entails gathering data and compiling a health history through patient interviews, a physical examination, and analysis of diagnostic and laboratory results as well as other sources of data such as health records and research. Providing patient-centered care requires collaboration among the patient, the family, and other members of the health-care team to explore the determinants of health as they relate to the patient (Box 10.1). Collecting data from multiple sources provides a holistic perspective of the patient's past and current health status and may identify factors that could influence the patient's health trajectory.

Assessment is an ongoing process that nurses use every time they interact with a patient. There are four types of assessments, which are primarily based on the context of the patient's needs. An initial assessment is completed most often when the nurse meets the patient for the first time. The nurse explores the presenting problem as well as contributing factors and could include a physical assessment, a health history, and psychosocial assessments. A focused assessment gathers specific details about the presenting concern. This could include assessments that are specific to one aspect of health, such as the mental status exam, and diagnostic tests

TABLE 10.1	The Nursing Process in Action		
Component	**Description**	**Activities**	**Purpose**
Assessment	Collect data Organize data Validate data Document data	Establish database • Consult with patient to obtain health history • Conduct a physical assessment • Review patient medical records • Review relevant literature • Consultations with support persons • Consultations with health-care professionals Update data Communicate data	Establishing a database of information about the patient's response to health concerns or illness and his or her ability to manage his or her health-care needs
Diagnosing	Analyze data Identify health problems, risks, and strengths Formulate diagnostic statements	Interpret and analyze data • Cluster or group data • Identify gaps in information • Identify inconsistencies Determine patient strengths Identify patient risks and problems Formulate nursing diagnoses and collaborative problem statements Document nursing diagnoses on the nursing care plan	Identifying patient strengths and any health problems that could be prevented or resolved by collaborative care and by independent nursing interventions
Planning	Prioritize problems and diagnoses Formulate goals and design health outcomes Select nursing interventions Write nursing interventions	Set goals and priorities or health outcomes in collaboration with the patient Collaborate with the patient to set goals and priorities/health outcomes Write a clear statement of goals/desired outcomes Consult with other health-care professionals Select dependent, independent, and collaborative interventions to achieve the stated goals. Consider the consequences of each nursing strategy and intervention Write nursing orders Write nursing care plan Communicate nursing care plan to other relevant health-care providers	Develop an individualized nursing care plan that specifies patient goals and the desired health outcomes, along with related nursing interventions
Implementing	Reassess patient Determine the nurse's need to assist Implement nursing interventions Supervise delegated care Document nursing activities	Reassess the patient to update the database of information Does the intervention require additional nursing support? Would assistance reduce stress on the patient? Does the nurse lack the knowledge or skills needed? Perform planned nursing interventions or Delegate planned nursing interventions Match the needs of the patient with caregivers who have the appropriate knowledge and skills Communicate the nursing actions that were implemented Document care Document patient responses to care Provide a verbal report if needed	Assist the patient in meeting the desired goals and health outcomes Promote wellness Prevent illness and disease Restore health Facilitate coping with altered functioning
Evaluations	Collect data related to outcomes Relate nursing actions to patient goals, outcomes Draw conclusions about problem status Continue, modify, or terminate the patient's care plan	Collaborate with patient in data collection Collect data related to the desired health outcomes Document achievement/success of health outcomes as well as any modification of the care plan Judge whether the goals/outcomes have been achieved How did nursing actions impact the outcomes? Was the care plan effective? Determine what additional plans of action might be required, if any Drawing from data, review and modify the care plan as determined or terminate nursing care	Determining whether to continue, modify, or terminate the plan of care

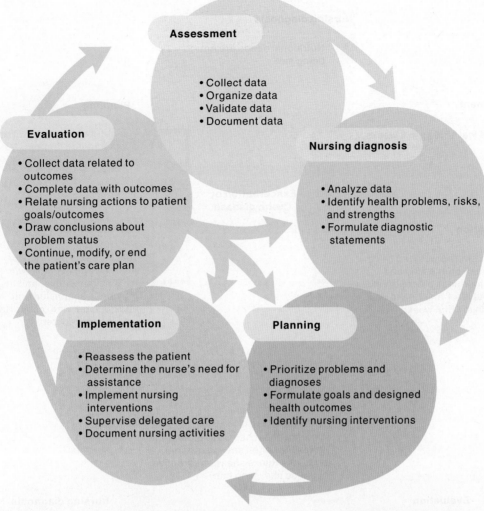

Assessment

- Collect data
- Organize data
- Validate data
- Document data

Evaluation

- Collect data related to outcomes
- Complete data with outcomes
- Relate nursing actions to patient goals/outcomes
- Draw conclusions about problem status
- Continue, modify, or end the patient's care plan

Nursing diagnosis

- Analyze data
- Identify health problems, risks, and strengths
- Formulate diagnostic statements

Implementation

- Reassess the patient
- Determine the nurse's need for assistance
- Implement nursing interventions
- Supervise delegated care
- Document nursing activities

Planning

- Prioritize problems and diagnoses
- Formulate goals and designed health outcomes
- Identify nursing interventions

Figure 10.1 The clockwise arrow indicates how the nursing process is typically used to provide patient care. While not depicted, counterclockwise arrows are "at play" and help us to understand how information acquired in one step of the nursing process informs the previous step. Note that evaluation relates to nursing diagnosis, planning, and implementation.

to either confirm or rule out abnormalities. After an initial assessment has been completed and treatment has been implemented, it may be necessary for the nurse to reevaluate the patient's status and identify whether the condition has improved, worsened, or stayed the same. This is called a *time-lapsed assessment* and may include all the previous methods of assessment. Lastly, in a trauma situation, the nurse would perform an emergency assessment. The purpose of this assessment is to ensure the patient has a patent airway, is breathing, and has adequate circulation and to identify the primary cause of the problem.

As a student nurse, determining what information you need, who to involve, and how best to gather data can be challenging. Some other questions you might ask yourself are as follows: What knowledge do I require to complete a thorough assessment? Would information from someone other than the patient or other sources enhance my assessment?

Throughout your undergraduate nursing education, you will learn about interpersonal relationships, therapeutic communication, principles of teaching and learning, diverse populations, pharmacology, physiology, pathology, and anatomy. As a student, you will learn what is considered normal pathology, physiology, normal laboratory results, and appropriate treatments for diseases and conditions. You will also learn how the determinants of health can positively or negatively affect the health status of your patient. The assessment step in the nursing process requires you to be knowledgeable in all of these areas.

Types of Data

Nurses collect two types of data: subjective and objective. **Subjective data** is the information you collect during an interview or conversation when you are listening to the

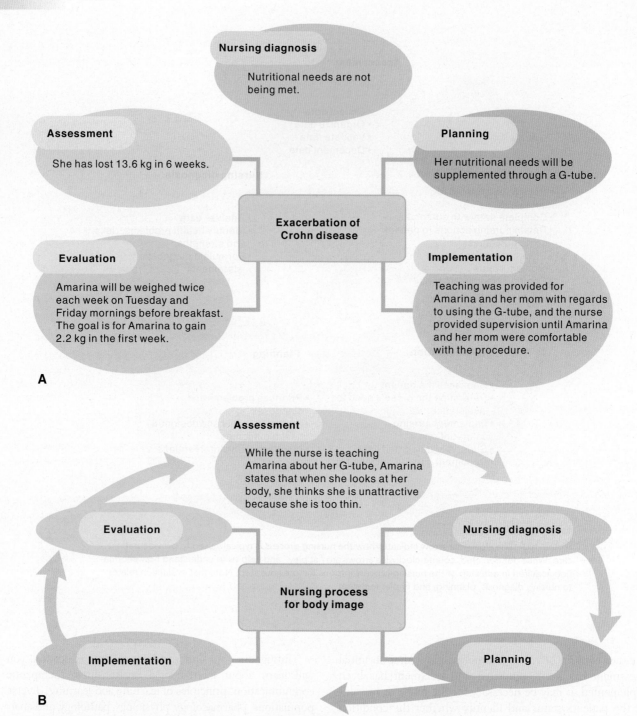

A

B

Figure 10.2 **A.** The patient in the initial case study experienced significant weight loss as a result of having Crohn disease. While learning how to supplement her nutrition through the G-tube, Amarina tells the nurse that she finds it hard to care for her G-tube because she feels too thin. This is new assessment data. **B.** The nursing process could be used to identify a nursing diagnosis, a plan, an intervention, and a means to evaluate a new set of outcomes. In addition, the outcomes of this nursing diagnosis will impact the nutritional plan, and the nurse may need to change the nursing diagnosis, plan, intervention, or evaluation to meet the new needs of the patient.

BOX 10.1 Determinants of Health

Income
Employment security
Environmental conditions
Education
Security
Supports
Housing
Food

Source: Public Health Agency of Canada. (2011). *Determinants of health*. Retrieved from http://www.phac-aspc.gc.ca/index-eng.php

experiences of your patient or family member. Examples include your patient's rating of pain, how often a particular symptom reportedly occurs, the patient's perspective of the impact of the illness, and a family member's comments about how well the patient is managing his or her treatment plan. **Objective data** is the information about the patient that you collect from examining the patient and from the patient's chart and medical records. This data is measurable and evaluated against a standard, which is considered the norm. Some examples include the results of a physical assessment, lab values, and diagnostic tests. Both subjective and objective types of data are essential when you explore the patient's concerns to ensure that your assessment data is comprehensive and holistic and reflects the reality of the patient's situation.

Sources of Data

The most common sources of data include the patient, his or her significant others, members of the interprofessional team, medical records, research, and literature. Some types of information are readily accessible, whereas others require permission from the patient or guardian before being collected or disclosed (Government of Alberta, 2012). Sometimes, an individual's health information is stored electronically and can be accessed by health-care providers quickly from various locations. This access may exist in some Canadian provinces where health-care services are controlled by a central governing authority (Government of Alberta, 2011). For each source, it is important to consider whether your request is relevant to the care you are providing and, if necessary, whether you have obtained proper consent. Collecting information from various sources will help you to identify areas where the data and the patient's response to care are congruent and where there are discrepancies that require further exploration. It is also essential to understand that data are not static but constantly changing. To monitor health status, the most recent data you have collected should be compared to baseline or previously collected data if it is available. For example, often, a difference in vital signs over time can signal a change in the patient's condition. You may also be able to identify patterns in the continuum of health and illness

for your patient. Perhaps your patient has had pneumonia during autumn for the past 2 years, or a 3-year-old has had two exacerbations of his asthma since the family bought a cat. Making these connections will help you to develop and deliver appropriate patient care.

Ways to Collect Data

There are four common ways that nurses collect patient data. They may conduct an interview, complete forms, perform an assessment, or review the patient's diagnostic and laboratory results. The methods you use depend on the purpose for collecting the information, the setting, and the acuity of the patient's illness. It is not uncommon for nurses to combine several methods when collecting data.

The Assessment Interview

To provide patient-centered care, it is essential to talk with the patient about his or her illness and current concerns. Patients can often provide the best details about their own health and illness experience. This information includes personal views of signs and symptoms, past medical history, ability to complete daily activities, lifestyle, relationships, desired outcomes, and willingness to participate in the treatment plan.

Establishing a respectful relationship with the patient entails coming to know the patient; what is at stake for him or her; and how the determinants of health affect the patient's health, well-being, and healing process (Public Health Agency of Canada, 2011). Creating this informed relationship will enable you to provide the best care possible that meets the unique needs of each individual patient and gives you a foundation for future advocacy.

The Interview

Most interviews begin with some predetermined questions and allow the interviewer to ask additional questions that are more specific to the patient's circumstances. Interviews provide an opportunity for the nurse and patient to exchange information and form a therapeutic relationship. They are usually done face-to-face but may occur over the phone in some settings. Nurses may have several predetermined questions based on the patient's diagnosis and general treatment options, and the order or nature of these may change in response to the patient's answers or behaviour. This type of assessment is ongoing, and the data can be collected or verified each time you interact with the patient. It is important to remember that every encounter provides an opportunity to assess your patient's condition in multiple dimensions. For example, you can assess your patient's cognitive status while interacting during morning care, assess the patient's skin while providing a bed bath, evaluate the patient's gait while ambulating, and gauge emotional responses to topics you are discussing. Developing a therapeutic relationship will help you to gather assessment data in a timely manner and encourage the patient to report changes in his or her health status as they become apparent. The expert nurse will use this data in conjunction with his or her own assessment findings to decide whether the plan of care needs to be changed.

To successfully develop a therapeutic relationship with your patient, you need to be respectful and trustworthy and use good nursing judgment. As a student nurse, you can be respectful by closing the patient's curtains when providing personal care, and you can develop trust by keeping your promises, such as returning to assess the effectiveness of a medication. Good nursing judgment occurs when the nurse is able to make decisions using his or her nursing knowledge and experience in conjunction with what he or she knows about the patient. For example, a nurse employed at a local drop-in centre works with patients who have addictions. She is aware of the harmful effects of using cocaine. Her patient is unable to stop using because of his physiological dependence, insecurity, and fear that he may no longer fit in with his peer group. In this scenario, the nurse may demonstrate good judgment by using a harm reduction approach based on respect for the patient and his right to make unhealthy choices. As a result of the trust developed in the therapeutic relationship, the nurse may be able to gradually engage the patient in behaviours that promote a healthier lifestyle (Sleeper & Thompson, 2008).

Throughout the patient interview, the nurse observes and uses both verbal and nonverbal communication. **Nonverbal communication** includes a person's facial expressions, gestures, posture, and attentiveness. **Verbal communication** includes what is said and the tone and rhythm of the person's voice. The interview may begin with **open-ended questions** that are used to elicit a broad range of detail. These types of questions encourage patients to provide additional information about their situation and can be very helpful if your patient is not easily engaged in conversation. In contrast, **closed-ended questions** are more specific and are used to limit the scope of the response or to focus on a specific area of interest, such as, "Do you have this pain every night?" Closed-ended questions are effective if you have a limited amount of time to gather information or if your patient is overinclusive. Other types of questions include **leading questions**, which suggest a direction for the conversation, and **neutral questions**, which provide an opportunity for the patient to respond according to his or her own perceptions.

Examples of other strategies that nurses use to gather and validate the accuracy of their data are restatement, paraphrasing, and clarification. **Restatement** simply repeats the patient's words, as when he says, "I am so lonely," and you reply, "You are lonely." **Paraphrasing** interprets the patient's words, such as, "You sound discouraged." **Clarification** seeks a bit more information to confirm your understanding, such as, "What is that sensation like?" Each of these techniques will elicit more information from the patient that will make your care more effective. These are just a few of the communication skills that you will learn in your nursing

program. Therapeutic communication skills are used to build rapport, gather information, teach, and counsel (Sleeper & Thompson, 2008). These skills include body posture, tone of voice, and ways of interacting. Being attentive to the patient helps the nurse use appropriate communication skills to build trust and demonstrate a caring attitude. The patient may feel more confident about the care received when the nurse is knowledgeable and able to communicate in a respectful and meaningful way.

Assessment Tools

Genograms and ecomaps are examples of a holistic approach to gather information about how the patient's relationships and lifestyle are connected to the patient's current situation. A **genogram** is a pictorial representation of the patient's family and health patterns (Fig. 10.3). The **ecomap** identifies various attachments the patient may have, such as relationships, school or employment, and recreation activities (Fig. 10.4). The ecomap also depicts how the patient values these attachments (Wright & Leahey, 2009). The scope of the initial nurse–patient conversation may be limited by various factors such as the location of the discussion, the acuity of the patient's condition, or whether the patient has been medicated. For example, a patient may seem hesitant sharing personal information if there is a roommate present or may be unable to converse if medicated by a paramedic prior to arriving at the hospital.

Examinations

Nurses conduct a physical and/or mental health examination to gather more information about areas of concern. For example, if the patient has abdominal pain not yet diagnosed (NYD), the nurse would use her physical assessment skills to gather the information required to make the diagnosis. This examination may include taking vital signs and a head-to-toe assessment. The nurse would use skills such as observation, auscultation, palpation, and percussion. Additional examinations may be required to evaluate a patient's report of pain or

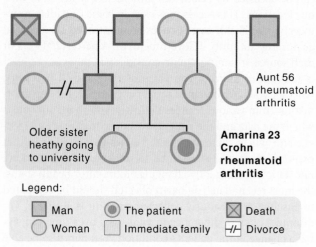

Figure 10.3 Amarina's family genogram.

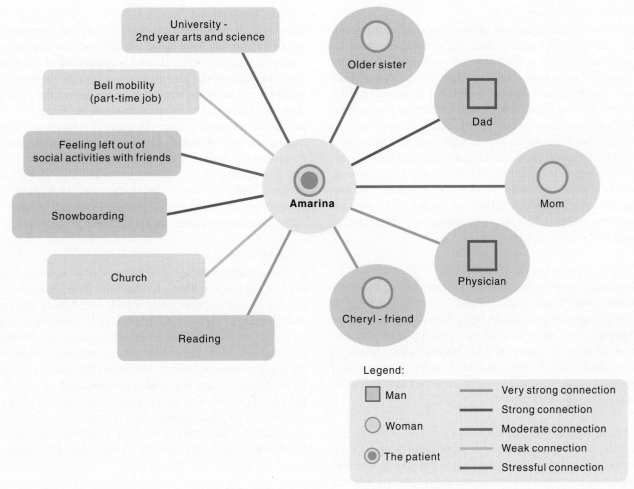

Figure 10.4 Amarina's ecomap.

to gather additional information about specific concerns. If the patient has a head injury, the nurse would perform a neurological assessment such as measuring the patient's level of consciousness, pupil reactions, motor responses, and reaction to painful stimuli (Gill, Windemuth, Steele, & Green, 2005). Some examinations are used to measure changes in functioning over time. For instance, the Mini-Mental State Exam is used routinely in the geriatric population to evaluate their level of cognitive functioning (Folstein, Folstein, & McHugh, 1975). Other examples include pain evaluation scales, fall risk evaluations, the Glasgow Coma Scale, and postnatal depression scales. Sometimes, nurses rely on more specific examination results of other professionals, such as psychologists, to inform their nursing assessments because the special examination is outside the nurse's scope of practice and knowledge.

A nurse's observational skills are important and can validate other findings, highlight discrepancies, and provide more information about the patient, such as coping abilities. During an examination, a nurse will observe for changes in the patient's behaviour, how he or she responds to touch (auscultation, percussion), and any notable smells. Box 10.2 lists additional details a nurse may notice.

BOX 10.2 Additional Nursing Observations

Sight

The colour of the patient's skin, urine, feces, and wound exudate

The presence of abnormal movements, tremors, difficulty initiating or terminating movement, unstable gait

The patient's level of consciousness

If ambulatory aids are required

The patient's response to touch (guarding, grimacing)

Smell

For example, the unique smells that are associated with infection, *Clostridium difficile*, or a gastrointestinal (GI) bleed

Touch

Noticeable changes in temperature and fluid volume (edematous, diaphoretic, etc.)

Sound

For example, those related to pain (groaning, moaning, crying), absent bowel sounds, abnormal lung sounds (crackles, wheezes, rubs)

Standardized Forms

Intake forms, checklists, and various other assessment forms are used to collect patient data. Some forms are used for specific tasks, such as the preoperative checklist. This form ensures the appropriate diagnostic and laboratory tests have been completed and that the patient has been prepared for surgery. This important information is collected for the operative team to ensure the safety of the patient during the operation. Other forms are more comprehensive. For example, a completed health history can include demographic information, the reason for seeking health care, patient expectations, present illness, past health history, family history, environmental and psychosocial history, spirituality, and a physical assessment. Figure 10.5 shows an example of a form used to complete a health history.

Diagnostic and Laboratory Results

Test results can provide valuable information about a patient's health status. Results may be within the standard range or may deviate from standard findings. Both types of results are important. For example, a patient with lupus may experience persistent symptoms and his lab results may be within the normal range. A physician usually orders diagnostic and laboratory tests; however, nurse practitioners may also order certain tests for their patients.

Interviewing Significant Others

Nurses collect information from significant others (family, partners, friends, and guardians) when the patient is unable to provide it or when the patient has given consent for others to be included in his or her care. Similarly, the nurse would also collect information from others if the patient is not old enough to give legal consent or if the patient is deemed mentally incompetent. The nurse might collect information such as symptoms, progress or trajectory of the disease or condition, allergies, current medications, and a health history from significant others instead of the patient. The nurse might also inquire about perceptions of how the patient is managing his situation, about previous patient experiences or responses to a disease or condition, the impact this disease or condition has had on the patient's daily life, and what has changed as a result. This secondhand information is important because often, significant others will notice functional changes in the patient before the patient becomes aware of them.

Interprofessional Team as a Source of Information

Patient care typically involves many disciplines at one time. As a result, it is important for nurses to include data from other team members such as physicians, social workers, licensed practical nurses, and spiritual care workers. Communicating with the team members involved in the patient's care is essential to the provision of consistent care. The interprofessional team often shares information and reviews the overall plan of care in meetings known as *case conferences*. In some settings, patients are invited to attend and participate in this discussion.

Clinical Records

Knowledge of the patient's past health history and corresponding treatments can help identify health and illness patterns, successful interventions, and new information, all of which are needed to address the patient's current concern. Nurses often begin by reviewing the admission assessment or the nursing database. This provides information about the events that led to the patient seeking care; the patient's perceptions, fears, and hopes; and the nurse's initial assessment and diagnosis. Reviewing the medical history gives the nurse a larger context and an overview of the patient's previous health and illness patterns. Preferably prior to providing care, other important areas to review are test results, treatments (including medications), and the most recent interprofessional progress notes.

Literature Review

It is important for nurses to be aware of new research affecting nursing practice. Being familiar with recent literature in nursing as well as other subjects such as infectious disease, pharmacology, and nonpharmacological treatments will help you maintain a current knowledge base and provide care that is supported by best practice standards. Some of the ways nurses stay current are to read the updates an employer provides regarding new equipment, medications, and policies. They can also attend in-services, workshops, and conferences or join a journal club. A nurse's licencing body also provides information on best practices, registration requirements, and opportunities for specialty certifications.

Documentation

Nurses are often the health-care providers who assimilate patient care data and convey this information to other team members involved in the patient's care. As a result, the nurse must be able to differentiate between significant and nonsignificant data. This skill can be difficult for novices because you are just learning what is considered a standard range for a particular assessment or test, or when the negative results are important to document. As a student, to ensure that safe patient care is provided, you also need to communicate your findings to your buddy (mentor) registered nurse and your instructor. For example, if your patient has chest pain, you immediately report your findings to both the registered nurse who is responsible for the patient and to your instructor and then document your assessment data. Your data may result in further assessment and interventions in response to this aspect of the patient's condition. When assessing your patient later, you may notice a change in your patient's vital signs, yet the data remains within what is considered a normal range. This information along with any other changes in your assessment data are all communicated to both your buddy registered nurse and your instructor.

There are many ways that assessment data can be recorded. How and where it is recorded will vary depending on the type of information and who has access to it. Most of the data nurses collect will be shared with one or

General Hospital

☐ FMC
☐ PLC
☐ RGH
☐ Other _____

HRN:

Name:

PHN: Gender:

Address:

CTAS CATEGORY	EMERGENCY ASSESSMENT and TREATMENT RECORD

Phone (H):

TRIAGE	Admission Date:		Time:		

Old chart Called	Mode of Arrival EMS	☐ Walk ☐ Carried ☐ W/G ☐ EMS	Triage	Location	Bed

PRESENTING COMPLAINT

VS   **SIGNATURE**

TIME: **INITIAL HISTORY AND PHYSICAL ASSESSMENT**

PAST MEDICAL HISTORY

PRESENT MEDICATIONS   **ALLERGIES & REACTIONS**

TEMP	PULSE		RESP	BLOOD PRESSURE		O₂ SAT	BLOOD SUGAR	WEIGHT	Last Tetanus	VISUAL ACUITY	
	Lying	Stand/Sit		Lying	Stand/Sit					Right	Left
						RA/O₂@ _____ L					

RESP
☐ N/P

AIRWAY
☐ Patent
☐ Obstructed
☐ Intubated
E.T.T. Size ____

RESPIRATORY
☐ Regular
☐ Shallow
☐ Laboured
☐ Indrawing

BREATH SOUNDS

CVS
☐ N/P

PULSE
☐ Regular
☐ Irregular
Capillary refill:
____ sec

SKIN COLOUR
☐ Pink
☐ Pale
☐ Mottled
☐ Other

SKIN QUALITY
☐ Warm   ☐ Dry
☐ Cool   ☐ Diaphoretic
☐ Hot
☐ Edema

Monitor ☐ No ☐ Yes – Rhythm _____ Pulses: _____

CNS
☐ N/P

EYES OPEN
4 Spontaneously   2 To Pain
3 To Speech   1 None
PUPILS
lt. Size ____ Reaction ____
rt. Size ____ Reaction ____

BEST MOTOR RESPONSE
6 Obeys Commands/Normal Movement
5 Localizes Pain/Withdraws To Touch
4 Withdraws To Pain
3 Flexion To Pain/Abnormal Flexion
2 Extension To Pain/Abnormal Extension
1 None

BEST VERBAL RESPONSE
5 Orientated/Coos, Babbles
4 Confused/Irritable Cry
3 Inappropriate Words/ Cries To Pain
2 Incomprehensible Sounds/Moans To Pain
1 None

GCS

1 2 3 4 5 6 7 8
(R) - Reacting
(S) - Sluggish
(F) - Fixed
(U) - Untestable

Motor Power _____
Sensation _____

BEHAVIOUR ☐ Co-operative ☐ Unco-operative ☐ Restless ☐ Combative ☐ Crying ☐ Agitated ☐ Non-communicative

GI
☐ N/P

ABDOMEN
☐ Soft   ☐ Rigid
☐ Distended   Last BM _____

GU/GYN
☐ N/P

URINARY ☐ Frequency ☐ Urgency ☐ Dysuria
☐ Hematuria ☐ Retention ☐ Incontinence
Bleeding ☐ No ☐ Yes Duration _____ Amount _____
LMNP _____ Gravida _____ Para _____ FHR _____ ☐ Discharge _____

MSK
☐ N/P

Color Sensation Movement Pulses Temperature Swelling Deformity Pain

INTEG
☐ N/P
EENT
☐ N/P

SIGNATURE   **INITIAL**

We routinely ask all patients about domestic abuse/violence in their lives. Is this a problem for you or your child(ren)?   Yes ☐ No ☐
Do you feel safe right now?   Yes ☐ No ☐ Other ☐ _____   Initial: _____

101070 R(2005/02)   **Legend**   N/P = not pertinent   CTAS = Canadian Triage & Acuity Scale

Figure 10.5 Health history form.

DIAGNOSTIC TESTS

Time _____
Drawn by _____

- [ ] CBC
- [ ] Electrolytes
- [ ] Glucose
- [ ] Creatinine
- [ ] Lipase
- [ ] CK/CKMB
- [ ] PTT/INR
- [ ] Blood Culture #1
- [ ] Blood Culture #2
- [ ] Type & Screen
- [ ] X-Match _____units
- [ ] ECG @ _____ @ _____

- [ ] ETOH
- [ ] ASA/ACETAMINO
- [ ] _____
- [ ] _____
- [ ] _____
- [ ] _____
- [ ] _____
- [ ] Extra tubes drawn

URINE DIP

@ _____
SG _____
pH _____
Leukocytes _____
Nitrate _____
Protein _____
Glucose _____
Ketone _____
Urobilinogen _____
Bilirubin _____
Blood _____
Pregnancy _____
R&M @ _____
C&S @ _____

Next of Kin Notified [ ] Yes [ ] No | Relationship/Contact Information

Site **A** Needle Size & Site	Initials					Site **B** Needle Size & Site	Initials				
Time	Bag #	Volume	Solution, Additives, & Rate	Init.	Abs.	Time	Bag #	Volume	Solution, Additives, & Rate	Init.	Abs.
				TOTAL						TOTAL	

Site **C** Needle Size & Site	Initials					OUTPUT			
Time	Bag #	Volume	Solution, Additives, & Rate	Init.	Abs.	Time	Urine (ml)	Other	Total (ml)
				TOTAL			TOTAL		

[ ] Refer to Neurological Observation Record

Time	T	P	R	BP	O₂ SAT	Medications	Continuing Assessments and Interventions
						[ ] Refer to Supplemental Care Record

DISPOSITION/DISCHARGE Time _____

Initials _____ | [ ] Teaching Sheet | Initials _____

TRANSFER INFORMATION

Report to (RN Name) _____ | Given by (RN Name) _____

		SIGNATURE	INITIAL	SIGNATURE	INITIAL
Report Time	Transfer				
	To _____ @ _____ hrs				
	UNIT TIME				

Figure 10.5 (continued)

more members of an interprofessional team, and therefore, it needs to be in a format that can easily be understood by all team members. Examples of this type of documentation include interprofessional progress notes, conference sheets, and care plans. The appearance and structure of these documents varies significantly between health-care agencies.

Organizing Data

The challenge for nursing students is putting all the pieces of data together to determine what is happening for that patient. It is similar to assembling pieces of a jigsaw puzzle to create a picture (Fig. 10.6). With increased knowledge and experience, you will be able to integrate all aspects of assessment with your nursing knowledge and clinical experience and your critical thinking and problem-solving skills to provide comprehensive and personalized patient care.

Nursing judgment refers to the process that nurses use to critically evaluate and interpret patient data and then make informed decisions about their patient's care (Levett-Jones et al., 2010). Understanding how your assessment data informs your nursing practice is similar to a three-dimensional picture. Your patient's situation could be seen as having three components: the parts of the problem and the interventions that are readily seen and are an immediate priority; the supporting data that is closely connected to the presenting concern, a secondary priority; and the issues that have an impact on the trajectory of the illness but are lower priority. Initially, a student nurse may only see the obvious aspects of the patient's situation such as a saturated dressing, an infected wound, or an increased temperature. However, there are underlying details affecting the patient's situation that are not as obvious; for example, the patient has a virus, he fell 2 weeks ago and has been less mobile, or aseptic technique was not used for the complex dressing change. There is a third layer of details that may not influence the immediate patient care provided but will have an impact on the long-term trajectory of the patient's well-being.

Through the eyes of a student

I was in my third year of nursing school, and I was caring for Mrs. Shea, who was diagnosed with chronic obstructive pulmonary disease (COPD) and retained carbon dioxide. She was supposed to be on 2 L of oxygen via nasal prongs at all times, but she consistently turned her portable oxygen up to 5 L, stating, "I need my oxygen to breathe." Throughout the day, I tried to teach her about her diagnosis and the danger of consistently increasing her oxygen to 5 L, but she kept saying her doctor knew best. I charted my interaction with Mrs. Shea, and then I left a note for her physician requesting that he write down how much oxygen Mrs. Shea should have on an official progress note that could be placed in her room.
(personal reflection of Lourdes, a 3rd year nursing student)

Through the eyes of a patient

*T*he nursing student wanted me to turn down my oxygen. She said having it too high was dangerous, but I know what I need to breathe. When my doctor came, she said I should not have my oxygen higher than 2 L because breathing in more oxygen means I will retain more carbon dioxide and eventually oxygen won't even help me breathe. She wrote it on the doctor's note paper and left it with me. I'm going to show the note to the nursing student when she comes tomorrow and let her know that her patient care was good.
(personal reflection of Mrs. Shea, Patient)

As you identify the links between the data you have collected and how these relate to the specifics of your patient's situation, you will determine which components of care are most pressing and need to be in the foreground. In Mrs. Shea's

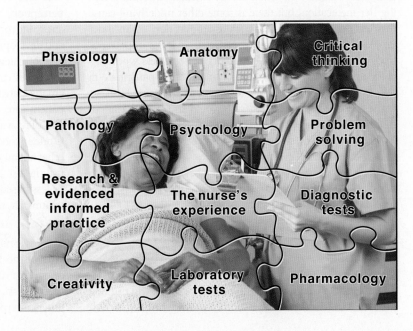

Figure 10.6 Like the pieces of a puzzle fit together, so does the data the nurse acquires through assessment, and when one piece or component is missing, the data is incomplete. If this happens, the nurse may be missing important details that contribute to the patient's care and his or her health may be jeopardized.

situation, it was important to consider how her beliefs about the roles of health-care providers influenced her participation in her care and the long-term effects on her health. The details that directly inform the priorities are part of the first and second layers of care. The details that may be important to other aspects of care such as discharge and follow-up care are of lesser immediate concern and thus are lower priorities. An experienced nurse will understand the clinical significance of the assessment data and be able to quickly **interpret** how this relates to the big picture, using his or her nursing knowledge, critical thinking, and problem-solving skills to make informed clinical decisions regarding patient care (Lunney, 2008). A nurse is constantly adapting and **prioritizing** in response to the changing health status of the patient, interpreting data, and identifying priority needs and nursing actions.

For example, Amarina is at a follow-up appointment with her gastrointestinal specialist. As the nurse, you do the preliminary assessment and notice that Amarina is pale, lethargic, and has lost a significant amount of weight. Her temperature is 37.5°C, her blood pressure is 100/60 mmHg, and her pulse is 70 beats/min. You also notice that she is withdrawn and does not maintain eye contact when she states that she needs to empty her ostomy appliance, within 15 minutes, after every time she eats. All of this data informs your immediate perception that Amarina's health status has deteriorated. As her nurse, you would inquire about the next layer of detail to better understand what additional factors are contributing to your patient that would help you provide safe and comprehensive patient care. In the case of Amarina, you would explore her nutritional intake (type and quantity) and review her medication regime, including the type of medication, the dose, the route, the time she takes it, the effectiveness, and any side effects that she may be experiencing. As you begin to identify the links between your assessment data, you may recognize that Amarina's weight loss is a result of diet that exacerbates the symptoms of Crohn disease, or she may not be adhering to the prescribed medication because the side effects are intolerable. Another possibility could be that Amarina has a healthy diet and is taking her medication, but there is some other underlying cause that has not been identified, such as an infection, so an order for blood work might be necessary. Details of lesser importance that would contribute to the trajectory of her illness would include an exploration of Amarina's motivation to participate in self-care and investment in the treatment plan because it relates to the need for additional surgery. It would also be important to discuss self-esteem with Amarina and provide nursing support for her mother. If these less immediate needs were not included in the patient care plan, Amarina's relationship with her mother may become less supportive, decreasing her ability to cope with her illness, and she may participate less in the treatment plan, resulting in future exacerbations of her Crohn disease.

Diagnosis

Formulating a **diagnosis** is the second phase of the nursing process and involves analyzing the data, identifying health problems and risks as well as strengths, and formulating diagnostic statements.

Identifying a diagnosis is not unique to the discipline of nursing. All members of the interprofessional team have a process for gathering information and formulating a diagnosis. A medical diagnosis relates primarily to the disease process, pathology, or condition and has implications for medical treatment. It tends to remain static during an episode of illness. A **nursing diagnosis** is a clinical judgment that describes the patient's response to actual and potential health problems (North American Nursing Diagnosis Association [NANDA] International, 2010), perhaps including more than one nursing diagnosis. This statement of nursing judgment refers to conditions that nurses are licensed to treat and will change over the course of the illness as patient responses change. To determine the nursing diagnosis, a nurse listens to the patient's story, looks for patterns in the data, and considers how these relate to the big picture.

There are four North American Nursing Diagnosis Association (NANDA) categories of nursing diagnoses: an actual diagnosis; a diagnosis based on potential risk; a wellness diagnosis; and a syndrome diagnosis, which describes a cluster of nursing diagnoses that are best understood together. A patient may have more than one type of nursing diagnosis. To write a standard nursing diagnosis, the nurse would choose a nursing diagnosis from the NANDA categories, select the type of diagnosis, identify the etiology (the probable stimulus for the patient response), and list the defining characteristics from the patient assessment data.

For example, a nurse is caring for a 14-year-old boy who is receiving chemotherapy and radiation for Hodgkin lymphoma (cancer of the lymph tissue). The nurse would talk with the patient and his family about how the treatment may alter his fertility and how this may affect future plans for fathering children. A holistic approach may result in more than one nursing diagnosis.

The NANDA International (2010) has grouped nursing diagnoses into 13 categories that reflect the topics of a holistic assessment. They are health promotion, nutrition, elimination and exchange, activity/rest, perception/cognition, self-perception, role relationships, sexuality, coping/stress tolerance, life principles, safety/protection, comfort, and growth and development (Table 10.2). Having a **taxonomy** (a codified way of categorizing and classifying information) for nursing diagnoses can be helpful to create a common understanding among patient care providers and enhance the continuity of patient care. Common diagnoses can also facilitate the collection of relevant data and consistency in how the treatment plan is understood and carried out by nurses and communicated to other members of the health-care team. Potentially, if nurses use the same terminology and definitions, then there would be less miscommunication about diagnoses and corresponding treatments, resulting in safer, more consistent patient care.

Limitations of Nursing Diagnoses

One of the limitations of using a standardized nursing taxonomy for diagnoses is that these are not widely used outside the professional practice of nurses, leading to confusion for other interprofessional team members about terminology

TABLE 10.2	North American Nursing Diagnosis Association Categories of Nursing Diagnoses for Holistic Assessment
Health promotion	Health awareness
	Health management
Nutrition	Ingestion
	Digestion
	Absorption
	Metabolism
	Hydration
Elimination and exchange	Urinary system
	Gastrointestinal system
	Integumentary system
	Pulmonary system
Activity and rest	Sleep or rest
	Activity or exercise
	Energy balance
	Cardiovascular–pulmonary responses
	Self-care
Perception and cognition	Attention
	Orientation
	Sensation or perception
	Cognition
	Communication
Self-perception	Self-concept
	Self-esteem
	Body image
Role relationships	Caregiving roles
	Family relationships
	Role performance
Sexuality	Sexual identity
	Sexual function
	Reproduction
Coping and stress tolerance	Posttrauma responses
	Coping responses
	Neurobehavioural stress
Life principles	Values
	Beliefs
	Value–belief action congruence
Safety and protection	Infections
	Physical injury
	Violence
	Environmental hazards
	Defensive processes
	Thermoregulation
Comfort	Physical comfort
	Environmental comfort
	Social comfort
Growth and development	Growth
	Development

Source: http://kb.nanda.org/article/AA-00236/37/English-/Frequently-Asked-Questions/Nursing-Diagnosis/Taxonomy/What-is-taxonomy-.html

and interventions. Further, a standardized nursing diagnosis, unless accompanied with specific patient data, cannot address the individuality of the patient who will respond differently to his or her health problem and interventions or account for a wide range of variables such as age, gender, culture, additional health concerns, spiritual beliefs, socioeconomic status, and psychosocial supports (Carrington, 2012).

A lack of consistent communication between health-care providers can lead to misunderstandings and misdiagnoses, which increase the risk to patient safety. A patient's safety can be further compromised if inappropriate interventions are used because assessment data are missed or interpreted incorrectly or a holistic approach to care is not embraced. Consider the surgical nurse who cares for Amarina after her next surgery. If his focus is on postoperative care and wound healing, he would not recognize the potential risk for depression related to a poor self-image. Another limitation is that standardized nursing diagnoses developed in the last decade may not accommodate the continuing expansion of the scope of nursing practice for nurse practitioners or nurses with advanced practice certifications who provide enhanced health services to individuals, groups, and populations.

Other Factors

Nurses are able to identify multiple diagnoses by exploring the relationship between the health problem and the patient's ability to cope in other areas. Changes in a patient's health status may affect his or her functioning in several domains. You may be given your patient assignment and asked to gather pertinent information and data prior to arriving in the clinical area. Although you have this background information, you will need to assess your patient using the nursing process. During this assessment, you learn that your patient may have financial concerns because it costs extra to travel from a rural community to the city for treatment. Or you may learn that the patient has very few support systems, has recently had surgery, and will be discharged with a colostomy or is living in the community but is not confident in administering his or her insulin. It is important to explore other domains of functioning with the patient because these can either facilitate or impede the patient's return to health.

Prioritizing Nursing Diagnoses

How does the nurse prioritize multiple nursing diagnoses? Prioritizing is being able to determine the most critical patient needs and what care will be given at what time (Kaplan & Ura, 2010). The nurse's knowledge, experience, and understanding of the patient and the Canadian Nurses Association's (CNA) Code of Ethics (2008) assist the nurse in prioritizing patient care, a process that occurs at all stages of care. Knowledge of pathology, physiology, pharmacology, and other pertinent information such as policies and procedures will assist you to identify situations where immediate, intermediate, or longer term intervention is required. Whenever possible, the patient should also be included in the discussion and planning of his or her care (Table 10.3).

Through the eyes of a student

I was in my third year of nursing school and working as an undergraduate nurse on a gastrointestinal surgical unit. One of the patients was an obese man with severe fluid retention. He was very diaphoretic as the two RNs and I helped him back to bed and positioned

(continued on page 178)

TABLE 10.3	Ineffective Self-Health Management Related to the Patient's Decreased Confidence to Administer Her Own Insulin	
The Patient's Measurable Action	**The Nurse's Measurable Action**
Immediate The patient will describe process to be used for giving herself insulin.	The nurse will describe the process for self-administering insulin.
Intermediate The patient will demonstrate appropriate self-administration of insulin three times.	The nurse will encourage the patient, reinforce her decision to learn how to self-administer her insulin, and praise her accomplishment.
Long Term The patient will express confidence in being able to self-administer insulin after discharge.	The nurse will ask the patient to describe how she will manage independently at home.

Through the eyes of a student (continued)

him on his side so I could complete his perineal care. I remember thinking he seemed to have lost control of his bowels, and this made it more difficult to ensure his skin was clean. I was almost done when one of the RNs shouted, "Roll him back." I didn't understand why they wanted to do this before I was done washing him up.

(personal reflection of Kate, a nursing student)

Through the eyes of a nurse

When we walked into the patient's room, I noticed the patient's colour was off. He looked a little gray. His legs were extremely edematous and felt cool and moist to touch. The floor was damp underneath his heels. He was weak when we transferred him to his bed, and his breathing was labored. Shortly after we positioned him on his side, his respirations became shallower, and then his eyes rolled back. I knew he was losing consciousness and that he could be having a myocardial infarction. His designated level of care included lifesaving measures. I shouted to the student that we needed to roll him back so we could immediately assess his cardiac status and prepare for CPR.

(personal reflection of Sarah, a nurse)

Planning

Planning is the third stage of the nursing process and includes the steps taken by the patient and family, nurse, and interprofessional team to identify health outcomes, formulate goals, prioritize appropriate nursing interventions, and coordinate necessary resources (Cardwell, Corkin, McCartan, McCullock, & Mullan, 2011). Nurses encourage patients, and if appropriate, their families, to actively participate in the planning process. Planning begins when the nurse first meets the patient and continues until the patient is discharged or care has been transferred.

There are three types of planning. Initial planning is usually part of the admission assessment and identifies what actions are required to move forward in providing patient care. Ongoing planning is continuous and involves adapting patient care in response to new information obtained through assessment and evaluation. Discharge planning anticipates and plans for the patient's needs as he or she transitions between health services as well as independent living. Effective discharge planning begins in the assessment phase when the nurse, based on the data collected, identifies the complexity of the patient's situation and the need for the services of other health professionals.

Prioritizing Patient Data

The planning phase of the nursing process begins with prioritizing the diagnoses (care needs) of the patient. By prioritizing care, the nurse is able to provide the right patient care at the right time. Nurses must use their theoretical and clinical knowledge as well as their experience to understand the factors influencing what care will be provided first. These factors include the acuity of the patient care situation, the patient's wishes, and available resources. Prioritizing also requires an understanding of how various aspects of care are connected. In addition, an experienced nurse will know when the priorities may need to be reordered as a result of a change in his or her patient's status.

For example, the goal of care for Amarina in the opening case study was for her to independently manage her nutritional needs and medication at home. However, Amarina's nurse would recognize that the care plan and goals for this admission would need to be revised as she has lost a significant amount of weight and has recently required assistance to care for her colostomy (Fig. 10.7).

Setting Nursing Priorities

When setting priorities, it is important to consider the nurse's scope of practice, the patient's needs and capabilities, and related professional policies and guidelines. Nurses must practice within the guidelines outlined by their licensing body. These documents identify entry to practice competencies, which describe the skills and attributes that all nurses must demonstrate in their clinical practice. There may be situations when

Date	Nursing Diagnosis	Patient Outcomes	Interventions	Outcome Evaluation (Initials and Date)
5/08/13	Self-care deficit (nutrition) as evidenced by loss of weight in short period of time related to exacerbation of Crohn disease	Aramina will regain the lost weight within 8 weeks. Aramina and her mother will be able to demonstrate administration of a successful tube feed.	Provide nutrition through G-tube for feedings Ensure tube feeds are nutritionally balanced and enhanced to stimulate weight gain Administer tube feeds at regular intervals four times per day Teach and demonstrate process for administering tube feed, including reasons for G-tube and contents of feed Supervise actions by Aramina and her mother Refer to social services for discharge planning and access to required supplies at home	
05/08/13	Risk of impaired skin integrity and infection related to poor nutritional status and presence of G-tube	Aramina will not develop an infection in the G-tube insertion site. Aramina and her mother will demonstrate how to cleanse and monitor the insertion site.	Cleanse and monitor G-tube insertion daily to prevent infection Teach Aramina and her mother how to cleanse and monitor the insertion site by demonstration and supervision.	

REVIEW DATES		
DATE	SIGNATURE	INITIALS
5/15/13	Tanja Holtz	TH, Nursing Student

Figure 10.7 Sample care plan.

advanced competencies or additional skills are required for patient care and an advanced practice nurse or a member of the interprofessional team may be necessary care providers. There are also models that describe what a person needs to survive and attain personal goals, such as Maslow's hierarchy of needs. Maslow grouped the needs of a person into five categories, stating that the needs in one category must be met before a person is able to move on to the next category. The five categories of needs are physiological, safety, love and belonging, esteem, and self-actualization. Although nurses spend considerable time planning care related to the first two categories, care planning could start in any category based on the patient's needs.

Prioritizing patient care is also influenced by the policies and guidelines of the health organization. For example, before Amarina has surgery to remove the rest of her colon, she will need to have the procedure and the risks and benefits explained to her, and she will need to sign a consent form. A patient's care is successfully prioritized when it meets the most pressing needs of the patient at any given time and follows the nurse's legal responsibilities as outlined in the nurse's scope of practice and the health-care system's policies and guidelines.

Synthesizing Information

How well a nurse mobilizes knowledge is essential to identifying relevant patient concerns and prioritizing them appropriately. **Synthesis** is the process of combining assessment data, nursing knowledge, and clinical experience to determine the provision of care. The ability to know the significance of particular information (or data) is not simply a matter of having been in a similar situation; rather, the nurse connects all the theoretical knowledge, moral-ethical reasoning, research, policies and procedures, an understanding of previous outcomes, and the patient's preferences to engage in evidence-informed decision-making and nursing practice (Canadian Nurses Association [CNA], 2010).

For example, in Amarina's situation, the nurse would note that she had lost a significant amount of weight (13.6 kg) in 2 months, has had to supplement her nutrition through a G-tube, and is not independently taking her medication or caring for her colostomy. The nurse may also inquire about Amarina's rheumatoid arthritis and the implications that an inflammatory exacerbation would have on the management of her Crohn disease. The nurse may also explore Amarina's motivation for self-care by asking, "Do you compare yourself to your sister?" This behaviour may discourage her from setting realistic expectations and striving for what her personal best could be. Although the nurse would identify Amarina's nutritional needs as the immediate priority, because all pieces of information are interconnected, the nurse would also address Amarina's psychosocial needs. Without building Amarina's confidence that she is able to set and accomplish life goals, she may remain disengaged from any plan to become well.

Frequently, nurses collaborate with others to plan effective care. The health-care team may include the patient, physician, other health-care providers, and family members. Collaboration provides an opportunity to develop a holistic care plan. In the example of Amarina, she may still need the assistance of her mother in the short term to ensure she is taking her medication, caring for her colostomy, and meeting her nutritional requirements. Her physician or nurse practitioner would be involved in prescribing medication and ordering tests. Other professionals who might also be involved in her care are ostomy nurses, surgeons, social workers, and a psychologist or psychiatrist.

Setting Goals

After the priorities of care have been determined, measurable goals can be established to assist the patient to move toward wellness. The patient, nurse, physician, and other team members may collaboratively participate in goal setting to provide holistic and comprehensive care. Part of goal setting includes outlining the expected outcomes so that progress can be reviewed and evaluated and new goals set. For goals to be successful, there are several factors the nurse must consider. You want to have realistic goals that are mutually agreeable to both the nurse and the patient. SMART is a common acronym that is used to help define the key components of writing clear, achievable goals (Table 10.4). The goals should be specific for your patient's needs, must be stated as patient outcomes or behaviour, and identify how much time is needed for the goal to be completed or reassessed. Outcomes can be expressed as an attitude, acquired knowledge, a demonstration of a skill, or specific physical manifestations, all of which may be observed directly or reported in test results. Goals for patient outcomes must reflect the patient status or activities, not the activity of the nurse. For example, if the desired outcome is for the patient to change her own colostomy bag, the goals will outline the necessary steps the patient must accomplish, rather than the nurse's actions such as providing the dressing supplies, which will not evaluate the patient's knowledge or ability.

The nature of the goal and whether it is short term, intermediate, or long term depends on the complexity of the desired goal, available resources, and, in some situations, the patient's readiness to participate. For example, consider the case of a 15-year-old girl who was recently diagnosed with Type 1 diabetes. She has spent several sessions with the diabetic nurse learning how to properly administer her own insulin but states that she is unable to "poke herself" with a needle. In this situation, the patient is not ready to assume

TABLE 10.4	Characteristics of SMART Goals	
	Successful Goal	Unsuccessful Goal
S The goal is **Specific** to your patient.	Describes the desired patient response or behaviour e.g., The patient will . . .	Describes the activities of the health-care provider e.g., To provide . . .
M The goal is **Measurable**.	Uses concrete and specific language to describe changes in behaviour or progress with respect to the goal. e.g., The wound will be 3 mm smaller in diameter than 7 days ago. He will walk 40 steps in 1 minute (endurance). She will swim 200 m three times a week (frequency).	Uses words that do not specifically measure the degree of change e.g., increasing, more, less, growing . . . He will walk more.
A The goal is **Achievable**.	Assumes that the appropriate resources are available and an adequate amount of time is allocated for the goal to be completed	The goal is not realistic in terms of time, resources, or patient motivation.
R The goal is **Realistic/ Relevant**.	Larger goals are divided into smaller tasks that must be accomplished in sequential order.	A broad goal is identified with no regard for smaller tasks that may need to be achieved prior to being able to complete the larger goal.
T The goal is **Timed**.	Describes the amount of time allotted to either achieving the goal or to when the progress toward the goal will be reviewed; works best for short-term and intermediate goals	If the accomplishment of the goal has not progressed as expected, and there is too much time between when the goal was set and when it is evaluated, there may be additional complications, and it may be harder to get back on track.

Source: Bovend'Eerdt, T. J. H., Botell, R. E., & Wade, D. T. (2009). Writing SMART rehabilitation goals and achieving goal attainment scaling: A practical guide. *Clinical Rehabilitation, 23*, 352–361.

the responsibility of administering her own insulin, and the goal would need to be reviewed. Situations where the patient expresses hesitancy offer an opportunity for nurses to use creative problem-solving strategies to find solutions that encourage and support patient participation.

Through the eyes of a student

Mr. Davies had abdominal surgery 36 hours ago for an obstructed bowel. He wanted to go to the bathroom to void instead of using the urinal. I examined his dressing and noted that it was dry and intact. I took his vital signs and they were normal, and then I took his oxygen saturation level, which was 88% on room air. I thought that Mr. Davies might become dizzy and simply provided him with a urinal. I also gave him an incentive spirometer and encouraged him to take some deep breaths.

(personal reflection of a nursing student)

Through the eyes of a nurse

I was doing a round on my patients and stopped to see how Mr. Davies was doing. He had been recovering well since his surgery. He requested to go to the washroom to void so I checked his vital signs, which were stable, and his oxygen saturation level, which was 88% on room air. This was below the preferred 90%, but I knew that ambulating would be beneficial for the prevention of postsurgery deep vein thrombosis as well as pneumonia. We agreed that he would sit on the side of the bed to determine if he could walk to the washroom. Mr. Davies was not dizzy sitting on the edge of the bed and was able to walk to the washroom, void, and return to bed. Mr. Davies did not voice any concerns about pain, and his gait was steady, and he stated that he did not feel light-headed. After he was settled back to bed, his oxygen saturation was 95% on room air.

(personal reflection of a nurse)

In this example, the registered nurse and patient agreed on the plan to ambulate to the washroom so the patient could void and return to his bed. The nurse believed this goal was realistic based on her assessment of the patient and her knowledge of the importance to ambulate a postsurgical patient. A specific distance was determined based on his need to void. His progress was evaluated by what the patient stated (no pain, no dizziness), what the nurse observed (his gait was steady), and the measurements the nurse obtained (oxygen saturation was 95% on room air).

Developing Care Plans

It is imperative to communicate the plan for achieving the goals to ensure continuity of patient care. Nursing care plans are documents that outline the care that is provided for the patient, family, or community. The care plan is holistic and has a nursing diagnosis, a nursing intervention, and a nursing outcome that is patient-focused. A nursing care plan will reflect the needs of the patient, based on his or her involvement and the nurse's assessment data and clinical judgment, the nurse's scope of practice, and the health-care agency guidelines and policies. The level of involvement of various disciplines often determines the format that is used to plan and communicate goals. If the setting and achieving of goals is predominantly determined by nursing, a nursing care plan may be developed. Goals may also be listed in a Kardex or an admission database. As the care becomes more complex, the number of health-care disciplines involved increases. In these situations, the nursing care plan may be embedded in a larger document. For example, a critical pathway may be developed by a health organization to be used as a case management tool for all patients with a particular diagnosis or a treatment such as surgery. Critical pathways require all disciplines to be familiar with the goals and interventions of the other disciplines in order to best deliver and coordinate care (Fig. 10.8).

Implementation

Implementation is the fourth phase in the nursing process. In the implementation phase, the nurse makes an intentional effort to achieve the goals related to the patient's health status and documents the care provided (Clement, 2011). Implementing involves reassessing the patient, determining in what ways the nurse needs assistance, implementing the nursing interventions, supervising any delegated care, and documenting all the nursing activities.

Goals are like a road map. Like cities, towns, and landmarks or points of interest, goals help us determine where we are going, but they do not provide the means to get there. Interventions or nursing actions help us to move from one point to another. They are the result of the collaborative actions of the nurse and patient to develop and implement a plan to promote wellness and modify patient outcomes. **Interventions** are planned nursing actions taken to address patient or family needs, working toward previously established collaborative goals for patient or family outcomes. These actions are based on evidence-based research and best practice standards that incorporate nursing knowledge, such as pharmacology, physiology, pathology, anatomy, and laboratory and diagnostic tests, as well as skills related to interpersonal relationships, therapeutic communication, and the principles of teaching and learning.

Implementation Skills

Nurses can intervene in various ways depending on the setting and their role. A wide variety of skills may be required, depending on the patient situation. These skills may include, but are not limited to, psychomotor dexterity, therapeutic communication techniques, analysis of similar clinical events, or the ability to articulate concepts. When providing direct patient care, the nurse might intervene by educating the patient and family

Clinical Pathway – Minimally Invasive Bowel Resection

	Pre-Admission	Day of Admission	Post-op on day of admission
Consult	• Anesthetist		
Tests	• Blood test • Electrocardiogram if required • Chest X-ray if required	• Blood test if required	
Medication		• Antibiotic	• Patient Controlled Analgesia (IV PCA) • Antibiotic (prevent infection) • Anti-nausea medications • Anticoagulant (blood thinner) • Patient's own medications if required
Assessment & Treatment	• Measure legs for support stockings (TEDs)	• Intravenous • TED stockings	• Vital signs (Blood Pressure, Heart & Respiratory Rate, Temperature, Bowel & Breath Sounds) • Oxygen if needed • Intravenous • Abdominal incisions • Drain/drainage (if present) • TED stockings
Activity			• Sit at side of bed
Nutrition		• Nothing by mouth	• Sips of clear fluids
Elimination			• Urinary catheter (if present)
Patient Teaching/	• Pre-op instructions • Bowel preparation • Skin preparation	• Pre-op instructions	• Deep breathing and coughing exercises • Ankle exercises
Discharge Planning	• Plan for a hospitalization of 4 days including day of surgery		

Figure 10.8 Example of a critical pathway.

Clinical Pathway – Minimally Invasive Bowel Resection

	Post-op Day 1	Post-op Day 2	Post-op Day 3 Discharge Day
Consult			
Tests	• Blood test	• Blood test	• Blood test if required
Medication	• IV PCA • IV Toradol (non-steroidal anti-inflammatory) • Anti-nausea medication • Anticoagulant • Patient's own medications if required	• IV PCA discontinued and oral pain medication started • Anti-nausea medication • Anticoagulant • Patient's own medications if required	• Oral pain medication • Anti-nausea medication • Patient's own medications if required
Assessment & Treatment	• Vital signs • Oxygen if needed • Intravenous • Abdominal incisions • TED stockings	• Vital signs • Oxygen if needed • Intravenous discontinued if drinking well • Abdominal incisions • Drain removed (if present) • TED stockings	• Vital signs • Abdominal incisions • TED stockings
Activity	• Sit in chair 2 times	• Walk in hall 3 times at least	• Activity as tolerated
Nutrition	• Surgery diet • Eat what you feel you can manage	• Surgery diet	• Surgery diet
Elimination	• Urinary catheter removed (if present)	• Up to bathroom	• Passing gas per rectum
Patient Teaching/	• Deep breathing and coughing exercises • Ankle exercises • Pain management • Activity	• Deep breathing and coughing exercises • Ankle exercises • Pain management • Activity	• Deep breathing and coughing exercises • Ankle exercises • Pain management • Activity
Discharge Planning		• Confirm plan to be picked up from hospital tomorrow by 10:00 a.m.	• Discharge

Figure 10.8 *(continued)*

about a procedure the patient will be having or how to care for an incision after discharge. The nurse may also track a patient's intake and output to ensure adequate nutrition, prevent dehydration, or as part of another assessment. Direct interventions would also include lifesaving measures such as cardiopulmonary resuscitation (CPR) or first aid. Nurses also intervene when they counsel patients and families in outpatient settings such as well-baby clinics, participate in community visits such as home care, or teach coping skills in a chronic pain clinic. Nurses complete indirect interventions when they are away from the clinical area focusing on groups of patients or events, such as participating in developing policies, identifying reasons for medication errors, or assessing quality of patient care.

When nurses select interventions, it is another opportunity to involve patients in their own care and support their abilities. Patients who are included in their own care report increased satisfaction with the care provided and an increased sense of well-being (Loh et al., 2007). Being able to successfully implement patient-specific interventions is key to promoting health and healing.

Nurses may use the **Nursing Interventions Classification (NIC)** as a guide to selecting implementation options. This internationally recognized list of nursing actions uses standardized labels and descriptions (Bulechek, Butcher, Dochterman, & Wagner, 2013). The main benefit of using standard language is that it promotes a common understanding among nurses. It provides a method to link diagnoses and interventions and identifies nursing skills that are required to implement nursing interventions and to identify planning resources. Limitations include the fact that nursing-based language may not transfer to other disciplines and that NIC may not include the full scope of care that the nurse provides. In addition, the NIC is not used in all settings and locations, and not all nurses are educated in how to use the NIC. Ultimately, patients benefit most from a holistic approach to their care implemented by caregivers who effectively communicate as a team.

RESEARCH

NURSING ASSESSMENT TOOLS/MODELS FOR DIVERSE ETHNO-CULTURAL NURSING CARE

There are an increasing number of diverse ethno-cultural groups in high-income nations, therefore increasing the need for competent and culturally responsive health care. The purpose of this review was to identify nursing assessment tools and/or models that could support effective and efficient nursing care of people from diverse ethno-cultural groups.

Review
Studies have shown that when the needs of diverse ethno-cultural groups are not met, there are increased risks associated with patient safety, a patient accesses health-care services more often, there is increased frequency of miscommunication resulting in simple and life-threatening errors, and there is decreased adherence with follow-up treatment. These unmet needs could result in higher health-care costs and additional legal liability for health-care agencies and individual health-care providers. This review identifies eight models/tools nurses could use to provide culturally relevant and comprehensive care and explores aspects such as communication, social determinants of health, and patient-centered care. The tools/models include frameworks for nursing assessment, intervention, and evaluation and have been used to guide research. The review concluded that by using tools/models that support ethno-cultural care, nurses can develop an awareness and sensitivity to the health-care needs that exist among people from varied ethno-cultural backgrounds and life journeys. The result would be patient care that supports positive patient outcomes and is professionally and fiscally responsible.

Nursing Implications
This review highlights the value of the nursing process to provide comprehensive, patient-centered care. The nurse's assessment is critical to understanding the context of the patient's concerns and lived experience, including cultural dimensions important to health and healing. The nursing process assists the nurse to understand patient care as a holistic process that includes various assessments, nursing diagnoses, and interventions, followed by the essential evaluation of the effectiveness in meeting patient needs.

Higginbottom, G. M. A., Richter, M. S., Mogale, R. S., Ortiz, L., Young, S., & Mollel, O. (2011). Identification of nursing assessment models/tools validated in clinical practice for use with diverse ethno-cultural groups [Review]. BMC Nursing, 10, 16. Retrieved from www.biomedcentral.com/1472-6955/10/16

Some interventions will focus on the signs and symptoms of the diagnosis, whereas others will be more specific to altering risk factors. Your focus will be determined when you prioritize your diagnoses and goals. Sometimes, there is more than one intervention for a particular goal. Determining which intervention will work best requires the nurse to consider other factors. The nurse must be competent in the skills that are required to implement the intervention, able to access the appropriate resources, and able to problem solve when the resources are unfamiliar or unavailable.

Discharge Planning

Acknowledging what the patient brings to the care planning process and his or her ability to participate is important. It is particularly important to consider what barriers may exist when creating a discharge plan because these may not be readily apparent while the patient is in hospital (Alspach, 2011). For example, if the patient is cognitively impaired, the goal of independence may not be realistic.

The nurse provides the necessary teaching and ensures that the patient can accomplish the task or goals independently by observing the patient completing the task. Patients may face limitations related to their illness. If the acuity of the patient or the complexity of his or her circumstances increases prior to discharge, so might the intervention, and it may be necessary to delay his or her discharge from hospital until home care is arranged. The nurse may need to consult other nurse specialists and health-care providers for their skills and expertise and may be able to do this independently or invite the physician to request a consultation.

One way nurses provide holistic care is to determine what types of resources are needed. It might be equipment such as an intravenous (IV) pole, a fetal monitor, or a dressing tray. Perhaps additional health-care workers are needed to safely ambulate a patient who has recently had a stroke. Perhaps the patient is in need of a nurse who is competent in a particular skill. Some competencies, such as drawing blood, irrigating central lines, and administering total parental nutrition, require additional education and supervised practice.

In addition to considering what resources are needed, it is important to consider if the cost of the resources is affordable by the patient. In Canada, the publicly funded universal health insurance system ensures that many medical and other health-care services are provided at no direct cost to the patient. Each province and territory, however, has unique policies limiting coverage by excluding certain services, procedures, or supplies. Patients may need to pay part or all of the cost, particularly if they do not have supplementary health-care insurance. As the cost of health care increases and funding does not increase by the same increment, many facilities limit supplies, purchase cheaper supplies, and ask families to provide or purchase some types of equipment and supplies.

Discharge planning can be complex. After Amarina's initial colostomy surgery, the nurse would have taught her how to care for her stoma and how to change her appliance. This would have included several opportunities for Amarina to demonstrate her ability to complete this task successfully. The nurse's evaluation of Amarina's ability would include her willingness to learn how to care for her colostomy, her level of skill (dexterity), and her ability to seek and accept help. The nurse may need to arrange for an ostomy nurse to provide care for Amarina at home. Evaluating Amarina's coping skills, her ability to meet her nutritional requirements, and to safely administer her own medication are also part of discharge planning. The nurse would also confirm that Amarina has the financial resources to buy her ostomy supplies.

Evaluation

Evaluation is the final phase of the nursing process. **Evaluation** is necessary to determine the effectiveness of our actions and occurs when the nurse reviews and measures whether the care goals were met, identifies any unintended outcomes, and determines if any changes to the plan are required to accomplish any unmet goals (Kloseck, 2007). In order to evaluate whether the goal was met, you must have a clear understanding of the expected outcomes, including how they will be measured.

For example, if one of the goals is that the patient will not acquire postoperative pneumonia because he properly uses an incentive spirometer every hour while awake, then you will assess both the patient's lungs as well as the patient's use of the incentive spirometer. You will use both subjective and objective data from and about the patient to evaluate the actual outcomes of the goal. For subjective input, you will need to talk with the patient about his perceptions of his illness and use of the spirometer. For objective data, you will use your physical assessment skills, take the patient's vital signs, and gather lab and x-ray results to identify and measure the presence or absence of the pneumonia. Test results and the nurse's examination findings are best understood in relation to one another. Understanding how the data fits together not only helps you identify if the goal has or has not been met or if the goal needs to be readjusted or changed but also provides rationale for the outcome.

To evaluate the effectiveness of the care plan, the nurse would review the patient's response to all of the interventions and the resources that were used. For example, even though the nurse visited the patient daily, this patient's health status may have deteriorated. Sometimes, the intended outcomes are not achieved, the outcomes are different, or there are unanticipated outcomes. Each of these outcomes can have a positive or negative impact on the patient's future and are important to include in the evaluation process. In this way, the circular and continuous nature of the nursing process is demonstrated. Initial assessment leads to interpretation of data to decide what is most important, analysis of the data helps you to prioritize both needs and actions, planning identifies the most appropriate actions, implementing the plans includes actions you and your patient take, and evaluation identifies new assessment data that will influence priorities and planning in the next cycle of the nursing process. Look again at Figure 10.1, which illustrates how the evaluation step is related to the other steps in the nursing process. Experienced nurses are continuously moving through these cycles, even as they provide care.

Through the eyes of a student

My patient's name was Amarina, and she had surgery for Crohn, which resulted in an ileostomy. She was underweight, probably due to having several exacerbations of Crohn disease over the last 2 years. She was reluctant to have an ileostomy but agreed because of the significant deterioration in her health over the last year. After surgery, she needed to learn how to care for her stoma. She was very uncomfortable when I started to teach her how to care for the stoma and ostomy appliance and asked if she could just get some written instructions. I acknowledged that it was normal for her to feel uneasy or afraid. I told her that when she demonstrated how to care for her ileostomy, she had better chances of the stoma remaining healthy and free from infection after discharge. I also reinforced the benefits of her remaining independent. *(personal reflection of a nursing student)*

Through the eyes of a patient

I was really embarrassed about having this ileostomy. I was worried about it leaking and the maintenance. When the student nurse told me she was going to teach me how to care for my ileostomy, I wanted nothing to do with it. Eventually, I agreed. She encouraged me to practice and encouraged me each time I got another step right. By the end of it, I was feeling pretty proud. I felt in charge of my body; something I had not felt in a long time.

(personal reflection of a patient)

In this example, the goal to have the patient change her ileostomy appliance was achieved; however, there are additional outcomes that need to be evaluated. The young woman expressed pride that she was able to change the appliance on her own and that she felt in control of her body. These feelings may contribute to a healthy sense of self-esteem and confidence, which may facilitate an easier transition back to her peer group. The nurse could note in the evaluation that the patient felt supported in the learning process and was able to identify personal successes in other areas.

Identifying additional or different outcomes for the intervention helps the patient and nurse to determine why or how the intervention was or was not successful. Considering these factors in the evaluation is critical because valuable information is obtained about how you and the patient can formulate future goals or revise current goals so that patient outcomes can be achieved. Other questions to consider when revising current goals and evaluating the outcome of the collaborative goals include the following: Is the objective/goal still relevant? (Has the patient's health status, finances, etc., changed?); Is the intervention still consistent with the current health needs? (Have we understood the patient/other health-care providers correctly?); Are the goals sustainable? (Are the appropriate resources available, e.g., funds, people, materials, equipment, transfer of care?). See Box 10.3.

BOX 10.3 **Additional Questions to Evaluate the Outcomes for Collaborative Goals**

Assumption: The goal was stated in terms of observable (measurable) patient behaviour with a single focus and a time frame.

1. Was the stated goal met?
   a. According to whom? (the patient, family, nurse, other care providers)
2. Are there any other approaches to meeting this goal that may be more effective?
3. If there were unintended outcomes, were these helpful?
   a. How?
   b. For whom?
4. What should the next set of goals be?

One important guide to describing nursing outcomes is the **Nursing Outcomes Classification (NOC)** system, an internationally recognized taxonomy with criteria for measurable or desirable outcomes as a result of interventions performed by nurses (Moorhead, Johnson, Maas, & Swanson, 2013). This common terminology and classification system also facilitates comparison and analysis between similar patients in similar situations so nurses can make decisions about how to use their resources most effectively. The NOC is also aligned with NANDA and the NIC, making research on nursing practice much more accurate and generalizable.

As a nurse, you determine the goal is accomplished only after you have discussed and evaluated the completed goals with your patient. You need to document your evaluation and discussion with the patient and indicate that the goal is met so that the intervention is discontinued. This note tells the team that no additional time needs to be spent on this goal. The nurse would then reassess the patient's status and determine with the patient how best to prioritize the remaining goals or create a new goal. Nurses will also evaluate the process of care with the patient by reviewing its efficiency: Did the care provided complicate the patient's progress, did it duplicate care provided by others, or did it conflict with other services or programs that were already being used by the patient? Inefficient, duplicate, or ineffective care would create unnecessary stress and costs for the health-care system and, perhaps, for the patient and family.

Code of Ethics

To ensure that patients have equal opportunity to receive quality nursing care, the CNA (2008) has developed a code of ethics (see Box 4.3). Although all registered nurses are required to practice according to the code of ethics, individual nurses have their own values and beliefs. Sometimes, it is difficult to put one's own beliefs aside as you provide care. Ethics are involved in every step of the nursing process because choices are constantly being made by the nurse that will either support or undermine the patient's goals. These choices that arise as you provide patient care include sources of data, decisions regarding what is the most important data, interpretation of data, priorities identified, interventions selected, and criteria used for evaluation of outcomes. If the views and priorities of health professionals are more important, the patient will leave the encounter with less self-confidence and less trust in the health-care system. To ensure that every contact with health professionals is supportive of patients, nurses are wise to use the nursing process to understand the patient's hopes, fears, goals, and priorities. Knowing that information before patient care begins will make it easier to reinforce the patient's knowledge and skills regarding his or her health condition, its management, and the incorporation of new behaviours into his or her daily life.

The Nursing Process in the 21st Century

As we become more of a global community, there are new challenges for nurses. We will rely more on the use of technology to help us with our assessments, access resources to provide services, implement treatment plans, store information, and communicate with others. A registered nurse's role, as identified in 2006 by the College and Association of Registered Nurses of Alberta (CARNA), may continue to be to promote, maintain, and restore holistic health. Nevertheless, how we access patients and populations, gather data, understand the issues, and engage with the interprofessional team will change. For example, nurses are currently able to attend workshops, conferences, in-services, and interprofessional meetings through video conferencing and webinars. Data can be obtained or added, and medications can be verified with the electronic chart at the patient's bedside using electronic mobile devices. As health-care costs become more of a concern, nurses may rely more on technology when using the nursing process. We may conduct initial visits and family interviews or perform wound assessments via video conferencing using a patient's computer or phone, particularly if patients live in a remote area or are unable to leave their residence. With the creation of centralized electronic charts, nurses could potentially access a patient's data quickly from various locations and could easily search for historical data related to the current concern. As a result, the amount of time nurses now spend gathering this data from the patient would decrease, the historical data would be consistent each time the patient accesses the health-care system, and more time could be spent exploring other aspects of his or her holistic health.

Technology in Patient Care

Some examples of how the nursing process can act as a framework to incorporate technology into care are discussed in this section.

Assessment

Technological tools can assist in many aspects of the nursing process. Traditionally, nurses have palpated for pedal pulses, and although this continues to be a valuable skill, nurses may also use a Doppler in more complex situations to obtain additional assessment data. Another way nurses use technology in their assessments is when they use digital thermometers. This tool decreases the time and labour needed to sterilize equipment, the results are obtained quickly, and there is less exposure to mercury (Fadzil, Choon, & Arumugam, 2010). The nurse can use video conferencing or Skype to interview patients and their families, to conference with members of the interprofessional team, or for educational purposes. A home care nurse may even be able to use a patient's e-mailed photo to assess a wound prior to a home visit to determine what supplies will be needed.

Planning

Internet access permits nurses to use current research regarding best practice guidelines and alternative therapies, refer patients to appropriate community resources, and provide various patient educational materials. Computer programs could be used to generate patient care plans, leading to a more consistent approach to care.

Diagnosis

Digital information can be assimilated quickly to formulate diagnoses. However, only the data that is entered will be available for consideration, so it is imperative that nurses use their critical thinking skills to determine if information is missing or if there are other possibilities to provide comprehensive patient care. The type of software program might also be used to cue nurses to collect additional assessment information.

Implementation

Nurses will need to understand the purpose of using technology as well as its limitations. For example, multiple IV fluids can be programmed into one IV pump, eliminating the need for multiple pumps and more than one IV pole. This feature makes it easier for the patient to mobilize; however, the technology does not recognize if the medications are correct or if the pump has been programmed correctly. The nurse's knowledge and critical thinking skills are essential to ensure patient safety.

Evaluation

With the use of technology, nurses are able to track multiple aspects of a patient's care simultaneously. For example, pulse, heartbeat, respirations, oxygen saturation levels, and blood pressure can all be displayed on one monitor. Perhaps in the future, this information can be linked to a database, which would then provide a list of possible reasons for what might be happening as well as potential interventions. In addition, technology may also change the way we involve patients in evaluating treatment outcomes. Patients could potentially provide ongoing feedback to the health-care team and adjust their health-care goals, if necessary, in real time using computer programs or secure e-mail. This approach may reduce the amount of time a patient spends at follow-up appointments or possibly the number of follow-up appointments that are required.

The Nursing Process in a Changing Environment

Increasingly, nurses will be required to think differently about the increasing complexity of the patient's concerns. Variables such as environmental factors, a change in how the family unit is defined, and economics will change the structure in which health care is provided and also the types of knowledge and interventions that nurses will need to include in the nursing process. Carper (1978) described the types of knowing that nursing will need to use to best understand the complexity of patient care. The four patterns of knowing are empirics (the science of nursing), esthetics (the art of nursing), ethics (moral-ethical reasoning in nursing), and personal experience (Carper, 1978).

Within the context of the patient's story, there may be multiple concerns that are related or that form patterns. The Outcome-Present-State Test (OPT) Model of Reflective Clinical Reasoning (Pesut, 2008) is a nonlinear process and advocates that nurses help patients make the transition from a state of illness to health by understanding the context of their story and by simultaneously considering the relationships among the nursing diagnoses. Exploration of these patterns can lead to increased insight into the patient's concerns and even identify a central issue that can act as a leverage point within the patient's story. This type of model acknowledges the complexity of our humanness and the presence of multiple concerns that may be related. In the future, there will be an increasing number of theories and tools that could be used to assist the nurse in applying all steps of the nursing process.

Traditionally, registered nurses have used their critical thinking skills to assimilate information from areas, such as anatomy, pathology, physiology, pharmacology, diverse populations, principles of teaching and learning, therapeutic communication, and interpersonal relationships. With the expansion of world economies and technology, our global community continues to grow, and the registered nurse will need to know the patient's story to understand the larger context of the concerns expressed. For example, the relative ease of travelling between countries has meant that many infectious diseases are not contained by geographical borders, such as severe acute respiratory syndrome (SARS) and avian influenza H5N1 (Mackenzie, 2011).

In the future, there will be an increasing push to find efficiencies in our health-care systems. As a result, the environment in which nurses provide care may become more digital and, as a result, potentially more portable. Nurses will be required to learn new technology quickly and adapt it seamlessly into their practice while being cognizant that each patient, family, or community is a unique entity with specific needs that are met within the context of a relationship. Being flexible, open to experimenting with new approaches to care for individuals, families, and changing populations as well as critically appraising the effectiveness of new technology will be valuable attributes for the 21st-century nurse.

Conclusion

Knowing your role as a nurse and your scope of practice helps to define how you will use the nursing process in your specific area of nursing. Your ability to use critical reasoning to integrate your theoretical knowledge and the knowledge you gain from experience will determine how effectively you use the nursing process. Each nurse incorporates personal strengths into practice in a different way. Often, this creativity is expressed in your unique approach and decisions related to patient teaching, problem solving, and implementing interventions related to your patient's situation.

The professional knowledge you gain through experience accumulates throughout your career and enables you to use the nursing process more efficiently. As you become more proficient at using the nursing process, you will be able to identify which assessments, specific to your patient, need to be done; complete them more quickly and accurately; integrate your data more thoroughly; identify an appropriate plan of care; successfully implement your nursing care; and evaluate its effectiveness.

As the occurrence of concurrent disorders (physical, mental health, addiction, psychological) increases, nurses will need to perform assessments and determine appropriate nursing diagnoses for multiple concerns and then plan and include separate interventions for each concern. However, the patient and nurse would also need to develop integrated solutions because each solution will have an impact on the other diagnoses as well as a synergistic effect. Working with patients who have multiple diagnoses requires the nurse to be able to implement the nursing process at various steps with multiple concerns simultaneously.

The five steps in the nursing process (assessment, diagnosis, planning, implementation, and evaluation) are used to provide safe, competent, and holistic care. The nursing process serves as a guide for both novice and expert nurse to gather information, identify priorities, plan and implement interventions, and evaluate the effectiveness of the care provided. These five steps prompt the student through the basic process of providing patient care. The nursing process can be used with conceptual systems such as NANDA and NIC that may allow care plans and processes to easily transfer to other care facilities or providers when the taxonomies are standardized. For the nursing student, the nursing process offers reassurance. It is a framework or heuristic device that helps students appreciate and understand the complexity of the care they provide. The nursing process provides a structure for care, a process for delivering that care, and a way of assessing the outcomes of care. For expert nurses, the "steps" of the nursing process are less distinct; their evidence-informed knowledge and past experiences become integrated, and they are able to process simultaneously all aspects of the care they provide that occur at different points in the nursing process. As your knowledge base increases and as you gain experience, these steps become integrated into your nursing practice. You will engage and enact the nursing process in a much more dynamic and fluid way.

In the opening case study, Tanja, a third-year nursing student, may have felt overwhelmed by the complexity of Amarina's health concerns and uncertain if she would be able to provide excellent patient care. As illustrated throughout the chapter, using the nursing process provides a systematic and rational method to approach Amarina's care. As a student, Tanja can collect pertinent and accurate assessment data from the patient, family, and several other sources so she can understand the context of Amarina's health concerns and begin to provide patient-centered care. Tanja considers Amarina's wishes and uses her communication skills and her knowledge of pharmacology, physiology, pathology, and anatomy to identify appropriate nursing diagnoses to meet Amarina's immediate, intermediate, and long-term health goals. This includes her nutritional needs, the need for surgery, and teaching on the importance of continued self-care and building supportive relationships. By using the nursing process, Tanja is able to provide holistic patient care by identifying nursing diagnoses and interventions that meet Amarina's physical, emotional, and cognitive needs. Tanja has also learned that the steps of the nursing process overlap and can occur simultaneously. She is able to provide Amarina's nutrition through a G-tube while discussing what type of support Amarina would like from her mother. Being able to organize her time and evaluate her care throughout her shift means that she can provide the right care at the right time. By using the nursing process, Tanja provides safe, holistic, and comprehensive care, and Amarina has the opportunity to experience positive health outcomes.

Critical Thinking Case Scenarios

▶ Now that you have learned how to apply the nursing process to the care you provide to patients, consider the following questions as they relate to the opening case study about Amarina.

1. List the assessment data from the case study and describe how each point relates to Amarina's care.
2. Formulate two nursing diagnoses for Amarina: one diagnosis relating to her physical health and one diagnosis related to her emotional well-being.
3. Amarina's physician has decided to hospitalize Amarina against her will. Describe an alternative intervention that would include Amarina in the decision-making process. Speculate on the effectiveness of these two interventions.
4. List the areas in order beginning with what is most pertinent that you would explore with Amarina to create a comprehensive care plan. Include your rationale for each area you have chosen.

▶ Jane Black is a 32-year-old mother of three who has just been admitted to the hospital unit on which you are working today. She is 22 weeks pregnant and has recently been diagnosed with diabetes. Her husband brought her to the hospital because she was drowsy, having difficulty focusing, was exceptionally thirsty, and was having to void frequently. Mr. and Mrs. Black brought their three children to the hospital because they did not have anyone to care for them. They have two girls, 3 and 7 years old, and a 5-year-old boy. Mrs. Black is a stay-at-home mom, and her husband

is a long-distance truck driver who is scheduled to leave in 2 days. Mr. Black is concerned about who will care for his children if his wife is still in the hospital when he leaves and asks when she will be discharged. In talking to Mr. Black, you discover that they live in a three-bedroom apartment.

1. List the five steps of the nursing process and give an example for each step that you could implement in this situation.
2. List three determinants of health and develop a question for each one that you could ask either Mr. or Mrs. Black.
3. List the people from the multidisciplinary team that you would include in caring for this family.
4. Create a care plan that would address Mrs. Black's diabetes.

▶ Lily, a home care nurse, visits her patient Jim Starblanket once daily at 9 AM to ensure he is taking his medications from his bubble pack. Mr. Starblanket has high blood pressure and has been treated for depression since his wife died 6 weeks ago. After 1 month, Lily observes that Mr. Starblanket has lost 8 lb, and he has not gone to the seniors' centre for the past two Tuesdays. She also notices that there is a cup beside Mr. Starblanket's bubble pack with several of his pills in it. Lily decides to complete a Mini-Mental State Exam, and Mr. Starblanket scores poorly on the exam.

1. What additional data would you collect?
2. List two nursing diagnoses for Mr. Starblanket and describe how they may be related.
3. What additional nursing knowledge or experience might be helpful to create a care plan for Mr. Starblanket?
4. How would you use the nursing process to decide whether Mr. Starblanket needs to be taken to the hospital emergency department?

Multiple-Choice Questions

1. Mr. Jones has returned to the unit after surgery for a bowel obstruction. You take his vital signs and determine that the dressing is intact. Mr. Jones states he is in a lot of pain, feels nauseated, and requests medication for both. The subjective data is:
   a. Mr. Jones' blood pressure, pulse, and respiratory rate
   b. Mr. Jones' dressing is securely attached, there is no redness around the edges of the wound, and there is no drainage evident through the dressing.
   c. Mr. Jones states he is in a lot of pain.
   d. Mr. Jones had a bowel obstruction.

2. Sheila is a second-year university student and came to the health centre for help with her nausea. The nurse in the health centre indicated that her human chorionic gonadotropin (hCG) levels were significantly increased and that she is pregnant. She is not currently

dating anyone and pays for her education and living expenses with her student loan. Which of the following would represent objective data?

a. She feels nauseated.

b. Her hCG levels are significantly increased.

c. She is not currently dating anyone.

d. She pays for her education and living expenses with her student loan.

3. Completing a health history, reviewing the physical assessment data and lab results, reviewing the literature, and documenting the data are part of this step of the nursing process.

a. Evaluation

b. Identifying a nursing diagnosis

c. Planning

d. Assessment

4. Synthesizing your data would include the following:

a. Predicting what could happen to your patient

b. Planning for your patient's discharge

c. Using your nursing knowledge and experience to identify patterns in the data

d. Evaluating whether your plan of care is working

5. A nursing diagnosis:

a. Is formulated with the multidisciplinary team

b. Identifies the patient's response to actual and potential health problems

c. Relates primarily to the disease process

d. Is only for short-term interventions

6. What factors determine the priority of the care provided to the patient?

a. The patient's wishes, the acuity of the situation, and the available resources

b. The nurse's experience and theoretical knowledge

c. The nurse's workload

d. The patient's response to the current treatment

7. Lisa gave birth to her daughter Britney 24 hours ago. Lisa is coping well with caring for her daughter and is eager to breast-feed but is finding it difficult. Both Lisa and Britney will be discharged in 2 hours. What is the most pertinent intervention for Lisa?

a. Refer Lisa to a public health nurse for a home visit today and give her the number of the lactation clinic.

b. Keep Lisa and Britney in the hospital until a lactation consultant can see them.

c. Make an appointment for Lisa and Britney with their family doctor.

d. Provide teaching to Lisa about the benefits of breast milk.

8. Identifying that your patient has a knowledge deficit related to wound care would occur during which step of the nursing process?

a. Assessment

b. Diagnosis

c. Planning

d. Implementation and evaluation

9. The nurse saw a psychiatric patient brought in by a family member in the emergency department. The patient's speech is random and nonsensical. Laboratory tests have been ordered, and the patient's medical history has been accessed on the computer. What else would you do as part of your assessment?

a. Let the patient rest in a secure room.

b. Continue talking to the patient.

c. Speak with family to obtain collateral information.

d. Offer the patient medication to decrease her anxiety.

10. Luke was diagnosed with an aggressive type of lung cancer. He chose to move to a hospice because he didn't want to be a burden to his partner. It may be necessary to reevaluate Luke's living arrangements based on which of the following:

a. His financial situation remains constant.

b. He has been given 3 weeks to live.

c. He is able to access all the resources he needs from either the hospice or home.

d. He misses being close to his partner for support.

REFERENCES AND SUGGESTED READINGS

Alspach, J. G. (2011). The patient's capacity for self-care: Advocating for a predischarge assessment. *Critical Care Nurse, 31*(2), 10.

Bakken, H. S., & Mead, C. N. (1997). Nursing classification systems: Necessary but not sufficient for representing "what nurses do" for inclusion in computer-based patient record systems. *American Medical Informatics Association, 4*(3), 222–232.

Bulechek, G. M., Butcher, H. K., Dochterman, J. M., & Wagner, C. (2013). *Nursing intervention classification* (NIC; 6th ed.). St. Louis, MO: Mosby.

Canadian Nurses Association. (2008). *Code of ethics for registered Nurses* (2008 centennial edition). Retrieved from http://www.cna-aiic.ca/cna/documents/pdf/publications/Code_of_Ethics_2008_e.pdf

Canadian Nurses Association. (2010). *Evidence-informed decision-making and nursing practice*. Retrieved from http://www.nanb.nb.ca/PDF/CNA-Evidence_Informed_Decision_Making_and_Nursing_Practice_E.pdf

Cardwell, P., Corkin, D., McCartan, R., McCullock, A., & Mullan, C. (2011). Is care planning still relevant in the 21st century? *British Journal of Nursing, 20*(21), 1378–1382.

Carper, B. A. (1978). Fundamental patterns of knowing in nursing: ANS/Practice Oriented Theory, Part 1. *Advances in Nursing Science*, *1*(1), 13–23.

Carrington, J. M. (2012). The usefulness of nursing languages to communicate a clinical event. *Computers, Informatics, Nursing*, *30*(2), 82–88.

Cauldwell, M., Beattie, C., Benita, C., Denby, W., Ede-Golightly, J., & Linton, F. (2007). The impact of electronic patient records on workflow in general practice. *Health Informatics Journal*, *13*(2), 155–160.

Clement, I. (2011). *Textbook of nursing foundations*. New Delhi, India: Jaypee Brothers.

College and Association of Registered Nurses of Alberta. (2006). *CARNA entry-to-practice competencies for the registered nurses profession*. Retrieved from http://www.nurses.ab.ca/carna-admin/Uploads/Entry-to-Practice%20Competencies.pdf

College of Nurses of Ontario. (2012). *Entry-to-practice competencies for Ontario registered practical nurses*. Retrieved from http://www.cno.org/Global/docs/reg/41042_EntryPracRPN.pdf

Fadzil, F. M., Choon, D., & Arumugam, K. (2010). A comparative study on the accuracy of noninvasive thermometers. *Australian Family Physician*, *39*(4), 238–239.

Folstein, M. F., Folstein, S. E., & McHugh, P. R. (1975). Mini-mental state: A practical method for grading the cognitive state of patients for the clinician. *Journal of Psychiatric Research*, *12*(3), 189–198.

Gill, M., Windemuth, R., Steele, R., & Green, S. (2005). A comparison of the Glasgow Coma Scale to simplified alternative scores for the prediction of traumatic brain injury outcomes. *Annals of Emergency Medicine*, *45*(1), 37–42. doi:10.1016/j.annemergmed 2004.07.429

Government of Alberta. (2011). *Alberta netcare electronic health record*. Retrieved from http://www.albertanetcare.ca

Government of Alberta. (2012). *Alberta's freedom of information and protection of privacy act (FOIP Act)*. Retrieved from http://www.servicealberta.ca/foip

Huckabay, L. M. (2009). Clinical reasoned judgment and the nursing process. *Nursing Forum*, *44*(2), 72–78.

Kaplan, B., & Ura, D., (2010). Use of multiple patient simulators to enhance prioritizing and delegating skills for senior nursing students. *Journal of Nursing Education*, *49*(7), 371–377.

Kloseck, M. (2007). The use of Goal Attainment Scaling in a community health promotion initiative with seniors. *BMC Geriatrics*, *7*, 16. doi:10.1186/1471-2318-7-16

Levett-Jones, T., Hoffman, K., Dempsey, J., Jeong, S. Y., Noble, D., Norton, C. A., . . . Hickey, N. (2010). The 'five rights' of clinical reasoning: An educational model to enhance nursing students' ability to identify and manage clinically 'at risk' patients. *Nurse Education Today*, *30*(6), 515–520.

Loh, A., Simon, D., Wills, C. E., Kirston, L., Niebling, W., & Harter, M. (2007). The effects of a shared decision-making intervention in primary care of depression: A cluster-randomized controlled trial. *Patient Education and Counseling*, *67*(3), 324–332.

Lunney, M. (2008). Critical need to address accuracy of nurses' diagnoses. *The Online Journal of Issues in Nursing*, *13*(1). doi:10.3912/OJIN.Vol13No01PPT06

Mackenzie, J. S. (2011). Responding to emerging diseases: Reducing the risks through understanding the mechanisms of emergence. *WHO: Western Pacific Surveillance and Response Journal*, *2*(1), 1–33.

Moorhead, S., Johnson, M., Maas, M. L., & Swanson, E. (2013). *Nursing outcomes classification (NOC): Measurement of health outcomes* (5th ed.). St. Louis, MO: Elsevier.

North American Nursing Diagnosis Association International. (2010). *NANDA-I Nursing Diagnoses: Definitions and Classification 2009–2011*. Retrieved from http http://www.nanda.org/NursingDiagnosisFAQ.aspx

Ohno-Machado, L. (2011). Electronic health records and computer-based clinical decision support: Are we there yet? *Journal of American Information Association*, *18*(2), 109. doi:10.1136/amiajnl-2011-000141

Pesut, D. J. (2008). Thoughts on thinking with complexity in mind. In C. Lindberg, S. Nash, & C. Lindberg (Eds.), *On the edge: Nursing in the age of complexity* (pp. 211–238). Bordentown, NJ: Plexus Press.

Public Health Agency of Canada. (2011). *Determinants of health*. Retrieved from http://www.phac-aspc.gc.ca/index-eng.php

Sleeper, J. A., & Thompson, C. (2008). The use of hi fidelity simulation to enhance nursing students' therapeutic communication skills. *International Journal of Nursing Education Scholarship*, *5*(1), 1–12.

Whitley, G. G., & Gulanick, M. (1996). Barriers to the use of nursing diagnosis language in clinical settings. *International Journal of Nursing Terminologies and Classifications*, *7*, 25–32.

Wright, L. M., & Leahey, M. (2009). *Nurses and families: A guide to family assessment and intervention* (5th ed.). Philadelphia, PA: F.A. Davis.

Nursing Theory and Theories Used in Nursing

LAURIE CLUNE AND DAVID GREGORY

Elizabeth Shannon is a nursing student in the first year of a degree program. She has overheard senior students making comments such as, "Theory is boring," "You will never use theory," and "You don't use theory in the real world." Elizabeth wonders whether learning about theory is necessary to practice nursing.

CHAPTER OBJECTIVES

By the end of this chapter, you will be able to:

1. Define the terms *concept*, *variable*, *theory*, and *hypothesis*.
2. Discern how Nightingale's work influenced the development of nursing knowledge.
3. Define the nursing metaparadigm concepts: person, health, environment, nursing, and social justice.
4. Describe selected nursing theorists and their views of the metaparadigm.
5. Compare types of critical social theories used in knowledge generation and nursing practice.
6. Describe how critical social theories influence how nurses understand, research, and theorize about phenomena.

KEY TERMS

Concept   An idea that we conceive (in our minds) to represent the world around us. Typically, a concept is a general abstract notion or idea about particular things that we see, hear, feel, taste, and touch (ideas about concrete things; e.g., "obesity"). Notions or ideas can also be about things that are abstract (things that we cannot claim to experience through our senses; e.g., the notion of "spirit").

Critical Social Theories (CST)   Theories suggesting that social reality historically produces power imbalances that can be critically examined. Knowledge, applied to critically analyze and challenge these realities, can serve to emancipate (free) people from the social forces of domination, oppression, or marginalization by others in power. The intent of CST is to bring about positive changes in the conditions that affect people's lives.

Grand Nursing Theories   Theories offering a general orientation or philosophical stance about nursing.

Hypotheses   Specific statements used by researchers to predict a relationship between or among variables. They serve as the link or bridge between theory and research and, as such, are used to test theory. A standardized process (the scientific method) is used to accept or reject hypotheses and ultimately confirm or disconfirm theory.

Metaparadigm   A set of concepts or ideas that is important to the discipline of nursing. The metaparadigm includes those concepts that are central or core to nursing: person, health, nursing, and environment. Recently, the concept of "social justice" is suggested as an element of nursing's metaparadigm.

Midrange (or middle range) Nursing Theories   Theories informed by practice and research and offer general direction for everyday nursing practice.

Nursing Practice Theories   Theories concerned with specific nursing situations and focused interventions.

Nursing Theories   Theories focused on nursing and the care of people. Typically, they address elements of the metaparadigm. These theories can exist at different levels of understanding or abstraction.

Social Justice   A concept that concerns fairness in society and states that all people, regardless of financial or social circumstances, ethnic origin, gender, religion, age, impairment, and sexuality, should have equal chances to succeed in life. Social justice is both a goal and process. Full and equal participation of all groups in a society is the goal of social justice. The process for its attainment should be inclusive and affirming of human potential to create change and address oppression.

Theory   Sets of ideas (concepts, variables) used to describe, explain, or predict the physical and social worlds. Theory takes concepts and suggests relationships within, between, or among them. In nursing, theory informs practice (what we do and how we do it) and, at the same time, practice informs, challenges, or confirms theory (our nursing realities compared to and contrasted with theory).

Variables   A change observable in characteristic, number, or quantity; can also be measured or counted by a researcher. "Weight" is an example of a variable; it can be quantified or measured. There are also categorical variables that are qualitative. They describe a quality or characteristic of something. For example, "hunger" can be reported as ravenous, peckish, or not hungry at all. These variables (weight, hunger) may be present in a concept (obesity).

Setting the Stage: Concepts and Theory

This chapter is designed to acquaint you, a student engaged in baccalaureate nursing education, with a basic understanding of concepts and theory. A brief account of the evolution of nursing knowledge is offered by taking a historical journey through nursing milestones. It is important to note this chapter is by no means an exhaustive discussion of theory. Other resources can provide you with more comprehensive descriptions of specific theories. This chapter provides an overview of the development of knowledge and theory in nursing. It will also assist you to understand that nursing (practice, research, education, and administration) makes use of many theories. Although some theory has its roots in nursing (i.e., developed by nurses for nursing), many other theories have been imported from other disciplines into nursing. These imported theories are most often adapted and revised to ensure a "good fit" with nursing.

What Is a Concept?

A **concept** is a general idea or mental notion that represents some aspect of our experiences and our world. Our understanding and sense of some concepts can change over time. For example, the concept of "heart disease" was originally applied to men; more recently, we have come to understand that heart disease greatly affects women. Based on research, we have come to know that heart disease is a lived experience and that gender (a **variable** and a concept) has an impact on that experience. Concepts are important in that they serve as the building blocks of theory.

Nurses use concepts to describe patient situations and circumstances. Examples of concepts used by nurses are environment, quality of life, empowerment, empathy, fatigue, resilience, spirituality, hope, caring, compliance, denial, and family-centered care (Lubkin & Larsen, 2013). These concepts are not understood universally, and how they are understood is influenced by context. The meaning of a concept can be different for each person; this is why concepts need to be clearly defined in practice and with research.

Grief is a concept that is abstract; having different meaning for different people. There are various definitions of grief (Table 11.1) (Wright & Hogan, 2008).

What Is Theory?

A **theory** comprises several concepts used to explain a phenomenon (what we are interested in understanding). Theory helps us to organize knowledge, make sense of ideas, and promote new discoveries to advance the practice of nursing (Meleis, 2012). Typically a body of knowledge, which is created through research, supports or helps to refine the theory. A theory can be tested. Is it right? Does it reflect reality? Does it accurately describe, explain, or predict things that we are concerned about? The research process is used to test theory. The research process is discussed in Chapter 12 (Nursing Research). You are likely familiar with the concept of **hypothesis**. Hypotheses suggest relationships between and among concepts in a theory. In quantitative research, and through the application of statistics, hypotheses formally test such relationships as suggested by theories. In qualitative research, one can suggest a hypothesis; however, it is not formally tested through statistical processes. Rather, people's stories and accounts of their experiences can help us to better understand concepts, the relationships between and/or among concepts, and whether or not the theory reflects the social realities revealed in participants' interviews.

Understanding the Place of Theory and Knowledge Development in Nursing

In this section, we want you to understand that theory is very much a part of nursing practice. Theory is not something you solely learn in a course (or the classroom) and then not use again. Theory and practice are inextricably linked. Nurses engage in practice, education, administration, and research using theory. Theory is developed from these areas, and importantly, practice, education, administration, and research also inform theory. And so, theory does not exist in isolation of nursing practice; it is intimately connected to it. Theory informs practice; and in a pas de deux, nursing practice contributes to theory formation and/or theory testing. Research connects theory to practice and practice to theory. Theory is not something removed from practice; it is very much a part of the real world of nursing (practice, research, education, and administration). See Figure 11.1 for an illustration of these relationships.

TABLE 11.1	Definitions of Grief	
Author	Grief Definition	Model
Kübler-Ross (Freeman, 2005)	Grief is described as a reaction to a personal trauma or change.	Five stages of grief: denial, anger, bargaining, depression, and acceptance
Bowlby (Worden, 2005)	Grief is something that happens when an affectionate attachment is lost or broken.	Phases of mourning: numbing, yearning and searching, disorganization, reorganization
Lindermann (Freeman, 2005)	Grief is a process of healing.	Grief work tasks: emancipation from the bondage of the deceased, readjustment to the environment in which the deceased is missing, and formation of new relationships
Rando (1993)	Grief is a process of mourning.	Six R model of mourning: phases an individual progresses through to recognize, react, recollect, readjust, relinquish, and reinvent

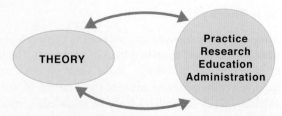

Figure 11.1 The relationship between theory and practice, research, education, and administration.

To appreciate knowledge development in nursing, consideration of the historical trends and the context of the profession's evolution is also warranted.

Historical Overview of Nursing Knowledge Development

To understand knowledge development and theory used in nursing, you need to consider the historical development of nursing. In England, during the 1800s, poor, uneducated women tended to the needs of wealthy people in their homes. They were called "nurse" or governess. This role, in part, was to provide domestic help, look after the children in the home, and tend to the needs of the sick. Formal education or training was not needed to assume such positions. Furthermore, these nursing jobs were viewed in society as being undesirable.

In the 19th century, women began to move off farms and into cities as a result of urbanization and industrialization (McPherson, 1996a). This shift resulted in women seeking paid employment in cities. To secure better employment and wages, women sought education. Nursing, as a profession, became more acceptable as a result of nurses seeking formal training, education, and authority (Hegge, 2013). This resulted in a gradual and positive shift in the social perception toward nursing. A formal education in nursing allowed women to gain knowledge in anatomy, elimination, and reproduction. Nurses learned how to care for the sick bodies of strangers, mostly men—diseased, injured, or ill from epidemics such as cholera, the battlefield, industrial accidents, and the effects of poverty (Hegge, 2013; Nelson & Rafferty, 2010) (Fig. 11.2).

Florence Nightingale: How Practice Influences Theory Development

Florence Nightingale (Fig. 11.3), considered the foundress of modern nursing, discovered that unsanitary conditions lead to infections and the spread of diseases and contributed to high death rates among soldiers. In 1854, Nightingale was asked by the military to organize a corps of nurses to tend to these men. She found the hospitals to be infested with bugs and rodents, the water supply contaminated, and bodily waste everywhere (Nelson & Rafferty, 2010). Nightingale and her group of nurses

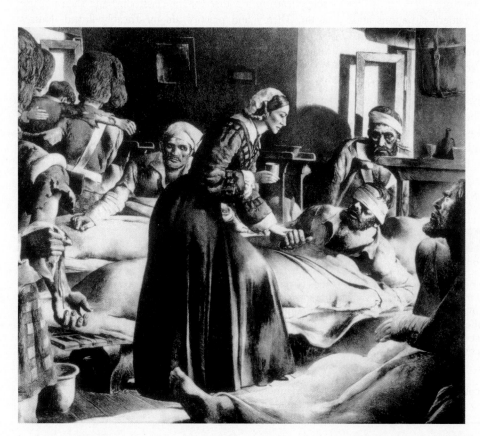

Figure 11.2 Nineteenth century nurse working in a ward.

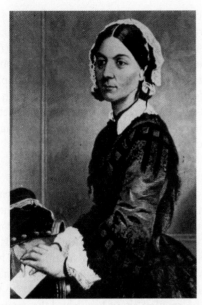

Figure 11.3 Florence Nightingale.

scrubbed walls and floors, established standards for sanitation, prepared cooked food for the patients, washed the laundry, and required fresh air for all patients (McPherson, 1996b). Her seminal report, based on her experiences in the Crimea war hospitals, *Notes on Matters Affecting the Health, Efficiency and Hospital Administration in the British Army* (published in 1858), provided the catalyst for radical changes in hospital care.

Nightingale devoted all of her time tending to the soldiers. In the night, she moved through the hallways carrying a lamp while making rounds. Soldiers named Nightingale the "Lady with the Lamp" (Bates, Dodd, & Rousseau, 2005; Nelson & Rafferty, 2010). Nightingale frequently checked on patients; this action influenced their recovery (see Box 11.1 for a modern-day "take" on Nightingale's rounds.). Her efforts to clean up the war hospital paid off as the death rate decreased by two thirds once Nightingale led the hospital care. Nightingale recognized that a change

in the patient's environment improved his or her health and recovery. Prior to her interventions, most deaths in the Crimea were related to poor sanitation rather than casualties in battle.

Assumptions of Nightingale's Practice Approach to Care

Based on the collection and analysis of data assembled about morbidity (sickness) and mortality (death), Nightingale posited four theoretical assumptions about nursing and health care:

- The nurse and patient relationship is important.
- The environment has a direct effect on the patient's well-being.
- Environmental factors such as fresh air, potable (drinking) water, cleanliness, and light contribute to good health and recovery. The absence or diminishment of these factors can lead to illness and poor health.
- A nurse can act to modify the environment and influence patient outcomes.

Nightingale was a systematic thinker and generator of nursing knowledge; she was a leading statistician during her day and pioneered data visualization of statistics. She developed an environmental approach for nursing care. Nightingale's work from the mid-19th century still influences nursing practice today (Hegge, 2013; Nelson & Rafferty, 2010; Nightingale, 1860).

Through the eyes of a patient

I had abdominal surgery yesterday. Throughout the night, my student nurse, Amy, checked me frequently. She did my vital signs, helped me to the bathroom, and checked the dressing covering my surgical incision. There was some fresh blood on the dressing so Amy wanted to check my incision and change the dressing. Prior to the procedure, she washed her hands, opened a sterile dressing tray, placed a sterile towel by my wound, and put on sterile gloves. I said, "This is a very technical procedure." Amy told me, "This is a sterile procedure. I want to look at your incision and make sure it is not bleeding or showing signs of infection. An infection could make you stay in hospital longer." I did not get an infection because each day the nurses checked my incision and changed my dressing. I went home as planned.

(personal reflection of a surgical patient)

BOX 11.1 Hourly Rounding: The Ottawa Hospital

As part of the Ottawa Hospital Model of Nursing Clinical Practice, nurses engage in hourly rounding. This practice enables nurses to assess and address pain, patient positioning, and toileting with each patient on an hourly basis as appropriate. Patient safety is promoted by reducing pressure ulcers and falls and improving optimal pain management. This intervention also fosters teamwork, encourages consistent patient care and concern, and enhances the therapeutic relationship between nurse and patient. For more information, access The Ottawa Hospital's "Model of Nursing Clinical Practice" (http://www.ottawahospital.on.ca/wps/portal/Base/TheHospital/OurModelofCare/ProfessionalModels/ModelofNursingClinicalPractice)

Think There are several different kinds of knowledge and theory used by Amy when caring for her surgical patient. Can you identify what knowledge or theory she used or applied in conducting the dressing change? Think of the theory guiding assessment, pathophysiology, asepsis, therapeutic communication, and patient education.

The Metaparadigm Framework

The term **metaparadigm** is used when describing a global framework or the way a professional discipline looks at the world (Kuhn, 1970). The primary phenomena or concepts that are of interest and importance to a profession are described by the metaparadigm.

The Metaparadigm of Nursing

Nursing has a metaparadigm that is used to describe the key concepts central to the discipline of nursing (Fawcett & Desanto-Madeya, 2012). Since the 1970s, the concepts of *person*, *health*, *environment*, and *nursing* have been used to describe nursing (Fig. 11.4). It is interesting to note that Nightingale's writings suggest the concepts of the metaparadigm. These concepts of the metaparadigm are used as a framework to organize guiding principles, beliefs, and values of nursing practice.

Some people incorrectly use the term *metaparadigms* (plural) of nursing. The profession of nursing has one metaparadigm that traditionally includes the four concepts.

The Concept of Person

The concept of person, like all concepts, is subject to dynamic changes in understanding over time. Recently, the notion of person has expanded to include "human being" as various societies define person differently and not necessarily in alignment with Euro-Western concepts (Lee & Fawcett, 2013). Persons can be individuals (the patient, the client), groups of people, families, and communities—regardless of setting. Nurses interact with persons for the express purpose of nursing care. The nurse–patient relationship is predicated on the presence of a person or persons; this is where healing partnerships take place. Persons are also considered holistically by nurses. Each person, family, and community has distinct physical, psychological, social, spiritual, cultural, and developmental characteristics. Furthermore, persons

live their lives within the context of systems (e.g., family system, partners/spouses, friends, and social systems), and this dimension of personhood is of importance to nurses and nursing practice. Relevant aspects of a person should be considered when nursing care is provided. For example, a nurse who provides care to a person who identifies with a particular religion should establish how such religious beliefs might influence his or her health choices and healing practices within the context of nursing care.

The Concept of Health

Health is a subjective term that is determined by each person or community. The concept of health includes the physical, psychosocial, relational, and spiritual aspects of an individual, family, or community. Often, the notion of health is described as it relates to a wellness–illness continuum. The English word *health* arises from the Old English word *hale*, meaning wholeness, being whole, sound, or well. See Chapter 8 for further information about health and the determinants of health, that is, those factors that shape or influence health.

Across the lifespan, an individual's expectations and definition of health changes. For example, the ability to walk two flights of stairs before becoming winded may indicate exceptional good health for a 90-year-old. For an 18-year-old, this may indicate that the person is in poor health.

The Concept of Environment

This concept explains the full context of health care and of nursing specifically. It is the totality of all things that impact a person (client, patient, family, community), and includes both the external and internal environments. Home life, mental state, addictions, physical pain, chances of relapse, rewarding work, sociocultural circumstances, religious beliefs, attitude toward death and suffering, and a host of other variables come to define the context of recovery and health. These factors impact not only a patient's health circumstances but also his or her recovery. For example, in the Ontario town of Walkerton, the water supply became contaminated with *Escherichia coli* because of runoff from a nearby farm. Almost 2,300 people became ill, and 7 people died as a result of this environmental tragedy (Schuster et al., 2005).

The Concept of Nursing

The concept of nursing includes attributes, characteristics, and actions of the nurse in relationship with the patient and the nature of care provided. Nursing is profoundly relational, and it is this relational stance that nurses recognize that patients and families are "experts" regarding their own lived lives. Relational nursing practice means being aware of the consequences of exercising power over another. It means entering into a partnership with patients and families where therapeutic and comfort caring occur, where ethical space is created, and culturally safe relationships with clients and health-care team members are enacted (College of Nurses of Ontario, 2009).

The practice of a nurse in Canada is guided by the Canadian Nurses Association's (CNA) Code of Ethics. Each

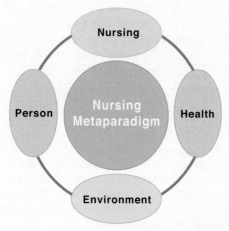

Figure 11.4 The traditional metaparadigm of nursing.

nurse, in all practice settings including hospitals, hospices, physicians' offices, rehabilitation facilities, and communities, has the ethical responsibility to

- Provide safe, compassionate, competent, and ethical care
- Promote health and well-being
- Promote and respect informed decision-making
- Preserve dignity
- Maintain privacy and confidentiality
- Promote justice
- Be accountable (Canadian Nurses Association, 2008, p. 8)

A Fifth Concept: Social Justice

The knowledge and practice of nursing have changed since the 1970s and the introduction of nursing's metaparadigm. Nurses today work in various places, including the community, a patient's home, a homeless shelter, on a street health bus, in a factory, university or college, school, places of care in community health as well as hospitals, hospices, long-term care settings. As a result, nursing care has changed and so has the very nature of nursing knowledge, and a new concept, **social justice**, has emerged as central to the metaparadigm of nursing (Schim, Benkert, Bell, Walker, & Danford, 2007) (Fig. 11.5).

Social justice means ensuring the allocation of life resources in a way that benefits the marginalized or vulnerable (such as the poor, or people with disabilities), and constrains the self-interest of the privileged, such as the wealthy and able bodied. The term *resources* includes access to health-care services as well as clean water, food security, housing, employment, income, safety services, and inclusion (Canadian Nurses Association, 2009). Nurses have taken on an advocate role, speaking up for the disadvantaged or vulnerable members of society. Instead of focusing solely on an individual, nurses taking a social justice approach consider how issues influence the entire population. For example, when setting up a breastfeeding support group in a community, a public health nurse considers if all mothers will have access to the location. Setting up a group in a location that can be reached only by mothers who have access to a car will disadvantage other mothers who do not own a vehicle and must rely on public transportation.

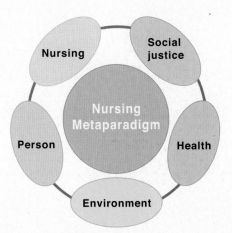

Figure 11.5 Social justice as another metaparadigm concept for nursing.

Nursing Theorists and Nursing Theories

Nursing theories are specific to nursing and address relationships among the major concepts that make up the metaparadigm of nursing. Nursing theories distinguish nursing from other health disciplines and communicate the distinct features of nursing practice. Each nursing theory offers a distinct approach to care. In this next section, you will find a brief summary of the themes outlined in selected nursing theories as well as their approaches to the metaparadigm. Please refer to other sources for a more detailed description of the theory.

Nursing Theories

Nursing theory represents the body of knowledge that is used to describe or explain various aspects or phenomena found in nursing practice. There are different kinds of nursing theories that range from philosophical accounts (or orientations) to **grand nursing theories**, **midrange theories** (narrower in scope, serving as bridges between grand nursing theories and practice), and **nursing practice theories** (developed for use within specific nursing care situations). Examples of grand nursing theories include those proposed by Nightingale, Roy, Watson, and others. Middle-range theories include, for example, Merle Mishel's Uncertainty in Illness Theory, Nola Pender's Health Promotion Model, and Pamela Reed's Self Transcendence Theory. Middle-range theories "emerge at the intersection of research and practice, when theory guides practice, practice generates research questions, and research informs understanding of theory and practice" (Liehr, 2005, p. 154). Practice-level theories (nursing practice theories) provide a framework for nursing interventions or activities—and suggest outcomes or the impact of nursing practice (Parker & Smith, 2010) (Table 11.2).

The changing health-care environment, with the advent of a greater use of technology, informatics, community health practice, and attention to the sociopolitical and economic factors shaping health care, has sparked a shift in how nurses use theory to generate new knowledge.

It is important to understand that each theoretical approach has strengths and limitations. A nurse may use different theoretical approaches in the care of a patient based on the context of his or her everyday life. For example, a nurse may use Watson's theoretical approach when caring with a palliative patient and apply Roy when caring with a rehabilitation patient. Select the theory (or aspects of theories) that best suits your practice situation and your developing sense of what it means to be a nurse and engage in nursing practice. Many nursing programs have students write a paper to identify their own approach or theory regarding nursing practice. You will need to review Table 11.2 and engage in further reading to meet the expectations of such an assignment. As you gain practice experience and progress through your nursing program, the middle-range theories and the nursing practice theories will become increasingly relevant to you.

(text continues on page 201)

TABLE 11.2   A Sample of Nursing Theorists and Nursing Theories

Theorist	Year Theory Developed	Country	Highlights of the Theory	Approach to the Metaparadigm
Hildegard Peplau (1909–1999) A psychiatric nurse	1952	United States	Introduced in 1952, Peplau's theory focuses on therapeutic relationships between the nurse and patient. This approach was particularly useful in mental health settings. In the 1950s, patients were seen by nurses in a very objective way. Peplau's approach challenged nurses to form a relationship with patients. The nurse–patient relationship involved four phases: 1. **Orientation:** The patient seeks help, and the nurse tries to understand the patient's problem and needs by forming a trusting relationship with the patient. The parameters of the relationship must be established. 2. **Identification:** The patient begins to identify problems to be worked on within relationship. The nurse's role is to help the patient recognize his or her dependent and interdependent role. Through this relationship, the nurse helps the patient to identify and become responsible for his or her health situation and behaviours. 3. **Exploitation:** The patient's trust of the nurse–patient relationship reaches its fullest potential. The patient uses the nurse's knowledge and services to help solve his or her problems. As a result, there is a shift in the balance of power from the nurse to the patient. 4. **Termination:** The patient has had his or her needs met which can now result in the termination of the nurse–patient relationship. The patient has become self-reliant, and the services of the nurse are no longer required.	Person: A person is described as the subject of his or her own experiences rather than the object of care. Health: includes interpersonal and intra-personal experiences Environment: includes the person's interpersonal experiences and the relationships he or she has in life Nursing: The environment of the patient is used to assist in recovery. A nurse takes on many roles during the relationship with a patient: *stranger, resource, teacher, counselor, surrogate, active leader, and technical expert.*
Virginia Henderson (1897–1996) Defines nursing	1966	United States	Henderson's unique contribution is she defined nursing in a way that made it distinct from medicine. Nurses care for patients until patients can care for themselves. Patients need the following 14 fundamental elements: 1. To breathe normally 2. To eat and drink adequately 3. To eliminate body wastes 4. To move and maintain desirable postures 5. To have sleep and rest 6. To select suitable clothes—dress and undress 7. To maintain body temperature within normal range by adjusting clothing and modifying environment 8. To keep the body clean and well groomed and protect the integument 9. To avoid dangers in the environment and injuring others 10. To communicate with others in expressing emotions, needs, fears, or opinions 11. To worship according to one's faith 12. To work in such a way that there is a sense of accomplishment 13. To play or participate in various forms of recreation 14. To learn, discover, or satisfy the curiosity that leads to normal development and health and use the available health facilities	Person: a physical being with various needs. A person is in relationships with others in order to meet these needs. Health: is defined by having the 14 fundamental elements Environment: the physical surroundings of the patient. A nurse manages the patient's environment by helping him or her to perform the 14 fundamental elements independently. Nursing: to assist a person who is unable to meet one or more of the 14 basic needs. "The unique function of the nurse is to assist the individual, sick or well, in the performance of those activities contributing to health or its recovery (or to peaceful death) that he would perform unaided if he had the necessary strength, will or knowledge" (Henderson, 1966, p. 15).

Sister Callista Roy (1938–) Adaptation model of nursing	1976	United States	Roy defines *adaptation* as, "The process and outcome whereby the thinking and feeling person uses conscious awareness and choice to create human and environmental integration" (Roy, 1997, p. 44). A person is a biopsychosocial being who is in constant interaction with a changing environment. To respond positively to environmental changes, a person must adapt. There are four modes of adaptation: physiological needs, self-concept, role function, and interdependence. The goal of nursing is to facilitate adaptation.	Person: interacts with his or her physical and social environments, the world, and God. A person must adapt to environmental stimuli. Health: In an environment, a person must interact and adapt. Environment: stimuli that is constantly changing Nursing: promotes the patient's adaptation in experiences such as health, quality of life, and death with dignity. This is done through the nurse's assessment of behaviours and factors that influence a person's adaptive abilities and by interventions to enhance the environment.
Jean Watson (1940–) Theory of human caring	1979	United States	The nurse, through the establishment of a caring relationship with the patient, can treat the body, mind, and spirit. When the nurse and the patient come together, they experience a caring moment. It is through the caring moment connection between the two that transformation and healing can occur. These moments are shaped by the nurse's attitude and competence. Watson identifies 10 Caritas Processes: 1. Embrace altruistic values and Practice loving kindness with self and others. 2. Instill faith and hope and honor others. 3. Be sensitive to self and others by nurturing individual beliefs and practices. 4. Develop helping – trusting- caring relationships. 5. Promote and accept positive and negative feelings as you authentically listen to another's story. 6. Use creative scientific problem-solving methods for caring decision making. 7. Share teaching and learning that addresses the individual needs and comprehension styles. 8. Create a healing environment for the physical and spiritual self which respects human dignity. 9. Assist with basic physical, emotional, and spiritual human needs. 10. Open to mystery and allow miracles to enter (Watson & Woodward, 2010).	Person: The physical body is restricted in space and time, but the mind and soul are not. Health: When there is a high level of physical, mental, and social functioning, the person can adapt to changes. Nursing: A human science of a person's health and illness experience is mediated by the professional, personal, scientific, ethical, and human transaction of a nurse. Environment: the internal and external influences that shape one's health

(continued on page 200)

TABLE 11.2   A Sample of Nursing Theorists and Nursing Theories (continued)

Theorist	Year Theory Developed	Country	Highlights of the Theory	Approach to the Metaparadigm
Margaret Campbell (1923–1992) University of British Columbia (UBC) Model of Nursing	1972	Canada	This model is a behavioural system approach to orient nurses in understanding the patient as an individual experiencing various critical periods throughout the life cycle. An individual has nine basic human needs or subsystems: achieving, affective, ego-valuative, excretory, ingestive, protective, reparative, respiratory, and satiative. When something happens to one subsystem, all are affected.	Person: An individual with nine basic needs. These needs are met by coping mechanisms. Health: stability of the needs Nursing: activities that help an individual learn and maximize his or her coping abilities to manage critical situations in his or her life cycle Environment: anything outside an individual's system
F. Moyra Allen (1921–1996) McGill model of nursing	1986	Canada	This model promotes a collaborative family-centered approach to care. Nurses engage with the person/family to maintain, strengthen, and develop health teaching by promoting a supportive learning environment. Together, the nurse and person set goals and build on strengths.	Person: the family of other social group Health: a social process that can be described, measured, and modified Nursing: the response of a professional to individuals seeking healthy living Environment: a social context where learning takes place

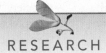

RESEARCH

EDUCATIONAL INNOVATION: A THEORIZED APPROACH TO APPLYING CARPER'S FUNDAMENTAL PATTERNS OF KNOWING WITH HIGH-FIDELITY SIMULATION

Nursing theory is actively used in contemporary education and research. For example, a group of educators at Ryerson University's Daphne Cockwell School of Nursing engaged in designing an approach to simulation using Barbara Carper's fundamental patterns of knowing (Table 11.3).

Carper's theory (1978) proposes four ways of knowing: (1) empirics (the science of nursing), (2) esthetics (the art of nursing), (3) personal knowledge in nursing, and (4) ethics (moral knowledge in nursing). These different types of knowing were used in the scenario development to frame the scenario, learning objectives, and debriefing experiences of nursing students.

Outcomes

Carper's work supported framing learning objectives, templates, and scripts and debriefing that expanded students' ways of thinking and doing in simulation. This approach within the context of high-fidelity simulation better represented the real world of nursing. In particular, students acknowledged relational cues and engaged in interpersonal communication, thereby gaining insight into the client's story and the contextual details of the patient scenario.

McGovern, B., Lapum, J., Clune, L., & Martin, L. S. (2013). Theoretical framing of high-fidelity simulation with Carper's fundamental patterns of knowing in nursing. Journal of Nursing Education, 52(1), 46–49.

TABLE 11.3 Carper's Ways of Knowing

The scenario: A woman in labour delivers full-term baby. The mother is 24 years old and lives in her parents' basement with her boyfriend. Throughout the pregnancy, the mother has smoked and used illicit drugs.

Way of Knowing as Defined by Carper	Definition	Practice Questions to Encourage Various Ways of Knowing
Empirics	Scientific, factual, and objective data used to explain a phenomenon	The vital signs of the mother are taken. The student nurse is asked to assess these empirical values in comparison to normal expected values.
Esthetics	Subjective knowledge developed from personal experiences	Student nurse is asked to consider ways of forming a relationship and demonstrating empathy with the mother.
Personal knowing	Knowledge that emerges from an interaction between the nurse and the patient	The student nurse is asked to reflect on his or her personal values and beliefs about health, illness, families, and childbirth. The student nurse is asked to consider how personal values may influence the interaction with the mother.
Ethics	The moral knowledge that a nurse possesses; what is right and wrong	The student is asked to consider how conflicting value judgments about what is right and wrong may influence the nurse–patient relationship.

Theories Used by Nursing

Considerable development of nursing theory has occurred within the discipline of nursing over a relatively short period of time, that is, within the last 50 years. The literature reveals grand, middle or midrange, and nursing practice theories. It is important that nursing develop its own body of knowledge that is unique to the discipline of nursing (this is one characteristic of a profession). There are also many theories that have been imported from other disciplines and used within nursing.

In the next section, we examine how the concept of disability is understood by biomedical theory and then by critical social theory, including feminist theory. Exploring disability through these different theoretical lenses illustrate how theories potentially influence or shape nursing practice concerning people living with disabilities. Theories are not without consequences; they advance a particular way of understanding the world, including people in it.

Think Think about the non-nursing courses you have completed as part of your program of studies. Can you identify theories from these courses that are relevant, or indeed have a presence within nursing? Consider your liberal arts and humanities courses. What about knowledge and theory from the basic and natural sciences (biology, microbiology, chemistry) and the social sciences (ethics, anthropology, sociology, psychology, women's studies)? Can you apply concepts and theories from these disciplines in your patient care situations?

Theories at Work: Contrasting Biomedical, Critical Social Theory, and Feminist Theory Perspectives on Disability

Critical social theories (CST) are used to address social and political conditions that cause oppression. These conditions influence the health and health care provided to Canadians. Such theories emphasize the need for emancipation, that is, liberation from oppression and the improvement of the human condition.

There are many theories that take a critical social approach; some include feminist theory, queer theory, anti-oppressive practice, and critical race theory. Central to each critical approach is a commitment to investigating the objective appearance of the world and exposing the underlying social relationships that create inequity in social, economic, and power relations. History produces and reproduces social ways of being. One who challenges the status quo in the social world is taking a critical social approach.

Disability as Understood Through the Lens of Biomedical Theory

In health care, the dominant way of viewing disability is from biomedical theory. A person is labelled as abled (normal) or disabled (abnormal) through an assessment of his or her biophysical functioning. Disability is viewed as a biologic problem experienced by the individual; it is pathological or dysfunctional. Health professionals such as physicians, nurses, and physiotherapists decide if a person has a disability. *Disability* is defined as a loss or limitation of one's functioning. For example, a patient with impaired mobility who requires a wheelchair may be considered disabled or impaired. Biomedical theory suggests that disability can be cured through corrective surgery and physical and occupational rehabilitation. It is through such processes that the disabled person can have normal functioning. Biomedical understanding of disability has been criticized by many in the disability community. Disability theorist, Paul Longmore (2005), suggests, "Telethons . . . are the single most powerful cultural mechanism defining the public identities of people with disabilities in our society today." Telethons are a sociopolitical way of disadvantaging people with disabilities. Disability activists believe that telethons exploit people with disabilities and portray businesses that donate large amounts of money to these events as good corporate citizens. Telethons portray people with disabilities and illnesses as needy and requiring the charity of others in order to cope with their conditions. The public develops assumptions and attitudes about people with disabilities because of what they see on telethon events.

Disability as Understood by Critical Social Theory

An alternate way to consider the concept of disability is from a critical social approach. From this perspective, people become disabled by the social, environmental, and attitudinal barriers that prevent a person from participating in all aspects of society. CSTs of disability suggest that it is systemic barriers, negative attitudes, and social exclusion that disable people. CST is concerned with equality and the changes required of society to enable people living with disabilities. Disability oppression is rooted in degradation, dependency, and powerlessness (Charlton, 1998). Charlton's (1998) seminal work, *Nothing About Us Without Us*, offered the first theoretical overview of disability oppression noting similarities and differences paralleling racism, sexism, and colonialism.

Through the eyes of a patient

*I*n my family, there are both little and average-sized people. Renovations were being done to the deck of the family room. Because three people in my family were little, they wanted to lower the railings to accommodate and make a safe environment for everyone. This deck would be little people friendly.

The building inspector arrived to review the structure and make sure it met the building safety codes and laws. Building codes require that the deck design must meet certain specifications to be considered safe. When the inspector saw the deck and railings he said that the structure was unsafe because the railings were too low. The standard railing height, according to the building code, must be at a level appropriate for average-sized people. Having a railing to fit little people was unacceptable. The inspector could not pass the structure because it failed to meet the building code.

(personal reflection of a family member)

You can see the way society is socially organized and controlled, in this case, through building codes that do not meet the needs of all people. The code is designed around what is considered average or normal, a policy that excludes the safety of little people. When environments are changed, people regardless of their age or ability can be advantaged.

Disability as Understood Through Feminist Theory

Feminist theories emerged out of the feminist movement and the fight for equal rights for women. This perspective seeks to understand the nature of gender inequality through the examination of women's (or vulnerable group) roles and everyday experience in society.

In the late 20th century, various feminists began to argue that gender roles are socially constructed, meaning that our society tells us through social expectations or norms what is acceptable and expected for male or females, and these signals are evident throughout the lifespan. See Table 11.4, which lists some common social cues, unspoken rules, and social expectations concerning gender.

There are interesting parallels between being female and having a disability. Both groups can be marginalized. Being female can become problematic when the sociocultural (society) context creates disadvantage for women. Similarly, disability can be viewed as a disadvantage because of social, cultural, attitudinal, and environmental barriers (Hiranandani, 2005). Both disability and gender can be socially constructed to

TABLE 11.4	Social Constructs	
Life Stage	Female	Male
Birth Childhood	• Wear pink clothing • Play with dolls • Take dancing lessons and modern dance such as ballet	• Wear blue clothing • Play with trucks • Play sports such as football, lacrosse, and hockey
Adolescent Adult	• Will be successful in languages and the arts • Will work in occupational roles such as nurse, primary school teacher, and hair stylist • Will be responsible for child care • Will take on household chores such as cooking and cleaning	• Will be successful in math and sciences • Will work in occupational roles such as firefighter, police officer, coal miner, doctor, and business executive • Will take on household chores such as cutting the grass or shovelling the snow
Older adult	• Will live longer than her husband • Will engage in hobbies such as knitting and sewing	• Will be cared for by his wife • Will engage in hobbies such as woodworking

marginalize people (women and people living with a disability). "A feminist analysis of disability is important because more than half of disabled people are women . . . and because the feminist movement has questioned the most deep-seated issues about cultural representations of the body" (Hiranandani, 2005, Feminist theories section, para. 3).

The Social Organization of Knowledge

Dr. Dorothy Smith, PhD, a Canadian sociologist and feminist, believes that the world is socially organized in ways that advantage some and disadvantage others. As a lecturer at the University of California, Berkeley, from 1964 to 1966, she noticed that the expectations of her as a professor and mother were different from those applied to her male colleagues in the same professional positions and roles as fathers. Smith was the only woman teaching in a faculty of 44. She, and other women's movement activists speaking out at this time, found women were experiencing inequities not only in the university but also in society.

Smith (1987, 2005) developed a sociologic approach for understanding women and marginalized people. Beginning from the standpoint of women and what happens in their everyday lives, Smith believes we can see how the world is socially organized to place people in positions of power or oppression. Many nurses have used Smith's approach to examine issues of nursing and health care.

To be honest, I was somewhat afraid of theory. I felt that I would not understand what it is all about. But theory isn't something to be frightened of anymore. Theory is all around me, and it is a part of everything that I do as a future nurse. I encounter theory in all of my classes and in the clinical setting. I use it when I prepare for my patient assignments. I also make use of it when I am providing care with my patients. Nursing theory was supposed to be boring, but I found it interesting. I especially liked the McGill model of situational nursing care. Even though I am just a nursing student, I can see how this approach to nursing will make me a better nurse as I become more experienced.

Elizabeth Shannon, nursing student

Critical Thinking Exercises

▶ The metaparadigm of nursing (person, environment, health, and nurse) has been enhanced to include social justice due to changes in how nurses practice. Can you think of other elements, such as ethics, for example, that might be considered in the future?

▶ Nurses use many theories to inform their practice each day. Can you name some other types of theories that shape nursing practice?

▶ You are on a nursing unit when a staff member says, "Nursing theory is just for academics. It has nothing to do with the reality of nursing practice." How would you respond to this comment?

Multiple-Choice Questions

1. A theory is:
   a. Composed of sets of ideas (concepts, variables) used to describe, explain, or predict the physical and social worlds
   b. A set of concepts that have relationships within, between, or among them
   c. Used to inform nursing practice
   d. All of the above

2. The metaparadigm of nursing includes the following concepts:
   a. Nursing, people, critical social theory, environment, wellness
   b. Nursing, person, environment, health, social justice
   c. Nursing, health, person, environment
   d. Environmental theory, ethics, health, social justice

3. Social justice is:
   a. An approach best suited when working with marginalized or vulnerable people
   b. An approach best suited to working with rich and able-bodied people
   c. An approach used in every practice setting
   d. An approach to be used in a community practice setting

4. List the four ways of knowing as described by Carper.
  a. Empiric, altruistic, personal, ethical
  b. Ethics, abstract, personal knowing, empirical
  c. Personal knowing, ethics, esthetic, experiential
  d. Ethics, personal knowing, esthetics, empirics

Suggested Lab Activities

● Break into small groups. In each group:
  a. Create your own definition of the nursing metaparadigm: person, environment, health, nursing, and social justice.

  b. Consider: Why did you define the concepts of the metaparadigm in this way? What life experiences shaped your definition?

  c. Select a nursing theorist and compare and contrast the theorist's definition of the metaparadigm with your definitions. What observations can you make between your definitions of metaparadigm concepts and those of the nurse theorist?

● Look up one midrange theory in nursing. Discuss how this theory illustrates a connection between theory, practice, and research.

REFERENCES AND SUGGESTED READINGS

Bates, C., Dodd, D., & Rousseau, N. (2005). *On all frontiers: Four centuries of Canadian nursing.* Ottawa, ON: University of Ottawa Press.

Canadian Nurses Association. (2008). *Code of ethics for registered nurses* (2008 centennial edition). Retrieved from http://www.cnaaiic.ca/CNA/documents/pdf/publications/Code_of_Ethics_2008_e.pdf

Canadian Nurses Association. (2009). *Ethics in practice for registered nurses.* Ottawa, ON: Author.

Carper, B. A. (1978). Fundamental patterns of knowing in nursing. *Advances in Nursing Science, 1*(1), 13–24.

Charlton, J. (1998). *Nothing about us without us: Disability oppression and empowerment.* Berkeley, CA: University of California Press.

College of Nurses of Ontario. (2009). *National competencies in the context of entry-level registered nurse practice.* Toronto, ON: Author.

Fawcett, J., & Desanto-Madeya, S. (2012). *Analysis and evaluation of nursing models and theories: Contemporary nursing knowledge.* Philadelphia, PA: F. A. Davis.

Freeman, S. (2005). *Grief and loss. Understanding the journey.* Belmont, CA: Thomas Learning Academic Resource Centre.

Hegge, M. (2013). Nightingale's environmental theory. *Nursing Science Quarterly, 23*(3), 211–219.

Henderson, V. (1966). *The nature of nursing: A definition and its implications for practice, research, and education.* Riverside, NJ: MacMillan.

Hiranandani, V. (2005). Towards a critical theory of disability in social work. *Critical Social Work, 6*(1). Retrieved from http://www1.uwindsor.ca/criticalsocialwork/towards-a-critical-theory-of-disability-in-social-work

Kuhn, T. (1970). *The structure of scientific revolutions* (2nd ed.). Chicago, IL: University of Chicago Press.

Lee, R. C., & Fawcett, J. (2013). The influence of the metaparadigm of nursing on professional identity development among RN-BSN students. *Nursing Science Quarterly, 26*(1), 96–98.

Liehr, P. (2005). Looking at symptoms with a middle-range theory lens. *Advance Studies in Nursing, 3*(5), 152–157.

Longmore, P. K. (2005). *The hands that feeds. Charity telethons and disability activism.* Toronto, ON: Ryerson University. Retrieved from http://www.ryerson.ca/ds/focusBoxes/charity_telethons.html

Lubkin, I., & Larsen, P. (2013). *Chronic illness: Impact and intervention* (8th ed.). Burlington, MA: Jones & Bartlett Learning.

McPherson, K. M. (1996a). *Bedside matters: The transformation of Canadian Nursing, 1900–1990.* Toronto, ON: Oxford University Press.

McPherson, K. M. (1996b). Carving out a past: The Canadian Nurses' Association war memorial. *Histoire Sociale/Social History, 29*(58), 417–429.

Meleis, A. I. (2012). *Theoretical nursing: Development and progress* (5th ed.). New York, NY: Lippincott Williams & Wilkins.

Nelson, S., & Rafferty, A. M. (2010). *Notes on Nightingale: The influence and legacy of a nursing icon.* New York, NY: Cornell University Press.

Nightingale, F. (1860). *Notes of nursing: What it is, and what it is not.* New York, NY: D. Appleton.

Ottawa Hospital. (n.d.). *Model of nursing clinical practice.* Retrieved from http://www.ottawahospital.on.ca/wps/portal/Base/TheHospital/OurModelofCare/ProfessionalModels/ModelofNursingClinicalPractice

Parker, M., & Smith, M. (2010). *Nursing theories and nursing practice* (3rd ed.). Philadelphia, PA: F. A. Davis.

Rando, T. A. (1993). *Treatment of complicated mourning.* Champaign, IL: Research Press.

Roy, C. (1997). Future of the Roy model: Challenges to redefine adaptation. *Nursing Science Quarterly, 10*(1), 42–48.

Schim, S., Benkert, R., Bell, S., Walker, D., & Danford, C. (2007). Social justice: Added metaparadigm concept for urban health nursing. *Public Health Nursing, 24*(1), 73–80.

Schuster, C. J., Ellis, A. G., Robertson, W. J., Charron, D. F., Aramini, J. J., Marshall, B. J., & Medeiros, D. T. (2005). Infectious disease outbreaks related to drinking water in Canada, 1974–2001. *Canadian Journal of Public Health, 96*(4), 254–258.

Smith, D. E. (1987). *The everyday world as problematic: A feminist sociology.* Boston, MA: Northeastern University Press.

Smith, D. E. (2005). *Institutional ethnography: A sociology of the people.* Lanham, MD: AltaMira Press.

Watson, J., & Woodward, T. (2010). Jean Watson's theory of human caring. In M. E. Parker & M. Smith (Eds.), *Nursing theories and nursing practice* (3rd ed., pp. 351–369). Philadelphia, PA: F. A. Davis.

Worden, J. W. (2005). *Grief counseling and grief therapy: Handbook for mental practitioners* (3rd ed.). New York, NY: Springer Publishing.

Wright, P. M., & Hogan, N. S. (2008). Grief theories and models: Application to hospice nursing practice. *Journal of Hospice & Palliative Care Nursing, 10*(6), 350–357.

Nursing Research and Evidence-Informed Practice

DONNA K. CILISKA AND LINDA PATRICK

Erika is a second-year nursing student with a clinical placement on a medical unit. She finds many practices on this unit that are not the same as the practices on a similar unit where she was placed last year. For example, the nurses in her current placement teach patients with diabetes that it is acceptable to give insulin injections through clothing, whereas the nurses on the other unit taught patients about exposing and cleansing the skin before injecting. Erika can see the potential benefits to the patient of both routines. But which routine is correct? Can it really be okay to inject through clothing?

CHAPTER OBJECTIVES

By the end of this chapter, you will be able to:

1. Differentiate between doing research and using research.
2. Explain the stages of evidence-informed practice.
3. Formulate a searchable question.
4. Describe the search process to locate preappraised literature, including nursing practice guidelines and systematic reviews.
5. Apply research findings to clinical practice after critically appraising their applicability.
6. Locate relevant preappraised research and appraise applicability to current practice.
7. Reflect on the effectiveness of your own practice.

KEY TERMS

Critical Appraisal The careful review of research literature with an assessment of its value or quality and usefulness to inform clinical practice.

Evidence In the context of this chapter, refers to the information derived from clinical research.

Evidence-Informed Practice (EIP) Professional practice should be based on the best available research evidence and applied in conjunction with patient preferences, context, available resources, and practitioner expertise.

Knowledge Translation (KT) The Canadian Institute of Health Research (CIHR, 2013, para. 1) defines knowledge translation as "a dynamic and iterative process that includes synthesis, dissemination, exchange and ethically sound application of knowledge to improve the health of Canadians, provide more effective health services and products and strengthen the healthcare system."

Mixed Methods Use of both quantitative and qualitative research methods in one study.

Nursing Research The process of using research to answer a nursing question as a support to nursing practice.

Qualitative Research Studies involving feelings, perceptions, or observations that are described and not measured.

Quantitative Research Studies involving measurement of variables.

Reflection Thinking about an idea or something you have read or seen with thoughtful consideration to the meaning.

Situational Analysis The collection of information with the intent of trying to understand the bigger context or meaning. This process of analysis or thinking is used to make decisions; in this chapter, it specifically refers to the barriers and supports that will influence the outcome of the proposed changes.

What Is Evidence-Informed Practice?

As a student in a nursing program, you are already familiar with the many hours spent reading and learning the basics in many different subject areas. This required reading is a preparation in becoming a knowledgeable, safe, and competent nurse able to meet the entry-level competencies of the profession and become registered by writing the Canadian Registered Nurse Exam (CRNE). There is an expectation in professional practice that in order to maintain your competency as a practicing nurse, you will engage in continuous learning and professional development throughout your nursing career.

Nurses have embraced evidence-based practice—the notion that decisions about practice should include the best available **evidence**, which is the information derived from clinical research, along with patient preferences, expert opinion, resource availability, and other contextual information. Often, that means that a large number of randomized trials have been synthesized into a recent, high-quality systematic review, but sometimes, there is no research to answer a question, and we have to rely on the other sources of information to make a decision.

It is not hard to understand why evidence-based practice is valued as an ideal. Billions of dollars are spent annually on health-related research. However, it takes an estimated 15 years to get research into recommended policy (Antman et al., 1992) and the minority of patients to get the recommended care (Schuster, McGlynn, & Brook, 1998). In addition, 30% to 40% of patients do not get treatments of proven effectiveness (Grol, 2001) and 20% to 30% of patients received acute care that was not needed or was potentially harmful (Schuster et al., 1998). We have an ethical imperative to give the best care possible and to use the results of high-quality research.

Emphasis on Research Evidence

Many different practitioners now use the term *evidence-based*, including dentists, veterinarians, psychologists, engineers, managers, and pastoral counselors. However, in health care, there has also been a negative reaction to the term. Even though the model clearly incorporates multiple factors, some people believe that the term *evidence-based practice* connotes blind application of research findings. And so there is a move to use the term **evidence-informed practice (EIP)**, and this chapter has adopted this terminology. However, you will still see both terms, and many textbooks and some journals still use the *evidence-based* nursing term. Later in the chapter, the EIP model will be applied. Refer to Figure 12.1, Evidence-informed decision-making.

The Difference Between Using Research and Conducting Research

It is important to distinguish using and applying research from conducting research. There is considerable confusion for some and an inappropriate interchangeable use of the

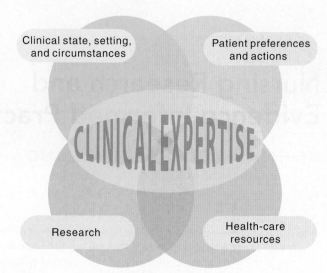

Figure 12.1 Evidence-informed decision-making.

terms. However, they are very different. A researcher will consider a clinical question and decide on a methodology to collect and analyze information from patients in order to answer that question. EIP is about applying the research that others have done. It means searching in the research literature to find an answer to your clinical question, then deciding if the methods of the research were such that you could be confident in the findings, and then deciding if the research can be applicable to your patient population.

The Steps of Evidence-Informed Practice

The listing of the seven steps of EIP as shown in Box 12.1 makes the process seem linear and deceptively simple. The process of research and collecting EIP begins with reflection. **Reflection** allows you to learn from your experiences, to think about how you react to situations, and how patients react to your interactions with them. Reflection is a skill that contributes to lifelong learning about yourself and about your practice. Reflection is a necessary stage to get to the question formulation (Fineout-Overholt & Johnston, 2005). It is important to take time to think about your patients not

---

BOX 12.1   **The Steps of Evidence-Informed Practice**

The steps of EIP are:

0. Reflection
1. Framing the question
2. Searching for research literature
3. Critical appraisal of research literature
4. Synthesis of findings from divergent literature
5. Adaptation of findings to practice
6. Implementation of practice change
7. Evaluation

only in terms of individuals you encounter but also your patient population as a whole. This is best done when you have a quiet time outside of work.

Step 1: Framing the Question

Related to the opening scenario, reflect on busy patients' lives and the fact that they are giving themselves insulin injections possibly four times a day. That means that two injections a day are probably done outside the home. Does that mean that these patients go off to a public washroom and set up their skin cleansing equipment and insulin and syringe and expose some part of their skin, cleanse the skin, inject, and then pack it all up? What if the public washroom is not very clean? What do they do with the information you have taught them about the proper way to prepare for the injection? Your teaching may not fit the reality of your patients' busy lives and may be disregarded. Is there an alternative? Can injections safely be done discreetly, at their desk or at the restaurant, without causing skin infections? This example scenario will be followed in the coming sections as we explore the steps for determining EIP. Refer to Box 12.2, Evidence-Informed Practice—Framing the Question.

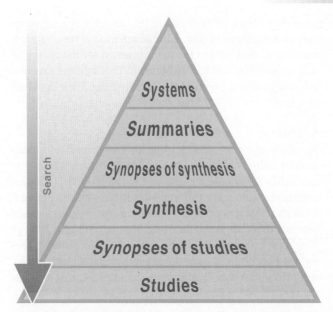

Figure 12.2 The 6S pyramid. (Adapted from DiCenso, A., Bayley, L., & Haynes, R. B. [2009]. Accessing pre-appraised evidence: Fine-tuning the 5S model into a 6S model. *Evidence-Based Nursing, 12,* 99–101. doi:10.1136/ebn.12.4.99-b)

BOX 12.2 Evidence-Informed Practice— Framing the Question

Now you are wondering if insulin injections can safely be done through clothing. Can that be part of your teaching approach? You use the PICO formulation for formatting questions about interventions:

P – patients, populations, or participants
I – intervention
C – comparison
O – outcomes

Using PICO, the question that arises from the scenario could be formulated as:

P – patients with diabetes mellitus who inject insulin
I – injecting insulin through clothing
C – usual skin exposure, cleansing and injection
O – infections, abscesses, lumpiness

For questions of causation, the **I** is changed to **E** for exposure. For example, if you are concerned that cell phone use by preteens causes brain tumors, the question would be formulated as:

P – preteens
E – cell phone use
C – landline only use
O – brain tumors

Finally, if you are wondering about what it is like for patients to experience an illness, surgery, recovery, or to live with diabetes mellitus and have to inject insulin several times a day, the question is formulated as the same **P**, but **S** stands for situation.

P – patients who need to inject insulin several times a day
S – coping with diabetes

Step 2: Searching for Research Literature

After the question is clearly formulated, you will be much more efficient in the search for relevant literature. Refer to the 6S pyramid shown in Figure 12.2, which shows the hierarchy of preappraised evidence. This includes systems, summaries, synopses of the syntheses, syntheses, synopses of studies, and studies. As you will see, the level of detail and specificity increase as you move down toward the base of the pyramid on information sources. Understanding the types of literature and what they contain is necessary to use the 6S pyramid.

Systems

At the top of the pyramid, we have systems that could be electronic systems with sophisticated links to patient records that prompt practitioners regarding guidelines for care: what tests to order or what interventions need to be done. For example, for a patient with Type 2 diabetes, the patient records with the recommended guidelines for care would prompt the caregiver that blood work, eye exam, foot exam, and diet review need to be done. The systems level also includes guidelines. You can access guidelines from the Web; some of the most useful sites that are currently available are provided at the end of the chapter.

Summaries

Summaries are usually text-based and are related to a specific disease or condition. An example includes the website Clinical Evidence (www.clinicalevidence.com). Unfortunately, you must subscribe either individually or via an institution to use this site. You may want to check the library at your school to see if they have a subscription to this resource or a subscription to something similar. Your librarian is a very valuable resource to steer you in the right direction for the most current information and how to access it. This will also save you valuable time and energy as you learn to balance the demands of school.

Synopses

Synopses are brief reports (one to two pages) of preappraised individual studies or systematic reviews which give key methodologic details and results, along with an expert commentary on issues of applying the results in practice. Examples of synopses are found in the evidence-based journals (e.g., Medicine, Nursing, Dentistry, Health Policy). There are currently 23 such journals. Some of these sites are open access, and some require individual or institutional subscription. Again, it is highly recommended that you use the services of the librarian at your school.

Syntheses

Syntheses include systematic reviews of all studies that could be found on a particular focused question. These include The Cochrane Library and the Agency for Healthcare Research and Quality (AHRQ) Evidence-based Practice Center reviews. Both groups have similar, rigorous methods for reviews, and links to the sites are provided at the end of the chapter.

Studies

Studies are the base of the pyramid where the greatest range of information is found on individual studies related to a particular focused question. There are several searchable databases that would help you find individual studies. The most used sites in Canada include MEDLINE, PubMed, and CINAHL, but there are many other specialized databases. PubMed provides a full citation and abstract as well as links to any full-text articles that are free to the public.

Erika searched using the 6S pyramid as her guide. In her placement, there are no evidence-based systems in place, so she checked the National Guideline Clearinghouse; although there were many guidelines about diabetes care, she found nothing specifically about injecting insulin through clothing. She then searched for a preappraised synopsis in the *Evidence-Based Nursing* journal and found an abstract of a single study that injecting insulin through clothing was safe and convenient.

Step 3: Critical Appraisal of Research Literature

How do you know if the information you find at any of the previous search sources is methodologically good enough to use? Can you trust the findings enough to consider applying to a patient population? Unfortunately, even peer-reviewed publications may have used questionable research methods. Unless you have found a preappraised article (such as a synopsis from an evidence-based journal), you must assess the methods of the source of information. This process of judging the quality of the methods is known as **critical appraisal**. Critical appraisal skills are quickly built with practice. Nurses can take courses at the undergraduate, graduate, and continuing education level. There are key quality criteria for any of the resources found in the 6S pyramid. In addition, there are many tools that have been developed to help you structure the critical appraisal.

An internationally accepted standard for critiquing guidelines derives from the Appraisal of Guidelines for Research and Evaluation (AGREE) collaboration (http://www.agreetrust.org/); the tool can also be found at their website. Although the AGREE tool may look intimidating simply given the number of pages, its length is a consequence of the explanations given for every criterion, explanations or scoring, and space for notes regarding your scoring. It is self-explanatory and, depending on the guideline, can usually be completed in well less than an hour.

Most of the available tools for appraising systematic reviews and primary studies are built from key criteria developed by the Evidence-Based Medicine Working Group for the series published in the *Journal of the American Medical Association* (*JAMA*), later collected in a book (Guyatt & Rennie, 2002). A good example is the Critical Appraisal Skills Program (CASP) of the Public Health Resource Unit in the United Kingdom. They have a series of tools with explanations of criteria that are freely accessible online for personal use. The criteria for assessing systematic reviews asks you about factors such as the clarity of the review question, if the search was thorough, the size and precision of the effect, and if the interventions described in the review could be applied to your population or patients. The criteria for intervention studies ask you about factors such as how bias was controlled (if the participants were randomized), the size and precision of the effect, and if the interventions could be applied to your population or patients.

Step 4: Synthesis of Findings From Divergent Literature

A focused search on the top levels of the 6S pyramid for the question regarding injecting insulin through clothing might yield 1 guideline, 2 systematic reviews, and 12 individual studies. Should you read and critically appraise them all? Using the 6S pyramid, start with the reading of the guideline; if it is relevant, you would go on to apply the AGREE tool to appraise the guideline. If you and your colleagues conclude that this guideline is of sufficient quality to be useable, that may conclude the synthesis stage. However, if you conclude it is not a good guideline, you need to proceed to the critical appraisal of the systematic reviews using the AGREE tool.

Systematic Reviews

One way to approach multiple systematic reviews of the same topic is to look first at those with the most recent date of searching. The date of publication may not be relevant, but in the methods under search strategy, it will detail the years included in the search. Then the critical appraisal can be ordered chronologically, starting your appraisal with the review with the most recent searches. This offers some confidence in how up-to-date is the publication. If you find a systematic review that is recent and of high quality, the only need to continue the search would be to look for any other primary studies published after the search dates in the systematic reviews. Were their results similar to the results reported in the systematic review, or have the more recent studies potentially altered the conclusions?

Primary Studies

In order to get the details of more complex intervention (almost anything beyond drug therapy), looking up the primary studies that were included in the guideline or systematic review is required, because these syntheses cannot include the detail that a clinician would need to actually perform the interventions. What if you find no research evidence at any level of the 6S pyramid? Some health-care questions have not yet been answered by research. Expert opinion is the best evidence.

Step 5: Adaptation of Findings to Practice

Research evidence comes from studies of particular samples of populations. You will find that all critical appraisal tools include a question related to applicability, "Can I use this research with my patients (or population)?" In every instance, you must consider the inclusion/exclusion of participants in the study. To answer this question, you need to look at the description of the participants in the study or studies and know the characteristics of your own patient population. For our question about injecting insulin through clothing, there may be different results depending on general hygiene of patient participants.

In addition, you must consider how this research evidence fits with external factors such as the magnitude of health issue in local setting; cost of implementing the intervention, including staff, education, equipment, space, and costs to the patients; availability of personnel to perform the intervention; organizational expertise and capacity; and acceptability of the intervention to patients (Buffett, Ciliska, & Thomas, 2007).

Erika assesses each patient for level of hygiene and uses that information in deciding if she can suggest the patient to inject through his or her clothing. There are no cost implications for staff (beyond their in-service education about this change in practice), and most patients would find it more convenient to be able to inject through their clothing.

Step 6: Implementation of Practice Change

Implementation of EIP is never a solitary activity in nursing. It requires that you interact with other nurses, other health-care professionals, managers in health-care institutions, and with patients. Looking back to our opening scenario, you have now framed the question; searched for, found, and appraised the research evidence; determined it is good enough to use; and you have concluded that for patients with good general hygiene, it is safe for them to inject insulin through their clothing. Now it is necessary to consider how to make this part of the education program for people with diabetes and for nurses to include this in their practice. This stage is also sometimes referred to as **knowledge translation** and the Knowledge to Action Framework (Graham et al., 2006).

As part of the change process, it is recommended that you assess both barriers to practice change and supports from the perspective of individuals involved, the organization, the broader social context, and the actual change you are trying to implement. This structured assessment of barriers and supports is called a **situational analysis**. The analysis will help you plan for strategies to implement change. As with any planned change, it is important to consider both how to build support as well as how to break down barriers. See Box 12.3 for five key questions to assist in planning for knowledge exchange.

The responsibility to educate the staff about practice changes will most likely be delegated to the clinical educator in an organization. After years of teaching about skin exposure and cleansing, it will be difficult for some staff to accept this change. It is important for the clinical educator to anticipate the arguments that some staff will present and the difficulty any change in practice represents to some staff. A smooth adoption of new practices will occur if the staff is engaged in discussion and provided with the evidence to support the changes.

BOX 12.3   Five Key Questions

Lavis, Posada, Haines, and Osei (2004) and Lavis, Robertson, Woodside, McLeod, and Abelson (2003) proposed five key questions to assist in planning for knowledge exchange. Answering these questions will form the basis of an implementation plan.

1. **What (is the message)?** This translates or transforms research findings into an actionable message.
2. **To whom (the audience)?** Be specific when defining who will need to get the message. Understand who are making the decisions.
3. **By whom (the messenger)?** Is the messenger credible and is there a chance for the audience to partner with the messengers?
4. **How (transfer method)?** What is the budget? What is the preferred mechanism for learning new information? Is the audience actively engaged in selected the mechanism? Is the transfer mechanism evidence-based? Is the intervention tailored to overcome the audience's identified barriers?
5. **With what expected impact (evaluation)?** What does the knowledge translation, synthesis and exchange (KTSE) project hope to change?

Step 7: Evaluation

It is important to monitor and evaluate any changes in patient outcomes, so that positive effects can be supported and negative ones remedied. Monitoring the effect of an EIP change on health-care interventions can help the nurse identify which patients are most likely to benefit from the intervention and can highlight flaws in implementation. Because clinical results can differ from those reported in the research literature, ongoing monitoring could help determine why.

As an example of the evaluation process, a hospital EIP group reviewed the literature on skin preparation for venipuncture and concluded the literature favored chlorhexidine. They created a hospital-wide policy, got their ordering/stores department to replace the alcohol swabs with chlorhexidine on the venipuncture preparation trays, had some strategies to communicate these changes to staff, and behold, the staff switched to using chlorhexidine for skin prep.

Some staff will resist teaching patients about injecting insulin through clothing—they have taught about skin exposure and preparation for several years and they are not going to change now! Changing the written policy and having a staff educational session may help to change practice, but what about those staff members who still resist?

If the practitioners follow the policy, is there an impact on the patient population? Five years later, is there any difference in the rate of injection site problems with the patients who come to your clinic? A chart audit before and after would allow you to evaluate that. For those who like logical progressions, a nice sequence is shown in Box 12.4.

Every step in this sequence is a fruitful area for program evaluation or a more formal funded research project. Studying how policy development and implementation take place and factors that affect each stage would increase our understanding about the policy process. We do not know very much about uptake of policy directives or how they get adapted at the clinical unit level. As an outcome, you could evaluate both skin problems in the patient population and the actual teaching practice of the staff.

Erika now has a beginning understanding of evidence-informed practice. She framed a clear question about the safety of injecting insulin through clothing, conducted an efficient search, appraised the results, and made a decision to implement the change of practice. The clinical educators are considering barriers and supports to the implementation in clinic and are planning the implementation and evaluation.

BOX 12.4   Steps in Evaluation

Introduce Policy ▶ Change Practitioner Behavior ▶ Impact Population Outcome

---

Various provincial nursing certification bodies have slightly different requirements, but all have expectations that nurses will practice in an evidence-based way. This means that practicing nurses must understand and use the principles and skills outlined earlier. The legal system uses the standard of usual care rather than best evidence in deciding health-care cases, but hopefully, these two principles will converge because more nurses and health-care organizations use best evidence as the standard of care. This will also allow for nurses to meet the ethical accountability of giving the best care for patients.

Conducting Research Versus Using Research

Thus far, we have only been talking about using research. Using research will be the primary expectation of you as a graduate of a baccalaureate nursing program in Canada. At some point, you may be asked to participate in research, either to collect information for a study or to be a participant, that is, the subject of a research question. If you go on to graduate school, you may be involved in conducting research. It is an exciting business to have clinical questions about your practice and to be able to work toward answering those questions. If no research exists to answer your questions, you might take them to your organization's research committee and see if you can get someone else interested in conducting the study. In order for you to be an informed consumer of research, it is useful to understand the conduct of research.

What Is Nursing Research?

Nursing research is the process of using research to answer a nursing question as a support to nursing practice. Nursing research primarily falls into two methods of inquiry: qualitative and quantitative research. Sometimes, the term is used to indicate that a nurse has conducted the research. Nursing-relevant research also appears in many non-nursing journals. For example, the answer to the opening scenario question (injecting insulin through clothing) appeared in a medical journal. There are specific steps to conduct research, as outlined in Box 12.5.

BOX 12.5   The Steps in Conducting Research

1. Define question.
2. Conduct literature review.
3. Develop methods, information, and consent letters.
4. Get ethics approval.
5. Collect data.
6. Analyze data.
7. Write report.
8. Disseminate report.

Approaches to Research

There are many different kinds of questions that come up when providing nursing to patients. What caused the condition? What is the usual progression of this disease? Is it contagious? How will the patient be affected 20 years from now? Could this have been prevented? How can it successfully be treated now? What are the side effects or potential harms of treatment? How can further harm be minimized (secondary prevention)? What is it like to live with this condition or with the treatment? How can people learn to live (cope) with this condition? The most suitable approach for a research study will be determined by the question being asked.

Qualitative Versus Quantitative Approaches

For years in nursing, there has been a tension between qualitative and quantitative research. Which type of research best represents nursing research? **Quantitative research** is simply any study that involves some measurement—how long, how many, blood values, alive/dead, affected/unaffected, and recovered/not recovered. **Qualitative research** involves the participants' own perspective (through their words, photos, videos, or art) used to describe their experience. From the list of questions, it is clear that neither qualitative nor quantitative research alone is sufficient to fully inform nursing practice; rather, both are required. In fact, more frequently of late, both appear together in studies called **mixed methods**, where the two major types of research are conducted simultaneously or sequentially. See Box 12.6 for more information about the types of research designs.

The key to deciding whether to use quantitative or qualitative methods, or both, rests with the questions being asked. The data collection techniques (whether by measurement of variables, interviews, observations, or photovoice) and subsequent analysis (such as tests of statistical significance or identifying themes or basic processes) will depend on the research design chosen. Each research question dictates a particular type of design, which dictates a particular type of data collection and analyses.

BOX 12.6 Types of Research Designs

1. Quantitative
   - Systematic reviews
   - Randomized trials
   - Cohort studies
   - Interrupted time series
   - Cross-sectional studies
   - Case control

2. Qualitative
   - Phenomenology
   - Grounded theory
   - Ethnography
   - Case study

Finally, researchers have an ethical duty to study participants, funders, and society to disseminate their research findings so that others (patients, practitioners, researchers, and policy makers) can use the research for improving patient care. Dissemination is traditionally done through professional conferences and journals but may also involve community meetings and interactive processes like deliberative dialogue.

You will learn more about the intricacies of the research process in a separate research course as part of your baccalaureate preparation in nursing. If you have the opportunity to be a research assistant while attending school, you may find this to be a valuable experience, especially if you are thinking about graduate school and conducting your own research in the future.

Ethical Considerations

No data can be collected from or about individuals unless the researcher has received ethics approval. Researchers must disclose to participants the research purpose, question, methods of data collection, and potential gains and harms from participating in the research. In addition, the researchers must state steps that will be taken to protect participants' identity and data after collection. Information must be given to and reviewed with all potential participants and then signed consent received. An ethics committee reviews the entire research proposal along with the letters of information and consent forms.

Nursing Research in Canada

How do nurse researchers in Canada get their career underway? How does nursing research get funded? Conducted? Published?

The doctoral degree is a basic preparation for most nursing research careers. Nurse researchers today can expect to complete a postdoctoral fellowship and then progress to a junior scientist, a midcareer scientist, then a senior scientist; at each level, there would be funding for career support. The completion of a postdoctoral fellowship would mean at least 8 years of education and training beyond a baccalaureate degree. Most nurse researchers have academic appointments and some also have clinical appointments that help to keep their research questions grounded in reality and ready for application upon completion.

In Canada, there are few specific funds for nursing research. Some provinces and the Canadian Health Services Research Foundation have had specific competitions for nursing research. Agencies like the provincial nursing associations and the Canadian Nurses Foundation have some limited funds for nursing research. Otherwise, nurse researchers compete with all other health-care researchers through competitions within the Canadian Institutes of Health Research or other disease-specific foundations like the Canadian Diabetes Association or Heart and Stroke Foundation of Canada. Rejection of first-time proposals is common for any researcher (nursing or otherwise), and the

BOX 12.7 Examples of Nursing Research Using Various Methodologies

1. Jack, S. M., Jamieson, E., Wathen, C. N., & MacMillan, H. L. (2008). The feasibility of screening for intimate partner violence during postpartum home visits. *Canadian Journal of Nursing Research, 40*(2), 150–170.

2. Dobbins, M., DeCorby, K., Robeson, P., Husson, H., & Tirilis, D. (2009). School-based physical activity programs for promoting physical activity and fitness in children and adolescents aged 6–18. *Cochrane Database of Systematic Reviews*, (1), CD007651. doi:10.1002/14651858.CD007651

3. Kerr, L. M. J., Harrison, M. B., Medves, J., Tranmer, J. E., & Fitch, M. I. (2007). Understanding the supportive care needs of parents of children with cancer: An approach to local needs assessment. *Journal of Pediatric Oncology Nursing, 24*(5), 279–293.

4. Maheu, C., & Thorne, S. (2008). Receiving inconclusive genetic test results: An interpretive description of the BRCA1/2 experience. *Research in Nursing & Health, 31*(6), 553–562. doi:10.1002/nur.20286

5. Ratner, P. A., Johnson, J. L., Bottorff, J. L., Dahinten, S., & Hall, W. (2000). Twelve-month follow-up of a smoking relapse prevention intervention for postpartum women. *Addictive Behaviors, 25*(1), 81–92.

comments from the first rejection are invaluable for revision and resubmission. Because development of knowledge in any field depends on research, higher levels of funding for all disciplines would be desirable, but nurses must have the level of research skills to compete with all disciplines. Box 12.7 has examples of nursing research that you may find interesting.

Publishing Findings

Where do research results get published? For optimum dissemination, nurse researchers publish where the target audience is most likely to read. Sometimes that means an online or clinical journal short results or application piece, with the full study report published in a research-oriented journal. To ensure greater accessibility, more nurse researchers are publishing in open-access journals, which means that regardless of library access, potential users of the research can acquire the full-text article.

RESEARCH

VOICES AND PHOTOGRAPHS OF RURAL PRECEPTORED NURSING STUDENTS

Olive Yonge, RN, PhD, Faculty of Nursing, University of Alberta; Florence Myrick, RN, PhD, Faculty of Nursing, University of Alberta; Linda Ferguson, College of Nursing, University of Saskatchewan; and Quinn Grundy, doctoral student, University of California at San Francisco.

Preceptored rural placements are an educational strategy designed to address rural nursing shortages (Bushy & Leipert, 2005; Edwards, Smith, Courtney, Finlayson, & Chapman, 2004; Van Hofwegen, Kirkham, & Harwood, 2005). Paradoxically, the challenges that face rural nursing such as isolation, lack of updated resources, and a unique community structure may become assets to student learning and provide a rich variety of experiences (Van Hofwegen et al., 2005), including interprofessional team experiences for patient-centered care. Students reporting high levels of confidence and competence in their abilities have a greater tendency to choose a rural placement, reflecting the perception that rural nursing is a specialty of its own (Edwards et al., 2004). Bushy and Leipert (2005) suggest that incorporating rural theory and practice perspectives into nursing curricula, inviting rural practitioners as guest lecturers to speak to students, and exposing students to the rural context through short-term placements are strategies to increase familiarity and confidence, thus encouraging more students to choose a rural placement for their senior precepted experiences.

The research question for this project was, "What is the story of teaching and learning during a rural preceptorship as depicted through individual narration and photo methods?"

The incorporation of visual data is frequently used in research, especially in the fields of sociology and anthropology; however, it is rarely presented as a photo-elicitation study or incorporated into rigorous formal methodology. Interestingly, we live in an increasingly visual society, yet we have no visual record of the world from a research perspective (Emmison & Smith, 2000; Harrison, 2002).

Method

Four students who had chosen rural placements for their preceptorships in the final year of their baccalaureate nursing program and their preceptors ($n = 5$) were recruited. At four of the six rural sites documented, the participants further delegated coworkers, friends, and family members to take pictures using the cameras we provided. At the time of recruitment, we provided all participants with a verbal explanation of the photovoice study, its purpose, and ethical clearance; we required them to sign a written consent to release to the rights and ownership of the data produced; and we advised them they would be free to withdraw at any time.

During a preliminary session at each acute care site, research team members led a discussion on digital cameras, the ethics of photography, and power structures within photography with participants (Wang & Burris, 1997). This discussion covered protocols such as obtaining consent from individuals being photographed, criteria used to evaluate a photograph, ownership of images, and audiotaping participants' commentary as well as the operation of camera equipment and basic photographic techniques. In addition to the students and preceptors already recruited, these information sessions were open to and attended by other professionals at each site, from physicians to cleaning staff, all of whom agreed to take part on both sides of the camera. We emphasized that everyone who gave consent was welcome to take his or her turn at collecting data.

Part of our strategy was to guide participants in picture taking to disclose the goals of the research project, including our hope to produce a recruitment tool. At the preliminary session, we provided a slideshow of images from rural health-care settings to clarify the nature of the project and inspire participants without leading them in a particular direction. We encouraged them to indulge their creative or playful inclinations and to photograph as much as possible, with the assurance that they would have a later opportunity to remove sensitive or compromising images. Finally, we encouraged participants to "become photojournalists for [their] rural hospital, to show the rest of the health-care world what rural health care is like."

Data Collection, Analysis, and Validation

Each Alberta preceptorship took place in a single, rural acute care setting, while Saskatchewan preceptorships were divided between acute and community care, yielding six health-care sites (together with their surrounding rural communities and landscapes) for potential data collection by four students, five preceptors, and one clinical instructor, plus coworkers, family members, and friends who agreed to take part. We supplied each student, preceptor, and clinical instructor with an inexpensive 10–12 megapixel digital camera ($n = 10$; either Nikon COOLPIX S3000 or Fujifilm Z33WP), which participants were free to keep afterward, in addition to an honorarium.

In keeping with the principles of participatory action research, participants were responsible for choosing what they thought was worthy of a photograph (Collier, 1967). In this regard, digital technology was advantageous; participants were able to review their photographs at leisure and remove any they did not wish to share with the researchers. This also constituted the first stage of data analysis because participants were able to reflect at length on the meanings of their images prior to meeting with us.

Following the endpoint discussions at each site, we imported the data (photographs, audio, and transcripts) into NVivo 8 for coding and thematic analysis. For validation, we created a PowerPoint slideshow of the participants' images, captioned with their comments and organized into our conceptual categories, which we presented to participants at the various sites. Seeing their own photographs, and those from the other sites, in the context of our thematic framework, participants supplied us with two types of validation: (a) internal replication, wherein participants supported or amplified their own statements made on previous occasions; and (b) external replication, wherein participants expressed agreement with the statements made by participants at other sites. These validation discussions were also audiorecorded and imported into NVivo 8, enabling further refinement of our categories and ultimately the construction of a rural nursing paradigm.

Reflections of the Researchers

In this study, photovoice was transformative both for researchers and for participants. At the outset, it was little anticipated how profound an effect the process of taking and discussing photographs would have in terms of reflexivity for everyone involved. For the students and preceptors, photovoice awakened a vital critical spirit and self-awareness that might otherwise have remained suppressed by the demands of the rural health-care environment. For the researchers, photovoice occasioned a reappraisal of certain aspects of design, agenda, and ethics.

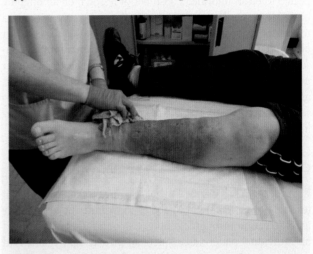

References

Bushy, A., & Leipert, B. (2005). Factors that influence students in choosing rural nursing practice: A pilot study. *Rural and Remote Health, 5*, 387. Retrieved from http://rrh.deakin.edu.au

Collier, J., Jr. (1967). *Visual anthropology: Photography as a research method.* New York, NY: Holt, Rinehart, & Winston.

Edwards, H., Smith, S., Courtney, M., Finlayson, K., & Chapman, H. (2004). The impact of clinical placement location on nursing students' competence and preparedness for practice. *Nurse Education Today, 24*, 248–255.

Emmison, M., & Smith, P. (2000). Researching the visual: Images, objects, contexts and interactions in social and cultural inquiry. London, United Kingdom: Sage.

Harrison, B. (2002). Seeing health and illness worlds—Using visual methodologies in a sociology of health and illness: A methodological review. *Sociology of Health & Illness, 24*(6), 856–872.

Van Hofwegen, L., Kirkham, S., & Harwood, C. (2005). The strength of rural nursing: Implications for undergraduate nursing education. *International Journal of Nursing Education Scholarship, 2*(1), 1–13.

Wang, C., & Burris, A. (1997). Photovoice: Concept, methodology, and use for participatory needs assessment. *Health Education and Behavior, 24*(3), 369–387.

Acknowledgments

The authors gratefully acknowledge the contributions of all primary participants as well as their coworkers, friends, and family members who agreed to take part. The authors would like to acknowledge the work of research assistants Jim Cockell, MA, and Judy McTavish, BScN.

Funding: The authors would like to acknowledge the Social Sciences and Humanities Research Council (SSHRC) of Canada for funding this research project.

Conclusion

The primary focus of this chapter has been on consuming research and the steps nurses use to do so. Underlying the sources of literature is the research process: Research questions are asked and answered and published. It is important to keep the distinction in mind that as a practicing nurse, you will be expected to be an informed consumer of research on an ongoing basis. However, there are no minimum competencies required related to the development of research proposals or the conduct of research without a graduate degree. To be an informed consumer of research, you have to keep up with reflecting on your practice, asking questions and conducting literature searches, assessing the strengths of the studies you find, making decisions about their applicability to your practice, and then creating a plan for implementation and evaluation.

Critical Thinking Case Scenario

▶ Your team has decided they are going to change the usual teaching of patients with diabetes to include the acceptability of injection through clothing. Of course, this will depend on individual patient assessment of their usual hygiene and environments where they would be doing the injections. Develop a beginning implementation plan targeted to all the nursing staff in the hospital, related to this change in practice, using the questions by Lavis et al. (2003).

1. What (is the message)?
2. To whom (the audience)?
3. By whom (the messenger)?
4. How (transfer method)?

Multiple-Choice Questions

1. Professional practice should be based on the best available research evidence and applied in conjunction with:
   a. Patient preferences
   b. Context
   c. Available resources
   d. All of the above

2. Meta-analysis should always be based on:
   a. Systematic reviews
   b. Randomized controlled trials
   c. Qualitative data
   d. Each individual study

3. Evidence-informed practice begins with:
   a. A physician's order
   b. A request from a family member
   c. Reflection by the nurse
   d. Consulting hospital policies

4. An internationally accepted standard for critiquing guidelines is:
   a. The ALIGN tool
   b. The ARGUE tool
   c. The AGREE tool
   d. The ACCESS tool

5. No data can be collected from or about an individual unless the researcher has:
   a. Permission from a physician
   b. Received a written order to collect information
   c. Read the hospital policies on data collection
   d. Received ethics approval

6. Most nurse researchers in Canada have basic preparation at the:
   a. Doctoral level
   b. Master's level
   c. Baccalaureate level
   d. Postdoctoral level

7. Newly graduated BScN-prepared nurses will primarily:
   a. Participate in research
   b. Conduct research
   c. Use research
   d. Study about research

8. Photovoice research does not require a consent form because you are just taking pictures.
   a. True
   b. False

9. A study that combines qualitative and quantitative data collection approaches would fit the definition of a mixed-methods study.
   a. True
   b. False

10. Primary studies collect original data and systemic reviews _____ the results of primary studies.
    a. Summarize
    b. Criticize
    c. Analyse
    d. Duplicate

Suggested Lab Activities

● Develop one or two clinical questions about an intervention you find interesting. You will be looking for quantitative research. Use the 6S pyramid and conduct a search at each level of the pyramid that is available to you (e.g., you may not have access to the top *System* level). Use the same search terms at each level. Compare your results across the pyramid.

● Repeat number 1 with a question about patient experience of, or coping with, a particular condition. You will be looking for qualitative research. Again, use the same search terms and compare results across the pyramid.

● Practice rating a guideline:

a) Download the AGREE tool (http://www.agreetrust.org/).

b) Search for a guideline about diabetes care.

c) Try out the AGREE tool to rate the guideline you found in b) earlier.

● Practice rating a systematic review:

a) Download the tool to appraise systematic reviews: http://www.phru.nhs.uk/learning/casp_s.review_tool.pdf

b) Search for a relevant systematic review or meta-analysis regarding diabetes care.

c) Try out the CASP review tool to rate the systematic review you found in b) earlier.

REFERENCES AND SUGGESTED READINGS

Antman, E. M., Lau, J., Kupelnick, B., Mosteller, F., & Chalmers, T. C. (1992). A comparison of results of meta-analyses of randomized control trials and recommendations of clinical experts. Treatments for myocardial infarction. *Journal of the American Medical Association, 268*(2), 240–248.

Brown, S. (1998). Injecting insulin through clothing was safe and convenient [Abstract]. *Evidence-Based Nursing, 1,* 12.

Buffett, C., Ciliska, D., & Thomas, H. (2007). *Can I use this evidence in my program decision? Assessing the applicability and transferability of evidence.* Hamilton, ON: National Collaborating Centre for Methods and Tools. Retrieved from http://www.nccmt.ca/pubs/2007_12_AT_tool_v_nov2007_ENG.pdf

Canadian Institutes of Health Research. (2013). *Knowledge translation—Definition.* Retrieved from http://www.cihr-irsc.gc.ca/e/39033.html

Catallo, C., Jack, S. M., Ciliska, D., & MacMillan, H. L. (2013). Minimizing the risk of intrusion: A grounded theory of intimate partner violence disclosure in emergency departments. *Journal of Advanced Nursing, 69*(6), 1366–1376.

DiCenso, A., Virani, T., Bajnok, I., Borycki, E., Davies, B., Graham, I., . . . Scott, J. (2002). A toolkit to facilitate the implementation of clinical practice guidelines in healthcare settings. *Hospital Quarterly, 5*(3), 55–60.

Fineout-Overholt, E., & Johnston, L. (2005). Teaching EBP: Asking searchable, answerable clinical questions. *Worldviews on Evidence-Based Nursing, 2,* 157–160.

Fleming, D. R., Jacober, S. J., Vandenberg, M. A., Fitzgerald, J. T., & Grunberger, G. (1997). The safety of injecting insulin through clothing. *Diabetes Care, 20,* 244–247.

Graham, I., Logan, J., Harrison, M. B., Straus, S. E., Tetroe, J., Caswell, W., & Robinson, N. (2006). Lost in knowledge translation: Time for a map? *The Journal of Continuing Education in the Health Professions, 26*(1), 13–24.

Grol, R. (2001). Successes and failures in the implementation of evidence-based guidelines for clinical practice. *Medical Care, 39*(8, Suppl. 2), II46–II54.

Guyatt, G., & Rennie, D. (Eds.). (2002). *Users' guides to the medical literature: A manual for evidence-based clinical practice.* Chicago, IL: American Medical Association.

Lavis, J. N., Posada, F. B., Haines, A., & Osei, E. (2004). Use of research to inform public policymaking. *Lancet, 364,* 1615–1621.

Lavis, J. N., Robertson, D., Woodside, J. M., McLeod, C. B., & Abelson, J. (2003). How can research organizations more effectively transfer research knowledge to decision makers? *The Milbank Quarterly, 81*(2), 221–248.

MacMillan, H. L., Wathen, N., Jamieson, E., Boyle, M. H., Shannon, H. S., Ford-Gilboe, M., . . . McNutt, L. A. (2009). Screening for intimate partner violence in health care settings: A randomized trial. *Journal of the American Medical Association, 302*(5), 493–501.

Registered Nurses Association of Ontario. (2002). *Toolkit: Implementation of clinical practice guidelines.* Toronto, ON: Author. Retrieved from http://www.rnao.org/Page.asp?PageID=924&ContentID=823

Schuster, M. A., McGlynn, E. A., & Brook, R. H. (1998). How good is the quality of health care in the United States? *The Milbank Quarterly, 76*(4), 517–563.

Culture and Cultural Safety: Beyond Cultural Inventories

COLLEEN VARCOE AND ANNETTE J. BROWNE

Jaswinder arrives early for her second shift on a medical oncology unit. This is the third 4-week clinical rotation of her first year of nursing school. Jas introduces herself to the charge nurse who is helping her clinical instructor decide student assignments. Jas hopes to have the same two women she provided care to yesterday because she spent considerable time last night reviewing their medications. However, Jas is dismayed to overhear the charge nurse decide that she should be assigned to two new patients, Mr. Singh and Mr. Bopal, saying, "It would be great to have someone of the same culture looking after them who can talk to them." Jas headed off to greet her patients with concern, feeling out of her depth, and worried about how she will provide care to patients who do not speak English.

CHAPTER OBJECTIVES

By the end of this chapter, you will be able to:

1. Critically appraise how culture is understood in predominantly liberal, multicultural Western societies, including Canada.
2. Evaluate how nursing conventionally has used the idea of culture in practice.
3. Reflexively examine your own culture and social location as a basis for considering difference and social advantages and disadvantages in relation to health and health care.
4. Consider the implications of using each of three different but overlapping approaches to culture in nursing and health care: cultural sensitivity, cultural competence, and cultural safety.
5. Analyze how life opportunities, choices, beliefs, and preferences are shaped by structural conditions, such as citizenship policies and laws, social policies, access to material wealth, and practices such as racism and other forms of discrimination.
6. Recognize that being able to communicate, particularly across language barriers, is integral to promoting culturally safe health-care environments.
7. Begin to practice nursing based on a critical awareness of different understandings and approaches to culture.

KEY TERMS

Biomedicine   Refers to the application of the principles of natural sciences such as biology and chemistry to understanding, treating, and promoting human health. Biomedical models are important but insufficient to understanding and responding to health-related issues because they are tied to conceptions of health as located in individuals, peoples' physical bodies, and microlevel interactions but leave unexamined the underlying social and structural dynamics that actually produce health and health inequality.

Colonization and Colonialism   The takeover of a minority population (often indigenous) by another nation and the resulting unequal relationships between them.

Corporatism   The use of a business model in shaping health care so that economics and profitability are the primary determinants rather than the promotion of human health.

Culture   Is a process that happens between people; we continuously participate in and create culture, and culture is constantly in flux. No two persons share any given cultural affiliation in identical ways.

Democratic Racism   Rather than using overt racial categories and ideas of racial or biologic inferiority/superiority, democratic racism uses *cultural differences* as a euphemism for racial differences to explain health, social, and economic inequities.

Diaspora   Refers to the migration and dispersion of people from their countries of origin and to the intricate ties that migrant communities maintain with their homeland.

Ethnicity   Refers to a group that shares a heritage, language, culture, or religion but is a very ambiguous and dynamic concept that can encompass many different aspects such as race, origin or ancestry, identity, language, nationality, and religion. In Canada, ethnicity is often used as a polite term for race.

Individualism   The valuing of individuals over the collective that is common to liberal democracies. Individualism is based on the idea that society is essentially an equal playing field, that people have fairly similar choices, and that individual rights are of greatest importance.

Neocolonialism   Comprises new, evolving, and ongoing colonial policies and practices that continue to govern, oppress, and subordinate certain groups. Whereas European colonial rule involved occupation of countries and lands, often through military means, neocolonialism involves more indirect forms of control through economic and cultural dependence, without the development of infrastructure in the subordinated lands as was characteristic of European colonialism.

Race   A way of categorizing people by primarily physical characteristics such as skin colour or hair texture. The concept of race has no basis in biologic reality and is therefore meaningless, independent of its social definitions.

Racialization   Categorizing people by racial characteristics and the resulting negative social, economic, and political effects.

Reflexivity   Means continuously scrutinizing your own knowledge and the basis of your practice and always checking your assumptions and "blind spots."

Visible Minority   People who are identified according to the federal Employment Equity Act as non-white in colour (non-Caucasian).

Understanding Culture: The Canadian Context

Canadians often pride themselves on living in a fair, tolerant, multicultural society. However, our colonial history, our ever-changing immigration policies, and the inequities that structure relationships among the diverse groups of people within Canada present significant challenges to fairness and tolerance. As a nation, Canada was built on colonial conquest, both of Aboriginal people and indigenous lands, and conquest of people around the globe who were subjugated to British and French rule.

Colonization and colonialism refer to the processes in which a population (often indigenous) is taken over and governed by a nation-state (such as Canada) such that power and authority are exercised in ways that consciously and unconsciously subordinate that population (Bourassa, McKay-McNabb, & Hampton, 2004). Colonization is not only a fact of past history; the processes of colonialism continue into the present in Canada and other countries (Furniss, 1999). In the changing world of economic globalization, Canada now has neocolonial relations with much of the world and its citizens. **Neocolonialism** refers to new, evolving, and ongoing colonial policies and practices that continue to govern, oppress, and subordinate certain groups. Whereas European colonial rule involved occupation of countries and lands, often through military means, neocolonialism involves more indirect forms of control through economic and cultural dependence, without the development of infrastructure in the subordinated lands as was characteristic of European colonialism. Groups affected by colonialism and neocolonialism experience oppression that has been shown to have detrimental effects on health (Adelson, 2005; Bourassa et al., 2004; Brownridge, 2008). For example, consistent with research on African **diaspora** in the United Kingdom and the United States, Nova Scotians descended from African ancestors have been shown to have higher incidence of circulatory disease, diabetes, and psychiatric disorders that cannot be explained by socioeconomic characteristics, distance to health care, recent immigration, or language, suggesting that experiencing oppression and discrimination explain the differences (Kisely, Terashima, & Langille, 2008).

As a part of former European colonial rule, and in alignment with other Western powers, Canada is a liberal capitalist democracy in which economic productivity is highly valued and in which the emphasis is on individual accomplishment. **Individualism** is the valuing of individuals over the collective that is common to liberal democracies. Individualism is based on the idea that society is essentially an equal playing field, that people have fairly similar choices, and that individual rights are of greatest importance. From an individualistic perspective, people are viewed as essentially separate, rational beings that can be understood apart from their social, economic, political, or historical contexts (Browne, 2001). Because individualism is so intricately woven into our society, it is often difficult to recognize the extent to which it shapes our social and political assumptions and our assumptions about culture. For example, common nursing concepts such as self-care and self-management as they relate to people with chronic illnesses are infused with individualism in ways that overlook the networks of relationships and informal caregiving that support people with such illnesses and obscure the complexities of their lives (Paterson, Russell, & Thorne, 2001; Peter et al., 2007). These individualistic values shape Canadian health and social policy, including multiculturalism policy and immigration policy, and shape how culture is understood in Canada, which in turn shapes people's experiences of culture.

Multiculturalism in Canada

Multiculturalism and respect for diversity is official policy of the Canadian federal government supported by a framework of policies and laws including the Canadian Multiculturalism Act (Government of Canada, 1988). This Act recognizes the freedom of all Canadians to preserve, enhance, and share their cultural heritage and promotes "the full and equitable participation of individuals and communities of all origins in the continuing evolution and shaping of all aspects of Canadian society and assist[s] them in the elimination of any barrier to such participation" (Government of Canada, 1988, C. 31, p. 838). However, many Canadians face considerable barriers to participating in society fully—such as participating through employment, obtaining resources adequate for safe shelter and adequate nutrition, civic engagement, playing a role in shaping policies that affect them, and voting—and face discrimination daily, including barriers to accessing health care. The intention to promote equity within multiculturalism in Canada is undermined by numerous other policies. For example, although Canada's historically explicitly racist immigration laws have been reformed (Walker, 2008), the reformed laws currently are structured to favour the most highly educated and wealthy people from other countries (depleting the resources of those countries) and in ways that disadvantage women in particular. For example, Canadian immigration law permits three classes of immigrants: family class immigrants, refugees, and economic immigrants. People admitted through the economic category are primarily skilled workers or business people and their accompanying spouses or dependents, with the laws structured so that spouses and dependents are bound economically to their sponsor with significant gendered effects. These laws directly shape the dynamics of intimate partner violence, particularly when women experience abuse but have no ability to exist economically outside of their dependence on male sponsors (Guruge & Collins, 2008; Hyman, Forte, Du Mont, Romans, & Cohen, 2009). To take another example, the federal Indian Act (Department of Justice Canada, 1985), which has been in effect since 1885 with some revisions since, remains the current law in Canada. In part, this law recognizes the unique status of First Nations people. However, until amendments made in 1960, in many ways, the Indian Act restricted people who were identified as status First Nations—including restriction from voting in federal elections and from leaving reserves without written permission—with serious effects on their ability to earn a living, obtain education, stay connected to family members, and participate in political decision-making.

Although the intention to uphold equity and extend respect to all persons is enshrined in various Canadian laws and policies and is part of Canada's national image, this intention is also undermined by prevailing attitudes. Throughout Canadian society, there are anti-immigrant sentiments and anti-Aboriginal sentiments that are often reflected in the media and in everyday public conversations. For example, immigrants are often subtly portrayed in the media as vectors of disease (Adeyanju & Neverson, 2007), such as during the recent severe acute respiratory syndrome (SARS) outbreak. Henry and Tator (2006) call the Canadian tendency to espouse equity and social justice, yet practice discrimination— **democratic racism**. Rather than using overt racial categories and ideas of racial or biologic inferiority/superiority, democratic racism uses *cultural differences* as a euphemism for racial differences to explain health, social, and economic inequities. So, differences in health or economic status between recent immigrants and the general Canadian population are explained as resulting from cultural differences instead of examining the social and economic dynamics that might shape such divergence. For example, a large population-based study of cancer screening showed that most immigrants and ethnic minority groups in Canada have markedly lower rates of Pap smear testing compared to the Canadian population as a whole, differences not explained by age, education levels, language spoken at home, or other demographic characteristics (McDonald & Kennedy, 2007, p. 333). The researchers

explained the differences as "cultural, perhaps arising from differences in beliefs about the necessity or nature of the procedures, differences in referrals from physicians, cultural/communication barriers and low health motivation, or traditions of modesty among certain ethnic minority groups" but did not consider how discrimination, racism, or structural barriers such as lack of access to English language courses, medical coverage, transportation, child care, lack of familiarity with the Canadian health-care system, and so on, might shape these barriers. Thus, democratic racism is subtle and unlikely to be challenged because commitments to democratic, liberal principles such as justice, equality, and fairness mask discrimination and hold minority groups and their cultures accountable for their health outcomes and the health-care inequities they may experience.

Nursing Values

Democratic racism helps to explain how espoused Canadian values can conflict with peoples' experiences of discrimination and the ongoing discriminatory practices and policies that give rise to experiences of discrimination. Democratic racism also clearly conflicts with the values of nursing. Nurses are obliged to uphold fairness, dignity, and respect for all persons. As the Canadian Nurses Association Code of Ethics states:

- When providing care, nurses do not discriminate on the basis of a person's race, ethnicity, culture, political and spiritual beliefs, social or marital status, gender, sexual orientation, age, health status, place of origin, lifestyle, mental or physical ability, socio-economic status or any other attribute.
- Nurses refrain from judging, labelling, demeaning, stigmatizing, and humiliating behaviours toward persons receiving care, other health-care professionals, and each other.
- Nurses make fair decisions about the allocation of resources under their control based on the needs of persons, groups or communities to whom they are providing care. They advocate for fair treatment and for fair distribution of resources for those in their care. (Canadian Nurses Association, 2008, p. 17)

These ethical ideals are made explicit in nursing because there are dynamics in our society that can make it challenging to uphold them. As we continue to discuss in this chapter, nurses need to be critically reflexive and aware of how our own social positioning, culture, and attitudes influence our views of and practices with various people. In order to do so, we need to examine what is meant by culture and how we approach differences.

Traditional Understanding of Culture

In Canadian society, and within our health-care system, culture often is defined simplistically as the values, beliefs, and practices common or inherent to a group of people.

Understanding culture in this way is problematic when trying to understand individuals because of the following:

- *Identifying a person's culture depends on associating them with a particular group, whereas most people affiliate with multiple groups.* For example, a person might identify as Iranian-Canadian, but depending on the context, that person's status as a Francophone or member of the Bahá'í Faith community might be most salient. Any of these identities or "cultures" might be more or less relevant depending on the situation.
- *People affiliate with multiple groups, which may imply diverse or even conflicting values and beliefs.* For example, Daniel emigrated from Ireland in his 20s. Raised Catholic, he found himself conflicted between the teachings of his religion, his sexual orientation, and his membership in a gay community with very liberal values.
- *Ascribing assumed group values to individuals suggests a static set of values, beliefs, and practices that do not change over an individual's life.* When he was in his early 20s, Daniel strongly identified with the values embedded in his Irish-Catholic background. However, over the years in Canada, many of his values changed significantly.
- *Culture is often narrowly conflated with ethnicity* or with notions of race or racialized characteristics.

Ethnicity and Race

Often, ethnicity is identified as the most relevant grouping that defines a person's culture. **Ethnicity** refers to a group or "community maintained by a shared heritage, culture, language, or religion" (Henry & Tator, 2006, p. 350) but is a very ambiguous and dynamic concept that can encompass many different aspects such as race, origin or ancestry, identity, language, nationality, and religion. In Canada, ethnicity is often used as a polite term for race. **Race** is defined as " . . . a socially constructed category used to classify humankind according to common ancestry and reliant on differentiation by physical characteristics such as colour of skin, hair texture, stature and facial characteristics. The concept of race has no basis in biological reality and, as such has no meaning independent of its social definitions" (Henry & Tator, 2006, p. 351). Although skin color, eye shape, and hair texture are genetically determined and reflect heredity and ancestry, research has determined that those features do not signify any meaningful biologic groupings. In fact, there is as much biologic and genetic variation within groups of so called races as there is between groups. Nevertheless, race continues to operate as a way of categorizing people socially, and social categorization is often done *as though* there is a biologic basis to race.

Ethnicity is often used as a substitute for the idea of race. In the United States, race and ethnicity are frequently used interchangeably to categorize people (e.g., as Hispanic, Asian, Black, White). In Canada, people are frequently classified by themselves or others as East Indian, French-Canadian, Jewish, Chinese, and so on, and this classification is used to identify the person's culture, ethnicity, or race. This emphasis on ethnicity or race as a basis for understanding culture leads to people attempting to apply general assumptions about groups to individuals; for example, by making assumptions about what people eat, how families function, or how death is ritualized. However, culture is actually much more complex.

Culture as Process: Contemporary Understandings

Culture is a process that happens between people; we continuously participate in and create culture, and culture is constantly in flux. No two persons share any given cultural affiliation in identical ways. Most Canadians identify with multiple cultures beyond those based on ethnicities, nationalities, or places of birth: Canadian culture, Western culture, Francophone or Anglophone culture, professional cultures (such as the culture of health care or nursing), religious cultures, recreational cultures (e.g., hockey culture), age-based cultures, and so on. People also participate simultaneously in multiple cultures and religions.

In nursing, defining culture simplistically as the values, beliefs, and practices common or inherent to a group of people is particularly limiting because such an understanding overlooks power and structural conditions. Attempting to use such an understanding as the basis for practice in relation to individuals or groups is problematic for several reasons. First, this understanding suggests that a nurse can know another person's culture by determining to which group the person belongs. Second, using culture, ethnicity, or race as the primary category of interest for some people (such as those from racialized groups) overlooks the complexity of the individual's life, may overlook more salient features of a person's experience, and sets the conditions for discrimination. This chapter is based on the premise that meaningful knowledge about an individual person cannot be gained simply by identifying the groups to which that person belongs. Thus, nursing requires a much more complex understanding of culture as a basis for upholding the ethical obligations of nursing, including promoting fairness, recognizing and addressing inequities, and practicing respectfully with all people.

Cultures are shaped by sociohistorical, political, and economic contexts and by power dynamics within those contexts. Understanding culture as an ongoing, dynamic process requires considering how contexts and power dynamics operate. For example, in Canada, certain family housing patterns (such as extended families of multiple generations and couples living in one household) often are thought of as cultural and judged against a presumed norm of the nuclear family without considering the contexts and power dynamics that shape both living patterns and how they are evaluated. In British Columbia, it became so commonplace to comment that "East Indians" tend to live in large family groupings that a certain large style of home (the "Vancouver Special") became associated with immigrants from India. Economics and standards of living influence changing housing options. The nuclear family only recently emerged with the rise of relative affluence. Although an increasingly affordable option in the post–World

War II era, it is becoming an increasing less viable option for many people. This chapter is based on the premise that nurses must develop an understanding of how contextual factors and power dynamics shape people's lives so that any person's culture is understood as much more than a simple stereotype based on ethnicity or notions of race.

By focusing on *knowing* about various perspectives on culture—what the idea means and why culture is often confused with race or ethnicity—we consider the consequences for nursing of practicing based on different understandings of culture. We then discuss the *thinking* required to consider your own multiple cultures and your own social location—that is, how you are positioned by where you were born, the resources you have, the education you received, the values you hold, your physical appearance, and so on. This will provide a basis for analyzing what shapes values, beliefs, and practices and for self-reflection about and responding to differences between yourself and others. By differences, we are referring to multiple distinctions that exist between everyone in our society, not just those that differ from the assumed dominant norm. We ask you to consider differences in light of power dynamics and to challenge any presumed superiority of one difference over another. We discuss how a broad understanding of culture can be helpful to nurses working across multiple variations: not just differences of habits and preferences (related to diet, rituals, parenting practices, and so on) but also differences created by histories, inequities in the distribution of social resources, and social practices such as racism and other forms of discrimination based on age, gender, class, ability, sexual orientation, and so on. We then consider what *being* a respectful nurse involves when working with patients from all backgrounds and across multiple differences. Finally, we discuss the skills required for *interacting* and *understanding* across differences.

Think Deaf culture is an excellent example to use in considering the presumed superiority or inferiority of differences. Most deaf people do not consider deafness to be a disability. In fact, many members of the deaf community in Canada view themselves as a culture. The Canadian Association of the Deaf (2012) takes the following position:

> Deaf Culture is a healthy sociological community of Deaf people. "The medicalization of deafness" is the treatment of deafness as a defect that must be fixed at any cost. The two approaches cannot be compatible. (para. 1)

What do you think is the dominant view of deafness in Canadian society? How have you thought about deafness?

Traditional Understanding of Culture in the Health-Care Context

Each health-care provider, each nursing student, and each patient comes with his or her own unique cultural experiences and affiliations. However, it is likely that many will have learned to think of culture as something they "have" and to equate their own cultures with their ethnicities rather than thinking of culture as a dynamic and constantly shifting process in which we all participate. People in Canada who are Euro-Canadian English speakers often think of themselves as "not having a culture" in part because they relate closely to the dominant culture, which is so pervasive that it becomes almost invisible. For example, people descended from those who emigrated from England, Scotland, Ireland, or other parts of Europe may not think of what they eat, believe, or do as being "cultural." However, those same people may see "others" from racialized groups as necessarily having culture, reflecting the common confusion of culture with ethnicity or race.

Racial Categories

Racialization is the process of categorizing people into racial categories that are constructed as different and unequal in ways that lead to negative social, economic, and political impacts (Galabuzi, 2001; Miles, 1989). For example, people descended from those who emigrated from China may think of themselves as belonging to some extent to Chinese culture in part because in Canada, they are subjected to ongoing discrimination. When a person is routinely identified primarily by a racial category (which is not routinely the case if you are a member of a dominant group—such as being Caucasian in many Canadian contexts), the category is always in the foreground. Categorizing people based on ethnicity is usually done to racialized groups and thus is generally a racializing process. For example, in Canada, the term **visible minority** applies to persons who are identified according to the federal Employment Equity Act "as being non-Caucasian . . . or non-white in colour (Employment Equity Act, 1995, § 3). Under the Act, Aboriginal persons are not considered to be members of visible minority groups". Used in this way, visible minority is a racializing category because it attempts to classify people by skin colour or other physical characteristics. Racializing is also a form of othering, that is, projection of assumed cultural characteristics, differences, or identities onto members of particular groups, a process that divides people into "us and them" (Varcoe & McCormick, 2007). As Ahmad (1993, p. 18) explains, by "defining the Other (usually as inferior) one implicitly defines oneself against that definition (usually as normal or superior)." Often, people are unaware that they are engaging in othering; as such, these conscious and unconscious practices contribute to labeling, stereotyping, alienation, marginalization, and stigmatization (Peternelj-Taylor, 2004). As you will see as you continue in this chapter, such processes have harmful consequences, including making erroneous assumptions, applying stereotypes, and obscuring the importance of taking the patient's actual needs and perspectives into account.

In the opening scenario when Jas was assigned to two new patients, it was on the basis of a racializing process. Based on her name, or perhaps her appearance, the charge nurse assumed she was "from the same culture" as the two particular patients and further assumed they would all speak the same language. First, although Jaswinder's ancestors were from India, her grandparents immigrated to Canada over 50 years ago. She and her parents were born in Canada and speak only English. Further, she knew that the two patients to whom she was assigned spoke different languages from each other, being recent immigrants from West Africa and Pakistan. The charge nurse's assumptions were wrong about Jas's and the patients' cultures and languages; in the process, the charge nurse did not enhance care for any of the patients (including the two women for whom Jas cared yesterday), and she failed to prioritize Jas's learning.

The Nursing Student Perspective

Nursing students are in positions of less power relative to their instructors and other staff. This is especially challenging when dealing with approaches to culture that confuse culture and ethnicity and perpetuate racialization. For students who are themselves from racialized groups, challenging discrimination is particularly difficult because such students may be seen by others as promoting their own special interests, or as defensive or overly sensitive, rather than taking an ethical and professional stance against discrimination. In a study of nursing students and clinical instructors, Paterson, Osborne, and Gregory (2004) showed that teachers' overt messages regarding equality may be contradicted by students' experiences. They found that discourses of equality and cultural sensitivity in clinical nursing were accompanied by clinical teachers' unspoken messages that constructed difference as problematic and as being *less than* the expected norm. Teachers encouraged adherence to one acceptable norm. For example,

> ... The cultural etiquette of students, particularly those whose country of origin was not in North America or Europe, was often not understood or appreciated by clinical teachers ... when teachers demanded that students be more active and open in their participation ... they discounted the cultural norms that prohibit such behaviour. (Paterson et al., 2004, p. 7)

Cultural diversity was constructed as a problem through complex and contradictory experiences of difference and expectations that everyone conforms to similar norms. Paterson et al. (2004) argued that both teachers' and students' experiences were shaped by broader social understandings of difference and diversity that tend to privilege dominant norms.

Through the eyes of a patient

I wish they wouldn't shout at me. "Mr. Singh, Mr. Singh." I am not deaf. My English is not good, but I am not deaf! Yesterday, they moved me beside this other old man—I think the nurses think we are from the same country or speak same language, and now they give me this new nurse. I can tell she is a student, and I think I need a real nurse.

(personal reflection of a patient, Mr. Singh)

Different Approaches to Culture in Nursing and Health Care

Different understandings of culture lead to different approaches in health care. In this chapter, we discuss three different but overlapping approaches: cultural sensitivity, cultural competence, and cultural safety. Each approach has a different degree of attention to analyses of power and structural conditions and to the significance of social and historical contexts and a different emphasis on individual rather than collective responsibility. At one end of the continuum, cultural sensitivity emphasizes that individual health-care providers should become sensitive toward individual patient differences from dominant norms. There is not necessarily any requirement for dominant norms or practices to be adapted or changed; the health-care provider helps the patient to adapt or makes accommodations for individuals regarding the differences. For example, nurses in different settings teach patients and family members to comply with rules regarding when they are allowed to participate in care, when they can visit, and so on (Varcoe, Rodney, & McCormick, 2003) and make exceptions for particular patients. This approach is based on viewing culture as a characteristic of people or as something held by groups of people. On the other end of the continuum, based on a more dynamic understanding of culture, cultural safety emphasizes critique of structural conditions and requires changes to dominant norms and ways of being, with an emphasis on collective responsibility. Changes are then made at the level of practice and policy (informal and formal, at health-care unit levels and beyond) to enhance care for all patients, not just those categorized as different from presumed norms. The notion of cultural competence is used in myriad ways—both ways that are congruent with the ideas of cultural sensitivity and ways that are congruent with cultural safety.

Cultural Care Theories

Nursing has been a leader in promoting the importance of culture in health care and in developing approaches to addressing culture in health care. Over the past four decades,

Dr. Madeleine Leininger, a nurse-anthropologist, developed a culture care theory within the broader field of transcultural nursing (Leininger, 2002a, 2002b). Leininger's work has been drawn upon extensively in nursing and other health-care professions, and her initial conceptualizations of culture have been highly influential in nursing and health care. Based on her work, nurses have endeavoured to integrate the concept of culture into their care for individuals they see as different from themselves. Leininger (2002a) describes her work on transcultural nursing "as a great breakthrough in caring for the culturally different" (p. 189), implying a norm by which others are defined as different. Nurses ascribing to Leininger's perspectives strive for cultural sensitivity by attending to patients' values, beliefs, attitudes, and behaviours. Leininger's work has been instrumental in helping nurses to recognize the significance of culture, and in this chapter, cultural sensitivity is recognized as an important starting place for developing awareness about the importance of culture.

Increasingly, nursing scholars have recognized that the concept of culture applies to all patients and that nurses themselves are cultural beings. They have also recognized the importance of examining how these factors intersect with the broader social determinants of health and how those determinants, along with power relations, shape peoples' lives. Dr. Leininger's work has been extended and developed by numerous scholars to take these broader contexts into account. For example, Stebnicki and Coeling (1999) used Leininger's theoretical perspective as a basis for exploring nursing practice with deaf patients, including taking into account how stereotypes about deaf people contribute to underemployment, unemployment, and limited educational opportunities.

Concepts of Culture in Canadian Nursing Contexts

Canadian nursing scholar Rani Srivastava (2007) built upon Leininger's work, using attention to power to consider culture in ways that directly consider racism and inequity. Her work promotes consideration of power dynamics and how histories shape people's experiences of culture, encouraging nurses to develop competence in relation to diverse individuals. Several Canadian scholars also have been leaders in promoting a critical conceptualization of culture that involves explicit attention to power, contexts, and structural inequities and an analysis of the role of nursing in addressing these factors. Dr. Joan Anderson (Anderson et al., 2003; Anderson & Reimer Kirkham, 1999; Anderson, Tang, & Blue, 2007) has played a leading role in transforming our understanding of culture as a dynamic process that is inextricably linked to political, social, historical, and economic contexts. In her work, Anderson emphasizes the importance of shifting the focus of analysis away from "cultural others" and onto the roles and responsibilities of nurses in disrupting inequitable policies, practices, and power relations in health care. Dr. Diana Gustafson also has promoted a critical conception of culture, arguing that attending to culture requires nursing to work

toward transforming the social practices and relations that institutionalize the dominant approach to social and human differences (Gustafson, 2005, 2008).

In summary, there are three approaches to culture in nursing and health care that are evolving and overlapping and are understood differently by various authors. For the purposes of this chapter, we emphasize the contrast between cultural sensitivity and cultural safety.

Cultural Sensitivity

As we discussed in the opening of this chapter, culture is often thought of as something that belongs to people or groups rather than something that happens between people. When culture is thought of as something that belongs to people, including values, beliefs, and practices, it is thought of as something static, permanent, and unchanging. Understanding culture without taking context and power dynamics into account suggests that culture is primarily a matter of personal preference or something that is inherent to particular groups. Using this view of culture in health care, the obligation of nurses is to find out what a person's culture is and to be sensitive to, and tolerant of, differences from the presumed norm, with tolerance often implying a tolerating majority and a tolerated minority. This approach has been supported by the proliferation of cultural inventories in various textbooks and assessment tools, which were intended to help nurses understand what people from various cultures value, believe, and do. For example, some health-care settings have developed information sheets designed to provide information about specific cultures. In one hospital, information sheets were developed to convey ideas about Chinese culture, including various religious practices, word meanings, food preferences, child-rearing practices, and privacy preferences, particularly for women. Although such inventories can alert nurses to a range of values, beliefs and practices, and the need to be respectful of peoples' preferences, the limitations of these inventories include the following:

- *The diversity within any group often exceeds the diversity between groups.* For example, there is no one religion common to people who identify as Chinese. Similarly, Chinese languages include many different dialects, and Chinese-speaking people cannot necessarily understand one another when they are from different geographical areas.
- *People often disagree with the classifications to which other people assign them* (Varcoe, Browne, Wong, & Smye, 2009). For example, the most recent Canadian census found that an increasing number of people prefer to self-identify as Canadian instead of classifying themselves as a member of another ethno-cultural group (e.g., African, Iranian, etc.) (Thomas, 2005).
- *Many people claim membership in a group but do not subscribe to all the practices associated with that group.* For example, a person may identify culturally as Jewish but not engage in the religious practices of Judaism or may associate with multiple groups to varying degrees.

- *Inventories of cultural values, beliefs, and practices can be stereotypical and can lead nurses to make erroneous assumptions about individuals.* For example, a nurse might falsely assume that every person, as Canadian-Italian Catholic, would be against abortion or birth control or homosexuality.
- *People from racialized groups, in particular, may find the process of being categorized by ethnicity offensive* (Varcoe et al., 2009). In a study (Varcoe et al., 2009) of patients' perspectives about being asked their ethnicity, patients responded:

> I feel extremely highly discriminated towards by asking such a question. Patient #48

> I'd be [offended] if this was asked of me. It's just another means to divide. Patient #21

> Because its, its, its not a good question, its not a good question at all, it doesn't relate to my health, this sort of question, it makes me really angry. Patient #41 (p. 1663)

- *Cultural sensitivity focuses attention on and tightens emphasis on individuals, often in isolation of, and overlooking, the broader context of people's lives.* For example, viewing families whose living arrangements include many generations living together in one home living as a cultural choice overlooks the economic circumstances that often makes doing so necessary.
- *Sensitivity often implies (a) that there is a preferred norm outside of which sensitivity and tolerance are required, (b) that minorities are tolerated by a dominant majority (implying superiority of the majority), and (c) that nurses have only a passive responsibility to be sensitive but not necessarily engage in change.*

Think In your first clinical experience in maternity, the nurse with whom you are working begins explaining to you that some women are more difficult than others to manage in labour. She tells you that native women are very stoic, so that it is difficult to assess their pain, whereas some others (she lists Latinas, Russians, East Indians, and several other groups) are very loud, so that you have to disregard much of their behaviour. She tells you, "If they're screaming, take it with a grain of salt."

How is this nurse understanding culture? What approach is she taking to culture? What are the limitations of this approach? What can you do or say?

Cultural Competence

Cultural competence is a term that is used in different ways, sometimes meaning developing competence in understanding different cultures, so that nurses become familiar with the beliefs, values, and practices of various groups of people. At other times, cultural competence is used in a way that is more compatible with a more critical understanding of culture, meaning that nurses should develop competence not only in learning about others but also in learning about themselves and about the contexts that shape experiences

of culture and health care. For the purposes of this chapter, we emphasize the contrasts between cultural sensitivity and cultural safety, understanding that cultural competence is an idea that can be used in ways compatible with either.

Cultural Safety

When culture is thought of as something that happens between people and groups, it can be seen as dynamic and ever-changing. Further, it can be seen as something that we can *create*. In the early 1990s, Maori leaders in nursing education in New Zealand developed cultural safety as an alternative concept to cultural sensitivity (Papps & Ramsden, 1996; Ramsden, 1993, 2000, 2002). Because the concept arose out of the bicultural relationship between Maori people and the descendants of British colonists, in New Zealand, the concept focuses exclusively on the relationship between indigenous peoples and descendants of early settlers. In Canada, this concept has been used to include all peoples. As the idea of cultural safety is being developed in Canada, it is founded on a critical understanding of culture that recognizes that cultures are dynamic and constantly shifting in relation to power dynamics in our society and historical, economic, political, and local trends (Browne et al., 2009; Reimer-Kirkham et al., 2009).

The central ideas of cultural safety are that

- *Cultural safety does **not** refer to the cataloguing of culture-specific beliefs but rather it is how a group "is perceived and treated that is relevant rather than the different things its members think or do"* (Polashek, 1998, p. 452). For example, the historical and ongoing discrimination against Nova Scotians descended from African people enslaved in the United States has significant effects on their health and well-being and shapes what might be seen as their culture.
- *The social, economic, and political positions of groups within society influence health and health care.* For example, the way in which Aboriginal people are treated in Canada and how policies differently affect their citizenship rights, their opportunities for education, the quality of life on reserves, their employment, and so on, are important for understanding their health and health-care experiences. Power imbalances contribute to health-care inequities; recognizing and addressing such inequities is assumed to be a central feature of nursing's mandate (Browne et al., 2009).
- *Individual and institutional discrimination in health care creates risks for patients, particularly when people from a specific group perceive they are "demeaned, diminished or disempowered by actions and delivery systems" including by those who typically hold the power in health-care contexts (namely, health-care providers)* (Ramsden & Spoonley, 1994, p. 164). For example, the consequences of racial discrimination have been linked to hypertension and cardiovascular disease for African-American people (Krieger, Sidney, & Coakley, 1998); for Aboriginal people in Canada, discrimination and colonization have been linked to diabetes (Poudrier, 2007) and intimate partner violence (Bourassa et al., 2004; Varcoe & Dick, 2008).

- *Critical reflexivity is essential to good nursing practice. Healthcare providers must "reflect on their own personal and cultural history and the values and beliefs they bring in their interaction with clients, rather than an uncritical imposition of their own understandings and beliefs on clients and their families"* (Anderson et al., 2003, p. 198).
- *Promoting safety requires actions that (a) recognize, respect, and nurture the unique and dynamic cultural identities of all people/families and (b) safely meet peoples' needs, expectations, and rights given the unique contexts of their lives.*

In Anticipation of Cultural Safety in the Practice Context

There are two beginning skills toward practicing in a culturally safe manner: First, cultural safety always begins with self-reflection on how our biases, assumptions, norms, and ways of being influence our viewpoints, interactions, and practices. Second, cultural safety requires being able to critically analyze the culture of health.

Self-Reflection: How Are You Socially Positioned?

We are all socially and culturally positioned by where we were born, where we live, what resources we have, how we appear physically, and what abilities and opportunities we have. In individualistic Western societies, however, we are encouraged to think of our social positions as personal accomplishments (or failings). For example, if we can afford an education, we are encouraged to think of this as an accomplishment by our parents or ourselves and as primarily a product of hard work—not a product of the opportunity to have employment in the first place or the consequence of family supports and public funding that enabled us to achieve an education. If we speak one of Canada's official languages as our first language, we are not encouraged to think of doing so as a privilege or an accident of birth and place of residence. Examining our own social positions, our advantages and disadvantages, is the first step in being able to analyze how we may be different from others, our assumptions about difference, and how differences affect us all—and to work effectively as a nurse across those differences.

Applebaum (2001) argues that analyzing your own social or cultural position or "locating one's self" is more than just listing your group affiliations. To say that you are a White, Jewish, lower middle class, English-speaking man is not sufficient to examine privilege and disadvantage. Furthermore, just listing group affiliations suggests that you are responsible for your own social position. Applebaum also argues that locating one's self for people who are in positions of privilege should not be "confessional," in the sense of feeling guilty and wanting absolution, and that it amounts to more than self-criticism. It is not useful to feel guilty that

you are a white woman from a highly educated, upper middle class, English-speaking family. It is also not useful to divide individuals or groups into advantaged/ disadvantaged categories, because each of us has various advantages and disadvantages that operate differently depending on social and cultural contexts. To some extent, we are positioned by our membership in preexisting groups, but these are shaped by historical, social, economic, political, and cultural factors. Therefore, it is more useful to consider *what shapes your social position.* How are you advantaged or disadvantaged by history? For example, we are all affected by the colonization of Aboriginal people in Canada and appropriation of traditional Aboriginal lands; we are all affected by changing immigration policies, taxation policies, shifts in the economy, global politics, and so on.

Think What are three dominant groups to which you belong? Are you, for example, highly educated? English speaking? What other privileged group do you affiliate with? How do these shape your opportunities in life? Your beliefs and values? What are three relatively subordinate groups to which you belong? Are you, for example, female? Gay? Part of a religious minority? How do these shape your values, beliefs, and opportunities? What are the risks and benefits of examining the privileges and disadvantages associated with these affiliations?

Critically Analyzing the Culture of Health Care and Nursing

As a nurse, you are part of the culture of health care, and you are both shaped by that culture and can participate in shaping it. Examining the culture of health care, how it shapes your practice, and how it shapes patients' experiences is as important as finding out about individual patients' preferences.

Health care is dominated by biomedicine, corporatism, and liberal individualism. Nursing, as part of Western health care, is also dominated by similar ideas and is widely considered to be predominantly white and feminized. **Biomedicine** refers to the application of the principles of natural sciences such as biology and chemistry to understanding, treating, and promoting human health. Biomedical models are important but insufficient to understanding and responding to health-related issues because they are tied to conceptions of health as located in individuals, peoples' physical bodies, and microlevel interactions but leave unexamined the underlying social and structural dynamics that actually produce health and health inequality (Weber & Parra-Medina, 2003). **Corporatism** refers to the primacy of a business model in which the dynamics of the marketplace and management and organizational theories shape health care so that economic and political values dominate (Varcoe & Rodney, 2009). As described earlier, **individualism** is the valuing of individuals over the collective that is common to liberal democracies, a valuing that operates in concert with corporatism to hold individuals responsible for not only their own economic well-being but also their health, regardless of their life circumstances.

Nursing has been described as dominated by whiteness, not just in terms of the ethnic composition of nursing but also in terms of the dominant values, beliefs, practices, and norms that characterize the profession (Allen, 2006; Phillips & Drevdahl, 2003; Puzan, 2003). The dominant values of nursing align with the values of those who dominate Western societies more generally based on race, class, and other forms of privilege. Puzan (2003) argues that talking about presumed racial characteristics is common practice in relation to non-white people, whereas doing so with respect to white people is so unfamiliar that the idea of discussing whiteness in relation to nursing may seem foreign. However, she says, "the presumed neutrality of whiteness conceals its authority to define knowledge, membership, and language, as well as its ability to stipulate and enforce the rules and regulations of everyday concourse and discourse. 'Acting white' and 'performing whiteness' is necessary for survival within the nursing establishment, regardless of color" (Puzan, 2003, p. 194). Even though the ethnic composition of nursing is diversifying, one can still see the dominance of whiteness in health care and nursing, especially in contrast to the ethnic composition of janitorial, food services, security, and other nonprofessional services. Whiteness intersects with employment and educational opportunities, and these in turn shape dominant nursing practices.

The Case of Visiting Hours

One common example of how dominant values operate in nursing is the way in which visiting hours, over which nurses generally have control, are set and differentially enforced. Visiting hours have been, and in many contexts continue to be, based on assumptions that families are available to visit outside of normal work hours, and that female family members are available to provide care. Increasingly under health-care reform, family members are expected to provide care to enable early discharge from health-care facilities. Visiting hour policies are often enforced differently, depending on the particular circumstances of the given patient.

Consider the following situation involving two different patients, and ask yourself: Who is being served by the policies? Which approach to culture does the nurse's actions represent? How do you explain the difference in how the two patients were treated? How do you think that patients or their family members might explain the difference? How do you think the culture of health care is shaping practice? Do you think language differences might have played a role? How might cultural safety guide the nurse?

What could he do differently? What could the student working with the nurse do or say?

Mrs. Dhaliwal, age 72 years, had a total hip replacement yesterday. Mrs. Dhaliwal emigrated from the Punjab state of India over 20 years ago; she speaks little English. This morning, both of her daughters came in at about 8 AM, although visiting hours are 2 PM to 8 PM. The nurse caring for Mrs. Dhaliwal talked to the daughters and discovered that they both work full time starting later in the morning and live about 2 hours from the hospital. The daughters were both very anxious to be with their mother as much as possible and explained that in their family, they see it as their duty as daughters to care for her. The nurse (Chris) gave permission for the daughters to visit outside of usual hours and left a note on the chart to alert other staff that he had done so. At noon, a leader from Mrs. Dhaliwal's temple (she is a devout Sikh) visited, along with several members of her temple. Chris explained the visiting hours to the temple leader and asked him to leave and to remind other temple members of the visiting hours. Chris expressed frustration to the nursing student with whom he was working, saying "These people seem to think the whole community has to visit—it is exhausting for the patient, and we can't get any work done."

Another patient Chris is caring for, 74-year-old Mrs. Kellet, had reconstructive back surgery yesterday and is in the same four-bed room as Mrs. Dhaliwal. Mrs. Kellet emigrated from England as a young woman. Her daughter and Mrs. Kellet's elderly sister also came in before 8 AM. Chris talked to the daughter and found that she works full time evening shifts and cares for both Mrs. Kellet and her sister, who live with her. The daughter explained that this is the only way she will get to see her mother. Chris also gave permission for the daughter to visit outside of usual hours and left a note on the chart to alert other staff that he had done so. At noon, Mrs. Kellet's minister (she is a devout Anglican) visited, along with several members of Mrs. Kellet's bible study group. Talking to Mrs. Kellet, the nurse realized how important these visits were to her. Chris explained the visiting hours to the minister but left him to conduct a prayer with Mrs. Kellet, later asking if he could encourage his parishioners to visit a few at a time and later in the afternoon.

Anticipating the Practice of Culturally Safe Care

Nurses practice within a complex web of relationships and contexts (Hartrick Doane & Varcoe, 2005). As discussed in this chapter, the practice of any nurse is shaped by his or her own values and beliefs, colleagues, and the wider culture of health care in which care is provided. Students are also influenced by the values of their nursing programs and their instructors, values that may be at odds with some values of practice settings. Although students have relatively less power within practice settings, they can still have a significant impact on the practice of others and can always strive to examine their own values and those of the nursing profession and practice in congruence with those values.

NURSING GUIDELINE 13.1: TOWARD CULTURALLY SAFE CARE

Practice Reflexivity

Reflexivity involves practitioners holding up for scrutiny their own and others' knowledge claims, taken-for-granted assumptions, and practices (Taylor & White, 2001). Acting reflexively means continuously scrutinizing your own knowledge and the basis of your practice and always checking your assumptions and "blind spots." In relation to striving to practice in a culturally safe manner, some of the following questions can help you as a nurse to practice reflexivity. Ask yourself:

- What am I assuming and why? What knowledge supports or contradicts my assumptions, and what knowledge might I be missing?
- Why am I applying this ethnic category to this particular patient? Are there alternative ways to describe this patient?
- What is my basis for liking or disliking this patient? What is my basis for approving or disapproving of this patient's or family's actions or decisions?
- When I think of something as cultural, what economic, political, or other social influences might be operating?

When considering the knowledge claims, perspectives, or assumptions of colleagues, you can apply similar questions and look for ways to engage in dialogue. Dialogue is central to the process of reflexivity. Engaging in reflexive approaches requires a commitment to creating opportunities for reflection and dialogue to consider the complexity and specificity of individuals, relationships, and contexts. If you find yourself making unwarranted assumptions, stereotyping, or being judgmental, it is useful to talk with colleagues, teachers, or students. Similarly, if you think that your colleagues are making unwarranted assumptions, stereotyping, or being judgmental, rather than judging them, it is important to engage in dialogue.

- *Develop tolerance for the discomfort of not knowing how to be or act or what to say.* In some situations, being willing to remain silent or watchful can be appropriate. The discomfort that we may encounter—particularly when we are used to filling up conversational spaces—can be instructive because it requires us to step outside of our comfort zones and reflect on how our usual ways of being may need to shift.

Ingrid just graduated from nursing school, moved to a new community, and started her new job. One of her patients is Mrs. Dumont, a Cree woman from a nearby rural setting. Ingrid wanted to be responsive to the patient's needs during the discharge planning process, but in her nursing program, she did not provide care to many Aboriginal patients. The woman was about to be discharged from hospital with crutches and had two small children at home. Because it was a weekend, Ingrid called in the on-call, after-hours social worker to assess Mrs. Dumont's discharge planning needs. After spending a few minutes with Mrs. Dumont, the social worker was baffled because Mrs. Dumont had already arranged for a live-in nanny for at least a few weeks so that she could return to work as soon as possible. Ingrid realized that she had made several assumptions, including the idea that a First Nations person would necessarily need a social worker. The problem lies not with the nurse's best intentions—she was working to ensure that patients are adequately supported as they prepare for the transition from hospital to home (Browne, 2007). Rather, the problem lies with the taken-for-granted assumptions that are applied to members of a group in ways that shut down curiosity about or interest in a patient's individual circumstances. Although the services of a social worker may be vital to many patients' well-being, in this case, presumptions precluded the nurse from directly assessing her patient's unique circumstances (as part of routine discharge planning). Ingrid told the social worker she felt embarrassed; the social worker spent time with Ingrid and made several suggestions to her regarding how she could better get to know the Cree community in the area and suggested that she begin by talking openly with Mrs. Dumont.

The Nursing Student Perspective

Students are routinely under scrutiny in clinical practice; instructors, other staff, and patients are continuously observing and providing feedback. For the most part, such scrutiny is well intentioned and supportive. However, students generally feel that they need to show that they know what they are doing. Trying to convey competence sometimes can get in the way of what is most needed.

Susan, a student nurse, was keen to show her instructor that she was aware of the importance of communicating clearly with Mrs. Chen, who was recovering from abdominal surgery. Mrs. Chen's mother tongue was Cantonese, although she could speak with Susan and others using some English phrases, such as "water please." In her efforts to show her instructor that she was interested in and able to communicate with Mrs. Chen despite their language differences, Susan spoke to Mrs. Chen in a loud voice using single-word phrases; for example, "water?" Part way through her shift, after seeing her with Mrs. Chen, Susan's instructor said that most people understand a second language better than they speak it and suggested that Susan might get an interpreter to help staff assess Mrs. Chen's understanding. Susan realized she had been talking to Mrs. Chen in an overly loud voice and as though she was a child and in the process had overlooked calling for an interpreter, who was readily available.

Applying Cultural Safety in the Practice Context

Interacting with and understanding culture as it relates to nursing involves both interacting with and understanding patients and colleagues. Cultural safety requires developing skills to challenge stereotypes, assumptions, and generalizations and shifting the way we interact and practice with others from the stance of expert to a stance of inquiry (Hartrick Doane & Varcoe, 2005).

Interacting With and Understanding Patients

Working toward cultural safety by interacting with and understanding patients requires you to do the following:

- *Practice from a stance of inquiry and active listening.* Seeking to better understand every patient and every situation will always lead to more respectful practice.
- *Practice nonjudgmental acceptance of people.* Because nurses are required to extend respect to all persons, nonjudgmental acceptance and unconditional positive regard are requirements of practice. It is important to remember that even if you disagree with a patient's behaviours or perspectives, you are obligated to be respectful; it does not mean that you accept or condone the behaviour. However, you will need to remain aware of your own judgments in order to continue to care for patients in ways that meet their needs, given the context of their situation. If you are unable to care for particular patients because of your judgments, you will need to discuss this with your instructor or supervisor and, in some cases, ask your colleagues to provide the care required.
- *Anticipate where you will be most judgmental and how you will practice in those circumstances.* Every nurse will encounter situations in which his or her ability to be nonjudgmental will be challenged. For example, one nurse, Carol, found it very difficult to be accepting of people with serious alcohol problems. In part because her mother had such problems, she found herself being very disapproving and judgmental. As she practiced trying to be respectful and interested regardless of people's alcohol histories, she found that in response, they opened up to her, and she felt less judgmental.
- *Pay attention to when people say they are being discriminated against.* Like pain, discrimination is what the patient says it is. Whether or not you can see discrimination, if people feel demeaned, humiliated, disrespected, or treated unfairly, it is their experiences that matter. It is often tempting to dismiss claims of people who feel discriminated against by assuming that they are being overly sensitive, overly reactive, or attempting to gain advantage by making such claims. Indeed, people who experience discrimination on a daily basis may not be able to distinguish intentional from unintentional unfairness. For example, Chris may not have meant to be unfair in treating Mrs. Dhaliwal and Mrs. Kellet differently, but Mrs. Dhaliwal and her supporters are more likely to have perceived his actions as discriminatory. As nurses, we will develop better relations with all patients if we take claims of discrimination seriously, without defensiveness, and with an understanding of the contexts in which experiences of discrimination arise.

- *When you are uncomfortable and don't know what to say or do, or feel you have done the wrong thing, be honest with others.* People generally are very forgiving if your intentions are good.
- *Ensure that people have the opportunity to communicate in the language that they are able to speak and understand.* Many health-care agencies have trained interpreters on call; some have full-time interpreter phone lines. Whenever possible, trained interpreters ought to be used to communicate with people who understand and speak a language other than the language you understand and speak. If an agency does not have accessible interpreters, nurses should draw attention to the need and lobby for such service.

Working With Language Interpreters

To create a culturally safe health-care environment for people who speak a language that is different from the dominant language spoken in any given health-care setting, it is essential to seek and make use of interpreter services. Relying on family members, children, friends, or untrained workers is not appropriate and ought not to be used as substitutes for trained interpreters. Many hospitals and agencies in Canada have on-call interpreter services available. Here are some general strategies for working with people through the use of an interpreter (Jarvis & Browne, 2014, p. 63):

- Before locating an interpreter, identify the language the person speaks at home. Be aware that it may differ from the language spoken publicly.
- Whenever possible, use a trained interpreter, preferably one who knows health-related terminology.
- Be aware of gender differences between interpreter and patient. In general, an interpreter of the same gender is preferred.
- Permit sufficient time. When using interpreters, conversations often take significantly more time.
- To ensure confidentiality and privacy, avoid using visitors or family members who may be visiting other patients as interpreters.

Interacting With and Understanding Colleagues

Working toward cultural safety by interacting with and understanding colleagues requires you to do the following:

- *Develop skills to challenge stereotypes, assumptions, and generalizations.* General communication skills apply, including using *I* statements such as "I am trying not to use racial categories"; modeling respectful behaviour, such as when a nurse refers to the Korean man in bed 2, saying "Oh, you mean Mr. Kim"; and posing questions such as "Are you saying that you think violence against women is more prevalent in that (specific) community or group of people?" and respectfully disagreeing. Although you are in the position of student, you can find ways of disagreeing without risking being seen as confrontational; for example, "I think violence against women is pervasive in all communities; however, some communities or groups are featured in the media more often than others." Further, develop knowledge or topics regarding which harmful assumptions are commonly made, such as issues that carry stigma. For example, what do you know about the prevalence of violence, the causes of substance use, factors that lead to poverty and homelessness, or factors that contribute to sexually transmitted infections?

- *Counter unwarranted assumptions of others, even when comments are seemingly innocuous.* This will help you to develop and practice the types of responses you can provide. For example, jokes are often a way that stereotypes and assumptions are expressed. Be prepared to respond to jokes by respectfully pointing out another point of view.
- *Challenge the use of racial and ethnic categories whenever they are being used.* Categorizing people based on racial categories is a daily feature of Canadian life and requires persistence and practice to unlearn. It is important to distinguish between the practices of identifying one's self ("I am Cree, from Kapuskasing") and respecting those identities ("The man in room 2 is Cree") versus categorizing others ("Take this dressing tray to the Asian woman in room 4").
- *Draw attention to the larger context that shapes health and health-care inequities and peoples' experiences of discrimination.* Take every opportunity to point to factors that shape inequities and develop your knowledge base to do so. For example, judgments about people's diets often need to be questioned in light of the influence of income. Given the high levels of poverty and food insecurity in Canada, problematic behaviours in children often are influenced by hunger. Wonder aloud about poverty, racism, discrimination, and so on. Replace assumptions based on stereotypes with assumptions based on knowledge about context— for example, you can assume that people from racialized groups will likely have experienced discrimination or that a large proportion of people from all cultures and groups will have experienced violence.
- *Develop strategies to create a culturally safe environment for all patients (not just particular patients).* When you encounter a challenging situation, ask yourself what could be done at a unit or organizational level to improve practice. For example, rather than just advocating for particular patients to have interpreters, could signs be posted in various languages most pertinent to your setting that welcome people and advise them that interpreters are available? Posting small signs on doors or walls with commonly used phrases in commonly spoken languages can make people feel welcome and can convey an interest in people.
- *Engage colleagues beyond your immediate clinical situation.* Take opportunities to get to know social workers, interpreters, porters, lab technicians, and administrative staff. Even as a student, having relationships with a range of care providers will expand your resources for providing more culturally safe care and increase your opportunities to influence the quality of care patients receive.

Through the eyes of a nurse

I am so embarrassed by my profession sometimes. This is such a tragedy. Last year, I looked after a man with a seizure disorder who had been discharged without treatment. He was Aboriginal, and when the emergency physician followed up with the previous hospital, they said they thought he had been drinking. The man had been drinking, but he also had a series of seizures! Working with Rebecca made me realize that I have to do something more than just provide good care to my own patients. If I don't speak up, how can I expect students like Rebecca to?

(personal reflection of a nurse)

SUMMARY

The world increasingly is characterized by heightened racial and ethnic tensions, accompanied by a growing gap between the wealthy and the very poor and between north and south. As throughout history, ethnicity and race figure in the dynamics of resource distribution—between countries, between groups, and within social institutions such as health care. Nurses are morally obligated to uphold and advocate for fairness, so rather than collude with interpretations of culture that sustain unequal and unfair treatment of certain people, nurses must develop and draw upon a complex understanding of culture as it is shaped by power dynamics and broader contexts. With such values and knowledge, nurses can provide more competent, ethical care and can contribute, one patient at a time, and one health-care setting at a time, to a fairer, more just world.

Critical Thinking Case Scenario

▶ Rebecca is a student nurse in her fourth year of her baccalaureate program. She is currently doing a final preceptorship in the overflow unit attached to an emergency unit in a large community hospital. The unit is primarily for patients who are admitted to the hospital through the emergency but awaiting beds. However, because the emergency is very busy this evening, Lise, the nurse with whom Rebecca is working, is assigned to care for a woman who has just arrived. The woman, Ms. Rose Johns, gave birth 2 days ago. She is admitted accompanied by her foster mother

(Mrs. Edna Wiens), who is furious. Ms. Johns had stroke-like symptoms about 7 hours ago but was discharged from the emergency unit of a hospital in another suburb of the city. Mrs. Wiens angrily explains that at the previous hospital, the staff repeatedly asked Ms. Johns how much she had been drinking—"just because she's native." Despite protests from both of them, Mrs. Wiens says the physician suggested she "go home and sleep it off." While assessing Ms. Johns, Lise listens and expresses empathy. "I can understand why you would be feeling angry. You must have been so worried." Ms. Johns is sent for an emergency CT scan immediately. After transferring Ms. Johns to radiology, Lise tells Rebecca that this is not the first time that an Aboriginal patient has come to this hospital after being dismissed elsewhere because the symptoms were assumed to have been due to alcohol use. Lise says that she is quite frustrated and feels she needs to do something. Lise went on to explain to Rebecca how quickly nurses and doctors in the emergency department assume that Aboriginal patients are likely to have used alcohol and how that sometimes obscures their ability to accurately assess or diagnose the patient's actual health condition. As one of the most pervasive and enduring stereotypes in Canada, assumptions about Aboriginal people as "prone" to alcoholism can affect the ability to provide needed health assessments and care (Browne, 2005). In reaction to Ms. Johns' situation, Lise and Rebecca decided to make this the focus of the next "lunch and learn" session on their unit to encourage dialogue and critical thinking among their colleagues.

1. What challenges should Lise and Rebecca anticipate in the "lunch and learn"?
2. What strategies might help them make the session more effective?
3. What are the limitations to this solution, and what else might they do?

Multiple-Choice Questions

1. Nurses are ethically obligated to:
   a. Learn about the beliefs and practices of the cultural groups with whom they work.
   b. Treat patients with respect regardless of ethnic origin, religion, or sexuality.
   c. Advocate for fair treatment and fair distribution of resources for those in their care.
   d. Provide care for everyone regardless of whether the care conflicts with the nurses' own moral commitments.
   e. Understand and support patient's health practices regardless of the potential for negative health consequences.
      a. a, b, d, e
      b. a, c
      c. b only
      d. b, c

2. Providing culturally safe care requires:
   a. Critical self-examination of one's own biases and assumptions
   b. Knowledge of cultural practices of other groups
   c. Countering stereotypes
   d. Knowledge of factors that influence inequity
   e. Advocating for systemic change
      a. a, b
      b. a, c, d
      c. a, c, d, e
      d. c, d

3. Interpreters are required for patients who do not speak Canada's official languages:
   a. Only when issues of consent or life-threatening situations arise
   b. When any health-care decisions are being made
   c. Only when family members are not available
   d. When it is not possible to find a staff member who speaks the patient's language

4. Democratic racism refers to:
   a. The process of voting on policies related to racism
   b. The process of conveying racism to proponents of democracy
   c. The process of espousing equity while practicing discrimination
   d. The process of addressing issues of racism in society

5. Which of the following are true of cultural inventories when used in health-care settings?
   a. Cultural inventories can alert nurses to a range of values, beliefs, and practices.
   b. Cultural inventories counter the formation of stereotypes about cultural groups.
   c. Cultural inventories are essential to culturally safe care.
   d. Cultural inventories can contribute to assumptions about cultural groups.
   e. Cultural inventories provide quick reference so individual's behaviours can be understood.
      a. a, b, e
      b. a, d
      c. b, c
      d. c, d, e

Suggested Lab Activity

● In communications labs, practice countering common stereotypes and assumptions. Generate a list of phrases commonly heard, and then practice different responses. Role-play various responses, allowing each student to develop his or her own style of responding and evaluating the effectiveness of different responses.

REFERENCES AND SUGGESTED READINGS

Adelson, N. (2005). The embodiment of inequity: Health disparities in aboriginal Canada. *Canadian Journal of Public Health. Revue Canadienne De Santè Publique, 96*(Suppl. 2), S45–S61.

Adeyanju, C. T., & Neverson, N. (2007). "There will be a next time"; Media discourse about an "apocalyptic" vision of immigration, racial diversity, and health risks. *Canadian Ethnic Studies, 39*(1–2), 79–105.

Ahmad, W. I. U. (1993). Making black people sick: 'Race', ideology and health research. In W. I. U. Ahmad (Ed.), *'Race' and health in contemporary Britain* (pp. 11–33). Buckingham, England: Open University Press.

Allen, D. G. (2006). Whiteness and difference in nursing. *Nursing Philosophy, 7*(2), 65–78.

Anderson, J. M., Perry, J., Blue, C., Browne, A. J., Henderson, A., Khan, K. B., . . . Smyve, V. (2003). "Rewriting" cultural safety within the postcolonial and postnational feminist project: Toward new epistemologies of healing. *Advances in Nursing Science, 26*(3), 196–214.

Anderson, J. M., & Reimer Kirkham, S. (1999). Discourses on health: A critical perspective. In H. Coward & P. Ratanakul (Eds.), *A cross-cultural dialogue on health care ethics* (pp. 47–67). Waterloo, ON: Wilfrid Laurier University Press.

Anderson, J. M., Tang, S., & Blue, C. (2007). Health care reform and the paradox of efficiency: "Writing in" culture. *International Journal of Health Services, 37*(2), 291–320.

Applebaum, B. (2001). Locating oneself: Self, "I" identification and the trouble with moral agency. *Philosophy of Education Year Book,* 412–422.

Battiste, M., & Youngblood Henderson, J. (2000). *Protecting indigenous knowledge and heritage: A global challenge.* Saskatoon, SA: Purich.

Bourassa, C., McKay-McNabb, K., & Hampton, M. R. (2004). Racism, sexism, and colonialism: The impact on the health of aboriginal women in Canada. *Canadian Woman Studies, 24*(1), 23–29.

Browne, A. J. (2001). The influence of liberal political ideology on nursing science. *Nursing Inquiry, 8*(2), 118–129.

Browne, A. J. (2005). Discourses influencing nurses' perceptions of First Nations patients. CJNR. *Canadian Journal of Nursing Research, 37*(4), 62–87.

Browne, A. J. (2007). Clinical encounters between nurses and First Nations women in a Western Canadian hospital. *Social Science & Medicine, 64*(10), 2165–2176.

Browne, A. J., Varcoe, C., Smye, V., Reimer-Kirkham, S., Lynam, M. J., & Wong, S. (2009). Cultural safety and the challenges of translating critically oriented knowledge in practice. *Nursing Philosophy, 10,* 167–179.

Brownridge, D. A. (2008). Understanding the elevated risk of partner violence against aboriginal women: A comparison of two nationally representative surveys of Canada. *Journal of Family Violence, 23*(5), 353–367.

Canadian Association of the Deaf. (2012). *Deaf culture vs. medicalization.* Retrieved from http://www.cad.ca/deaf_culture_vs._medicalization.php

Canadian Nurses Association. (2008). *Code of ethics for registered nurses* (2008 centennial edition). Ottawa, ON: Author.

Department of Justice Canada. (1985). *Indian act.* Retrieved from http://laws.justice.gc.ca/en/ShowFullDoc/cs/I-5//20090805/en

Employment Equity Act, S.C. 1995, c. 44. Retrieved from http://laws-lois.justice.gc.ca/eng/acts/E-5.401/page-1.html#h-3

Furniss, E. (1999). *The burden of history: Colonialism and the frontier myth in a rural Canadian community.* Vancouver, BC: University of British Columbia Press.

Galabuzi, G. E. (2001). *Canada's creeping economic apartheid: The economic segregation and social marginalization of racialised groups.* Toronto, ON: Centre for Social Justice Foundation for Research and Education.

Government of Canada. (1988). *Canadian multiculturalism act.* Ottawa, ON: Queen's Printer for Canada.

Guruge, S., & Collins, E. (2008). *Working with immigrant women: Issues and strategies for mental health professionals.* Toronto, ON: Centre for Addiction and Mental Health.

Gustafson, D. L. (2005). Transcultural nursing theory from a critical cultural perspective. *Advances in Nursing Science, 28*(1), 2–16.

Gustafson, D. L. (2008). Are sensitivity and tolerance enough? Comparing two theoretical approaches to caring for newcomer women with mental health problems. In S. Guruge & E. Collins (Eds.), *Working with immigrant women: Issues and strategies for mental health professionals* (pp. 39–63). Toronto, ON: Centre for Addiction and Mental Health.

Hartrick Doane, G., & Varcoe, C. (2005). *Family nursing as relational inquiry: Developing health-promoting practice.* Philadelphia, PA: Lippincott Williams & Wilkins.

Henry, F., & Tator, C. (2006). *The colour of democracy: Racism in Canadian society* (3rd ed.). Toronto, ON: Nelson Thomson.

Hyman, I., Forte, T., Du Mont, J., Romans, S., & Cohen, M. M. (2009). Help-seeking behavior for intimate partner violence among racial minority women in Canada. *Women's Health Issues, 19*(2), 101–108.

Jarvis, C., & Browne, A. J. (2014). The interview. In A. J. Browne, J. MacDonald-Jenkins, & M. Luctkar-Flude (Eds.), *Physical examination and health assessment by Carolyn Jarvis* (2nd Canadian ed., pp. 45–65). Toronto, ON: Elsevier.

Kisely, S., Terashima, M., & Langille, D. (2008). A population-based analysis of the health experience of African Nova Scotians. *CMAJ: Canadian Medical Association Journal, 179*(7), 653–658.

Krieger, N., Sidney, S., & Coakley, E. (1998). Racial discrimination and skin color in the CARDIA study: Implications for public health research. *American Journal of Public Health, 88*(9), 1308–1313.

Leininger, M. (2002a). Culture care theory: A major contribution to advance transcultural nursing and practices. *Journal of Transcultural Nursing, 13*(3), 189–192.

Leininger, M. (2002b). *Transcultural nursing: Concepts, theories, research, and practice* (3rd ed.). New York, NY: McGraw-Hill.

McDonald, J., & Kennedy, S. (2007). Cervical cancer screening by immigrant and minority women in Canada. *Journal of Immigrant and Minority Health, 9*(4):323–334.

Miles, R. (1989). *Racism.* London, United Kingdom: Routledge.

Papps, E., & Ramsden, I. (1996). Cultural safety in nursing: The New Zealand experience. *International Journal for Quality in Health Care, 8*(5), 491–497.

Paterson, B. L., Osborne, M., & Gregory, D. (2004). How different can you be and still survive: Homogeneity and difference in clinical nursing education. *International Journal of Nursing Education Scholarship, 1*(1), 1–13.

Paterson, B. L., Russell, C., & Thorne, S. (2001). Critical analysis of everyday self-care decision making in chronic illness. *Journal of Advanced Nursing, 35*(3), 335–342.

Peter, E., Spalding, K., Kenny, N., Conrad, P., McKeever, P., & Macfarlane, A. (2007). Neither seen nor heard: Children and homecare policy in Canada. *Social Science & Medicine, 64*(8), 1624–1635.

Peternelj-Taylor, C. (2004). An exploration of othering in forensic psychiatric and correctional nursing. *Canadian Journal of Nursing Research, 36*(4), 130–146.

Phillips, D. A., & Drevdahl, D. J. (2003). "Race" and the difficulties of language. *Advances in Nursing Science, 26*(1), 17–29.

Polashek, N. R. (1998). Cultural safety: A new concept in nursing people with different ethnicities. *Journal of Advanced Nursing, 27*(3), 452–457.

Poudrier, J. (2007). The geneticization of aboriginal diabetes and obesity: Adding another scene to the story of the thrifty gene. *Canadian Review of Sociology & Anthropology, 44,* 237–261.

Puzan, E. (2003). The unbearable whiteness of being (in nursing). *Nursing Inquiry, 10*(3), 193–200.

Ramsden, I. (1993). Cultural safety in nursing education in Aotearoa (New Zealand). *Nursing Praxis in New Zealand, 8*(3), 4–10.

Ramsden, I. (2000). Cultural safety/Kawa Whakaruruhau ten years on: A personal overview. *Nursing Praxis in New Zealand, 15*(1), 4–12.

Ramsden, I. (2002). *Cultural safety and nursing education in Aotearoa and Te Waipounamu* (Unpublished doctoral dissertation). University of Wellington, Wellington, New Zealand.

Ramsden, I., & Spoonley, P. (1994). The cultural safety debate in nursing education in Aotearoa. *New Zealand Annual Review of Education, 3,* 161–174.

Reimer-Kirkham, S., Varcoe, C., Browne, A. J., Lynam, M. J., Khan, K. B., & McDonald, H. (2009). Critical inquiry and knowledge translation: Exploring compatibilities and tensions. *Nursing Philosophy, 10*(3), 152–166.

Srivastava, R. H. (2007). *The health care professionals guide to clinical cultural competence.* Toronto, ON: Elsevier.

Stebnicki, J. A., & Coeling, H. V. (1999). The culture of the deaf. *Journal of Transcultural Nursing, 10*(4), 350–357.

Taylor, C., & White, S. (2001). Knowledge, truth and reflexivity: The problem of judgment in social work. *Journal of Social Work, 1*(1), 37–59.

Thomas, D. (2005). "I am Canadian." *Canadian Social Trend, 76,* 1–7.

Varcoe, C., Browne, A., Wong, S., & Smye, V. (2009). Harms and benefits: Collecting ethnicity data in a clinical context. *Social Science & Medicine, 68*(9), 1659–1666. doi:10.1016/j.socscimed.2009.02.034

Varcoe, C., & Dick, S. (2008). Intersecting risks of violence and HIV for rural and Aboriginal women in a neocolonial Canadian context. *Journal of Aboriginal Health, 4,* 42–52.

Varcoe, C., & McCormick, J. (2007). Racing around the classroom margins: Race, racism and teaching nursing. In L. Young & B. Patterson (Eds.), *Learning nursing: Student-centered theories, models, and strategies for nurse educators* (pp. 439–446). Philadelphia, PA: Lippincott, Williams & Wilkins.

Varcoe, C., & Rodney, P. (2009). Constrained agency: The social structure of nurses work. In B. S. Bolaria & H. D. Dickinson (Eds.), *Health, illness and health care in Canada* (4th ed., pp. 122–150). Toronto, ON: Nelson.

Varcoe, C., Rodney, P., & McCormick, J. (2003). Health care relationships in context: An analysis of three ethnographies. *Qualitative Health Research, 13*(7), 957–973.

Walker, B. (Ed.). (2008). *History of immigration and racism in Canada: Essential readings.* Toronto, ON: International Press.

Warry, W. (2007). *Ending denial: Understanding aboriginal issues.* Peterborough, ON: Broadview Press.

Weber, L., & Parra-Medina, D. (2003). Intersectionality and women's health: Charting a path to eliminating health disparities. *Advances in Gender Research, 7,*181–230.

Improving Patient and Nurse Safety: Learning From Past Experiences

LYNN SHERIDAN AND RONI L. CLUBB

Mr. Smith, a long-term care (LTC) facility resident, is totally dependent on the health-care team for his activities of daily living (ADL) because of stroke-related physical impairments. His communication ability and cognitive abilities are intact. Today, Angela, a new staff member, has been assigned to care for Mr. Smith. Angela is an experienced acute care nurse who was assigned a "buddy shift" with a staff member last week in lieu of the formal employee staff orientation session. During morning report, Angela is told to use the mechanical lift to transfer Mr. Smith to his wheelchair. Following report, she looks for a procedure to follow because she is unfamiliar with all the different mechanical lifts in the facility. Unable to find one, she enlists help from an experienced care aide, and together, they set a plan to transfer Mr. Smith at 10 AM. However, during morning care, Mr. Smith requests to be up at 9:30 AM for an unexpected family visit. Angela asks another caregiver to enter the room to help her with the transfer. They transfer Mr. Smith using the procedure shown to Angela on her "buddy shift" day. During the procedure, Mr. Smith slides from the sling and falls to the floor.

How could this accident have been prevented? What system failure caused Mr. Smith to fall? What risk assessments should be considered? How should the organization respond to this event? We address these and other questions as we progress through this chapter.

CHAPTER OBJECTIVES

By the end of this chapter, you will be able to:

1. Describe the systems approach to patient safety.
2. Determine how practice standards inform safe competent patient care.
3. Apply nursing practice standards to decrease risk of patient safety events.
4. Discuss the nurse's role in advancing patient safety and reducing patient harm.
5. Describe the benefits of reporting incidents.
6. Determine how interprofessional collaboration sustains a safety culture.
7. Discuss the challenges of nursing practice as it relates to patient safety.

KEY TERMS

Adverse Event An unfavourable occurrence that is a direct result of the provision of care or health-care services and is unrelated to the patient's medical condition.

Contributing Factor An influential care occurrence with the potential to lead to a negative patient safety event.

Critical Incident A grave patient safety outcome, such as loss of life, limb, or organ function.

Disclosure A caregiver communication process, delivered by a caregiver, to inform the patient of a safety event.

Engineering Controls Physical controls or barriers that isolate or remove a hazard.

Good Catch Also called *near miss*, an event with the potential to cause harm that is discovered before an injury occurs.

Harm A patient care outcome with detrimental effects on the patient's health status.

Incident An event, process, practice, or outcome that creates a hazard for patients.

Near Miss See *good catch*.

Patient Safety A set of practices designed to promote positive patient outcomes by reducing and intercepting harmful acts.

Risk Management An organizational strategy designed to reduce and manage all adverse events.

Root Cause Analysis A thorough review of a patient safety event to identify the multiple causes and contributing factors that caused the patient harm. The process concludes with specific system change recommendations to minimize the potential for similar events in the future.

System Failure A faulty organizational process, operation, or structure that places the patient and/or health-care worker in danger of harm.

Patient Safety Overview

Nurses strive to deliver quality patient care but at times find situations that make safe care delivery very difficult. What is the nurse to do in such a situation? In this chapter, we provide insights into the present reality for nurses striving to keep their patients and themselves safe in today's Canadian health-care system. We provide strategies for you, your peers, and other health-care professionals to use to promote patient and personal safety.

Why should a nursing student learn about **patient safety**? The answer is simple: Patient safety is a big problem both in our country and globally. *Patient safety* is defined as "the reduction and mitigation of unsafe acts within the health-care system, as well as through the use of best practices, shown to lead to optimal patient outcomes" (Davies, Hebert, & Hoffman, 2003, p. 12). Approximately 1 in 13 Canadians in acute care institutions experience an adverse event: an injury, complication, or some other potentially negative outcome not related to the reason the patient sought hospitalization (Leeb, Zelmer, Wester, & Pulcins, 2005). In your student clinical sites, potentially 1 in 9 patients will contract an infection, be given the wrong medication, or the wrong dose of a medication during their hospital stay (Leeb et al., 2005). A national research project by Baker et al. (2004) found that 7.5% of all patients experience adverse events, and of those adverse events, approximately 35% were considered preventable. Some were so severe that patients died as a consequence. The statistics cited are equivalent to an airplane carrying 200 passengers crashing every 3 days. You and your classmates will make a tremendous contribution to patient safety, but first, you need to understand why these events happen and what you, a student nurse, can do to prevent or minimize them by intervening before an adverse event occurs.

Understanding Patient Safety: A Systems Perspective

The initial step in patient safety is to acknowledge that unsafe events happen while vulnerable people are in our care. Understanding the challenges and roadblocks to safe practice that occur daily in the nurse's workplace can decrease the likelihood of incidents. An **incident** includes events, processes, practices, or outcomes that are noteworthy by virtue of the hazards they create for or the harms they cause to patients (Canadian Patient Safety Institute [CPSI], 2008b). Some obstacles can be controlled by the nurse; others cannot and require a system response. Many contributing factors are invisible to the practitioner at the bedside: They may be hidden within the overall system. We expect a system that keeps everyone safe—patients, staff, and families. Patient safety is the responsibility of the whole health-care system, which needs to be designed to allow everyone to do their work in a safe, caring, and competent manner. Even the nurse with 25 years of experience cannot perform perfectly if the system is not set up to deliver safe care. Absolute perfection is not possible.

A system that is grounded in patient safety is ready to recognize and act on the warning signals that indicate that harm is a potential outcome. **Harm** is a product of unsafe acts or safety events. From a patient safety perspective, harm occurs as a result of the health-care interaction unrelated to the reason the person entered the health-care system. Harm can occur to a patient and/or staff member or even to family members. Harm can impact any dimension of health—physical, emotional, social, and/or spiritual well-being. Think of how each of these dimensions of well-being would be affected if, for example, the wrong limb were accidentally removed in a surgical amputation procedure. Harm can also occur to a staff member; for example, a back injury or verbal abuse. An early warning patient safety system needs to be in place and practiced by all members, like an early warning earthquake system, with one exception: The health-care system will require many different types of warning systems; some formal, and others informal. Some will be in response to major events, whereas others will become a part of everyone's daily practice. Safe practice within the system can only happen if the people in health care are committed to this broad understanding of patient safety on a shift-to-shift, hour-by-hour, and minute-by-minute basis. This type of safety commitment requires the inclusion of the student nurse for effective functioning.

The Nursing Student's Perspective

What is expected of you regarding patient and staff safety? It is anticipated that students will make mistakes, so nursing programs must have checks and balances in place to minimize those events. It is always important that you are prepared and knowledgeable about the care you will provide. Practicing within your professional standards and competency base is expected. You will need to ask questions, especially if you are concerned or perplexed about any aspect of patient care. Your instructor and the nurses on the unit are prepared for you to ask a lot of questions. Ask for clarification if you are not sure of what you read or how to perform a task. Report anything that seems not quite right to your instructor. It will be necessary to get assistance with problem solving in patient care situations that appear confusing to you. Use your critical thinking skills and resources to problem-solve for a safe resolution.

Think *Mr. Smith Event—Student's Perspective*
Reflect on Angela's patient care responsibilities for Mr. Smith.

What type of preparation is required specific to the mechanical transfer?

What agency protocols need to be researched prior to transferring a patient?

What level of understanding is required by Angela in relation to the transfer equipment?

How should Angela communicate with Mr. Smith prior to, during, and after the transfer?

What other safety precautions should Angela undertake during the transfer?

The Nurse's Perspective

You will acquire an understanding of the complex nature of nurses' work over the length of your nursing program. You will be exposed to many clinical settings and learn from nurses who have been engaged in their nursing careers for many years. They have witnessed many patient safety events, some with good outcomes and some with unfortunate outcomes. Listen and learn from their stories.

Nursing students contribute to the system in their clinical education by discovering and communicating potential safety concerns on the unit. Because you are a visitor for a brief time on the unit, you will see the nursing routine differently than someone who has been working on the unit for a long time. You have the power to stop a patient safety event from occurring simply by asking questions and talking about confusing aspects of care. Asking questions of your instructor or the staff on the unit can be intimidating. (See Box 14.1 for suggestions on determining who to approach with your questions.) However, do not let fear stop you from asking your questions. It is better to ask for clarification than to put a patient at risk for harm.

Safety Systems

Baker and Norton (2001) identified three interdependent components in their safety system model: measurement, systems tools and change strategies, and culture. The components require a reliable system to measure the nature and

---

BOX 14.1 Approaching Expert Nurses on Patient Care Issues

Staff Member
1. Choose a staff member who is knowledgeable on the specific care of the patient.
2. A full-time staff member usually is more knowledgeable on unit practices than a casual member.
3. Do not interrupt a staff member who is in the middle of a procedure (e.g., medication administration). Wait until he or she acknowledges your presence.
4. Introduce yourself complete with program information.
5. Outline the care dilemma briefly but succinctly.
6. Offer your perspective first and ask for his or her advice at the end.
7. Be courteous and respectful.

Clinical Instructor
1. Write down the questions you want to discuss.
2. Take your research information with you if relevant.
3. Present your query with factual information; integrate your research information and patient assessment data.
4. Indicate that you are perplexed by the care issue and state the reasons why.
5. Offer your solution to demonstrate you have reflected on the care issue.
6. Ask for a follow-up consultation to discuss the evaluation of the strategy chosen for implementation.

---

type of problems that occur, a learning culture, and an effective system to reduce error (McKelvey, 2001). Measurement information must be used to work toward system and culture change (Baker & Norton, 2001). In 2002, the National Steering Committee on Patient Safety took up the challenge to build a safer system by developing documents, strategies, and tools.

The Patient's Perspective

Many events occur when health-care professionals disregard a patient's comment related to a patient care activity that is unfamiliar to the patient or out of the patient's ordinary routine. Remember to listen to your patients; they have health-care experience as well but from the opposite side of the health-care interaction. What could Mr. Smith have said to the nurses if he believed they were using the wrong lift or performing the procedure incorrectly? Would the nurses have listened if they were in a hurry?

The Family's Perspective

When the family arrives to visit Mr. Smith, they could encounter a man in pain, distressed, and potentially angry. The family would be upset and feel helpless in this situation. The family would most likely seek the nurses out for an explanation of Mr. Smith's behaviour. What should the health-care team disclose? **Disclosure**, "the process by which an adverse event is communicated to the patient by healthcare providers" (CPSI, 2008b, p. 8), is covered later in the chapter.

The Institution's Perspective

The long-term care (LTC) facility is also impacted by Mr. Smith's event. The reputation of the facility and the reputation of the staff who work at this facility have all been compromised. Would this impact the community's view of the LTC facility? If you were a nurse working on the unit, how would you feel? If you were the unit manager, what would you do? The worst response for the institution as a whole is to try and hide the fact that the event happened or to blame the nurses. The best response is to investigate why it happened, strategize on how to prevent this from occurring again, and support all those affected by the event.

Conceptual Models

Many conceptual models explain how safety events happen in an organization. All the models have one focal point, the system, and do not focus on the person(s) directly involved in the event. We briefly explore the models known as the Swiss Cheese Model, the Domino Theory, and the Iceberg Model.

James Reason, a well-known safety expert, developed the Swiss Cheese Model (Reason, 2000a) to understand the journey of a safety event through the health-care system;

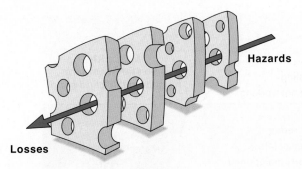

Figure 14.1 Swiss Cheese Model.

it illustrates how safety events occur in organizations. The Swiss Cheese Model represented in Figure 14.1 depicts several system layers that a harmful event passes through before it reaches the patient.

The safeguards the system has in place are represented by slices of Swiss cheese, and the holes in the cheese help you visualize a weakness in the safeguard layers. The presence of weaknesses or holes in the system layers is how the harmful event is able to pass through the various system layers. In a patient safety event, the harmful event travels through the holes without detection. The holes in the layers would not always line up perfectly to allow the event to pass through. But it only takes once for the holes to line up in a row to permit the conditions for an unsafe act to occur. Therefore, it takes multiple failures to occur in several layers in an organization to lead to patient harm. Many patient safety events are now viewed as systems failures. Systems failure is a fault, breakdown, or dysfunction in how an organization is structured or operates (Runciman et al., 2009). Simply, the safeguards that were built into the system fail on occasion, producing harm. One intervention at any one layer would stop the event's passage and keep the patient safe.

Think *Mr. Smith Event—Swiss Cheese Analysis*
Draw a Swiss Cheese Model to illustrate Mr. Smith's event trajectory.

1. Start with a drawing of a block of Swiss cheese, similar to Figure 14.1.
2. Slice the model into the various mishaps that occurred generic to his fall.
3. Line up the holes to draw the harm outcome (fall) for Mr. Smith.

A second model of understanding how safety events occur is based on a theory developed by W. H. Heinrich in 1931 called the Domino Theory. The safety event takes on the form of falling dominos. Each time it passes through a system layer or a subsystem of the organization, the momentum of the fallen dominos cause more dominos to fall. If the domino effect is not stopped, it can eventually end in harm or even death of a patient. It only takes one intervention anywhere to halt the dominos from falling.

In order to understand Mr. Smith's event more clearly, we must look deeper than the surface or visible factors, and

consider the invisible factors. The Iceberg Model is one way to identify potential invisible factors that led to this event. Figure 14.2 represents Mr. Smith's adverse event using the Iceberg Model. In this figure, we see the two employees, Mr. Smith, and the mechanical lift above the water line as the tip of the iceberg. The visible factors above the water, the wrong sling and the malfunction of the emergency stop button, appear to be the direct cause of the incident. Focusing on only the visible part of the iceberg does not allow the examination of the submerged iceberg portion.

A deep sea diver can see things lurking below the surface and would be able to describe the submerged portion. Unsafe acts or potential pitfalls represented as contributing factors are uncovered with deeper investigation. **Contributing factors** are the "reason(s), situations factor(s), or latent condition(s) that played a role in the genesis of an adverse event" (Davies, Hebert, & Hoffman, 2003, p. 55). An investigation is done through data collection, communication with the health-care team, and continuing to ask why, until new responses are exhausted. After the data collection phase, contributing factors can be identified and the root causes, which are generally system failures, are found. A **system failure** is a faulty organizational process, operation, or structure that places the patient and/or health-care worker in danger of harm. The use of critical thinking, deep sea diving questioning, and identification of root causes allows for recommendations for improvement that are distributed to all health-care providers.

In Mr. Smith's example, the worst case scenario would be to look only at the portion of iceberg above the water, or at the caregivers directly involved in the transfer. By isolating these individuals, disciplinary action is a potential outcome and would characterize a blame culture. The nurse needs to advocate for a different non-blame approach, one that looks below the surface of the water so the entire iceberg can be understood. A system-wide holistic approach will help the organization learn from the event and remedy the factors that allowed the event to occur. If learning does not take place, the system cannot correct itself. If no action is taken to understand and fix the problems, the same incident may reoccur with another patient and caregiver.

Through the eyes of a student

I am caring for Mr. Smith today, and my chart research identified that he was traumatized last week because of a fall from a mechanical lift. I know I will have to be very careful today and follow the correct patient moving procedure that I learned in lab. I can't help wondering about what I might not know. I am a bit anxious but realize I have a lot of resources on the unit, including the policy and procedure manual. I can ask my instructor, the other nurses, and my peers for guidance if I have questions. Mr. Smith can answer some questions too. I hope he is feeling okay and not anxious about the transfer.

(personal reflection of a nursing student)

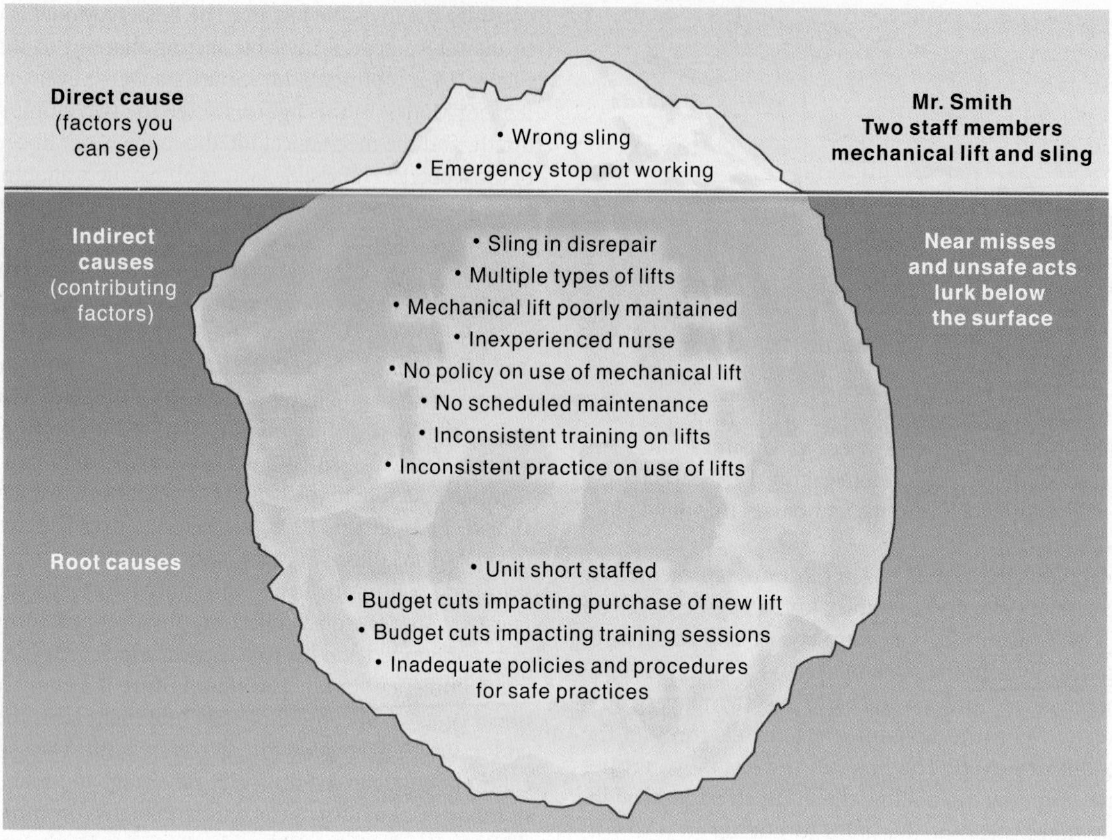

Figure 14.2 Mr. Smith's adverse event using Iceberg Model.

Practice Standards

Being a competent nurse requires adherence to professional standards produced by national nursing associations and provincial nursing regulatory bodies. Standards may come in the form of codes of ethics, competencies or professional standards, position statements, or best practices. See Table 14.1 for selected examples of patient and nurse safety statements issued by professional nursing associations.

Codes of Ethics

The Canadian Nurses Association (CNA, 2008) Code of Ethics for Registered Nurses provides a framework for all nurses delivering patient care. The CNA provides guidance for seven nursing values and ethical responsibilities, including providing safe, compassionate, competent, and ethical care; the provinces and territories articulate and monitor competencies and standards related to patient safety as well. See Box 14.2 for an abbreviated version of the CNA subcategories related to patient safety. The Registered Psychiatric Nurses of Canada (RPNC, 2010) Code of Ethics and Standards also contains patient safety values and statements, as found in Box 14.3.

Position Statements

Patient safety position statements can be found in international, national, provincial, or jurisdictional organizations. "The International Council of Nurses (ICN) believes that

the enhancement of patient safety involves a wide range of actions in the recruitment, training and retention of health care professionals, performance improvement, environmental safety and risk management, including infection control, safe use of medicines, equipment safety, safe clinical practice, safe environment of care, and accumulating an integrated body of scientific knowledge focused on patient safety and the infrastructure to support its development" (International Council on Nursing [ICN], 2012, p. 1). The ICN document lists patient safety responsibilities for nurses and nursing associations. The CNA patient safety position states that "patient safety cannot be achieved without system accountability and system competence" (CNA, 2009, p. 2). The Canadian Association of Schools of Nursing (CASN) patient safety and nursing education position statement calls for schools to "foster learning environments (classroom and clinical) which promote 'self disclosure'" (CASN, 2006, p. 5) working in collaboration with agency partners. CASN encourages schools to use measurement tools as well as establish and analyze data sets of adverse events related to patient safety. Within nursing curriculum, CASN also advises the inclusion of the following six competencies:

- Assess the safety and quality of care and apply prevention measures;
- Adopt a system approach to patient safety;
- Recognize, report, and manage risks, adverse events, and near misses;

TABLE 14.1	Nursing Association Examples of Patient Safety Statements
Patient Safety Standards and Competency Example Statements	**Nursing Association**
Demonstrates responsibility and accountability to the public by providing safe, competent care	Prince Edward Island (Association of Registered Nurses of Prince Edward island [ARNPEI]) http://www.arnpei.ca/default.asp?id=190&pagesize=1&sfield=content.id&search=110&mn=1.45
Advocates for practice environments that have organizational and human support systems and resources allocation necessary to provided safe, competent care	Alberta (College and Association of Registered Nurses of Alberta [CARNA]) http://www.nurses.ab.ca/CarnaAdmin/Uploads/new_nps_with_ethics.pdf
Nursing administrator role is to advocate for a quality practice environment to support nurses in providing safe, competent care.	Ontario (RNAO) http://www.rnao.org/Storage/38/3297_Policy_Statement_on_Patient_Safety.pdf
Requires nurse to have relationships fostering an environment in which patients and nurses are safe from abuse	
Nursing researcher role is to ensure the safety and well-being of the patient above all other objectives, including the search for knowledge.	
Appropriately supervises students	
Communicates and collaborates with patients, the nursing team, and members of the health-care team for the delivery of safe, competent care	Northwest Territories and Nunavut (Registered Nurses Association of Northwest Territories and Nunavut [RNANT/NU]) http://www.rnantnu.ca/Portals/0/Documents/Standards_Nrsing_Prac_2006.pdf
Registered nurse in an educator role provides a safe practice setting, which enables students to apply their knowledge.	British Columbia (College of Registered Nurses of British Columbia [CRNBC]) http://www.crnbc.ca/downloads/128.pdf
Reports unsafe practice to appropriate person or body	Newfoundland and Labrador (Association of Registered Nurses of Newfoundland and Labrador [ARNNL])
Knowing where to find key information	http://www.arnnl.nf.ca/PDF/Education/Competencies_required_for_entry_level_RN_08_13.pdf
Protects patients through recognizing and reporting unsafe practices when patient and staff safety and well-being are potentially or actually compromised	
Questions, recognizes, and reports near misses, errors (own and others), and takes action to minimize harm arising from adverse events	Nova Scotia (College of Registered Nurses of Nova Scotia [CRNNS])
Uses safety measures to protect self and colleagues from injury or potentially abusive situations (e.g., appropriate needle disposal or patient abuse)	http://www.crnns.ca/documents/Patient%20Safety%202007.pdf
Has knowledge of body mechanics, safe work practices, and management of aggressive and violent behaviour	
Applies safety principles, infection control measures, and appropriate protective devices	
Questions, recognizes, and reports near misses, errors (own and others), and takes action to minimize harm arising from adverse events	
Questions, recognizes, and reports near misses, errors (own and others), and takes action to minimize harm arising from adverse events	Manitoba (College of Registered Nurses of Manitoba [CRNM]) http://cms.tng-secure.com/file_download.php?fFile_id=143
Knowing where to find key information	
Uses health-care resources appropriately to ensure a culture of safety (e.g., patient-lifting devices, safer sharps, safe disposal of sharps, and safe staffing levels)	
Uses a systems approach to patient safety and participates with others in the prevention of errors, near misses, and adverse events	Saskatchewan (Saskatchewan Registered Nurses Association [SRNA]) http://www.srna.org/nurse_resources/standards_competencies.pdf
Uses technology appropriately, ensuring patient safety	

- Communicate about risks and adverse events;
- Learn from an adverse event; and
- Maintain the dynamics of the culture of safety (CASN, 2005).

Nova Scotia has a joint position statement on patient safety developed in collaboration with other health-care professionals. The statement outlines the provincial position on patient safety and identifies the role of the individual health-care

professional, the health-care professional regulators, the agencies or organizations, the government, and the patients and their families (College of Registered Nurses of Nova Scotia, 2007). The Registered Nurses Association of Ontario (RNAO, 2004) policy statement describes patient safety as a priority in public accountability for individual nurses, administrators, organizations, professional associations, and all levels

> **BOX 14.2** Canadian Nurses Association Code of Ethics Safety-Related Value Statements
>
> **Providing Safe, Compassionate, Competent and Ethical Care**
>
> Nurses guided by ethical practice standards interact with patients and their families as well as communities, groups, populations, and other members of the health-care team to meet this care value.
>
> Nurses question and intervene to address unsafe or incompetent practice or conditions that interfere with their ability to provide safe, competent care.
>
> Nurses admit mistakes and take all necessary actions to prevent or minimize harm arising from an adverse event. They work with others to reduce the potential for future risks and preventable harms.
>
> Nurses in collaboration with other health-care providers adjust priorities; inform patients, families, and employers of adjustments as a result of inadequate resources. These could be staffing levels or supplies not being available.
>
> Nurses safeguard the health and safety of people during job action.
>
> Nurses have a duty to care during communicable disease outbreaks using appropriate safety precautions.
>
> Nurses support, use, and engage in research that promotes safe, competent care.
>
> Nurses work to prevent and minimize risk of violence to protect themselves and others.
>
> Source: Canadian Nurses Association. (2008). *Code of ethics for registered nurses* (2008 centennial edition). Ottawa, ON: Author.

> **BOX 14.3** Registered Psychiatric Nurses of Canada Code of Ethics Safety-Related Value Statements
>
> **Safe, Competent, and Ethical Practice to Ensure the Protection of the Public**
>
> Strives to maintain a level of personal health, mental health, and well-being in order to provide competent, safe, and ethical care.
>
> Ensures that one neither initiates nor participates in any practice that is considered harmful to the welfare of others.
>
> Accepts responsibility and accountability for one's own actions taking all necessary steps to prevent or minimize harm.
>
> **Quality Practice Environments**
>
> Contributes to promoting and maintaining safe practice environments.
>
> Ensures that safe and competent practice is a priority by advocating for human and material resources.
>
> Source: Registered Psychiatric Nurses of Canada. (2010). *Code of ethics and standards of psychiatric nursing practice*. Edmonton, AB: Author.

of government. It also states registered nurses are a key link in the health-care system for the protection of patients, family, or community. It identifies high-quality patient care and nursing, quality work environments, and multilevel accountability as key factors in patient safety.

Interprofessional Patient Safety Competencies

As nursing practice has moved toward an interprofessional model of function, patient safety thinking has also moved to collaborative practice. A CPSI project has developed a framework for patient safety flexible enough to be used for all health-care providers. This framework identifies six domains: Contribute to a culture of patient safety; work in teams for patient safety; communicate effectively for patient safety; manage safety risks; optimize human and environmental factors; and recognize, respond to, and disclose adverse events (Frank & Brien, 2008).

Occupational Health and Safety Legislation

Occupational Health and Safety (OH&S) has federal and jurisdictional legislations that describe what employers must have in place to protect their workers. Although patient safety is not included in these legislations, the precautions covering health-care providers indirectly protect the patients. Additionally, Protection for Health Care Workers Part XXXI of the Saskatchewan *Occupational Health and Safety Regulations* (Gov-

ernment of Saskatchewan, 1996b) identifies more specific requirements. In 2005, the requirement for protection from exposure to blood and body fluid was added. Legislated engineering controls include a movement to needleless systems, and where that is not possible, requiring needles with engineered protective devices to prevent needle poke, the use of regulated sharps containers, infection control measures for spill cleanup, vaccinations, and worker training on hazards. **Engineering controls** are physical controls or barriers that isolate or remove the hazard (Government of Saskatchewan, 1996a, amended 2007). Ontario and Manitoba have similar legislated engineering control measures for needles. Respirators that protect from severe acute respiratory syndrome (SARS); hemoagglutinine-1 and neuroaminidase-1 (H1N1), proteins found on the surface of the virus; and other such diseases were included under respiratory protection devices in 2007. Saskatchewan health regions are fitting nurses and other health-care workers for N95 masks to comply with this legislation. By mid-2009, no other jurisdiction had this OH&S legislation in place, but many health regions and authorities are incorporating this measure to protect their workers. In response to a review of reported back injuries to nurses, the 2007 update also included specific requirements for patient transferring, lifting, and repositioning. Nova Scotia and New Brunswick legislation mentions lifting and moving a person but without the detail included in the Saskatchewan legislation. Finally, Saskatchewan provides legislation outlining requirements for supervisors in health-care facilities to adequately train and supervise workers on hazards. Saskatchewan also includes legislation on violence and harassment for the protection of nurses and other health-care professionals as well as patients. You can expect to see more jurisdictions including similar legislation for protection of health-care workers.

Think Clinical days are busy, and often, the mundane aspects of care can become rushed when we feel pressured for time. Sometimes, the student can be lured into performing tasks that deviate from best practices but from the student's perspective appear to be the norm for the clinical setting. Harm is lurking beneath the waters when aspects of procedures are taken as care "short cuts." A nursing student emptying a catheter bag without wearing safety glasses, the procedure used by nurses on the unit, could result in an infected or blood-streaked urine splash to the eye, necessitating the commencement of the body fluid exposure protocol. Deviations from best practice may be modeled in the care setting. Be sure to discuss these with your instructor because it may be your novice perspective which can lead to misunderstandings of staff performance.

Understanding Patient Safety: Foundations for a Culture of Safety

Two forces shape the culture of any organization: the organizational framework and the behaviours demonstrated by the employees in the organization (CPSI, 2008b). For a culture of safety to flourish, both forces must be committed to patient safety. The organizational framework needs to be structured with safety in mind. For example, funding should be available to put safety mechanisms in place; the organizational leaders must make safety a priority and empower their staff members to engage in safety projects. The second force is at the foundational level—employee's behaviour. If safety culture is to flourish, then everyone needs to be on board—the housekeeping staff, the kitchen staff, and the security staff as well as the professional staff. A safety culture will not survive and strengthen unless everyone in the organization thinks safety at all times. Therefore, the contributions of students to a culture of safety are important. A commitment to patient safety is a foundational, professional value that is played out daily in patient care and is a value the student is expected to demonstrate quickly in the clinical setting. The student's inquisitive nature and constant questioning will advance the patient safety culture by uncovering the factors beneath the surface of the iceberg.

The Connection Between Organizational Culture and Harm

How can culture lead to harm? Let's consider Mr. Smith's event from a culture perspective. Many nursing units have two ways of operating. One way is to follow policy and procedure, and the other way is to do it like everyone else does on the unit. Many times, how skills are applied on the units does not stem from bad employees but rather flows from outdated policies and from conditions that do not allow staff to follow policy. We know from the Mr. Smith case study that Angela wanted to do the procedure correctly, so she engaged the help of an expert. However, when confronted with Mr. Smith's request to get up earlier, she accommodated his request by asking an available staff member to enter the room for assistance. Do we know if this individual was aware of Angela's novice status with the lift? What do you think the likelihood is of the staff transferring everyone the same way because it has become routine? Doing routine tasks can become monotonous, and harm can occur if nurses do not think through all safety implications in the planning stage.

Through the eyes of a nurse

Many student nurses struggle in organizing their patient's care, especially if the nursing unit or the patient population is new for them. I see many students running in and out of the patient's room because they have forgotten equipment, and I wonder if they need some tips on how to organize their care. Also, some students fail to recognize what is absolutely important to know or do right away for a patient and what can wait until later in the shift. A pen-and-pencil plan is necessary, and the ability to adjust the plan as the day unfolds is critical for safe patient care to develop.
(personal reflection of a nurse)

The Nursing Student's Perspective

All nursing students continually work on developing and refining the organizational skills of nursing practice. A recent study performed by Gregory, Guse, Dick, Davis, and Russell (2009) found that an important source of student nurse clinical transgressions stemmed from the student's inability to set patient priorities. Failure to collect important patient data impacted the student's ability to make clinical judgments that guide the priorities for patient care. Subsequently, the inability to set patient priorities directly impacts the student's ability to follow through the necessary patient care. These aspects of patient care will gradually develop; but, like any other skill development, you need a road map on how to execute these skills in the practice setting. Each new clinical opportunity will contribute to your ability to prioritize patient care. Be sure you take as much time to develop these organizational skills as you do your psychomotor skills. Boxes 14.4 and 14.5 provide some practical guidance on how to prepare for these situations.

Characteristics of a Culture of Safety

Reason (2000b) identified several interdependent subcultures that are characteristic of safety culture. The subcultures that he refers to are a(n):

- Reporting culture
- Informed culture
- Flexible culture
- Learning culture

BOX 14.4 Organize Before Skill Performance

1. Identify the nursing skills to be performed the night before.
2. Review the procedure.
3. Make a pocket-sized shopping list of the equipment to be gathered prior to the procedure.
4. Write the location of the equipment next to each item.
5. Write any questions you have for your instructor or the staff members that will enable safe performance of the skill.
6. Ask the questions after report to the appropriate nurse or to your instructor.
7. Visualize in your head your successful performance of the skill. Do you see yourself using your therapeutic communication skills when you interact with the patient?
8. List the clinical observations to be made during the procedure. Star the essential observations to chart.

If these subcultures are healthy within the organization, then a *just* culture is at work. In a just culture, reporting becomes the norm. In order for adequate reporting to occur, the culture must trust that the reporting behaviour will not result in punishment. A just culture becomes an informed culture when it becomes continuously aware of what is on the verge of unacceptable danger and what is indeed relatively safe (Reason, 2000b). The fine line, or what Reason describes as the *edge*, can only be understood by a system that learns through reporting. The culture becomes informed through applied knowledge gained from analyzing adverse event reports. Thus, an informed culture is an outcome of a reporting culture. In order for the culture to learn and then make the necessary adjustments to the system, the culture must be flexible. A flexible culture and learning culture are elements that hinge on the establishment of a reporting and informed culture (Reason, 2000b). The flexibility component is evident by the processes that demonstrate teamwork

BOX 14.5 How to Identify Patient Priorities

1. Listen to morning report. Ask yourself the following questions:
   What has changed?
   Are the changes detrimental to the patient's health status or do they indicate progress?
   What information follows your research about the patient's conditions and what data have no immediate link to the medical condition?
2. If the patient's status has changed, write down the pieces of information you need to gather now.
3. Perform your assessment. What pieces of information are congruent with report and the patient's status and what pieces of data do not make sense to you?
4. Report your findings to the primary nurse or your instructor. Seek assistance with the assessment findings you do not understand.
5. Change your plan based on what you have discovered. You may wish to discuss this with the primary nurse or your instructor.

using shared accountability principles, open communication practices, and reflect shared power among members.

How does one contribute to a culture of safety on a daily basis? What role does the nursing student play? It starts with you keeping patient safety in the forefront of your mind. Every decision, every plan you put in motion, and every act is framed in safety. When a red flag goes up in your mind, you must stop, reflect, and communicate your concerns to another. Patient safety has to permeate every aspect of your nursing practice.

Enhancing a Culture of Safety

The need for health-care provider education on identifying hazards, errors, and unsafe practices to decrease adverse events and patient risks and enhance an incident reporting system is now coming to the forefront (Collins, 2007; Johnstone & Kanitsaki, 2007). Including patients and families' unique perspectives in these processes can further move the patient safety agenda forward. In the following sections, we explore aspects that contribute to the development and enhancement of the culture of safety.

Risk Management

Risk management is the practice of minimizing untoward events by planning for their occurrence by placing safeguards to offset the danger. The development of policies, procedures, and processes is the foundation of a risk management program. These include, but are not limited, to "risk identification, risk factors, effectiveness of risk management for behaviour modification, statistical risk, likelihood of negative outcome, risk [vs] safety" (O'Bryne, 2008, p. 3) and focus on systems, not individuals or intent. Quality improvement and patient safety are seen as part of health-care risk management and are both being incorporated into health-care accreditation standards (Canadian Council on Health Services Accreditation, 2005; Unruh, Lugo, White, & Byers, 2005). To meet these requirements, health-care facilities are implementing near miss incident analysis, electronic order entry (Unruh et al., 2005), and an incident reporting system to establish a culture of patient safety toward improving quality of care (Burkoski, 2007). Electronic order entry allows health-care providers to use technology such as computers to order tests, medications, and consultations. These orders are then visible to and easily read by other members of the patient's health-care team. You can expect to see more evidence of health-care provider technology education to identify hazards, errors, and unsafe practices and enhance an incident reporting system during your clinical rotations.

Quality Improvement

Quality improvement has long been known as a good business case approach. Health care is a more recent convert to quality improvement, partially spearheaded by accreditation requirements. Improved patient outcomes resulting from quality improvement are now being combined with quality improvement in patient safety initiatives. Five provincial organizations (BC Patient Safety and Quality Council, Health Quality Council of Alberta, Saskatchewan Heath Quality Council, Manitoba Institute for Patient Safety, and Ontario Health Quality Council) along with the Health Council of Canada have safety initiatives that reflect the movement. So what is quality improvement? From a patient's perspective, it is based on how he or she feels about the service he or she receives when interacting with the system; feeling cared about as well as cared for results in trust, improved follow through with recommended treatments, and improved health outcomes (Chilgren, 2008). From the organization's perspective, it means focusing more on quality improvement programs, aligning patient safety with vision and mission statements (Chilgren, 2008), and learning from one another (McAlearney, 2008), leading to improved outcomes (Grote, 2008), including patient safety.

Reporting

Reporting all types of patient safety events, either real or potential, is absolutely imperative and becomes the signature of safety cultures. Types of events to report are numerous and generally fall under the following classifications: adverse event, critical incident, and good catch. An **adverse event** is an event that results in harm to a patient that is unrelated to his or her medical condition. An adverse event is directly related to the care and/or services provided to the patient. A **critical incident** is an adverse event that results in a significant physical impairment or loss of life. A **good catch** or **near miss** is an event that is caught before it reached the patient. Near misses occur in greater numbers than adverse events, and critical incidents are just a fraction of adverse events. In a true culture of safety, all these events need to be reported to ensure that their contributing factors will be examined.

Saskatchewan, Manitoba, and Quebec have mandatory reporting of critical incidents. In these provinces, it is compulsory for institutions to report and to subsequently act on all critical incidents. Specific legislative statutes set the reporting route and dictate the process (CPSI, 2008a). Reporting starts with the transfer of information from the frontline workers to the hospital administration. In the case of Mr. Smith, Angela would initiate the report to her unit manager.

The name of this report will vary from one health-care system to another. Some facilities use printed forms and others will have electronic forms. Some nursing programs will also want their students to report the event to the school. Most reporting systems are anonymous to encourage the reporting of events by removing the possibility of blame. The institutional process and policy dictates how the report moves through the organization. However, in most institutions, a patient safety event will fall to the risk assessment department or the quality improvement department.

Some provinces have critical incidents legislation requiring incidents be reported to the appropriate arm of the provincial government. As you learn about the particular process in the institutions you practice in during your student experiences, you will become an important source of information for the reporting system.

Nurse managers have the responsibility to follow up on patient care issues, including incidents. In the case of Mr. Smith's fall event, an incident report completed by Angela and the care aide was given to the nurse manager on the unit. As part of the root cause analysis investigation, the nurse manager talks to a number of staff and discovers that staff has been holding on to the loops whenever moving patients since Mr. Smith's incident. This puts staff members in a very awkward position, risking back injuries. How can the nurse manager improve staff and patient safety? Requiring three staff members to move patients allows for more options of holding loops while using good posture. The mechanical lift company looks at reengineering the lift to prevent this problem. Mechanical lifts now have a safety loop installed to prevent the loop from slipping off. Focusing on the root cause as well as the visible direct cause resulted in improvements to the mechanical lift for all health-care facilities.

The initial formal communication needs to happen as close to the incident as possible and should be done within 2 days of the event (CPSI, 2008b). The format used is an apology as well as disclosure of what is known at the time about the incident. All people who are on the receiving end of an adverse event deserve to be told that an unintended event has happened, whether it is obvious or not. Mr. Smith's event cannot be hidden, he did fall and harm did occur.

Who apologizes and discloses the information will vary in different care settings and will be dependent on the type of incident. Most practitioners will want to apologize immediately if an event occurred while the patient was in their care. Some events will require a full spectrum of communication to the patient and family from the organization's leadership team as well as the frontline workers directly involved in the event. For example, critical incidents will require the organization's leader to provide ongoing communication. The patient and/or the family may become part of the investigation that follows.

Disclosure Process

How do you know who should communicate what? Most institutions will have a policy and procedure outlining the disclosure process. The CPSI has guidelines for institutions to use when setting disclosure policy and procedures. Institutional procedure will outline the participants in the disclosure process, and these members will vary from setting to setting and fluctuate with the type of event. A plan should be discussed prior to meeting with the patient because it is important that all facts are understood by those who will participate. Generally, patients want to know the following:

- How the incident was handled
- Future plans to minimize the event from occurring again
- Regret the event occurred (CPSI, 2008b)

Anticipation of the patient's reaction and a plan for support should also be considered prior to patient communication. The disclosure should be expressed using blame-free vocabulary and terminology the patient can understand. The apology should be sincere and express sympathy for the patient's situation. Using the words "I'm sorry for" reflects a caring response to the harm the patient has experienced (CPSI, 2008b). Apologizing does not imply that the practitioner was at fault nor does it imply that the institution is legally liable. The apology simply acknowledges regrets for the harm caused to the patient and a commitment to include them in further developments. If an event occurs during your clinical time as a student, ask for permission to observe the session. Permission should be routed through your clinical instructor, the institution, and the patient. Nurses are well positioned to participate in the disclosure interaction because therapeutic communication skills are key to the delivery of the apology and disclosure.

Think *Mr. Smith Event—Patient/Family's Perspective*
Reflect on the institution's responsibility to Mr. Smith and his family.

Does Mr. Smith deserve an apology? If yes, by who?
What information should be disclosed to Mr. Smith and his family?
Should they be kept apprised of the investigation findings?
How can they have input into system improvements?
Do you believe Mr. Smith would want the caregivers involved in the event to be disciplined?

Interprofessional Communication

Creating and sustaining a culture of safety requires efforts from the whole health-care community. In order to continuously create a safe environment, the team needs to work collaboratively and use a shared voice to identify pitfalls and solutions to safety concerns. At the core of creating and sustaining a culture of safety are relationships that are equalitarian and respectful. When a patient safety event occurs, the team cannot be fractured into "us versus them" approaches. This type of behaviour will not be of any benefit to those involved, including the patient or institution. In fact, it will be a negative influence on how the event is analyzed, understood, and remedied. Let's take Mr. Smith as an example again. A reaction to the fall that pitted the care aides against the nurses would be

dysfunctional. It would not allow the team to identify the contributing factors in the case. Assigning blame must be avoided.

Authority Gradient: Contributing to Safety Barriers

It is widely accepted that system flaws threaten patient safety. Some system flaws are easy to identify, whereas others are very difficult to pinpoint because they operate under the safety radar of the organization as part of the submerged iceberg. Power imbalances on the health-care team are a direct cause of potentially divisive system failures. A power gradient exists in health-care settings today and is categorized as an organizational communication flaw (Manasee, 2003). The perception that one person is better or more knowledgeable than another based on rank or title is classified as an authority gradient and represents a barrier to communication (Manasee, 2003). Blocks in the communication process among the health-care team members are fertile ground where harm can occur.

A very good example of a power gradient consequence is taken from the aviation industry. The worst airplane disaster in history prior to September 11, 2001 occurred between two airliners on Tenerife island runway. The conditions were very poor; visibility was foggy, and the messages from air traffic control were confusing. The copilot voiced concern to the pilot regarding the decision to take off—he believed permission had not been obtained. The pilot failed to listen to the copilot's objections and collided with another aircraft, killing 585 people (Manasee, 2003).

Health-care teams can learn from this aviation tragedy. For example, a surgical team can cause patient harm if the team functions like the crew in the Tenerife accident. Consider a patient who has consented for his right kidney to be removed. That patient is put to sleep by the anesthetist believing the team members will perform their jobs to the best of their ability. What if the surgeon begins to make an incision on the left side of the patient's body and a team member, either the anesthetist or the nurse, questions the surgeon? What if the surgeon dismisses it out of hand, believing he knows better than the others, and continues to operate and removes the left kidney? Remember, the patient is asleep and cannot advocate for himself. The outcome is a critical incident, and now, the patient will be left without a healthy kidney because a communication flaw was at work in the operating room. In this example, the flaw is an authoritarian attitude that has devastating results.

Power or authority gradients are well entrenched in health care. Hierarchical structures within the culture serve as a barrier to patient safety and communication (Fancott, Velji, Almone, & Sinclair, 2006). Power imbalances exist between disciplines and in the family of nursing groups as well. Do you think there are power imbalances between student nurses and registered nurses? Do you think patient harm can result if a health-care team member dismisses your concerns out of hand, simply because you are a student? This is an unfair situation for a student to be put in and violates the notion of a safety culture. Realistically, however, you must think about how you will handle a situation where you encounter someone who believes he or she can exert power over you.

If patient safety is to be improved, the health-care team will need to share the responsibility for patient safety; by doing so, the safety culture in the organization is advanced. Respect for each member's contribution on a daily basis serves as a litmus test for equalitarian health team relationships. Leadership support of interprofessional collaborative practices, conflict-management education programs, and policies and procedures that provide an avenue for conflict resolution are other indicators in the health-care system illustrating a desire to balance the power gradient.

Investigation

There are several different approaches to investigating a safety event. The one approach that is consistent in Canada and endorsed by CPSI is **root cause analysis (RCA)**. RCA is a quality improvement tool that uses a systematic approach in improving patient safety and reducing harm. The intended outcomes of RCA are to identify the various factors that contributed to the event, determine risk reduction strategies, and develop a plan of action in response (CPSI, 2006). A RCA is useful across care settings and is primarily used to investigate critical incidents. An overview of the RCA process can be seen in Figure 14.3.

The RCA will require the expertise of an interprofessional team made up of frontline personnel familiar with the situation. If we take Mr. Smith's fall as a case example, a team composed of an RCA facilitator, care aide, nurse, member responsible for mechanical lift training, mechanical lift expert (preferably one who is knowledgeable in the ongoing operation and maintenance), unit manager, and a patient representative is a good place to start. All of these individuals would come together with their unique body of knowledge and understanding of the situation. The team will be asked to answer several questions that are aimed at getting the root cause of the safety event. Overarching questions such as "Why did this happen?" "What can we do to reduce the chance of this happening again?" and "What is our plan to redesign the system so it doesn't happen again?" can be asked. This gives you a sense of the direction the analysis takes. The team will

be expected to keep the detailed information learned during the course of investigation or RCA in confidence.

Uncovering and recognizing system issues that contributed to the safety event are central to the work of the RCA team. Think back to the iceberg image of a safety event. The RCA team will dive deeply to identify submerged factors that led to the event. To accomplish a deep dive, they need access to all levels of the institution and many different experts to answer their probing questions. Once causation factors are identified, the team will develop actions to address the root causes uncovered during the analysis. A report will be created and submitted to the leadership team of the organization. The findings are normally reported to the patient and/or family, the staff involved in the incident, and the government body as indicated by provincial legislation.

The RCA of Mr. Smith's fall could uncover system issues that can be fixed. These are diagrammed in Figure 14.3. Hypothetically, the RCA could unveil the following two direct causes: wrong sling used for the transfer and the malfunction of the emergency stop button. Further investigation could reveal multiple contributing factors, such as lift sling in disrepair, multiple mechanical lifts and slings on the nursing unit, mechanical lift in disrepair, no policy or procedure on routine maintenance on the mechanical lifts, inconsistent training for frontline staff on the use of mechanical lifts, short staffing on the nursing unit, and budget cuts to equipment purchases. Once recommendations are made to remedy the safety pitfalls, the system can begin the work of creating safety.

Disseminating the Learning Lessons

Communication on what was learned from the RCA will need to be shared with those who could benefit from the information. One of the characteristics of a safety culture is to share the information within the institution where the incident occurred and also with the broader health-care community. The organization can decide what to share with other health-care centres in their region. In Mr. Smith's example, the information would most likely be shared with other care facilities using mechanical lifts. If critical incident reporting is managed by a provincial body, the province will decide what information should be shared with other provinces and other countries.

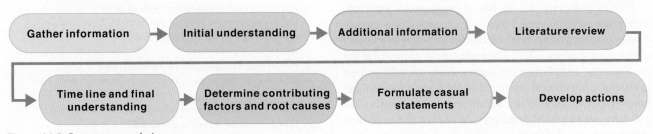

Figure 14.3 Root cause analysis process.

Human Factors Engineering

Human factors engineering is a scientific discipline dedicated to designing systems that meet the needs of the intended user population. This discipline examines the design with humans in mind—does the machine or workplace really take into account the person who will work with it or work within the particular space? You may be asking yourself, "How appropriate is human factors in the world of patient safety?" Well, think about the equipment you have worked with thus far in the nursing lab or in the clinical area. Has it all been logical? Does the way you interact with this equipment make sense? Also, what about your workspace? Has the space you work within allowed you to transfer a patient from the bed to a wheelchair safely? Have you had difficulty toileting a patient in the bathroom because of the layout of the bathroom space? What elements have been good or bad about these workspaces? Does the design of the space make your job any easier or does it create more challenges for you in providing patient care?

Nurses' work is complex. Nursing practice requires not only psychomotor and affective skills but also complex thinking processes so a course of action can be determined. The structure of the nurse's working environment complicates the nurse's ability to make clinical decisions using clinical reasoning skills by adding an additional factor to consider. Caring for multiple patients in environments that are fast-paced and unpredictable is the present reality for most nurses. Human factor engineering research can aide nurses in their quest to overcome these types of variables.

How Staffing Impacts Patient Safety

The nursing shortage in Canada has resulted in nurses working in understaffed conditions or on too many consecutive shifts. Many nurses are overworked, stressed, or fatigued, which increases the risk for adverse events. An employer strategy to address chronic nurse understaffing is the enforcement of mandatory overtime. The effects of extended hours beyond the normal work day or normal work week, in combination with the demands of responsibilities outside of the workplace, are conditions that create a sleep-deprived nursing workforce. A tired nurse often lacks the attentiveness for normal nursing duties and puts the nurse and the patient at risk for errors (Collins, 2007). "In fact, prolonged wakefulness can degrade performance, leaving a healthcare provider with the equivalent of a blood alcohol concentration of 0.1% which is above the legal limit for driving" (Dawson & Reid, as cited in Institute for Safe Medication Practices, 2005). The detrimental effects of fatigue are listed in Box 14.6.

Nurses' work requires the use of psychomotor skills, affective reasoning, complex thinking processes, and clinical decision-making skills, all of which are affected by fatigue and distractions (Collins, 2007). The reality of the nurse's working environment complicates the nurse's ability to make expert decisions using clinical reasoning skills. Caring for multiple patients in environments that are fast paced and unpredictable and have issues related to access to resources and unreliable information are common characteristics of many nursing

---

BOX 14.6   Effects of Fatigue

- Slowed reaction time
- Reduced accuracy
- Diminished ability to recognize significant but subtle changes in a patient's health
- Inability to deal with the unexpected
- Lapses of attention and inability to stay focused
- Compromised problem solving and decision-making
- Impaired communication skills
- Inability to recall
- Short-term memory lapses
- Reduced motivation
- Irritability or hostility
- Indifference and loss of empathy
- Intrusion of sleep into wakefulness
- Decreased energy for successful completion of required tasks
- Decreased learning of new activities
- Reduced hand-eye coordination

Source: Institute for Safe Medication Practices. (2005). *Medication safety alert: An exhausted workforce increases the risk of errors.* Horsham, PA: Author. Retrieved from http://www.ismp.org/Newsletters/acutecare/articles/20050602.asp

---

work settings (Potter et al., 2005). Multitasking is a skill that is difficult to do safely in a chaotic environment. One can only juggle so many tasks before a mistake is imminent. There are many tasks that require full undivided attention, especially when you are performing these skills for the first few times in the clinical environment. How will you keep your focus? What processes or behaviours can you develop to keep your mind on the matter at hand? Some general strategies to use in high-risk situations are outlined in Box 14.7.

Leape et al. (1995) cited other staffing problems that contribute to medication errors. These include lack of expert nurses to mentor novice nurses and work environments that isolate the nurse (Leape et al., 2005). Inadequate staffing also makes it difficult for nurses to step away from patient care to participate in continuing education, quality improvement, and risk management initiatives.

BOX 14.7   Strategies to Minimize Risk From Fatigue or Distractions

1. Recognize the critical times that require a quiet, distraction-free space. Examples include high alert medication preparation and sterile skill performance.
2. Prepare high alert medications in the closed medication room and not in the hallway at the medication cart.
3. Control distractions when performing sterile procedures or other treatments by closing the door and turning down the volume on the television.
4. Follow procedures. Focus on each step one at a time. Do not eliminate steps in a process because you are tired or in a hurry.
5. Abort a procedure if a critical step has been omitted.
6. Come to clinical rested and prepared.

Students and Medication Safety

The number one type of safety event reported by nurses is the medication event. Therefore, it stands to reason that medication administration will also be of concern for student nurses. In fact, a recent study by Gregory et al. (2009) found that medication error was the most frequent type of safety transgression performed by student nurses.

The frequency of medication error increases when one patient is cared for by two individuals (Institute of Safe Medication Practices [ISMP], 2008)—the nurse on the unit and the student nurse. Often, miscommunication will occur, and doses can be missed and/or double doses can be given. Be sure you communicate well with the nurse who is also assigned to care for your patient while you are on the unit, both verbally and through timely charting. Keeping the nurse updated on the patient's status as well as what aspects of care you have delivered is key for keeping the patient safe from harm.

Culture of Safety in Canada

Health Canada has a system to collect and assess adverse reaction reports on various health products. Information is collected on prescription and nonprescription drugs, biologics (select blood products and vaccines), natural health products, and radiopharmaceuticals. Dissemination of the findings can be accessed by subscribing to the *MedEffect e-Notice and Canadian Adverse Reaction* newsletter. The website is listed in Table 14.2.

Canadian Medication Incident Reporting and Prevention System (CMIRPS) is a collaborative effort among three agencies: Health Canada, Institute of Safe Medication Practices (ISMP) Canada, and Canadian Institute for Health Information (CIHI). The intent of CMIRPS is to manage the risks associated with medication use. ISMP Canada releases an electronic medication safety alert newsletter, entitled *Nurse Advise-ERR*, to nurses who subscribe. The ISMP Canada website is listed in Table 14.2.

Safer Healthcare Now!

The Safer Healthcare Now! campaign is the largest healthcare improvement effort made to date in Canada. In April 2005, the campaign was launched by CPSI and during the reporting period 2005 to 2008, had enrolled 1,100 teams working in more than 300 health-care organizations across the county (Safer Healthcare Now!, 2009). The campaign presently consists of nine initiatives aimed at reducing adverse events and harm. In 2005, the campaign started with six target interventions (listed 1 to 6), and in 2008, three additional interventions were added (7 to 9).

1. Preventing adverse drug events through medication reconciliation: acute care and LTC
2. Improving care for acute myocardial infarction patients
3. Preventing surgical site infections
4. Preventing central line-associated bloodstream infections
5. Deploying rapid response teams
6. Preventing ventilator-associated pneumonia
7. Preventing venous thromboembolism
8. Preventing antibiotic-resistant organisms, specifically methicillin-resistant *Staphylococcus aureus* (MRSA)
9. Preventing falls and injuries from falls

Medical Device Incident Reporting

Health Canada is interested in adverse events that result from issues with medical equipment. Medical devices are put through a rigorous pre-market evaluation before they are released to the Canadian public. However, even after this process, events can occur that give cause for concern and necessitate investigation. Safety surveillance is ongoing, and Health Canada has the ability to recall medical devices should a safety trend develop.

Canadian Adverse Event Reporting and Learning System

The need for a central pan-Canadian reporting and learning system was identified by CPSI in 2004. In recent years, consultations across the country have taken place with the goal to bring to fruition a national system that would coordinate the collection of information about adverse events. The intent of the Canadian Adverse Event Reporting and Learning System (CAERLS) is to go beyond the collection phase of event information and to provide analysis and formulate appropriate actions that would address key results (CPSI, 2008a). The development of the CAERLS is a priority for CPSI over the 5-year period from 2008 to 2013. In early 2009, consultation with stakeholders was completed and has now expanded to a more broad consultation process.

Expansion of Safer Healthcare Now! Initiatives

Following the success of the campaign thus far, two pilot projects were initiated. It is the intent to extend these projects to a national campaign should the pilot projects be successful. The first project is entitled "High-Risk Medication Delivery in Paediatrics" and will determine the scope of the issues related to high-risk medication delivery in acute care settings. The paediatric project will also identify the best practices for sustainable change related to high-risk medication delivery. The second project is an extension to home care settings of the highly successful medication reconciliation intervention.

TABLE 14.2	National Safety Surveillance Systems	
Organization	**Web Address**
Adverse Drug Reaction Reporting and Medical Incident Reporting	http://www.hc-sc.gc.ca/dhp-mps/index-eng.php
Institute of Safe Medication Practices Canada	http://www.ismp-canada.org/

Mentorship

The CNA identified mentoring as a valuable way to integrate nurses into new roles in all four domains: direct care, education, administration, and research (CNA, 2004). New nurses benefit from the experience of the mentor, and the mentor benefits from the new nurse who is fresh from school with many new ideas and awareness of current best practices. Mentoring has become more formal in many health-care institutions. The Saskatoon Health Region provides an example, where every new grad has two mentoring options: formal mentoring or buddy with whom he or she shares the workload for an extended period of time. A learning partnership with one experienced nurse for advice on a wide variety of issues helps build confidence and competence.

Through the eyes of a nurse

Going from student to grad nurse is a big jump. One of my biggest fears is to experience a code. A code is called when a health-care professional comes across a patient who is not breathing or who has no heartbeat. This is something I haven't experienced as a student, and I was worried that I wouldn't know what to do or that I would make a mistake with serious consequences. The thought of a code caused me some anxiety. I was able to discuss this with my mentor, and she answered my questions and gave me feedback that helped calm my fears. She helped me to realize that I'm never really alone on the unit, that there are always other nurses available to help me. I feel that I am a safer nurse having someone available to me to talk about anything I may need.

(personal reflection of Kaylin Loster, graduate nurse)

Workplace Hazardous Materials Information System

The Canada-wide Workplace Hazardous Materials Information System (WHMIS) legislated in 1988 identifies the duties of suppliers, employers, and workers to protect worker from hazardous controlled products (Government of Canada, 2011). It is based on three main parts: labels, material safety data sheets (MSDS), and required workplace education sessions (Ontario Ministry of Labour, 2008). The suppliers must label containers and supply MSDS to all workplaces that purchase their product (Government of Canada, 2011). See Figure 14.4 for an example of a supplier label.

Any workplace-specific container, such as a bottle of 10% bleach solution used to wipe up blood and body fluid spills, must have a workplace label attached. Workplace labels must include the name of the product, safe handling information, and a statement that the MSDS is readily available for workers to review (Canadian Centre for Occupational Health and Safety, 2014). Employers must provide education sessions on WHMIS, ensure workers have access to MSDSs, and monitor compliance with labeling. Education sessions must include general WHMIS education on the label and the location and

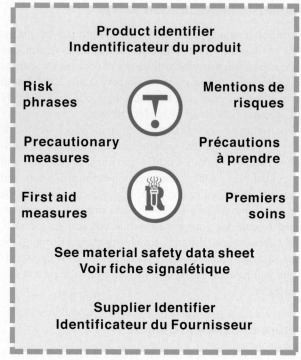

Figure 14.4 Sample supplier label.

use of MSDS as well as information on specific hazardous workplace materials. Specific education on each hazardous product a worker uses must include safe work procedures for handling, use and storage, and emergency procedures to follow in the event of an exposure or spill. MSDSs provide information on the specific product including type of hazard, health risks, and precautionary and first aid measures. Refer to Table 14.3 for hazardous symbols.

Canada is in the process of moving to the Globally Harmonized System (GHS) that will result in the MSDS expanding to 16 sections. In addition, the controlled products list will be expanded to include many products currently exempt, including some household products. The hazard symbols may also change to match the Transportation of Dangerous Goods symbols. It is important to keep yourself up-to-date with these upcoming changes.

Final Perspectives on Patient Safety

The publication of the *Canadian Adverse Events Study* (Baker et al., 2004) set off a chain of events to address the alarming picture of patient safety in the country. The CPSI has been instrumental in coordinating safety efforts across the nation. Preliminary efforts have been focused on collecting information through reporting and disseminating the learning trends so health-care organizations can make necessary changes. Throughout the system transformation, nurses have been taking an active role and will continue to be front and centre in advancing patient safety.

TABLE 14.3	Workplace Hazardous Materials Information System Hazard Symbols

	Class A—Compressed gas	Contents under high pressure Cylinder may explode or burst when heated, dropped, or damaged.
	Class B—Flammable and combustible material	May catch fire when exposed to heat, spark, or flame May burst into flames
	Class C—Oxidizing material	May cause fire or explosion when in contact with wood, fuels, or other combustible material.
	Class D, Division 1 Poisonous and infectious material: Immediate and serious toxic effects	Poisonous substance; a single exposure may be fatal or cause serious or permanent damage to health.
	Class D, Division 2 Poisonous and infectious material: Other toxic effects	Poisonous substance; may cause irritation Repeated exposure may cause cancer, birth defects, or other permanent damage.
	Class D, Division 3, Poisonous and infectious material: Biohazardous infectious materials	May cause disease or serious illness Drastic exposures may result in death.
	Class E—Corrosive material	Can cause burns to eyes, skin, or respiratory system
	Class F—Dangerously reactive material	May react violently causing explosion, fire, or release of toxic gases, when exposed to light, heat, vibration, or extreme temperatures

Source: Canadian Centre for Occupational Health and Safety. (2009). *Workplace Hazardous Materials Information System (WHMIS): WHMIS hazard symbols.* Retrieved from http://www.ccohs.ca/products/posters/pdfs/whmisSymbols.pdf

SUMMARY

In the past decade, the national effort to improve the culture of safety has touched all nurse workplace settings. Creative ideas were generated by interest groups, and nurses were and remain instrumental to strategy implementation. Reporting of all incidents including near misses is an essential component of this safety culture. Several reporting mechanisms are in place and have implications for student input. Using RCA analysis such as the Swiss Cheese Model, the Domino Theory, and the Iceberg Model to investigate these reports will uncover direct as well as indirect causes and contributing factors. During your student nursing practice experience, implement the necessary steps to keep your patients safe. A few strategies have been presented to you in this chapter, such as arriving to clinical experiences well rested and prepared; prioritizing your care, keeping safety in the forefront; and always report near misses, events, and critical incidents.

The learning that occurs after a patient safety event is widespread and touches many layers of the health-care system. By using Mr. Smith's example, one can see the positive outcomes possible by approaching his fall from a safety perspective. The following list captures the potential strategies to minimize a fall from a mechanical lift in the future:

- Installment of ceiling mechanical lifts
- Dedicated lift slings for each patient
- Limited number of portable lift types in a facility to avoid operation confusion
- Regular lift service maintenance
- Regular safety walk-arounds on the unit by the health-care team and administrator

Students can actively advance the culture of safety in the institutions they frequent during their program of study. By viewing the work environment through a safety lens, students can serve as an early warning system to a future patient safety event.

Critical Thinking Case Scenarios

▶ You have just finished doing your research on Bridgette, your patient for tomorrow's clinical day. Bridgette is a more complex patient than you have cared for before. She has been diagnosed with multiple sclerosis (MS), Type 1 diabetes mellitus, and hypertension (high blood pressure). Her vital signs are done every morning. Her blood sugar is tested four times a day as her short-acting insulin dose has just recently been increased. Her long-acting insulin has remained the same for quite some time. Bridgette has an open sore on her left foot that requires dressing changes twice daily. She is not able to bathe in the whirlpool tub until the wound has healed, so she requires a bed bath. Her MS causes a very unsteady walking gait so she uses a quad cane for short distances and a wheelchair for longer distances. The nurse's notes reveal she gets quite tired after physiotherapy, scheduled for 10:00 AM, so her gait is more unsteady at that time.

- Prioritize the patient care that you will be providing for Bridgette.
- Identify the potential patient safety risks for this patient.
- Describe precautions or strategies you will use to minimize these risks.

▶ You have been helping a fellow student transfer their immobile patient from bed to chair. This task has taken longer than you both anticipated but is completed at 9:55 AM. You go to Bridgette's room to take her blood pressure only to discover she has already left for physiotherapy. You as yet have not done the dressing change.

- How does this change your planned care for the day?
- Have you put Bridgette at any undue risk?

1. Discuss MS, including symptoms, treatment, and patient care assessment of mobility, ADL, cognitive function, and safety issues.
2. Discuss Type 1 diabetes, including causes, symptoms, medications, complications, and safety issues.
3. Discuss wound care and the impact Type 1 diabetes has on wound healing.
4. Discuss high blood pressure, including causes, monitoring requirements, treatment options, and safety concerns.

Multiple-Choice Questions

For Questions 1 and 2, refer to the following situation.

During equipment collection for a dressing change, the nurse gathers hydrogen peroxide instead of normal saline. The nurse notices the odor of the solution as it is poured into the dressing tray. The nurse stops and discards the tray and returns to the cart where the solutions are stored. The nurse notices that the two solutions, hydrogen peroxide and normal saline, are stored side by side on the cart.

1. The incident outlined in the given scenario is best described as which type of safety event?
   a. Critical incident
   b. Sentinel event
   c. Good catch
   d. Negligent behaviour

2. The fact that the two solutions were stored side by side on the collection cart is an example of which patient safety term?
   a. Root cause
   b. Contributing factor
   c. Best practice
   d. Adverse event

3. Later that same day, a student nurse runs to the cart to retrieve normal saline in response to a colleague's eye splash—but she accidently takes hydrogen peroxide from the cart. What should the student nurse do?
   a. Keep it to herself as disclosure is admitting incompetence.
   b. Nothing because there was no harm done; it has been reported already.
   c. Fill out the hospital's event report.
   d. Wait for her clinical experience mark before disclosing.

For Questions 4 to 6, refer to the following situation.

A nursing manager makes a unilateral decision to have the footrests welded to all wheelchairs on the unit because many footrests are disappearing from the unit. The manager is unable to replace them due to budget constraints. Since the footrest welding, several nurses have hurt their backs transferring patients from the wheelchair to the bathroom because the wheelchairs cannot easily be maneuvered into the patient bathrooms.

4. The budget constraint factor can be explained using a systems theory approach as which type of factor?
   a. System communication failure
   b. System design flaw
   c. System defense breakdown
   d. System forcing function

5. The unit nurses approach the unit manager with their safety concerns in relation to the wheelchairs. The unit manager responds in an authoritarian style, accusing them of poor nursing judgment. The unit manager's response is an example of what type of system characteristic?
   a. Authority gradient
   b. Power balance
   c. Missed patient care
   d. Best practice

6. The occupational health and safety committee reviews all the back injury reports. They request the manager meet with the wheelchair sales representative to look at a solution that allows for safe patient transfer while keeping the chair rests attached to the chair. What strategy are they using?
   a. Following safe work practices
   b. Using appropriate PPE

   c. Being fiscally responsible
   d. Exploring safe engineering controls

7. An Aboriginal patient requests to visit the Aboriginal centre for a healing ceremony during his hospital stay. The nurse immediately denies his request stating she is too busy to transport him to the centre in the hospital. Which type of harm has the patient experienced?
   a. Physical
   b. Social
   c. Cultural
   d. Spiritual

8. Which of the following factors explains why competent health-care professionals are involved in adverse events?
   a. They are incompetent.
   b. They are negligent.
   c. They are human.
   d. They are indifferent.

9. Which of the following is the best definition of *patient safety*?
   a. A way of monitoring health professionals' work
   b. A way of decreasing unsafe acts
   c. A way of improving patient satisfaction
   d. A way of assigning responsibility to nurses only

10. WHMIS in composed of what three required areas?
    a. MSDS training, workplace label training, and use personal protective equipment (PPE)
    b. Workplace labels, worker training, and safe working practices
    c. Supplier labels, MSDS, and education sessions
    d. Use of PPE, safe working practices, and worker training

Suggested Lab Activities

● Caring for patients with multiple health issues can make it difficult for nursing students to prioritize care in advance. Doing thorough patient research on medical conditions, medications, surgical procedures, ADL abilities, and health promotion activities can help prepare you for the unexpected. The student nurse, Mary, arrives for the clinical experience prepared to assess her stable patient and complete the teaching for discharge home alone by the end of the week. Morning report identifies the patient had an unsettled night with frequent urination and generalized pain. Assessment starts with the following questions:

- What doesn't fit with the patient's history?
- This patient usually sleeps well throughout the night— that is new.
  a. Is it related to her urinary frequency or is it something else?
  b. Why was she up?

c. Was anything else different about last night?

d. Did she get her sleeping pill?

e. Is she worried about something?

f. Is she anxious about going home or excited about going home?

- The pain is also new. She hasn't needed pain killers for 3 weeks.

a. What is the source of the discomfort?

b. How is her breathing?

c. Are the symptoms of insomnia, pain, and frequent bathroom visits related?

- What assessments does Mary need to perform to answer these questions?

Vital signs and pulse oximetry readings are done now rather than when scheduled at 10:00 AM. An abdominal assessment is completed. A pain assessment which includes checking the medication record is also done. The patient's self-report of how she feels is an important assessment to include.

Assessment reveals the following patient data. The patient has a low-grade fever, a slight elevation in heart rate, but no change in blood pressure or respiratory status. The patient self-report reveals vague muscle and joint aches and reports awakening with abdominal cramps throughout the night. She passed one loose stool between the night nurse's last assessment and Mary's assessment. After consultation with the primary nurse also caring for the patient, he or she decides to send a stool for culture and immediately put the patient on contact precautions. Mary changes her assessment plan and incorporates assessing and maintaining hydration status into her care. She also knows to start implementing a fall prevention strategy as a precaution because the patient may get progressively weaker. Changing the planned care in response to the patient's condition ensured that the patient's safety became the priority and not the discharge at the end of the week.

● Complete an incident/accident investigation form that follows your school of nursing format for the following scenario.

I was rushing to finish up my clinical rotation for the day as postconference was to start in a few minutes. My last task was to empty Mr. Smith's catheter bag, measure the urine, and document the amount. I was excited because I had not done this procedure before. I put on my gloves, retrieved the measuring container from the patient's bathroom, and proceeded to empty the catheter bag. I noted the urine was quite concentrated with blood streaks throughout. I opened the tubing to empty the urine from the bag into the measuring container and felt fluid splash into my left eye. I immediately closed the tubing and asked the first nurse I saw to help me flush out my eye. Once the eye was flushed for 15 minutes, we initiated the blood and body fluid exposure protocol. My instructor and I went over the procedure for

emptying catheter bags. Did I just forget to wear my safety glasses for this procedure or was I rushed and missed this important step? I keep asking myself this over and over in my head—why did I perform this task so differently than how I had practiced it in the lab? I'm concerned now about getting an infection. I wish I could have those 5 minutes back—I would do things differently.

Following my eye splash incident, my instructor and I worked at completing a report. We identified that the direct cause for the injury was not wearing the proper PPE, safety glasses. However, as we investigated why I was not wearing the PPE, other causes were uncovered. Safety glasses were not in my pocket, and none were readily available in the patient room. I had not reviewed and collected all the equipment required for this skill before actually performing it. I recalled seeing nurses do this task without wearing this PPE. I did not follow best practice by consulting the unit policy and procedure. Recommendations for improvement included a review of the unit policy and procedure in postconference for the nursing students. The unit manager made a notation in the communication book for all nurses to review the policy along with a copy of the policy, complete with signing sheet for nurses to initial once they had reviewed it. I hope they read it as I see a lot of nurses avoiding the PPE step. I will fill out my nursing program's safety event form now on my own. I feel good that my exposure has helped others understand how important it is to protect ourselves as well as patients.

● Identify a near miss or a real patient safety event that occurred with your current clinical group. Complete the institution form to report the near miss or event as a clinical group.

● Do a safety walkabout with your clinical group on your current clinical unit. Identify the hazards in the nurse's workplace that may contribute to a patient safety event.

● For this activity, students should divide into groups of four. Read the RNAO's *Executive Summary on Nurse Fatigue and Patient Safety* available on the CNA website at http://www.cna-aiic.ca/CNA/documents/pdf/publications/Fatigue_Safety_2010_Summary_e.pdf . Discuss the system level recommendations, the organizational level recommendations, and the individual level recommendations to manage fatigue and prevent negative patient safety events.

● For this activity, students should break into small working groups. Read and then discuss *Harm Reduction and Currently Illegal Drugs: Implications for Nursing Policy, Practice, Education, and Research* available on the CNA website at http://www.cna-nurses.ca/CNA/issues/harm/default_e.aspx

REFERENCES AND SUGGESTED READINGS

Baker, G., & Norton, P. (2001). Making patients safer! Reducing error in Canadian healthcare. *HealthcarePapers, 2,* 10–31.

Baker, G., Norton, P., Flintoft, V., Blais, R., Brown, A., Cox, J., . . . Tamblyn, R. (2004). The Canadian adverse events study: The incidence of adverse events among hospital patients in Canada. *Canadian Medical Association Journal, 170,* 1678–1686.

Burkoski, V. (2007). Identifying risk: Limitations of incident reporting. *Canadian Nurse, 103*(3), 12–14.

Canadian Association of Schools of Nursing. (2006). *Position statement: Patient safety and nursing education.* Ottawa, ON: Author.

Canadian Centre for Occupational Health and Safety. (2014). *WHMIS general.* Retrieved from http://www.ccohs.ca/oshanswers /legisl/intro_whmis.html

Canadian Council on Health Services Accreditation. (2005). *Patient safety in Canadian health services organizations: Results of a national survey.* Ottawa, ON: Author.

Canadian Nurses Association. (2004). *Achieving excellence in professional practice: A guide to preceptorship and mentoring.* Ottawa, ON: Author.

Canadian Nurses Association. (2008). *Code of ethics for registered nurses* (2008 centennial edition). Ottawa, ON: Author.

Canadian Nurses Association. (2009). *Patient safety.* Ottawa, ON: Author.

Canadian Patient Safety Institute. (2006). *Canadian root cause analysis framework.* Edmonton, AB: Author.

Canadian Patient Safety Institute. (2008a). *Building a safer system: The Canadian adverse event reporting and learning system consultation paper.* Edmonton, AB: Author.

Canadian Patient Safety Institute. (2008b). *Canadian disclosure guidelines.* Edmonton, AB: Author.

Canadian Patient Safety Institute. (2008c). *The Safety Competencies.* Edmonton, AB: Author.

Chilgren, A. (2008). Managers and the new definition of quality. *Journal of Healthcare Management, 53*(4), 221–229.

College of Registered Nurses of Nova Scotia. (2007). *Joint position statement on patient safety.* Halifax, NS: Author. http://www.crnns.ca/documents/Patient%20Safety%202007.pdf

Collins, S. E. (2007). Setting a new standard of patient care: Potential legal implications of patient safety research. *Journal of Nursing Law, 11*(2), 87–92.

Davies, J., Hebert, P., & Hoffman, C. (2003). *The Canadian patient safety dictionary.* Ottawa, ON: Royal College of Physicians and Surgeons of Canada.

Dyck, D. (2007). *Occupational health and safety: Theory, strategy and industry practice.* Markham, ON: LexisNexis Canada.

Fancott, C., Velji, K., Almone, E., & Sinclair, L. (2006). Exploration of patient safety phenomena in rehabilitation and complex continuing care [Special issue]. *Healthcare Quarterly, 9,* 135–140.

Frank, J., & Brien, S. (2008). *The safety competencies: Enhancing patient safety across the health professions.* Ottawa, ON: Canadian Patient Safety Institute.

Government of Canada. (2011). *Controlled products regulations.* Retrieved from http://laws-lois.justice.gc.ca/eng/regulations/SOR-88-66/index.html

Government of Saskatchewan. (1996a). *The occupational health and safety regulations, 1996, amended 2007.* Regina, SK: Author.

Government of Saskatchewan. (1996b). *The occupational health and safety regulations, 1996.* Regina, SK: Author. Retrieved from http:// www.qp.gov.sk.ca/documents/English/Regulations/Regulations /O1-1R1.pdf

Gregory, D., Guse, L., Dick, D. D., Davis, P., & Russell, P. (2009). What clinical learning contracts reveal about nursing education and patient safety. *Canadian Nurse, 105*(8), 20–25.

Grote, K. (2008). The "new economics" of clinical quality improvement: The case of community-acquired pneumonia. *Journal of Healthcare Management, 52*(4), 246–258.

Institute for Safe Medication Practices. (2005). *Medication safety alert: An exhausted workforce increases the risk of errors.* Horsham, PA: Author. Retrieved from http://www.ismp.org/Newsletters/ acutecare/articles/20050602.asp

Institute of Safe Medication Practices. (2008). Error-prone conditions that lead to student nurse-related errors. *Nurse Advise-ERR, 6*(4), 1–3.

International Council of Nurses. (2012). *Position statement: Patient safety.* Geneva, Switzerland: Author. Retrieved from http://www .icn.ch/images/stories/documents/publications/position _statements/D05_Patient_Safety.pdf

Johnstone, M. J., & Kanitsaki, O. (2007). Clinical risk management and patient safety education for nurses. *Nurse Education Today, 27*(3), 185–191.

Kalisch, B. J., Landstrom, G. L., & Hindshaw, A. S. (2009). Missed nursing care: A concept analysis. *Journal of Advanced Nursing, 65*(7), 1509–1517.

Leape, L., Bates, D., Cullen, D., Cooper, J., Demonaco, H., Gallivan, T., . . . Amy Edmondson. (1995). System analysis of adverse drug events. ADE Prevention Study Group. *Journal of the American Medical Association, 274*(1), 35–43.

Leape et al. (2005). Leeb, K., Zelmer, J., Wester, G., & Pulcins, I. (2005). Safer care—Measuring to manage and improve [Special issue]. *Healthcare Quarterly, 8,* 86–89.

Manasee, H. (2003). Not too perfect: Hard lessons and small victories in patient safety. *American Journal Health-System Pharmacy, 6,* 780–787.

McAlearney, A. (2008). Using leadership development programs to improve quality and efficiency in healthcare. *Journal of Healthcare Management, 53*(5), 319–331.

McKelvey, M. (2001). Professional must recognize personal responsibility. *HealthcarePapers, 2,* 56–58.

O'Bryne, P. (2008). The dissection of risk: A concept analysis. *Nursing Inquiry, 15*(1), 30–39.

Ontario Ministry of Labour. (2008). *Workplace hazardous materials formation system (WHMIS): A guide to the legislation.* Retrieved from http://www.labour.gov.on.ca/english/hs/pdf/whmis.pdf

Potter, P., Wolf, L., Boxerman, S., Grayson, D., Sledge, J., Dunagan, C., & Evanoff, B. (2005). An analysis of nurses' cognitive work: A new perspective for understanding medical errors. *Advances in Patient Safety, 1,* 39–51.

Reason, J. (2000a). Human error: Models and management. *British Medical Journal , 320,* 768–770.

Reason, J. (2000b). Safety paradoxes and safety culture. *Injury Control and Safety Promotion, 7,* 3–14.

Registered Nurses Association of Ontario. (2004). *Position statement: Patient safety.* Toronto, ON: Author. Retrieved from http:// rnao.ca/policy/position-statements/patient-safety

Registered Psychiatric Nurses of Canada. (2010). *Code of ethics and standards of psychiatric nursing practice.* Edmonton, AB: Author.

Runciman, W., Hibbert, P., Thomson, R., Van Der Schaaf, T., Sherman, H., & Lewalle, P. (2009). Towards an international classification for patient safety: Key concepts and terms. *International Journal for Quality in Health Care, 21*(1), 18–26.

Safer Healthcare Now! (2009). Retrieved from http://www.safer-healthcarenow.ca/EN/Pages/default.aspx

Unruh, L., Lugo, N. R., White, S. V., & Byers, J. F. (2005). Managed care and patient safety risks and opportunities. *The Health Care Manager, 24*(3), 245–256.

Educative Nursing Practice: A Role for Professional Nurses

BARBARA L. PATERSON AND LYNNE E. YOUNG

Edwin Hamme is a fourth-year nursing student who is working with a preceptor in the final clinical practicum in his undergraduate nursing education program. One morning, he commented to his preceptor, "I need to find time to teach Mr. Fraser about his new diet." Edwin's preceptor answered, "I wouldn't stress about it, Edwin. It's my experience that you can work really hard to teach patients something, but they either don't do what you have told them or they don't remember what you've said." Edwin thought about what his preceptor said. He found himself wondering why he had learned about the importance of teaching patients in his program if what the preceptor said was true.

CHAPTER OBJECTIVES

By the end of this chapter, you will be able to:

1. Discern how professional nursing practice has evolved with respect to educative nursing practice.
2. Describe the major theories that have influenced educative nursing practice.
3. Appreciate the importance of and the place of a personal vision of educative nursing practice.
4. Understand the common features of learning.
5. Discuss how the Educative Nursing Practice Framework supports your growth as an educative practitioner in the clinical and classroom settings.
6. Apply the Educative Nursing Practice Framework in your clinical practice.

KEY TERMS

Andragogy   A term coined by Malcolm Knowles to describe a theory of adult learning.

Critical Incident Reflections   Thoughts about events or situations that are particularly moving, stressful, or confusing for the purpose of increasing one's understanding and awareness.

Educative Nursing Practice Framework   A tool to assist nurses to make decisions about what and how to teach patients or to determine why teaching was not successful in assisting a patient to learn new content or skills.

Emotionality   A negative response to learning when what has to be learned is viewed as risky, a loss, or frightening.

Incremental Fluctuation   A rhythm of learning in which students initially embrace alternative perspectives and challenge previously held assumptions but then fall back temporarily to past ways of thinking or sensing situations or phenomena.

Learning Climate   The context or the atmosphere in which learning takes place that has a profound effect on a patient's ability to learn.

It includes the physical climate, such as the temperature, ventilation, and noisiness of the room, and the effectiveness of aids to learning and equipment.

Learning Theories   Five main schools of thought or paradigms that have influenced educative nursing practice to date—behaviourism, cognitivism, humanism, constructivism, and andragogy—each giving rise to a number of other learning theories. What all learning theories have in common is the belief that learning brings about change; however, how this change happens is open to debate among theorists.

Personal Vision of Educative Nursing Practice   What you believe, value, and understand about the purposes of educative nursing practice and how to be a nurse educator. A personal vision of educative nursing practice assists you to organize your teaching so you know not only what you are doing but also what you want to accomplish (i.e., your goals) and how you will know if you achieved them.

Social Constructivism   A theory, attributed to the work of Lev Vygotsky, of how knowledge develops through social interaction.

History of Educative Nursing Practice

The vignette that begins this chapter highlights the challenges in enacting the educative role of nursing practice. Part of understanding why the preceptor may have answered Edwin as she did is found in an analysis of the history of educative nursing practice.

The educative nursing practice role has only recently been recognized as important enough to warrant teaching nurses the skills and knowledge that are integral to such a role. The shift to an educative role for nursing is a key marker of the shift in nursing from task orientation to professional status. Prior to and into the 1960s, nurses' work was largely task-oriented, directed at routine patient care, and also chores such as cleaning floors, carrying trays, and cleaning equipment. As health-care technology evolved, nurses undertook new and complex tasks; for example, managing blood transfusions and ventilators. At the same time, in response to the increasingly complex hospital workplace, the concept of progressive patient care was adopted, which is the progression from intensive care unit (ICU) to intermediate care, self-care, long-term care, and home care (Donahue, 1985). In light of this change in health-care services, philosophical understandings of nursing evolved from viewing nursing as a task-oriented occupation to understanding nursing as a professional practice. Theories of nursing that advanced nursing as a professional practice focused on the nurses' role in fostering health and healing; the teaching and learning process enacted with patients and families was a cornerstone of this concept of new nursing (Pearson, 2003).

In the United States, in the 1960s, Lydia Hall advanced the core, care, cure theory of nursing. Central to her theory was teaching and learning, distinctly in contrast to the task orientation of nursing (Alfano, 1971). In the 1970s, Dr. Moyra Allen at McGill University in Montreal lead the development of the McGill Model of Nursing, a vision of nursing in which health promotion is the primary goal of nursing. According to the McGill model, because health is a learned process, the goal of nursing is to engage the patient and family in the process of learning about and acquiring healthier ways of living (Gottlieb & Rowat, 1987). Subsequently, numerous nurse theorists have advanced ways of thinking about nursing expressed in conceptual models or theories that feature the educative role of nursing.

Consistent with the perspective that the health professional is the expert in health, the educative role of nursing initially placed the nurse in the role of expert. In recent years, as paradigmatic discourses, theorizing, empirical studies, and wisdom shaped understandings about the educative role of nursing in new ways; it is now understood that the patient and/or the family are the experts in the situation, an insight particularly relevant in cases of managing chronic illness. Thus, current models of nursing and health-promoting nursing practice emphasize that in the educative role, the nurse and the patient and/or family share expertise. The patients' and families' expertise developed through years of living with a chronic condition. The nurses' expertise based on knowledge was acquired through study of the literature on nursing, medical, and other sciences; reflection on practice in light of theories and research; and so on. This awareness has deepened thinking about the educative role of the nurse, shifting the focus of current models to the relational nature of practice, including teaching and learning.

Dr. Rosemarie Parse's (1992) human becoming theory suggests that the goal of nursing is to foster through relationship the quality of life of those in nurses' care from the perspective of those living it. Hall, like Parse, emphasized the importance of the relationship between the nurse and the patient and/or family (Tomey & Alligood, 2006). Thus, since the turn to the new nursing, nurse theorists envision that the relationship between the nurse and those in his or her care is therapeutic and fosters health, healing, and, in Parse's theory, quality of life. At times, this relationship fosters new insights and information that have therapeutic outcomes; this is what we mean by educative nursing practice.

Theories and Educative Nursing Practice

In the vignette at the beginning of this chapter, the preceptor indicates that she does not think teaching patients is a priority because of her past experiences with patients who do not seem to learn. Rather than basing her educative nursing practice role on experience alone, it is important for the preceptor to consider different theoretical explanations for why the patients responded as they did to her teaching.

Historically, nursing has relied on theories from other disciplines to inform patient teaching. In more recent years, nurse theorists have contributed theoretical perspectives that are unique to nursing; however, teaching and learning in educative nursing practice continues to reflect the influence of theories from psychology and education. Later in this chapter, we focus on a framework, developed by the authors, that encompasses the foundations of nursing practice as critical to understanding educative nursing practice.

There are five main schools of thought or paradigms that have influenced educative nursing practice to date: behaviourism, cognitivism, humanism, constructivism, and andragogy. Each has given rise to a number of **learning theories**. The only thing that all learning theories have in common is the belief that learning brings about change; however, how this change happens is open to debate among theorists.

There is an old fable about a group of blind people who are asked to describe an elephant. One who is holding the trunk says an elephant is like a snake. Another who has his hands on the elephant's side says that an elephant is like a house. Yet another who is holding a tusk says an elephant is like a spear. All are correct, and yet, they do not completely describe an elephant. So it is with learning paradigms and theories. There are many schools of thought about what learning is and how it happens. Rather than selecting only one favourite learning theory, nursing students will gain a more complete picture of what teaching and learning entails by examining various learning theories. Becoming familiar with learning theories enables the student to ensure a fit between the theoretical assumptions about teaching and learning that informs an education strategy and the theoretical assumptions the student holds about nursing practice. When enacting an educative role, the nursing student determines the best fit between nursing theory and education theory relative to the situation and the needs of the learner.

Behaviourism

One of the earliest schools of thought that shaped the way in which nurses teach patients is behaviourism, particularly as it was described in the 1930s by Burrhus Frederick (B. F.) Skinner, a behavioural psychologist. According to Skinner (1984), learning occurs when teachers reinforce or reward the consequences of learning. Accordingly, it is solely the teacher's responsibility to provide the reinforcements that will determine the learner's motivation to learn. In behaviourist ways of educating, the teacher explains or demonstrates something, and then the learner tries to repeat it. The teacher provides praise and corrective feedback until the learner gets it right (Box 15.1).

There are several criticisms of behaviourism as a foundation for educative nursing practice. Behaviourism assumes that the teacher is in control; the student remains passive. Behaviourism also assumes that there is a standard checklist of teaching components that can be applied to every patient. In addition, although frequent feedback from the teacher can be motivating to some patients, other patients may find this irrelevant or annoying.

Still, behaviourism has led to practices that nurses continue to use in teaching patients. For example, many nurses believe that it is important to identify what patients need to learn in terms of observable and measurable behavioural objectives (e.g., the patient will be able to identify how diuretics [medication that causes the kidneys to excrete more urine] work). However, not all learning can be directly observed and measured.

BOX 15.1   Tenets of Behaviourism

- The goal of teaching is to change the learner's behaviour.
- The behaviour to be changed should be broken down into small incremental steps to be evaluated by criteria that can be observed and measured by the teacher.
- If a behaviour is reinforced, it is likely to occur again.
- Reinforcers are intrinsic (the learning itself may be rewarding) or extrinsic (rewards given by someone else, such as marks or praise provided by the teacher).
- Reinforcers can be positive (rewarding learning by providing something, such as praise) or negative (rewarding learning by removing something that is difficult for the learner, such as pain).
- The teacher's job is to determine what reinforcers will be most effective in motivating the patient to learn.

Nurses often use standardized teaching plans or read from prepared teaching manuals in order to be consistent in their teaching, a notion supported by behaviourists. Although such standardized tools help to remind nurses what should be covered in teaching patients, the danger is that these tools promote the one-size-fits-all approach to patient teaching.

Behaviourism has also supported nurses viewing themselves as the experts who know best what the patient needs. Nurses often approach patients with a list of what they should learn, and they proceed to teach accordingly. They assume that if they talk, the patient will learn. Nurses may give patients, and sometimes family members, pamphlets or manuals for the patient to read, assuming that what is read will be learned.

The emphasis of behaviourism on measurable and observable indicators of behavioural change has been immensely popular with nurses who like ticking off a list of components that must be covered while assuming that doing so means that they have done their job as an educator. It also appeals to nurses who want evidence of work completion. What we know from patients and nurses is that this popular checklist approach is minimally effective because it precludes what is important about teaching and learning; that is, the skill of the nurse in opening a space for meaningful conversations with the patient and his or her family about health-related situations. Nonetheless, having a list of relevant items to guide an educative conversation is useful to the nurse in terms of determining what the patient and his or her family members know already and what they want to know about topics relevant to the situation.

The notion of reinforcement in behaviourism is applicable to educative nursing practice. It is important that nurses recognize that patients will have varied notions of what reinforces their learning and that what is reinforcing for one may not be effective for another. For example, nurses often believe that patients who have a chronic disease want to learn how to manage their disease to prevent related complications. But many people do not see the prevention of complications as a reinforcer worth considering. People who have been diagnosed with Type 2 diabetes but feel perfectly well often do not really believe they have the disease, let alone believe they must prevent disease-related complications. Some people decide that the disease is not their priority, especially if they have a family member who is also ill and needing their attention. Others may believe that there is nothing they can do that will prevent disease-related complications. This is common among people who have seen many people in their group develop complications of the disease (e.g., Aboriginal people who live with diabetes).

Cognitivism

Cognitive theories consider that learning derives from the way the brain works, a view that was developed by critics of behaviourism who saw behaviourism as too simplistic view of learning. Cognitivists view the human brain as though it is a computer in which data (information) is stored, processed, and then produces specific learning responses. Learners, according to this view, are logical, rational beings who learn best when actively involved in developing mental structures for processing information. As you read previously, the behaviourist view does not explain why people organize and make sense of the information they receive. Cognitive learning theories focus on the functions of the brain that are involved in the processing of information, such as thinking, memorizing, comprehending, and problem solving. For Hartley (1998), a cognitive theorist, learning is more than acquiring habits. Learning involves expectations, drawing inferences, and making connections (Box 15.2).

Cognitive theories have influenced educative nursing practice in several ways. Most importantly, they have highlighted how people sort and store information in short- and long-term memory. Nurses who teach patients with impaired short-term memory draw on cognitive theories to identify strategies to improve the patient's ability to remember by storing new learning in their long-term memory. For example, nurses might relate new learning to something that the patient has experienced many years before, such as using a diary or chart to keep track of medication regimens. However, critics of cognitivism point out that the theory is insufficient to explain all learning; learning is more than rational thinking and often involves language and emotion (Smith, 1999).

Humanism

Humanism is a philosophical school of thought that holds that the dignity and autonomy of people as sacred. Humanism is centered on the learner as a unique experiencing person. Learning is understood in humanist theories as a process that has potential to foster the self-actualization of the learner in terms of deepening emotions, attitudes, and insights (Elias & Merriam, 1995).

Humanism has historical roots with Carl Rogers (1902–1987), a modern theorist often cited in the nursing education literature. Central to humanistic education theories is the belief that the educative relationship must be enacted in ways that promote individual freedom and respect for the learner's individuality and honour the right of learners to determine the nature of their learning. In humanistic educative nursing practice, teaching is focused on what patients say they need and want. The nurse's role is that of a facilitator of the patient's learning.

Humanistic theorists describe teaching as a process in which the teacher is a facilitator, helper, and partner to the learner in the learning process (Rogers & Freiberg, 1993). In this theory, learners are active participants in their learning and, at times, teach the teacher (Box 15.3).

The emphasis on relational practice as a key component of nursing can be partially traced to the work of Rogers. Rogers's influence in nursing is best recognized whenever nurses engage patients in respectful conversations about their experiences of health and illness to elicit understanding of what the patient needs and wants to learn. In addition, his influence is shown in therapeutic groups designed and facilitated by nurses, such as groups on psychiatric units.

There are several reasons why humanistic theories have become so popular in nursing. These theories resonate with the essence of nursing as a caring profession that respects the individuality of people and supports the principles of democracy. Although the current emphasis on relational practice in nursing can be traced to several theorists, humanism could be considered a significant influence on this development in theorizing nursing. However, humanism is not without criticism.

Several critics have suggested that not all people older than the age of 18 years are capable or desirous of determining their learning goals or how best to learn. They point to situations in which patients want to be told what to do by nurses, not explore what they might do. Still, other critics highlight the emphasis on group learning as a problem in humanistic theories. Not all people benefit from group learning because many people are intimidated in groups.

Constructivism

A central belief in the theory of constructivism is that people develop knowledge and meaning by building and reflecting on their experiences. Reflecting on experiences enables learners to generate their personal principles and mental models to make sense of their experiences. In a constructivist view, learning is adapting mental models to fit new experiences, and teaching entails helping learners to discover their mental models.

Constructivist learning is a highly personal experience whereby learners actively apply what they have learned and understood from past and current experiences to real-world situations. Nurses who teach patients in a constructivist way

BOX 15.4   Tenets of Constructivism

- Learning is an active, not passive, process.
- Learning entails searching for personal meaning; therefore, all learning should begin with the content or issues that are relevant to the learner.
- Requiring learners to memorize the right answer or to give back to the teacher what he or she has said is not appropriate.
- Learning requires understanding of the whole, not isolated, parts or facts.
- Students are the best judge of what and how well they have learned.
- Learning is best when it occurs in real-world settings and situations.

act as a facilitator of learning by encouraging them to discover meaningful knowledge for themselves while they attempt to solve real-life problems. For example, during a teaching/learning session on managing a child's epilepsy, the nurse might engage parents in a conversation about how they could handle their child's epileptic seizure while visiting a theme park rather than only providing the parents with a list of do's and don'ts (Box 15.4).

Some critics of constructivism say that the theory does not take into consideration that the teacher may have expert knowledge that could be beneficial to the learner. However, what constructivist teachers do is draw on their own expertise to help learners discover knowledge. Teachers draw on and foster the learner's curiosity and needs to help the learner acquire meaningful knowledge. Another criticism of constructivism is that teaching this way is too unstructured and flexible for novice learners who require structure and predictability in their learning because they have few mental models to draw on.

Social constructivism is a genre within constructivist theories attributed to Lev Vygotsky (1896–1934; Young & Maxwell, 2007). Like constructivists, social constructivists hold that learning is an active, not passive, process. Vygotsky took this one step further, proposing that new knowledge is formulated in social interactions and that the use of language plays a key role in acquiring new understandings. Nurses who draw on this theoretical perspective might lead group sessions with patients (and their family members) following myocardial infarction using a social constructivist design that fosters engagement in conversation. For example, small groups might share tips for heart-healthy eating and then report back to a large group.

The appeal of constructivism and social constructivism for many nurses is that teaching begins with the patients' perspectives on the situation. When guided by this perspective, patients are viewed as partners with the nurse in the learning process because together, they identify what the patient needs and wants to learn as well as how they best learn it. It also requires that the nurse choose teaching strategies that are tailored to the patient's unique needs and interests. This dialogical process is appealing to nurses who emphasize caring relationships in their nursing practice because it requires that they know the patient as a person.

Andragogy

Andragogy is a term first used by Malcolm Knowles to label his theory of adult learning. Knowles articulated what he understood to be unique to adult learning (andragogy) to differentiate adult learning from learning in children (pedagogy; Knowles, Holton, & Swanson, 2005). Knowles believed that adults learn in distinctly different ways from children (Box 15.5).

If you notice similarities with humanism, that would be an accurate perception because Knowles drew on humanistic theories in the development of his theory of andragogy. Basically, andragogy highlights the need for educators of adults to focus on the process of learning, not the content they teach. Since Knowles' introduction of the term *andragogy*, there has been much debate about the attributes of an adult student (e.g., Is one an adult learner at age 18 years? Are all adult learners self-directed?) and whether children actually do learn in different ways than adults. In addition, several critics have pointed out that self-direction in learning is not a worldwide concept; some cultural communities actually promote adults as passive students and teachers as experts. However, the theories of adult learning continue to influence nurses in their educative practice, primarily because the theories resonate with the need to address adults in a distinct way from children and because every nurse has witnessed that readiness is critical to learning. Andragogy reminds nurses that adults have many priorities in their lives; if they seem not to want to learn something, it may be because other things are more pressing, and the person has decided to attend to those instead.

Nurses who integrate andragogy in their educative nursing practice do not assume that everything they teach will be relevant to adult patients nor do they assume that its relevance will be immediately visible to the patient. They explain why they believe the content might be relevant and ask the patient for his or her perspective about its relevance. Such nurses shy away from asking patients to memorize things or repeat what the nurse has said. Instead, the nurse takes into account that every adult is different. They consider the patient's unique background, preferred way of learning, and past experiences in planning the learning activity. They also encourage adults to discover some things through experience, but they are there to offer guidance and encouragement as necessary.

BOX 15.5   Tenets of Andragogy

- Adults learn as they experience things, even mistakes.
- Adults are most interested in the things that are relevant to them in their jobs or personal lives.
- Adults should be involved in planning and implementing their learning experiences.
- Adults are more interested in solving real-life problems than they are in learning for the sake of having more knowledge.
- Adults take responsibility for their own learning.
- Adults learn when they are ready to learn.

Developing a Personal Vision of Educative Nursing Practice

Nurses who are skilled educators are able to respond to the unique needs of their patients and the patients' significant others. This means that they need a clear understanding, or a personal vision, for their educative nursing practice. A **personal vision of educative nursing practice** is what each nurse believes, values, and understands about the purposes of educative nursing practice and how to be a nurse educator. Being clear about your perspective on educative nursing practice assists you to organize your teaching so you know not only what you are doing but also what you want to accomplish (i.e., your goals) and how you will know if you achieved it. Consequently, in the next sections of this chapter, we speak to you directly, as a beginning nurse who is developing your own personal vision of educative nursing practice.

If the preceptor in the case study at the beginning of this chapter had a clear personal vision of educative nursing practice, she would have been better able to help patients learn what they wanted to learn. Such a vision works much like a global positioning system (GPS) in a car, giving guidance about where the car is going and how to get there. Nurses who understand their views on patient teaching are unlikely to be swayed by whatever is commonplace or popular among their nursing colleagues, regardless of whether this is the most effective way to teach patients. In the history of educative nursing, we as nurses have often adopted new ways of teaching patients, such as developing contracts or using standard teaching plans for all patients and in all situations. These ways are often abandoned a few years later, despite the fact that they are at times effective for particular patients. Having a personal vision of educative nursing practice helps you to understand why you choose certain methods of teaching particular patients and to avoid the atheoretical adoption–rejection cycle that has occurred from time to time in the nursing profession.

A personal vision is important for you because inevitably someone or something might cause you to question why you teach in the way you do. When something that has worked in the past with other patients is not effective in teaching a new patient, a vision statement will help you to articulate what you believe about educative nursing practice and to reflect on whether those beliefs are appropriate. You are less likely to feel confused and inadequate if you have a clear statement of what you believe and value in your educative nursing practice. A personal vision of educative nursing practice will ensure that those you teach experience your educative nursing practice as well-thought-out and thorough.

A personal vision of educative nursing practice should be based on *knowing*. That includes learning about teaching and learning, including learning theories, research about how people learn, and knowing about yourself as a learner. For example, researchers have discovered that most educators teach because they would like to learn. A nurse who likes to memorize the steps of a procedure in order to learn it will tend to teach procedures to patients as a series of steps to be memorized. However, if nurses know about research and learning theories that highlight that people learn in different ways, they will ask patients about how they prefer to learn and plan the teaching accordingly. For example, some people do not like to learn by memorizing; they may prefer to play with the equipment and to watch the procedure to learn it. Knowing this will reinforce the need to incorporate different learning styles in the nurse's personal vision of educative nursing.

One of the best ways to develop your personal vision of educative nursing practice is to remember your experiences of learning, particularly the ways you responded when you needed to learn something that was new and difficult. Nurses who have forgotten what it is like to be a student tend to underestimate how frightening some of the things that they teach can be and how difficult it is to learn them. It is also important to reflect on what behaviours by teachers helped you to feel comfortable in learning and what behaviours may have hindered your learning.

Through critical reflection in watching and doing, you will learn about educative nursing practice, and as a result, you will further develop a personal vision of educative nursing practice. As you interact with patients, nurses, and others in care settings, you will have many opportunities to observe how nurses perform educative nursing practice and how patients respond. You will also have opportunities to teach patients and their significant others. Reflecting critically about these occasions allows you to add to or refine your personal vision of educative nursing practice as you come to understand about what works well and why, as well as what is not as effective and why, in educative nursing practice. If you reflect following each of these occasions, you will begin to develop an understanding of the common "rhythms of learning" (Brookfield, 1991, p. 31), such as the most common signs of frustration and anxiety in learning and what nurses can do to help patients who are experiencing them.

Critical incident reflections are useful tools to help you to develop your personal vision of educative nursing practice. These are either written or oral reflections on a critical incident that has occurred in the course of your educative nursing practice (i.e., something that has been surprising, rewarding, or distressing to you). The critical incident can be something that happened to you or it can be something that you observed or heard about from someone else. Box 15.6 provides some questions to help you reflect on a critical incident.

You can translate much of what you know about being a learner yourself to developing a personal vision of educative nursing practice. For example, as a nursing student, some of your professors may require you to write in a journal about your learning in a course or in the clinical setting. These journals/diaries are records of your reflections on the good, bad, and the confusing in that learning as you experienced it. You might write about a time in which you felt very good about yourself as a student and why you felt that way. You might also write about what you learned about educative nursing practice in that situation. After you have a collection

BOX 15.6   Questions to Foster Critical Reflection About a Critical Incident

What happened in the critical incident?

How did it compare with your previous experiences?

Where and when did the critical incident take place?

Who was there?

What else was happening at the time in the immediate surroundings?

What emotions did you or others in the critical incident experience or express during or after the incident?

What was it about this critical incident that was surprising, rewarding, or distressing to you?

What did you learn about teaching or learning in this critical incident?

of entries in your diary, you will likely see some patterns or trends in how you respond and what you are learning. For example, one of the things that nursing students often see as they review their entries is that in the beginning, they tended to focus on what they as students were experiencing, whereas with time and experience, they are more often able to see what the patient is experiencing in the situation. That's progress! Although not everyone is a writer and some people are reluctant to put down in writing their personal thoughts and feelings, the learning journal/diary can be a powerful way for you to critically reflect on what you have observed or experienced, particularly if your nursing professors read your journal/diary entries and provide their own reflections.

Sometimes, a nursing professor may ask you to write your autobiography as a student. The professor may ask you to reflect on how you have spent your life as a student, including the high and low points in that journey. Reflecting on your experiences as a learner has significant implications to your personal vision of educative nursing practice. It will help to make you more aware of how learners respond and how what you do as an educator may affect patients and their significant others. It would be important in your learning autobiography to recall when you had most surprised yourself as a student and what helped you in those situations. For example, was there something you avoided learning and then at one point, embraced the topic? for example, the Kreb's cycle? What was the turning point? What or who helped you to risk learning about this? You could review the comments and evaluations you receive as a student and reflect on what meaning these have for you. Most importantly, you could use an autobiography to reflect on how your beliefs and values about teaching and learning have been shaped by your personal experiences as a student.

Lastly, you can develop your personal vision of educative nursing practice by sharing insights and experiences with nurses, nursing professors, and nursing students. Through these exchanges, you will develop an understanding of what features of educative nursing practice are effective in most situations and which are unique to particular patients, situations, or contexts—a skill foundational to being a critically reflective educator.

Understanding the Common Features of Learning

As a critically reflective educator, you should be aware of some features of learning that are common across cultures, ages, and socioeconomic backgrounds. The first of these is what Brookfield (1991) calls "the Impostor Syndrome." We call it "the everyone else is smarter than me, and it's only a matter of time before the educator finds out" syndrome. This syndrome occurs to most students when they enter a new learning situation. The student feels like an impostor, someone who really shouldn't be learning such difficult content. What is interesting about this syndrome is that it is common across people of all walks of life. We have seen it in doctorate students and undergraduate students alike, and we have even seen it in ourselves.

The Impostor Syndrome makes learners want to hide their secret (i.e., their impostor status) from the educator. This results in all kinds of interesting behaviour. For example, some students experiencing this syndrome will be very quiet, afraid that if they talk, they will expose themselves as impostors. Others talk all the time, emphasizing how smart they are, to cover up their impostor status. One way that nurses can help patients who are experiencing the Impostor Syndrome is by making a statement that let the patient knows that this is a very common but temporary response ("I often find that people in their first class about dialysis are feeling that they won't be able to learn everything about dialysis. But within an hour, they learn that everyone else in the class is feeling the same thing, and they go on to learn everything they need to know").

Emotionality is another common feature of learning. If you ask patients to tell you about their learning experiences in a hospital or other care setting, they will usually describe it in emotional terms (e.g., "I was a basket case," "I was so anxious," "I felt so relieved"). They talk about "feeling the hairs in the back of my neck stand up" or being "red faced with embarrassment." Emotionality is particularly evident when patients assess their learning as a threat. Sometimes, patients see learning as a threat because what has to be learned is viewed as risky, a loss, or frightening. Thus, some people may avoid or tune out of teaching sessions if they are not emotionally ready to hear what the nurse has to say.

One of the emotions that patients experience in learning that we almost never talk about is grief brought on by the losses, changes, and/or challenges of illness. When people learn about diet for heart disease, for example, they often experience grief for the times when they did not have to think about ordering whatever they wanted in a restaurant. They may mourn the loss of a favorite food that is not on their prescribed diet. At times, emotionality about learning can cause the person to react in anger or frustration. Nurses are well advised to spend some time with patients before, during, and after teaching them to explore how the patient is feeling about the learning.

Another common feature of learning is **incremental fluctuation**. People rarely progress in a straight path in their learning, particularly if what they have to learn is complicated and involves many new skills and new knowledge. The best way to explain incremental fluctuation is to think of the cartoons in which a character is running so fast that suddenly he realizes that he has run off the cliff and is suspended in air over a huge chasm. His response is to defy gravity and to quickly run back to the edge of the cliff. When we are learning many new things, it is often exciting. We may learn in great leaps, and for a while, we are thirsty for more. But all of a sudden, we can become overwhelmed at how much we are learning and how much there is to learn. Our response may be to temporarily take a break by returning partway back (note that we didn't say *all* the way back) to our old self. It may seem as if we have forgotten what we have learned, but we are merely regrouping, getting enough energy to continue in our learning. This is an important concept for you to remember if you ever find yourself being inconsistent in your learning or you encounter patients who seem to know things 1 day and then forget the next. Sometimes, the best thing that can happen in such cases is for the educator to encourage the learner to accept incremental fluctuation as a natural course of learning.

Through the eyes of a nurse

*T*his is such a small thing really, but what I have learned is to never assume that what I am teaching is no big deal for that patient. As a nurse, you get used to things and when you have to teach something, like emptying a colostomy bag, to a patient, you tend to think, "Oh, this is nothing" because you've seen it a hundred times. And to you, it's nothing. But to the patient, it means so much more than emptying a bag. It means, "Will I ever be normal again? Will my wife love me the same way? Will my cancer come back?" I try to remember always that what I am teaching is often a very emotional thing for patients.

(personal reflection of Rebecca C., BSN [nurse on gastroenterology surgical unit])

Through the eyes of a student

I think about the teachers that have made me believe I could learn anything. They seemed to have such faith in me, even when I didn't have faith in myself. And they always let me know that I wasn't stupid when I didn't get it right away. One of my teachers always says when I am learning a new skill, "No student gets that until they have done it at least five times." So I don't feel badly when I make mistakes the first or second time. And if I get it on the third time, I feel like a genius. I use the same approach with patients.

(personal reflection of Simon R., fourth-year nursing student)

Learning Climate

Another common feature of learning is the influence of the **learning climate**. The learning climate is the context or the atmosphere in which learning takes place. It can have a profound effect on a patient's ability to learn. The learning climate includes the physical climate, such as the temperature, ventilation, and noisiness of the room. It also includes that the necessary aids and equipment are in place and in good working order. When you are teaching patients, you don't want to have to spend several minutes running to replace faulty equipment before you begin. If you are planning learning activities, such as skill practice or small group discussions, you will need to consider if you have the space and the right facilities. If you are teaching in a space that is too cluttered, this may affect the patient's ability to focus on what you say, and it may be awkward to do the learning activities you have planned. Privacy is also very important. If a patient in a two-bed room is concerned about the patient in the next bed listening, he may be less attentive to what you teach than if the patient is alone.

The psychosocial aspects of the learning climate are those that affect how the learners feel about being themselves with you and how comfortable they are with you. If they do not trust you, they do not feel accepted, or they feel judged, patients and their families will often be reluctant to open up to you about their needs and preferences in learning (Box 15.7).

Educative Nursing Practice Framework

Educative nursing practice is a key role for professional nurses. In this role, nurses who are guided by nursing and education theories in their practice are more thoughtful and flexible and more likely to shape the teaching/learning session to be attuned to the needs of the patient and his or her family members in a particular situation and thus be more effective in enacting

---

BOX 15.7   How to Communicate Trust, Respect, and Acceptance to the Learner

- Be honest and open about your own mistakes.
- Be well prepared for your teaching.
- Be punctual for your teaching.
- Ask for feedback and be receptive to the learner's feedback about what and how you taught.
- Encourage learners to challenge and question you.
- Avoid sarcasm and insults.
- Accept different beliefs and perspectives.
- Ask for and show appreciation of the learner's past experiences and knowledge by drawing on it and indicating when you have learned something from the learner.
- Include the learner in decisions about what should be taught/learned and how learning should occur.

Source: Hammond, M., & Collins, R. (1991). *Self-directed learning: Critical practice*. London, United Kingdom: Kogan Page.

the role in a way that enhances the health, well-being, and/ or quality of life of those in the nurses' care. Such a textured practice in the context of the demanding life of a nurse is challenging. To assist you with your transition to professional practice, explore the following conceptual tool, the **Educative Nursing Practice Framework**.

When one is a beginning nurse, there is a tendency to assume that educative nursing practice is merely learning how to teach and then teaching every patient in the same way. The fact is that every patient's needs are unique. An example of how important this awareness is in educative nursing practice is the use of a script to teach all patients with chest pain about their medication. The nurse might deliver the script flawlessly and then walk away from the patient feeling confident that the patient has learned everything that is necessary to know. However, if that patient was worried about being off work and the impact on his or her financial situation or if he or she could not understand many of the words the nurse used, very little learning will occur. Educative nursing practice is not a formula that can be applied across the board to every patient and in every situation.

The Situated Clinical Decision-Making Framework by Gillespie and Paterson (2009) has been adapted specifically for educative nursing practice. This framework helps you reflect on your educative nursing practice and encourages your development as an expert educator in your nursing practice. Following each opportunity you have to teach a patient or family member, use this tool to help you to figure out what went well and what didn't and why. The framework is based on constructivist and humanist theories of learning in which respect, reflection, and collaboration are important concepts.

Some of the assumptions that underlie this framework are the following:

- Educative nursing practice is a dialogical (or conversational) and a reciprocal process between the nurse and the patient.
- Nurses bring themselves, including their history as learners, their values, and their preconceptions, to their educative nursing practice.
- Educative nursing practice entails building and sustaining caring relationships between the nurse and the patient as well as between the nurse and others (e.g., significant others, health-care practitioners). This requires compassion, thorough listening, assessment, authentic engagement, the application of principles of teaching and learning, and organized care based on nursing priorities.
- Nurses may draw on formal and informal theories of learning and evidence, alone or in combination, in educative nursing practice.
- Educative nursing practice entails knowing how the social, cultural, political, ideological, economic, historical, and physical context of the clinical situation or clinical setting affects how learning occurs and is assessed.
- Reflection is critical to the nurse's development as a skilled educator in educative nursing practice.
- Educative nursing practice occurs in clinical settings in which the nurse works with others in a community of practice.

The Educative Nursing Practice Framework emphasizes that educative nursing practice is a journey of exploration and discovery in which nurses determine what they know about the profession, the person, the content, learning, and the self to decide in collaboration with the patient and others (e.g., the family, other nurses) how and what to teach. More than book study of theories and content alone, it requires that the nurse be open to learning from patients and their significant others as well as other health-care practitioners. Nurses bring their interpersonal and communication skills to the teaching situation, with a recognition that not all patients prefer to learn in the same way. In addition, using this framework requires that nurses be continually reflective about the process and content of their educative nursing practice and about how the context has affected it.

Central to the Educative Nursing Practice Framework is *caring* through compassion, generous listening, assessment, authentic engagement, application of the principles of teaching and learning, and organized care based on nursing priorities. Caring provides the interpersonal *context* in which educative nursing practice occurs.

Another central component of the Educative Nursing Practice Framework is knowing. *Knowing* means more than learning from textbooks. It means continually seeking new ways of understanding and reflecting on what one knows and what one needs to understand. Reflection in this context entails thinking in critical and systematic ways about what one plans to do or has done in relation to educative nursing practice (Box 15.8).

BOX 15.8   Knowing in the Educative Nursing Practice Framework

Knowing About Learning
Knowledge of learning theories, how to apply relevant learning theories to particular clinical situations, teaching approaches/ strategies, how to assess learning outcomes

Knowing the Profession
Knowledge of standards of practice, competencies, skills, and roles of nurses

Knowing the Self
Knowledge of individual strengths, limitations, skills, experience, assumptions, preconceptions, learning, and other needs

Knowing the Case
Knowledge of what is needed in typical cases and typical patient responses

Knowing the Patient
Knowledge of a patient's clinical profile, including factors related to ability and motivation to learn, and documented past teaching

Knowing the Person
Knowledge of a patient's history, needs, wants, preferences, fears, and available supports in relation to learning

Skilled educative practitioners draw on knowing about learning, the self, the profession, the case, the patient, and the person. *Knowing about learning* requires that the nurse understand learning theories and be able to apply those that are relevant to particular clinical situations. The nurse will know about various ways to teach as well as to evaluate learning. *Knowing the self* entails the nurse reflecting on his or her strengths, limitations, preconceptions, past history as a learner, and values/assumptions in relation to learning, including his or her emotional comportment relative to the patient and the situation. The nurse acknowledges what he or she knows, does not know, and cannot know about the content that is to be taught. *Knowing the profession* helps the nurse decide what is appropriate for him or her to teach and how to act within the boundaries of the profession. *Knowing the case* is useful because it helps the nurse know what is typical in certain educative clinical situations, such as what people typically need to know and what typical responses are to specific learning situations or approaches. *Knowing the patient* involves understanding the patient's clinical profile. Most of this information comes from the patient's chart, such as level of consciousness, the diagnosis, and the teaching that has been documented to date. *Knowing the person* means finding out about what the person wants, needs, and prefers in relation to learning as well as his or her supports, past history as a learner, and concerns about learning the content.

According to the Educative Nursing Practice Framework, educative nursing practice involves a process of clinical decision-making in which the nurse identifies cues, makes judgments and then decisions, and then assesses the outcomes. This process of decision-making occurs within the content of the relationship that the nurse has with the patient and his or her significant others, the clinical setting, and society (Box 15.9).

Cues in the decision-making of educative nursing practice indicate that the patient has a need to learn something. A cue may be a physician's order to teach the patient, a patient's request, a nurse's assessment that the patient does not understand something that is vital to his or her well-being, or an indication from someone else, such as a family member, that the patient has a learning need. When a nurse attempts to make a judgment about what needs to be learned and how this learning deficit should best be met, the nurse seeks for information from the patient and others that would answer these questions. The nurse also tries to determine how urgent the learning insufficiency is.

At this point, the nurse determines who else should be consulted or involved. He or she decides what should be done, how it should be done, and who should be involved. In addition, nurses consider the timing of the teaching (e.g., "Should it be in the early morning or later in the day?" "Can it wait until tomorrow?"). When the nurse has made a decision, he or she needs to determine who else will be required to validate that this is the best decision. As a general rule, the patient is always involved in such a validation (e.g., "So how does this plan seem to you? Does anything need to be changed?"). The final decision includes the feedback of those with whom the nurse has consulted. Evaluation of the outcomes entails determining what the patient has learned and whether the patient has been able to use that learning in his or her life. It means finding out if there needs to be more teaching or if there are different ways of learning that might have been more appropriate.

The following sections of this chapter show how the components of the Educative Nursing Practice Framework relate to one another. Notice that the decision-making process is located within a house that is made up of knowing, caring, and context (Fig. 15.1). In the next sections of this chapter, case scenarios based on actual situations represent some common challenges in educative nurse practice. After reflecting on each scenario, you will have a better idea about why in the case study that began this chapter, the preceptor told the nursing student that teaching patients does not always achieve what nurses want, such as a change in the patient's lifestyle. You will also be able to identify ways to ensure that your educative nursing practice is effective.

BOX 15.9   Decision-Making Process in Educative Nursing Practice

Cues
- Observations
- Statements from patient or others
- Laboratory and assessment data
- Intuition

Judgments
- What learning needs to occur?
- What adjustments/revisions to the learning climate need to be made?
- How should teaching/learning occur?
- What data/evidence supports this?
- Do I need more information? From whom?
- Whom should I involve/consult with?
- What priority is this?

Decisions
- Should I wait?
- Should I try something?
- Who else should I involve or consult with?
- Is this the best decision?

Evaluation of Outcomes
- Did the desired learning occur?
- Can/does the patient apply the learning?
- Should I make other decisions?
- Do I need more information? From whom?
- Whom should I involve/consult with?
- What further teaching/learning should occur?

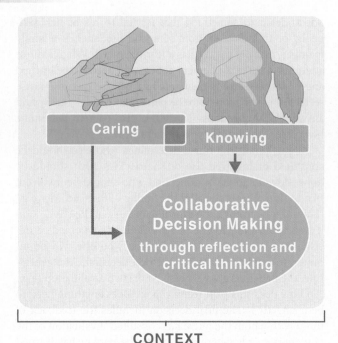

CONTEXT

Figure 15.1 Schematic of Educative Nursing Practice Framework.

Applying the Framework

Allison Barnes is a third-year nursing student on a busy surgical unit in the hospital. She is assigned to care for Mrs. Chung, a 49-year-old woman who has recently emigrated from mainland China. Mrs. Chung is to undergo a cholecystectomy (removal of the gallbladder) later that day. Allison has used her medical-surgical nursing textbook and the unit standard preoperative teaching plan to outline how she will teach Mrs. Chung about her surgery and her postoperative care. She also develops a checklist of content so that she can make sure she covers the important aspects of preoperative teaching when she talks with Mrs. Chung. Allison sits with Mrs. Chung in her hospital room and goes through her plan, step-by-step, speaking slowly and respectfully to Mrs. Chung. Every few minutes, Allison stops and asks, "Did you understand that? Do you have any questions?" Mrs. Chung thanks Allison for her thorough teaching. However, an hour later, as Mrs. Chung is about to leave the unit for the operating room, she asks Allison, "Will I be able to pass water if I don't have a bladder anymore?" Later, when Allison discusses the situation with her clinical teacher, she says, "I just don't understand it. I covered everything I was supposed to. She said she understood. But now I realize that she didn't know what a gallbladder was!"

You will remember that a central component of the Educative Nursing Practice Framework is knowing. This includes the knowledge that the nurse brings about learning theories and how to apply these to the teaching/learning situation. In the preceding scenario, Allison has relied on behavioural and cognitive theories of learning to plan and implement Mrs. Chung's preoperative teaching. Behavioural theories emphasize the need to clearly identify what the person is supposed to learn and to describe those things in directly observable and measurable ways. Cognitive theories indicate that if the content to be learned is divided into small chunks of information, the content will be easier to learn than if it is given as whole. Consequently, Allison spent considerable time making a checklist, derived from standardized teaching plans and her textbook. This was a helpful strategy because it helped her to plan the teaching so that she didn't miss any of the important content. However, other theories, such as constructivism or humanism, might have been helpful in this situation.

Constructivist theories of learning highlight that learners bring their past experiences as well as their personalities, preferences, beliefs, and values to learning new things. They also describe learning as a process that occurs in a relationship between teacher and learner. If Allison had considered constructivist theories of learning, she would have considered that learning is a dialogical process that occurs between her and Mrs. Chung. Allison is to be commended for her respectful comportment toward Mrs. Chung; however, if she had considered humanistic theories of learning in more depth, she would have recognized that her role as an educator was to help Mrs. Chung articulate what she wanted to learn. She would have begun by asking Mrs. Chung what she knew and felt about her surgery, instead of assuming that a standardized teaching plan and her textbook would provide this information. She would have also asked Mrs. Chung what she wanted to know about her surgery. If she had asked these questions, she may have discovered Mrs. Chung's misconceptions about the gallbladder.

One constructivist theory of learning that is applicable to this situation is Vygotsky's Social Development Theory, a social constructivist theory. Vygotsky described learning as a process in which the quality of the interaction between the teacher and the student is critical. Vygotsky also emphasized that it is important that learners play an active role in determining what they want to learn and how they want to learn it. Allison assumed that she knew what Mrs. Chung wanted and needed. Clearly, her assumptions were incorrect.

Vygotsky was one of the first theorists to suggest that people bring their cultural and social understandings and ways to learning. He emphasized that some students have learned that to ask questions or to say that they don't know something is not polite or is too risky (i.e., it may expose the patient's lack of understanding). It is possible that if Allison had known that Mrs. Chung was someone who rarely interrupts or asks questions, she would not have assumed that, when Mrs. Chung said she understood what Allison had taught, this was in fact so. She might have found some different way of determining what Mrs. Chung had understood, such as asking her to explain the surgery in her own words.

Allison obviously knew her limitations as a novice nurse (i.e., knowing the self) because she consulted her textbook and the standardized teaching plans. However, these are sources of information that are generalized; they are not designed to be specific to individual patients' needs and desires. They provide information that is relevant to knowing the case, not knowing the patient, or knowing the person. According to Vygotsky, if Allison had known Mrs. Chung as a person (i.e., she had a relationship with Mrs. Chung), it is possible that Mrs. Chung would have told her about her understanding of her surgery the moment Allison began her teaching. It is apparent in this scenario that Allison may have missed some important cues that might have indicated that Mrs. Chung did not understand her surgery.

Some common cues that signify that learners might have something else on their minds than what you are talking about include restlessness, frequently looking away from you, diminished eye contact, and failure to laugh or smile when prompted. Other cues may have been available in the patient's chart. For example, if Allison read in Mrs. Chung's chart that she had difficulty understanding English and she knew (knowing the case) that the anaesthetist may not have known that during his preoperative visit, she may have realized that Mrs. Chung had not understood everything the anaesthetist had said. As it is possible that Allison had never met Mrs. Chung before, Allison would have been well advised to talk to Mrs. Chung and to some nurses that knew the patient better than she did before planning her teaching. Because she used only the cues that she received from the textbook and the teaching plans, Allison was unable to make correct judgments about what teaching Mrs. Chung actually needed. Consequently, she missed addressing Mrs. Chung's greatest concern.

The part of the Educative Nursing Practice Framework that Allison seems to have overlooked entirely is evaluation. If Allison had considered how each item in her teaching checklist would be assessed, she may have picked up that Mrs. Chung did not understand her surgery. What is clear is that asking patients if they understand is not a sufficient way to evaluate learning. Asking patients if they liked the teaching is also not an effective evaluation method. Learners may think they understand something but later discover they did not truly understand it. Some patients may be reluctant to tell the nurse they did not understand or did not like the session because they fear being impolite or looking stupid.

Evaluation requires that the nurse do some thinking before the teaching begins about what learning should occur during the teaching session and how that learning should be measured. For example, if Allison had planned to teach Mrs. Chung how to do postoperative deep breathing and coughing exercises, she could ask Mrs. Chung to demonstrate how she would do the exercises and say how often she would do them. Generally, asking patients to demonstrate a skill or to tell you what they would do in certain situations are the most common ways of evaluating educative nursing practice. However, you could also videotape a patient doing the skill you had taught, and then together, you could analyze the videotape for what the patient did

correctly or incorrectly. Remember that evaluation should occur for a period after the teaching/learning has occurred. The best way of evaluating learning is to assess if the patient was able to use that learning when they needed to, not just immediately after the teaching session. For example, Allison should assess whether Mrs. Chung is actually doing her deep breathing and coughing exercises after her surgery—this is the true test of the effectiveness of a teaching session.

Applying the Educative Nursing Practice Framework reveals that Allison could have improved her educative nursing practice by

- Considering additional learning theories
- Knowing the person
- Looking for cues by consulting Mrs. Chung, the chart, and other nurses prior to beginning teaching
- Making more accurate judgments and decisions
- Evaluating the teaching/learning more comprehensively

Paul Perley is a second-year nursing student who is to teach how to give insulin by injection to Mr. Bastien, a 67-year-old who has been recently diagnosed with insulin-dependent diabetes. Paul organizes his teaching so that he begins with simple tasks (e.g., how to take the cap off the needle) and then progresses to more complex ones (e.g., actually administering the insulin). He demonstrates the skill first and then asks Mr. Bastien to repeat it. He provides a great deal of affirmation ("Well done!" "That's the way!") whenever Mr. Bastien performs the skill correctly. Mr. Bastien is awkward in handling the equipment. He cannot seem to manage filling the syringe with saline. He is obviously frustrated about the mistakes he is making. He says, "It's useless. I am so clumsy." Paul talks to his clinical teacher and the nurse who is caring for Mr. Bastien. The nurse says, "Do you know that his granddaughter also has diabetes? That is what is written in his medical history in his chart. She and Mr. Bastien are very close. Maybe we could involve her as his teacher." Paul talks to Mr. Bastien and his granddaughter when she visits. He tells them that he thinks that the granddaughter will be able to show Mr. Bastien "tricks of the trade" that Paul does not know. Mr. Bastien enjoys learning how to give insulin with his granddaughter's coaching. In a short time, he is able to administer insulin to himself independently.

Knowing about learning is evident in this scenario. Paul has drawn from all five schools of thought about learning: behaviourism, cognitivism, constructivism, humanism, and andragogy. For example, in keeping with constructivism, humanism, and andragogy, Paul seems to understand that his telling is not sufficient to help Mr. Bastien learn the skill. He provided practice time, as well as explanations of the skill, in his teaching. He has drawn from cognitivism to break the skill down into manageable chunks and progresses from the simple to the more complex to help Mr. Bastien learn the new skill. Constructivism informed the need to include opportunities for Mr. Bastien to observe and model the behaviours that Paul demonstrated. Involving the granddaughter increased the relevance of the learning for Mr. Bastien (andragogy) and enhanced his motivation (constructivism and humanism). In addition, Paul applied many of the principles of behaviourism (e.g., he offered praise as reinforcement). Despite this, Paul disregarded some of these theories. For example, it is not apparent that he has consulted with Mr. Bastien about what he wants and needs to know; this is central to all but behaviourism and cognitivism. Additionally, Paul might have considered another theory. One example is Weiner's Attribution Theory (Weiner, 1986).

Weiner's Attribution Theory (Weiner, 1986) is a useful constructivist theory to consider when someone seems unable to master a new concept or skill. According to this theory, when we have trouble learning, we tend to blame either ourselves or another person. If patients want to learn something but have difficulty, they often blame themselves (internal attribution) and think there's nothing that can be done about it (e.g., "I am clumsy and so I'll never be able to handle a syringe properly"). Then, it becomes a self-fulfilling prophecy—they don't learn. However, if a nurse offers another attribution (explanation), such as, "All people have trouble at first, but when I show you some tricks, you'll learn it right away," the person is apt to change their initial attribution from internal and uncontrollable to internal and controllable. In most cases, they learn what they wanted to learn.

Paul received many cues in this scenario. He observed Mr. Bastien's frustration, and he received information from the clinical teacher and the nurse. We cannot tell in this scenario how much Paul knows about Mr. Bastien as a case, patient, or person. However, we get glimpses into how Paul knows himself when he recognizes that he needs to talk to someone with more experience to discuss what to do to assist Mr. Bastien in his learning. Paul should be commended for acknowledging that he had come to the end of his kit bag of strategies to help Mr. Bastien. Because of his willingness to be open about his limitations, the clinical teacher and the nurse were able to point Paul to new directions that ultimately proved to be successful. We have to wonder, though, if Paul wouldn't have discovered the need to involve Mr. Bastien's granddaughter before he began his teaching if he had simply spent time trying to know Mr. Bastien as a person.

Applying the Educative Nursing Practice Framework reveals that Paul could have improved his educative nursing practice by

- Considering additional learning theories
- Being congruent with the learning theories he uses
- Knowing the person

The next scenario is different than those previously presented because the framework will be used to identify a plan for teaching/learning and not as an analysis of a nurse's educative nursing practice.

Betty Billingsley is a fourth-year nursing student who is currently completing a clinical rotation in community health. She visits Bob Wilson and his family in their home. Bob is a university student who had a major car accident. His brain injury has left him unable to care for himself. He can no longer walk or talk. He requires complete care from his family. During her visit, Bob's mother says, "I just don't understand why the hospital staff didn't prepare us for what this was going to mean to us as a family. They didn't teach us anything. They didn't give us any information." Betty is aware that the hospital staff on the unit in which Bob was a patient is well known for their comprehensive family teaching prior to the patient's discharge. When she checks with the unit, one nurse says, "I remember distinctly that they attended the discharge planning conference in which physicians, nurses, psychologists, physiotherapists, and social workers taught them about Bob's care and the services that are available. We also gave them a manual of educational information to take home. I just don't know why they would say that when we worked so hard to teach them what they needed to know."

As in many cases in educative nursing practice, cues are evident in this scenario that the family has a need for teaching/learning. However, the cues seem to contradict one another. The staff of the hospital unit say that Bob's family was taught the things they needed to know to take Bob home and cope well with his needs. Bob's family members, on the other hand, say they did not receive this teaching.

Let's suppose that Betty consults the Educative Nursing Practice Framework for guidance. Betty would be aware that establishing an effective learning climate (context) is integral to educative nursing practice. She would reflect on the physical, social-cultural, and emotional context that may have been present during the Wilsons' time in the discharge planning conference. Because she was not there at the time, she will need to consult staff who had been present and the Wilson family themselves. For example, one aspect of an effective learning climate is the quality of interpersonal relationships between the educators and the students. Betty may want to inquire if the Wilsons knew any of the professionals present at the discharge planning conference beforehand and the nature of their relationship with them.

In her use of the Educative Nursing Practice Framework, Betty would review what she knows about learning that might be applicable to this situation. For example, she might consider andragogy and the principles of relevance and readiness. She might ask herself, "Was the family ready to hear what the staff said in the discharge planning conference? Was what they said relevant to the Wilsons?" She may review the content of the discharge planning conference in an attempt to answer these questions. She might also ask Bob's family about their experience at the discharge planning conference.

Betty could think about what she knows about herself in relation to this scenario. She might recall discharge planning conferences she had attended where patients and their families had participated actively in planning the patient's discharge from hospital. She may ask if Bob's family had participated actively or if they had been quiet. This could indicate that she needed more information about Bob's family's role in the conference. As well, Betty would need to admit that she was relatively inexperienced in relation to discharge planning and people with brain injuries. She should consider whom to consult for more information and advice about how she might proceed in this situation. Betty would also think about what she knows about the profession and a nurse's role in such a situation. She might consult her professional standards or ask her clinical teacher about the nurse's role as a family advocate and how this will influence her educative nursing practice.

Drawing on the framework, Betty would consider what she knew about cases like the one Bob's family presented. If she had little experience with such cases, she could consult nurses who were more experienced. She might also read relevant literature. For example, Paterson, Kieloch, and Gmiterek (2001) found that many families did not recall what had been taught during discharge planning conferences because they were too anxious about taking the person home and therefore could not listen to what the professionals were saying. As well, the things that the staff discussed were not relevant to them (e.g., the staff talked about the injured person eventually returning to school but the injured person could not talk and did not recognize family members) and the health-care professionals used medical jargon that the families did not understand. Betty could draw on this research in two ways: (1) to reflect on whether such factors accounted for the contradictory reports about teaching that had been provided to Bob's family, and (2) to plan with Bob's family the teaching/learning they desired (e.g., she would ask what they were most interested in learning and she would avoid medical jargon).

Knowing the patient would assist Betty to understand what his family might find relevant to learn as well as to appreciate the stressors that might cause them to feel anxious. For example, reading about the extent of Bob's injury and the physicians' notations about his prognosis in his chart, as well as nurse's notes about interactions with the family, can provide a context that will be useful in planning and implementing the teaching/learning.

Knowing the person in this scenario means more than knowing Bob; it includes knowing how the family relates to one another, what their needs are in relation to Bob's injury, and what supports they need and have. It means knowing that Bob's mother prefers to learn alone because she becomes anxious if her other son finds fault with what she does. It means knowing that a family friend is such a vital source of support that the family and their friend prefer that he is included in all the teaching. It means knowing that although three members of the family want to know how to catheterize Bob, one of them never wants to know that skill.

All forms of knowing provide cues that Betty can use to plan and implement teaching of Bob's family. She can use the cues to reflect on whether she needs more information or should consult more sources. She can then make decisions to provide the learning the family needs in the way they wish it to occur. It may mean that she is not the right one to do the teaching—a person who is an expert in specific content might be called for. It also may mean that she teaches in collaboration with others, perhaps a member of another patient's family whose loved one experienced a brain injury.

After Betty has enacted her teaching/learning, she could use the Educative Nursing Practice Framework to reflect on whether she could have improved it or whether additional teaching/learning is required. Such an evaluation is essential to her becoming the critically reflective educator she needs to be.

Educative Nursing Practice in Action

As emphasized previously in this chapter, educative nursing practice is a process, not a formula to apply across the board to every patient and in every situation. Educative nursing practice turns on the knowledge and requisite skills that the nurse has acquired through study, practice, reflection, and life experience as this relates to knowing about learning, knowing about the profession, knowing the self, knowing the case, knowing the patient, and knowing the person. Listening and being well informed and organized are essential strategies for enacting this framework. Nonetheless, there will always be times when the nurse does not have sufficient information or experience to fully practice knowing as she enacts the educative role.

Attentiveness

Listening and observing with intention are foundational skills required for the educative role in nursing practice. This means that you need to listen for what those in your care say they need to know in terms of information or skills. What do they know already? What previous experiences has the learner had that could be used to foster learning in this situation? Be attentive to the patient's readiness to learn. Is the patient still anxious having received a frightening diagnosis, or is she able to hear what you have to say? Consider the patient's health literacy level. Does the patient seem to understand the terms you use, or do your words elicit quizzical expressions and/or blank stares? Watch for signs about how the patient takes up what you have offered in terms of information. How does the patient seem to learn best? It is also important to observe how you come across in terms of respecting the knowledge of the learning and your own knowledge. Are you paternalistic or compassionate? Is it a two-way or one-way conversation? Listen for what additional information is required by the patient based on the new information he has acquired when learning with you. What more does the learner wish to know? Consider and listen for clues about for who else should attend the session. Is there a spouse, family caregiver, or significant other who should be present?

Being Well Informed and Organized

To be effective in the educative role, it is foundational for the nurse to be clear in his or her mind about the subject matter. Thus, to ensure that you as a nurse are well prepared for a teaching session, study various sources on the topic—empirical, theoretical, and critical—prior to enacting this role. Even though educative nursing practice does not adhere to a formula, there is core knowledge that is required when teaching in particular substantive areas of practice; for example, diabetes, oncology, or orthopedic surgery. As knowledge is ever-changing in this fast-paced world, keeping current with new developments is essential. Thus, being organized in the educative role requires that you build time into your life to update your knowledge base in the substantive areas of your practice. Some groups of nurses form research teams or journal clubs as a way of staying current with new knowledge. Others attend rounds and professional conferences or enroll in courses to stay current in their field. Thus, being organized about the educative role in nursing is a lifelong matter.

The educative role in nursing is enacted in various ways and in a range of settings, from just-in time learning, to one-on-one sessions, to teaching in groups. Enacting this role in various ways requires that the nurse is well organized with regard to managing time and teaching materials. The educative role for many nurses, especially those on fast-paced units, is enacted not as a discrete task but rather is integrated into nursing; for example, during medication administration, carrying out procedures such as dressings, or coaching the patient and her family in the use of intravenous patient controlled analgesia (IV PCA). For such teaching, the nurse must have a solid base of knowledge clearly organized in her mind, have the capacity to think quickly, and know where to access teaching tools (e.g., handouts or pamphlets) in a moment's notice. In settings where formal teaching is required, the organized nurse will set aside ample time to engage the patient and his or her family, or a group of learners, in an authentic educative conversation—allowing time for assessment, interaction, evaluation of, and reflection on what was learned. Further, a skilled nurse will enable interactions during the teaching session in which learners learn from each other.

No matter what the setting, similar principles guide educative nursing practice:

- Be knowledgeable about the substantive area.
- Be respectful, warm, and engaging.
- Listen to what the patient wants to learn.
- Attend to how the patients learn best.
- Build on their previous experiences.
- Tailor the session to accommodate patient preferences.
- Select effective teaching tools.

- Keep teaching tools organized.
- Evaluate what the patient has learned.
- Reflect on your teaching.
- Document the learning goals achieved.

Not Knowing

In educative nursing practice, there will be moments in which knowing as we have set it out in the framework is impossible, or only partially possible. Sensitivity, silence, and authenticity are the strategies that will sustain a nurse through these challenging moments. As nurses, it may not be possible to know the patient; for example, when a person is unconscious or near death. In such situations, a highly tuned sensitivity in combination with silence may open spaces for the patient, family, and nurse to connect in meaningful ways to acquire important new insights. Another area of not knowing that often faces beginning nurses pertains to not knowing the substantive area well enough to be effective in the educative role. Such moments will require that the student nurse be authentic regarding his or her capacity to enact the educative role. As humbling and frustrating as this can be, it is such moments that point us to areas where we need to deepen our knowledge, thereby opening new paths that can be defining moments for us in our professional journey.

Tools for Educative Nursing Practice: Examples, Issues, and Complexities

The nurse will use various approaches in the educative role: distributing pamphlets and fact sheets, arranging videos/ DVDs with or without a workbook, one-on-one teaching, and group sessions to foster learning. A common practice in nursing units, clinics, and health units is using a manual as a guide to provide patients with information. Examples of manuals are the *Cardiovascular Patient Education Resource Manual* edited by Gershendon and the Diabetes and Cardiovascular Disease Toolkit produced by the American Diabetes Association and the American Heart Association (copies of the toolkits are available at http://professional.diabetes.org and http://www.heart.org). Such manuals cover a range of topics: understanding symptoms; managing medications; and reducing risk, including lifestyle risks—all very important topics for someone newly diagnosed with diabetes or heart disease. Toolkits such as these are available in print and CD-ROM. The Diabetes and Cardiovascular Disease Toolkit comes with educational handouts in PDF format that nurses can use during education sessions. However, these tools are based on theoretical positions on teaching and learning consistent with the view that the learner is an empty vessel that needs to be filled. This is in opposition to theories reviewed earlier in this chapter that current teaching and learning theories and empirical research suggest are effective in supporting adult learning with the potential to change behaviour.

Through the eyes of a nurse

We had this patient. He kept coming back onto our unit with blood pressure readings that were through the roof. Every time he came back to us, we trotted down to his room with the patient teaching manual and ticked off the topics we had covered on his chart. After about his fourth admission, I decided to put aside the manual as we didn't seem to be getting anywhere. I used the time to sit and chat "about nothing" with him and his wife. As we chatted, the conversation turned to what he loves to eat. Well, I almost fell off my chair when I learned that he loves pickles and eats a jar a day. The man had no idea that a jar of pickles had a dangerously high level of salt! After this, I wanted to get rid of the manual, but the pressure [in the hospital] to use it to guide practice is such a deterrent.

(personal reflection of Brenda M., cardiac nurse educator)

Selecting an approach to teaching and learning in the educative role is complex and challenging. In everyday practice, approaches that are in common practice are often taken up uncritically and delivered with minimal awareness of the complexity of teaching and learning. The impact of factors such as demographic characteristics such as age and gender and environmental factors such as hospital policies are not always considered in the selection of approaches; this is despite evaluation research on health-related educational interventions pointing directly to the importance of considering such influences.

The research literature abounds with studies demonstrating the importance of matching the delivery method to a specific patient group. For example, nurses are frequently called on to educate for changes in lifestyle behaviours in primary prevention settings, and nursing students are frequently assigned to such a challenge in the upper years of their program. In one study (Mullen et al., 1997), a meta-analysis that looked at evaluation research focusing on various health promotion practices such as breast and testicular self-examination, the researchers concluded that although the answer to primary prevention of lifestyle risk behaviours requires attention not only to patient education but also to individual and environmental factors, interventions that used media and personal communication were most effective in fostering changes in smoking and weight.

Innovative new approaches to supporting patients in making lifestyle changes include e-tools such as the Heart & Stroke Foundation of Canada, *My Heart & Stroke Healthy Weight Action Plan*, an Internet-based program that offers persons who may be overweight with the opportunity to assess their weight relative to normative standards and provides information tailored with respect to age, gender, and ethnicity. This strategy is consistent with key findings in the evaluation research of educational interventions that speak to the importance of tailoring educational approaches with attention to demographic factors. The program draws on research that has demonstrated that self-monitoring is

an effective strategy to support weight loss (Wing & Hill, 2001); thus, the education strategy used in the tool is tailored to the targeted behaviour. The educational intervention is self-paced and provides users with opportunities to read more or less material in each session. The language used is at a level of health literacy appropriate for most readers. Each session provides readers with a featured article. The articles are written in plain language and provide empowering information such as what a measured portion in the Canada's Food Guide looks like—for example, one portion of bread is the size of a CD case. There are several astute features in this program: The instructions are clear, the program uses first person, the user can access the science behind the advice, there is a built in tool that is a log for monitoring weight and food intake, the program guides users to meet challenges and glitches, and so on. Such a tool is most commendable in its incorporation of theory and empirical research on patient education. Go to the website and read *My Heart & Stroke Healthy Weight Action Plan* (https://ehealth.heartandstroke.ca/heartstroke/hwap2/index.asp) to view a well-designed educational tool.

An innovative approach to educative practice targeting adolescents with diabetes and their parents is described by Løding, Wold, and Skavhaug (2008). Because this was an educational intervention for a group, the underlying pedagogy is Vygotsky's social learning theory. The group intervention was envisioned to augment individual sessions. The educators drew on theories about group communication in the design. For example, at the outset of the first meeting, they set rules for group process to deal with issues such as confidentiality, verbal abuse, and absenteeism. Each session began with warm-up exercises that were unrelated to diabetes, and the topic for each session emerged through a process of consensus. The teen group covered a wide range of topics from "Me and My Diabetes" to "Diabetic Ketoacidosis" to "Living on My Own." At the end of the sessions, each person had a chance to hold the floor, with the group leaders summarizing the discussion. The group leaders were equal members of the group rather than teachers. The authors concluded that a group intervention such as this has potential to improve physiological indicators of diabetes while not diminishing self-reported quality of life.

As a nursing student, you will have opportunities to develop knowledge and skills for educative nursing practice. You will be challenged in several ways in enacting this role, but meeting the challenges with a high level of professionalism and curiosity, humility and sensitivity, creativity, and good humour will stand you in good stead as you develop competence.

Conclusion

In this chapter, we have presented theories and strategies to guide your educative nursing practice. Educative nursing practice is a key role for professional nursing that is guided by nursing and education theories. In this chapter, we provided a brief overview of key education theories that nurses draw on in the educative role: behaviourism, cognitivism, humanism, constructivism, and andragogy. With a view to encouraging

BOX 15.10   Practical Tips for Patient Teaching

Is the Patient Ready to Learn?
Find out if your patient believes and understands his diagnosis. Keep his age and literacy level in mind. Are there any health-related factors (e.g., pain, worry, anxiety) that may impact his ability to learn?

Time to Teach
Introduce yourself. Speak clearly and purposefully. Determine with the patient what it is that she needs and wants to know. Ask the patient if someone else should be included the teaching sessions; for example, a spouse or partner. Allow reasonable time for demonstration and return demonstrations (as appropriate).

Assessing Outcomes
Assess learning and teaching during the session. Is the patient attentive? What does the patient's body language say? Is the conversation interactive or is it one way? Reflect on the session. How did you feel? Did the teaching go as planned? How do you know that learning occurred? Document the session and your teaching.

Organization
Organize your teaching resources in advance of encountering the patient and his or her family. Keep teaching resources current (e.g., handouts, videos, and fact sheets) and keep teaching aids simple.

Information
Use teaching aids developed at no more than a Grade 5 reading level. (There are readability formulas you can use to calculate the readability of any teaching material. Search the Internet using the search terms *readability calculation*.) Look for the teachable moment (i.e., the moment that presents itself as a valuable opportunity to teach something that the patient wants to learn). Offer information in manageable doses to allow time for processing (don't overwhelm people with volumes of information). This mistake can occur as part of discharge planning; that is, great volumes of information are presented just prior to the patient/family leaving the unit. This is likely not the best time for the patient as he or she will be thinking about going home.

Communication
Remember that patients require privacy when the teaching/learning sessions address sensitive or intimate topics. When other patients in the room can hear the session, the patient may develop anxiety and thus become unable to focus his attention on learning. Use effective body language—good eye contact, tone of voice, and touch—as appropriate and where relevant. Adapt your session if the patient suffers any barriers to learning such as hearing or vision impairments or cognitive deficits. Assist the patient with making links between new learning and previous experiences. Ask open-ended questions to evaluate the extent to which learning has taken place.

Source: Adapted from Southern California Renal Disease Council. (1997). *Patient teaching tips.* Retrieved from http://www.esrdnetwork18.org/pdfs/QI%20-%20Tools%20&%20Forms/Patient_Teaching_Tips.pdf

students to "make this theory real" in practice, we challenged readers to develop a vision for their educative role, offering ideas for how to go about doing so and rationale for why this is important. The Educative Nursing Practice Framework was then presented as a tool to guide decision-making when enacting the educative role: knowing (i.e., about learning, profession, case, self, patient, and person), caring, and context. Three case studies were presented to illustrate the framework relative to the education theories presented earlier in this chapter. This chapter concluded with a discussion of strategies and tools for enacting the educative role in nursing practice (Box 15.10). In reading this chapter, considering the ideas, and rising to the challenges, we hope you have developed new skills and knowledge for educative nursing practice.

Critical Thinking Activities

▶ Return to the case study at the beginning of this chapter. Now that you have a thorough grasp of educative nursing practice, how would you respond to the preceptor if you were Edwin? What learning theories would you draw on for your answer?

▶ Think about two situations in which you or another nurse were required to teach a patient, one that was effective and one that did not result in the learning you or the nurse had hoped for. Use the Educative Nursing Practice Framework to analyze both situations to identify what insights are evident from these situations that could enhance your own educative nursing practice.

▶ Some hospitals across the globe are suggesting that nurses are too busy to teach patients. They have established teaching programs on various topics that patients can watch on television or on computers. Nurses in these hospitals have a limited educative nursing practice role. If you were a nurse in such a hospital, how could you present your personal vision of educative nursing practice and your knowledge of relevant learning theories to debate such a stance?

Multiple-Choice Questions

1. Mr. George Bulman has received extensive teaching about his prescribed diet from the dietitian. He tells you that he understood everything the dietitian taught him. However, he continues to eat foods that are contraindicated in his prescribed diet. Which of the following is the best explanation for such behaviour?
   a. Understanding what is required does not necessarily translate to changes in behaviour.
   b. People may not be ready to apply the new knowledge they have learned.
   c. The foods one chooses have personal and social meaning.
   d. Sometimes people think they understand something, but they do not really understand it.

2. Marilyn Ng is a third-year nursing student who is to teach Billy Boyle about injecting insulin. Beforehand, she read extensively and consulted her clinical instructor about what she should teach Billy. She made a detailed plan. However, when she began to teach him, Billy said, "This is all too overwhelming. I can't deal with so many things at once." Which of the following would have helped Marilyn to avoid such a scenario and to improve her educative nursing practice?
   a. Knowing the case
   b. Knowing the self
   c. Knowing about the patient
   d. Knowing about the person

3. Amrit Singh is 67 years old. She has approached you because she would like to know how to prevent her recurrent bladder infections. Which of the following statements demonstrate that you are applying the principles of andragogy in your response?
   a. "I can certainly tell you a few things that might help you to prevent bladder infections."
   b. "Let's start with the most simple techniques and then I will introduce some more complicated ones."
   c. "Let's talk for a while about what you know already and what you would like to happen in this session."
   d. "I will look this up in some resources we have in the department and get back to you."

4. Jolene Bennett, a third-year nursing student, is assigned to the cardiovascular unit. It is her first day, and she is feeling nervous because she is new to cardiovascular nursing. Jolene's preceptor urges her to teach a patient who has just had a primary percutaneous coronary intervention (PCI) about lifestyle risks for coronary heart disease using the materials on the unit. What should Jolene do first?
   a. Go into the patient's room to introduce herself.
   b. Find out what teaching materials are available on the unit.
   c. Brush up on PCI.
   d. Ask if she could have another assignment.

5. Joshua Longman has been placed on an orthopedic unit for his final practicum. He is responsible for discharging two patients on this particular day. Both need to be taught how to give themselves a heparin injection. The patients will leave the hospital in an hour. What education theories will be particularly relevant to his teaching?
   a. Behaviourism, constructivism, humanism
   b. Andragogy, cognitivism, humanism
   c. Social constructivism, andragogy, attribution
   d. Humanism, social constructivism, andragogy

Suggested Lab Activities

● Pretend that you are a nurse working in a hospital unit who is about to teach a patient and her family about how to administer an anticoagulant by subcutaneous injection in her home after she is discharged from the hospital. Set up the furniture and other elements of the teaching environment to foster learning. Consider such things as lighting, comfort, privacy, temperature, etc.

● Teach a classmate a lab skill (e.g., administering an intravenous medication, assessing neurological signs) with which he is unfamiliar. Use the Educative Nursing Practice Framework to implement and evaluate your teaching.

REFERENCES AND SUGGESTED READINGS

Alfano, G. (1971). Healing or caretaking—Which will it be? *Nursing Clinics of North America, 6,* 273.

Brookfield, S. D. (1991). *The skillful teacher.* San Francisco, CA: Jossey-Bass.

Donahue, M. P. (1985). *Nursing: The finest art.* Toronto, ON: C. V. Mosby.

Elias, J. L., & Merriam, S. B. (1995). *Philosophical foundations of adult education* (2nd ed.). Malabar, FL: Krieger.

Gillespie, M., & Paterson, B. L. (2009). Helping novice nurses make effective clinical decisions: The situated clinical decision-making framework. *Nursing Education Perspectives, 30*(3), 164–170.

Gottlieb, L., & Rowat, K. (1987). The McGill Model of Nursing: A practice derived model. *Advances in Nursing Science, 9*(4), 51–61.

Hartley, J. (1998). *Learning and studying. A research perspective.* London, United Kingdom: Routledge.

Holer, S. (2004). Tips for better patient teaching. *Nursing2004, 34*(7), 32hn7–32hn8.

Knowles, M. S., Holton, E. F., III, & Swanson, R. A. (2005). *The adult learner: The definitive classic in adult education and human resource development* (6th ed.). Burlington, MA: Elsevier.

Løding, R. N., Wold, J. E., & Skavhaug, A. (2008). Experiences with a group intervention for adolescents with type 1 diabetes and their parents. *European Diabetes Nursing, 5,* 9–14.

Mullen, P. D., Simons-Morton, D. G., Ramírez, G., Frankowski, R. F., Green, L. W., & Mains, D. A. (1997). A meta-analysis of trials evaluating patient education and counseling for three groups of preventive health behaviors. *Patient Education and Counseling, 32,* 157–173.

Parse, R. (1992). Human becoming: Parse's theory of nursing. *Nursing Science Quarterly, 5,* 35–42.

Paterson, B., Kieloch, B., & Gmiterek, J. (2001). 'They never told us anything': Postdischarge instructions for families of persons with brain injuries. *Rehabilitation Nursing, 26*(2), 48–53.

Pearson, A. (2003). A blast from the past: Whatever happened to the 'new nursing' and 'nursing beds'? *International Journal of Nursing Practice, 9,* 67–69.

Rogers, C., & Freiberg, H. J. (1993). *Freedom to learn* (3rd ed.). New York, NY: Merrill.

Skinner, B. F. (1984). Selection by consequences. *Behavioral and Brain Sciences, 7*(4), 477–481.

Smith, M. K. (1997, 2004). *Carl Rogers and informal education, the encyclopaedia of informal education*. Retrieved from http://www.infed.org/thinkers/et-rogers.htm

Tomey, A., & Alligood, M. R. (2006). *Nursing theorists and their work* (6th ed.). St. Louis, MO: Mosby/Elsevier.

Weiner, B. (1986). *An attributional theory of motivation and emotion*. New York, NY: Springer-Verlag.

Wing, R. R., & Hill, J. O. (2001). Successful weight loss maintenance. *Annual Review of Nutrition, 21*, 323–341.

Young, L. E., & Maxwell, B. (2007). From rote to active learning: Constructivism in the context of teaching theories. In L. E. Young & B. Paterson (Eds.), *Teaching nursing: Developing a student-centered learning environment* (pp. 1–25). Philadelphia, PA: Lippincott Williams and Wilkins.

Ways of Thinking: Critical Thinking in Nursing

CHRISTY RAYMOND-SENIUK AND JOANNE PROFETTO-MCGRATH

Chris is a first-year nursing student. During the past term, Chris received feedback that she needs to enhance her critical thinking. Chris is not clear exactly what critical thinking is and how she should proceed to further develop it as she progresses through her nursing program.

CHAPTER OBJECTIVES

By the end of this chapter, you will be able to:

1. Compare different definitions of critical thinking.
2. List common components of critical thinking.
3. Recognize indicators of critical thinking.
4. Describe methods that have been used to measure critical thinking.
5. Differentiate ways to engage in critical thinking, such as reflection and critical reading.
6. Recognize the link between critical thinking and evidence-based practice.
7. Engage in forming arguments for or against certain positions.

KEY TERMS

Context The environment, situation, or occasion that impacts a related thought or topic.

Critical Thinking A combination of skills and dispositions to maximize one's ability to purposely reflect and think deeply.

Deductive Reasoning Using generalizations to create specific conclusions.

Dispositions Personal traits or qualities.

Evidence-Based Practice The use of various types of knowledge to guide one's practice in the clinical setting toward the goal of quality patient care outcomes.

Inductive Reasoning When specific events, or findings from those events, are used to form broader generalizations.

Perfections of Thought Originally coined by Paul (1990), these are traits or goals that describe clear, concise, exemplary thinking.

Reflective Skepticism Positive, respectful examination, analysis, and questioning of a specified topic or issue.

Reflective Thinking A consecutive, successive thought process, prompted by uncertainty or perplexity, where consequence and grounds for the belief is thoroughly examined.

Thinking Outside of the Box Thinking that is considered unconventional or against commonly engrained traditions. Thinking outside the box is often used synonymously with creative thinking or creating a new perspective, in contrast to "thinking inside of the box," which is thinking that follows traditional pathways or perspectives. Thinking inside the box is often representative of the "status quo" or usual ways of thinking about things.

In order to explore the meaning and application of critical thinking in nursing, this chapter is organized using a questioning approach. Questioning is one method that fosters critical thinking, and it provides a creative way to guide our exploration of this concept. The history of philosophy highlights the value that has been placed on questioning to further human thought. For example, questioning can be linked to Socrates, who believed that knowledge was constantly changing and an interacting element of life. Knowledge can be further developed through questioning what we experience as well as examining others' positions and philosophical perspectives. The questions posed in this chapter will help to enrich and extend your knowledge about critical thinking.

Think

"Sometimes questions are more important than answers." Nancy Willard

Think about your nursing education so far. Do you feel you have more questions than you do answers? This quote offers the important insight that questions stimulate our thinking process. Without questions, we would not necessarily think about things in order to gain a resolution or deeper understanding. Questioning helps us attain a deeper level of understanding rather than accepting things superficially. Once you are in the clinical setting, you will appreciate that there are many more questions than answers. Looking for answers implies a search for one best path. Looking for questions implies a wealthier and more holistic journey of understanding, which one needs in order to learn the role of nurse. Try searching for questions versus answers in your next clinical experience.

Think

"The power to question is the basis of all human progress." Indira Gandhi

Although your nursing education helps with learning how to perform the skills and abilities of a nurse, thinking more broadly is at the heart of nursing practice. Although we often think nursing is about the patient, thinking critically is about seeing the big picture. This big picture involves thinking about mankind and their abilities to think and use cognitive processes. Human beings have developed and gained important knowledge and insights through our curiosity and questioning of our practices, thought processes, and theories. Without questioning, this progress may not have occurred. Innovations and groundbreaking ideas would have not emerged without questioning, thinking, and challenging the status quo. Challenge yourself to think broadly during your nursing career. Cultivate your curiosity and challenge the status quo around you.

What Is Thinking?

Thinking can mean many different things to different people. For example, we may think about what food we will consume or what tasks we need to do before we leave for work and also about the human suffering and starvation happening in the world. The common feature of thinking is that there is conscious engagement about an idea, thought, or perceived problem. John Dewey (2007) stated that "a being without

capacity for thought is moved only by instincts and appetites" (p. 11). Thus, the nature of rational thinking for a higher purpose is an important component of human thought processes. When the mind engages with the content of our thought processes, there are many things that can happen. Some thoughts will only be acknowledged and then will leave our conscious awareness, whereas some thoughts will prompt further work. This additional work might include processes such as reasoning to reach further conclusions.

What Is Reasoning?

Two types of reasoning, inductive and deductive reasoning, are often associated with reasoning methods. **Inductive reasoning** refers to specific events used to form broader generalizations. **Deductive reasoning** refers to generalizations used to create specific conclusions. Reasoning processes are helpful to solve problems, make decisions, or gain deeper understanding about a particular topic of interest. Think about other thinking processes that you engage in. Compare your ideas to Box 16.1, which outlines some common thought processes along with their respective definitions.

What Is Critical Thinking?

The distinction between thinking and critical thinking is based on the reason, content, and process of thinking. Everyone has fleeting thoughts about random things. However, critical thinking is a purposeful process that is reflective, consecutive, and goes beyond recognition of an initial thought. General thinking that is not classified as critical thinking tends to be biased and uninformed by a significant level of past knowledge or experience. Dewey (2007) added that critical thinking includes the basis and consequences of thought; therefore, the outcome of thinking is as much a part as the initial impetus that brought the thought to the forefront of one's mind. As well, reflection is a key element of critical thinking: the ability to *think about thinking* and evaluate its purpose and process. We are thus able to look on our thinking without biased emotion and assess the quality and purpose of the thinking.

Critical thinking can be different things in different situations or contexts. However, in nursing, critical thinking can be described as a mode of thinking about any subject, content, context, or issue in which the thinker endeavors to improve the quality of his or her thinking by applying intellectual standards to the thinking process. It is based on intellectual values that transcend subject matter: clarity, accuracy, precision, consistency, relevance, sound evidence, good reasons, depth, breadth, and fairness. As well, critical thinking involves an individual's **dispositions**, or habits of mind including "confidence, contextual perspective, creativity, flexibility, inquisitiveness, intellectual integrity, intuition, open-mindedness, perseverance, and reflection" (Scheffer & Rubenfeld, 2000, p. 357).

Critical thinking is an important part of people's everyday personal and professional lives. Nurses and student nurses can use critical thinking to process the constant stream of

BOX 16.1   Common Thought Processes

Decision-making—process of reaching a conclusion about a course of action. Includes identifying a decision to be made; weighing alternative options; selecting options; and making a choice, direction, or action.

Distinguishing—finding and acknowledging existing differences between entities, objects, facts, or other elements of thought.

Evaluating—systematic intentional determination or comparison of level or worth against a determined or stated measure.

Hypothesizing—creation and/or acknowledgment of a supposed alternative, outcome, or explanation based on previous knowledge or suspected conclusion.

Making inferences—reaching conclusions using knowledge or suppositions that are known or assumed to be correct or true.

Memorization—deliberate committing or storing of facts or other cognitive schema to memory for the purpose of recall or use at a later time.

Metacognition—thinking about thinking, knowing about knowing, or cognition about cognition. A reflective act that considers one's own knowledge about how knowledge and other cognitive processes are handled within one's capacity to know and think.

Organizing—classifying objects of cognition into predetermined or purposeful categories.

Planning—conscious process of thinking ahead about actions, thought, or goals and the necessary processes to achieve them.

Predicting—forecasting based on various sources of knowledge or personal thought.

Problem solving—attempting to solve an identified problem through various potentially cyclical stages, including identification of the problem, understanding of the problem, creation of possible solutions, exploring the stated solutions, choosing one solution, implementing the chosen solution, and evaluating the implemented solution.

Rationalization—engaging in a process of seeking and providing reason through various processes in order to come to an optimal conclusion.

Reflection—looking inwards or being introspective about various aspects of human process, thought, action, or essence.

Synthesis—combining simpler objects of thought to create a larger more substantial one or moving from general to more particular thoughts.

Translating—changing items of thought into other formats through a comprehension of meaning and then transformation.

Understanding—reaching a state of comprehension where concepts are attached to thoughts in order to better manage and deal with them using other cognitive processes.

---

information and knowledge needed to effectively and competently care for patients in various settings. The skills of processing knowledge and thinking analytically can also benefit one's personal life. Relationships with others can be strengthened when one is able to think critically about events and to communicate understanding and empathy. More broadly, critical thinking skills and abilities benefit society as a whole. Critical thinking by individuals about larger purposes and the consequences of others' actions promote understanding and support stronger decision-making about global issues.

Critical Thinking in Nursing

Critical thinking is a term and a process that is often used in nursing contexts. Its importance is identified and promoted everywhere. Professional nursing associations and accrediting boards cite critical thinking as an important skill in nursing. For example, the College and Association of Registered Nurses of Alberta (CARNA) states that "the registered nurse demonstrates critical thinking in collecting and interpreting data, planning, implementing and evaluating all aspects of nursing care" (College and Association of Registered Nurses of Alberta [CARNA], 2005, p. 3). As well, the Association of Registered Nurses of Newfoundland and Labrador (ARNNL) state that each registered nurse "searches for, interprets, and uses information from a variety of sources; uses comprehensive assessment, [and] critical thinking . . . to provide competent nursing services relevant to the area of practice (Association of Registered Nurses of Newfoundland and Labrador [ARNNL], 2007, p. 10). Many other provincial associations include critical thinking as an important practice standard that nurses are expected to demonstrate when providing nursing care in various contexts. In their *Position Statement on Baccalaureate Education and Baccalaureate Programs*, the Canadian Association of Schools of

Nursing (CASN) also emphasizes the responsibility baccalaureate schools of nursing have in providing "the foundation for sound clinical reasoning and clinical judgment, critical thinking and a strong ethical component in nursing" (Canadian Association of Schools of Nursing [CASN], 2004, p. 1)

The diagram in Figure 16.1 illustrates a connection between knowledge and knowing, critical thinking, and the

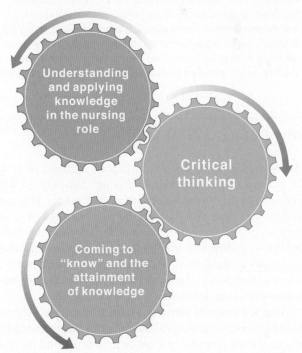

Figure 16.1 From knowing to being: critical thinking in the process of nursing.

application of thinking and knowing to the role of a nurse. The role of the nurse encompasses a myriad of knowledge, concepts, and facts necessary to function effectively. Competent nursing practice involves thinking about and deciphering pertinent knowledge related to a specific nursing encounter, applying that pertinent knowledge within a nursing role, and understanding how broader contextual concepts relate to that nursing encounter and the broader concept of nursing and the nursing role. Critical thinking helps to transform knowledge into understanding and prompts action, or nursing practice, which is supported by the nurse's understanding of the knowledge and the nursing encounter. Without critical thinking, a deeper understanding of knowledge would not occur, leaving nursing care essentially ineffective.

There are many resources such as textbooks and articles as well as several organizations that are devoted solely to the development of critical thinking. One such organization is the Foundation for Critical Thinking, which holds annual conferences and has a wide selection of published resources. Let's look at the opening statement from the Foundation for Critical Thinking website and address some questions that arise from that statement: "The Center for Critical Thinking and Moral Critique and the Foundation for Critical Thinking, two sister educational non-profit organizations, work closely together to promote essential change in education and society through the cultivation of fair-minded critical thinking."

Think "Critical thinking is essential if we are to get to the root of our problems and develop reasonable solutions. After all, the quality of everything we do is determined by the quality of our thinking" (The Critical Thinking Community, 2009)

Are these claims for promoting essential change necessary or even true? Who is the intended audience for this statement? Is this centre widely accessed or used to promote critical thinking by various populations? Asking questions about what you see on the Internet is an important aspect of thinking critically. Just as there are many questions that we could ask about this organization, there are many questions we ask in general about critical thinking.

Why Define Critical Thinking?

The answer depends on several factors, such as, what is the purpose of defining critical thinking? The purpose will guide you to choose certain definitions over others. This can change with time and fluctuate between settings. If your purpose for defining critical thinking is to develop the skills and foster the dispositions of critical thinking, you may wish to consider all the definitions and determine in what aspects you need to improve. Using certain aspects from each definition may be more useful than using only one definition.

What is the setting where you wish to apply your critical thinking? This can be a clinical, laboratory, or classroom setting in your nursing program, or it can be in your personal life and relationships. There are many definitions suitable for certain contexts. Two nursing specific definitions, one by Alfaro-LeFevre

(2009) and another from Scheffer and Rubenfeld (2000), are explored on the following pages. These definitions are general enough to be used in most nursing environments (e.g., clinical, classroom, or lab settings). We will also explore Facione's (1990) definition, developed for the American Philosophical Association (APA), which may be more applicable to developing critical thinking skills and attributes in one's everyday life.

It might seem logical that if all of these organizations, programs, and authors are emphasizing the importance of critical thinking in nursing, it must be a well-known and comprehensively understood concept. Actually, critical thinking is not a commonly understood concept and there is a lack of consensus regarding its definition. Despite the demands to have it, demonstrate it, and improve it as a nursing student, critical thinking is defined in many different ways, is not easy to develop, and is difficult to demonstrate within one's nursing practice.

To understand what critical thinking is, it is helpful to examine some of the more prominent definitions. Given the complexity of critical thinking and the abundance of definitions to describe it, it is sometimes difficult to choose which one to use.

American Philosophical Association Definition of Critical Thinking

One of the most popular critical thinking definitions comes from outside nursing. The APA commissioned a Delphi study to create a definition and measure of critical thinking.

What Is the Delphi Method?

In a Delphi technique, experts collaborate to create a definition through a process of consensus. Over a period of time, the experts respond to various questions presented, and their opinions are then tabulated. Gradually, the questioning leads to deeper inquiry into specific components of the concept being defined. Eventually, consensus is achieved, and an understanding and definition are put forth to the wider academic community for consideration. The benefits of a Delphi technique include the collaboration of well-known experts in the topic. As well, the experts include individuals from a wide geographical area. A drawback of the Delphi method is its expense. If experts are convened, then there are location costs. However, if the experts are accessed via distance, then time spent communicating with all of the experts can be extensive and costly. The Delphi method can also take years to complete.

A Definition of Critical Thinking

In 1990, Peter A. Facione led the APA conference in a Delphi process attempting a definition of critical thinking. Upon completion of the process, they released this statement.

Expert Consensus Statement Regarding Critical Thinking and the Ideal Critical Thinker:

We understand critical thinking to be purposeful, self-regulatory judgment which results in interpretation, analysis, evaluation, and inference, as well as explanation of the evidential, conceptual, methodological, criteriological, or contextual considerations upon which that judgment is based. CT is essential as a tool of inquiry. As such, CT is a liberating force in education and a powerful resource in one's personal and civic life. While not synonymous with good thinking, CT is a pervasive and self-rectifying human phenomenon. The ideal critical thinker is habitually inquisitive, well-informed, trustful of reason, open-minded, flexible, fair-minded in evaluation, honest in facing personal biases, prudent in making judgments, willing to reconsider, clear about issues, orderly in complex matters, diligent in seeking relevant information, reasonable in the selection of criteria, focused in inquiry, and persistent in seeking results which are as precise as the subject and the circumstances of inquiry permit. Thus, educating good critical thinkers means working toward this ideal. It combines developing CT skills with nurturing those dispositions which consistently yield useful insights and which are the basis of a rational and democratic society. (Facione, 1990, p. 3)

The definition of critical thinking developed through the APA includes skills and dispositions or attributes that individuals need to demonstrate to support critical thinking. The combined skills and attributes are a common theme in most definitions to be examined. The skills identified in the definition are depicted in Figure 16.2 and represent overall cognitive judgment. The specific attributes listed in the Facione (1990) definition are illustrated in Figure 16.3. The attributes collectively represent an overall critical spirit that individuals should have in order to search for and process knowledge.

Even though memorizing definitions can be important in certain situations, it will be the underlying discussion of the definitions of critical thinking that will bring us to more fruitful conclusions. The questions that are pertinent when you read the definition by Facione (1990) include the following:

- Is this definition correct and does it make sense from your perspective?
- How can you apply this definition to your studies as a nursing student?

The process of coming to understand which definition is right for your context can be confusing. If you are not sure if this definition is correct or applicable to you, it is important to look at other definitions before selecting one to incorporate into your practice.

Scheffer and Rubenfeld's (2000) Nursing-Based Definition of Critical Thinking

Reading various definitions helps to clarify how critical thinking is viewed in nursing. Scheffer and Rubenfeld developed one such definition in collaboration with nursing scholars, using a Delphi technique (Scheffer & Rubenfeld, 2000). They created a nursing-focused definition, as follows:

Critical thinking in nursing is an essential component of professional accountability and quality nursing care. Critical thinkers in nursing exhibit these habits of the mind: confidence, contextual perspective, creativity, flexibility, inquisitiveness, intellectual integrity, intuition, open-mindedness, perseverance, and reflection. Critical thinkers in nursing practice the cognitive skills of analyzing, applying standards, discriminating, information seeking, logical reasoning, predicting and transforming knowledge. (p. 357)

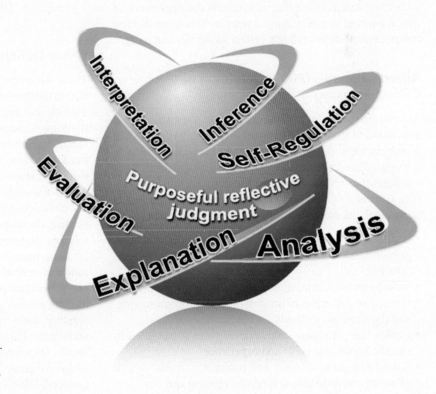

Figure 16.2 Critical thinking skills (Image © Insight Assessment 2010; used with permission). Facione, P. A. (2013). Critical thinking: What it is and why it counts. *Insight Assessment*. Millbrae, CA: Author.

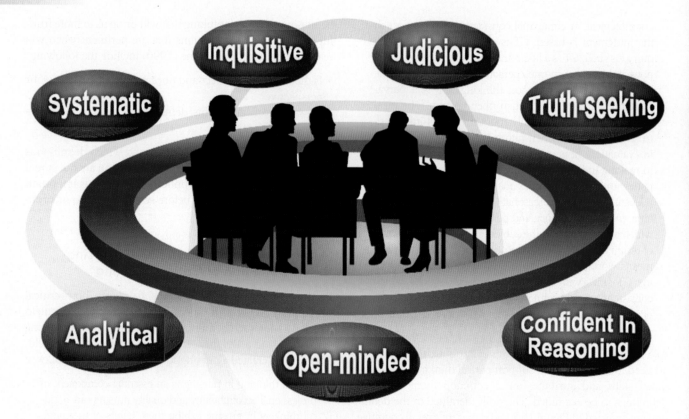

Figure 16.3 Attributes of critical thinking (Image © Insight Assessment 2010; used with permission). Facione, P. A. (2013). Critical thinking: What it is and why it counts. *Insight Assessment*. Millbrae, CA: Author.

This definition also identifies both skills and dispositions as important components of critical thinking. The link that Scheffer and Rubenfeld (2000) make between critical thinking and quality nursing care is interesting as it reflects the importance of critical thinking in quality nursing practice. This is one of a few critical thinking definitions that pertain specifically to nursing.

Alfaro-LeFevre's (2009) Definition of Critical Thinking

Another definition for nursing comes from the many scholarly works of Rosalinda Alfaro-LeFevre, who has published numerous tools and textbooks related to critical thinking in nursing. Alfaro-LeFevre (2009) describes critical thinking as a process that results in clinical judgment in nursing practice. Critical thinking and clinical judgment in nursing is purposeful, informed, outcome-focused thinking that:

- is guided by professional standards, ethics codes, and laws, carefully identifies the key problems, issues, and risks involved;
- includes patients, families, and caregivers early in the process;
- is based on principles of nursing process, problem solving, and the scientific methods;
- applies logic, intuition, and creativity and is grounded in specific knowledge skills and experience;
- is driven by patient, family, and community needs, as well as nurses' needs to give competent, efficient care;

- calls for strategies that make the most of human potential and compensates for problems created by human nature; and
- requires constantly reevaluating, self-correcting, and striving to improve (Alfaro-LeFevre, 2009, p. 7).

Other Definitions of Critical Thinking

There are several other critical thinking definitions in addition to the three provided in this chapter so far. Many authors discuss the availability of multiple definitions of critical thinking. Gordon (2000) found that nursing scholars were similar to non-nursing scholars in their definition of critical thinking. More specifically, nurse scholars agreed on the skills and dispositions found in Facione's (1990) definition with a few additions. The additional concepts nurse scholars considered part of critical thinking included problem solving, decision-making, and planning, whereas non-nurse scholars disagreed with these additions. The disagreement by some regarding the inclusion of these skills in the definition of critical thinking stems from the relationship that exists between problem-solving, decision-making, and the nursing process with critical thinking. Critical thinking may enhance these processes; however, it is not synonymous with them. There are many things that critical thinking may entail. Therefore, critical thinking may extend beyond the additions nurse educators felt defined critical thinking in Gordon's (2000) study.

Another aspect to consider when examining critical thinking is its link with creative and good thinking. Facione (2010) believed that critical thinking is not the same as good thinking. Good thinking is broader and includes other types of thinking such as creative thinking. *Creative thinking* can be defined as "thinking that leads to new insights, novel approaches, fresh perspectives, and whole new ways of understanding and conceiving things" (Facione, 2000, p. 12). Creative thinking is often visible by its results, such as artistic creations or creative innovations. The main premise behind creative thinking is that it allows individuals to see the world in new ways and to think in an unstructured way, or what some call **thinking outside of the box**. In nursing, the inclusion of creativity as a recognized disposition is different from other definitions. Therefore, in nursing, creative thinking might very well be linked to how nurses think critically and manage their environments. Although Facione (1990) described creative thinking as being different from critical thinking, these may be linked in nursing.

Seymour, Kinn, and Sutherland (2003) identified two different versions of creative thinking in nursing: one that occurs from a blank slate for the purpose of developing a creative outcome and the other as a reflective view that draws or reflects on past knowledge and experience in order to think creatively about how to deal with future situations. In both cases, creativity drives new ideas and innovative solutions.

Where does this leave our student, Chris, who wants to know more about what critical thinking means? There is no magic answer that defines critical thinking, but the answer lies within the very process of thinking critically. Thinking about what critical thinking means is an important step in deciding what critical thinking means to you in the specific context in which you find yourself. If critical thinking can be defined in one way, it defeats the very purpose of what it proposes to do (i.e., represent deep thinking).

Exploring Various Definitions of Critical Thinking

There are some similarities in how different authors define critical thinking. Those similarities (e.g., the inclusion of skills and dispositions or attributes) provide a starting point to understanding critical thinking broadly. If critical thinking is context specific, the context would need to be considered prior to choosing one critical thinking definition over another.

Comparing the Definitions

If one compares the three definitions presented in this chapter, the nursing-specific definitions of critical thinking include some of the components not present in the definition by Facione (1990). More specifically applicable and relevant to nursing settings, both Alfaro-LeFevre (2009) and Scheffer and Rubenfeld (2000) include intuition as an important component in nursing specific definitions of critical thinking. Alfaro-LeFevre (2009) included patients, families, and communities as a component of that definition, which are not included in any other definition. Another difference in the definitions provided by Facione (1990), Scheffer and Rubenfeld (2000), and Alfaro-Lefevre (2009) is the inclusion (or omission) of skills and dispositions related to critical thinking. Facione (1990) as well as Scheffer and Rubenfeld (2000) identified skills and dispositions in their definition, whereas Alfaro-Lefevre (2009) does not include any attributes as part of her definition, although she does discuss them in her various publications. One similarity among the three definitions is the inclusion of cognitive processes such as decision-making, problem identification, and problem solving.

These differences and similarities reflect the varied perceptions associated with critical thinking. Although this may be confusing, the definitions' diversity can precipitate some interesting conversations and thinking. More specifically, questions that one might ask after reading and reflecting on these critical thinking definitions are the following:

- Should critical thinking be defined in only one way to be a valuable concept?
- Do the differences among definitions preclude us from using any of the definitions in some situations?
- What underlies the differences between definitions of critical thinking?
- How do I learn to think critically thinking if there is no consensus definition?

The answers to these questions lie in the differences you perceive in the definitions and your thoughts on these questions. There is no one right answer, just as a person's use of critical thinking does not lead to finding the one right answer to a complex situation. The existence of various definitions is not specific to critical thinking. There are multiple definitions for many concepts and terms used in nursing. For example, the term *caregiver* can refer to many different individuals and differs based on the setting being referenced. In the same way, critical thinking can be viewed differently, depending on the situation to which it is being applied. Would Alfaro-LeFevre's (2009) definition be appropriate for someone who needs to create a wholesome meal and is making decisions at the grocery store as to what should be purchased to make a meal? The answer could be yes or no, depending on the individual who is doing the shopping. Therefore, the use of critical thinking is very independent and related to an individual's perception of the context. Consider the questions posed in Box 16.2.

After comparing the various definitions in this chapter, some generalizations can be made, offering an idea of what critical thinking might look like and some possible behaviours that might assist in demonstrating one's ability to think critically.

What is one's personal perspective on critical thinking? Critical thinking definitions have similarities and differences. However, they are developed by individuals or groups based on their own ideas of what critical thinking should be. This diversity displays the nature of human perception and preferences. If you like one particular definition of critical thinking, examine why you are drawn to it over another. Why do you like it? Is it the language? How do we decide which definition to use? Do we have to choose one definition over another?

Recognizing Critical Thinking at Work

If the variety of definitions is not enough to challenge someone trying to investigate what critical thinking is, what it looks is also difficult to capture. Given that critical thinking is a complex skill, this is not surprising. The interactive, curiosity triggered, and intraspective nature of critical thinking help to further distinguish what it entails.

Critical Thinking Is Interactive

Although some aspects of critical thinking can be carried out in isolation (e.g., evaluation or analysis of an idea or piece of knowledge), critical thinking is also an interactive process. More specifically, ideas, thoughts, and knowledge created by other people can be engaged through a thinking process. The interactive nature of critical thinking was supported by hooks (2010). Many components of critical thinking require the individuals' engagement with content, thought, and other people. Although being passive is usually more comfortable than deep thinking, critical thinking involves the sharing of ideas and perspectives. Thinking can be uncomfortable when it stretches our perspectives and challenges our assumptions and beliefs. Being interactive and seeking others' opinions, perspectives, and thoughts is a starting point.

What effect does **context** have on critical thinkers? Individuals interact within contexts or environments when they are thinking critically. Contexts or environments in nursing can include many different physical spaces that individuals find themselves in. These spaces are filled with many factors, both concrete and less tangible (e.g., tense environments which cause one to feel tension). The contexts or environments that individuals interact with, or are affected by, are the medium in which certain types and kinds of knowledge are created. Thought and knowledge may be deemed domain specific with some overlap between contexts. For example, nursing knowledge can be quite specific. However, some concepts are common among disciplines. Education may use some of the communication knowledge that nursing uses. Nursing also draws on some of the foundations from psychology and sociology when working with patients. Individuals may use context-specific as well as general knowledge when thinking critically. This is evident in the wide breadth of knowledge a nurse is able to draw on and demonstrate (use of concepts from pathophysiology to understand disease processes).

Critical Thinking Is Triggered by Curiosity

Critical thinking is educated thought triggered by curiosity and inquisitiveness (Paul, 1990.) Does this statement mean one has to be educated to think critically? Perhaps more importantly, a critical thinker has evidence or knowledge that supports what the individual says. Therefore, the individual has learned or is aware of the knowledge related to a particular topic and can use that knowledge to support his or her ideas. Is it accurate to assume that one who thinks critically retrieves evidence, analyzes it, and then applies it to an appropriate situation? One way to think about educated thought is to use the work of Paul (1990). He identifies **perfections of thought** as one aspect of critical thinking. These perfections of thought include goals of thinking and showcase the purposeful nature of trying to think more effectively (Paul, 1990). The perfections of thoughts identified by Paul (1990, p. 51) include:

- Clarity
- Precision
- Specificity
- Accuracy
- Relevance
- Consistency
- Logicalness
- Depth
- Completeness
- Significance
- Fairness
- Adequacy for the purpose at hand

These perfections of thought require diligent practice and can be used as standards to judge thinking in order to reach fair and just conclusions amidst a hectic and sometimes unjust world (Paul, 1990). Although they are not meant to be used as a checklist, they offer standards and goals aimed at developing one's ability to think critically.

Think   Think of someone whose thinking does *not* meet many of these standards. Possibly this individual thinks just enough for social acceptance, has some illogical ideas about how the world operates, or demonstrates that he or she only thinks about things that are potentially irrelevant to others (e.g., their own issues and circumstances).

The second aspect of Paul's (1990) statement indicates that critical thinking is triggered by curiosity and inquisitiveness. Browne and Keeley (2010) identify that a primary value of a critical thinker includes curiosity. This curiosity sparks the thinking process so that one can really think about what he has read and heard. Brookfield (1987) identified triggers in the critical thinking process as events (usually traumatic ones) that initiate questioning of one's assumptions. However, critical thinking can also be spurred by the sincere engagement with life that most critical thinkers demonstrate.

Critical Thinking Involves Self-Direction and Self-Awareness

The idea that critical thinking involves self-direction and self-awareness refers to the dispositions discussed earlier in the chapter. These dispositions are explored in some of the critical thinking definitions. Being self-aware entails being attentive to one's inner qualities such as being inquisitive or open-minded as well as having a good grasp of one's biases and values as they relate to certain situations and contexts. A critical thinker is genuinely aware of how his or her emotions affect his or her thinking. Being self-directed refers to being able to initiate thinking and actions without cues or interference from others. In addition to being self-directed and self-aware, critical thinking involves self-discipline to limit the influence of emotions and biases, thereby promoting clarity of thought and truth seeking.

Is it skepticism or cynicism? If an individual analyzes, examines, and questions in a respectful manner, then it is more appropriate to call this type of thinking **reflective skepticism**. This reflective, yet respectful, skepticism is an important aspect of critical thinking. However, **reflective thinking** can be mistaken for negative cynicism if it is perceived as disrespectful or not valuing the ideas and opinions of others. Someone who is respectful uses reflective skepticism and is aware of his or her thinking and the way others perceive his or her. This combination of self-awareness and reflective skepticism is important for critical thinking. How can you ensure the questions you ask are viewed as skeptical versus cynical?

Think Some individuals believe that those who ask many questions, examining ideas, and analyzing perspectives are cynical. Think of individuals whom you have met who question everything. How do their actions make you feel? Do you think others are being cynical when they ask lots of questions? In the clinical setting, questions from experienced nurses may make you feel like you are being scrutinized. However, questions are an important tool of communication when working in teams. Nurses need to know what care you have provided the patient. As well, your instructor will also use questions to uncover how you have completed certain nursing skills. You can also use questions to further your own learning and seek out information from peers and other health-care team members.

Critical Thinking Indicators

If we understand critical thinking to be an interactive activity where one's knowledge is evident in a self-directed and self-reflective process, the list of indicators by Alfaro-LeFevre (2009) might assist us in applying some of these to our practice. See Box 16.3 for a detailed list of these indicators.

BOX 16.3 Alfaro-LeFevre (2009) Critical Thinking Indicators

- **Self-aware**: clarifies biases, inclinations, strengths, and limitations; acknowledges when thinking may be influenced by emotions or self-interest
- **Genuine**: shows authentic self, demonstrates behaviours that indicate stated values
- **Self-disciplined**: stays on task as needed, manages time to focus on priorities
- **Healthy**: promotes a healthy lifestyle, uses healthy behaviours to manage stress
- **Careful and prudent**: knows own limits, seeks help as needed, suspends or revises judgment as indicated by new or incomplete data
- **Confident and resilient**: expresses faith in ability to reason and learn, overcomes disappointments
- **Honest and upright**: seeks the truth, even if it sheds unwanted light; upholds standards; admits flaws in thinking.
- **Curious and inquisitive**: looks for reasons, explanations, and meaning; seeks new information to broaden understanding.
- **Alert to context**: looks for changes in circumstances that warrant a need to modify thinking or approaches
- **Analytical and insightful**: identifies relationships, expresses deep understanding
- **Logical and intuitive**: draws reasonable conclusions ("if this is so, then it follows that . . . because . . . "), uses intuition as a guide to search for evidence, acts on intuition only with knowledge of risks involved
- **Open- and fair-minded**: shows tolerance for different viewpoints, questions how own viewpoints are influencing thinking

- **Sensitive to diversity**: expresses appreciation of human differences related to values, culture, personality, or learning style preferences; adapts to preferences when feasible
- **Creative**: offers alternative solutions and approaches, comes up with useful ideas
- **Realistic and practical**: admits when things aren't feasible, looks for user-friendly solutions
- **Reflective and self-corrective**: carefully considers meaning of data and interpersonal interactions, asks for feedback; corrects own thinking, alert to potential errors by self and others, finds ways to avoid future mistakes
- **Proactive**: anticipates consequences, plans ahead, and acts on opportunities
- **Courageous**: stands up for beliefs, advocates for others, don't hide from challenges
- **Patient and persistent**: waits for right moment; perseveres to achieve best results
- **Flexible**: changes approaches as needed to get the best results
- **Empathetic**: listens well, shows ability to imagine others' feelings and difficulties
- **Improvement oriented**: identifies learning needs; finds ways to overcome limitations, seeks out new knowledge
- **Patient**: promotes health; maximizes function, comfort, and convenience
- **Systems oriented**: identifies risks and problems with health-care systems; promotes safety, quality, satisfaction, and cost containment

Source: Alfaro-LeFevre, R. (2009). *Evidence-based critical thinking indicators.* Available at www.AlfaroTeachSmart .com. Used with permission. Copyright 2009.

Use the indicators created by Alfaro-LeFevre (2009) to identify which ones you think you do very well, which ones you think you do satisfactorily, and which ones you think you need to improve upon. This list will help to initiate a self-reflective process; an important step to identify what a critical thinker looks like. More importantly, this reflection will help you identify where you are in your development as a critical thinker.

 Think Does one need to exhibit all of the indicators listed in order to be a critical thinker? If one exhibits only a few indicators, are they considered to be critical thinkers? How do we decide that an individual is or isn't a critical thinker? Indicators are often not clear all-or-none principles of a specific skill such as critical thinking. Although checklists provide us with a concrete way to evaluate whether we have specific components of critical thinking, a checklist cannot fully represent the level of our critical thinking in every situation.

What Is Strong Critical Thinking?

Facione (1990), Paul (1990), and Browne and Keeley (2010) believe that identifiable traits exist in both weak and strong critical thinkers. According to Paul (1990), the difference between weak and strong critical thinking is the focus of one's activities or actions. For example, if the thinking serves only the individual, then it is considered a weak sense of critical thinking (also called *sophistic critical thinking*). If the thinking includes the "interests of diverse persons" (Paul, 1990, p. 51), then the critical thinking can be deemed to be strong sense of (or fair-minded) critical thinking. Browne and Keeley (2010) add that weak critical thinkers are "unconcerned with moving toward truth or virtue" (p. 8). As well, weak sense critical thinking is evident when one resists thinking that is incongruent with the traits of the person who is doing the thinking. Conversely, strong sense critical thinking includes asking critical questions regarding all claims, including our own beliefs and perspectives (Browne & Keeley, 2010). Another perspective comes from Facione (2010), who states that a weak critical thinker is "muddle-headed about what he or she is doing, disorganized and overly simplistic" (p. 10) and tends to settle for the status quo if a good reason is stated. Alternatively, strong critical thinkers are orderly, clear, diligent, and persistent and like to have a rationale for actions versus doing something just for the sake of conformity (Facione, 2010). Do these two descriptions provide clear explanations of excellent critical thinking in nursing? Let's read what some of your colleagues might say.

Through the eyes of a nurse

Critical thinking to me is deep thinking where I get to the answer from relevant evidence. I see critical thinking in the clinical setting as the nurse's ability to think outside the box and provide quality patient care that is specifically for that patient. Finding creative solutions to care for patients with complex problems is at the heart of critically thinking as a nurse.
(personal reflection of a nurse)

Through the eyes of a student

Critical thinking is confusing, and everyone defines it differently. I am not sure how to show that I am thinking critically except to apply my knowledge to the situation and hope my nursing instructor likes it.
(personal reflection of a nursing student)

Through the eyes of a nurse

Critical thinking is a buzzword that encompasses what it means to think as a nurse: using all of your knowledge, experience, and intuition to ensure your patients get the best care in an environment filled with so much to know and apply to one's nursing practice.
(personal reflection of a nurse)

Critical thinking is evidenced by different behaviours in different people. The individual nature of dispositions and skills, along with the setting in which critical thinking occurs, affects the appearance of this complex concept.

Is Critical Thinking Measurable?

Measuring critical thinking is another challenging endeavour. How do we know people are thinking critically—can we measure it? According to the research literature, attempts have been made to measure nursing students' and nurse educators' critical thinking. Students' critical thinking in all stages of progression in their nursing program has been documented in various studies (Adams, 1999; Brunt, 2005a). Nurse educators have been shown to have critical thinking skills and dispositions (Raymond & Profetto-McGrath, 2003). The results of various studies examining nursing students' critical thinking have been inconclusive. (Adams, 1999; Brunt, 2005a). The inconclusive results might be linked to the measurement tools used. More specifically, the measurement tools commonly used have been designed using Facione's (1990) definition. That definition was created outside nursing; therefore, the tools do not reflect the nursing context and nursing-specific components of critical thinking. The applicability of these tools to nursing has been questioned because of their non-specific content. See Table 16.1 for descriptions of the most currently used tools for measuring critical thinking. It is also possible that self-reporting assessment tools are not accurate measures of critical thinking.

Tools to Measure Critical Thinking

There are a few commonly used self-reporting tools to capture individuals' levels of critical thinking. Based on the mixed research results in the literature, it is unclear whether

TABLE 16.1	Comparisons of Three Main Critical Thinking Measurement Tools		
Assessment Tool	**What Is Being Measured?**	**Who Is This Measure Intended For?**	**Comments**
Watson-Glaser Critical Thinking Appraisal (WGCTA)	Skills of inference, recognition of assumptions, deduction, interpretation, and evaluation of arguments	General adult population and postsecondary students	80 items and takes approximately 60 minutes to complete Computer and pencil-and-paper versions
California Critical Thinking Disposition Inventory (CCTDI)	Dispositions of truth seeking, open-mindedness, analyticity, systematicity, confidence, inquisitiveness, and maturity	General adult population	75 items Likert scale and takes approximately 20 minutes to complete Computer and pencil-and-paper versions
California Critical Thinking Skills Test (CCTST)	Skills of analysis, evaluation, inference, explanation, interpretation, deductive reasoning, and inductive reasoning	Varied versions available Elementary–doctoral level education	34 items multiple choice and takes approximately 45 minutes to complete Available online.

the completion of a nursing education program positively impacts nursing students' critical thinking.

The Watson-Glaser Critical Thinking Appraisal (WGCTA) was developed by Watson and Glaser (1980) and is an 80-item self-reporting tool that participants are given 40 minutes to complete. The tool measures the critical thinking skills of inference, recognition of assumptions, deduction, interpretation, and evaluation of arguments. The California Critical Thinking Disposition Inventory (CCTDI) was created by Facione and Facione (1992) and is based on the Delphi definition of critical thinking that was part of the research commissioned by the APA. The inventory is a 75-item self-reporting tool that uses a Likert scale format and takes 20 minutes to complete. The tool measures the dispositions of truth seeking, open-mindedness, analyticity, systematicity, confidence, inquisitiveness, and maturity. The California Critical Thinking Skills Test (CCTST) is a 34-item self-reporting measurement tool that was developed by Facione (1992). Each item has four possible responses with one correct answer. The CCTST reports scores for seven subscales including: analysis, evaluation, inference, explanation, interpretation, deductive reasoning, and inductive reasoning. This test was originally developed for college-level students in various disciplines.

The Need for a Nursing-Specific Tool

Brunt (2005b) noted that the three tools listed in Table 16.1 are non-nursing specific. The literature calls for the development of a nursing-specific tool in light of the mixed results obtained from studies using these measurement tools (Adams, 1999; Brunt, 2005a). The complexity of critical thinking makes its measurement a difficult task. Not only is an individual's ability for critical thinking in a constant state of development, it also can appear different in various settings. How should your critical thinking best be measured?

There have been many studies investigating critical thinking in nursing students over the past 10 years. In one

such Canadian study, Profetto-McGrath (2003) obtained some interesting results showing the improvement of critical thinking in students when measured in all 4 years at a western Canadian nursing program. See Research box for a description of the research that was completed.

RESEARCH

THE RELATIONSHIP OF CRITICAL THINKING SKILLS AND CRITICAL THINKING DISPOSITIONS OF BACCALAUREATE NURSING STUDENTS

Study

Critical thinking is an important aspect of nursing practice. This study researched the critical thinking skills and dispositions of baccalaureate nursing students in a 4-year baccalaureate nursing program in western Canada. The CCTST and the CCTDI were the measurement tools used for this study. Participants were conveniently sampled. Out of 649 students in the baccalaureate program, 228 students across all 4 years of the program agreed to participate. The self-reporting, pencil-and-paper measurement tools were administered during regularly scheduled class time. The results from this study showed that the mean total score for the CCTST was 17.4 (standard deviation was 4.0) for all students. Year 1 students attained a mean score of 17.1; year 2, 17.7; year 3, 16.7; and year 4, 17.9. Overall, year 4 students scored relatively higher than the other 3 years. Interestingly, the year 3 students had the lowest overall mean score. There was, however, an increase from the year 1 mean score to the year 4 mean score. Despite the differences of scores between years of the program, there were no statistically significant differences found. The total mean score for the CCTDI for all 4 years was 312.3 (standard deviation was 36.4). Year 1 total mean

(continued on page 282)

THE RELATIONSHIP OF CRITICAL THINKING SKILLS AND CRITICAL THINKING DISPOSITIONS OF BACCALAUREATE NURSING STUDENTS (CONTINUED)

score was 304.2, year 2 was 315.4, year 3 was 313.5, and year 4 was 312.7. Year 2 students had the highest overall mean score for the study with year 1 having the lowest overall mean score on the CCTDI. Again, there were no statistically significant differences between the scores from the 4 years of the program. However, the correlation of nursing students' critical thinking skills and critical thinking dispositions were significantly and positively correlated (χ^2 9.37, $p = .014$, power .80). The results from this Canadian study indicate that from the sample, critical thinking skills increased from year 1 to year 4. As well, it was reported that most students (85.5% of the sample) scored 280–350 on the CCTDI indicating that they had a positive inclination to think critically. This positive inclination is an important finding as dispositions are a necessary element in the development of students' critical thinking.

Nursing Implications

Nursing students' dispositions and skills to think critically are important components to further develop their critical thinking in nursing practice. Measuring and knowing students' dispositions and skills to think critically in nursing education help educators to create quality learning experiences at various levels of baccalaureate nursing education. These results also offer a Canadian perspective on the critical thinking levels using the previously mentioned assessment tools, which will inform future research in this area. This research also emphasizes important areas that require further investigation, including students' fluctuating levels of critical thinking within their nursing program, and the need to understand which educational activities best promote critical thinking in student populations.

Profetto-McGrath, J. (2003). The relationship of critical thinking skills and dispositions among baccalaureate nursing students. *Journal of Advanced Nursing, 43(6)*, 569–577.

Why Do We Need Critical Thinking?

Critical thinking is valuable to our everyday lives and personal relationships, but it can also enhance our abilities to manage in nursing contexts and increase our contributions to a democratic society. The purposes of critical thinking can be categorized into social, economic, political, ethical, and moral aspects. Figure 16.4 represents the purposes of thinking critically.

Critical Thinking as a Tool for Personal Growth

By using critical thinking in our everyday relationships, we are better able to reflect and adjust our thinking, perceiving, and actions as the relationship grows.

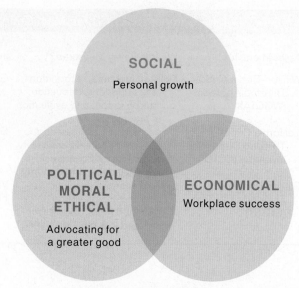

Figure 16.4 Purposes of thinking critically.

Brookfield (1987) asserts that critical thinking is an important aspect of personal relationships. Through a complex process of analyzing, understanding, being open-minded, and thinking holistically about a situation, critical thinking can assist us to navigate complex situations in relationships.

The notion that critical thinking is a constantly evolving individual process supports the belief that we are constantly developing and transforming. The more experiences we gain, the more knowledge we have to reflect on and think about. Being aware of and attuned to our own and others' perceptions and thoughts through a mutual process of understanding helps to strengthen our relationships. When we achieve a genuine mutual understanding with others, we can acknowledge the differences and/or similarities regarding our perceptions, thoughts, and ways of thinking. Think back to a situation when you experienced an issue within a personal relationship. Was this issue related to a difference in values, assumptions, and/or perceptions about a certain aspect of your relationship? Was there a difference of opinion about an incident or how a situation was handled? When we hold our opinions so tightly that we are unable to understand others' perspectives and how they feel about certain things, an emotional distance is created. Critical thinking helps to bring awareness about one's own and others' feelings and thinking. More specifically, critical thinking acts as an impetus for effective communication by fostering open and honest dialogue between people. This can be termed *intellectual empathy*, which is defined by The Critical Thinking Community (2013) as imagining putting oneself in another's place. Intellectual empathy involves authentically understanding another's perspective, thereby fostering an understanding of the reasoning or logic behind another person's actions or thought processes.

Critical Thinking as a Tool for Economic and Workplace Success

Critical thinking has been identified as an important skill for nurses to have throughout their careers (Mundy & Denham, 2008). It is instrumental for nurses to function within fast-paced health-care settings and when working with acutely ill patients or those with complex health needs in the community. By thinking through situations using analysis, interpretation, evaluation, and reflection, nurses can enhance their understanding of the complex factors that impact patients and their families. Critical thinking can be used to effectively plan and implement nursing care. It is believed that nurses' patient specific in-depth thinking can facilitate a better understanding of individual patient contexts, which should then foster better patient outcomes. Critical thinkers also engage in reflective practice to continually advance their professional skill development in areas of clinical judgment, clinical reasoning, and clinical decision-making. Additionally, nurses who are critical thinkers can question the status quo when needed. This questioning is important to make nursing care more effective, the daily routines more efficient, and the health-care system more responsive to patients and their families. Think about what nursing would be like today if nurses had not questioned how to further nursing knowledge and practice. By questioning and challenging previously held assumptions and beliefs, critical thinkers can attempt to change situations and contexts. Nurses advocate for patients and families and critically question ethical issues that arise in the process of care. Without critical thinking, nurses would not be able to navigate through the many difficult situations they face. As with personal relationships, critical thinking in nursing can enhance communication and understanding between individuals and groups.

Critical Thinking as a Tool to Advocate for the Greater Good

Humanity is defined as the "quality of being humane" (Princeton University, 2010), and as individuals, we all have the potential to be so. It can be easier to understand the benefits of using critical thinking in our professional and personal lives; however, critical thinking is also important for citizens to understand and act on political, moral, and ethical issues faced by society. We may think that the act of voting during elections completes our political responsibility. Although this is an important aspect of individual engagement within society, with the help of critical thinking, we can do more.

First, critical thinking is a purposeful tool to help us understand situations abroad, including international complexities. Brookfield (1987) agrees that critical thinking helps individuals feel connected and part of wider events and "happenings" (p. 53). Although we may not be directly impacted by a war in a far-off country, the reasons, the perspectives, and the injustices for the innocent all impact us as a human race. Despite our tendencies to be focused on our own contexts most of the time, other individuals, contexts, and realities, need to be considered. These considerations help us to avoid repeating similar mistakes and crises worldwide.

Secondly, part of critical thinking is the action that follows the thinking. Understanding that our actions and lives affect the contexts of others around the globe is an important starting point to use critical thinking to foster the greater good. Informed societies can act as a collective force and are powerful change agents of the future. Engaged and thoughtful societies acknowledge inequities of others and change their actions, individually or collectively, to help society recognize and make changes. Ford and Profetto-McGrath (1994) constructed a model where the role of critical thinking is to use knowledge to envision new possibilities. This envisioning process can bring about emancipatory results, or results that address power struggles that have created an oppressive effect on some individuals or groups. Effecting change can start with small efforts, such as buying fair trade coffee and tea at a local market, or can lead to larger organized efforts, such as Greenpeace's efforts to protest unfair environmental practices that are impacting our planet. Either way, critical thinking triggers understanding, which, in turn, can lead to actions that foster fairness, equality, and morality in the world.

Recall our scenario where Chris is confused about how to better develop her critical thinking through the educational experiences available to her in her nursing program. Understanding the various purposes of critical thinking is important to capture the breadth of the concept. Critical thinking is not only about developing the right skills to be a good nurse. It also serves to develop effective skills to better engage in society and to foster healthy and happy relationships in one's personal life. We are individuals who traverse many contexts. Within these varied contexts, critical thinking can strengthen our ability to function effectively, morally, ethically, and politically. For Chris, this means understanding that developing critical thinking in one aspect of her life may also affect other aspects. Now, it is time to apply all of this information and consider specific approaches and strategies that can develop one's critical thinking.

Developing Critical Thinking

How can individuals develop their critical thinking abilities? Critical thinking can be developed in different ways, but the two main approaches we suggest are internal and external processes.

Internal Processes

The development of critical thinking is ongoing, yet difficult to capture in simple steps. Through the practice of reflecting on your own values, assumptions, and thinking processes, critical thinking can be enhanced and understood. Reflection is at the heart of developing critical thinking. It is the activity in which individuals stop and think about events, situations, or interactions, either in the moment or after they have occurred.

Dewey (1933) defined *reflective thoughts* as "active, persistent, and careful consideration of any belief or supposed form of knowledge in the light of the grounds that support it and the further conclusions to which it tends . . . it includes a conscious and voluntary effort to establish belief upon a firm basis of evidence and rationality" (p. 9). Dewey (1933) identified that reflective thought starts with a feeling of unknowing or discomfort. This unknowing or discomfort triggers a process whereby one considers a phenomenon, situation, context, or occurrence in depth. Dewey (1933) also acknowledged the importance of the active or self-directed nature of reflective practice.

Reflecting on Values

Individuals hold values and beliefs at the core of their thought processes. Think about what values you have. See Box 16.4 for examples of values that you might hold. There may be other values that you have that are not included in the box. By examining one's values, it is possible to acknowledge and understand the framework or frame of reference from which your thinking stems. For example, if we value being kind and caring, then our thinking will likely follow these values and thus be reflected through our thinking. If we value wealth, our thinking will also be impacted by this value, possibly in a negative way that detracts from seeking the truth over making more money.

Understanding ourselves is an important element in developing critical thinking. If we are aware of our own values and the lens that we create using our thoughts and perceptions, we can better understand others' values. More specifically, if

we are aware of our own values, we can perceive when the values that others have are dissimilar to ours. By understanding when others' values are not the same as ours, the potential for an emotional reaction is lessened. Awareness of our values is a key part of critical thinking and lays the foundation for understanding the values that others hold.

Reflecting on Assumptions

Assumptions are created from our experiences throughout our lives. Have you ever assumed something was a certain way, only to find out your assumptions were wrong? Brookfield (1987) identifies assumptions as "self-evident rules about reality" (p. 44). Assumptions shape how one views the world on all levels, including personal and political. You might think some of these assumptions are individual, but other people may hold similar assumptions. An example of an assumption in one's personal life is that we should marry and have children. This assumption is not true for everyone, yet some believe that this is the way life should unfold. How one understands society and the possible influence of culture helps to determine what assumptions one may hold. In order to be self-aware and understand how one's thoughts are formed, it is necessary to be aware of one's assumptions and whether these assumptions are based in truth or reason.

One way to explore your assumptions is to ask yourself why you think and act the way you do. Think of how you got ready this morning. Why did you do it that way? At times, we believe we should get ready 15 minutes ahead of an anticipated event so that we are prepared in case of unexpected circumstances. We brush our teeth a certain way because we were taught to brush that way by our parents or dental hygienist. Are these assumptions based on truth, experience, others' advice, or our culture? Another way to elicit your assumptions is to think back to a tragic event in your life. Why was the event tragic to you and what were your thoughts about the situation? Is a particular event tragic to us because we assume certain things are not supposed to happen? There are many ways to reflect on your assumptions and related outcomes with the goal of becoming more self-aware of those rules or realities that guide your thinking about facts, events, and actions.

Reflecting on Thinking

How do individuals reflect on their own thinking? This can be difficult to do. However, thinking about your thinking is a necessary step to understand how one arrives at thoughts and conclusions. For example, thinking can be deemed to be rational and deductive based on facts and knowledge. As such, thinking is a cognitive process that uses facts to reach conclusions and solve problems. Thinking can also be creative, unconventional, and filled with emotion compared to what we call "in the box" thinking. Miller and Babcock (1996) remind us that thinking can result from outside influences that are not easily recognized. Ask yourself these questions that can initiate the reflective process about thinking: How would you describe your thinking? Are you

BOX 16.4   Common Values

Accomplishment	Creativity
Equity	Hard work
Individuality	Loyalty
Privacy	Punctuality
Speed	Tradition
Accuracy	Diversity
Excellence	Honesty
Knowledge	Money
Power	Safety
Teamwork	Unity
Challenge	Decisiveness
Fun	Innovation
Justice	Merit
Perfection	Individuality
Tolerance	Wisdom

divergent, that is, able to examine many ideas and alternatives; or are you more convergent and thus able to generate one best solution or idea? What prompts your thinking? Are there certain triggers that initiate your thinking process? Is it hard to turn your thinking off? By asking and thinking about these questions, you can become more aware of your thinking triggers, patterns, and processes.

External Processes

In addition to internal processes that assist us in identifying our values, assumptions, and thinking, there is also a need to use some external techniques to strengthen our critical thinking.

Engaging in Critical Questioning

Riddell (2007) believed that critical questioning can trigger reflection and self-directed analysis of the content or idea being questioned. Critical questions which are specific to "events, situations or people" (Riddell, 2007, p. 122) assist individuals to explore events or ideas in more depth. Brookfield (1987) stated that critical questioning is one of the most effective means of externalizing ingrained assumptions (p. 93). Brookfield (1987) also suggested that questions should be (a) specific to situations, events, or people without being general or vague; (b) move from particular to general to elicit themes; and (c) be conversational to avoid the perception of interrogation.

Think *Examples of Critical Questions*

1. Thinking about the care that patient A received, why might the nurse caring for this patient have administered an injection 30 minutes earlier than scheduled?
2. Given that medication X that was administered 30 minutes early, what might the nurse have been thinking when she gave the medication?
3. Imagine you were the nurse caring for patient A. What might have impacted your thinking about the care you gave this patient?

Asking yourself critical questions prior to providing nursing care is an important safety aspect of nursing practice. If you don't ask certain questions such as, "What will happen to patient X if Y occurs?" and "How do I know whether I am providing safe care?" you will not consider important information that will better direct your nursing care, thus making your care less effective and potentially unsafe for the patient.

Individuals can pose critical questions in order to examine what assumptions, values, and beliefs are underlying the thought process in a specific situation. Questions can be asked of others or directed internally to oneself. The benefit of questions that prompt reflection is the resulting thinking process. The outcomes of reflection can include understanding, awareness, and knowledge for future reference. For example, if it is known that unit culture and busyness can affect nurses' abilities to think, this information might prompt thinking about how being busy and rushed can affect patient care.

Writing to Develop and Communicate Thought

Writing is an important way to organize and communicate thought processes. Critical thinking can be better developed through analytical, argumentative, and reflective writing, all of which can foster systematic and higher level thought through the process of developing ideas and supporting them with credible, relevant sources. Bean (2011) added that "writing is both a process of doing critical thinking and a product that communicates the results of critical thinking" (p. 4). Writing displays the ability of the mind to actively engage in a problem with depth and comprehensiveness. As well, writing fosters "the generation of ideas and the production of one's own arguments" (Bean, 2011, p. 21).

Using Research to Inform Thinking and Action

Another way to inform one's nursing practice is to use research and engage in evidence-based practice to foster critical thinking skills and dispositions. In fact, critical thinking skills and dispositions support using research in one's practice. Profetto-McGrath, Hesketh, Lang, and Estabrooks (2003) found that the use of research was correlated with critical thinking dispositions in a sample of nurses studied. This relationship seems logical as the dispositions of being inquisitive, a truth seeker, analytical, judicious, and systematic could prompt one to use research and build arguments accordingly. Knowledge and evidence, especially that which results from research, needs to be part of the equation. To use research, an individual needs to understand the research to be applied and the context where it will be applied. Profetto-McGrath (2005) identified problem-based learning, reflective journals, role modeling, and journal clubs as effective means of developing critical thinking to support evidence-based practice in nursing.

Evidence-Based Practice

Evidence-based practice is a term heard often amongst nurses and in health-care settings. The term **evidence-based practice** arose from use in the medical field and is related to the need for care that is well supported by research findings. Evidence can be defined in various ways, including (a) support for a position or argument, (b) information to support beliefs, or (c) a basis for making inferences (Upshur, 2001). In addition, Rycroft-Malone et al. (2004) also outlined that evidence can be research, individuals' experiences from the clinical setting, and contextual information. With the variation in the definitions of evidence, it is not surprising there are many differing opinions on what constitutes the best evidence. These differences, although reflective of reality and the variation in existing views of evidence, make understanding evidence difficult. Sackett et al. (1996) stated that "evidence based medicine is the conscientious, explicit, and judicious use of current best evidence in making decisions about the care of individual patients. The practice of evidence based medicine means integrating individual clinical expertise with the best available external clinical evidence from systematic research" (p. 71). Evidence-based practice links research to practice by providing a solid base of knowledge from which care decisions can be made. Effective, efficient, and well-researched care is the goal of evidence-based practice. Evidence-based practice in nursing stems from the medical origination of evidence-based practice and emphasizes the use of research and other sources of knowledge to inform nursing practice. However, locating and using current evidence to inform the multitude of nursing actions is difficult. The challenges associated with the use of knowledge are an important research topic that will help inform the complex process of transferring knowledge into practice.

Other Sources of Evidence

Research is only one form of evidence that can be used to inform the thinking process. There are additional forms of evidence, some of which are more controversial than others. For example, think about the various websites available from which to access and obtain information. When assessing the best form of evidence to answer a nursing-based question, would information from Wikipedia or a peer-reviewed journal article be more appropriate? Depending on the information being sought, the applicability of evidence can vary. Some may consider intuition, anecdotal evidence, and personal experience to be valuable forms of knowledge.

Evaluating Sources of Evidence

Evaluating sources of evidence is another activity that fosters critical thinking skills. By actively analyzing and interpreting research, one engages in the process of critical thinking. If someone doesn't question and think about the source of the information he is accessing, who is responsible if he applies that information, which is potentially false? In nursing, applying false information (e.g., bathing in bleach is an effective way to eliminate microorganisms on the skin) could result in serious consequences for the nurse and patient. Evidence-based practice initiatives seek to explore the best possible interventions based on the most current and available research. Critical thinking exists throughout the processes of acquiring, questioning, and using research knowledge.

Reading Critically

Another skill that can foster one's critical thinking skills and dispositions is reading critically. Although we read a lot in nursing programs, the way we read is as important as what we read. Browne and Keeley (2010) identified reading critically as reacting with systematic evaluation to what one has read. Critical reading includes reading with concentration as well as thinking about and asking critical questions of the content presented. Reading, understanding the meaning behind what is written, and then questioning and analyzing

what has been read is an important process that uses and further fosters critical thinking. To read critically, an organized approach to interpreting and evaluating the prose may include reviewing the following questions:

1. What is the type of literature you are reading? Is it a fictional piece, scholarly article, research review, blog, tweet, anecdotal record, descriptive article, or news story?
2. What is the source or authorship of the literature? Is the author an expert or someone with limited experience? Is this known? What are the credentials of the author (both formal and informal)? Does the author have the authority to be stating what he or she is discussing?
3. What is the audience for the literature? Is the piece appropriately written for this audience? How did you come to find the piece?
4. What is the purpose of the literature? Is it to inform, produce controversy, spark dialogue, report objective findings, or meet objectives for a class assignment? Is the purpose obvious or covert?
5. What is the quality and structure of the literature? Is the grammar, spelling, and overall writing structure coherent and clear? Is the structure formal, a story format, informal, or random ideas? Is the reading clear and does it depict coherent thought and/or substantiated argument(s)?
6. What is the foundation for the ideas or arguments produced? Is there justification for the ideas or information presented? Is there clear evidence or rationale presented to support the prose? Can you evaluate the foundation or evidence of the piece?
7. What is your reaction to the literature? What are your thoughts and feelings when reading it?

Think Think back to the last thing you read in this chapter. Did it make sense to you? What questions arose in your mind as you read it? Was it from a credible source? Was the language understandable and appropriate? Is the information applicable to your practice and, if so, how? How was the information created, and how old is it? These are just some of the questions that you could ask yourself as you read in order to read critically. Asking questions about what you find on the Internet is an important aspect of thinking critically. The answers to these questions will foster reflection, which in turn results in a deeper understanding of what you read.

By fostering an application type mindset when reading large quantities of information, reading critically assists students to prepare for exams. Important conclusions can be drawn when you ask yourself: What does this information mean to me and my practice as a nurse? For example, by reading an article on skin care and ulcer prevention, it might be understood that turning a patient will prevent the development of pressure sores. If you were to apply this information, you would need to think about the setting and how this might be accomplished. You might ponder how frequently turning would be necessary. You could then imagine that certain situations would require more turning of patients than others where the patients were more easily mobile. If an exam question asked about how one might apply ulcer prevention principles in a long-term care setting, your thought process might lead you to an answer relating turning and skin care.

Applying Thinking to Practice

Applying knowledge in practice (and clinical) experiences can also strengthen critical thinking. Critical thinking in a nursing practice course requires learning, understanding, and application of new knowledge. Because action and doing are important aspects of critical thinking, nursing practice courses provide real situations and contexts in which to use critical thinking.

Through the eyes of a student

I seriously had no idea how to use the textbook knowledge I had gained until I stepped foot in the clinical setting. I had practiced in the labs and done the written work as well as anyone had. However, when you are face-to-face with a real live patient, there are thinking processes that engage in a way that they just can't and don't in class or lab settings.

(personal reflection of a nursing student)

Through the eyes of a nurse

*C*ritical thinking is such an important way of nursing care. It is how we think and process the vast amounts of knowledge and pieces of information that affect nursing care and the work we do. Although some can easily say they are using critical thinking, it appears so different for each person and in each context. This makes critical thinking difficult to capture but rightfully so—it is a complex process that aids in traversing complex terrain.

(personal reflection of a nurse)

Some authors have identified experience as an important component of critical thinking. According to Kataoka-Yahiro and Saylor (1994), without experience to reflect on and apply knowledge to, critical thinking can be limited. Critical thinking remains hypothetical without the ability to engage in actual decision-making and problem solving in a clinical setting. Although the experiences of asking questions and fostering understanding through discussion are important and valuable to developing certain skills and dispositions in critical thinking, the application in real time appears to solidify the reasons for which we think critically as a nurse.

Where Do We Go From Here?

What's next? We have looked at the various questions that may surround a beginning discussion of critical thinking. You will continue to hear and read about critical thinking throughout your program of study and in your practice as a nurse. There is much to learn about critical thinking; more than one chapter can cover. You may find that this chapter leads you to more questions. How will you think of critical thinking when you hear the term now? Are you a critical thinker? How do you plan to develop your critical thinking? Where do you go from here?

In our opening scenario, Chris was asking what critical thinking is and how she could develop it further. We have examined various definitions of critical thinking, presented how critical thinking might look in practice, identified the need to think critically, and have also explored how one might develop critical thinking skills and dispositions. Critical thinking is a complex concept. It does not have clear boundaries and borders that look identical in every situation. It can be hard to capture due to its constant state of development in individuals. However, without critical thinking in nursing, effective decisions, complex care modalities, and the individualized nature of nursing care would not be actualized.

Critical Thinking Exercises

Refugees

▶ During the past few years, the arrival of refugees into Canada off our western shoreline has increased in frequency. The arrival of the refugees sparks debate regarding the intent of those providing transportation to our country. Is the intent to bring refugees here to allow the spread of international terrorism, or are the boatloads of individuals legitimately here to seek safety and shelter from their homeland? Debate the pros and cons of the arrival of refugees into Canada and identify your personal stance on the issue. Reflect on the values and assumptions you have regarding this issue.

Knowledge

▶ Think about how you have come to know things in your nursing program or career. Answer the following questions about that knowledge. What is a valuable source of knowledge you trust to provide the information? Identify three sources of knowledge that have informed the choices you have made today. What values influence the knowledge you perceive as valuable? What role does knowledge play in your nursing practice and how can you ensure you are using the best possible knowledge to inform your nursing care of patients?

The Real World

▶ Take the following quote and identify the initial thoughts you have on it, the pros and cons of the quote, and the additional information you might need to understand the full meaning of the quote.

Quote: "I think nursing school doesn't prepare you for much of the real world. Who needs half the stuff you are expected to memorize in your classes?"

Multiple-Choice Questions

1. Which of the following is true regarding the definition of critical thinking?
   a. No definition exists for this complex term.
   b. A definition exists but is limiting to nursing practice.
   c. Many definitions exist; however, it is difficult to choose one.
   d. Definitions are endless, and none capture what the concept includes.

2. What are the two main and most popular components of critical thinking found in different definitions?
   a. Dispositions and skills/abilities
   b. Skills/abilities and contextual awareness
   c. Contextual awareness and dispositions
   d. Intuition and skills/abilities related to higher thinking

3. Which of the following best describes the interactive nature of critical thinking?
   a. Individuals are curious beings and need to seek out the truth.
   b. Groups work better together when one or more are critical thinkers.
   c. Relationships flourish when one or both partners are critical thinkers.
   d. Individuals interact with others and the environment as part of critical thinking.

4. Which of the following identifies the three main purposes of critical thinking?
   a. Social, economic, and political/moral/ethical
   b. Psychological, social, and ethical
   c. Psychological, ethical, and physiological
   d. Social, psychological, and political/moral/ethical

5. Which of the following is a benefit of critical questioning?
   a. Leads to more questions that further complicate the issue
   b. Engages the thinker in a process of directing their actions
   c. Triggers reflection and analysis of a given situation
   d. Offers insight into the values one holds related to a given situation

REFERENCES AND SUGGESTED READINGS

Adams, B. L. (1999). Nursing education for critical thinking: An integrative review. *Journal of Nursing Education, 38*(3), 111–119.

Alfaro-LeFevre, R. (2009). *Critical thinking indicators: Evidence-based version.* Stuart, FL: Author. Retrieved from www.AlfaroTeachSmart.com

Association of Registered Nurses of Newfoundland and Labrador. (2007). *Standards for nursing practice.* St. John's, NL: Author.

Bean, J. C. (2011). *Engaging ideas: The professor's guide to integrating writing, critical thinking, and active learning in the classroom* (2nd ed.). San Francisco, CA: Jossey-Bass.

Brookfield, S. D. (1987). *Developing critical thinkers: Challenging adults to explore alternative ways of thinking and acting.* San Francisco, CA: Jossey-Bass.

Browne, M. N., & Keeley, S. M. (2010). *Asking the right questions: A guide to critical thinking.* Upper Saddle River, NJ: Prentice Hall.

Brunt, B. A. (2005a). Critical thinking in nursing: An integrative review. *The Journal of Continuing Education in Nursing, 36*(2), 60–67.

Brunt, B. A. (2005b). Models, measurement, and strategies in developing critical thinking skills. *Journal of Continuing Education in Nursing, 36*(3), 255–262.

Canadian Association of Schools of Nursing. (2004). *CASN position statement on baccalaureate education and baccalaureate programs.* Ottawa, ON: Author.

College and Association of Registered Nurses of Alberta. (2005). *Nursing practice standards.* Edmonton, AB: Author.

The Critical Thinking Community (2009). *Our mission.* Retrieved from http://www.criticalthinking.org/pages/our-mission/405

The Critical Thinking Community (2013). *Valuable Intellectual Traits.* Retrieved from http://www.criticalthinking.org/pages/valuable-intellectual-traits/528

Dewey, J. (1933). *How we think: A restatement of the relation of reflective thinking to the educational process.* Boston, MA: Heath.

Dewey, J. (2007). *How we think.* Stilwell, KS: Digireads.

Facione, P. A. (1990). *Critical thinking: A statement of expert consensus for purposes of educational assessment and instruction. Executive summary: The Delphi report.* Millbrae, CA: California Academic Press.

Facione, P. A. (1992). *The California critical thinking skills test manual.* Millbrae, CA: California Academic Press.

Facione, P. A. (2010). *Critical thinking: What it is and why it counts.* Millbrae, CA: California Academic Press.

Facione, P. A., & Facione, N. C. (1992). *The California critical thinking disposition inventory: Test manual.* Millbrae, CA: California Academic Press.

Ford, J. S., & Profetto-McGrath, J. (1994). A model for critical thinking within the context of curriculum as praxis. *The Journal of Nursing Education, 33*(8), 341–344.

Gordon, J. M. (2000). Congruency in defining critical thinking by nurse scholars and non-nurse scholars. *Journal of Nursing Education, 39*(8), 340–351.

Hooks, B. (2010). *Teaching critical thinking: Practical wisdom.* New York, NY: Routledge.

Kataoka-Yahiro, M., & Saylor, C. (1994). A critical thinking model for nursing judgment. *The Journal of Nursing Education, 33*(8), 351–356.

Lipe, S. K., & Beasley, S. (2004). *Critical thinking in nursing: A cognitive skills workbook.* Philadelphia, PA: Lippincott Williams & Wilkins.

Miller, M. A., & Babcock, D. E. (1996). *Critical thinking applied to nursing.* St. Louis, MO: Mosby.

Mundy, K., & Denham, S. (2008). Nurse educators-still challenged by critical thinking. *Teaching and Learning in Nursing, 3,* 94–99.

Paul, R. (1990). *Critical thinking: What every person needs to survive in a rapidly changing world.* Rohnert Park, CA: Center for Critical Thinking and Moral Critique.

Princeton University (2010). "Humanity". WordNet. Princeton University. Retrieved May 29, 2010 from http://wordnet.princeton.edu

Profetto-McGrath, J. (2003). The relationship of critical thinking skills and critical thinking dispositions of baccalaureate nursing students. *Journal of Advanced Nursing, 43*(6), 569–577.

Profetto-McGrath, J. (2005). Critical thinking and evidence-based practice. *Journal of Professional Nursing, 21*(6), 264–371.

Profetto-McGrath J., Hesketh, K. L., Lang, S., & Estabrooks, C. A. (2003). A study of critical thinking and research utilization among nurses. *Western Journal of Nursing Research, 25*(3), 322–337.

Raingruber, B., & Haffer, A. (2001). *Using your head to land on your feet: A beginning nurse's guide to critical thinking.* Philadelphia, PA: F.A. Davis.

Raymond, C. L., & Profetto-McGrath, J. (2003). Nurse educators' critical thinking: Reflection and measurement. *Nurse Education in Practice, 5,* 209–217.

Riddell, T. (2007). Critical assumptions: Thinking critically about critical thinking. *The Journal of Nursing Education, 46*(3), 121–126.

Rycroft-Malone, J., Seers, K., Titchen, A., Harvey, G., Kison, A., & McCormack, B. (2004). What counts as evidence in evidence-based practice? *Nursing and Health Care Management and Policy, 47*(1), 81–90.

Sackett, D. L., Rosenberg, W. M., & Gray, J. A. (1996). Evidence based medicine: What it is and what it isn't. *British Medical Journal, 312,* 71–72.

Scheffer, B. K., & Rubenfeld, M. G. (2000). A consensus statement on critical thinking in nursing. *Journal of Nursing Education, 39*(8), 352–359.

Seymour, B., Kinn, S., & Sutherland., N. (2003). Valuing both critical and creative thinking in clinical practice: Narrowing the research-practice gap? *Journal of Advanced Nursing, 42,* 288–296.

Upshur, R. E. (2001). The status of qualitative research as evidence. In J. M. Morse, J. M. Swanson, & A. J. Kuzel (Eds.), *The nature of qualitative evidence* (pp. 5–26). Thousand Oaks, CA: Sage.

Watson, G., & Glaser, E. M. (1980). *Watson-Glaser critical thinking appraisal manual.* Cleveland, OH: Psychological.

Transforming Nursing Education Using Simulation

COLETTE FOISY-DOLL, LEANNE J. WYROSTOK, AND JUDY A. K. BORNAIS

Megan is a first-year nursing student who just learned that she will be participating in a clinical simulation experience next week as part of her nursing fundamentals course. She is both excited and nervous and wonders what simulation will be like and how she can best prepare for it. She has heard from others that simulation can be stressful but fun and that cameras are sometimes used to record group and individual performances. Her instructor has sent the students online resource materials to review prior to attending the clinical scenario. Megan is aware that the scenario will require that she apply knowledge and skill she has acquired by attending class and completing assigned readings and nursing skills practice. In addition, all students will be asked to write a short reflective journal on how they prepared for this first simulation experience. Megan begins by preparing and reflecting on the reasons why she feels anxious. She identifies that she is concerned about the possibility of performing poorly in front of her peers. She worries about her lack of familiarity with the simulation process and equipment in the room and reluctantly offers that she lacks confidence in her abilities. In addition, Megan is uncomfortable with the idea of seeing herself on camera. To prepare for her first simulation event, Megan has referred to course learning objectives and a list of required preparatory activities. She will review a simulation orientation video and information package prepared by faculty, complete assigned readings and video reviews on related content and skills, and answer preparatory reflection questions in advance of simulation event day. In doing so, she understands that she will optimize learning outcomes for both herself and her peer group.

CHAPTER OBJECTIVES

By the end of this chapter, you will be able to:

1. Define simulation-based learning and identify the associated methods and tools used to develop and create simulated clinical experiences and clinical scenarios.
2. Describe the present context of simulation and the major changes that have occurred in health care and education that have influenced the growth in simulation-based learning.
3. Discuss the advantages and disadvantages of simulation in health-care education.
4. Identify the challenges of incorporating simulation technologies into health-care education.
5. Describe the roles of the student and teacher in simulation-based learning.
6. Explain the importance and relevance of the presimulation, intrasimulation, and postsimulation phases.

KEY TERMS

Clinical Scenario The plan of an expected and potential course of events for a simulated clinical experience. The clinical scenario provides the context for the simulation and can vary in length and complexity, depending on the objectives. The scenario design includes: participant preparation, briefing, patient information, and participant objectives (Meakim, Boese, Decker, Franklin, Gloe, Lioce, Sando, & Borum. 2013).

Computer-Based Simulation The use of computer-assisted or web-based platforms for learning. The student may be a passive (computer animation) or an active (decision choices) participant. Also referred to as *screen-based simulation*.

Cueing Information provided that helps the participant progress through the clinical scenario to achieve stated objectives (National League for Nursing Simulation Innovation Resource Center [NLN-SIRC], 2013).

Debriefing   An activity that follows a simulation experience and is led by a facilitator. Participants' reflective thinking is encouraged, and feedback is provided regarding the participants' performance while various aspects of the completed simulation are discussed. Participants are encouraged to explore emotions and question, reflect, and provide feedback to one another. The purpose of debriefing is to move toward assimilation and accommodation to transfer learning to future situations (Meakim et al., 2013).

Facilitator   An individual who provides guidance, support, and structure during simulation-based learning experiences (Meakim et al., 2013).

Feedback   Information given or dialogue between participants, facilitator, simulator, or peer with the intention of improving the understanding of concepts or aspects or performance (Meakim et al., 2013).

Fidelity   Believability, or the degree to which a simulated clinical experience approaches reality; as fidelity increases, realism increases. The level of fidelity is determined by the environment, the tools and resources used, an many factors associated with the participants. Fidelity can involve a variety of dimensions, including a) physical factors such as equipment, and related tools; b) psychological factors such as emotions, beliefs, and self-awareness; c) social factors such as participant and instructor motivation and goals; d) culture of the group; and e) degree of openness and trust, as well as participants' modes of thinking (Meakim et al., 2013).

High Fidelity   Experiences using full-body, computerized human patient simulators, virtual reality, or standardized patients that provide a high level of interactivity and realism for the student (NLN-SIRC, 2013).

Human Patient Simulators (HPS)   Lifelike manikins equipped with computer software that is accessed via an externally connected communicating/controlling device, such as a laptop, personal digital assistant (PDA), or even a telephone. The HPS populates practice laboratories as well as on- or off-site training areas to mimic patients in various health-care settings. HPS offer a high level of interactivity with the student.

Hybrid Simulation   The concurrent use of two or more simulation modalities to enhance realism. Such as, with the use of standardized patients in conjunction with simulation technology to enhance the realism of a clinical scenario and foster participant learning outcomes.

Low Fidelity   Experiences incorporating case studies, role-playing, the use of partial task trainers, models, or static manikins to immerse students in a clinical situation or practice a specific skill (NLN-SIRC, 2013).

Manikin   Full or partial body representation of a patient for learning purposes.

Moderate (Midlevel) Fidelity   Experiences that are more technologically sophisticated, such as computer-based, self-directed learning systems simulations in which the participant relies on a two-dimensional focused experience to problem-solve, perform a skill, and make decisions or the use of more realistic manikins having breath sounds, heart sounds, and/or pulses (also called *intermediate fidelity*; NLN-SIRC, 2013).

Moulage   Techniques used to simulate injury, disease, aging, and other physical characteristics specific to a scenario. Moulage supports the sensory perceptions of the participants and supports the fidelity of the simulation scenario through the use of makeup, attachable artifacts, (e.g. penetrating objects), and smells (Meakim et al., 2013).

Pedagogy   The art and science of instructional methods. The study of teaching methods, including goals of education and the ways those goals can be achieved (Meakim et al., 2013).

Prebrief   An information session held prior to the start of a simulation activity in which instructions or preparatory information about the clinical situation are given and/or received and questions are addressed. Orientation to the equipment, environment, manikin, roles, and time allotment are also provided (also called *Prebriefing*.).

Problem Solving   Refers to the process of selectively attending to information in the patient care setting, using existing knowledge and collecting pertinent data to formulate a solution. This complex process requires different cognitive processes, including methods of reasoning and strategizing, in order to manage a situation (Meakim et al., 2013).

Prompt   A cue given to a participant in a scenario (Meakim et al., 2013).

Psychomotor Skills   The ability to carry out physical movements efficiently and effectively, with speed and accuracy. Psychomotor skill is more than the ability to perform; it includes the ability to perform proficiently, smoothly, and consistently under varying conditions and within appropriate time limits (Meakim et al., 2013).

Reflective Thinking   The engagement of self-monitoring that occurs during or after a simulation experience. Considered an essential component of experiential learning, it promotes the discovery of new knowledge with the intent of applying this knowledge to future situations. Reflective thinking is necessary for metacognitive skill acquisition and clinical judgment and has the potential to decrease the gap between theory and practice. Reflection requires the creativity and conscious self-evaluation to deal with unique patient situations (Meakim et al., 2013).

Role   A responsibility or character assumed in a simulation-based learning activity (Meakim et al., 2013).

Simulated Clinical Experience/Encounter (SCE)   The process where participants use their assessment, psychomotor, critical thinking, and/or problem-solving skills during the pre-, intra-, and postsimulation phases of a replicated clinical situation.

Simulation   A pedagogy using one or more typologies to promote, improve, or validate a participant's progression from novice to expert (Meakim et al., 2013).

Simulation-based Learning Experience   An array of structured activities that represent actual or potential situations in education and practice and allow participants to develop or enhance knowledge, skills, and attitudes or analyze and respond to realistic situations in a simulated environment or through an unfolding case study (Meakim et al., 2013).

Simulator   An environment, manikin, device, computer program, or system that recreates essential elements and cues to encourage experiential learning in conjunction with specific educational objectives.

Standardized/Simulated Patient   An individual who is trained to portray a patient with a specific condition in a realistic, standardized, and repeatable way (Association of Standardized Patient Educators [ASPE, 2011]).

Simulation in Nursing Education

Simulation (health care) education is a powerful experiential learning process that can involve patient actors, computer-based virtual platforms, the use of human patient simulators, and task training devices. Additionally, simulation education is characterized by the emergence of associated teaching and learning methods that are grounded in reflective learning processes for the student.

Although many may think of simulation as a new concept, the techniques have been around for many decades, if not centuries. Most people have probably experienced simulation very early in life. For example, when a child pretends to be a schoolteacher, firefighter, or rescue hero, he or she acts the part and takes on the various facets of these roles. This depiction of role-play is a rudimentary form of simulation.

This chapter will focus on the evolution of simulation as a revolutionary **pedagogy**: as an art and science that is challenging traditional teaching and learning approaches and, in doing so, is transforming the face of nursing education.

The Evolution of Simulation in Health Care

Very early principles of simulation can be traced back to the work of Herophilus, one of the early anatomists, in approximately 300 BC (Schiavenato, 2009; Wiltse & Pait, 1998). Most writers identify the inception of modern simulation as dating back to the 1930s when the army used link trainers for flight simulation (Harder, 2009; Scherer, Bruce, Graves, & Erdley, 2003). For decades, simulation has been used in aviation and nuclear power industries to allow risk-free practice and to teach, train, and/or evaluate critical thinking skills (Haskvitz & Koop, 2004; Issenberg et al., 1999; Satish & Krishnamurthy, 2008). Simulation in health care drew heavily on the success and principles involved in simulation training and teaching from both of these industries. Reports from the 1920s identify nurses participating in basic simulation as they practiced giving injections into oranges. Modern health-care simulation tends to identify its origin in the 1960s with the development of human patient simulators (Grenvik & Schaefer, 2004). Most students are familiar with **low-fidelity** simulators such as Resusci-Anne **manikins** that are used in the training of cardiopulmonary resuscitation (CPR). Generally, a **simulator** can be defined as an environment, manikin, device, computer program, or system that recreates essential elements and cues to encourage experiential learning (Fig. 17.1). One of the first reported simulation manikins in nursing was "Mrs. Chase," a life-sized, hard, plastic human model that was first used in the classroom in 1911. The idea of the Mrs. Chase manikin was first conceived by the principal of a hospital-based nursing school that wanted to offer students a means by which they could better transition theory into practice. By the 1950s, Mrs. Chase was being used extensively in nursing programs

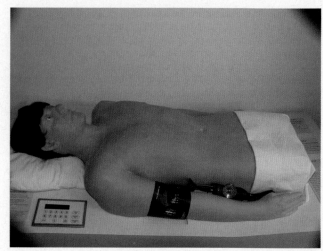

Figure 17.1 Harvey simulator. (Photo courtesy of David P. Bornais)

for clinical nursing skills practice (Hiestand, 2000; Seropian, Brown, Gavilanes, & Driggers, 2004).

In the 1960s, patient simulators expanded to include more realistic features, the ability to move, and animated sounds. Early simulators included "Harvey," a cardiopulmonary simulator conceived in 1967. The 1960s also brought *Resusci-Anne*, a resuscitation tool, and *Sim One*, the first computer-controlled simulator that was used for anesthesiology training (Schiavenato, 2009). In the past 10 years, significant strides in the development of simulation technologies have given rise to the **high-fidelity** human patient simulator: a complex, realistic, computer-driven manikin that is designed using physiological modeling. Over the past 10 years, nursing education programs have experienced a distinct shift toward nursing curricula that emphasize active learning (Gates, Parr, & Hughen, 2012; Jeffries, 2007). In current health-care education and clinical practice contexts, simulation-based learning is now widely accepted as an effective method for the teaching and learning of professional competencies, including leadership and interprofessional teamwork (Conrad, Guhde, Brown, Chronister, & Ross-Alaolmolki, 2011; Dillon, Noble, & Kaplan, 2009; Kyle & Bosseau-Murray, 2008; Lapkin, Levett-Jones, Bellchambers, & Fernandez, 2010; Norman, 2012). When underpinned with best practices in education and correctly executed, simulation-based education enables a "student-centered approach in which students . . . solve problems and think critically" (Jeffries, 2010, as cited in Institute of Medicine [IOM], 2000, p. 20; Laschinger et al., 2008). In simulation, students are given an opportunity to realize their potential in a low-risk, experiential learning environment that permits observation and experimentation of new behaviours prior to engaging in *real* clinical practice situations. Moreover, clinical simulations can foster building relational and teamwork competencies required for effective interprofessional collaborative practice (Dillon et al., 2009). Many health-care education institutions around the world have embraced simulation-based learning, resulting in a significant rise in the number of simulation programs and centres. In fact, Bremner, Aduddell, Bennett, and VanGeest (2006) have described the inclusion of high-fidelity simulation as "one of the most important issues in nursing education today" (p. 170).

Simulation Strategies

Simulation-based learning often employs interactive, computerized manikins that mimic human physiology and that are realistic and engaging. **Simulation-based learning experiences**, therefore, involve "an array of structured activities that represent actual or potential situations in education and practice and allow participants to develop or enhance knowledge, skills, and attitudes or analyze and respond to realistic situations in a simulated environment or through an unfolding case study" (Meakim et al., 2013, p. S9). They require that students employ active rather than passive learning and provide them with immediate physiological feedback. **Feedback** is considered one-way communication provided to a participant from an instructor, simulator, or other participants regarding understanding of concepts or performance of skills. Dunn (2010), medical director of the Multidisciplinary Simulation Center of the Mayo Clinic, asserted that the traditional system of passive educational experiences in the form of lectures to seated audiences is no longer justifiable. He stated that simulation-based technologies might qualify as a "mechanism for transformational improvement" in continuing health-care education (Dunn, 2010). Similarly, Tanner (2006), a distinguished nurse scholar and author, stated that the clinical nursing education models of the past 40 years are no longer relevant. The development of new approaches to clinical education that integrate simulation is necessary to effect radical transformation (Benner, Sutphen, Leonard, Day, & Shulman, 2009).

Simulation activities can be designed to meet either group or individual learning objectives. Based on the identified learning objectives, the appropriate educational resources are then chosen. Simulation is particularly useful for students in the

integration of knowledge and skill. Students in simulation are provided opportunities to demonstrate skill performance, prioritization of care, and time management in a realistic and lifelike situation. Learning encounters in highly contextualized environments are, therefore, designed to allow the student to manipulate learned concepts and to repeat skills without undue stress until proficiency is achieved. In this controlled simulated environment, the focus is on the students and the teachable moments of a **clinical scenario**, often simply referred to as *scenario*. The scenario comprises the expected and/or potential course of events for a simulated experience. The scenario provides the context for the simulated experience and varies in length and complexity depending on the objectives (Issenberg, McGaghie, Petrusa, Gordon, & Scalese, 2005; Meakim et al., 2013). The educator has the flexibility to introduce or lessen contextual elements and alter the pace of the scenario depending on the individualized needs of the student and the desired learning outcomes.

Megan, our questioning nursing student, wonders why simulation is becoming more prevalent in nursing educational settings.

Present Context

The current interest in simulation accompanies three major changes occurring in health care and education. Firstly, cost containment issues in health care settings have resulted in the decreased availability of suitable clinical learning sites, with fewer skilled supervisors available to mentor students. Secondly, technological advances requiring an enhanced skill set by healthcare providers, combined with increasing patient acuity, result in a greater demand for a well-equipped workforce. This is a major driver for change. Thirdly, in light of the risk-laden, health-care environment and increases in untoward patient events, the traditional educational practice of using real patients for learning is being met with increased scrutiny (Frank & Brien, 2008). The U.S. Institute of Medicine's (IOM, 2000) seminal report, *To Err is Human: Building a Safer Health System*, and subsequent Canadian Patient Safety Institute (CPSI, 2008) reporting on errors in Canadian health-care systems have brought to light the critical need for sweeping changes to current health-care educational models for harm reduction and prevention.

The CPSI is a national body that provides leadership and coordination for health-care institutions and professionals. This organization is working toward building a culture of patient safety and quality improvement throughout the Canadian health-care system. Aligned with CPSI Safety Competencies Framework recommendations, today's health disciplines in postsecondary institutions share a common educational vision to address patient safety (Frank & Brien, 2008). The current educational trend of incorporating critical thinking into educational programs has also been identified as an impetus for developing new, effective teaching strategies in nursing education (Vandrey & Whitman, 2001). These teaching strategies assist students to better integrate knowledge into nursing practice.

The inculcation of nursing values involves a process that supports students in the acquisition of nursing knowledge, technical skills, and relational and reflective practice abilities as essential components of nursing education. To that end, simulation-based learning has been cited as an excellent teaching strategy for the learning of nursing competencies (Benner et al., 2009; Jeffries, 2007). The Canadian Association of Schools of Nursing (CASN) concluded that simulated clinical learning offers "significant advantages over traditional educational methods. Benefits include the provision of a safe environment for both patient and student during training in high risk procedures. . . . " (CASN, 2007, p. 2).

Internal stakeholders such as nursing regulatory bodies, professional associations, nurse educators, practicing nurses, and even nursing students have called for enhanced graduate competencies across all levels of nursing education in order to meet the growing demands in health care. Collectively, these stakeholder positions underscore the need for transformation of nursing curricula and significant advancements in nursing education (Benner et al., 2009; Canadian Nurses Association [CNA], 2010). External stakeholders such as other health disciplines, patient safety groups, and nongovernment organizations also recognize the vital roles of nurses where all stakeholders, including the recipients of health care, stand to benefit from better-prepared nurses. Institutional administrators and nurse educators are thereby commissioned with the task of providing educational programs that prepare graduate nurses for increasingly diverse and complex professional practice roles.

A growing number of schools of nursing are expanding their simulation programs to include interprofessional participants, so that students from nursing, medicine, pharmacy, respiratory therapy, prehospital care, social work, and other disciplines learn and practice together in teams. Simulation exists not only in undergraduate nursing programs but also in postgraduate nurse practitioner programs, critical care certifications, and continuing education programs. Nursing students engage in simulation within small groups, in classrooms, and in nursing labs (Fig. 17.2). Students who participate in simulation in undergraduate nursing programs gain important experience that will serve them well in their future practice. For example, simulation strategies are being used in hospitals for new employee orientations, skills certification, team training, and other ongoing professional development activities. The opportunities for simulation experiences are as extensive as the types of simulation available. See "Through the Eyes of a Student" for student comments illustrating how simulation has been woven into their nursing education programs.

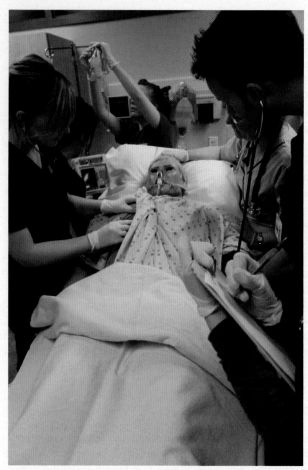

Figure 17.2 A typical group size for a simulation experience. (Photo courtesy of The Faculty of Nursing, University of Calgary)

Through the eyes of a student

*T*he high-fidelity simulators are used in every year of our nursing program. The scenarios are just like real-life cases, and you have the chance to be the nurse and handle the scenario that you are given.

(personal reflection of Matthew, a fourth-year nursing student)

Simulation and Simulation Modalities

In order to fully appreciate the importance of simulation in nursing education, it is essential to understand the distinction between the terms *simulator* and *simulation*. Very simply stated, a simulator (the tool) can be used when creating a simulation (the learning event).

Simulation is commonly defined as a way to imitate or pretend. When applied to nursing, simulation has been further defined as "a pedagogy using one or more typologies to promote, improve, or validate a participant's progression from novice to expert" (Meakim et al., 2013, p. S9).

Many individuals erroneously think of simulation in terms of the *human patient simulator*; however, the stand-alone simulator

Through the eyes of a student

I found the heart/lung simulator really helpful to learn and recognize different respiratory and heart sounds. Practicing on this simulator made a big difference in my confidence when I listened to the real thing on patients.

(personal reflection of Angela, a first-year nursing student)

is only one of many tools that may be used to create simulated learning events. Students and practicing nurses can actively engage in learning events involving assessment, clinical decision-making, planning, implementing, and evaluation. The simulation is the *entire learning process* that aims to replicate clinical reality for learning. As previously stated, simulation is a recognized, pedagogical approach where students interact with various techniques, tools, or devices. These common approaches used to simulate clinical reality in health care are clustered into broader categories better known as *simulation modalities*. Simulation modalities type or classify a simulation activity or tool. Simulation literature identifies core simulation modalities as the use of **standardized/simulated patients**, virtual reality, and **computer-based simulation** platforms and the use of low-, moderate-, and high-fidelity patient simulators (Bushell & Gaba, 2007; CPSI, 2008; Ellaway, Kneebone, Lachapelle, & Topps, 2009). Students participate in learning events using one or a blend of these modalities (otherwise known as **hybrid simulation**) that come to life in **simulated clinical experiences/encounters (SCEs)**.

Standardized Patients

According to the Association of Standardized Patient Educators (ASPE), "a standardized or simulated patient (SP) is an individual (sometimes a paid actor) who is trained to portray a patient with a specific condition in a realistic, standardized and repeatable way" (ASPE, 2011, para. 1). The use of SPs supports the assimilation and integration of theoretical knowledge to practice where educators and SPs are "co-creators of an imaginary world that needs to feel, smell, sound, and look as if it were in the real world of an actual patient being seen and treated by a real [health-care provider]" (Wallace, 2007, p. 5). Therefore, when an SP portrays an actual patient, a clinical reality unfolds. The encounter challenges the student to think critically and problem-solve when performing activities such as a health history and conducting assessments. SPs bring a face-to-face human interaction into a controlled, safe learning environment.

Computer-Based Simulation

Screen-based simulation uses computer-assisted or web-based platforms that provide students with a wide variety of educational opportunities (Brindley, Suen, & Drummond, 2007). For example, students can view computer animations that help explain human physiology or assessment. One program allows participants to observe the flow of blood through the heart while listening to the heart sounds that are produced during the contraction and relaxation of the ventricles. Other screen-based computer simulations allow students to assess a health-care situation and make clinical decisions. Students are then given computer-generated feedback on their decisions while simultaneously observing the results of their actions on the screen. Screen-based technology has now evolved to include immersive simulation environments that project three-dimensional (3D) images. Using this dynamic, highly interactive approach, the student dons special eyewear that allows them to view and manipulate 3D images that appear suspended before them in midair (Alverson, Caudell,

& Goldsmith, 2008). Screen-based computer technologies are scalable and fall on a continuum ranging from small individual 3D computer stations to IMAX sized lecture halls. Currently, 3D anatomy programs are being widely used in nursing education.

Virtual Reality Simulation

Key concepts taught in nursing education can be integrated into a multitude of virtual reality simulation learning platforms that replicate real-world experiences using computer-based programs. Many of today's students are fluent in virtual reality simulation and the use of social network platforms such as computer gaming and communal virtual learning spaces. These platforms provide a balance of experiential learning for individuals and groups and a forum for student and educator interface. Students find themselves in a virtual learning space where they can participate in codesigning their learning experiences (Hetzel-Campbell & Daley, 2009; Prensky, 2007; Skiba, 2007).

Advancing technology has given rise to a wide variety of interactive learning platforms; the most sophisticated of which can sense human movement, pressure, and touch and allow for human to computer live interfacing (Fig. 17.3). One such example is a computer-based, virtual intravenous (IV) training haptic system. While students physically manipulate the haptic device, the computer program interprets their movements and provides them with sensory cues such as a realistic

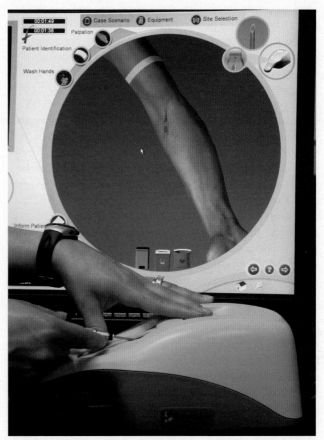

Figure 17.3 A virtual reality IV simulator. Students can palpate and feel for a vein and then insert the IV cannula. The touch pad and computer recognize and register the depth of the needle and insertion technique. (Photo courtesy of David P. Bornais)

vein pop as the needle enters the vein. A **cue** or **prompt** is information that helps the participant progress through the scenario. The haptic program monitors the student's choice of equipment, the order of the procedure, and timing of its use, all the while detecting the needle angle and accuracy of the user's insertion technique. Immediate, on-screen visual feedback such as swelling or bleeding helps to prepare students for real-life experiences. The use of computerized technology in virtual reality readily supports student practice and assists in the refinement of advanced procedural skills such as pelvic and rectal exams, cardiac catheterizations, bronchoscopies, and colonoscopies among others (Gaba & Raemer, 2007).

Other virtual reality learning platforms include computer-based programs featuring virtual patients that are modeled on human behaviours through the use of artificial intelligence and voice recognition technologies. Predetermined pathways of typical responses are built into computer programs and produce an endless array of realistic, timely verbal patient responses. This high-tech approach, therefore, enables the virtual person to produce real-time spontaneous verbal interaction in discussion with students. It is now feasible for an SP interview and assessment to occur with a virtual SP in the virtual world.

Specialty Environments

Imaging science technologies are increasingly influencing educational environments in health care to include *distributable simulation environments* that are accessible to individuals and teams who may be separated by distance (Alverson et al., 2008). Transdisciplinary teams composed of engineers, computer scientists, graphic and sound artists, information technology (IT) and network specialists, and educators have collaborated to create amazing virtual learning innovations. In specialized environments called *Cave Automatic Virtual Environments* (CAVEs), students can interact with 3D images by dissecting, rotating and manipulating, and moving them. The CAVE is a theatre room that creates immersive environments through the use of multiple high-resolution projection screens and cameras. A student who is immersed in the photo-realistic environment experiences the perception of actually being in that setting. The student wears an interactive human tracking device and a handheld wand that permits complete immersion and interaction with the images on the screen. In that space, the student can experience limitless movement in any direction, and sensory elements such as sounds, smells, temperatures, and sensations can be injected to heighten the sense of realism.

Multiuser virtual social spaces such as Second Life are increasingly being adopted for use in health-care and nursing education. Educators have the ability to create endless contextual realities including entire university campuses, hospitals, classrooms, and even simulation labs using these programs. In Second Life®, all participants create avatars (a virtual representation of themselves in the virtual world) that enter virtual worlds where they can engage in active learning in either asynchronous (independent) sessions or synchronous learning with other student avatars in groups (Skiba, 2007). One Second Life site has built an entire simulation centre that even includes debriefing rooms: rooms designated for active reflection and discussion where students can debrief as avatars online after participating in a virtual clinical scenario.

Think You are a nursing student, and your teacher has announced that you will be using Second Life simulation in one of your courses. In Second Life, you will build your avatar, a virtual representation of yourself as a student nurse, and enter a simulation lab to participate in patient care scenarios. Students find this as an exciting and enticing way to learn, but the downside is that it necessitates learning and developing proficiency with an additional layer of technology. What resources do you have available to you in your institution that could assist you in quickly adapting to this new learning environment? Can you describe how this social network platform might be helpful to you in your nursing education? Is it possible to learn serious concepts using gaming and other virtual platforms? What are the ethical implications, if any, to using these approaches?

Levels of Simulator Fidelity

Fidelity in simulation is defined as the "level of believability, or the degree to which a simulated clinical experience approaches reality; as fidelity increases, realism increases. The level of fidelity is determined by the environment, the tools and resources used, and many factors associated with the participants. Fidelity can involve a variety of dimensions, including a) physical factors such as equipment, and related tools; b) psychological factors such as emotions, beliefs, and self-awareness; c) social factors such as participant and instructor motivation and goals; d) culture of the group; and e) degree of openness and trust, as well as participants' modes of thinking" (Meakim et al., 2013). Others have defined fidelity as the extent to which a real event or skill can be recreated for learning (Waldner & Olson, 2007). The following section identifies low-, moderate-, and high-fidelity simulators and their applications.

Low-Fidelity Simulators

Low-fidelity simulators provide the opportunity for students to focus on the rote performance of particular **psychomotor skills**. Static manikins, homemade devices, and partial task trainers such as IV insertion arms, central venous line chest models, and a catheterization pelvis are tools commonly associated with low-fidelity simulation (Fig. 17.4).

Because low-fidelity tools are less complex, they are particularly useful for novice students who require repetitive practice to strengthen skills such as dexterity with instruments, time efficiency, organization of supplies, and fluidity of movement. Students work at developing mastery with various components of a basic psychomotor skill so that when challenged by more complex care situations, they are better able to perform. Although low-fidelity tools lack realism and detail and are rarely animated or integrated with computers (Hyland & Hawkins, 2009), they also tend to be less expensive, require less maintenance, offer limited or no interaction with the learner, and are more portable.

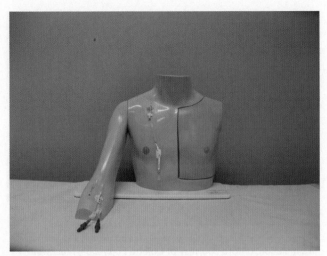

Figure 17.4 Low-fidelity central line task trainer. (Photo courtesy of David P. Bornais)

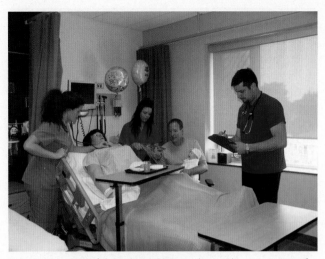

Figure 17.6 High-fidelity METI ECS simulator (Photo courtesy of Judy A. K. Bornais)

Moderate-Fidelity Simulators

Moderate (Midlevel) fidelity (also called *medium fidelity*) simulators provide more realism than their low-fidelity counterparts; with minimal programming and operational needs, responses from the simulator can heighten the level of interactivity with the student. An example of a moderate-fidelity simulator would be a chest auscultation model that has audible breath sounds, heart sounds, and a palpable apex (Fig. 17.5; Seropian et al., 2004; Waldner & Olson, 2007).

High-Fidelity Patient Simulators

High-fidelity simulators, also commonly referred to as **human patient simulators (HPS)**, offer the most technologically advanced form of realism with a sophisticated level of interactivity (Fig. 17.6). In order to heighten the perception of reality and suspend any disbelief in the student, simulation activities attempt to replicate all elements of a clinical situation including believable props, personnel, and interactions (Seropian, 2003). Full-scale (sometimes referred to as *full-mission*) simulation attempts to replicate complex learning events using real places and real people. An example is a mass-casualty scene that takes place outdoors using real ambulances complete with props, makeup, emergency response teams, nurses, and bystanders. There are many applications for the use of high-fidelity simulators; often, full-scale simulations are orchestrated with the use of high-fidelity simulators.

High-fidelity simulators are computer-generated manikins capable of realistic physiological and verbal responses. These simulators may be programmed to allow students to experience a wide range of clinical conditions and observe the outcomes of their interventions and clinical decisions (Nehring & Lashley, 2004). An SCE can be standardized and enacted by multiple students, which enhances consistency in education and evaluation (Ravert, 2002). However, this advanced technology comes with a hefty price tag with costs that can range from $35,000 to $250,000 Canadian dollars (CDN) per simulator.

Through the eyes of a student

*E*ach year during clinical practicums, students from the nursing faculty are put into real-world situations where people's lives are at stake. For a student, this creates much anxiety. What's great about the simulation lab is that it helps relieve this anxiety by showing you what areas of your practice need improvement. It also gives students a chance to understand what a nurse's real responsibilities entail. All too often, students walk into a care situation with the idea that someone else is going to lead the way. In the simulation lab, we learn that we are at the front line of health care and must be leaders. In order to do this, we must practice our skills in this lab so that we can provide the best care possible in the real world.

(personal reflection of Russell, a third-year nursing student)

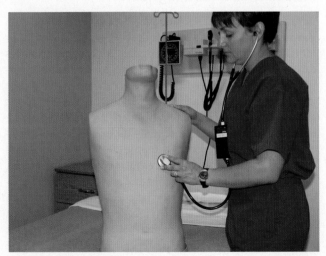

Figure 17.5 Moderate-fidelity heart and lung simulator. (Photo courtesy of David P. Bornais)

Advantages of Simulation

There are many reasons to incorporate simulation technology into current health education programs. A major advantage is that simulation fosters the students' ability to apply their knowledge; gain and improve skills; and formulate best-practice clinical decisions in a controlled, safe, and realistic environment without risk to actual patients. Having an opportunity following the simulation event to review and analyze decisions and actions (or lack of action) is essential to further learning. Although not a replacement for actual clinical experiences with real patients, simulation provides a meaningful bridge between theory and practice (Rauen, 2004).

Student Preparedness

A major advantage to simulation is its potential to improve students' preparedness and comfort in managing real medical emergencies they may confront in clinical practice, without the potential of an adverse consequence to a human being (Feingold, Calaluce, & Kallen, 2004). Students can be exposed to complex clinical situations that are low in frequency and high in acuity. For example, all students in a nursing program may not have exposure to a patient experiencing an acute myocardial infarction during a clinical practicum nor would they likely be the first provider assigned to carry out initial assessments or interventions during an actual event. In fact, in the hospital setting, the student would most often be relegated to an observational role. However, through the use of simulation, it is quite feasible for every student to have the opportunity to manage the immediate needs of the patient in cardiac crisis (Fig. 17.7).

Through the eyes of a student

In clinical, we had a patient come in that was experiencing an acute MI (heart attack) and I felt like I knew exactly what was going on and felt like I knew exactly what to do. Because of the sim lab and class, I was able to assist in caring for the patient, who actually had a very favorable outcome. It seemed to me like a pretty textbook case because I have become so familiar with MI through lecture and the application of lecture in the sim lab. Actually, the "real-life" MI was almost exactly the same as the clinical scenario. I had numerous compliments from the staff in the ER and was even recommended for preceptorship there. I wouldn't have been able to perform the way I did without the faculty's help.

(personal reflection of Ryan, a third-year nursing student)

Students are set up to "think on their feet, not in their seat" (Rauen, 2004, p. 46). They engage in a process that supports and guides them in all aspects of patient care. Reinforcing

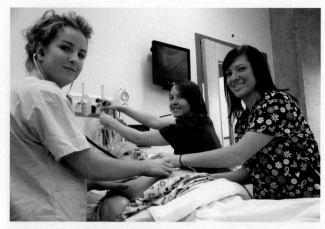

Figure 17.7 Students actively caring for an acutely ill patient in simulation. (Photo courtesy of Colette Foisy-Doll, MacEwan University, Edmonton, AB)

prior learning, students are given opportunities to practice skills such as critical thinking, focused communication, and the identification of appropriate nursing interventions. The high emotional engagement of the student produces indelible mental images that are thought to increase knowledge retention and improve clinical judgment abilities (Dillard et al., 2009; Fanning & Gaba, 2007). The urgent need for astute and time-efficient problem solving and follow-up can be both challenging and exhilarating for students. Ultimately, simulations have the potential to bolster their confidence and competence prior to being placed on a clinical unit (Alinier, Hunt, Gordon, & Harwood, 2006; Jeffries, 2007).

Although some students experience discomfort at having to perform skills in front of their peers, Jamison, Hovancsek, and Clockesy (2006) reported a diminished level of anxiety, greater self-confidence, and improved critical thinking in response to simulation activities. A study involving novice baccalaureate nursing students found benefits from simulation training including enhanced practicality, confidence, and comfort prior to clinical exposure (Bremner et al., 2006).

Flexibility as a Teaching Tool

Additional advantages include the adaptability of simulation activities to be designed to meet specific course objectives or individual learning needs. Appropriate educational resources can be chosen in relation to those criteria. Simulation is particularly useful for remediation whether there is a knowledge integration deficit, an inability to perform a skill correctly, or challenges with implementing planned care in a prioritized, efficient manner. Students repeat skill exercises until proficiency is reached (Haskvitz & Koop, 2004). The educator has the flexibility to alter contextual elements and scenario events, allowing the simulation to unfold to achieve the desired learning outcomes. For example, the practical skill of initiating an IV could initially be introduced, practiced, and mastered in a basic skills lab using a combination of student partner and task trainers. This process allows for repetitive practice that is free of time constraints. The use of peer partners is advantageous for practice elements such as patient teaching, organization, and the proper application of the tourniquet. Simulated IV arms and flashback units (task trainers) are specifically used for accurate cannula insertion and taping. Higher order learning involving this same skill could be facilitated for the student through an integrated scenario in real time using a high-fidelity patient simulator. For example, students could partake in a scenario of an anxious, postpartum patient experiencing a hemorrhage where the skill of IV initiation is required to be performed in a knowledgeable, skillful, and time-efficient manner to prevent deleterious consequences. It also calls on the student to remain composed under pressure.

Feedback and Debriefing

Instructor-guided reflection and feedback are the most salient features of simulation-based strategies to promote effective learning (Alinier et al., 2006; Issenberg et al, 2005). **Debriefing** is a process that involves critical self-reflection as an integral aspect of simulation and is considered an essential dimension of professional growth (Cannon-Diehl, 2009). Best practice in simulation offers that "all simulation-based learning experiences should include a planned debriefing session aimed toward promoting reflective thinking" (Decker et al., 2013, p. S27). Guided debriefing is a process used by the facilitator during debriefing that reinforces the critical aspects of the experience and encourages insightful learning, allowing the participant to assimilate theory, practice, and research to influence future actions (NLN-SIRC, 2013). **Reflective thinking** is the *engagement of self-monitoring* that occurs during or after an experience. It is also considered an essential component of experiential learning and promotes the discovery of new knowledge with the intent of applying this knowledge to future situations. Following a scenario affords students dedicated time and psychological space for reflection-on-action (Schön, 1983). This time is structured to allow students to openly discuss their successes as well as to rethink actions, reactions, and care decisions. Mistakes are considered "puzzles to be solved and not errors to be punished" (Rudolph, Simon, Dufresne, & Raemer, 2006, p. 10). In other words, when students are not formally evaluated in simulation, they are freed to make mistakes and learn from them without the pressure of a grade or the risk of endangering a real person. Participants seem to learn whether they are engaged in the observer role or active role during the simulation (Girzadas et al., 2009; Jeffries, 2005). In simulation-based learning, it is important to employ a structured debriefing process that addresses the perspectives of all participants and supports the culture of productive peer feedback while striving for high performance standards.

There is great benefit to creating an interprofessional team environment where students from various disciplines can practice integrating relational and clinical knowledge and skills while engaging in professional dialogues with one another (Gaba & Raemer, 2007). Collaborating on complex, multifaceted scenarios in real time enhances cooperation, communication, and leadership abilities (Lasater, 2007).

Think Studies show that when health professionals are educated together, they gain valuable knowledge and an increased understanding of each other's skills and scopes of practice. The results are improved team functioning, increased patient safety, better patient care outcomes, and overall increases in job satisfaction. At a time when the Canadian health system is suffering from a shortage of providers, interprofessional education and subsequent improved collaborative practice can also contribute to system efficiency, shorter wait times, and better access to health services (Canadian Interprofessional Health Collaborative [CIHC], 2007; CPSI, 2008). Can you think of the various disciplines that make up health-care teams? Knowing that most team errors involve miscommunication, think of one patient safety-focused interprofessional scenario you would create to benefit both teams and patients. Explain the theme and the sequence of events as you envision them unfolding.

Present-day students are technologically savvy in the digital language of computers, gaming, and the Internet. They have an intuitive ability to adopt new systems for communicating, sharing, searching, analyzing, and reporting information but often lack the prerequisites for learning engagement and motivation (Prensky, 2005, 2007). For educators to have relevance, it is essential to find alternatives to traditional methods of educating in order to engage students in meaningful ways. Students expect and, in some instances, demand rapidly paced challenges and modern tools to facilitate their learning (Rothgeb, 2008). The sophisticated computer interface and programmability of the patient simulator appeals to the contemporary student.

Limitations of Simulation

Although advances in technology have spurred much enthusiasm in academic circles, there continue to be various challenges to incorporating high-end simulation within health education programs. The significant expense of high-fidelity simulation, SP, and virtual learning programs coupled with the need for resource heavy support and related infrastructure can be daunting. Recent global economic downturns and fiscal constraints in health care and education have resulted in the need for judicious resource allocation in both sectors. For the student, this means that, although simulation has been found to be beneficial, funding inequities and regional disparities in program resources may limit nursing students' access to high-fidelity simulation. As a result, some nursing programs are exploring collaborative sharing models, such as simulation centre consortia, as a means of promoting access to high-end simulation experiences for their students (Harder, 2009; Jeffries & Battin, 2012). However, it is important to note that in lieu of the use of high-fidelity simulators, both low- and moderate-fidelity trainers have proven efficacy in supporting high-fidelity clinical simulation experiences for students. For example, PartoPants are very inexpensive obstetrical birthing simulator scrub pants that are designed to recreate a wide variety of live birth scenarios. This low-cost, low-tech birth simulator alternative has been used successfully in high-fidelity obstetrical simulations (Cohen, Cragin, Rizk, Hanberg, & Walker, 2011). Ultimately, simulators are simply tools that must be properly used in order to achieve powerful learning. The use of a high-fidelity simulator alone does not, in and of itself, equate to high-fidelity simulation outcomes. Rather, powerful simulation-based learning is generated through application of the entire simulation-based learning process.

A major limitation to incorporating simulation into health care and education is the financial expense of purchasing the equipment (Rothgeb, 2008). Costs vary in accordance with the inherent features and functionality of patient simulators; however, current manufacturers are just beginning to address this issue by offering innovative financing options such as leasing.

Other physical resources include adequate space to accommodate the manikins, participants, and observers; diagnostic instruments; suctioning and compressed air capability; equipment such as IV pumps and stretchers; props to realistically "makeup" or **moulage** an SP or patient simulator to enhance the realism of the simulation experience; and consumables such as gloves, dressing supplies, and simulated medications. The added expense of the information technology/audio visual (IT/AV) equipment needed to digitally record and archive simulation activities for real-time and postsimulation viewing is another major consideration, as are operating, servicing, and replacement costs over time. The physical space and money required for building simulation centres can create internal competition for sought-after real estate and funding in institutions. Increasingly, administrators are exploring creative ways to acquire simulators in order to develop and sustain their programs (Gaba, 2004). Strategies to help mitigate such challenges include partnerships between educational institutions and hospitals to secure joint funding, develop cost-sharing arrangements, and carry out collaborative user training (Jeffries & Battin, 2012).

Challenges for Nurse Educators

Human resources are essential to the success of using alternative learning approaches; however, the costs associated with the development and training of simulation educators and staff is substantial. In today's educational settings, reduced resources and increased student numbers are the norm (Howard, 2011; Medley & Horne, 2005). Although there is generally strong educator support for the value and benefits of simulations for learning, time-intensive professional development for educators has been cited as a major disadvantage (Nehring, Lashey, & Ellis, 2002). Too often, there is little formal instruction provided for users of simulation. Experimentation with advanced technology and best-practice scenario development is time-consuming and often frustrating. Additional time for setup and low student to instructor ratios (usually 4:1 per scenario) can be limiting factors (Feingold et al., 2004). Delivering the full scope of simulation that is grounded in best practice and current

evidence requires educators who are knowledgeable in simulation and teaching and learning principles (Howard, 2011). These people are often referred to as *simulation champions*. Elements such as curriculum design, knowledge of quality educational experiences, scenario development, evaluation and assessment, expert facilitation skills, and research require an in-depth knowledge of simulation.

In addition, educators using simulation must possess a broad knowledge base in nursing and other disciplines, including areas such as psychomotor skills, pathophysiology, pharmacology, and clinical practice standards, and they must also be technologically savvy. This role is certainly a challenging one to fill. Efforts to create standardized certification programs for educators are underway. However, there is currently no universally adopted certification process and no commonly adopted set of competencies to prepare nurse educators for this pedagogy (Jeffries, 2008). Over and above this, modalities such as SP and virtual learning programs require that educators develop expertise in these additional areas. If teachers are to adopt these educational tools and related pedagogies successfully, they must be adequately supported through a systematic adoption process across the curriculum (Howard, 2011; Kardong-Edgren & Oermann, 2009). Currently, several international simulations in health-care organizations are in the process of developing educator certification and credentialing programs, whereas some institutions have initiated graduate-level certificate courses specializing in simulation.

Challenges for Students

For students participating in simulation activities, a lack of familiarity with the simulator and a fear of what lies ahead are natural concerns. The apprehension associated with working in front of peers under the close supervision of a simulation educator also has the potential to limit its effectiveness. Anxiety may be further exacerbated if the simulation activity is used for evaluation and grades are attached to performance. However, when the activity is accompanied by the heightened (but not debilitating) emotional engagement of the student, significant learning outcomes may be achieved (Fanning & Gaba, 2007). To optimize learning, students should receive a thorough orientation to the simulator and the simulation environment as well as a review of the process and associated learning objectives. It is important to note that students will experience increased benefit from the simulation by preparing for the scenario the same way they would prepare to care for a real patient. Nursing students have identified anxiety and lack of realism as limitations in both simulators and certain aspects of simulation events (Bremner et al., 2006). A recent study identified that these barriers for nurses were further influenced by their prior simulation exposure, years of experience, and area of professional practice (Decarlo, Collingridge, Grant, & Ventre, 2008).

Creating challenging, evidence-based simulations is a complex and detailed process that requires immense planning, coordination, and follow-through. However, having the most well-orchestrated event and employing the most current technology does not ensure that realism will be created for the student. As such, educational scholars and clinical experts are increasingly working together to develop realistic scenarios that reflect current practice and exchanging their time and expertise. Additionally, educators are cognizant of the need to provide comprehensive orientation and ongoing support to students as a means of lessening anxiety and promoting a safe environment for experiential learning where mistakes are made and lessons are learned (Jeffries, 2007).

The Process of Simulation

There are many accepted approaches to the design and delivery of simulation experiences, but it is imperative that simulation-based learning be grounded in best practices in education (Jeffries, 2007). Simulation events can be described as being composed of a presimulation, intrasimulation, and postsimulation phase (Durham & Alden, 2008). In simulation event design, adaptations are often needed relative to students' needs, their level of education, their prior exposure to clinical practice, and the identified learning objectives. The number of learning objectives tends not to exceed three or four to promote realistic time frames for achieving said outcomes. Each objective should be relevant for the participants and linked to program curriculum, competency standards, or criterion for performance evaluation and overall program outcomes (Alinier, 2010). Scenarios developed for undergraduate students may involve a significant amount of preparatory work in advance of the event, whereas an expert professional may not be exposed to any preparatory period whatsoever. Scenarios may be tailored by educators based on their clinical expertise and previous practice experiences, be derived from journal articles or other published case studies, or be entirely fabricated. Fully preconfigured scenarios in the form of software programs are also available for purchase and are used as is or can be adapted to meet specific learning goals. Moreover, entire scenario-curriculum packages can be adapted so as to align with an existing nursing curriculum. Scenarios are designed to match and challenge the students' level of competency and then are positioned in the overall curriculum base where scenario designers have the flexibility to enhance, modify, or reposition them accordingly. To make them more relevant, case information such as patient demographics, prescribed interventions, baseline physical data, best-practice guidelines, and protocols from regional health-care systems may be added.

Common elements found in SCEs may be represented through the use of templates proposed by simulation industry companies such as Medical Education Technologies, Inc.'s (now CAE Healthcare, Inc., 2011) *Program for Nursing Curriculum Integration*, and Laerdal, Inc. and the National League for Nursing's Simulation Scenarios. Other simulation scholars have also developed and adapted useful templates based on their extensive experience in simulation (Alinier, 2010; Diekmann & Rall, 2008).

Recently, book publishers, such as Lippincott Williams & Wilkins, have developed simulated case presentations that assist the student to prepare for simulation. The student, therefore, may be required to answer questions and review assessments and skills online prior to participating in simulation. Additionally, simulation scholars and users throughout the world have created useful frameworks. As a result, there have been various hybrid models for scenario development that have evolved over time.

Elements of a Simulated Clinical Experience

The variable elements of an SCE (sometimes referred to as *scenario*) are the case and curricular information, fidelity of realism, the patient information, and the flow of the scenario progression.

Case/Scenario Information

The case information situates the student within the scenario by describing the context or setting and may include additional participants such as health-care providers or family members. The site where simulation is enacted may be actual or contrived. Locations can vary from the acute primary care setting to a battlefield. Other possibilities include trauma/accident scenes, extended care facilities, the community, or a home setting. For example, students may encounter a patient being admitted to an acute care medical unit for surgery or enter an apartment to carry out a postpartum home visit for a mother and her newborn baby. Alternately, the use of portable simulators permits the student to be exposed to an emergent event in a hallway, a bathroom, or even out on the street.

Curricular Information

The primary component of scenario design is the development of specific, realistic, and relevant learning objectives. In fact, this key factor impacts all planning decisions from the type of simulation used to the selection of the appropriate educational tools. Scenario setup involves the development and dissemination of support materials for both simulation educators and students. The information provided in advance of the simulation differs for the educator who facilitates and should not be viewed by the student. Policies, guidelines, and confidentiality agreements for use in simulation are established to preserve the integrity of the curriculum.

Realism in Simulation

Creating realism or levels of fidelity in simulation learning requires careful planning of equipment and supporting objects or props (Taekman, 2008). The higher the level of fidelity, the more the event has the potential to be perceived as reality. Fidelity has been further categorized into *physical*, *environmental*, and *psychological modes* (Hetzel-Campbell & Daley, 2009; Rehmann, Mitman, & Reynolds, 1995), and, more recently, explores the *sociological mode* of fidelity in simulation (Sharma, Boet, Kitto, & Reeves, 2011).

Physical Fidelity

Physical or *equipment fidelity* concerns the degree to which the high-fidelity simulator approximates the appearance and life-like actions of a human, such as blinking and breathing. The physical layout of the room and room contents such as medical charts, supplies, diagnostic instruments, equipment, and personal items of the patient (e.g., bedside greeting cards, flowers) all contribute to creating this reality (Figs. 17.8A and 17.8B).

Environmental Fidelity

Environmental fidelity is the second dimension of realism referring to the aspects of the event that provide sensory cues to the participants in support of critical thinking about the unfolding situation in order to make clinical decisions or predictions. Rudolph, Simon, and Raemer (2007) describe this dimension as *conceptual fidelity* in which clinical reasoning skills are called on and *if-then* type relationships are made. For example, *if* the breath sounds are diminished, *then* the pulse oximetry measurement will be affected.

Psychological Fidelity

The third element of realism, *psychological fidelity*, is considered the most crucial aspect for engaging participants in simulation and relates to the *holistic experience of the situation* (Beaubien & Baker, 2004). The patient's ability or inability to speak and respond to the student profoundly impacts perceived reality during an event. The ultimate goal in designing effective scenarios is that students are meaningfully engaged on an emotional level that allows for "higher level processing and improvisation, activates pertinent stored knowledge and anchors important lessons for the future" (Rudolph et al., 2007, p.163).

Sociological Fidelity

Sociological fidelity examines how to best recreate sociological factors in SCEs such as the hierarchy, power relations, culture, gender, conflict, and identity aspects of a given situation (Sharma et al., 2011). This concept is key when recreating realistic SCEs that promote critical thinking and effective functioning, while taking into account the social fabric of practice within interprofessional teams or for teams within singular disciplines (Dieckmann, Gaba, & Rall, 2007). More research is needed to discern the impact that each of the dimensions of fidelity has on desired learning outcomes in immersive simulation-based learning.

Patient Information

Patient data pertaining to demographics such as gender, race, age, and ethnicity; physical findings; pertinent health history; current diagnosis; medical and nursing treatment regimens; and diagnostic reports need to be detailed. The patient's current health status and presenting condition should be clearly described.

Scenario Progression

Scenario progression highlights the flow or unfolding of the SCE and can be broken into smaller subsections or mini scenarios, called *states* (Taekman, 2008). In each state, the students interact with the simulator, and their interventions (actions or inactions) produce what are termed triggers (Fig. 17.9). For example, a stand-alone SCE may be entitled Cardiac Arrest, whereas the smaller states that progress within the scenario are entitled state 1, onset of chest pain; state 2, patient condition worsens; state 3, relief of pain; and state 4, patient stabilizes.

Triggers are catalyst-type behaviours or events that are often tied to student action or inaction within an SCE. These triggers will cause the patient to move from one state to another. For example, student actions such as medication administration, timely assessments, and nonpharmacological interventions in the previous cardiac arrest scenario will trigger states to progress. If the student administers morphine to the patient for chest pain, he moves to an improved state. These care interventions and actions are communicated to the simulator through internal simulator recognition systems such as sensors or alternately are manually inputted by a computer operator. When designing the flow of the scenario (progression of states), baseline and fluctuating physical findings and all possible simulator responses need to be considered. Some simulator platforms allow the instructor to define

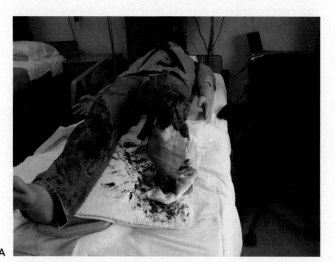
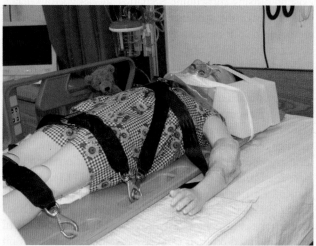

A   B

Figure 17.8 **A** and **B.** Creating realism in simulation. (Photo courtesy of Judy A. K. Bornais)

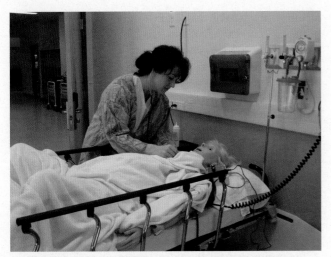

Figure 17.9 Creating a realistic environment helps students engage in the scenario. (Photo courtesy of Colette Foisy-Doll, MacEwan University)

and manipulate physiological responses on the fly, even when using a preconfigured scenario. This means that the operator has the option of controlling the timing and progression of the event in response to the actions of the student. For instance, Mrs. B. is a postpartum patient who presents in an initial state of early hemorrhage. Students must carry out focused assessments, prioritize patient needs, and perform interventions in a timely and holistic manner. Early in this scenario, the student should summon appropriate support, tend to the patient's emotional needs, reposition the patient, administer oxygen, and modify IV therapy. In response to the accuracy and timeliness of these interventions, Mrs. B. will progress to a worsened or improved state. It is imperative that all nonstudent participants involved in the scenario be informed about the range of possible patient outcomes that may occur in the unfolding of the event (Seropian, 2003). Current research and best practices in education and health-care delivery underpin the entire simulation development process.

Presimulation Activities

The presimulation phase involves preparation for both educators and students. The context of the desired learning experience and previous theory and clinical course learning should be taken into consideration (Schiavenato, 2009). The simulation learning process supports synthesis and consolidation of theoretical and practice concepts and related skills.

Preparation of Nurse Educators

Today's educators are faced with increasingly complex and demanding workloads. In addition, the continuous stream of new technologies requires that educators possess specific knowledge and skill sets (Krautscheid, Kaakinen, & Warner, 2008). Ideally, devoted teams of educators who understand the benefits of simulation to teaching provide a contextual framework for these learning experiences throughout the curriculum. This student-centred pedagogical approach entails the

need for comprehensive orientation and education programs. Therefore, all those who teach using simulation must receive adequate instruction on how to use it (Kardong-Edgren & Oermann, 2009). In some cases, where no technical support is provided, this may include hands-on technological training. It is essential that the educator understands the simulation delivery options and, when applicable, is capable of manipulating the simulator interface and multimedia equipment. Professional development through simulation learning opportunities is now readily accessible through conferences, online courses, workshops, and interest group meetings.

Prior to a simulation session, educators should be provided with a comprehensive instructor guide that directs the teaching process (Jeffries, 2005). This guide includes information on flow, timing, and salient instructor points in addition to group size; patient scripts with verbal prompts, sensory cues, and room; and simulator equipment requirements. This supports the SCE unfolding in a consistent, organized, and logical fashion. The voice of the patient may be that of the simulation assistants, technicians, or educators. Given their extensive theory base, practice backgrounds, and lived experience, faculty members can be optimally effective in this role. Moreover, clinical nurse educators who are facilitating their own student groups can gain insights into how students perform individually and as team members. The educator can assess students' leadership qualities, relational practices, clinical reasoning, decision-making abilities, and skill performance (Durham & Alden, 2008).

A rehearsal or dry run of the SCE prior to student participation helps to illuminate problems with the flow of the scenario or the programming of the simulator. This rehearsal allows for refining and modifying the scenario and/or a participant **role** prior to implementation. Ultimately, it serves to enhance the simulated learning experience, diminish the likelihood of problematic events, and increase consistency between educators teaching the same scenario (Kesten, Brown, Hurst, & Briggs, 2010).

Preparation of the Student

Students benefit from an introduction to the simulation process and need to have a clear understanding of their roles and responsibilities within an event. In most settings, participants are required to sign agreements pertaining to confidentiality, preservation of the integrity of the scenarios, and media releases. When research is conducted, separate consent forms are generated. If performance evaluations are carried out, specific criteria must be provided to the student in advance. Upon arrival to the simulation suite, students should participate in a **prebrief**, a hands-on orientation session. This serves to increase student familiarity with the simulator functions, the surrounding environment such as visual and auditory props (telephone, call bell, overhead pager), and relevant equipment. In addition, this introduction is helpful in decreasing initial anxiety (Durham & Alden, 2008). Supporting text materials should include detailed case information, patient data, relevant history, a clear set of learning objectives, and thought-provoking questions. Students also need to know the configuration of the event including group size, the roles they are asked to assume, and the allotted time frame.

One of the most essential elements of student preparation includes eliciting a commitment from students to respond to sensory cues as though they are real. These cues include props, actual physical findings via the simulator (e.g., empty inhaler at the bedside, oozing bandage, tears, and diaphoresis), and verbal prompts by the patient. In turn, the simulation developers along with the scenario facilitators commit to creating as real a situation as possible given the known constraints. The **facilitator** is an individual who guides and supports participants to understand the common objectives and assists participants to achieve them. Together, these elements form the basis of what is coined a *fiction contract* (Rudolph, Simon, Raemer, & Eppich, 2008). Inherent in this agreement is a stance of mutual respect and the belief that all participants enter into the simulation process with a desire to fully engage and do their very best. Adequate preparation helps set the stage for the students' optimal participation in the presimulation, intrasimulation, and postsimulation phases. In some instances, as with senior students or post-licensure groups of students, there may not be any preparatory period. The occurrence of a crisis may be used to challenge their immediate clinical decision-making abilities, spurring them into action at a moment's notice.

Intrasimulation

The *intrasimulation* phase follows preparation for the event and commences once the student enters the patient care setting. Authenticity in learning encounters can be heightened by asking students to engage in realistic verbal interaction with the SP or simulator while performing comprehensive, holistic, and evidence-based care. When successfully implemented, the event can feel so real that it elicits poignant human emotions. A heightened sense of emotion is tied to an increased ability to remember and later applies the concepts that have been lived and learned during the event. According to the classic Yerkes-Dodson Law (Yerkes & Dodson, 1908), a positive correlation exists between the level of emotional arousal of the students and their ability to perform. If a student is understimulated or on the contrary too anxious, his or her performance is compromised, and his or her learning retention wanes. This law, now supported by current evidence, is a process that is often illustrated graphically as an inverted U-shaped curve that depicts how performance increases and then decreases with fluctuations in arousal (Raglin & Turner, 1993).

Active and Observational Student Roles

Students may be the sole participants in a simulated event or may assume one of several different active roles in pairs or groups. Active nurse roles that may be assumed in an SCE include being an assessment, resource, medication, or procedure nurse. One other example could be the role of a lead communication nurse. The lead communicator assumes responsibility for information dissemination between team members, the patient, and family. Communication by phone, paging system, and chart and using an organizing tool such as Situation, Background, Assessment, Recommendation (SBAR) are key aspects of this role.

A student may also be given the role of observer. The observer can be assigned to watch certain strategic aspects of the simulation, such as communication both within the team and between the team and patient/family. Observers may be assigned to identify and make notes about when pertinent clinical decisions are made or to critically appraise the enactment of procedures and assessments. Constructive observer feedback significantly contributes to the quality of the debriefing session and aids in the closure of performance gaps. Participants all seem to learn, whether engaging in active or observational roles during the simulation (Jeffries, 2005).

Environmental fidelity is an important consideration in the intrasimulation phase. Heightened realism in physical spaces such as the patient room and equipment enhance the participant's ability to engage in the scenario without interruption in flow and sequence (Fig. 17.10).

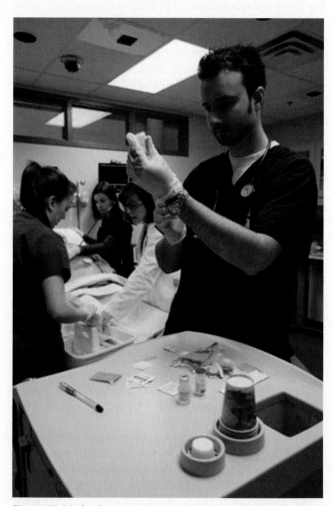

Figure 17.10 Student engaging in a simulation experience. Note that each student is carrying out a particular role in this scenario, such as primary assessment nurse, medication nurse, and so on. (Photo courtesy of The Faculty of Nursing, University of Calgary)

For example, the primary nurse may need to call for assistance, making the presence of a functional call bell at the bedside a particularly important feature. The student is then able to proceed without having to pause or pretend. The inclusion of that one small piece of equipment (the call bell) can significantly impact the student's *suspension of disbelief* (Halamek et al., 2000). Other enhancements to environmental fidelity might include a beginning shift report; patient charts that include x-rays, CT scans, and lab results; and relevant ancillary equipment such as telephones and pagers.

As the students encounter problems during the event, they may be given the option of calling a huddle or time-out. These timed reprieves involve suspending the clock during the event where the simulator goes to sleep. Students can have a quick team discussion of the patient's case. Scenarios can focus on individual and/or team performance roles where either formal or informal feedback can be provided. During the event, the student will then pay particular attention to those performance indicators that are related to specified learning objectives. For instance, if the goal of the scenario is to provide individual performance feedback on interaction with the patient, the student will pay particular attention to gathering appropriate patient information from the chart, introducing himself or herself to the patient, addressing the patient respectfully, and displaying appropriate affective messages through empathetic responses. The student nurse may also give thought and attention to his or her professional attire and appearance, recognizing that these can impact initial patient impressions at the bedside. Students will want to ensure their attire is clinically appropriate and consistent with dress code regulations.

If the objectives for the scenario are to address team behaviours, team functioning, and related outcomes, the focus during the event shifts to relating how individual behaviours contributed to or detracted from predetermined performance indicators of teamwork (Fig. 17.11).

Additional areas of focus for discussion and critique of team performance might include leadership, effective resource management, delegation, communication, process, organization, timing, responsibility, autonomy (the extent to which each member carries out the full scope of practice within a scenario), decision-making, critical thinking, **problem solving**, and group dynamics.

Operator Role

Simulation operators, whether they are educators or other staff, are able to effectively record the event as it unfolds while simultaneously providing annotations on the recording at strategic points during the event. Annotations are written comments appearing on the video screen that can be accessed and viewed on video playback by students, peers, or educators for post-encounter reflection. It is true that not all simulation centres are staffed with dedicated simulation operators who are technical experts, but as technical capabilities continue to increase, so will the demand for expert staff. Along with educator annotations, students may also be

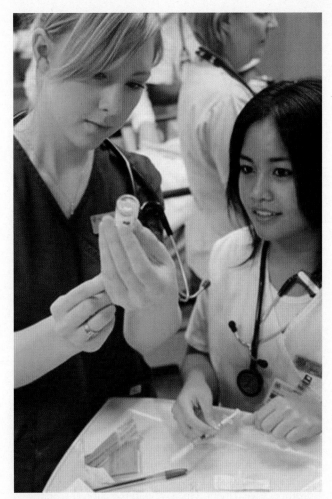

Figure 17.11 Students working in collaboration during simulation. (Photo courtesy of The Faculty of Nursing, University of Calgary)

asked to input computer annotations when reviewing video recordings for self-reflection or peer feedback purposes.

Recording objective data is imperative to the debriefing process, regardless of whether the data is digitally captured or manually recorded by a participant. Advancements in technology have been specifically applied to the simulation experience and have resulted in the creation of very sophisticated systems. Also, digital video capture systems have the potential to interface with the simulator, capturing physiological data as the event unfolds. This data capture capability adds significantly to the bank of rich data that is available for review in the postsimulation phase.

Another role of the operator is to orchestrate the mechanics of the event, keeping track of timing, initiating, and ending recordings; sometimes providing the patient voice; and tending to outside observers or trainees who may have questions and comments. In many simulation centres, there exist additional layers of support personnel such as simulation technicians, event managers, or runners to assist.

Nurse Educator Roles in the Intrasimulation Phase

Educators can assume various roles during the intrasimulation phase. They possess clinical experience that allows them to be highly effective as the patient's voice or as actors;

many are also trained as technologically skilled simulator operators. They may choose to formally assess student performance during an SCE. When using this approach, the process and related evaluation criteria should be made known to the students in advance of the event. Formative feedback provides performance review information aimed at helping the student to increase self-awareness and plan for performance improvements. Observations are made and then discussed in the debriefing session during the postsimulation phase. Summative feedback is usually accompanied by an assigned grade, sometimes a pass/fail, and is related to the student's ability to meet specific behavioural objectives for that learning event. Feedback approaches in undergraduate nursing programs tend to be more formative in nature, structured primarily for use in a debriefing approach (McGaghie, Issenberg, Petrusa, & Scalese, 2010). A four-step, evidence-based model for collecting and delivering feedback provides an effective method of data collection during an event (Rudolph et al., 2008). The steps are

1. Note salient performance gaps.
2. Clearly describe the performance gap.
3. Investigate the basis for the gap.
4. Offer suggestions to help close the gap.

Through the eyes of a student

I really enjoyed our second-year simulation experience. I found it hard to understand what it meant to "put all the pieces together" of how to care for a postoperative patient. Once we had the clinical scenario, it all came together.

(personal reflection of Mikayla, a second-year nursing student)

Through the eyes of a nurse

*A*s a faculty member, it is difficult to explain to students how all the pieces fit together in one patient scenario. Students are often worried about one particular skill and may not see the bigger picture. Simulation takes the focus off one skill and transforms the learning into a multidimensional, holistic, and realistic experience.

(personal reflection of J. Bornais, nursing faculty member)

Learning in a Simulation Environment

Certain aspects of simulation education present nurse educators with an opportunity to rethink assumptions about how students learn best in a simulated environment. Among the questions that arise are the following: Is there a place for didactic teaching inside a simulation room? Should the educator be present inside the room participating in the event or is it better for student learning if the educator remains outside the simulation room? Is educator participation in the simulation event room better suited to a certain level of student or type of learning objective? Answers to these questions should be driven by research, the learning objectives, and the desired outcomes of the event. When a facilitator adopts an in-room coaching stance during the intrasimulation phase, the results can be very effective. Modeling a *reflection-in-action* approach during the event, educators can show critical thinking, problem solving, and troubleshooting in the presence of the student (Schön, 1983). Simulation technologies are designed to accommodate this teaching approach, providing an option to stop and restart the event at any point, allowing for timely expert input and coaching. Information is shared between the student and the teacher as the scenario unfolds; theoretical concepts and practice assumptions may be periodically questioned and clarified. Teaching tools such as slide presentations, patient diagnostic findings, and other data can be displayed on a large screen monitor inside the simulation room where all participants readily have access to information. This approach can be helpful in providing a psychological safety net for simulation neophytes who often experience heightened levels of performance anxiety. If the educator is role-playing in an event (e.g., physician role), it is important that they remain "in character" throughout the scenario to avoid confusion and interruptions for the students.

Often in simulation sessions, the educator chooses to remain outside the simulation room or as simply an observer within the room. Students may be assigned specific roles and then proceed to engage with the simulated patient, just as they would in an actual health-care setting. These types of events typically proceed without interruption, and students simply carry on without the active participation of the educator inside the room. This approach allows students to work through the processes of problem solving, critical thinking, and troubleshooting without interruption. However, if the educator acts as the patient voice, verbal cues may be subtly offered that assist the students in assessing, decision-making, and problem solving. For example, because a high-fidelity simulator is not equipped to demonstrate movement during a motor power check, the operator may state, "The nurse that performed that check on me an hour ago said I was very strong!"

Postsimulation

The postsimulation phase optimally transpires immediately after the intrasimulation event. It is important to recognize that a very significant portion of learning in simulation is derived from postsimulation discussion sessions, commonly known as the debriefing period. Debriefing is considered to be the most important aspect of simulation because it provides an opportunity for students and educators to review the events that occurred during the scenario. An ideal starting point for the debriefing session involves the participants sharing the positive aspects of the experience. Ensuring that the learning objectives for the simulation are addressed and the linkages between learned concepts and practice are made are also essential components of the debriefing session (Jeffries, 2007; Rauen, 2001). Furthermore, clarification and reinforcement of important content allows the students to consolidate their learning and identify strategies to improve their future performance. Debriefing should occur immediately following the simulated experience to capture the emotions, feelings, and insights while they are fresh in the minds of the participants. A delay in the opportunity to debrief may result in content being forgotten or distorted over time (Jeffries, 2007).

In advance of the debriefing session, the instructor sets the tone for the session, ensuring that participants feel safe to share their insights, feelings, and observations. Equally important is creating a safe atmosphere that fosters equal participation from students, so that the input from all participants becomes part of the learning. It has been shown that valuing and ensuring participation and engagement in debriefing leads to "deeper levels of learning and increases the likelihood of transfer to the clinical setting" (Center for Medical Simulation, 2009, para. 1; Fig. 17.12). During debriefing, students should have an opportunity to reflect on their assessments, clinical decision-making ability, feelings, communication behaviours, and nursing interventions. Henneman, Cunningham, Roche, and Curnin (2007) referred to this as the reflective thinking session.

Schön's (1983) classic work on reflection in learning highlights a similar process using the phrase *reflection-on-action* to describe the opportunity for students to critique their interactions after participating in simulation events in order to create new understandings to apply to future learning. Conversely, *reflection-in-action* refers to the students' lived experience while actively thinking on their feet in a simulation event and describing what was happening for them in the heat of the moment. Regardless of the term used, post-simulation reflections allow students to critically assess their actions, inactions, successes, and challenges in order to learn from them.

During the debriefing period, participants may be assigned specific roles to help solicit feedback from all participants and foster a productive discussion. Common roles include timekeeper, observer, and team facilitator. During debriefing, the instructor also plays a significant role. Instructors guide the reflective thinking process, ensuring that successes and challenges of the encounter are addressed, misperceptions are clarified, and incorrect or unsafe practices are illuminated and rectified. A review of nursing skills and relational practices as well as the rationale for assessments and intervention decisions are usually discussed to consolidate participants' understanding of the purpose and implications of their actions. This is also an opportunity for the facilitator to identify and close gaps in knowledge or skills and help students integrate correct behaviours into their practice (Beaubien & Baker, 2004; Durham & Alden, 2008). Using this process strongly supports the development of self-reflection, a competency of the CNA (2010).

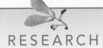

RESEARCH

A study by Lasater (2007) explored the relationship between critical thinking and simulation. The study looked at students' simulation experience followed by a focus group. Four dimensions were studied: (1) students' self-report of confidence in their clinical judgment skills, (2) students' aptitude for critical thinking, (3) qualitative observations of students' clinical judgment skill during simulation, and (4) students' experiences of learning in a focus group.

Participating students reported that "simulation served as a bridge to bring the information from the classroom and the psychomotor skills learned in lab together . . . and they felt the simulation was a superior method to just reading about a particular disease or condition" (Sanford, 2010, p. 1008).

Nursing Implications

When students come prepared to fully engage in simulated learning, many insights can be derived from retrospective reflection on the actions and thinking processes employed in patient care. How can engaging in experiential learning contribute to the development of critical thinking skills? How would you, as a nursing student, demonstrate critical thinking ability in a simulated learning environment?

Lasater, K. (2007). High-fidelity simulation and the development of clinical judgment: Students' experiences. Journal of Nursing Education, 46, 269–276.

Sanford, P. G. (2010). Simulation in nursing education: A review of the research. The Qualitative Report, 15(4). Retrieved from http://www.nova.edu/ssss/QR/QR15-4/sanford.pdf

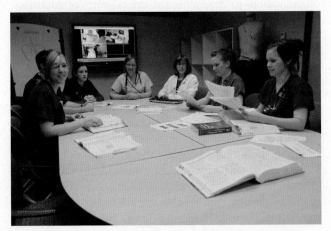

Figure 17.12 A debriefing session with students and faculty. (Photo courtesy of The Faculty of Nursing, University of Calgary)

Following the scenario and debriefing, students may have an opportunity to repeat the simulation. Although not always feasible, repeating a scenario allows for immediate performance improvement and further consolidates the learning from the previous encounter.

In the postsimulation phase, several facets of evaluation must be considered. During preliminary event planning stages, time and consideration must be devoted to selecting or creating valid and reliable tools for the evaluation of students (Adamson & Kardong-Edgren, 2012; Davis & Kimble, 2011; Society for Simulation in Healthcare [SSH], 2012). Educators facilitating simulation should be evaluated as well as the scenario event and its ability to meet the stated learning objectives. Additionally, evaluation surveys and user data are helpful in informing simulation centre operations. Mechanisms for both formal and informal feedback and for research activities require that permissions be obtained well in advance of the event implementation. Ethics approval boards for research proposals are one example of such a mechanism. Valuable information can result from simulation research findings that form the basis for future change. Simulation research finding can drive change within a nursing program and can also influence initiatives at the local, national, and international level.

Student Evaluation

There has been much debate whether student feedback in a simulated learning environment should be formative or summative in nature. As a result, both approaches are addressed in this chapter.

Formative Evaluation

Formative evaluation involves the provision of verbal or written feedback that is intended to encourage objective, critical review of performance without the assignment of a grade (Oermann & Gaberson, 2009). Psychomotor skills, clinical judgment, and decision-making abilities as well as relational skills and confidence may be evaluated (Bambini, Washburn, & Perkins, 2009). The digital video playback and annotation capabilities that are used during the simulation offer an enhanced platform for self-assessment and/or peer review. Current recording management systems include an option for simultaneous video playback with an accompanying written checklist or a series of open-ended questions that may be submitted by the student as part of the formal evaluation. Students who are identified as needing extra help or practice may then set up a learning contract or remediation plan as part of their formative evaluation process. The teacher and/or the student develop a plan for acquiring the necessary knowledge and skills by identifying one or more learning objectives and outlining the learning criteria to be met within a prescribed time frame. In this context, the debriefing session can serve as a powerful vehicle where teacher and student cocreate new insights; deepen understanding of actions and reactions; and explore student values, beliefs, and attitudes (Rudolph et al., 2008).

Summative Evaluation

Summative evaluation typically occurs at the completion of a course and accompanies the assignment of a final grade. In nursing education, this grade can be tied to either a singular event such as an Objective Structured Clinical Examination (OSCE) or a pass/fail final clinical course mark. Summative evaluation can also be a compilation of many singular criteria such as tests, papers, or assignments used in theory classes for evaluation. Multiple issues have arisen relative to grading student performance in simulation. One of the most significant issues is the limited research correlating the performance of the student in a simulated environment with their actual clinical performance. Among other concerns are student performance anxiety, the fact that patient simulators do not provide an exact representation of a real-life encounter, the variable skill level of the controller/facilitator, and the quality of the evaluative tools. However, summative evaluation has been successfully applied to the acquisition of specific psychomotor skills such as intubation where competence can be clearly assessed and graded (Hotchkiss, Biddle, & Fallacaro, 2002).

High-stakes summative evaluation is a process that involves a major consequence for the student. Often, this test forms the basis for an impacting grading decision such as being assigned a passing or failing grade in a course (Meakim et al., 2013). Increasingly, this type of assessment is being used for post-licensure testing and certainly could contribute to decisions to hire or fire employees. Dr. Howard, current president of International Nursing Association for Clinical Simulation and Learning (INACSL, President's Message, 2013b), notes that as this type of testing becomes more prevalent, so too must adherence to strict educational standards in simulation.

Although the use of simulation has the potential to contribute significantly to educational reform, competency testing using simulation should not occur until standardized, reliable testing processes have been developed (Decker, Sportsman, Puetz, & Billings, 2008). Current simulation methods used in assessment and evaluation of competence have not been rigorously tested for reliability and validity (Adamson & Kardong-Edgren, 2012; Jeffries, 2007). More research is needed to support the use of competency testing (both low and high stakes), to validate the usefulness of simulation, to determine the critical roles of educators/facilitators, and to determine best approaches for meeting learning outcomes (Adamson & Kardong-Edgren, 2012; Medley & Horne, 2005).

Event Evaluation

As scenarios are implemented, it is imperative that feedback be collected from all participants on the quality of the experience and the impact of the experience on learning and retention. It is very important that standardized validated tools be used—these tools that are scientifically proven to be effective for performance assessment and that promote a rigorous, systematic, and reliable approach to evaluation processes (Adamson & Kardong-Edgren, 2012). See Box 17.1 for questions that can be used to evaluate the simulated experiences.

BOX 17.1 Questions to Ask When Evaluating Simulation Experiences

What were the strengths of the learning experience?

What actual or potential problems did students experience with the scenario?

Which aspects of simulation did the students perceive to be most valuable to their learning?

Was the use of simulation effective in attaining the desired learning outcomes?

How effective was the scenario as a teaching strategy?

Were learning objectives clearly stated, realistic, and achievable for the simulation event?

Did the simulation event promote critical thinking in the students?

Were students able to reason and make accurate clinical decisions during the simulation?

Was the event at an appropriate level for the students? Was it challenging? Was it overstimulating?

If psychomotor and assessment skills were involved in the scenario, how well were they performed?

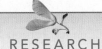

RESEARCH

In the fall of 2011, the NCSBN launched a national landmark, multisite, longitudinal study involving students from 10 schools of nursing from across the United States.

Nursing Implications

Using a standardized simulation curriculum at all sites, the study is exploring the differences in students who spend up to 10%, 25%, and 50% of the time normally spent at clinical sites in SCEs (NCSBN, 2011). The findings from this study are certain to impact future replacement of clinical hours with simulation. It will be fascinating to uncover findings to burning questions such as specific benefits or drawbacks of replacing clinical time in health-care settings with simulated learning.

National Council of State Boards of Nursing. (2011). NCSBN national simulation study. Retrieved from https://www.ncsbn.org/2094.html

Summarizing Simulation in Nursing Education

Although there may be an increasing prevalence of simulation in both education and health-care organizations, there are still gaps in accessibility to high-fidelity simulation equipment; many smaller schools are unable to afford them (Rauen, 2001). However, as simulation innovations continue to evolve, so do the learning opportunities for nurses, both pre- and post-licensure. According to the CPSI's *Patient Simulation Needs Assessment*, the number of simulation programs is growing in Canada as "more and more health practitioners recognize the value of simulation training" (CPSI, 2008, p. 5). In the field of medicine, licensing examinations have included the OSCE that employs simulations using both SPs and patient simulators. It is conceivable that nursing regulatory bodies may 1 day also use simulation as part of their licensing requirements. Ongoing competency validation and recertification in health care has already employed the use of simulation. In fact, certification courses such as the American Heart Association's Pediatric Advanced Life Support (PALS) and Advanced Cardiac Life Support (ACLS) have used high-fidelity simulation for teaching and evaluation for well over a decade (Cannon-Diehl, 2009; Decker et al., 2008). It is reasonable to speculate that funding to hospitals and health-care agencies in the years to come might be dependent on positive patient outcomes linked to simulation education.

The evolution of simulation within nursing education programs has already led to the replacement of clinical hours in the United States and Canada. Although controversial, the National Council of State Boards of Nursing (NCSBN) in the United States published the results of a national survey that found 16 of 44 states allowed up to 25% of clinical hours to be replaced using high-fidelity simulation (Cannon-Diehl, 2009).

With the increasing shortage of adequate practicum placements and the higher patient acuity within hospital organizations, the trend to use simulation as a substitution for clinical hours may occur in Canada and other parts of the world as well.

Think

In 2010, Sigma Theta Tau International Honor Society of Nursing, a national, nonprofit organization that supports the development of nursing knowledge and professional development along with CAE Healthcare, Inc. (formerly Medical Education Technologies, Inc., [METI]), a leading company in the production of patient simulators and health-care education tools, awarded grant money that supports research on simulation-based education. Brewer (2011) conducted an extensive literature on HPS in nursing education, noting that it holds great promise as a valid educational method for the future, but that improvements are needed to maximize the use of HPS, including the development of valid tools and additional research.

Imagine that your instructor has decided to apply for this research grant and has come to you for input on a research topic. Assemble a group of your classmates and, based on what you have learned in this chapter, make a list of potential research topics you could submit when applying for this research grant.

Brewer, E. (2011). Successful techniques for using human patient simulation in nursing education. Journal of Nursing Scholarship, 43(3), 311–317.

A View to the Future With Simulation

As nursing education and health-care organizations focus on patient safety outcomes, the use of simulation is likely to continue to flourish. In fact, with the growing public interest in preventable errors and patient safety, it may no longer be an option for nursing students to learn and practice their clinical skills on real patients. Success in aviation safety through simulation and crew resource management techniques, and now for many applications of simulation in health care, confirms the benefits of using simulation to prepare for high-risk events. Educators are able to standardize experiences for all students and do so without placing patients in jeopardy. Health-care organizations and teaching institutions can effectively use simulation for training purposes in developing problem-solving and crisis management skills, particularly when applied to new and potentially hazardous procedures and equipment (IOM, 2000, p. 179). Patient safety organizations, such as the CPSI as well as the Agency for Healthcare Research and Quality, liability insurers, the IOM, and the public will no doubt drive the future of simulation in health care.

Standards of best practice for simulation in nursing education were recently published, and the formulation of accompanying best-practice guidelines is on the horizon (INASCL, 2013a). Moreover, leaders from public and private agencies, associations, and organizations unite at the Society for Simulation in Healthcare (SSH) simulation summits for ongoing discussions on global standards for simulation-based learning.

Although there are numerous advocates of simulation, health-care education is largely driven by evidence-informed research. Therefore, it is not surprising that many aspects of simulation methods and technology are currently being investigated. Numerous studies have examined its effectiveness and ability to improve student confidence, competence, and learning (Jeffries, 2007; Prion, 2008). Although an abundance of studies exists, few have been able to assess how simulation experiences and learning translate into competency at the point of care in the clinical setting. Many questions remain unanswered. Which simulation tools are required to achieve specific desired outcomes? How much exposure to simulation is required to achieve the desired learning outcomes? What features of simulation and types of simulation experiences yield the most effective learning outcomes? Despite the unanswered questions, it is clear that simulation technology is here to stay. With future research, established standards of practice for simulation, and advances in simulator technology, one can be assured that simulation will continue to change, evolve, and transform the future of health care.

Following her first simulation experience, Megan said, "Even though we were orientated to the simulator and the environment, I thought my heart was going to beat out of my chest when I walked into the patient's room. I fumbled for my stethoscope and dropped my pen on the floor because I was so nervous . . . but I did remember to thoroughly clean it before I used it. I managed to settle down when the patient began to speak to me. He was really kind and cooperative, and I honestly forgot that I was talking to a plastic person!

I had practiced the skills that I was supposed to carry out, but I found it quite challenging having to concentrate on performing them correctly in the right order as well as attend to him in a holistic way. When I watched my performance on the videotape during the debriefing session, I noticed lots of things that I did right, even though I forgot to lower the side rails of the bed. I will be more conscious of that in the future, for sure. I was grateful for having a skilled and experienced instructor guide our discussion, and the observations of my peers were also of great benefit to my learning how to "think like a nurse." I certainly understood how thorough advanced preparation facilitated my learning and performance in the simulation lab. Even though participating in simulations does make me feel nervous, all in all, I appreciate that simulation helped me to feel more confident that I will be able to capably care for my real patients during clinical . . . and I am really looking forward to that!"

Multiple-Choice Questions

1. Which phase of a simulation session is most integral for learning?
   a. Preparation
   b. Scenario enactment
   c. Follow-up debrief
   d. Two weeks postsimulation

2. What advantages to simulation as a learning tool have been documented in the literature?
   a. Increases student preparedness for real clinical experiences
   b. Allows the students to improve their memorization skills
   c. Provides opportunity to practice with only small risks to patients
   d. Exposes students to sophisticated high-fidelity simulation equipment that makes them more positive about their education

3. What factors limit the use of high-fidelity simulation as a teaching strategy?
   a. Educator inexperience
   b. Small class sizes
   c. Low cost of the simulators
   d. Frequent breakdown in technology

4. Which of the following statements is accurate about the future of simulation in nursing?
   a. Simulation in nursing appears bleak at best.
   b. Simulation in nursing will likely to be self-limiting.
   c. Simulation in nursing will need more research in order to move forward.
   d. Simulation in nursing will continue to play an important role in nursing education.

5. Which simulation tool would be the most suited to be used for repetitive practice of a skill in isolation?
   a. A standardized patient
   b. A low-fidelity simulator
   c. A computer-based virtual reality program
   d. A high-fidelity patient simulator

6. Which of the following best describes intrasimulation?
   a. It is the preparation the student completes before the simulated event and is essential in learning process.
   b. It is the briefing period of simulation when the educator ensures the learning objectives were met in the simulated event.
   c. It occurs once the learner enters the simulated learning environment.
   d. It is when the students have an opportunity to discuss the simulated event and reflect upon their actions and clinical decisions.

REFERENCES AND SUGGESTED READINGS

Adamson, K. A., & Kardong-Edgren, S. (2012). A method and resources for assessing the reliability of simulation evaluation instruments. *Nursing Education Perspectives, 33*(5), 334–339.

Alinier, G. (2010). Developing high-fidelity health care simulation scenarios: A guide for educators and professionals. *Simulation & Gaming, 42*(1), 9–26.

Alinier, G., Hunt, B., Gordon, R., & Harwood, C. (2006). Effectiveness of intermediate-fidelity simulation training technology in undergraduate nursing education. *Journal of Advanced Nursing, 54*(3), 359–369. doi:10.1111/j.1365-2648.2006.03810.x

Alverson, D., Caudell, T., & Goldsmith, T. (2008) Creating virtual reality medical simulations. In H. Riley (Ed.), *Manual of simulation in healthcare.* Oxford, England: Oxford University Press.

Association of Standardized Patient Educators. (2011). *Terminology Standards.* Retrieved from http://www.aspeducators.org/node/102

Bambini, D., Washburn, J., & Perkins, J. (2009). Outcomes of clinical simulation for novice nursing students: Communication, confidence, clinical judgment. *Nursing Education Perspectives, 30*(2), 79–82.

Beaubien, J. M., & Baker, D. P. (2004). The use of simulation for training teamwork skills in health care: How low can you go? *Quality and Safety in Health Care, 13*(Suppl. 1), i51–i56.

Benner, P., Sutphen, M., Leonard, V., Day, L., & Shulman, L. S. (2009). *Educating nurses: A call for radical transformation.* San Francisco, CA: Jossey-Bass.

Bremner, M. N., Aduddell, K., Bennett, D. N., & VanGeest, J. B. (2006). The use of human patient simulators: Best practices with novice nursing students. *Nurse Educator, 31*(4), 170–174.

Brindley, P. G., Suen, G. I., & Drummond, J. (2007). Part two: Medical simulation—How to build a successful and long-lasting program. *Canadian Journal of Respiratory Therapy, 43*(5), 31–34. Retrieved from http://ezproxy.macewan.ca/login?url=http://search.ebscohost.com.ezproxy.macewan.ca/login.aspx?direct=true&db=rzh&AN=2009765224&site=eds-live&scope=site

Bushell, E., & Gaba, D. M. (2007) *Health services/technology assessment text (HSTAT) AHRQ evidence report* (Report No. 45). Retrieved from http://www.ncbi.nlm.nih.gov/books/bv.fcgi?rid=hstat1.part.88879

CAE Healthcare, Inc. (2011). *Program for nursing curriculum integration.* Retrieved from http://caehealthcare.com/images/uploads/brochures/PNCI_White_Paper.pdf

Canadian Association of Schools of Nursing. (2007). *Clinical placement projects: Project 3: Inventory of the use of simulated clinical learning experiences and evaluation of their effectiveness.* Retrieved from http://casn.ca/en/Clinical_Education_73.html

Canadian Interprofessional Health Collaborative. (2007). *Briefing documents.* Retrieved from http://www.cihc.ca/resources-files/CIHC_BriefingDocument_Mar2.07.pdf

Canadian Nurses Association. (2010). *Competencies for professional practice.* Retrieved from http://www.cnaaiic.ca/CNA/nursing/rnexam/competencies/default_e.aspx

Canadian Patient Safety Institute. (2008). *Patient simulation needs assessment.* Retrieved from http://www.patientsafetyinstitute.ca/English/education/simulation/Documents/Patient%20Simulation%20Needs%20Assessment%20-%20May%202008.pdf

Cannon-Diehl, M. R. (2009). Simulation in healthcare and nursing: State of the science. *Critical Care Nursing Quarterly, 32*(2), 128–136.

Center for Medical Simulation. (2009). *DASH—Debriefing assessment for simulation in healthcare.* Retrieved from http://www.harvardmedsim.org/debriefing-assessment-simulation-healthcare.php

Cohen, S. R., Cragin, L., Rizk, M., Hanberg, A., & Walker, D. M. (2011). PartoPants™: The high-fidelity, low-tech birth simulator. *Clinical Simulation in Nursing, 7*(1), e11–e18. doi:10.1016/j.ecns.2009.11.012

Conrad, M. A., Guhde, J., Brown, D., Chronister, C., & Ross-Alaolmolki, K. (2011). Transformational leadership: Instituting a nursing simulation program. *Clinical Simulation in Nursing, 7,* e189–e195. doi:10.1016/j.ecns.2010.02.007

Davis, A. H., & Kimble, L. P. (2011). Human patient simulation evaluation rubrics for nursing education: Measuring The Essentials of Baccalaureate Education for Professional Nursing Practice. *Journal of Nursing Education, 50*(11), 605–611. doi:10.3928/01484834-20110715-01

Decarlo, D., Collingridge, D., Grant, C., & Ventre, K. (2008). Factors influencing nurses' attitudes towards simulation-based education. *Simulation in Healthcare, 3*(2), 90–96.

Decker, S., Fey, M., Sideras, S., Caballero, S., Rockstraw, L., Boese, T., . . . Borum, J. C. (2013). Standards of best practice: Simulation standard VI: The debriefing process. *Clinical Simulation in Nursing, 9*(6S), S27–S29. doi:10.1016/j.ecns.2013.04.008

Decker, S., Sportsman, S., Puetz, L., & Billings, L. (2008). The evolution of simulation and its contribution to competency. *The Journal of Continuing Education in Nursing, 39*(2), 74–80.

Dieckmann, P., Gaba, D., & Rall, M. (2007). Deepening the theoretical foundations of patient simulation as a social practice. *Simulation in Healthcare: The Journal of the Society for Simulation in Healthcare, 2*(3), 183–193.

Diekmann, P., & Rall, M. (2008). Designing a scenario as a simulated clinical experience: The TupASS scenario script. In R. R. Kyle & W. B. Murray (Eds.), *Clinical simulation: Operations, engineering and management.* San Diego, CA: Academic Press.

Dillard, N., Sideras, S., Ryan, M., Carlton, K. H., Lasater, K., & Siktberg, L. (2009). A collaborative project to apply and evaluate the clinical judgment model through simulation. *Nursing Education Research, 30*(2), 99–104.

Dillon, P. M., Noble, K. A., & Kaplan, W. (2009). Simulation as a means to foster collaborative interdisciplinary education. *Nursing Education Perspectives, 30*(2), 87–90.

Dunn, W. (2010). *Mayo Clinic Multidisciplinary Simulation Center: Director's message.* Retrieved from http://www.mayo.educ/simulationcenter/directors=message.html

Durham, C. F., & Alden, K. R. (2008). Chapter 51: Enhancing patient safety in nursing education through patient simulation. In R. G. Hughes (Ed.), *Patient safety & quality: An evidence-based handbook for nurses.* Retrieved from http://ezproxy.macewan.ca/login?url=http://search.ebscohost.com.ezproxy.macewan.ca/login.aspx?direct=true&db=eda&AN=43740407&site=eds-live&scope=site

Ellaway, R. H., Kneebone, R., Lachapelle, K., & Topps, D. (2009). Practica continua: Connecting and combining simulation modalities for integrated teaching, learning and assessment. *Medical Teacher, 31*(8), 725–731. doi:10.1080/01421590903124716

Fanning, R., & Gaba, D. (2007). The role of debriefing in simulation-based learning. *Simulation in Healthcare, 2*(2), 115–125. doi:10.1097/SIH.0b013e3180315539

Feingold, C. E., Calaluce, M., & Kallen, M. A. (2004). Computerized patient model and simulated clinical experiences: Evaluation with baccalaureate nursing students. *Journal of Nursing Education, 43*(4), 156–164.

Forbes, M. O., & Hickey, M. (2009). Curriculum reform in baccalaureate nursing education: Review of the literature. *International Journal of Nursing Education Scholarship, 6*(1), 1–15.

Frank, J. R., & Brien, S. (Eds.). (2008). *The safety competencies: Enhancing patient safety across the health professions.* Ottawa, ON: Canadian Patient Safety Institute.

Gaba, D. M. (2004). The future vision of simulation in health care. *Quality and Safety in Health Care, 13*(Suppl. 1), i2–i10. doi:10.1136/qshc.2004. 009878

Gaba, D. M., & Raemer, D. (2007). The tide is turning: Organizational structures to embed simulation in the fabric of healthcare. *Simulation in Healthcare, 2,* 1–3.

Gates, M. G., Parr, M. B., & Hughen, J. E. (2012). Enhancing nursing knowledge using high-fidelity simulation. *Journal of Nursing Education, 51*(1), 9–15. doi:10.3928/01484834-20111116-01

Girzadas, D. V., Delis, S., Bose, S., Hall, J., Rzechula, K., & Kulstad, E. (2009). Measures of stress and learning seem to be equally affected among all roles in a simulation scenario. *Simulation in Healthcare, 4*(3), 149–154. doi:10.1097/SIH.0b013e3181abe9f2

Grenvik, A., & Schaefer, J. J., III. (2004). Medical simulation training coming of age. *Critical Care Medicine, 32*(12), 2549–2550.

Halamek, L., Kaegi, D., Gaba, D., Sowb, Y., Smith, B. C., Smith, B. E., & Howard, S. (2000). Time for a new paradigm in pediatric medical education: Teaching neonatal resuscitation in a simulated delivery room environment. *Pediatrics, 106*(4), e45. doi:10.1542/peds,106.4.e45

Harder, N. B. (2009). Evolution of simulation use in health care education. *Clinical Simulation in Nursing, 5,* 169–172. doi:10.1016/j.ecns.2009.04.092

Haskvitz, L. M., & Koop, E. C. (2004). Students struggling in clinical? A new role for the patient simulator. *Journal of Nursing Education, 43*(4), 181–184.

Henneman, E. A., Cunningham, H., Roche, J. P., & Curnin, M. E. (2007). *Human patient simulation: Teaching students to provide safe care.* Retrieved from http://ezproxy.macewan.ca/login?url=http://search.ebscohost.com.ezproxy.macewan.ca/login.aspx?direct=true&db=edswsc&AN=000249638500009&site=eds-live&scope=site

Hetzel-Campbell, S., & Daley, K. (2009). *Simulation scenarios for nurse educators.* New York, NY: Springer Publishing.

Hiestand, W. (2000). Think different. Inventions and innovations by nurses, 1850 to 1950. *American Journal of Nursing, 100*(10), 72–77.

Hotchkiss, M. A., Biddle, C., & Fallacaro, M. (2002). Assessing the authenticity of the human simulation experience in anesthesiology. *American Association of Nurse Anesthetist Journal, 70*(6), 470–473.

Howard, V. M. (2011). President's message: Simulation faculty development. *Clinical Simulation in Nursing, 7*(6), e203–e204.

Huang, Y. M., Pliego, J. F., Henrichs, B., Bowyer, M. W., Siddall, V. J., McGaghie, W. C., & Raemer, D. B. (2008). 2007 simulation education summit. *Simulation in Healthcare, 3*(3), 186–191.

Hurley, K. F. (2005). *OSCE and clinical skills handbook.* Toronto, ON: Elsevier Saunders.

Hyland, J. R., & Hawkins, M. C. (2009). High-fidelity human simulation in nursing education: A review of literature and guide for implementation. *Teaching and Learning in Nursing, 4*(1), 14–21.

Institute of Medicine. (2000). *To err is human: Building a safer health system.* Washington, DC: National Academies Press.

International Nursing Association for Clinical Simulation and Learning. (2013a). Standards of best practice: Simulation. *Clinical Simulation in Nursing, 9*(6S). doi:10.1016/j.ecns.2013.05.010

International Nursing Association for Clinical Simulation and Learning. (2013b). Standards of best practice: Simulation. President's message. *Clinical Simulation in Nursing, 9*(6S). doi:10.1016/j.ecns.2013.05.010

Issenberg, S. B., McGaghie, W. C., Hart, I. R., Mayer, J. W., Felner, J. M., Petrusa, E. R., . . . Ewy, G. A. (1999). Simulation technology for health care professional skills training and assessment. *JAMA: The Journal of the American Medical Society, 282,* 861–866.

Issenberg, S. B., McGaghie, W. C., Petrusa, E. R., Gordon, D. L., & Scalese, R. J. (2005). Features and uses of high-fidelity medical simulations that lead to effective learning: A BEME systematic review. *Medical Teacher, 27*(1), 10–28.

Jamison, R. J., Hovancsek, M. T., & Clockesy, J. M. (2006). A pilot study assessing simulation using two simulation methods for teaching intravenous cannulation. *Clinical Simulation in Nursing Education, 2*(11). Retrieved from http://www.inacsl.org

Jeffries, P. R. (2005). A framework for designing, implementing, and evaluating simulations used as teaching strategies in nursing. *Nursing Education Perspectives, 26*(2), 96–103.

Jeffries, P. R. (Ed.). (2007). *Simulation in nursing education. From conceptualization to evaluation.* New York, NY: National League for Nursing.

Jeffries, P. R. (2008). Getting in S.T.E.P. with simulations: Simulations take educator preparation. *Nursing Education Perspectives, 29*(2), 70–73.

Jeffries, P. R., & Battin, J. (2012). *Developing successful health care education simulation centers: The consortium model.* New York, NY: Springer Publishing.

Kardong-Edgren, S., & Oermann, M. H. (2009). A letter to nursing program administrators about simulation. *Clinical Simulation in Nursing, 5*(5), 161–162.

Kesten, K. S., Brown, H. F., Hurst, S., & Briggs, L. A. (2010). Acute care for advanced practice nurses. In N. W. Nehring & F. R. Lashley (Eds.), *High-fidelity patient simulation in nursing education* (pp. 233–272). Toronto, ON: Jones and Bartlett.

Krautscheid, L., Kaakinen, J., & Warner, J. R. (2008). Clinical faculty development: Using simulation to demonstrate and practice clinical teaching. *Journal of Nursing Education, 47*(9), 431–434.

Kyle, R. R., & Bosseau-Murray, W. (2008). *Clinical simulation: Operations, engineering and management.* San Diego, CA: Academic Press.

Lapkin, S., Levett-Jones, T., Bellchambers, H., & Fernandez, R. (2010). Effectiveness of patient simulation manikins in teaching clinical reasoning skills to undergraduate nursing students: A systematic review. *Clinical Simulation in Nursing, 6*(6), e207–e222. doi:10.1016/j.ecns.2010.05.005

Lasater, K. (2007). High-fidelity simulation and the development of clinical judgment: Students' experiences. *Journal of Nursing Education, 46*, 269–276.

Laschinger, S., Medves, J., Pulling, C., McGraw, D., Waytuck, B., Harrison, M., & Gambeta, K. (2008). Effectiveness of simulation on health profession students' knowledge, skills, confidence and satisfaction. *International Journal of Evidence-Based Healthcare, 6*(3), 278–302. doi:10.1111/j.1744-1609.2008.00108.x

McGaghie, W. C., Issenberg, S. B., Petrusa, E. R., & Scalese, R. J. (2010). A critical review of simulation-based medical education research: 2003-2009. *Medical Education, 44*(1), 50–63. doi:10.1111/j.1365-2923.2009.03547.x

Meakim, C., Boese, T., Decker, S., Franklin, A. E., Gloe, D., Lioce, L., . . . Borum, J. C. (2013). Standards of best practice: Simulation standard I: Terminology. *Clinical Simulation in Nursing, 9*(6S), S3–S11. doi:10.1016/j.ecns.2013.04.001

Medley, C. F., & Horne, C. (2005). Using simulation technology for undergraduate nursing education. *Journal of Nursing Education, 44*(1), 31–33.

National League for Nursing Simulation Innovation Resource Center. (2013). *SIRC glossary.* Retrieved from http://sirc.nln.org/mod/glossary/view.php?id-183

Nehring, W., & Lashley, F. R. (2004). Current use and opinions regarding human patient simulators in nursing education: An international survey. *Nursing Education Perspectives, 25*(5), 244–48.

Nehring, W. M., Lashley, F. R., & Ellis, W. (2002) Critical incident nursing management using human patient simulators. *Nursing Education Perspectives, 23*(3), 128–132.

Norman, J. (2012). Systematic review of the literature on simulation in nursing education. *ABNF Journal, 23*(2), 24–28.

Oermann, M. H., & Gaberson, K. B. (2009). *Evaluation and testing in nursing education.* New York, NY: Springer Publishing.

Prensky, M. (2005, September/October). Engage me or enrage me. *EDUCAUSE Review.* Retrieved from http://net.educause.edu/ir/library/pdf/erm0553.pdf

Prensky, M. (2007). Changing paradigms: From "being taught" to "learning on your own with guidance". *Educational Technology.* Retrieved from http://www.marcprensky.com/writing/Prensky-ChangingParadigms-01-EdTech.pdf

Prion, S. (2008). A practical framework for evaluating the impact of clinical simulation experiences in prelicensure nursing education. *Clinical Simulation in Nursing, 4*(3), e69–e78. doi:10.1016/j.ecns.2008.08.002

Raglin, J. S., & Turner, P. E. (1993). Anxiety and performance in track and field athletes: A comparison of the inverted-U hypothesis with zone of optimal function theory. *Personality and Individual Differences, 14*(1), 163–171.

Rauen, C. A. (2001). Using simulation to teach critical thinking skills: You just can't throw the book at them. *Critical Care Nursing Clinics of North America, 13*(1), 93–103.

Rauen, C. A. (2004). Simulation as a teaching strategy for nursing education and orientation in cardiac surgery. *Cardiovascular Surgery, 24*(3), 46–51.

Ravert, P. (2002). An integrative review of computer-based simulation in education process. *CIN: Computers, Informatics, Nursing, 20*, 203–208.

Rehmann, A., Mitman, R., & Reynolds, M. (1995). *A handbook of flight simulation fidelity requirements for human factors research.* Wright-Patterson AFB, OH: Crew Systems Ergonomics Information Analysis Center.

Rothgeb, M. K. (2008). Creating a nursing simulation laboratory: A literature review. *The Journal of Nursing Education, 47*(11), 489–494.

Rudolph, J. W., Simon, R., Dufresne, R. L., & Raemer, D. B. (2006). There's no such thing as "nonjudgmental" debriefing: A theory and method for debriefing with good judgment. *Simulation in Healthcare, 1*(1), 49–55.

Rudolph, J. W., Simon, R., & Raemer, D. (2007). Which reality matters? Questions on the path to high engagement in healthcare simulation. *Simulation in Healthcare, 2*(3), 161–163.

Rudolph, J. W., Simon, R., Raemer, D., & Eppich, W. (2008). Debriefing as formative assessment: Closing performance gaps in medical education. *Academic Emergency Medicine, 15*, 1010–1016.

Satish, U., & Krishnamurthy, S. (2008). Role of cognitive simulations in healthcare. In H. Riley (Ed.), *Manual of simulation in healthcare.* Oxford, England: Oxford University Press.

Scherer, Y., Bruce, S., Graves, B., & Erdley, W. (2003). Acute care nurse practitioner education: Enhancing performance through the use of clinical simulation. *AACN Clinical Issues, 14*(3), 331–341.

Schiavenato, M. (2009). Reevaluating simulation in nursing education: Beyond the human patient simulator. *Journal of Nursing Education, 48*(7), 388–394.

Schön, D. (1983). *The reflective practitioner: How professionals think in action.* New York, NY: Basic Books.

Seropian, M. (2003). General concepts in full-scale simulation: Getting started. *Anesthesiology Analog, 97*, 1597–1605.

Seropian, M., Brown, K., Gavilanes, J., & Driggers, B. (2004). An approach to simulation program development. *Journal of Nursing Education, 43*(4), 170–174.

Sharma, S., Boet, S., Kitto, S., & Reeves, S. (2011). Interprofessional simulated learning: The need for 'sociological fidelity'. *Journal of Interprofessional Care, 25*, 81–83. doi:10.3109/1356 1820.2011.556514

Skiba, D. (2007). Nursing education 2.0: Second life. *Nursing Education Perspectives, 28*(3), 156–157. Retrieved from http://nlnjournals.org/doi/full/10.1043/1094-2831%282007%2928%5B156%3ANESL%5D2.0.CO%3B2

Society for Simulation in Healthcare. (2012). *Council for accreditation of healthcare simulation programs: Accreditation standards and measurement criteria.* Retrieved from http://ssih.org/search/search&keywords=accreditation%20standards&rx=0&y=0

Taekman, J. (2008). *Duke university simulation development template, 2008.* Retrieved from http://simcenter.duke.edu/support.html

Tanner, C. A. (2006). Thinking like a nurse: A research-based model of clinical judgment in nursing. *Journal of Nursing Education, 45*(6), 204–211.

Vandrey, C. I., & Whitman, K. M. (2001). Simulator training for novice critical care nurses. *American Journal of Nursing, 101*(9), 24GG–24LL.

Waldner, M. H., & Olson, J. K. (2007). Taking the patient to the classroom: Applying theoretical frameworks to simulation in nursing education. *International Journal of Nursing Education Scholarship, 4*(1), 1–14.

Wallace, P. (2007). *Coaching standardized patients.* New York, NY: Springer Publishing.

Wiltse, L., & Pait, T. (1998). Herophilus of Alexandria (325-255 B.C.). The father of anatomy. *Spine, 23*, 1904–1914.

Yerkes, R. M., & Dodson, J. D. (1908). The relation of strength of stimulus to rapidity of habit-formation. *Journal of Comparative Neurology and Psychology, 18*, 459–482.

chapter
18

Family Nursing and Community Health Nursing

SEANNA CHESNEY-CHAUVET AND
MELANIE J. HAMILTON

The Cortez family is Cecilia's first appointment today at the clinic. Gemma is a 10-year-old girl with cerebral palsy. Her parents divorced 5 years ago, and her mother has since remarried. Gemma lives mainly with her mother, Annie; stepfather; grandmother; and siblings but visits her father on alternating weekends and some holidays. Everyone in the household was born in Canada except for the stepfather, Jose, who was born in Chile. This family actively practices two faiths. Gemma and her mother practice in the Mormon faith, and her stepfather is Catholic. Gemma has two older stepbrothers from her stepfather's first marriage and one younger sister, who was born after her Mom and stepfather were married. All seven members live together in a four-bedroom condo complex in a small urban city, about 100 km from the nearest tertiary hospital. Gemma has many appointments with the outpatient clinic because of her cerebral palsy and has been admitted to the hospital three times this year.

CHAPTER OBJECTIVES

By the end of this chapter, you will be able to:

1. Identify the current demographic trends and realities in Canadian families.
2. Discuss the impact of health determinants on family health and explain the impact that family relationships have on health.
3. Understand the relationships among negative/stressful family realities and health.
4. Explain the focus of care in family nursing.
5. Identify the foundational beliefs of family nursing.
6. Articulate why the McGill Model of Nursing and the Calgary Family Assessment Model are appropriate to guide the practice of family nursing.
7. Describe the philosophy of Family-Centered Care (FCC).
8. Identify the Canadian community health nursing standards.
9. Describe and discuss the many roles and settings of the community health nurse in promoting and maintaining the health of Canadians.
10. Understand some of the agencies involved in policy development for Canadian community health nursing.
11. Identify how two community health nursing programs reflect the concepts of family nursing.

KEY TERMS

Calgary Family Assessment Model (CFAM) A framework in nursing that can assist nurses to assess a family, to use as an organizing framework or a template which can assist families to resolve issues.

Caregiver Stress The state of emotional, mental, or physical or strain/exhaustion related to caregiving.

Community A group of people who share a geographical and social environment.

Community Health Nursing Nursing that occurs in and with a community with the goal of promoting health from a strengths-based perspective.

Cultural Safety Founded by Maori nurses in New Zealand. Assumes a critical understanding of culture that recognizes people are dynamic and constantly shifting in relation to power dynamics in society.

Cultural safety is concerned with historical, economic, political, and power forces within nursing and within society. Such forces have an impact on nurses and the practice of nursing.

Family A group of people who feel united and support each other.

Family-Centered Care (FCC) A philosophy of care that encompasses a respectful, compassion, and culturally responsive, collaborative approach to patients and their family. This approach attends to the needs, values, beliefs, as well as cultural preferences of patients and their families.

Family Nursing Nursing that focuses on families as a holistic unit and cares, supports, and guides a family's experiences during times of health and/or illness.

Family Violence Any form of violence that one family member inflicts on another. The types of violence include physical, emotional, sexual, and financial.

McGill Model of Nursing (MMN) An approach to nursing where the nurse works with a family as they strive toward health. The main focus is health promotion.

Patient-Centered A widespread philosophy that supports the active involvement of the patient and his or her family regarding the

decision-making options for care and treatment in the health-care setting. Health-care professionals support patients and families by providing them with full context information, risks, and benefits about their situation.

Shift Work A practice of organizing work that occurs over 24 hours. A work day is divided into parts such as days, evenings, or nights. Most workers' schedules include a rotation where they would work more than one type of shift over a period of time.

This chapter introduces you to the world of families and communities and to the opportunities available for a nurse interested in working with them. We explore the diverse concept of family and the changes families undergo through the lifespan, along with factors that impact a family's health and how family nursing can empower a family to move toward healthy goals. Working with families allows nurses to share in the experiences of birth, life, grief, loss, pain, joy, and hope. Each family is unique, and they live and connect within an equally unique **community**. A family nurse uses a unique focus working with each family toward their goals for health. A family nurse's approach includes bringing a nonjudgmental approach and initiating positive relationships with family members. This chapter introduces Canadian family nursing frameworks and models to explore ways to assess and plan care for families.

Much of family nursing is embedded in **community health nursing**; therefore, this chapter also introduces the concepts of community and community health nursing, including the many roles of a community health nurse and how policy and programs impact the lives of Canadian families and communities.

Nursing Focus and the Unit of Care

When a nurse begins to work with a patient, there is a moment when he or she pauses to silently ask some questions. Who is the patient? What is the context for this patient? What is my focus? What is the patient's focus? Finally, who am I and what do I bring to this relationship? The nurse's questions and the patient and the family's answers will help novice and experienced nurses authentically enter into health-care relationships with families.

When a nurse sees the patient as an individual and then considers the individual's context within the home with his or her family or in a hospital setting, the nursing care approach is called **patient-centered**. Although families are indeed part of patient-centered care, the focus is on the individual patient and a health-care system that is integrated. When a patient moves from one part of the health-care system to another (e.g., from hospital to long-term care), the system may fail the patient. When we consider family nursing, the family is the unit of care. Rather than a focus on the individual (patient), the nurse views the whole family as the focus of his or her care. A community health nurse considers the "community" as the focus/unit of care to promote

the prevention of disease, maintenance of health, and the overall health and well-being of the community.

What Is Family Nursing?

Nursing has seen family as an integral part of healing and health as far back as Florence Nightingale (Neils, 2010). Nursing curricula in Canada historically included family nursing as an important type of nursing, and graduate nursing programs often include family nursing as a specialty or area of focus (Moules & Johnstone, 2010; St. John & Flowers, 2009). **Family nursing** focuses on families as a holistic unit where nurses provide care and support and guide a family's experiences during times of health and/or illness. This type of nursing is rooted in mutual respect and grounded in a shared therapeutic relationship.

What Is Community Health Nursing?

The community health nurse (CHNs) partners with clients and holds the following values, ". . . caring, principles of primary health care, multiple ways of knowing, individual and community partnerships, empowerment, and social justice" (The Community Health Nurses of Canada, 2008, p. 2). The goal is to improve the health of Canadians within the context of the community (Canadian Public Health Association [CPHA], 2010). The foundation of community health nursing is a strengths-based approach that seeks to recognize and support the development of strengths that exist in a person, family, and community. This approach always starts from a place of identifying and mobilizing strengths rather than looking to what is wrong and not working (chnc.ca, 2013; Gottlieb, Gottlieb, & Shamian, 2012).

Community Health Nursing Roles and Settings

Community health nurses in Canada work in various settings, with diverse populations and people. They work in patient homes, public and community health centres, hospitals, parish communities, and mental health clinics, just to name a few. They work for governments, provincial health authorities, and not-for-profit agencies. The work is often independent and in partnership with other disciplines. These disciplines include licensed nurse practitioners, communicable disease experts, parish nurses, forensic nurses, childbirth educators, and lactation consultants. CHNs work with clients in the areas of public health, primary health care, health promotion, disease and injury prevention, health protection, health surveillance, population health assessment, and emergency preparedness and response. The roles of a CHNs include advocate, educator, researcher, consultant, collaborator, policy developer, case manager, leader, and caregiver. Although the roles, settings, and titles may change, the work is consistently grounded in the focus on capacity building (chnc.ca, 2013). Just as a family nurse works with and not for a family, the community health nurse works with a community.

Who Am I and What Do I Bring to the Relationship?

It is essential for a family nurse to understand cultural safety and cultural humility and engage in authentic self-reflection prior to working with any family. **Cultural safety** urges us as nurses to critically examine our own beliefs, biases, and power over others who look or act different from us and for whom we engage in nursing care. From this self-reflection, we gain an understanding of who we are as a person and as a health-care provider and how our perspectives about others influence our nursing care (refer to Chapter 25 for more on self-reflection). There is also an obligation to explore and understand the social inequities and power imbalances that exist within the health-care environment (Bourque Bearskin, 2011; Browne et al., 2009). Cultural humility creates space for the family or community to share about their culture and how it might impact the health-care relationship or situation (Fahey et al., 2013). From this place of awareness, the nurse and the family move toward an open and honest place in which to begin a relationship. These approaches help novice and experienced nurses authentically enter into health-care relationships with families. Refer to Chapter 13 to learn more about culture and cultural safety.

Cecilia prepared for clinic by looking up cerebral palsy, including the possible disabilities that can occur. She reflected on how having a child with a disability meant a lifelong commitment for the parent, writing in her journal about all the challenges. Would the family have to live somewhere special? How many extra costs would the

family have? Is it difficult to go on vacation? And what about the siblings? Would they feel burdened when their sibling needed so much extra care and attention?

When Gemma and her mom entered the clinic, Cecilia was surprised. Gemma had special braces and crutches and walked in on her own steam, laughing and smiling. Cecilia realized at that moment that her research was focused in the wrong direction. She had reflected on the extra work and the burden that a disability could cause in a family. She hadn't thought of a child with cerebral palsy as a happy child with a diagnosis. Her preconceived ideas were not allowing her to see who this family really was. Gemma was full of potential, and it was Cecilia's job to get to know the patient and her family and what they might want for her future.

What Is a Family

There are many ways of describing and defining **family**. Families are structured in many different ways and composed of individuals in a wide range of relationships. One definition of family from the Vanier Institute of the Family (2013) is "any combination of two or more persons who are bound together over time by ties of mutual consent, birth and/or adoption or placement and who, together, assume responsibilities for variant combinations of some of the following:

- Physical maintenance and care of group members
- Addition of new members through procreation or adoption
- Socialization of children
- Social control of members
- Production, consumption, distribution of goods and services
- Affective nurturance—love." (para. 1)

This definition encompasses the unique compositions of families and reminds us that families are not merely human beings cohabitating in a home but have tasks, responsibilities, and goals, and they in turn grow, transition, and age (Table 18.1). It is also important to understand that a family

TABLE 18.1	Distribution (Number and Percentage) and Percentage Change of Census Families by Family Structure, Canada, 2001–2011						
	2001		2006		2011		Percentage Change
Census Family	Number	Percentage	Number	Percentage	Number	Percentage	2006 to 2011
Total census families	8,371,020	100.0	8,896,840	100.0	9,389,700	100.0	5.5
Couple families	7,059,830	84.3	7,482,775	84.1	7,861,860	83.7	5.1
Married	5,901,420	70.5	6,105,910	68.6	6,293,950	67.0	3.1
Common-law	1,158,410	13.8	1,376,865	15.5	1,567,910	16.7	13.9
Lone-parent families	1,311,190	15.7	1,414,060	15.9	1,527,840	16.3	8.0
Female parents	1,065,360	12.7	1,132,290	12.7	1,200,295	12.8	6.0
Male parents	245,825	2.9	281,775	3.2	327,545	3.5	16.2

Sources: Statistics Canada. (n.d). *2011 Census. Previous Censuses, Archived 2001, 2006.* Retrieved from http://www12.statcan.gc.ca/census-recensement/index-eng.cfm; CBC News Canada. (2012). *Census shows new face of the Canadian family.* Retrieved from http://www.cbc.ca/news/canada/census-shows-new-face-of-the-canadian-family-1.1137083

does not have to include children. Child-free couples also feel bonded and committed to each other.

Defining Family Through Nursing Models

Nursing models and theories provide definitions of the family that help to inform nursing practice. The McGill Model of Nursing defines family as those people who surround and support the individual (Gottlieb & Gottlieb, 2007). When the family nurse considers the needs of the patient, he or she includes all the people that the patient identifies as family. The nurse allows the patient and the family to define who they are. A nurse might assume that the family consists of those living together in the home, yet with further investigation, she might discover this not the case. Remember that in family nursing, the family is the focus of care, therefore gaining an understanding of who is the family is essential to effective and holistic care.

For example, when caring for a young single mother, a nurse might assume that the baby's father and the grandparents are the family unit that are to be included in the plan of care. Depending on experience, level of support, history, and social relationships, the notion of family for that young mother might be her friends and a neighbour. Therefore, the unit of care is who she believes are and holds as her family. This way of viewing family helps nurses to see families as unique and not defined by our biologic relatives or geographical housemates. Biology originates the family, but social and psychological connections clarify the client's real family. However, there are limitations when nonlegal family members encounter the health-care system. For example, issues concerning privacy (who can legally obtain and receive patient information) can surface.

Within the Calgary Family Assessment Model, Wright and Leahey (2013) define *family* as a "group of individuals who are bound by strong emotional ties, a sense of belonging, and a passion for being involved in one another's lives." (p. 54). Wright and Leahey stress that the family is who they say they are (see Table 18.1).

There are five critical attributes to the concept of family:

1. The family is a system or unit.
2. Its members may or may not be related and may or may not live together.
3. The unit may or may not contain children.
4. There is a commitment and attachment among unit members that includes future obligation.
5. The unit's caregiving functions consist of protection, nourishment, and socialization of its members.

Family Composition

Statistics Canada reported there have been many changes in Canadian families and their living arrangements since the 1960s. The nuclear family is no longer the norm. Instead, Canadians are now increasingly living alone, in a remarriage, have stepchildren, may be empty nesters, or have multiple generations sharing one household (Box 18.1). With more diversity in family structure comes more complexity (Canadian Press, 2012a; Ministry of Industry, 2012).

BOX 18.1 Facts on Families

- 67% of Canadian couples are married.
- The divorce rate as of 2008 was 210.8 per 100,000.
- 58.3% of mothers are working.
- One-person households make up 27.6% of all homes.
- 39.2% of families are parents with children.
- Common-law families are 16.7%.
- 1 in 10 children lives in a reconstituted arrangement (stepfamilies).
- Same-sex couples have increased 42.4% since 2006, making up 0.8% of couples in Canada in 2011.
- Lone-parent families make up 16.3% (8 out of 10 are mothers).
- In 2011, there were 29,590 foster children younger than the age of 14 years.
- 42.3% of adult children ages 20–29 years still live at home.
- 4.8% of children aged 14 years and younger live full-time with their grandparents.

Source: Ministry of Industry. (2012). *Statistics Canada. Portrait of families and living arrangements in Canada. Families, households and marital status, 2011 Census of Population.* Ottawa, ON: Author.

Some key terms and definitions of common types of families in Canada are as follows:

Nuclear family: Two parents (opposite or same sex) and their children. Traditionally, this meant the parents were married but now also includes common-law parents.

Lone-parent family: One parent and his or her children.

Step and blended family: A family created through marriage or other circumstances that includes children from a previous marriage or relationship of one parent or both.

Multigenerational family: Members from multiple generations living together.

Boomerang family: Adult children return to the home in which they were parented/raised.

Adoptive family: Parents have adopted one or more children.

Foster family: Children in the home have been placed with the parent(s) by an agent of the government, usually a social worker, to provide a safe and nurturing home.

See Figure 18.1.

Lone Parents

Lone parents may be widowed, separated, divorced or single (Canadian Press, 2012b). Some of the differences between lone-parent families and nuclear or blended families may include parental styles, financial status, living conditions, and number of familial transitions. Lone parents may face a multitude of stresses, including working long hours or more than one job, the need for more education and income, and increased risk of poverty (which may be a result of addictions or mental illness) (Safaei, 2012).

Nurses consider the following when caring for a lone-parent family unit:

- Income
- Education

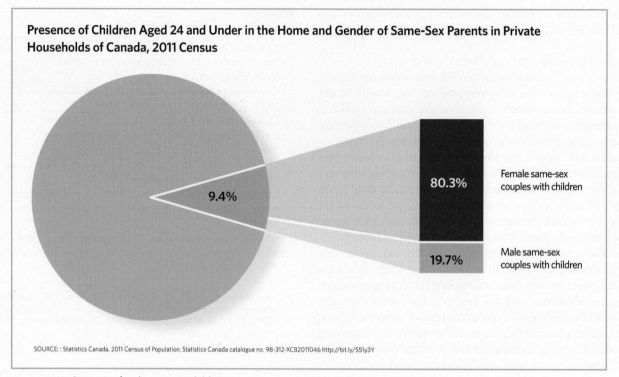

Figure 18.1 Same-sex families raising children.

- Mental health
- Social relationships
- Social support and programming

Stepfamilies

One of the greatest challenges of stepfamilies is coordination of the needs of all family members. Ministry of Industry (2012) classifies stepfamilies as simple or complex (Fig. 18.2.). Simple stepfamilies are composed of biologic or adopted children predating the relationship from only one of the spouses. There are three types of complex step-

families: those with at least one child from each parent with no children from both, at least one child to both parents with one or more from only one parent, and children from both parents and at least one child from each parent's previous relationship. Nurses should be aware that accompanying blended families are stresses that may include legal proceedings, custody arrangements (managing time between two households), financial strains, and emotional strains for adults and children (what to call their new parents, official documents for school) (Canadian Press, 2012c; Vanier Institute of the Family, 2010c).

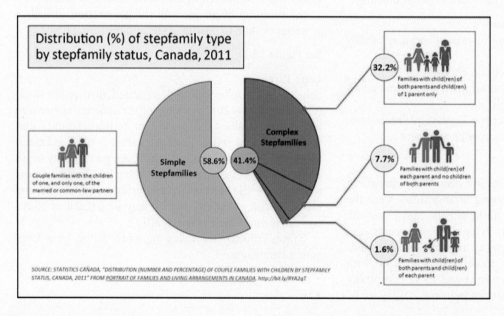

Figure 18.2 Blended families.

Multigenerational Families

According to Ministry of Industry (2012), there is an increasing number of Canadians who are choosing to live in multigenerational households. There are several reasons for this increase. Some grandparents want to spend more time with their grandchildren, there are adult children returning home (what some call the *boomerang children*), or multiple generations may live together out of necessity (sick family member, financial assistance). With the increase in life expectancy, more older adults are moving in with family members rather than into assisted living facilities. In 2006, there were about 515,000 grandparents living with their grandchildren.

The benefits of shared accommodation include shared finances, emotional support, assistance with child care, assistance with eldercare, learning cultural traditions and heritage, and building solid family ties. Reciprocal care allows grandparents to assist their adult children to care for their grandchildren and at the same time, the adult children can care for their aging parents. The challenges of shared accommodation include close proximity to family members, limited space and privacy, and conflicting ideas regarding parenting (Loney, 2012; Ministry of Industry, 2012).

Changes in composition of families may be temporary or permanent (Wright & Leahey, 2013). Permanent changes can include the addition of a new person to the family such as a new baby, a spouse, or the death of a family member. Temporary changes could include a live-in caregiver or aging parents. In Canada, the need for both parents to work has caused a shift in family composition. There are families who rely on live-in caregivers to assist with the care of children and aging parents (Box 18.2 and Table 18.2). There are also transient compositions, most common with blended families, where children from previous relationships spend time with both sets of families.

During the initial conversation or interview with a patient, a nurse might ask the following questions to assess family composition: Who is in your family? Who lives with you? Is there anyone in your family who does not live with you?

BOX 18.2 Canada's Seniors: Living Arrangements

According to the Vanier Institute of the Family (2010b), at some point in the next 5–10 years, the number of people aged 65 years and older will exceed the number of children younger than 15 years of age (see Table 18.2). An increase in life expectancy and the aging of the baby boomers generation have contributed to the increasing older adult population. In 2011, an estimated 5.0 million Canadians were 65 years of age or older, a number that is expected to double in the next 25 years to reach 10.4 million seniors by 2036. By 2051, about 1 in 4 Canadians is expected to be 65 years or older.

The living arrangement of seniors plays an important role in health and social policy. Most individuals want to stay in their home as long as possible; however, the home can also pose potential hazardous risks and situations. Changes that are part of the normal aging process, such as declining vision, hearing, sense of touch or smell, and bone density can increase the risk of injury. Injuries can also be more of a problem for seniors because, as the body ages, it takes longer to heal and recover from injury. Aging affects each individual differently. Some seniors experience physical limitations that seriously affect their level of activity, whereas others are able to remain quite active. The natural process of growing older, however, generally includes changes in abilities.

TABLE 18.2 Living Arrangements of Seniors by Age Group, 2006

	Aged 65–74 Years			Aged 75 Years and Older			Aged 65 and Over		
	Men (%)	Women (%)	Total (%)	Men (%)	Women (%)	Total (%)	Men (%)	Women (%)	Total (%)
In a collective dwelling	2.1	2.2	2.1	9.2	16.2	13.5	5.1	9.3	7.5
In private households									
In census family with spouse/common-law partner, and/or children	79.9	65.3	71.3	67.3	34.3	47.2	74.6	48.6	59.9
In other family situations	1.8	4.9	3.4	2.8	6.9	5.3	2.2	74.6	59.9
Alone	13.9	26.8	20.7	18.8	40.4	32	16	33.8	26
In other situations	2.3	2.5	2.4	1.9	2.1	2	2.1	2.3	2.2
Total	100	100	100	100	100	100	100	100	100

Collective dwelling is dwelling used for commercial, institutional, or communal purposes, such as a hotel, a hospital, or a work camp. Over 90% of seniors living in collective dwellings live in a health care–related facility such as a nursing home, residence for seniors, or long-term care facility. Census family refers to a married couple (with or without children of either or both spouses), a couple living common-law (with or without children of either or both partners), or a lone parent of any marital status with at least one child living in the same dwelling. A couple may be of opposite or same sex. Other family situations include living with a parent or another census family. Other situations refer to individual living with another relative(s) or nonrelative but not with a census family.

Source: Statistics Canada. (2013). *Living arrangements of seniors by age group.* Retrieved from http://www12.statcan.ca/census-recensement/2006/as-sa/97-554-XWE2006054/96-553-XCB2006018-eng.cfm

Through the eyes of a patient

I was really worried about my mom. Her house is so big, and she is starting to struggle with the upkeep and daily household tasks. We were having coffee last week, and she mentioned she was having trouble getting in and out of the bathtub. She is 75 years old and wants to stay where she is. I asked her if she thought about some supports to keep her safe in the home. Two weeks later, a home care registered nurse came and completed an assessment for mom. She set mom up with safety features such as grab bars in the bathroom and improved lighting and suggested we remove all of her floor rugs to reduce her risk of falls. Mom is happy with the safety improvements. These small modifications allow her to remain in her community with her friends and the home where our large family gathers together every Sunday for family dinners.

(personal reflection of a family member)

W hat are some of the stepfamily challenges that may impact Gemma and her family?

Changing Family Structures and Nursing

It is essential to consider family structure or composition when building a relationship. It is important to know who plays a significant role in the day-to-day lives of families. You will also want to establish how the family functions.

- Who in the family has the financial responsibilities and social responsibilities?
- How are family members involved in child rearing and parenting?
- It is important to understand how families make decisions about health and health care.

As you gain the family's trust, it is helpful to discuss their perceptions about their health. We address perceptions on health later in the chapter.

Family Roles

When considering the structure of the family, it is important to assess the roles of each family member within the family (Box 18.3). Think about your own family, what are your roles within your family? Now, think about the roles your family members play. Is there someone in your family who is more of a nurturer, who takes on more of a lead with finances, or with health matters? Now, think about some other roles that may be challenging for family members. Consider family roles when assessing the family unit. When families access health services, nurses support the family unit during varying levels of health, illness, and crisis. Remember that

BOX 18.3   Family Roles

- Provider
- Housekeeper
- Child care
- Socialization (interacting within the family/community)
- Caregiver in illness

certain family roles may be impacted in stressful situations and that another family member might have to take on additional or new roles. For example, a stay-at-home mother may now have to work outside the home to support her family after her husband is injured in a motor vehicle accident and is prevented from working. Nurses can help the family unit cope and adapt when these situations arise. Ensure that you keep in mind that family roles constantly change and may not always be what they seem.

W hat do you think might happen within the family or at home while Gemma and Annie are in the hospital? What are some additional roles that Jose might have to assume while his wife and Gemma are away? What questions could you ask Jose and the rest of the family that would help you understand what they are going through?

Working With Families

Working with a family is a privilege and should be met with this in mind. Nurses work to create a positive and trusting relationship, but this takes time and skill. Families take a chance on you when welcoming you into their home or intimate relationships. Although definitions and terms will help you understand the various types and demographics that make up our family landscape in Canada, there is much more to know before beginning to work with a family. What else does a nurse need to know? How do we begin to form a relationship of respect and trust? How do we begin to work with families to maintain their health or move them toward their health potential?

Life Stages of the Family

Understanding human development is an important part of understanding family members to help them as they strive for health (Gottlieb & Gottlieb, 2007). Scholarly work has been conducted in the area of development tasks and life stages of families. It is essential for a nurse to consider not only the composition of the family but also where they are in their life journey.

Smith and Hamon (2012) provide an overview of family theories, including family development theories and the work of Duvall. Such theories suggest that a family moves through various developmental and functional stages. Family development theory necessarily considers "family dynamics, family development, the family life cycle, change, stages and tasks, norms, and the life course perspective" (Griffore, 2012, p. 102). Carter and McGoldrick (2005) also explored family stages but included a stage of "leaving home" to reflect the stage where an adult may live on his or her own or with a partner for an extended period of time without children. They also discuss the process of divorce and the ways in which families adjust to life after divorce as significant phases for a family.

However, if a stage-based theory outlines normative milestones, then a family that does not follow such stages might be labeled nonnormative or abnormal. In Canada, "nonnormative" families may outnumber the "normative," which effectively calls into question how normative the norm ever was. Despite the limitations associated with stages theories, they do provide a vocabulary and a common way of describing families. As a family nurse, you will encounter families that may or may not follow the expected journey that is reflected in the literature.

Health Challenges in Life

A nurse working with families must not only understand the unique family, what life stage are they at, and what developmental tasks they are possibly working through but also what health challenges are present. Families continually not only face opportunities to create and enhance their health but also face challenges that could shift their state to one of poor health. These health realities can impact not only the present state of the family but also the future health of the family.

For example, an unattached young adult can seek healthy sexual behaviours as he or she explores dating, relationships, and sexual intercourse. This same adult could also be uninformed about sexual risks and lack knowledge about safer sex. He or she can engage in behaviours that result in a sexually transmitted infection or unexpected pregnancy. Or, a family with adolescents may be dealing with body image challenges. This situation can serve as an opportunity to promote family fitness and healthy nutrition. However, it can also challenge a family and the adolescent and result in poor dietary habits. And so you can see that working with families is complex. It is important that you assess possible health opportunities and challenges within a family. This is why nurses work in partnership with families and draw on their existing strengths, potential, and capacities. The nurse, in partnership with families, is poised to address health and social challenges in the life of the family.

Factors Impacting a Family's Health

Nurses take time to discuss perceptions of health within the family, considering family patterns. Each family member may perceive health differently and therefore may place

---

BOX 18.4 Families and Healthy Behaviours

- Emotional support
- Physical affection
- Support with academics/schooling
- Exercising together
- Positive communication
- Participating in recreational and leisure activities
- Support for healthy eating
- Building social relationships

---

different value on health. Some of these differences may include healthy eating, physical activity, natural and homeopathic treatments, risk-taking behaviours, and poor health choices (smoking, drugs, or alcohol). Some of these health perception differences can impact the way a family functions. If one family member is trying to lose weight and another keeps buying cookies and potato chips, you can see they are at odds with one another's individual health behaviours and beliefs (Box 18.4). The Public Health Agency of Canada (PHAC, 2013) explains there are many factors that influence the health of Canadians. We can use the social determinants of health to illustrate key factors that impact family health.

Social Determinants of Health

The Canadian Nurses Association (CNA, 2005) supports the idea that social determinants of health have a significant impact on individuals and groups related to health. As a nurse, these social determinants of health may help you assess for family risk and strengths. Social determinants of health were covered in depth in Chapter 2; here, we review in brief.

Income and Social Status

According to the PHAC, income and social status may be the most important determinants of health. Most Canadians (73%) in high-income groups report their health as good or excellent, as opposed to only 43% of Canadians in the lowest income bracket (PHAC, 2013). Individuals and families in higher income and social statuses are able to access better housing in safer communities, buy healthier foods, and may have better health-care habits. Individuals and families in lower income brackets are more likely to die earlier and/or experience more illnesses due to poor health habits and not seeking medical care.

Personal Health Practices and Coping Skills

Personal health practices is a largely neutral term for practices that can prevent disease, promote self-care, and make healthy choices that enhance health or choices that lead to illness and poor health. For example, in Canada, smoking, coronary heart disease, drinking and driving, and drinking and unsafe sex are personal health-care practices than can be linked to illness and death.

Personal life choices are influenced by the socioeconomic environments in which people live, learn, work, and play (PHAC, 2013). Lifestyle choices can impact at least five areas:

- Personal life skills
- Stress
- Culture
- Social relationships and belonging
- A sense of self control

Coping With Stress

Stress is a common everyday experience in most families. It can be social or physiological circumstances that contribute to short- or long-term stress. If excessive stress is not addressed, it may have detrimental effects on health. Drawing on the classic work of Selye (1974), stress can be defined in both positive (good stress, *eustress*) and negative (bad stress, *distress*) forms. Eustress, or positive stress, is the optimal amount of stress that can provide us with the energy to perform a task well, such as public speaking, engaging in competition, or completing a job interview. Exercise and physical activity can also be considered a positive stressor, although overtraining can lead to injury. Distress occurs when stress is not resolved through coping or adaptation. It can lead to anxiety and mental and physical problems.

Coping skills support a healthy lifestyle, allowing individuals and families to interact with the world around them and to deal with stressful events and challenges they may encounter in their everyday life. Family members can support each other through stressful situations by developing effective coping skills. PHAC (2013) indicates that coping skills need to be developed to foster healthy lifestyles. Family members can assist each other to solve problems, make healthy lifestyle decisions, and face stressors. Evidence shows those individuals who have family supports are more likely to adopt and sustain healthy behaviours and lifestyles (Tables 18.3 and 18.4).

Social and Physical Environments

Social environments are largely responsible to including health and well-being of individuals and families (PHAC, 2013). Lifestyles can be thought of as a broad description of individual or family behaviour within the social environment and personal and private lives.

The physical environment where a family, lives, works, or plays can also impact health. Families who live in lower economic housing environments may be exposed to poorer indoor and outdoor air quality. Families may have to rely more on public transportation, which may impact their ability to partake in healthy behaviours (e.g., longer commutes, less time for exercise of home meal preparation, or seeking regular health-care appointments).

Both social and physical environments are influenced by poverty and income inequality. Poverty directly harms the health of those with low incomes. Income inequality affects the health of all Canadians through the weakening of social infrastructure and the destruction of social cohesion

TABLE 18.3	Stress Inventory: Holmes and Rahe Stress Scale

To measure stress according to the Holmes and Rahe Stress Scale, the number of Life Change Units that apply to events in the past year of an individual's life are added, and the final score will give a rough estimate of how stress affects health.

Life Event	Life Change Units
Death of a spouse	100
Divorce	73
Marital separation	65
Imprisonment	63
Death of a close family member	63
Personal injury or illness	53
Marriage	50
Dismissal from work	47
Marital reconciliation	45
Retirement	45
Change in health of family member	44
Pregnancy	40
Sexual difficulties	39
Gain a new family member	39
Business readjustment	39
Change in financial state	38
Death of a close friend	37
Change to different line of work	36
Change in frequency of arguments	35
Major mortgage	32
Foreclosure of mortgage or loan	30
Change in responsibilities at work	29
Child leaving home	29
Trouble with in-laws	29
Outstanding personal achievement	28
Spouse starts or stops work	26
Begin or end school	26
Change in living conditions	25
Revision of personal habits	24
Trouble with boss	23
Change in working hours or conditions	20
Change in residence	20
Change in schools	20
Change in recreation	19
Change in church activities	19
Change in social activities	18
Minor mortgage or loan	17
Change in sleeping habits	16
Change in number of family reunions	15
Change in eating habits	15
Vacation	13
Christmas	12
Minor violation of law	11

Score of 300+: At risk of illness.
Score of 150–299: Risk of illness is moderate (reduced by 30% from the above risk).
Score <150: Only have a slight risk of illness.
The American Institute of Stress. (n.d.). *Holmes-Rahe stress inventory*. Retrieved from http://www.stress.org/holmes-rahe-stress-inventory

(Raphael, 2002). "Living in poverty can cause stress and anxiety which can damage people's health; and low income limits peoples' choices and militates against desirable changes in behaviour" (Benzeval, Judge, & Whitehead, 1995, p. xxi).

TABLE 18.4	Stress Inventory for Non-Adults

A modified scale based on Holmes and Rahe stress scale (1967) was been developed for non-adults. Similar to the adult scale, stress points for life events in the past year are added and compared to the rough estimate of how stress affects health

Life Event	Life Change Units
Death of parent	100
Unplanned pregnancy/abortion	100
Getting married	95
Divorce of parents	90
Acquiring a visible deformity	80
Fathering a child	70
Jail sentence of parent for over one year	70
Marital separation of parents	69
Death of a brother or sister	68
Change in acceptance by peers	67
Unplanned pregnancy of sister	64
Discovery of being an adopted child	63
Marriage of parent to stepparent	63
Death of a close friend	63
Having a visible congenital deformity	62
Serious illness requiring hospitalization	58
Failure of a grade in school	56
Not making an extracurricular activity	55
Hospitalization of a parent	55
Jail sentence of parent for over 30 days	53
Breaking up with boyfriend or girlfriend	53
Beginning to date	51
Suspension from school	50
Becoming involved with drugs or alcohol	50
Birth of a brother or sister	50
Increase in arguments between parents	47
Loss of job by parent	46
Outstanding personal achievement	46
Change in parent's financial status	45
Accepted at college of choice	43
Being a senior in high school	42
Hospitalization of a sibling	41
Increased absence of parent from home	38
Brother or sister leaving home	37
Addition of third adult to family	34
Becoming a full-pledged member of a church	31
Decrease in arguments between parents	27
Decrease in arguments with parents	26
Mother or father beginning work	26

Score of 300+: At risk of illness.
Score of 150–299: Risk of illness is moderate (reduced by 30% from the above risk).
Score <150: Slight risk of illness.
Source: Bronstad, D. (n.d।). *Childhood stress and grief*. Retrieved from http://www.stages-of-grief-recovery.com/childhood-stress.html

What are some social determinants of health that could apply to Gemma's family?

• What if Gemma's stepfather did not speak or read English?
• What challenges might religious differences bring?
• What are some personal health practices that could affect the health of the family?

• What would happen to Gemma and her family if they had trouble accessing health care as a consequence of their physical environment?

Complex Family Relationships

Not all family relationships are straightforward or healthy. In Canada, there are many factors that contribute to challenges in family dynamics. This section briefly highlights some common issues that may impact the family unit. Family violence, shift work, Canadian residential schools, and caregiver stress are larger challenges that nurses might encounter when interacting with families.

Family Violence

Family nurses work with all kinds of families during all types of healthy and unhealthy situations. For some families, it is the relationships, the behaviours, and the choices that create an unhealthy reality for the family members. Some families suffer from **family violence**, and the ramifications are long lasting and harmful. The Government of Canada defines *family violence* as "when someone uses abusive behaviour to control and/or harm a member of their family, or someone with whom they have an intimate relationship" (Government of Canada, n.d., para. 1). A family nurse, with the focus on the family as a whole and the relationships within, can identify families at risk for family violence. Table 18.5 outlines the different types of abuse and definitions of the terms commonly used.

Family Violence and Impact on Health
Family violence affects all members of the family. Our health and justice systems are also burdened with the impact of family violence. The victims of abuse suffer the long-lasting physical and psychological scars and need the support of the health-care system. The justice system endeavours to keep victims safe and prosecute the offenders (Cunningham & Baker, 2007).

The collateral damage of family violence cannot be ignored. Children who witness family violence can be considered to "suffer the same consequences as those who are directly abused" (Royal Canadian Mounted Police [RCMP], 2012, p. 5). These children can experience behaviour problems, difficulties with peers, mood disorders, and inappropriate responses to social situations including sexual and violent behaviour. These behaviours and feelings may carry forward into adulthood. Some victims become abusers, either toward others or themselves (RCMP, 2012).

It is important to understand the types of violence; the statistical reality in Canada; and the impact that violence has on families, children, and society. Health-care professionals are in a key position to recognize abuse and help the families

TABLE 18.5	Types of Family Violence
Nature of Abuse	**Definitions**
Intimate partner violence	Violence toward an intimate partner with no bias toward gender; can occur male to female, female to male, male to male, or female to female
Child abuse	All abuse that is directed toward a child including sexual, physical, emotional, neglect
Emotional abuse	Abuse targeted at hurting the emotional and psychological person through insults, isolation, control, damaging property, and hurting pets; children witnessing violence is also considered emotional abuse.
Economic abuse	Abuse that controls the finances and economic well-being of the person
Spiritual abuse	Abuse that controls or punishes for a religious or spiritual belief or tradition
Physical abuse	Abuse that physically hurts and may cause injury (slap, punch, push, etc.)
Elder abuse	Physical, emotional, financial, spiritual, sexual abuse against an elderly person

Source: Cunningham, A., & Baker, L. (2007). *Little eyes, little ears: How violence against a mother shapes children as they grow.* Ottawa, ON: Family Violence Prevention Unit and Public Health Agency of Canada. Retrieved from http://www.phac-aspc.gc.ca/ncfv-cnivf/sources/fem/fem-2007-lele-pypo/index-eng.php; Royal Canadian Mounted Police. (2012). *The effects of family violence on children: Where does it hurt?* Retrieved from http://www.rcmp-grc.gc.ca/cp-pc/chi-enf-abu-eng.htm

find safe and appropriate resources. Nurses are legally obligated to report any suspected, witnessed, or reported abuse against children, women, men, or seniors. However, family nurses also are prepared to help victims identify an abuser, leave an unsafe home, protect themselves and their children, and eventually support the family as they embark on a path of healing.

In Alberta, the Victorian Order of Nurses Canada runs a unique program titled "People In Crisis Program." Nurses working in this program provide nursing services to women and children who have fled from abusive situations and have sought safety in shelters and transitional housing. They are a visible and therapeutic presence for women living in shelters in Edmonton. They also work closely with the issue of elder abuse and in health promotion and awareness campaigns (Victorian Order of Nurses Canada, 2012). Because of their focus on care and the environment in which they work, family and community health nurses are in unique positions to directly influence individuals, families, communities, and governments in the area of family violence.

In working with Gemma, what would you do if she told you that her stepfather hits her mom sometimes? What questions would you ask? What actions would you take?

The Impact of the Canadian Residential School System

Canadian residential schools (in existence between 1878 and the mid-20th century) left a devastating and far-reaching legacy (Fig. 18.3). An estimated 150,000 Aboriginal children were placed in residential schools as a part of the Canadian government's plan to assimilate the Indian people. Tragically, many of the schools were not a safe haven of learning for the children. After having been forcibly removed from their homes, many of the children experienced isolation, all forms of abuse, substandard living conditions,

and a poor education. These victims have suffered and continue to suffer long-lasting negative effects. Nurses working with Aboriginal families see the impact the schools have had on a whole generation of people. The generations of residential students often lacked not only a childhood but also any remnant of parenting, nurturing, or Aboriginal family life. How does a person parent when he or she never experienced a sense of mothering, fathering, or family in his or her childhood? Any role modeling from a parent was impossible because an entire generation of parent–child interactions were eliminated. This discussion is only a small piece of the tragic legacy of Canada's residential schools. Nurses working with Aboriginal families need to bring this knowledge, true compassion, and an openness to understand the many layers and complexities in working with people to rebuild their family life (http://www.legacyofhope.ca; Smith, Varcoe, & Edwards, 2005).

Families Working Shift

Shift work is very common in Canada's labour market. Rotating and irregular schedules are the most common type of shift work. Nursing, paramedics, other health-related professions, police officers, and correctional officers are a few examples of careers that require shift work. There are also many jobs in industry that require family members to work shifts, such as factory workers, sales clerks, and trades. A nurse may also see members of a family working away from home for a period of time. This may include rig workers, pilots, construction/trades, and salespeople, for example. According to the Vanier Institute of the Family (2010d), 28% of workers aged 19 to 64 years worked a shift schedule in 2005. Shift work can provide a family with the opportunity to balance both work and family obligations; however, this same type of work can cause role overload and lower levels of satisfaction with work. Families may be impacted by a member who works varying hours in many of ways including lack of child care in the evenings, night, and weekends (Fig. 18.3).

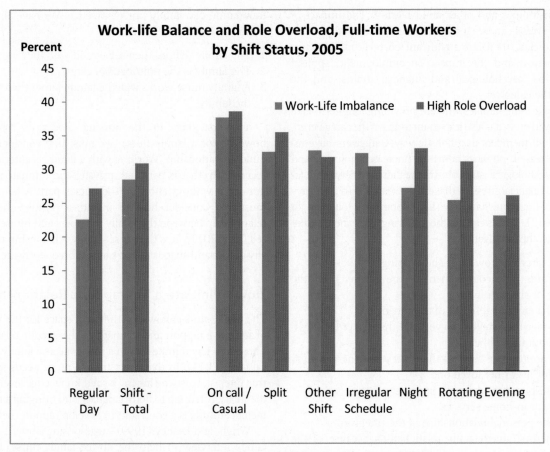

Figure 18.3 Work–life balance and role overload, full-time workers by shift status, 2005. (Source: Williams, C. [2008, August]. Work-life balance of shift workers. *Perspectives on Labour and Income.* Retrieved from http://www.statcan.gc.ca/pub/75-001-x/2008108/article/10677-eng.htm)

Through the eyes of a nurse

I love my job as a registered nurse. I have worked on the same unit since before I was married. I never minded working various hours, including days, nights, and weekends. Since I had children, I have found there is more stress working in a position with shift work. It is harder to find child care that starts at six in the morning. I hate having to wake up my kids to drop them off so early. I work full-time, and it is hard to get time off. I often miss my children's school events, sports games, and dance recitals. I am exhausted after working a night shift and then having to get up and still clean the house, do laundry, and make meals before I go back to work. My husband is very helpful but also puts in long hours at his job. Sometimes, he has to travel, and I am more dependent on family and friends to take care of my children during the night. I wish I had more of a work–life balance.

(personal reflection of a nurse)

Caregiver Stress

The Canadian Caregiver Coalition (2008) indicates there are over 2.85 million Canadians caring for family members with long-term health issues, including care for spouses, children, parents, and other members of their extended family. Family members who need support include children, aging parents, individuals with long-term or chronic illness, and those with debilitating medical conditions or injuries.

The health-care challenges in Canada have contributed to the need for family members to assist in providing care for their loved ones. Caregiving includes support of activities of daily living (ADL) such as personal care (bathing, dressing, toileting), meal assistance, or assistance with mobility or instrumental activities of daily living (IADL) such as grocery shopping, laundry, housekeeping, meal preparation, shopping, handling finances, transportation to and from medical appointments, and medication management. The Canadian Caregiver Coalition (2008) reports that 15.6 million hours per week are spent caring for persons with chronic conditions.

Nurses are aware that family members caring for their loved ones are most likely to also have employment responsibilities outside the home in addition to their home life responsibilities and other child rearing. The impact of **caregiver stress** can be far reaching. As McDaniel and Allen (2012) indicate, there are significant correlations between caregiver stress and the impact on employment, spousal relationships, psychological and financial strains, and the health of the caregiver.

When assessing families who are providing long-term care for their loved ones, it is also important to assess the caregiver(s), looking at all members in a holistic way. Caregivers have reported increased physical ailments (increased injuries and illness), psychological stressors (depression, anxiety, and fatigue), and financial stressors that are associated with the heavy demands of their caregiving role (Lilly, Robinson, Holtzman, & Bottorff, 2012). Nurses can use the following assessment strategies to assist the caregiver:

- Ask the caregiver how he or she is doing.
- Offer words of encouragement to the caregiver for the work he or she is doing.
- Assess the emotional health of the caregiver:
  - Encourage the caregiver to verbalize his or her feelings.
  - Ask about mental health.
- Discuss appropriate services that may assist the caregiver to care for his or her loved one:
  - Offer respite care whenever possible.
- Arrange for in-home services.
- Assess the personal relationships of the caregiver:
  - Are there strained family relationships because of the caregiving?
- Assess the stressors of the caregiver.
- Assess the personal health of the caregiver:
  - Are they partaking in unhealthy behaviours such as smoking and drinking?
  - Assess for physical ailments such as headaches, back pain, and frequent illnesses.
- Assess the caregiver's leisure activities:
  - Does he or she have time for personal interests and hobbies?
- Assess their nutrition, physical activity, and sleep patterns.

List some of the stresses that Annie or Jose might be experiencing while caring for Gemma. What are some supports you as a nurse could offer the Cortez family?

Working With Families

Now that we've defined the key concepts of family, let's look at family-centered care and the applied role of the family nurse. Working with families includes establishing a positive initial rapport, developing a therapeutic relationship, and collecting appropriate data and information with the family. Although each nurse might approach these aspects differently, there are foundational beliefs that are the foundation of a family nurse's practice. We have already explored three of these beliefs:

1. The family defines themselves and who they are.
2. The family is the unit/focus of care.
3. A family nurse works *with* the family rather than doing *for* the family.

The first stage in the nursing process is assessment; however, for a family nurse, we must first consider how to build a relationship. Working with a family is entering into a relationship that is personal, private, and intimate and does not occur without effort on the nurse's part. A family nurse must first consider how to initiate a positive therapeutic relationship between the family members and himself or herself (Bell, 2011). It is the nurse–family relationship that actually guides and shapes the care and subsequently the nursing.

How to Initiate a Therapeutic Relationship

The family nurse allows for time and space for the initiation of a positive rapport and ultimately a therapeutic relationship. Those first few minutes when a nurse meets a family are critical (Bell, 2011). In that short time, a nurse needs to convey true interest, trustworthiness, a solid knowledge level, and authenticity. Attention to body language and bringing a nonjudgmental attitude is a good start to develop rapport (Bell, 2011).

Wright and Leahey (1999) suggest using a brief 15-minute family interview to help the novice family nurse. Having a framework helps the novice nurse to have a place to start when beginning to work with families. This interview provides this structure. The 15-minute family interview consists of "manners, therapeutic conversation, family genogram [and in some situations, an ecomap], therapeutic questions, and commendations" (Wright & Leahey, 1999, p. 261). The first element, *manners*, reminds nurses to properly introduce themselves to everyone in the family. Therapeutic conversation reveals that all conversation with a family has the potential to convey trust and move the family toward health. Some key questions can help the nurse to begin to create a family genogram. Wright and Leahey (1999) suggest starting with easier questions such as, "Who are your family members? What are their ages?"

Then, as the interview progresses, the nurse can move to deeper questions such as, "Which of your family members have health concerns? Which family members contribute to your stress?" These questions may be asked within the family interview and can then be asked again within a one-to-one interaction. A nurse should not be surprised to learn that the answers may differ among family members. These open-ended, probing but respectful questions help to build a picture or map of the family in which you are working (Bell, 2011; St. John & Flowers, 2009) (For more on interviewing and open-ended questions, see Chapter 26.) The therapeutic questions are those that address universal issues in the health relationship including information sharing, family needs, and how the nurse can best work with the family. Finally, the 15-minute interview calls on the nurse to offer commendations to the family. The nurse looks for strengths in the individual and in the family and sincerely shares them at the end of the interview. These are not trivial compliments but real strengths the nurse sees in the family that they can build on for what is to come.

Assessing Family Health

Nursing assessments of the family include asking family members about their views on health. These assessments may be asked within the community and acute care setting. It is important to consider the family's own understandings and meaning of health, so the nurse has a reference point in understanding the family's thoughts, ideas, and readiness to learn.

- Start by asking family members their own perception of the meaning of health.
- Take the time to listen to each family member.
- Do not be surprised if certain members of the family have different opinions or views.
- Ask family members if they have cultural or religious practices that impact health in their family.
- Remember to inquire about homeopathic or natural remedies that may be used within the family.
- Ask if family members are in agreement or supportive for healthy behaviours or whether there is disparity or conflict.

For example, you meet George and his wife Martha. George has been diagnosed with a heart condition. His physician has told him to eat a heart-healthy diet that includes limited fat, increased fruits, vegetables, and fibre. He tells you that when he explains this to Martha, she refuses to change her cooking habits, and she is going to continue to fry her meats in oil and cook with cream. How are their needs and actions impacting each other's health?

This example illustrates that not all family members view health in the same way. As a nurse, how can you assist both George and Martha? What are some broader concerns inherent in Martha's stance regarding her cooking?

Gathering Data/Assessment

Nursing frameworks, models, and theories are available to help shape the assessment of a family. Two Canadian models, the **McGill Model of Nursing (MMN)** and the **Calgary Family Assessment Model (CFAM)**, provide good choices for family assessment. Nursing students and novice nurses can benefit from using a model as a guide while building their professional experience and confidence with family assessments.

McGill Model of Nursing

MMN, developed by Dr. Moyra Allen at McGill University, reflects the belief that nurses are the "primary promoters and facilitators of family health" (Gottlieb & Rowat, 1987, p. 52). The model was developed during a time of health-care delivery and role changes in the 1970s. The following assumptions are espoused in the model:

- The client is the family, and the family is the client. The nurse views the individual through the lens of the family and as the individual influences the family so does the family influence the individual. The family is the unit of care for a nurse using the McGill model (Gottlieb & Rowat, 1987; Wright and Leahy, 2013).
- The nurse views the family from a perspective of their strengths rather than deficits.
- Nursing is grounded in health promotion, and the nurse works as a collaborator with the family. The nurse allows the family to lead and always works with them as a partner.
- Health is multidimensional and can coexist with illness. We learn about health and how to cope within our family unit. Families strive for what they see as their health goals and their unique coping methods and development shape this journey toward health (Gottlieb & Rowat, 1987).

The assessment phase for a family nurse using the MMN is an open-ended and unstructured phase (http://www.mcgill.ca/nursing/about/model/). The nurse creates a safe climate in which the family feels comfortable to share and talk. It is not only a time when the nurse uses questions tailored to gathering information but also a time to support the family in identifying their strengths and goals.

In other approaches to assessment, there is a reliance on information surrounding the diagnosis and treatment (Gottlieb & Gottlieb, 2007). In contrast, this model encourages family nurses to see the individual and the family as primary sources. Using this approach with families in the community and their home makes sense for a family nurse because the MMN sees health as occurring and transforming within the family and the family environment. The strengths-based nature of this model also lends itself to the acute care environment. Hospitals today are busy with a high acuity level and heavy workloads. The idea of seeing the patient as a family unit and with the perspective of building on the strengths they possess has the potential for empowering the family of the acutely ill patient. Can you see some basic similarities between the MMN and the underlying principles of the 15-minute interview?

Calgary Family Assessment Model

CFAM can be used by nurses to assess a family. CFAM is a multidimensional framework consisting of three major categories: family structural components, family development, and family functioning (Wright & Leahey, 2013). The model is based on a theory of foundation involving systems, cybernetics, communication, and change. CFAM is particularly useful for nursing students and novice nurses to assess families. According to Wright and Leahey (2013), families "present themselves or are encountered by nurses while coping or suffering with an illness, loss and/or disability or are seeking assistance to improve their quality of life" (p. 53). The nurse uses the family assessment to understand the interactions among all the members within a family. Take the time to discuss who is in the family and what the connection is among these members.

Through the eyes of a nurse

I had been working with Healthy Beginnings for few years, but this home visit was very challenging for me. Melody lived in a situation complicated with poverty and an unhealthy relationship with the baby's father. I knew from experience that breast-feeding would be a cost-effective and convenient method of feeding for her and Grady. However, she was very nervous about it, and by the end of the visit, she told me that she really didn't want to breast-feed. She shared that the idea was daunting for her, and she would feel much more comfortable bottle-feeding the baby. She also knew that it would be easier for her to return to school if others could feed the baby. She looked so frightened, and I knew that she felt alone and unable to cope with the initial demands and stresses of breast-feeding. I knew that choosing to bottle-feed had its own stresses including a financial cost and constant cleaning of supplies. She was adamant about this, though, and I decided that supporting her in this goal was important. Melody was using this issue to take control of her situation, and I knew that it was my role as a partner and collaborator to support her in this decision. I commended her on knowing what she wanted to do. We sat down and developed a plan that helped her transition from breast-feeding to formula.

(personal reflection of a nurse)

Family-Centered Care

The term **family-centered care (FCC)** originated in the 1960s specifically addressing areas in maternity nursing (Dokken & Ahmann, 2006). As the FCC approach evolved, maternity care practices, family support for children with chronic illnesses, and changes in early intervention practices were addressed, and adverse effects of the hospitalized child were reduced. FCC brought increased visiting hours on pediatric units, focus on developmentally appropriate care for each child, and encouraged parental involvement in care decisions. Today, the FCC philosophy has been adopted for children's nursing and is recognized by most national and international pediatric nursing organizations (Coyne, O'Neill, Murphy, Costello, & O'Shea, 2011). FCC is considered the ideal system of care to structure the involvement of parents and families in health care.

FCC approach is grounded in a mutually beneficial partnership between the patient, the family, and health-care providers (Institute for Patient- and Family-Centered Care, n.d.). FCC applies to all ages and stages of life, encompassing families from birth to death. The well-being of individuals and family members includes not only physical support for health care but also addresses emotional, social, and developmental support.

Core Concepts of Family-Centered Care

Four core concepts developed by the Institute for Patient- and Family-Centered Care guide the practice of FCC.

- Respect and dignity. Health-care practitioners listen to and honour patient and family perspectives and choices. Patient and family knowledge, values, beliefs, and cultural backgrounds are incorporated into the planning and delivery of care.
- Information sharing. Health-care practitioners communicate and share complete and unbiased information with patients and families in ways that are affirming and useful. Patients and families receive timely, complete, and accurate information in order to effectively participate in care and decision-making.
- Participation. Patients and families are encouraged and supported in participating in care and decision-making at the level they choose.
- Collaboration. Patients and families are also included on an institution-wide basis. Health-care leaders collaborate with patients and families in policy and program development, implementation, and evaluation; in health-care facility design; and in professional education as well as in the delivery of care.

When speaking with a family who is hospitalized, some of the questions you may want to ask include the following:

1. Have you ever been admitted to the hospital before?
2. What are some things we can do to help your stay?
3. Is there anything that we do that has not worked in the past?
4. What is your loved one's routine?
5. Are there any cultural or religious considerations we should be aware of?
6. Do you have any questions for the health-care team?

Do not forget the importance of initiating a positive rapport before entering the nurse–family relationship. One way to remember is

K-Knock.
I-Introduce yourself.
D-Explain your professional designation.
S-State to the family what you are doing and why.

Many hospitals in Canada follow the patient- and family-centered care philosophy. More and more health-care centres are applying the FCC model to adult patients as well. As FCC evolves, some hospitals are even creating FCC networks, which allow health-care professionals to partner with families both at the bedside and at the operational level of the hospital. Families are now sitting on interview panels, policy and procedure committees, and are actively involved in teaching FCC.

A Family-Centered Care Exemplar

The Stollery Children's Hospital in Edmonton, Alberta, Family Centred Care Network (FCCN) has over 400 members, which include families, health-care professionals, and senior leaders. Some of the responsibilities of the FCCN at the Stollery include the following:

- Sharing the power of their story at
  - New staff orientation
  - Education of health professionals
  - Grand rounds
- Reviewing and providing input on
  - Policy and procedures
  - Documentation for families
  - Design and improvement of facilities and services
- Supporting other families through peer support opportunities
- Providing tours for families
- Participating in selection of new senior level staff and physicians
- Serving on other committees and special projects

There are two formal groups that work on FCC at the Stollery—the Family Centred Care Council and the Neonatal Intensive Care Unit Family Advisory Care Team (NICU FACT). The Family Centred Care Council sets priorities for network activities, and the NICU FACT is a unit-specific

group. Both groups are built on a collaborative model, with half the membership drawn from families who have experience with their children receiving care at the hospital and the other half including representatives from senior management, staff, and physicians. These two groups have a screening and interview process for membership and are governed by terms of references (Alberta Health Services, 2013a) (Fig. 18.4).

Within Stollery Children's Hospital, there is a family room, providing a quiet environment and resources for families. The goal of this space is "to support families before, during and after their hospital experience by building capacity in families, health professionals and hospital staff for informed, collaborative decision-making and care of the pediatric patient" (http://www.albertahealthservices .ca/5510.asp, 2013, para. 6). Figure 18.5 is a 10-year-old patient's illustration of her hospital stay. Figure 18.6 shows a typical private room at the hospital. As a nurse, it is essential to remember that families should be involved in all the care decisions for their loved one.

The Role of Family in Family-Centered Care

One of the most important concepts of FCC is that family members remain with their loved ones as they navigate through the health-care system. Examples include a parent or guardian spending the night with a child, a partner assisting his partner during birth, or a family member staying with an aging parent or spouse. As FCC has evolved, family members' roles have broadened to include advocacy for one's children or family members, peer support to other families, and involvement in day-to-day medical and

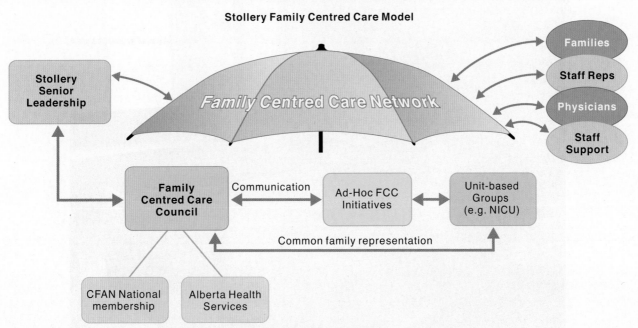

Figure 18.4 Alberta Health Services. (n.d.). *Family centred care at the Stollery Children's Hospital.* (Source: http://www.albertahealthservices.ca/ps-1009669-fcc-introducing-fcc.pdf.)

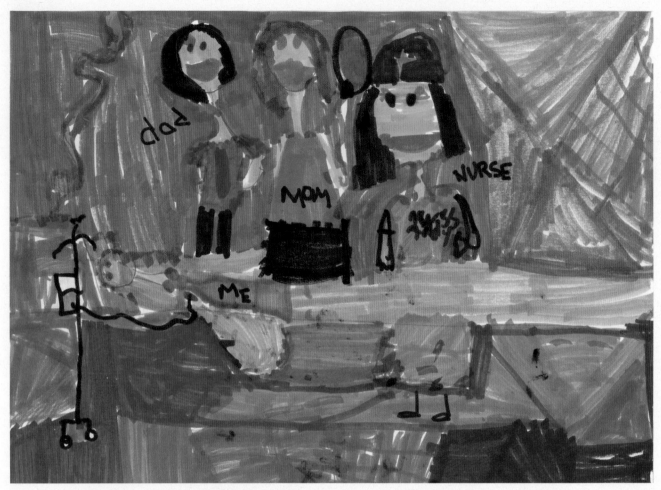

Figure 18.5 Child's drawing of family in hospital.

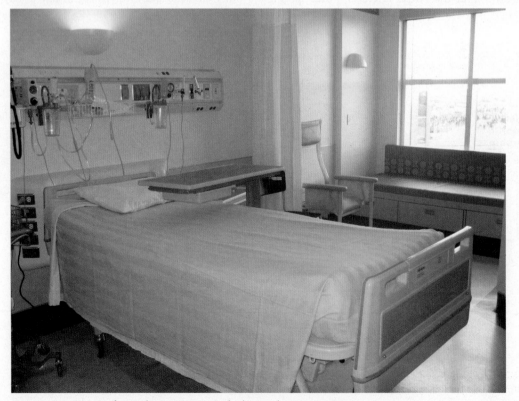

Figure 18.6 Picture of typical private room at the hospital.

nursing decisions (see Box 18.5). Nurses should remember that FCC does not just include parents or guardians but also other members such as siblings, grandparents, or other family relations. In FCC, nurses acknowledge "the family as a complete unit, and encompasses care of the family as a whole and the effect the sick child has on the family" (Coyne et al., 2011, p. 2564).

Through the eyes of a patient

This is the fourth time I have taken my daughter, Rosie, to the hospital in 6 months. We have been admitted for 2 days now. I always feel so lucky that we have a hospital specifically for children, with a private room and a bed for me to stay with my daughter. But today, I am really frustrated. On morning rounds, eight health-care professionals came into the room to discuss Rosie's case. No one introduced themselves. I also wish they would ask Rosie how she is doing. Instead, they talk over her head. She is 9 years old and quite capable of answering their questions herself. I am becoming more comfortable advocating for Rosie during her hospitalizations and standing firm about what is best for Rosie, but I am afraid the nurses and physicians will get mad at me when I stand my ground. We know what works best for Rosie, we live with her every day, and her medical team only sees her when she is sick. How can I balance asking questions, providing my own care for Rosie, and participating in decisions about her care without being an overbearing, bossy parent? How can I get the health-care professionals to see that we are a team?

(personal reflection of a parent)

Ronald McDonald House

Having a family member who is sick can be one of the most stressful and exhausting times of the family's life. It is even more stressful when the family must travel for health services. Sometimes, hospitalizations, clinical visits, and medical tests and procedures require families to be away from home for days, weeks, or even months. Although the family member is sick, especially in the case of a child being ill, not only do family members have to care for their hospitalized child but they also have other responsibilities such as caring for the other children at home, keeping their source of income, and managing the responsibilities of everyday life. For some advice for health-care professionals when interacting with family members, see Box 18.5.

Ronald McDonald houses (RMH) all across Canada provide families in need with a home away from home. When children are in a nearby hospital, the RMH offer support and programs to lessen the burden and stresses for families. One unique aspect of staying at an RMH is that there are many other families who can also offer support. In Canada, there are 14 houses that offer a place for

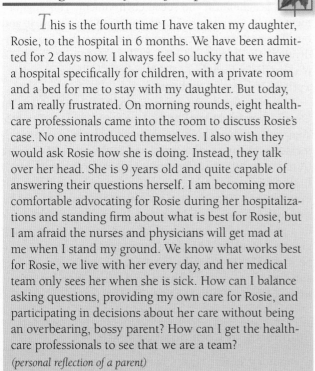

BOX 18.5 Advice for Health-Care Professionals

Advice for health-care professionals when interacting with family members:

Family Involvement
- Family is the focus of the care.
- Respect the role of each family member.
- Listen to what the family member has to say (families are the experts in the care of their loved one).
- Some family members are intimidated by health-care professionals, allow them the opportunity to tell their story.
- When giving information, use words and explanations they understand.
- Ask a family member what he or she thinks is going on with his or her loved one.
- Recognize that family members have different coping strategies.
- Acknowledge the impact of the hospitalization on the whole family unit.

Partnerships
- Ensure you are explaining what and why you are doing at all times.
- Ask a family member what has worked and not worked in previous situations or hospitalizations.
- Encourage family members to participate as much as they feel comfortable.
- Empower family members.
- Incorporate all teaching and training to include the family unit.

Negotiation
- Continue to assess the patient and family's needs.
- Ask family members how much they want to participate in the patient's care.

Adapted from Coyne, I., O'Neill, C., Murphy, M., Costello, T., & O'Shea, R. (2011). What does family-centred care mean to nurses and how do they think it can be enhanced in practice. *Journal of Advanced Nursing, 67*(12), 2561–2573.

---

over 10,000 Canadian families to stay each year (Ronald McDonald House, 2013).

Community Health Nursing

Having explored definitions, key concepts, the impact of complex relationships, and family nursing, we introduce community health nursing with a view toward understanding some of the key connections between family and community health nursing.

The field of community health nursing, such as that of family nursing, is as diverse and complex as the communities it serves. Entire nursing textbooks are dedicated to the study of this field. This chapter introduces the field with some key connections between family and community nursing. Although they are different fields of practice and study, they have some commonalities which serve to help the beginning nurse understand the foundations of both (Box 18.6).

BOX 18.6   What Do Community Health Nurses Do?

- Promote, protect, and preserve health and prevent disease and injury.
- Promote, protect, and preserve the environment that contributes to health.
- Advocate for healthy public policy.
- Lead in the integration of comprehensive and multiple health promotion approaches that build the capacity of clients.
- Respect the diversity of clients and caregivers, focus on the linkages between health and illness experiences and enable clients to achieve health.
- Provide evidence-informed care in various settings such as the client's home, school, office, clinics, on the street, communal living settings, or workplace.
- Cooperate, coordinate, and collaborate with various partners, disciplines, and sectors.
- Recognize that healthy communities and systems that support health contribute to health for all.
- Engage a range of resources to support health by coordinating care and planning services and programs.
- Work with a high degree of autonomy to initiate strategies that will address the determinants of health and positively impact people and their community.

Source: Community Health Nurses of Canada. (2011). *Professional practice model and standards of practice.* Retrieved from http://www.chnc.ca /documents/CHNC-ProfessionalPracticeModel-EN/index.html#/2/

History

Canada has a long history in community health nursing (CHN) dating back to the late 1890s in response to the health threat realities of tuberculosis, poor sanitation, poverty, and the subsequent mortality rates. Urban initiatives led to the establishment of public health officials and public health nurses. Public health in the early 1900s worked to reduce infant mortality, improving the maternity care of women and the lives of infants and children. Over time, public health clinics, well-child clinics, and school health programs grew from urban centres to rural areas, although each province developed at its own pace. Public health nursing today continues to be grounded in communicable disease control, promoting the health of women and infants, building capacity in communities, and focusing on the social determinants of health (McKay, 2009).

The history of home care or how we think of home care today comes from a long tradition of visiting nurses. In 1897, the Victorian Order of Nurses (VON) was established as a home visiting care service, beginning as a voluntary service funded by charitable organizations. Early in the 20th century, visiting nurses had a full clientele; although through the ensuing decades, hospital-based care grew. In the 1970s, the rising costs of hospital care in turn drove the need for home care. Early discharge from hospitals and the growing demand for home care resulted in provincial and local funding for an organized home care service. In some provinces, as home care became centrally funded, the VON took on

this new role and in other provinces their focus shifted to other community health needs (Grypma, Wolf, & Reimer-Kirkham, 2012).

What Is a Community?

Understanding what a community is and how the health of a community affects the health of families and individual citizens is critical. *Community* is defined as group of people who share a geographical and social environment. This environment can be temporary or fixed, and people can move in and out. The health influences that exist reverberate from the individual, the family, and back to the community. Examples of community include a neighbourhood, a homeless shelter, a school, a campsite, and even a city.

For example, if you are a community health nurse in Ontario, you might work at the Jane Street clinic in Toronto. Your work might include counseling patients on sexual health including offering birth control and confidential HIV testing (http://www.toronto.ca/health/sexualhealth/sh_clinics.htm). In this role, you would engage in relationship building, for example, to foster trust in your patient that came to you for a sexual concern. In Edmonton, Alberta, you might work in a public health centre facilitating a new mom's network group. In working with these moms and babies, you would be fostering the strengths in the new families and offering anticipatory guidance, support, and information for various topics (Alberta Health Services, 2013b).

Standards of Community Health

Community health nurses have five standards that guide practice. The standards of practice guide the CHNs as they work with Canadians to protect and promote their health. Attention to caring, primary health-care principles, an integrated knowledge base, partnerships with clients and communities, and empowerment are the underpinnings that shape the ways a CHNs works (Community Health Nurses of Canada, 2003/2008).

The five standards of the community health nurse include the following:

1. Promoting health
2. Building individual and community capacity
3. Building relationships
4. Facilitating access and equity
5. Demonstrating professional responsibility and accountability (Community Health Nurses of Canada, 2003/2008)

You may see the titles *community health nurse* and *public health nurse* used interchangeably in literature and government documents. PHAC uses them together to describe the work of these nurses (CPHA, 2010). Yet, others define *public health nursing* as one group fitting within the broader group community health nurses. Does the title *public health nurse* identify the nurse's client or does it signify the overarching health goal? Is a community health nurse focused on the health of the community first and the individual second? Or is it that both of these terms suggest that the nurse cares for the patient and/or family with the parallel and intersecting knowledge that the effect on the community must also be considered? These are interesting questions that are debated regularly in the community health nursing domain.

Agencies That Influence Canadian Community Health Nurses

Today, community and public health nursing in Canada is shaped and governed by a number of bodies and policies. Provincial and federal legislation dictates the mandate and scope of many programs and initiatives. Other agencies impacting public health include the World Health Organization, PHAC, and Health Canada (e.g., see Box 18.7).

World Health Organization

The World Health Organization (WHO) is committed to improving the health of people globally (WHO, 2007). The following outlines the mandate for WHO:

> is the directing and coordinating authority for health within the United Nations system. It is responsible for providing leadership on global health matters, shaping the health research agenda, setting norms and standards, articulating evidence-based policy options, providing technical support to countries and monitoring and assessing health trends. (http://www.who.int/about/en/index.html)

It is through this mandate that WHO directs policy for public health programs. United Nations members are obligated to follow the goals and to institute programs and policy that reflect the evidence-based direction of WHO. For instance, in response to the global threat of chronic diseases as a result of tobacco use, WHO instituted a treaty that sets the standards for tobacco control (WHO, 2007). As a response to this and to our own chronic disease reality in Canada, Health Canada has responded with legislation, tobacco product labeling and programs geared toward reducing tobacco users in Canada (Health Canada, 2013). As an example, in Saskatchewan, the Green Light Project focuses on the Métis community with the following goals:

- To increase the number of smoke-free homes within Métis communities; and,
- To reduce the number of people exposed to the harmful effects of environmental tobacco smoke.

Participants sign up for a green light bulb (or sticker), which is placed at the door or front porch. The green light signals that the home is smoke-free. In addition, educational workshops and peer counsellors to work in their own communities and promote smoke-free homes (http://www.mn-s.ca/green-light-project.htm).

BOX 18.7 Age-Friendly Communities

In 2006, the World Health Organization (WHO) developed the Global Age-Friendly Cities Project. This project brought together cities from around the world that were interested in supporting healthy aging by becoming more age-friendly. These cities gathered information from seniors, senior-care providers, and other groups and individuals with an interest in age-friendly communities. This information helped to identify eight key areas of community life in which communities can become more age-friendly. These areas are as follows:

- Outdoor spaces and buildings
- Transportation
- Housing
- Social participation
- Respect and social inclusion
- Civic participation and employment
- Communication and information
- Community support and health services

In 2007, federal, provincial, and territorial Age-Friendly Rural and Remote Communities Initiative piloted the WHO program in Canada. Policies, services, and structures related to the physical and social environment were designed to help seniors "age actively." The communities were set up to assist seniors to live safely, enjoy good health, and stay involved.

Some examples of an age-friendly community include the following:

- Keeping sidewalks well lit and in good shape
- Ensuring buildings have automatic door openers and elevators
- Providing seniors with community programming and activities, which may include visiting museums or libraries; taking courses; or volunteering for service clubs, charities, or civic duties

The PHAC also reports that in an age-friendly community, community members must

- Recognize that seniors have a wide range of skills and abilities.
- Understand and meet the age-related needs of seniors.
- Respect the decisions and lifestyle choices of seniors.
- Protect those seniors who are vulnerable.
- Recognize that seniors have a lot to offer their community.
- Recognize how important it is to include seniors in all areas of community life.

Source: Public Health Agency of Canada. (2012). *Age-friendly communities.* Retrieved from http://www.phac-aspc.gc.ca/seniors-aines/afc-caa-eng.php

---

The Public Health Agency of Canada

PHAC informs citizens and health professionals of current evidence, policy and trends from the a leadership perspective designed to protect and promote the health of Canadians (http://www.phac-aspc.gc.ca/about_apropos/index-eng.php). PHAC promotes the health of all Canadians with the following roles:

- Promote health,
- Prevent and control chronic diseases and injuries,
- Prevent and control infectious diseases,

- Prepare for and respond to public health emergencies,
- Serve as a central point for sharing Canada's expertise with the rest of the world,
- Apply international research and development to Canada's public health programs, and
- Strengthen intergovernmental collaboration on public health and facilitate national approaches to public health policy and planning.

Provincial and Territorial Health Departments

Provincial and territory health departments look to the PHAC for leadership and strategy in their own implementation of health policy. For example, in the document, *Curbing Childhood Obesity: A Federal, Provincial and Territorial Framework for Action to Promote Healthy Weights* (Public Health Agency of Canada, 2011), governments use this document to support and build their own programs to reduce the issue of childhood obesity in their province, territory, and at the community level. In the province of Manitoba, the Healthy Eating Campaign supports school initiatives to improve the eating habits and nutritional knowledge in their students (http://www.gov.mb.ca/healthyschools/campaigns/index .html#.Ub847-e1F_c). In Edmonton, Alberta, the Healthy Beginnings Postpartum program is unique in its approach and is an example of the blending of family and community nursing.

Two Community Health Programs

CHN is a field of nursing encompassing programs, roles, and settings. Within many community health programs, the fields of family nursing and community health nursing work together for the benefit of the patient. Two program examples are highlighted.

Healthy Beginnings Postpartum Program

The Healthy Beginnings Postpartum Program (HBPP) through Alberta Health Services, piloted in 1992, came about when discharges from hospitals after birth were changing from 5 to 7 days to 2 or 3 days. HBPP sought to bridge the gap between the hospital and the community by having experienced nurses visit the families within 24 hours of discharge, thus establishing an opportunity to connect with new families and introduce them to the public and community health system. The program was successful and expanded to include every mother who gave birth in the Edmonton region. Mother and newborn's health is assessed and monitored, and the family is introduced to the benefits and the many services of the community health system. When HBPP nurses visit a new family, they see the whole family as the focus rather than just the mom or just the newborn. For the most part, the new family is healthy, as birth is a health state, and the nurse is able to develop a therapeutic relationship, nurture the family's strengths, and help support the family as they learn to care for their new baby and transition into

a larger family. Once the infant is 2 months old, the family shifts into the well-child clinic program at the public health centre.

The program offers

- health assessment of mom and baby;
- breast-feeding support and education;
- counselling;
- education and support about parenting and newborn care;
- referrals; and
- 24-hour telephone hotline.

(Source: http://www.albertahealthservices.ca/services.asp ?pid=service&rid=580)

Child Health Clinic

At Vancouver Coastal Health's Child Health Clinic, parents bring their infants and children to appointments with nurses who assess the child's growth and development, answer questions, offer support, teach about immunizations and aftercare, and administer the appropriate vaccines according to the provincial guidelines. The appointments are an opportunity for the nurse to connect with families and support them in their parenting and offer anticipatory guidance in the areas of nutrition, safety, sleep, dental health, development (physical, social, emotional), and overall health. These appointments also serve to promote the provincial immunization policies and provide the nurse with opportunity to connect the families to needed and appropriate resources.

Through the eyes of a nurse

When I graduated from nursing school, I worked in the neonatal intensive care unit, and I loved working with moms, dads, grandparents, siblings, and all the visitors that cared for the newborn. Over time, I felt I became very skilled at helping to see a family's strengths and understanding their concerns. I was adept at helping them to plan for their newborn's discharge and the challenges that discharge might bring. When I took a job in public health in a child health clinic, I wondered how I would care for the family as a whole with time constraints and the full agenda that needs to be fulfilled during the appointment. It took me awhile, but I came to understand that by paying attention to those first moments as I greeted a family when they entered my clinic room, I could establish a positive and therapeutic working relationship quickly. When I worked the fall influenza clinics, I was able to use my grounding in family nursing to establish relationships, see my patient in the context of their family, and to see and build on the strengths that I saw and the strengths they communicated to me.

One 5-year-old boy coming to receive his influenza vaccine told me how scared he was of needles. I asked him about his family and his siblings, and he shared that his big sister was bossy and sometimes told him what to do. I asked him what he did to handle it, and he replied that he squeezed his teddy bear really tight when he was upset. I smiled and reminded him that he was smart to bring that teddy, and I urged him to use that same technique during the needle. He was a skeptical but was willing to try, and when it was over, he commented, "Wow, that even worked on needles." I patted him on the hand and told him he was really good at handling tough situations. He nodded and cuddled up to his teddy and his mom as they left my station.

I believe strongly that no matter where my profession might take me, I will be able keep family as my focus and leave each patient and family feeling cared for, empowered, and more equipped to move towards their health goals.

(personal reflection of a nurse)

Cecilia took the time to learn as much about the family and their concerns as possible. She recognized Jose's desire to be a good father to all his children. With his very limited English, it was clearly very challenging for Gemma's father to come to the clinic. She arranged for an interpreter and reading materials in Spanish. She helped the family work together with the interprofessional team. Cecilia's efforts helped strengthen the Cortez family, reinforcing their skills in working together and supporting their goals for health in the future.

Critical Thinking Exercises

▶ Think for a moment, if you were to become ill, and a nurse asked you who your family was. What would you answer? Who are those closest to you that you consider to be your supports and your family? Do they reach beyond family members? Would you include family members?

Now consider how you would feel if you were admitted into the hospital and saw the following sign:

Visiting Hours 12-8pm
Immediate Family Only
Must be over the age of 14

Why do you think a hospital would have this policy? Would all members of who you consider your family be included in this policy? Now, consider if you were the nurse—how can you advocate for patients where this policy may exclude the people most important to them?

▶ Think back to your upbringing and try to recall a health habit your parents instilled in you (e.g., the importance of breakfast, regular exercise). Is this a habit you continue now? Why? Were there any unhealthy habits that your family had? Do you continue these? Why? Do you think individuals change their health habits easily? What might be some motivators for a change in a health habit?

▶ You have been approached by a patient's mother who tells you that she likes to do all the care and medications for her child. She admits to you that she is pretty nervous having others interrupt her routine and that she has had some bad experiences with health-care workers in the past. How can you work together with the mom to provide safe and competent care?

Multiple-Choice Questions

1. Which of the following is not a core concept of FCC?
   a. Respect and dignity
   b. Collaboration
   c. Physician-led
   d. Participation

2. The unit of care in family nursing is:
   a. The child
   b. The relationships in the family
   c. The family
   d. The individual in the context of the family

3. Cultural safety and humility include which of the following?
   a. Trying to become a member of a culture
   b. Reading enough about a culture to feel like an expert
   c. Understanding the best thing for a culture is to try to blend in.
   d. Self-awareness is key to working with other people.

4. A family nurse would consider which of the following to be incongruent with his or her nursing beliefs?
   a. Listening to the family
   b. Helping the family to identify their strengths
   c. Developing a plan of care that the nurse feels is best for the family
   d. Helping to make arrangement for the family member to stay overnight with a sick child.

Suggested Lab Activities

● Divide into small groups and discuss the following questions:
   a. Would a nurse in VON People in Crisis program be a family nurse or a community health nurse? Could he or she be both?
   b. When working with a family with addiction issues, how can you help the family identify their strengths?

c. How does reflecting and being honest with your own beliefs and biases toward people who are different (culture, socioeconomic status, etc.) help initiate a therapeutic relationship with a family?

d. Compare your family with one that is different (e.g., a same-sex family). What are some of the challenges each might face?

● Please gather in small groups and consider the following critical thinking questions related to Canada's residential school system.

• If you had been parented in a different family, do you think you would be a different person? If so, in what ways?

• What if these parents struggled to know what it meant to be a parent? What if their childhood was unhealthy and abusive?

• If you had your family life destroyed by a government program, what would your level of trust be toward a nurse who works for the government?

● Divide into pairs and have one of you role-play that you are a patient of a family nurse in a community setting. As the patient, decide who your family is, either real or imagined. Then let the other student role-play being the nurse to find out "who your family is," your strengths, and what goals you are working toward.

● Self-reflection activity: Imagine if you were to move to another part of Canada that is different from what you know and what you have experienced. What challenges do you think you would face if you became sick? What would it be like to be in the hospital and your caregivers didn't speak English? How would you feel with your family and supports living so far away?

REFERENCES AND SUGGESTED READINGS

Alberta Health Services. (n.d.). *Family Centred Care at the Stollery Children's Hospital.* Retrieved from http://www.albertahealthservices.ca/ps

Alberta Health Services. (2013a). *Family centre care network.* Retrieved from http://www.albertahealthservices.ca/5516.asp-

Alberta Health Services. (2013b). *New moms network.* Retrieved from http://www.albertahealthservices.ca/services.asp?pid=service&rid=7822

Bell, J. M. (2011). Relationships: The heart of the matter in family nursing. *Journal of Family Nursing, 17*(3), 3–10.

Benzeval, M., Judge, K., & Whitehead, M. (1995). *Tackling inequalities in health: An agenda for action.* London, United Kingdom: Kings Fund.

Bourque Bearskin, R. L. (2011). A critical lens of culture in nursing practice. *Nursing Ethics, 18*(4), 548–559.

Browne, A. J., Varcoe, C., Smye, V., Reimer-Kirkham, S., Lynam, M. J., & Wong, S. (2009). Cultural safety and the challenges of translating critically oriented knowledge in practice. *Nursing Philosophy, 10,* 167–179.

Canadian Caregiver Coalition. (2008). *Caregiver facts.* Retrieved from http://www.ccc-ccan.ca/content.php?doc=43

Canadian Nurses Association. (2005). Social determinants of health and nursing: A summary of the issues. *CNA Backgrounder.* Retrieved from http://www.cna-aiic.ca

Canadian Press. (2012a). *Census shows new face of the Canadian family.* Retrieved from http://www.cbc.ca/new/canada/story/2013/09/19/census-data-families-households.html

Canadian Press. (2012b). *More Canadian single dads head rise in lone-parent families.* Retrieved from http://www.cbc.ca/news/canada/story/2012/09/19/census-single-parent-families.html

Canadian Press. (2012c). *Stepfamilies make up 12.6% of Canadian families.* Retrieved from http://www.cbc.ca/news/canada/story/2012/09/19/census-stepfamilies.html

Canadian Public Health Association. (2010). *Public health ~ Community health nursing practice in Canada: Roles and activities.* Ottawa, ON: Author. Retrieved from http://www.cpha.ca/uploads/pubs/3-1bk04214.pdf

Carter, B., & McGoldrick, M. (2005). *The expanded family life cycle: Individual, family, and social perspectives.* New York, NY: Allyn & Bacon.

Community Health Nurses of Canada. (2008). *Canadian community health nursing standards of practice.* Retrieved from http://www.chnc.ca/documents/chn_standards_of_practice_mar08_english.pdf (Original work published 2003)

Community Health Nurses of Canada. (2011). *Canadian community health nursing: Professional practice model & standards of practice.* Retrieved from http://www.chnc.ca/documents/chnc-standards-eng-book.pdf

Coyne, I., O'Neill, C., Murphy, M., Costello, T., & O'Shea, R. (2011). What does family-centred care mean to nurses and how do they think it can be enhanced in practice. *Journal of Advanced Nursing, 67*(12), 2561–2573.

Cunningham, A., & Baker, L. (2007). *Little eyes, little ears, how violence against a mother shapes children as they grow.* Ottawa, ON: Family Violence Prevention Unit and Public Health Agency of Canada.

Dokken, D., & Ahmann, E. (2006). The many roles of family members in "family-centred care"—Part 1. *Pediatric Nursing, 32*(6), 562–565.

Fahey, J. O., Cohen, S. R., Holme, F., Buttrick, E. S., Dettinger, J. C., Kestler, E., & Walker, D. (2013). Promoting cultural humility during labor and birth: Putting theory into action during PRONTO obstetric and neonatal emergency training. *The Journal of Perinatal and Neonatal Nursing, 27*(1), 36–42.

Gottlieb, L. N., & Gottlieb, B. (2007). The developmental/health framework within the McGill model of nursing: "Laws of nature" guiding whole person care. *Advances in Nursing Science, 30,* 43–57.

Gottlieb, L. N., Gottlieb, B., & Shamian, J. (2012). Principles of strengths-based nursing leadership for strengths-based nursing care: A new paradigm for nursing and healthcare for the 21st Century. *Canadian Journal of Nursing Leadership, 25*(2), 38–50.

Gottlieb, L. N., & Rowat, K. (1987). The McGill model of nursing: A practice-derived model. *Advances in Nursing Science, 9*(4), 51–61.

Government of Canada. (n.d.). *About family violence.* Retrieved from http://www.justice.gc.ca/eng/cj-jp/fv-vf/about-apropos.html

Griffore, R. (2012, September). Book review. [Review of the book *Exploring family theories* (3rd ed.), by S. R. Smith & R. R. Hamon]. *Family & Consumer Sciences Research Journal, 41*(1), 102–104.

Grypma, S., Wolf, D., & Reimer-Kirkham, S. (2012) Returning home: Historical influences on home healthcare in Canada. *Home Healthcare Nurse, 30*(8), 453–460.

Health Canada. (2013). *Health concerns.* Retrieved from http://www.hc-sc.gc.ca/hc-ps/tobac-tabac/res/index-eng.php

Holmes, T., & Rahe, R. (1967). The social readjustment rating scale. *Journal of Psychosomatic Research, 11,* 213–218.

Institute for Patient- and Family-Centered Care. (n.d.). *Bibliographies/supporting evidence.* Retrieved from http://www.ipfcc.org/advance/supporting.html

Legacy of Hope Foundation. (2011). *100 years of loss.* Retrieved from http://www.legacyofhope.ca/downloads/100-years-colour.pdf

Legacy of Hope Foundation and Aboriginal Healing Foundation. (2011). *Hope and healing.* Retrieved from http://www.legacyofhope.ca/downloads/hope-and-healing.pdf

Lilly, M. B., Robinson, C. A., Holtzman, S., & Bottorff, J. L. (2012). Can we move beyond burden and burnout to support the health and wellness of family caregivers to persons with dementia? Evidence from British Columbia, Canada. *Health & Social Care in the Community, 20*(1), 103–112. doi:10.1111/j.1365-2524.2011.01025.x

Loney, S. (2012). *The multi-generational home makes a comeback.* Retrieved from http://www.theglobeandmail.com/life/relationships/the-multi-generational-home-makes-a-comeback/article570274/

McDaniel, K. R., & Allen, D. G. (2012). Working and care-giving: The impact on caregiver stress, family-work conflict and burnout. *Journal of Life Care Planning, 10*(4), 21–32.

McKay, M. (2009). Public health nursing in early 20th century Canada. *Canadian Journal of Public Health, 100*(4), 249–250.

Ministry of Industry. (2012). *Statistics Canada. Portrait of Families and Living Arrangements in Canada. Families, households and marital status, 2011 Census of Population.* Ottawa, ON: Author.

Moules, N. J., & Johnstone, H. (2010). Commendations, conversations, and life-changing realizations: Teaching and practicing family nursing. *Journal of Family Nursing, 16*(2), 146–160. doi:10.1177/1074840710365148

Neils, P. E. (2010). The influence of Nightingale rounding by the liaison nurse on surgical patient families with attention to differing cultural needs. *Journal of Holistic Nursing, 28,* 235–243. doi:10.1177/0898010011036886

Public Health Agency of Canada. (2011). *Curbing childhood obesity: A federal, provincial and territorial framework for action to promote healthy weights.* Retrieved from http://www.phac-aspc.gc.ca/hp-ps/hl-mvs/framework-cadre/2011/overview-resume-eng.php

Public Health Agency of Canada. (2013). *What makes Canadians healthy or unhealthy?* Retrieved from http://www.phac-aspc.gc.ca/ph-sp/determinants/determinants-eng.php

Raphael, D. (2002). *Poverty, income inequality, and health in Canada.* Toronto, ON: The Centre for Social Justice Foundation for Research and Education.

Ronald McDonald House. (2013). *About the Ronald McDonald House charities.* Retrieved from http://www.rmhccanada.com/

Royal Canadian Mounted Police. (2012). *The effects of family violence on children: Where does it hurt?* Retrieved from http://www.rcmp-grc.gc.ca/cp-pc/chi-enf-abu-eng.htm

Safaei, J. (2012). Socioeconomic and demographic determinants of mental health across Canadian communities. *The Internet Journal of Mental Health, 8*(1). Retrieved from http://www.ispub.com/IJMH/8/1/14282

Selye, H. (1974). *Stress without distress.* Philadelphia, PA: J. B. Lippincott Company.

Shessler, J. B., Wilder, B., & Byrd, L. W. (2013). Reflective journaling and development of cultural humility in students. *Nursing Education Perspective, 33*(2), 96–99.

Smith, D., Varcoe, C., & Edwards, N. (2005). Turning around the intergenerational impact of residential schools on Aboriginal people: Implications for health policy and practice. *Canadian Journal of Nursing Research, 37*(4), 38–60.

Smith, S., & Hamon, R. (2012). *Exploring family theories* (3rd ed.). New York, NY: Oxford University Press.

St. John, W., & Flowers, K. (2009). Working with families: From theory to clinical nursing practice. *Collegian, 16,* 131–138.

Vancouver Coastal Health. (2013). *Child health clinic.* Retrieved from http://www.vch.ca/403/7676/?program_id=10449

Vanier Institute of the Family. (2010a). *Canada's racial and ethnic diversity.* Retrieved from http://www.vanierinstitute.ca/modules/news/newsitem.php?ItemId=130#.UcnFyKH4C70

Vanier Institute of the Family. (2010b). *Canada's seniors: Living longer, together.* Ottawa, ON: Author. Retrieved from http://www.vanierinstitute.ca/research_topics_seniors

Vanier Institute of the Family. (2010c). *Children growing up in step-families.* Retrieved from http://www.vanierinstitute.ca/modules/news/newsitem.php?ItemId=146#.UcnEHaH4C70

Vanier Institute of the Family. (2010d). *Families working shift.* Retrieved from http://www.vanierinstitute.ca/modules/news/newsitem.php?ItemId=144#.UcnC9qH4C70

Vanier Institute of the Family. (2013). *Definition of family.* Retrieved from http://www.vanierinstitute.ca/definition_of_family#.Ucm8rqH4C70

Victorian Order of Nurses Canada. (2012). *Programs and services.* Retrieved from http://www.von.ca/NationalDirectory/branch/pages.aspx?BranchId=11&section=programs&cat=4

World Health Organization. (2007). *Working for health. An introduction to the World Health Organization.* Geneva, Switzerland: Author.

Wright, L. M., & Leahey, M. (1999). Maximizing time, minimizing suffering: The 15-minute (or less) family interview. *Journal of Family Nursing, 5,* 259–273. doi:10.1177/107484079900500302

Wright, L. M., & Leahey, M. (2013). *Nurses and families: A guide to family assessment and intervention* (6th ed.). Philadelphia, PA: F. A. Davis.

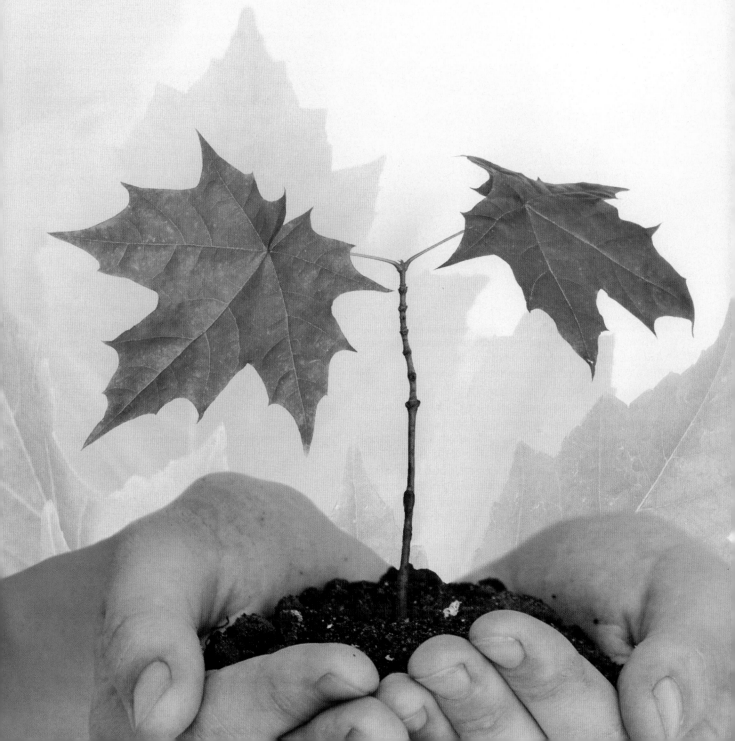

three
Being

Principles of Asepsis

B. NICOLE HARDER

Nadine is a nursing student starting her first clinical rotation in a long-term care facility. Although she has worked as a community health representative in the past and has helped nurses with wound care and other skills, she is now concerned about her ability to maintain asepsis as she practices as a student nurse. Nadine has learned the different kinds of asepsis and how to prevent the spread of infection, but there seems to be so many things to remember. With microorganisms such as influenza present in many facilities, she wants to be sure that she is not the cause of transmission.

CHAPTER OBJECTIVES

By the end of this chapter, you will be able to:

1. Identify common terms related to principles of asepsis.
2. Understand the difference between medical and surgical asepsis.
3. Understand how practice standards inform aseptic technique.
4. Understand how the chain of infection relates to nursing practice.
5. Use the principles of asepsis during hand washing and infection control.
6. Describe principles of patient safety and documentation related to asepsis in nursing practice.
7. Discuss principles of culture, communication, and comfort related to the practice of asepsis.

KEY TERMS

Acute Inflammation   Inflammatory response that is relatively short, lasting anywhere from a few minutes to several days. Signs of acute inflammation include redness, swelling, heat, pain or discomfort, and loss of function.

Asepsis   The absence of bacteria, viruses, and other microorganisms; also commonly used to refer to practices that promote or induce asepsis in medicine to prevent infection.

Chronic Inflammation   Inflammatory response that can last from days to years. Characteristics of chronic inflammation are primarily due to infiltration with macrophages, lymphocytes, and fibroblasts, leading to persistent inflammation, fibroblast proliferation, and scar formation. As a result, the risk for deformity and potentially decreased mobility is considered greater than in acute inflammation.

Communicable   Contagious, simply by virtue of being able to be transmitted between people.

Contact Transmission   Microorganism transfer—either direct, which occurs when microorganisms are transferred by physical contact with an infected or colonized patient, or indirect, which involves transfer of microorganisms via an object.

Iatrogenic Infection   Nosocomial infection that results from a diagnostic or therapeutic treatment.

Immunocompromised   Patients whose immune system is weakened; as a result, they more easily contract disease while in hospital.

Inflammatory Response   The body's response to contact with disease-causing microorganisms.

Nosocomial Infection   Infection that is acquired by patients while they are institutionalized or hospitalized.

Pandemic   Outbreaks of specific diseases or illnesses on a global scale.

Pathogen   Microorganisms that can cause infection; they are present on both living beings and inanimate objects.

Personal Protective Equipment (PPE)   The selection of gowns, gloves, masks, and/or face protection used while interacting with patients.

Reservoir   An environment that supports the life of a microorganism and allows it to remain in its current state or, perhaps, even multiply. This reservoir can be a multitude of places, including both living and nonliving objects.

Resident Flora (Resident Microbiota)   Microorganisms that cannot be removed due to their location in the deep layers of the epidermis; also found on the surface of the skin. These can only be removed with vigorous scrubbing and by using hand hygiene products containing antimicrobial agents.

Sterile   Free of all contaminants, not just those that can cause disease. A surgical field is sterile, ideally.

Transient Flora (Transient Microbiota)   Microorganisms that colonize on the superficial layers of the skin and are more amenable to removal by routine hand washing.

Virulent   Able to produce disease.

In this chapter, we discuss the concepts associated with the foundational knowledge regarding the principles of asepsis as well as the chain of infection, including the spread of infection. In the application section of the chapter, we discuss how asepsis relates to various patient situations and the integration of skills. We also look at what it means to be the nurse responsible for patient care and patient safety and ensuring that you have done your best to prevent the spread of infection.

The Basic Concepts of Asepsis

To begin, you need to understand the basics of asepsis. The term **asepsis** means the absence of bacteria, viruses, and other microorganisms, but it is commonly used to refer to practices that promote or induce asepsis in medicine to prevent infection. So, the word *asepsis* means both the state of as well as the process of creating an environment free of contaminants. Elimination of infection is the goal of asepsis, not creating a sterile field. Ideally, a surgical field is **sterile**, meaning, it is free of all contaminants, not just those that can cause disease.

As nursing students prepare to enter the clinical setting, often the first thing they are told is to "wash your hands." This demand is put not only to nursing students but essentially to all individuals who work in health care. The reason for washing our hands is clear—to prevent the spread of infection. Although scientific knowledge of microorganisms and infectious diseases has increased, the primary means to prevent the spread of disease still begins with hand washing.

Understanding and applying the principles of asepsis includes understanding and skills such as the following:

- The manual dexterity skills required to apply sterile gloves
- Knowing about the microorganisms that you are dealing with and how to prevent them from spreading
- Knowing where to find information and apply it to your understanding of asepsis
- The importance of caring and compassion as well as patient safety when applying the principles of asepsis

What Are the Principles of Asepsis?

We mentioned hand washing, but is this all that asepsis is about? Although it is an important part of asepsis, there is much more that is included in this area. There are different expectations and principles, depending on whether you are talking about medical or surgical needs. Four basic principles of asepsis are highlighted here, some of which will be covered in greater depth later in the chapter.

1. All articles used in a surgical operation have been sterilized previously. When preparing the surgical equipment that is to be used for an operation, always remember that the equipment is already sterilized and therefore is free from pathogen, so never touch them with your bare hands. Sterile instruments should only be touched with sterile gloves. When you have sterile gloves on, you can only touch other sterile items. Touching anything else (such as outside packaging) will render your gloves unsterile.

2. If in doubt about the sterility of anything, consider it unsterile. If you think that you may have contaminated a glove, assume that you did and obtain a new set of sterile gloves.

3. The edge of anything that encloses sterile contents is not considered sterile.
   - Never touch the rims of bottles/containers of sterile content. Consider the rims of bottles unsterile.
   - There is a 1-inch border (3 cm) around the perimeter of your sterile field. This area is not sterile.

4. Moisture may cause contamination. Be sure to avoid spilling cleaning solutions such as sterile water on the sterile field. Moisture can wick bacteria and easily transmit microorganisms.

What Is Medical Asepsis?

Both medical and surgical asepsis involve keeping an area contaminant-free. However, there are several differences that you should know. Medical asepsis is also commonly known as *clean technique*. As the term implies, the goal of medical asepsis is to keep the area as clean as possible in order to reduce the transmission of disease. This transmission generally occurs between people, whether it is between the nurse and patient, visitor and patient, or patient and patient. This is why you are asked to wash your hands—to prevent transmission of disease from nursing students to the patients. You must also wash your hands between contacts with patients in order to prevent transmission of disease between patients. Your skin will never be sterile, but it can be clean. Taking vital signs from your patient is something that can be done with clean technique.

What Is Surgical Asepsis?

Surgical asepsis, or sterile technique, is a technique used when you want no transmission of microorganisms to the patient. This is most commonly used in the operating room or with any procedures that involve an open wound, sterile cavities in the body, or any other invasive procedures that involve a break in the skin. Instruments used in any of these situations have been previously sterilized and should not be in contact with anything that is not considered sterile. A good example of this is to think about what happens in the operating room. All the instruments are sterile, and the team wears sterile gloves to use the instruments during surgery. Another example is inserting a urinary catheter. The catheter itself must remain sterile, so the nurse uses sterile gloves to manipulate the catheter.

Routine Practices

Routine practices are the basic precautions that a healthcare provider takes to prevent infections from occurring. These were formerly known as *universal precautions* as well as *standard precautions*; you may still hear these terms.

Although germs are always present, routine practices are used to minimize the spread of infection between people. How microorganisms are transmitted is described in another section of this chapter; however, it is important to know that even though you cannot see the infectious agents, they can still be present. For that reason, you want to treat each patient as well as yourself as potentially having an infectious agent that can be transmitted. We will talk about the ways microorganisms can be transmitted as well as how you can prevent the spread of microorganisms.

World Health Organization Practice Standards

In 2009, the World Health Organization (WHO) published their *WHO Guidelines on Hand Hygiene in Health Care*. This document began development in 2004 and included over 100 international experts who contributed to the guidelines. These guidelines provide health-care workers (HCWs), hospital administrators, and health authorities with a thorough review of evidence on hand hygiene in health care and specific recommendations to improve practices and reduce transmission of pathogenic microorganisms to patients and HCWs. The *Guidelines* are intended to be implemented in any situation in which health care is delivered either to a patient or to a specific group in a population. Therefore, this concept applies to all settings where health care is permanently or occasionally performed, such as home care by birth attendants. While ensuring consistency with the *Guidelines*' recommendations, individual adaptation according to local regulations, settings, needs, and resources is desirable.

The *Guidelines* provide the reader with useful information and research study results surrounding hand hygiene and providing care for individuals in various settings. The *Guidelines* are easily accessed through the WHO website.

The Chain of Infection

In order to understand how to prevent infection, it is important to know how infection is transmitted in the first place. With millions of microorganisms living in our environment, it can be overwhelming to think of what may or may not cause an infection. Most microorganisms are harmless and are not the cause of infection. Those that can cause infection are called **pathogens** and are present on both living beings and inanimate objects. The presence of a pathogen in itself does not mean that an infection or disease will occur. In order for disease or infection to be present, the pathogen must first enter a host and be able to live and replicate within the host. How the pathogen is transmitted from person to person is dependent on the type of pathogen. However, simply by virtue of being transmitted between people, the pathogen is considered contagious, or **communicable**, and can be further transmitted to others.

The chain of infection is a commonly accepted model that describes how microorganisms are transmitted (Fig. 19.1).

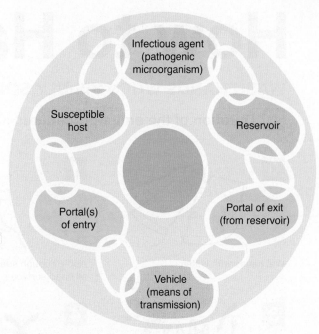

Figure 19.1 Chain of infection.

According to the chain of infection, the following needs to occur before a microorganism can be considered a pathogen. Each link must be present and in sequential order for an infection to occur.

1. An infectious agent or pathogen
2. A reservoir or source for pathogen growth
3. A portal of exit from the reservoir
4. A mode of transmission
5. A portal of entry to the host
6. A susceptible host

It is important for nurses to know how the chain of infection works in order to break the chain and keep infection from developing.

Infectious Agents

Infectious agents include literally hundreds of microorganisms that are capable to causing an infection. Although there are many microorganisms, they typically fall under the more specific categories of bacteria, virus, fungi, or protozoa. Many of these microorganisms live on both inanimate or body surfaces and do not cause infection. Some of these, regardless of how much hand washing or scrubbing that we do, cannot be removed due to their location in the deep layers of the epidermis. These **resident flora (resident microbiota)** live under the superficial cells of the stratum corneum and are also found on the surface of the skin. These can only be removed with vigorous scrubbing and by using hand hygiene products containing antimicrobial agents. **Transient flora (transient microbiota)** are microorganisms that colonize on the superficial layers of the skin and are more amenable to removal by routine hand washing (Fig. 19.2). Because of

How to Handwash?

WASH HANDS WHEN VISIBLY SOILED! OTHERWISE, USE HANDRUB

🕐 **Duration of the entire procedure:** 40-60 seconds

0
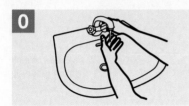
Wet hands with water;

1
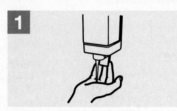
Apply enough soap to cover all hand surfaces;

2
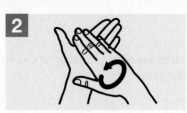
Rub hands palm to palm;

3
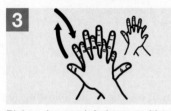
Right palm over left dorsum with interlaced fingers and vice versa;

4
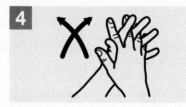
Palm to palm with fingers interlaced;

5
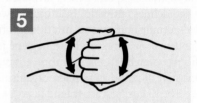
Backs of fingers to opposing palms with fingers interlocked;

6
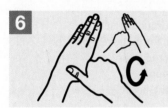
Rotational rubbing of left thumb clasped in right palm and vice versa;

7
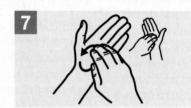
Rotational rubbing, backwards and forwards with clasped fingers of right hand in left palm and vice versa;

8
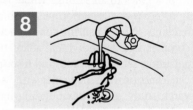
Rinse hands with water;

9
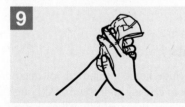
Dry hands thoroughly with a single use towel;

10
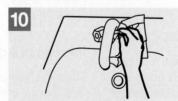
Use towel to turn off faucet;

11
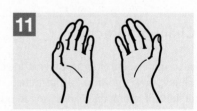
Your hands are now safe.

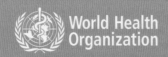

World Health Organization | **Patient Safety** A World Alliance for Safer Health Care | **SAVE LIVES** Clean **Your** Hands

May 2009

Figure 19.2 Guidelines on hand washing from the World Health Organization (WHO). (Source: World Health Organization [WHO]. [2009]. *How to Handwash*. Retrieved from http://www.who.int)

their location, they are also very easily transmissible between people, and the need for hand washing becomes even more apparent.

When transient flora is passed from one person to another or from a nurse to a patient, the transference of the microorganism does not mean that infection will necessarily occur. Factors that influence disease or infection transmission include the following:

- Type of organism
- Number of organisms present
- Source of transmission and destination
- Size and virulence of microorganisms

What this means is that you need to have enough of the microorganisms present, it needs to be **virulent** (able to produce disease), and you need to have a host who is able to receive the disease. Transferal is not enough. The host must be susceptible (as is often the case with people who are already sick) and able to have the microorganisms affect them in a negative way. Imagine, for example, that you are working on a surgical unit. Your patient has had surgery and has an open wound. This is a desirable destination for the microorganisms. Previously, you just finished changing the dressing of a patient with pseudomonas and have some of this microorganism on your hands. You do not wash your hands between patients. With the amount of pseudomonas on your hands, the virulence of that microorganism, and the open wound on your new patient, you have the perfect combination for the transmission of disease.

A Reservoir: Source for Pathogen Growth

In order for infection or disease to occur, the microorganism needs to be housed somewhere while it waits for its opportunity to infect someone or something. This house or **reservoir** must be an environment that supports the life of the microorganism and allows it to remain in its current state or, perhaps, even multiply. This reservoir can be a multitude of places, including both living and nonliving objects. It is important to remember that simply housing a microorganism does not mean that someone will be infected. For example, many people can be considered carriers of a disease (e.g., flu virus) but not have any symptoms of infection. It is not until they transmit the microorganism to a receptive host who is susceptible that the virus multiplies and makes the individual symptomatic.

A Portal of Exit From the Reservoir

To have a microorganism transmit from one person to another, something has to happen. In our example earlier, where you as a nurse did not wash hands between patients, the microorganism was transmitted by exudates or material from the first patient's wound. This exudate from the wound is considered the portal of exit. The most common portals of exit include the mucous membranes (i.e., mouth, nose, vagina, rectum) or breaks in the skin (e.g., wounds).

Blood and body fluids are considered portals of exit and can carry microorganisms as well. Different microorganisms are transmitted through various fluids, including blood, vaginal secretions, semen, stool, urine, vomitus, saliva, mucus, wound exudate, and sputum. What this means is that the nurse must assume that any and all body fluids have the potential to carry microorganisms, and all are considered a portal of exit.

Modes of Transmission

Now that we have ascertained that there are microorganisms all around us and understand their potential to infect an unsuspecting host, we now have to determine how they get from point A to point B. In our situation earlier, you did not wash your hands between patients, which led to the transmission occurring through touch or direct contact. This is one of the most common modes of transmission; however, several other modes are also responsible for diseases and infections. It is the nurse's responsibility to understand these modes of transmission to avoid contamination.

Contact Transmission

Contact transmission may be either direct or indirect. Direct transmission occurs when microorganisms are transferred by direct physical contact with an infected or colonized patient. This is one of the most common modes of transmission. Indirect contact involves transfer of microorganisms via an object. This may occur when hands are not washed between patients, through contact with contaminated gloves, medical equipment or instruments, or other objects.

Droplet Transmission

Droplet transmission involves large droplets (greater than or equal to 5 microns in size) that come from the respiratory tract during coughing or sneezing or during procedures such as suctioning. These droplets are propelled a short distance (less than 1 m) through the air and land on the nasal or oral mucosa of the new host. Environmental surfaces or objects also become contaminated when droplets land on them; for example, doorknobs.

Airborne Transmission

Airborne transmission involves microorganisms being carried by dust or other small particles in the air. Microorganisms that are less than 5 microns in size remain suspended in the air and are widely dispersed by air currents. Susceptible hosts who may be some distance away from the source are exposed to microorganisms through inhalation.

Common Vehicle Transmission

Common vehicle transmission involves a contaminated source that may result in a large-scale outbreak; for example, the *Escherichia coli* contamination and recall of packaged meat that occurred in Canada in 2012. Common vehicles for transmission can be food, medication, intravenous fluid, or equipment.

Vector-Borne Transmission

Vectors refer to carriers such as mosquitoes, skunks, or mice who transmit microorganisms. Examples of vector-borne transmission are West Nile virus, rabies, or Hantavirus.

A Portal of Entry to the Host

Once the microorganism has left its initial reservoir and is transported through a mode of transmission, it needs a place to land or a portal of entry. Just as the microorganism leaves the body or host through a portal of exit, these same areas can serve as a portal of entry. Again, these are areas such as mucous membranes and breaks in the skin. Once the microorganism has entered the host, it attempts to start infecting the host. Its success or lack of success depends on the response from the host.

A Susceptible Host

We are all in contact with microorganisms on a daily basis and do not always become sick. Susceptibility depends on various factors, such as the virulence of the microorganisms or the resistance or immunity that the host might have. If you think of your own health, how many times have you been around people who were coughing or sneezing? Did you become ill each time this happened? Although you may have been exposed and all of the other links in the chain were in place, if you were not susceptible to that particular microorganism at that particular time, you did not become infected. This is just one example of how one link in the chain of infection can have an impact on whether or not disease and illness is transmitted.

Normal Defense Mechanisms

Knowing how the chain of infection works is important but so is knowing about our normal defense mechanisms. When talking about the susceptibility of the host, it is important to note that susceptibility is not just something that occurs by chance. There are normal defense mechanisms that allow the human body to protect itself from the microorganisms it comes into contact with every day. The better known response that occurs in the body is called the *inflammatory response*. The body recognizes the difference between the self and the nonself. The self includes agents that are part of the genetic makeup of the being. The nonself includes agents that are foreign to the being and are referred to as *antigens*. Antigens are the foreign proteins that are present to the body and trigger a response from the immune system to defend itself from these nonself agents. These responses can be specific or nonspecific. Specific responses occur when specific pathogens are encountered and can lead to serious illness or death if the immune system does not engage. Nonspecific responses occur regularly and protect against microorganisms regardless of previous exposure. The nonspecific responses include the skin and normal flora, mouth and mucous membranes, elimination tracts and acidic environments, and inflammation.

Skin and Normal Flora

Intact skin is the first line of defense against infection. The skin serves as a protective barrier against microorganisms. It is important to remember that intact skin alone may not always be sufficient. Nearly 10^6 skin *squames* (a scale or flake of skin) containing viable microorganisms are shed daily from normal skin, so it is not surprising that patient gowns, bed linen, bedside furniture, and other objects in the immediate environment of the patient become contaminated with patient flora. This demonstrates the importance of hand washing. Each individual also carries normal flora on skin called *resident flora*. It is important to note that although resident flora is less likely to be associated with infections, it can cause infections in sterile body cavities, the eyes, or on non-intact skin. The hands of some HCWs may become persistently colonized by pathogenic flora such as *Staphylococcus aureus*, gram-negative bacilli, or yeast.

Mouth and Mucous Membranes

Mucous membranes also serve as a protective barrier against microorganisms. Mucous membranes produce a thick secretion called *mucus*, which serves to protect the body. Mucus is a viscous solid containing antiseptic enzymes such as lysozyme and immunoglobulins that project the epithelial cells in the respiratory, gastrointestinal, and urogenital tracts. In the respiratory tract, mucus protects the lungs by trapping infectious agents that enter primarily through the nose during normal respiration. In the nares, the nasal mucosa traps small particles and infectious agents and prevents them from entering the respiratory system. These all serve to protect the individual from coming into contact with microorganisms that may cause infection.

Inflammation

The **inflammatory response** is the body's response to contact with disease-causing microorganisms. Inflammation is commonly divided into two basic categories: acute or chronic. Acute inflammation is relatively short, lasting anywhere from a few minutes to several days. Chronic inflammation is longer and can last for a few days up to years.

Acute Inflammation

Acute inflammation includes several cardinal signs specific to this type of inflammation. These signs include redness, swelling, heat, pain or discomfort, and loss of function. Along with these cardinal signs, the individual may be febrile. These signs may not be present when internal organs are involved.

Acute inflammation involves both vascular and cellular changes. Immediate vascular changes include vasoconstriction followed rapidly by vasodilation of the arterioles and venules that supply the area. This is what causes the redness and warmth. There is also an increase in capillary permeability, which causes swelling or edema to the area. Edema is responsible for pain and decreased mobility. Cellular changes that occur during the inflammation response include movement of phagocytic white blood cells (WBCs), primarily granulocytes and monocytes, to the affected area. These WBCs migrate from the blood vessel and into the intracellular space where they destroy microorganisms and other small particles.

Chronic Inflammation

Chronic inflammation is different in that the inflammation can last from days to years. Characteristics of chronic inflammation are primarily due to infiltration with macrophages, lymphocytes, and fibroblasts, leading to persistent inflammation, fibroblast proliferation, and scar formation. As a result, the risk for deformity and potentially decreased mobility is considered greater than in acute inflammation.

Applying the Principles of Asepsis

The nursing student perspective is an important starting point for this discussion because thoughts, opinions, and knowledge changes throughout the process of learning about asepsis. By understanding the applicable perspectives and context of asepsis in nursing, you can better prepare to apply the principles while engaging in any psychomotor skill, even in a hectic, constantly changing, and complex patient care environment.

The following sections on applying the principles of asepsis emphasize specific concepts and knowledge. Even the simplest skill requires an understanding of asepsis. Although there are many topics that are relevant to this skill, patient susceptibility, recognizing which microorganisms are present, and types of hand hygiene products are important. In addition to hand hygiene products, personal protective equipment is reviewed in the context of asepsis.

Nadine knows that it is important to pay attention to asepsis and prevent the transmission of infection, but there are so many things to remember, and she doesn't want to be the one who causes the transmission of a microorganism. From her work as a community health representative, she has helped nurses and watched them apply principles of asepsis, but she is not sure how some microorganisms are transmitted and some are not. She wants to know what she needs to do to keep her patients healthy.

Nursing students have a unique perspective when it comes to the principles of asepsis. Some students may worry that they won't know what to do when their patient has a specific virus or microorganism or, worse, that they won't know when they have contaminated something. Asepsis is involved in every skill that nurses perform and is often a source of stress for students when they are being closely supervised by faculty and practicing nurses. Both students and faculty members need to work together to reduce the stress of skills such as wound care or isolation precautions to a realistic level. Students then need to work toward effective and efficient application of aseptic technique that follows both agency policies and procedures and provincial regulations and standards.

Through the eyes of a nurse

As the students care for more complex patients, I am concerned about their ability to maintain asepsis. They seem to have a pretty solid understanding of the importance of hand washing, even if I do have to remind them every once in a while. It seems, though, that when the patient is sicker and the skills are more complex, they are more concerned about the steps of the skill and forget about the principles of asepsis. If they could just remember that the principles of asepsis are important with everything that they do with their patients, I think the steps of the skills would be less overwhelming for them. And I know that they will make mistakes in the beginning, which is why it is important to guide them through the first few skills and then help them problem-solve through their skill application. Once the light bulb goes on and they see how asepsis fits with their skills, I think that is when they are able to be more independent. Faculty need to help them with this problem solving and not just tell them that something is wrong. *(personal reflection of a nurse)*

The Nurse's Perspective

Nurses are often more comfortable than nursing students with applying the principles of asepsis. This makes sense because asepsis is a part of most actions that a nurse does; through repeated practice and application, asepsis has become a daily part of a nurse's work. However, a nurse should never become complacent with something as familiar as asepsis. With new microorganisms that often surface, combined with facilities that have rapid patient turnover and a busy environment, being complacent and taking shortcuts with asepsis can mean the difference between transmitting infections from patient to patient, or keeping them as free from infection as possible. All nurses, regardless of how long they have practiced, need to be reminded of the necessity of asepsis and how to prevent transmission of some of the newly identified microorganisms in our environment. In addition, the practicing nurse should also keep in mind the professional regulations and policies that exist both on a provincial and agency level. Not all patients have the same infections, and although most infections are treated the same, this isn't always the case.

Through the eyes of a nurse

*I*t is so different applying aseptic technique as a nurse compared to when I was a student nurse. I am so used to just washing my hands and keeping sterile and clean separate that I do not always have to think about it. It just becomes routine. With students, you sometimes have to remind them to wash their hands before doing any task, even something as straightforward and routine as vital signs. Watching them perform wound care or when they first enter isolation rooms, the look of concentration makes me wonder if they are just going through the steps or if they really understand how asepsis fits into what they do. After asking a few questions, it becomes evident that they understand what asepsis is, but they just need a little more time to put it all together. The good part of having students on our units is when we get less common microorganisms or infections in our facility. The students are so savvy in finding the information that they often have the latest reports from the government agencies before I do. I then see my role in helping them apply this information to practice. *(personal reflection of a nurse)*

Nosocomial Infections

Patients come to institutions such as hospitals to get better, not worse; and applying the principles of asepsis uniformly and consistently with all patients can make the difference in the patient's health status. Infections that are acquired by patients while they are institutionalized or hospitalized are called **nosocomial infections**. Those acquired outside of health-care facilities are called *community acquired*. Nosocomial infections are especially common in hospitals, not surprisingly because hospitals have a high population of individuals who are both ill and with high acuity. As such, many patients may already be **immunocompromised** and easily contract disease while in hospital. Nosocomial infections represent a serious public health problem, and significant attempts have been made to decrease their incidence. **Iatrogenic infections** are nosocomial infections that result from a diagnostic or therapeutic treatment. Infection resulting from urinary catheterization is an iatrogenic nosocomial infection that has experienced a significant decrease in rates, primarily because of strong educational programs.

Nosocomial infections are classified as either exogenous or endogenous in nature. If you recall our earlier discussion, we all have both resident and transient flora that live on the surface of our skin. Exogenous infections can occur when transient flora are introduced to the susceptible host. An example of this would be the *Salmonella* organism present in chicken eggs and subsequently ingested by a susceptible host. Endogenous infections can occur when resident flora become altered and proliferate. The equilibrium has been disturbed, and infection can occur. An example of an endogenous infection could be the *Candida* yeast that is part of the normal vaginal

flora. External use of detergents or douches, or internal disturbances (hormonal or physiological), can disturb the normal vaginal flora, leading to candidiasis, an endogenous infection.

Patient Susceptibility

Although routine practices must be considered for all patients, patient susceptibility to infection will determine what, if any, additional measures may apply. This means that various individuals can be at greater or lesser risk of contracting an infectious disease. We can all think of a time when we were stressed and were more likely to catch a viral illness such as a common cold. It is these differences that make patients more susceptible to contracting disease.

Age

Think back to the many times that you have likely heard of the very elderly and very young being more susceptible to contracting a particular disease. The elderly and the very young have various susceptibilities to contracting infection. The very young are born with only the antibodies provided by the mother, which means that they have an immature and developing immune system. Their WBCs are unable to produce immunoglobulins necessary to fight infection. One way to boost immunity is to breast-feed infants, as they continue to receive antibodies from the mother through breast milk. As children age, they begin to develop their own immune system and are better able to fend off infection. However, as their immune system continues to mature, they are still susceptible to viral illnesses and frequently develop common colds.

The elderly are also susceptible to contracting illnesses, however, for different reasons. The immune system becomes less efficient with age, in large part due to the decrease in T cell and B cell production. These cells are mature lymphocytes and are the most abundant lymphocytes found in the human body. Their primary function is to support the immune system in recognizing and responding to infectious agents. Along with changes to the integumentary, respiratory, and urinary systems, this all increases the susceptibility of the older adult to contracting illnesses and disease.

Stress

Stress has unique physiological effects on the human body. As people experience stress, the body attempts to compensate by releasing cortisol. Although stress is not the only reason that cortisol is secreted into the bloodstream, it has been termed the *stress hormone* because it's also secreted in higher levels during the body's fight or flight response to stress and is responsible for several stress-related changes in the body.

If a short-term stressor is experienced, it can actually boost the immune system. It seems that the fight or flight response prompts the immune system to ready itself for infections resulting from bites, punctures, scrapes, or other challenges to the integrity of the body. However, chronic, long-term stress suppresses the immune system. The longer the stress period, the more the immune system shifts from the adaptive changes seen in the fight or flight response to more negative changes, first at the cellular level and later in broader immune function. The most chronic stressors (i.e., stress that seems beyond a person's control or seems endless) result in the most global suppression of immunity. Almost all measures of immune system function drop across the board. Higher and more prolonged levels of cortisol in the bloodstream (e.g., those associated with chronic stress) have been shown to have negative effects, such as the following:

- Impaired cognitive performance
- Suppressed thyroid function
- Blood sugar imbalances such as hyperglycemia
- Decreased bone density
- Decrease in muscle tissue
- Higher blood pressure
- Lowered immunity and inflammatory responses in the body, slowed wound healing, and other health consequences

The immune systems of the elderly or those already sick are more subject to stress-related changes.

Nutritional Status

Nutrition is a fundamental element in healthy human development and is essential for healing and immunity. Individuals with poor nutritional intake are at greater risk of delayed wound healing and lowered immunity to infectious microorganisms. Inadequate stores of proteins, carbohydrates, fats, vitamins, and minerals all negatively influence immunity. Protein deficiencies prolong the inflammatory phase of healing, whereas carbohydrates are necessary as an energy source for WBCs. Fats are essential components of cell membranes and are needed for the growth of new cells. Vitamins and minerals are necessary for various stages of healing and immunity (see also Chapter 34, Ensuring Nutrition).

Known Microorganisms

Presence of disease has a significant impact on immunity. For example, individuals with the human immunodeficiency virus (HIV) are already immunocompromised, and the introduction of additional infectious microorganisms can have disastrous consequences. Several other diseases or treatment for diseases (e.g., chemotherapy) can also weaken the immune system. The nurse needs to think of not only the disease that the individual has but also the treatment that the patient is receiving. For example, corticosteroids are commonly prescribed for individuals with chronic bronchitis or chronic obstructive pulmonary disease (COPD). Remembering that the respiratory mucosa is one of the lines of defense in the body, an individual with chronic bronchitis likely has an impairment in the ability to fight infection in this area. Add to that a corticosteroid, which is known to have the potential to suppress immunity. Imagine that this same individual is assigned to a nursing student who, while she has a cold and does not want to miss clinical for fear of a decrease in clinical grades, coughs into the air near the patient, potentially spreading infectious droplets. Given that the patient already has a respiratory illness and is taking inhaled corticosteroids, what do you think is the impact of this simple action of coughing by the nursing student?

The body also needs an adequate supply of blood flow and oxygen delivery for healing to occur. Diseases that affect either arterial or venous vascularity impair healing and increase susceptibility to infection. When dealing with blood flow, any type of bleeding or trauma will also have a negative effect on the ability to fight infection.

Products for Hand Hygiene

There are numerous products available related to hand hygiene. Among these products are non-antimicrobial soaps and alcohol-based antiseptics. We often think of soap and water; however, with the introduction of waterless hand hygiene products, the nurse must have an understanding of what is available and when to use each product.

Hand hygiene is the umbrella term for hand washing with soap and water as well as the use of alcohol-based hand rubs. The purpose of routine hand hygiene and hand washing in patient care is to remove dirt and organic material as well as any microorganisms that may be present due to direct patient contact or with the environment. Although we often think of water as a significant means to wash our hands, water alone is often not enough to remove substances that may be present on the hands.

Plain (non-antimicrobial) soaps are detergent-based products that are available in various forms including bar soap, tissue, leaf, and liquid preparations. Their cleansing activity can be attributed to their detergent properties that result in the removal of lipids and dirt, soil, and various organic substances from the hands. Plain soaps have minimal, if any, antimicrobial activity; although, hand washing with plain soap can remove loosely adherent transient flora. For example, hand washing with plain soap and water for 30 seconds reduces more than twice the bacterial counts on the skin compared to washing for only 15 seconds. In several studies, however, hand washing with plain soap failed to remove pathogens from the hands of nurses and other HCWs.

Most alcohol-based hand antiseptics contain either ethanol, isopropanol or n-propanol, or a combination of two of these products. Concentrations of alcohol are given as either percentage of volume (% v/v), percentage of weight (% m/m), or percentage of weight/volume (% m/v). Alcohol solutions containing 60% to 80% alcohol are most effective, with higher concentrations being less potent. Alcohols have excellent germicidal activity against gram-positive and gram-negative bacteria (including multidrug-resistant pathogens such as methicillin-resistant *Staphylococcus aureus* [MRSA] and vancomycin-resistant *Enterococcus* [VRE]), *Mycobacterium tuberculosis*, and various fungi; however, they have virtually no activity against bacterial spores or protozoan oocysts and very poor activity against some non-enveloped (nonlipophilic) viruses. Some enveloped (lipophilic) viruses such as herpes simplex virus (HSV), HIV, influenza virus, and the respiratory syncytial virus (RSV) are susceptible to alcohols when tested in the laboratory setting.

The efficacy of alcohol-based hand hygiene products is affected by several factors including the type of alcohol used, concentration of alcohol, contact time, volume of alcohol used, and whether the hands are wet when the alcohol is applied. Small volumes (0.2 to 0.5 ml) of alcohol applied to the hands are no more effective than washing hands with plain soap and water. In recent studies, it has been found that 1 ml of alcohol was significantly less effective than 3 ml. The ideal volume of product to apply to the hands is not known and may vary for different formulations. In general, however, if hands feel dry after being rubbed together for less than 10 to 15 seconds, it is likely that an insufficient volume of product was applied. Alcohol-impregnated towelettes contain only a small amount of alcohol and are not much more effective than washing with soap and water.

Alcohols are not good cleansing agents, and their use is not recommended when hands are dirty or visibly contaminated with materials such as blood. When a relatively small amount of blood is present however, ethanol and isopropanol may reduce viable bacterial counts on hands. But this does not mean that there is no need for hand washing with water and soap whenever such contamination occurs. For more details on hand hygiene products, see Table 19.1.

Glove, Gown, and Mask

Using gloves, gowns, and masks is part of **personal protective equipment (PPE)**. The type of PPE chosen depends on the clinical situation and the type of interaction required with the patient. The selection of gowns, gloves, masks, and/or face protection should include consideration of the following issues: probability of exposure to blood and/or body fluids, amount of blood and/or body fluids likely to be encountered, and the probable route of transmission.

Gloves

Gloves are the most commonly used PPE in health-care institutions. These are often seen in hallways and in patient rooms. However, the use of gloves should be considered as an additional measure, not as a substitute for hand hygiene. When indicated, the nurse should put on gloves directly before the task/procedure to be performed and then remove the gloves immediately following completion of task at the point of use and before touching clean environmental surfaces.

There also is concern regarding the overuse of gloves. Overuse of gloves has been linked to a decrease in compliance with hand hygiene. Gloves are not required for routine activities where contact is limited to intact skin, activities such as taking a blood pressure. Gloves must be changed between care activities and procedures with the same patient; for example, never use the same pair of gloves to empty a drain and perform wound care, even if on the same patient.

TABLE 19.1	Hand Hygiene Products	
Products	Indications	Special Considerations
Plain soap, bar soap, liquid, granules	For routine care of patients/residents For washing hands soiled with dirt, blood, or other organic material	May contain very low concentrations of antimicrobial agents to prevent microbial contamination growth in the product Bar soap should be on racks that allow water to drain; small bars that can be changed frequently are safest.
Waterless antiseptic agents: - rinses - foams - wipes - towelettes	Demonstrated alternative to conventional agents For use where hand washing facilities are inadequate, impractical, or inaccessible (e.g., ambulances, home care, mass immunizations) For situations in which the water supply is interrupted (e.g., planned disruptions, natural disasters)	Not effective if hands are soiled with dirt or heavily contaminated with blood or other organic material Follow manufacturer's recommendations for use. Efficacy affected by concentration of alcohol in product Hand creams should be readily available to protect skin integrity.
Antiseptic agents	May be chosen for hand scrubs prior to performance of invasive procedures (e.g., placing intravascular lines or devices) When caring for severely immunocompromised individuals; based on risk of transmission (e.g., specific microorganisms) Critical care areas such as intensive care nurseries or operating rooms When caring for individuals with antimicrobial resistant organisms	Antiseptic agents may be chosen if it is felt important to reduce the number of resident flora or when the level of microbial contamination is high. Antiseptic agents should be chosen when persistent antimicrobial activity on the hands is desired. They are usually available in liquid formulations. Antiseptic agents differ in activity and characteristics. Routine use of hexachlorophene is not recommended because of neurotoxicity and potential absorption through the skin. Alcohol containers should be stored in areas approved for flammable materials.

Note: Disposable containers are preferred for liquid products. Reusable containers should be thoroughly washed and dried before refilling, and routine maintenance schedules should be followed and documented. Liquid products should be stored in closed containers and should not be topped up.

Source: World Health Organization. (2009). *WHO guidelines on hand hygiene in health care.* Geneva, Switzerland: Author. Retrieved from http://whqlibdoc.who.int/publications/2009/9789241597906_eng.pdf

Gloves should be long enough to fit over the cuff of a gown, if a gown is worn (e.g., isolation precautions or when likelihood of exposure is high). Clean, nonsterile gloves of appropriate size should be worn when contact with blood, body fluids, secretions, and excretions, mucous membranes, draining wounds, or non-intact skin is likely. They should also be worn for handling items visibly soiled with blood, body fluids, secretions, or excretions or when the nurse has open lesions on the hands. Hand hygiene should be performed after removing gloves. Single-use disposable gloves should be discarded after use.

Gowns

Routine use of gowns is not recommended nor is it necessary. Use gowns to protect uncovered skin and prevent soiling of clothing during procedures and patient care activities likely to generate splashes or sprays of blood, body fluids, secretions, and excretions. The sleeves should extend to the wrist and be cuffed for a snug fit. A disposable impervious/water repellent apron may be used under the gown to prevent contamination of clothing from leakage of large volumes of blood, body fluids, secretions, or excretions. The nurse should remove the gown after completion of the patient activity, when leaving the room, or when gown is heavily soiled/wet. Gowns should only be worn once, and disposable gowns are to be discarded after each use.

Masks

Standard surgical or procedure masks are worn to protect the mucous membranes of the nose and mouth during procedures and patient care activities that are likely to generate splashes, sprays or aerosols of blood, body fluids, secretions, or excretions. Masks are to be worn within 1 m (3 ft) of a patient who is coughing possibly due to a respiratory infection. The nurse should discard a mask if it is crushed, wet, has dangled around the neck, or become contaminated and should perform hand hygiene immediately after mask removal.

N95 Face Piece Respirators

The N95 face piece respirators are another form of PPE. This specially designed mask is used to reduce airborne particle exposure. Disposable N95 respirators are an item of PPE worn by nurses and other HCWs who are likely to be exposed to patients with airborne, communicable diseases such as tuberculosis, acute respiratory syndrome, and, in some cases, H1N1 (swine flu). Respirator fit testing and annual retesting is currently a requirement in many workplaces and health authorities in Canada. The fit-testing process involves selecting the correct size and type of respirator (mask) for each nurse and ensuring that they know how to use it correctly. Many faculties and schools of nursing are requiring nursing students to be fit-tested for the N95 respirator. In preparation for a fit test, the person being tested is asked not to eat, drink (except water), smoke, or chew gum for a minimum of 30 minutes prior to the test. Anything that reduces the sense of taste will adversely affect the test process. Men who are required to be fit-tested must be cleanly shaved because facial hair can interfere with the fit of the mask. The process can take approximately 20 minutes as individuals complete a sensitivity test followed by a return demonstration of the correct way to don, wear, and remove the mask. Individuals are not given a mask rather they are given a card indicated the style and size of mask which should be worn in the future.

Eye Protection

Another type of PPE includes eye protection, worn to protect the mucous membranes of the eyes during procedures and patient care activities that are likely to generate splashes, sprays, or aerosols of blood, body fluids, secretions, or excretions. Eye goggles are common types of eye protection. Prescription eyeglasses are not considered eye protection because they do not provide adequate protection from splashes or sprays. Eye protection should fit over prescription glasses.

Face Protection

Face protection is worn to protect the mucous membranes of the eyes, nose, and mouth during procedures and patient care activities that are likely to generate splashes, sprays, or aerosols of blood, body fluids, secretions, or excretions. Face protection should fit over prescription glasses and be an appropriate size for the wearer. It should be large enough to protect mucous membranes of the face (eyes, nose, and mouth). Face shields are common types of face protection.

Implementing Skills of Asepsis

This section emphasizes the actual skills involved in implementing the principles of asepsis. The steps of each process are outlined with applicable concepts and issues integrated into each skill. The skills associated with asepsis include hand hygiene and donning PPE. These are often required prior to implementation of other skills. It is important to master and remember these core skills.

Nadine says, "I have watched many practicing nurses put on sterile gloves and perform wound care, and I have even helped some of them put the patient in the correct position! I know how important it is to keep items sterile, but I don't always know when I contaminate something. I tried to memorize where my hands have been, who and what I've touched, but it just didn't help. I couldn't remember where my hands had been. I stopped trying to memorize their last location, and decided that I just needed to treat every surface I touched as though it were dirty and that helped me to remember how to apply the principles of asepsis. I knew that I needed to break the chain of infection and that proper hand hygiene combined with an understanding of the modes of transmission would help me do just that."

Hand Hygiene

The performance of hand hygiene is important and equally as important is the selection of appropriate agents to be used during hand hygiene (Skill 19.1).

Think *Are You Spying on Me?*

Often, nurses will become aware of other health-care professionals who enter patient rooms or engage in patient care without washing their hands. They may be certain that these persons have not washed their hands, but what should the nurse do? Think about what is best for the patient and what is necessary to prevent the spread of disease and illness. It is acceptable and even necessary for the nurse to bring this to other health-care professionals' attention and to remind them of the need to wash their hands.

Isolation Precautions

Prior to applying any type of PPE, the nurse must first conduct a risk assessment. In these situations, the risks being assessed are for both the patient and the nurse. Many institutions have policies surrounding the use of PPE, and these policies should be consulted as part of the risk assessment. In addition, infection control manuals are available at each institution and should be consulted when dealing with particular microorganisms. These sources clarify for the nurse which particular type of precautions should be taken (Skill 19.2).

Gloves

Gloves are worn in an isolated environment to prevent the spread of microorganisms between patients as well as between the nurse and the patient. Gloves should be used in addition to hand hygiene and must be discarded after a single use. Gloves are worn in this environment because the nurse will be touching items in the room that may be contaminated. Remember, infectious agents are not usually visible.

Think *To Glove or Not to Glove*

When is it required to wear gloves, and when is it not? This can be an easy question to answer. Whenever the nurse will be potentially in contact with blood or other body fluids, either from the patient or from the nurse herself, she should wear gloves. If the activity does not include the potential spread of microorganisms, gloves are not necessary. Activities such as obtaining a blood pressure do not require gloves; however, the nurse should be aware of institutional policies because some places may even require gloves for something such as obtaining a blood pressure, typically for reasons other than blood and body fluid contamination.

Gowns

Gowns should be worn to prevent soiling of clothing during procedures—any activities likely to generate splashes of bodily fluids, etc., and when recommended by infectious diseases departments. The nurse should always consult the infectious diseases manual for specific information.

Masks

The purpose of standard surgical/procedure masks is to protect the mucous membranes of the nose and mouth during procedures and patient care activities that are likely to generate splashes, sprays, or aerosols of blood, body fluids, secretions, or excretions. They are also used to prevent the transmission of some microorganisms that are transmitted via the respiratory system.

Sterile Gloves

Certain procedures require that the nurse wear gloves that are sterile (Skill 19.3). It is important to remember that this is different from wearing clean gloves for the purpose of personal protection. Sterile gloves are used for procedures such as catheterization or when you are entering or accessing a sterile part of the body. In these situations, sterile gloves are to protect against microorganisms because the skin is no longer a barrier that is able to provide protection. Think of changing the dressing of someone with a burn or when a patient is in the operating room.

Preparing a Sterile Field

Setting up a sterile field requires an understanding of where your hands have been and what can or cannot be touched. Although it may appear easy, opening a sterile drape and creating a sterile field requires that the nurse pay particular attention to the areas of the field that are considered sterile and those that are not considered sterile (Skill 19.4).

Think *Oh No! Now, What Do I Do?*

When preparing a sterile field, the nurse needs to be aware of where his or her hands and fingers are at all times. He or she also needs to be aware of any potential contamination of the sterile field and know what to do in that situation. Think of what you might do if you inadvertently contaminated your sterile field. Possibilities include discarding the current sterile field and starting from the beginning, or depending on what was contaminated; it may mean simply removing the instrument and replacing it with a sterile one. If the nurse has set up an extensive field such as in the operating room, there may be other possibilities as well. The main priority, however, is recognizing when something is contaminated and being able to think through the possibilities of what to do next in order to ensure sterility of the equipment and field that will be in contact with the patient.

Professional Practice

In this section, we outline concepts that are associated with the principles of asepsis. We also offer observations related to the role of the nurse. Interprofessional communication, teaching and learning concepts, the role of culture in applying the principles of asepsis, and comfort measures are highlighted.

Through the eyes of a patient

*I*t was one of those really busy days when all the nurses looked like they were just running. I was alone in my hospital room yesterday, but sometime during the night, another patient was assigned to my room. From what I could tell, my new roommate was really sick and several nurses were in and out of the room. First thing in the morning, my nurse came in to change the dressing on my knee from the knee replacement I had a few days ago. The nurse started to get the supplies ready and was interrupted when my neighbour called the nurse over. I couldn't see what happened over there as the curtain was drawn between us. When the nurse was done, she came back over to me to finish changing my dressing. I didn't see where the nurse went and I don't know if she washed her hands between us or not. I was worried. I had such a horrible infection 2 years ago when I had my other knee operated on and I really didn't want to go through that again. I told my nurse from the day before about the previous infection that I had, and the nurse told me about how infection can be transmitted and how important it was to perform proper hand washing, especially if I or anyone else was going to be touching my incision. That nurse also made it obvious every time she washed her hands or told me if she washed her hands outside of my hospital room. I felt comfortable with this. I didn't know what was wrong with my roommate, but he sounded pretty sick and I didn't want to catch what he had, and I especially didn't want another infection in my knee. I worried the entire time that the nurse changed my dressing and wondered if I was going to get an infection. I worried for many days after that as well. I was literally sick with worry!

(personal reflection of a patient)

Communicating With the Patient

Communication is important between the nurse and the patient. The scenario demonstrates how important something seemingly this simple can be. How might the nurse avoid this type of situation? By using the sink in the room to wash or using the alcohol-based rubs that are often located in patient rooms as well, the nurse could have made it apparent to the patient that she had washed her hands. If nothing was available in the room and if the nurse had washed her hands out of the patient's view, it would have been very easy to simply tell the patient. Alternatively, if the nurse were changing a dressing, using PPE such as gloves would have provided protection for both the nurse and the patient and would have been clearly visible as well. With many media spots indicating the importance of hand washing, patients are very aware of the importance of this step in preventing infection from spreading. Patients can also be uncomfortable questioning their health-care providers about hand washing for fear of appearing to question the care that they are receiving. It is up to the nurse to either make this step visible or to state to the patient that this step has been taken.

Patient Teaching

The teaching of patients regarding the chain of infection and the role of asepsis is very important both for patients in hospital or in the community. The greater public should know this information and the protective measures because adherence could keep people infection free and out of health-care institutions. Patient visitors should also be aware of asepsis, especially if they are visiting people who are more susceptible to contraction of infection. Ensuring that people are aware of proper hand washing procedures, cough and sneeze etiquette, or even when to stay home from visiting those who are more susceptible to contracting illness or disease can help prevent the spread of harmful microorganism. There are a few considerations for patient education to ensure clients/patients have the information they need.

Consider the developmental age of the patient and the best medium to convey information (e.g., an elderly patient might not be able to read a piece of written information in small type). Children should be taught of proper hand washing procedures at a young age and should be aware of proper cough and sneeze etiquette. This is often done through media presentations.

What is the patient's condition at the time of teaching? Patients are often not feeling well if they are in the hospital. It is very difficult to review information related to the spread of disease with patients when they are acutely ill. It is important to include family or support individuals in the teaching to ensure that the information is received and can be recalled as needed once the patient returns home. This information is equally important for family members because they would not want to be responsible for spreading disease to their loved ones.

What type and how much depth of information you are going to give to the patient? This is an important point as too much medically based information might not be appropriate for some patients. It is also not helpful to simply reiterate textbook knowledge. Try to speak to a patient in plain language using common phrases.

Choose the setting and allow time to review the information with the patient and to confirm his or her understanding. The setting plays an important role in relaying information to patients about asepsis. Because hand washing is a simple step, it is often assumed that minimal time is required to teach it. Incorporate asepsis into other teaching that you need to do but ensure that information is complete. For example, what can a person do if there is no running water available?

Cultural and Social Considerations

Culture and social context are important aspects to consider when addressing asepsis. The role of culture affects all areas of being, including rules and beliefs related to touch and hand hygiene. Every patient (and nurse and nursing student for that matter) lives within a cultural and social context. The ways in which patients live their lives will have an impact on how their asepsis is understood and carried out. Although it is impossible to be aware of all cultural and social implications with patients and their families, two core ideas may help guide your practice as you consider these aspects of patient care. Hand hygiene can be practiced for hygienic reasons, ritual reasons during religious ceremonies, and symbolic reasons in specific everyday situations. Personal hygiene is a key component of human well-being regardless of religion, culture, or place of origin.

The Concept of Visibly Dirty Hands

The Public Health Agency of Canada, the U.S. Centers for Disease Control and Prevention (CDC) guidelines, and the present WHO guidelines recommend that health-care professionals wash their hands with soap and water when they are visibly soiled. Otherwise, hand rubbing with an alcohol-based rub is recommended for all other opportunities for hand hygiene during patient care because it is faster, more effective, and better tolerated by the skin (Fig. 19.3). Infection control practitioners find it difficult to define precisely the meaning of "visibly dirty," and it is necessary to give practical examples while schooling health-care professionals in hand hygiene practices. In a transcultural perspective, it could be increasingly difficult to find a common understanding of this term. In fact, actually seeing dirt on hands can be impeded by the colour of the skin: It is, for example, more difficult to see a spot of blood or other proteinaceous material on very dark skin. According to some religions, the concept of dirt is not strictly visual but reflects a wider meaning that refers to interior and exterior purity.

The cultural issue of feeling cleaner after hand washing rather than after hand rubbing was recently raised within the context of a widespread hand hygiene campaign in Hong Kong. A cultural preference for hand washing may be at the root of the lack of long-term sustainability of hand hygiene compliance achieved during the severe acute respiratory syndrome pandemic. From a global perspective, these considerations highlight the importance of making every possible effort to consider the concept of visibly dirty in accordance with racial, cultural, and environmental factors and to adapt it to local situations with an appropriate strategy when promoting hand hygiene.

Alcohol-Based Hand Rubs

According to scientific evidence arising from efficacy and cost-effectiveness, alcohol-based hand rubs are currently considered the gold standard approach for hand hygiene. In some religions, alcohol use is prohibited or considered an offence requiring a penance because it is considered to cause mental impairment. As a result, the adoption of alcohol-based formulations as the standard for hand hygiene may be unsuitable or inappropriate for some nurses either because of their reluctance to have contact with alcohol or because of their concern about alcohol ingestion or absorption via the skin. Even the simple denomination of the product as an alcohol-based formulation could become an obstacle in the implementation of WHO recommendations.

It is important to discuss hand hygiene with patients and their families to see how culture and social contexts may impact asepsis. Not all cultures have the same beliefs and practices; therefore, it is imperative to understand each patient's specific application of culture in order to holistically care for that patient.

Providing Comfort Measures

In terms of asepsis, the primary comfort that the patient would derive from the nurse practicing aseptic technique would be the lack of infection or illness. However, think back to the patient scenario earlier. The patient was obviously worried about whether the nurse had washed her hands. A simple verbal reassurance or making the hand washing visible to the patient would have put that patient at ease. Informing patients of your hygiene practices puts them at ease in knowing that their care provider is taking their well-being seriously.

Interprofessional Communication

Interprofessional communication regarding asepsis usually follows the premise that one individual has not engaged in adequate adherence to asepsis and another professional has observed this. For example, if you were a nurse in the operating room and observed the surgeon or another member of the team contaminate himself or herself in any way, it would be your responsibility to inform the other

How to Handrub?

RUB HANDS FOR HAND HYGIENE! WASH HANDS WHEN VISIBLY SOILED

Duration of the entire procedure: 20-30 seconds

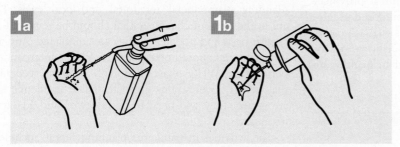

Apply a palmful of the product in a cupped hand, covering all surfaces;

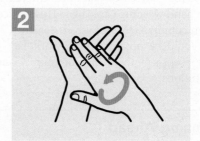

Rub hands palm to palm;

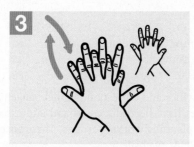

Right palm over left dorsum with interlaced fingers and vice versa;

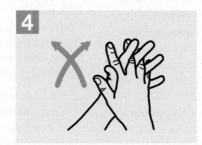

Palm to palm with fingers interlaced;

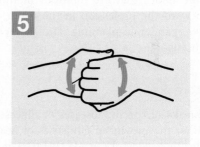

Backs of fingers to opposing palms with fingers interlocked;

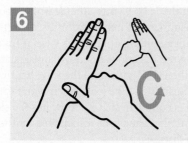

Rotational rubbing of left thumb clasped in right palm and vice versa;

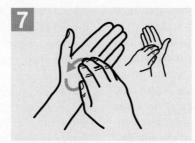

Rotational rubbing, backwards and forwards with clasped fingers of right hand in left palm and vice versa;

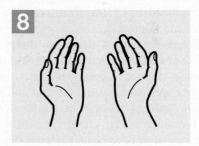

Once dry, your hands are safe.

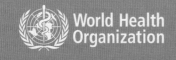

World Health Organization | **Patient Safety** A World Alliance for Safer Health Care | **SAVE LIVES** Clean **Your** Hands

May 2009

Figure 19.3 Guidelines on hand rub from the World Health Organization (WHO). (Source: World Health Organization [WHO]. [2009]. *How to Handrub*. Retrieved from http://www.who.int)

team member of this to ensure that he or she does not introduce harmful microorganisms to the patient. Although this situation is fairly straightforward, think of what would happen if a nurse saw another nurse enter a room to engage in a task and knew that he did not wash his hands. It can be uncomfortable but necessary to ask the nurse if he has washed his hands.

Recognizing the challenges that are currently being seen in the workplace and with the public, the College of Registered Nurses of Manitoba entered into a province-wide hand washing campaign. This was composed of television commercials, bus advertisements, as well as posters that could be posted around workplace facilities to promote asepsis both in the community and in health-care institutions.

Planning Ahead

In this section, we explore other issues that are prominent in the context of the principles of asepsis. These are the issues that are forefront in nursing and serve to forward the profession in the realm of asepsis. Outbreaks, pandemic planning, and new equipment needs are discussed.

Outbreaks

Outbreaks of specific diseases or illnesses are reportable to either the provincial ministries of health, to the Public Health Agency of Canada (PHAC), or to both. On the PHAC website, there is a list of which diseases are reportable; each individual disease has a particular set of guidelines, many of which are designed for each province, and are downloadable. PHAC then traces these reported incidences and informs health-care professionals and the public about outbreaks of illnesses or diseases in a particular area. Outbreaks are considered to have occurred when a disease is present in greater numbers than would otherwise be expected in a particular time and place. This could be two cases, or it could be 2,000. However, once the numbers become high enough, epidemiologists may consider the outbreak to be an epidemic. Should the number continue to rise and become global, the WHO may classify the outbreak as a **pandemic**. According to the WHO, a pandemic can be identified when three conditions have been met:

- emergence of a disease new to a population;
- agents infect humans, causing serious illness; and
- agents spread easily and sustainably among humans.

A disease or condition is not a pandemic merely because it is widespread or kills many people; it must also be infectious. For instance, cancer is responsible for many deaths but is not considered a pandemic because the disease is not infectious or contagious.

Pandemic Planning

The WHO has created phases of pandemics and monitors outbreaks and categorized these accordingly. In Canada, we have adopted the same phases as the WHO and have created pandemic planning to coincide with these phases.

Planning for a pandemic involves the consideration of what activities are necessary for optimal management of each stage of the pandemic. This section provides a list of planning activities that were developed to facilitate planning at provincial, territorial, and local levels. These are in the form of checklists that should be reviewed on a regular basis and updated as they are completed. Any planning activities should take place during the interpandemic period (i.e., WHO phases 1 and 2) with the recognition that, when novel strains are detected or pandemic alerts are issued, they will need to be reviewed and adapted as necessary.

The activities in pandemic planning should include the following:

- Surveillance
- Vaccine programs
- Antivirals
- Health services
- Emergency planning and response
- Public health measures
- Communications

Many of these activities and corresponding federal activities and responsibilities have been discussed and addressed by various pandemic planning working groups. These are easily accessible on the PHAC website.

Nadine is currently on a unit that has recently admitted several patients with the H1N1 virus. After learning about asepsis and the transmission of microorganisms, Nadine now has a better understanding of how this virus is transmitted. After reading the infectious disease manual, she also knows more about the H1N1 virus and the way that this particular virus is transmitted. She feels much better caring for her patients and is confident that she now has the skills and abilities to ensure that she is not responsible for the spread of infectious diseases.

Conclusion

Understanding medical and surgical asepsis is somewhat complex. The nurse needs to understand the process of how infectious agents are transmitted, the factors that can affect transmission, and the best modality to use to prevent the spread of transmission. All of this decision-making is done in the context of what the patients' needs are. Teaching patients about the prevention of transmission of microorganism will help them stay healthier in the long term.

SKILL 19.1 Hand Hygiene

Reviewing Pertinent Information

Step

Review the patient chart to identify any issues related to immunity or susceptibility for infection.

Review policies and procedures for your area to identify if special or additional considerations should be given to hand hygiene.

Rationale

All patients should be considered at risk for infection, and routine practices should be taken with all patients.

Some areas such as burn units or neonatal units have particular criteria surrounding hand hygiene. These are precautions in addition to routine practices.

Preparing for Hand Hygiene

Step

Gather supplies needed:
- Appropriate soap or antiseptic agent
- Paper towels or air dryer
- Sink with warm running water

Inspect hands for breaks or cuts in skin.

Inspect hands for heavy soiling.

Inspect nails for length and any chipped polish.

Rationale

It is important to get organized prior to performing hand hygiene. Organization can reduce time looking for supplies midway through hand washing.

Open cuts or wounds can be portals of exit for microorganisms and can put both the nurse and the patient at risk for infection.

Bulky matter should be washed and removed first and then proceed to routine hand washing practices.

Nails should be short and filed due to the potential harbouring of microorganisms under the nails. Chipped or old polish can be a contaminant.

Hand Hygiene

Step

Remove jewelry before hand wash procedure, including watch. If possible, watch can be pushed up above the wrist.

Turn warm water on.

Rinse hands under warm running water and dispense soap into palm.

Rationale

Jewelry can harbour microorganisms between the item and the surface of the skin.

Warm water generally cleanses better than cold water.

This allows for suspension and washing away of the loosened microorganisms.

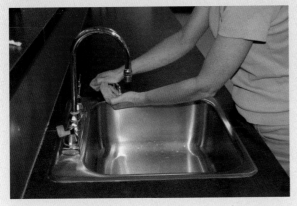

Figure 1 Getting soap.

Using friction, cover all hand surfaces, including palms, back of hands, fingernails, web spaces, and fingers, with soap.

The minimum duration for this step is 10 seconds; more time may be required if hands are visibly soiled. For antiseptic agents, 3–5 ml is required. Frequently missed areas are thumbs, under nails, backs of fingers, and hands.

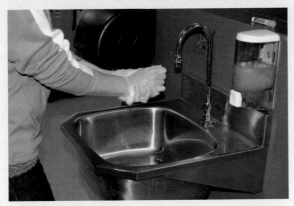

Figure 2 Lathering hands.

(continued on page 358)

SKILL 19.1   Hand Hygiene (continued)

Hand Hygiene (continued)

Step	Rationale
Rinse under warm running water.	This step is to wash off microorganisms and residual hand washing agent.

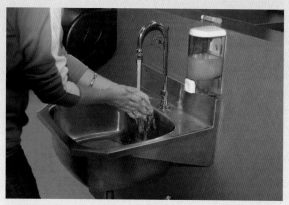

Figure 3 Rinsing hands.

Step	Rationale
Dry hands thoroughly with single-use towel or forced air dryer.	Drying achieves a further reduction in number of microorganisms. Reusable towels are avoided because of the potential for microbial contamination.
Turn off faucet.	Avoid recontaminating hands.

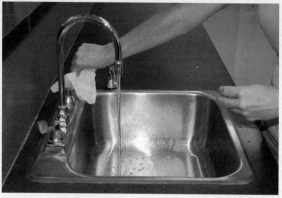

Figure 4 Turning off the tap.

Step	Rationale
Do not use fingernail polish or artificial nails.	Artificial nails or chipped nail polish may increase bacterial load and impede visualization of soil under nails.

Engaging in Evaluation

Step	Rationale
Inspect hands.	This is to ensure that the hands are clean and free of visible contaminants after washing. Also, inspect hands again to observe for any cuts or open areas.

Documenting Effectively

Step	Rationale
Hand hygiene is expected for all activities that nurses engage in with their patients. Documentation is not routinely required for this activity.	

SKILL 19.2 Isolation Precautions: Personal Protective Equipment

Reviewing Pertinent Information

Step	Rationale
Identify patients at risk or situations that present risk.	Immunocompromised patients are at greater risk of contracting illness and disease. Situations that present the opportunity of microorganism transmission should also be identified.
Review the infectious disease control manuals and/or hospital policy regarding the PPE required.	Some microorganisms or infectious diseases require specific equipment to be worn. In other circumstances, routine practice is all that is required. Nurses must know the difference.

Preparing for PPE

Step	Rationale
Gather supplies needed: • Gowns • Standard masks • Clean gloves	Having supplies available reduces the need to go back and forth to the supply room. Gloves, gowns, and masks are the most common types of PPE currently in use.
Identify the order of applications of the gloves, gown, or mask.	The type of PPE required will dictate the order of application.

Donning PPE—Masks

Step—Application

Remove mask from box.
Place mask over mouth and nose.

Loop first strap over one ear or tie top straps of mask to the top of head.

Rationale

The mask must cover both the mouth and nose to prevent transmission via the respiratory tract.
Tying the top strap prevents the mask from dropping forward onto the face or neck and to ensure correct placement of the mask.

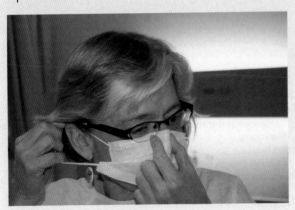

Figure 1 **Nurse donning mask.**

Loop the second strap over other ear or tie bottom straps behind head.	This secures the mask in place.
Ensure fit by molding mask to face at the bridge of the nose.	The soft piece over the bridge of the nose is formed to individually fit the nose and create a seal.

Step—Removal

Leave area/exit room prior to removing mask.

Use both hands to pull loops from behind ears or undo ties beginning with the bottom tie.
Pull mask away from face using ties or loops.
Discard into garbage.

Perform hand hygiene.

If the patient is in isolation, this step must be performed prior to removing the mask.
The bottom tie must be removed first to prevent the mask from dropping onto the face or neck.
This is to prevent self-contamination.
Masks generally do not require special disposal unless contaminated with blood or body fluids.
This must be done upon completion of any skill.

Donning PPE—Gloves

Step—Application

Remove appropriate-sized gloves from box.

Apply gloves and adjust if necessary by interlacing the fingers.
Ensure that gloves are pulled up over the cuffs of the gown if applicable.

Rationale

The nurse must ensure that the gloves are the appropriate size to allow for the best fit and protection.
Interlacing the fingers provides a better fit.
This creates a continuous barrier between the gloves and gown.

(continued on page 360)

SKILL 19.2   Isolation Precautions: Personal Protective Equipment (continued)

Donning PPE—Gloves

Step—Removal	
Using one gloved hand to grasp glove at opposite wrist.	This is to prevent self-contamination.
Remove glove with that hand.	This is to prevent self-contamination.
Slide the other hand inside the wrist to remove the other glove.	This is to prevent self-contamination.
Discard the gloves.	Unless visibly soiled by blood and body fluids, special disposal is not required.
Perform hand hygiene.	This is required upon completion of any skill.

Donning PPE—Gowns

Step—Application	**Rationale**
Put on long-sleeve gown with opening at the back.	This creates a barrier to the front, which is the area that is generally facing the patient.
Tie the neck and then waist ties.	The gown is more secure upon tying the neck ties. Then proceed to the waist ties.

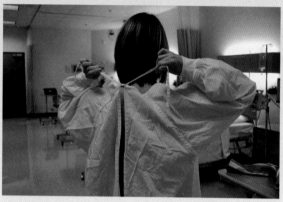

Figure 2 Nurse donning gown (tying neck tie).

Step—Removal	
Remove the gown prior to exiting area/patient room.	If the patient is in isolation, this step must be performed prior to removing the mask. This is generally done at the entry to the room.
Perform hand hygiene.	Hand hygiene should be performed prior to touching the neck or waist ties to prevent self-contamination.
Untie neck ties.	This allows the gown to fold over itself and prevent self-contamination.
Untie waist ties.	
Place the fingers of one hand under the opposite cuff and pull cuff over hand.	This is to prevent self-contamination.
Using the gown-covered hand, pull the gown down over the other hand.	This is to prevent self-contamination.
Pull the gown down off the arms, being careful that hands do not touch the outside of the gown.	This is to prevent self-contamination.
Hold the gown away from clothing and roll it downward with the contaminated side inside in a way that minimizes air disturbance.	This is to prevent self-contamination as well as spread via airborne routes.
Dispose of the gown into the garbage or appropriate receptacle.	
Perform hand hygiene and use paper towel to open door.	Hand hygiene should be performed following the performance of any skill.

Engaging in Evaluation

Step	**Rationale**
Inspect hands and other areas of the body.	This is to ensure that the hands and body are clean and free of visible contaminants after removal of PPE and hand hygiene.

Documenting Effectively

Step	**Rationale**
Donning PPE is required for any situation where there may be contact with blood or body fluids or if indicated by the infectious diseases manual. Formal documentation is not routinely required for this activity; however, it may be indicated on a flow sheet.	

SKILL 19.3   Donning Sterile Gloves

Reviewing Pertinent Information

Step	Rationale
Review patient chart to determine if sterile gloves are required. Review institution policy and procedure manuals to determine if sterile gloves are required.	Some instances do not require sterile gloves, and the skill can be performed using clean gloves.
Look for patient or nurse allergies to latex.	Most sterile gloves are made of latex; however, if allergies are present, alternative kinds of sterile gloves are available.

Preparing for Application of Sterile Gloves

Step	Rationale
Gather supplies needed: • Sterile gloves of appropriate size made of either latex or other components	Sterile gloves typically fit much tighter to the hand. Nurses should know their glove size to ensure an appropriate fit. If latex allergies are present, gloves made of either silicone or neoprene are available.

Donning Sterile Gloves

Step—Application	Rationale
Check the sterile package for the date or any evidence of contamination.	Packages that have expired or have been visibly tampered with cannot be guaranteed to be sterile and should not be used.
Prepare a large, clean, dry area for opening the package of gloves.	For ease of application, appropriate space is required.
Perform hand hygiene and remove rings.	Donning gloves does not replace hand hygiene. Rings can puncture sterile gloves and render them useless.
Open the outer wrap by holding onto the folded flaps. Proceed by opening the inner glove wrapper, exposing the cuffed gloves with the palms up and close to the body.	By holding the outer wrapper only, this ensures that the inside area of the sterile gloves remain sterile.

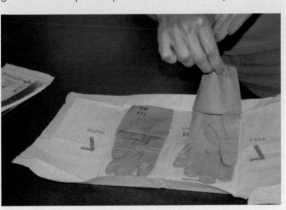

Figure 1 Picking up the first sterile glove.

Don the first glove by grasping the inside of the cuff with thumb and forefinger. Slip your other hand into the glove.	The inside cuff will later be in contact with the skin and can be touched at this point. Do not touch the outer portion of the gloves with a bare hand.
Hold the gloved hand away from the body.	This prevents accidental contamination with contact to the body.

(continued on page 362)

SKILL 19.3   Donning Sterile Gloves (continued)

Donning Sterile Gloves

Step—Application

Don the second glove by putting the gloved hand under the cuff of the second glove. Be careful not to contaminate the gloved hand with the ungloved hand as the second glove is being put on.

Rationale

Putting the sterile gloved hand into the cuff will mean that you are touching the outside of the glove. Both of these areas are sterile.

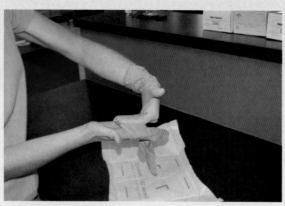

Figure 2 **Picking up the second sterile glove.**

Interlace fingers to position gloves without contaminating glove cuffs.

Handle only sterile items with gloved hands.

This fits the gloves firmly on the hand and around the fingers.

The moment sterile gloves touch any item that is not sterile, the gloves are no longer considered sterile.

Step—Removal

Remove first glove by grasping outside with the other gloved hand.

Pull glove of one hand down over the other hand. This removes the first glove. Hold the first glove in the opposite hand.

Place the ungloved hand inside the cuff.

Pull the glove down over the hand and over the first glove that is being held in the second hand.

Pull the gloves inside out while removing the second glove.

Put contaminated gloves in appropriate disposal unit.

Perform hand hygiene.

Rationale

This allows for removal without accidental spreading of microorganisms.

Pulling the glove over itself prevents spread of material. Holding it in the second gloved hand allows for neat disposal of both gloves.

This prevents self-contamination.

This creates a little ball of dirty gloves and prevents the spread of microorganisms.

Hand hygiene should be performed upon completion of any skill.

Engaging in Evaluation

Step

Inspect hands.

Rationale

This ensures that the hands are clean and free of visible contaminants after hand hygiene.

Documenting Effectively

Step

Donning sterile gloves is required for any situation where there is contact with other sterile areas, such as during surgery or in performing urinary catheterization. Formal documentation is not routinely required for this activity; however, it may be indicated on a flow sheet.

Rationale

SKILL 19.4 Preparing a Sterile Field

Reviewing Pertinent Information

Step
Check the chart, supplies package, or institution policy to determine if a sterile field is required.

Rationale
Sterile fields can be part of a skill (e.g., urinary catheterization or wound care). In some situations, separate fields are required (as in the operating room).

Preparing to Create a Sterile Field

Step
Gather supplies needed:
• Sterile drape

Rationale
This skill addresses the creation of a sterile field. Other items can be added depending on the skill being performed.

Creating a Sterile Field

Step
Inspect for tears, holes, and expiry dates of the sterile drape prior to opening the drape.
Place the drape pack on a clean, dry surface.

Rationale
Packages that have expired or been visibly tampered with cannot be guaranteed to be sterile and should not be used.
Sterile drapes establish an aseptic barrier that minimizes the passage of microorganisms between nonsterile and sterile areas. Wet areas wick through the drape and render them unsterile.

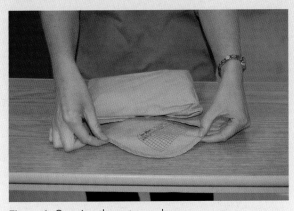

Figure 1 Opening the outer package.

Unfold the drape by grasping the outside of the wrapper. To open the sterile package, open away from you then laterally toward you. Do so touching only the outside margins.

The inside of the outer wrapper becomes the table drape and the base of the sterile field. Care must be taken so that the inside or sterile portion of the wrapper does not touch any part of the nonsterile surface.

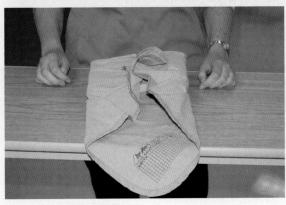

Figure 2 Opening away from body.

(continued on page 364)

SKILL 19.4 | Preparing a Sterile Field (continued)

Creating a Sterile Field

Step	Rationale

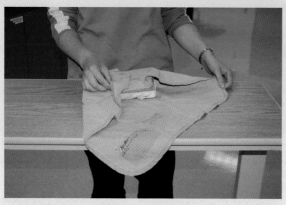

Figure 3 Opening laterally.

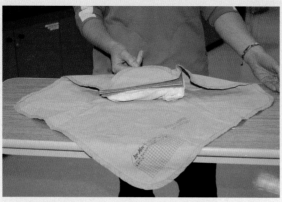

Figure 4 Opening toward the body.

Step	Rationale
When opened, the edges of the drape are considered non-sterile. Any areas below the level of the table or other flat surface are also considered nonsterile.	Your fingers have touched the edges, and therefore, all edges are considered nonsterile (1 in. margin). Areas below waist level are not continually visible and, therefore, are also considered nonsterile.

Engaging in Evaluation

Step	Rationale
Inspect for tears or holes immediately, before additional items are placed on the sterile field.	If any visible holes or tears are located, the drape is no longer considered sterile.

Documenting Effectively

Step	Rationale
Formal documentation is not generally required; however, in documenting other skills, sterility is often referred to or documented (e.g., catheterization performed using sterile technique).	

Critical Thinking Case Scenarios

▶ You are the nurse assigned to Ms. Whittaker, a patient in a room on isolation precautions. In order to enter her room, the nurse must use glove, gown, and mask. Ms. Whittaker requires her abdominal dressing to be changed. You have prepared all of your supplies ahead of time because you know that you cannot easily leave the room if you have forgotten anything. When you get into the room, Ms. Whittaker tells you that she is really thirsty and would like to have some ice water. She says that she buzzed the nurses' desk just before you came in. A few minutes later, a health-care aide carrying a pitcher of ice water comes to the room and stands by the door. She is not wearing any gloves, gown, or mask. She asks you to come and get the water quickly as she just wants to stay in the room "for a few seconds."

1. What should you do in this situation?
2. What factors affect your decision-making in this circumstance?

▶ A nurse has set up a sterile field in preparation of performing wound care. While she is introducing 2 × 2s into the field, one falls off to the side of the field and into the 1-in. margin.

1. What should the nurse do to maintain sterility of the field?

▶ This is the first day that the nursing student has been assigned to Mr. Hahn, who has an infection with a known microorganism. The nursing student knows that Mr. Hahn has isolation precautions; however, he is uncertain exactly what steps need to be taken for his infection.

1. Where could the nursing student find this information?
2. What should the nursing student do to protect himself, Mr. Hahn, and the other people they may be in contact with?

▶ When washing his hands, the nurse notices that he has several small open areas around the cuticles of his fingers. The nurse knows that this is likely due to the dry hands that he has been recently experiencing. He is caring for several patients who are elderly.

1. How can the nurse prevent the spread of microorganisms in this situation?

Multiple-Choice Questions

1. Direct contact:
   a. Involves transfer of microorganisms by an object.
   b. Involves a contaminated source that may result in a large-scale outbreak.
   c. Involves physical contact with an infected or colonized patient.
   d. Is one of the most common modes of transmission.
   e. C and D

2. When washing hands, which of the following points are important to remember?
   a. Use warm, not hot, water.
   b. Lather and rub hands together for 10 to 15 seconds.
   c. Using friction, cover all areas of the hands including fingernails, web spaces, thumbs, and palms.
   d. Turn faucet off using a clean disposable towel.
   e. All of the above

3. Alcohol-based hand rub may be used instead of soap and water if hands are not visibly soiled.
   a. True
   b. False

4. Infectious agents, reservoirs, and modes of transmission are links in the chain of infection.
   a. True
   b. False

5. The nurse determines what PPE to wear by considering which of the following?
   a. Whether the patient is known to have Hepatitis or HIV
   b. Probability of exposure to blood and/or body fluids
   c. Amount of blood and/or body fluids likely to be in contact with
   d. Probable mode of transmission
   e. B, C, and D

Suggested Lab Activities

● In pairs, have the students work through the third Critical Thinking Case Scenario earlier. Create an isolation room by drawing the curtains around the bed and pinning an isolation precautions sign on the outside of the curtain. Have all the necessary isolation equipment available, including standard masks, clean vinyl gloves of various sizes, isolation gowns, and the infectious diseases or isolation precautions manual. In the critical thinking scenario earlier, the patient has a known microorganism; however, you can create several stations by naming different microorganisms for each station (e.g., MRSA, *Clostridium difficile*). At each station, have the students do the following:

• Look up the named microorganism to understand what type of precautions are required.
• Create the necessary isolation precautions sign for the room.
• Select the appropriate equipment.
• Don the appropriate equipment in the order listed in their isolation manual.
• Enter and exit the room according to procedure.

● Obtain some "dot" type stickers. These can be the small round type that are used as stickers to label files, usually the size of a hole-punched piece of paper. After the students have entered the lab and sat down, give them each 10 dots and have them reenter the lab and attempt to put the dots on surfaces that they remember touching upon entering the lab. Common areas (e.g., door knobs) will likely have many dots. Discuss with the students the importance of hand hygiene, especially related to touching surfaces, and the implications of potential transmission of microorganisms from those surfaces to their patients.

● Have the students watch a video on applying sterile gloves. You can even create this video yourself and post it on a shared network either within your institution or using an outside application. Request that the students watch the video prior to attending their lab. During the lab, give each student a pair of sterile gloves of the required size or have these available with their lab kits. Watch the students don sterile gloves, first by grasping the inside of the cuff and then applying the second glove by scooping the cuff on the outside with their gloved hand. Ensure that they are using appropriate technique and correct any incorrect application of the sterile gloves.

SUGGESTED READINGS*

Bottone, E. J., Cheng, M., & Hymes, S. (2004). Ineffectiveness of handwashing with lotion soap to remove nosocomial bacterial pathogens persisting on fingertips: A major link in their intra-hospital spread. *Infection Control and Hospital Epidemiology, 25,* 262–264.

Brett, D. W. (2006). Impact of exudates management, maintenance of a moist wound environment, and prevention of infection. *Journal of Wound, Ostomy, and Continence Nursing, 33*(6 Suppl.), S9–S14.

Carlet, J., Fabry, J., Amalberti, R., & Degos, L. (2009). The "zero risk" concept for hospital-acquired infections: A risky business! *Clinical Infectious Diseases, 49,* 747–749.

Dugall, H., & Watson, R. (2009). What is the relationship between nurses' attitude to evidence based practice and the selection of wound care procedures? *Journal of Clinical Nursing, 18,* 1442–1450.

Eninger, R. M., Honda, T., Adhikari, A., Heinonen-Tanski, H., Reponen, T., & Grinshpun, S. A. (2008). Filter performance of N99 and N95 facepiece respirators against viruses and ultrafine particles. *Annals of Occupational Hygiene, 52*(5), 385–396.

Gasnik, L. B., & Brennan, P. J. (2009). Isolation precautions for antibiotic-resistant bacteria in healthcare settings. *Current Opinions in Infectious Diseases, 22,* 339–344.

Gould, D. (2009). Isolation precautions to prevent the spread of contagious diseases. *Nursing Standard, 23*(22), 47–55.

Halcomb, E. J., Fernandez, R., Griffiths, R., Newton, P., & Hickman, L. (2008). The infection control management of MRSA in acute care. *International Journal of Evidence-Based Healthcare, 6,* 440–467.

Harrison, W., Griffith, C. J., Ayers, T., & Michaels, B. (2003). Bacterial transfer and cross-contamination potential associated with paper-towel dispensing. *American Journal of Infection Control, 31,* 387–391.

Kirby, J. P., & Mazuski, J. E. (2009). Prevention of surgical site infection. *Surgical Clinics of North America, 89,* 365–389.

Lark, R. L., VanderHyde, K., Deeb, G. M., Dietrich, S., Massey, J. P., & Chenoweth, C. (2001). An outbreak of coagulase-negative staphylococcal surgical-site infections following aortic valve replacement. *Infection Control and Hospital Epidemiology, 22,* 618–623.

Larson, E. L., Eke, P. I., Wilder, M. P., & Laughon, M. P. (1987). Quantity of soap as a variable in handwashing. *Infection Control, 8,* 371–375.

Pittet, D., Dharan, S., Touveneau, S., Sauvan, V., & Perneger, T. V. (1999). Bacterial contamination of the hands of hospital staff during routine patient care. *Archives of Internal Medicine, 159,* 821–826.

Ranasinghe, S., Lee, A. J., & Birnbach, D. J. (2008). Infection associated with central venous or epidural catheters: How to reduce it? *Current Opinion in Anaesthesiology, 21,* 386–390.

Riggs, M. M., Sethi, A. K., Zabarsky, T. F., Eckstein, E. C., Jump R. L., & Donskey, C. J. (2007). Asymptomatic carriers are a potential source for transmission of epidemic and nonepidemic Clostridium difficile strains among long-term care facility residents. *Clinical Infectious Diseases, 45,* 992–998.

Smith, S. M. (2009). A review of hand-washing techniques in primary care and community settings. *Journal of Clinical Nursing, 18,* 786–790.

Souweine, B., Lautrette, A., Aumeran, C., Benedit, M., Constantin, J., Bonnard, M., . . . Traore, O. (2009). Comparison of acceptability, skin tolerance, and compliance between handwashing and alcohol-based handrub in ICUs: Results of multicentric study. *Intensive Care Medicine, 35,* 1216–1224.

Stein, R. A. (2009). Lessons from outbreaks of H1N1 influenza. *Annals of Internal Medicine, 151,* 59–62.

World Health Organization. (2009). *WHO guidelines on hand hygiene in health care.* Geneva, Switzerland: Author. Retrieved from http://whqlibdoc.who.int/publications/2009/9789241597906_eng.pdf

Zoutman, D. E., & Ford, B. D. (2008). A comparison of infection control program resources, activities, and antibiotic resistant organism rates in Canadian acute care hospitals in 1999 and 2005: Pre- and post-severe acute respiratory syndrome. *American Journal of Infection Control, 36*(10), 711–717.

---

*These sources were consulted during the creation of this chapter.

Health Assessment Across the Lifespan

JUDY A. K. BORNAIS

Megan Jones is a 21-year-old university student who has come to student health services with a cough and pain in her right ear. She started with a cold 10 days ago but is now finding herself extremely fatigued, with a fever, sore throat, cough, and earache. She has been asked to wait in the examination room for you. Your colleague already obtained her vital signs when she first arrived. Her temperature was 37.7°C; her blood pressure was 134/88 mmHg; her pulse was 88 beats/min, regular, 2+, and elastic; and her respirations were 22 breaths/min, shallow and laboured.

CHAPTER OBJECTIVES

By the end of this chapter, you will be able to:

1. Describe the importance and purpose of performing a thorough physical examination of your patient.
2. Identify the importance of a subjective data assessment to determine the type and systems to be included in the physical examination.
3. Identify the equipment and supplies required prior to beginning a physical assessment.
4. Explain special considerations the nurse should take when beginning a health assessment.
5. Describe the four types of assessments and databases based on the patient's symptoms.
6. Define and differentiate between the four essential assessment techniques used during the physical examination of body systems.
7. Identify the essential components required in specific system assessments.
8. Identify the steps required to perform system-based assessments.
9. Identify common or expected findings of the assessment of each body system.
10. Explain what health assessment findings tell you about your patient.
11. Identify concerning signs and symptoms and unexpected findings when conducting a physical examination.
12. Articulate and reflect on the importance of health assessment in caring for a patient and family.

KEY TERMS

Adventitious Abnormal sounds that are heard on auscultation. This may include sounds that are heard in an unusual place or manner.

Ascites Abnormal accumulation of fluid in the abdominal peritoneum that is observed as protuberant or distended.

Auscultation Listening to the sounds made by the various body structures as a diagnostic method.

Bronchial Breath sounds that are loud and of a harsh or blowing quality, heard on auscultation of the chest, made by air moving in the large bronchi, and barely, if at all, modified by the intervening lung; duration of the expiratory sound is as long as or longer than that of the inspiratory sound, and its pitch as high as or higher than that of the inspiratory sound; may be heard over a consolidated lung, above a pleural effusion due to an underlying compressed lung, and rarely over a pulmonary cavity; whispered pectoriloquy is another manifestation that usually can be elicited when bronchial breathing is present.

Bronchovesicular Breath sounds that are intermediate in intensity and pitch and are often auscultated over the major bronchi. Inspiration and expiration are almost equal in duration in bronchovesicular breath sounds.

Bruits An abnormal auscultatory sound similar to a heart murmur that can be blowing, harsh, musical, or rumbling; have a low, medium, or high pitch; and range in intensity from very faint to very loud.

Bursa A closed sac or envelope lined with synovial membrane and containing synovial fluid, usually found or formed in areas subject to friction (e.g., over an exposed or prominent body part or where a tendon passes over a bone).

Central Nervous System Consists of the brain and spinal cord.

Cranial Nerves (CNs) Are those nerves that emerge from, or enter, the cranium or skull, in contrast to the spinal nerves, which emerge from the spine or vertebral column. The 12 paired CNs are the olfactory (CN I), optic (CN II), oculomotor (CN III), trochlear (CN IV), trigeminal (CN V), abducent (CN VI), facial (CN VII), vestibulocochlear or acoustic (CN VIII), glossopharyngeal (CN IX), vagal (CN X), spinal accessory (CN XI), and hypoglossal (CN XII).

(continued on page 368)

Crepitus   A cracking or grating sound during movements.

Cyanosis   A dark bluish or purplish discolouration of the skin, nail beds, lips, or mucous membrane due to deficient oxygenation of the blood, evident with reduced hemoglobin in the blood.

Dermatome   The area of skin supplied by cutaneous branches of a single cranial or spinal nerve.

Distention   The act or state of being distended or stretched.

Dull   A dull sound, similar to a muffled thud, is produced when organs such as the heart, liver, and spleen are percussed.

Erythema   An intense redness of the skin. It is often a result of excess blood in the tissue and occurs when the superficial capillaries are dilated.

Flat Percussion Note   Soft, short sound produced over dense tissue such as bone or muscle.

Glasgow Coma Scale   A measure used to assess level of consciousness and reaction to stimuli in a neurologically impaired patient based on performance in three categories: eye opening, verbal response-performance, and motor responsiveness. Lower scores predict poorer outcomes.

Hyperresonance   Percussion note that is higher in pitch than resonance and is created when lung tissue is hyperinflated.

Inspection   Involves intentional observing along with close assessment of the patient.

Jaundice   Is a yellowing of the skin, indicating elevated bilirubin blood levels as can be seen in patients with acute hepatitis and liver failure.

Ligament   A band or sheet of fibrous tissue connecting two or more bones, cartilages, or other structures, or serving as support for fasciae or muscles.

Muscle Strength   Assesses a patient's ability to move actively against resistance. A scale for grading muscle strength is used to denote the variability in a patient's strength.

Objective Data   What the nurse detects during the examination and includes all physical exam findings.

Ophthalmoscope   A device for studying the interior of the eyeball through the pupil.

Otoscope   An instrument for examining the ear.

Pallor   The skin has lost its red-pink tones and has taken the colour of the underlying connective tissue. This generalized pallor is often a result of inadequate oxygenation to the tissue.

Palpation   The use of touch, feeling, or perceiving by the sense of touch to examine and acquire objective data of the patient's physical condition.

Percussion   Involves tapping or controlled striking of the body surface. The act of percussing elicits sounds produced in the body. The different sounds, also known as *percussion notes*, allow the nurse to determine the density of the underlying tissue.

Peripheral Nervous System   The part of the nervous system external to the brain and spinal cord from their roots to their peripheral terminations. This includes the ganglia, both sensory and autonomic, and any plexuses through which the nerve fibres and all the peripheral nerves run.

Point of Maximal Impulse (PMI)   The point on the chest wall at which the maximal cardiac impulse is seen and/or palpated.

Range of Motion   The measured beginning and terminal angles, as well as the total degrees of motion, traversed by a joint moved by active muscle contraction or by passive movement.

Reflexes   Represent an involuntary reaction of the autonomic nervous system to a stimulus applied to the periphery such as percussion of a partially stretched tendon (deep tendon reflex) or to stroking of the skin with a blunt object (cutaneous reflex).

Resonance   Hollow-sounding percussion note heard over air-filled lungs.

Stethoscope   An instrument originally devised by Laënnec for aid in hearing the respiratory and cardiac sounds in the chest but now modified in various ways and used in auscultation of any of vascular or other sounds anywhere in the body.

Striae   Commonly known as *stretch marks*, are bands of thin, wrinkled skin, initially red or blue (recent) but becoming purple and white or silver (old), that occur commonly on the abdomen, buttocks, and thighs and result from atrophy of the dermis and overextension of the skin; the most common causes are puberty and/or during and following pregnancy, or weight gain, and also associated with ascites.

Subjective Data   Information that the patient reports. It may include data about symptoms that the patient describes and the reason for seeking care and can include individual and family histories, past and current medical conditions, social history, etc. It is subjective in nature.

Symmetry   Equality or correspondence in form of parts distributed around a centre or an axis, at the extremities or poles, or on the opposite sides of any body.

Tendon   A nondistensible fibrous cord or band of variable length that is the part of the muscle (some authorities, however, consider it as part of the muscle complex), which connects the fleshy (contractile) part of muscle with its bony attachment or other structure.

Tympany   The loudest of the percussion notes; heard over gas-filled tissues such as the stomach and bowels.

Vesicular   Breath sounds that are soft and low-pitched and are found over the lung fields near sites of air exchange. In vesicular breath sounds, inspiration lasts longer than expiration.

Assessment: An Essential Component of the Nursing Process

The goal of any health assessment is to obtain data from your patient. The goal may be to acquire baseline data on the patient's current health state or to reassess/evaluate the patient's condition after treatment or intervention. As a result of the assessment, the nurse should be able to identify the patient's needs and decide on mutually agreed-upon goals. Assessment is essential when looking at the overall plan for the patient. Without appropriate assessment, the greatest plan will not be effective. The more thorough you are in your physical assessment, the easier it is for a diagnosis to be made and an effective plan/intervention to be initiated. Prior to beginning any physical examination, you will need to prepare for the assessment.

Through the eyes of a nurse

*H*aving worked in labour and delivery, the operating room, and in diabetes education, I can't emphasize enough how important my assessment skills were to provide great patient care. I think health assessment is critical to what I do every day as a nurse. I even have a health assessment textbook with at work should I need to look anything up. Every patient will teach you something. Knowing health assessment makes me a better nurse every day. If you don't know what to assess, then you can't get the path to wellness started. Knowing the content in my health assessment textbook has saved a lot of lives.

(personal reflection of Danielle Laing, BScN, RN, CDE)

Preparing for the Assessment

Prior to the patient's arrival, there are steps to take to help ensure an efficient and thorough assessment that considers the patient's comfort and dignity. This includes preparing yourself as the nurse: ensuring you are dressed appropriately with hair off your face and collar and clean and trimmed nails, wearing appropriate identification so patients know who you are, and washing or sanitizing your hands to prevent the spread of infection. Gathering the appropriate equipment and supplies, setting the environment, and ensuring privacy are also essential components to help ensure an efficient and thorough assessment. There is nothing more frustrating for the nurse and the patient than to have the exam interrupted so that the nurse can leave the room to gather necessary equipment and supplies.

Equipment and Supplies

In order to provide the best experience for the patient, the nurse gathers all of his or her equipment that might be needed prior to beginning the physical examination. A good starting point is to gather the following equipment that is used in most system assessments: sterile/clean gloves, alcohol swabs, and a penlight. In order to protect yourself and your patient, there are times when you will need to wear either clean gloves or sterile gloves. Always keep in mind the standard precautions when performing a physical assessment. It is a good idea to bring in alcohol swabs for cleaning your instruments prior to using them on a patient. A penlight is used in many different ways during the physical assessment—from using the light to assess the patient's skin to examining the reactivity of your patient's pupils. Several other pieces of equipment and supplies are required for specific exams, and these will be indicated with the assessment for the specific system.

Preparing the Setting

Prior to beginning your assessment, ensure you are familiar and comfortable with the room and its layout. Check where the light switch is located in case you need to dim the lights for an ophthalmoscopic exam. Know where the garbage is located for discarding tongue depressors or gloves. Locate the sink or hand sanitizer so you are not looking for these during the exam. Decide where to place the supplies you will be using during the physical assessment. Will you place your supplies on an overbed table or a counter? Consider placing a clean paper towel on the table or counter before placing your supplies. You want to minimize the movement you will need to reach for supplies, so think about your setup prior to beginning the physical examination.

Special Considerations

An essential component of the physical examination is ensuring you always provide your patient with privacy. Most of us would not be comfortable exposing our body to strangers.

Similarly, patients may feel very vulnerable and uncomfortable having their body exposed. To respect your patient's right to privacy, pull curtains or close doors and be aware of draping. Whenever possible, keep unexamined body parts covered until they need to be examined. The type of assessment required will determine the extent of the skin to be exposed. Some assessments require your patient to wear a gown, whereas others can occur without the patient removing any of his or her normal clothing. Beforehand, consider the type of assessments you will need to perform and decide in advance whether or not you should ask your patient to put on a gown and if you will need a drape.

Always explain to your patient what you will be performing as part of your assessment and ensure you have your patient's consent.

Megan Jones, the university student, has come to student health services with a cough and pain in her right ear. What additional questions might you want to ask Megan? Which equipment and supplies do you think you need in order to perform an assessment on Megan? Are there any special considerations that might be taken into account before beginning your assessment? How might you start your assessment and obtain Megan's consent?

One example of how you might obtain the patient's consent is to introduce yourself and say, for example, "I will be the registered nurse working with you today. In order to assess your ears, I will begin by checking the outside of the ear and then examining your ear canal with an instrument called an *otoscope*. Is that alright with you?" As you proceed with your exam, it would be important to explain what you are doing as you go along. This is also an excellent time to incorporate health teaching into your examination.

Depending on the type of assessment, and particularly when you are providing an invasive exam (e.g., a gynecological exam), a patient may want someone with her in the examination room. It is always a good idea to offer the option to have someone with the patient during the assessment. As you perform the examination, reassure, support, and explain what the next steps involve so the patient is informed.

For some physical exams, it is important to have the patient void prior to commencing your assessment. For example, when performing the abdominal examination, your patient needs to be relaxed and comfortable. A full bladder makes it difficult for the patient to relax while you palpate the abdomen. Try to anticipate what might help facilitate your assessment and ask this of your patient prior to beginning the exam.

Through the eyes of a student

I have thoroughly enjoyed learning about health assessment this year. Having the opportunity to apply the knowledge and skills learned from class on classmates has been a new experience for me. Taking vital signs, listening
(continued on page 370)

to heart and lung sounds, and developing my communication skills are only a few pieces of the experience. I have learned about the signs and symptoms of certain diseases, have expanded my knowledge on how the body functions as an integrated whole, and I'm extremely eager to learn more as I continue on my path to becoming a nurse.

(personal reflection of Puneet Bhardwaj, first-year nursing student)

Types of Assessments

Essentially, there are four types of assessments: the emergency assessment, the problem-centered assessment, the follow-up assessment, and the baseline or comprehensive assessment. The type of data the nurse needs to collect is dependent on the patient's presenting symptoms and the clinical situation.

Determining which physical assessments to perform depends largely on the subjective data assessment and the patient's presenting symptoms. The importance of the health history to drive the physical assessment cannot be overstated. A robust subjective data assessment along with effective interviewing techniques is essential to determine the appropriate physical assessments to perform. **Subjective data** is information that the patient reports. It may include data about symptoms that the patient describes and the reason for seeking care and can include individual and family histories, past and current medical conditions, social history, etc. It is subjective in nature.

In addition to the subjective data obtained from the patient or his or her significant others, the depth of the physical exam should be dictated by the nurse's clinical judgment based on information provided by other health-care providers, lab and diagnostic tests, and findings from the actual physical assessment—what the nurse observes. As a student performing a health assessment, you should ask yourself, "Should I be spending more or less time on this system?" "Are there other systems which might be affected or involved?" "What type of data do I require to perform appropriate care?"

Emergency Assessment

An emergency assessment is warranted in urgent situations often when lifesaving measures are required. Data is needed in a very timely manner, and the assessment is focused on determining the problem in order to ensure critical interventions are implemented to help stabilize the patient.

Think Imagine you are walking down the street and see a person riding a bike get struck by a car that was turning the corner. The person on the bike was not wearing a helmet and was thrown over the handlebars and hits his head on the curb. What questions would be important to ask the person who struck the curb? What assessments and actions should you take?

In this type of emergency situation, it would not be appropriate for the nurse to ask the person who struck his head about whether or not he received his flu vaccination or to perform a peripheral vascular assessment. The priority for the initial assessment is to assess for life-threatening problems. Oftentimes, nurses assess and perform interventions concurrently. For example, the nurse in the given scenario should ensure the person's airway is patent and that he is breathing, while supporting and protecting his cervical spine. The nurse should assess for bleeding and put pressure on any significant bleeds; he or she should then assess for level of consciousness and disability such as broken bones while stabilizing the injured limb, etc. Clearly, the focus of the emergency assessment is to stabilize any life-threatening problems.

Problem-Centered Assessment

A problem-centered assessment is used in home care, primary care, long-term care facilities, and hospitals when nurses are trying to determine the status of a patient's symptoms or concerns. It focuses on one or two main systems and is broader than the emergency assessment but much less inclusive than the comprehensive assessment. In the problem-centered assessment, the nurse collects subjective data that is relevant to the presenting problem and focuses the assessment on the patient's concerns. Recall the example of Megan Jones, with a cough and pain in her right ear. The subjective data collection for Megan should include an assessment of her cough, ear pain, history of respiratory illness, and immunizations. The physical examination should include a general survey; a set of vital signs; and an examination of the ears, nose, sinuses, throat, lymph nodes, and respiratory system. The nurse assesses more than simply the ear and cough knowing that the nose, sinuses, and throat are connected to the ears and respiratory system. By making certain that the relevant systems are assessed, the nurse helps ensure that appropriate treatment can be provided.

Follow-Up Assessment

Like a problem-focused assessment, the follow-up assessment can occur in virtually all health-care settings. The follow-up assessment allows the nurse to compare the patient's current state to his or her previous health status. It can occur as a follow-up to a treatment or intervention to evaluate if implementing them worked. It can also occur after an initial assessment and diagnosis of a chronic disease to evaluate how the patient is doing. In the follow-up assessment, the nurse should ask himself or herself, "Is the patient better or worse compared with the last assessment?" "Are further assessments or treatments required?" Think again of Megan Jones, who, following her problem-focused assessment, was started on an antibiotic for her ear infection and pneumonia. In a follow-up assessment, she would return to the student health services after completing the course of antibiotics to ensure that the pneumonia and ear infection were cleared up. If the assessment during the follow-up visit found that she was completely recovered, no further follow-up for these resolved symptoms would be required.

Baseline or Comprehensive Assessment

A comprehensive assessment entails a complete health history along with a full physical examination. It is intended to establish a baseline of the patient's past and current health status and serves as a comparison for all future assessments. Establishing a baseline assessment makes it easier for the nurse to identify when a change has occurred. Comprehensive assessments are typically completed on an annual basis during a primary care visit or upon admission to a home care service, hospital, or long-term care facility. In a primary care setting, during a comprehensive assessment, the nurse may be seeing a patient for the first time as a wellness visit. As a result, the nurse would want to include an assessment of the patient's health history including illnesses, vaccinations, medical treatments, surgeries, and current medications. Family history of any illness or conditions would also be important in order to identify possible risk factors for the patient. The visit would also include lifestyle, health promotion, and self-care behaviours along with coping patterns, social supports, functional abilities, strengths, and the patient's perception of health along with current health goals.

In a facility such as a hospital, the comprehensive health history assessment may include information about the patient's home environment and activities of daily living. For example, if a patient presented in the emergency department with a broken hip, it would be important to assess what type of home the patient lived in. If the patient lived in a two-storey home with no bathroom on the first floor, then it would be essential for the nurse to begin planning for discharge and the possibility of alternative home arrangements until the patient is able to navigate the stairs.

The physical assessment of the comprehensive examination should include all body systems in a systematic fashion and typically follows a head-to-toe approach. This includes a general survey and mental status assessment followed by an assessment of the skin, hair, and nails; head and neck; eyes; ears; nose, mouth, and throat; thorax and lungs; cardiac; peripheral vascular and lymphatics; breast and axillae; abdomen; anus, rectum, and prostate; genitourinary; musculoskeletal; and neurological (Box 20.1). Each of the system assessments will be explained in detail later on in this chapter.

Sequence of the Assessments

The order of the physical examination should always be based on the needs and type of patient (infant, child, adult, or elderly). Some examiners merge systems to decrease position changes and make the exam more patient-friendly. It is always important to ask yourself, "Who is the patient and what would be best for him or her?" For example, while examining a child with a cough and ear pain, it might be best to move from the least invasive and painless portion of the assessment such as listening to the child's lungs and looking in his or her throat to the more invasive or pain-inducing assessment of palpating the ear and examining the ear using an otoscope. If, on the other hand, the patient is the university student who came to the student health services with a cough and pain in her ear, it would be reasonable to assess her in a head-to-toe format beginning with the ears. Although the specific order of the assessment may change, it is important that the nurse follow a consistent approach to the assessment to help ensure that all components of the examination are included and none are omitted or forgotten. Regardless of the order of the assessment, essential assessment techniques are used in virtually all system assessments.

Essential Assessment Techniques

Four essential assessment techniques are used in physical exams. These include inspection, palpation, percussion, and auscultation. These four techniques are used by nurses and other health-care professionals to thoroughly examine and acquire objective data on the patient's physical condition. **Objective data** is what the nurse detects during the examination and includes all physical exam findings.

Inspection

Inspection involves intentional observing along with close assessment of the patient. Inspection requires the integration of the nurse's senses. Inspection can be broken into general and local inspection.

General Inspection
The general inspection begins with the first moment of interaction between the nurse and the patient. In the general inspection, the nurse uses his or her sense of sight, hearing, and smell. Think of the first time you met someone that you were interested in dating. You would have noticed his or her approximate age, the person's hair, the colour of the eyes, the smile, what he or she was wearing, etc. These observations mirror the basics of general inspection. However, when a nurse completes the general inspection, he or she is intentionally observing for specific characteristics of the patient. The general inspection, sometimes also referred to as the *general survey*, includes observing the patient's physical appearance, behaviour, mobility, and body structure. To assess the patient's physical appearance, the nurse examines the patient's face for symmetry and his or her skin colour (Does he or she look pale, jaundiced, or cyanotic?) and looks for signs of distress. **Symmetry** refers to equality or correspondence in form of parts distributed around a centre or an axis, at the extremities or poles, or on the opposite sides of any body. In this example, do both sides of the face seem equal

BOX 20.1   Head-to-Toe Framework for Completing Physical Assessment

General Assessment
General survey
Vital signs and anthropometric measurements

Mental Status Assessment
Level of consciousness
Orientation to person, place, and time
Cognition
Orientation
Mood
Language and memory

Skin, Hair, and Nails
Inspect the hair.
Assess skin colour, moisture, temperature, texture, mobility, and turgor.
Observe for the presence of edema, lesions, or skin breakdown.
Inspect the nails.

Head and Neck
Inspect the head and scalp.
Assess the trachea and thyroid.
Palpate the lymph nodes.

Eyes
Inspect and examine the eyes.
Test visual acuity.
Assess visual fields and extraocular muscles.

Ears, Nose, Mouth, and Throat
Inspect and examine the ears.
Test auditory acuity.
Inspect and examine the nose.
Inspect and examine the oral cavity and teeth.
Grade the tonsils.

Thorax and Lungs
Inspect and palpate the posterior and anterior thorax.
Auscultate the five lung lobes.
Assess oxygen saturation.
Percuss as necessary.

Cardiac
Inspect and palpate the precordium.
Auscultate the heart and carotids.
Assess for jugular venous distention.

Peripheral Vascular
Palpate peripheral pulses.
Assess capillary refill.
Inspect for edema.
Assess for PAD and PVD.

Breast
Inspect and palpate the breasts.
Inspect and palpate the lymph nodes in the axillae.

Abdominal
Inspect, auscultate, and palpate the four quadrants.
Percuss for general tympany.
Palpate and percuss the liver, spleen, and bladder.
Assess bowel elimination.

Genitalia
Inspect female genitalia.
Inspect male genitalia.
Assess urinary elimination.

Musculoskeletal
Observe posture.
Assess gait and balance.
Evaluate mobility and ability to perform activities of daily living (ADL).
Assess joints.
Evaluate muscle strength and grade.

Neurological
Assess CNs.
Test sensory function.
Assess cerebellar and vestibular function.
Evaluate motor function of the upper and lower extremities.
Percuss deep tendon reflexes.

with corresponding parts distributed equally on opposite sides of the face?

The nurse assesses the patient's apparent age and health status (Does he or she look older or younger, or unwell?). The patient's behaviour is assessed by his or her appearance and hygiene (Is he or she dressed appropriately or is there some concern with neglect or cognitive challenges?). Are there any odors coming from the patient? Is the patient alert and is he or she responding appropriately to questions? The nurse assesses the patient's level of consciousness by asking the patient if he or she can state his or her name, if he or she knows where he or she is, and if he or she knows the date. The nurse would then document the patient as alert and oriented ×3 (oriented to person, place, and time) if he or she was able to answer all three questions correctly.

The third component of the general survey is mobility. The nurse would assess the patient's mobility by examining the patient's gait. For example, does he or she walk with a limp or with a wide stance? Lastly, the patient's body structure is assessed by examining the patient's body size, shape, and structure (emaciated or overweight) and the patient's posture (Is he or she sitting relaxed or in a guarded position due to pain or distress? Is he or she rigid? Hunched in pain?). As part of the assessment of body structure, the nurse should assess the patient's weight in respect to height.

Local Inspection

Local inspection follows the general inspection and is the direct observation of a particular area or system. In the local inspection, the nurse examines the body part or region for specific criteria. For example, if a patient fell and presented with a scrape and concerns over a possibly broken arm, the nurse would inspect for the colour, symmetry, alignment, and movement, comparing the affected to the unaffected arm. The nurse would look for swelling as well as the shape and integrity of the skin around the scrape and injury.

Within each system assessment of this chapter, the important components of inspection will be identified. Regardless of the system being assessed, there are some general guidelines for local inspection. For a thorough inspection to occur, exposure of the body part being examined is necessary. As an example, if a nurse wanted to inspect a patient's back as part of a screening for abnormal moles, the nurse should ask the patient to remove her shirt to ensure proper visualization of the back. Local inspection also requires good lighting in order to properly assess body parts. Lighting may be direct or oblique. Consider the questionable moles earlier. To determine if the moles were cause for concern, the nurse should obtain good direct lighting to illuminate the skin. Direct lighting is from a light source placed directly over the area being examined, such as that from an overhead light, a gooseneck lamp, a penlight, or a dermascope. Oblique lighting, also known as *tangential lighting*, casts shadows on the region being illuminated (Stephen, Skillen, Day, & Bickley, 2010), permitting the detection of contour, movements, and pulsations.

Palpation

Palpation is the use of touch to examine and acquire objective data of the patient's physical condition. Palpation requires a systematic and calm approach by the nurse. Remember to always drape the patient appropriately and explain what you will be doing before you begin.

Because palpation uses parts of the nurse's hands, warm the hands by rubbing them together or washing in warm water prior to touching the patient. Different parts of the examiner's hands can be used to elicit information about the patient as illustrated in Table 20.1 and Figure 20.1.

Determining which part of the hand the nurse should use during palpation is dependent on the type of data the nurse requires. Although the fingertips and pads contain numerous nerve endings, practice by the nurse is required to gain attunement to understand the sensations being palpated. In order to effectively palpate tissues and organs in the body, the nurse may need to vary the amount of pressure used during palpation. There are two types of pressure that can be exerted during palpation: light and deep.

Light Palpation

Light palpation is used in virtually all assessments. With light palpation, the skin of the patient is depressed to a depth of approximately 1 cm. This allows the nurse to detect the characteristics of the skin surface as well as structures located superficially under the skin. To perform light palpation, the nurse places the finger pads of his or her dominant hand against the patient's skin and gently pushes in a circular motion to detect any lesions, lumps, masses, tenderness, or areas of inflammation. Figure 20.2A illustrates this technique.

For example, the technique of light palpation is used during the breast assessment. During the breast examination, the nurse should palpate in small concentric circles applying light pressure initially to assess the consistency of the breast tissue and for any tenderness or nodules.

Deep Palpation

Deep palpation may use one hand or two hands. The use of two hands during palpation is termed *bimanual palpation*. In deep palpation, the nurse uses firm pressure to palpate structures that are 3 to 4 cm below the skin surface (Fig. 20.2B). Unlike with light palpation, deep palpation uses discontinuous pressure to maintain tactile sensitivity. The different techniques for light and deep palpation are illustrated in Figure 20.2.

TABLE 20.1	Parts of the Examiner's Hand for Palpation		
Area of the Hand	**Sensitive to Detect**	**Used to Determine**	**Example**
Fingertip	Finer tactile discriminations	Pulsatility and elasticity, turgor and fluid content, and thickness of the skin and tissues as well as vascularity	Obtaining the patient's rate, rhythm, and elasticity
Finger pad	Tactile discrimination: texture, moisture, contour, and consistency	Pulsatility and elasticity, turgor and fluid content, and thickness of the skin and tissues as well as vascularity	Obtaining information about the location, size, consistency, and mobility and tenderness of an enlarged lymph node during the assessment of the head and neck
Dorsum	Temperature variations	Temperature	Obtaining a comparison of temperature of the lower legs during a PV assessment
Ulnar edge of the hand	Temperature variations and vibrations	Temperature and vibrations that originate from the body organs and structures	Obtaining information about the vibrations felt while assessing tactile fremitus during the respiratory assessment
Ball of the hand	Vibrations	Vibrations that originate from the body organs and structures	Assessing for thrills on the anterior chest during the cardiac assessment

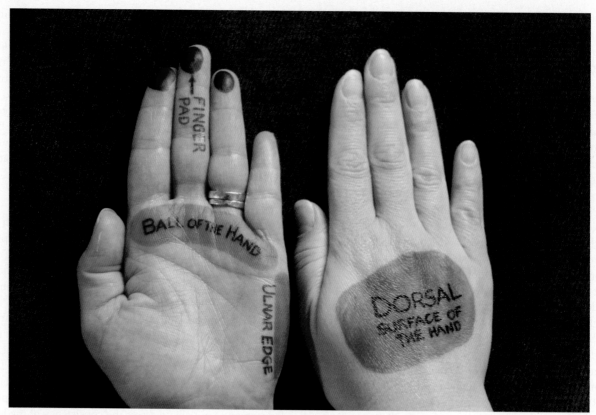

Figure 20.1 Visual of the parts of the hand for palpation. (Photo courtesy of David P. Bornais)

Several types of movements are used during palpation to elicit different information for the assessment. The common movements of deep palpation include the following:

- Circular motions—Accentuate the qualities of the underlying structures
- Dipping motion—By making a quick depressing movement with the fingers, the nurse can detect contour, elasticity, mobility, and guarding.
- Direct pressure—By placing the hand perpendicular to the skin and pressing downward, the nurse can assess for blanching, tenderness, resistance, and guarding.

- Gliding motions—The nurse places the finger pads of the nondominant hand over the interphalangeal joints of the three middle fingers of the dominant hand to examine the underlying tissue in both the vertical and horizontal directions.
- Grasping motion—By pinching or grasping the surface structures, the nurse is able to detect the consistency, shape, and location of an organ or mass.

Keep in mind that tender areas should ideally be palpated last to avoid causing any pain and guarding, which might impact the remainder of the examination. Throughout deep palpation, the nurse should be observing the patient for any

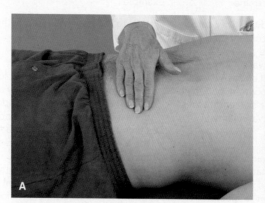
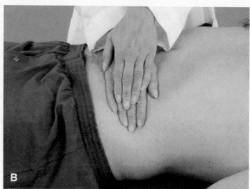

Figure 20.2 Technique for palpation. **A.** In light palpation, light pressure is applied by placing the fingers together and depressing the skin and underlying structures about 1/2 in. (1 cm). **B.** Deep palpation is used with caution. The skin and underlying structures are depressed about 1 in. (2 cm). (Photos by B. Proud)

signs of pain or discomfort. A novice nurse performing deep palpation is cautious to avoid injury to the patient. Similarly, nursing students should only perform deep palpation when supervised by a qualified instructor. Avoid deep palpation in patients with acute abdominal pain and if there is potential to cause internal injury. For example, if a patient has a suspected spleen injury, the nurse should not use deep palpation to determine the size of the spleen, risking splenic rupture (Handen, Lux, & Stossel, 2003, p. 7).

Percussion

Percussion involves tapping or controlled striking of the body surface. The act of percussing elicits sounds produced in the body. The different sounds, also known as *percussion notes*, allow the nurse to determine the density of the underlying tissue. For example, percussing over gas- or air-filled space creates a sound commonly described as bell-like or as a low-pitched, drum-like note.

Tympany, the loudest of the percussion notes, is heard over gas-filled tissues such as the stomach and bowels. **Resonance** sounds hollow and is percussed over air-filled lungs. **Hyperresonance** is higher in pitch than resonance and is created when lung tissue is hyperinflated. A **dull** sound, similar to a muffled thud, is produced when organs such as the heart, liver, and spleen are percussed. A **flat percussion note** is a soft, short sound produced over dense tissue such as bone or muscle. Understanding and recognizing the different percussion notes allows the nurse not only to determine the density of the underlying tissue but also to assess the location and estimate the size of body organs.

There are two ways to percuss the body: directly and indirectly.

Direct Percussion

Direct percussion requires the examiner to tap with his or her finger directly against the body part being examined. In our example of the university student with a cough and pain in her ear, the nurse should use direct percussion to examine the sinuses. To do this, the nurse should tap briskly with his or her plexor (middle) finger over the surface of the patient's frontal and maxillary sinuses to assess for any pain or tenderness.

Indirect Percussion

Indirect percussion is used more commonly than direct percussion in the physical examination. Indirect percussion involves the nurse striking his or her own hand or finger which is placed against the patient's skin surface. One form of indirect percussion is used when percussing the lungs for resonance. The nurse should extend the middle finger of his or her nondominant hand and place it over the area (lung field) being examined. It is important to lift the other fingers of the nondominant hand so that they do not rest on the patient's skin and dampen the sound created during percussion. With his or her dominant hand, the nurse should strike above the interphalangeal joint of the middle finger, which is firmly placed against the patient's skin (Fig. 20.3).

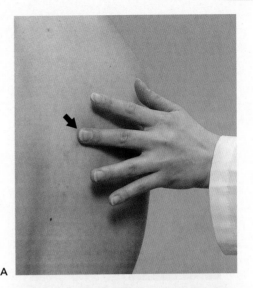

A

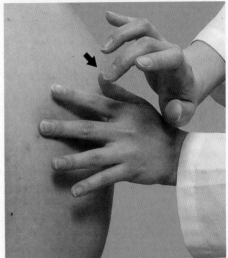

B

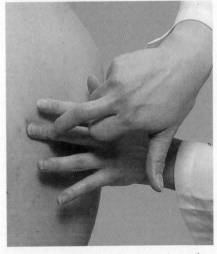

C

Figure 20.3 Indirect percussion. Percussion is used to access the location, shape, size, and density of tissues. **A.** The nondominant hand is placed directly on the area to be percussed, and the middle finger is placed firmly on the body surface *(arrow)*. **B.** The tip of the middle finger of the dominant hand *(arrow)* strikes the joint of the middle finger of the opposite hand **(C)**.

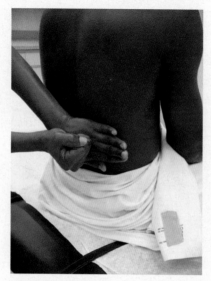

Figure 20.4 Indirect percussion for costovertebral angle tenderness.

Two brisk taps of the middle finger (known as the *plexor*) are commonly used to percuss and elicit sounds. Indirect percussion is also used to assess for costovertebral angle tenderness (Fig. 20.4). In this example, the nurse would place the entire nondominant hand against the patient's flank area. With his dominant hand, the nurse would make a fist and strike his nondominant hand to assess for any tenderness from the patient's kidney area.

Both forms of indirect percussion, like many other assessment skills, take practice to become proficient. To help improve your ability to percuss with the plexor finger, ensure the motion comes from the wrist and is firm and rapid. Picture the pecking motion of a chicken's beak; a similar quick, firm, and rapid approach is required during indirect percussion to elicit a clear percussion note. Remember to prepare in advance; your nails should be short and smooth before attempting this assessment to avoid hurting yourself (and your patient) and to make good contact.

Auscultation

Auscultation involves listening to the sounds made by the various body structures as a diagnostic method. In some cases, the nurse can auscultate without the aid of a stethoscope. The act of listening without a stethoscope is considered *direct auscultation* or auscultation with the unaided ear. However, in many situations, the nurse is not able to hear the sounds produced by the body without the aid of a stethoscope. The **stethoscope** is an instrument originally devised by Laënnec to aid in hearing the respiratory and cardiac sounds in the chest but now is modified in various ways and used in auscultation of vascular or other sounds anywhere in the body.

One of the most valuable pieces of equipment for the nurse to have during the physical assessment is a good-quality stethoscope. A good-quality stethoscope conducts the sounds created by the body and also blocks environmental noises. A stethoscope should have a single thick tubing, which helps

block environmental noise. The length of the tubing is important. Short tubing, 30 to 35 cm, helps to increase transmission of sound and also decreases the amount of tubing that might come in contact with patient's clothing or the surrounding area. When tubing touches or brushes against clothing or objects, it creates a noise that can be heard through the stethoscope. This extraneous noise is called *artifact*, and it can detract from the nurse's ability to hear the sound produced by the body. One of the most important components of the stethoscope is the end known as the *chestpiece* or *endpiece*. Nurses should ensure they have a stethoscope that has both a bell and a diaphragm on the endpiece (Fig. 20.5).

The bell part of the stethoscope is used to hear low-pitched tones such as vascular sounds (e.g., heart sounds and murmurs). The diaphragm or flat-disc endpiece is used to assess high-pitched sounds (e.g., lung sounds). Try to remember "di-high" for determining when to use the diaphragm. Along with a bell and diaphragm, a good-quality stethoscope also has two earpieces which should fit snugly into the ears and should be tilted slightly forward so that the sound is transmitted at the correct angle into the ear canal. When using your stethoscope to auscultate, remember to always disinfect it between patients to avoid the spread of pathogens.

Despite having a quality stethoscope, it can sometimes be difficult for the nurse to hear sounds produced in the body. A few helpful tips can assist the nursing student during auscultation:

- minimize distractions and quiet the environment,
- close your eyes when auscultating to help concentrate on the sense of hearing and block out environmental stimuli,
- hold the stethoscope as still as possible to avoid creating any artifact,
- become familiar with the sounds you are trying to auscultate,
- learn the best endpiece to use to hear different sounds, and
- know how to apply the endpiece to the skin (e.g., apply the bell lightly to skin to hear low sounds; firmly applying the bell to the skin will make it function like a diaphragm to pick up high-pitched instead of low-pitched sounds).

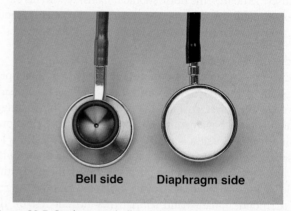

Bell side   **Diaphragm side**

Figure 20.5 Stethoscope bell and diaphragm. Use the bell of the stethoscope to detect low-pitched sounds. Hold the bell lightly against the body part being auscultated. Use the diaphragm of the stethoscope to detect high-pitched sounds. Hold the diaphragm firmly against the body part being auscultated.

TABLE 20.2	Auscultation Sounds					
Tone	Intensity	Pitch	Quality	Duration	Location
Blood pressure	Soft to loud	High	Swooshing or knocking	60–100/min	Arm
Abdominal sounds	Soft to loud	High	Gurgly, intermittent	5–35/min	Abdomen
Heart sounds	Moderate	Low	Lub-dub, rhythmic	60–100/min	Anterior thorax
Lung sounds vesicular	Soft	Low	Rustling, wispy	Inspiration > expiration, 12–20/min	Anterior and posterior thorax

Although the stethoscope helps conduct sound, the nurse needs practice in order to become proficient and ascertain the different sounds. The sounds auscultated over the various body parts sound differently, and descriptors of these sounds will be explained in this chapter under each specific system. All sounds are described according to their quality, intensity, pitch, and duration (Table 20.2).

Health Assessments by Systems

The remaining sections of this chapter will include a breakdown of the basic system assessments using a head-to-toe approach. The requirements to complete the specific physical examination for each system assessment will be included within the section.

Mental Status

The mental status of the patient is assessed during the health history assessment. The patient's response to the nurse's questions will provide some initial impressions of whether the patient is able to appropriately follow the conversation and answer questions. If there are concerns over the patient's ability to recall events, if he or she is unable to follow the conversation, or if the responses are incomprehensible, it may be necessary to assess the patient's mental status more formally using the Montreal Cognitive Assessment or the Mini-Mental State Examination (MMSE). The Montreal Cognitive Assessment is a newer test than the MMSE and has shown high sensitivity and specificity for identifying mild cognitive impairment.

Skin and Nail Assessment

Assessment of the skin and nails starts during the general survey and continues throughout the physical examination. Virtually, every system that is assessed has a component of the skin or nail assessment included with it. If the nurse is preparing to complete a comprehensive skin assessment, this would include examining all parts of the body, including assessing between the fingers and toes as well as the palms and soles of the feet. An optimal skin assessment requires good lighting and should include privacy and warmth for the patient.

Of the four essential assessment techniques used in physical assessments—inspection, palpation, percussion, and auscultation—only inspection and palpation are used during the objective assessment of the skin and nails. The nurse uses these assessment techniques to assess the patient's skin for colour, moisture, temperature, texture, mobility, and turgor, and the presence of edema or lesions. The colour of the skin can provide the nurse with information about the patient's current health status. The generalized abnormal skin colours include pallor, cyanosis, erythema, and jaundice.

Pallor

When a patient is pale (called **pallor**), the skin has lost its red-pink tones and has taken the colour of the underlying connective tissue. This generalized pallor is often a result of inadequate oxygenation to the tissue. The best places to assess for pallor are in areas with the least pigmentation. These include the mucous membranes of the mouth, the palms of the hands, and nail beds as well as the soles of the feet. In Caucasian individuals, the skin appears white (sometimes referred to as *bloodless*), whereas in black-skinned individuals, the skin appears more ashen gray. Consider the patient who has been in a car accident and has lost a significant amount of blood. As the patient begins to go into shock from the blood loss, he or she may experience peripheral vasoconstriction and a decrease in tissue oxygenation. Examination of the patient's skin and nails during early blood loss may reveal nails that appear pale as well as pallor of the hands, feet, and face (Guly et al., 2011).

Cyanosis

Unlike the white or ashen grey colour of pallor, **cyanosis** is a dark bluish or purplish discolouration of the skin, nail beds, lips, or mucous membrane due to deficient oxygenation of the blood. Central cyanosis often indicates alterations in circulation with decreased tissue perfusion and hypoxia and is best assessed in the lips, oral mucosa, and tongue (Baernstein, Smith, & Elmore, 2008).

Erythema

Erythema is an intense redness of the skin. It is often a result of excess blood in the tissue and occurs when the superficial capillaries are dilated. An example is the face of the patient who is hot and flushed often appears red. A patient who has a fever or local inflammation may present with erythema.

Jaundice

Jaundice is a yellowing of the skin, indicating elevated bilirubin blood levels as can be seen in patients with acute hepatitis and liver failure. Jaundice can be first noted in the hard

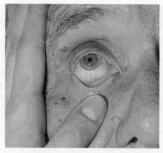

Figure 20.6 Jaundice seen in the sclera of the eyes and the yellow tone of the skin.

and soft palate of the mouth, the sclera of the eyes, and then in the skin.

To accurately assess the colour of the patient's skin, the nurse should inspect the entire area of the skin, paying special attention to the face, the eyes, and the mucous membranes of the mouth. To inspect the mouth, the nurse should use a light source (such as a penlight) to illuminate the membranes of the cheek and hard and soft palate. To examine the sclera, ask the patient to look up while you gently place your thumbs below the patient's lower eyelids and slide the lower lids downward (Fig. 20.6).

Assessing Temperature

Along with assessment of the patient's skin colour, the nurse should assess the skin for moisture and temperature. If a patient is experiencing hyperthermia or an elevated temperature from heavy exercise, sunburn, or fever from an infection, his or her skin will likely be hot and moist. On the other hand, a patient experiencing hypothermia will often be cold and dry. To assess the temperature of the skin, the nurse should use the dorsal surface of his or her hands (Fig. 20.7). Assessing the skin temperature of a patient who injured his or her left wrist would involve placing the dorsal surface of the hands on both of the patient's hands and moving upward along the forearm comparing the temperature of one side to the other.

Palpating the skin will provide the nurse with information about the skin's temperature as well as moisture. Upon palpation, the skin may feel dry, wet, or oily.

Mobility and Turgor

Inspection of the texture, mobility, and turgor of the skin will provide the nurse with important information about the patient's overall status. Normally, a patient's skin should appear smooth and firm. Rough patches may be related to overuse, or thyroid or skin conditions. Mobility and turgor relate to the skin's ease of rising and its ability to promptly return to place within 1 to 2 seconds when released. To assess mobility and turgor, the nurse would lift a fold of skin, ideally at the clavicle and release the skin, noting the time it takes to return to place (Fig. 20.8). Poor skin turgor is often seen in patients who are dehydrated, whereas decreased mobility can be seen in patients who are edematous.

Inspection for edema is included in the assessment of the skin. Edema is caused by the accumulation of fluid in the intercellular spaces. This can occur when a patient has an injury with local swelling, which is usually unilateral and localized to the area of injury. Patients can present with general or bilateral edema because of kidney failure or cardiovascular dysfunction such as in venous insufficiency or in congestive heart failure. To assess for edema, the nurse begins by inspecting the skin, looking for areas of swelling or areas where the skin is taut and glistening. If edema is present, the nurse would palpate the area by pressing the thumb or fingers firmly against the skin. Any indentation is considered *pitting edema* (Fig. 20.9) when the indentation persists after the pressure is released and is graded on a scale from 1+ to 4+ (Table 20.3). When peripheral edema is present in the feet or legs, the nurse should assess at the dorsum of the foot and ankle malleolus as well as along the tibia. If edema is present in the lower legs, the nurse should consider measuring and comparing the size of the legs using a measuring tape.

Lesions

Inspecting and palpating any lesions that may exist on the body is another component of the skin assessment. If a lesion or lesions are present, the nurse should assess the

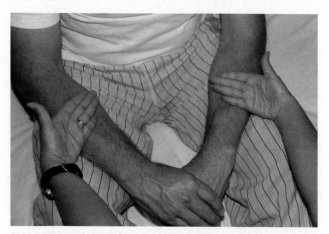

Figure 20.7 Palpating for temperature. (Photo courtesy of Mikayla Bornais)

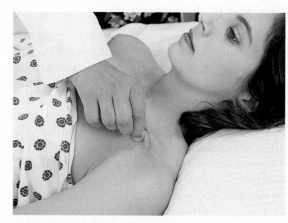

Figure 20.8 Assessing skin turgor.

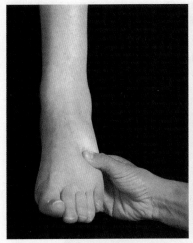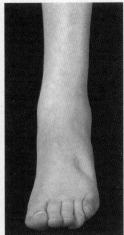

Figure 20.9 A 3+ pitting edema.

characteristics of the lesion, such as location, pattern or shape, border, colour, diameter (size), evolution and elevation, and presence of any exudate. The location and pattern of distribution over the body can help the nurse with identifying some skin disorders that present with typical patterns. For example, eczema in adults often presents on the skinfolds or flexor surfaces of the body such as behind the knees, ankles, and antecubital fossa. A patient may have contact dermatitis localized to a specific area with a pattern of redness and vesicles where contact occurred with the allergen. Common patterns and shapes of lesions include linear, clustered, annular, geographic or serpiginous, or wormlike.

The shape and size of the skin lesion can help when differentiating the different types. Common primary skin lesion types include macules, patches, papules, plaques, nodules, cysts, wheals, vesicles, pustules, and burrows. See Table 20.4 for examples of primary skin lesions.

Lesions are often categorized as primary or secondary. Primary skin lesions are visible changes of the tissue of the skin. Some primary lesions are present at birth, such as a mole or café au lait spot. Other primary lesions develop over the course of a person's lifetime. Some examples include lesions associated with viruses (e.g., warts, herpes zoster) or those that occur during an allergic reaction (wheals and hives,

which can occur with contact dermatitis) (Jones & Statler, 2011). Other primary skin lesions can occur in response to environmental agents such as vesicle or bulla from a sunburn. Secondary skin lesions are changes in the tissue of the skin that often develop from primary skin lesions, either as a natural progression or as a result of a person manipulating (e.g., scratching or picking at) a primary lesion (Goodheart, 2009). A patient with wheals might scratch, developing a crust or a scar.

Nails

Assessment of the nails is often included in the cardiovascular and respiratory assessment. Assessment of the nails includes inspection for the colour of the nail, shape and contour, and consistency. Palpation of the nails for capillary refill is included in the assessment. Inspection of the nail should reveal a smooth surface that is flat or slightly curved. The lunula (little moon) appears as a crescent-shaped marking at the base of the nail with the nail bed appearing pinkish in colour, because it is highly vascular. When inspecting the nail, the nurse examines the index finger from the side (its profile), noting the angle of the nail bed to the skin. The angle should be less than 180° (Myers & Farquhar, 2001). The nurse palpates the nail base which should feel firm. A spongy nail base with an angle greater than 160° indicates clubbing that can occur with emphysema and chronic bronchitis (Spicknall, Zirwas, & English, 2005). Along with shape and contour of the nail, the nurse assesses its consistency, which should appear smooth and uniform. Lastly, the assessment of the nails includes palpation for capillary refill. This is done by holding the person's hand level with the heart and depressing the nail until it turns whitish. The nurse then releases the pressure and assesses how long it takes until the original colour returns to the nail. Normally, colour should return within 1 to 2 seconds. A delayed return in colour of longer than 2 seconds can indicate cardiovascular or respiratory dysfunction (Guly et al., 2011).

Head and Neck

Regions of the head take their names from the underlying bones of the skull. For example, the frontal area is located over the frontal bone. Knowledge of the anatomy of the head and neck muscles is important for assessing the appropriate regions. The two main neck muscles that are important in the assessment of the head and neck are the sternomastoid and the trapezius muscles (Fig. 20.10).

The neck houses the trachea and upper esophagus, routes by which the body accesses oxygen and nourishment. The neck also contains the thyroid, the largest endocrine gland. The head and neck also contain a large number of lymph nodes, which play a large role in the immune process. Examination of the head and neck should begin with a thorough subjective assessment followed by inspection of the head.

TABLE 20.3	Grading Scale for Edema	
Grading	Definition	Appearance
1+	Mild pitting	Slight indentation but no perceptible swelling
2+	Moderate pitting	Indentation subsides rapidly
3+	Deep pitting	Indentation remains for a short time and the area appears swollen
4+	Very deep pitting	Indentation persists for some time and the area appears swollen

TABLE 20.4 Primary Skin Lesions

Macule

Flat, circumscribed, discoloured, <1 cm diameter
Examples: freckles (shown), tattoo, stork bite

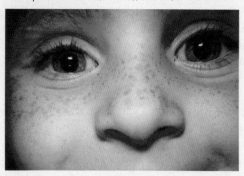

Patch

Flat, circumscribed, discoloured, >1 cm diameter
Examples: vitiligo (shown), melasma, tinea versicolor

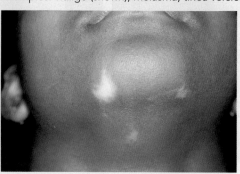

Papule

Raised, defined, any colour, <1 cm diameter
Examples: wart, insect bite, molluscum contagiosum (shown)

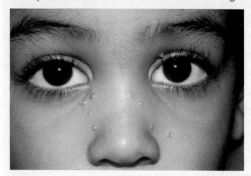

Plaque

Raised, defined, any colour, >1 cm diameter
Examples: psoriasis (shown), lichen sclerosus

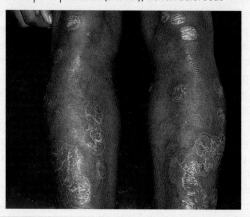

Wheal

Raised, flesh-coloured or red edematous papules or plaques,
    varies in size and shape
Example: urticaria (shown)

Nodule

Solid, palpable, >1 cm diameter, often with some depth
Example: basal cell carcinoma (shown)

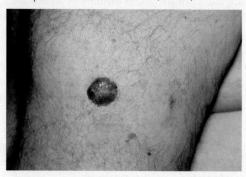

Tumor

Large nodule
Examples: large nevus, basal cell carcinoma, lipoma (shown)

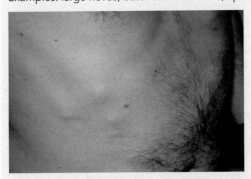

Vesicle

Fluid-filled, <1 cm diameter
Examples: herpes simplex, chickenpox (shown)

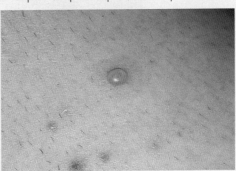

Bulla

Fluid-filled, >1 cm diameter
Examples: second-degree burns, bullous impetigo (shown)

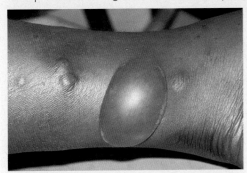

Pustule

Purulent, fluid-filled, raised of any size
Examples: pustular acne (shown), folliculitis

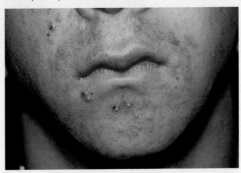

Cyst

Distinct and walled-off, containing fluid or semisolid material, varies in size
Examples: epidermal cysts (shown), cystic acne

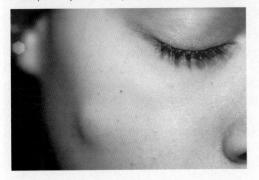

Inspection and Palpation of the Head

Initial inspection involves inspecting the hair and scalp for quantity, texture, distribution of hair, pattern of hair loss, foreign bodies, scaliness, lumps, or lesions of the scalp. Inspection of the head also involves examining the size of the head and palpating the contour of the skull for any deformities, depressions, lumps, and/or tenderness.

Inspection and Palpation of the Face

Inspection of the face is included in the examination of the head and neck. This involves assessing for the patient's skin colour. Note the inclusion of the skin assessment within the assessment of the head and neck; skin is included with virtually every other system assessment. The nurse assesses if there are any colour changes in the patient's face, the sclera, conjunctiva, lips, hard palate, and soft palate, noting any rashes, lumps, or lesions. The nurse assesses the patient's facial expressions for signs of pain or distress, for any involuntary movements, edema, lesions, or masses. In addition, the nurse assesses for facial symmetry by asking the patient to smile, frown, raise his or her eyebrows, and puff out his or her cheeks, noting that both sides move symmetrically, providing data about the cranial nerve VII (the facial nerve).

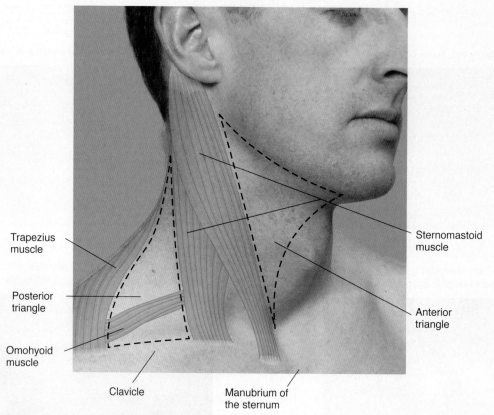

Trapezius
muscle

Posterior
triangle

Omohyoid
muscle

Clavicle

Manubrium of
the sternum

Sternomastoid
muscle

Anterior
triangle

Figure 20.10 Location of the neck muscles.

Palpation of the face involves palpating the temporomandibular joint located in front of the tragus of the ear. The nurse places three fingers on the joint and feels as the patient opens and closes his or her mouth. The joint should move smoothly without any clicking, deviation, or tenderness. The nurse palpates the temporal area located above the cheek bone between the lateral canthus of the eye and the top of the ear. A pulsation may be palpated at the temporal artery, but it should not be hard or tender. Note the parotid, submandibular, and sublingual glands are located on the sides of the face. The parotid gland is superficial to and behind the mandible and is only visible and palpable when enlarged. The submandibular gland is located inferior to the mandible and underneath the base of the tongue, whereas the sublingual gland lies in front of the submandibular gland under the mucous membranes that cover the floor of the mouth.

Inspection and Palpation of the Neck

Assessment of the neck includes inspection and palpation. The nurse examines the position of the head to determine if it is midline and erect. This provides the nurse with information about the muscles of the neck. Inspection of the neck muscles includes assessment to determine if the muscles of the neck are relaxed and symmetrical, observing for any masses, lesions, scars, or enlargement in the neck. This involves inspecting and palpating the 10 lymph node regions of the head and neck.

Lymph Nodes

Inspection of the lymph nodes requires the nurse to study one side compared with the other, noting any swelling or enlargement. Skill 20.1 details this assessment.

Position of the Trachea

Follow inspection of the lymph nodes with inspection and palpation of the trachea to ensure it is midline. Begin by inspecting the trachea for any deviations. Place your index finger in the groove between the trachea and the sternomastoid muscle on the one side of the trachea mid-way between the clavicle and mandible. Use the thumb of the same hand and place it on the opposite side of the trachea deviating it to the right and left and comparing side to side. The space should be symmetrical.

Thyroid Gland

The thyroid sits below the cricoid cartilage and above the suprasternal notch. Begin by standing in front of the patient and ask him or her to tilt his or her head back slightly to allow for better viewing of the area. Next, ask the patient to take a sip of water and watch as the thyroid gland moves upward during the swallowing. The thyroid gland should rise with swallowing and appear symmetrical with no visible masses or bulges. Next, move to stand behind the patient and ask the patient to lower his or her chin to relax the sternomastoid muscle and allow for easier palpation. Place your index, middle, and ring finger on either side of the cricoid cartilage and palpate along the thyroid gland, assessing

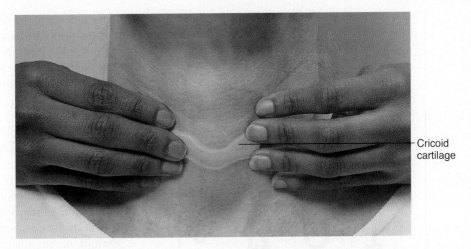

Cricoid cartilage

Figure 20.11 Palpating the thyroid gland.

for any enlargement, nodules, or masses. Next, place your fingers just below the cricoid cartilage. Ask the patient to take another sip of water and feel for the thyroid isthmus that lies across the trachea below the cricoid cartilage as it rises up under your finger pads. With the patient's chin still lowered, ask him or her to move his or her head slightly to the left. Displace the trachea to the left with fingers of your right hand and palpate the left thyroid gland with your left hand, noting the size, shape, and consistency of the gland (Fig. 20.11).

Repeat with examination of the right lobe, identifying any masses, nodules, or tenderness. If the thyroid gland feels enlarged, auscultate over the area with the bell of the stethoscope listening for any soft rushing or whooshing sounds known as *bruits*. A **bruit** may sound similar to a heart murmur that can be blowing, harsh, musical, or rumbling; have a low, medium, or high pitch; and range in intensity from very faint to very loud (Roach, Roddick, & Bickley, 2010). A bruit is created by turbulent blood flow that can occur in an enlarged thyroid gland.

Range of Motion of the Neck and Muscle Strength

Continue with inspection of the neck by asking the patient's ability to move in flexion, extension, rotation, lateral bending, protraction, and retraction. To assess flexion, ask the patient to touch his or her chin to his or her chest. For extension, have him or her look up at the ceiling. Rotation involves turning the head to the side looking over the shoulder. Lateral bending involves looking straight ahead and tilting the head so that the ear moves toward the shoulder. Protraction involves pushing the chin forward, and retraction involves pulling the chin inward. Observe as the patient moves in each of these directions, noting symmetry from side to side and full range of motion. **Range of motion** refers to the total degrees of motion a joint can move either by active muscle contraction or by passive movement. Next, assess the muscle strength of the spinal accessory nerve (cranial nerve XI) by gently placing your hands on both of the patient's shoulders. Ask him or her to shrug his or her shoulders upward against your hands, noting if he or she has equal strength on both sides of his or her trapezius muscles. Next, place your hand

on the patient's left cheek with your palm on his or her chin. Ask the patient to turn his or her head to his or her left side against your hand. Continue with the opposite side, noting the patient's strength of his or her sternomastoid muscles.

Assessment of the neck can include inspection and palpation for pulsations, but this portion of the assessment will be included with the cardiac system when the patient is in the supine position.

Eyes

Several items are required to perform a thorough examination of the eyes. In addition to the standard items used in physical examinations such as gloves, alcohol wipes, and a penlight, to assess the eye, the nurse will also need a Snellen eye chart, a handheld visual screener or Jaeger card, as well as an opaque card or occluder, an applicator stick, and an ophthalmoscope. An **ophthalmoscope** is a device for studying the interior of the eyeball through the pupil.

Visual Acuity

Examination of the eyes usually begins with a general screening for visual acuity. Begin by testing central visual acuity or central vision by using the Snellen eye chart. Ask the patient to stand 6.1 m or 20 ft from the chart. Because this is a screening, if the patient needs glasses for distance or contacts, he or she should use them. You will need to assess the vision of one eye at a time. Ask the patient to cover one eye by using an opaque card or occluder and begin reading starting from the largest letter, the E at the top of the first line (Fig. 20.12).

Have the patient continue reading each line until either he is no longer able to read a line or he makes more than three mistakes on any one line. Document the patient's visual acuity in each eye. The number 20/20 constitutes perfect vision. The patient can see at 20 ft what a person with normal vision can see at 20 ft. The larger the denominator, the worse the patient's vision. As an example, if a patient sees 20/100, he can read at 20 ft what a person with perfect vision can read at 100 ft. He needs to be 80 ft closer to the chart to read the line compared with someone with normal vision.

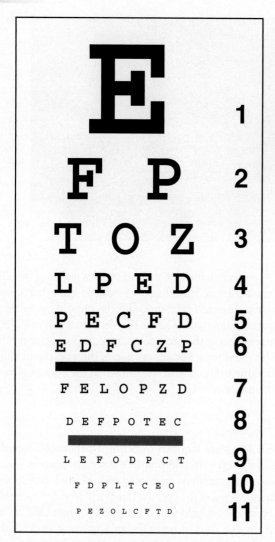

E	1
F P	2
T O Z	3
L P E D	4
P E C F D	5
E D F C Z P	6
F E L O P Z D	7
D E F P O T E C	8
L E F O D P C T	9
F D P L T C E O	10
P E Z O L C F T D	11

Figure 20.12 Snellen eye chart.

a time and read the chart until he or she is no longer able to read the print. The words on the Jaeger chart get smaller as one progresses down the chart. Document the lowest section the patient is able to read. Note that the visual acuity for near vision is out of 14. Normal vision is 14/14 bilaterally.

Visual Fields

Once you have completed assessing for visual acuity, assess for peripheral vision loss, which is commonly seen in macular degeneration. To screen for peripheral vision loss, perform the confrontation test. The specificity of confrontation tests is high, and identification of field defects using the confrontation test warrants further investigation (Pandit, Gales, & Griffiths, 2001). Stand at eye level, approximately 60 to 90 cm from the patient (arm's length), and ask the patient to cover her right eye while you cover your left eye. This allows you to assess for visual loss in one eye at a time. With the patient looking straight ahead, ask her to let you know when she sees your fingers moving. Using your right hand, start superiorly, above the patient's left eye, and move diagonally toward your waist. When the patient acknowledges that she saw your wiggling fingers, move to the next point. Note, as the examiner, you should be able to see the movement of your fingers at approximately the same point in time as the patient. Moving to the horizontal plane, at eye level, start with your arm outstretched and begin wiggling your fingers as you move toward midline (Fig. 20.14).

Next, move to the inferior position (arm at approximately 45° to the leg). Wiggle your fingers as you move your arm in a diagonal toward the patient's right eye; stop when she sees your fingers. Repeat the three directions on the patient's temporal side to determine possible borders of vision loss. Then have the patient switch eyes. Note, a temporal defect in one eye suggests a nasal defect in the other.

Examination of the Eye

Begin by examining the position and alignment of the eyes by standing above the patient. Looking from above and behind the seated patient's head, assess for any protrusion of the eyes. Next, move to the front of the patient and assess for protrusion. Inspect the eyebrows and eyelashes

To assess near vision in patients reporting difficulty reading print, or those older than 40 years of age who are at risk for presbyopia, consider using a pocket screener, the Jaeger chart (Fig. 20.13).

Ask the patient to hold the Jaeger chart 35 cm (14 in.) from his or her eye. Instruct the patient to cover one eye at

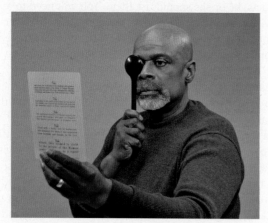

Figure 20.13 Assessing visual acuity using the Jaeger chart.

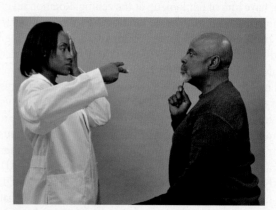

Figure 20.14 The confrontation test used to assess peripheral vision loss.

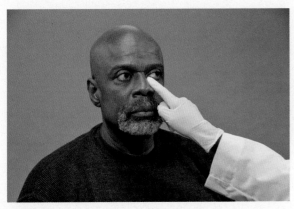

Figure 20.15 Palpating the lacrimal apparatus assessing for discharge.

Pupil Gauge (mm)

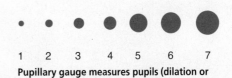

| 1 | 2 | 3 | 4 | 5 | 6 | 7 |

Pupillary gauge measures pupils (dilation or constriction) in millimeters (mm).

Figure 20.17 Pupil size measurements.

for symmetry, quantity, and distribution of the hairs. If the patient is reporting any redness or discharge from the eyes or eyelashes, evert the upper eyelid with an applicator stick and assess for colour, any swelling, or lesions. Ask the patient to close her eyelids and ensure adequacy of the closed eyelids. Ectropion (eyelids turned out) and entropion (eyelids turned in) may impede closing of the eyelids.

Assess the eyes for tearing and discharge. Begin by inspecting the lacrimal gland and sac for swelling. Next, with gloves on, depress the nasolacrimal sac using your index finger, observing for any discharge from the puncta (Fig. 20.15).

Fluid released from the puncta indicates a blocked duct. After assessing the lacrimal apparatus, assess the patient's conjunctiva and sclera. Instruct the patient to look up and then, using your thumbs, slide the lower lid down along the body orbital rim (Fig. 20.16) and ask the patient to look left and right, noting the colour and vascular pattern, checking for redness, swelling, exudates, or foreign bodies.

Assess the cornea and lens of the eye for lesions, scarring, or opacities. Begin by asking the patient to look straight ahead and, using oblique lighting, either from an ophthalmoscope split light or a penlight, shine the light from the lateral side of the eye across the cornea to the inner canthus. Repeat on the other eye. The cornea should be smooth and clear and the lens translucent. Continue examining the structures of the eye as you assess the iris. The iris is the

coloured area (blue, brown, hazel, green) around the pupil. When assessing the iris, begin by looking to see that the colour is evenly distributed and smooth. Next, shine your penlight or ophthalmoscopic light directly from the temporal side across the iris looking for a shadow on the medial side of the iris. Normally, no shadow should be present, but in cases of narrow-angle glaucoma, a shadow is often observed.

Assessing the Pupils

When it comes to the pupil, the eye tells us a great deal about the neurological status of the patient. The examination of the patient's pupils involves inspecting the pupils for size and shape and assessing for symmetry. Pupils are normally 4 to 5 mm (Fig. 20.17), round, and within 0.5 mm in size of each other. Variances of greater than 0.5 mm between pupils are suggestive of central nervous system concerns.

In addition to assessing for size, shape, and symmetry, the nurse should assess the pupils' reactivity to light. When exposed to bright light, the pupil of the eye constricts as a result of the circular muscles of the iris contracting. When we enter a dark room on the other hand, our pupils dilate. As part of the eye examination, the nurse should assess that the pupillary light reflex is intact. Where possible, dim the lights in the room and instruct the patient to look into the distance. Bring a light from the lateral side of the right eye to the middle of the right pupil. Note the direct reaction of constriction of the right pupil to the light. Repeat on the right eye, noting the consensual reaction of the left (opposite) eye, which should constrict simultaneously with the direct constriction of the right eye. Repeat these two steps with the left eye. Next, check that the pupils accommodate. To assess accommodation, instruct the patient to begin looking at an object in the distance; while the patient is staring at a distant object, bring a finger or pencil from below the patient's line of vision to approximately 30 cm in front of the patient. Ask the patient to focus on the object; the pupils should constrict and converge, indicating that the patient can accommodate from far to near focus (Fig. 20.18). Normally, the (P) pupils are (E) equal, (R) round, and (R) reactive to (L) light and (A) accommodation; the nurse would record this as PERRLA.

Assessing Extraocular Muscle Function

Movements of the eye are controlled by the coordinated movement of six extraocular muscles and by three cranial nerves that supply them. Tests can be used to assess the strength of these muscles as well as provide information

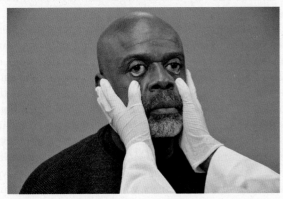

Figure 20.16 Inspecting the conjunctiva and sclera.

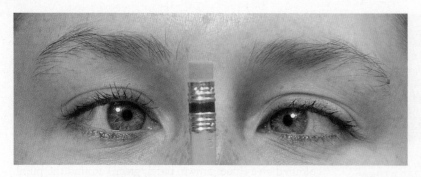

Figure 20.18 Constriction and convergence of the pupils.

about the cranial nerves (III, IV, and VI). The three tests are the Hirschberg test, the cover test, and assessment of the six cardial directions of gaze.

To assess the corneal light reflex, known as the *Hirschberg test*, instruct the patient to look straight ahead. Using a penlight, shine the light directly in front of the patient at eye level from a distance of approximately 30 to 60 cm away (1 to 2 ft). Inspect the location of the reflection of light on both corneas. The reflection of light should appear in the same place in both eyes. Asymmetry could be a result of weakness or dysfunction of the extraocular muscles.

The cover test is used to assess for extraocular muscle weakness. Begin by sitting at eye level to the patient and instruct the patient to look straight ahead and focus on a near object, such as your nose. Inform the patient that you will be covering one eye at a time but request that he or she continues to focus on the fixed point (your nose). Move an opaque card or eye cover from the lateral side of the patient's right eye to completely cover the right eye. Inspect the uncovered eye (left eye) for any movement. Then remove the opaque card from the right eye while watching the right eye for any movement. If a patient is unable to remain fixed on your nose and his or her eye deviates, it is known as *refixation*. Repeat by covering and uncovering the left eye. Normally, the patient is able to maintain his or her gaze and stay focused on a near object. In cases where patients have problems with extraocular muscle function resulting in weakness (or *strabismus*) as well as in cases of abnormalities in cranial nerves III, IV, and VI, the patient's covered eye drifts to a relaxed position. When the relaxed position is a drift inward toward the bridge of the nose, it is known as *esotropia*. *Exotropia* is the outward turning of the eye during the cover test.

The six cardinal directions of gaze allow the nurse to test cranial nerves III, IV, and VI. Begin by instructing the patient to look straight ahead while you hold your finger approximately 45 cm away from the patient's face. Ask the patient to follow your finger with his or her eyes only, keeping his or her head erect. Move your fingers to the right superior position (the direction of 2 o'clock on a clock) while watching that both eyes follow the direction of the finger symmetrically. Note any *nystagmus* or shaking of the eyes as they follow your finger. Next, move in a diagonal to the left inferior position (7 o'clock) without stopping and then return to the midway point. Next, assess eye movement in the horizontal plane moving to right lateral position (3 o'clock) and move your finger to the 9 o'clock position, noting the eye movement. Finally, move your finger to the left superior position (11 o'clock) and bring your finger in a diagonal to the 5 o'clock position. The eyes should move symmetrically in a smooth fashion in all directions.

Ophthalmoscopic Exam

Inspection of the internal structures of the eye necessitates the use of the ophthalmoscope (Nursing Guideline 20.1).

Ears, Nose, Mouth, and Throat

The ear, nose, mouth, sinuses, and throat are all interconnected. Therefore, assessment of one of the systems should include examination of the others. Think back to the case of our nursing student with an earache and a cough. The nurse should conduct an assessment of her ear, nose, sinuses, and throat as well as lymph nodes and respiratory system.

Examining the Ear

Let's begin with the examination of the ear. Examination of the ear should begin with the subjective data assessment, noting any difficulties with hearing, and follow with inspection and palpation of the external ear, inspection of the ear canal and tympanic membrane, and assessment of hearing acuity. The ear is divided into three parts: the external ear, middle ear, and inner ear. The external ear, also known as the *auricle*, has six anatomical landmarks: the helix, antihelix, external auditory meatus, tragus, antitragus, and lobule (Fig. 20.19).

These landmarks serve as the typical reference points when examining and documenting findings. The ear canal is included in the external ear and is separated from the middle ear by the tympanic membrane. The middle ear is a tiny air-filled cavity located inside the temporal bone that contains the malleus, incus, and stapes. These three bones transmit sound. The middle ear also opens to the eustachian tube, which connects the middle ear with the nasopharynx and allows for the passage of air. The inner ear contains the cochlea, which is the central hearing apparatus, and the vestibule and semicircular canals, which make up the vestibular apparatus, important for equilibrium.

NURSING GUIDELINE 20.1: USING THE OPHTHALMOSCOPE

1. Begin by dimming the lights to allow the pupils to dilate and allow for better visualization of the internal structures of the eye.
2. Turn the ophthalmoscope on and adjust the light to the small, round beam of white light.
3. Turn the wheel of the ophthalmoscope (also known as the *lens disc*) to the 0 diopter.
4. Hold ophthalmoscope in your right hand to examine patient's right eye with your right eye and in your left hand to examine patient's left eye with your left eye.
5. Ask the patient to focus on a distant object.
6. Stand directly in front of patient. Place your hand on the patient's head. Stand approximately 40 cm away and at an angle of 15° lateral to patient's line of vision.
7. Shine the ophthalmoscope light toward the patient's right pupil. This allows the nurse to visualize the patient's red reflex that looks like an orange glow.
8. While looking through the viewing hole on the ophthalmoscope, follow the red reflex as you move inward toward the nasal aspect of the visual field until you are approximately 6–10 cm away from the patient's forehead.
9. Move the ophthalmoscope wheel from 0 to + black numbers (on some ophthalmoscopes, this might be green numbers). Adjust the wheel until the anterior ocular structures come into focus. Inspect for transparency.
10. After visualizing the anterior structures, adjust the wheel from + black numbers to the − red numbers to focus on structures progressively more posteriorly. Adjust the wheel until the structures come into focus. It should be possible to visualize paired retinal vessels with smooth crossings. Inspect the veins and arteries and follow them peripherally in each of four directions, noting any irregularities, lesions, or pooling of blood. With the patient's pupils dilated, and with much practice with the ophthalmoscope, the nurse should be able to visualize the optic disc which is on the nasal side and a yellowish-orange colour. The optic disc should be round or oval in shape with distinct and sharply demarcated margins.
11. Adjust the ophthalmoscope aperture to the green light to make viewing the macula easier. Move toward the temporal side to examine the macula. The macula is light sensitive and is darker than the optic disc, with a light reflective middle known as the *fovea*. It is often difficult for the novice nurse to view the macula. Be careful not to spend too long attempting to view the internal structures of the eye without providing the patient with a break. Remember the light from the ophthalmoscope can be glaring and irritating when held in the same position for an extended period of time.
12. Repeat the same procedure in the left eye.

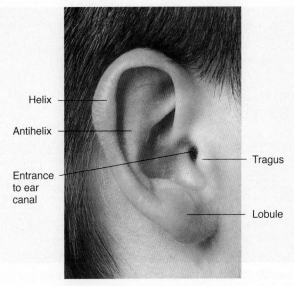

Figure 20.19 Parts of the external ear.

Inspection and Palpation of the External Ear

The examination of the external ear begins with inspection for size and shape. As with previous systems, it involves comparing one side to the other to determine if they are equal in size or if there is any swelling or enlargement. The condition of the skin of the external ear, including all of the six anatomical landmarks, is inspected for colour, consistency, lesions, lumps, or deformities. Palpate the external ear beginning with the pinna, moving along the helix to the lobule, assessing for pain or tenderness. Then, press against the tragus, occluding the ear canal, and move to the mastoid bone behind the ear and palpate it; no pain should be produced.

Otoscopic Examination

After inspection of the external ear, begin the otoscopic examination. The **otoscope** is an instrument used for examining the ear. The position of the patient's head and ear as well as the examiner's hand is important for the otoscopic examination. First, examine the unaffected ear prior to examining the affected ear. Ask the patient to slightly incline his or her head away from you toward his or her opposite shoulder. This allows for the nurse to have a view of the ear canal at the correct angle. Gently pull the pinna of the patient's ear up and back to straighten the ear canal and enhance visualization. Do not release traction on the ear until you have completed the exam and removed the otoscope. For the novice examiner, it is prudent to hold the otoscope upside down so that the examiner's free fingers or back of hand are resting on patient's cheek bone. Proper placement of the examiner's hand helps to steady the otoscope and prevent the speculum tip from being pushed too far into the ear canal, causing pain or damage. Use the largest ear speculum on the otoscope tip that the ear canal can accommodate. Insert the speculum gently into the ear canal while looking through the viewer. Avoid touching the very sensitive inner bony section of ear

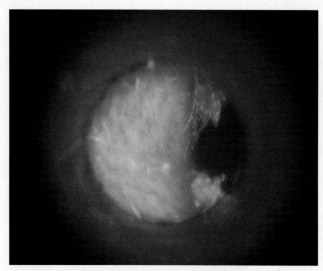

Figure 20.20 The ear canal with cerumen present. (Photo courtesy of Judy Bornais)

canal with the speculum. Direct the tip downward along the angle of the ear canal, inspecting for redness, swelling, lesions, foreign bodies, and any discharge. It is common to see cerumen (ear wax) in the ear canal (Fig. 20.20).

Inspect the eardrum through the tympanic membrane. The tympanic membrane should normally be a translucent pearly grey in colour, and the cone of light should clearly be reflected in the anterior inferior quadrant; if you are looking in the right ear, the cone of light should be at 5 o'clock and at 7 o'clock in the left ear. Note the position of the eardrum, which should be flat and not bulging and slightly pulled in at the centre (Fig. 20.21). Inspect the integrity of the membrane for any perforations and note the small bones of the ear, the handle, and short process of the malleus as well as the incus (Bluestone & Klein, 2007).

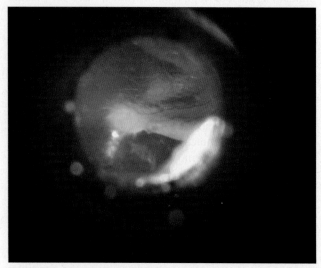

Figure 20.21 A normal tympanic membrane with the cone of light, malleus, and incus visible along with some cerumen in the ear canal. (Photo courtesy of Judy Bornais)

Assessing Auditory Acuity

Examination of the ear should include testing for hearing. As part of your assessment, you should be noting the patient's ability to hear and respond to questions during your subjective data assessment. To further assess hearing, ask the patient to stand with his or her back to you and cover one ear at a time by placing a finger against the tragus to occlude the ear canal. Stand at arm's length (0.6 m) behind the patient and quietly exhale before whispering a combination of numbers and letters (e.g., T-2-B) or a two-syllable word. Ask the patient to repeat what he or she heard. If the patient is able to correctly repeat the combination, hearing is considered normal. If a patient incorrectly identifies the combination or word, repeat the test using a different two-syllable word. The patient is considered to pass the hearing screening test if he or she is able to repeat at least three out of a possible six numbers/letters or three of six two-syllable words correctly (Glasziou, Papinczak, & Pirozzo, 2003). Test each ear separately starting with the unaffected ear first. If hearing loss is detected, use the Weber and the Rinne test to try to distinguish if the hearing loss is conductive or sensorineural. To conduct the Weber test, gently tap a tuning fork against the palmar surface of your hand to activate the vibration (Fig. 20.22). While holding the base of the tuning fork between your thumb and finger, place the vibrating tuning fork in the midline of the person's skull and ask if sound is equal in both ears or better in one.

Normally, during the Weber test, the patient would hear the vibrations equally in both ears. For sound lateralized to the affected ear, suspect unilateral conductive hearing loss. Like the Weber test, the Rinne test also uses a vibrating tuning fork (Fig. 20.23). Begin by placing the base of the vibrating tuning fork against the patient's mastoid process.

Instruct the patient to inform you when he or she no longer hears the sound from the tuning fork. When the sound stops, quickly invert the tuning fork so that the vibrating end is in front of the ear canal and ask the patient if he or she can hear sound from the tuning fork. This allows for discrimination of air versus bone conduction. Normally, a patient should hear the sound twice as long through air compared with bone. If bone conduction is equal or greater than air conduction, suspect conductive loss.

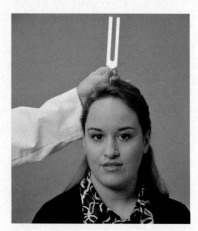

Figure 20.22 The Weber test.

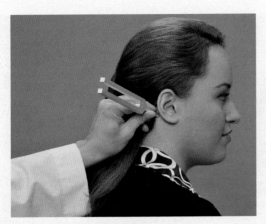

Figure 20.23 The Rinne test.

Nose, Sinuses, Mouth, and Throat

The nose is the first segment of the respiratory system. The nurse considers the connection with the lungs when there are concerns with the nose, sinuses, mouth, or throat. Begin your assessment by examining the external nose, checking for symmetry, deformities, and that it is midline on the face. The nose is mostly cartilage with only the upper one third consisting of bone. Palpate, beginning at the bridge of the nose where the bone is present. Use your thumb and forefinger to palpate along the nose to the nares. There should be no tenderness or pain on palpation. Next, ask the patient to breathe in and out through the nose, occluding one nostril at a time checking for patency and airflow. It is important to determine if there are any alterations in airflow from either nostril, especially prior to inserting a nasogastric tube. Next, inspect the internal nose. Examine the mucosa for colour, swelling, discharge, bleeding, exudate, ulcers, polyps,

or foreign bodies. Check the nasal septum for any deviation, inflammation, or perforations. A perforation in the right nare will appear as a white light shining through the left nare. Normally, when shining the light in the right nare, only a reddish glow should be visible in the left nare. Next, examine the turbinates in each nostril. The parasinuses are air-filled pockets within the cranium. There are four pairs of paranasal sinuses but only two are accessible to examination, the frontal and maxillary sinuses (Fig. 20.24) (William & Simel, 1993).

The ethmoid and sphenoid sinuses are smaller and located more deeply within the skull and are not accessible to examination. Begin by inspecting the area above the forehead over the frontal sinuses and the maxillary sinuses for any redness or swelling. Then palpate the sinuses by pushing with the thumbs of your hands against the area (Fig. 20.25).

Follow palpation with percussion of the frontal and maxillary sinuses by directly tapping along the frontal and maxillary sinuses using the tip of your first two fingers. Normally, the patient should feel pressure but no tenderness or pain on palpation or percussion.

Mouth and Pharynx

Examination of the mouth includes the lips, teeth, gums, buccal mucosa, tongue, hard palate, soft palate, tonsils, and uvula. Begin by inspecting the lips for colour, symmetry, moisture, lumps, ulcers, cracking, or scaliness. Wearing a pair of gloves and holding a light and a tongue depressor, begin by shining the light on the teeth, gums, and buccal mucosa (the *cheek*). Look at the overall oral health of the patient, the presence, colour, and position of teeth, and the bite: Do the teeth align to allow for proper chewing? Assess the gums, which should be pink and moist, and check for any dental caries. If the patient wears dentures, have him or her remove the dentures so you may examine the gums

Frontal sinus

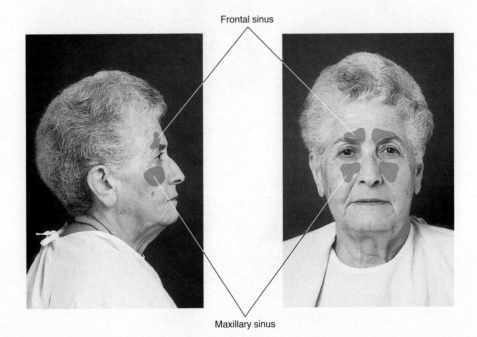

Figure 20.24 The frontal and maxillary sinuses.

Maxillary sinus

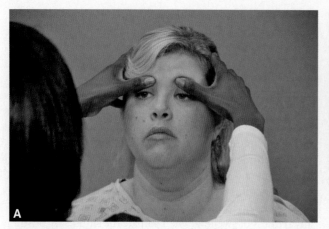
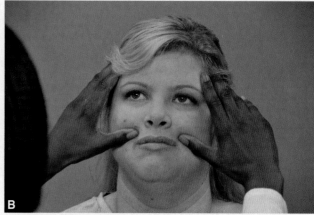

Figure 20.25 Palpating the sinus area. A. Palpating the frontal sinus. B. Palpating the maxillary sinus.

and mucosa underneath the dentures. Inspect the roof of the mouth. The hard palate is made of bone and should appear whitish in colour, whereas the soft palate is posterior to the hard palate and is made up of a muscle that is much pinker. Next, inspect the tongue. While holding gauze, gently grasp the tongue and move it from side to side as well as toward the roof of the mouth looking for colour, lesions, nodules, or ulcers. While shining the light on the uvula, ask the patient to stick out his or her tongue and say, "aah." Normally, the uvula should rise midline symmetrically. Continue to examine the oropharynx, noting the tonsils, which should appear pink and symmetrical without exudate, swelling, ulceration, or tonsil enlargement. In a healthy adult, the tonsils should be graded as +1 to +2 (Newland, 2003). See Figure 20.26 for grading of the tonsils.

Respiratory System

The nurse assesses current symptoms and past history of respiratory infections as part of the subjective data collection. What would be important subjective data questions to ask a patient seeking care for a cough? Consider asking when the cough started: Was it gradual or sudden? Ask the patient to describe the cough: Is it a hacking cough, dry, barking, congested, or productive cough? It would be important to ask if the patient is bringing up any sputum when he or she coughs, and if so, what colour is it, is there any odour to the sputum, and what is its consistency? Is there a specific time the cough occurs or is continuous throughout the day? In what part of his or her chest does he or she feel the cough? How much is he or she coughing? Does anything make it

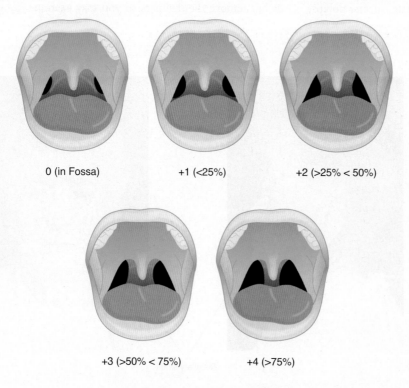

0 (in Fossa)   +1 (<25%)   +2 (>25% < 50%)

+3 (>50% < 75%)   +4 (>75%)

Figure 20.26 Grading of the tonsils.

better or worse? Does he or she have any associated symptoms with the cough such as shortness of breath, wheezing, chest pain, temperature, sore throat, and runny nose? Knowing whether the patient smokes is important and if he or she is exposed to any environmental factors that may be contributing to the cough. Once the subjective data is collected, the nurse should then proceed with the physical examination.

Anatomical Landmarks and Reference Lines of the Chest and Lungs

Knowledge of the anatomical landmarks and imaginary reference lines is important for the nurse to understand when performing the respiratory assessment and completing appropriate documentation. During the assessment, these lines and landmarks define the specific areas being assessed. Figure 20.27 shows the location of the five lung lobes and the reference lines anteriorly, posteriorly, and from the lateral view.

Whether you are assessing Megan, or a patient in an acute care setting, a general respiratory assessment should occur every time you assess a patient. As with the other assessments, begin with inspecting and observing the patient.

Inspection of the Respiratory System

Although you may have already taken the patient's vital signs, as part of the respiratory assessment, you should observe the rate, rhythm, depth, and effort the patient takes to breathe. Assess if the patient is experiencing respiratory difficulty, and if so, has it compromised his or her level of consciousness? Inspect for any signs of respiratory difficulty such as the patient's position (a tripod position is often assumed when people are in respiratory distress). Observe the patient's facial expression. Does he or she appears as though he or she is struggling to breathe? Is he or she tachypneic or bradypneic? Listen to the patient's breathing; normal breathing should be silent, automatic, symmetric, and effortless (known as *eupneic*).

Inspect the neck and thorax, looking for the use of any accessory muscle to aid in breathing. Inspect to see if the trachea is midline or if it is displaced. Inspect the colour of the patient's lips for cyanosis and the nails for colour, clubbing, and capillary refill. Finally, observe the shape and configuration of the patient's chest.

Figure 20.28 shows the shape and configuration of the adult thorax, normally oval in shape and twice as long (traverse diameter) as it is wide (anteroposterior [AP] diameter). In certain conditions such as chronic obstructive pulmonary disease (COPD), the AP diameter increases, and the patient may present with a barrel chest with an AP to traverse diameter closer to a 1:1 ratio.

The remainder of the respiratory assessment should be performed in sections, usually beginning with the posterior chest and moving to the anterior chest assessment.

Posterior Chest Assessment

Begin the posterior chest assessment by standing midline behind the patient and inspecting the chest. Note the shape of the thoracic cage and the way in which it moves while the patient breathes. Normally, the chest should expand equally on both sides and there should not be any retraction of the intercostal spaces (ICSs) during inspiration. Assess if the thoracic cage is uniform in colour and look for the presence of any lesions or bruises. Inspect that the spine is midline and the scapulae are symmetrical and look for any deformities, asymmetry, or irregular curvatures. Normally, the spine should have three curvatures in the cervical, thoracic, and lumbar area.

Palpation

Begin the palpation of the posterior chest with general palpation. Place the finger pads along the chest wall making small concentric circles. Start palpating above the scapula in the upper lobes of the lungs and progress laterally to the midaxillary line. Move side to side comparing findings bilaterally ending at the base of the lungs.

Figure 20.29 illustrates the locations for the sequence of general palpation of the posterior chest. While palpating, assess for any areas of tenderness, pain, or abnormalities. Abnormalities may consist of lesions, lumps, masses, or subcutaneous emphysema (a coarse, crackling sensation similar to rice crispy cereal under the skin created by air entering the subcutaneous tissue). During palpation, note the moisture and temperature of the skin. Following general palpation, proceed with palpation for symmetric chest expansion.

Palpation for Chest Expansion. Palpating to assess for symmetrical chest movement can be performed by testing for chest expansion.

Using the common landmarks of C7/T1, palpate down the spinous process to T9 or T10. Alternatively, find the floating rib at the midaxillary line and follow it to the spine and palpate up the spinous process to T9 or T10. Now, place your thumbs at the level of T9 to T10. Wrap the palmar surface of your hands on the chest wall with your fingers loosely grasping the lungs (Fig. 20.30). Your fingers should lie almost horizontally and be parallel to the rib cage. Slide the thumbs of your hands inward to create a loose skinfold between your thumbs and the spine. Ask the patient to take a deep breath and observe the distance between your thumbs as they move apart when the patient inhales. Feel for symmetry and for the extent of expansion and contraction of the rib cage beneath your hands. It is normal for your thumbs to move apart approximately 5 to 10 cm symmetrically.

Palpation for Tactile Fremitus. *Tactile fremitus* refers to the vibrations that are felt under the ball of the hand (refer to Figure 20.1) when a patient speaks. Normally, when a patient speaks, sound is generated in the larynx and transmitted throughout the bronchial tree to the chest wall and can be felt as vibrations. Fremitus varies among individuals, but symmetry is the key. Tactile fremitus is performed when the nurse is concerned that an obstruction or consolidation of lung tissue exists. The nurse instructs the patient to say and repeat the word "ninety-nine" as the nurse moves the

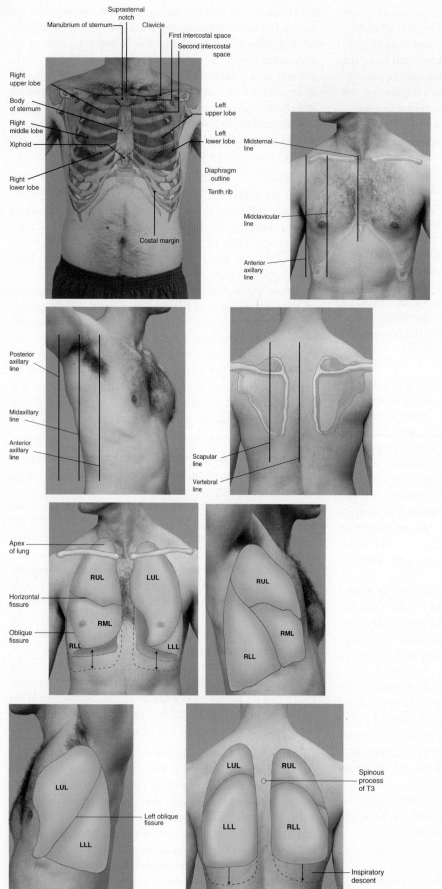

Figure 20.27 Views of the lungs and reference lines of the chest.

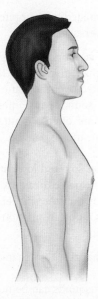

Normal adult chest

Figure 20.28 Normal traverse to AP diameter (2:1) of the adult.

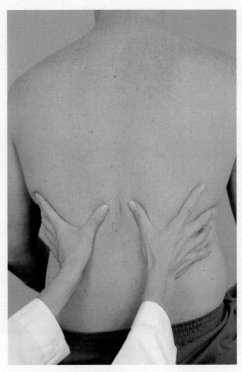

Figure 20.30 Testing for chest expansion posteriorly.

ball of her hands, feeling for vibrations across the posterior chest comparing side to side (Fig. 20.31). Fremitus is usually more intense along the main bronchus and less intense at the base of the lungs. As an example, pneumonia would cause increased vibrations, and the sound would be more intense over the area of pneumonia.

Percussion

The predominant percussion note over the lung fields is resonance, created by air in the underlying lung tissue. Fluid-filled or solid lung tissue has different percussion tones. By percussing the lung fields and comparing side to side, the nurse can assess for obstructions, consolidations, or changes in the underlying lung tissue. Using the indirect percussion technique described at the beginning of this

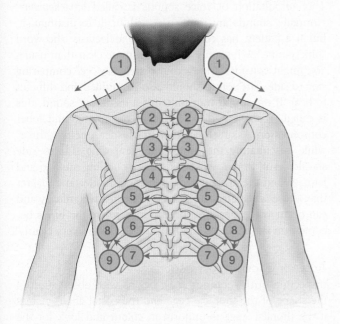

Figure 20.29 Locations for general palpation of the posterior chest.

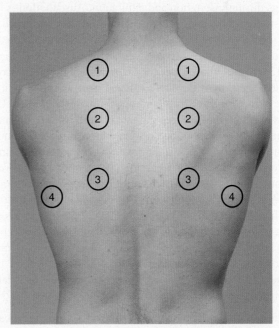

Figure 20.31 Location and sequence of palpating tactile fremitus posteriorly.

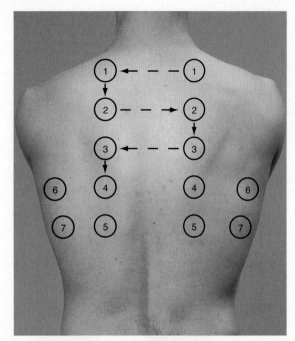

Figure 20.32 Location and sequence of percussing and auscultating the posterior chest.

chapter (see Fig. 20.3), percuss from side to side, listening for changes in percussion notes (Fig. 20.32). Note that percussion should occur between the ICSs, avoiding the ribs and the bony scapular area, both of which will produce a flat sound.

Auscultation
Auscultation of the lungs involves listening with a stethoscope to the sounds created by the movement of air into the lungs during inspiration and expiration. Auscultation is the most important examination technique for assessing airflow through the respiratory passage and lungs and for determining abnormalities (Ponte, Moraes, Hizume, & Alencar, 2013). To auscultate, place the diaphragm of the stethoscope against the skin of the chest wall and instruct the patient to take slow deep breaths in and out through the mouth. Use a systematic sequence (see Fig. 20.32) and listen for a complete cycle of inspiration and expiration in each location, comparing side to side. Along with listening to the sounds generated by breathing, listen for any unexpected or adventitious sounds. **Adventitious** breath sounds are abnormal sounds heard on auscultation. This may include sounds that are heard in an unusual place or manner. If breath sounds are too soft or difficult to hear, ask the patient to breathe deeper, but be aware of any discomfort or changes in patient's condition due to hyperventilation. You may need to allow the patient to rest during the assessment if he or she feels faint or light-headed.

Breath Sounds. Three common breath sounds are heard in specific locations in the lungs: *bronchial, bronchovesicular,* and *vesicular.* These breath sounds are heard in specific

places and are differentiated by their pitch, intensity, and duration of inspiration versus expiration.

- **Bronchial** sounds are loud and high-pitched, and expiration is longer than inspiration. If audible, bronchial sounds are auscultated over the manubrium.
- **Bronchovesicular** sounds are intermediate in intensity and pitch and are often auscultated over the major bronchi. Inspiration and expiration are almost equal in duration.
- **Vesicular** sounds are soft and low-pitched and are found over the lung fields near sites of air exchange. It takes more time to move air down to the smaller airways, and therefore with vesicular sounds, inspiration (moving air in) lasts longer than expiration.

Table 20.5 summarizes the characteristics of breath sounds.

Unexpected breath sounds can be normal breath sounds (bronchial, bronchovesicular, or vesicular) heard outside of their usual locations or adventitious breath sounds such as crackles (sometimes called *rales*), wheezes, rhonchi, pleural fiction rubs, and stridor. Table 20.6 explains in more detail the different adventitious breath sounds.

You may find clinically that patients who have been in bed for prolonged periods of time present with audible crackles with their first breath after sitting up. These sounds are produced by collapsed alveoli when opening. Consider asking the patient to cough to see if the crackles disappear. Fine and coarse crackles as a result of pathology do not disappear after a cough (Wipf et al., 1999).

If you detect abnormal breath sounds, such as bronchial or bronchovesicular sounds in the wrong locations, ask the patient to say "ninety-nine" while you listen with your stethoscope across the chest wall comparing side to side. This auscultation of voice sounds is called *bronchophony.* Normally, sounds are muffled and difficult to distinguish, but if a patient has consolidation or atelectasis, the word "ninety-nine" will sound louder and more clear than usual. You might consider asking your patient say "ee" comparing side to side. The sound should also be muffled and difficult to hear. If the sound transmitted is a nasal "ay" sound, this is called *egophony* and can occur in pneumonia and lobar consolidation. Asking the patient to whisper "one-two-three" while auscultating the lungs and comparing side to side should result in the whispered voice sounding muffled and faint. When the auscultated sounds are louder and clearer than those whispered, it is called *whispered pectoriloquy* and can occur with consolidation of lungs where the lungs become firm and inelastic and transmit the sound very clearly.

Anterior Chest Assessment
Inspection of the anterior chest begins with observation of the shape of the thoracic cage and the costal angle. Assess if the thoracic cage is uniform in colour and look for the presence of any lesions or bruises. Look for any deformities or asymmetry. Observe the movement of the chest wall,

TABLE 20.5	Characteristics of Normal Breath Sounds			
Location	Description	Ratio of Inspiration to Expiration	Intensity	Pitch
Bronchial	Blowing, hollow sounds over the trachea	Inspiration / Expiration	Expiration is markedly longer and louder	Expiration is higher
Bronchovesicular	Intermediate sounds over first and second anterior ICSs and posteriorly between scapula	Inspiration / Expiration	Medium and similar	Medium and similar
Vesicular	Soft and breezy sounds over all lung area except airways	Inspiration / Expiration	Inspiration markedly longer and louder	Inspiration is higher

Scapula

Intercostal space

looking for symmetry on both sides with no retraction of the supraclavicular area or ICSs.

Palpation

Begin the palpation of the anterior chest with general palpation. Place the finger pads along the chest wall making small concentric circles. Start palpating above the clavicles at the apices of the lungs and move from side to side comparing findings bilaterally, ending below the costal angle and moving laterally to the midaxillary line. While palpating, assess for any areas of tenderness, pain, or abnormalities. Abnormalities may consist of lesions, lumps, masses, or subcutaneous emphysema. During palpation, note the moisture and temperature of the skin. If during inspection the trachea did not appear midline, palpate it to determine if it is deviated. Following general palpation, proceed with palpation for symmetric chest expansion.

Palpation for Chest Expansion. To palpate for symmetrical chest movement anteriorly, place your thumbs along each costal margin near the sternum and place your fingers laterally on the rib cage (Fig. 20.33).

Create a loose skinfold between your thumbs and ask the patient to take a deep breath and observe the distance between your thumbs as they move apart when the patient inhales. Feel for symmetry and for the extent of chest movement.

Palpation for Tactile Fremitus. Palpate both sides of the chest using the ball of the hand to feel for vibrations when your patient says, and repeats, "ninety-nine" as you move your hands from the lung apices to the base and laterally comparing side to side (Fig. 20.34).

Fremitus is usually decreased or absent over the precordium because of the heart and is felt the greatest between the second and third ICSs over the large airways. When palpating a female patient for fremitus anteriorly, it may be helpful to ask her to displace her breasts because fremitus is often decreased over breast tissue.

Percussion

Percussion over the anterior chest follows the same technique as percussion of the posterior chest. Begin at the apices of the lungs, above the clavicle, and percuss

TABLE 20.6	Adventitious Breath Sounds		
Unexpected Sound	Description	Mechanism	Associated Conditions
Fine crackles (rales)	High-pitched, soft, brief crackling sounds that can be simulated by rolling a strand of hair near the ear or stethoscope	Deflated small airways and alveoli will pop open during inspiration. In early congestive heart failure (CHF), small amounts of fluid in the alveoli may cause fine crackles.	Late inspiratory crackles are associated with restrictive disease (e.g., fibrosis and heart failure). Early inspiratory crackles occur with obstructive diseases (e.g., asthma and COPD).
Coarse crackles (rales)	Low-pitched, moist, longer sounds that are similar to Velcro slowly separating	Small air bubbles flow through secretions or narrowed airways.	Pulmonary fibrosis, pulmonary edema, COPD
Wheeze (high-pitched or sibilant)	High-pitched musical sounds heard primarily during inspiration	Air passes through narrowed airways and creates sound similar to that of a vibrating reed. Note if inspiratory or expiratory.	Asthma, bronchitis, emphysema
Rhonchi (gurgle, low-pitched wheeze, sonorous wheeze)	Low-pitched snoring or gurgling sound that may clear with coughing	Airflow passes around or through secretions or narrowed passages.	Pneumonia
Pleural friction rub	Loud, coarse, and low-pitched grating or creaking sound similar to a squeaky door during inspiration and expiration; more common in the lower anterolateral thorax	Inflamed pleural surfaces lose their normal lubrication and rub together during breathing.	Pleuritis
Stridor	Loud, high-pitched crowing or honking sound louder in upper airway	Laryngeal or tracheal inflammation or spasm can cause stridor, as can aspiration of a foreign object.	Epiglottitis, croup, partially obstructed airway; can indicate an emergency requiring immediate attention

the anterior and lateral chest comparing both sides (Fig. 20.35).

Remember to only percuss between ICSs, listening for resonance. Anteriorly, you will hear dullness over the heart and the upper border of the liver. Note that in the midclavicular line by the fifth ICS, you are likely to hear tympany because of the stomach.

Think   Why do you need to auscultate the lungs anteriorly if you auscultated them posteriorly? Remember the anatomical location of the lobes of the lungs. Posteriorly, your patient has predominantly lower lobes with only a small amount of upper lobes to T3. If you only auscultate the posterior chest and not the anterior chest, you will miss a significant amount of the upper lobes and the entire right middle lobe.

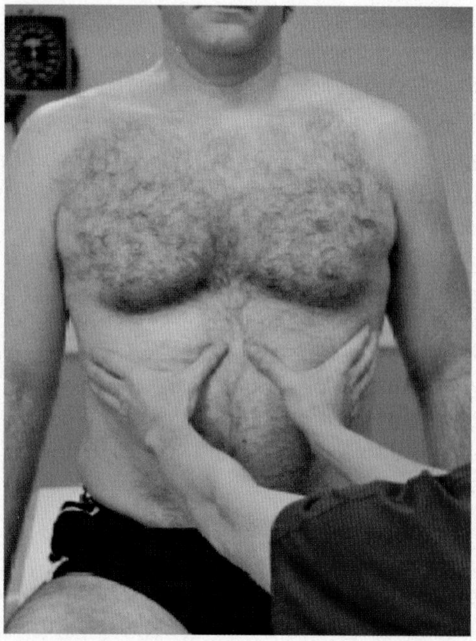

Figure 20.33 Testing for chest expansion anteriorly.

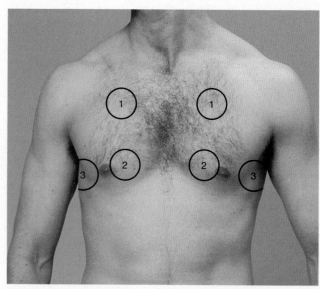

Figure 20.34 Location and sequence of palpating tactile fremitus anteriorly.

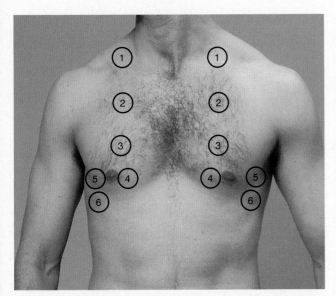

Figure 20.35 Location and sequence of percussing and auscultating the anterior chest.

Auscultation

Auscultation of the lungs anteriorly involves listening with the stethoscope, using a systematic sequence beginning at the apices of the lungs and moving laterally (refer to Fig. 20.35). Remember to listen for a full cycle of inspiration and expiration in each location, comparing side to side while the patient takes deep breaths through the mouth. Once again, displacement of the breast tissue may be necessary. Along with listening to the breath sounds, listen for any unexpected or adventitious sounds. If indicated, listen for transmitted voice sounds using the same technique as used with the posterior chest assessment.

Oxygenation

The final component of the respiratory assessment involves assessing the patient's oxygenation. This may have been completed with vital signs, but it is an important component of the respiratory assessment. Oximetry is used to monitor oxygen saturation levels in patients at risk for hypoxemia, including patients undergoing surgery, cardiac stress testing, mechanical ventilation, heavy sedation, or lung function testing, or who have multiple trauma (Pagana & Pagana, 2010). A patient's oxygen saturation should ideally be greater than or equal to 95% (Radford, County, & Oakley, 2004, p. 81). When assessing a patient's oxygen saturation with a pulse oximeter, remember to include in your document if the patient is on oxygen or if the reading was assessed on room air.

Cardiovascular System

Assessment of the cardiovascular system includes assessment of the patient's blood pressure, heart rate, carotids, jugular veins, and precordium, which includes the heart. As part of the assessment of the cardiovascular system, the nurse must consider the patient's blood pressure and heart rate because these provide the nurse with important information about the heart's pumping ability. Significant deviations from normal blood pressure and heart rate can be one of the first signs that there is a serious problem in the cardiovascular system. It is important to have a blood pressure from both arms, comparing any pressure differences between them. A significant difference in blood pressure between the right and left arm can suggest serious heart ischemia. Assessment of the blood pressure in lying, sitting, and standing positions can be important as part of the cardiac assessment. The patient's radial pulses can provide important information about the electrical activity of the heart if the rhythm is regular or irregular. Comparing the patient's heart rate at the radial pulse versus the apical pulse is important to determine any pulse deficits. As with other assessments, to perform the assessment of the cardiovascular system, the nurse will need to inspect, palpate, percuss, and auscultate.

Carotids

Carotid arteries are located on both sides of the neck, between the patient's trachea and the sternomastoid muscles (Fig. 20.36).

The carotids are the only arteries supplying oxygenated blood to the brain. Special care is required when assessing the carotids to ensure the oxygen supply to the brain is not cut off during palpation; doing so for any significant period of time may result in brain damage.

Inspection

With the patient sitting in the upright position, begin by inspecting the carotids for any movement. Examine both the right and left carotid arteries from the clavicle up to the level of the patient's jaw. Carotid arteries have a biphasic waveform, meaning they have a double stroke which corresponds with S_1 and S_2.

Palpation

With the patient's head elevated, gently place your index, middle, and ring fingers on the right then the left carotid arteries and palpate the carotid upstroke. The carotid artery is usually a strong pulsation. As the major artery to the brain, the carotids often continue to be palpable even with the patient's cardiac output (heart rate vs. stroke volume) is diminished. If you recall when you learned cardiopulmonary resuscitation (CPR), it was the carotid artery that you assessed for a pulse, not the radial artery. This is because when the cardiac output is low, whether because the body is in shock or hypovolemic, the body shunts blood away from the periphery to the central organs—the heart, lungs, and brain. When palpating the carotids, never palpate the right and left carotid arteries simultaneously. Doing so can result in a lack of oxygen to the brain and result in the patient passing out. It is important that you do not push hard or massage the carotids during palpation because doing so can affect the patient's heart rate and blood pressure. Palpate the strength of the pulse and grade it on a 0 to 4 scale as you would a peripheral pulse. Compare the right to the left carotid; they should be equal bilaterally without any thrills. A thrill, a vibrating sensation similar to the purring of a cat, can often be

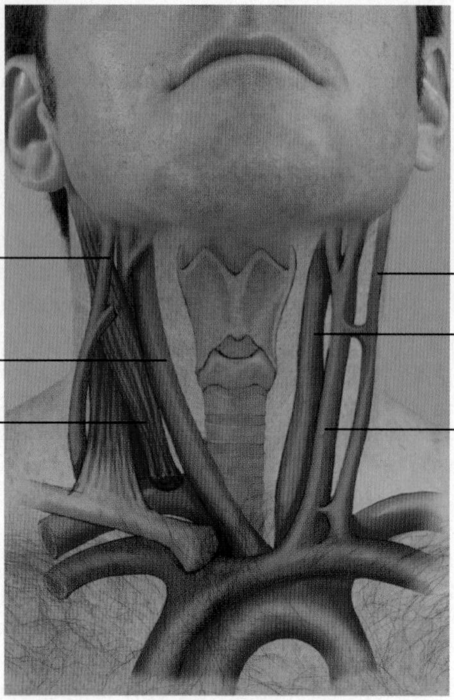

Figure 20.36 Anatomy of the neck vessels.

felt when there is turbulent blood flow in the carotid, often caused by atherosclerosis. A thrill is often present when a bruit is auscultated.

Auscultation

Auscultation of the carotids allows the nurse to detect possible narrowing of the carotids from atherosclerosis. With the patient in an upright position, instruct him to inhale, exhale, and hold his breath on the exhalation. Holding the exhalation ensures that breath sounds do not obscure any vascular sounds or bruits (whooshing or swooshing sounds) that are caused by turbulent blood flow. While the patient is holding the exhalation, listen with the bell of the stethoscope, along the carotid in three places: along the clavicle, below the jaw, and halfway between the clavicle and the jaw. Be sure to let the patient know that if he feels the need to breathe, do so. You may have to have the patient inhale, exhale, and hold the exhalation more than once to auscultate each carotid. If arterial occlusion exists, you may hear a bruit. Note that if you do not hear a bruit, this does not mean there is no occlusion. Carotids that are greater than 75% occluded do not result in bruits (Eskandari, Pearce, & Yao, 2010, p. 8). A carotid ultrasound can confirm if a carotid is truly occluded. If a bruit is present on auscultation, this is a significant finding and should be reported to the physician. Normally, no sound should be audible through the stethoscope.

Jugular Vein

Internal and external jugular veins are found on both the left and right side of the neck. These jugular veins drain blood from the head and neck directly into the superior vena cava which flows directly into the right atrium. The right internal jugular vein lies more medially to the superior vena cava than the right external jugular vein and the left internal and external jugular veins. With no valve between the right atrium and the superior vena cava and the right internal jugular vein, the right internal jugular vein reflects pressure in the right atrium. The jugular venous pressure (JVP) is thus best estimated from the right internal jugular vein because of its more direct anatomic channel into the right atrium, and therefore, the right internal jugular vein is the preferred blood vessel for assessing JVP (Cook & Simel, 1996).

Inspection and Palpation

To inspect the right internal jugular vein, instruct the patient to lie flat on the bed or examination table. Gravity allows for venous drainage; a patient sitting upright prevents visualization of the JVP if it is not distended. On the other hand, having the patient in the supine position generally results in the external neck vessels distending, which enhances visualization. The experienced examiner will not need to begin with the patient in the supine position because he or she will be comfortable with locating the internal jugular vein. For the novice examiner, beginning in the supine position will allow the jugular veins to distend and be more visible. Remove any large pillows that might cause the patient's neck to flex, tightening the sternomastoid muscles, which may affect the ability to visualize the JVP. Ask the patient to turn his or her head gently to the left. Shine a gooseneck lamp or a penlight over the right side of the neck and identify the uppermost point of the flickering venous pulsations. Sometimes, it is challenging for the novice examiner to determine if the pulsation he or she is viewing is the carotid or the internal or external jugular vein. To help you determine which vessel you are

TABLE 20.7	Comparison of Distinguishing Features Between the Carotid and Internal Jugular Vein
Internal Jugular Vein	**Carotid**
Rarely palpable	Palpable
Two waves/elevations	One wave
Pulsation eliminated by light pressure on the vein	Pulsation not eliminated by pressure
Level of pulsation changes with position	Level of pulsation unchanged by position

viewing, palpate the vessel. Unlike the carotid, the internal jugular vein is rarely palpable and if palpable disappears with light pressure. Table 20.7 will help decipher which vessel you are examining by distinguishing between inspection and palpation of the carotid and internal jugular vein.

Once you have determined the location of the internal jugular vein, keep an eye on the pulsation as you raise the head of the bed to a semi-Fowler position (30° to 45° angle). Did the pulsation disappear? If the pulsation is no longer visible, simply chart, "JVP not elevated" and no further examination of the jugular vein is required. However, if the pulsation is still visible, you will need to measure its height. Place a centimeter ruler upright at the location of the sternal angle (bony ridge located along the sternum parallel to the second ribs). Locate the height of the jugular venous pulsation and draw a horizontal line from the top of the JVP to the ruler located at the sternal angle. Be sure that where the rulers meet, you have a right angle (90° angle) (Fig. 20.37).

Measure the height on the vertical ruler at the sternal angle. This measurement is the distance of the pulsation above the sternal angle in centimeters. Ideally, measurements should be less than 3 cm above the sternal angle. Elevations above 3 to 4 cm are associated with fluid volume overload. One example is when the right side of the heart cannot compensate for the excessive fluid and it backs up the superior vena cava and is visible in the internal jugular vein. This is found in right-sided congestive heart failure.

Assessing the Precordium

The patient's precordium refers to the area of the anterior chest and includes the patient's great vessels and heart.

Inspection of the Precordium

With the patient disrobed and in the supine position, move to be eye level with the patient's chest and examine the entire anterior chest for any lesions, masses, or movements. Heaves or thrills appear as forceful movements of the chest wall. Note any such movement. Inspect the apical area for pulsations. The apex of the heart is usually located at the fourth or fifth left ICS, midclavicular line. A pulsation in this area that occurs with ventricular contraction is called the **point of maximal impulse** or **PMI**. The PMI may not be visible in all individuals, particularly those with large breasts. It is easier to visualize in children and adults with a thin chest wall. Lastly, inspect the precordium for colour. The colour of the chest wall should be uniform throughout and consistent with the rest of the skin. No cyanosis or redness should be present.

Palpation of the Precordium

Palpation of the precordium will require the use of several parts of the hand. Begin by palpating with the pads of the index, middle, and ring finger. Palpate for any lesions, masses, or tender areas. Palpate from right to left, beginning at the right anterior axilla line at the second ICS to left anterior axilla line. The second ICS can be located by finding the sternal angle which is consistent with the second rib and moving below the second rib to the space; this is the second ICS. Then move to the third, fourth, and fifth ICS, palpating in concentric circles for any lesions, masses, or tenderness. At the fifth ICS, midclavicular line, place your finger pads flat along the anterior chest, palpating for any pulsations. This is the location of the left ventricular area and the location of the PMI. During contraction of the left ventricle, the apex beats can be felt as a light tap against your fingers on the chest wall. If your patient has large breasts, ask her to raise the breasts so that you are able to place your hands in the correct location without obstruction from the breast tissue. Note that the PMI many not be palpable in all individuals. If you are not able to palpate the PMI, ask the patient to roll to the left lateral decubitus position. This allows the heart to move closer to the chest wall and can make palpation of the apex more apparent (Fig. 20.38). The PMI should only occupy one ICS, the fourth or fifth, and be at or medial to the midclavicular line (Fig. 20.39). PMIs that are displaced to the left or down can indicate an enlarged heart (Ostovan, Shahrzad, Taban, & Moniri, 2013).

Next, use the ball of your hands or the ulnar edge of the hand. The ball and ulnar surface of the hands are most sensitive for detecting vibrations. Palpate across the precordium in five main areas: the aortic, pulmonic, sternum, tricuspid, and mitral area (Fig. 20.40).

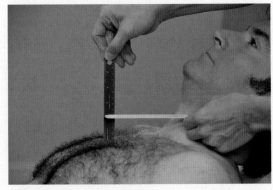

Figure 20.37 Estimating JVP.

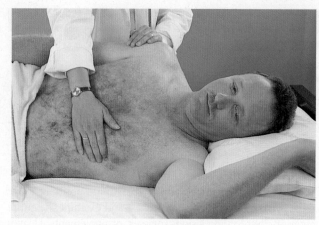

Figure 20.38 The left lateral decubitus position.

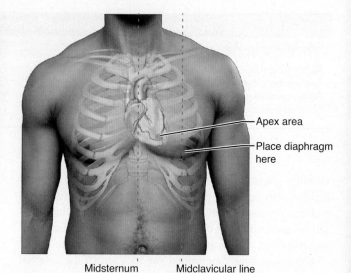

Apex area

Place diaphragm here

Midsternum   Midclavicular line

Figure 20.39 The location of the apex or PMI.

To do this, hyperextend your fingers so that the ball of your hands are directly touching the anterior chest. Ask the patient to inhale, exhale, and hold his or her breath (the same techniques used with the carotid auscultation). Push gently against the chest, feeling for any heaves, thrills, lifts, or pulsations. Begin at the second ICS, right midclavicular line, the aortic area. Following the same technique, move to the pulmonic area at the second ICS, left midclavicular line. Next, move to the third ICS sternal border palpating over Erb point. Move to the fourth ICS sternal border for the tricuspid area ending at the mitral area at the fifth ICS, left midclavicular line. No pulsations or movements should be felt aside from the PMI.

Auscultation of the Precordium

Accurate and clear auscultation is critical in the cardiovascular assessment, and practice is needed to help train your ear to the different heart sounds that are auscultated. To make listening easier, ensure the room is quiet and the

stethoscope is placed against the chest wall without any interference from clothing, hair, or shivering. Begin by using the diaphragm of the stethoscope placed in the second ICS, right midclavicular line, and follow the same pattern used during palpation. Listen for normal heart sounds: S_1 and S_2. S_1 occurs when the left ventricle starts to contract and ventricular pressure rapidly exceeds left arterial pressure. This results in the closure of the mitral valve, producing the first heart sound. S_2 occurs at the beginning of diastole, once the left ventricle has ejected most of its blood and the ventricular pressure begins to fall below aortic pressure. This pressure change causes the closing of the aortic valve producing the second heart sound. S_1 is heard louder than S_2 at the apex, and S_2 is heard louder than S_1 at the base. Sometimes, it can be difficult to determine which sound is S_1 and S_2. Try to

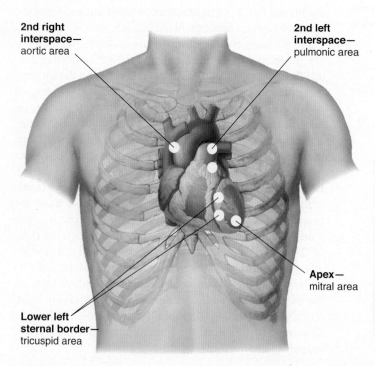

2nd right interspace— aortic area

2nd left interspace— pulmonic area

Apex— mitral area

Lower left sternal border— tricuspid area

Figure 20.40 Anatomical sites for palpation and auscultation.

palpate the radial pulse while auscultating the heart sounds. The S_1 normally coincides with the artery pulse.

Once you have listened in all five locations with the diaphragm, switch the stethoscope to the bell and listen in the same five locations for abnormal heart sounds: S_3, S_4, and murmurs. To listen with the bell, ask the patient to inhale, exhale, and hold the exhalation while you listen. Normally, you should only hear an S_1 and S_2. An extra heart sound in most cases needs further investigation because it can indicate fluid overload, hyperthyroidism, or problems with ventricular compliance. An S_3 sounds like a gallop, and the S_3 sound is heard immediately after the normal S_2 heart sound. An S_4 heart sound occurs immediately before the S_1 and, like the S_3, is best heard at the apex when the patient is positioned in the left lateral decubitus position. Figure 20.41 illustrates the location of the S_3 and S_4 heart sounds in relation to S_1 and S_2 as well as in the cardiac cycle.

Murmurs may also be auscultated with the bell of the stethoscope but are challenging for novice practitioners to hear. Murmurs are vibrating sounds that occur when there is turbulent blood flow and sound like a blowing or swooshing sound. They can be caused by a partial obstruction of blood flow through a heart valve that can occur due to a hardening or stenosis of the valve. Murmurs are also caused by leaky or incompetent valves that allow blood to flow backward causing increased blood flow. Murmurs can be caused by blood flowing into a dilated heart chamber as well as blood flowing between abnormal openings in the chambers of the heart. Recall blood normally flows between chambers of the heart through either the atrioventricular valves or the semilunar valves. Some murmurs have no underlying pathology and are known as *innocent murmurs*. As a nursing student, if you auscultate a murmur, try to identify the location on the chest wall, its timing in the cardiac cycle (systole or diastole), as well as its pitch, intensity, and if it is loud or soft. To best determine the characteristics of the murmur, you may wish to move the patient to an upright and leaning forward position or the left lateral decubitus position. Both of these positions move the heart closer to the chest wall and may make it easier to distinguish between the abnormal heart sounds.

Peripheral Vascular

Along with the heart and major blood vessels, the peripheral vessels help supply oxygenated blood to the tissue and along with the lymphatic system help return waste products back to the major vessels. The peripheral vascular (PV) assessment includes inspection and palpation of the skin,

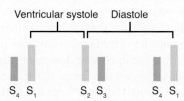

Figure 20.41 Occurrence of S_3 and S_4 in relation to S_1 and S_2 and the cardiac cycle.

pulses, veins, and tissue. Often, components of the PV assessment are included along with other system assessments, although it can also occur independently. As an example, if a patient injures her right arm playing soccer, assessment of the skin for swelling, pulse for circulation, and the nail bed for capillary refill would all be included with the musculoskeletal assessment. Knowing when and how to include the PV assessment into the various system assessments takes practice, but realizing the alterations in PV predicts other cardiovascular events, such as heart disease and stroke, is critical.

Inspection

Begin the PV assessment by noting the size and symmetry of the limbs and inspect for any swelling or edema. Assess skin for colour and edema (previously discussed) (refer to Table 20.3 and Fig. 20.9). If edema is present, measure the circumference of each limb, checking for symmetry and grade the pitting edema. To assess for pitting edema press firmly but gently with your first three fingers for at least 5 seconds over the dorsum of each foot, behind the medial malleolus and over the tibia looking for any depression or "pitting" caused by pressing your fingers over each area. While assessing the colour of the skin, check for any associated hair loss, which is often present with peripheral arterial disease. Inspect the veins, noting any swollen, varicose, or twisted vessels; look for any lesions and note their shape, colour, and location. In completing the PV assessment, it is important to examine the legs in three positions—lying, sitting, and standing—looking for colour changes with position changes. Determining the perfusion to the extremities is included in the PV assessment and requires assessing the nails for capillary refill and palpating the skin and pulses.

Palpation

Along with inspection, palpation for temperature and turgor can help the nurse determine proper perfusion to the peripheral tissue. To assess temperature, use the dorsal surface of your hand. Temperature that is warm or cool bilaterally may be normal, but unilateral red and warm or hot areas may indicate local infection. In the back of the calf, if red, hard, and hot, this may indicate a deep vein thrombosis. Also of concern is unilateral coolness and pallor, which may indicate decreased blood flow and, if this is associated with cyanosis and an absent pulse, may be an emergency situation requiring immediate notification of the physician. Palpation also occurs when feeling for a pulse.

Arterial Pulses

Arteries carry oxygenated blood and nutrients to the tissue. As the heart pumps, every heartbeat generates a pulse wave that can be felt over superficial bone. There are 10 locations where peripheral pulses can be felt.

- The carotids and femoral pulses are locations of larger vessels and should be used when palpating a patient who is unstable or shutting down peripherally; for example, when the patient has lost a great deal of blood and it is difficult to assess the patient's pulses peripherally.

TABLE 20.8	Grading Scale for Pulses
Grade	Description
0	Absent
1+	Diminished, thready, easily obliterated
2+	Normal, not easily obliterated
3+	Increased, full volume
4+	Bounding, hyperkinetic

- Three additional pulse sites are located in the arms: the brachial, radial, and ulnar pulses.
- Four pulses are palpated below the waist: the femoral, popliteal, posterior tibial, and dorsalis pedis (also known as the *pedal pulse*).
- The last two pulse sites are the temporal area located along the temporal artery lateral to the eyes.

Assessing the pulses includes determining the rate, rhythm, force, and elasticity. The force or strength of the pulse is graded on a 0 to 4+ scale (Table 20.8).

When assessing pulses, it is important to always compare the pulses bilaterally to determine alterations from one side to the other, which can indicate differences in perfusion. Pulses should be symmetrical, regular, 2+, springy, and elastic.

Peripheral Arterial and Peripheral Vascular Disease

Peripheral arterial disease (PAD) is caused by atherosclerotic occlusions of lower extremity arteries and affects approximately 1 million Canadians. The patient presents with skin that is glistening and shiny, with no hair, or if present, uneven hair distribution; the extremity is usually cool to touch with faint or absent pulses. Often, the patient will also have decreased capillary refill as a result of the arterial disease. The extremities are usually pale, particularly on elevation, and when dependent, they are a dusky red colour. In patients with intermittent claudication, a triad of classic symptoms occurs: sharp calf pain with exercise that results in the exercise being stopped and the disappearance of pain within 5 to 10 minutes of resting. Assessing postural changes and using the ankle-brachial index can be done to assess for PAD (Anderson et al., 2013).

Peripheral vascular disease (PVD) differs in clinical presentation from PAD. Alterations in venous circulation can occur with varicose veins (when veins become dilated) and when veins have incompetent valves (blood pools resulting in edema).

Unlike in PAD where there is little or no edema, in PVD, there is often marked edema. In PVD, patients often report dull, aching leg cramps and present with warmth to the extremities, brown pigmentation to the skin (from the leaking of red blood cells into the tissue), chronic pain, and weepy ulcers which are very slow to heal.

Breast Assessment

There has been a significant amount of research on breast cancer in the last two decades, which has resulted in clinical practice changes (Warner, 2011) (see research review, "Research on Breast Self-Examinations"). According to the Canadian Task Force on Preventative Health Care (2011), although no longer routinely recommended as part of the yearly screening guidelines for breast cancer, the clinical breast examination (CBE) is still an important part of the examination when concerns arise with patients and their breasts. The sensitivity of the CBE is estimated at only 54% for detecting breast cancer, but a study by Barton, Harris, and Fletcher (1999) found that sensitivity increases when the examiner uses standard exams and when the duration of the exam is longer (vs. shorter). The CBE includes inspection and palpation of the breast tissue. It is important that the nurse is aware that women and girls may feel apprehensive and/or embarrassed to have their breast tissue examined. Develop a therapeutic nurse–patient relationship, ask permission prior to beginning the examination, and explain what you will be doing are all important when conducting a CBE to help patients feel more comfortable. Begin by asking the patient to sit forward, disrobed to the waist or with a gown draped over the shoulders and the opening at the front. Start by inspecting both breasts, comparing one side with the other.

Inspection

Ask the patient to place her arms on the sides, and inspect both breasts. It is normal for one breast to be slightly larger than the other, but they should be symmetrical and round. Inspect the skin looking for localized areas of redness, bulging, or dimpling of the skin. Normally, breast should be free of edema and lesions, with even colour and texture throughout. Inspect the nipples and areola area for size, lesions, and the shape and direction in which they point. Nipples should be symmetrical, pointing in the same direction without any fissure, ulceration, bleeding, or other discharge. Examine the lymph area under the axillae and the supraclavicular nodes, looking for bulging, discolouration, or edema. Ask the patient to raise her hands above her head while you examine for retraction—the fixation of the underlying tissue to the chest wall is seen in carcinoma (Fig. 20.42).

Ask the patient to place her hands back on her hips and lean forward, examining for fixation of the skin or protrusion of any lymph nodes. Next, ask the patient to lie flat on her back with one arm placed on her forehead or above her head and a small pillow placed under the side to be examined. Provide a blanket or place the patient's gown over the breast not being examined to provide privacy.

Palpation

Begin by palpating one breast at a time, starting from below the clavicle and the anterior axillae line palpating in a straight line toward the sixth or seventh rib. Use the finger pads of the index, middle, and ring finger, making small circular movements as you palpate in a vertical pattern. According to Barton et al. (1999), the vertical stripe pattern is the best validated technique for detecting abnormalities (Fig. 20.43).

Continue to palpate in circular movements up and down the breast tissue feeling for any lumps, masses, tenderness, or abnormalities, ensuring you move from the starting point to the end point in a systematic fashion. Be sure to examine the entire breast, including the nipples, periphery, and the axillary tail of Spence. Note the upper outer quadrant of the breast is

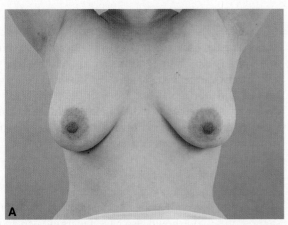
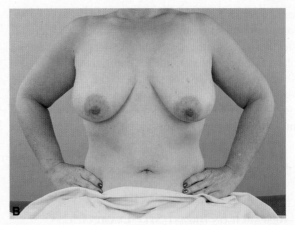

Figure 20.42 Maneuvers for retraction during inspection of the breast. Figure A: Arms are over her head. Figure B: Arms are pressed firmly on her hips.

the most common site of breast cancer so pay particular attention to this area (Lee, 2004). Drape the breast just examined, move the small pillow under the unexamined breast, and ask the patient to lift her arm and place her hand on her forehead or above her head. Repeat the palpation of the unexamined breast using the vertical technique. Note that in women with large breasts, it may be necessary to displace the breast tissue in order to adequately assess the area. You may find it helpful to ask the patient to turn on her side to help displace breast tissue and allow for proper palpation. Once you have completed palpating both breasts with the patient supine, ask the patient to sit up and begin examination of the axilla and lymph nodes (Fig. 20.44). Have the patient raise her left arm and support the weight of her left arm with your left arm so that her left hand can hang freely. Using small circular movements, begin at the tail of Spence and examine the lymph nodes of the axilla moving toward the apex of the axilla. Cup the fingers of your right hand so that your fingers are as high as possible toward the apex of the axilla, directly behind the pectoral muscles.

Examine the entire axilla area as well as the underside of the upper arm from the lateral lymph nodes to the epitrochlear lymph node along the upper part of the humerus, feeling for any enlarged and palpable nodes. Repeat with the other arm. Compression of the nipple with the index finger is no

longer considered part of the routine screening for breast cancer but is considered a special technique used when there is concern of breast cancer. If your patient reports abnormal discharge from her nipple, perform this special technique by compressing the areola with index finger while watching for discharge to appear through any of the duct openings on the nipple's surface. If discharge appears, note the colour, consistency, quantity, and the exact location it is released.

The CBE is an ideal time for the nurse to educate the patient about breast cancer. Some patients may ask about breast self-examination; knowing and understanding the latest research is important (see research review on breast

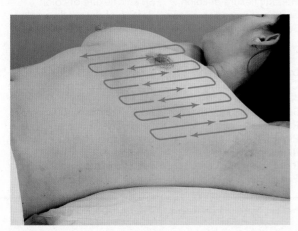

Figure 20.43 Vertical stripe pattern for palpation of the breast.

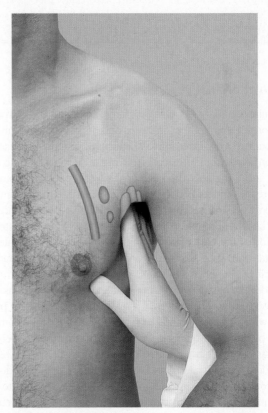

Figure 20.44 Palpation for the axilla and lymph nodes during the clinical breast examination.

self-examinations). As a nurse, if a patient is wanting to know how to perform breast examinations at home, it is important to let her know that there is no right or wrong way to examine her breasts as long as she examine the entire area. This should include feeling from below the breast to the collarbone including the nipple as well as her axillae (Canadian Cancer Society, 2014). Let your patients know that most changes are not cancerous but report any unusual changes to their doctor.

RESEARCH

RESEARCH ON BREAST SELF-EXAMINATIONS

A Cochrane summary on regular self-examination for early detection of breast cancer did not find a beneficial effect of regular breast self-examination in term of improvement in breast cancer mortality. In addition, women who were assigned to the control group, those who conducted regular breast self-examinations, were almost twice as likely to undergo a biopsy of the breast compared with women who did not conduct breast self-examination (BSE) (Kosters & Gotzsche, 2008). Other research has found that breast awareness provided women with some acknowledgement of the part they can play in being empowered to fight breast disease (McCready, Littlewood, & Jenkins, 2005).

Kosters, J. P., & Gotzsche, P. C. (2008). Regular self-examination or clinical examination for early detection of breast cancer. Cochrane Database of Systematic Reviews, (2), CD003373.

McCready, T., Littlewood, D., & Jenkins, J. (2005). Breast self-examination and breast awareness: A literature review. Journal of Clinical Nursing, 14(5), 570–578.

Abdominal

Examination of the abdomen requires thoughtful and purposeful consideration of the structures and organs contained in the abdominal cavity. Direction for the focus of your physical examination comes from your acquisition of comprehensive subjective data, including your thorough analysis of reported symptoms. Due to the number of body systems contained in the abdominal region, assessment is complex and challenging. Patient concerns may be related to one or more of any of the following systems: cardiovascular, endocrine, gastrointestinal, hematologic, integumentary, musculoskeletal, neurologic, reproductive, respiratory, or urinary. Reported symptoms might be associated with psychosocial or mental health causes rather than body systems.

You conduct an emergency assessment when a patient presents with direct abdominal trauma or abdominal pain accompanied by other symptoms (Seller, 2007). You perform a focused assessment when a patient reports concerns such as bowel or bladder function, nausea and vomiting, or changes in abdominal contour. Follow-up abdominal assessments are used to determine the effects of treatment and interventions. Comprehensive abdominal assessments are required for baseline data.

Landmarks for Abdominal Assessment

The abdomen is divided into four quadrants or nine regions, using imaginary lines to aid in identifying and communicating examination findings accurately and clearly. The upper and lower quadrants are created by drawing one imaginary vertical and horizontal line through the umbilicus. These imaginary lines are used for describing and documenting the location of structures and organs. Table 20.9 presents the structures that are located in each quadrant.

Equipment and Supplies

Aside from the equipment identified as common to all assessments—alcohol wipes, clean gloves, penlight, and stethoscope—you should also have a marking pen and measuring tape for the abdominal assessment.

Assessment Techniques

All four examination techniques are used for the abdominal assessment in the sequence of inspection, auscultation, percussion, and palpation. To avoid artificially changing the frequency of bowel sounds and subsequently misinterpreting and inaccurately reporting your findings, always auscultate before you percuss or palpate the abdomen.

Ensure that your patient has emptied his or her bladder. Place a pillow under the patient's head and perhaps under the knees for comfort and support, especially for a frail patient. Identify areas of abdominal pain so that you examine those areas last. Warm your hands by rubbing them together and then warm your stethoscope in your hands. Ensure that you have short fingernails. For any unvocalized signs of discomfort, watch your patient's facial expressions during the examination.

TABLE 20.9	Structures in the Four Abdominal Quadrants
1 – Upper Right Quadrant	**3 – Upper Left Quadrant**
Liver	Left lobe of the liver
Gallbladder	Stomach
Duodenum	Spleen
Head of pancreas	Body of pancreas
Right adrenal gland	Left adrenal gland
Upper lobe of right kidney	Upper lobe of left kidney
Hepatic flexure of colon	Splenic flexure of colon
Section of ascending colon	Section of descending colon
Section of transverse colon	Section of transverse colon
2 – Lower Right Quadrant	**4 – Lower Left Quadrant**
Lower lobe of right kidney	Lower lobe of left kidney
Cecum of large intestine	Sigmoid colon of large intestine
Appendix	
Section of ascending colon	Section of descending colon
Right ovary	Left ovary
Right fallopian tube	Left fallopian tube
Right ureter	Left ureter
Right spermatic cord	Left spermatic cord
Part of uterus (if enlarged)*	Part of uterus (if enlarged)*

*The uterus and urinary bladder are located in the lower midline in the suprapubic region.

Inspection

Standing at the patient's right side, observe the abdomen, first obliquely from the side and the foot of the bed and then horizontally across the abdomen as you bend down. Inspect the skin for scars, dilated veins, lesions, petechiae, striae, and position of the umbilicus. Dilated veins may indicate liver disease or venous obstruction. **Striae**, commonly known as *stretch marks*, are bands of thin, wrinkled skin, initially red or blue (recent) but becoming purple and white or silver (old), that occur commonly on the abdomen, buttocks, and thighs and result from atrophy of the dermis and overextension of the skin; the most common causes are puberty and/or during and following pregnancy, or weight gain and also associated with ascites. Use your penlight tangentially as you examine for pulsations, bulges, and asymmetry. Visible movements may be seen in naturally thin patients, and at times, an aortic pulsation may be seen in thin or anxious patients. Observe the abdominal contour for a flat, round, protuberant, or scaphoid (hollowed) shape. **Ascites** presents as protuberance or distention caused by accumulated fluid in the abdominal peritoneum. If distention is present, for example, from decreased peristalsis, the skin may appear taut and the abdomen larger than usual. **Distention** is the state of being distended or stretched. Ask the patient if clothes are fitting more tightly.

Auscultation

By performing auscultation immediately after inspection, you ensure that the pressure from your fingers or hand does not alter the motility of the intestines. Auscultation may detect changes related to inflammation, obstruction, or vascular disease (bruits). Skill 20.2 outlines the techniques of auscultation of the abdomen for bowel, vascular, and friction sounds.

Usually, bowel sounds are 5 to 34 clicks or gurgles per minute (Harder, Skillen, & Bickley, 2010). In addition to the expected bowel sounds of clicks and gurgles, listen for bruits (which could indicate occlusive disease of arteries). A bruit may sound similar to a heart murmur that can be blowing, swooshing, harsh, musical, or rumbling; have a low, medium, or high pitch; and range in intensity from very faint to very loud (Roach et al., 2010). Listen over the spleen and liver for friction rubs (they sound like two pieces of leather rubbing together). Be alert to high tinkling sounds known as *borborygmi*. Borborygmi are hyperactive bowel sounds and indicate increased intestinal peristalsis such as diarrhea or obstruction, or hunger (stomach growling). You may hear borborygmi before a meal, sounds associated with diarrhea, or indications of early intestinal obstruction.

Percussion

Percussion is used to identify the distribution and location of tympany and dullness in the abdomen. It is helpful for identifying the presence of tenderness or abdominal masses that are solid or fluid-filled before you palpate. Percussion detects dullness from an enlarged liver in the right midclavicular line and possibly the midsternal line. A dull percussion note is a thud-like sound that is medium in pitch and

in intensity. Percussion detects the tympany of the gastric bubble in the left upper quadrant (LUQ) and the tympany of the nonenlarged spleen in Traube space or in the left anterior axillary line. Tympany is musical or drumlike, loud, and high-pitched. Assess midline for a distended bladder by percussing downward from the umbilicus to the symphysis pubis. When the bladder is distended, you will detect dullness superior to the symphysis pubis. Otherwise, you will percuss tympany.

Use the lightest blow of the striking middle finger (plexor) on the pleximeter finger (middle finger of the opposite hand) in order to elicit a clear percussion note.

Palpation

Use light palpation to identify an area of tenderness, any muscular resistance, and masses. Palpate each quadrant, leaving any reported area of tenderness to examine last. To promote relaxation, ask the patient to keep arms at the sides, knees flexed, and to breathe through the mouth (if necessary because of anxiety). Depress the abdomen about 1 to 2 cm as you palpate all four quadrants. Use a smooth, light, dipping motion for light palpation and observe the patient's facial expression for signs of undisclosed discomfort. If you discover an abdominal mass, use deep palpation to determine its size, shape, mobility, location, tenderness, consistency, pulsatility, and relation to respiration. Do not mistake fecal matter, a distended bladder, or a pregnant uterus for an alarming mass. Avoid deep palpation over a tender area or in a patient who reports severe abdominal pain of sudden unknown onset.

Collaboration and Delegation

After a surgical intervention, inform the surgeon and other health professionals such as a registered dietitian when the patient's bowel sounds have returned and the patient is passing flatus postoperatively. This positive development generally warrants a change (improvement) in the patient's diet.

Anus, Rectum, and Prostate

Examination of the rectum involves inspection and palpation. With the patient in either the left lateral position or standing with feet facing inward, begin by inspecting the area of the anal verge, which should be smooth, shiny, darkly pigmented, and free of inflammation, lesions, or hemorrhoids. Ask the patient to bear down and inspect the anal opening to ensure there are no protrusions or fissures. Next, explain to the patient that you are going to begin the internal examination. Using gloves, place lubricant on the index finger and place it against the anal verge. Initially, the external sphincter will constrict and tighten, but then it will relax. Wait until the sphincter relaxes before inserting your fingertip into the anal canal. Insert in the direction pointing toward the umbilicus. Note any tenderness, nodules, internal hemorrhoids, or irregularities. When examining the male patient, rotate your index finger counterclockwise so that you can examine the posterior surface of the prostate gland. Let the patient know that you are examining his prostate and that he might feel the need to void. The prostate gland is heart-shaped with a median sulcus between two lateral lobes and feels rubbery. Palpation of the prostate gland should not cause discomfort, and no nodules should be palpable. As you remove your finger from the rectum, examine the colour and consistency of stool on the glove. There should be no traces of blood present.

Female Genitalia

Before beginning the examination of the female genitalia, it is important to explain to the woman what you will be doing and obtain her consent. With the patient in the lithotomy position, ask her to bend her knees and allow her legs to spread apart so that you are able to visualize the external structures. For inspection of the female genitalia, it is important to have good light (e.g., a gooseneck lamp) for better visualization. Inspect the labia majora and the labia minora as well as the clitoris and vaginal opening. The area should be free of any inflammation, lesions, and foreign bodies. It should be pink with some pigmentation, and any secretions should be clear or white and odorless. Examination of the internal reproductive organs is considered an advanced skill and is not part of the basic health assessment unless the nurse is specially trained and working in a sexually transmitted disease (STD) or gynecological clinic or in the labour and delivery unit.

Male Genitalia

As with examination of the female genitalia, it is important to explain to the male patient what you will be doing before you begin the examination. With the patient in a semi-Fowler or lying position, inspect the shaft of the penis, as well as the foreskin, glans, and urethral opening. If the patient is uncircumcised, it will be necessary to gently retract the foreskin of the penis to examine the glans and urethral opening. Note any lesions or discharge. Next, examine the scrotum and testes. It is not uncommon for one scrotal sac, typically the left, to be slightly larger. Using a gloved hand, inform the patient that you will begin the examination of the testicles. Place a scrotal sac in between your fingers and your thumb and palpate by gently rolling along the testes. Each testicle should feel rubbery but smooth and should be freely moveable. The testicle feels almost like a soft boiled egg. Repeat the examination on the other testicle. As you perform the exam, consider teaching the patient about the importance of testicular self-examinations and how to conduct the examination. Examination of the testicles should not cause any pain, and there should not be any swelling or nodules present upon palpation.

 ## Musculoskeletal System

The musculoskeletal system provides structure and support for other systems, permits erect posture, and makes body movements possible. At any stage of life, this system may require assessment because of changes associated with growth, development, lifestyle, occupation, and aging. Muscles, joints, and bones are assessed in the head, neck, torso, and extremity examinations. In the event of a potential fracture, dislocation, or rupture, you conduct an emergency assessment. Commonly, you undertake a focused musculoskeletal assessment when a patient reports symptoms such as muscle pain, swollen joints, weakness, stiffness, or impaired mobility. Follow-up assessments are used to evaluate for improvement, deterioration, or new symptoms associated with a joint, muscle, or bone concern. Comprehensive musculoskeletal assessments contribute to baseline data and the diagnosis of systemic disorders. Subjective data always guide the type of assessment you perform.

Landmarks for Musculoskeletal Assessment

Landmarks are depicted using the anatomical position, wherein the patient is imagined to be standing straight, looking forward, feet together with great toes and heels touching, arms at sides, and palms facing anteriorly (Skillen & Bickley, 2010).

This position has been adopted internationally to facilitate written or verbal description of observations with their landmarks (Moore & Dalley, 2006). In this position, the term for a surface may be related to its function, such as *flexor*, which might indicate the surface of a flexed arm or *extensor* indicating an extended leg. *Medial* and *lateral* are used to define a location of a finding on an extremity as being closer to or farther away from the midline of the body. Body surfaces, structures, and functions determine how you landmark when assessing the musculoskeletal system. Landmarks for joints vary according to their type, function, and structure. The three primary types of joints are slightly moveable (cartilaginous), nonmoveable (fibrous), or freely moveable (synovial). Slightly mobile joints are located between the vertebrae and midline in the symphysis pubis. Nonmoveable joints are located in the sutures of the skull. Freely mobile ball-and-socket joints (shoulders, hips) permit flexion, extension, adduction, abduction, internal rotation, and external rotation. Other movements of mobile joints include supination, pronation, inversion, and eversion. Joints have articular and nonarticular structures that include bursae, **ligaments**, **tendons**, synovial fluid, bones, muscles, fasciae, nerves, and skin. Be mindful of these structures as you conduct your assessment.

Equipment used in the musculoskeletal assessment includes clean gloves in case of discharge or skin lesions, a marking pen, a measuring tape in case of swelling or atrophy, and a grading scale.

Assessment Techniques

After collection of subjective data that includes a symptom analysis of a patient's concern, inspection and palpation are the examination modes used to assess the structures of the musculoskeletal system. Always begin with inspection to avoid missing important observations. Ask the patient to point to the area(s) of concern. Take advantage of body symmetry to help you sharpen your observations regarding shape, size, and movement and any differences. Watch the mobile patient for gait, posture, and ease of movement.

Inspection

Standing at the right side of the bedridden patient or in front of the seated, mobile patient, the collected subjective data may direct you to examine the upper extremities. Inspect the arms and hands and compare sides. Alternatively, you may need to inspect the legs and feet and compare sides (for full exposure, the patient might have to stand or lie down). Be alert to changes in the skin, hair, or nails that indicate conditions of the patient's integumentary, PV, or peripheral nervous systems. Pitting of the nails is associated with psoriasis, a condition of the skin. Varicose veins are convoluted, enlarged peripheral veins frequently seen in the lower leg. If the peripheral arterial circulation is impaired, you will observe pale, shiny, and hairless skin. Muscle atrophy (wasting) may be seen in a patient with diabetes whose peripheral nerves have been affected.

Concentrating on the musculoskeletal system, inspect for the symmetry of alignment, muscle bulk and contours, and joint size. Be alert to the symmetrical joint deformities of the hands in rheumatoid arthritis. Nodules on the joints of some fingers often indicate an osteoarthritic process. Redness and/or swelling may be seen with inflammation of a soft tissue structure such as the olecranon bursa of the elbow or the Achilles tendon at the ankle. A **bursa** is a closed sac or envelope lined with synovial membrane and containing synovial fluid, usually found or formed in areas subject to friction (e.g., over an exposed or prominent body part such as the elbow). Watch the patient for the degree and ease of moving the extremities. Look for involuntary movements such as tremors, fasciculations, or tics. Listen for **crepitus**, a cracking or grating sound, during movements. This may be heard when the patient has osteoarthritis, or inflamed joints or tendons.

Assess the patient's range of motion and note any limitations of movement. First, demonstrate the expected movements and instruct the patient to move each joint through its range of motion. Remember that joints vary in their level of mobility.

TABLE 20.10	Grading Scale for Muscle Strength
Grade	**Description**
0	No detectable muscle contraction
1	Barely detectable contraction; no joint movement
2	Complete range of motion or active body part movement with gravity eliminated (joint supported)
3	Complete range of motion or active movement against gravity
4	Complete range of motion or active movement against gravity and some resistance
5	Complete range of motion or active movement against gravity and full resistance

When examining the spine, estimate the degree of the patient's forward and lateral flexion, extension, and rotation. When examining the extremities, compare sides and note any differences as the patient moves through the range appropriate for the joint. For example, expect shoulders and hips to be fully mobile.

Palpation

Use light palpation to identify and localize areas of tenderness, muscular resistance, or soft tissue changes around a joint. Screen for crepitus by palpating large moving joints such as shoulders and knees. Palpate each joint. Assess muscle tone of the extremities using passive range of motion before evaluating muscle strength. **Muscle strength** assesses a patient's ability to move actively against resistance. In accordance with patient ability, grade muscle strength against resistance or gravity (Table 20.10 and Box 20.2). Look for symmetry but expect that strength may be slightly greater on the dominant side. Do not force a joint during passive range of motion if the patient reports pain or if you detect resistance. Skill 20.3 covers this procedure.

BOX 20.2 Important Lifespan Considerations for the Musculoskeletal System

Newborn and Infant

Newborns have little or no voluntary control over muscular movements. Most motor activity is a mass response to stimuli.

Muscle tone is assessed by holding the infant under the shoulders and observing flexion and extension of the arms and legs.

Head and chest circumference measurements are used to monitor growth and development.

All infants should be assessed for congenital hip dislocation.

Toddler and Preschooler

Young children are often fearful of strangers. Spend time becoming acquainted with the child. Consider making the examination of the musculoskeletal system a game.

Use approved screening tools to assess psychomotor skills.

School-Aged Child and Adolescent

Older children are modest and may or may not want a parent to be present during the examination. Let the child or adolescent make the choice.

Provide privacy and protect modesty.

Explain what you plan to do and enlist cooperation.

Screen for scoliosis (lateral curvature of the spine).

Older Adult

Prevent chilling of the older adult.

Assist to obtain a comfortable position when arthritic joints reduce mobility.

Avoid long, tiring examinations; conduct your examination over shorter episodes.

Expect muscle strength to be decreased in the older patient.

Assess for risk of falls.

Avoid assessing flexion greater than 90° and adduction in the patient with a hip replacement.

Assess for risks from osteoporosis.

<table>
<tr><td>

BOX 20.3   Equipment and Supplies Used in the Neurological Assessment

Clean gloves in case of discharge or skin lesions
Cotton balls
Glasgow Coma Scale and grading scale for reflexes
Marking pen
Penlight
Pungent scents (e.g., alcohol, cloves, coffee)
Small familiar objects (e.g., key, coin, paper clip)
Tongue depressors (splintered)
Tuning fork 128 Hz
Reflex hammer
Vials of warm and cool water

</td></tr>
</table>

Collaboration and Delegation

When the musculoskeletal assessment indicates that a patient has muscle weakness or impaired gait and balance, consult with other health professionals such as the physician, physiotherapist, or occupational therapist regarding the benefit of assistive devices.

 ## Neurological Assessment

The complex neurologic system controls the mind, body, spirit, and emotions. Every system or regional assessment that you perform is an examination of some aspect of the nervous system whether it is mental status, speech, cranial nerves, sensory pathways, motor pathways, or reflexes. All types of assessments are guided by subjective data. You conduct an emergency assessment when an individual develops the symptoms and signs of a stroke, suffers a head or spinal injury, or experiences a seizure. You choose a focused assessment when a patient reports symptoms such as tremors, weakness, tingling, headache, dizziness, or sudden vision/hearing loss. Follow-up assessments are required for evaluating the response to treatment, progression or reduction in symptoms, or new associated symptoms. A comprehensive neurological assessment involves the entire body and contributes to baseline data and the diagnosis of nervous system disorders (Box 20.3). As you conduct your assessment, ask yourself three questions: "What is the mental status of the patient?" "Are my findings symmetric on the patient's left and right sides?" "If asymmetric, does the cause lie in the peripheral nervous system (cranial, spinal, or peripheral nerves) or in the central nervous system?" (Anderson & Bickley, 2010). The **central nervous system** consists of the brain and spinal cord, whereas the **peripheral nervous system** is the part of the nervous system external to the brain and spinal cord from their roots to their peripheral terminations. It includes the ganglia, both sensory and autonomic, and any plexuses through which the nerve fibres and all the peripheral nerves run (Box 20.4).

Landmarks for Neurological Assessment

Landmarks for the nervous system vary according to the category of neurological assessment. Are you assessing the central nervous system or the peripheral nervous system? Do you want to evaluate the cranial nerves, spinal nerves, or peripheral nerves? Are you assessing function such as sensory response, motor response, or reflexes, or do you want to assess voluntary (purposeful motor actions) as opposed to involuntary function (glands, organs, smooth muscles)?

BOX 20.4   Important Lifespan Considerations for the Neurological Assessment

Newborn and Infant	**Toddler and Preschooler**	**School-Aged Child and Adolescent**	**Older Adult**
Infants are born with several protective reflexes: rooting (to suckle), sucking (for swallowing and gagging), Moro (when startled by loud noise or sudden movement), and tonic neck (position when sleeping or relaxed). As the neurologic system matures, these reflexes disappear. Infants have a positive Babinski response (toe up) to testing of the plantar reflex. This can persist up to 2 years of age and disappears in association with established walking. Newborns have little or no voluntary control over muscular movements. Most motor activity is a mass response to stimuli.	Young children are often fearful of strangers. Spend time becoming acquainted with the child. Make the examination of the neurologic system a game. Use approved screening tools to assess psychomotor skills. By 2–3 years of age, children are standing and walking.	Older children are modest and may or may not want a parent to be present during the examination. Let the child or adolescent make the choice. Provide privacy and protect modesty. Explain what you plan to do and enlist cooperation. Myelinization of nerve fibres is completed in adolescence to establish gait, learning abilities, and motor activities.	Prevent chilling of the older adult. Assist to obtain a comfortable position if neurologic impairments reduce mobility. Avoid long, tiring examinations; conduct your examination over shorter episodes. Expect diminished position sense and response to sensory testing, reduced vibratory sense in toes, slower psychomotor skills, and short-term memory changes. Expect deep tendon reflexes to remain intact, but be slightly weaker, and information processing to slow. Assess impact of pharmaceuticals on neurologic function.

TABLE 20.11	Glasgow Coma Scale	
The GCS is a tool for assessing a patient's response to stimuli. Scores range from 3 (deep coma) to 15 (normal).		
Eye opening response	Spontaneous	4
	To voice	3
	To pain	2
	None	1
Best verbal response	Oriented	5
	Confused	4
	Inappropriate words	3
	Incomprehensible sounds	2
	None	1
Best motor response	Obeys command	6
	Localizes pain	5
	Withdraws	4
	Flexion	3
	Extension	2
	None	1
Total		3–15

Source: Teasdale, G., & Jennett, B. (1974). Assessment of coma and impaired consciousness. A practical scale. *Lancet, 304*, 81–84.

Consider organizing your thinking in terms of mental status, cranial nerves, sensory pathways, motor pathways, and reflexes. You assess mental status during the health history. Level of consciousness is evaluated using the quantifiable Glasgow Coma Scale (Table 20.11). The **Glasgow Coma Scale** assesses level of consciousness and reaction to stimuli in patients based on performance in three categories: eye opening, verbal response-performance, and motor responsiveness.

The 12 paired cranial nerves are assessed together. **Dermatomes** is the area of skin supplied by cutaneous branches of a single cranial or spinal nerve guides your assessment of the sensory pathways. Sensory receptors in the skin transmit sensations of pain, temperature, touch, vibration, discrimination, and position to spinal cord tracts and the brain. Motor pathways are important for coordination, gait, balance, and muscle tone assessments, which are assessed when examining the extremities. **Reflexes** represent an involuntary reaction of the autonomic nervous system to a stimulus applied to the periphery such as percussion of a partially stretched tendon (deep tendon reflex) or to stroking of the skin with a blunt object (cutaneous reflex).

Referring to the anatomical position, when comparing the right and left sides of the patient, you use terms such as *ipsilateral* (on the same side) and *contralateral* (on the opposite side) to report findings. If referring to different areas on one extremity, you use the term *distal* to refer to a finding far from the trunk of the body and *proximal* to a finding closer to the trunk of the body (Skillen & Bickley, 2010). Other terms of movement are used when testing deep tendon reflexes at the ankle (Achilles tendon). You *dorsiflex* the foot and watch for *plantar flexion* (Stephen, Day, & Skillen, 2013). When testing the patellar reflex of the *flexed* knee, you watch for *extension*.

Assessment Techniques

Guided by subjective data and symptom/sign analyses, you use inspection, palpation, and percussion to examine the neurologic system. Pay attention to the body region(s) and side(s) affected and observe the patient's movements. Begin by assessing the 12 paired cranial nerves (Skill 20.4). **Cranial nerves (CNs)** are those nerves that emerge from, or enter, the cranium or skull, in contrast to the spinal nerves, which emerge from the spine or vertebral column.

Inspection

Inspect the mobile patient for gait, coordination, balance, and body position while walking (motor system) and inspect the patient for involuntary movements and muscle bulk. When inspecting the extremities, remember to watch for changes in the skin, hair, or nails that can indicate conditions of the patient's integumentary or PV systems. An unusual body position or movement alerts you to potential neurological damage. Note any rhythmic repetitive movements such as tremors, dyskinesias (bizarre movements of the face and mouth), or tics, which are brief and irregular. You may see atrophy of muscles of the hands if ulnar and median nerves (peripheral nerves) are damaged (Skill 20.5).

Inspect for coordination of muscle movement, which is dependent on the integrity of cerebellar, vestibular, sensory, and motor systems. To assess motor system pathways, instruct the patient to perform rapid alternating movements, point-to-point movements, shallow knee bends, tandem walking, hopping, and heel walks and toe walks. Assess position sense (sensory system) using the Romberg test. To perform the Romberg test, ask the patient to stand with his or her feet together and eyes closed. Stand behind the patient observing the patient for the potential to fall. Count for 30 seconds. Normally, a patient may sway mildly, but significant swaying is abnormal. An uncoordinated gait may be related to loss of position sense, alcohol intoxication, or a cerebellar disorder.

Although assessment of tone and strength will detect disorders in the muscles during the musculoskeletal examination, the neurological assessment can detect weakness from central or peripheral nerve lesions. If subjective data lead you to examine the CNs, assess their motor and sensory functions and observe for symmetry and/or strength of response. This involves inspection and/or palpation. Bell palsy and trigeminal neuralgia are detected with this focused assessment. Bell palsy is a one-sided paralysis with loss of motor control (CN VII). Trigeminal neuralgia is a painful sensory condition (CN V). Five CNs have only motor functions, four have both motor and sensory functions, and three have just sensory functions. In contrast, most peripheral nerves contain both motor and sensory fibres.

Palpation

To assess the sensory system pathways, touch is required. Peripheral neuropathy usually shows up first in the feet and/or hands because the peripheral nerves are the longest nerves in the body. Patients may report tingling, numbness, and/or pain. It is frequently associated with diabetes and with ulnar or median nerve entrapment.

Always test corresponding (symmetrical) areas with the patient's eyes closed. Use the splintered tongue depressor to test superficial pain sensation, the vials of water for temperature detection, and a wisp of cotton ball to test light touch. Set the tuning fork vibrating and test the most distal joints of the arms and legs for the patient's ability to detect vibration. The sense of vibration is often lost in diabetes and alcoholism. Disorders of the sensory cortex may be detected using tests for tactile discrimination. Use a small familiar object to test stereognosis in the palm of each hand, your light touch on each hand simultaneously to test for extinction, and a blunt object to draw a number on the palm of each hand for graphesthesia. Expect intact and symmetrical findings for all tests of sensation. Careful mapping of loss of sensation helps determine where the causative neurologic lesion is located.

Touch is required for testing superficial (cutaneous) reflexes such as the abdominal and plantar reflexes. Using a blunt object, stroke each side of the abdomen lightly toward the umbilicus. Observe for muscle contraction and movement of the umbilicus toward the stimulus. In the presence of peripheral and central nervous system disorders, the abdominal reflex can be absent. Using the same blunt object, stroke the sole of the foot from the heel to the ball of the foot. Expect the toes to flex (negative Babinski). A positive Babinski response occurs when the great toe dorsiflexes (points up), indicating neurologic damage.

Percussion

Test the deep tendon reflexes using percussion. Swinging a reflex hammer loosely in an arc, tap a slightly stretched tendon for the response and compare sides. Expect the response to be equal. Skill 20.6 explains and illustrates the procedures. Because each deep tendon reflex is associated with specific spinal segments, an unexpected response alerts you to the area of impairment. See Table 20.12 for grading the reflex response.

Collaboration and Delegation

When the neurological assessment indicates that a patient has weakness; impaired gait, coordination, or balance; or reduced sensation or motor function, consult with health professionals such as the neurologist, physiotherapist, or occupational therapist regarding the benefit of a detailed neurological examination and evaluation for the use of assistive devices.

TABLE 20.12	Grading the Reflex Response
Grade	Description
0	No detectable response
1+	Sluggish, minimal response
2+	Immediate, strong response (expected)
3+	Brisker than expected
4+	Very brisk response, hyperactive, clonus observed

Let's return to the opening case study of Megan Jones who had a cough and ear pain. After assessing her vital signs, Megan should have had a focused health history and physical assessment completed on her ears, nose, mouth, throat, sinuses, and respiratory system. The assessments completed would allow the nurse to document his findings and report any concerning findings to the primary care practitioner.

Health assessment is one of the foundations of the nursing process, and so knowing what is normal and what is a cause for concern is imperative for the nurse and has significant implications for the health of his or her patients. Thus, it is critical as a nursing student and future nurse that you keep abreast of changes and incorporate new guidelines and best practice recommendations into your nursing practice. Entire research centres are focusing on nursing best practice to "bring together the best knowledge to nursing and health care to enhance practice and system outcomes" (Nursing Best Practice Research Centre [NBPRC], 2013, para 1). Understanding how to best learn health assessment skills is also important for nursing students (see research review, "Using Standardized Patients to Improve Health Assessment Skills Among First-Year Nursing Students").

RESEARCH

USING STANDARDIZED PATIENTS TO IMPROVE HEALTH ASSESSMENT SKILLS AMONG FIRST-YEAR NURSING STUDENTS

A Canadian study by Bornais, Raiger, Krahn, and El-Masri (2012) looked at having students work with standardized patients to learn health assessment skills. Standardized patients are people who are trained to act as a real patient both in the history they provide and the physical presentations they exhibit. In the study, after controlling for baseline differences between the students, those who practiced health assessment skills on standardized patients performed significantly better on their objective structured clinical examinations (OSCEs) compared with students who only practiced on their peers (Bornais et al., 2012).

Bornais, J. A. K., Raiger, J. E., Krahn, R. E., & El-Masri, M. M. (2012). Evaluating undergraduate nursing students' learning using standardized patients. Journal of Professional Nursing, 28(5), 291–296.

The role of the nurse is likely to expand in the future—to provide nurses with opportunities to work to their full scope of practice. In order for nurses to truly function to their full scope of practice, they must be proficient and knowledgeable in how to complete a physical assessment on a patient.

SKILL 20.1 Lymph Node Assessment

Purpose

To determine the presence or absence of any enlarged lymph nodes. Normally, lymph nodes are either nonpalpable, or if they are palpated, they should be mobile, small, discrete, and nontender. Any palpable lymph node should be assessed for its size, shape, mobility, consistency, and tenderness. Because lymph nodes filter fluid before it is returned to the vasculature, any local enlargement of the lymph nodes requires examination of the surrounding tissue for the source of the problem.

Equipment

Stethoscope

Preparation

- Provide for patient privacy.
- Ensure the room is warm and quiet.
- Explain to the patient what you plan to do and how long it will take.
- Obtain patient consent.

Lymph Node Assessment Procedure

Step

1. Perform hand hygiene in front of the patient.

2. Identify the patient.
3. Close door or bed curtains and explain the procedure to the patient.
4. Begin palpating the lymph nodes using the pads of the index, middle, and ring fingers moving in gentle circular movements. Palpate the lymph nodes on both sides of the patient's face and neck comparing one side with the other.
5. Follow a standard pattern of lymph node assessment. The following sequence is commonly used to palpate the lymph nodes:
   1. *Preauricular* lymph nodes, which are located in front of the ear
   2. *Posterior auricular* located superficial to the mastoid process
   3. *Occipital* located on the posterior side at the base of the skull
   4. *Tonsillar* lymph nodes located at the angle of the mandible
   5. *Submandibular* located between the angle and tip of the mandible
   6. *Submental* located below the chin, midline, and a few finger widths behind the tip of the mandible. To assess the submental lymph node, it is best to palpate using only the index and middle finger of one hand while supporting the top of the head with the other hand.
   7. *Superficial cervical* located superficial to the sternomastoid
   8. *Posterior cervical* located along the anterior edge of the trapezius muscles
   9. *Deep cervical* lymph nodes appear in a chain pattern deep within the sternomastoid muscle. To examine these lymph nodes, it is easiest to ask the patient to tilt his or her head toward your hand as you hook your middle and index finger on one side of the sternomastoid muscle and the thumb on the other side. This relaxes the muscle and makes for easier palpation.
   10. *Supraclavicular* lymph nodes are located above the clavicle in the grove formed by the angle between the clavicle and the sternomastoid muscle. To facilitate palpation of the supraclavicular lymph nodes, it is easiest to ask the patient to place his or her hands on his or her hips and lean forward rounding his or her shoulders and elbows forward. This accentuates the angle and allows for easier palpation.
11. Document the results of lymph node assessment.

Rationale

Reduces microbe transmission and reassures patients that you are minimizing their risk of infection

Ensures correct patient receives the indicated assessment

Promotes patient privacy, reduces patient anxiety, increases patient cooperation, and promotes learning

Lymph nodes follow specific drainage patterns. Comparing one side with the other allows the nurse to determine if there are any changes or enlargements.

A standard pattern of lymph node assessment ensures that all of the lymph node areas are examined. Figure 1 shows the location of the 10 lymph nodes located in the head and neck.

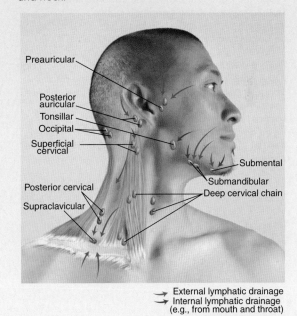

→ External lymphatic drainage
→ Internal lymphatic drainage (e.g., from mouth and throat)

Figure 1

Documentation provides a record of the assessment and communicates the findings from the assessment to other health care professionals.

SKILL 20.2   Auscultating the Abdomen

Purpose

To determine the presence or absence of intestinal peristalsis, bruits, or friction rubs.

Equipment

Stethoscope

Preparation

- Provide for patient privacy.
- Ensure the room is warm and quiet.
- Explain to the patient what you plan to do and how long it will take.
- Obtain patient permission.
- Attend to any immediate patient need first; for example, comfort measures for pain, need to urinate.
- Turn the suction off during auscultation if the patient has a nasogastric tube.
- Stand at the right side of the patient.
- Auscultate before percussing or palpating to avoid altering bowel motility.

Abdominal Assessment Procedure

Step	Rationale
1. Perform hand hygiene in front of the patient.	Reduces microbe transmission and reassures patients that you are minimizing their risk of infection
2. Identify the patient.	Ensures correct patient receives the indicated assessment
3. Close door or bed curtains and explain the procedure to the patient.	Promotes patient privacy, reduces patient anxiety, increases patient cooperation, and promotes learning
4. Ask when the patient ate last.	Bowel sounds may increase shortly after eating or if a meal is long overdue.
5. Ask the patient to urinate before you conduct your examination.	An empty bladder promotes patient comfort and accurate observations.
6. Examine the patient in the supine position.	The supine position helps relax the abdominal muscles and spread adipose tissue.
7. Drape the patient to expose the abdomen from the xiphoid process to the symphysis pubis.	Full exposure permits a thorough and accurate examination.
8. Imagine a vertical and a horizontal line crossing the umbilicus to create four quadrants (see Table 20.9).	Landmarking facilitates identification of underlying abdominal structures and communication of findings to other health professionals.
9. Place the warm diaphragm chestpiece of a stethoscope in the right lower quadrant and listen for the pitch, frequency, and duration of bowel sounds for 1 minute.	Active bowel sounds are clicks and/or gurgles that occur at a rate of 5–34 per minute.
10. Listen in the other three quadrants for active bowel sounds.	Bowel sounds are expected to be heard in each quadrant.
11. If you do not hear bowel sounds, listen for 5 minutes in each of the four quadrants before concluding that the abdomen is silent.	Bowel sounds are irregular and require longer assessment before concluding they are absent and not hypoactive. Both hypoactive and absent bowel sounds indicate decreased intestinal motility.

Abdominal Assessment Procedure (continued)

12. Listen with the bell chestpiece of the stethoscope for bruits over the aorta, renal arteries, and iliac arteries (see Figure 1).

Bruits suggest vascular occlusive disease and are heard better with the bell.

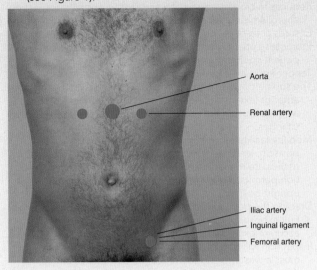

Figure 1

13. Listen with the bell for friction rubs over the liver and the spleen (see Table 20.9). Note their relationship with respiration.
14. Proceed with percussion and palpation of the abdomen or cover the patient's abdomen and ensure the patient is comfortable.
15. Document the results of auscultation.

Friction rubs indicate inflammation of the peritoneal surface of the organ. Friction rubs may change with inspiration and expiration.

Avoids chilling the patient, preserves patient dignity, and promotes patient comfort

Establishes a baseline and communicates observations to other health professionals

---

SKILL 20.3	Palpating Muscle Strength: Lower Extremities

Purpose

To assess the strength and symmetry of muscles of the legs for gait, posture, balance, and self-care activities of the patient.

Equipment

Grading scale, measuring tape in case of swelling

Preparation

- Provide for patient privacy.
- Ensure the room is warm and quiet.
- Explain to the patient what you plan to do and how long it will take.
- Obtain patient permission.
- Attend to any immediate patient need first; for example, comfort measures for pain, need to urinate.
- Stand at the right side of the bedridden patient or in front of the seated patient.

(continued on page 414)

SKILL 20.3   Palpating Muscle Strength: Lower Extremities (continued)

Procedure for the Musculoskeletal Assessment

Step	Rationale
1. Perform hand hygiene in front of the patient.	Reduces microbe transmission and reassures patients that you are minimizing their risk of infection
2. Identify the patient.	Ensures correct patient receives the indicated assessment
3. Close door or bed curtains and explain the procedure to the patient.	Promotes patient privacy, reduces patient anxiety, increases patient cooperation, and promotes learning
4. Ask the patient if there are any areas of tenderness.	Tender areas are examined last in the examination sequence.
5. Examine the bedridden patient in the supine position.	The supine position permits you to lift the legs to examine the anterior (extensor) and posterior (flexor) surfaces of the legs without causing the patient undue discomfort from position changes.
6. Examine the mobile patient in the seated and standing positions.	Mobility facilitates an efficient examination. In the seated position, landmarks are more easily visualized and soft tissues are more relaxed for palpation. The standing position permits you to see any changes that occur only in the upright position.
7. Drape the bedridden patient to cover the perineum but fully expose the legs.	Draping the perineum protects dignity and promotes comfort. Full exposure of the extremities permits a thorough and accurate examination.
8. Perform palpation after inspection.	Inspection will detect swelling, inflammation, deformities, muscle wasting, and asymmetry of soft tissues and joints that you may miss if doing palpation directly.
9. Assess muscle tone for *slight* residual tension before assessing muscle strength.	Avoids misinterpreting increased residual tension/spasticity/rigidity of the muscle as strength rather than tone
10. Test each leg by supporting the limb and moving the hip, knee, and ankle through a passive range of motion.	The slight residual tension of muscle tone is best assessed using passive stretch to evaluate the resistance of the muscle.
11. Assess strength of specific muscle groups by having the patient extend and flex at the corresponding joints of the legs against resistance provided by your hands.	Absence of symmetry of the same muscle groups can indicate impairment. Tests the quadriceps femoris, hamstring muscles, gastrocnemius, anterior and posterior tibial muscles, toe extensors and flexors, iliopsoas, gluteus maximus, gluteus medius, and gluteus minimus.
12. Assess the standing patient by asking the patient to hop on each foot, perform shallow knee bends separately, walk on heels, and walk on toes.	Tests strength of muscle groups working together
13. Document the results of palpation for muscle strength.	Establishes a baseline and communicates observations to other health professionals

SKILL 20.4   Assessment of the 12 Cranial Nerves

Purpose

To assess the 12 paired CNs.

Equipment

Cotton balls, penlight, pungent scents (e.g., alcohol, cloves, coffee), clean gloves, tongue depressor, tuning fork

Preparation

- Provide for patient privacy.
- Ensure the room is warm and quiet.
- Explain to the patient what you plan to do and how long it will take.
- Obtain patient permission.

Procedure for Assessing the 12 Cranial Nerves

Step	Rationale
1. Perform hand hygiene in front of the patient.	Reduces microbe transmission and reassures patients that you are minimizing their risk of infection
2. Identify the patient.	Ensures correct patient receives the indicated assessment
3. Close door or bed curtains and explain the procedure to the patient.	Promotes patient privacy, reduces patient anxiety, increases patient cooperation, and enhances learning
4. Ask the patient if he or she has had any altered sense of smell. If the patient has noticed alterations, ask the patient to identify different mild aromas such as vanilla, coffee, orange, or peppermint using one nostril at a time.	Assesses CN I (olfactory nerve) which is not routinely assessed unless the patient reports alterations in the sense of smell. An olfactory tract lesion may compromise the ability to discriminate odors.
5. Ask the patient to read the Snellen eye chart.	CN II (optic nerve) is assessed by testing visual acuity using the Snellen chart. Patients with difficulty reading the chart may have problems with CN II.
6. Assess the patient's pupils for PERRLA and for the six cardinal positions of gaze.	CN III (oculomotor nerve) functions to control pupillary reflex and extraocular eye movement. CN IV (trochlear nerve) controls lateral and downward movement of the eyeball, and CN VI (abducens nerve) controls lateral movement of the eyeball. The intactness of CNs III, IV, and VI are assessed using these two tests.
7. Instruct the patient to close his or her eyes. Brush a cotton swab across the patient's forehead, down the cheek, and across the chin. Ask the patient to inform you where he or she has been lightly touched (see Figure 1).	Assessing the sensation of touch along the three branches (ophthalmic, maxillary, and mandibular) of the trigeminal nerve provides the nurse with information about CN V (trigeminal nerve) which controls sensation of the cornea, skin of the face, and nasal mucosa.

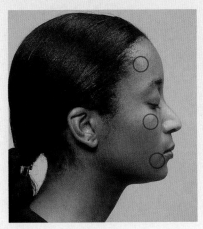

Figure 1

(continued on page 416)

Procedure for Assessing the 12 Cranial Nerves (continued)

8. Ask the patient to tightly clench his or her teeth as you palpate over the jaw for the masseter muscle and the temporal muscle. Assess for symmetry (see Figure 2).

CN V has a motor function that is assessed by observing the face for muscle atrophy, symmetry, and movement.

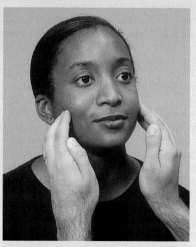

Figure 2A

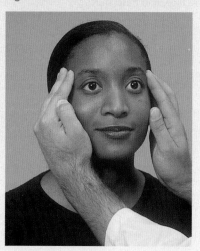

Figure 2B

9. Instruct the patient to smile, frown, raise his or her eyebrows, and puff out his or her cheeks.

CN VII (facial nerve) has a sensory and motor component. Movement and strength of the facial muscles are controlled by CN VII. If CN VII is intact, the patient should not have difficulty with these movements. If a patient does, however, have difficulty with these motor functions, assess the sensory component of CN VII by asking the patient to identify different tastes (sweet, salt, sour) on the tip and sides of his or her tongue. CN VII controls the taste of the anterior two thirds of the tongue. This provides important information about the intactness of CN VII.

10. Assess the patient's ability to hear. If hearing loss is present, perform the Weber test by placing the tuning fork in the middle of the patient's head.

CN VIII (acoustic nerve) is involved with the patient's ability to hear.

11. Ask the patient to stick out his or her tongue and say "aah." Using a tongue depressor and a light source, observe the movement of the soft palate, uvula, and the pharynx.

The motor component of CNs IX (glossopharyngeal nerve) and X (vagus nerve) is involved with swallowing and allows the soft palate to rise symmetrically and the uvula to remain midline. Injury to the vagus or glossopharyngeal nerve causes the uvula to deviate from midline.

Procedure for Assessing the 12 Cranial Nerves (continued)

12. From behind, look for symmetry, atrophy, or fasciculations of the trapezius muscles. Instruct the patient to shrug both shoulders upward against resistance by your hands (see Figure 3A). Ask the patient to turn his or her head to each side against your hand (see Figure 3B).

CN XI (spinal accessory nerve) controls movement of the trapezius and sternomastoid muscles which should be equal and strong.

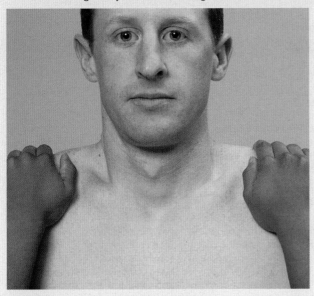

Figure 3A

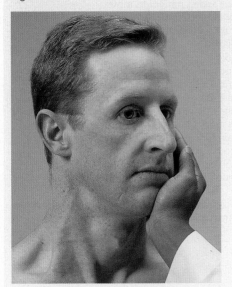

Figure 3B

13. Ask the patient to say "light, tight, and dynamite" and to stick out his or her tongue.

CN XII (hypoglossal nerve) supplies the intrinsic and extrinsic muscles of the tongue. Lesions of the hypoglossal nerve may result in fasciculations, asymmetry, atrophy, or deviations of the tongue from midline.

14. Document the results of palpation for muscle strength.

Establishes a baseline and communicates observations to other health professionals

SKILL 20.5   Inspecting the Neurologic System: Upper Extremities

Purpose

To assess coordination (cerebellar function), position sense, and muscle bulk of the arms for patient safety and self-care activities.

Equipment

Grading scales, marking pen, measuring tape in case of swelling, penlight

Preparation

- Provide for patient privacy.
- Ensure the room is warm and quiet.
- Explain to the patient what you plan to do and how long it will take.
- Obtain patient permission.
- Attend to any immediate patient need first; for example, comfort measures for pain, need to urinate.
- Stand at the right side of the bedridden patient or in front of the seated patient.

Procedure for the Neurological Examination

Step	Rationale
1. Perform hand hygiene in front of the patient.	Reduces microbe transmission and reassures patients that you are minimizing their risk of infection
2. Identify the patient.	Ensures correct patient receives the indicated assessment
3. Close door or bed curtains and explain the procedure to the patient.	Promotes patient privacy, reduces patient anxiety, increases patient cooperation, and enhances learning
4. Ask the patient if there are any areas of tenderness.	Tender areas are examined last in the examination sequence.
5. Examine the bedridden patient in the supine position.	The supine position permits you to lift the arms to examine the anterior (extensor) and posterior (flexor) surfaces passively without asking patient to move.
6. Examine the mobile patient in the seated position.	Mobility facilitates an efficient examination. In the seated position, landmarks are more easily visualized and soft tissues more relaxed.
7. Drape the bedridden patient to cover the chest but fully expose the arms.	Draping protects dignity, promotes comfort, and prevents chilling. Full exposure of the upper extremities (hands to shoulders) permits a thorough and accurate examination.
8. Perform local inspection of the arms.	Local inspection is a focused scrutiny for specific characteristics related to the neurologic system which could be missed if palpation was done directly.
9. Inspect for asymmetry, atrophy, deformity, tremors, fasciculations, irregular movements, muscle bulk, and position at rest of the arms.	May indicate impairment in the central nervous system or peripheral nervous system
10. Instruct patient how to perform a series of rapid alternating movements.	Assesses coordination (cerebellar function)
11. Have patient pat thigh as rapidly as possible by alternating the palm and the dorsum of the hand. Test hands separately. Compare sides (see Figure 1).	Difficulty may indicate cerebellar disorders. Testing separately avoids bilateral matching of speed by the patient.

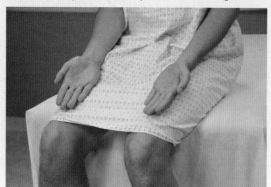

Figure 1

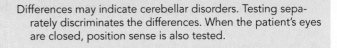

Procedure for the Neurological Examination (continued)

12. Ask patient to touch the tip of his or her nose and then extend his or her arm to touch the tip of the examiner's finger. Have the patient continue to do this while the examiner's finger is moved each time (see Figure 2). After several tries, instruct patient to close eyes and repeat while the examiner keeps his or her finger stationary. Test each arm separately. Compare sides.

Differences may indicate cerebellar disorders. Testing separately discriminates the differences. When the patient's eyes are closed, position sense is also tested.

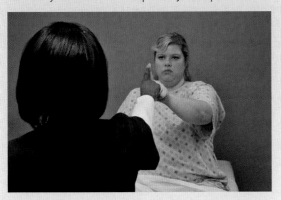

Figure 2A

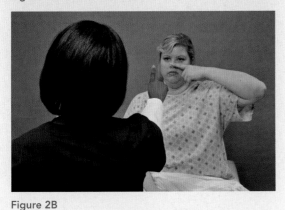

Figure 2B

13. Document the results of inspection of the upper extremities.

Establishes a baseline and communicates observations to other health professionals

---

SKILL 20.6 Assessment of Deep Tendon Reflexes

Purpose

To assess the deep tendon reflexes of the patient as part of the neurological assessment.

Equipment

Tuning fork, deep tendon reflex grading scale

Preparation

- Provide for patient privacy.
- Ensure the room is warm and quiet.
- Explain to the patient what you plan to do and how long it will take.
- Obtain patient permission.

(continued on page 420)

SKILL 20.6   Assessment of Deep Tendon Reflexes (continued)

Procedure for Assessing the Deep Tendon Reflexes

Step

1. Perform hand hygiene in front of the patient.

2. Identify the patient.

3. Close door or bed curtains and explain the procedure to the patient.

4. Assess the biceps reflex. Place patient's flexed arm, palm down, on thigh. Place your thumb on biceps tendon in the antecubital fossa. Strike thumb with reflex hammer (see Figure 1).

Rationale

Reduces microbe transmission and reassures patients that you are minimizing their risk of infection

Ensures correct patient receives the indicated assessment

Promotes patient privacy, reduces patient anxiety, increases patient cooperation, and enhances learning

Expected response

A normal response upon percussion of the biceps reflex is flexion at the elbow.

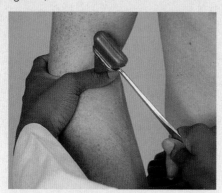

Figure 1A

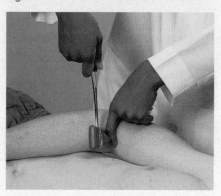

Figure 1B

Procedure for Assessing the Deep Tendon Reflexes (continued)

Step	Expected response
5. Assess the triceps reflex. Support patient's flexed arm. Strike triceps tendon just above the olecranon process (see Figure 2).	A normal response upon percussion of the triceps reflex is extension at the elbow.

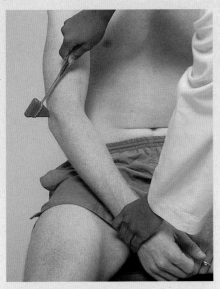

Figure 2A

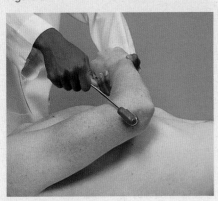

Figure 2B

6. Assess the patellar reflex. With the patient sitting, legs hanging loosely, or with the patient supine, knee flexed. Strike the patellar tendon just below patella (see Figure 3).

A normal response upon percussion of the patellar reflex is extension of the lower leg at the knee.

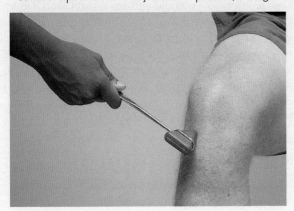

Figure 3

(continued on page 422)

SKILL 20.6   Assessment of Deep Tendon Reflexes (continued)

Procedure for Assessing the Deep Tendon Reflexes (continued)

Step

7. Assess the Achilles reflex. Have the patient's knee flexed while you slightly dorsiflex the foot. Strike Achilles tendon 3 cm above heel with reflex hammer (see Figure 4).

Expected response

A normal response upon percussion of the Achilles reflex is plantar flexion at the ankle.

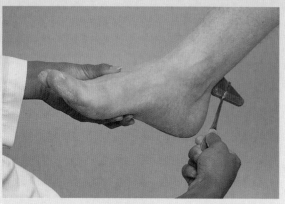

Figure 4A

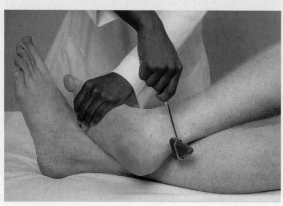

Figure 4B

8. Document the results of palpation for muscle strength.

Rationale

Establishes a baseline and communicates observations to other health professionals

Critical Thinking Case Scenarios

▶ Imagine you are a nurse working in a primary care office when a patient arrives with concerns over a cough and shortness of breath. What subjective data questions would you want to ask this patient? What physical examinations should you perform?

▶ Imagine you are working as a nurse in an emergency department and a patient arrives with slurred speech and reports weakness on her right side. What cerebellar assessments would you perform?

▶ Your patient has a family history of macular degeneration. What eye assessments would be important to perform? Which tests might be abnormal?

▶ You are working in a breast screening clinic and a patient, Mrs. Smith, asks about her risk factors for breast cancer.

Mrs. Smith is 52 years old and has a sister who had breast cancer at 48 years of age. Mrs. Smith began menstruating at 11 years, had her first child at 32 years, and she has not yet experienced menopause. She is Caucasian, nonsmoking, and has two to three glasses of wine each night. She is from an affluent family, she is sedentary, and she has a BMI of 30. She has had three benign breast biopsies. What are Mrs. Smith's risk factors for breast cancer?

Multiple-Choice Questions

1. The nurse is performing inspection. Which of the following would he be doing?
   a. Assessing of the skin for warmth
   b. Determining liver size
   c. Smelling wound drainage
   d. Checking reflexes

2. A nurse is auscultating the abdomen of a patient who has arrived at the emergency room. Which of the following is essential for the nurse to communicate immediately to the attending physician or nurse practitioner?
   a. Abdomen is protuberant.
   b. Borborygmi are present throughout abdomen.
   c. High tinkling sounds are heard in left upper quadrant.
   d. Twenty clicks and gurgles are heard per minute in the right lower quadrant.

3. A nurse prepares for conducting an abdominal assessment by visualizing the structures of each quadrant. Which of the following structures would the nurse expect to be in the right lower quadrant?
   a. Adrenal gland, body of pancreas, liver, and ureter
   b. Adrenal gland, section of transverse colon, part of uterus, and gallbladder
   c. Appendix, lower lobe of kidney, cecum, and section of ascending colon
   d. Appendix, section of transverse colon, hepatic flexure of colon, and duodenum

4. When a nurse is assessing the neurologic system of a middle-aged adult, what is one of the most essential techniques?
   a. Percuss any reported weak areas.
   b. Assess deep tendon reflexes using a reflex hammer.
   c. Examine the dominant side of the body first and then the opposite side.
   d. Conduct all examinations with the patient supine, sitting, and standing.

5. When a nurse is assessing the musculoskeletal system of an older adult who has had a previous knee replacement, what is one of the most essential techniques?
   a. Compare sides for symmetry and strength.
   b. Start with palpation of any reported tender areas.

c. Conduct the examination only with the patient standing.
   d. Examine the entire side of the body with the knee replacement first.

6. Over which part of the lungs are bronchovesicular sounds normally auscultated?
   a. Over the trachea
   b. Over the peripheral lung fields
   c. At the first and second ICSs lateral to the sternum
   d. At the third and fourth ICSs lateral to the sternum

7. Which of the following is the most common site of cancerous breast tumors?
   a. Upper inner quadrant
   b. Upper outer quadrant
   c. Lower inner quadrant
   d. Lower outer quadrant

8. It is normal to palpate the apical impulse in the:
   a. Second ICS on the right adjacent to the sternum
   b. Second ICS on the left adjacent to the sternum
   c. Fourth ICS on the left at the sternal border
   d. Fifth ICS on the left at the midclavicular line

9. Which of the following findings describes normal healthy lymph nodes?
   a. Rubbery, discrete, mobile, and nontender
   b. Small, firm, nonmobile, and tender
   c. Small, soft, mobile, and nontender
   d. Large, firm, mobile, and tender

10. Which vessel is best for assessing JVP?
    a. The right internal jugular vein
    b. The left internal jugular vein
    c. The right carotid artery
    d. The left carotid artery

REFERENCES AND SUGGESTED READINGS

Anderson, J. A., Halperin, J. L., Albert, N. M., Bozkurt, B., Brindis, R. G., Curtis, L. H., . . . Shen, W. K. (2013). Management of patients with peripheral artery disease (compilation of 2005 and 2011 ACCF/AHA guideline recommendations): A report of the American College of Cardiology Foundation/American Heart Association Task Force on Practice Guidelines. *Circulation*, 127(13), 1425–1443. Retrieved from http://circ.ahajournals.org/content/early/2013/03/01/CIR.0b013e31828b82aa.citation

Anderson, M. C., & Bickley, L. S. (2010). The nervous system. In T. C. Stephen, D. L. Skillen, R. A. Day, & L. S. Bickley (Eds.), *Canadian Bates' guide to health assessment for nurses* (pp. 683–758). Philadelphia, PA: Lippincott Williams & Wilkins.

American Medical Association. (n.d.). *Point of maximal impulse* [Video reference]. Retrieved from http://archinte.ama-assn.org/content/vol166/issue19/images/data/2132/DC1/kress_166_19_2132.mov

Baernstein, A., Smith, K., & Elmore, J. (2008). Singing the blues: Is it really cyanosis? *Respiratory Care*, 53(8), 1081–1084.

Barton, M. B., Harris, R., & Fletcher, S. (1999). Does this patient have breast cancer? The screening clinical breast examination: Should

it be done? How? *Journal of the American Medical Association*, 282(13), 1270–1280.

Bluestone, C. D., & Klein, J. O. (2007). *Otitis media in infants and children* (4th ed.). Hamilton, ON: BC Decker.

Canadian Cancer Society. (2014). *Screening for breast cancer*. Retrieved from http://www.cancer.ca/en/cancer-information/cancer-type/breast/screening/?region=on#Knowing_your_breasts#ixzz2qhEVFjwK

Canadian Task Force on Preventative Health Care. (2011). Recommendations on screening for breast cancer in average-risk women aged 40–74. *CMAJ*, 183(17), 1991–2001.

Cook, D. J., & Simel, D. L. (1996). Does this patient have abnormal central venous pressure? *Journal of the American Medical Association*, 275(8), 630–634.

Eskandari, M. K., Pearce, W. H., & Yao, J. S. T. (2010). *Carotid artery disease: Modern trends in vascular surgery*. Shelton, CT: People's Medical Publishing House.

Glasziou, P., Papinczak, T., & Pirozzo, S. (2003). Whispered voice test for screening for hearing impairment in adults and children: Systematic review. *British Medical Journal*,

327(7421), 967. Retrieved from http://go.galegroup.com /ps/i.do?id=GALE%7CA110456753&v=2.1&u=wind05901 &it=r&p=AONE&sw=w&asid=10f380150978c821a7c0b9c 6361e4bf6

Goodheart, H. P. (2009). *Goodheart's photoguide to common skin disorders: Diagnosis and management* (3rd ed.). Philadelphia, PA: Lippincott Williams & Wilkins.

Guly, H. R., Bouamra, O., Spiers, M., Dark, P., Coats, T., & Lecky, F. E. (2011). Vital signs and estimated blood loss in patients with major trauma: Testing the validity of the ATLS classification of hypovolaemic shock. *Resuscitation, 82*(5), 556–559.

Handen, R. I., Lux, S. E., & Stossel, T. P. (2003). *Blood: Principles and practice of hematology* (2nd ed.). Philadelphia, PA: Lippincott Williams & Wilkins.

Harder, N., Skillen, D. L., & Bickley, L. S. (2010). The abdomen. In T. C. Stephen, D. L. Skillen, R. A. Day, & L. S. Bickley (Eds.), *Canadian Bates' guide to health assessment for nurses* (pp. 509–561). Philadelphia, PA: Lippincott Williams & Wilkins.

Jones, P. E., & Statler, P. M. (2011, May). How many skin lesions can you identify? *The Clinical Advisor*, pp. 35–48.

Lee, A. H. (2004). Why is carcinoma of the breast more frequent in the upper outer quadrant? A case series based on needle core biopsy diagnoses. *Breast, 14*(2), 151–152.

Moore, K. L., & Dalley, A. F. (2006). *Clinically oriented anatomy* (5th ed.). Philadelphia, PA: Lippincott Williams & Wilkins.

Myers, K. A., & Farquhar, D. E. (2001). Does this patient have clubbing? *JAMA, 286*(3), 341–347. doi:10.1001/jama.286.3.341

Newland, D. (2003). Pediatric otolaryngology. In M. Layland & T. Lin (Eds.), *The Washington manual survival guide series: Otolaryngology survival guide*. Philadelphia, PA: Lippincott Williams & Wilkins.

Nursing Best Practice Research Centre. (2013). *About*. Retrieved from http://nbprc.ca/

Ostovan, M., Shahrzad, S., Taban S., & Moniri A. (2013). Idiopathic right atrial enlargement. *Asian Cardiovascular and Thoracic Annals*. Advance online publication. doi:10.1177/0218492312463148

Pagana, K. D., & Pagana, T. J. (2010). *Mosby's manual of diagnostic and laboratory tests*. St. Louis, MO: Mosby.

Pandit, R. J., Gales, K., & Griffiths, P. G. (2001). Effectiveness of testing visual fields by confrontation. *The Lancet, 358*, 1339–1340.

Ponte, D. F., Moraes, R., Hizume, D. C., & Alencar, A. M. (2013). Characterization of crackles from patients with fibrosis, heart failure and pneumonia. *Medical Engineering & Physics, 35*(4), 448–456. doi:10.1016/j.medengphy.2012.06.009

Radford, M., County, B., & Oakley, M. (2004). *Advancing perioperative practice*. Cheltenham, United Kingdom: Nelson Thornes.

Roach, S., Roddick, P., & Bickley, L. S. (2010). The cardiovascular system. In T. C. Stephen, D. L. Skillen, R. A. Day, & L. S. Bickley (Eds.), *Canadian Bates' guide to health assessment for nurses* (pp. 423–478). Philadelphia, PA: Lippincott Williams & Wilkins.

Seller, R. H. (2007). *Differential diagnosis of common complaints* (5th ed.). Philadelphia, PA: Saunders/Elsevier.

Skillen, D. L., & Bickley, L. S. (2010). The physical examination: Objective data. In T. C. Stephen, D. L. Skillen, R. A. Day, & L. S. Bickley (Eds.), *Canadian Bates' guide to health assessment for nurses* (pp. 91–111). Philadelphia, PA: Lippincott Williams & Wilkins.

Spicknall, E. E., Zirwas, M. J., & English, J. C. (2005). Clubbing: An update on diagnosis, differential diagnosis, pathophysiology, and clinical relevance. *Journal of the American Academy of Dermatology, 52*(6), 1020–1028.

Stephen, D. L. Skillen, R. A. Day, & L. S. Bickley (Eds.). *Canadian Bates' guide to health assessment for nurses* (1st ed., pp. 91-111). Philadelphia, PA: Wolters Kluwer Health/Lippincott Williams & Wilkins.

Stephen, T. C., Day, R. A., & Skillen, D. L. (Eds.). (2013). *A syllabus for adult health assessment*. Edmonton, AB: Faculty of Nursing, University of Alberta.

Stephen, T. C., Skillen, D. L., Day, R. A., & Bickley, L. S. (2010). *Canadian Bates' guide to health assessment for nurses*. Philadelphia, PA: Lippincott Williams & Wilkins.

Stephen, T. C., Skillen, D. L., Day, R. A., & Jensen, S. (2012). *Canadian Jensen's nursing health assessment*. Philadelphia, PA: Lippincott Williams & Wilkins.

Warner, E. (2011). Breast-cancer screening. *The New England Journal of Medicine, 365*(11), 1025–1032.

William, J. W., & Simel, D. L. (1993). Does this patient have sinusitis? Diagnosing acute sinusitis by history and physical examination. *JAMA, 270*(10), 1242–1246.

Wipf, J. E., Lipsky, B. A., Hirschmann, J. V., Boyko, E. J., Takasugi, J., Peugeot, R. L., & Davis, C. L. (1999). Diagnosing pneumonia by physical examination: Relevant or relic? *Archives of Internal Medicine, 159*(10), 1082–1087. doi:/10.1001/archinte.159.10.1082

Measuring Vital Signs

EM M. PIJL-ZIEBER AND PETER KELLETT

Tracy is a first-year student preparing for her nursing skills lab session on vital signs. She is excited to be learning about how to take vital signs because she knows this is often the first step in a thorough assessment. To prepare, Tracy decides to read through the material carefully, learn the expected values, and apply as much of this learning as possible during the lab the next day. Tracy knows that these skills take practice to perfect, and fairly soon, she is confident that she will be able to assess vital signs accurately in the clinical setting.

CHAPTER OBJECTIVES

By the end of this chapter, you will be able to:

1. Apply relevant nursing practice standards and legal considerations in the measuring, documenting, and interpreting of vital signs.
2. Think critically about the factors affecting the accurate measurement of vital signs, including home monitoring and the use of technology.
3. Be a skilled practitioner who integrates skills, assessments, and knowledge related to the measurement of vital signs into daily practice.
4. Interact with health-care professionals and engage with patients in communicating about vital signs.
5. Understand the challenges of nursing practice as they relate to the measurement of vital signs, including complex cases, advanced interpretations, and discerning errors in measurement.

KEY TERMS

Ambulatory Blood Pressure Monitoring (ABPM) Involves the use of a non-invasive blood pressure monitoring device to take blood pressure readings over a 24-hour period while patients engage in their usual activities.

Aneroid Without liquid; that is, an aneroid sphygmomanometer does not use a liquid such as mercury.

Apex of the Heart The tip of the heart that can be auscultated to obtain an apical heart rate by placing the stethoscope over the left fifth intercostal space on the midclavicular line. Located inferiorly to the base of the heart.

Apical Pulse Pulse taken at the apex of the heart (fifth intercostal space, midclavicular line).

Apnea Temporary cessation of ventilation or breathing.

Arrhythmia A deviation in the heart's regular rhythm.

Atrioventricular (AV) Node The part of the cardiac conduction system of the heart that regulates heart rate. This cluster of cells is located in the centre of the heart between the atria and ventricles.

Auscultate The technical term that means to listen to the internal sounds of the body, usually by means of a stethoscope.

Auscultatory Gap A silent interval in the middle of the Korotkoff sounds during which the pulse wave can still be felt.

Axillary (Armpit) Temperature The temperature measurement obtained from the skin in the axilla (armpit) that is somewhat protected from the surrounding or ambient air.

Brachial Pulse The pulse of the brachial artery that can be palpated in the antecubital fossa (inside the elbow). It is commonly used for assessing blood pressure and also for assessing the peripheral pulse in infants.

Bradycardia Heart rate below 60 beats/minute in an adult.

Bradypnea Respiratory rate less than 10 breaths/minute. *Brady* means slow; *pnea* refers to breathing or respiration.

Cardiac Cycle The process of filling and emptying the heart's chambers. One cardiac cycle encompasses an entire heartbeat. The two phases of the cardiac cycle are diastole and systole.

Cardiac Output The volume of blood pumped out of each ventricle each minute. It is a factor of the heart rate in beats per minute and the stroke volume (SV), which is the volume of blood pumped from the left ventricle with each beat. Cardiac output changes according to the body's needs.

Core Temperature Measures the temperature of the core thermal compartment, which consists of the vital organs of the trunk and head. Core body temperature more closely represents the temperature of the vital organs, which are highly perfused, tightly regulated, and not influenced by external factors.

Cyanosis A bluish colour of the skin and mucous membranes that may occur when there is a large amount of deoxygenated hemoglobin in the blood.

(continued on page 426)

Diaphoresis   Excessive perspiration or sweating.

Diastole   The brief rest period following systole when the chambers dilate and fill with blood.

Diastolic Pressure   The lowest arterial pressure present during diastole.

Dorsalis Pedis Pulse   A peripheral pulse that can be palpated on the top (dorsal surface) of the foot.

Dysrhythmia   An irregular rhythm that can be further described as being regularly irregular or irregularly irregular.

Eupnea   Normal respiration rate. *Eu* means good; *pnea* refers to breathing or respiration.

Expiration or Exhalation   Air leaving the lungs when a person breathes out.

Homeostasis   *Homeo* means similar, and *stasis* means standing still. When one aspect of a body system changes, other aspects (and sometimes even other body systems) respond to accommodate the change and return the body to optimal conditions and balance.

Hypertension   Blood pressure elevated above expected levels.

Hyperventilation   Breathing faster or deeper than necessary. It can be brought about voluntarily or can result from physiological or emotional processes.

Hypotension   Blood pressure below expected levels.

Hypoventilation   Breathing shallower and slower as in respiratory depression.

Hypoxia   Low oxygen levels in the body tissues.

Inspiration or Inhalation   Air entering the lungs when a person breathes in.

Korotkoff Sounds   Sounds corresponding with changes in blood flow through an artery as the pressure is released from a sphygmomanometer cuff.

Orthopnea   Type of dyspnea (difficulty breathing) in which breathing is easier when the patient sits or stands.

Orthostatic Hypotension   A temporary drop in blood pressure related to assuming an upright position.

Oxygen Saturation   Represents the percentage of hemoglobin binding sites (the part of the red blood cell that carries oxygen) that are occupied by oxygen. The result is expressed as a percentage (%). Conveniently measured noninvasively by a pulse oximeter.

Perfusion   The transport of gases to and from peripheral capillaries.

Peripheral Gas Exchange   The transfer of gases between tissue capillaries and the tissues.

Peripheral Pulse   A pulse palpated at a peripheral site (e.g., radial pulse).

Peripheral Temperature   Refers to the temperature of the peripheral compartment, which consists of extremities (arms and legs), the skin, and peripheral tissues.

Posterior Tibial Pulse   A lower limb pulse that can be palpated on the medial side of the ankle behind and slightly below the medial malleolus.

Pulmonary Gas Exchange   The exchange of gases in the lungs through diffusion between the alveoli and pulmonary capillaries.

Pulse Deficit   When the apical and peripheral or radial pulses differ. A pulse deficit may indicate atrial fibrillation, atrial flutter, premature ventricular contractions, or varying degrees of heart block.

Pulse Oximetry   A noninvasive monitoring of oxygen saturation, expressed as a percentage, via a clip-like device that transmits a beam of light through body tissue to a receiver. The oximeter device measures oxygen and counts pulse rate, hence the term *pulse oximeter*.

Pulse Pressure   The difference between systolic and diastolic pressure or the change in blood pressure when the heart contracts.

Pulse Wave   The pressure wave that is produced throughout the arterial network when the heart contracts.

Radial Pulse   The pulse of the radial artery that can be palpated at the wrist over the radius. It is the site most often used for assessing pulse rate because it is relatively easy to find and palpate, and convenient for both the nurse and the patient.

Sinoatrial (SA) Node   The main pacemaker of the heart. Located at the wall of the right atrium, it initiates the electrical impulses that cause the heart to beat.

Sphygmomanometer   A device to measure blood pressure in conjunction with a stethoscope that consists of a manometer and a cuff that constricts and gradually releases the arterial blood flow so that the pulse can be auscultated to determine systolic and diastolic blood pressure. *Sphygmo* refers to pulse, and a *manometer* is a device that measures pressure.

Syncope   Temporary loss of consciousness, generally related to insufficient oxygen to the brain.

Systole   The phase of heart contraction in which blood is ejected into the aorta and the pulmonary artery.

Systolic Blood Pressure   The highest arterial pressure present during systolic contraction.

Tachycardia   Heart rate exceeding 100 beats/minute in an adult.

Tachypnea   Respiratory rate exceeding 18 breaths/minute. *Tachy* means fast; *pnea* refers to breathing or respiration.

Temporal Artery Thermometer   A noninvasive way to measure temperature by using a scanner probe to obtain infrared readings of temporal artery blood flow from the skin of the forehead.

Thermoregulation   The ability of the human body to maintain its body temperature within the boundaries that support optimal conditions. This is one aspect of homeostasis. The regulation of body temperature is controlled by the hypothalamus.

Tympanic Membrane Thermometers   A thermometer that detects heat radiation from the tympanic membrane using an infrared sensor.

Ventilation   The mechanical process of the lungs which brings oxygen into and expels carbon dioxide from the body. Ventilation includes inhalation and exhalation.

White Coat Hypertension   A phenomenon often seen in health-care settings in which a patient's blood pressure reading is high in health-care settings but normal otherwise.

Vital Signs—A Foundational Nursing Skill

This chapter begins by looking at the larger context of vital signs from the perspective of nursing students and practicing nurses and from a legal and regulatory perspective to establish the foundations on which the rest of the chapter will be built. Then, we explore specific foundational concepts that inform the actual application of your newly acquired vital signs measurement skills. Measurement of vital signs is a skill applied by many different health-care professional groups.

The next section addresses interprofessional communication of vital signs. In addition, we discuss effective approaches to teaching patients and family members about vital signs using a patient-centred approach. The chapter concludes with the most challenging and important aspect of vital sign measurement, which is the application of your knowledge and critical thinking skills in the interpretation of vital signs data and subsequent clinical decision-making. Throughout the discussion, we illustrate the development of an increasingly rich understanding of vital signs and their implications for practice as a person transitions from student to nurse.

What Are Vital Signs?

Vital signs traditionally refer to a group of important clinical measurements including temperature (T), pulse (P), respiratory rate (R), and blood pressure (BP). Often, oxygen saturation is included as part of vital sign assessment as well as pain assessment (see Chapter 30). Vital signs tell us about the health status of a patient; they are interrelated with each other and an important part of a comprehensive patient assessment. When examined together, vital signs provide a snapshot of a patient's thermoregulatory, respiratory, and cardiovascular status, which are all essential components for body functioning and maintenance of homeostasis. Vital signs assessments can identify the patient's degree of wellness, the presence of an acute medical problem, how ill a patient is and how well his or her body is adapting to the illness, and the presence of chronic health problems.

Vital Signs in Context

Measuring vital signs is one of the first skills you will learn; it is an early acquired skill set because it is fundamental to assessing the health status of patients. As a student, you will be gradually taking on the role of the practicing nurse. In the clinical setting, your findings will matter, and you will increasingly learn how to interpret vital signs, how vital signs relate to each other, and how they factor into the planning of patient care. It is essential for nurses to measure vital signs accurately and to combine their knowledge of vital signs and physiology along with critical reasoning to enhance their assessment of patient status and in provision of patient care.

Through the eyes of a nurse

I always assess vital signs before administering any medication. I remember when I was a fairly recent graduate and still getting used to the fact that my assessments really mattered. One of my patients was scheduled to receive a beta-adrenergic blocker medication, which slows the heart rate to decrease the workload on the heart muscle and thus lowers BP. I knew that an apical heart rate was a key assessment that is necessary before administering this class of medication. I determined her apical heart rate was 40 beats/minute, which was below the acceptable limit for administering this particular medication according to my drug guide. I withheld the medication, and after consulting with the hospital pharmacist and patient's physician, we decided not to administer beta-adrenergic blocker until the following day. If I had not done this key assessment and had administered the medication, the patient's heart rate might have decreased to a dangerously low level.

(personal reflection of Sophie, BN, RN)

Vital Signs in the Context of Professional Nursing Practice

Canadian nursing practice is regulated by provincial and territorial colleges or professional associations, which license nurses and seek to protect the public by ensuring all nurses meet nursing practice standards. These provincial and territorial associations also collaborate under the umbrella of the Canadian Nurses Association (CNA) to ensure that practice standards are consistent across the country. Although there are slight variations in the actual wording of practice standards related to patient assessment among these jurisdictions, all jurisdictions require nurses to complete and document accurate and appropriate patient assessments and to use this data in the planning, implementation, and evaluation of patient care. Accurate measurement, interpretation, and documentation of vital signs are fundamental components of a thorough patient assessment. Therefore, it is essential that nurses strive to not only measure vital signs accurately but also consistently use their knowledge of vital signs and physiology in conjunction with critical thinking to inform their assessment of patient status and subsequent nursing care.

Tracy is assigned to a patient with peripheral vascular disease who recently had vascular surgery to restore adequate circulation to his right leg. Pedal pulse checks are essential every hour for the first 8 hours and every 2 hours after that to ensure the patient's right leg receives adequate blood supply. When preparing for clinical practice, Tracy notes that close monitoring of the pedal pulse, skin colour, temperature, pain, and sensation in the patient's right leg are essential elements of her plan of care for this patient and to assess for postoperative complications. Failure to adequately monitor the patient's circulation status may not only contribute to an unfavourable clinical outcome but may also place Tracy and the hospital at risk of malpractice litigation.

As a nurse, you will assess and document vital signs not only in accordance with medical and nursing directives but also within the context of evidence-informed practice. Keep in mind that the "ordered" frequency of vital signs is the minimum requirement and that you may increase your vital signs assessment schedule based on your assessment findings and clinical judgment. Measuring vital signs is not just a task that merely has to be completed and recorded. The application of professional nursing knowledge and critical thinking in understanding the significance of vital sign findings and their implications for nursing care are key components in the delivery of effective and appropriate nursing care. Box 21.1 highlights when to assess vital signs.

Vital Signs: The Basics

This section explores physiological concepts as they relate to temperature, pulse, respiration (including oxygen saturation), and blood pressure. A recurring theme will be homeostasis.

- According to policy and standard procedure on the unit
- Upon admission to the unit
- When the patient's status changes
- Before and after invasive diagnostic procedures or treatments
- Before, during, and after a blood transfusion
- After surgery, especially during the initial postoperative period (often this means q 15 min × 1 h, q 30 min × 2 h, q 1 h × 1, and then q 4 h × 4)
- Before and after giving medications that impact cardiovascular and respiratory function
- Before and after nursing interventions that impact vital signs—such as after ambulation following surgery

Homeostasis is the body's balancing act that keeps all of the body systems operating in their optimal conditions. In addition, both the external and internal environments may be changing, but the body is always seeking to bring itself back to a state of balance. Homeostasis is like a dance in which both partners seek to be balanced with the other for optimum performance. Following each section on physiology, we will explore the method of measuring each vital sign.

Through the eyes of a nurse

I was doing a rotation on a surgical floor. My patient, Mary, was being visited by her 56-year-old husband. Mary suddenly said, "I don't feel so good." I noticed she looked very pale, maybe even a little gray. I helped her back to bed, and then I took her vital signs—her respirations were increased and shallow, and her heart rate was fast and irregular. Mary was starting to sweat (diaphoresis). I had a bad feeling. I actually wondered if she was having a silent heart attack (MI, or myocardial infarction). I called my instructor over, and we called the resident on call STAT and Mary was transferred to CCU where she was diagnosed with an MI. It felt good to know that my assessment made a life-and-death difference!

(personal reflection of Julia, new graduate nurse)

Temperature

The concept of body temperature, in a general sense, refers to the degree to which the body is hot or cold. Temperature measurements inform us how well the body can generate and dispel heat and how well these processes are kept in balance to best support body functions and wellness. Alterations in body temperature can indicate the presence of infection, an inflammatory response, deteriorating patient status, or thermoregulatory disorders (Moran et al., 2007). Although taking temperature measurements is part of routine patient care, it is more than just a ritual; alterations in body temperature affect decisions regarding tests, diagnosis, and treatment and form a basic part of initial and ongoing patient assessment.

Regulation of Temperature

To ensure optimal conditions are present for cells to function and survive, the human body needs its core temperature to be within a specific narrow range that allows minor fluctuations. Although the body is set, much like a thermostat, to optimal core temperature (approximately 36.5° to 37.5°C), small fluctuations of 0.2° to 0.4°C can occur without the body mounting a response to bring it back to normal (Braine, 2009; Sessler, 2008).

The temperature control system is complex and involves numerous feedback systems. The hypothalamus is responsible for regulating body temperature (**thermoregulation**). The body's cold and warm temperature receptors (thermoreceptors) send messages to the hypothalamus, which responds in such a way as to restore homeostasis. To maintain homeostasis and optimal body temperature, the body takes specific actions to bring the internal environment back to normal range (Sessler, 2008). For example, in the event that your body is too warm, heat loss is promoted through increasing capillary blood flow through vasodilation, which causes flushing and ultimately brings blood closer to the surface of your body to dissipate heat. Heat loss is also promoted through sweating, which is the body's only mechanism to dissipate heat in an environment that is warmer than core temperature.

If the body is too cold, the hypothalamus triggers heat production and conservation. The metabolic rate of body cells increases heat production. When you are very cold, your blood vessels constrict (become narrow) to keep blood flow away from the skin so that your body can conserve energy, keeping blood closer to the warm core of your body and away from the cold environment. You may also start shivering, an involuntary contraction of muscles which generates more heat; this is also controlled autonomically in direct response to low body temperature (Braine, 2009; Sessler, 2008). Box 21.2 lists some important normal (not related to illness) alterations and differences in temperature regulation.

- Older people may have less ability to conserve and generate heat due to reduced muscle mass and decreased ability to shiver (Woodrow, 2005).
- Older people may have less ability to feel cold due to degeneration of nerves (Woodrow, 2005). They may also be more sensitive to environmental temperature fluctuations.
- Babies and very young children do not shiver and tend to be sensitive to environmental temperature fluctuations (Sessler, 2008).
- Young individuals have a more rapid response to changes in environmental temperature.
- Exercise temporarily increases body temperature.
- In women, core body temperature tends to fall just prior to ovulation and rises during the luteal phase, by approximately 0.5°C (Braine, 2009; Sessler, 2008).
- Circadian (daily) rhythm causes the temperature to typically lower 0.5°–1°C between 2 AM and 4 AM and to be the highest between 6 PM and 10 PM (Braine, 2009).

Normal and Altered Body Temperature

Normal body temperature varies between people but is typically considered to be 37°C, if measured orally (by mouth). The normal range is between 36.5° and 37.5°C in most people. Table 21.1 indicates normal body temperature standards at various measurement sites. Figure 21.1 indicates the range of body temperature and the implications for health and illness.

Through the eyes of a nurse

As a new public health nurse (PHN) conducting newborn assessments in the home, I learned early on that I could not always assess vital signs in the order they appeared on the flow sheet: temperature, pulse, and then respiration. I found that babies tended to cry when I took their temperature, mainly because they were exposed and cold, and then I was unable to take an accurate apical pulse or respiration because they were crying so hard. So, I started with a 1-minute count of both heart and respiratory rates by just slipping my stethoscope under the baby's clothing while she was still content in her mother's arms. Much later in the assessment, prior to disrobing the baby, I slipped the thermometer under the baby's clothing and held it firmly in place in her axilla. Changing the order in which I took vital signs and completed my other newborn assessments was the key to successful home visits.

(personal reflection of Penni, BN, RN)

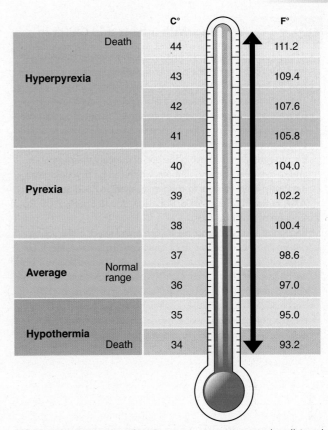

Figure 21.1 The range of body temperature (measured orally) and the implications for health and illness.

Measuring Body Temperature

There are two measures of temperature used in clinical practice: peripheral and core. The **peripheral temperature** measures the temperature of the peripheral compartment, which consists of extremities (arms and legs), the skin, and peripheral tissues. The core thermal compartment consists of the vital organs of the trunk and head (Hooper & Andrews, 2006). **Core temperature** more closely represents the temperature of the vital organs, which are highly perfused, tightly regulated, and not influenced by external or environmental factors (Moran et al., 2007; Sessler, 2008).

TABLE 21.1	Average Body Temperatures
Site of Measurement	**Mean Temperature (Range)**
Core	36.5°–37.5°C
Oral	37.0°C (35.5°–37.5°C)
Tympanic	36.5°C (35.5°–38.0°C)
Rectal	37.5°C (36.6°–38.0°C)
Axillary	36.0°C (34.7°–37.3°C)
Temporal artery	35.0°C

Source: Canadian Paediatric Society. (2007). Temperature measurement in paediatrics. *Position Statement: Canadian Pediatric Society*; Health Canada. (2001). *Pediatric clinical practice guidelines for nurses in primary care*. First Nations & Inuit Health Branch; Sessler, D. I. (2008). Temperature monitoring and perioperative thermoregulation. *Anesthesiology, 109*(2), 318–338.

Although core monitoring provides the most accurate information on patient temperature, it is invasive, inconvenient, often unavailable, and generally reserved for critical care and intraoperative settings. Instead, there are various sites used in the clinical setting that are considered near core; that is, yielding a measurement close to that of the core temperature. These peripheral sites include oral (sublingual or under the tongue), axilla (armpit), tympanic membrane (ear), rectum, and temporal artery (forehead). Peripheral temperatures are easy to access, convenient, and minimally invasive; however, they are often considered unreliable because they can be influenced by external factors, such as environmental temperature. There is considerable debate in health care around which method of temperature measurement is the most accurate; that is, which best reflects the gold standard of pulmonary artery temperature (Moran et al., 2007). There is even disagreement concerning the level of accuracy that is clinically necessary (Sessler, 2008). Ultimately, we must use our judgment as we apply this skill in clinical practice.

The measurement of temperature using a thermometer is only one part of temperature assessment. The thermometer reading must be considered in the context of the broader physical assessment and previous assessment findings. For example, what is the patient's skin temperature like? Is it cold or hot to touch? What is the patient's level of comfort? Is he shivering? Is he thirsty? Is the patient's fever resolving

BOX 21.3   Working With Infants and Children

- If the patient is brought in from home with a reported fever, note the values obtained by the parents and ask the parent or caregiver how the temperature was taken at home (El-Radhi & Barry, 2006). The method used may result in a falsely high or falsely low reading.
- Educate and support parents or caregivers in the accurate measurement of vital signs, the actions to take in response to altered vital signs, and the correct use of tympanic thermometers. Encourage parents to avoid the use of mercury thermometers and to avoid rectal temperatures, which can be psychologically if not physically harmful to children (Canadian Paediatric Society, 2007; El-Radhi & Barry, 2006; Robinson, Jou, & Spady, 2005; Royal College of Nursing, 2007).
- Recognize and provide for the psychological needs of the young patient and his or her parents or caregivers. Explain to patients (as appropriate for age), parents, and caregivers why and how vital signs will be assessed and encourage parents or caregivers to assist (where appropriate for age of patient) (Royal College of Nursing, 2007).
- Recheck very high and very low temperatures. Accurate body temperature measurement is especially crucial in pediatric patients who are critically ill and younger than 3 months of age (El-Radhi & Barry, 2006).

- For children younger than 2 years of age, pull the pinna gently down and back to straighten the ear canal. For individuals older than 2 years of age, pull the pinna up and back.
- The Canadian Paediatric Society (2007) recommends the following temperature measurement techniques for the pediatric population:

Age	Recommended Technique
Birth to 2 years	Although rectal temperatures are considered definitive, axillary temperatures are safer and used for screening low-risk children.
Older than 2 years to 5 years	Although rectal temperatures are considered definitive, axillary, tympanic, or temporal artery thermometry is preferred for screening low-risk children.
Older than 5 years	Oral thermometry is considered definitive. However, axillary, tympanic, or temporal artery is most commonly preferred for screening low-risk children.

or is it getting worse? The numbers on the thermometer are important, but it is your other observations and what the patient tells you that will complete the clinical picture. If the temperature reading is incongruent with the rest of your assessment, double-check the measurement with a different thermometer or a different route.

In terms of measurement devices, each method of thermometry has its benefits and drawbacks in terms of accuracy, convenience, ease of use, and patient comfort. Accuracy is affected by where on the body the temperature is taken, the type of measurement device, the nurse's technique and knowledge, and a wide variety of patient factors such as anatomical and physiological differences and mental and functional competence (Giantin et al., 2008). It is also difficult to compare measurements from the same patient when different instruments are used. Box 21.3 lists some tips for working with infants and children.

Think You can probably recall a time when you were a child and your parent would feel your forehead to see if you had a fever. Although such an assessment does not deliver an actual number, tactile assessment does provide important information and under an expert hand can actually be surprisingly accurate in determining if the patient is febrile (El-Radhi & Barry, 2006; Lockwood, Conroy-Hiller, & Page, 2004). In fact, mothers' tactile assessment of fever has been shown to be more accurate than nurses' and physicians' tactile assessment of fever (El-Radhi & Barry, 2006). Can you think of reasons why health-care providers often minimize parents' knowledge of their own children?

Oral Temperature

In health-care settings, oral temperature measurement is considered to be a consistent and reliable measure of core body temperature (Hooper & Andrews, 2006; Lawson et al., 2007). Oral temperature measurements are convenient with the advent of digital, electronic thermometers. Oral thermometers measure the heat that radiates from sublingual blood vessels and the floor of the mouth, which forms a temperature pocket between these vessels (Latman, 2003).

Oral thermometry is appropriate for a patient who is able to close his or her mouth around the thermometer or probe. An oral temperature is not appropriate for a patient who is unconscious or confused, intubated, recovering from mouth or nose surgery, very young, or unable to follow directions (Canadian Paediatric Society, 2007; Giantin et al., 2008; Lawson et al., 2007). In addition, hot or cold foods and ice chips can falsely raise or lower findings if consumed within the 30 minutes prior to temperature measurement. An oral temperature reading should be interpreted with caution for a patient who has smoked within 15 to 30 minutes prior to taking an oral temperature (Hooper & Andrews, 2006; Lawson et al., 2007; Lockwood et al., 2004) or who is receiving oxygen by mask (Hooper & Andrews, 2006; Lawson et al., 2007; Lockwood et al., 2004). Other sources of error for oral thermometry include misplacement of the probe (Latman, 2003) and small fluctuations in oral temperature related to local vasoconstriction and vasodilation. See Skill 21.1 for step-by-step instructions on taking an oral temperature.

Tympanic Membrane Temperature

Tympanic membrane thermometry is used almost exclusively in many health-care settings. Tympanic membrane (eardrum) temperatures are commonly preferred because the reading is immediate (within seconds) and there is little discomfort for the patient. Tympanic membrane thermometers (depicted in Fig. 21.2) detect heat radiation from the tympanic membrane using an infrared sensor. It does not touch the tympanic membrane but measures the temperature of the thermal radiation emitted from the tympanic membrane and ear canal. The thermometer then converts this measurement so that what you read on the thermometers is an estimation of core body temperature (Hooper & Andrews, 2006).

The infrared tympanic membrane thermometer is perhaps not only the most highly debated but also the most widely used measure of temperature. It tends to be more variable than oral and rectal temperatures (Casa et al., 2007; Lawson et al., 2007), and many practitioners doubt its accuracy and suggest that it should not be used for assessing the critically ill (Casa et al., 2007; Hooper & Andrews, 2006; Moran et al., 2007). In general, this method of thermometry, when compared with oral thermometry, produces highly variable intra-patient and interpatient measurements (between patients and within the same patient) and errors that tend to increase with higher temperatures (Giantin et al., 2008). Slight differences (0.05°C) in tympanic temperatures between a patient's left and right ear are not unusual (Bickley, 2009; Lockwood et al., 2004). Box 21.4 lists the potential sources of error in infrared tympanic membrane thermometry. The Canadian Paediatric

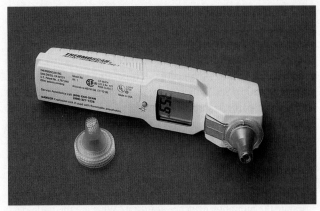

Figure 21.2 Tympanic thermometer with probe cover.

Society (2007) advises that tympanic thermometry is too inaccurate compared with rectal thermometry to be used with confidence in children or patients who are critically ill and who require accuracy in monitoring. Furthermore, a tympanic membrane temperature assessment is not appropriate for a patient who is experiencing extremes in environmental temperatures and localized heating and cooling (Lockwood et al., 2004), has considerable cerumen (earwax) in the ears, especially if it is impacted (Lockwood et al., 2004), or is elderly and being screened for fever (Giantin et al., 2008).

To obtain an accurate temperature reading using a tympanic thermometer in patients older than 2 years of age, the ear canal must be straightened by pulling the pinna up and back (called

---

BOX 21.4 Sources of Error in Infrared Tympanic Membrane Thermometry

Improper Technique
- Having an ineffective seal against the outer ear (Canadian Paediatric Society, 2007; Lawson et al., 2007; Sessler, 2008)
- Reaching for the opposite ear instead of that which is closest to you (Lawson et al., 2007)
- The patient talking or yawning during the procedure can change the shape of his or her external auditory canal (Latman, 2003).
- Inconsistently applying the "ear tug" on the external ear (Canadian Paediatric Society, 2007; Hooper & Andrews, 2006; Latman, 2003; Lockwood et al., 2004; Mackechnie & Simpson, 2006)

Anatomical Features
- Tympanic temperatures represent an average of the temperature of the tympanic membrane, the air within the ear canal, and heat radiated from the wall of the ear canal (Canadian Paediatric Society, 2007; Casa et al., 2007), so there are many sources of error.
- The auditory canal of different individuals can vary in size, shape, structure, and relationship with the tympanic membrane (Hooper & Andrews, 2006; Latman, 2003; Sessler, 2008).
- The position of the tympanic membrane in relation to the detector is also different between individuals (Latman, 2003).
- The eternal auditory canal lengthens and its diameter increases with age, and the angle of the tympanic membrane shifts.

Thus, neonates, children, and adults must be considered differently in the assessment of tympanic membrane temperature (Latman, 2003).
- The probe must be small enough to enter the ear canal; a small meatus, as seen in neonates and young children, can result in falsely low readings (Canadian Paediatric Society, 2007).
- The presence of a bolus of cerumen between the lens and the tympanic membrane can impact accuracy.

Equipment
- A dirty lens can alter the reading (Lawson et al., 2007; Mackechnie & Simpson, 2006).
- Instrument temperature can negatively impact accuracy. When bringing the thermometer from a cold to a warm environment for use, allow it to adjust to the new environment before using (15 minutes) (Mackechnie & Simpson, 2006).
- Improper instrument calibration or incorrect manufacturer's conversion/offset to accommodate low tympanic temperatures (Canadian Paediatric Society, 2007; Casa et al., 2007; Hooper & Andrews, 2006)
- Variations among different brands in terms of design, technology, offsets, and operating instructions, leading to reliability and accuracy issues (Canadian Paediatric Society, 2007)

the "ear tug" technique) so that the sensor has a direct and consistent view of the tympanic membrane (Latman, 2003; Lockwood et al.,2004; Mackechnie & Simpson, 2006). If the ear canal is not straightened, the temperature reading can be as much as 2°C lower than actual temperature (Mackechnie & Simpson, 2006). See Skill 21.1 for step-by-step instructions on taking a tympanic membrane temperature.

Think Tympanic thermometry is the most widely used method of assessing temperature. However, research has shown this method to be unreliable at times. What factors do you think contribute to the continued reliance on this method despite the mounting evidence against it? What are the trade-offs?

Axillary Temperature

The **axillary (armpit) temperature** is derived from skin in an area that is somewhat protected from the surrounding or ambient air. The axilla is the preferred site for temperature measurement in infants and young children because it is relatively easy, safe, and convenient, and it does not require a lot of cooperation. In addition, this site is commonly used when oral and rectal sites cannot be used.

Electronic axillary thermometry readings tend toward high accuracy (Giantin et al., 2008). However, they are consistently lower than core body temperature (approximately 0.5°C lower than oral, and 1°C lower than rectal) and this difference must be accounted for in interpretation of the findings. The accuracy of axillary temperature readings is impacted by the placement of the thermometer, if the patient has bathed within the last 30 minutes, or if the patient is experiencing vasoconstriction (e.g., after surgery), vasodilation (e.g., with sepsis), or sweating (which cools the body as the sweat evaporates) (El-Radhi & Barry, 2006). See Skill 21.1 for step-by-step instructions on taking an axillary temperature.

Temporal Artery Temperature

A **temporal artery thermometer** is a noninvasive way to measure temperature. It uses a scanner probe to obtain infrared readings of temporal artery blood flow; because this artery is superficial, the temperature of the skin over the temporal artery is a fairly accurate measure of body temperature. The temporal artery arises from the carotid artery, which leads directly from the aorta. In fact, it is the only such artery that is close enough to the skin surface to provide the necessary access to take an accurate temperature measurement. The temporal artery is not significantly affected by changes in thermoregulation, has a high perfusion rate, and is readily accessible because it is ideally located at the front portion of the forehead. Readings are negatively affected by **diaphoresis** (excessive perspiration or sweating) and by airflow across the face. Its accuracy in monitoring core body temperature is the subject of considerable debate (Hooper & Andrews, 2006; Lawson et al., 2007; Sessler, 2008). Temporal artery thermometry is often used with infants because no cooperation is required and it is noninvasive. Avoid taking a temperature from an area affected by scar tissue, open sores, or abrasions. If the forehead is not a desirable site to obtain this temperature, the region behind and below the level of the ear may be used, if it is not covered. See Skill 21.1 for step-by-step instructions on taking a temporal artery temperature.

Rectal Temperature

The rectal temperature is thought by many nurses to be the most accurate representation of actual core body temperature. However, given the potential for discomfort and embarrassment, and the risk of damaging (perforating) rectal tissue, it is only used when greater accuracy is needed or when no other options are available. Another possible risk of rectal temperatures is vagus nerve stimulation which, although rare, can result in a slowed heart rate (**bradycardia**) and **syncope** (temporary loss of consciousness). Watch for these signs and listen to what your patient is telling you, such as that he or she feels "funny" or feels he or she may faint. If you suspect vagus nerve stimulation, remove the thermometer immediately and assess the patient's BP and pulse. Notify the nurse who is supervising and make a note in the patient's chart and care plan. Use other routes of thermometry in the future with the patient.

Due to higher risks of damage to delicate rectal tissue and for rectal perforation in children and infants, rectal temperatures are not used with the young pediatric population unless a definitive temperature is required or other methods are not available (Canadian Paediatric Society, 2007). This route is also not appropriate for patients who have had rectal surgery or other conditions affecting local blood flow, patients with diarrhea or rectal disease, patients with a low white blood cell count, patients with certain cardiac conditions or following cardiac surgery, and patients with spinal cord injuries. Additionally, this route should be avoided with patients who may be impaired mentally or functionally or who may not cooperate with the procedure, which may create an unsafe situation for the patient (Giantin et al., 2008).

Factors that can affect the accuracy of a rectal temperature are few in comparison with other routes. The primary consideration is to make sure that a rectal temperature is not contraindicated in the patient and to ensure that the thermometer is not placed in fecal material. In addition, it is important to note that rectal temperatures do not change as rapidly as core temperatures (Canadian Paediatric Society, 2007; Sessler, 2008). Thus, the patient may have a normal rectal temperature, and yet, he or she is developing a fever. See Skill 21.1 for step-by-step instructions on taking a rectal temperature.

Think There are a wide variety of practice standards in the measurement of vital signs. For example, the frequency and preferred route of measurement and accepted normal values parameters vary between institutions, research findings, and health-care professionals. In addition, it has been suggested that the practice of measuring vital signs may have more ritualistic than diagnostic value (Lockwood et al., 2004). Why do you think there is such variation in practice and beliefs about assessing vital signs?

Pulse

Pulse refers to the effect of the beating of the heart on the body's arteries. With each heartbeat, the force of the left ventricle's contraction forces blood into the aorta and arteries, which are elastic, muscular, and compliant. When we take a patient's pulse, it is the force of the contraction that is felt as a pulse wave at a peripheral arterial site.

A **pulse wave** is the pressure wave that is produced throughout the arterial network when the heart contracts. Assessing a patient's pulse can tell us a great deal about the patient's cardiovascular system and his or her general state of health. Alterations in heart rate (HR) and pulse can indicate anything from emotional state to physical fitness level to underlying processes such as cardiovascular disease. Pulse rates, like other vital signs, need to be interpreted in light of other assessment findings and the rest of the patient's clinical picture. In addition to pulse rate, we also assess the rhythm and amplitude of the pulse. As you will see, this information, as part of a comprehensive patient history and assessment, can yield nurses valuable information to guide patient care.

Regulation of Heart Rate

The **sinoatrial (SA) node** is the main pacemaker of the heart. Located in the wall of the right atrium, it initiates the electrical impulses that cause the heart to contract (beat). In most adults, the SA node causes the heart to beat between 60 and 100 beats/minute.

The autonomic nervous system (ANS) controls the triggering of the SA node. Sympathetic nerve stimulation increases the activity of the SA node and enhances **atrioventricular (AV) node** conduction to increase the HR within seconds. For example, when you exercise, your heart speeds up so that it can keep up with the body's demand for oxygen. The parasympathetic portion of the ANS decreases activity of the SA node and slows AV node conduction; thus, it decreases the HR.

The AV node is located in the centre of the heart, between the atria and ventricles. The volume of blood pumped out of each ventricle each minute is called the **cardiac output** (CO). It is a factor of the HR (beats per minute) and the stroke volume (SV), which is the volume of blood pumped from the left ventricle with each beat. CO changes according to the body's needs. In this sense, CO can be seen as the goal of the heart beating in the first place.

$$HR \times SV = CO$$

An increase in CO is generally demanded by the body in times of stress or exertion. The only way to increase CO is by increasing the HR or the SV—how fast it's pumping or how much it's pumping out. If the heart muscle is ineffective or the patient is hemorrhaging, the SV may be low—it cannot put out the required volume because there is not enough volume to begin with. To compensate, it must increase the HR to maintain the CO required for body tissues. If the SV is high, the heart does not have to work as hard to keep up the CO, so the HR slows down to compensate. If the HR is increased,

as in the case of **tachycardia**, the filling time of the heart is decreased. This decreases the SV and thus the CO.

The **cardiac cycle** is the process of filling and emptying the heart's chambers. One cardiac cycle encompasses an entire heartbeat. The two phases of the cardiac cycle are **diastole** and **systole**. Diastole is the relaxation phase of the ventricles when they fill with blood. Systole is the contraction of the ventricles when they empty of blood. The heart valves close in response to the contraction of the heart's chambers to prevent backflow of blood. The closure of valves is what produces the heart sounds that we count when we listen to the **apex**, or tip, of the heart. The normal heart sounds similar to *lub-dub*, which represents one cardiac cycle or one heartbeat. The first heart sound correlates with the beginning of ventricular systole and is commonly referred to as *lub*. It results from the closing of the AV (tricuspid and mitral) valves. Sometimes two sounds can be heard, one representing each valve. Lub is a low-pitched sound that extends longer than the second heart sound (Weber, 2006). The second heart sound, or *dub*, marks the beginning of ventricular diastole. It results from the closing of the semilunar (aortic and pulmonic) valves when the intraventricular pressure begins to fall. This dub sound is a sharper and shorter sound than the first heart sound because the semilunar valves tend to close much more rapidly than the AV valves. Sometimes, dub may also be heard as two distinct sounds (Weber, 2006).

The second part of the cardiovascular system is composed of the body's blood vessels. The arterial network carries oxygenated blood from the heart to the capillaries of the body. It is a high pressure system, and therefore, the arterial walls are thick, elastic, and muscular. These qualities allow it to handle the considerable pressure of each heartbeat. When the heart contracts, it produces a pressure or pulse wave throughout the arterial network (Marieb & Hoehn, 2007). This is called the arterial or **peripheral pulse**, characterized by alternating expansion and recoil of elastic arteries. Peripheral pulse is a factor of the force of the heart's contractions, the regularity of the heart's contractions, the elasticity of the arteries (how much they flex when blood is pumped through them), the overall pressure and resistance within the cardiovascular system, and the volume of blood being pumped. These factors directly influence pulse and BP assessment findings.

Normal and Altered Pulse

Pulse is described in terms of its rate, rhythm, amplitude or strength, and equality. Most adults have a resting pulse between 60 and 100 beats/minute. However, many factors influence what a patient's usual resting pulse is. For example, athletes often have slow but very effective and strong pulses because their hearts are conditioned. Pulse rates also vary across the lifespan. Table 21.2 provides pulse rate ranges across the lifespan. Bradycardia is a sustained HR of less than 60 beats/minute, and **tachycardia** is a sustained HR of greater than 100 beats/minute.

The pulse should have a regular rhythm. If the pulse is irregular, assess if there is a pattern to the missed beats. An irregular rhythm is also called **dysrhythmia** and can

TABLE 21.2	Age-Related Variations in Pulse, Respirations, and Blood Pressure		
Age	Pulse (beats/min)	Respirations (breaths/min)	Blood Pressure (mmHg)
Newborn	80–180	30–80	73/55
1–3 years	80–140	20–40	90/55
6–8 years	75–120	15–25	95/75
10 years	75–110	15–25	102/62
Teens	60–100	15–20	102/80
Adults	60–100	12–20	<130/85
>70 years	60–100	15–20	<130/85

Adapted from Drouin, D., & Milot, A. (Eds.). (2007). *Hypertension therapeutic guide* (3rd ed.). Montreal, QC: The Quebec Hypertension Society; Taylor, C., Lillis, C., Lemone, P., & Lynn, P. (2008). *Fundamentals of nursing: The art and science of nursing care* (6th ed.). Philadelphia, PA: Lippincott Williams & Wilkins.

be described as regularly irregular or irregularly irregular. Pulse also needs to be assessed to determine its amplitude or strength. Peripheral pulses should have a resilient quality that give a bounce to each pulse. Pulses can be described as strong, thready, bounding, or weak on a scale of 0 to 3+, with normal amplitude designated 2+ (Weber, 2006). Table 21.3 lists common terms used to quantify and describe pulse qualities. Finally, when assessing peripheral pulses, note how equal they are on the opposite side of the body. Peripheral pulses should be of equal strength bilaterally. Unequal pulse strength can indicate a clinically significant issue that requires further investigation.

Abnormal findings need to be interpreted in light of the patient's health status and baseline rates and qualities. In older patients, be aware of any medications they are

TABLE 21.3	Terms to Quantify and Describe Pulse Qualities	
	Term	Description
Rhythm	Regular	Normal finding
	Irregular	Abnormal finding
	Regularly irregular	
Pulse amplitude or strength	0 Nonpalpable or absent	Not palpable
	1+ Diminished, weak, and barely palpable	Easy to obliterate
	2+ Strong	Obliterate with slight pressure
	3+ Full, increased	Obliterate with moderate pressure
	4+ Bounding	Unable to obliterate or requires significant pressure to obliterate

Source: Skillen, D. L. (2012). General survey and vital signs assessment. In T. C. Stephen, D. L. Skillen, R. A. Day, & S. Jensen (Eds.), *Canadian Jensen's nursing health assessment: A best practice approach* (pp. 91–124). Philadelphia, PA: Lippincott Williams & Wilkins; Weber, J. (2006). *Health assessment in nursing* (3rd ed.). Philadelphia, PA: Lippincott Williams & Wilkins.

taking, particularly those that affect HR or SV (Wolf, 2007). **Arrhythmias**, or irregular heartbeats, are also more common in older people (Woodrow, 2005).

Assessing Pulse

There are two ways we can assess HR and pulse: at the apical site, directly over the apex of the heart using a stethoscope, or at a peripheral site (commonly the radial pulse). When we assess the **apical pulse**, we can determine the rate, rhythm, and strength of the actual heart itself. See Figure 21.3 for a labeled picture of a stethoscope, showing the relevant parts. Listening to the apical pulse with a stethoscope is called *auscultation*.

When we assess a peripheral pulse, we can determine how well the heartbeat translates to sites further away from the heart and how well the heart is able to pump blood around the body.

There are numerous sites on the body at which you can palpate or feel a peripheral pulse so that you may assess it (Fig. 21.4). The peripheral pulse rate is determined by the number of pulsations felt over a peripheral artery during 1 minute. Peripheral sites, such as the radial pulse, are usually sufficient for patients who are well. The **radial pulse** is the pulse of the radial artery, which can be palpated at the wrist over the radius. In general, the information we gather from taking a radial pulse is a reliable indicator of what is actually happening with the heart. The radial pulse is more convenient for the nurse and comfortable for the patient because exposing the chest is not required as it is for the apical pulse.

Keep in mind that both peripheral and apical assessments of pulse yield different but related information about the patient's cardiovascular and other body systems. When assessing a peripheral pulse, remember that if a patient's heart is having problems, this may not always translate to a peripheral site. In addition, when we compare both the apical and peripheral pulses at the same time, we can find if there is a discrepancy between the two. This is known as a **pulse deficit**, the difference between the apical and peripheral/radial pulses that may

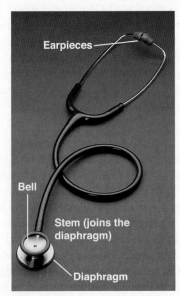

Figure 21.3 The parts of a stethoscope.

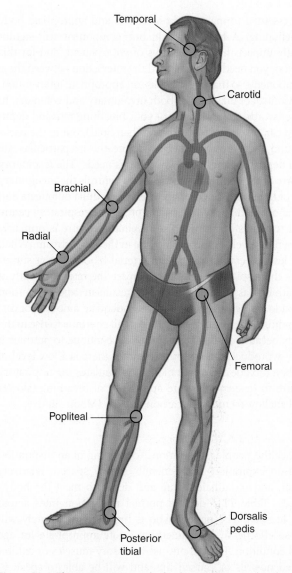

Figure 21.4 The various sites on the body to assess peripheral pulse.

and continue to monitor the patient. Always assess pulse in the context of other findings, such as the patient's baseline pulse rate, recent pulse trends, and other assessments findings.

The technique for palpating a peripheral pulse is not complicated. However, you need to be aware that your thumb has a pulse, and therefore, you should not use it to assess a pulse. Instead, use the pads of your index and middle finger, curved over the patient's wrist, to palpate the pulse. Remember to press gently but firmly so you don't obliterate the pulse. Palpate peripheral pulses for either 30 or 60 seconds. Research indicates that 15-second counts, which are very common in health-care settings, are the least accurate, and 60-second counts are the most accurate, especially if the patient has an irregular pulse. If the pulse is rapid or difficult to palpate, measure it apically using a stethoscope (Lockwood et al., 2004). The step-by-step instructions for assessing the apical and radial pulse are outlined in Skill 21.2.

Apical Pulse

The apical pulse is assessed using a stethoscope directly over the apex of the heart. The apical pulse is preferred over a peripheral pulse in patients who have an irregular HR (arrhythmia or dysrhythmia), have a very slow HR (bradycardia) or a very fast HR (tachycardia), are taking cardiac medications, have a pulse deficit (radial and apical pulses differ), or have a radial pulse that is difficult to palpate or inaccessible due to a cast or dressing. Apical pulses are also preferred for infants or young children and for adults who have an established cardiac history.

The apex of the heart is in the left fifth intercostal space on the midclavicular line. Place the stethoscope over the apex, as shown in Skill 21-2. **Auscultate** (listen) with a stethoscope and count the apical pulse for either 30 or 60 seconds. Box 21.5 outlines tips for assessing pulse in children and infants.

In the vital signs lab, Tracy works with a partner to try and locate all the various pulse sites. She has some difficulty palpating the brachial pulse and the dorsalis pedis. Her lab partner consults the nursing fundamentals textbook she brought along, while Tracy consults her tablet computer for the notes she made last night. They try again to locate the brachial pulse, in the antecubital fossa, and the dorsalis pedis pulse, on the dorsum of the foot—and they are successful. Tracy notices that other students in the lab are also having trouble palpating these pulses and offers to help them out. She starts to gain confidence in her ability to assess the various pulse sites.

Respirations and Oxygenation Status

The purpose of breathing is twofold: to bring oxygen into and to remove carbon dioxide from the body. The survival of every cell in the body depends on the delivery of adequate amounts of oxygen through the bloodstream. Carbon dioxide is a by-product of cellular metabolism and must also be removed from

indicate atrial fibrillation, atrial flutter, premature ventricular contractions, and varying degrees of heart block (Weber, 2006).

Peripheral Pulses

There are numerous sites on the body for assessing peripheral pulse, as shown in Figure 21.4. Commonly, the radial pulse is palpated to assess peripheral pulse. The **brachial pulse**, the pulse of the brachial artery, is used for assessing the peripheral pulse in infants and also used in assessing BP. It can be palpated in the antecubital fossa (inside the elbow). The posterior tibial and dorsalis pedis pulses are used to assess the quality of circulation to the lower extremities. The **posterior tibial pulse** can be palpated behind and slightly below the medial malleolus. The **dorsalis pedis pulse** can be palpated on the dorsal aspect of the foot. When assessing the peripheral pulse rate, also assess its rhythm and amplitude. If you find that the pulse is irregular, assess the patient to find out what other physiological events are occurring, notify the nurse who is supervising, and chart your assessment. Recheck the pulse

BOX 21.5 Tips for Assessing Pulse and Respiration in Children and Infants

Pulse

- Assess the apical pulse of children younger than 2 years of age.
- Double-check digitally derived data with listening or palpating.
- Count pulse for 60 seconds.
- Note if the brachial pulse rate differs from the apical rate.
- Consider HR in relation to age, clinical state, and other assessment findings.
- Consider the patient's emotional status (especially fear) in determining the meaning of elevated pulse rates.

Respiration

- Count the respiratory rate for 1 full minute.
- Use a stethoscope against the chest to count when the respiratory rate is rapid.
- Count respirations when the patient is at rest, not when the patient is agitated, crying, or otherwise distressed.
- Infants and children younger than 6 or 7 years of age primarily breathe abdominally, not thoracically.
- Consider respiratory rate in relation to age, clinical state, and other assessment findings.
- Consider the patient's emotional status (especially fear) in determining the meaning of elevated respiration rates.
- Remember that fever can increase the respiratory rate in children.

Source: Aylott, M. (2006). Observing the sick child: Part 2a. Respiratory assessment. *Pediatric Nursing, 18*(9), 38–44; Lockwood, C., Conroy-Hiller, T., & Page, T. (2004). Vital signs. *JBI Reports, 2*, 207–230; Royal College of Nursing. (2007). *Standards for assessing, measuring and monitoring vital signs in infants, children and young people.* London, United Kingdom: Author.

the bloodstream or a toxic environment is created. A balance of oxygen and carbon dioxide is necessary in certain amounts in the body in order for it to function properly, and the task of the respiratory system is to monitor and regulate the levels of each so that an optimal internal environment is maintained.

As nurses, we need to understand the cause of changes in respiration. A change in respiratory rate and depth can occur in response to changing demands of the body, a respiratory problem, or a problem in another body system. In fact, respiratory rate is considered to be a strong predictor of adverse events, particularly in the presence of other signs of deteriorating physiological function (Cretikos et al., 2008; Lockwood et al., 2004).

Regulation of Respiration and Oxygenation

Respiration has four components: ventilation, pulmonary gas exchange, gas transport, and peripheral gas exchange. **Ventilation** simply means that air is entering and leaving the lungs. Air entering the lungs is called **inspiration** or **inhalation**, and air leaving the lungs is called **expiration** or **exhalation**. **Pulmonary gas exchange** is the exchange of gases in the lungs through diffusion between the alveoli and pulmonary capillaries. **Perfusion** is the transport of gases to and from peripheral capillaries. Finally, **peripheral gas exchange** is the transfer of gases between tissue capillaries and the tissues (Moore, 2007). All components of respiration

are essential to maintain homeostasis and appropriate body functioning. A breakdown in one component will significantly impact the health status of your patient, and for this reason, you need to understand the interaction between these components so that you can plan an appropriate intervention.

Control of breathing is both involuntary and voluntary. In other words, you can control your breathing rate and depth (you can take a deep breath and then hold), but in the background, there is a constant drive to breathe at a particular rate and depth, depending on your body's needs. The respiratory centre in the central nervous system controls the involuntary act of breathing. Specifically, it is the medulla oblongata and pons of the brainstem that comprises the respiratory centre and regulates breathing. The respiratory centre is primarily driven by levels of carbon dioxide in the bloodstream. When the level of carbon dioxide in arterial blood rises, it stimulates the respiratory centre to increase the rate and depth of breathing (faster and deeper). This results in expelling carbon dioxide. If the lungs cannot expel adequate amounts of carbon dioxide, carbon dioxide levels will continue to rise in the body because cellular respiration will continue to produce it as a byproduct. On the other hand, if there is a low level of carbon dioxide in arterial blood, it stimulates the respiratory centre to decrease the rate and depth of breathing (slower and shallower) to retain carbon dioxide (Moore, 2007).

Normal and Altered Respirations

In healthy people, respirations (consisting of an inspiration and an expiration) are generally evenly spaced, relatively quiet, and of sufficient rate and depth to meet the body's needs. Table 21.2 depicts normal respiration rates across the lifespan. The patient who is breathing adequately will do so effortlessly and quietly at a rate appropriate for age and condition. He will not use accessory muscles or exhibit flared nostrils or pursed lips and will be able to speak in full sentences. He will have healthy colour and be conscious and alert when roused. He will also be able to breathe without effort when lying down and not be limited to upright or tripod positions (**orthopnea**) (Moore, 2007; Weber, 2006).

With some illnesses and conditions, breathing rates become faster or slower than the body requires or respiration may become laboured and noisy. All of these altered respiratory patterns may impact the ability of the body to function properly because the amount and frequency of oxygen entering and carbon dioxide leaving the body is altered. Table 21.4 outlines the different major types of breathing patterns. Table 21.5 lists factors that influence respirations.

Assessing Respiration and Oxygenation Status

Assessing respirations at a basic level involves counting respirations and determining if the respirations are adequate. In addition to counting respirations, we assess the rate, rhythm, depth, and pattern of breathing and listen for any adventitious (added) sounds. Checking a patient's oxygenation status requires the use of a pulse oximeter, a machine that measures the percentage of hemoglobin carrying oxygen to body tissues.

TABLE 21.4	Major Types of Breathing Patterns		
Description	**Rate**	**Pattern**	**Possible Causes**
Normal or eupnea	12–20 breaths/minute, regular		
Bradypnea	<10 breaths/minute, regular		Medications such as CNS depressants Brain trauma Postanesthesia
Tachypnea	>24 breaths/minute, shallow		Exercise Trauma Stress Fever Respiratory disorders
Apnea	Breathing temporarily stops and then starts up again		Sleep disorders Narcotic overdose
Hypoventilation	Slow and shallow		Overdose of CNS depressants Respiratory muscle weakness Brain damage
Hyperventilation Kussmaul	Fast and deep		Fear Anxiety and panic Extreme physical exertion Metabolic acidosis Diabetic ketoacidosis Aspirin overdose
Cheyne-Stokes respiration	Alternating periods of apnea and increasingly deep, rapid breathing		Cerebral injury Left ventricular failure End of life Some elderly individuals have this breathing pattern during sleep.
Biot's or ataxic respiration	Irregular, vary in depth and rate with periods of apnea		Meningitis Severe brain damage

CNS, central nervous system.

Source: Bickley, L. S. (2009). *Bates guide to physical examination and history taking* (10th ed.). Philadelphia, PA: Lippincott Williams & Wilkins; Moore, T. (2007). Respiratory assessment in adults. *Nursing Standard, 21*(49), 48–57; Weber, J. (2006). *Health assessment in nursing* (3rd ed.). Philadelphia, PA: Lippincott Williams & Wilkins.

Assessing Ventilation

Counting respirations (assessing ventilation) involves watching the chest rise and fall and counting each cycle as one breath. In addition to counting breaths for 30 or 60 seconds, we also assess the rate, rhythm, depth, and pattern of breathing and notice any sounds associated with breathing or the presence of coughing or sputum production. Because patients become self-conscious about their breathing when they know it is being counted or assessed, it is helpful to count respirations directly after pulse while you are still holding the patient's wrist and looking at your watch. Box 21.5 highlights tips for assessing respirations in infants and children.

Normal and Altered Oxygen Saturation

Although assessing the rate, rhythm, and quality of ventilation provides valuable information about one component of respiratory status, it is also beneficial to assess the effectiveness of gas exchange, gas transport and perfusion, and peripheral gas exchange. You can do this by assessing the patient's colour. For example, a blue (**cyanosis**) or pale (pallor) tone of the skin and mucous membrane can indicate poor oxygenation (**hypoxia**) in body tissues (Moore, 2007). Cyanosis may be noticeable when oxygen saturation is below 85% and is generally a late sign of respiratory dysfunction. Central cyanosis affects the area around the core and lips, whereas peripheral cyanosis affects the extremities.

TABLE 21.5	Some Factors That Influence Respirations
Factor	Example
Age	Children's respiratory rate is generally higher and then decreases as age increases toward adulthood.
Gender	Females tend to use their intercostal muscles (between the ribs) more than males, who tend to breathe more diaphragmatically.
Exercise	With exercise, breaths deepen and increase in rate to bring in more oxygen and blow off more carbon dioxide to accommodate the needs of body cells.
Acid–base balance	Alkalosis results in slower breathing to retain carbon dioxide. Acidosis results in faster breathing to blow off carbon dioxide.
Anxiety	Anxiety causes faster breathing and can result in hyperventilation and potentially leading to respiratory alkalosis.
Acute pain	Acute pain can cause faster and more shallow breathing.
Anemia	Anemia is characterized by fewer oxygen-carrying hemoglobin molecules. Less oxygen carried means more breaths must occur to ensure the body gets enough oxygen.
Altitude	Changing from low to high altitude requires faster breathing because there is less oxygen at higher altitudes. Changing from high to low altitude requires slower breathing because there is more oxygen closer to sea level.
Alterations in the central nervous system	Lesions can affect the brain's ability to sense, interpret, and act on carbon dioxide levels in the blood. A spinal cord injury at or above the fourth cervical vertebrae will require the patient to be on a ventilator.
Medications	Some medications, such as narcotics and other central nervous system depressants, can cause respiratory depression.
Anesthesia	Respiratory rate and depth is usually decreased in the postanesthesia period.
Lung conditions	Lung conditions, such as emphysema and asthma, can limit ventilation and/or gas exchange.
Body position	Lying down makes breathing harder, whereas sitting upright and slightly forward makes breathing easier.
Overdose	Narcotic overdose can result in hypoventilation because opiates can reduce respiratory drive and respiratory response to oxygen and carbon dioxide levels (Cretikos et al., 2008).
Pregnancy	Fluid retention and displacement of the diaphragm can make breathing more shallow (Moore, 2007).
Obesity	Obesity can decrease lung expansion (Moore, 2007).
Circulatory problems	Pulmonary edema can impair gas exchange (Moore, 2007).
Chest trauma	Chest pain and chest wall injury such as rib fractures decreases the ability to take deep breaths (Moore, 2007).

In people with dark skin, cyanosis may be seen in the lips, gums, around the eyes, and nail beds.

You can also assess peripheral oxygen saturation using **pulse oximetry**, which measures **oxygen saturation**, the approximate percentage of hemoglobin binding sites (the part on the red blood cell that carries oxygen) that are occupied by oxygen. Oxygen saturation, determined by a pulse oximeter, is expressed as a percentage (%). A pulse oximeter is a noninvasive device that measures oxygen saturation and also counts pulse rate. When you hear nurses talking about a patient's *sats*, they are talking about his or her oxygen saturation. You may also see the abbreviation "SpO_2" preceding the percent score; this means that the measurement was taken from a peripheral site (most likely the patient's finger) using the noninvasive sensor probe of an oximeter or pulse oximeter. The sensor of the oximeter, located in a clip-like device, transmits a red, infrared light beam through body tissue to a photodetector or receiver, which then sends a signal to a computerized unit that displays the calculated oxygen saturation (SpO_2) and the average pulse rate. The wavelengths are altered by the amount of hemoglobin saturated with oxygen (Bianchi et al., 2008; Booker, 2008; Moore, 2007). The probe can be applied to any relatively translucent area of the body that has a pulsating blood flow; in adults, the fingertip is most commonly used.

Determining SpO_2 levels, through pulse oximetry, is not always part of taking vital signs. However, it is included in this chapter at an introductory level because it is often part of a basic respiratory assessment. Taken and interpreted correctly, in conjunction with other assessment findings, SpO_2 can help nurses know if a patient is getting enough blood circulation and oxygen to his or her body tissues. It is important to remember, however, that oximetry does not provide information into how well the patient is ventilating and thus is not a replacement for counting and assessing the rate and depth of respirations nor does it provide information on how much actual oxygen is in the blood or in the tissues (Cretikos et al., 2008; DeMeulenaere, 2007). Oximetry findings, like other assessment findings, should be interpreted with the larger clinical picture in mind and in light of other assessment findings (Cretikos et al., 2008; Moore, 2007).

Assessing Oxygen Saturation

Pulse oximetry can provide you with adjunct information on the respiratory status of the patient. It does not replace respiratory assessment or counting respiratory rate. Because the sensor transmits light through body tissue to obtain a reading, both the finger and the sensor must be clean to avoid obstructing the light beam. The probe is designed for use on the fingertip, although occasionally other translucent areas are used, such as the earlobe. Several patient factors can contribute to inaccurate oximetry results: dark nail polish, acrylic fingernails, heavy soiling or blood on the fingertip, and some health conditions.

Step-by-step instructions for assessing both respirations and oxygenation are in Skill 21.3. Keep in mind that although respirations are considered part of routine vital signs, pulse oximetry is not always considered part of the routine measurement of vital signs. It has been included in this section because both skills contribute to a more comprehensive and accurate clinical picture.

Blood Pressure

Blood pressure (BP) refers to the pressure exerted on the arterial walls by the force of the heart's contractions. The level of this pressure varies in response to the different phases of the cardiac cycle and physiological influences on BP regulation (Bell, 2008; Skillen, 2012). **Systolic blood pressure** refers to the arterial pressure during the phase of heart contraction or systole. Following the contraction of the ventricles, a wave of blood passes through the arteries, and the pressure during systole effectively represents the highest pressure exerted on the arterial walls (Skillen, 2012). The **diastolic pressure** represents the lowest pressure present in the arteries that occurs during the brief rest period, called *diastole*, between systolic cardiac contractions (Skillen, 2012). Blood pressure measurements are recorded as a fraction with systolic pressure over diastolic pressure (e.g., 120/80 mmHg). In addition, a third BP value that is often reported is the **pulse pressure**, or the difference between the systolic and diastolic pressures (e.g., BP 120/80 mmHg: 120 − 80 = pulse pressure = 40). Pulse pressure represents the force that the heart generates each time it contracts; interpreted in consideration of other physical assessment findings, the pulse pressure can provide valuable information about the patient's risk profile for various health conditions, as well as information about the cardiovascular system's functioning.

Adequate BP is essential for: the perfusion of all body tissues with oxygenated blood; transportation of essential nutrients; and, removal of waste materials by the liver, the kidneys, and the lungs. In other words, without adequate BP, the human body cannot survive. Alternately, high BP (**hypertension**) in the vascular system over a sustained period of time can contribute to vascular wall damage, atherosclerosis, and vascular disease that can damage many organs and body systems. Hypertension has been shown to significantly increase the risk of stroke (cerebrovascular accidents [CVA]), heart attack (myocardial infarction [MI]), heart and kidney disease/failure, and even sexual problems, and is also related to some forms of dementia (Hypertension Canada [HC], 2013).

According to Hypertension Canada (HC, 2013), over 5 million Canadians suffer from high BP, and hypertension is the leading risk for death in North America. Blood pressure naturally tends to increase as a person ages and may be influenced by heredity, but this process may be accelerated if a person's lifestyle includes elements such as a diet high in saturated fat, inactivity, and high stress (HC, 2013).

Regulation of Blood Pressure

Blood pressure is influenced by HR, the volume of CO, total blood volume, and the amount of resistance in the vascular system. Central blood volume and arterial pressure are primarily influenced by neural and hormonal mechanisms (Bell, 2008). It is helpful for nurses to develop a good understanding of these physiological processes in order to interpret the significance of their patient's BP readings and articulate this information in simple terms when providing patient education on BP.

Neural control of the cardiovascular system involves both the sympathetic and parasympathetic branches of the ANS. An individual's HR, arterial resistance, and venous tone are regulated by the medulla oblongata in response to feedback that it receives from stretch receptors (baroreceptors) in the heart and arteries. Based on this information, the medulla oblongata stimulates the sympathetic or parasympathetic branches of the ANS (Bell, 2008). If there is sympathetic autonomic stimulation, HR, CO, and systemic vascular resistance (SVR) increase due to stimulation of cardiac and vascular muscle, effectively raising the BP. Alternately, if the parasympathetic branch is stimulated, HR, CO, and SVR lower due to decreased stimulation of cardiac and vascular muscle, and the result is lower BP.

Hormonal influences on the cardiovascular system are also impacted by baroreceptor reflexes. If baroreceptors in the renal arteries detect a decrease in arterial pressure, the result is increased sympathetic nervous stimulation of the kidney and release of the hormone renin, which activates the renin-angiotensin-aldosterone system (RAAS) (Bell, 2008). Angiotensin increases vascular resistance to raise BP, whereas aldosterone causes the kidneys to retain salt and water, resulting in increased blood volume and a rise in BP. Baroreceptor identification of low BP also causes the hypothalamus to influence the posterior pituitary to release arginine vasopressin (AVP). AVP is a vasoconstrictor and also causes the kidneys to save water, therefore increasing BP in two ways. On the other hand, an increase in arterial pressure results in decreased AVP release and increased excretion of water by the kidneys. Although hormonal effects on BP can be significant, their effect on BP can take hours to days, as compared to ANS effects that occur in seconds to minutes (Bell, 2008).

Normal and Altered Blood Pressure

Patients frequently ask what constitutes a normal BP reading, but there is not a magic number that represents normal BP at all times, in all cases. Blood pressure, like other vital signs, is constantly changing from 1 minute to the next depending on body position, activity level, psychological state, and internal physiological processes. In addition, it is also important to interpret a patient's BP within the context of his or her individual norms, especially in the case of an elderly patient or one who consistently demonstrates high or low BP values (Wolf, 2007).

For example, if an elderly patient consistently has an average BP reading of 160/90 mmHg, an isolated reading of 110/70 mmHg might be a significant change for them despite the fact that 110/70 mmHg would be considered quite normal in the average adult patient. Interpretation of BP readings must therefore be informed by individual patient medical history and in the context of a wide range of current assessment data.

Table 21.6 outlines the recommended classification of BP according to the Canadian Hypertension Society and the World Health Organization (WHO). For the average adult, it is desirable to have a consistent BP reading below 130 mmHg systolic and 85 mmHg diastolic. In patients with high vascular risk conditions, such as diabetes, the target BP should be ideally below 130 mmHg systolic and 80 mmHg diastolic (Canadian Hypertension Education Program [CHEP], 2012; Culleton et al., 2008; Kaplan, Mendis, Poulter, & Whiteworth, 2003). Readings above 130/85 mmHg become increasingly undesirable, with hypertension being diagnosed if these levels exceed 140 mmHg systolic and/or 90 mmHg diastolic over several office visits (CHEP, 2012). Table 21.6 also lists the systolic and diastolic ranges for Grades 1, 2, and 3 hypertension. If average systolic BP remains consistently above 140 mmHg while average diastolic BP remains below 90 mmHg diastolic, the patient may be diagnosed with isolated systolic hypertension (ISH). Table 21.2 presents normal (average) and altered BP readings across the lifespan.

A phenomenon often seen in health-care settings is **white coat hypertension**, characterized by BP readings that are high in health-care settings but normal otherwise (Drouin & Milot, 2007). It is estimated that this phenomenon is present in 10% to 30% of patients with suspected hypertension (Drouin & Milot, 2007). Be aware of this potential effect on the accuracy of patients' BP readings and advocate for the use of home or **ambulatory blood pressure monitoring (ABPM)** to determine your patient's true status when a diagnosis of hypertension is being considered. Ambulatory monitoring involves the use of a noninvasive BP monitoring device to take BP readings over a 24-hour period while patients engage in their usual activities in their usual environment.

Equipment for Measuring Blood Pressure

In most clinical settings, a sphygmomanometer and stethoscope are used to indirectly auscultate BP. A **sphygmomanometer** is a device used to measure BP. It consists of a manometer, which measures pressure in millimeters of mercury (mmHg), and an inflatable cuff that constricts and gradually releases the arterial blood flow so that the pulse can be auscultated to determine systolic and diastolic BP. *Sphygmo* refers to pulse, and a *manometer* is a device that measures pressure. The unit, mmHg, refers to the amount of pressure to raise a column of mercury 1 mm. Noninvasive BP measurements require a cuff to be applied to the patient's upper arm. Direct (invasive) BP measurement is used in critical care areas, using an intraarterial vascular line and a pressure monitor. Noninvasive techniques, however, are preferred.

There are several types of sphygmomanometers. The most accurate way to measure BP in a noninvasive way is the mercury sphygmomanometer. Mercury-based devices do not require calibration unlike other nonmercury devices for measuring BP (Schell, 2006). Unfortunately, mercury is a well-known toxic substance and environmental hazard, so there is a movement to replace mercury sphygmomanometers in health-care settings with other devices such as aneroid sphygmomanometers and automatic BP monitors (Schell, 2006). Figure 21.5 depicts labeled pictures of mercury and aneroid sphygmomanometers. Despite the fact that mercury is increasingly rare (if not obsolete) in health-care settings in North America, millimeters of mercury (mmHg) continue to be the standard units by which BP is measured.

Aneroid sphygmomanometers use a manometer that does not contain mercury. These sphygmomanometers are easily distinguishable from mercury sphygmomanometers because rather than a mercury column, they have a dial to measure the pressure of the cuff inflation.

Automatic noninvasive BP monitors determine BP using an oscillometric technique rather than auscultation. These devices are often used in cases where frequent BP readings are required or ongoing regular monitoring of BP is necessary, such as in critical care areas. Oscillometric devices determine BP by monitoring changes in the amplitude of arterial wall pulsations (Schell, 2006). These devices

TABLE 21.6	Classification of Blood Pressure		
Category	Systolic (mmHg)		Diastolic (mmHg)
Normal	<130	and/or	<85
High normal	130–139	and/or	85–89
Grade 1 HTN	140–159	and/or	90–99
Grade 2 HTN	160–179	and/or	100–109
Grade 3 HTN	≥180	and/or	≥110
Isolated systolic HTN (ISH)	>140	and/or	<90

HTN, hypertension.

Source: Adapted from Drouin, D., & Milot, A. (Eds.). (2007). *Hypertension therapeutic guide* (3rd ed.). Montreal, QC: The Quebec Hypertension Society; Kaplan, N., Mendis, S., Poulter, N., & Whiteworth, J. (2003). 2003 World Health Organization (WHO)/International Society of Hypertension (ISH) statement on management of hypertension. *Journal of Hypertension, 21*(11), 1983–1992.

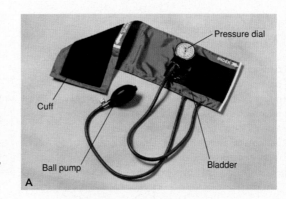
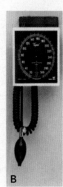

Figure 21.5 **A.** Aneroid sphygmomanometer with an adult cuff, with parts labeled. **B.** Wall-mounted aneroid sphygmomanometer, with cuff tucked behind dial.

(depicted in Fig. 21.6) are becoming very popular because they are easy to use, and they do not require auscultation skills. The accuracy of these devices is a topic of ongoing debate (Schell, 2006) as oscillometric devices can be compromised by an irregular HR and if the patient is moving during measurement (Stebor, 2005). Many noninvasive BP monitor manufacturers suggest that these devices should not be used in individuals with irregular HRs because of the difficulty in detecting pulse amplitude (Schell, 2006). To promote patient safety, when using an oscillometric monitor, if you find that the patient's BP reading is extremely high or low, confirm the BP using the auscultatory method as well.

Oscillometric devices are increasingly accessible, easy to use, and affordable, and as such, they are often used by patients at home. If used correctly, self-monitoring of BP using an approved monitor is a useful adjunct to readings obtained in a clinic setting and is comparable to readings obtained from an ambulatory BP monitor (Drouin & Milot, 2007). As a nurse, you may still want to confirm these home readings.

It is likely that aneroid sphygmomanometers and automatic BP monitors will be the norm in most Canadian health-care settings in the coming years. As a nurse, it is important to be familiar with using each device and to keep in mind the potential strengths and limitations of each method of BP measurement. Remember that mercury-free

devices require regular calibration in order to maintain their accuracy (Schell, 2006).

Measuring Blood Pressure

Blood pressure is most commonly measured using both a sphygmomanometer (either mercury or aneroid) and stethoscope and requires a combination of auscultation (listening to) and palpation of the brachial artery. The most common site of BP measurement is the upper arm, using the brachial artery to auscultate the BP by placing the diaphragm of the stethoscope over the artery in the antecubital fossa. Alternate sites for measuring BP include the thigh, the popliteal artery, and the forearm, which is more commonly used with oscillometric automatic BP monitors. Research suggests that if BP is measured in sites other than the upper arm, measurement accuracy may be adversely affected (Lockwood et al., 2004). See Box 21.6 for sites to avoid when measuring BP. Steps to prepare the patient for BP measurement are listed in Box 21.7.

A sphygmomanometer consists of an inflatable and airtight cuff attached by one tube to a manometer to measure the air pressure applied by the cuff, with a second tube attached to a valve and bulb that is used to inflate the cuff. In order for a sphygmomanometer to accurately measure a patient's BP, it is important to use the correct size of cuff. The inflatable bladder must cover 80% of the upper arm's circumference, and the cuff width should be at least 40% of the circumference of the arm. If a cuff is too narrow, the result may be an overestimated BP, whereas a cuff that is too wide for the patient can lead to underestimation of BP (Lockwood et al., 2004). The cuff must be placed over the brachial artery, without bulky

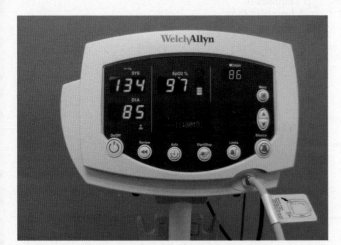

Figure 21.6 Oscillometric sphygmomanometer.

BOX 21.6 **Sites to Avoid When Measuring Blood Pressure**

Avoid measuring BP using an arm that

- Has a dialysis graft to prevent damage to the graft.
- Is on the same side as a mastectomy because it can contribute to the development of lymphedema in the arm.
- Is painful or swollen.
- Has an IV infusing because it could contribute to the IV site becoming infiltrated.

BOX 21.7   Preparing the Patient for Blood Pressure Measurement

- Ensure the patient has not had caffeine in the past hour.
- Ensure the patient has not smoked in the past 15–30 minutes.
- Ensure the patient has not exercised in the past 30 minutes.
- Ensure the patient has not taken medication or substances that are stimulants (often present in decongestants).
- Ensure the patient has emptied his or her bladder.
- Ensure the room is warm and calm.
- Remove tight or restrictive clothing from the patient's arm or forearm.
- Help make the patient comfortable and reduce any anxiety.
- Ensure the patient is free from acute anxiety, stress, or pain.
- Ask the patient to not speak during the reading.
- Position the patient:
  - Calmly seated for 5 or more minutes.
  - Make sure his back is supported.
  - Ensure the patient's arm is at the level of his or her heart and supported.
  - Ensure the patient's legs are not crossed.

Source: Drouin, D., & Milot, A. (Eds.). (2007). *Hypertension therapeutic guide* (3rd ed.). Montreal, QC: The Quebec Hypertension Society.

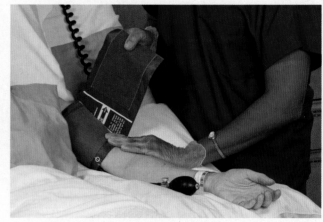

Figure 21.7 Correct placement of the BP cuff.

clothing underneath the cuff (Fig. 21.7). When the sphygmomanometer cuff is inflated to a pressure greater than the arterial BP, blood flow to the brachial artery and the lower arm is temporarily occluded, and no sounds will be auscultated over the brachial artery. As the cuff pressure is slowly lowered, you will listen for the sound of blood flow returning to the brachial artery (Phase I sounds). These sounds are called

Korotkoff sounds, and they pass through five phases while you auscultate the BP until they are no longer heard. The cuff pressure when the first sound is heard represents the highest pressure present in the brachial artery, or the systolic pressure. This is the point when the pressure in the artery is first able to overcome the pressure exerted by the sphygmomanometer cuff, and blood flow starts to return to the brachial artery below the cuff. Korotkoff sounds will continue to be heard as the pressure in the cuff continues to decline until they become muffled (Phase V) and eventually cease to be heard at the level that represents the lowest pressure in the artery (diastolic pressure). Refer to Figure 21.8 for a visual representation of this process. Step-by-step instructions for measuring BP are outlined in Skill 21.4.

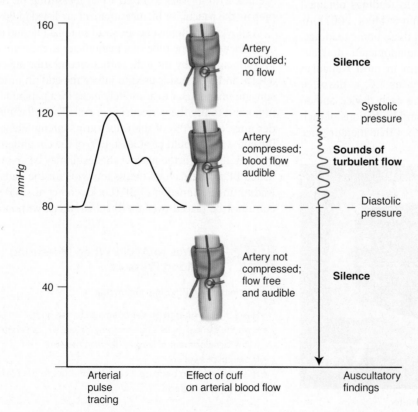

Figure 21.8 Auscultation of BP.

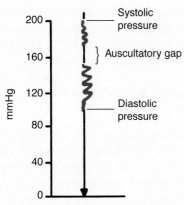

Figure 21.9 Illustration of the auscultatory gap.

Occasionally, patients may have a silent interval in the middle of the Korotkoff sounds we use to determine systolic and diastolic BP, and if undetected, this can result in underestimation of systolic BP. In order to avoid missing this **auscultatory gap**, it is recommended that you initially estimate systolic BP using palpation and then inflate the cuff to 20 to 30 mmHg above this level when auscultating BP so that you are sure to capture the true systolic value (Fig. 21.9).

Hypotension is a condition in which blood pressure is abnormally low. **Orthostatic hypotension** is a drop in BP that occurs with a change in position from lying to sitting, or sitting to standing. Patients who are older than 65 years of age, have diabetes, or are being treated with medications to lower BP (antihypertensives) are particularly at risk for orthostatic changes in BP, so you should first check their BP in the usual seated position, and then 1 to 5 minutes after, they stand in order to check for the presence of orthostatic hypotension (Drouin & Milot, 2007).

When the time comes to practice auscultating BP, Tracy wonders if she will be able to determine the same systolic and diastolic readings as her lab partner. She wants to do this skill correctly but has heard that at first, it can be difficult to get accurate readings. Tracy read last night in her textbook that it is easier to hear the Korotkoff sounds clearly if she avoids touching the stethoscope tubing and stays as still as possible to eliminate extraneous noises. Tracy keeps practicing on her friends and gains more confidence in the accuracy of her BP readings.

Through the eyes of a nurse

When I was a student, I quickly became disenchanted with taking vital signs once I felt I had mastered the skill. I guess I thought that the clinical experience was about *my* clinical experience and what new things I could learn. Sometimes, I think students on my unit feel this way. I want to tell them that the clinical experience isn't about them—it's about being a part of the collective

assessment and care on a day-to-day basis. Therefore, vital signs are not a task to be abandoned or left to others once we feel comfortable with the skill.

The other important thing for nursing students to remember is that they will increasingly be able to recognize and understand deviations in vital signs assessment as they increasingly are familiar with normal findings. It may seem boring to take four dozen BP measurements from healthy college students during a college health fair. But knowing what normal is like helps us recognize when something is not right. So my advice to nursing students is to take every opportunity to hone your skills as part of patient care and as part of developing expertise.

(personal reflection of Hannah, BN, RN)

RESEARCH

BLOOD PRESSURE TARGETS IN PATIENTS WITH DIABETES

Hypertension is a common issue in patients with diabetes and significantly contributes to the development of both the macrovascular and microvascular complications of diabetes. For example, people with diabetes have a 2 to 7 times greater risk of cardiovascular problems, and the United Kingdom Prospective Diabetes Study (UKPDS) noted that the risk of microvascular disease increases by 13% for each 10 mmHg rise in diabetic patient's systolic BP (Culleton et al., 2008). In addition, the risk of MI and death also rose by 12% for each 10 mmHg increase in systolic BP (Culleton et al., 2008).

Because of the poor outcomes associated with high BP in people with diabetes, the Canadian Diabetes Association Clinical Practice Guidelines Expert Committee (2008) recommends that target BP levels in diabetic patients should be below 130/80 mmHg. The evidence for this recommendation is based on several major research studies including the UKPDS, the Hypertension Optimal Treatment (HOT) trial, the Appropriate Blood Pressure Control in Diabetes (ABCD) randomized control trial, and the Pittsburgh Epidemiology of Diabetes Complications Study (Culleton et al., 2008). The UKPDS and HOT trial found that clinically significant reductions in both microvascular and macrovascular complications, cardiovascular death, and diabetes-related death were seen in the lowest BP groups (Culleton et al., 2008). The ABCD study also noted a direct relationship between higher systolic BP levels and death, coronary artery disease, nephropathy, and proliferative nephropathy (Culleton et al., 2008). Finally, the Pittsburgh Epidemiology of Diabetes Complications Study reported statistically significant relationships between cardiovascular complications and mortality as systolic BP levels rose

(continued on page 444)

BLOOD PRESSURE TARGETS IN PATIENTS WITH DIABETES (CONTINUED)

above 115 mmHg and diastolic BP levels rose above 80 mmHg (Culleton et al., 2008).

This is but one example of how research informs health-care professional's practice around vital sign interpretation.

Culleton, B., Drouin, D., LaRochelle, P., Leiter, L. A., McFarlane, P., & Tobe, S. (2008). Treatment of hypertension. Canadian Journal of Diabetes, 32, s115–s118.

Communicating and Teaching About Vital Signs

The nurse has an important role to play in communicating with other health professionals, teaching patients about their health, and administering comfort measures. After completing a thorough evaluation of vital signs, these findings must be communicated and documented. There are often many opportunities to help patients understand what vital signs measurements mean and why they are important.

Communication With Other Health Professionals

Nurses and nursing students must communicate their vital signs findings with other health professionals. As a student, you are required to inform the nurse who is responsible for your patient about his or her status, particularly in the case of abnormal findings. Furthermore, you will report findings to your instructor. This communication promotes patient safety, quality care, and better outcomes. Remember: Your assessment findings matter! Chart and/or report them in a timely fashion.

There are two primary ways in which we communicate vital signs assessments: through the patient's chart or record and through verbal report. You may record vital signs on a vital signs flow sheet (Fig. 21.10), and you may also write

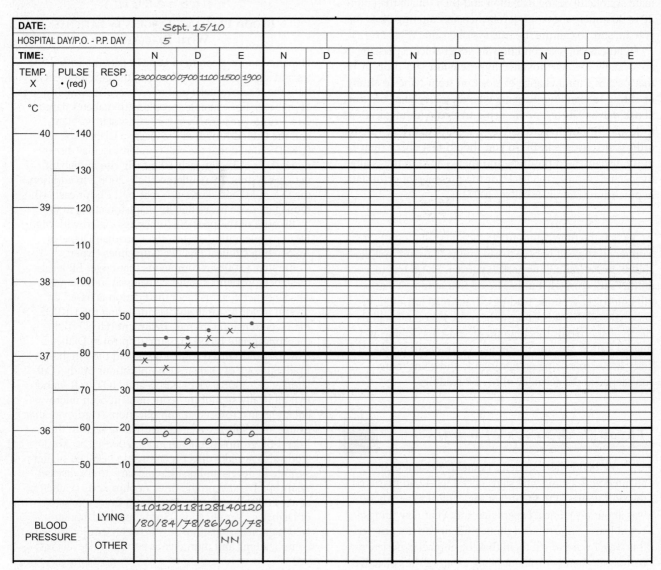

Figure 21.10 Sample vital signs flow sheet.

TABLE 21.7	Abbreviations Used in Vital Signs Charting
Abbreviation	**Definition**
T	**Temperature**
C	Celsius
F	Fahrenheit
P	**Pulse**
bpm	Beats per minute
R	**Respirations**
SpO_2	Oxygen saturation as measured by pulse oximetry
O_2	Oxygen
BP	**Blood pressure**
mmHg	Millimeters of mercury
HTN	Hypertension
Q	Every
Min	Minute
H	Hour

your findings in the nurses' notes or interdisciplinary chart. Table 21.7 lists some of the common abbreviations used in vital signs charting. (A more extensive list of abbreviations can be found in Chapter 23.) You will need to report changes in vital signs and notify your colleagues to monitor them more frequently if the patient is unstable or his or her health status is changing. Box 21.8 contains important information to share verbally when you talk to the nurse in charge about vital signs.

BOX 21.8 Information to Share Verbally When You Talk to the Nurse in Charge About Vital Signs

When reporting vital signs findings to the registered nurse:
1. Introduce yourself, what year you are in, and for whom you are responsible.
2. In your verbal report, include the following:

• Patient's name and room number
• Vital signs in this order: temperature, pulse, respiration, and BP. If measuring SpO_2, include this information also.
• Any other relevant information, particularly in the case of abnormal findings:
  • Temperature (condition of skin—cool or warm to touch, any measures taken to reduce or increase body temperature)
  • Pulse (rate, rhythm, amplitude, whether the patient is receiving medications that alter pulse)
  • Respiration (rate, ease, quality, sounds, whether the patient is receiving oxygen therapy)
  • Blood pressure (presence of auscultatory gap, whether the patient is receiving medications that alter BP)
  • Your plan of care related to vital signs findings
  • When you plan to measure vital signs next

3. Ask the nurse if he or she has any questions.

If the facility uses electronic charting you may also enter them directly into an electronic record. (See Fig. 21.11 for an example of an electronic health record you may use.)

Working Collaboratively

As a nurse, you will be working alongside other health-care workers, particularly practical nurses and unregulated health-care workers (e.g., health-care aides, nursing assistants, and personal care attendants) throughout your nursing career. As a student, it is unlikely you will delegate vital signs to other health-care workers. Still, it is important to remember that you are responsible for having accurate knowledge of your patient and of his or her vital signs. Provide leadership by acknowledging the important contributions of all caregiving staff and support them by using an empowering and collaborative approach to patient assessment and care. All caregivers have an important role to play in the provision of optimal patient care.

Patient Teaching

Teaching patients about their health, illness, and healing is an important part of nursing. As a nursing student, you may have mixed feelings about patient teaching. You may think, "What do I know that I can teach them?" If you are assessing a patient's vital signs, you may think, "What is there to teach?" You may have to suspend your disbelief in your abilities or in the value of this information. As a student, all of the theory is fresh in your mind as you approach a patient. What better approach is needed for patient teaching than the thorough, systematic, and theory-based you have been exploring as a nursing student?

Teaching is a wonderful way in which to interact with your patients. In the student role, you may have the time to teach or you may more easily recognize teachable topics that other care providers have overlooked due to familiarity. Professionals deal with this information every day; however, for patients, this may be new information. Does the patient understand why you take vital signs, and what normal values are? As a student, you have a unique relationship with your patients—a learning and caring relationship—and this can help patients understand that your role is not limited to basic care. Patient teaching is a dialogue, and the patient can actually be empowered by the sharing of information and mutual learning that can occur. Patient teaching is a great habit to adopt now, and to integrate into all that you do.

So, when is teaching pertaining to vital signs appropriate?

• Many patients will know what vital signs consist of but may not know why we need this information and what it tells us.
• Many patients measure their own vital signs at home, especially temperature, pulse, and BP. They need to know the correct technique, accurate interpretation of findings, and when they should call 911, their physician, or telehealth or nurse line.

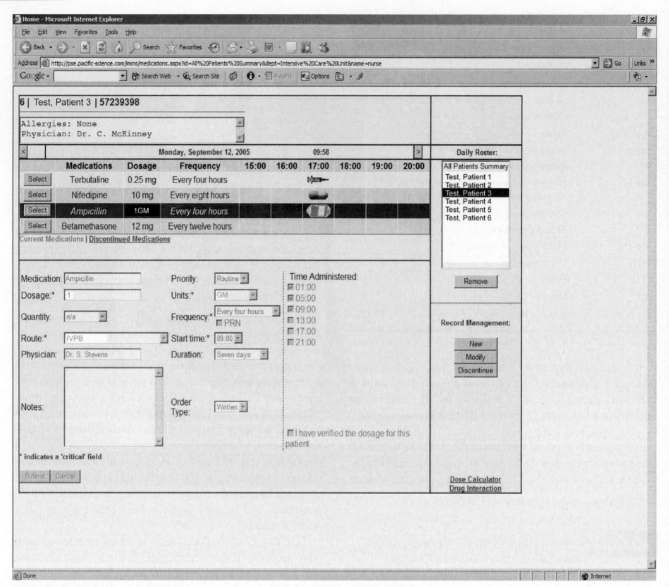

Figure 21.11 Electronic health records are increasingly being used across all health-care settings.

- Patients on medications that alter vital signs—especially for BP or HR—need to monitor and interpret their own vital signs accurately.
- Parents often do not know what course of action to pursue when their child has a fever. This is a significant area of teaching in emergency and pediatric departments.

Through the eyes of a patient

I was recently admitted to the hospital, during which time my heart medications were changed. I was fortunate to have a nursing student, Gurvir, participate in some of my care. I like the way Gurvir took the time to explain procedures and medications to me. He treated me like I knew something, even though I am not a health professional. This meant a lot to me. One of the medications I was put on was digoxin. I didn't know anything about it, so I asked Gurvir. He explained in *everyday language* that digoxin is a medication that slows down the heart and strengthens my heart's contractions. Then, it occurred to me that I'd heard that digoxin comes from a plant, so I asked Gurvir about that. He said he didn't know but would check and get back to me. Gurvir came back half an hour later and said that indeed, digoxin is a purified extract from the foxglove plant. He then thanked me for asking such a great question because he had learned something, too! My advice to nursing students is to not worry if you don't know something but to just let the patient know that you will find out and get back to him or her. None of us knows everything, and we are all learning all the time. As a patient, it feels good to know that I was part of a student's education.

(personal reflection of a patient)

In teaching patients about vital signs, it's helpful to capitalize on teachable moments. These are moments when the teaching is highly relevant to what is happening for the patient. Perhaps you are taking a patient's BP; you can ask him, "So, do you know what I'm measuring when I take your blood pressure?" Or, when you get the BP reading, you can tell the patient the results and then ask him, "Do you understand what these numbers mean?" For obvious reasons, teachable moments do not include situations when the patient's condition is poor or deteriorating. A patient in a respiratory crisis is not going to really care about respiratory homeostasis—better to wait until he or she has stabilized and in a learning frame of mind. Box 21.9 lists common teaching areas for vital signs.

Adults tend to want to learn when it will help them solve a problem. As nurses, we can capitalize on a mutual problem as we engage the patient in his or her own care. For example, we can engage the patient in a discussion around a vital sign deviation: "Phil, your pulse is still high. What I'm thinking about is that your body is compensating for something I can't see. Sometimes, a high pulse can mean several different things, so I'm going to need to find out." It's also beneficial for adult patients to build on what they already know. For example, you can build on a mother's previous experience when teaching her how to better use a tympanic thermometer. You could say, "So, Mary, you've used a tympanic thermometer for your son's temperature reading. That's good. You're getting some good measurements. Why don't you try pulling on the ear like this to make the readings a little better?"

Finally, always document the teaching you have done. This alerts other members of the interdisciplinary team and enables them to build on your teaching. It also protects you in the event that the patient's learning (or lack thereof) becomes a critical antecedent to a change in health status.

Comfort Measures

All patients seek comfort. As nurses, it is easy to fall into the trap of focusing on the skill but not on care and comfort, especially as we attend to routine tasks such as vital signs. Remember that patients are vulnerable people who are experiencing imbalance at this moment in their lives due to illness. When taking vital signs, make sure the patient is comfortable before, during, and after assessing his or her vital signs; return them to a position of comfort after assessing vital signs. Whenever possible, choose less invasive techniques of measurement. Use a therapeutic and gentle approach when touching the patient; remember that the patient is a person, not merely a source of vital signs data. Finally, if you have raised the patient's bed, make sure you return it to a safe height to prevent the patient from falling and injury and return side rails to the appropriate level for that patient.

Putting It All Together: Vital Signs and Patient Care

Now that you have some background information about the various vital signs, and how they are measured correctly, it is time to apply this knowledge to your nursing practice decisions. Vital signs are valuable in terms of understanding your patient's status, and they inform numerous clinical decisions you make on an ongoing basis.

BOX 21.9 **Common Teaching Areas for Vital Signs**

Temperature
- What is the range of normal body temperature?
- What is abnormal body temperature? When should a patient be concerned? When should a patient seek medical attention for abnormal temperature?
- If the patient is young, do his or her parents know how to take accurate measurements of temperature? Do his or her parents know how to medicate and treat a fever?
- What is the correct technique for taking a temperature at home?
- What other signs and symptoms can be present with fever?
- What should a patient do if he or she thinks his or her thermometer is wrong?
- How should thermometers be stored in the home?
- What are common sources of error in home thermometry (especially with tympanic thermometers)?
- How can patients and their families prevent the spread of infection when sharing thermometers?
- How are glass thermometers used? How should they be stored and handled?

Pulse
- What is pulse and what does it indicate?
- What is a normal pulse?

- How do cardiac medications affect pulse?
- How can pulse be checked?

Respirations
- What is a normal respiratory rate?
- If the patient is young, do his or her parents know what a normal respiratory rate is? Do they know what to look for in terms of rate, depth, and adventitious breath sounds? Do they know when to seek medical attention?

Blood Pressure
- What is BP?
- What does the systolic versus the diastolic pressure mean?
- What is high BP?
- How do BP medications work?
- How can a patient take an accurate BP at home? What is the correct use of home BP monitors?
- When should a patient seek medical attention for altered BP?
- What other signs and symptoms can be present with high (or low) BP?
- What should a patient do if he or she thinks his or her automatic BP monitor is wrong?

Vital Signs and Medications

Many medications have the potential to affect your patient's vital signs, and measuring vital signs is often a key step in determining the effectiveness of certain medications. Sometimes, the effect of medication on a vital sign is a desired or therapeutic effect. For example, beta-adrenergic blockers are medications that intentionally slow the HR to decrease cardiac muscle workload and oxygen demand, and they also lower a patient's BP by decreasing CO. In this case, the desired effect is lowered HR and lowered BP, so if these changes are noted in response to this medication, then the medication is deemed effective. Sometimes, even a significant deviation from normal values may be a desirable therapeutic outcome.

Alternately, sometimes, the effect on vital signs represents an undesirable side effect of a medication. Opiate pain medications are primarily administered to manage moderate to severe pain in patients; however, if the dose is too high, an undesirable effect can be slower respirations resulting in the patient being unable to maintain adequate oxygenation.

Baseline vital signs can be used to determine if it is safe to administer a particular medication. It is important to know your patient's current BP in the context of his or her BP history before administering any antihypertensive medication. If an individual's BP is already below an acceptable level, then administering an antihypertensive has the potential to lower BP to dangerously low levels.

The examples provided in this section represent only a small sample of all the possible medication and vital signs interactions. It is your responsibility as a nurse to be familiar with your patient's medications, anticipate potential effects on your patient's vital signs, and monitor for these possible outcomes. In Table 21.8, several common classes of medications and their potential influences on vital signs are identified.

Vital Signs and Health Conditions

Vital signs are significant indicators of your patient's status in several essential areas, including thermoregulation, cardiovascular functioning, and respiratory and oxygenation status. Vital signs can inform many aspects of the nursing management of your patient's condition, which is why regular vital signs are an essential part of your regular patient assessment. It would be impractical to explain all the possible influences of vital sign data on the management of your future patients, but the following examples are provided to illustrate how vital signs might influence your care.

Imagine that you are caring for a patient who is suffering from a serious wound infection and a fever of 39°C. The patient is receiving intravenous antibiotics to treat the infection; he may also receive acetaminophen (Tylenol) to lower his fever so he is more comfortable. In making the decision about whether to give the patient acetaminophen or not, you will measure his body temperature to determine if administering this medication is appropriate. If you give acetaminophen for fever, you will also need to measure the patient's temperature about 30 minutes after administering the medication to determine if the medication was effective in lowering the fever and continue to monitor the patient's body temperature to determine if subsequent doses of acetaminophen will be needed in the near future. As the wound infection resolves due to the antibiotics, you may notice that your patient is no longer suffering from a fever, and this provides evidence that the infection is resolving and that the current approach to treatment is working.

In another example, imagine that you are caring for a patient following abdominal surgery. In the immediate postoperative period, your patient's BP was noted to be 130/80 mmHg and her pulse was 80 beats/minute. Two hours after the patient is returned to the surgical floor,

TABLE 21.8	Some Examples of Medication Classes and Potential Vital Signs Effects
Medication Class	**Potential Effect on Vital Signs**
Opiate analgesics (e.g., morphine)	Lowered respiratory rate, lowered pulse, lowered BP, or orthostatic hypotension
Cardiac glycosides (e.g., digoxin)	Lowered HR, lowered BP
Beta-adrenergic blockers (e.g., Betalol)	Lowered HR, lowered BP
Antihypertensives (e.g., calcium channel blockers, angiotensin-converting enzyme inhibitors, angiotensin receptor blockers, etc.)	Lowered BP, possible elevated HR, potential for orthostatic hypotension
Antipyretics (e.g., acetaminophen, acetylsalicylic acid [ASA])	Potential to lower body temperature to normal if the patient has a fever

Please note there are numerous medication effects on vital signs, and you should note potential vital signs effects as part of your medication research.

Source: Karch, A. M. (2008). *2009 Lippincott's nursing drug guide.* Philadelphia, PA: Lippincott Williams & Wilkins.

however, she starts to complain about increasing abdominal pain and your postoperative vital signs assessment indicates that her BP has dropped to 100/60 mmHg and her pulse has increased to 100 beats/minute. You decide to contact the surgeon to assess the patient because increased pain accompanied by decreasing BP and increasing pulse rate could indicate that your patient has postoperative internal bleeding. In your nursing practice, always remember that vital signs can provide you with useful information about your patient, especially when considered within the context of the entire patient assessment and medical history. As you research different medical conditions, consider what vital signs are the most important to monitor for your patient and incorporate this knowledge into your plan of care. For special situations in which a patient has tested positive for an antibiotic-resistant organism (ARO), see Box 21.10.

Frequency of Vital Sign Measurement

Vital signs are usually assessed on a routine schedule in most health-care settings, and frequency may be further indicated by a patient's physician or a protocol. However, keep in mind that these guidelines represent only the minimum frequency that vital signs should be completed. As the nurse coordinating the care for the patient, it is sometimes necessary to change the frequency of vital sign measurement based on the patient's changing condition. For example, your patient might have vital signs assessment scheduled every 4 hours, but if his BP or pulse is unstable, you may want to check these vital signs more frequently. Likewise, you may use vital signs to assess the effectiveness of a treatment approach or a medication, requiring you to check them at a time other

than the routine scheduled time. Nurses use their clinical judgment and discretion in assessing vital signs as needed as part of a comprehensive plan of care.

Technology and Vital Sign Measurement

The health-care environment has seen an infusion of technological innovation over the past few decades. Nurses will see even more application of technology in coming years in the forms of new equipment, treatment approaches, computer based record keeping, and information systems.

Consider the use of technology in the measurement of vital signs: electronic and tympanic thermometers, non-invasive BP monitors, pulse oximeters, vital signs monitors, and remote monitoring devices. In many cases, the addition of these new technologies to measure vital signs has helped health-care professionals to deliver care more efficiently, easily, and comprehensively. The increased use of electronic health records has also meant that vital signs measurements can be entered into the electronic flow sheet so that health professionals can readily see vital signs trends, and this data can be used as part of informed clinical decision-making.

With the increase in telehealth, telemedicine, and videoconferencing technologies, it is possible for a patient's vital signs and condition to be monitored at a distance, so that expertise and support from major health-care centres can be shared with rural and remote health-care facilities (Whitten, 2006). Technology for continuous and/or remote measurement of vital signs and other physiological data includes both wireless applications, which enable remote vital sign monitoring on mobile smart phones and telemetry devices that monitor patients' vital signs and other parameters and transmit this information to a remote location such as a nurses' station.

BOX 21.10 **Vital Signs Assessment and Antibiotic-Resistant Organisms**

Antibiotic resistant organisms (AROs) such as methicillin-resistant *Staphylococcus aureus* (MRSA) and vancomycin-resistant enterococci (VRE) are increasingly a part of health-care clinical realities. These organisms are not always more virulent, but they are resistant to antibiotic treatment. In addition to standard precautions (taken for all patients), hand hygiene is the most effective way to prevent the transmission of organisms. If a patient in an acute care setting or other high-risk situation has tested positive for an ARO, special isolation precautions will need to be taken to protect other patients. When assessing an ARO-positive patient's vital signs,

- Follow isolation and/or ARO precautions, as per the agency.
- Make sure there is a dedicated stethoscope, BP cuff, thermometer, IV pole, and other patient care items to remain in the patient's room for the duration of the isolation period. If equipment cannot be dedicated, ensure that it is cleaned and disinfected as appropriate to the item prior to reuse with another patient.
- Avoid taking the patient chart into the patient's room.

Avoiding Overreliance on Technology

You may be wondering why you are still expected to learn how to do vital signs manually with the presence of automated machines that can do some of these functions for you. Sole reliance on technology to assess a vital signs such as pulse will mean that you will only obtain a rate without any knowledge of other pulse qualities, such as rhythm, quality, and amplitude. Clearly, you would be missing important assessment data if your patient has an irregular heartbeat or develops arrhythmias that you do not pick up because you only used a machine to assess the pulse. Additionally, you should double-check abnormal pulse and BP readings manually if you doubt your findings (Schell, 2006). For example, you may find that a patient's BP is very low when taken with an automatic machine, when the patient normally has a much higher BP. In a situation like this, you should take a manual reading to confirm your findings. Always keep in mind that technology is a very useful tool when used correctly, but it does not replace the need to apply your specialized nursing knowledge and judgment in the usage and interpretation of vital signs data (Dragon, 2006). Furthermore, as nurses, we cannot overlook the importance of human touch, even in something as fundamental and routine as vital signs. When you do use higher technological instruments, remember to focus on the patient, not the equipment.

Now that Tracy has obtained the fundamental skills and knowledge required to assess vital signs, she feels confident and excited to continue working on accurate assessment in the clinical setting. She commits herself to take vital signs whenever possible in the clinical setting, so she learns the nuances of accurate vital signs measurement. Tracy is also excited to learn more nursing skills. She realizes that with diligence and practice, she can be successful in performing any nursing skill that comes her way. She has also learned that performance of the nursing skill is only one part of the puzzle. It also takes good understanding of the related principles and physiology, critical thinking, and nursing judgment in order to use these skills effectively in her nursing practice.

Conclusion

Throughout this chapter, you have learned a great deal about the four core vital signs and oximetry and how to measure these in your nursing practice. Although you will soon become proficient in the measurement of vital signs to a point where the process will become routine, always remember that the measurement of the vital signs values is only the first step.

Vital signs assessment is a skill that requires practice to both gather the data and interpret the data. The use of technology cannot replace understanding the subtle nuances of vital signs assessment. Nurses need to know when and how to use technology, know its limitations, and know when to confirm unusual findings manually or with low-tech equipment.

Using your specialized nursing knowledge and judgment to interpret your patients' vital signs in the context of their other assessment findings, treatment plan, and medical history, ensures that this data becomes a valuable tool in the delivery of safe and effective patient care.

SKILL 21.1	Measuring Temperature

Reviewing Pertinent Information

Step	Rationale
Review the patient's chart and the patient care plan. • Check how often temperature is to be measured. • Check the patient's record to see if temperature is altered, if signs and symptoms are present that would require more frequent checks, and if the patient is receiving treatment for altered body temperature. • Check to see which method of measurement is being used with the patient and if the patient's condition is best suited to a particular method. • Determine the most appropriate route to measure the temperature. • Check to see if the patient has received medication that might affect temperature, such as an antipyretic.	It is important to know if the patient requires routine screening and monitoring or if the patient has an altered temperature or signs and symptoms that require increased monitoring of temperature. It is also important to be consistent in how a patient's temperature is measured because each method may yield slightly different results.
Review patient allergies.	Some patients may be allergic to latex and other substances associated with taking vital signs. Avoid exposing patients to allergens.
Review the applicable thermoregulatory principles and temperature norms you expect based on the patient's chart, expected physiological norms for the patient's age and gender, and expected measurement based on the chosen route and device.	Knowing the thermoregulatory mechanism can aid in monitoring for altered temperature. This information is also useful when teaching your patient.
Make sure you understand how to use the measuring device effectively. Some units do not need to be turned on and turn on automatically once a probe cover is attached. Some methods of thermometry are more susceptible to nurse error.	Being familiar with the measuring device eliminates the possibility of error, thus enhancing patient safety and patient care.

Preparing for Measuring

Step	Rationale
Perform hand hygiene.	Hand washing prevents the spread of microorganisms to the supplies being used and prevents further spread to the patient.
Gather supplies needed:	Organization will make sure the procedure is comfortable for the patient and efficient for you.
• Disposable gloves (only if you will be contacting blood or body fluids or if you are taking a rectal temperature)	
• Digital oral thermometer, digital rectal thermometer, or tympanic membrane thermometer	
• Water-soluble lubricant (for rectal temperature only)	
• Probe cover	
• Note pad and pen	
Prepare the equipment:	Transmission of heat radiation through a dirty sensor can alter the reading, especially with tympanic membrane temperatures.
• Ensure the thermometer is charged and ready for use.	
• Ensure sensory components are free of debris, clean, and ready for use.	
Prepare the patient:	
• Introduce yourself, if the patient may be unfamiliar with you.	Introducing yourself establishes your role as professional care provider and increases the patient's comfort level.
• Confirm the patient's identity by checking the patient armband and then asking the patient to verify name.	Checking patient identification helps ensure you are taking the correct patient's temperature.
• Oral: Check with the patient to ensure he or she has not consumed hot or cold foods in the last 15 minutes.	Ensuring the patient has not consumed hot or cold foods in the last 15 minutes contributes to accuracy of the reading.
• Axillary: Check with the patient to ensure he or she has not bathed in the last 15 minutes.	
• Temporal artery: Ensure the patient is not diaphoretic and that the temporal artery region is accessible to you and not impacted by a wound or scar tissue.	
• Tympanic: See Box 21.4 for potential sources of error in tympanic membrane thermometry.	
• Check for latex allergies (indicated on the armband).	
• Explain the measurement process and purpose of temperature measurement and provide an explanation if a more invasive route than that with which the patient is familiar is used.	Explaining the purpose of the procedure and why it's important fosters patient collaboration and integration into the care and diagnostic process.
• Adjust the bed or chair height and create privacy by drawing the curtains or closing the door.	Adjusting the bed height can help prevent back injuries.
• Provide patient teaching about temperature measurement.	Patients who are more knowledgeable about the process are usually more comfortable asking questions.
	Teaching can provide the necessary understanding that will foster more effective outcomes through patient participation.

Measuring Oral Temperature with a Digital Thermometer

Step	Rationale
Apply disposable gloves if you will be in contact with blood or body fluids.	Gloves will protect the patient from surface organisms from the nurse's hands and will protect the nurse from possible body secretions that may come into contact with the nurse's hands during the procedure.

(continued on page 452)

SKILL 21.1   Measuring Temperature (continued)

Measuring Oral Temperature with a Digital Thermometer (continued)

Step

Withdraw the oral probe and apply a disposable probe cover, which should snap into place (see Figure 1) . If required, push the "on" button and wait for the "ready" signal on the thermometer. (Some units turn on when the probe cover is attached—follow manufacturer's directions.)

Rationale

Covering the probe prevents contamination and prevents the spread of infection between patients.

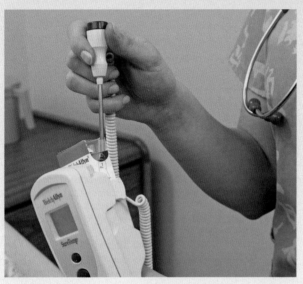

Figure 1

Note: Some digital thermometers have two probes: one for oral temperatures and one for rectal temperatures. Do not use these interchangeably.

Ask the patient to open his or her mouth. Place the probe under the patient's tongue in the left or right posterior sublingual pocket (see Figure 2). Ask the patient to close his or her lips around the probe.

Taking oral temperature from the left or right sublingual pocket results in a more accurate temperature measurement, whereas under the centre of the tongue results in lower readings.

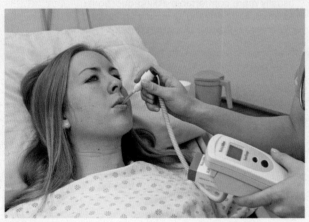

Figure 2

Measuring Oral Temperature with a Digital Thermometer (continued)

Step

Hold the probe until the thermometer beeps.

Remove the probe from the patient's mouth. Note the temperature reading.

Dispose of the probe cover into the garbage by pressing the release button (see Figure 3).

Rationale

Holding the probe ensures it does not move out of place.

The thermometer will beep when it has completed the measurement.

Making a note of the temperature reading is important because most devices have an auto-off function, and the reading may be lost.

Helps prevent the spread of microorganisms

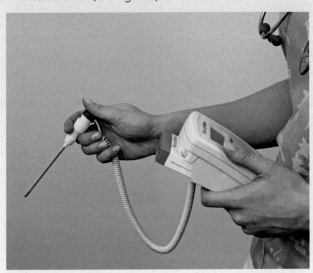

Figure 3

If you raised the bed, lower it now to make the environment safe for the patient.

Return the probe to the holder and return the thermometer to its charging unit (if applicable).

Perform hand hygiene.

Helps prevent falls

Ensures it is ready for next time it is needed

Hand washing prevents the spread of microorganisms.

Measuring Tympanic Membrane Temperature with an Infrared Digital Thermometer

Step

Apply disposable gloves if you will be in contact with blood or body fluids.

If required, visually or with an otoscope, inspect the ear and tympanic membrane for obstructions, debris, or cerumen. It may also be advantageous to view the placement of the tympanic membrane with an otoscope prior to taking the temperature.

Apply a disposable probe cover, which should snap into place. If required, push the "on" button and wait for the "ready" signal on the thermometer. (Some units turn on when the probe cover is attached—follow manufacturer's directions.)

Rationale

Gloves will protect the patient from surface organisms from the nurse's hands and will protect the nurse from possible body secretions that may come into contact with the nurse's hands during the procedure.

A common source of error with tympanic thermometry is an obstructed tympanic membrane. Ensuring there are no obstructions increases the accuracy of the measurement.

Covering the probe prevents contamination and prevents the spread of infection among patients.

(continued on page 454)

SKILL 21.1   Measuring Temperature (continued)

Measuring Tympanic Membrane Temperature with an Infrared Digital Thermometer (continued)

Step

Stand at the patient's side at which you will take the temperature. Gently pull the adult patient's pinna (external ear) up and back to straighten the ear canal (see Figure 4). Place the probe into the ear canal as far as it will go but without hurting the patient. Insert the probe into the ear firmly, so that the opening is sealed. Angle the probe toward the patient's jaw. (For a child younger than 2 years old, pull the pinna down and back to straighten the ear canal.)

Rationale

Pulling up and back on the pinna and aiming the sensor toward the patient's jaw results in a more accurate temperature measurement.

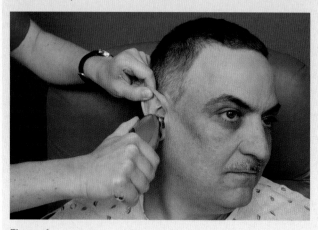

Figure 4

Step	Rationale
Activate the trigger to get the measurement.	A reading will not be taken until the trigger is activated.
Remove the probe from the patient's ear. Note the temperature reading. If the temperature is too high or too low or not what you were expecting based on previous readings or the patient's condition, recheck the temperature in the other ear. Accept the higher reading as the more accurate reflection of core body temperature.	Making a note of the temperature reading is important because most devices have an auto-off function, and the reading may be lost.
Dispose of the probe cover into the garbage by pressing the release button.	Helps prevent the spread of microorganisms
If you raised the bed, lower it now to make the environment safe for the patient.	Helps prevent falls
Return the thermometer to its charging unit (if applicable).	Ensures it is ready for next time it is needed
Perform hand hygiene.	Hand washing prevents the spread of microorganisms.

Measuring Axillary Temperature with a Digital Thermometer

Step	Rationale
Apply disposable gloves if you will be in contact with blood or body fluids.	Gloves will protect the patient from surface organisms from the nurse's hands and will protect the nurse from possible body secretions that may come into contact with the nurse's hands during the procedure.
Assist the patient to a lying (supine, on his or her back) or sitting position. Move clothing away from his or her shoulder.	Increases access to the axilla
Withdraw the oral probe and apply a disposable probe cover, which should snap into place (see Figure 1). If required, push the "on" button and wait for the "ready" signal on the thermometer. (Some units turn on when the probe cover is attached—follow the manufacturer's directions.)	Covering the probe prevents contamination and prevents the spread of infection between patients.

Measuring Axillary Temperature with a Digital Thermometer (continued)

Step	Rationale
Raise the patient's arm and inspect the armpit/axilla for lesions or excessive perspiration. Place the probe in the patient's axilla and return the patient's arm to his side, holding the probe in place (see Figure 5).	Taking axillary temperature from a sustained exposure to local arteries results in a more accurate temperature.

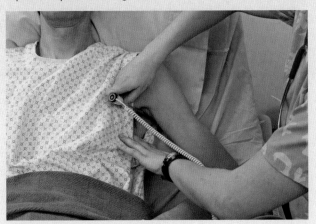

Figure 5

Step	Rationale
Hold the probe until you hear it beep.	Holding the probe ensures it does not move out of place. The thermometer will beep when it has completed the measurement.
Remove the probe from the patient's axilla. Note the temperature reading. Restore patient's clothing.	Making a note of the temperature reading is important because most devices have an auto-off function, and the reading may be lost. Maintain patient comfort and dignity by restoring the patient's clothing.
Dispose of the probe cover into the garbage by pressing the release button (see Figure 3).	Helps prevent the spread of microorganisms
If you raised the bed, lower it now to make the environment safe for the patient.	Helps prevent patient falls
Return the probe to the holder and return the thermometer to its charging unit (if applicable).	Ensures it is ready for next time it is needed
Perform hand hygiene.	Hand washing prevents the spread of microorganisms.

Measuring Temporal Artery Temperature with a Digital Thermometer

Step	Rationale
Apply disposable gloves if you will be in contact with blood or body fluids.	Gloves will protect the patient from surface organisms from the nurse's hands and will protect the nurse from possible body secretions that may come into contact with the nurse's hands during the procedure.
Determine at which part of the patient's forehead to take the temperature. Only obtain a temperature from the side of the head exposed to the environment.	Covered areas tend to insulate the area and can result in falsely high readings.
Remove the protective cap and inspect the lens for cleanliness. Apply a disposable probe cover, which should snap into place. If required, push the "on" button and wait for the "ready" signal on the thermometer. (Some units turn on when the probe cover is attached—follow the manufacturer's directions.)	Covering the probe prevents contamination and prevents the spread of infection between patients.

(continued on page 456)

SKILL 21.1   Measuring Temperature (continued)

Measuring Temporal Artery Temperature with a Digital Thermometer (continued)

Step

Inspect the forehead for excessive perspiration. Position the thermometer flush against the forehead, in the centre, halfway between the hairline and eyebrows (see Figure 6). Press the "scan" button and lightly slide the thermometer straight across the forehead. (If there is perspiration on the forehead, take the temperature behind the ear lobe by first pushing away any hair and exposing the area.

Rationale

Midline on the forehead, the temporal artery is about a millimeter below the skin. Measuring in other sites, such as the side of the face, would result in falsely low readings.

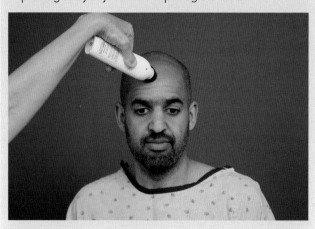

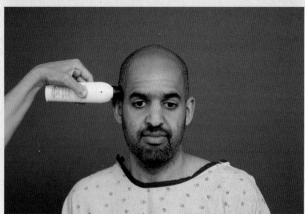

Figure 6

Then, place the thermometer on the neck under the ear lobe, in the soft round depression [see Figure 7].)

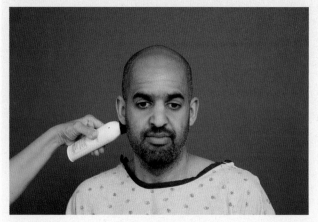

Figure 7

Measuring Temporal Artery Temperature with a Digital Thermometer (continued)

Step	Rationale
Hold the probe in place over the forehead until a reading is obtained, as indicated by the thermometer. Then, release the "scan" button and remove the thermometer from the forehead.	Holding the probe ensures it has opportunity to gather the required temperature data.
Remove the probe from the patient's forehead and note the temperature reading. If you need to take the temperature again, wait about 30 seconds before measuring to avoid excessive cooling of the skin.	Making a note of the temperature reading is important because most devices have an auto-off function, and the reading may be lost.
Dispose of the probe cover into the garbage by pressing the release button. Replace the cap.	Helps prevent the spread of microorganisms; the cap protects the lens when thermometer is not in use.
If you raised the bed, lower it now to make the environment safe for the patient.	Helps prevent falls
Return the probe to the holder and return the thermometer to its charging unit (if applicable).	Ensures it is ready for next time it is needed
Perform hand hygiene.	Hand washing prevents the spread of microorganisms.

Measuring Rectal Temperature with a Digital Thermometer

Step	Rationale
Apply disposable gloves.	Gloves will protect the patient from surface organisms from the nurse's hands and will protect the nurse from possible body secretions that may come into contact with the nurse's hands during the procedure.
Assist the patient onto his or her side, with his or her upper leg flexed at the hip and knee. Rearrange bed linens to keep the patient covered, exposing only the anal area.	Keeping the patient covered will keep him or her more comfortable.
Withdraw the rectal probe and apply a disposable probe cover, which should snap into place (see Figure 8). If required, push the "on" button and wait for the "ready" signal on the thermometer. (Some units turn on when the probe cover is attached—follow manufacturer's directions.)	Covering the probe prevents contamination and prevents the spread of infection between patients.

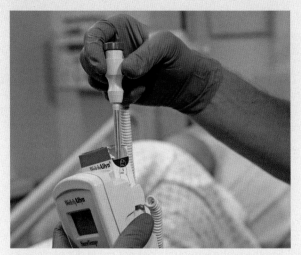

Figure 8

Note: Some digital thermometers have two probes: one for oral temperatures, and one for rectal temperatures. Do not use these interchangeably. The figure shows a digital thermometer with a rectal probe (red) being used.

(continued on page 458)

SKILL 21.1 Measuring Temperature (continued)

Measuring Rectal Temperature with a Digital Thermometer (continued)

Step	Rationale
Apply water-soluble lubricant to the probe cover, up to about 4 cm (see Figure 9).	Lubrication makes insertion easier and less traumatic to rectal tissue.

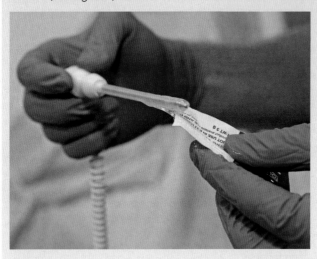

Figure 9

Step	Rationale
Separate the patient's buttocks to expose the anus with your nondominant hand. Encourage the patient to breathe slowly and relax.	Separating the buttocks exposes the anus. Encouraging the patient to breathe and relax helps relax the anal sphincter.
Gently insert the probe into the patient's anus, in the direction of the umbilicus, approximately 3–4 cm in an adult (in an infant 1.25 cm and 2.5 cm in a child). Never force the thermometer if you meet resistance; instead, withdraw the thermometer (see Figure 10).	Gentle insertion, without resistance, protects the rectal tissue from trauma.

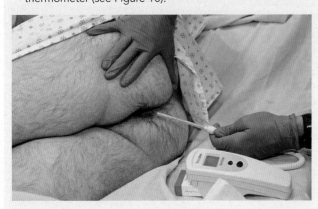

Figure 10

Step	Rationale
Hold the probe until you hear it beep.	Holding the probe ensures it does not move out of place. The thermometer will beep when it has completed the measurement.
Remove the probe from the patient's rectum. Note the temperature reading.	Making a note of the temperature reading is important because most devices have an auto-off function, and the reading may be lost.
Wipe the patient's anal area with a tissue to remove lubricant or feces. Discard tissue.	Cleaning the patient makes him or her feel more comfortable and promotes hygiene.
Dispose of the probe cover into the garbage by pressing the release button.	Helps prevent the spread of microorganisms
If you raised the bed, lower it now to make the environment safe for the patient.	Helps prevent falls
Return the probe to the holder and return the thermometer to its charging unit (if applicable).	Ensures it is ready for next time it is needed
Remove and discard gloves and perform hand hygiene.	Hand washing prevents the spread of microorganisms.

Engaging in Evaluation

Step	Rationale
Assess patient response to temperature measurement. How well did the patient tolerate the procedure?	Noting the patient's response to the procedure is important for notifying future health-care providers of areas of difficulty a patient may have with the assessment.
Determine if the temperature is within a normal range or if it is altered. If the patient is currently being treated for an altered body temperature, determine if the treatments are effective.	Ensures that the temperature measurement is evaluated in light of previous findings
Assess patient for other signs and symptoms that indicate altered body temperature: • Cool or hot to your touch • Sweating (diaphoresis) • Shivering	Ensures that the temperature measurement is considered in light of other physical signs

Documenting Effectively

Step	Rationale
Document temperature in a timely manner: • Document your findings on the vital signs flow sheet, indicating the date and time of the measurement, the route used, and the temperature in *C. • Document your findings in the nurses' notes or interdisciplinary notes, including any other observations, signs, or symptoms indicative of altered body temperature or change in body temperature (including a return to normal). Also note any treatments you administered for altered body temperature and what the physiological response was, and how the patient responded to the assessment (e.g., tolerated well).	Documentation is the key communicative method among health-care professionals. The more complete the documentation, the better able other health-care team members understand the patient's condition. The correct diagnosis and treatment of patients relies heavily on communication of assessment findings.

SKILL 21.2   Assessing Radial and Apical Pulse

Reviewing Pertinent Information

Step	Rationale
Review the patient's chart and the patient care plan. • Check how often pulse is to be assessed. • Check for any baseline HR, if available. • Check the patient's record to see if cardiovascular status or HR is altered, if signs and symptoms are present that would require more frequent checks, and if the patient is receiving treatment for altered cardiovascular status or HR. • Check to see if the patient has received any treatment that might affect HR.	It is important to know if the patient requires routine screening and monitoring or if the patient has an altered cardiovascular status or signs and symptoms that require increased monitoring.
Review patient allergies.	Some patients may be allergic to latex and other substances associated with taking vital signs. Avoid exposing patients to allergens.
Review the applicable cardiovascular principles and norms you expect based on the patient's chart, expected physiological norms for the patient's age and gender, and expected results based on patient status.	Knowing the mechanisms of cardiovascular physiology and the impacts of disease processes can aid in monitoring for altered HR and pulse. This information is also useful when teaching your patient.

Preparing for Assessing

Step	Rationale
Perform hand hygiene.	Hand washing prevents the spread of microorganisms.
Gather supplies needed: • Gloves (only if you will be contacting blood or body fluids) • A watch • Note pad and pen	Organization will make sure the procedure is comfortable for the patient and efficient for you.

(continued on page 460)

SKILL 21.2   Assessing Radial and Apical Pulse (continued)

Preparing for Assessing (continued)

Step	Rationale
Prepare the patient:	
• Introduce yourself, if the patient may be unfamiliar with you.	Introducing yourself establishes your role as professional care provider and increases the patient's comfort level.
• Confirm the patient's identity by checking the patient armband and then asking the patient to verify name.	Checking patient identification helps ensure you are taking the correct patient's pulse rate.
• Check for latex allergies (indicated on the armband).	Explaining the purpose of the procedure and why it's important fosters patient collaboration and integration into the care and diagnostic process.
• Adjust the bed or chair height and create privacy by drawing the curtains or closing the door.	Adjusting the bed height can help prevent back injuries.
• Provide patient teaching about cardiovascular status.	Patients who are more knowledgeable about the process are usually more comfortable asking questions.
	Teaching can provide the necessary understanding that will foster more effective outcomes through patient participation.
Note: Respirations are almost always counted immediately after the patient's pulse is taken and before you let go of the patient's pulse site. Basically, we pretend we are still taking the pulse, but really, we have moved on to counting respirations, so that the patient is unaware we are assessing respiration.	Patients who are aware that we are assessing their respirations become self-conscious about their breathing, which negatively impacts accurate assessment.
• Consider the presence of conditions that would put the patient at risk of altered pulse.	
• Assess patient for the presence of signs and symptoms of altered cardiac function.	
• Assess patient for the presence of factors that impact pulse rate, amplitude, and rhythm (see Table 21.3).	

Assessing Radial Pulse

Step	Rationale
Apply disposable gloves if you will be in contact with blood or body fluids.	Gloves will protect the patient from surface organisms from the nurse's hands and will protect the nurse from possible body secretions that may come into contact with the nurse's hands during the procedure.
Choose the patient's arm that is closest to you and that does not have any constrictive devices above the site. (If counting respirations is to follow, ensure you are able to visualize the rise and fall of the chest. This may mean that bed linens need to be moved. However, keep the patient as covered as possible, without compromising your ability to assess rate and depth of respirations. See Figure 1 to see the location and appropriate method to find and palpate the radial pulse. Count respirations immediately following pulse, without letting go of the patient's wrist.) Keep the patient's lower arm at a comfortable position, either across the abdomen if he or she is lying down or bent at the elbow if he or she is sitting. Keep the lower arm in a natural position.	Using the arm closest to you represents better body mechanics than reaching across the patient. Constrictive devices above the site of pulse assessment can alter the accuracy of assessment.
	Balances the need for correct assessment with the need for privacy and dignity

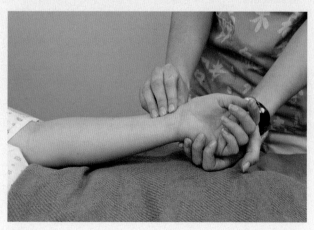

Figure 1

Assessing Radial Pulse (continued)

Step	Rationale
With your dominant palm down, gently grasp the patient's wrist and place the pads of your index and middle fingers over the radial artery (in the groove along the thumb side of the inner wrist) to locate the radial pulse. Press over the radial artery until you detect maximal pulsation. Each pulsation is one beat. If the rhythm is regular and the rate is within a normal range, count the pulse for 30 seconds. Multiply the number of pulsations by 2 to get the rate in beats per minute. If the rhythm is irregular or rate outside of a normal range, count for 1 full minute. Record your findings and compare to previous baseline and established norms.	The index and middle fingers lack a significant pulse (unlike the thumb) so it is relatively easy to distinguish the patient's pulse. By pressing just enough so you detect pulsation, you are not obliterating the pulse but able to assess it fully.
While you are palpating and counting the radial pulse, pay attention to	These are important qualities to assess, in addition to counting a rate.
• the rhythm of the pulsations. Is it regular or irregular? • the amplitude of the pulsations. How strong are they? See Table 21.3 for words nurses use to describe these.	
Perform hand hygiene.	Hand washing prevents the spread of microorganisms.

Assessing Apical Pulse

Step	Rationale
Apply disposable gloves if you will be in contact with blood or body fluids.	Gloves will protect the patient from surface organisms from the nurse's hands and will protect the nurse from possible body secretions that may come into contact with the nurse's hands during the procedure.
Ensure you are able to visualize the chest directly. This may mean that bed linens and gown need to be moved to expose the sternum and left chest. However, keep the patient as covered as possible, without compromising your ability to assess the apical rate.	Balances the need for correct assessment with the need for privacy and dignity
Locate the anatomical landmarks and find the point of maximal impulse (PMI) or apical impulse (see Figure 2).	Using the arm closest to you represents better body mechanics than reaching across the patient. Constrictive devices above the site of pulse assessment can alter the accuracy of assessment.

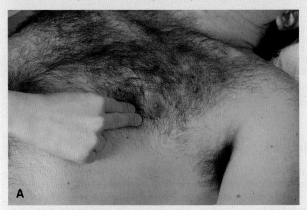

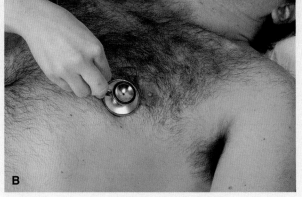

Figure 2

(continued on page 462)

SKILL 21.2   Assessing Radial and Apical Pulse (continued)

Assessing Apical Pulse (continued)

Step	Rationale
Warm the diaphragm of the stethoscope in your palm for a few seconds. Then, place it over the assessment site and auscultate for the lub-dub of the heart sounds. If the rhythm is regular and the rate is within a normal range, count the pulse for 30 seconds. Multiply the number of pulsations by 2 to get the rate in beats per minute. If the rhythm is irregular, the rate outside of a normal range, or the patient receiving cardiovascular medication, count for 1 full minute. While you are auscultating and counting the apical pulse, pay attention to • the rhythm of the heart sounds. Are they regular or irregular? Is the irregularity regular or irregular? • any other heart sounds you notice If you cannot find the pulse, ask the patient to lie in a left lateral position. This moves the heart toward the left chest wall and moves the apical impulse further to the left (Weber, 2006).	Warming the stethoscope makes the procedure more comfortable for the patient. Assessing other qualities, in addition to counting, yields important information about the patient's cardiovascular system and health status.
Compare radial pulse to apical pulse. Note any discrepancy (pulse deficit).	A pulse deficit can indicate various heart conditions.
Assist the patient to restore his or her gown and bed linens. Return the bed to a safe height for the patient.	Restoring clothing contributes to patient dignity. Restoring bed height helps prevent falls.
Record your findings and compare to previous baseline and established norms.	Ensures your evaluation is shared with other caregivers Ensures your assessment is interpreted in light of previous findings and norms
Perform hand hygiene. Clean stethoscope chestpiece with an equipment wipe.	Hand washing prevents the spread of microorganisms. Cleaning the chestpiece between patients prevents the spread of microorganisms.

Engaging in Evaluation

Step	Rationale
Assess patient response to pulse assessment. How was the procedure for the patient? Was the patient able to cope with the procedure or was it painful?	Noting the patient's response to the procedure is important for notifying future health-care providers of areas of difficulty a patient may have with the assessment.
Determine if the pulse rate, rhythm, amplitude, and equality are within normal ranges or if it is altered. If the patient is currently being treated for altered HR or cardiovascular disease status, determine if the treatments are effective. Assess patient for other signs and symptoms that indicate altered cardiovascular status.	Ensure interpretation of pulse occurs in the context of the cardiovascular system and relevant treatments.

Documenting Effectively

Step	Rationale
Document pulse in a timely manner: • Document your findings on the vital signs flow sheet, including the date and time, beats per minute, and note unexpected or new findings by flagging the documentation and recording in the nurses' notes. • Document your findings in the nurses' notes or interdisciplinary notes, including any other observations, signs, or symptoms indicative of altered cardiovascular status (including a return to normal if previously abnormal). As well, record any treatments you administered for altered cardiovascular status and what the response was.	Documentation is the key communicative method among health-care professionals. The more complete the documentation, the better able other health-care team members understand the patient's condition. The correct diagnosis and treatment of patients relies heavily on communication of assessment findings.

SKILL 21.3   Assessing Respirations and Oxygenation

Reviewing Pertinent Information

Step	Rationale
Review the patient's chart and the patient care plan. • Check how often respirations and oxygenation are to be assessed. • Check for any baseline respiratory rate and oxygenation data, if available, both on room air and on oxygen (if applicable). • Check the patient's record to see if respiration or oxygenation status is altered, if signs and symptoms are present that would require more frequent checks, and if the patient is receiving treatment for altered respiration or oxygenation status. • Check to see if the patient has received any treatment that might affect respiration or oxygenation status. • Review any related laboratory values (arterial blood gases [ABGs], SpO_2, and complete blood count [CBC], with particular attention to the hemoglobin values)	It is important to know if the patient requires routine screening and monitoring or if the patient has an altered respiration or oxygenation status or signs and symptoms that require increased monitoring.
Review patient allergies.	Some patients may be allergic to latex and other substances associated with taking vital signs. Avoid exposing patients to allergens.
Review the applicable respiration and oxygenation principles and norms you expect based on the patient's chart, expected physiological norms for the patient's age and gender, and expected results based on patient status.	Knowing the mechanisms of respiration and the impacts of disease processes can aid in monitoring for altered respirations. This information is also useful when teaching your patient.

Preparing for Assessing

Step	Rationale
Perform hand hygiene.	Hand washing prevents the spread of microorganisms.
Gather supplies needed: • Disposable gloves (only if you will be contacting blood or body fluids) • A watch • Note pad and pen • Pulse oximeter with finger probe	Organization will make sure the procedure is comfortable for the patient and efficient for you.
Prepare the patient: • Introduce yourself, if the patient may be unfamiliar with you. • Confirm the patient's identity by checking the patient armband and then asking the patient to verify name. • Check for latex allergies (indicated on the armband). • Adjust the bed or chair height and create privacy by drawing the curtains or closing the door. • Provide patient teaching about respiratory and oxygenation status.	Introducing yourself establishes your role as professional care provider and increases the patient's comfort level. Checking patient identification helps ensure you are measuring the correct patient's respiration rate or oxygenation data. Explaining the purpose of the procedure and why it's important fosters patient collaboration and integration into the care and diagnostic process. Adjusting the bed height can help prevent back injuries. Patients who are more knowledgeable about the process are usually more comfortable asking questions. Teaching can provide the necessary understanding that will foster more effective outcomes through patient participation
Note: It is helpful if the patient is unaware that you are assessing his or her respiration rate. If the patient becomes aware that you are counting his or her respirations, he or she will become self-conscious about his or her breathing, and the rate will change. For this reason, respirations are almost always counted immediately after the patient's pulse is taken and before you let go of the patient's pulse site. Basically, we pretend we are still taking the pulse, but really, we have moved on to counting respirations.	

(continued on page 464)

SKILL 21.3   Assessing Respirations and Oxygenation (continued)

Assessing Respiratory Rate

Step	Rationale
Apply disposable gloves if you will be in contact with blood or body fluids.	Gloves will protect the patient from surface organisms from the nurse's hands and will protect the nurse from possible body secretions that may come into contact with the nurse's hands during the procedure.
Ensure you are able to visualize the rise and fall of the chest. This may mean that bed linens need to be moved. However, keep the patient as covered as possible, without compromising your ability to assess rate and depth of respirations.	Balances the need for correct assessment with the need for privacy and dignity
• Watch the rise and fall of the patient's chest. Each complete respiratory cycle (one inspiration and one expiration) counts as one breath. Once you have observed one full cycle, check your watch and begin counting the rate for the required time.	Ensures that full cycles are being observed and counted
While you are watching the rise and fall of the chest, pay attention to • the depth of the respirations • if there is any sound associated with breathing • the pattern or rhythm of breathing See Table 21.4 for words nurses use to describe these.	Ensures that your assessment of respiration is not limited to counting breaths per minute but rather considers the adequacy and ease of ventilations
If the rhythm is regular, count respirations for 30 seconds. Multiply the number of breaths by 2 to get the rate per minute. If the rhythm is irregular, count for 1 full minute. Record your findings and compare to previous baseline and established norms.	Sixty-second observations always provide greater accuracy.
Perform hand hygiene.	Hand washing prevents the spread of microorganisms.

Assessing Pulse Oximetry/Oxygenation Status

Step	Rationale
Apply disposable gloves if you will be in contact with blood or body fluids.	Gloves will protect the patient from surface organisms from the nurse's hands and will protect the nurse from possible body secretions that may come into contact with the nurse's hands during the procedure.
If required, push the "on" button and wait for the "ready" signal on the oximeter (follow manufacturer's directions).	
If the patient is on oxygen therapy, note • if it is continuous or intermittent, • how recently it has been started prior to measuring oximetry, • what the rate of flow is, and • the route of delivery (mask or nasal prong/cannula).	Considers the assessment findings in light of existing treatment
Ask the patient to provide a finger. Ensure that the site is warm and has good circulation, free of soiling (including dried blood), and free of nail polish. Ensure the skin is intact. Do not take pulse oximetry on the same limb as the patient's BP is being done.	Taking oximetry readings from a site that is warm, has good circulation, is free of nail polish and soiling will result in a more accurate reading. Pulse oximetry readings can be hindered by constriction above the site, as in taking BP simultaneously on the same limb.

Assessing Pulse Oximetry/Oxygenation Status (continued)

Step
Place the probe over the finger. Position it securely and
symmetrically and not too tightly. Figure 1 shows how to
correctly position the probe.

Rationale
If the probe is too tight, it may obstruct the blood flow and
reduce accuracy of the readings.

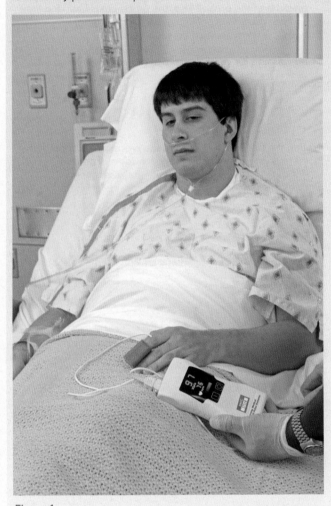

Figure 1

Check to ensure the oximeter is providing a reading.
It should be recognizing a pulse wave that corresponds
with the radial pulse. Once the oxygen level registers and
stabilizes (up to 5 minutes), make note of the number. It will
be provided as a percentage. If the number is not what you
expected or if it is unusually high or low, recheck using a
different finger (or toe).

Correct positioning should result in accurate readings.
Checking your findings in conjunction with other assessment
findings ensures that findings are considered in context,
to enhance patient safety and outcomes.

(continued on page 466)

SKILL 21.3   Assessing Respirations and Oxygenation (continued)

Assessing Pulse Oximetry/Oxygenation Status (continued)

Step	Rationale
If the SpO$_2$ is to be monitored continuously, reposition the probe every 1 or 2 hours.	Prevents skin breakdown at the site of measurement from pressure of the probe. Also, the probe emits heat and light and can cause burns if left in place for too long.
Remove the probe.	
Decontaminate and return the probe to the holder and return the thermometer to its charging unit (if applicable).	Ensures it is ready for next time it is needed.
Perform hand hygiene.	Hand washing prevents the spread of microorganisms.

Engaging in Evaluation

Step	Rationale
Assess patient response to respiratory and oxygenation assessment.	
How was the procedure for the patient? Was the patient able to cope with the procedure or was it painful?	Noting the patient's response to the procedure is important for notifying future health-care providers of areas of difficulty a patient may have with the assessment.
Determine if the respiration rate, depth, and pattern is within a normal range or if it is altered. Determine if the oxygenation is within a normal range or if it is altered. If the patient is currently being treated for altered respirations or oxygenation, determine if the treatments are effective.	Ensures the assessment findings are considered in the context of the patient, norms, and treatments
Assess patient for other signs and symptoms that indicate altered respiratory status. • Bluish colour (cyanosis) of lips or mucous membranes • Restlessness • Difficult breathing (dyspnea) • Adventitious breath sounds	Ensures that assessment findings are considered in light of other findings

Documenting Effectively

Step	Rationale
Document respiration and oxygenation in a timely manner: • Document your findings on the vital signs flow sheet, including the date and time, breaths per minute, oxygen saturation as a percentage, and whether the patient was receiving oxygen therapy, the route (nasal prongs [NP], nasal cannula [NC], or mask), and the rate of flow; if the patient is not on oxygen, document as on room air (on "RA"). • Document your findings in the nurses' notes or inter-disciplinary notes including any other observations, signs, or symptoms indicative of altered respiratory status or change in body oxygenation (including a return to normal if previously abnormal). Also document any treatments you administered for altered respiratory or oxygenation status and what the response was to the assessment itself and any treatments given.	Documentation is the key communicative method among health-care professionals. The more complete the documentation, the better able other health-care team members understand the patient's condition. The correct diagnosis and treatment of patients relies heavily on communication of assessment findings.

SKILL 21.4 Measuring Blood Pressure (Brachial)

Reviewing Pertinent Information

Step	Rationale
Review the patient's chart and the patient care plan. • Check how often BP is to be assessed. • Check baseline BP readings, if available. • Check the patient record to see if cardiovascular status or BP is altered, if signs and symptoms are present that would require more frequent checks, and if the patient is receiving treatment for altered cardiovascular status or BP. • Check to see if the patient has received any treatment/medications that might affect BP. Review patient allergies.	It is important to know if the patient requires routine screening and monitoring or if the patient has an altered cardiovascular status or signs and symptoms that require increased monitoring.
	Some patients may be allergic to latex and other substances associated with taking vital signs. In particular, many BP cuffs contain latex. Avoid exposing patients to allergens.
Review the applicable cardiovascular principles and norms you expect based on the patient's chart, expected physiological norms for the patient's age and gender, and expected results based on patient status.	Knowing the mechanisms of cardiovascular physiology and the impacts of disease processes can aid in monitoring for altered BP. This information is also useful when teaching your patient.

Preparing for Assessing

Step	Rationale
Perform hand hygiene.	Hand washing prevents the spread of microorganisms.
Gather supplies needed: • Disposable gloves (only if you will be contacting blood or body fluids) • Sphygmomanometer (make sure you select the correct cuff size for your patient). The inflatable bladder must cover 80% of the upper arm's circumference, and the cuff width should be at least 40% of the circumference of the arm. • Stethoscope (if an electronic/digital machine is being used this is not necessary) • Note pad and pen	Organization will make sure the procedure is comfortable for the patient and efficient for you.
Prepare the patient: • Introduce yourself, if the patient may be unfamiliar with you.	Introducing yourself establishes your role as professional care provider and increases the patient's comfort level.
• Confirm the patient's identity by checking the patient armband and then asking the patient to verify name.	Checking patient identification helps ensure you are taking the correct patient's BP.
• Check for latex allergies (indicated on the armband).	Explaining the purpose of the procedure and why it's important fosters patient collaboration and integration into the care and diagnostic process.
• Adjust the bed (preferably into an elevated semi- or high-Fowler's position) or ensure the patient is seated comfortably with his or her back supported, legs uncrossed, for at least 5 minutes before measuring BP with the arm supported at the level of the heart.	Adjusting the bed height can help prevent back injuries, and correct patient posture helps to ensure BP readings are accurate.
• Create privacy by drawing the curtains or closing the door. • Provide patient teaching about cardiovascular status.	Patients who are more knowledgeable about the process are usually more comfortable asking questions.
• Consider the presence of conditions that would put the patient at risk of altered BP. • Assess patient for the presence of signs and symptoms of altered cardiovascular function.	Teaching can provide the necessary understanding that will foster more effective outcomes through patient participation.
• Assess patient for the presence of factors that impact BP (see Box 21.7). • Determine the most appropriate site to measure blood pressure. See Box 21.6 for possible sites to avoid.	Being aware of the factors that affect the accurate measurement of BP and sites to avoid helps to ensure that BP measurement will be carried out accurately and without harm to the patient.

Measuring Blood Pressure

Step	Rationale
Apply disposable gloves if you will be in contact with blood or body fluids.	Gloves will protect the patient from surface organisms from the nurse's hands and will protect the nurse from possible body secretions that may come into contact with the nurse's hands during the procedure.

(continued on page 468)

SKILL 21.4   Measuring Blood Pressure (Brachial) (continued)

Measuring Blood Pressure (continued)

Step	Rationale
Assist the patient to assume a comfortable lying or sitting position. Support the patient's forearm closest to you at the level of the patient's heart, with his palm upward (see Figure 1). Expose the brachial artery. Move loosened clothing above where the cuff will be placed. If a sleeve is too tight to be moved about the cuff site, you may need to ask the patient to slip his arm out of the sleeve.	Using the arm closest to you represents better body mechanics than reaching across the patient. Constrictive devices above the site of assessment can alter the accuracy of assessment.

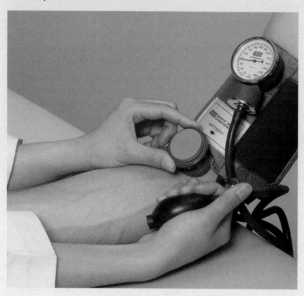

Figure 1

Step	Rationale
Palpate the brachial artery. Place an appropriately sized cuff on the upper arm, with the centre of the bladder directly over the brachial artery (some cuffs identify this centre point with an arrow labeled "artery") and the tubing should be pointing toward the wrist. Place the lower edge of the cuff 2–3 cm above the antecubital fossa; the cuff should be applied smoothly and snugly around the upper arm.	Correct sizing and placement of the cuff will improve the accuracy of the BP measurement.
Ensure that the needle on an aneroid manometer or the mercury in a mercurial manometer is at zero.	If the manometer is not reading "zero" before applying pressure to the cuff, the accuracy of the reading will be affected. Note: An aneroid manometer should be calibrated every 6–12 months by referencing it against a mercury manometer to ensure its accuracy.
Estimate the patient's systolic pressure manually using palpation. Palpate the brachial or radial artery pulse. Tighten the screw valve on the pump, without cinching it closed. Inflate the cuff while palpating the artery. Make a mental note of the level (mmHg) at which the pulse disappears. Deflate the cuff promptly and wait 15–30 seconds. (If reading a mercury manometer, read the level in the column at eye level to ensure an accurate reading.)	Provides an estimate of the systolic pressure and helps to avoid the potential for error from an auscultatory gap Waiting 15–30 seconds allows the blood to circulate through the arm and ensures the auscultated BP is not impacted by the previous cuff inflation.
Position the stethoscope in your ears with the earpieces tilted slightly forward.	Correct placement of the stethoscope in your ears assists you to auscultate the BP clearly.
With your nondominant hand, place and hold the bell or diaphragm of the stethoscope over the brachial artery. Make sure it does not touch clothing or the cuff. Keep your fingers as still as possible and avoid touching the tubing of the sphygmomanometer or the stethoscope. With your dominant hand, hold the pump, tighten the valve, and inflate the cuff until the pressure is 20–30 mmHg above the estimated systolic pressure.	Although BP can be auscultated using the bell or the diaphragm, many experts suggest that the bell is better to hear the low-pitched Korotkoff sounds. Inadvertently touching the stethoscope or sphygmomanometer tubing can create artifact noise that makes it hard to hear the Korotkoff sounds clearly. Inflating the cuff to a level that is 20–30 mmHg over estimated systolic pressure temporarily occludes blood flow in the arm.

Measuring Blood Pressure (continued)

Step	Rationale
Gently open the valve with the thumb and forefinger of your dominant hand (the hand that is holding the pump). Slowly allow the cuff to deflate at a rate of 2–3 mmHg per heartbeat or per second. Note the mmHg at which the first clear (even if faint) Korotkoff (Phase I) sound appears. This is the systolic pressure. Continue slowly deflating the cuff. Note the mmHg at which the Korotkoff sounds become muffled (Phase IV) and can no longer be heard. This level is the diastolic pressure. If the sounds do not disappear, use Phase IV as the diastolic reference.	Deflating the cuff slowly improves the accuracy of the BP reading and assists you to hear the first and last Korotkoff sounds.
Release the remaining air quickly.	Allows the complete restoration of blood flow to the lower arm
If you are concerned that the reading is not accurate, wait 30–60 seconds before repeating it. Make sure the cuff is completely deflated before attempting a second BP.	Allows circulation to return to normal in the arm before repeating BP measurement
Remove the cuff and return the equipment. Sanitize the equipment as required.	Ensures the equipment is available for use by another person Sanitizing the equipment prevents the spread of infection.
Record your findings as measured to 2 mmHg without rounding and compare to previous baseline and established norms.	Recording finding immediately and to the nearest 2 mmHg ensures that the accurate measurement is retained in the patient record.
Perform hand hygiene. Clean the stethoscope chestpiece with an equipment wipe.	Hand washing prevents the spread of microorganisms. Cleaning the chestpiece between patients prevents the spread of microorganisms.

Engaging in Evaluation

Step	Rationale
Assess patient response to BP assessment. How was the procedure for the patient? Was the patient able to cope with the procedure or was it painful?	Noting the patient's response to the procedure is important for notifying future health-care providers of areas of difficulty a patient may have with the assessment.
Determine if the BP is within a normal range or if it is altered. If the patient is currently being treated for altered BP or cardiovascular disease, determine if the treatments are effective.	Interpreting the BP within the context of normal values and the patient's individual history enables you to determine its significance.
Assess patient for other signs and symptoms that indicate altered BP or cardiovascular status. For example, • Headache, flushing, dizziness (elevated BP) • Weakness, dizziness or syncope on standing (low BP or orthostatic hypotension) • Peripheral edema, pulmonary edema, distended jugular venous pressure (cardiac failure, circulatory overload)	Interpreting BP readings in the context of other cardiovascular signs and symptoms contributes to a comprehensive assessment of patient status.

Documenting Effectively

Step	Rationale
Document BP in a timely manner: • Document your findings on the vital signs flow sheet, including the date and time, the systolic and diastolic pressures (expressed as a fraction) to the nearest 2 mmHg, and the position the patient was in during measurement. Note unexpected or new findings by flagging the documentation and recording in the nurses' notes. • Document your findings in the nurses' notes or interdisciplinary notes. Include any other observations, signs, or symptoms indicative of altered BP or cardiovascular status (including a return to normal if previously abnormal). Include any treatments you administered for altered BP or cardiovascular status and what the response was. Finally, document the patient's response to BP measurement.	Documentation is the key communicative method among health-care professionals. The more complete the documentation, the better able other health-care team members understand the patient's condition. The correct diagnosis and treatment of patients relies heavily on communication of assessment findings.

Critical Thinking Case Scenarios

▶ Mrs. Ferguson underwent a left radical mastectomy (surgical removal of the breast and surrounding lymph nodes) 2 days ago to treat breast cancer. She has a large surgical incision on the left side of her chest and has been having incisional pain when she moves. What are the key vital signs to monitor in Mrs. Ferguson? Why? What is the influence of Mrs. Ferguson's surgical history and current condition on your approach to vital sign measurement and potential findings?

1. What is the potential influence of surgery and a surgical incision on temperature, pulse, respirations, BP, and SpO_2 level?
2. Are there any considerations related to performing vital signs on an individual that has had a mastectomy?
3. How might the pain from the chest incision affect the vital signs?

▶ Mr. Brown has been admitted to hospital due to a chest infection (pneumonia) and has a history of chronic obstructive pulmonary disease (COPD) secondary to smoking one pack of cigarettes per day for the past 30 years. COPD is caused by damage to the airways and lungs over time, which affects the ability of the lungs to exchange oxygen effectively, and can lead to excessive mucous production and even air trapping in the lungs. What influence might Mr. Brown's condition have on his vital signs? Why?

1. What effect would COPD have on Mr. Brown's respiratory rate and/or his SpO_2?
2. Can chronic lung disease contribute to changes in pulse and BP?
3. How frequently would you monitor Mr. Brown's temperature?
4. What effect might cigarette smoking have on Mr. Brown's vital signs?

▶ You are scheduled to do a home visit with Mrs. White who has had three myocardial infarctions (heart attacks, also abbreviated "MI") in the past 2 years that have severely damaged her heart muscle and contributed to the development of congestive health failure and an irregular heartbeat (arrhythmia). Congestive heart failure is characterized by congestion of the heart with blood and ineffective cardiac contraction, which can lead to fluid in a patient's lungs (pulmonary edema) and peripheral swelling (edema), especially in the legs and feet. As part of your assessment of Mrs. White's condition, you plan to take her vital signs. Based on her history and condition, what are the main things you need to consider in completing her vital signs? Consider the potential effect on temperature, pulse, respirations, BP, and SpO_2, and how you will assess and record these vital signs.

1. When assessing Mrs. White's pulse, what qualities are you going to consider given the fact she has a history of a cardiac arrhythmia?
2. How might congestive heart failure affect the HR and BP readings?
3. What effect do you think congestive heart failure might have on respirations?
4. Is the monitoring of body temperature important for someone with congestive heart failure?

Multiple-Choice Questions

1. Which of the following set of vital signs would be considered to be normal for a healthy 50-year-old male?
   a. T = 37.5°C, P = 90 beats/min, R = 20 breaths/min, BP = 150/95 mmHg
   b. T = 39°C, P = 55 beats/min, R = 22 breaths/min, BP = 130/70 mmHg
   c. T = 36.5°C, P = 120 beats/min, R = 18 breaths/min, BP = 100/60 mmHg
   d. T = 37.2°C, P = 85 beats/min, R = 16 breaths/min, BP = 125/75 mmHg

2. What would be the best approach to obtain an accurate BP in a patient with a known auscultatory gap?
   a. Use the auscultatory method with a manual sphygmomanometer.
   b. Use the palpatory method to estimate the systolic pressure prior to auscultating the BP with a manual sphygmomanometer.
   c. Use an oscillometric automatic BP machine and an appropriately sized thigh cuff.
   d. Use an ABPM to decrease the influence of white coat syndrome on the auscultatory gap.

3. Which of the following pulse rates would be indicative of tachycardia?
   a. 96 beats/min
   b. 55 beats/min
   c. 110 beats/min
   d. 85 beats/min

4. The accuracy of respiratory rate assessment can be affected if the patient becomes self-conscious about the fact his or her respirations are being counted. An effective strategy to deal with this problem is:
   a. Count the respirations first before the other vital signs so that temperature, pulse, and BP measurement will not affect the patient's respirations.
   b. Count the respirations while still holding the patient's wrist following assessment of pulse rate, so that the patient is not aware that you are counting his or her respirations.
   c. Rely on the patient's self-reported respiratory rate.
   d. Wait until the patient is sleeping to count his or her respiratory rate.

5. Mr. Smith has the following vital signs: T = 37.4°C, P = 90 beats/min, R = 18 breaths/min, BP = 145/90 mmHg, SpO$_2$ = 96%. Based on these vital signs, what is Mr. Smith's pulse pressure?
   a. 90 mmHg
   b. 72 mmHg
   c. 55 mmHg
   d. 145 mmHg

6. Mrs. Harris is being treated for hypertension and has been experiencing a sudden drop in BP and dizziness when she stands after being seated. While explaining the reason for these symptoms, you explain that this phenomenon is called:
   a. Orthostatic hypotension
   b. White coat hypotension
   c. Orthostatic hypertension
   d. Systolic hypertension

7. When using a tympanic thermometer to take the temperature of a 1-year-old girl, what is the correct technique for straightening the ear canal to obtain the most accurate temperature reading?
   a. Pull the pinna gently up and back.
   b. Pull the pinna gently up while the child is lying down.
   c. Pull the pinna gently down while the child is seated in their parent's lap.
   d. Pull the pinna gently down and back.

8. When assessing an infant's peripheral pulse rate, the most appropriate peripheral pulse site to assess is the:
   a. Radial pulse
   b. Popliteal pulse
   c. Dorsalis pedis
   d. Brachial pulse

Suggested Lab Activities

● Students can explore the factors that will affect the accuracy of temperature measurement in small groups by first taking temperature using incorrect technique and comparing these temperature readings with readings obtained using correct technique.
   a. First, take someone's temperature with a tympanic thermometer without carefully placing the probe properly into the ear canal and straightening the ear canal with an ear tug (up and back). Then, take the same person's temperature using correct placement of the probe in the ear canal. Did you notice any difference in the readings?
   b. Using an electronic thermometer and the oral temperature probe, first take a fellow student's temperature with the probe placed anywhere in the mouth other than under the tongue. Record the reading and then repeat the process with the same person under the following conditions: with the probe placed properly under the tongue and mouth closed,

with the probe under the tongue and the mouth open, and finally after drinking a cold glass of water. What differences did you note with the incorrect techniques as opposed to the correct technique?
   c. Using an electronic thermometer with the oral temperature probe, take a volunteer's axillary temperature using the correct technique and dwell time. Take the same person's axillary temperature without placing the probe properly in the axilla. Did you notice any difference in the two readings?
   d. Using a volunteer, take an oral temperature, axillary temperature, and tympanic temperature using correct technique in all cases. Is there any difference in the temperature reading based on the site used? What implications might this have for your interpretation of temperature readings?

● Students will practice assessing a patient for the presence of orthostatic hypotension by auscultating a student's BP following changes in body position.
   a. Have a student lie down flat on a bed or stretcher for 5 minutes and then take the BP using correct technique and record the results.
   b. Have the student move to a seated position and measure the BP again. Was there any change?
   c. Finally, have the student stand and repeat the BP reading one more time. Was there any change in the BP reading?

Please note: Younger adults who are not receiving medication to treat BP are not as susceptible to orthostatic hypotension because their BP compensatory mechanisms react quite quickly, so an actual change in BP may not always be noted during this exercise.

● Students can assess the potential effect of several activities on temperature, pulse, BP, and respirations.
   a. Take a baseline set of vital signs (T, P, R, BP, SpO$_2$) on a volunteer while he or she has been at rest for at least 5 minutes.
   b. Have the volunteer do some kind of aerobic exercise (running, brisk walking, jogging on the spot, jumping jacks, etc.) for 5 minutes. Retake all the vital signs. What changes did you note? If there are changes in the vital signs, theorize about why these changes happened.
   c. If possible, ask the volunteer to drink a hot cup of coffee. After 5 minutes, recheck their vital signs. Were there any changes in any of the vital sign readings? Why?
   d. Ask the volunteer to meditate or take slow deep breaths with his or her eyes closed in a quiet environment for 5 to 10 minutes. Following this period, take the volunteer's vital signs. Were there any changes in the vital signs? Why or why not?

● Current recommendations suggest that a patient's BP should be taken with his or her arm in a supported position, at approximately the level of the heart. Students can examine the influence of arm position on BP readings by first taking a student's BP with his or her arm in a supported position, then with the arm raised, and then with the arm hanging by the students side. Did arm position affect BP readings for the student?

a. In a group of three students, have two students take the third student's radial pulse simultaneously on both sides. One student should determine the pulse based on a 15-second count, whereas the other should take the pulse rate based on a count for a full minute. Was there a difference in the HR determined using the two approaches? What are the implications of taking a patient's pulse for 15 seconds as opposed to 30 seconds or a full minute?

REFERENCES AND SUGGESTED READINGS

Bell, D. R. (2008). Control mechanism in circulatory function. In R. A. Rhoades & D. R. Bell (Eds.), *Medical physiology: Principles for clinical medicine* (3rd ed., pp. 305–318). Philadelphia, PA: Lippincott Williams & Wilkins.

Bianchi, J., Zamiri, M., Loney, M., McIntosh, H., Daw, R. S., & Douglas, W. S. (2008). Pulse oximetry index: A simple arterial assessment for patients with venous disease. *Journal of Wound Care, 17*(6), 253–260.

Bickley, L. S. (2009). *Bates guide to physical examination and history taking* (10th ed.). Philadelphia, PA: Lippincott Williams & Wilkins.

Booker, R. (2008). Pulse oximetry. *Nursing Standard, 22*(30), 39–41.

Braine, M. E. (2009). The role of the hypothalamus, part 1: The regulation of temperature and hunger. *British Journal of Neuroscience Nursing, 5*(2), 66–72.

Canadian Diabetes Association. (2008). 2008 Clinical practice guidelines for the prevention and management of diabetes in Canada. *Canadian Journal of Diabetes, 32*(Suppl. 1), S1–S201.

Canadian Hypertension Education Program. (2012). *2012 CHEP recommendations for the management of hypertension.* Retrieved from http://www.hypertension.ca/chep-recommendations

Canadian Paediatric Society. (2013). *Temperature measurement in paediatrics. Position Statement.* Retrieved from: http://www.cps.ca/documents/position/temperature-measurement

Casa, D. J., Becker, S. M., Ganio, M. S., Brown, C. M., Yeargin, S. W., Roti, M. W., . . . Maresh, C. M. (2007). Validity of devices that assess body temperature during outdoor exercise in the heat. *Journal of Athletic Training, 42*(3), 333–342.

Cretikos, M. A., Bellomo, R., Hillman, K., Chen, J., Finfer, S., & Flabouris, A. (2008). Respiratory rate: The neglected vital sign. *Medical Journal of Australia, 188*(11), 657–659.

Culleton, B., Drouin, D., LaRochelle, P., Leiter, L. A., McFarlane, P., & Tobe, S. (2008). Treatment of hypertension. *Canadian Journal of Diabetes, 32*, s115–s118.

DeMeulenaere, S. (2007). Pulse oximetry: Uses and limitations. *The Journal for Nurse Practitioners, 3*(5), 312–317.

Dragon, N. (2006). Patient care in a technological age. *Australian Nursing Journal, 14*(1), 16–19.

Drouin, D., & Milot, A. (Eds.). (2007). *Hypertension therapeutic guide* (3rd ed.). Montreal, QC: The Quebec Hypertension Society.

El-Radhi, A. S., & Barry, W. (2006). Thermometry in paediatric practice. *Archives of Disease in Childhood, 91*(4), 351–356.

Giantin, V., Toffanello, E. D., Enzi, G., Perissinotto, E., Vangelista, S., Simonato, M., . . . Sergi, G. (2008). Reliability of body temperature measurements in hospitalised older patients. *Journal of Clinical Nursing, 17*(11), 1518–1525.

Hooper, V. D., & Andrews, J. O. (2006). Accuracy of noninvasive core temperature measurement in acutely ill adults: The state of the science. *Biological Research for Nursing, 8*(1), 24–34.

Hypertension Canada. (2013). *Hypertension: The silent killer.* Retrieved from https://www.hypertension.ca/

Kaplan, N., Mendis, S., Poulter, N., & Whiteworth, J. (2003). 2003 World Health Organization (WHO)/International Society of Hypertension (ISH) statement on management of hypertension. *Journal of Hypertension, 21*(11), 1983–1992.

Latman, N. S. (2003). Clinical thermometry: Possible causes and potential solutions to electronic, digital thermometer inaccuracies. *Biomedical Instrumentation and Technology, 37*(3), 190–196.

Lawson, L., Bridges, E. J., Ballou, I., Eraker, R., Greco, S., Shively, J., & Sochulak, V. (2007). Accuracy and precision of noninvasive temperature measurement in adult intensive care patients. *American Journal of Critical Care, 16*(5), 485–496.

Lockwood, C., Conroy-Hiller, T., & Page, T. (2004). Vital signs. *JBI Reports, 2*, 207–230.

Mackechnie, C., & Simpson, R. (2006). Traceable calibration of blood pressure and temperature monitoring. *Nursing Standard, 21*(11), 42–47.

Marieb, E. N., & Hoehn, K. (2007). *Human anatomy and physiology* (7th ed.). San Francisco, CA: Benjamin Cummings.

Moore, T. (2007). Respiratory assessment in adults. *Nursing Standard, 21*(49), 48–57.

Moran, J. L., Peter, J. V., Solomon, P. J., Grealy, B., Smith, T., Ashforth, W., . . . Peisach, A. R. (2007). Tympanic temperature measurements: Are they reliable in the critically ill? A clinical study of measures of agreement. *Critical Care Medicine, 35*(1), 155–164.

Robinson, J. L., Jou, H., & Spady, D. W. (2005). Accuracy of parents in measuring body temperature with a tympanic thermometer. *BMC Family Practice, 6*(3), 1–8.

Royal College of Nursing. (2007). *Standards for assessing, measuring and monitoring vital signs in infants, children and young people.* London, United Kingdom: Author.

Schell, K. A. (2006). Evidence-based practice: Noninvasive blood pressure measurement in children. *Pediatric Nursing, 32*(3), 263–267.

Sessler, D. I. (2008). Temperature monitoring and perioperative thermoregulation. *Anesthesiology, 109*(2), 318–338.

Skillen, D. L. (2012). General survey and vital signs assessment. In T. C. Stephen, D. L. Skillen, R. A. Day, & S. Jensen (Eds.), *Canadian Jensen's nursing health assessment: A best practice approach* (pp. 91–124). Philadelphia, PA: Lippincott Williams & Wilkins.

Stebor, A. D. (2005). Basic principles of noninvasive blood pressure measurement in infants. *Advances in Neonatal Care, 5*, 252–261.

Weber, J. (2006). *Health assessment in nursing* (3rd ed.). Philadelphia, PA: Lippincott Williams & Wilkins.

Whitten, P. (2006). Telemedicine: Communication technologies that revolutionize healthcare services. *Generations, 30*(2), 20–24.

Wolf, L. (2007). How normal are "normal vital signs"? Effective triage of the older patient. *Journal of Emergency Nursing, 33*(6), 587–589.

Woodrow, P. (2005). Recognising acute deterioration. *Nursing Older People, 17*(5), 31–32.

Principles and Practice of Medication Administration

CHRISTY RAYMOND-SENIUK, NADINE MONIZ, AND DAVID GREGORY

Jonathan is a second-year nursing student starting his first medical-surgical clinical placement. He reads the course outline and wonders what it will be like giving medications. Jonathan is worried about the difficulty of this skill and wonders how he might learn the steps necessary to master this skill.

CHAPTER OBJECTIVES

By the end of this chapter, you will be able to:

1. Appreciate the student and nurse perspectives related to medication administration.
2. Understand how practice standards inform medication administration practice.
3. Describe basic pharmacological principles.
4. Describe principles of patient safety and documentation related to the administration of medications in nursing practice.
5. Use the process of medication administration for various administration routes and procedures.
6. Discuss how culture, communication, and comfort impact the practice of medication administration.

KEY TERMS

Adverse Drug Event A patient injury that occurs after receiving the wrong medication or after not receiving a required medication.

Ampoule A small, sealed, and sterile glass container that generally holds a single dose of a liquid.

Aspiration Pulling back on the syringe plunger after needle insertion but before injection.

Automated Dispensing Cabinet Computerized system that stores and provides drugs and supplies to users.

Controlled Substances Drugs or medications that have some potential for abuse or dependence and are regulated and monitored provincially and federally.

Gastrointestinal (GI) Tube A tube inserted through the nose or into the stomach; sometimes used to feed a patient or administer medications to a patient.

High-Alert Medications Drugs that have a significant impact on human health if given incorrectly.

Human Factors Design A branch of engineering dedicated to understanding and correcting poor work design equipment.

Independent Double Check A safety check done by a second nurse and completed without prompting or communication between the nurses used to verify that a process done by the first nurse is correct.

Intradermal Inside the dermal layer of the skin below the epidermis.

Intramuscular (IM) Inside a muscle.

Medication Administration Record (MAR) A document that keeps track of medications that are prescribed and administered to patients. MARs may be handwritten, computer-generated from the pharmacy medication profile, or fully electronic (eMAR).

Needleless An intravenous (IV) administration system of tubing that includes blunt-end cannulas and valve systems to connect tubing together without using needle connectors.

Needle Shield A protective cover that fits over the needle of a syringe.

Needlestick Injuries Injuries from the syringe of a needle.

Patient Identification The places that identify an individual patient (e.g., the patient's wrist band) and used to verify patient's name and hospital identification number.

Patient Safety Reducing the risk of patient harm associated with healthcare system factors.

Pharmacology The science related to the preparation, properties, uses, and effects of drugs.

PRN Medication A medication given to a patient as needed after the patient is assessed by a nurse.

Puncture The act of piercing, typically with a sharp-pointed implement, such as a needle.

Rights of Medication Administration Safety checks a nurse completes before and during medication administration that include the right medication, right dose, right time, right route, right patient, right patient education, right documentation, right to refuse, right assessment, and right evaluation.

(continued on page 474)

Subcutaneous The loose connective tissue between the skin and muscle.

Therapeutic Effect The body's expected or intended response to a medication.

Three Checks in Medication Preparation A three-level safety comparison designed to prevent medication error. The nurse compares the medication to the medication order and patient identity three times to prevent a medication error.

Transdermal A medication route in which a drug is applied topically through the skin and the absorbed into the bloodstream.

Vial A small glass or plastic container with a rubber seal on top that holds liquid medication or solutions.

When the public is asked what a nurse does, they might answer that nurses give needles. This simplistic account does not do justice either to nursing or to the art and science of medication administration. Giving medications encompasses caring, compassion, critical thinking, and strict attention to patient safety. Some nursing students cannot wait to give medications, whereas other nursing students may fear this skill. This chapter focuses on the knowledge, skills, and best practice guidelines you need to be competent, safe, and efficient while administering medications.

In this chapter, we discuss core knowledge concepts associated with giving medications to patients. We discuss the critical thinking associated with medication administration; this involves integrating knowledge associated with the skills and concepts in relation to giving medications. We also think about being a responsible nurse who administers medications according to specific steps and processes and who adopts a holistic approach to patient care. Finally, we integrate all these concepts as they apply to interacting with and understanding patients and interprofessional colleagues when giving medications.

Medication administration entails the following:

- Knowing: You have to know your medications and why they are being prescribed. This includes knowing the side effects, incompatibilities, concentrations, and so forth. Why are these particular medications relevant to the care of your patient?
- Thinking: You cannot just memorize things, you've got to understand them; moreover, you'll need to bring previous knowledge to bear on your current patient care situations.
- Manual dexterity: This becomes easier with practice; drawing up medications may seem difficult at first—but you will get the hang of it; the adage "Practice Makes Perfect" applies here.
- Caring: A powerful synthesis of compassion, thorough assessment skills, application of patient safety principles, and organized care based on nursing priorities.

The Nurse and Student Perspectives

Let's begin with the nursing student's perspective—an important starting point for learning about thoughts, opinions, and knowledge development that will come about as you develop this important skill. You can also check the changes to knowledge and thinking within "The Nurse's Perspective" section. The practice standards and legal aspects are reviewed to give you a more complete picture of the complexity of safe

medication administration. By understanding the perspectives and contexts of medication administration in nursing, you will be prepared to administer medications in hectic, constantly changing, and complex patient care environments.

Jonathan, our second-year nursing student, said, "As a new student, I am afraid of giving the wrong medication to an individual and causing them harm. I know I need to be extra diligent with medication administration, but how do I ensure I do not make a mistake in the busy health-care setting? I think you really have to know a lot before you give any medication. What sort of things do I need to know?"

The Nursing Student's Perspective

Nursing students may have many perspectives when it comes to medication administration. Some students have fears concerning the extent of knowledge needed to give medications and initially worry about the skills involved in administering medications safely. Medication administration is one of the most closely supervised skills engaged in by nursing instructors. Expressing concern about safe and accurate medication administration is natural; these healthy fears may assist you to adequately prepare for medication administration (Box 22.1). Fear is not helpful when it immobilizes you at

---

BOX 22.1 **Preparing for Medication Administration**

Students can feel more confident if they have thoroughly prepared for administering medications by looking into the following areas before administering any medications:

- Preparing—knowledge and understanding regarding specific medications
- Practicing in the skills lab to ensure that the student has a baseline sense of comfort with his or her skills
- Understanding the rationale for the use of specific medications with particular patients
- Comprehending the administration of medications within the context of the patient's entire care plan
- Incorporating medication administration within the context of overall nursing care priorities and planned nursing work for the morning, afternoon, and/or entire shift or setting
- Understanding that medication administration has several phases: preparation, patient encounter and medication administration, evaluation, and documentation

the time of administration. Both students and faculty members should work together to reduce the stress of medication administration to a realistic level so as to ensure that the skill is carried through (Box 22.2). Students must work toward safe medication administration that follows agency policies/procedures and provincial regulations and standards.

Through the eyes of a nurse

I am always nervous on Day 1 when students are giving medications for the first time. I think that there is so much stress in the medication room; this tension doesn't really help a student learn. The students who spend most of their time copying and memorizing the drug book and not really thinking about their patients and why they need the medication are often the most nervous. It is really important that students are prepared and understand the rationale for the medications they are administering as well as basic information about how they work and possible side effects. Learning medications takes time, and nursing instructors have the ability and capacity to really foster calmness in a student.

(personal reflection of a nurse)

The Nurse's Perspective

Nurses are more comfortable than nursing students when it comes to medication administration. Being a nurse means that one is accountable for his or her own actions, and fears typically associated with medication administration usually subside as the nurse gains ongoing experience and expertise. However, there are always new medications and new information and uses for older medications. This means that one is constantly learning about medications and the numerous reasons for administration. The practicing nurse needs to know when the medication being administered is a new one and then assume responsibility for looking up any new information before giving a medication to a patient. The practicing nurse always considers professional standards and policies that exist both on a provincial and agency or unit level.

Through the eyes of a nurse

*I*t is so different administering medications as a nurse compared to when I was a student. At first, I asked others to double-check my medications for me just as my instructor often did in my clinical rotations. I was a little nervous when I administered medications on my own as new graduate nurse. I soon learned that I had to know all I could about the medications I was administering, and if I didn't feel I knew enough, then I would look them up. It becomes easier once you know your patients and the medications they are receiving.

(personal reflection of a nurse)

BOX 22.2 Reducing the Stress of Medication Administration in the Clinical Setting: A Partnership Between Faculty Members and Students

Students can experience much anxiety in the clinical settings when it comes to administering medications. Faculty members and students can both work together to help reduce the potential stress by engaging in one or more of the following activities:

1. Communication is key. Faculty, students, and staff members need to be on the same page when it comes to the activities surrounding medication administration. Faculty and students can communicate with staff to make this happen more smoothly. Faculty need to communicate with students about what is expected of them regarding medication administration in a specific setting. As well, students need to be aware of knowledgeable about the medication administration policies and procedures of both the agency and the learning institution.
2. Working together to make it happen safely. Patient care can be exceptionally hectic in today's health-care settings. Students and faculty need to work together through teamwork to ensure that patients receive the highest level of care. If shifts become hectic, students need to request the assistance of others to ensure they are administering medications safely. As well, faculty members need to assist students to deliver this care through assistance and guidance where possible.
3. Knowing when it isn't working. Faculty members need to assist students in evaluating their medication administration practices to ensure that they are safe and effective. Students need to recognize when they are not able to give medications safely and to inform their faculty member and appropriate staff members in a timely fashion.
4. Celebrating the successes. Students and faculty members need to celebrate when students have successfully completed their assigned medication administration and review what principles and practices went well, so that students can continue to grow in their medication administration practices for future experiences.

Practice Standards

Each province and territory in Canada grants responsibility for the regulation of nursing to professional colleges and/or nursing associations (e.g., Yukon Registered Nurses Association, Saskatchewan Registered Nurses Association, College of Nurses of Ontario, College of Registered Nurses of Nova Scotia). Professional colleges and associations ensure protection of the public through the establishment of nursing practice standards and competencies and some provincial regulatory bodies specifically address medication administration. Standards and competencies outline prerequisites for safe, competent, and ethical nursing care, and all licensed and registered nurses are accountable to the provincial standards for nursing practice. It is important to understand that nurses are held directly accountable for administering medications competently and safely. Nurses are often the last person to check for medication safety before the patient actually takes a drug.

Provincial regulatory bodies are responsible for defining the scope of practice for nurses. Several regulatory bodies have developed specific standards related to medication administration. For example, the College and Association of Registered Nurses of Alberta outlines medication administration in the document *Medication Administration: Guidelines for Registered Nurses* (College and Association of Registered Nurses of Alberta, 2005) and other provinces such as the College of Registered Nurses of British Columbia and the College of Nurses of Ontario have practice standard documents for medication administration, some of which include online learning modules related to medication administration.

Safe Medication Administration

Critically thinking and focusing your attention toward medication safety will improve medication administration. It is important to realize that you are directly responsible for your own practice. There are ways that you can actively prevent medication errors. For example, you cannot assume that a medication ordered by another health-care professional is always a safe dose for a patient. Avoiding assumptions and implementing specific error prevention strategies during medication administration is a key way to prevent errors. Another strategy is to complete safety checks such as the **three checks in medication preparation** step. Another consideration might be to critically think about the effects of certain medications. For example, you must always consider that mixing two or more medications together could be lethal or could result in unexpected reaction for a patient. Sometimes, nurses or nursing students make medication errors. Medication errors (also known as **adverse drug events**) happen for many reasons. For example, an adverse drug event might occur when a nurse gives the wrong medication to a patient, gives two incompatible medications, forgets to give a medication, or gives a medication at the wrong time. Some students may not realize that giving a medication 30 minutes late may actually be considered an adverse drug event.

Not all adverse drug events can be foreseen or prevented by the nurse; however, safety can be enhanced by being aware of key safety danger points. Some medications, known as "high-alert" medications, are more prone to be given incorrectly. Confusing or unclear drug labeling can also contribute to errors. Taking shortcuts, such as not using proper monitoring equipment, may impact drug safety and not clarifying unclear orders might contribute to unsafe medication administration (*The Patient Safety Education Program*, 2011c).

can greatly increase the ability of health-care providers to be aware of and put actions into place that can reduce the possibility of such adverse events.

In a recent international study on adverse events related to health care, 10% of those Canadians who responded indicated they had experienced a wrong medication being administered during provision of health care. Thus, 1 in 10 hospitalized adults with health problems reported receiving a wrong medication or dose. One of the difficulties that health-care providers experience is knowing exactly which medications a patient is taking or has been prescribed. Many individuals have multiple doctors and health-care providers; it is very common for a health-care provider to be unaware of the full list of medications a patient may be receiving.

To reduce the risk of the adverse drug events that stem from incorrect prescriptions and wrong doses of medication, medication reconciliation has been initiated in some Canadian hospitals. This initiative is a response to the high rate of adverse drug events that have taken place in Canadian hospitals and health-care settings. Medication reconciliation is a comprehensive way to track all medications a patient is taking, so that even through admissions to acute care facilities and care in the community, all medications are known and communicated among health-care providers. The reduction in medication errors can be as high as a 70% improvement. In fact, over 15% decreases in adverse drug events have been seen with the implementation of this program in some Canadian facilities. Nursing admission time has also been noted to decrease by about 20 minutes by having medication reconciliation in place. Pharmacist involvement also has been shown to decrease by 40 minutes per discharge per patient with this process in place. Overall, this is one example of how the research has shown medication prescribing and administration practices were resulting in an increase in adverse events for patients. The medication reconciliation initiative is working to reduce the number and frequency of mediation related adverse events through better communication at various levels of health care and more comprehensive understanding of the medications a patient is receiving.

Safer Healthcare Now! (2007). Getting started kit: Medication reconciliation prevention of adverse drug events how to guide. *Retrieved from http://www.saferhealthcarenow.ca*

Canadian Institute for Health Information. (2007). Patient safety in Canada: An update. Analysis in Brief. *Ottawa, ON: Author.*

RESEARCH

MEDICATION RECONCILIATION

Adverse events in medication administration can result in serious consequences for both the patient and health-care provider. Understanding medication prescription and administration practices, policies, and procedures

When errors occur, **patient safety** is your primary concern. For patient safety reasons, it is very important that you take *immediate* steps to resolve and report the error. Some Canadian health-care systems, in a quest to learn from mistakes and then make systems better, have implemented new approaches to patient safety. This new approach includes a movement from blaming individual nurses for errors to looking at nurses within health-care systems and the role individuals and systems play when errors occur. This systems-focused thinking is sometimes referred to as a "no blame culture" approach to patient safety where individuals feel safe in reporting errors. A shift to systems thinking does not mean that a nursing student is not accountable for making an error. If you give the wrong medication, you are required to directly communicate what happened to your clinical instructor, preceptor, or a member of the health-care team that you are assigned to follow for the day. Because there may be many reasons why an error occurs, communication of that error helps individual nurses and systems learn how to prevent future errors from occurring (*The Patient Safety Education Program*, 2011a).

Drug Regulation and Legislation

Drug regulation in Canada is a very complex process involving federal and provincial legislative bodies. They are concerned with the introduction of new drugs into the market, the production and regulation of controlled foods and medications, and the distribution of drugs within Canada. There are statutes and laws at federal and provincial levels across the country. At the federal level, Health Canada reviews, approves, and regulates food and drugs for quality and safety. New drugs are approved for sale after they have been scientifically reviewed. The Government of Canada amended the Food and Drug Act (2012b) and added stricter requirements for the labeling of food additives and nutritional claims on foods and items labeled as natural health products. Provincial governments share responsibility for regulating drugs by managing health-care services, regulating health-care personnel and their scopes of practice, and through consideration of financial details of drug distribution within provincial health-care systems (Government of Canada, 2012a).

For safety reasons, some drugs are more regulated than others. There are two key concepts students should know about the legal and legislative aspects of drug control. Federally and provincially, there is distribution control and management of therapeutic drugs and pharmaceutical agents. There is also control of particular substances believed to result in addiction and/or potential abuse, and these are referred to as **controlled substances**. The Controlled Drugs and Substances Act (1996 and amended in 2012; Government of Canada, 2012a) lists different levels of drug regulation within Canada. For example, Schedule 1 medications are drugs that require a prescription. Schedule 2 medications are drugs that are located behind a pharmacy counter. Box 22.3 provides further explanation for the scheduled medications.

In the hospital, controlled substances are kept under lock and key, and nurses are responsible for administering them only to the individuals for whom they are prescribed. Each dose is recorded on the agency's (or unit's) narcotic sheet or via an electronic medication system as well as on the patient's **medication administration record (MAR)** so an

---

BOX 22.3 Canada's Drug Schedule

Schedule 1—Drugs that can be sold to a consumer with a prescription and direct intervention from a licensed pharmacist within a pharmacy. These drugs are subject to all of the same considerations as drugs listed in Schedule F of the national Food and Drug Regulations (Canada).

Schedule 2—Drugs that can be sold to a consumer without a prescription but are kept behind the counter of a pharmacy.

Schedule 3—Drugs that can be sold to a consumer without a prescription and in an open area that allows for self-selection within a pharmacy.

Unscheduled—Drugs not included in Schedule 1, 2, or 3 that can be sold to a consumer from any retail outlet.

Controlled Drugs—Drugs included in Schedule F (Part I and II) from the Food and Drug Regulations (Canada) and in the Controlled Drugs and Substances Act (formerly the Narcotic Control Act and Schedule G to the Food and Drug Regulations).

Source: Alberta College of Pharmacists. (2007). *Understanding Alberta's drug schedule*. Edmonton, AB: Author.

---

accurate inventory is maintained. Typically, nurses engage in a count of these controlled substances both at the beginning and end of each shift to ensure that the remaining inventory balances out with the medication that was administered and/or wasted.

Through the eyes of a nurse

I can remember as a student looking at the controlled drug cabinet thinking that this must be really important, as students are not often allowed to enter the locked cabinet without a faculty member or registered nurse overseeing everything that students had to do in the narcotic cupboard.

(personal reflection of a nurse)

Nurses are responsible to their provincial practice standards and the Code of Ethics for Registered Nurses (Canadian Nurses Association [CNA], 2008), and nurses who abuse medications or struggle with addictions (e.g., alcohol, prescribed medications, or controlled substances) are held professionally accountable for their personal fitness to practice. The Canadian Nurses Association (CNA) states that substance abuse is a threat to safe nursing care because it impairs judgment and decision-making (CNA, 2008, p. 1).

Critical Thinking and Medication Administration: A Vital Combination

Medication administration requires a combination of skill, critical thinking, and clinical decision-making. Nurses must use their knowledge of pharmacology; technology; physical medication administration techniques; documentation; dosage calculations; medication preparation; and implementation of critical safety checks, such as the **rights of medication administration** and **patient identification**, when administering any medication.

Pharmacology

Pharmacology is a complex science, and this chapter is designed to review the essential concepts and principles you need to safely administer medications. Essential concepts of pharmacology include classification of medication names, drug preparations, effects of medications, medication actions, consideration of medication side effects, and specific pharmacological factors related to medication administration.

Classification and Identification of Medications

Medications typically have three assigned names: the chemical name, generic name, and trade name. An example of the chemical, generic, and trade names of a drug is the popular over-the-counter drug Tylenol. Tylenol is a trade name, acetaminophen is a generic name, and N-(4-hydroxyphenyl) acetamide is a chemical name. Drugs are given a chemical name initially, and this name describes the chemical components and molecular structure. Generic names are shortened chemical names given to drugs because they are easier to remember than chemical names. Generic drugs are copies of brand name drugs and contain the same medicinal ingredients as brand name drugs. Health Canada is responsible for regulating the safety of generic drugs. A drug's trade name is determined by drug companies for marketing purposes. The trade name signifies that the drug's name is a registered trademark of the company. For safety purposes, nurses should know both generic and trade names because often patients and health-care professionals use these names interchangeably (Government of Canada, 2012a).

Drug identification numbers (DINs) are 8-digit numbers assigned by Health Canada to prescription and over-the-counter medications prior to marketing. The DIN identifies approved medications that can be sold and marketed in Canada. The DIN indicates that a medication has passed testing and review specifications and can be legally marketed and sold in Canada. The DIN is used to track and monitor medications in Canada (Health Canada, 2001).

Importance of Knowing Drug Names

You may wonder why it is important to know both the trade and generic names and why one name isn't used for consistency. These are important questions to ask, with many possible answers. Although the production of medications helps patients, we know that pharmaceutical companies seek profit from the medications they produce and distribute. Generic drugs are often less expensive than the same trade drug, even though both have the same medicinal ingredients and are indicated for the same use(s). Although the two names, generic and trade, assigned to medications might confuse nursing students and nurses, it is very important to be aware that there

are two names and to know both the trade and generic names of any given drug in order to safely administer medications to patients. When talking to patients about their medications, it is recommended that nurses should use the trade and generic names of the drug because the patient may recognize either one of the names (*The Patient Safety Education*, 2011c).

Drug Preparations

Drugs are available in many forms or preparations such as creams, tablets, capsules, tincture, suppositories, or elixirs. The drug form determines how the drug must be given to a patient (commonly referred to as the *route of administration*). More information about routes and types of medications and drug administration is covered later in this chapter.

The Effects of Medications

Medications can have a **therapeutic effect** (which is the drug's desired effect) or an adverse effect (an unintended effect of a drug). If a patient experiences an excessive or unintended reaction to a medication, this is called an adverse drug event. For example, a patient may be allergic or have a serious immune reaction to a medication. This is very serious because patients who experience an allergic reaction may experience anaphylaxis—a potentially life-threatening, hypersensitive reaction.

Medication Actions

Pharmacokinetics is the study of medications and how they travel to each body system. It involves the processes of drug absorption, distribution, metabolism, and excretion of all medications. Absorption occurs as a medication enters the bloodstream and begins to cause an effect within the body. Sometimes, a medication is broken down but not absorbed by the body (also known as the *first-pass effect*). Factors that inhibit the absorption of medication include the route of drug administration (e.g., via the gastrointestinal [GI] route compared to the intravenous [IV] route), presence of food in the GI tract, health status of the body when the medication was given, and the presence of other medications that may alter medication absorption. After absorption, medication is distributed to various locations in the body via the bloodstream. Factors affecting the distribution of a drug include the drug's chemical formulation and preparation, its use in the body, and the drug's ability to bind or penetrate body proteins or tissues. Drug metabolism (also known as *biotransformation*) occurs after the drug has reached its site of action. It then undergoes a chemical alteration within the body, where medications are broken down. During biotransformation, drugs become inactive within the body and dissolve into more soluble compounds. Drugs are metabolized in the liver, kidneys, muscle, lungs, plasma, and the intestinal mucosa, and each medication's chemical composition of the drug determines how and where the medication is metabolized. Excretion of the medication out of the body can occur through different body systems such as the

GI tract and kidneys. If an organ system is compromised (e.g., liver or kidney failure), this can impact how a drug is metabolized and excreted. Acutely ill patient tends to have different reactions to medications than those without acute illness or coexisting health concerns. It is important to assess and monitor physiological and psychological responses to the medications among these patients because their ability to metabolize and excrete medication may be compromised.

The Onset, Peak, and Duration of Medications

When giving a medication, nurses must know when to expect a therapeutic response from the drug. The *onset* of a medication is the time it takes for a medication to start producing a therapeutic response within the body; the *peak* of a medication is the time it takes for a medication to reach its maximum therapeutic response, and the *duration* is the length of time the medication will usually exhibit a therapeutic response. Knowing this information is important for clinical decision-making. For example, as a nursing student, your nursing care plan may include interventions such as mobilization of a postoperative patient. If this patient requires an analgesic prior to mobilization, it is important for you to understand the mechanism of the drug you are giving by considering the medication's onset and then actively planning the patient's walk while the medication is most effective. When it comes to onset, peak, and duration of medications, medication knowledge and understanding the timing of medication is truly power in terms of therapeutic effect, safe administration, and effective clinical decisions. Figure 22.1 visually depicts these important concepts.

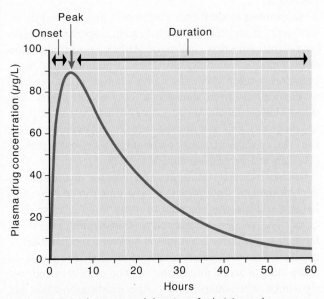

Figure 22.1 Peak, onset, and duration of administered medication. When medications are administered, the start of the drug action (or onset), the peak serum drug level, and the duration of drug action are important factors to consider. The variation in administering one dose versus repeated doses changes the concepts of onset, peak, and duration.

Pharmacological Factors for Consideration

Body systems that have been frequently exposed to medications often exhibit tolerance to specific medications. Tolerance means that a medication has a reduced effect on the individual when frequently administered.

Also, other medications and foods can alter the effects of additional medications administered. For example, grapefruit and/or its juice can have tragic consequences for patients who are taking the drug atorvastatin (Lipitor). Remember that there is a lot of information about which medications or food substances interact when exposed to each other, and pharmacology texts, drug handbooks, online resources, and pharmacists are excellent resources to help you understand food and drug interactions.

Think — *Implications of Food Intolerances on Medication Administration*

Patient allergies and intolerances of food can cause catastrophic events post administration. These allergies should be well documented before medication administration. The most frequently experienced allergies in food such as peanuts, shellfish, soy, eggs, nuts, and dyes as well as intolerances to such items as gluten, lactose, and soy can be experienced with medication administration as many contain these very items. Although there are no concrete guidelines to ensuring that patients do not have certain allergies or intolerances to medications prior to their administration, it is important for the practitioner to know the food allergies and intolerances that the patient has in order to question whether the medications are appropriate for that individual. As well, it is important to know which medications pose an allergy or intolerance risk in order to better screen patients for potentially serious reactions. Although many parents of small children and adults know food items to which they are allergic, many do not often mention the intolerances they have to certain foods or ingredients. Asking patients about allergies as well as intolerances will elicit more useful information than just questioning about allergies alone.

Age and Gender Factors

Specific pharmacological considerations must include certain patient populations such as pregnant women, pediatric, and older adults. The Canadian Agency for Drugs and Technologies in Health (CADTH) regulates medications to ensure their general safety and effectiveness. All prescription and over-the-counter medications are tested to see if they are safe and effective before they become available to the public. Pregnant women usually are not included in these tests because of the possible risks to the unborn baby (Table 22.1). Children are smaller; have less surface area than adults; and have immature body systems that affect absorption, distribution, metabolism, and excretion of drugs. Similarly, older adults may have altered physiological needs due to changes of body systems that affect drug absorption. Older adults may also be taking multiple medications or natural health

TABLE 22.1	Current Categories for Drug Use in Pregnancy
Category	Description
A	Adequate, well-controlled studies in pregnant women have not shown an increased risk of fetal abnormalities.
B	Animal studies have revealed no evidence of harm to the fetus, however, there are no adequate and well-controlled studies in pregnant women. **or** Animal studies have shown an adverse effect, but adequate and well-controlled studies in pregnant women have failed to demonstrate a risk to the fetus.
C	Animal studies have shown an adverse effect and there are no adequate and well-controlled studies in pregnant women. **or** No animal studies have been conducted and there are no adequate and well-controlled studies in pregnant women.
D	Studies, adequate well-controlled or observational, in pregnant women have demonstrated a risk to the fetus. However, the benefits of therapy may outweigh the potential risk.
X	Studies, adequate well-controlled or observational, in animals or pregnant women have demonstrated positive evidence of fetal abnormalities. The use of the product is contraindicated in women who are or may become pregnant.

Retrieved from U.S. Food and Drug Administration. (2001, May–June). Pregnancy and the drug dilemma. *FDA Consumer Magazine*. Retrieved from http://www.fda.gov/fdac/features/2001/301_preg.html#categories

products. The number and types of medications and natural health products a person takes can significantly increase his or her risk for serious drug interactions.

Medication Administration in Community Settings and Homes

Home care nurses might not directly supervise patients taking medications in homes; however, they still need to teach patients safe medications use. Nurses should ensure patients know the name, purpose, and instruction of each prescribed medication. They need to be informed of the drug's therapeutic and side effect, or problem, with other medication and substance and the importance of adherence (*The Patient Safety Education*, 2011c). Nurses facilitate additional medication safety strategies outside hospitals that might include measures such as medication reminders communicated over the phone or teaching patients how to use specialized medication dispensers. Medication dispensers, labeled by time and day of the week, sometimes have timers and alarms to help patients with medication schedules or alert a patient that they have taken or missed a medication dose. Nurses help patients fill the medication dispensers and answer questions about the medications and their side effects. Home care nurses may delegate medication administration to health-care aides who have special medication administration education. Even though medication administration may be delegated to others, home health nurses are still responsible to monitor medication safety including the therapeutic effects of medications and possible side effects of drugs. For nurses, patient safety and drug administration has the same focus whether drugs are administered in hospitals, communities, or homes.

Technology and Medication Administration

Canadian health-care facilities have many types of medication administration systems including paper-and-pen medication systems and **automated dispensing cabinets**. In Canada, written processes are still most common, but automated dispensing cabinets are becoming more common. These automated systems, designed by **human factors design** engineers, store and dispense drugs and supplies electronically when users enter identifiers and passwords.

Dispensing medications is a complex process, and therefore, written and electronic medication dispensing systems have significant safety challenges. Medication administration in hospitals typically includes verbal communication, interpretation, written processes such as transcription, retrieval of medications from drawers or electronic systems, and dispensing protocols. Many people are involved in dispensing processes, and as a nursing student, you will need to be alert that mistakes that may occur at any level of this process (*The Patient Safety Education*, 2011c) (Fig. 22.2).

Nurses interpret, transcribe, and dispense medication orders for patients. Interpreting handwriting can be very challenging and has the potential to result in an adverse drug event. The process of rechecking transcription orders by more than one nurse is a common and very important safety mechanism in the written process of medication systems. In many clinical areas, nurses and nursing students need two signatures when dispensing certain medications that are more commonly involved in adverse drug events. Similarly, even though computerized drug dispensing systems were designed to make medication administration safer, these systems also have major safety challenges. For example, medication systems are stocked by people; if the wrong

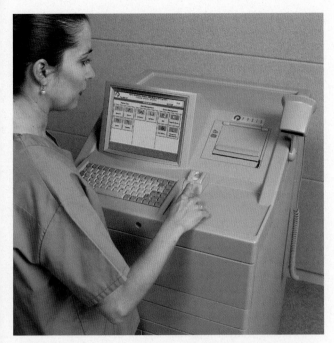

Figure 22.2 Automated medication dispensing machine. Automated medication administration machines are becoming more common in acute care settings. These machines offer dispensing that is tailored to each patient and reduces the chance for medication errors.

medication or wrong dose of a drug is introduced into the system, dire consequences are possible. For example, if you assume a medication cart is stocked correctly and then miss completing your medication safety checks, a potentially fatal adverse drug event might happen (*The Patient Safety Education*, 2011b).

Electronic devices and software applications are used across Canada to deliver patient care, and nurses are expected to understand and use technology in patient care situations. For example, medication ordering and transcribing is one area where nurses use technology. Some physicians and nurse practitioners may write patient medication orders on hard copy carbon-based paper, whereas others may use personal digital systems or computer-based ordering methods to prescribe medications. One role of a nurse is to interpret and transcribe ordering information into computer ordering systems. To fulfill this role, nurses use telephones and computer operating systems when receiving patient drug orders from physicians or nurse practitioners. As well, nurses use various technologies to document medication administration, the results of medication administration, and to track adverse drug events (Table 22.2).

Medication Administration Areas and Medication Carts

For nurses in acute or community health centres, organizing, preparing, and giving medications takes place in medication rooms or around medication carts. Medication rooms are sometimes the busiest places in a hospital besides the cafeteria at lunchtime. Familiarizing yourself with the environment where medication preparation occurs will help alleviate some stress when it comes to preparing for medication administration. You will need to know where to find things:

• Where to find information about the medications you are preparing. This information may be found in manuals, books, or through online resources. For example, the annual Compendium of Pharmaceuticals and Specialties

TABLE 22.2	Advantages and Disadvantages of Technological Systems	
	Advantages	Disadvantages
Training or orientation	Allows for more complex functions that all individuals are able to complete according to their areas of responsibility	Time-consuming and requires some direction and tutorage from a qualified individual
Preparation	Checking of the medications dispensed needs to take place; less time obtaining medications from various sources; can decrease the questioning whether a medication was taken out of the machine or not	Can be time-consuming if there are not enough medication administration systems; technological issues and machine trouble may cause more time delays; may give a false sense that the machine has already fully prepared the medications, whereas the same preparation and checking of the medication dispensed should take place
Administration	Remains the same	Remains the same
Documentation	Does not decrease the charting that the nurse is responsible for; documentation might be easier through a computer-based system. Unit based drug counting for controlled substances may be a bit easier with the computerized machines.	May give a false sense that the medications dispensed are already documented; if the machine is "down," then it will take more time and communication.
Overall organization	May save some time by avoiding retrieving medications from various sources	May take more time if the technology fails or if individuals relay on the machine to complete some of the checking, thereby causing mistakes

(CPS; Canadian Pharmacists Association, 2012) is a manual containing all Canadian medications on the market today. Some health-care facilities have intranets with online drug information. In addition, drug manuals or medication books may be located in the medication preparation area.

- The place where you prepare the medications before giving them to patients. Common preparation areas include medication rooms, medication carts (small, mobile carts that hold drugs and supplies), or a patient's kitchen table. If a medication cart is used, controlled substances are not stocked on the cart.
- Where to find medications. On most patient care units, fridges are available for medication storage for drugs that must be kept cool. Patient-specific medications, which are not commonly used by the general patient population on a care unit, may be stored in patient-specific cubbies or drawers located in the medication room, or on the medication carts. Drugs that are classified as controlled substances are found in locked cupboards. Controlled drugs are closely monitored, counted daily, and often require two signatures before they are given to patients.
- Where to find reminders, information, and charts that might assist in medication administration. Some units display safety reminders and information notices in poster formats on walls or fridges. These information items might draw your attention to important new knowledge or safety concerns about certain medications. Another example might be medication charts about the onset, peak, and duration of common drugs used in the patient care unit or a chart that displays IV medication compatibilities. For safety purposes, make sure to ask if this information is current and correct.
- Medications

Think · *Beware the Cart!*

Although medication carts are a great convenience, medication administration can sometimes be difficult from carts, and often, medication administration becomes a process bound by time limits and busy units with high acuity. As well, make sure carts do not go into the patient rooms because they become a vehicle for bacterial and viral transmission between patients. The areas in which carts are left should be monitored; this can be a safety hazard if unauthorized persons have access to the medications in the cart. For example, a child visiting a family member could access some medications if the cart is left in an open area while the health-care professional is giving the medications to a patient in the room. Make sure carts are stored in a secure location when not in use.

Promoting Patient Safety

Nurses are directly responsible for patient safety when dispensing medications. There are specific steps that nursing students can take to reduce the risk of medication errors. These include the following:

- Review a patient's medical history, allergies, diagnosis, current medications, and treatment plan prior to medication administration. This information can be found on the patient chart and by interacting with the patient.
- Know the medication you are preparing: Understand why the drug is being given, the therapeutic effects, side effects, safe dosages, and common indications of adverse reactions to the drug.
- Check the patient's order: Before giving a drug, make sure the medication ordered for the patient is correct.
- Check the rights of medication administration. Ensure that the right dose is being prepared for the right person in the right form or ordered route and that the drug will be administered at the right time.
- Check the patient identification before giving the medication.
- Document giving the medication carefully and completely.

Nursing student Jonathan says, "I never knew how much thinking was involved when giving medications! It seems to be such a complex skill. Of course, patient safety is so important, and I understand the nurse's role in medication administration is a key part in keeping patients safe. I know that I need to practice safely at all times—I just need to understand how to do that!"

Completing Medication Safety Checks

Safety checks (i.e., the rights of medication administration) assist nurses in making sure they are giving medications safely. Actively thinking about each safety check will increase the likelihood that medications will be given correctly. Organization, focus, and concentration are fundamental components of the overall administration process. As a nursing student, applying safety checks such as the rights of medication administration is universally expected when giving drugs to your patients (Vihos & Buckner, 2010).

The foundational five rights of medication administration include the following:

1. Right drug
2. Right dose
3. Right patient
4. Right time
5. Right route

The four rights that are also used in the clinical setting are as follows:

1. Right documentation
2. Right reason
3. Right to know
4. Right to refuse

BOX 22.4 Known Error Points in Medication Administration

- Shortcuts and working around specific safety procedures when preparing medications—For example, pre-pouring medications to save time is unsafe, and it fails to ensure that the safety checks are being done. Shortcuts such as this can contribute to errors being made in medication administration.
- Failure to read and interpret patient drug orders—If drug orders are unclear, they must be clarified prior to administration. If a medication order is incomplete, illegible, or does not make sense in terms of volumes or dosage forms (e.g., administering more than two capsules or ampoules of a drug), then the drug order needs clarification before giving it to the patient.
- Mistakes in calculations—Rechecking calculations with a second or third person can prevent errors.
- Failing to check with the patient and family before giving a medication—Patients and their families need to be listened to

when giving medications. If a family member questions or has a concern about a medication or its effect—stop and recheck the medication.
- Multiple interruptions while preparing medications interfere with concentration and safety checks
- Failure to correctly identify a patient before giving a medication—Checking an armband and patient identification must be completed.
- Failing to question, ask, or seek clarification about medications—Nursing students need to check with their instructors or assigned nurses for advice or questions about medication administration if they are unsure about any step in the medication administration process. All nurses must clearly and assertively communicate with all health-care professionals, when seeking clarification about any medication order.

Sources: Davis, R. E., Sevdalis, N., Jacklin, R., & Vincent, C. A. (2012). An examination of opportunities for the active patient in improving patient safety. *Journal of Patient Safety, 8*, 36–43; Emanuel, L. L., Taylor, L., Hain, A., Combes, J. R., Hatlie, M. J., Karsh, B., . . . Walton, M. (Eds). (2011). *The patient safety education program. Module 12c: Interventional care: Medication safety.* Ottawa, ON: Canadian Patient Safety Institute; Murphy, M. (2012). Mentoring students in medicines management. *Nursing Standard, 26*(44), 51–56.

Within health-care systems, patients require an original medication order written by physicians or nurse practitioners before the patient receives a prescribed drug. Patients are sometimes prescribed many medications, which can be confusing when preparing medications. Choosing the wrong medication could have widespread consequences to your patient. Remember to exercise caution during when choosing medications, especially **high-alert medications**. Confusion occurs when giving medications because some packaging is difficult to read, and some drugs have similar sounding or confusing names. Both nursing students and nurses need **independent double checks** to be completed with high-alert medications. As a student, high-alert medications will need to be checked by your nursing instructor or your assigned nurse. For graduate nurses, independent double checks requirements are mandated by the health-care systems and the different institutions they work within. Before beginning the medication administration process, assemble basic supplies (medication cups, your list of medications, your drug information book, or medication cards), try to make a space to complete your medication administration safely, and remember to bring key knowledge about your patient and the drugs you are preparing to the actual preparation process (Box 22.4).

The importance of the foundational five rights is that it provides a framework for nurses to follow to ensure that they are giving the correct dose of medication to the correct patient. If done consistently, it provides a solid foundation for medication administration for all nurses, which can contribute to minimizing medication administration errors. Some jurisdictions have added additional rights to these core seven rights we discuss here. Check with your lab and clinical instructors regarding your local medication administration rights and policies. Box 22.5 outlines some important safety tips concerning medication preparation and administration.

Right Drug

The first step to ensuring you have the right drug for your patient is to verify the medication order. Compare the original written order (written by the physician or nurse practitioner) to the order you have received either in a paper copy format from the written MAR or from a computer printout of a patient's medication order that you have in front of you. After carefully verifying the patient medication order (and this must be done for each patient), you are ready to begin the process of pouring medications.

As you begin the process of pouring medications, a key step is to complete three checks of medication preparation, which involves comparing the label of the drug you select to the actual medication order sheet in front of you. The three checks of medication preparation will help you choose

BOX 22.5 Medication Preparation and Administration Safety Tips

- Prepare medications for patients one at a time.
- Focus, concentrate, and minimize interruptions from other nursing students and nurses.
- Systematically complete all independent three checks of medication safety and the seven rights of medication administration
- Leave drugs dispensed in individual packages in the packages when placing them into medication cups; check the drug name on the package right before giving it to the patient.
- Do not pre-pour medications and leave medications unattended in the medication room or in the patient room. Only administer medications that YOU have chosen, checked, and prepared.
- If a patient or family member questions the medication you have chosen, listen, and recheck the medication name and order.
- Be extra vigilant with high-alert medications.
- Always check patient identification prior to giving medications (Government of Canada, 2012a; Vihos & Buckner, 2010).

the right medication from the cupboard or medication cart. When comparing the label of the drug to the ordered medication look carefully at the drug label three times as follows: first, before you remove the drug from the cupboard or medication cart; second, when you remove the drug from its container; and third, when you return the drug to its original spot in the cupboard or medication drawer (Institute for Safe Medication Practices [ISMP], 2013).

Right Dose

Medications might be dispensed in individual unit doses from pharmacy that directly coincide with the medication order. However, sometimes, medications are stocked in bulk, in individual doses containers or in multiple-dose strengths in bottles, **vials** or **ampoules** on medication carts or in cupboards. If medications are not stocked in individual dose units, nurses need to calculate and prepare the correct dose of a drug for their patients. As a nursing student, your first consideration about the drug dose is whether the ordered medication is a safe dose for the patient. If you are unsure about what constitutes a safe dose, always check the resources provided within the clinical area before dispensing. Make sure the dosage ordered is the most current order written by the physician or nurse practitioner. Remember to recheck orders every time you give a medication as orders often change throughout the clinical day. Next, if a medication requires calculation in terms of the number or amount of drug needed, you will use formulas to calculate the amount of drug that should be given. It is always recommended to double-check your calculations with your instructor or your assigned nurse to ensure the correct dose is being calculated and given to the patient. You should consider the logic of your calculation—for example, in terms of the amount of pills or liquid being given to a patient—and ask yourself if the dosage makes logical sense. Completing a calculation that indicates a patient should get a liter of medication or 10 pills is highly questionable and should be considered a potential mistake that needs to be rechecked.

Right Person/Patient

As a nursing student, you may be assigned to one or more patients, and verifying the identity of each patient will prevent errors. Each time you give a drug, make sure that you are giving the ordered drug to the right patient by requesting or verifying two forms of identification. One way to identify a patient is to check the patient identification wristband and compare the patient's name and identification number with the medication record or patient label. In some settings, the patient identification is typed on a wristband that includes identifying information; sometimes, identifying information is contained within a barcode that nurses scan before giving a medication. In some facilities and within community and home care settings, patients may not wear wristbands. Using two forms of identification is still safest. For example, the nurse can ask a family member to say and spell the patient's name; this could

be used to identify a patient before administering his or her medications. It is unsafe to just ask the question, "Are you Mr. Smith?" because there are many people with the same or similar sounding names. If you have any doubts about a patient's identity, it would be prudent to ask a second nurse to verify a patient's identity before giving a medication.

I [CI] walked to both sides of the bed looking for a wristband on the patient and could not find one. She [student] was proceeding to administer the IV medication and had inserted the syringe into the buretrol when I said, "Mr. X you seem to have lost your wristband." She [student] then stopped. The patient then stated, "But I am Mr. X" and I verified the patient's birthdate with the patient. Student then proceeded to give the medication. This was once again an unsafe administration of medication; the patient was put at risk because she [student] did not check patient identification. (Gregory, Guse, Davidson Dick, Davis, & Russell, 2008, p. 161)

During administration of the medications she [student] had to be reminded to check the ID bracelet before administering the medications. This is not an uncommon mistake for students to make, the first time they do this new skill. (Gregory et al., 2008, p. 201)

Right Time

Correct timing of the medication being administered is imperative for the effectiveness of the medication and regimen. It is common practice that there is a 30-minute window on either side of the scheduled medication administration time and is considered within the scheduled administration time. Anything outside this time window is considered too early or too late and should be documented accordingly. Drugs that are administered outside of this time schedule can have serious effects for the patient and can contribute to an adverse event. Administration times can be set by numerous individuals: pharmacists, nurses, and physicians. When using a computer-generated MAR, the computer can default to certain set times of the day.

These administration times should be followed closely because the patient's active treatment in the hospital may be dependent on it. Administration times are done with the entire patient care picture taken into consideration. If the patient has multiple medications, the medications should be given so as to not interact with each, contradict the action of another medication, and that they complement the medication's peak and half-life. The patient situation should also be considered when administering medications. If the nurse realizes that the patient may not tolerate a large quantity of medications at a particular time of the day, it is the nurse's responsibility to communicate with the pharmacist in order to come up with a solution that best meets the needs of the patient. In another situation, if a patient is feeling overwhelmed with the volume of medications being given to them, the nurse could stagger its administration over an hour or two. For example, if a patient has many medications ordered at 8 AM and 9 AM, these medications can safely be given from 7:30 AM until 9:30 AM (within 30 minutes on either side of the ordered time). Breaking up the administration over this 2-hour time frame might make medication administration more tolerable for the patient. Administration times for those patients in their own homes can be determined by the patient and home care nurse to meet the needs of patients and their individual schedules.

Right Route

Medications that are ordered via one route need to be administered by that route only. Medication routes cannot be interchanged and careful consideration should be given when one medication order addresses differing routes for the same medication. Sometimes, medications can be administered by different routes; however, the strength and amount of medication needed for each route often differs. Consult the orders and drug literature carefully to decide whether a medication ordered for multiple routes has the correct dose and route prescribed.

Challenges to giving the medications via the correct route are often associated with patient factors that are out of the control of the nurse. If a medication is due to be given intravenously and there is no IV site, then the nurse needs to call and have the order changed, and in the interim, a new route or new IV site should be obtained.

Another challenge is the many different medication forms that are available on the unit. Confusion can occur when medications are available in various routes, and the nurse has to ensure that he or she chooses the correct dosage strength and formulation for the route ordered. For example, morphine is available for parenteral injection, IV administration, oral consumption in pill or liquid form, or suppositories for rectal administration. Ensuring the right preparation is chosen is imperative. The following two incidents illustrate the importance of the right route.

> You almost gave heparin in your patient's abdomen when it had a large incision and 2 drainage tubes. When I suggested giving it in the arms you were going to give it intramuscularly. This was unsafe. (Gregory et al., 2008, p. 162)

> One student . . . administered Dilaudid subcutaneously and not orally; the second event occurred when the same student gave a pump bolus instead of oral medication for breakthrough pain. (Gregory et al., 2008, p. 201)

Additional Rights Associated With Medication Administration

There are four additional rights (nine in total) that have been brought forward in the literature. Although not the foundational rights (i.e., the five rights), they are important to think about when administering medications. These include right documentation, right reason, right to know, and right to refuse. Right documentation entails ensuring that the documentation for each medication is completed thoroughly in a timely fashion for each medication administered. The right reason involves knowing that the medications are being given for the right indication the patient is experiencing. In addition, it is making sure that the intention of the nurse administering the medication is to alleviate or assist with the indicated use for that medication (e.g., the medication for nausea is given as ordered for nausea not for the sleep effects it may have for the patient).

The right to know means that the patient has the right to know what medications he or she is taking. The individuals receiving the medication should have an understanding of the reasons why they are receiving the medication whenever possible. Finally, the right to refuse means that patients have the right to refuse medications if they so choose. If a patient refuses medication, then he or she also has the right to know what those effects may be for him or her and his or her health status. The nurse or student needs to document the patient's refusal of the medication including the date, time, medication, and reason for refusal. When a medication is refused, it is important to communicate this to the health-care team, inclusive of the charge nurse, pharmacist, and physician, so that there is awareness amongst the entire health-care team, about what decisions the patient is making. The right to know and the right to refuse work hand in hand, as the patient has to know the right information in order to make the most informed decisions regarding his or her treatment.

Orders

An order is a written direction given by a nurse practitioner, physician, or designate regarding a treatment or medication that is to be given to the patient. Orders can be written for treatments or for medications.

In Canada, the person ordering the medication or treatment must be a recognized individual with prescribing authority. This can be a nurse practitioner, physician, dentist, or other designate such as a medical resident. Nurses can transcribe orders when they are given verbally, when it is not possible to obtain written orders. Note that students cannot take verbal orders.

There are many different types of medication orders that can be written. There are routine orders that indicate what medication or treatment a patient should receive and when. There are also STAT (Latin, *statim*, which means immediately) orders that are urgent and need to be attended to immediately. There are orders that outline "prn" (Latin, *pro re nata*, "for the thing born" or as needed) medications and orders that are standing orders where they are preestablished based on the patient's condition and standardized treatment protocol.

Abbreviations

There are many abbreviations that need to be considered before reading and interpreting orders for patient medications. Knowing these abbreviations and understanding the specific agency and site policies surrounding approved abbreviations is an important first step in medication administration. There are so many abbreviations that it is difficult to memorize them all. Some practice settings are even coming out with special educational imperatives to highlight the discouraged use of some abbreviations to improve patient safety. Even if you have memorized all of the abbreviations, it is often that you find yourself stumbling across new ones that you have never seen before. Box 22.6 lists common abbreviations used with medication administration.

 Think *Think First—Look-Alike Abbreviations and Their Mistaken Meanings*

There can be many abbreviations that look like other abbreviations in the health-care setting. The following are the most contested abbreviations.

U or IU—means international unit however can be misread as IV or intravenous if not clearly written. It is suggested that the whole word unit should be written out.

QD, QD, or QOD—means every day and every other day. These abbreviations can be misread as qid or four times per day. It is suggested to write daily, every day, or every other day to alleviate the confusion

@, >, <—symbols are often mistaken for numbers or letters. Best to avoid them if at all possible.

1.0 or other decimal numbers can be misread as 10 times the dose ordered. It is suggested that we never use decimal points for whole numbers.

.1 or other numbers requiring a decimal point with no zero preceding the decimal can be misread without the decimal. It is suggested to always use zeros before a decimal point to emphasize the less than whole unit amount.

Sources: Institute for Safe Medication Practices Canada. (2006). Eliminate use of dangerous abbreviations, symbols, and dose designations. ISMP Canada Safety Bulletin, 6(4); Cowell, J. (2007). Improving patient safety by eliminating unsafe abbreviations from medication prescribing. Alberta RN, 63(8), 8–9.

What Are the Parts of a Medication Order?

A medication order requires that certain parts be specified by the individual writing the order. The essential parts of any medication order are the correct patient identifying data, the date and time, the medication, the dose, the route, and the frequency. Additional information that may be provided for any medication order includes the dual trade and generic drug names and the indication for use. Approved abbreviations should be used in the medication order.

What Do I Do With an Order?

Orders are transcribed and communicated to a pharmacy representative by the charge nurse or nurse in charge of processing the patient care orders. This process and the people involved (e.g., charge nurse) will vary from practice setting to practice

---

BOX 22.6   Common Abbreviations Associated With Medication Administration

Timing/Frequency

qd	every day
qam	every morning
qod	every other day
bid	twice a day
tid	three times a day
qid	four times a day
hs	at bedtime
ac	before meals
pc	after meals
OD	in left eye
OS	in right eye
OU	in both eyes
PRN or prn	as needed (*pro re nata*)
q2h	every 2 hours
q4h	every 4 hours
q6h	every 6 hours
q8h	every 8 hours
STAT	immediately

Route

po	orally
sl	sublingually
pr	per rectum/rectally
IV	intravenous
IM	intramuscular
SC or sc	subcutaneous
supp	suppository
susp	suspension
tab	tablet
gtt	drop

Common Intravenous Solutions

NS	normal saline
D5NS	5% dextrose in normal saline
D10	10% dextrose
½ NS	0.45% normal saline

Medication Measurement

ml	millilitre
u	unit
mg	milligram
IU	international unit
SI	standard international (units)

Other

c	with
s	without

---

setting. You will want to find out the specific process used on your unit. To stay abreast of any changes in medications for their patients, students should be looking at patient charts to see whether new medications are ordered. It is important that students know how to read orders and interpret abbreviations correctly, thus ensuring safe medication administration.

What Do I Do if the Order Changes?

If an order changes, it is important to know when the change occurred, what the change was, and the reason behind the change. If a medication was discontinued because of an allergic reaction then a prompt response to the change is required immediately. Some medication transcription processes can take time, and by the time it is entered into the computer system or communicated to pharmacy, the patient may have received another dose. Nurses and students need to be monitoring medication orders to ensure they identify when a change occurs.

Dosage Calculations

Once an order is received and the medication is prepared for administration, it is important to know how to calculate how much of the medication the patient should receive. Drug calculations can be intimidating. Calculations are not as hard as they look especially if you understand the principles behind the calculation. Remember to always to think and make use of common sense, when determining medication dosages.

- First—Don't stress but think.
- Second—Use a formula that works for you. There are a few to choose from, but the bottom line is you are asking yourself to complete a dosage ratio where you "need this much" and the pill comes "in this dosage."
- Third—Double-check your math.
- Fourth—Perform a "Does this dose make sense?" check.

Pill-Form Medication Calculations

Nurses are often faced with deciding how much of a tablet or how many tablets needed to give of a certain medication. For example, you are asked to give 150 mg of drug X to a patient. Each tablet contains 75 mg. How many tablets do you need? Determine the correct dosage using the four steps listed previously as a guideline to administering medications in pill form:

1. Common sense is telling me that if one tablet is 75 mg, then two tablets would equal the 150-mg dose.
2. Use a formula because sometimes you are so busy that thinking, and common sense may elude you. One such formula is

Unit Dose of Medication / Per Unit Quantity of Medication = Dose Desired (x) / Quantity Desired (x)

This formula is setting up a ratio that examines the form that the medication comes in (unit dose of medication per unit quantity of medication, e.g., 75 mg per one tablet) and then uses that information to discover how many tablets to administer of the oral medication. If each tablet is 75 mg, then how many do I need to administer the 150-mg dose required? Cross multiplication in a medication calculation question is fairly simple.

$$\frac{75 \text{ mg}}{1 \text{ tab}} = \frac{150 \text{ mg}}{x \text{ tabs}}$$
$$75 \text{ mg} \times x \text{ tabs} = 150 \text{ mg} \times 1 \text{ tab}$$
$$75 \text{ mg} \times x \text{ tabs} = 150 \text{ mg}$$
$$x \text{ tabs} = 150 \text{ mg divided by } 75 \text{ mg}$$
$$x \text{ tabs} = 2$$

For this equation, you would take the 150 mg and multiply that by the one tablet (to equal 150). Then, you would take the 150 mg and divide that by the 75 from the previous calculation to get two tablets.

3. Double-check your math—very important! Always recheck that you have multiplied correctly prior to proceeding because setting up cross multiplication can be a bit tricky.
4. Does this make sense?—Yes, it is the same thought you may or may not have had from the first step. It makes sense that if each pill is 75 mg, then I would need two of these to make up the 150-mg dose required in this order.

 Think *What if Your Patient Vomits the Medications You Just Gave Him or Her?*

Many students have had this experience where they have just given a lot of medications orally to a patient and the patient then vomits them shortly after administration. The first thing to remember is to tend to your patient. Often, students get really frantic when medication administration doesn't go as planned, and the patient then is often left out of the equation. When tending to your patient, assess the vomit and see whether the medications or particles of the medication can be seen. Knowing what each medication looks like is really helpful in this situation!

After assessing your patient and the vomit, you need to tell the charge nurse, your buddy nurse, and/or your instructor about the incident. The following information will decide the actions to take:

- What medications were administered
- What percent of and what medication was seen to be vomited

Usually, the physician is notified, and the decision to readminister, hold additional doses, or assess the patient further is made based on the given factors. As a student, prompt assessment and communication is necessary in these situations.

Liquid-Form Medication Calculations

Liquid medication calculations are similar to that of the tablet calculations. If you have a medication that is 50 mg per 5 ml of liquid, how much liquid do you need if the order is for 150 mg? The same questions and formula can be used for liquid medications as follows:

1. Think—If 5 ml has 50 mg in this situation and we need 150 mg (which is 3 times the unit dose), then it would be common sense to need 3 times the unit amount, which is 5 ml. Thus, the total amount should be 15 ml.
2. Calculate

Unit Dose of Medication / Per Unit Quantity of Medication = Dose Desired (x) / Quantity Desired (x)

$$\frac{(x) \, 50 \text{ mg}}{5 \text{ ml}} = \frac{150 \text{ mg}}{x \text{ ml}}$$

FIRST   SECOND

$$\frac{50 \text{ mg}}{5 \text{ ml}} \quad \frac{150 \text{ mg}}{x \text{ ml}} \qquad \frac{50 \text{ mg}}{5 \text{ ml}} \quad \frac{150 \text{ mg}}{x \text{ ml}}$$

$$150 \text{ mg} \times 5 \text{ml} = \qquad 750 \text{ mg} / x \text{ ml divided by}$$
$$750 \text{ mg} / x \text{ ml} \qquad 50 \text{ mg} = 15 \text{ ml}$$

3. Double-check your math—very important! Always recheck that you have multiplied correctly prior to proceeding because setting up cross multiplication can be a bit tricky.

4. Does this make sense?—Yes, it is the same thought you may or may not have had from the first step. It makes sense that if there are 50 mg in 5 ml, then I would need 15 ml to make up the 150 mg dose required in this order.

Notice, if you include the units as you cross multiply, they end up cancelling each other out and leaving the units you require for the answer.

Preparing to Administer Medications

Before administering medications, it is important to prepare adequately. This preparation consists of not only knowing how to calculate medication doses and important pharmacological principles but also the comprehension on how these all fit together. Why does one need to contemplate the pharmacology of a medication before administering it, if he or she knows the correct procedure to give it to the patient? The answer is found in the context of medication administration for that particular patient and his or her specific clinical situation. It is also found in the nurse's situation before giving medication to a patient and whether he or she is focused on integrating all the knowledge of pharmacology, medication technology, medication safety checks, and dose calculations. In addition, the nurse and nursing student need to assess and evaluate the patient, consider whether or not the medication needs to be altered or its form changed, and be organized prior to giving medications.

Assessment and Evaluation

It is the responsibility of the nurse and student to assess the patient before, and evaluate the patient after, medication administration. Areas to consider when assessing prior to medication administration include the following:

- Reason or need for medication (e.g., pain, infection, shortness of breath, cardiovascular function, diabetes, psychological well-being);
- Patient status prior to medication administration related to each medication required (e.g., if a blood pressure medication is to be given, then the patient's blood pressure should be known prior to medication administration);
- Patient perspective on the medications being administered (e.g., Is the patient aware of the medication that is being given and what the patient's thoughts about taking the medication?); and
- Potential change that the medication may have on the patient's health status.

Thinking ahead to evaluation is important even in the assessment phase of the process. Table 22.3 outlines the most common, but not exclusive, areas of evaluation that should be completed after a medication has been administered.

Altering Medication Administration Strengths and Forms

Altering a medication's form is sometimes a dangerous endeavor if the medications are not meant to be altered or changed. There has been a lot of pressure to gain expedience in medication administration, and mixing crushed medications has been one way that some have thought to save time. Some medications should never be crushed because

TABLE 22.3	Common Areas of Evaluation	
Type of Medication	**Type of Evaluation to Consider**	**Other Points**
Pain medication/analgesic	• Pain rating and evaluation of pain levels after administration • Potential side effects from the specific medication including respiratory status and cognitive status • Possibly elimination patterns because some medications in this category can cause constipation and urinary retention	Ongoing assessment not just a one-time evaluation after administration should be done for all medications because they may have durations that last beyond the evaluation time period. All medications require that the nurse check for allergic reactions or sensitivities to the medication. Severe allergic reactions are possible.
Antibiotic	• Allergies and allergic reactions • Signs of infection • GI upset depending on the route of medication administration	
Cardiovascular medication includes blood pressure and heart function medications	• Blood pressure as indicated • Heart rate as indicated • General perfusion status (capillary refill and colour)	
Respiratory medications including inhalation medications	• Respiratory status and ease of breathing • Breath sounds (auscultation) • Oxygen saturation levels	

BOX 22.7 Medications That You Cannot Crush

The following medications should not be crushed before administration:

- Extended- or sustained-release capsules that are meant to release over a period of time (sometimes indicated with an "ER," "XR," "LA," or "SR" after their names, although there are MANY abbreviations that could follow a medication that indicate extended release)
- Enteric-coated medications—for example, acetylsalicylic acid (ASA)
- Capsules that contain tiny particles or powder encased in a plastic covering. Usually, these capsules that contain active medicinal ingredients are extended-release or are damaging to the esophagus or stomach and thus should not be crushed prior to medication administration.
- Certain analgesic medications for pain
- Medications that could damage or irritate the esophagus
- Other indicated medications such as Accutane, vitamin C, potassium supplements, Theo-Dur and theophylline sprinkles, Prozac, Colace liquid gels, Sinutab, Claritin D, sublingual preparations (discussed later), Nitro-Bid

There are other medications other than those listed here that cannot be crushed without serious repercussions to the patient. Always check with your pharmacist, medication drug guides, or the CPS for relevant information prior to crushing any medication.

this may alter the medication's effect. Mixing medications or changing the form of medications is not a safe practice in which to engage. It is wise to consult with a pharmacist or look up the medications to see if they are compatible with other medications. You need to ask yourself if they can be mixed together, or if they can be changed from their original physical form. See Box 22.7 for a list of medications that generally cannot be crushed.

Organization

It is important to keep yourself organized so that you are better prepared to administer medications. One way to do this is to use an organizational technique to prepare for the required and expected (although in nursing, you need to expect the unexpected!) medication administration times during your shift using a structured worksheet.

One organizational technique is to create a care plan work sheet at the start of the shift. It consists of a list of medications and their times of administration. This care plan worksheet can also list all patient treatments and care modalities. As a nursing student, two of the key challenges you will face are

1. organizing your nursing care and
2. determining your patient care priorities.

The care plan worksheet will be invaluable to you as you develop these skills, critical thinking abilities, integrated with medication administration.

Table 22.4 illustrates the use of the care plan worksheet and how medications can be highlighted according to the hour they are due to be administered. You can also write the actual medications on the worksheet as well. The nurse or student updates the care planning worksheet throughout the day to reflect any changes in orders or medications. Notice how care planning worksheet starts 1 hour later than the usual nursing shift start time (7 AM). This is because nurses are usually responsible for giving medications up to and including the hour they are finished with their shift. The same reciprocal action is seen at 3 PM; the nurse working until 3 PM is responsible for giving the 3 PM medications before leaving.

Skills of Medication Administration

This section emphasizes the actual skills of medication administration. The steps of each process are outlined with applicable concepts and issues being integrated into each skill. Forms of medications, equipment, and routes of administration are discussed.

Jonathan says, "When I first gave medications on a busy surgical unit, I was frightened. I felt I was expected to memorize all the little details about the medication so that I could tell my instructor prior to giving the meds. I stayed up late memorizing the medications, and I thought about all the details throughout the morning shift report. In the end, I drew a blank and couldn't recite my medication side effects when asked by my clinical instructor. I realized that memorizing doesn't help you learn why the patient is receiving the medication—which is what nursing instructors often want you to know about medications. Next time, I will spend more time thinking and less time panicking!"

TABLE 22.4	The Patient Care Worksheet							
	0800	0900	1000	1100	1200	1300	1400	1500
Patient A	MEDS × 4		MEDS × 2	MEDS × 1				MEDS × 3
Patient B		MEDS × 6			MEDS × 5	MEDS × 1		MEDS × 4

Administering Oral Medications

Oral medications are those that are taken by mouth and include those administered through a **gastrointestinal (GI) tube**. These can be medications that come in pill, tablet, capsule, wafer, gummy troches, lozenges, or in elixir (liquid) form. Some oral medications are to be taken whole, whereas some can be crushed for ease of administration or can be split, depending on the dose required. Be aware that not all pills can be split or crushed. Those that cannot be split or crushed can cause harm to the patient if they are split or crushed. Refer back to Box 22.7 for medications that generally should not be crushed. See Table 22.5 for common forms of oral medications. See Skills 22.1 and 22.2 for step-by-step instructions on administering oral medications.

Splitting and Crushing Oral Medications

Nurses are often seen splitting and crushing medications, and student nurses are told to do the same. However, these directions are not directly in the patient care orders. So how does a student nurse know when and how to do this? Crushing is usually done when the patient has a hard time swallowing pills and needs them crushed and mixed with a palatable medium, such as applesauce, for ingestion. Splitting is done when your medication calculations indicate ½ or a pill is required or when the pill is too large to be taken easily by the patient. There are some medications that can be dissolved in water or juice before administration. It is imperative to check with the pharmacist to see whether some medications can be crushed, split, or dissolved for ease of

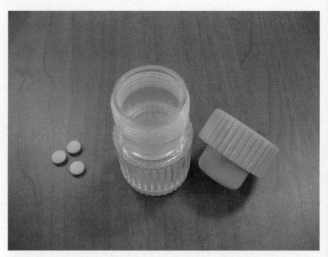

Figure 22.3 Pill crusher. Pill splitters and crushers are pieces of equipment that can be used to cut scored tabs or crush medications requiring a different form for administration. It is important to ensure that these pieces of equipment stay clean and uncontaminated.

administration or whether a liquid alternative is available. Enteric coated, long acting, sublingual, buccal, and capsules usually cannot be crushed, split, or dissolved. When numerous medications are crushed, they should not be mixed with one another, in case of them reacting adversely together, and have an adverse effect occur to the patient.

Medications can be crushed using various techniques specific to the setting and the equipment available. When crushing a medication, first attempt to crush your medication within its packet. This is done easily with individually dosed pills (Fig. 22.3). If the pill must be removed from its packet or container and placed in the device, ensure the device is cleaned before and after each medication is crushed. Cleaning the device between medications is important because contact between medications should be avoided in case that there is an interaction. To split a medication, take the medication without touching it and place it in the splitter with the scored aspect of the pill in line with the cutting mechanism. If the pill does not align with the cutting mechanism, tap the device to align the pill. Again, clean the device before and after use because any remaining residue or powder could interact and cause an adverse effect in the patient.

Think   *To Touch or Not to Touch . . .*

What if you saw a nurse on the unit take a few pills from a bottle in the palm of his or her hand and then pick out two and place them in a patient pill or medication cup. Do you think touching medications with your hands, even washed hands, is okay?

Here is what is at debate with this issue. Some nurses suggest that oral medication administration is not a sterile technique but rather a clean technique. If you wash your hands, then

TABLE 22.5	Common Medication Preparations
Preparations	**Description**
Capsule	Gelatinous container to hold powder or liquid medicine; capsules can also contain medication that is time released.
Enteric coated	Coating that causes drug absorption in intestines rather than the stomach; prevents stomach irritation
Liquid	A pourable form of oral medication that can come in the form of suspension, elixir, emulsion, or syrup
Powder	Finely ground drug; frequently mixed with liquid before administration
Tablet	Compressed hard disk of powdered medication; may be scored for easy breaking; may be sugar-coated or have film coating for cohesion

Adapted from Craven, R., Hirnle, C., & Jensen, S. (2013). *Fundamentals of nursing: Human health and function.* Philadelphia, PA: Lippincott Williams & Wilkins.. Table 19-2, p. 401.

they are technically clean, and you should be able to touch medications. However, one cannot tell what microorganisms they are harbouring on his or her skin, and even despite thorough hand washing, there is no way to guarantee that a potentially harmful microorganism is on the very fingers used to touch the medications. This is also of great concern to patients who have compromised immune systems.

When dispensing medications from a bottle, it is best practice to tap the medication needed into the cap of the bottle and then release the ordered amount into the pill or medication cup. This then promotes the no-touch technique of medication administration where the nurse's microorganisms found on his or her hands are not transferred to the patient or to the remaining medication in the bottle. When taking medications from packages, it is imperative that you do not touch the medications because they are being placed in the pill or medication cup.

As well, when you are splitting medications, although probably easier, do not touch the medication to align it with the cutting surface. Use tapping the splitter if at all possible. Even though something is clean technique, hands are not clean even despite washing them.

Medication Cups

Pill cups, both paper and plastic, are used to carry medications to the patient so that nurses do not touch medications with their hands (Fig. 22.4). The patient may wish to touch the medication by taking it out of the medication cup when it is given to her. Pill cups can also act as barriers between medications if one medication requires administration before another or if special instructions are required for its administration. Beware that all little white pill cups look alike. Make sure that once the pills are poured into the medication cup, you do not lose sight of that pill cup. The pill cup should be labeled appropriately with a patient label or have some form of patient identification.

Think *Cutting Tablets*

What do you do if you require a ½ tablet? Can you cut the medication in half? Luckily, many medications are "scored," meaning they have lines on them indicating they can be cut in half. Medications that are not scored are often not guaranteed to have ½ the medication in any one ½ of the tablet. Therefore, you should be cutting only the tablets that are scored. If you require a ½ tablet after completing your medication calculation but do not have scored tablets, check with another nurse or pharmacy whether there is another dose of tablet that you should be using. Always be cautious and ask! TAKE NOTE: Capsules and enteric-coated medications often cannot be cut in half or crushed.

Pouring Liquids

Plastic liquid cups are used for the pouring and administration of liquid medications. When pouring liquids, it is important to ensure you complete your three medication checks. Liquids are poured into appropriate plastic liquid medication cups with calibrations or measurements on the side. When pouring medication, ensure the label is placed against your palm to avoid spilling medication down the label, making it potentially unreadable. Pour the liquid into the liquid medication cup at eye level. The liquid will form a curved line with the lowest portion near the middle of the medication cup. When reading the calibrations or measurements on the medication cup, the upper portion of the lowest aspect of the curve (meniscus) is where the measurement is taken (see Fig. 22.5 for clarification). In order to ensure dosing accuracy, a nurse can use a syringe (without a needle) to draw up liquid volumes of 10 ml or less. This is especially important in the area of pediatric nursing. When you are done, replace the lid securely on the medication bottle and double-check the label again to make sure the medication is the correct one.

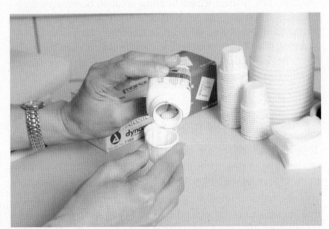

Figure 22.4 Pill cups/medication cups. Medication pill cups are an important component of medication administration. There are plastic cups that have calibrations on them for measuring liquids; there are paper cups for pill administration.

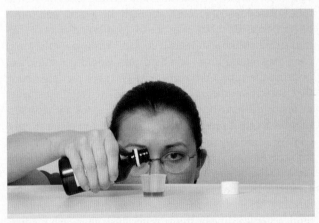

Figure 22.5 Reading calibration on a medication cup. When pouring liquid medications, ensure you are eye level with the measurement lines on the cup in order to better visualize the amount you have poured.

Think *Think Before You Administer Medication—
Three or More Checks Is Best!*

Medications should be checked at least three times before administering them to a patient. These three checks enable nurse to ensure the medication is the correct one for the intended patient. The first check occurs when the nurse retrieves the medication and looks at the medication label to ensure it is the correct drug. The second check happens when the nurse compares the medication and dose to the patient's medication record just before pouring or preparing the drug for administration. The third check takes place when the nurse returns the medication to the shelf or rechecks the wrapper to make sure the medication is the correct drug and dose. After these checks have been completed, it is crucial that the nurse ensure that the person for whom the medications were checked and prepared for is the individual that receives them. Checking a patient's wristband is the final check in a carefully orchestrated process that decreases the chances of medication errors.

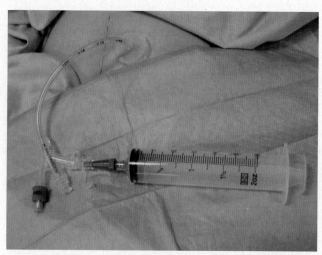

Figure 22.6 Administering medication via a GI tube, syringe, and adapter.

Sublingual and Buccal Medications

Oral medication can come in sublingual and buccal forms. Sublingual medications are placed under the tongue or sprayed under the tongue for absorption versus being swallowed. There is controversy whether these medications should be left to dissolve or whether patients can chew them. Sublingual medications are usually used for relaxation, to decrease anxiety, and for vasodilation. Examples of sublingual medications include lorazepam (Ativan) and nitroglycerin.

Buccal medications are those that are placed in the inner aspect of the cheek or the buccal mucosa for absorption. Although buccal medications are not commonly seen in health-care settings, examples of medications that may use this route include benzocaine as an anesthetic agent and fentanyl for pain relief.

Administering Gastrointestinal Tube Medication

There are many medications that can be administered via a GI tube. GI tubes include tubes that are placed nasogastrically (e.g., decompression tubes and feeding tubes) as well as tubes placed percutaneously through the gastric wall (often referred to as GI tubes) (Fig. 22.6). Medications that are administered via these tubes may require crushing, or they may come in a liquid form. Standard pills would get stuck and obstruct the tube. Although most GI tubes are large bore, they come in numerous diameters and are certainly smaller in diameter than the esophagus. These tubes are also susceptible to great pressure changes, which can result in tube damage if too much pressure is used to force medications through the tube. The size of the selected syringe impacts the pressure that is injected from the syringe. A syringe 10 ml or greater is recommended for medication administration and flushing. Medications that are given via the GI tube route require a sterile saline or sterile water flush after each medication is administered. The amount and type of flush depends on various patient factors including age, fluid restrictions, and is always indicated on the patient care orders.

 Think *Nasogastric (NG) Tubes and Feeding Tubes—
Can We Administer Medications in These?*

Medication administration policies and procedures vary between institutions. Some agencies will allow medications to be administered into NG and small-bore feeding tubes, and others do not. The pros, cons, and other considerations are listed as follows:

NG tubes in Canada are mainly used for stomach decompression versus GI access for feeding. They are however large-bore durable tubes that can be used for feeding. It is important to note that some NG tubes do have a port for air release; however, a patient in need of decompression is not likely to be a great candidate for enteral feeds.

In Canada, small-bore feeding tubes are used for enteral feeds. These small-bore tubes are more susceptible to collapsing and becoming plugged than the large-bore feeding tubes. You can administer medications through these feeding tubes; however, the nurse must take into consideration, the viscosity, the amount, and the pressure being exerted by the syringe size and how these factors can cause the tube to obstruct or collapse. It is important to use adequate flushing solution between medications, medications that can come in a liquid formulary or finely crushed and dissolved medications to prevent occluding the feeding tube. Larger syringes exert less pressure; therefore, using syringes larger than 10 ml will reduce potential pressure damage to the tube.

Topical Medication Administration

Topical medications are those that are placed on the surface of the skin or other tissue areas for absorption. These areas include **transdermal** applications, eye and ear medications, and vaginal and rectal routes. When administered, transdermal medications are placed in areas that are free from hair, lacerations, incisions, and other open areas. Each medication has a specific targeted region for application; be sure you read where the medication is intended to be placed prior to administering it. Wear gloves when administering topical medications to avoid absorbing any of the medication through your own skin.

Transdermal medications are specifically placed on the dermal tissue or skin (Fig. 22.7). These medications are usually time released and require exact application and removal times. An example of this type of application is a nitroglycerin patch that is applied in the morning and removed in the afternoon, usually 12 hours later.

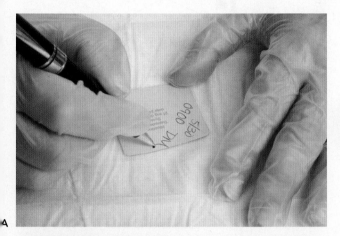

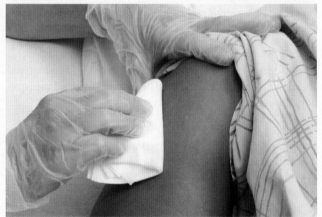

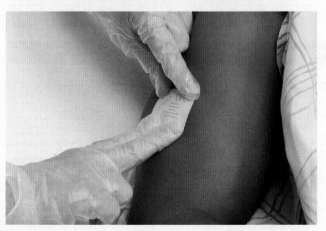

Figure 22.7 Preparation and application of a transdermal patch. **A.** Prepare the transdermal patch for application by writing the date and time of the application on the patch. **B** and **C.** When applying the transdermal patch, ensure the skin is clean, dry, and intact.

Administering Eyedrops and Ointments

Eyedrops are used for various reasons. These drops can aid in eye examinations by altering the pupil dilation or constriction, decrease intraocular pressure with glaucoma patients, treat infection, or assist with eye lubrication. See Skills 22.3 and 22.4 for guidelines on administering eyedrops and eye ointments.

Administering Eardrops

Eardrops are often used to relieve pain, decrease swelling, loosen earwax, and treat infections. Whether for medication administration or ear assessment, nurses need to know how to effectively straighten the external auditory canal in patients/patients of all ages (Nursing Guidelines 22.1, Administering Eardrops).

NURSING GUIDELINES 22.1: ADMINISTERING EARDROPS

Administering eardrops requires that the medication is deposited and can reach the inner ear area for absorption. First, put on gloves and wipe the ear canal with a moistened cloth or gauze pad to ensure that there is no debris blocking the outer canal.

- For adults—Pull the pinna up and back or up; out and back is also acceptable.
- For children older than the age of 3 years—Pull the pinna straight back.
- For children and infants younger than age of 3 years— Pull the pinna down.

After positioning the pinna, usually drops are placed in the outer ear and allowed to run into the internal ear canal. Placement of medication directly into the inner canal can cause pain and discomfort; therefore, allow the medication to gently reach this area for absorption. After medication has been administered into the ear canal, place a clean cotton ball into the external canal to prevent the medication from running out of the ear with movement and have the patient lay on the opposite side for approximately 15 minutes to promote absorption.

Administering Vaginal Suppositories and Creams

Vaginal medications are inserted into the vagina and are absorbed through the vaginal wall. Some medications that are inserted into the vagina act locally within the body cavity to fight infection (e.g., Monistat for vaginal yeast infections). Vaginal medications can come in tablet, cream, or suppository form. Procedures for inserting each form of medication vary slightly (Skill 22.5).

Administering Rectal Suppositories

Rectal medications are those inserted into the distal end of the intestines through the rectum. Medications are absorbed through the intestinal (rectal) wall and carried through the bloodstream. Medications that are inserted rectally must be well lubricated prior to insertion in order to decrease trauma and potential tissue damage. Rectal suppositories are commonly used for regulating bowel elimination. Rectal suppositories are also used for pain relief and general muscle relaxation (Skill 22.6).

Administering Parenteral Medications

Parenteral medication administration involves giving medications into other routes besides the GI tract (*Stedman's Medical Dictionary*, 2005). This can include IV (into the vein), **subcutaneous** (into subcutaneous tissue, the lowermost layer of the integumentary system), **intradermal** (into the space between the dermis and epidermis), and **intramuscular (IM)** (into the muscle) administration (Fig. 22.8). In this chapter, we focus on parenteral administration of medications into the subcutaneous, intradermal, and IM areas. The purpose of giving medications via the parenteral route can depends on (a) the patient situation and whether the parenteral route better meets their medication needs (e.g., someone vomiting should receive medication through the parenteral route vs. the oral route), (b) the type of medication ordered (e.g., some medications cannot be given orally), and (c) the urgency of the need for the medication (e.g., a severe infection may respond more favorably to medications administered parenterally vs. topically or orally).

When considering the parenteral route for the medication ordered, it is important to consider maximum fluid volumes for each specific parenteral site. Deciding how much fluid volume a particular site can tolerate is a balancing act where the size of the patient, the amount of tissue available, and the volume of medication to be administered are carefully considered. Slim older adults patients would not tolerate the maximum dose allowed in the various sites; thus, assessment alterations need to be made. See Table 22.6 for the guidelines for administering parenteral medications.

Equipment Required for Injections

There are various syringes and needles that suit different purposes in medication administration. It is important to select the right size syringe and needle before administering any

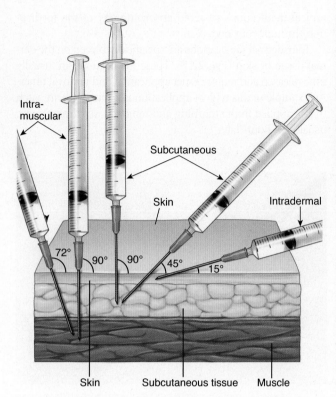

Figure 22.8 Parenteral medication administration. Different types and angles of parenteral administration.

medication to ensure that the medication being administered correctly in the right location. The quality of the administration starts with the equipment used.

Syringes

There are different types of syringes to choose from for injectable medications. There are syringes that are already assembled with needles attached and those that require appropriate needle selection. Syringes vary by the amount of fluid they hold or by the purpose they serve. The different types include 50- and 100-unit insulin syringes that are

TABLE 22.6	Guidelines for Parenteral Medication Administration		
Site	Maximum Amount/ Volume Injected	Age-Related Variations	Notes
IM: deltoid	0.5–1 ml	Not usually used for infants	Some institutions will allow up to 2 ml of fluid in each injection; however, check with agency policy because the potential for underlying nerve damage exists with larger amounts.
IM: vastus lateralis	0.5–2 ml	Decreased amount in younger populations	Used most frequently in infant and young children
IM: ventral gluteal	0.5–3 ml	Decreased amount in younger populations	Used most frequently in adults Some institutions will allow up to 5 ml in one injection; however, check with agency policies because this amount is not frequently injected.
Subcutaneous sites	Up to 1 ml	Decreased amount in younger populations	Some institutions will allow up to 2 ml; however, discomfort and tissue damage may occur with a larger amount.

marked with units as opposed to milliliters for ease of drawing up insulin and 1-ml, 3-ml, 5-ml, and 10-ml syringes. You
may use a 20-ml syringe for drawing up a medication that will
be inserted into an infusion pump or to insert a crushed and
dissolved medication into a GI tube; however, a 20-ml syringe
is not commonly used for injecting medications into patients.

Needles

There are various needles to choose from for parenteral medication administration. If a needle is not attached to your
syringe, then an appropriate one must be selected. When
selecting a needle, consider the gauge (the diameter of the
opening from which medications will be delivered to the
patient) and the length to ensure that the medication will
be deposited in the correct anatomical space (subcutaneous
tissue or IM space) (Box 22.8). Decisions on needle size
must be made for each person on the basis of the size of the
muscle, the thickness of adipose tissue at the injection site,
the volume of the material to be administered, and injection
technique. The gauge of needle is decided based on viscosity
of the medication (thicker medications may require smaller
gauged [wider lumen] needles, e.g., no. 18 gauge) and what
the needle is being used for (a no. 18 gauge needle is helpful for drawing up thick medications however would not
be used for an injection). So in this case, after drawing up
the medication with a no. 18 gauge needle, you would then
switch to a needle whose length and gauge is appropriate for
administering the medication (Fig. 22.9).

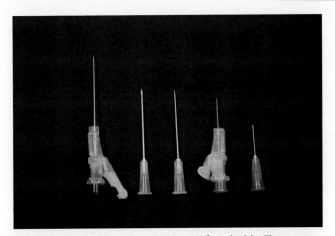

Figure 22.9 Needles with and without safety shields. There are
many different types and sizes of needles that can be used to
inject and draw up medication. Some needles come with white
plastic safety shields that extend over the needle after an injection
to prevent needlestick injuries.

Needleless Components

Some institutions have switched to **needleless** or needle-
free components, systems that allow the nurse or nursing student to draw up medications without the use of
needles. However, giving an injection requires you to switch
to a regular needle before administering the medication.
Figure 22.10 shows how a needleless components are used
to administer medications into existent patient access lines
(e.g. an intravenous line). There are needleless syringe ends
as well as needleless entry ports that are used in the clinical
setting.

Additional Equipment Used With Injections

A sharps container is an important piece of equipment as
all sharp objects including the syringes that are attached
to the needles are disposed of in a proper puncture-proof
receptacle. Gloves and alcohol or chlorhexidine swabs are
also needed.

BOX 22.8   General Needle Gauges and Lengths

The gauge of a needle refers to the diameter of the needle
shaft. It correlates with the size of the needle opening. The
smaller the gauge, the larger the diameter of the needle shaft.
The larger the diameter of the needle shaft, the more viscous
the medication that can be administered to the patient. Understandably, the smaller gauged needles can result in more tissue
damage on insertion. Usual gauges vary from no. 18 to 28,
whereas no. 18 is larger and no. 28 is a smaller diameter.

Subcutaneous injection needles

- Usually ½" to ⅝" length (12 to 16 mm)
- Some obese patients may require 1" needle length (25 mm).
- No. 24 to 26 gauge

IM injection needles

- Commonly use 1" to 1½" needle length (25 to 40 mm)
- Some obese patients may require 2" needle length (50 mm).
- Smaller adult and children may require a shorter needle.
- No. 20 to 22 gauge

Intradermal injection needles

- Commonly use ¼" to ⅝" needle length (6 to 16 mm)
- No. 25 to 27 gauge

Insulin injection needles (excluding insulin pen needles)

- Usually use ½" needle length (12 mm)
- Some obese patients may require 1" needle length (25 mm)
- No. 25 to 29 gauge

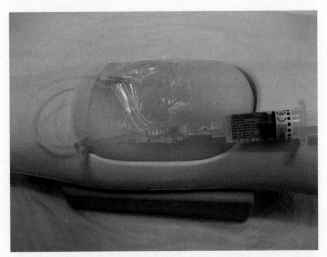

Figure 22.10 Needless equipment used to connect syringes with
needless ports attached to the patient intravenous line.

Think

The Use of Gloves With Injections . . .
Should We or Shouldn't We?

The use of gloves with injections is a debate that is still ongoing in the clinical settings. Some nurses observe that the gloves hamper the awareness that is necessary to avoid contaminating the needle during injections. Gloves may also decrease one's spatial awareness, thereby potentially causing **needlestick injuries**. Other nurses suggest that gloves are imperative to guard against contact with blood and other body fluids during the injection. The third alternative is that a gloved nondominant hand should be used (the hand that will most likely come into contact with the patient during the procedure) and a bare dominant hand holds the syringe. The answer lies in the policies that the agency has put forth for its employees and the individual nurse's practice. Nurses have to decide what their preference is, and if gloves are not worn, protection against unforeseen exposure to blood and body fluids may be limited.

Preventing Needlestick Injuries

Needlestick injuries occur when a needle **punctures** the skin and breaks the skin integrity. In the health-care setting, these injuries can happen to anyone that comes into contact with needles. This can include cleaning staff, physicians, nurses, students, lab technicians, therapists, and many others. The risk with needlestick injuries includes transmission of blood-borne diseases and contact spread bacteria, such as HIV, hepatitis B and C, bacteria, viruses, and fungi.

Frequency

The Canadian Centre for Occupational Health and Safety (2005) reported that needlestick injuries happen far too frequently in health-care settings, and these injuries remain an ongoing issue. In data reported in 2000 from the Centre for Occupational Health and Safety, nurses comprised more than 70% of the total needlestick cases. Needlestick injuries occur most often with percutaneous (including IM or subcutaneous routes) injections but can occur at any stage of the medication administration process.

Outcomes and Interventions

The outcomes from needlestick injuries are often fear, stress, possible infection, and ultimately a loss in work hours. Often after a needlestick injury, the injured individual needs to bleed out the affected area to remove any surface organisms that might be present. After administering first aid practices, the injured individual needs to report the incident through the appropriate channels and with the site-designated occupational health and safety individual. Once the incident has been reported, the source individual's blood should be drawn and sent for screening of blood-borne pathogens. In some areas, the injured individual's blood is also taken as a precaution; however, this is not always necessary until the results are known. If the source blood is negative, then the risk of transmitting the more serious diseases is obviously decreased. If the source blood tests positive for any of the blood-borne pathogens and diseases, then further testing of the injured

individual's blood needs to take place. Once the status of the injured individual is known, then protocols for management of the illness(es) are put into place. For example, prophylaxis treatment for HIV exposure can be implemented. Again, each site and setting has their own protocol for dealing with needlestick incidents. It is imperative that nurses and students know this protocol prior to finding themselves in the unfortunate circumstance of having a needlestick injury.

Having a needlestick injury is a very frightening situation. The injured person needs support and reassurance that everything that can be done is in fact being done. Each nursing program in Canada has a policy and/or protocol in place regarding such injuries, so your program will have a well-developed plan of action in place. Should you incur a needlestick injury or other injuries, inform your clinical instructor, buddy nurse, and/or preceptor right away.

Strategies to Prevent Needlestick Injuries

Prevention is a key strategy in reducing the number of needlestick injuries in Canada. Some strategies recommended by the Canadian Centre for Occupational Health and Safety (2005) are outlined as follows:

- Implement employee training program that focus on facts of needlestick injuries and prevention strategies.
- Follow recommended guidelines that treat all sharp objects as potentially contaminated, ensure all sharp objects are placed in puncture proof disposal units, and avoid recapping any needles.
- Use safe recapping procedures only in exceptional circumstances.
- Use effective disposal systems.
- Implement effective surveillance programs.
- Foster improved equipment design.

Avoiding Needle Contamination

The contamination of needles and syringes occurs when the sterile aspects of the needle and syringe come into contact with nonsterile surfaces. The parts on a needle that are sterile (Fig. 22.11) include the bevel, shaft, and hub. The sterile aspects of a syringe include the tip where the needle connects and the inner aspect of the plunger because it retreats into the sterile inner aspect of the syringe. The barrel and the finger pad on the plunger are the two areas that are not considered sterile. In order to keep needles and syringes sterile, take the following measures:

- Keep all sterile connection ends in plain sight when attaching needles to syringes. Always remove needles and syringes from the wrappers they are encased in. Connecting syringes and needles inside wrappers that impeded the view of the sterile connections can greatly increase the risk of contaminating without even knowing it!
- If your hands shake, anchor in your elbows closer to your body. This will decrease the shaking and lessen the chance of mistakenly touching sterile parts to nonsterile aspects. Don't worry, the hand shaking will eventually subside and disappear as you gain confidence and experience with the skill.

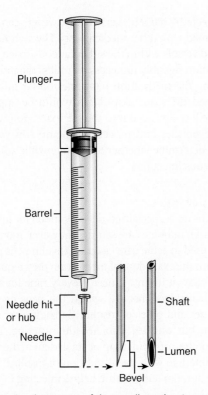

Figure 22.11 Sterile aspects of the needle and syringe: keeping it clean. All components of the needle and syringe need to be kept sterile when administering parenteral medications. The two exceptions to this rule are the barrel exterior (where a nurse grips the syringe) and the finger pad (top of the plunger) do not remain sterile when administering medications.

- Once the needle and syringe are connected, make sure to keep your fingers only on the cap, the barrel of the syringe, and the finger pad of the plunger. Touching other areas of the syringe will contaminate the sterile parts of your equipment.
- Practice maneuvering the syringe and plunger by only touching the nonsterile parts. This will take some time and practice to get it right.

Drawing Up From Vial

Drawing up medication from a vial can be a challenging skill for many nursing students. You will need to develop your manual dexterity skills. There are a few different ways to do this correctly. Vials can be plastic or glass and can contain many different medications that are administered parenterally. This skill will be described using the thinking and preparing steps of medication administration. The actual administration and evaluation steps are discussed with the relevant methods of administration (subcutaneous, IM, intradermal, and IV) found later in this chapter (Skill 22.7).

Once you have the skills for drawing up from a single vial, using two vials and mixing two medications will appear less of a challenge. Whenever mixing medications, it is imperative that you check the compatibility of the two medications being mixed (Skill 22.8).

Reconstituting Medications in Vials

Usually, the facility pharmacy will provide the medications already reconstituted for patient administration; however, there are circumstances where medications require reconstitution from a powder state to a liquid form. This requires adding diluent to the vial and ensuring the powder is fully dissolved in the diluent.

It is important to first read the directions on the vial and note the fully constituted strength or concentration of the medication when you are finished. This will be used to calculate the amount of the newly reconstituted medication you will need to administer. As well, always swab the top of vials with an alcohol swab to ensure the surface is clean prior to inserting any needles or needleless devices.

After reading the directions, draw up the required diluent (sterile normal saline or sterile water) and add it to the vial. Gently remove the syringe from the vial because a pressure buildup will form with the addition of the diluent. Roll the vial lightly between your hands for at least 20 seconds to dissolve the medication entirely. Inspect the liquid to make sure the powder has been dissolved. Label the vial with the new strength of medication as well as the date and time it was reconstituted. Usually, reconstituted medications outdate (expire) within 24 hours. However, check with pharmacy on the shelf life and storage requirements (usually refrigerated) of each reconstituted medication.

Drawing Up Insulin From Two Vials

Preparing an insulin injection is the most common application of drawing up medication from two vials. Typically, there is a short-acting insulin combined with a longer acting insulin drawn up in the same syringe. The short-acting insulin is the most pure—hence, it is clear in nature. The longer acting insulin is cloudy. A mnemonic (or memory aid) to remember is to always draw up "clear to cloudy." Another way to remember the order to draw up two insulins is that clear comes before cloudy in the dictionary; therefore, clear insulin should be drawn up first. This tells us that the clear insulin is drawn up first in the syringe, and then the longer acting insulin is drawn up second. This prevents contamination of the larger supply (the purer, short-acting insulin) with the cloudy longer acting type.

Drawing Up Medications From an Ampoule

Drawing up from an ampoule is a challenging skill for many nursing students, and there are a few different ways to do this. Ampoules are made from glass and can contain many different medications that are administered parenterally. Administration and evaluation steps are discussed with the relevant methods of administration (subcutaneous, IM, intradermal, and IV) found further in this chapter (Skill 22.9).

Drawing Up Medication From Two Ampoules

Drawing up medication from two ampoules uses the same principles as the technique for two vials in that you need to check compatibility of the medications and to decide which medication to draw up first. Usually, the more controlled medication is drawn up first to avoid any potential complications of drawing up more than needed. This usually means that the medication being drawn up first is a narcotic or controlled analgesic. The second medication is usually the lesser of the controlled medications. This includes antiemetics and drugs that are given with more controlled substances. An example of drawing up two medications from two ampoules would be morphine sulfate (the narcotic) and dimenhydrinate (antiemetic). They are considered compatible in the syringe together and could be administered in one injection. Depending on the amount of solution that being drawn up, the appropriate site of injection needs to be selected. Another consideration is being able to differentiate which medication caused a reaction, if the patient has an adverse event. If the patient were to react to the injection of morphine and Dimenhydrinate, it would be challenging to tell which medication caused the reaction. If the patient has received the medications on separate occasions, it would be safe to proceed with the injection; however, if it is the patient's first time receiving the medication, it may be prudent to give them separately, due to the possibility of a reaction. Because ampoules are an open medication container, there is no air that needs to be injected when withdrawing the medication.

Administering Intradermal Injections

Intradermal medications are administered into the dermal space using a needle and syringe. Most intradermal medications are diagnostic in purpose; for example, the tuberculin Mantoux testing and allergy testing where the medication is administered into the very superficial layers of the skin. Intradermal injections are usually done in specialized settings to test for sensitivity to allergens or disease exposure. Intradermal injections can be also used for local anesthesia (Skill 22.10).

Administering Subcutaneous Injections

Subcutaneous injections are common and used in various settings. Subcutaneous medications are administered parenterally into the subcutaneous tissue using a needle and syringe. There are various medications that can be delivered via this route; examples include insulin, pain medication, and anticoagulants. With this route of delivery, they are absorbed and take effect more quickly than oral medications. Once these medications are administered, they cannot be retracted (Skill 22.11).

Aspiration During Administration

Should **aspiration** be done with subcutaneous injections? The purpose of aspirating is to determine whether the needle has struck a vein or capillary. Injecting directly into a capillary or vein can be potentially life-threatening to the patient when injecting a subcutaneously dosed medication into the patient's blood supply. The applicable principle here is that aspiration of the syringe should never be completed with medications that can cause tissue damage when aspirated

and reinjected—namely, heparin. However, can aspiration be performed with other medications? There should be minimal blood vessels within the subcutaneous space, thus making aspiration possibly unnecessary unless the individual administering the medication has gone too far into the more vascularized IM space. Aspiration would be appropriate if the needle has advanced into the IM space. You will want to check the policies and procedures manual in your clinical setting to determine whether to aspirate while administering subcutaneous injections.

Using Insulin Pens

Insulin pens are a specialized delivery mode for insulin. They are often seen in home care settings; however, more and more are being used in acute care facilities. Insulin pens provide the patient with the exact dose of medication they require without having to draw it up into a needle every time for administration. The cartridges that are within the pens come in various mixtures and types of insulin. Cartridges are stored in a refrigerator but warmed prior to administering. In order to prevent lipodystrophy (a lump or small dent in the skin which can then interfere with the absorption of insulin), the insulin should be at room temperature before injecting (Skill 22.12).

Administering Intramuscular Injections

IM injections are a common medication route for parenteral medication administration. Many medications can be administered intramuscularly versus subcutaneously because of the vascularity of IM sites and the ability of these sites to hold more medication than the others. IM medications are administered into muscle tissue using a needle and syringes. These sterile liquids vary and can include pain medication (analgesics) and other antiemetics for nausea. As with subcutaneous medications, these types of medications are absorbed more quickly than oral routes. They are given in larger volumes than subcutaneous medications because the muscle is capable of holding and absorbing more medication fluid. Once these medications are given, they cannot be removed (Skill 22.13).

Intramuscular Sites

There has been a shift in the most commonly used IM site over the past 10 years. Previously, the dorsal gluteal, which offers larger tissue and muscle mass, was the preferred injection site. The use of this site has decreased because sciatic nerve complications have manifested in the clinical setting. The ventral gluteal site is now preferred, thereby decreasing the chances of injecting medications near the lower gluteal nerves. The ventral gluteal site does have an adequate muscle mass and can be easily identified by prominent bony landmarks, such as the greater trochanter and iliac crest. There are some circumstances where the dorsal gluteal site is preferred (or required); individual patient situations, surgeries, and preferences all need to be considered when selecting a site for an IM injection. As students, it is important to know your options regarding injection sites and the pros and cons of each. See pictures of commonly used IM sites for parenteral medication administration with Skill 22.13.

Z-Track Method

Some sources suggest that Z-tracking is the preferred method for all IM injections (Carter-Templeton & McCoy, 2008) (Fig. 22.12). However, the method is mainly used to administer irritating and viscous medications that require the tissue to be sealed after an injection so that medication does not leak out of the site and irritate the tissues outside of the IM space. The decision to consistently use the Z-track method with all IM injections should be based on nurse preference and the policies and procedures that guide a nurse's contextual practice. The procedure for the Z-track IM injection is as follows:

- After the site has been landmarked and swabbed with alcohol or the equivalent for 20 seconds, the nondominant hand displaces the tissues 5 to 10 cm (2 to 4 in.) in a lateral direction.
- Using your dominant hand, inject the needle at a 75 to 90° angle, using a darting motion.
- As the nondominant hand keeps the tissues displaced with the lateral aspect of the hand, it stabilizes the syringe in the injection site while the dominant hand injects the medication.
- Once the medication is fully injected, the syringe is removed, and the skin being displaced by the nondominant hand is released, causing the medication to become trapped in the IM space.

Administering Inhalation Medications

Inhaled medications are those that are administered into the lungs by the force of the patient's breath. These medications can be in the form of aerosolized liquid, powder, or gaseous form. Medications are inhaled from devices such as metered dose inhalers (MDIs) and dry powder inhalers (DPIs). These devices deliver medication in either an aerosol or powder format. The intended effect of these medications is often bronchodilation and/or to reduce inflammation of the airways (Skill 22.14). Often, you will see the use of a spacer with an inhaler. This is a cylindrical chamber that is placed on the end of a metered dose aerosol inhaler to assist with the distribution of the medication upon inhalation. This device decreases the chance of getting the dose delivered to the wrong oral location, thereby decreasing its effectiveness. Spacers should be washed at minimum every week to prevent the buildup of microorganisms and medication.

Another type of inhaled medication is nebulized liquid that is delivered to the lungs using compressed air or oxygen to break the liquid medication into smaller particles for easier disbursement in the lungs. These medications are used frequently to ease congestion, decrease wheezing, reduce inflammation, and dilate the bronchioles (Skill 22.15).

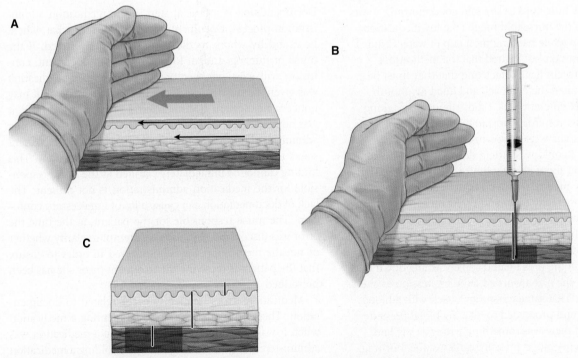

Figure 22.12 Z-track IM injection method. The Z-track method is one type of IM administration that enhances medication absorption into the muscle tissue. This type of injection technique is useful for viscous or irritating medications. **A.** displacing the skin to one side prepares the site for injection, **B.** injecting into the intramuscular space places the medication deep into the appropriate tissue, and **C.** releasing the traction that was used during the medication administration procedure ensures that the medication is kept within the desired location with minimal leakage out of the original needle entry point.

Critical Thinking and Medication Administration: Combining Knowledge and Skill

In this section, we offer observations related to the role of the nurse especially in regard to interprofessional communication, teaching and learning concepts, the role of culture in medication administration, and comfort measures.

Communicating With the Patient and With Health-Care Professionals

When administering medications, it is imperative that nurses and students communicate with other health-care professionals and with the patient about medication administration. Communication is crucial for quality patient care, patient safety, and decreasing medication errors in the health-care setting. During a busy shift, it is often challenging to take the time to communicate with others. However, limited communication creates the potential for students and nurses to precipitate medication errors (e.g., giving prescribed medications to the same patient twice).

Through the eyes of a patient

*I*t was really early in the morning when the nurse came into my room with a tray of little cups. She handed me one of the little cups as she said good morning. I was half asleep as the nurse told me to take my medications inside the cup while handing me a cup of water. I didn't have my glasses on but figured that the medications were for my recent heart attack and that they must be important. I tilted the cup back and filled my mouth with about six different pills. I didn't remember taking this many pills yesterday morning. I tried to wash down the pills but some were dissolving in the back of my throat before I could wash them down. It tasted horrible, and it took me about another hour to remove the bitter taste from my mouth. About an hour and a half later, I started feeling really dizzy and threw up some of the pills. The same nurse that gave me the pills stated that the only pill I was to get in the morning was a vitamin so that shouldn't have caused me to vomit. I told the nurse about all the pills I had trouble washing down that morning and she had a worried facial expression as she left the room. That same nurse came back with a blood pressure cuff and proceeded to take my blood pressure. I was worried there was something wrong as she had already taken my blood pressure earlier in the morning. After taking my blood pressure, the nurse told me that I had been given the wrong medications and that the medications I took could elevate my blood pressure. I was shocked and upset. How could this happen?
(personal reflection of a patient)

The "Through the Eyes of a Patient" illustrates how a patient can easily take the wrong medications when there is limited communication between the patient and nurse. How might the nurse have avoided this type of situation? The nurse could have waited a few moments until the patient was alert and oriented. The nurse could have made sure the medication was intended for this patient by checking the identification band and asking the patient her name. To ensure the patient is receiving the right medication, a nurse should explore the extent to which the patient is familiar with the medications he or she is being given. Patient teaching about the administered medications would also have empowered the patient to speak up and question the medications given to her that morning. Clear communication between the patients and nurses starts with the nurses. Patients are often unsure whether they can ask about the medications and administration procedures. It is up to the nurse to make sure the patient is comfortable asking questions about his or her care by providing the opportunity for this to occur. If a patient or his or her family member questions the medication you are about to administer, stop, and take stock of the situation. Listen to the patient's concerns and then check the medication orders. If these strategies are incorporated into your practice of administering medications, they will help decrease the occurrence of medication errors.

Documentation

Documentation is a crucial step in the medication administration process. Documenting communicates what, when, how, and by whom medications were administered. If the nurse or nursing student forgets or fails to document, confusion will exist whether or not a prescribed medication was given. Because nurses work in shifts, the next shift may notice a medication documentation error. For example, it was noticed that a medication was not documented as being administered during the previous shift. However, the patient states that she was sure she received the medication. This finding cannot be immediately clarified as the nurse responsible for the medication administration is not present. The lack of documentation can cause a lot of unnecessary confusion. The nurse responsible for the patient, at the time the error was discovered, will have to attempt to clarify whether or not the medication was administered in order to ensure that the patient is receiving the treatment he or she has been prescribed.

Medication errors frequently occur related to documentation. These errors include not documenting a medication when it was actually given, documenting a medication was administered when it actually was not, holding a medication and not indicating why the medication was held (not given), documenting medication administration on the wrong patient, and also documenting the wrong medication and dosage of the scheduled medication. Serious consequences can arise from not properly documenting medications that were administered. Patients can become seriously ill as a consequence of medication administration documentation errors. The nurse is responsible for ensuring that the documentation is entered in a timely fashion so that other health-care professionals are clearly able to understand and see that the medication was administered to a patient. The following should be documented for each regularly scheduled medications:

- Correct patient name and identification number
- The drug administered
- The dose administered
- The route administered
- The time administered
- The reason for administration
- Any patient monitoring required for the administration
- Signature and designation of the nursing student or registered nurse who administered the medication (please note this can be an electronic signature that is created when you log on to a computer program using your confidential password and access)
- The patient's reaction to the administered medication if applicable

Ideally, nurses should document immediately following administration of the medication. However, given the acuity of some patients, modification of this practice is necessary to ensure that all patients receive their medications on time. Nurses often administer medications for all patients under their care and then document the administration of these medications during a single charting session.

Nursing students are often told they must document immediately after they have administered their medications. Prompt documentation ensures that other health-care team members know that the medication was given, preventing the patient from possibly receiving another dose in error. Often, nursing students have a small enough patient assignment to follow best practice guidelines of always immediately after they have administered their medications.

Depending on the type of system used for documenting medications, you can expect to document the medication administration event on a paper-and-pen–created log or on a computer-based program that brings up each patient's medication to be administered. Not all MARs are always correct or fully up-to-date. You will want to check with the patient's chart/orders and talk with the nurse responsible for the patient to ensure that you have administered all of the necessary medications. Communication is critical to the health and well-being of your patients, and documentation is one step in that communication process.

Nursing students and other nurses are sometimes asked to document for other nurses who need some assistance with their workload. Although it is a nice gesture to assist your colleagues, this is not an appropriate or safe way to help them. You can only document the administration of medications that you have prepared and administered. If you document for someone else, you are in fact stating that you are taking responsibility for giving that medication. Do not document for others; instead, offer to assist that nurse with something else. Situations may indeed warrant others signing medications for others, such as an emergency code one or cardiac arrest. However, students should not be signing medications for other nurses under any circumstances.

Patient Teaching

Teaching patients about their medications is a very important aspect of administering medications. Patients should know what medication(s) they are receiving, why they are receiving the medication(s), and what the implication(s) of the medication(s) are. More specifically, the possible side effects, what to do if they experience side effects, and the therapeutic actions of the medication is important information to convey to patients. To ensure patients have the information they need, the nurse must consider factors that may influence patient teaching:

- Developmental age and the best medium for the information (e.g., an older adult patient might not be able to read information in size 10 font). Children as well as many adults may not comprehend the depth of medical information that you could provide; therefore, the information needs to be tailored for their specific life circumstances.
- A patient's condition at the time of teaching. Patients who are not feeling well may find it difficult to review medication information when they are acutely ill. Accordingly, it is important to include family or support individuals in the teaching to ensure that the information is understood and can be recalled as needed once the patient returns home and is feeling better.
- Type and depth of information you offer to the patient. This is an important point because medically focused information might not be appropriate for some patients. It is not helpful to simply reiterate textbook knowledge to a patient.
- Setting in which you review the information with the patient. The setting plays an important role in relaying information to patients about their medication regimens. Trying to relay information to patients in a busy and noisy hospital room just prior to discharge is sometimes the only time you may have to speak with the patient; however, it might not be the best setting and time for the uptake of information by the patient and his or her spouse, family members, or significant others.
- Holistic picture including all medications and how best to take the medications. Often, patients do not just have one medication when leaving hospital. Frequently, medications are given to counteract the side effects of the main medication ordered. A holistic review of the medication regimen is important; this is an opportunity to check for interactions and possible side effects that might make the patient more ill. Patients need to have a sense of the bigger picture regarding their medications as well as the specifics of each medication to better manage their medications safely once they leave the health-care setting.

Cultural Considerations

Culture is an important aspect to consider when administering medications to a patient. Every patient (and nurse and nursing student) lives within a cultural context or lifescape. The nature of these lifescapes will influence the extent to which prescribed medication regimens are followed (or not) at home. Although it is impossible to be aware of all cultural implications with patients and their families, the following ideas may help guide your practice as you consider cultural aspects of your patient(s) care:

- Dietary habits and preferences that might impact medication administration;
- Need for privacy during medication administration if any body parts or areas need to be exposed;
- Lifestyle and methods of integrating medication administration into that lifestyle after discharge;
- Spiritual beliefs related to taking medications; and
- Fasting and other rituals that might impact medication administration practices.

It is important to explore the given categories with the patients to better understand possible implications between their current life situation and medication administration.

Providing Comfort Measures

Ensuring that your patient is comfortable may not be an easy task, especially when as a student, you have enough to think about with medication pharmacology and getting the procedure right in front of other nurses and your instructor. Using other measures such as comfort measures, may not seem like a priority when you first start administering medications. Nevertheless, comfort measures are an important part of the administration experience for the patient. These measures are not necessarily time-consuming tasks but can be easily forgotten in the busy clinical environment. The following are some simple things you can do to make sure the patient's experience with medication administration is a comfortable one:

- When giving oral medications, ask the patient how he or she is doing on this medication and let him or her talk about his or her experiences;
- Offer the patient palatable drink or food (if possible and as appropriate) when administering his or her medications;
- Offer a warm blanket when you go into the patient's room in the morning (with his or her medications) or after administering an injection; and
- Use reassuring touch, as appropriate, when giving injections.

Thinking Beyond Medication Administration

In this section, we explore some more essential concepts surrounding medication administration. The administration of PRN or *as needed* medications, medication errors, incident reporting, and the need for lifelong learning are some of the concepts discussed.

Interpreting PRN Orders

PRN medications or *pro re nata* (for an occasion that has arisen) medications are those given on an as-needed basis according to the ordered dose, route, and frequency. PRN medications can be interpreted differently in different settings. For example, critical care areas use PRNs differently than medical or surgical hospital units. The practice of PRN administration is one in which physicians and nurses are interdependent—that is, physicians prescribe the medications; however, nurses make the clinical decisions to administer them. A significant percentage of adult inpatients, 63% to 82%, are prescribed PRN medications (Stein-Parbury, Reid, Smith, Mouhanna, & Lamont, 2008). More focus has been brought on PRN medications recently as some health-care settings and regions want more concrete or consensus guidelines regarding the use of PRN medications. For example, Baker, Lovell, Harris, and Campbell (2007) explored multidisciplinary consensus of best practice for PRN psychotropic medications within acute mental health settings. The study concluded that there is significant ambiguity surrounding how the medication orders are written and the interpretation of dosing and administration times that accompany PRN medication orders. There was also lack of consensus and standardization with regards to the appropriate documentation associated with the administration of PRN medications.

Orders for PRN medications can be complex due in part to the increasing number of PRN orders that are being written, or exist as standing orders, for each patient. If a patient has multiple orders, using multiple routes, the stage is set for medication errors to occur. An example demonstrates how the same ordered medication can have multiple routes, but it does not indicate that the different routes call for different medication strengths.

The order reads, *Morphine 10 mg IV, PO, IM, or SC q4h PRN*. With different absorption rates, this order does not specify if the dose of morphine should be altered according to the differing routes.

Another issue with PRN medications is how nurses interpret the orders with time and dose ranges. The following example is given to illustrate this issue.

The order reads, *Morphine 1–5 mg IV q4–6hr PRN*. This order implies that the nurse is to make a judgment about whether there should be 1 to 5 mg given to the patient every 4 or every 6 hours. Some nurses have given 1 mg and then 30 minutes later decided that they should have given 5 mg and proceeded to "top" the patient up. This "topping up" can result in the collision of the onset, peak, and duration of the medication—multiplying its effects and possibly causing respiratory depression and even respiratory arrest in some patients.

Documentation issues have also arisen with PRNs where inconsistent documentation about which PRN medications are used for what purpose, which medications are ineffective, and the resultant effects of the medications used. Clear and comprehensive documentation surrounding PRNs is required.

The following recommendations are pertinent when giving PRN medications. When interpreting orders,

- Request dose clarification for each route included in the order. Be knowledgeable about the safe doses for each possible route for a specific medication.
- If the order has a dose range, use your assessment skills to determine what the most appropriate dose is to be given. Once a dose is given, do not top up or give additional medication until the time frame has expired on the first dose given. If the patient is in pain after the dose has been administered and the dose has had time to take effect, then call the physician, let them know of the situation, and request a one-time order for an analgesic medication.
- If the order has a time range, ensure you are assessing the adequate length of time that is most effective for that particular patient.

When documenting orders, ensure that documentation always includes the following:

- Pre-dose administration assessment
- Time and date
- Dose
- Route
- Therapeutic effects
- Any adverse effects

Medication Administration Errors

Medication administration errors are said to occur as frequently as at least once per every five medication administration events (McBride-Henry & Foureur, 2006). This degree of incidence is concerning because not all medication errors are reported, and near-miss events are infrequently reported. How frequent are medication errors occurring and what role can nurses and students take to prevent these errors from resulting in patient harm? As a student, it is difficult to balance knowledge of medications with the task of administering medication. There is also an urgent need to decrease medication errors in the health-care system, and students are in a tough but pivotal role to reduce the number of errors that occur.

In a study conducted by Wolf, Hicks, and Farley (2006), the errors made by students mainly resulted in with no harm being done to the patient ($n = 921$, 70.6%). However, 25% of the time, there were incidents of the student medication administration error reaching the patient resulting in extra treatment or monitoring required ($n = 332$, 25.4%). With these statistics in mind, it is important to understand the student perspective for medication errors and what contributes to their occurrence. This study found that the major reason for errors was performance deficits ($n = 579$, 51%); the second most common reason was centered on procedures or protocols not being followed ($n = 362$, 32%). Other reasons included knowledge deficit, inadequate communication, system safeguard failures, and poor or inadequate documentation (Wolf et al., 2006).

Preventing Medication Errors

To avoid making errors in medication administration, ensure you are knowledgeable about the setting, have in-depth knowledge about the medication, know the medication administration practices and policies of the agency and your educational institution, and, most importantly, stay aware that you don't know everything. Although it may seem easier to administer a medication you are not sure about than admit to not knowing something, it is prudent to acknowledge your knowledge deficit and defer the skill until you have obtained that knowledge. Remember that your clinical instructor is there for you. If you are unsure about any aspect of medication administration, ask your clinical instructor or unit nurses for assistance or support.

Some ways to reduce medication errors in the student and nurse population include examining the role of workplace distractions that contribute to potential medication errors, human factors that contribute to medication errors, and to ensure better communication of the protocols and procedures that need to be followed. A recent study examined these factors and targeted initiatives in improving interdisciplinary teamwork, communication, and unit atmosphere to reduce medication errors. It was found that working explicitly with dosage calculation skills amongst nursing students can reduce the potential they have for making medication errors (Pape et al., 2005). Box 22.9 lists tips for preventing

BOX 22.9 Tips for Preventing Medication Errors

In order to better prevent against medication errors,

- Always be knowledgeable about the medications that are being given by looking them up if the information is not readily available from memory.
- Do not administer medications you do not know how to administer—ask for help.
- Double- and triple-check medication dosage calculations before giving a medication
- Know the patient who is receiving the medication—knowing the patient history and context will assist in prevention of giving the wrong medication.
- Know and understand the policies and procedures of the setting and also the educational institution where the student is from.
- Keep open and frequent communication between nurses, students, and instructors. This can prevent double and missed dosing of medications.
- Double-check patient identifying information by using an armband and also asking the patient to state his or her name EVERY time a medication is given.
- Checking the chart frequently for discontinued and stopped orders.
- Documenting the administration after the medication has been given. Although this can be time-consuming, reporting an incident of medication error is more time-consuming.
- Eliminate distractions as much as possible to help focus one on the task of medication administration.
- Foster and promote good team work on the unit.
- Report all incidences of medication errors so that more can be learned from them.

medication errors. Although it is expected that students will make mistakes, it is also expected that their nursing program will ensure that students are strongly positioned to be safe in the clinical setting (Gregory et al., 2008).

Writing Occurrence or Incident Reports

Occurrence or incident reports do not always mean that absolute harm has come to a patient; they can mean that an incident has occurred, from where little to significant harm has happened. Faculty members and nurses are looking out for students and want to help to prevent serious mistakes from occurring. As a student learning to give medications, you may cause a medication error and consequently have to fill out an incident report. Many students feel devastated when this happens, but it is important to use the experience to grow and mature as a novice clinician.

Incident reports will be filed for late medications, omitted medications, improperly administered medications, double administered medications, and also adverse medication patient reactions. The ethical thing to do if you think you have contributed to an error is to own up to it; this practice is in keeping with the Canadian Nurses Association's Code of Ethics for Registered Nurses (2003). The Canadian Patient Safety Institute has recently developed competencies for health-care professionals regarding such an event (2008). Students need to learn how to recognize, respond to, and disclose adverse events or errors. After ensuring that the patient is safe and not in harm's way, report the incident to the appropriate individuals, including your clinical instructor, faculty member, and the charge nurse. Being accountable and responsible for your actions is paramount in nursing. After the incident has been addressed, you need to reflect on the incident and ask yourself why it happened, what happened, and how you could have prevented the error. Others involved in the situation should also reflect on the same questions. Finally, for those students who do not demonstrate growth in their clinical practice or whose actions concerning medication administration are assessed as unsafe, clinical learning contracts or clinical enhancement plans can be implemented. These contracts identify where students are having difficulty. Moreover, they provide a plan of action to strengthen the student's knowledge and skills. The clear majority of students who enter into these contracts demonstrate success (Gregory et al., 2008).

Practicing Lifelong Learning

The world of medications is constantly changing; new medications, techniques for administration, and new knowledge are arising every day. The "Research Review" box offers an example of new and interesting ways research is being applied to the field of medication administration. This being said, it is up to each individual nurse to read and become familiar with new medications and techniques in order to keep abreast of changes and new innovations that are being integrated into health-care settings. These changes impact the way heath care is delivered and the way we practice as nurses. As you come to the end of this chapter and think "There was a lot to learn in this chapter," know that there is a lot more awaiting you in the world of nursing, as you embark to administer medications safely, competently, and effectively. Nurses are indeed knowledge workers!

Jonathan's perspective, "Finally, after learning about medication administration and completing the various skills associated with this very large concept, I felt immensely better about all that goes into medication administration. Although it may seem like common sense after you have applied it in the clinical setting, it is truly very intricate as you are learning it. I feel better equipped to be a good nurse and focus on giving quality patient care versus just worrying and being anxious about giving medications!"

SKILL 22.1	Administering Oral Medications

Reviewing Pertinent Information

Step	Rationale
Review the medication(s) ordered from the medication record or patient chart.	Important to know why the patient is receiving the medication, if the medication is appropriate for the patient's situation, and actual appropriateness of the dose and route ordered
Review patient allergies to medications and food products.	Some food products are found in medications and can cause an allergic reaction as well as medication allergic reaction to the active medicinal ingredient.
Review the applicable pharmacological principles of the medication including the onset and duration of action.	Knowing the pharmacological mechanism of action can aid in monitoring for therapeutic and adverse effects of the medication. This information is also useful when teaching your patient the expected outcome(s) of the medication.
Review pertinent lab results pertaining to the medication indication for your patient.	Lab and diagnostic results offer more information into why the patient is receiving the medication and if the medication is having a therapeutic or adverse effect.

Preparing for Administration

Step	Rationale
Wash hands.	Prevents the spread of microorganisms to the supplies being used and handled and prevents further spread to the patient
Gather supplies needed: • Medication • Appropriate medication cup • Liquid for swallowing medication if needed or mixing agent for crushed meds (jam, applesauce, etc.) if applicable. • Copy of patient identification information (can be a patient label, a copy of the medication record, or other piece of information that identifies the patient)	Important to get organized prior to administering medications to the patient; organization can save a potential medication error. Bringing patient identifying information (label, medical record, or other suitable alternative) can aid in the reminder to check patient identification and also provides a solid piece of material from which to ensure your patient's identity prior to administering medication.
Prepare the medication for administration by • Checking medication for expiry date • Checking the medication once when it is removed from its storage location and again for the second time to the patient's medication record; a third check is completed when the medication storage container or wrapper is returned to storage or discarded. • Leaving medication in its original wrapper and remove medication just prior to administering at the bedside.	Expiration dates can easily go unnoticed on some medications. Expired medications can be ineffective or cause unknown side effects from ingestion. Completing three medication checks can limit the chances of medication error.
Prepare the patient by • Checking patient identifying information using a two-step method; checking the patient armband and then asking the patient to verify his or her name. • Checking the medication against the armband • Explaining the administration process and purpose of medication(s) • Adjusting the bed height and creating privacy • Completing any necessary pre-administration assessments including the ability of the patient to take the medication via the prescribed route • Providing patient teaching about the administration and needed follow-up	Double-checking patient identification greatly decreases potential for error. Explaining the purpose of the medication and what will occur fosters patient collaboration and integration into the medication administration process. Checking the medication against the patient wristband is a crucial step in ensuring the right medications are given to the right patient. Patients who are more knowledgeable about the process are usually more comfortable asking questions. Some patients may not be able to take the medications via the route intended and may need to have the order reevaluated. Teaching can provide the necessary understanding that will foster more effective outcomes through patient participation.

Administering the Medication: Oral Medications

Step	Rationale
1. Position patient in a semi-Fowler to high Fowler position unless contraindicated. 2. Open medication package and allow medication to fall into medication cup without touching the medication. Repeat if there is more than one medication to administer. 3. Offer the medication cup to the patient with the applicable swallowing agent or liquid for swallowing. Note: Sublingual or buccal medications are not to be swallowed thus require administration separate from other oral medications. See next with the specifics of administering sublingual or buccal medications (see Figure 1).	Semi-Fowler or high Fowler position promotes ease of swallowing. Keeping the medications in the package allows you to remember which medications are which. This aids in patient teaching about each medication and fosters the administration of the correct medications to each patient. Patients can take their medications with water or regular liquid. Crushed medications can be added to applesauce, pudding, or jam-like food products for ease of administration.

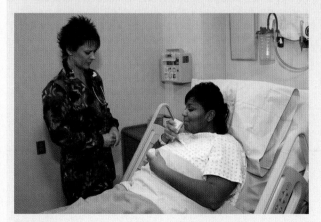

Figure 1

(continued on page 506)

SKILL 22.1   Administering Oral Medications (continued)

Administering the Medication: Oral Medications (continued)

Step	Rationale
4. Assist the patient as needed with swallowing the medications.	Some patients prefer you to drop the pills from the cup into their mouth if they have visual complaints or are unable to grasp the pills with their hands or fingers.
5. Assist patient to comfortable position.	Patient comfort
6. Wash hands.	Removes potential microorganisms from hands and stops cross-contamination between patients

Administering the Medication: Sublingual Medications

Step	Rationale
1. Position patient in a semi-Fowler to high Fowler position unless contraindicated.	Semi-Fowler or high Fowler position promotes ease of swallowing.
2. Prepare the medication a. Pill form—Open medication package and allow medication to fall into medication cup without touching the medication. Repeat if there is more than one medication to administer. b. Spray form—Double-check the label prior to administering.	Keeping the medications in the package allows you to remember which medications are which. This assists with patient teaching about each medication and fosters the administration of the correct medications to each patient.
3. Administer the medication a. Pill form—Offer the medication cup to the patient and ask him or her to place the medication underneath the tongue. b. Spray form—Ask the patient to lift his or her tongue and administer the ordered number of sprays.	Sublingual medications are to be placed under the tongue for faster absorption than regular oral medications.
4. Assist patient to comfortable position	Patient comfort
5. Wash hands.	Removes potential microorganisms from hands and stops cross-contamination between patients

Engaging in Evaluation

Step	Rationale
Assess the patient's response to medication administration.	How was the procedure for the patient? Was the patient able to cope with the procedure or was it painful?
Evaluate for specific therapeutic effects of the medication.	Monitoring for therapeutic effects will assist in ensuring the medication is working for the patient.
Monitor for adverse effects after administration.	Some medications do have adverse effects, and quick identification of these will prevent further potential complications for the patient.

Documenting Effectively

Step	Rationale
Document the medication administration in a timely manner and include the following: • Date and time • Medication administered • Route administered • Patient's response • Medication effects (therapeutic and adverse) • Other pertinent observations	Documentation is the key communicative method between health-care professionals. The more complete the documentation, the better other health-care team members are able to understand exactly what and how the medication was administered. The prevention of medication errors and adverse events relies heavily on communication.
	Regularly scheduled medications and as-needed medications are often logged in the patient MAR. These records can either be electronic or hard copy. PRN medications are often documented in the patient medication record and in the narrative documentation notes to ensure that the dose, route, reason for administration, and effect of the medication are noted. Regularly scheduled medications are often just logged in the MAR and not in the narrative nurses' notes. However, unusual observations and adverse effects should be adequately documented in the nurses' notes, for any scheduled medications.

SKILL 22.2 Administering Gastrointestinal Tube Medications

Reviewing Pertinent Information

Step	Rationale
Review the medication(s) ordered from the medication record or patient chart.	Important to know why the patient is receiving the medication, if the medication is appropriate for the patient's situation, and actual appropriateness of the dose and route ordered
Identify patient allergies to medications and food products.	Some food products are found in medications and can cause an allergic reaction as well as medication allergic reaction to the active medicinal ingredient.
Consider the applicable pharmacological principles of the medication including the onset and duration of action.	Knowing the pharmacological mechanism of action can aid in monitoring for therapeutic and adverse effects of the medication. This information is also useful when teaching your patient the expected outcome(s) of the medication.
Review pertinent lab results pertaining to the medication indication for your patient.	Lab and diagnostic results offer more information into why the patient is receiving the medication and if the medication is having a therapeutic or adverse effect.

Preparing for Administration

Step	Rationale
Wash hands.	Prevents the spread of microorganisms to the supplies being used and handled and prevents further spread to the patient
Gather supplies needed: • Medication • Nonsterile gloves • Pill crusher if needed • Water for mixing with crushed medications if needed • Liquid medication cups if needed • Two 60-ml syringes • 10-ml syringes as necessary • Appropriate adapters end to fit into the GI tube • Water, sterile water, or sterile saline for flushing as per agency policy • Copy of patient identification information (can be a patient label, a copy of the medication record, or other piece of information that identifies the patient)	Important to be organized prior to administering medications to the patient; organization can save a potential medication error. Bringing patient identifying information (label, medical record, or other suitable alternative) can aid in the reminder to check patient identification and also provides a solid piece of material from which to ensure your patient's identity prior to administering medication.
Prepare the medication for administration by • Checking medication for expiry date • Checking the medication once when it is removed from its storage location and again for the second time to the patient medication record; a third check is completed when the medication storage container or wrapper is returned to storage or discarded.	Expiration dates can easily go unnoticed on some medications. Expired medications can be ineffective or cause unknown side effects from ingestion. Completing three medication checks can limit the chances of medication error.
Some medications will come in liquid form and prefilled for direct administration into the GI tube. These prefilled syringes will need to have appropriate adapter ends attached to them prior to administration. If the medications are required to be crushed, the nurse will need to ensure the medication is crushable, then crush the medication and mix it with appropriate diluent (sterile water or sterile saline as per agency policy). Once the crushed medication is dissolved into the diluent, it should be drawn up into an appropriate sized syringe (10 ml or greater) for administration. A proper adapter is required for the syringe to fit into the GI tube.	Although prefilled syringes are much easier, ensure the syringe is large enough so that undue pressure will not be exerted on the tube. The smaller the syringe, the greater the pressure that it dispenses when liquid is pushed from it. Usually, the rule is a 10-ml syringe, and no smaller should be used to administer medications into a GI tube.
If the medication is a liquid and comes in a multiple-dose bottle, use a liquid medication cup and dispense the correct amount into the plastic cup. Then, draw up the medication using a 10–20-ml syringe (depending on amount of liquid needed/ordered) for administration into the GI tube. Again, a proper adapter is required for the syringe to fit into the GI tube.	Note: Do not put the syringe directly into the medication bottle because the outside of the syringe is not sterile and will cause cross-contamination of microorganisms.

(continued on page 508)

SKILL 22.2   Administering Gastrointestinal Tube Medications (continued)

Preparing for Administration (continued)

Step	Rationale
Prepare the patient by • Checking patient identifying information using a two-step method; checking the patient wristband and then asking the patient to verify his or her name • Checking the medication against the wristband • Explaining the administration process and purpose of medication • Adjusting the bed height and creating privacy • Completing any necessary pre-administration assessments and vital signs • Providing patient teaching about the administration and needed follow-up	Double-checking patient identification greatly decreases potential for error. Explaining the purpose of the medication and what will occur fosters patient collaboration and integration into the medication administration process. Checking the medication against the patient wristband is a crucial step in ensuring the right medications are given to the right patient. Patients who are more knowledgeable about the process are usually more comfortable asking questions. Teaching can provide the necessary understanding that will foster more effective outcomes through patient participation.

Administering the Medication

Step	Rationale
1. Position patient in a semi-Fowler to high Fowler position and put on nonsterile gloves.	Semi-Fowler or high Fowler position promotes ease of digestion and reduces risk of aspiration. Gloves protect from contact with any gastric contents.
2. Stop or place any GI tube feedings that may be running on hold and remove the line attached, ensuring the line end does not touch anything.	Will stop any of the feed solution from coming out the GI tube when you go to administer medications
3. Attach a 60-ml syringe to the GI tube and aspirate for stomach contents/residual. Residual over 100 ml should be reported if the patient is not being fed at that particular time. Any contents aspirated are then returned to the stomach. Clamp the tube.	Confirms placement and checks on residual amounts
4. Draw up 20-ml flush solution with the second 60 ml syringe and attach the syringe to the GI tube. Unclamp the tube and flush the GI tube with the solution. Clamp the tube when done.	Clears the tube of stomach contents and residual prior to medication administration
5. Remove 60-ml syringe and attach medication syringe. Unclamp the tube and using gentle pressure, depress the plunger and administer the medication into the tube. Clamp the tube when you are done.	Clamping in between medication and flush stops the tube from regurgitating the content just delivered by syringe.
6. Use a flush of 15–20 ml with the appropriate flush solution between medications. Clamp the GI tube when done.	Clears the tube of medication residual; ensures patency in the GI tube
7. Use a final flush of 20–30 ml after all medications have been infused.	Clears the tube of all medications and prevents occlusions from occurring
8. Clamp the tube and remove the syringe. Reattach the feeding tube as needed and unclamp the GI tube. If the GI tube is left unhooked, ensure clamp is on.	Leaves the tube clamped so medications cannot leak out
9. Leave patient in semi-Fowler position for at least 30 minutes after medication administration.	Fosters the digestion and absorption of the medications; prevents aspiration
10. Assist patient to comfortable position	Patient comfort
11. Remove gloves and wash hands.	Removes potential microorganisms from hands and stops cross-contamination between patients

Engaging in Evaluation

Step	Rationale
Assess the patient's response to medication administration.	How was the procedure for the patient? Was the patient able to cope with the procedure or was it painful?
Evaluate for specific therapeutic effects of the medication.	Monitoring for therapeutic effects will assist in ensuring the medication is working for the patient.
Monitor for adverse effects after administration.	Some medications do have adverse effects, and quick identification of these will prevent further potential complications for the patient.

Documenting Effectively

Step	Rationale
Document the medication administration in a timely manner and include the following: • Date and time • Medication administered • Route administered • Patient's response • Medication effects (therapeutic and adverse) • Other pertinent observations	Documentation is the key communicative method between health-care professionals. The more complete the documentation, the better able other health-care team members are able to understand exactly what and how the medication was administered. The prevention of medication errors and adverse events relies heavily on communication.

SKILL 22.3   Administering Eyedrops

Reviewing Pertinent Information

Step	Rationale
Review the medication(s) ordered from the medication record or patient chart.	Important to know why the patient is receiving the medication, if the medication is appropriate for the patient's situation, and actual appropriateness of the dose and route ordered
Identify patient allergies to medications and food products.	Some food products are found in medications and can cause an allergic reaction as well as medication allergic reaction to the active medicinal ingredient.
Consider the applicable pharmacological principles of the medication including the onset and duration of action.	Knowing the pharmacological mechanism of action can aid in monitoring for therapeutic and adverse effects of the medication. This information is also useful when teaching your patient the expected outcome(s) of the medication.
Review pertinent lab results pertaining to the medication indication for your patient.	Lab and diagnostic results offer more information into why the patient is receiving the medication and if the medication is having a therapeutic or adverse effect.

Preparing for Administration

Step	Rationale
Wash hands.	Prevents the spread of microorganisms to the supplies being used and handled, and prevents further spread to the patient
Gather supplies needed: • Medication bottle • Nonsterile gloves • Washcloth or normal saline and gauze • Tissue • Copy of patient identification information (can be a patient label, a copy of the medication record, or other piece of information that identifies the patient)	Important to get organized prior to administering medications to the patient; organization can save a potential medication error. Bringing patient identifying information (label, medical record, or other suitable alternative) can aid in the reminder to check patient identification and also provides a solid piece of material from which to ensure your patient's identity prior to administering medication.
Prepare the medication for administration by • Checking medication bottle for expiry date • Checking the medication bottle once when it is removed from its storage location and again for the second time to the patient's medication record; a third check is completed when the medication storage container or wrapper is returned to storage or discarded. • Verifying the order as to which eye or eyes it is being administered into	Expiration dates can easily go unnoticed on some medications. Completing three medication checks can limit the chances of medication error.

(continued on page 510)

SKILL 22.3   Administering Eyedrops (continued)

Preparing for Administration (continued)

Step	Rationale
Prepare the patient by • Checking patient identifying information using a two-step method; checking the patient armband and then asking the patient to verify his or her name • Checking the medication against the armband • Explaining the administration process and purpose of medication • Adjusting the bed height and creates privacy • Completing any necessary pre-administration assessments • Providing patient teaching about the administration and needed follow-up	Double-checking patient identification greatly decreases potential for error. Explaining the purpose of the medication and what will occur fosters patient collaboration and integration into the medication administration process. Checking the medication against the patient wristband is a crucial step in ensuring the right medications are given to the right patient. Patients who are more knowledgeable about the process are usually more comfortable asking questions, when privacy is provided. Completing an eye assessment for redness, swelling, discharge, and pain prior will offer a baseline from which the nurse can further assess the changes after medication administration. Teaching can provide the necessary understanding that will foster more effective outcomes through patient participation.

Administering the Medication

Step	Rationale
1. Put on nonsterile gloves.	Gloves will protect the patient from surface organisms from the nurse's hands and will protect the nurse from possible body secretions that may come into contact with the nurse's hands during the administration procedure.
2. Wet the clean washcloth with warm (not hot) tap water or soak the gauze in normal saline solution and gently clean the eye(s) from the inner canthus toward the outer canthus.	Cleaning the eye removes any discharge from the eye that may impede administration, distribution, and absorption of the medication. Use separate cloth to clean each eye to avoid transferring unwanted microorganisms between eyes.
3. Have the patient tilt his or her head back and look up toward a focal point on the ceiling.	Exposes the lower conjunctival sac for administration
4. Remove the medication cup from the eyedrop bottle; be careful not to contaminate the tip of the bottle by touching it to anything (including the outer aspect of the cap). Hold the bottle in your dominant hand.	Keeping the medication bottle tip clean ensures no contamination of the medication inside the bottle.
5. With your nondominant hand, gently pull the lower eyelid(s) down, exposing the lower conjunctival sac (see Figure 1).	Exposes the lower conjunctival sac and provides a pocketed area for administration

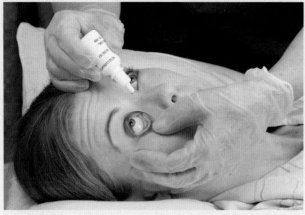

Figure 1

6. Invert the medication bottle and hold it about 7–10 cm above the eye for administration.	Ensures adequate distance as to not touch or damage the eye if the bottle moves suddenly
7. Administer the prescribed number of drops by gently squeezing the medication bottle.	Using gentle pressure will ensure you are able to deliver the exact amount of medication desired. Too much pressure will release more medication than ordered.
8. Release the lower lid from your nondominant hand, ask the patient to gently close his or her eyes, and place gentle pressure on the inner canthus to assist in medication absorption.	Allowing for medication absorption will assist in the distribution of medication to the affected areas.

Administering the Medication (continued)

Step	Rationale
9. Offer patient tissue if needed.	Administration can cause nasal discharge. It is important to not have the patient absorb any medication from the eye.
10. Assist patient to comfortable position.	Keeping the head tilted back for too long will be uncomfortable for the patient.
11. Remove gloves and wash hands.	Washing your hands removes any powder from gloves and potential microorganisms.

Engaging in Evaluation

Step	Rationale
Assess the patient's response to medication administration.	How was the procedure for the patient? Was the patient able to cope with the procedure or was it painful?
Evaluate for specific therapeutic effects of the medication.	Monitoring for therapeutic effects will assist in ensuring the medication is working for the patient.
Monitor for adverse effects post administration.	Some medications do have adverse effects, and quick identification of these will prevent further potential complications for the patient.

Documenting Effectively

Step	Rationale
Document the medication administration in a timely manner and include the following: • Date and time • Medication administered • Route administered • Site of administration (which eye or both eyes) • Patient's response • Medication effects (therapeutic and adverse) • Other pertinent observations such as a completed eye assessment prior to medication administration	Documentation is the key communicative method between health-care professionals. The more complete the documentation, the better other health-care team members are able to understand exactly what and how the medication was administered. The prevention of medication errors and adverse events relies heavily on communication.

SKILL 22.4   Administering Eye Ointments

Reviewing Pertinent Information

Step	Rationale
Review the medication(s) ordered from the medication record or patient chart.	Important to know why the patient is receiving the medication, if the medication is appropriate for the patient's situation, and actual appropriateness of the dose and route ordered
Identify patient allergies to medications and food products.	Some food products are found in medications and can cause an allergic reaction as well as medication allergic reaction to the active medicinal ingredient.
Consider the applicable pharmacological principles of the medication including the onset and duration of action.	Knowing the pharmacological mechanism of action can aid in monitoring for therapeutic and adverse effects of the medication. This information is also useful when teaching your patient the expected outcome(s) of the medication.
Review pertinent lab results pertaining to the medication indication for your patient.	Lab and diagnostic results offer more information into why the patient is receiving the medication and if the medication is having a therapeutic or adverse effect.

Preparing for Administration

Step	Rationale
Wash hands.	Prevents the spread of microorganisms to the supplies being used and handled and prevents further spread to the patient
Gather supplies needed: • Medicated ointment • Gloves • Washcloth or normal saline and gauze • Tissue • Copy of patient identification information (can be a patient label, a copy of the medication record, or other piece of information that identifies the patient)	Important to be organized prior to administering medications to the patient; organization can save a potential medication error. Bringing patient identifying information (label, medical record, or other suitable alternative) can assist in the reminder to check patient identification and also provides a solid piece of material from which to ensure your patient's identity prior to administering medication.

(continued on page 512)

SKILL 22.4   Administering Eye Ointments (continued)

Preparing for Administration (continued)

Step	Rationale
Prepare the medication for administration by • Checking medication for expiry date • Checking the medication once when it is removed from its storage location and again for the second time to the patient's medication record; a third check is completed when the medication storage container or wrapper is returned to storage or discarded. • Verifying the order as to which eye or eyes the ointment is being administered into	Expiration dates can easily go unnoticed on some medications. Expired medications may be ineffective or cause unknown side effects. Completing three medication checks can limit the chances of medication error.
Prepare the patient by • Checking patient identifying information using a two-step method; checking the patient armband and then asking the patient to state his or her name • Checking the medication against the armband • Explaining the administration process and purpose of medication • Adjusting the bed height and creates privacy • Completing any necessary pre-administration assessments • Providing patient teaching about the administration and needed follow-up such as not rubbing the eye while the ointment is absorbing and not wiping away the ointment from the eye for as long as possible	Double-checking patient identification greatly decreases potential for error. Explaining the purpose of the medication and what will occur fosters patient collaboration and integration into the medication administration process. Checking the medication against the patient wristband is a crucial step in ensuring the right medications are given to the right patient. Patients who are more knowledgeable about the process are usually more comfortable asking questions. Completing an eye assessment for redness, swelling, discharge, and pain prior will offer a baseline from which the nurse can further assess the changes after medication administration. Teaching can provide the necessary understanding that will foster more effective outcomes through patient participation.

Administering the Medication

Step	Rationale
1. Put on nonsterile gloves.	Gloves will protect the patient from surface organisms from the nurse's hands and will protect the nurse from possible body secretions that may come into contact with the nurse's hands during the administration procedure.
2. Wet the clean washcloth with warm (not hot) tap water or soak the gauze in normal saline solution and gently clean the eye(s) from the inner canthus toward the outer canthus.	Cleaning the eye removes any discharge from the eye that may impede administration, distribution, and absorption of the medication. Use separate cloth to clean each eye in order to avoid transferring microorganisms.
3. Have the patient tilt his or her head back and look up toward a focal point on the ceiling.	Exposes the lower conjunctival sac for administration
4. Remove the lid from the ointment tube; be careful not to contaminate the tip of the bottle by touching it to anything (including the outer aspect of the cap). Hold the tube in your dominant hand.	Keeping the tip of the medication tube clean ensures no contamination of the medication inside the bottle.
5. With your nondominant hand, gently pull the lower eyelid(s) down, exposing the lower conjunctival sac.	Exposes the lower conjunctival sac and provides a pocketed area for administration
6. Squeeze approximately 1–2 cm (½ in.) of medication from the tube.	Over squeezing of the medication will provide too much ointment for the eye.
7. Gently place the ointment into the lower conjunctival space; be careful not to touch the eye with the medication tube.	If the tube touches the eye, it can contaminate the medication tube and also potentially cause damage to the eye.
8. Release the lower lid from your nondominant hand, ask the patient to gently close his or her eyes, and move his or her eyes around under their eyelids to help absorb the thick ointment.	Allowing for medication absorption will assist in the distribution of medication to the affected areas.
9. Offer patient tissue if needed.	Administration can cause nasal discharge. Important to not have the patient soak up any medication from the eye.
10. Assist patient to comfortable position.	Keeping the head tilted back for too long will be uncomfortable for the patient.
11. Remove gloves and wash hands.	Washing removes any powder from gloves and potential microorganisms.

Engaging in Evaluation

Step	Rationale
Assess the patient's response to medication administration	How was the procedure for the patient? Was the patient able to cope with the procedure or was it painful?
Evaluate for specific therapeutic effects of the medication.	Monitoring for therapeutic effects will assist in ensuring the medication is working for the patient.
Monitor for adverse effects post administration.	Some medications do have adverse effects, and quick identification of these will prevent further potential complications for the patient.

Documenting Effectively

Step	Rationale
Document the medication administration in a timely manner and include the following: • Date and time • Medication administered • Route administered • Site of administration (which eye or both eyes) • Patient's response • Medication effects (therapeutic and adverse) • Other pertinent observations such as eye assessment completed prior to medication administration	Documentation is the key communicative method between health-care professionals. The more complete the documentation, the better other health-care team members are able to understand exactly what and how the medication was administered. The prevention of medication errors and adverse events relies heavily on communication.

SKILL 22.5   Administering Vaginal Suppositories

Reviewing Pertinent Information

Step	Rationale
Review the medication(s) ordered from the medication record or patient chart.	Important to know why the patient is receiving the medication, if the medication is appropriate for the patient's situation, and actual appropriateness of the dose and route ordered
Identify patient allergies to medications and food products.	Some food products are found in medications and can cause an allergic reaction as well as medication allergic reaction to the active medicinal ingredient.
Consider the applicable pharmacological principles of the medication including the onset and duration of action.	Knowing the pharmacological mechanism of action can aid in monitoring for therapeutic and adverse effects of the medication. This information is also useful when teaching your patient the expected outcome(s) of the medication.
Review pertinent lab results pertaining to the medication indication for your patient.	Lab and diagnostic results offer more information into why the patient is receiving the medication and if the medication is having a therapeutic or adverse effect.

Preparing for Administration

Step	Rationale
Wash hands.	Prevents the spread of microorganisms to the supplies being used and handled and prevents further spread to the patient
Gather supplies needed: • Medication • Water-soluble lubricant • Nonsterile gloves • Perineal pad • Washcloth • Perineal wash product • Copy of patient identification information (can be a patient label, a copy of the medication record, or other piece of information that identifies the patient)	Important to get organized prior to administering medications to the patient; organization can save a potential medication error. Bringing patient identifying information (label, medical record, or other suitable alternative) can assist in the reminder to check patient identification and also provides a solid piece of material from which to ensure your patient's identity prior to administering medication.

(continued on page 514)

SKILL 22.5   Administering Vaginal Suppositories (continued)

Preparing for Administration (continued)

Step	Rationale

Prepare the medication for administration by
• Checking medication for expiry date
• Checking the medication once when it is removed from its storage location and again for the second time to the patient's medication record; a third check is completed when the medication storage container or wrapper is returned to storage or discarded.
• Preparing the suppository for administration by either of the following:
  a. Suppository—Removing suppository from package and lubricating the rounded end of the suppository; place the lubricated suppository in a pill cup for transport to the patient room.
  b. Tablet or cream—Placing the tablet or prescribed amount of cream in the designated applicator and lubricating the outer aspects of the applicator
	Expiration dates can easily go unnoticed on some medications.
	Completing three medication checks can limit the chances of medication error.

Prepare the patient by • Checking patient identifying information using a two-step method; checking the patient armband and then asking the patient to verify his or her name • Checking the medication against the armband • Explaining the administration process and purpose of medication • Adjusting the bed height and creating privacy • Completing any necessary pre-administration assessments • Positioning the patient supine with legs apart, exposing the perineal area • Providing patient teaching about the administration and needed follow-up	Double-checking patient identification greatly decreases potential for error. Explaining the purpose of the medication and what will occur fosters patient collaboration and integration into the medication administration process. Checking the medication against the patient wristband is a crucial step in ensuring the right medications are given to the right patient. Patients who are more knowledgeable about the process are usually more comfortable asking questions. Teaching can provide the necessary understanding that will foster more effective outcomes through patient participation.

Administering the Medication

Step	Rationale
1. Put on gloves.	Gloves will protect the patient from surface organisms from the nurse's hands and will protect the nurse from possible body secretions that may come into contact with the nurse's hands during the administration procedure.
2. Perform perineal care using a wet washcloth and or perineal wash product, ensuring you are wiping the labia from anterior to posterior.	Cleaning the perineal area limits the bacteria potentially introduced into the vagina when inserting the suppository.
3. Using your nondominant hand, spread the labia to expose the vaginal opening.	Positioning allows for clear visualization prior to administration.

4. Administer the medication.
  a. Suppository—With the index finger of your dominant hand, gently insert the lubricated suppository rounded end first, into the vagina along the vaginal wall approximately 7–10 cm (3–4 in.).
  b. Tablet or cream in an applicator—With your dominant hand, gently insert the lubricated applicator approximately 7–10 cm (3–4 in.) into the vagina. Use the nondominant hand to stabilize the applicator while the dominant hand pushes gently on the plunger to release the medication. Gently remove the applicator.
	Insertion into the correct position allows for great absorption of the medication. Inserting the suppository too low in the vagina can cause it to fall out prior to the medication being absorbed. Insertion too far can cause discomfort and potential trauma to the cervix.

5. Release the nondominant hand from the labia.	Returns the perineum to its natural position
6. Use tissue to remove any excess lubricant from the perineum.	Promotes comfort
7. Offer the patient a perineum pad if needed.	Promotes comfort and absorbs excess discharge if present
8. Assist patient to comfortable position.	Keeping the legs apart for too long will be uncomfortable for the patient.
9. Remove gloves and wash hands.	Removes any powder from gloves and potential microorganisms

Engaging in Evaluation

Step	Rationale
Assess the patient's response to medication administration.	How was the procedure for the patient? Was the patient able to cope with the procedure or was it painful?
Evaluate for specific therapeutic effects of the medication.	Monitoring for therapeutic effects will assist in ensuring the medication is working for the patient.
Monitor for adverse effects after administration.	Some medications do have adverse effects, and quick identification of these will prevent further potential complications for the patient.

Documenting Effectively

Step	Rationale
Document the medication administration in a timely manner and include the following: • Date and time • Medication administered • Route administered • Patient response • Medication effects (therapeutic and adverse) • Other pertinent observations	Documentation is the key communicative method between health-care professionals. The more complete the documentation, the better other health-care team members are able to understand exactly what and how the medication was administered. The prevention of medication errors and adverse events relies heavily on communication.

SKILL 22.6   Administering Rectal Suppositories

Reviewing Pertinent Information

Step	Rationale
Review the medication(s) ordered from the medication record or patient chart.	Important to know why the patient is receiving the medication, if the medication is appropriate for the patient's situation, and actual appropriateness of the dose and route ordered
Identify patient allergies to medications and food products.	Some food products are found in medications and can cause an allergic reaction as well as medication allergic reaction to the active medicinal ingredient.
Consider the applicable pharmacological principles of the medication including the onset and duration of action.	Knowing the pharmacological mechanism of action can aid in monitoring for therapeutic and adverse effects of the medication. This information is also useful when teaching your patient the expected outcome(s) of the medication.
Review pertinent lab results pertaining to the medication indication for your patient.	Lab and diagnostic results offer more information into why the patient is receiving the medication and if the medication is having a therapeutic or adverse effect.

Preparing for Administration

Step	Rationale
Wash hands.	Prevents the spread of microorganisms to the supplies being used and handled and prevents further spread to the patient
Gather supplies needed: • Medication • Nonsterile gloves • Water-soluble lubricant • Absorbent pad • Tissue • Copy of patient identification information (can be a patient label, a copy of the medication record, or other piece of information that identifies the patient)	Important to be organized prior to administering medications to the patient; organization can save a potential medication error. Bringing patient identifying information (label, medical record, or other suitable alternative) can assist in the reminder to check patient identification and also provides a solid piece of material from which to ensure your patient's identity prior to administering medication.
Prepare the medication for administration by • Checking medication for expiry date • Checking the medication once when it is removed from its storage location and again for the second time to the patient's medication record; a third check is completed when the medication storage container or wrapper is returned to storage or discarded. • Removing suppository from package and lubricating rounded end; place lubricated suppository in a pill cup for transport to the patient's room.	Expiration dates can easily go unnoticed on some medications. Completing three medication checks can limit the chances of medication error.

(continued on page 516)

SKILL 22.6   Administering Rectal Suppositories (continued)

Preparing for Administration (continued)

Step	Rationale
Prepare the patient by • Checking patient identifying information using a two-step method; checking the patient armband and then asking the patient to verify his or her name • Checking the medication against the armband • Explaining the administration process and purpose of medication • Adjusting the bed height and creating privacy • Draping the patient by exposing only the perineum • Completing any necessary pre-administration assessments • Positioning patient in the left side-lying Sims position unless contraindicated • Providing patient teaching about the administration and needed follow-up	Double-checking patient identification greatly decreases potential for error. Explaining the purpose of the medication and what will occur fosters patient collaboration and integration into the medication administration process. Checking the medication against the patient wristband is a crucial step in ensuring the right medications are given to the right patient Patients who are more knowledgeable about the process are usually more comfortable asking questions. Teaching can provide the necessary understanding that will foster more effective outcomes through patient participation.

Administering the Medication

Step	Rationale
1. Put on gloves.	Gloves will protect the patient from surface organisms from the nurse's hands and will protect the nurse from possible body secretions that may come into contact with the nurse's hands during the administration procedure.
2. Using the nondominant hand, spread the buttocks to expose the anus.	Visualization of the anus prior to insertion ensures the suppository is inserted into the right location.
3. Using the index finger on the dominant hand, gently insert the lubricated suppository rounded end first approximately 7–10 cm (3–4 in.) into the rectum, along the rectal wall (see Figure 1).	Insertion of the suppository well into rectum promotes better absorption of the medication.

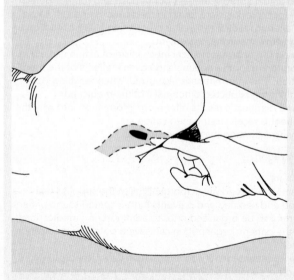

Figure 1

Step	Rationale
4. Remove index finger gently from rectum and release buttock.	Returns patient to normal position
5. Use tissue to remove any excess lubrication from the anus.	Patient comfort
6. Leave patient on his or her side for 5–10 minutes and replace covers over patient for privacy. Remove gloves.	Allows medication to absorb In removing gloves, there is no cross-contamination of fecal matter in preceding steps.
7. Ensure call bell is within reach.	Ensures patient has access to nurse if needed
8. Wash hands.	Removes any powder from gloves and potential microorganisms.

Engaging in Evaluation

Step	Rationale
Assess the patient's response to medication administration.	How was the procedure for the patient? Was the patient able to cope with the procedure or was it painful?
Evaluate for specific therapeutic effects of the medication.	Monitoring for therapeutic effects will assist in ensuring the medication is working for the patient.
Monitor for adverse effects after administration.	Some medications do have adverse effects, and quick identification of these will prevent further potential complications for the patient.

Documenting Effectively

Step	Rationale
Document the medication administration in a timely manner and include the following: • Date and time • Medication administered • Route administered • Patient's response • Medication effects (therapeutic and adverse)	Documentation is the key communicative method between health-care professionals. The more complete the documentation, the better other health-care team members are able to understand exactly what and how the medication was administered. The prevention of medication errors and adverse events relies heavily on communication.

SKILL 22.7 Drawing Up From a Vial

Reviewing Pertinent Information

Step	Rationale
Determine whether the vial is a single-use or multidose vial. Most medications are single use, whereas vials that contain normal saline and potassium can be for multiple doses.	It is important to know whether the vial can be reused or should be discarded after use.
Ensure the sterility of the medication is maintained. Vials contain sterile medication and need to be treated as sterile.	Reminding oneself that sterile technique must be used to access the vials is important to not contaminate the medication or the introduce microorganisms to the patient.

Preparing for Administration

Step	Rationale
Wash hands.	Prevents the spread of microorganisms to the supplies being used and handled and prevents further spread to the patient
Gather supplies needed for drawing up medication from a vial and find a clean surface on which to work. Supplies: • Syringe • Needle • Needleless needle and adapter if using a multiple-dose vial • Alcohol swabs or equivalent	Important to be organized prior to administering medications to the patient; organization can save a potential medication error.

Administering the Medication

Step	Rationale
1. Check expiry date on medication vial.	Ensures the medication is not expired and potentially dangerous for the patient
2. Calculate the dose needed from the vial.	Ensures the proper dose is removed from the vial (See how to calculate dosages covered earlier in the chapter.)
3. Remove plastic top off vial to expose the rubber membrane.	Gains access to the medication in the vial
4. Swab the rubber membrane with the alcohol swab for 20 seconds and allow to dry.	Even if the vial had never been accessed, it is always prudent to swab the top in case it came into contact with your fingers when removing the cap. Swabbing for 10 seconds provides for more effective removal of microorganisms versus shorter time frames.

(continued on page 518)

SKILL 22.7   Drawing Up From a Vial (continued)

Administering the Medication (continued)

Step	Rationale
5. Draw up the medication.	
a. If multiple-dose vial insert the needleless multidose adapter into the vial through the rubber membrane, using the syringe with a needleless needle, draw up air equal to the amount of medication needed. Swab the port of the multidose adapter port, insert the needleless needle into the multiple dose access port, and inject the air into the vial.	Multidose vials saves the vial from repeated punctures and possible degradation of the rubber membrane. They can be accessed repeatedly. These vials often have some preservatives in them to protect the medication from expiring because of frequent access.
b. If single-use vial, draw up the amount of air that equals the amount of needed solution and insert the needle through the rubber membrane and inject the air.	
6. Invert the vial upside down or on an angle on its side to withdraw the needed amount of medication from the vial.	The fluid level needs to be where the bevel of the needle or level of the multidose vial adapter is. If not inverted or tilted on its side, air will be withdrawn instead of fluid.
7. Remove the syringe and draw the fluid back while keeping the syringe with the needle end pointing up (see Figure 1).	Withdrawing all the medication from the needle will prevent contamination of the needle when attempting to expel air by drawing all the fluid that is potentially in the needle into the syringe.

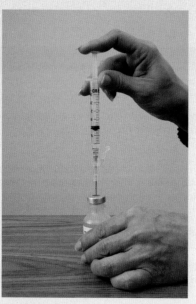

Figure 1

Step	Rationale
8. Push the remaining air from the syringe until fluid is almost at the top of the needle.	Removing air is necessary prior to administration of the medication to the patient.
9. Remove all air bubbles from the syringe by tapping gently on the syringe to dislodge them to the top of the syringe. Draw back on the syringe and expel the air out.	Removing air is necessary because it can cause harm to the patient.
10. If there is more fluid in the syringe than needed, do not discard the medication back into the vial. With all the air removed from the syringe, invert the syringe upside down and remove the excess fluid into a medication cup or other clean receptacle without contaminating the needle.	Letting the fluid drip out and over the needle contaminates the needle surface. Letting the fluid squirt into a garbage can or over a dirty sink poses sanitary concerns given the proximity of the needle to the dirty surfaces.
11. Recap the needle.	To prevent contamination of the needle prior to administration.
12. Obtain any co-signatures required for the medication that was just drawn up.	Some medications require co-signatures directly after preparation and prior to administration.
13. Label the syringe with the medication, dose, patient name, date, and time. Be careful not to place a label on the syringe, so it impedes the view of the medication amount.	Using a small label will prevent mistaken administration of the fluid or medication to another patient.

SKILL 22.8   Drawing Up and Mixing Two Medications

Reviewing Pertinent Information

Step	Rationale
Determine whether the vials are single-use or multidose vial. Most medications are single use, whereas vials that contain normal saline, potassium, and insulin can be for multiple doses.	It is important to know whether the vial can be reused or should be discarded after use.
Ensure the sterility of the medication. Vials contain sterile medication and need to be treated as sterile.	Reminding oneself that sterile technique must be used to access the vials is important to not contaminate the medication or the introduce microorganisms to the patient.

Preparing for Administration

Step	Rationale
Wash hands.	Prevents the spread of microorganisms to the supplies being used and handled and prevents further spread to the patient
Gather supplies needed for drawing up medication from a vial and find a clean surface on which to work. Supplies: • Vials of medication • Syringe • Needle • Alcohol swabs or equivalent	Important to get organized prior to administering medications to the patient; organization can save a potential medication error.

Administering the Medication

Step	Rationale
1. Check expiry dates on medication vials.	Ensures the medication is not expired and potentially dangerous for the patient
2. Calculate the doses needed from the vial.	Ensures the proper dose is removed from the vial (See how to calculate dosages covered earlier in the chapter.)
3. Remove plastic top off vial to expose the rubber membrane if not already removed.	Gains access to the medication in the vial
4. Swab the rubber membranes of both vials with the alcohol swab for 20 seconds and allow to dry.	Even if the vial had never been accessed, it is always prudent to swab the top in case it came into contact with your fingers when removing the cap. Swabbing for 10 seconds provides for more effective removal of microorganisms versus shorter time frames.
5. Determine the order in which you are to draw up the medication. In the syringe, draw up the amount of air that equals the amount of solution needed from the second vial. Insert the needle through the rubber membrane and inject the air. Remove the syringe.	By injecting air first into the second vial from which you will draw the medication from, there is no need to inject air into the vial after the first medication has been withdrawn.

(continued on page 520)

SKILL 22.8   Drawing Up and Mixing Two Medications (continued)

Administering the Medication (continued)

Step

6. In the syringe, draw up the amount of air equal to the amount of solution needed from the first vial and inject it into the vial (see Figure 1).

Rationale

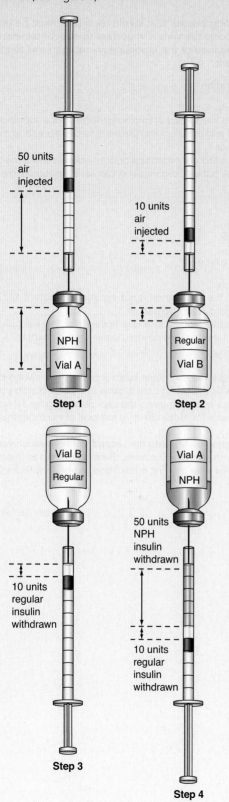

50 units air injected

10 units air injected

NPH
Vial A

Step 1

Regular
Vial B

Step 2

Vial B
Regular

10 units regular insulin withdrawn

Step 3

Vial A
NPH

50 units NPH insulin withdrawn

10 units regular insulin withdrawn

Step 4

Figure 1

Administering the Medication (continued)

Step	Rationale
7. Invert the first vial upside down or on an angle on its side to withdraw the needed amount of medication from the vial.	The fluid level needs to be where the bevel of the needle or level of the multidose vial adapter is. If not inverted or tilted on its side, air will be withdrawn instead of fluid.
8. Remove the syringe and draw the fluid back while keeping the syringe with the needle end pointing up.	Withdrawing all the medication from the needle will prevent contamination of the needle when attempting to expel air by drawing all the fluid that is potentially in the needle into the syringe.
9. Push the remaining air from the syringe until fluid is almost at the top of the needle.	Removing air is necessary prior to administration of the medication to the patient.
10. Remove all air bubbles from the syringe by tapping gently on the syringe to dislodge them to the top of the syringe. Draw back on the syringe and expel the air out.	Removing air is necessary because it can cause harm to the patient.
11. If there is more fluid in the syringe than needed, do not discard the medication back into the vial. With all the air removed from the syringe, invert the syringe upside down and remove the excess fluid into a medication cup or other clean receptacle without contaminating the needle.	Letting the fluid drip out and over the needle contaminates the needle surface. Letting the fluid squirt into a garbage can or over a dirty sink poses sanitary concerns due to the proximity of the needle to the dirty surfaces.
12. Recap the needle.	To prevent contamination of the needle prior to administration
13. Obtain any co-signatures required for the medication that was just drawn up	Some medications require co-signatures directly after preparation and prior to administration.
14. Swab the second vial again with an alcohol swab or equivalent and gently insert the needle into the second vial while stabilizing the plunger.	Swabbing the vial again reduces the risk of contamination after the needle was removed the first time. Stabilizing the plunger does not allow any seepage of medication from the syringe into the second vial in the presence of a possible pressure gradient difference between the syringe and the vial.
15. Invert the second vial and withdraw the exact amount of medication needed.	Exact measurement is crucial here because no medication can be expelled back into the vial once it has been withdrawn.
16. If air exists in the syringe, pull the needle out and draw back the fluid so all the fluid from the needle enters the barrel of the syringe. Push the plunger forward and expel only the air in the syringe without losing any of the medication.	Expelling air reduces the risk of injecting it into the patient.
17. If more medication is needed from the second vial, then repeat Steps 13–15 earlier.	
18. Obtain another co-signature if needed on the second medication.	Some medications require co-signatures at each stage of drawing up.
19. Label the syringe with the medication, dose, patient name, date, and time. Be careful not to place a label on the syringe so it impedes the view of the medication amount.	Using a small label will prevent mistaken administration of the fluid or medication to another patient.

SKILL 22.9   Drawing Up From an Ampoule

Reviewing Pertinent Information

Step	Rationale
Determine the appropriate ampoule to pick based on the concentration and dose needed.	Using an ampoule where you are going to use the whole dose within a reasonable amount of fluid is best.
Ensure the sterility of the medication. Ampoules contain sterile medication and need to be treated as sterile.	Reminding oneself that sterile technique must be used to access the ampoule is important to not contaminate the medication or the introduce microorganisms to the patient.

Preparing for Administration

Step	Rationale
Wash hands.	Prevents the spread of microorganisms to the supplies being used and handled and prevents further spread to the patient
Gather supplies needed for drawing up medication from a vial and find a clean surface on which to work. Supplies: • Medication ampoule • Gauze 2 × 2 • Syringe • Needle • Needleless needle and adapter if using a multiple dose • Vial • Alcohol swabs or equivalent	Important to be organized prior to administering medications to the patient; organization can save a potential medication error.

(continued on page 522)

SKILL 22.9   Drawing Up From an Ampoule (continued)

Preparing Medication

Step	Rationale
1. Check expiry date on medication ampoule if applicable.	Ensures the medication is not expired and potentially dangerous for the patient
2. Calculate the dose needed from the ampoule.	Ensures the proper dose is removed from the vial (See how to calculate dosages covered earlier in the chapter.)
3. Inspect the ampoule for any cracks, leaks, or precipitate inside the ampoule.	Precipitate in the ampoule could necessitate the need to use a filtered needle for withdrawing the solution. Note: Filtered needles are only used to withdraw solution and not for administration of medication to patients.
4. Remove any fluid that may be trapped in the head and neck of the ampoule by gently tapping the head of the ampoule or turning the ampoule in a circular fashion by rotating your wrists.	Places all available medication in the body of the ampoule; medication that is trapped in the head of the ampoule will then be wasted when the ampoule is opened, possibly leaving not enough medication in the ampoule for the dose required.
5. Wrap the head of the ampoule with an alcohol swab (still in its wrapper) or with a 2 × 2 gauze piece.	Using barrier protects the hands and fingers of the nurse from getting cut by the glass.
6. With a succinct clean motion away from the body, break the head of the ampoule off.	Clean breaks are needed to avoid getting pieces of glass in the ampoule.
7. Discard the head of the ampoule and the alcohol swab or gauze 2 × 2.	The alcohol swab package or the 2 × 2 gauze may contain pieces of glass and should be discarded.
8. Invert the ampoule upside down, tilted on its side or sitting vertically on a flat surface, and insert the needle and syringe into the ampoule (see Figure 1).	There are a few different positions to withdraw medication from an ampoule. The main principle is to ensure the bevel of the syringe is immersed in medication to avoid drawing up air.

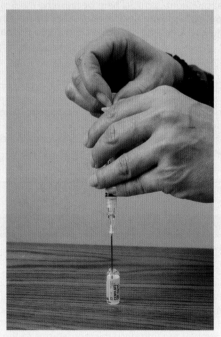

Figure 1-A

Preparing Medication (continued)	
Step	**Rationale**

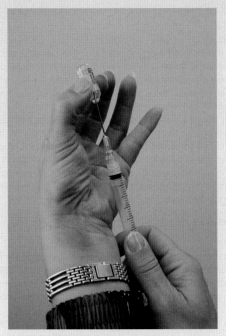

Figure 1-B

9. Being careful not to contaminate the syringe by touching the outer aspect of the neck of the ampoule, withdraw the required amount of medication.
10. Remove the syringe and draw the fluid back while keeping the syringe with the needle end pointing up.

11. Push the remaining air from the syringe until fluid is almost at the top of the needle.
12. Remove all air bubbles from the syringe by tapping gently on the syringe to dislodge them to the top of the syringe. Draw back on the syringe and expel the air out.

13. If there is more fluid in the syringe than needed, do not discard the medication back into the ampoule. With all the air removed from the syringe, invert the syringe upside down and remove the excess fluid into a medication cup or other clean receptacle without contaminating the needle.
14. Recap the needle.

15. Obtain any co-signatures required for the medication that was just drawn up.
16. Label the syringe with the medication, dose, patient name, date, and time. Be careful not to place a label on the syringe so it impedes the view of the medication amount.

The outer aspects of the neck may contain small pieces of glass. Touching the outer aspect of the ampoule would contaminate the syringe.
Withdrawing all the medication from the needle will prevent contamination of the needle when attempting to expel air by drawing all the fluid that is potentially in the needle into the syringe.
Removing air is necessary prior to administration of the medication to the patient.
Removing air is necessary because it can cause harm to the patient. Injecting air parenterally can cause discomfort, and air may potentially enter the bloodstream if the needle accidentally accesses a vessel.
Letting the fluid drip out and over the needle contaminates the needle surface. Letting the fluid squirt into a garbage can or over a dirty sink poses sanitary concerns due to the proximity of the needle to the dirty surfaces.

Recapping will prevent contamination of the needle prior to administration.
Note: Recapping should only occur after a medication has been drawn up—not after patient administration.
Some medications require co-signatures directly after preparation and prior to administration.
Using a small label will prevent mistaken administration of the fluid or medication to another patient.

SKILL 22.10   Administering Intradermal Injections

Reviewing Pertinent Information

Step	Rationale
Review the medication(s) ordered from the medication record or patient chart.	Important to know why the patient is receiving the medication, if the medication is appropriate for the patient's situation, and actual appropriateness of the dose and route ordered
Identify patient allergies to medications and food products.	Some food products are found in medications and can cause an allergic reaction as well as medication allergic reaction to the active medicinal ingredient.
Consider the applicable pharmacological principles of the medication including the onset and duration of action.	Knowing the pharmacological mechanism of action can aid in monitoring for therapeutic and adverse effects of the medication. This information is also useful when teaching your patient the expected outcome(s) of the medication.
Review pertinent lab results pertaining to the medication indication for your patient.	Lab and diagnostic results offer more information into why the patient is receiving the medication and if the medication is having a therapeutic or adverse effect.

Preparing for Administration

Step	Rationale
Wash hands.	Prevents the spread of microorganisms to the supplies being used and handled and prevents further spread to the patient
Gather supplies needed: • Gloves • Medication to be injected • Syringe (tuberculin) 1 ml • Needle—usually no. 25–27 gauge, ¼"–⅜" length • Alcohol swabs or equivalent • Copy of patient identification information (can be a patient label, a copy of the medication record, or other piece of information that identifies the patient)	Important to get organized prior to administering medications to the patient; organization can save a potential medication error. Bringing patient identifying information (label, medical record, or other suitable alternative) can aid in the reminder to check patient identification and also provides a solid piece of material from which to ensure your patient's identity prior to administering medication.
Prepare the medication for administration by • Checking medication for expiry date • Checking the medication once when it is removed from its storage location and again for the second time to the patient's medication record; a third check is completed when the medication storage container or wrapper is returned to storage or discarded. • Drawing up medication from vial or ampoule using the techniques discussed earlier in the chapter • Labeling medication with patient name, date, and time; be careful not to block the measurements on the side of the syringe.	Expiration dates can easily go unnoticed on some medications. Completing three medication checks can limit the chances of medication error.
Prepare the patient by: • Checking patient identifying information using a two-step method; checking the patient armband and then asking the patient to verify his or her name • Checking the medication against the armband • Explaining the administration process and purpose of medication • Adjusting the bed or chair height and creating privacy • Completing any necessary pre-administration assessments • Providing patient teaching about the administration and needed follow-up	Double-checking patient identification greatly decreases potential for error. Explaining the purpose of the medication and what will occur fosters patient collaboration and integration into the medication administration process. Checking the medication against the patient wristband is a crucial step in ensuring the right medications are given to the right patient. Patients who are more knowledgeable about the process are usually more comfortable asking questions. Teaching can provide the necessary understanding that will foster more effective outcomes through patient participation.

Administering the Medication

Step	Rationale
1. Put on nonsterile gloves.	Gloves will protect the patient from surface organisms from the nurse's hands and will protect the nurse from possible body secretions that may come into contact with the nurse's hands during the administration procedure.
2. Select site for the injection. (See diagram after procedure for commonly used sites for intradermal injections.)	Assessment and selection of the site prior to injection allows for proper site selection.
3. Swab the skin with the alcohol swab or equivalent for 20 seconds and let dry.	Removes microorganisms on the skin surface prior to injection

Administering the Medication (continued)

Step	Rationale
4. Pull the skin taut with the nondominant hand.	Stabilizes the skin for injection
5. With the dominant hand, keeping the needle bevel up, enter the skin at a 10–15° angle and forward the needle into the skin approximately 1 cm (⅛–¼ in.).	Intradermal needles need to enter the intradermal space. If the needle goes in at a steeper angle, it could enter the subcutaneous space. If the insertion is not deep enough, medication could leak from the site before it is absorbed. If the bevel faces down, the medication may be administered in the incorrect site.
6. Stabilize the needle against the skin with the nondominant hand while the dominant hand gently injects the medication into the skin (see Figure 1).	Ensures the needle remains in the intradermal site

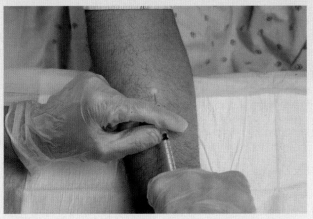

Figure 1

Step	Rationale
7. As the medication is being injected, notice the bleb or wheal being formed underneath the skin.	The lack of a bleb or wheal may indicate that the needle is in the subcutaneous space or that the needle was not inserted far enough.
8. Gently withdraw the needle and do not recap.	Intradermal injections can hurt more than subcutaneous or IM injections due to the sensitive nature of the site you are injecting.
9. Dispose of needle or engage **needle shield** immediately after withdrawal.	Ensure all sharps are disposed of immediately to reduce the risk for needlestick injuries.
10. Apply gauze over the injection site as needed; be careful not to apply pressure that will expel the medication.	Gauze can be placed over the site loosely if the site is bleeding slightly.
11. Instruct patient that he or she should not scratch or put pressure on the area for at least 15 minutes.	Medication requires time to absorb in this area.
12. Remove gloves and wash hands.	Removes any powder from gloves and potential microorganisms

Engaging in Evaluation

Step	Rationale
Assess the patient's response to medication administration.	How was the procedure for the patient? Was the patient able to cope with the procedure or was it painful?
Evaluate for specific therapeutic effects of the medication.	Monitoring for therapeutic effects will assist in ensuring the medication is working for the patient.
Monitor for adverse effects after administration.	Some medications do have adverse effects, and quick identification of these will prevent further potential complications for the patient.

Documenting Effectively

Step	Rationale
Document the medication administration in a timely manner and include the following: • Date and time • Medication administered • Route administered • Patient's response • Medication effects (therapeutic and adverse)	Documentation is the key communicative method between health-care professionals. The more complete the documentation, the better other health-care team members are able to understand exactly what and how the medication was administered. The prevention of medication errors and adverse events relies heavily on communication.

SKILL 22.11   Administering Subcutaneous Injections

Reviewing Pertinent Information

Step	Rationale
Review the medication(s) ordered from the medication record or patient chart.	Important to know why the patient is receiving the medication, if the medication is appropriate for the patient's situation, and actual appropriateness of the dose and route ordered
Identify patient allergies to medications and food products.	Some food products are found in medications and can cause an allergic reaction as well as medication allergic reaction to the active medicinal ingredient.
Consider the applicable pharmacological principles of the medication including the onset and duration of action.	Knowing the pharmacological mechanism of action can aid in monitoring for therapeutic and adverse effects of the medication. This information is also useful when teaching your patient the expected outcome(s) of the medication.
Review pertinent lab results pertaining to the medication indication for your patient.	Lab and diagnostic results offer more information into why the patient is receiving the medication and if the medication is having a therapeutic or adverse effect.

Preparing for Administration

Step	Rationale
Wash hands.	Prevents the spread of microorganisms to the supplies being used and handled, and prevents further spread to the patient.
Gather supplies needed: • Gloves • Medication to be injected • Syringe 1–3 ml, insulin syringe if administering insulin • Needle—usually no. 24–26 gauge, ½"–1" length • Alcohol swabs or equivalent • Copy of patient identification information (can be a patient label, a copy of the medication record or other piece of information that identifies the patient)	Important to be organized prior to administering medications to the patient; organization can save a potential medication error. Bringing patient identifying information (label, medical record, or other suitable alternative) can aid in the reminder to check patient identification and also provides a solid piece of material from which to ensure your patient's identity prior to administering medication.
Prepare the medication for administration by • Checking medication for expiry date • Checking the medication once when it is removed from its storage location and again for the second time to the patient's medication record; a third check is completed when the medication storage container or wrapper is returned to storage or discarded. • Drawing up medication from vial or ampoule using the techniques discussed earlier in the chapter • Labeling medication with patient name, date, and time; be careful not to block the measurements on the side of the syringe.	Expiration dates can easily go unnoticed on some medications. Completing three medication checks can limit the chances of medication error.
Prepare the patient by • Checking patient identifying information using a two-step method; checking the patient armband and then asking the patient to verify his or her name • Checking the medication against the armband • Explaining the administration process and purpose of medication • Adjusting the bed or chair height and creating privacy • Draping the patient and exposing only the area for injection • Completing any necessary pre-administration assessments • Providing patient teaching about the administration and needed follow-up	Double-checking patient identification greatly decreases potential for error. Explaining the purpose of the medication and what will occur fosters patient collaboration and integration into the medication administration process. Checking the medication against the patient wristband is a crucial step in ensuring the right medications are given to the right patient. Patients who are more knowledgeable about the process are usually more comfortable asking questions. Teaching can provide the necessary understanding that will foster more effective outcomes through patient participation.

Administering the Medication

Step	Rationale
1. Put on gloves.	Gloves will protect the patient from surface organisms from the nurse's hands and will protect the nurse from possible body secretions that may come into contact with the nurse's hands during the administration procedure.
2. Select site for the injection.	Assessment and selection of the site prior to injection allows for proper site selection.

Administering the Medication (continued)

Step	Rationale
3. Swab the skin with the alcohol swab or equivalent for 20 seconds and let dry.	Removes microorganisms on the skin surface prior to injection
4. Pull the skin together or gently pinch it together with the nondominant hand. It is also acceptable to pull the skin taut in individuals with a lot of subcutaneous tissue.	Stabilizes the skin for injection
5. With the dominant hand, inject the needle into the skin at a 45–90° angle. Those with more subcutaneous tissue will require the needle to be at a 90° angle, whereas those with little subcutaneous tissue will require the 45° angle (see Figure 1).	Subcutaneous needles need to enter the subcutaneous space. If the needle goes in at a lower angle than needed, it could enter the intradermal space; or if the angle is too steep, the IM space could be entered.

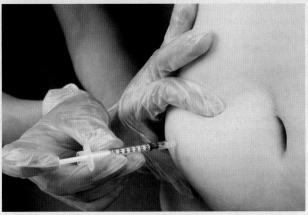

Figure 1

Step	Rationale
6. Stabilize the needle against the skin with the nondominant hand while the dominant hand gently injects the medication into the skin at a slow but steady rate.	Ensures the needle remains in the subcutaneous site and does not move upon injection
7. Gently withdraw the needle and do not recap.	If the needle is withdrawn abruptly, more pain can be caused to the patient.
8. Dispose of needle or engage needle shield immediately after withdrawal.	Ensures all sharps are disposed of immediately to reduce the risk for needlestick injuries
9. Apply gauze over the injection site as needed.	Gauze can be placed over the site loosely if the site is bleeding slightly.
10. Remove gloves and wash hands.	Removes any powder from gloves and potential microorganisms

Engaging in Evaluation

Step	Rationale
Assess the patient's response to medication administration	How was the procedure for the patient? Was the patient able to cope with the procedure or was it painful?
Evaluate for specific therapeutic effects of the medication.	Monitoring for therapeutic effects will assist in ensuring the medication is working for the patient.
Monitor for adverse effects after administration.	Some medications do have adverse effects, and quick identification of these will prevent further potential complications for the patient.

Documenting Effectively

Step	Rationale
Document the medication administration in a timely manner and include the following: • Date and time • Medication administered • Route administered • Patient response • Medication effects (therapeutic and adverse)	Documentation is the key communicative method between health-care professionals. The more complete the documentation, the better other health-care team members are able to understand exactly what and how the medication was administered. The prevention of medication errors and adverse events relies heavily on communication.

SKILL 22.12   Using an Insulin Pen

Reviewing Pertinent Information

Step	Rationale
Review the medication(s) ordered from the medication record or patient chart.	Important to know why the patient is receiving the medication, if the medication is appropriate for the patient's situation, and actual appropriateness of the dose and route ordered
Identify patient allergies to medications and food products.	Some food products are found in medications and can cause an allergic reaction as well as medication allergic reaction to the active medicinal ingredient.
Consider the applicable pharmacological principles of the medication including the onset and duration of action.	Knowing the pharmacological mechanism of action can aid in monitoring for therapeutic and adverse effects of the medication. This information is also useful when teaching your patient the expected outcome(s) of the medication.
Review pertinent lab results pertaining to the medication indication for your patient.	Lab and diagnostic results offer more information into why the patient is receiving the medication and if the medication is having a therapeutic or adverse effect.

Preparing for Administration

Step	Rationale
Wash hands.	Prevents the spread of microorganisms to the supplies being used and handled, and prevents further spread to the patient.
Gather supplies needed:	Important to get organized prior to administering medications to the patient; organization can save a potential medication error.

Gather supplies needed:
- Insulin pen
- Needles usually no. 29–31 gauge ⁵⁄₁₆ – ½" length (5–12 mm)
- Insulin cartridge
- Alcohol swabs or equivalent
- Gloves
- Copy of patient identification information (can be a patient label, a copy of the medication record, or other piece of information that identifies the patient)

Bringing patient identifying information (label, medical record, or other suitable alternative) can aid in the reminder to check patient identification and also provides a solid piece of material from which to ensure your patient's identity prior to administering medication.

Prepare the medication for administration by
- Checking medication cartridge for expiry date and adequate volume for the dose required
- Checking the medication once when it is removed from its storage location and again for the second time to the patient's medication record; a third check is completed when the medication storage container or wrapper is returned to storage or discarded.
- Loading the insulin pen with the corresponding needle and inserting the cartridge
- Dialing two units into the device and expressing the air from the cartridge; ensure the dose dial now reads zero.
- Dialing the required/ordered dose of insulin into the insulin pen for this administration (see Figure 1).

Expiration dates can easily go unnoticed on some medications.
Completing three medication checks can limit the chances of medication error.

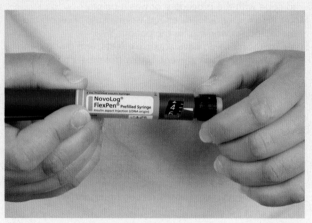

Figure 1

Preparing for Administration (continued)

Step	Rationale
Prepare the patient by: • Checking patient identifying information using a two-step method; checking the patient armband and then asking the patient to verify his or her name • Checking the medication against the armband • Explaining the administration process and purpose of medication(s) • Adjusting the bed height and creating privacy • Selecting the site for the subcutaneous injection • Completing any necessary pre-administration assessments such as blood glucose reading • Providing patient teaching about the administration and needed follow-up	Double-checking patient identification greatly decreases potential for error. Explaining the purpose of the medication and what will occur fosters patient collaboration and integration into the medication administration process. Checking the medication against the patient wristband is a crucial step in ensuring the right medications are given to the right patient. Patients who are more knowledgeable about the process are usually more comfortable asking questions. Teaching can provide the necessary understanding that will foster more effective outcomes through patient participation.

Administering the Medication

Step	Rationale
1. Put on gloves.	To protect from coming into contact with bodily fluids
2. Invert the pen approximately 10 times to mix the insulin in the cartridge.	Ensures the insulin inside the cartridge is mixed well
3. Swab the selected subcutaneous site with an alcohol swab or equivalent and allow to dry.	To reduce surface microorganisms
4. Remove the lid from the insulin pen.	Exposes needle
5. Using your nondominant hand, gently pinch the skin or pull it taut.	Some individuals will require you pinch the skin to ensure you have subcutaneous tissue, and others with more subcutaneous tissue will require it to be pulled taut to expose the site.
6. Inject the pen needle at a 45–90° angle into the subcutaneous tissue (see Figure 2).	Depending on the patient, the angle will vary.

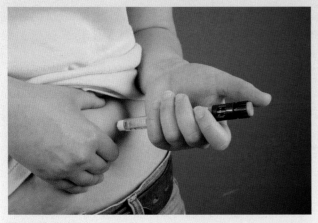

Figure 2

Step	Rationale
7. Have the nondominant hand stabilize the pen as the dominant hand depresses the pen plunger and releases the dose of insulin.	Stabilizing reduces pain and discomfort for the patient.
8. Remove the needle and discard into sharps. Check to make sure the entire dialed dose was given and the dial is now at zero.	Ensures dose was given and supplies are properly discarded
9. Assist patient to comfortable position.	Patient comfort
10. Remove gloves and wash hands.	Removes potential microorganisms from hands and stops cross-contamination between patients

(continued on page 530)

SKILL 22.12   Using an Insulin Pen (continued)

Engaging in Evaluation

Step	Rationale
Assess the patient's response to medication administration.	How was the procedure for the patient? Was the patient able to cope with the procedure or was it painful?
Evaluate for specific therapeutic effects of the medication.	Monitoring for therapeutic effects will assist in ensuring the medication is working for the patient.
Monitors for adverse effects post administration	Some medications do have adverse effects, and quick identification of these will prevent further potential complications for the patient.

Documenting Effectively

Step	Rationale
Document the medication administration in a timely manner and include the following: • Date and time • Medication administered • Route administered • Patient's response • Medication effects (therapeutic and adverse) • Other pertinent observations	Documentation is the key communicative method between health-care professionals. The more complete the documentation, the better other health-care team members are able to understand exactly what and how the medication was administered. The prevention of medication errors and adverse events relies heavily on communication. Insulin usually has its own medication administration sheet record in addition to the either computer-logged or hard copy–logged administration. Check with your agency policies for the applicable documentation that needs to occur with insulin administration.

SKILL 22.13   Administering Intramuscular Injections

Reviewing Pertinent Information

Step	Rationale
Review the medication(s) ordered from the medication record or patient chart.	Important to know why the patient is receiving the medication, if the medication is appropriate for the patient's situation, and actual appropriateness of the dose and route ordered
Identify patient allergies to medications and food products.	Some food products are found in medications and can cause an allergic reaction as well as medication allergic reaction to the active medicinal ingredient.
Consider the applicable pharmacological principles of the medication including the onset and duration of action.	Knowing the pharmacological mechanism of action can aid in monitoring for therapeutic and adverse effects of the medication. This information is also useful when teaching your patient the expected outcome(s) of the medication.
Review pertinent lab results pertaining to the medication indication for your patient.	Lab and diagnostic results offer more information into why the patient is receiving the medication and if the medication is having a therapeutic or adverse effect.

Preparing for Administration

Step	Rationale
Wash hands.	Prevents the spread of microorganisms to the supplies being used and handled and prevents further spread to the patient
Gather supplies needed: • Gloves • Medication to be injected • Syringe 3–5 ml • Needle—usually no. 20–22 gauge,1″–1½″ (25–40 mm) length; it is possible that a 2″ needle (50 mm) may be required for obese patients. • Alcohol swabs or equivalent • Copy of patient identification information (can be a patient label, a copy of the medication record, or other piece of information that identifies the patient)	Important to get organized prior to administering medications to the patient; organization can save a potential medication error. Bringing patient identifying information (label, medical record, or other suitable alternative) can aid in the reminder to check patient identification and also provides a solid piece of material from which to ensure your patient's identity prior to administering medication.

Preparing for Administration (continued)

Step	Rationale
Prepare the medication for administration by • Checking medication for expiry date • Checking the medication once when it is removed from its storage location and again for the second time to the patient's medication record; a third check is completed when the medication storage container or wrapper is returned to storage or discarded. • Drawing up medication from vial or ampoule using the techniques discussed earlier in the chapter • Labeling medication with patient name, date, and time; be careful not to block the measurements on the side of the syringe.	Expiration dates can easily go unnoticed on some medications. Completing three medication checks can limit the chances of medication error.
Prepare the patient by • Checking patient identifying information using a two-step method; checking the patient armband and then asking the patient to verify his or her name • Checking the medication against the armband • Explaining the administration process and purpose of medication • Adjusting the bed or chair height and creating privacy • Draping the patient and exposing only the area needed for injection • Completing any necessary pre-administration assessments • Providing patient teaching about the administration and needed follow up	Double-checking patient identification greatly decreases potential for error. Explaining the purpose of the medication and what will occur fosters patient collaboration and integration into the medication administration process. Checking the medication against the patient wristband is a crucial step in ensuring the right medications are given to the right patient. Patients who are more knowledgeable about the process are usually more comfortable asking questions. Teaching can provide the necessary understanding that will foster more effective outcomes through patient participation.

Administering the Medication

Step	Rationale
1. Put on nonsterile gloves.	Gloves will protect the patient from surface organisms from the nurse's hands and will protect the nurse from possible body secretions that may come into contact with the nurse's hands during the administration procedure.
2. Select site for the injection (see Figure 1).	Assessment and selection of the site prior to injection allows for proper site selection.

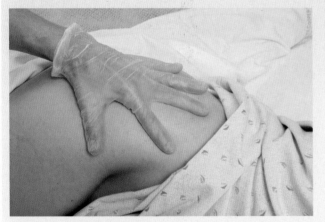

Figure 1

3. Swab the skin with the alcohol swab or equivalent for 20 seconds and let dry.	Removes microorganisms on the skin surface prior to injection
4. Pull the skin taut with the nondominant hand.	Stabilizes the skin for injection

(continued on page 532)

SKILL 22.13   Administering Intramuscular Injections (continued)

Administering the Medication (continued)

Step	Rationale
5. With the dominant hand, inject the needle into the skin at a 75–90° angle using a swift darting motion (see Figure 2).	IM injections need to enter the IM space. If the needle goes in at a lower angle than needed, it could enter the subcutaneous space.

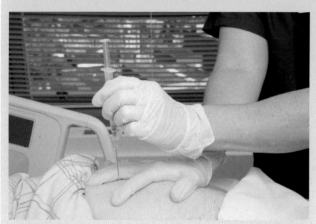

Figure 2

Step	Rationale
6. Stabilize the needle against the skin with the nondominant hand while the dominant hand gently injects aspirates to see if there is blood return in the syringe. If there is blood, then remove the needle and discard the syringe and medication according to agency policy. A new syringe will need to be prepared. If blood is not aspirated, proceed with the injection.	Aspiration is crucial to determine if the medication will be delivered into the IM space and not into a vessel where the medication could have serious effects for the patient. Stabilizing the needle ensures the needle remains in the IM site.
7. With the dominant hand on the plunger pad, inject the medication slowly into the IM space (see Figure 3).	Medication should be administered slowly but at a rate no longer than 10 seconds/ml.

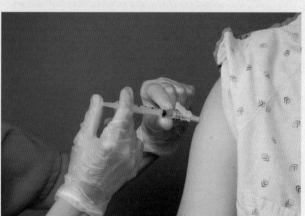

Figure 3

Step	Rationale
8. Gently withdraw the needle and do not recap.	If the needle is withdrawn abruptly, more pain can be caused to the patient.
9. Dispose of needle or engage needle shield immediately after withdrawal.	Ensures all sharps are disposed of immediately to reduce the risk for needlestick injuries
10. Apply gauze over the injection site as needed.	Gauze can be placed over the site loosely if the site is bleeding slightly.
11. Remove gloves and wash hands.	Removes any powder from gloves and potential microorganisms

Engaging in Evaluation

Step	Rationale
Assess the patient's response to medication administration.	How was the procedure for the patient? Was the patient able to cope with the procedure or was it painful?
Evaluate for specific therapeutic effects of the medication.	Monitoring for therapeutic effects will assist in ensuring the medication is working for the patient.
Monitor for adverse effects after administration.	Some medications do have adverse effects, and quick identification of these will prevent further potential complications for the patient.

Documenting Effectively

Step	Rationale
Document the medication administration in a timely manner and include the following: • Date and time • Medication administered • Route administered • Patient's response • Medication effects (therapeutic and adverse)	Documentation is the key communicative method between health-care professionals. The more complete the documentation, the better other health-care team members are able to understand exactly what and how the medication was administered. The prevention of medication errors and adverse events relies heavily on communication.

SKILL 22.14   Administering Medications by Inhalation

Reviewing Pertinent Information

Step	Rationale
Review the medication(s) ordered from the medication record or patient chart.	Important to know why the patient is receiving the medication, if the medication is appropriate for the patient's situation, and actual appropriateness of the dose and route ordered
Identify patient allergies to medications and food products.	Some food products are found in medications and can cause an allergic reaction as well as medication allergic reaction to the active medicinal ingredient.
Consider the applicable pharmacological principles of the medication including the onset and duration of action.	Knowing the pharmacological mechanism of action can aid in monitoring for therapeutic and adverse effects of the medication. This information is also useful when teaching your patient the expected outcome(s) of the medication.
Review pertinent lab results pertaining to the medication indication for your patient.	Lab and diagnostic results offer more information into why the patient is receiving the medication and if the medication is having a therapeutic or adverse effect.

Preparing for Administration

Step	Rationale
Wash hands.	Prevents the spread of microorganisms to the supplies being used and handled and prevents further spread to the patient
Gather supplies needed: • Medication/device containing medication in either aerosol or powder form • Mouth care supplies • Copy of patient identification information (can be a patient label, a copy of the medication record, or other piece of information that identifies the patient)	Important to get organized prior to administering medications to the patient; organization can save a potential medication error. Bringing patient identifying information (label, medical record, or other suitable alternative) can aid in the reminder to check patient identification and also provides a solid piece of material from which to ensure your patient's identity prior to administering medication.
Prepare the medication for administration by • Checking medication for expiry date • Checking fullness of medication device (see checking fullness of aerosol or MDIs) • Checking the medication once when it is removed from its storage location and again for the second time to the patient's medication record; a third check is completed when the medication storage container or wrapper is returned to storage or discarded.	Expiration dates can easily go unnoticed on some medications. Expired medications may be ineffective or cause unwanted side effects. Completing three medication checks can limit the chances of medication error.

(continued on page 534)

SKILL 22.14   Administering Medications by Inhalation (continued)

Preparing for Administration (continued)

Step

Prepare the patient by
- Checking patient identifying information using a two-step method; checking the patient armband and then asking the patient to verify his or her name.
- Checking the medication against the armband
- Explaining the administration process and purpose of medication(s)
- Adjusting the bed height and creating privacy
- Completing any necessary pre-administration assessments
- Providing patient teaching about the administration and needed follow-up

Rationale

Double-checking patient identification greatly decreases potential for error.

Explaining the purpose of the medication and what will occur fosters patient collaboration and integration into the medication administration process.

Checking the medication against the patient wristband is a crucial step in ensuring the right medications are given to the right patient.

Patients who are more knowledgeable about the process are usually more comfortable asking questions.

Teaching can provide the necessary understanding that will foster more effective outcomes through patient participation.

Administering the Medication

Step

1. Position patient in a semi-Fowler to high Fowler position if not contraindicated.
2. Shake the MDI prior to use (note that the DPIs do not need to be shaken).
3. For the MDIs, have the patient inhale and exhale fully. Upon the following inhalation, place the inhaler about 2–5 cm (1–2 in.) or two finger widths from the patient's open mouth and release one dose of the medication toward the posterior aspect of the throat as the patient inhales. Instruct the patient to hold breath for 5–10 seconds if possible after each dose is administered. Replace the cap on the MDI.
4. If using a DPI, have the patient inhale and exhale fully. Upon inhalation, with the device against the lips, have the patient inhale while inhaling in the powdered medication. Have the patient hold breath for 5–10 seconds if possible for each dose administered (see Figure 1).

Rationale

Semi-Fowler or high Fowler position promotes ease of breathing.

By shaking, you are ensuring that the medication is evenly distributed in the aerosol chamber.

The dose is delivered toward the posterior aspect of the throat so that it is inhaled into the lungs.

DPIs do not require that you aim the device at the back of the throat. The inhaling action administers the dose from the device into the lungs.

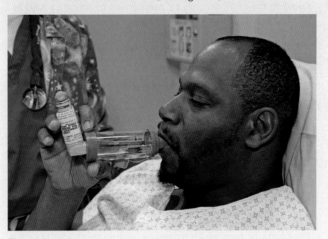

Figure 1

5. Provide mouth care.
6. Assist patient to comfortable upright position.
7. Wash hands.

To prevent an oral thrush infection

Patient comfort

Removes potential microorganisms from hands and stops cross-contamination between patients

Engaging in Evaluation

Step	Rationale
Assess the patient's response to medication administration.	How was the procedure for the patient? Was the patient able to cope with the procedure or was it painful?
Evaluate for specific therapeutic effects of the medication.	Monitoring for therapeutic effects will assist in ensuring the medication is working for the patient.
Monitor for adverse effects post administration.	Some medications do have adverse effects, and quick identification of these will prevent further potential complications for the patient.

Documenting Effectively

Step	Rationale
Document the medication administration in a timely manner and include the following: • Date and time • Medication administered • Route administered • Patient response • Medication effects (therapeutic and adverse) • Other pertinent observations	Documentation is the key communicative method between health-care professionals. The more complete the documentation, the better other health-care team members are able to understand exactly what and how the medication was administered. The prevention of medication errors and adverse events relies heavily on communication. Regularly scheduled medications and as-needed medications are often logged in the patient medication record. These records can either be electronic or hard copy. PRN medications are often documented in the patient medication record and in the narrative documentation notes to ensure that the dose, route, reason for administration, and effect of the medication are noted. Regularly scheduled medications are often just logged in the medication record and not in the narrative nurses' notes. However, unusual observations and adverse effects should be adequately documented in the nurses' notes, even for scheduled medications.

SKILL 22.15   Administering Nebulized Medications

Reviewing Pertinent Information

Step	Rationale
Review the medication(s) ordered from the medication record or patient chart.	Important to know why the patient is receiving the medication, if the medication is appropriate for the patient's situation, and actual appropriateness of the dose and route ordered
Identify patient allergies to medications and food products.	Some food products are found in medications and can cause an allergic reaction as well as medication allergic reaction to the active medicinal ingredient.
Consider the applicable pharmacological principles of the medication including the onset and duration of action.	Knowing the pharmacological mechanism of action can aid in monitoring for therapeutic and adverse effects of the medication. This information is also useful when teaching your patient the expected outcome(s) of the medication.
Review pertinent lab results pertaining to the medication indication for your patient.	Lab and diagnostic results offer more information into why the patient is receiving the medication and if the medication is having a therapeutic or adverse effect.

Preparing for Administration

Step	Rationale
Wash hands.	Prevents the spread of microorganisms to the supplies being used and handled, and prevents further spread to the patient.

(continued on page 536)

SKILL 22.15   Administering Nebulized Medications (continued)

Preparing for Administration (continued)

Step	Rationale
Gather supplies needed: • Medications • Sterile and appropriate diluent (sterile saline or water) • Stethoscope for lung assessment • Nebulizer tubing • Mask or mouthpiece for patient inhalation • Air compressor or oxygen hookup as appropriate • Gloves can be worn but do not necessarily need to if nurse is not coming into contact with bodily secretions. • Mouth care supplies • Copy of patient identification information (can be a patient label, a copy of the medication record, or other piece of information that identifies the patient)	Important to get organized prior to administering medications to the patient; organization can save a potential medication error. Bringing patient identifying information (label, medical record, or other suitable alternative) can aid in the reminder to check patient identification and also provides a solid piece of material from which to ensure your patient's identity prior to administering medication.
Prepare the medication for administration by • Checking medication and diluent for expiry dates • Checking the medication once when it is removed from its storage location and again for the second time to the patient's medication record; a third check is completed when the medication storage container or wrapper is returned to storage or discarded.	Expiration dates can easily go unnoticed on some medications. Completing three medication checks can limit the chances of medication error.
Prepare the patient by • Checking patient identifying information using a two-step method; checking the patient armband and then asking the patient to verify his or her name • Checking the medication against the armband • Explaining the administration process and purpose of medication(s) • Adjusting the bed height and creating privacy • Completing any necessary pre-administration assessments such as a lung assessment prior to medication administration • Providing patient teaching about the administration and needed follow-up	Double-checking patient identification greatly decreases potential for error. Explaining the purpose of the medication and what will occur fosters patient collaboration and integration into the medication administration process. Checking the medication against the patient wristband is a crucial step in ensuring the right medications are given to the right patient. Patients who are more knowledgeable about the process are usually more comfortable asking questions. Teaching can provide the necessary understanding that will foster more effective outcomes through patient participation.

Administering the Medication

Step	Rationale
1. Position patient in a semi-Fowler to high Fowler position unless contraindicated.	Semi-Fowler or high Fowler position promotes ease of breathing.
2. Unwrap the nebulization tubing and connect the patient mask or mouthpiece.	Checking the tubing ensures you have the right pieces and end connectors for effective administration.
3. Connect the tubing to the air or oxygen source (dependent on the agency policy and equipment).	Some agencies prefer to use air versus oxygen and vice versa. Check with your agency regarding the policy. Patients who are already on oxygen should be given oxygen with their treatments to prevent desaturation.

Administering the Medication (continued)

Step

4. Open the medication chamber and add medication to chamber with diluent if required. Close the medication chamber (see Figure 1).

Rationale

Usually, one medication is administered at once; however, there are some instances where medications can be mixed. Always check compatibilities prior to mixing. As well, all bronchodilators should be administered prior to anti-inflammatory nebulized medications to allow for maximum effect of both medications.

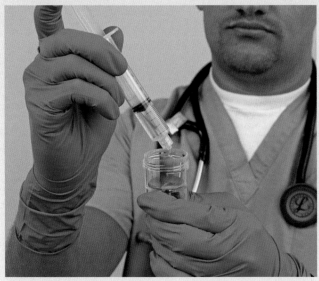

Figure 1-A

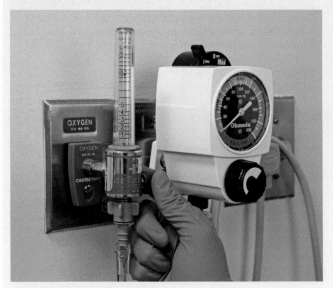

Figure 1-B

5. Turn on the air or oxygen until a fine mist is seen coming from the mouthpiece or mask.

If the air or oxygen is on too low, there will not be enough mist to nebulize the medications. Too much may actually force the line connections in the tubing to break apart. Usually, the rate of flow of oxygen or air is approximately 6 L/minute.

(continued on page 538)

SKILL 22.15 Administering Nebulized Medications (continued)

Administering the Medication (continued)

Step	Rationale
6. Assist the patient to don the mask or take the mouthpiece in the mouth. Instruct the patient to breathe slowly and deeply through the mouth as the medication is being administered (see Figure 2).	Patients can choose if they prefer a mask or mouthpiece. More cognitively aware patients can use mouthpieces; however, if the patient is drowsy, tired, or unable to hold a mouthpiece, a mask should be used.

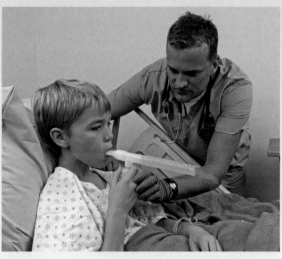

Figure 2

Step	Rationale
7. Repeat with additional medications.	There may be multiple medications that need to be administered, either concurrently or consecutively, using this route.
8. Provide mouth care.	To prevent an oral thrush infection, especially from steroidal nebulized medications
9. Ask patient to remain in upright position for about 15 minutes.	Patient comfort and ease of breathing
10. Wash hands.	Removes potential microorganisms from hands and stops cross-contamination between patients.

Engaging in Evaluation

Step	Rationale
Assess the patient's response to medication administration	How was the procedure for the patient? Was the patient able to cope with the procedure or was it painful?
Evaluate for specific therapeutic effects of the medication.	Monitoring for therapeutic effects will assist in ensuring the medication is working for the patient. It is important to complete a full lung assessment after the nebulized medication has been administered.
Monitor for adverse effects after administration.	Some medications do have adverse effects, and quick identification of these will prevent further potential complications for the patient.

Documenting Effectively

Step	Rationale
Document the medication administration in a timely manner and include the following: • Date and time • Medication administered • Route administered • Patient response • Medication effects (therapeutic and adverse) • Lung assessment pre- and post-medication administration • Other pertinent observations	Documentation is the key communicative method between health-care professionals. The more complete the documentation, the better other health-care team members are able to understand exactly what and how the medication was administered. The prevention of medication errors and adverse events relies heavily on communication. Regularly scheduled medications and as-needed medications are often logged in the patient medication record. These records can either be electronic or hard copy. PRN medications are often documented in the patient medication record and in the narrative documentation notes to ensure that the dose, route, reason for administration, and effect of the medication are noted. Regularly scheduled medications are often just logged in the medication record and not in the narrative nurses' notes. However, unusual observations and adverse effects should be adequately documented in the nurses' notes even for scheduled medications.

Critical Thinking Case Scenarios

▶ Mr. Jones is to receive his eyedrops at 8 AM in the morning. You are the nurse administering the eyedrops to his right eye. When you go to administer the eyedrops, some drops miss the eye and land on the Mr. Jones' cheek. What would you do in this situation and how would you justify your actions? What factors affect your decision-making in this circumstance?

▶ Mrs. Smith has a GI tube that medications could be administered through. What different kinds of medication can be administered through the GI tube and how does the nurse know which ones should be administered using this route? What should the nurse do if when administering medications through the GI tube, they are unable to push anything through the tubing as if there was a blockage?

▶ Mr. Hiddert is receiving an IM injection with two medications. The medication totals 4 ml. What is the best site for administration and what factors might affect your decision-making?

▶ Two types of insulin are often drawn up together. What is the correct procedure for drawing up two types of insulin? What would you do if you obtain too much of the second type of insulin in the syringe and you are over in the total amount of insulin the patient requires for injection?

▶ Medication administration is completed by various individuals and is part of many professional's scopes of practice. Discuss the various professionals that are administering medications in acute and non-acute settings. What is your role in medication administration and how would you work with the other health-care professionals to ensure that the patients you encounter do not receive incorrect medications or doses?

Multiple-Choice Questions

1. When practicing medication administration within a laboratory setting, the student develops which of the following?
   a. A baseline sense of comfort with the skills
   b. A sound knowledge base regarding medications
   c. A relationship of trust with the patient
   d. A new appreciation for the clinical setting

2. Which of the following describes the role of the regulatory body in relation to medication administration?
   a. The regulatory body provides guidelines that do not relate to medication administration.
   b. The regulatory body is not responsible for providing medication administration related standards.
   c. The regulatory body provides standards of practice that encompass medication administration.
   d. The regulatory body only disciplines those who make medication errors and is not responsible for setting guidelines surrounding practice.

3. Which of the following describes the generic name of a medication?
   a. The name given to the medication that is used to market the medication
   b. The name of the medication that describes its molecular ingredients
   c. The name of the medication that is used by pharmacists to classify the medication
   d. The name of the medication that is assigned by Health Canada

4. Which of the following are the five rights of medication administration?
   a. The right patient, drug, trade name, dose, and time
   b. The right patient, drug, dose, time, and route
   c. The right place, drug, route, time, and person administering the medication
   d. The right documentation, drug, dose, person, and time

5. If 50 mg of drug A was ordered and the medication came in a dose strength of 25 mg in 2 ml of oral liquid, how much liquid would need to be drawn up?
   a. 10 ml
   b. 2 ml
   c. 4 ml
   d. 5 ml

6. When giving an IM injection, what is the purpose of aspirating?
   a. To ensure you are not in a blood vessel
   b. To ensure you have adequate blood supply
   c. To foster absorption of the medication
   d. To create an air lock for a Z-track injection

7. When teaching a patient how to use a MDI, how far should the inhaler be from the patient's lips?
   a. 10 cm
   b. 2 finger widths
   c. 30 cm
   d. 5 finger widths

8. Which of the following is true when drawing up two types of insulin?
   a. Draw medication from the cloudy vial first.
   b. Insert air into the clear vial first.
   c. Withdraw medication prior to inserting air.
   d. Withdraw medication from the clear vial first.

Suggested Lab Activities

● Students can develop their application thinking skills by using some scenario-based activities that have the students complete the medication administration and documentation activities as they would in the clinical setting. The following scenario might be useful.

Mrs. Smith is a surgical day patient that has come in to the hospital to get a mass removed from her groin. She is on blood pressure medications that require 25 mg to be administered twice a day. The pills that are available come in 50 mg scored tabs. It is in the morning, and Mrs. Smith's pill is due to be given. The physician has cleared her to have this medication by mouth prior to the procedure. Practice splitting the medication and giving it to Mrs. Smith. Document the actions taken in the MAR.

● Invite students to discuss the following unexpected outcomes in pairs:

• What happens if the suppository is not inserted far enough into the rectum? How can this be prevented?
• What if you are inserting the suppository into the rectum of a child, how does the procedure vary?
• What should the nurse do if the patient has the immediate urge to defecate right after the insertion of the suppository?

● Have the students practice manual dexterity by

• Practicing with the various equipment
• Gain experience drawing up medications in pairs and provide each other with feedback
• Practice manual dexterity by using inject-a-pads with needle and syringes. Students can practice various routes of administration and compare the techniques, advantages, and disadvantages of each
• Landmarking on each other to experience human variation in how each site looks and can be landmarked

● Have the students practice manual dexterity by using the equipment required for both nebulized medication administration and inhaled medications using both the DPIs and MDIs. Use placebo MDIs and DPIs to teach each other how to use the inhalers properly. Using a spacer will also enhance the experience.

REFERENCES AND SUGGESTED READINGS

Baker, J., Lovell, K., Harris, N., & Campbell, M. (2007). Multidisciplinary consensus of best practice for pro re nata (PRN) psychotropic medications within acute mental health settings: A Delphi study. *Journal of Psychiatric and Mental Health Nursing, 14*, 478–484.

Brophy, K. M., Scarlett-Ferguson, H., & Webber, K. (2008). Clinical drug therapy for Canadian practice. Philadelphia, PA: Lippincott Williams & Wilkins.

Canadian Centre for Occupational Health and Safety. (2005). *OHS answers. What are needle stick injuries.* Retrieved from http://www.ccohs.ca/oshanswers/diseases/needlestick_injuries.html

Canadian Nurses Association. (2003). *Position statement: Patient safety.* Ottawa, ON: Author.

Canadian Nurses Association. (2008). *Position statement. Problematic substance use by nurses.* Ottawa, ON: Author.

Canadian Institute for Patient Safety. (2006). *Communication by nurses and physicians to prevent medication incidents.* Retrieved from http://www.patientsafetyinstitute.ca/uploadedFiles/News/Communication%20by%20Nurses%20and%20Physicians%20to%20Prevent%20Medication%20Incidents.pdf

Canadian Pharmacists Association. (2012). *Compendium of pharmaceuticals and specialities.* Ottawa, ON: Author.

Carter-Templeton, H., & McCoy, T. (2008). Are we on the same oate?: A comparison of intramuscular injection explanations in nursing fundamental texts. *MEDSURG Nursing, 17*(4), 237–240.

College and Association of Registered Nurses of Alberta. (2005). *Medication administration: Guidelines for registered nurses.* Edmonton, AB: Author.

Cowell, J. (2007). Improving patient safety by eliminating unsafe abbreviations from medication prescribing. *Alberta RN, 63*(8), 8–9.

Craven, R., Hirnle, C., & Jensen, S. (2013). *Fundamentals of nursing: Human health and function.* Philadelphia, PA: Lippincott Williams & Wilkins.

Emanuel, L. L., Taylor, L., Hain, A., Combes, J. R., Hatlie, M. J., Karsh, B., . . . Walton, M. (Eds). (2011). *The patient safety education program. Module 12c: Interventional care: Medication safety.* Ottawa, ON: Canadian Patient Safety Institute.

Government of Canada. (2012a). *Consolidation of controlled drugs and substances act.* Retrieved from http://laws-lois.justice.gc.ca

Government of Canada. (2012b). *Consolidation of processed products regulation.* Retrieved from http://laws-lois.justice.gc.ca

Gregory, D., Guse, L., Davidson Dick, D., Davis, P., & Russell, C. (2008). *The question of safety: An exploration of errors among undergraduate nursing students placed on clinical learning contracts.* Retrieved from http://www.uleth.ca/dspace/bitstream/10133/692/1/The_Question_of_Safety_Final_Report_Nov_03_08.pdf

Health Canada. (2001). *Drug identification number.* Retrieved from http://www.hc-sc.gc.ca

ISMP Canada (2013). *Definitions of Terms* available online @ Safe Medication Practices Canada (ISMP Canada)

Institute for Safe Medication Practices Canada. (2013). *Definitions of terms.* Retrieved from http://www.ismp-canada.org/

Karch, A. M. (2010a). *Focus on pharmacology* (5th ed.). Philadelphia, PA: Lippincott Williams & Wilkins.

Karch, A. M. (2010b). *2010 Lippincott's nursing drug guide.* Philadelphia, PA: Lippincott Williams & Wilkins.

McBride-Henry, K., & Foureur, M. (2006). Medication administration errors: Understanding the issues. *Australian Journal of Advanced Nursing, 23*(3), 33–41.

Pape, T. M., Guerra, D. M., Muzquiz, M., Bryant, J. B., Ingram, M., Scranner, B., . . . Welker, J. (2005). Innovative approaches to reducing nurses' distractions during medication administration. *The Journal of Continuing Education in Nursing, 36*(3), 108–116.

Springhouse. (2008). *Nursing drug interactions handbook.* Philadelphia, PA: Lippincott Williams & Wilkins.

Stedman's medical dictionary for the health professional and nursing (5th ed.). (2005). Philadelphia, PA: Lippincott Williams & Wilkins.

Stein-Parbury, J., Reid, K., Smith, N., Mouhanna, D., & Lamont, F. (2008). Use of pro re nata medications in acute inpatient care. *Australian and New Zealand Journal of Psychiatry, 42*, 283–292.

The Patient Safety Education Program. Module 1: Systems Thinking: Moving Beyond Blame to Safety. (2011a). Edmonton, AB: Canadian Patient Safety Institute.

The Patient Safety Education Program. Module 6: Technology: Impact on Patient Safety. (2011b). Edmonton, AB: Canadian Patient Safety Institute.

The Patient Safety Education Program. Module 12c: Interventional Care: Medication Safety. (2011c). Edmonton, AB: Canadian Patient Safety Institute.

Vihos, J., & Buckner, S. (2010). Medication administration. In J. C. Ross-Kerr & M. J. Wood (Eds.), *Canadian fundamentals of nursing* (Rev. 4th ed., pp. 675–773). Toronto, ON: Elsevier.

Wolf, Z., Hicks, R., & Farley Serembus, J. (2006). Characteristics of medication errors made by students during the administration phase: A descriptive study. *Journal of Professional Nursing, 22*(1), 39–51.

Effective Documentation

KELLY N. KILGOUR

Collin and Jane are second-year nursing students of a Baccalaureate of Science in Nursing program in Ottawa, Ontario. They are thrilled to be starting their first real clinical experience in the local acute care hospital. Both had a busy day on the rehabilitation unit where they have assessed their assigned patients, given personal care and medications, and even changed a dressing to an abdominal incision and an ostomy site. At 1300 hours, Collin and Jane approach their clinical professor and state, "We have done all our nursing care. What should we do now?" The clinical professor asks if they had documented the care that they have provided to their patients. Both Collin and Jane acknowledged that they forgot and will complete their patients' care flow sheets right away.

CHAPTER OBJECTIVES

By the end of this chapter, you will be able to:

1. Describe the purposes of documenting.
2. Recognize who is responsible for documenting patient care.
3. Understand when to document patient care.
4. Understand how legal and professional practice standards and agency policies guide documentation methods.
5. Describe and exercise the steps of writing late entries of a patient's care.
6. Identify and apply different documentation approaches and forms.

KEY TERMS

Abbreviations   Common short terms used to simplify many familiar long-syllable health-care terms.

Care Plan   A patient's plan of care is developed where the priority patient care diagnoses are identified and interventions are listed out in ink pen or through an electronic version by the entire interprofessional team.

Chart   A patient's record of care compiling the patient's admission sheet, code status, doctor's orders, interprofessional notes, consultations, and other relevant health-care forms. This is considered the bible resource of each individual patient's health-care decisions and services provided.

Charting by Exclusion   A documentation style focusing on the abnormalities or variances from the standard norms of patient's treatment, age, or population expectations. Often, charting by exclusion is completed in the progress notes only when the patient care flow sheets, treatment care pathways, or time lines show variances in standard care planning.

Charting by Inclusion   A documentation style describing each health-care professional's assessments and actions during their care shift. If any notation is missed, it is considered that the care service was not provided to the individual patient. This includes the patient's initial assessment, any physical or mental changes along with the nurse's actions, and the patient's outcomes.

Checklists   Standardized forms used to prepare the patient for a specific medical procedure, such as an operation, or hospital discharge.

Communication Sheet   An effective, informal form to correspond (1) to nurses about all important patient care appointments and special care needs for all patients on the unit and (2) to physicians about non-urgent issues or questions about a patient's care services. This form is commonly reviewed at the beginning of each shift as it is situated within the nursing station.

Documentation   Any chronologically written or electronic data entered into a patient's chart regarding all care services provided to the patient, including the assessment, interventions, patient's responses, and interprofessional patient planning meetings, by all health-care professionals caring for the patient.

Electronic Health Records   A patient health-care record stored, usually by health-care number, in an electronic form where health-care professionals can review and chart into a strictly secure computer format within the hospital or community settings. Greater interprofessional collaboration and efficiency in care can be gained with the electronic format usage rather than the standard reliance on patient charts and waiting for archived patient records to arrive.

Falsifying a Patient Record   Omitting information or making a false documentation in a patient's chart; considered professional misconduct under the Nursing Act, 1991.

(continued on page 542)

Flow Sheet   A checklist form of all standard routine or daily patient care provided during each shift of care. Abbreviations are used to provide descriptions with checkmarks and staff initials are all used to indicate completion of specific patient care services.

Focus Charting   A narrative charting style focusing on only one specific patient problem per entry. Focus charting requires the health-care professional to specify the problem focus of the entry, such as pain, constipation, or wound care, and often the discipline documenting, such as nursing or medical doctor (MD).

Group Documentation   A charting technique used when a health-care professional is working with a group of patients in an outpatient or community setting. Only the entire group assessments and interventions are documented because it is unnecessary to chart on each specific group member.

Incident Report   A long, double-sided form requiring an involved health-care professional, commonly a nurse, to complete when a possible or actual error and physical harm has occurred to a patient, a staff nurse, or a visitor for quality assurance tracking reasons.

Kardex   A working document written in pencil to highlight the patient's diagnoses, allergies and code status, current doctor's orders, medical procedures and tests, specialized diets, and mobility aids for the individual hospitalized patient. It provides a quick snapshot of patient's care services for nursing staff.

Late Entry   A documentation note written just beside or below the documentation date into the patient's chart when the entry should have been completed several hours or days earlier. This usually occurs when the writer forgot to document an intervention, wrote in the wrong patient's chart, or delayed in charting due to an emergent crisis.

Master Signature Record   A signature log where each health-care professional must print his or her name and title designation and provide a signature to identify his or her documentation throughout the unit and even the hospital.

Narrative Charting   A written paragraph highlighting the patient's assessment findings, the interventions completed, and the patient outcomes in chronological order during each health-care professional's shift.

Patient Care Worksheet   An informal piece of paper or an agency preprinted care assignment worksheet helping to organize a health professional's patient assignment. This tool is individually modified and colour enhanced to highlight the staff member's assigned patients and helps prioritize "to dos" at the start of a busy shift.

Progress Notes   A key documentation form permitting all health-care professionals to chart in a narrative paragraph style about their important assessments, interventions, and communications with the specific patient, the patient's family members, and other interprofessional team members.

Shift Report   An audiotape, direct verbal report, or brief summary report summarizing the key patient status and concerns on the unit from the nurses "going off" to the nurses "coming on" during shift change.

SOAP/SOAPIER   A problem-oriented documentation approach clearly guiding the writer to inscribe one step per charting line, which represents each SOAP or SOAPIER letter—**S**: Subjective assessment data, **O**: Objective assessment data, **A**: Assessment, **P**: Plan or **S**: Subjective, **O**: Objective assessment data, **A**: Assessment, **P**: Plan, **I**: Intervention, **E**: Evaluation, and **R**: Revision.

Timely Documentation   An entry into a patient's chart must be documented immediately after the health-care professional has completed the intervention or action to the patient so chronological order of the patient's chart is maintained. Generally, an entry within the hour from the intervention completion is considered timely documentation.

Transfer Record   A communication form highlighting key features of the patient's health information from one health-care agency to another.

The Art of Documentation

Among all the skills a nursing student will learn, documentation is the most essential yet the most difficult to grasp. Students often find real-life situational documenting far more challenging than what they expected. Their expectations are usually based on their observations of staff swiftly charting, as seen in Figure 23.1. The art of documentation appears easy until students experience charting for themselves. They frequently draw a blank when they need to write an abbreviation along with accurately and briefly describing the patient's assessment or the event and interventions that had occurred only a few hours ago.

Through the eyes of a nurse

*T*he challenges of documentation become more complicated as the number of patients in your care increases. Which patient had the rash? Was the hip replacement on the left or right for Patient C? However, documentation provides you a few minutes to finally sit down and reflect; and there will be times when you really appreciate these moments to sit!

(personal reflection of a nurse)

Correct

3/15/2014	0730 Client awake, alert, denies complaints, sitting up in bed watching TV, VS taken, IV infusing s̄ difficulty, IV site Ⓡhand s̄ redness, Ⓛhip drsg dry and intact . 0830 100% of full liquid breakfast taken. 0900 Partial bath at bedside, pt tolerated sitting in chair X 30 min without fatigue. 0930 Δ Drsg to Ⓛhip approx 50cc pink drng, sutures intact, 0 redness or edema at incision line, pt tol s̄ pain 1015 1000cc D5 ½ NS added to present IV to run at 125cc/hr. pt resting. 1100 To x-ray via stretcher. 1145 Returned from x-ray, back to bed for rest. 1200 Reg lunch taken 100%
	── MS Gorski RN

Figure 23.1 Example of an experienced nurse's charting notes.

What Is Documentation?

Documentation is "any written or electronically generated information about a client that describes the care or service provided to that client—and it is an integral part of nursing practice" (College of Registered Nurses of British Columbia [CRNBC], 2008, p. 1) and interprofessional documentation (College of Nurses of Ontario [CNO], 2009). Nursing documentation communicates the nurse's assessment, decisions, interventions, and the patient's outcome. Thus, the patient's medical chart or electronic health record is a pertinent record to accurately detail health-care observations and actions by the interprofessional health-care team in chronological order.

Documenting the Individual

Most documentation is recorded about an individual patient. This is seen in hospitalized or home care patients. Yet, the patient's individual or entire family may be recorded into the patient's chart if it concerns the patient's care. When would it be appropriate to record a patient's family or friend in the patient's chart? The answer is - when the family member helps or hinders the patient's health care. Some examples are the following:

- Primary family caregiver
- Substitute decision-maker or power of attorney
- Family abuser—concerns of physical and emotional harm to the patient
- Person providing illegal actions or providing addictive products to the patient which could harm his or her health (e.g. cocaine to a methadone patient)

Through the eyes of a student

*D*o I chart or don't I? What do I need to document in the progress notes? Considering the assessments and interventions that I completed for my patients, I think about anything different or extra I had to do for one particular patient versus another one. These are excellent charting points to enter into a patient's narrative progress note.

(personal reflection of a nursing student)

Documenting a Group

Public health nurses often provide health promotion interventions to a group of patients or a community as a patient. It is not realistic for the registered nurse to chart on each group member. Thus, the registered nurse will document on the group as a whole and only chart on individual members separately when he or she is concerned about a single person or specific interventions are initiated. When a single group member is documented other group members are not identified in the patient's chart. This maintains a separation between the group as a patient and the individual member as a patient. According to College of Nurses of Ontario (CNO, 2009) and College of Registered Nurses of British Columbia (CRNBC, 2007), **group documentation** includes the following:

1. The identified needs and goals of the group,
2. The criteria for patient participation,
3. The nurses' actions to help guide the group to meet their goals,
4. The outcomes of the group's actions, and
5. The evaluation of the group and its outcomes.

Although this documentation method is efficient, it is not commonly used in the hospital settings.

J ane returns from her break and checks on Mrs. Whoare, who has vomited twice this morning. Mrs. Whoare has a big smile on her face and states, "Did you hear the good news? The doctor says that I can get rid of this NG tube and can start eating again. It has been weeks since I've had a good roast beef sandwich! When can I get this tube out of my nose? Can you do it now?" What should Jane do and why should she document it?

Why Document?

Documentation has three purposes. It is an effective communication tool, a confirmation that suitable professional care has been provided, and a legal record of accountability.

Documentation for Effective Communication

The first purpose of documentation is a method for all health-care professionals to effectively communicate about the patient's care with each other. "The use of communication tools, typically in very rudimentary forms (e.g., pencil and paper), has long been in place to help health care providers determine the concerns and needs of our patients" (Henneman, 2009, p. 130). Documentation provides clear communication to the entire health-care team. It shows the writer's initial assessment; any changes from the original assessment, concerns regarding the patient's care; the plan of care, including discharge plans; interventions completed; and the treatment effectiveness or patient outcomes. In Jane's situation, she should first check the doctor's orders. If nothing is recorded in the chart and there are no apparent orders, then the physician has not clearly communicated that Ms. Whoare's nasogastric (NG) tube should be removed.

Documentation for the Confirmation of Suitable Professional Practice

The second purpose of documentation is confirming safe and suitable professional care has been provided to the patient. The documentation clearly displays each health-care professional's role and demonstrates, through professional practice, what interventions have been completed, which meets the standards of practice. In Jane's situation, she should chart Ms. Whoare's NG removal request along with her rationale to not remove the NG (i.e., patient vomiting twice in the morning and no doctor's order to remove).

Documentation may also provide important data to nursing researchers and hospital administration regarding workload management and patient care outcomes. Thus, nurses should be documenting their continuous nursing process of assessment, nursing diagnosis, planning, intervention, and evaluation for each patient. Interventions include reporting concerns to the attending physician or charge nurse and completing a referral of another health-care professional such as the social worker.

Documentation for Legal and Professional Standards

The final purpose of documentation is supporting legal and professional practice in relation to standards of care. The patient's **chart** is a "comprehensive record of care" (CRNBC, 2008, p. 1). Documentation endorses the accountability of your professional care within the expectation of the professional standards. It justifies the professional knowledge and expertise skill as expected by the professional standards of care (CNO, 2009). "Nursing care and the documentation of that care will be measured according to the standard of a reasonable and prudent nurse with similar education and experience in a similar situation" (CRNBC, 2007, p. 6). Documentation also details your professional nursing practice actions, that could be reviewed and possibly called into legal court. A Canadian nurse's documentation was first accepted as admissible legal evidence, without the testifying of the nurse, in the *Ares v. Venner* court case in 1970 (CRNBC, 2007). Over the past four decades, nursing documentation has evolved to be admissible evidence in the following circumstances: lawsuits, coroners' inquests, and professional disciplinary hearings. Because legal proceedings often occur several years later, the registered nurse or registered practical nurse will unlikely recall the patient; therefore, documentation supports the full practice and protects the nurse who has met the provincial professional standards. CRNBC (2008) states "documentation is generally accepted as evidence in legal proceedings. It establishes the facts and circumstances related to the care given and assists nurses in recalling details in a specific situation" (p. 1).

Document only the care you personally have provided for the patient and not the care others have completed. Other staff members are responsible to document their professional care for the patient and may not delegate documentation to another. There are only two exceptions to this rule. The first exception is a patient emergency, where a recorder of the care events takes charge of the minute-by-minute documentation. The second

exception is documentation information provided to you by a health-care volunteer, who does not have authority to record in the patient's chart. Thus, the volunteer will report patient care information, such as the patient vomiting, to the assigned nurse who must decide how she will intervene and document it. In this circumstance, the registered nurse should document that the information was reported to you and by whom, such as the hospital volunteer, along with his name.

Through the eyes of a student

*I*nitially, I found charting in the progress notes so awkward and frustrating. It took a long time to learn it. My clinical professor would edit, my draft progress notes over and over before I could enter it into my patient's chart. The sentences are unusually short and not written in a standard sentence format. Plus, I could never remember all the abbreviations. Now, it feels good when I am able to draft a progress note on a piece of blank paper and get someone like a clinical professor or another classmate to read it with no edits made. Once I got accustomed to this new writing style, and after a few entries, my frustration reduced, and my confidence and efficiency have greatly improved.

(personal reflection of a nursing student)

Signing Documentation

How do others know your documentation from other health-care professionals? Most health-care organizations require annual completion of a master signature record for specific unit verification. The **master signature record** is a signature log where each health-care professional must print her name, title designation, and provide a signature to identify her documentation throughout the unit and even the hospital. When documenting, always sign your name and add your title designation (SN for student nurse, RPN for registered practical nurse, LPN for licensed practical nurse, RN for registered nurse, MD for medical doctor, or R for resident doctor, along with the numerical year of the resident) after each entry. Have you tried writing out your signature and title? If not, it is best to practice so you become comfortable with your new role and signature. As a student, you should always include your year of study as well as the name of your school to present your affiliation. When there is not enough room to sign on the current line, draw a line on the current and half of the next line and then place your signature and title as shown in Figure 23.1. Once you have mastered your own professional signature, it is wise to verify specific organizations' official documentation guidelines before you start charting. Most organizations have specific guidelines for consistent documentation that support communication between health-care professionals, effective patient care, and fulfilling provincial standards for professional standards.

Documentation Guidelines

All health-care agencies maintain documentation policies that support their standardized health-care records within their own region. These agency policies provide guidelines to all health-care professionals based on committee accepted documentation practices expected within their specific health-care region, agency, and even, sometimes, particular units. Agency policies provide details of the following:

1. Different documentation methods utilized in the care settings
2. Documentation frequency
3. Procedure to record a late entry into a patient's chart
4. List of accepted abbreviations or a reference source
5. Procedure to take and record doctor's verbal and telephone orders, and
6. Process of patient health record storage and disposal.

Always review your agency policies on documentation and never rely just on what another health-care professional tells you about how to document. Table 23-1 displays a list of standard documentation fundamentals. Remember that you are responsible to adapt your documentation to meet the agency policies and professional practice guidelines so your practice complies with the legal and professional standards. When policies are outdated, nurses are encouraged to advocate for suitable revisions to maintain their professional standards of care.

Think Jane notices that Samantha, another nursing student, is charting with a sparkly pink gel pen. Jane comments to Samantha, "I thought only black and blue pens were allowed for any legal documents." Samantha responds, "I don't see what the difference is. This other person documented in red pen," as she points to another entry above hers. Is Jane's statement true or false?

Timing of Documenting—When Do You Chart?

Frequently, students try to fill out the patient's care flow sheet before actually completing the patient's full care. They recognize that they are using their time well when their patient still wants to sleep along with stating, "I know that I am going to wash her and toilet her so I am just documenting it ahead of time." Although this may seem like an innocent thing to do, it is not an ideal nursing practice. **Timely documentation** is part of the nurse's standards of care. The CRNBC places "documentation timely and appropriate reports of assessment, decisions about client status, plans, interventions, and client outcomes" (CRNBC, 2008, p. 10) as an important indicator or competent application of clinical practice knowledge in their professional standards. They note that "the timeliness of documentation will be dependent upon the setting. Settings in which the client acuity, complexity, and variability is high will require more frequent documentation than settings in which clients are less acute, less complex and/or less variable" (CRNBC, 2008, p. 10). Additionally, patient documentation will be more frequent, thorough, and descriptive when a patient is suddenly unstable, is more acutely ill, has multiple complex health problems, and displaying inconsistent or manipulative behaviour, including threatening to sue the health-care team.

Any practicing professional nurse, including a student nurse, who documents that he or she has completed care before he or she actually has fully done so, is illegally falsifying a record. **Falsifying a patient record** is considered professional misconduct under the Nursing Act, 1991 (Service Ontario Publications, 1993) because you are claiming that you have provided professional care when you have not. What would you do if the patient refuses your care after you have documented that you have done it? Health-care professionals are legally responsible to accurately document the completion of their care or an event after it has just occurred. Thus, documentation occurs at the moment of your completed action or soon afterward. The CRNBC emphasizes that "in a court of law, accurate, complete and timely documentation may lead to the conclusion that accurate, complete and timely care was given to the patient. The converse is also true. If it is not documented, it is questionable if it was really done" (CRNBC, 2008, p. 2).

Although both timely documentation and no documentation are understood in the legal system, an alternative documentation of a late entry is widely accepted. A **late entry** is a documentation note entered into the patient's chart several hours or days after the original intervention was completed. It happens after a patient has had a major crisis and you are finally able to document the event once the patient is physically stable. It also occurs when you have forgotten to acknowledge something in the chart. Late entries are not the end of the world. Everyone forgets to chart something sooner or later. Document the late entry into the patient's chart as soon as possible. Write "Late entry for (date and time)," record the current date and time that you are documenting this entry, and then chart your documentation. Because the chronological order of the documentation is interrupted and communication with other health-care professionals is delayed, nurses must write a late entry only when necessary.

Avoid Delaying Documentation

The typical working shift is busy. The ideal of sitting down to document every task and event right after it has occurred is not always possible. Thus, it is important to set time aside to chart after all morning care and medications have been completed, usually midmorning, midday, and again within the last hour of your care shift. Nonetheless, CRNBC (2008) reminds us that documentation delays may lead to the writer's cloudy memory of the patient's care events and possible omissions or errors in their documentation record; this must be kept in mind, especially for late entries. Most nurses make notes on their patient care worksheet to remind them

TABLE 23.1	Key Essentials to All Documentation
Documentation Essentials	**Rationale**
All documentation should be "clear, concise, factual, objective, timely, and legible" (CRNBC, 2008, p. 1).	Promotes effective documentation of all care provided and clear communication to the rest of the health-care team
Always verify and follow unit and agency policy on documentation.	Each health-care unit may document in a different manner.
Use black or blue pen for all documentation.	Red pen maybe used for transcribing of orders or recording of vital signs. Pencil may only be used on kardex where the patient's care interventions are being regularly modified. Also, yellow highlighting may indicate discontinuation or signaling of an important order. Verify with the unit staff and agency policy about their particular colour pen coding and its meaning. Never use red or other crafty gel pens for documentation on a legal document!
Make sure that the sheet clearly has the patient name, date of birth, and room number on the form. If it does not, write it on with pen or name plate it immediately.	Promotes clear patient identification on all forms; this prevents patient sheets being misplaced or accidentally placed in the wrong chart.
Always write neatly or print.	Allows others to easily read your documentation and care actions
Objectively describe the event: what you saw, smelled, and heard. Then, describe what your assessment and interventions were.	Being clear and concise in your data prevents others' presumptions about your care or you assuming that other health-care professionals will know what you mean. Remember: Subjective documentation belongs in your own self-reflection, not in a patient's chart.
Write the time that you are entering the documentation into the chart. If this is a late entry, write "Late entry for [date and time]."	Chronological order can be maintained.
Write in proportion to the documentation sheet.	Multiuse forms offer narrower writing areas which require lesser and smaller charting; for example, a flow sheet requires the writer to print small or only place a checkmark in a box as the one form is used for multiple days of care.
Only use unit- and hospital-accepted abbreviations that are understood by all staff.	Promotes consistent and effective documentation of care provided along with clear communication to the rest of the health-care team
Never leave a space blank or omit information, especially when the agency uses charting with inclusion. It is better to thoroughly document in the progress note and write N/A (not applicable) in the flow sheet.	If the documentation is blank or the progress notes have omitted the assessment or interventions, then it means that you never assessed or completed the care. This could be considered faulty practice. Also, blank spaces permit others to accidentally write within your documentation, where misrepresentation of your practice and assessment completion of the patient's care can occur. It is best to record all your assessment or inscribe that intervention was not needed because the patient is asymptomatic. This tells any reader that you considered it, and it was not fitting or needed for the patient at the time.
Always sign your name and add your title designation (SN for student nurse, RPN for registered practical nurse, LPN for licensed practical nurse, or RN for registered nurse) after each documented entry. If there is not enough room for your signature on the current line, draw a line on the current and half of the next line and then place your signature and title.	Clearly identifies your documentation as your own; if space on the entry line is too small for you to sign, it is common practice to sign on the next line. However, draw a line on any space without words so no free space is left open. Please see example Figure 23.1.
Your name and signature may need to be placed in a master signature record.	Maintains health-care professional name and signature verification and it is common practice within many agencies.
Errors are crossed out once or twice from the word or sentence that is wrong. Initial your error and enter the reason for error (except if it is a spelling mistake) and then continue your writing. See Figure 23.2 for an example.	Everyone makes mistakes in spelling or choice of words when writing. But, it is important that any reader can read what you accidentally wrote wrong so the error is clear and does not look falsified.
Always reread your charting.	Verifies your documentation is clear and concise
Never alter or delete someone else's documentation.	You are responsible for your patient care actions and documentations. They are responsible for theirs in the legal system.

of completed interventions during a hectic shift. The only exception of this rule is when you have called a physician on several occasions and unable to receive an answer from him. It is important to record your attempts to contact a physician and how you went about trying to get a response.

Documenting Amidst an Emergency Crisis

There are times when you need to document immediately; for example, when a patient is complaining of chest pain. After assessing the patient, taking his vital signs, and administering his nitroglycerin spray, record the vital signs immediately and continue this process for three consecutive nitroglycerin sprays. Frequent and immediate documentation often occurs when the vital sign demographics forms are with you at the bedside. However, never leave this form loose where it can get lost. It is counterproductive because you will be searching everywhere for this record when the physician is waiting to look at it.

During a crisis, such as a chest pain turning into a code blue, use a loose piece of paper or paper towel to write down key information, such as the time of patient's complaint, what his vital signs were, when the physician was called, and any medications given. When the emergency team or the attending physician arrives, clearly report the highlights of your assessment and vital signs from the notes. If the notes are clearly organized with findings beside the time taken, you may show them to the physicians to make your communication clear and efficient. This approach often facilitates the entire health-care team in their swift assessments and critical interventions. Always have the patient's chart and medication record handy for the response health-care team or attending physician to review the recent documentation. During a crisis, it is understood that there will not always be time to document the recent care provided. Just report to the team what has occurred and record vital signs as soon as possible. If a code is occurring, ask who should document the vital signs and medication administration. This is important because some teams expect the patient's assigned nurse to take a lead, whereas other teams prefer to take over during a crisis. They will designate a recorder. Once the crisis is over, sit down and document the event, your interventions, and the patient's response.

Correcting Documentation Errors

When you make an error, you must never completely cross out, leave a big black splotch, or make an obvious whiteout erasure. This leaves the reader wondering what was crossed out and raises a red flag about the credibility of the author or even implies falsification the documentation. Every student faces the problem of correcting an error at least once in the first month of health-care documentation. It is better to cross out the word or sentence that is wrong by striking through the word, sentence, or paragraph once or twice. Next, initial the change and enter the reason for the error (except if it is a spelling mistake), then continue writing the remaining documentation. See Figure 23.2 for an example. This correction should be made as soon as possible to avoid any documentation delays.

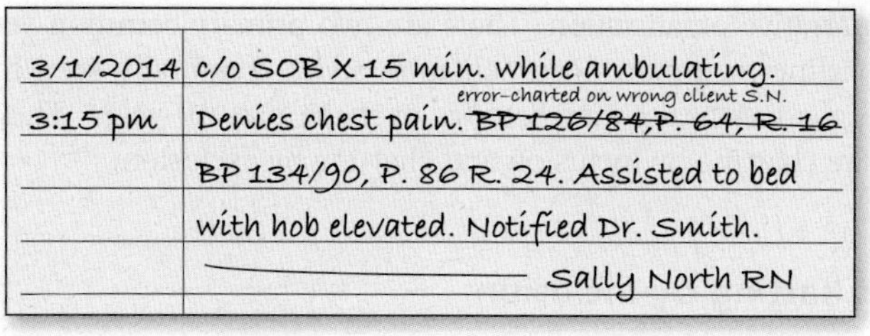

3/1/2014	c/o SOB X 15 min. while ambulating.
3:15 pm	~~error–charted on wrong client S.N.~~ Denies chest pain. ~~BP 126/84, P. 64, R. 16~~
	BP 134/90, P. 86 R. 24. Assisted to bed
	with hob elevated. Notified Dr. Smith.
	———————————— Sally North RN

Figure 23.2 Example of a correction to an error when charting a progress note.

Using Abbreviations

With all the multiple terms and conditions spoken and written in health care, **abbreviations** are common short terms used to simplify many familiar long syllable health-care terms. All documentation, whether paper, temporary, or electronic, relies on a system of abbreviations. Shortened terms are valued for saving space in written documentation and verbal conversation with other health-care professionals. Although many abbreviations are used throughout Canada and worldwide, nurses should never assume that one abbreviation is accepted in all health-care settings. For example, what does BS mean? It could be interpreted as bowel sounds or blood sugars. Both of these terms have very different meanings when read in a sentence. It is best to always verify the agency policy for accepted documentation abbreviations.

Standardized Abbreviations

Student nurses are exposed to many new terms and abbreviations. If you do not know an abbreviation that a health-care professional has stated, ask him or her what the term means as well as verify the agency's policies because there are no guarantees that a staff member is using it correctly. For instance, many hospitals have an approved documentation flow sheet abbreviations form (go to **thePoint** to see an example from The Ottawa Hospital). This flow sheet is often placed on the clipboard for easy staff reference. This abbreviation form standardizes common care terms so all health-care professionals will uniformly document on the patient's bedside flow sheet. It helps reduce subjectivity by providing more accurate measurement; for example, the measure of edema amount 0 (*none*) to 5 (*brawny*) when pressed on the patient's edematous extremity for 5 seconds. As a student, it is best to write these abbreviations down in your notepad and keep them nearby for a quick reference until you have them fully memorized.

Documentation Approaches

Although abbreviations are universally used in all charting documents, there are various documentation approaches. Documentation approaches, such as focus charting and problem-oriented medical records, are generally applied to narrative progress notes and help guide the writer with the narrative organization. There are two primary common yet distinct common documentation styles commonly seen in Canadian health-care settings over the past 10 years. They are charting by inclusion and charting by exclusion.

Charting by Inclusion

Charting by inclusion is continuous documentation of at least two recordings in the patient's progress notes per shift where the patient's initial assessment and any changes are continually recorded along with the nurse's actions and the patient's outcomes. Charting by inclusion involves a more head-to-toe documentation approach and often ends the notation with "the patient is resting comfortably." *If the nurse does not document it, she did not do it* is the accepted understanding for this documentation style. For example, the medication administration record nicely fits into charting by inclusion documentation approach.

Charting by Exclusion

Charting by exclusion focuses on charting about abnormalities or variances from the standard norms of the patient's treatment, age, or population expectations. Charting by exclusion is often completed in the patient's progress notes only when the patient care flow sheet, treatment care pathways, or timelines show some abnormalities. The nurse should enter a note, such as "see progress notes," and describe the specific concern along with interventions and patient outcomes in the progress notes. This documentation style upholds a new charting principle of "all documentation has been met with a normal or expected response unless documented otherwise" (CRNBC, 2007, p. 12); however, the medication administration record, as described in Chapter 22, does not apply to charting by exclusion. All medications must be recorded in the medication administration record.

Types of Documentation

Currently, health records are completed in two manners: hard copy (handwritten by pen) or electronic form. Although electronic documents have been developing over the past 10 years, most of our nursing documentation is still performed the rudimentary way, by hand, on paper for a hard copy. Regardless of the method, numerous types of health records are still completed in a similar manner. The forms range from helping the staff and unit function within its capacity (patient care worksheets, shift reports, and kardex), through to documenting in a patient's medical chart (narrative progress notes, and flow sheets), and even transfer records to other health-care centres. Common documentation forms are listed and further described in Table 23.2 so their appropriate usage is clear.

Patient Care Worksheets

The **patient care worksheet** is the first documentation form that student nurses learn to use. It is their own tool that highlights their assigned patients and helps organize their day. The worksheet can be as informal as a blank piece of paper with your notes or as formal as an agency preprinted care assignment worksheet. Regardless of the style, it is a working tool for staff to organize and prioritize their multiple patient care tasks throughout their shift. Here are a few common items that should be placed on the worksheet:

- Patient's name and room number
- Age
- Diagnosis
- Allergies
- Code status
- Attending physician's name
- Vital sign frequency: q4h, q8h, q shift, or q week
- Ambulation status: FWB, PWB, NWB
- Particular diagnostic testing with times
- Fluid input and output
- Last bowel movement
- Particular nursing interventions required: dressing change or suppository

These items help organize your day as well as provide a quick reference list to answer unexpected questions asked by attending physicians or senior nursing staff. This is one of the most useful documentation sheets that you will use from your first week as a student nurse through to an experienced registered nurse.

Temporary Hard Copy Documents

There are some forms used to communicate important patient care issues to other health-care professionals. These forms are the communication sheet, shift report, and patient kardex. The **communication sheet** is a form found in the nursing station that reports each patient's important inpatient or outpatient appointments to the assigned nurse, such as, "Patient has outpatient cancer agency appointment at 0900 hour," "Occupational therapist to complete swallowing assessment," and "NPO since midnight - OR at 0730 hours." This information affects how the assigned nurses will provide care to individual patients and how they will prioritize their schedules within the patient assignments. Another communication sheet tool is nonurgent notes to the attending physicians. This sheet is often available on a clipboard or in a communication binder with each physician's name on top. It permits all healthcare professionals to write down the specific patient needs or order requests that are not urgent (these orders can wait until the physician's next follow-up rounds on the unit). When using this communication sheet, make sure that the patient's name and room number along with the order request is clearly written.

TABLE 23.2	Common Documentation Forms		
Documentation Forms	Category	Formal or Informal Usage	Key Purpose
Patient care worksheet	Personal staff usage of assigned patients	✓ Informal or formal Personal usage: RN and RPN commonly use Availability: depends on unit	– Useful quick reference list and organizational tool – Organizes and prioritizes multiple patients' care throughout the shift (e.g., patient information, vital signs, ambulation status, fluid in & out, last bowel movement, & stat interventions)
Communication sheet	Informal unit usage of all patients	✓ Informal Unit usage for entire interprofessional health-care team Availability: usually found inside the nursing station on a clipboard or in a communication binder with physicians' names specified	– Communicates patient care issues to health-care professionals – Reports patient's important inpatient or outpatient appointments (i.e., physio appointments, planned discharge transfer, PICC line insertion) – Also, nonurgent patient needs or order requests are written in brief note to the attending physicians (e.g., upcoming renewal of medication and patient's weekend pass request)
Shift report	Informal unit usage of all patients	✓ Informal Unit usage for RN, RPN, and PSW Availability: always inside the nursing station	– Summarizes the patient status and care at shift change (night shift nurse to oncoming day shift nurse) – Key points from the shift report are often recorded on oncoming nurse's patient care worksheet. – Various methods from audiotape, direct verbal report, or brief summary shift report sheets
Kardex	Permanent medical record of individual patient	✓ Formal Unit usage for entire interprofessional health-care team Availability: in patient's chart or medication record	– Usually a one- to four-page document written primarily in pencil because document is frequently changed to with new orders. – Quick reference tool of the patient's daily care, but it never replaces the patient's progress notes, care plans, and order forms; similar to a recipe card – Highlights existing doctor's orders, upcoming procedures, and routine patient care (e.g., specialized diets, use of mobility aids) – Important to regularly update the kardex and verify the patient's order forms match the kardex information
Care plan	Permanent medical record of individual patient	✓ Formal Unit usage for entire interprofessional health-care team Availability: in patient's chart	– Interprofessional patient care plans which are commonly developed by the entire health-care team – Priority patient care diagnoses are identified and interventions are listed electronically or in pen.
Progress notes	Permanent medical record of individual patient	✓ Formal Unit usage for entire interprofessional health-care team Availability: in patient's chart	– A central collaborative document that shares detailed, chronological assessments and interventions among the entire health-care team simultaneously working and communicating together – May also chart important communications with the patient, their family members, and interprofessional team members (e.g., CPR status) – Narrative paragraph form but not written in standard English sentence structure – Common charting methods are narrative, focus, and SOAP/SOAPIER.

(continued on page 550)

TABLE 23.2	Common Documentation Forms (continued)		
Documentation Forms	Category	Formal or Informal Usage	Key Purpose
Flow sheet	Permanent medical record of individual patient	✓ Formal Unit usage for entire interprofessional health-care team Availability: on clipboard outside patient's room or in a binder on the medication cart	– Primary documentation form to record all routine or daily patient care – May check off or initial specific patient care completed and place an abbreviation for the assessment finding (e.g., bowel movements & chest auscultation) – For an abnormal finding, write "see progress notes" in flow sheet and then write a progress note. – There are specialized flow sheets for neurological, pain, wound care, and diabetic assessments. – Remember to maintain patient confidentiality due to flow sheets availability.
Checklist	Permanent medical record of individual patient	✓ Formal Unit usage for entire interprofessional health-care team Availability: in patient's chart	– Guides the completion of specific tasks before the patient leaves for a procedure (e.g., operation) or a hospital discharge – Similar to flow sheets, however, staff may collectively complete separate sections of the checklist – May be completed over several days; requires dating and initialing when each task is completed
Transfer record	Permanent medical record of individual patient	✓ Formal Unit usage for entire interprofessional health-care team; RN and social worker commonly complete Availability: in patient's chart	– A communication form used between two or more health-care professionals to share individual patient health information from one health-care agency to another (e.g., rehabilitation unit transfer or hospital discharge to long-term care facility or community health services) – Highlights patient information, physicians contact information, medications ordered and last gave, and specific care interventions (e.g., wound care instructions, neonate's birth and current weight) – Additional documentation (e.g., progress notes, flow sheets, and doctor's orders) are photocopied and attached to the transfer record for supplementary information.
Incident report	Permanent unit and agency record for quality assurance reasons when a possible or actual error or physical harm has occurred to a patient, visitor, or staff member	✓ Formal Agency usage for statistical tracking Availability: always inside the nursing station	– A quality assurance tracking tool completed for the administrative level when a possible or actual error or physical harm has occurred within the agency (e.g., missed or incorrectly administered medication and accidental falls) – Protected from legal court disclosure, thus, incident reports are separate from the patient's chart – Good practice to review the form with another colleague or the charge nurse to ensure all the form sections are correctly completed – Unit manager and physician must sign the completed incident report in acknowledgement of the incident, any aftermath interventions, and patient response outcomes.
Reflection	Personal staff usage	✓ Informal Personal usage; RN and RPN commonly use Availability: depends on staff usage	A reflective tool to promote individual staff professional development outside the clinical setting – Involves thoughtful writing about a key patient care event – May enhance the staff's critical thinking and emotional insights into their professional practice – Refer to Chapter 25 for further description.

CPR, cardiopulmonary resuscitation; PICC, peripherally inserted central catheter; PSW, personal support worker

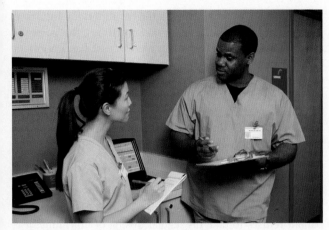

Figure 23.3 Verbal shift report between two nurses.

Shift Report

A **shift report** is a method to summarize the patient status and care from the end of shift nurses to the oncoming nurses. This report is shared in various methods from audiotape, direct verbal report, or brief summary shift report sheets. In the past few years, brief summary shift reports are frequently seen in practice; however, they do not replace the direct verbal report needed when a patient is acutely ill or requires complex care. Figure 23.3 displays a common direct verbal report between two nurses. Each assigned patient's primary care focuses are noted during the shift report, and key points are highlighted in the oncoming nurse's patient care worksheet. Some examples of items presented in a nursing shift report are the following:

- How well the patient slept
- How much or often the patient voided and last bowel movement
- Any isolation precautions
- Any irregular vital signs
- Any as-needed (prn) medications given and the reason
- Any new treatments started such as blood transfusion or fasting blood work
- Any abnormal behaviours such as seizures or fainting
- Any injuries to the patient such as a fall out of bed
- Any requested orders needed from the physician
- Reminder of any new code status or special appointments during the next shift

Kardex

A **kardex** is a working document that communicates existing doctor's orders, diagnostic tests or surgeries (completed or to be done), specialized diets, or the use of mobility aids for ambulation for the specific patient (CNO, 2002). It is commonly written in pencil because a kardex requires frequent modifications (erased and rewritten in pencil) throughout the patient's treatment of care. However, some of the information is written in ink pen such as the patient's name and other identifiers, attending physicians, allergies, and cardiopulmonary resuscitation (CPR) status. Regardless of it being primarily written in pencil, a kardex is still a legal document and considered part

of the patient's permanent medical record. The kardex is an excellent place for a quick reference of the patient's daily care, but it never replaces the patient's narrative progress notes, care plans, and order forms in the chart. An excellent sample of an established kardex, used by the Vancouver Coastal Health Authority, can be viewed on **thePoint**. Could you see how a surgical unit would use this working document differently than a medical unit? For example, a surgical unit frequently uses a kardex as they modify how often the patient's routine vital signs need to be taken—from every hour during the first shift on the unit to every 4 hours to 12 hours. They also use the kardex to highlight intravenous site changes and surgical drain and dressing removals. For a medical unit, a kardex is used to follow patient's last bowel movements, mobility transfers, wound care instructions, and even the next chemotherapy treatment. The kardex will also remind nursing staff when the next bath day for a patient who has been on a unit for a long period of time or awaiting a long-term care bed. In long-term care, the kardex will be used to remind staff to record a monthly patient weight as well as provide a reminder of when the influenza vaccine will be coming along with a consent form, which needs to be completed by the patient or his substitute decision-maker. When it is regularly updated, the kardex is a very useful documentation tool that helps guide the daily patient care. All nursing staff and unit clerks should regularly verify the patient's chart matches the kardex information. This important verification ensures that the kardex is up-to-date with the continuously changing documentation in the patient's chart.

Through the eyes of a student

*A*lways check the information on the kardex for accuracy. Often, a patient will change rooms because of isolation precautions, yet no one has changed this information on the kardex. As a student, I was very helpful to staff when I took the time to update the information on the kardex. However, you should inform your assigned nurse so she or he is aware that you have made some changes to the kardex.

(personal reflection of a nursing student)

Through the eyes of a student

*R*emember, a kardex never replaces the original documents in the patient's chart! It is only a quick reference guide or a "recipe card" to guide your patient's care.

(personal reflection of a nursing student)

Patient Care Plans

Another working document is the patient **care plan**. The care plan is commonly developed with an interprofessional team where the priority patient care diagnoses are identified and interventions are listed electronically or in ink pen. Most hospitals are promoting interprofessional treatment care plans. Go to **thePoint** to see a good example of The Ottawa Hospital *Interprofessional Patient Care Plan*.

 Think Have a look at a few patients' care plans. What do they remind you of in your own student assignments?

Progress Notes

A **progress note** is the key documentation form where you chart important patient assessments, interventions, as well as communications that you have had with the patients, their family members, and interprofessional team members. Although it is written in a narrative paragraph form, the sentences do not hold the standard English sentence structure. It is always good practice to enter a brief progress note because most patients have an issue or two that require monitoring or they would not require your care. Consider this list of common charted topics as a guide when charting:

- Pain—Any pain or discomfort? Consider chronic and acute pain, usage of prn analgesics, and headache
- Wounds or potential pressure sores—Is the dressing intact and scheduled for change tomorrow? Does the patient have a bony hip prominence that is very red which may lead to a pressure sore? Does the patient have a new skin tear from the adhesive tape?
  - Any prn medications administered? What were the reason and their effect?
  - Any drainage coming out of the patient? It is always good to record the type of drainage, its location, its odor, and (if there is one) the drainage tube in situ and if it is patent.
- Emotional talks—Did the patient talk about their health-care and spiritual values, express their code status/end of life wishes, or voice family abuse or issues?
- Preparation of patient's change of care—Did you complete an operating room (OR) checklist? Did you witness the consent of a procedure? Did you complete the transfer record form? If so, all these should be written in a brief progress note to acknowledge that they were completed or initiated.
- Other health-care professionals—Did the wound care nurse, palliative care specialist, or geriatric outreach team visit the patient? Did they make a note of their visit? Did the surgeon mention that your patient is planning to have his right leg x-rayed again, but the surgeon rushed off the unit before writing the order? It is good practice to verify if these professionals entered a progress note. If they did not, it is important to record their presence; however, your progress note is limited to what you were told by the physician. It is not your responsibility to chart on their actions.
- Patient's mood—Is the patient really happy today or notably shows improved health compared to past shifts? Alternatively, is the patient suddenly really quiet, distant, or depressed? What are the causes of the patient's mood change?

The progress notes can highlight important informed consent and CPR status changes. Sometimes, the narrative charting indicates that a patient has discussed an important care decision with the night shift registered nurse and is awaiting the physician or social worker to assist in the completion of the official paperwork such as CPR status or substitute decision-maker. At these times, documentation is integral to the entire interprofessional collaboration where the health-care team can efficiently and effectively work together to minimize duplication and repetition of the patient's care.

Another time, when progress notes are used, is any abnormalities in the patient's care. For example, when a patient refuses to take his regular dosing of morphine, it is important to document the patient's refusal, his rationale for the refusal, and what your intervention was, such as you tried to advise the importance or provided some patient education on the reasons to take his morphine medication, and, finally, you informed the patient to let you know if he changes his mind and would like his pill later. These notations are important as over time, they may reveal that the patient always refuses his 11 AM morphine dose, and the patient's physician should review this dosage. Although the nursing staff completes most of the documentation in the progress notes, the entire health-care team involved in this patient's care should review the patient's progress notes from the previous few days. Additionally, all health-care professionals document a summary of their assessments and recommendations within the progress notes. Physicians will highlight their quick assessment, query potential diagnoses and recommendations for ordering further medical tests or a referral to another specialty. An occupational therapist will highlight when he or she completes a swallowing assessment and his or her brief recommendations beyond the full consultation record (usually found in the very back or the very front of the patient's chart); other specialty consultants will similarly write notes. Progress notes are a central collaborative document that shares detailed assessments and interventions among the entire health-care team simultaneously working and communicating together.

Through the eyes of a student

As a student, I am always uncertain why a patient has been ordered a new antibiotic or diagnostic test. To find the answer, I review the doctor's order sheet of the new order and note the date of this order. Next, I search the progress notes for the specific order date and read the physician's narrative notes. There should be an explanation for the new order. This information enhances my understanding of my patient and the care that I am providing. Plus, it allows me to show critical thinking and stronger rationale for my nursing care plan assignments.

(personal reflection of a nursing student)

Charting Methods for Progress Notes

To write a progress note, there are three common charting methods that the agency may support in either charting with inclusion or charting with exclusion documentation approaches. The charting methods are narrative, focus, and SOAP.

Narrative Charting

Narrative charting is a paragraph written to highlight the patient's assessment findings, interventions completed, and patient outcomes in chronological order. Figure 23.4 provides a sample of narrative charting. The organization of the narrative paragraph includes the following:

1. Objective observations — typically head-to-toe assessments and then psychosocial assessments,
2. Subjective observations — thoughts or concerns on the objective findings including nursing diagnosis,
3. Intervention or action — actions taken, and
4. Outcomes — the patient's responses to the interventions.

Objective observations are written first to set the scene of the patient's current health state. These include diagnostic test records, such as electrocardiogram (ECG) monitoring strips, and patient's statements. When a diagnostic test is very small and cannot be easily three-holed punched into the patient's medical chart, it can be taped into the progress notes. For example, a patient's ECG monitoring strip. It is too small and narrow to stand alone in the patient's medical chart so it is documented into the progress note and taped in as objective data. Another excellent objective finding is derived from the patient's own words. The patients' statements best describe their perceptions and often help guide your assessment findings. "Use patient quotes to illustrate objective observations.

Correct

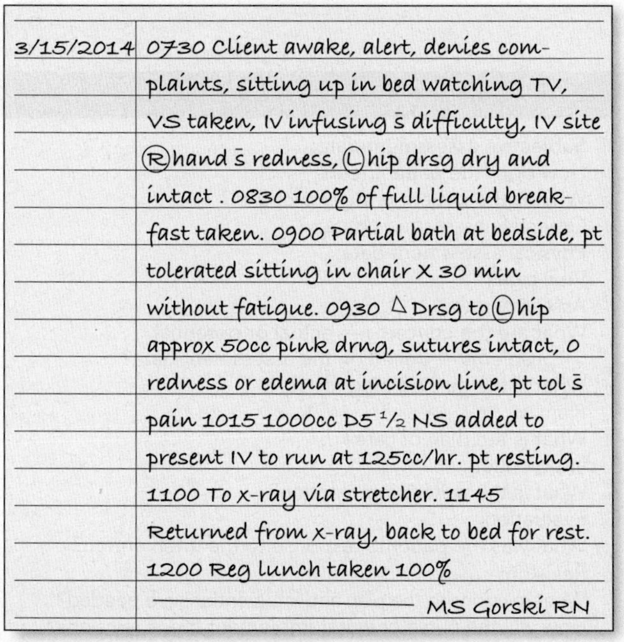

3/15/2014	0730 Client awake, alert, denies complaints, sitting up in bed watching TV, VS taken, IV infusing s̄ difficulty, IV site ®hand s̄ redness, Ⓛhip drsg dry and intact . 0830 100% of full liquid breakfast taken. 0900 Partial bath at bedside, pt tolerated sitting in chair X 30 min without fatigue. 0930 △ Drsg to Ⓛhip approx 50cc pink drng, sutures intact, 0 redness or edema at incision line, pt tol s̄ pain 1015 1000cc D5 ½ NS added to present IV to run at 125cc/hr. pt resting. 1100 To x-ray via stretcher. 1145 Returned from x-ray, back to bed for rest. 1200 Reg lunch taken 100% ———————————— MS Gorski RN

Figure 23.4 Example of narrative progress notes.

Avoid labeling patients or drawing subjective conclusions" (CRNBC, 2008, p. 2). Always quote your patient instead of paraphrasing because this demonstrates the ideal assessment data without your subjective labeling. For example, when a patient is describing her pain to be "burning hot like an iron," her quote is the best description of her pain. To accurately quote the patient's words write, "The patient states [fill in the quote here]." Avoid writing "the patient states" without accurately quoting her statement.

Additionally, any communication over the telephone needs to be documented in the progress notes. When speaking with a physician regarding a patient over the telephone, a registered nurse is expected to write out any new instructions on the doctor's order form. However, it is important that the nurse charts how she contacted the physician, what was the patient concern, paraphrase how the physician responded, and what the nurse's next actions will be. These steps would account for the full intervention. The patient outcomes can be charted during the intervention, but they should always be recorded at the end of the interventions when the patient's responses are fully known and assessed.

Think In the nursing station, Dr. Smith tells Collin, a fourth-year nursing student, that Mr. Alberto (Collin's patient) needs another x-ray to verify the pin placement in his tibia. Dr. Smith walks out of the nursing station. An hour later, Collin reviews Dr. Alberto's chart and notices that Dr. Smith did not write any notations in it. What should Collin do?

Focus Charting

Focus charting is a more simplified narrative charting approach. It is simplified by focusing on one specific problem per entry. So, if the patient had a bowel disimpaction prior to his dressing change and later had severe pain while ambulating, this period of time would be documented over three different focus chart entries. Focus charting requires the writer to specify the problem of the entry, such as constipation, wound care, and pain, along with the discipline documenting, such as nursing or MD. This charting method uses the organization of data, action, and response (DAR):

Data: objective and subjective findings in relation to the focus problem; this can include patient's mental or emotional status during the focus problem

Action: completed interventions

Response: the patient's physical and emotional reactions to the interventions

An example is shown in Figure 23.5.

SOAP or SOAPIER Charting

SOAP or SOAPIER is a problem-oriented documentation approach. It is quite similar to focused charting, but it requires greater written lines to fully complete the documentation. This charting method is organized as either SOAP or SOAPIER, depending on the agency's preference. Both styles are presented in their layout format for your comparison in Table 23.3

Date/Time	FOCUS	NOTE
2/13/06	Injection Instruction	**Data:** Referred to injection room for teaching re-injection technique as wife will be discharged and need IM injections of Compazine for nausea control. Husband states willingness to learn, yet states anxiety re-"sticking wife and causing her pain."
		Action: Demonstrate injection technique including drawing up medication in syringe, locating site, injecting medication, keeping record of medication administered. Have husband verbalize steps and then demonstrate technique.
		Response: Husband able to draw up medication correctly in syringe and verbalize steps to injection technique without cuing. Husband injected model, hands shook, and needed verbal cuing to aspirate.
		—J. Morales RN
2/14/06	Injection Instruction	**Response:** Husband demonstrated good technique giving wife injection, without cuing. Wife will be discharged in AM with visiting nurse follow-up. —J. Morales RN

Figure 23.5 Example of focus progress notes.

Each SOAP letter illustrates one documentation line for charting. This charting approach requires lots of progress note space and time to complete. Figure 23.6 gives a good example of SOAP charting where empty space is left after each charted sentence. It is wise to draw a line in any empty space so the next documenter does not accidentally write in your charted and signed entry.

Flow Sheets

Flow sheets are a typical documentation form. They are usually found inside a covered clipboard outside a patient's room or a binder on the medication cart. Because these forms are placed in a more public location, it is imperative that the clipboard or binder should be closed to cover the patient's data and maintain patient confidentiality. The flow sheet is a form that lists all routine or daily patient care. the**Point** displays detailed patient flow sheets from The Ottawa Hospital and the Vancouver Coastal Health Authority. When you compare the two different hospital flow sheets, you can see that nurses will check off or initial specific patient care completed and place an abbreviation for the assessment finding or standard intervention given, such as a patient's bathing method, urine output, and bowel movements. The flow sheet is the primary documentation form, whereas the narrative progress notes are supplementary. If there is no noted concern or problem in the flow sheet, then a progress note is not required. However, if there is a problem, such as low urinary output, the nurse should enter "see progress notes" on the flow sheet. The next step is to write a progress note focusing on the identified problem.

Specialized Flow Sheets

There are specialized flow sheets used for neurological, pain, wound care, and diabetic assessments. An example of a neurological vital signs record can be found on the**Point**. This

TABLE 23.3	SOAP Versus SOAPIER Format		
S	Subjective assessment data: How does the patient feel? What is the patient primary problem?	S	Subjective assessment data: How does the patient feel? What is the patient primary problem?
O	Objective assessment data: Physical assessment data, Vital signs	O	Objective assessment data: Physical assessment data, Vital signs
A	Assessment: What are the concerns — actual or potential problems — based on the assessment data? What is the nursing diagnosis?	A	Assessment: What are the concerns — actual or potential problems — based on the assessment data? What is the nursing diagnosis?
P	Plan: What interventions were acted upon? Does the plan require some revision? How has the plan of care changed?	P	Plan: What is the plan of care?
		I	Intervention: What is the writer's intervention?
		E	Evaluation: What was the patient's response to the intervention?
		R	Revision: What revisions to the plan and interventions are needed? How will the nurse or writer implement these revisions?

Correct

Problem	6/1/06	"S" My head hurts right in the back
#3	0900	of my eyes. Client describes pain
		worse bending over, like sinus
		headaches in past.
		"O" Eyes closed, lights dim, hesitant
		to move head when questioned.
		HR80 R20 P140/90 T98.6
		"A" HA probable 2° sinus pressure.
		"P" 1. Decongestant prn as ordered
		2. Warm wash cloth to eyes
		3. Monitor temp q 4°
		4. Assess pain after med and
		contact physician as
		indicated
		————————— MS Gorski RN

Figure 23.6 Example of SOAP progress notes.

neurological assessment form focuses on a patient's level of consciousness, Glasgow Coma Scale, and oxygen usage with any patient's brain injury or recent surgery. The Vancouver Coastal Health Authority interdisciplinary pain flow sheet, also found on thePoint, provides a thorough pain and sedation assessment. It is commonly completed when a patient is administered analgesics. The wound assessment and treatment flow sheet is another specialized form. This flow sheet guides the nurse to document the type of wound, its measurement, bed granulation, surrounding skin presence, and exudates description along with a small section to list the dressing treatment. Similar to the wound flow sheet, the incision and pin site assessment flow sheet requires the nurse to identify the type of wound (suture or staples), location of pins, exudate, and treatment plan provided. The last specialized flow sheet is the diabetic record, where the nurse can track the glucose level, medication administration, and insulin location site (listed based on the upper torso diagram). Examples of all of these specialized flow sheets can be found on thePoint. Although there are numerous flow sheets, each is used based on the patient's primary and secondary diagnoses. For example, a patient with diabetes who had brain tumor removal would have four different flow sheets: patient, neurological, diabetic, and wound care. These flow sheets will save the registered nurse time when documenting the progress notes while providing the ease in tracking the patient's improvement for a specific condition.

Checklists

Checklists are similar to flow sheets; however, they are specific for the patient's transition for a procedure, such as an operation, or a discharge from the hospital. These forms list all standard required items for the patient to be completed before he or she leaves the hospital unit. Look on thePoint for samples of a preoperative checklist and a discharge checklist from The Ottawa Hospital. What are the similarities and differences of these forms? How do they help guide the registered nurse through the process of transferring the patient off the hospital unit?

Both the preoperative and discharge forms specifically indicate items that the patient requires before he or she leaves the hospital unit. For example, recent blood work should be completed and included in the preoperative patient's medical chart, and all jewellery removed. Additionally, the patient should have all his or her discharge instructions, awareness of when to see his or her physician for a follow-up appointment, and any prescriptions given to him or her prior to discharge. This form guides the nurse on the steps to be completed before the patient may leave the unit. These checklists are nice because different nurses can collectively complete separate boxed items; this often occurs when the evening or night shift nurse has a quieter shift than the day shift nurse. Checklist items can be completed over a period of time and by different nurses as long as they are dated and initialed. When the checklist is completed and the patient is about to leave, nurses should record a notation in the progress notes about the checklist completion as well as the patient discharge by wheelchair (or taken to OR by a porter) as a final progress note before the patient leaves the unit.

Transfer Record

The **transfer record** is a communication form used between two or more health-care professionals to share patient health information from one health-care agency to another. Often, transfer forms are completed by the social worker or registered nurse from acute care hospital to inform the new health-care agency (e.g., a long-term care facility, community health service, palliative care unit, rehabilitation unit, or mental health hospital), who will be next providing the patient's care. The transfer record highlights the patient name, age, diagnosis, allergies, attending physicians' contact information, next of kin, medications, as well as pertinent medical problems and care interventions (go to thePoint to see an example). Additional documentation, such as progress notes, last 2 days of flow sheets, medication administration record, and doctor's orders, are frequently photocopied and attached to the transfer record as supplementary information.

Incident Reports

Incident reports are "administrative risk management tools to track trends and patterns about groups of clients over time" (CRNBC, 2007, p. 7). These reports are completed, for the administrative level only, for quality assurance reasons when a possible or actual error or physical harm has occurred to a patient, visitor, or staff member. Although the event and interventions are recorded in the patient's chart, if it is directly pertinent to the patient, the actual incident report is not part of the patient's health-care record. Incident reports are protected from legal court disclosure according to the British Columbia Laws, Evidence Act, Section 51 (1996). Thus, incident reports should never be referenced in the patient's progress notes because both are distinct forms and stored separately; this protects the incident report's quality assurance from malpractice lawsuits. If a nurse happens to document the incident report in the progress notes, then the incident report can be subpoena as evidence into legal court proceedings. According to the Evidence Act (British Columbia Laws, 1996), the patient and his or her family are not permitted to know about or receive a copy of the incident report.

For example, a medication was missed and thus was not given to the patient at the correct time or a patient experienced a skin tear when he fell out of bed. It is an objective assessment that a possible harm may have occurred to the patient. The patient's physician and the unit manager must sign the completed incident report in acknowledgement of the incident and any aftermath interventions and patient response outcomes. Next, the incident reports are compiled within the health-care organization. They are used statistically to report all incidents on each health-care unit and organization to the provincial and federal government to identify "quality improvement" concerns (CRNBC, 2008, p. 2). When an incident report must be completed, all important health-care professionals must be notified, such as the assigned registered nurse of the patient, the nurse in charge or unit manager, and the physician. When you have not completed an incident report in a long time or have never had to do so, it is good practice to review the form with another professional colleague or nurse in charge so you fully understand the form's sections. The form also requires the hospital and unit code number that identifies your location—ask your unit clerk or manager for it if you do not know it. Once the incident report is completed, ask someone to review it to verify that your statements are clear. If the incident involved a medication error, a photocopy of the medication administration record may be useful to highlight the error or the cause of the error. This photocopy should be attached to the incident report. Remember that the nurse still needs to document the actual patient event in the patient's progress notes. The incident report must neither replace nor be mentioned in the patient's progress notes.

Reflections

Reflections are a tool for individual professional improvement. For the purposes of this chapter, reflections involve thoughtful writing about a key patient care event, which engages the writer's greater critical thinking and emotional insights. All registered nurses and registered practical nurses are familiar with reflections of their professional practices. Student nurses are expected to complete clinical reflections to explore their growing health-care expertise. This is a very important

documentation technique outside of the health-care setting. Chapter 25, Reflection and Reflexivity: On Being a Nurse, will further discuss how a licensed nurse can explore his or her practice of care through reflections and how this documentation type promotes his or her best professional practices.

Collin, a fourth-year nursing student, has had a busy day caring for two patients on a medical oncology unit. He, finally, is able to chart his patient care of two patients, including one wound dressing changed of a gangrene right foot. He obtains the patients' charts and situates himself into a quiet meeting room beside the nursing station. While Collin is charting his wound dressing change, the unit clerk, Carole, hollers into the room, "Does anyone have patient charts 506 bed 2 and 505?" Collin realizes that the unit clerk wants the two charts that he is writing in. Carole comments, "I have been looking all over for these! Dr. Smith, the oncologist, is on the phone and I need the chart now!."

Documentation Etiquette

A student nurse often forgets that the patient's chart will be needed by other health-care professionals when he or she is focused on reviewing past documentation or writing his or her documentation in the chart. This is a simple oversight; however, it can cause significant inconvenience and annoyance for the unit clerk and physician as indicated in the earlier case scenario. It is important for all documenters to remember that the patient's chart is a communication tool shared with the entire health-care team. Many health-care professionals frequently review and document in a patient's chart (registered nurses, social worker, attending physicians, other consulting physicians, physiotherapist, occupational therapist, dietician, and pharmacist). Hence, there are four common documentation etiquette techniques appreciated in all health-care settings and students need to quickly learn them. They are the following:

1 Be considerate.
2 Communicate.
3 Replenish forms.
4 Keep the charts intact.

Each of the four documentation etiquette is described for greater clarity.

Be Considerate

The first etiquette technique is when another health-care professional needs the patient's chart, be considerate and hand over the patient's chart to others. This supports all health-care professionals, such as the unit clerk, physicians, registered nurses, and social workers, whom immediately require a patient's chart because they are often providing complex care interventions and consulting other health-care professionals. These health-care professionals will appreciate your consideration when you offer the chart to them. It is fair that you request for the chart back when they have finished with it.

Communicate

The second etiquette technique is when you take a chart to another room beyond the nursing station, it is recommended that you tell the unit clerk where the chart will be located and the length of time that it will be away from the unit station. Some hospital units have signs that can be placed in the chart's slot to communicate that the chart is out. If there is no such signage, create your own by placing a note on a blank piece of paper and then leave it in the chart's slot. This helps the unit clerk and others to more effectively find the chart instead of wasting time searching for it.

Replenish Forms

The third etiquette technique is regularly add additional documentation forms if they are getting low, their last or second last sheet, in the patient's chart. It is always helpful and appreciated when the patient's chart has enough documentation space for the next health-care professional to record his or her documentation. This is an easy, but extremely helpful, step to show your consideration and promote documentation efficiency for the entire interprofessional health-care team.

Keep the Charts Intact

The final etiquette technique is never remove individual documentation sheets from a patient's chart. It is so easy for one or two sheets of paper to go missing from a patient's chart. This frequently occurs when someone removes several single pages out of the chart. Over the past few years, hospitals are not permitting health-care professionals to remove any sheets from active patients' charts; thus, you have to maintain the entire chart as a whole. Several years ago, it was quite considerate to take the current progress notes out of a patient's chart to finish your documentation while another health-care professional used the same chart. However, individual sheets of the patient's chart have gone missing, which has caused significant stress to the student, unit clerk, and registered nurse because of the patient's chronological records are lost. The recent solution is no health-care professional may remove single pages from any patient's chart so less risk of legal errors in missing documentation may occur.

Strategies

Because students require additional time to collect their thoughts and write in a patient's chart, several documentation strategies are suggested. These strategies are available in Box 23.1. Since four documentation etiquette techniques and some strategies are established surrounding paper documentation, it is important to also explore the rules for electronic documentation.

BOX 23.1 Documentation Strategies for the Student

There are several strategies to help guide students through completing their novice documentation experiences:

- Always make a note of any important findings, during your assessment or when another health-care professional discusses the patient care with you, on a spare piece of paper. For example, vital signs will rarely be remembered an hour after taking them.
- Find a quiet spot to sit and write out your documentation.
- Give yourself time to write your documentation; do not wait until the end of the clinical shift because you will be rushed and flustered at this point.
- Complete personal care flow sheets right after you have completed the patient's care.
- Always write out a draft progress note on a rough piece of paper and have it edited by yourself as well as your professor or colleague for clarity, particularly if it is a notation about a complex patient or intervention. Once your progress note clearly describes the event and your actions, you can neatly chart it in the patients' chart.
- Keep the rough draft and rewrite it so you have a good example of a clear and concise progress note. However, remove the patients name from this draft due to confidentiality reasons.
- When you have a free moment, review other nurses' documentation. You will find some really poor and wonderfully skillful

documenters. Learn from the poor documentation—What are they not telling you? What questions do you have about their notation? What are you confused on? Borrow from the skillful documentation! What sentences make this documentation clear and concise? How does the writer clearly make the wound so visible? Jot down key sentences that you admire and practice them in your own draft progress notes. As you progress in your nursing career, you will gain your own documentation style.
- Document head to toe in your assessment or how the event chronologically started. This will allow you to focus one objective step at a time and organize your thoughts.
- Always directly quote the patients' or their family members' words if it best documents the assessment. This is far better than you paraphrasing or making presumptions of how they are doing. For example, patient states, "I am much better now that I have my pain medications."
- Never write the word *state* unless you are actually stating the person's actual words in verbatim and place them in quotations. Paraphrasing a patient's words is not exact; thus, they are not direct quotes.
- Always end your notation with how you intervened such as notified patient's assigned RN, or how the patient is responding since the intervention has been completed, such as patient resting comfortably in bed at present.

Electronic Documentation

Although documentation is becoming more technologically advanced, health-care settings have been slow to implement this type of electronic documentation into Canadian health-care professionals' regular practices. Electronic health records have been sluggish to fully evolve and interconnect between hospital and community health-care systems, a topic explored in more depth within Chapter 24. An **electronic health record** is "a collection of the personal health information of a single individual, entered or accepted by health care providers, and stored electronically, under strict security" (CRNBC, 2007, p. 14).

Technology is slowly advancing in Canadian health-care practices. In particular, how health-care professionals document will transform with greater technological advancement within the next 5 to 10 years. In the meantime, some electronic documentation, such as electronic health records, e-mails, and fax transmissions, has been effectively incorporated into health-care practices. These will be briefly reviewed to describe their integration into current nursing practices. It is important to note that early documentation principles are sustained regardless of paper or electronic documentation methods.

Guidelines for Electronic Health Records

Electronic health records are a digital repository of a patient's information about his or her health status and interactions within the health-care system. As electronic health records become implemented into practice, it is important that nurses frequently change their computer access passwords, select difficult to decipher passwords (e.g., capital and small letters, numbers and even symbols), avoid lending your computer identification or access to anyone, log off when not using the computer system, inform your supervisor if one suspects identification or computer access is stolen, and immediately retrieve any printed patient information. Because security is a significant consideration with computers, especially when it is portable as shown in Figure 23.7, most documentation into patient's electronic health record is deemed permanent and cannot be changed or deleted. If a nurse has made an error in their documentation, he or she must follow the agency policies to enter a correction entry into the patient's health record. However, agencies must provide policies to guide their users on how to handle electronic health records; for example, both the erroneous entry and the late entry correction will be permanently stored into the patient's electronic health record.

Agency Policies for Electronic Health Records

Agencies must provide policies to guide their users of how to handle electronic health records, provide printers securely away from the general public, and secure networks for data

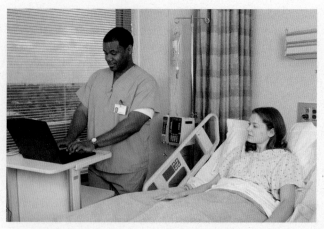

Figure 23.7 Use of a portable computer for documentation.

transmission between computer terminals. Agency policies should guide their users about the following:

- Entering late entries,
- Making corrections to documentation errors such as wrong patient entries,
- Averting the deletion of patient data,
- Identifying methods to highlight updates or changes to a patient's health record,
- Securing and backing up patient health information and new data, including preventive,
- Maintaining patient confidentiality,
- Recommending the frequency of the user password change,
- Processes to protect against system and electronic failures,
- Sustaining security of user passwords and system protection against virus and hackers (firewalls with encryption, and password usage), and
- Identifying the information technology support contact, including 24-hour, 7 days a week telephone and onsite support.

E-Mail

E-mails are considered an aspect of electronic documentation. E-mail has rapidly become an expedient and reliable way to share information within health-care agencies and between health-care professionals. Directors of nursing and unit managers commonly e-mail news and health-care changes to groups, such as nursing staff. This is an efficient method to pass messages about changing news in the agency regarding new directors, infection outbreaks, and modified polices or procedures. Nursing educators use e-mail to share local and regional educational workshops as well as conference information. For nursing staff working night shifts, when their working hours are opposite of the unit administration, e-mail has been helpful to communicate updates or concerns about the unit's function to the nursing manager or educator. Because there is no guarantee that your e-mail is completely secure, confidential, or encrypted, this is not a recommended method to communicate confidential patient health information. However, if e-mail is used to transfer patient health information, nurses must remember that these e-mails are considered equal to paper documentation. The e-mails can be printed and added to the patient's chart as a permanent record. Hence, e-mails could be called into legal court, and nurses need to remember that e-mail communication should maintain professionalism and confidentiality.

The CRNBC (2007) recommends the following eight e-mail confidentiality guidelines:

1. Attain written consent from the patient to transmit his or her health information via e-mail, including forwarding e-mails.
2. Confirm the recipient's e-mail address and check the correct spelling of the address before you click send.
3. Verify that the e-mail message is sent over a secure or encrypted network with user verification.
4. Verify or place a confidentiality warning at the top or bottom of the e-mail claiming, "Present information is confidential and only the intended recipient may read the message. This message may not be copied or forwarded to anyone else."
5. Prevent others from using your e-mail account.
6. Never allow another to use your password or user identification to access any computer.
7. Printers should be securely located away from public access.
8. Any printed information, including e-mails, must be obtained immediately after printing.
9. Nursing staff should advocate for confidential and secure computer systems. Many recommendations of the above e-mail confidentiality guidelines comply with the standard electronic health record guidelines. Since e-mail confidentiality guidelines have been established, patient health information and doctor's orders sent over faxed transmissions should be discussed.

Fax Transmissions

Occasionally, you may receive or be asked to send specific patient information to another health-care agency; for example, a consulting physician, dietician referral, or when updating the community health-care team pre-discharge. This often occurs in the community health setting, where health-care professionals work at community health offices afar and visit patients in their homes. These health-care professionals frequently need to verify the patient's prescription bottles to the faxed hospital discharge or transfer record. It is important that patient health information is transmitted in the most secure method because there is a high risk of accidentally breaching patient confidentiality. If a fax transmission is the method used to send the patient health information, you should always verify the fax number of the transmission recipient. You may have to telephone the recipient to clarify the fax number and if the fax is on. This protects patient' confidentiality and is far more time efficient, so you are not waiting for a delayed or rejected transmission. Next, the fax cover letter should be completed with the name of the recipient and the name of the sender along with written word "confidential" across the form. All patients' health information

are considered confidential between the patient, his or her designated substitute decision-maker, and the interprofessional health-care team in verbal, written, and electronic communication forms. So, the cover sheet should display confidential warnings such as "In the event of a misdirected fax, it will be confidentially and immediately destroyed without being read" (CRNBC, 2007, p. 15). Next, fax the document. If you are ever uncertain how to transmit a document to another health-care professional or agency, talk with your unit clerk or community health administrator assistant, who have great expertise dealing with confidential files. After you have faxed the document, you must always retrieve the transmission activity report to verify that the transmission was successful. If it was not and it was cancelled, resend the fax at a later time. Always keep the fax transmission in the patient's chart and document in the progress notes that you have sent a fax to the recipient. It is important to document this because your recipient may deny that he or she received anything from you. This provides evidence that you did fax the required documents. Also, it is good practice to call the recipient to verify that your fax was received.

When you receive a fax regarding a patient's health information, the faxed pages are considered original, not a duplicate or facsimile. Thus, you should date and time the receipt of the document, including your initials or signature. You may also write on this copy as long as your notation(s) comply with your agency documentation policies and the date, time, and signature are provided. CRNBC (2007) reminds us that faxed information sheets are deemed part of the patient's health record; thus, they can be called into legal court evidence. In the community, registered nurses frequently receive faxed doctor's orders. It is the nurse's responsibility to verify the accuracy of the physician's signature. If there is doubt, the nurse must substantiate if the order is authentic. He or she can telephone the physician's office and speak with the receptionist, whom could confirm the faxed document or directly contact the physician to verify. Never assume the faxed order is authentic, the nurse is the person implementing the order; therefore, the nurse is responsible for her assumptions. Although fax transmissions are occasionally used in practice, they are being slowly replaced with e-mail and other advanced technology along with electronic signatures.

SUMMARY

Effective documentation is essential to all health-care professional practice. It upholds the purposes of clear and concise communication to other health-care professionals regardless of the time of day; descriptively illustrates the ongoing function of assessment, intervention, and patient outcomes; and sustains legal and professional practice standards of care. Regardless of what setting you work within and what skills you have performed, you are expected to document in either charting by inclusion or charting by exclusion approach based on the agency's policies. As a novice documenter, such as the case studies featuring nursing students Jane and Collin, you will be challenged to organize periods of time to chronologically document in a timely manner, gain experience completing various forms, and become more proficient in your descriptive assessments with multiple patients' progress notes. Although documentation is an ongoing professional skill, it is also a special art of nursing. With every new documentation entry, nursing students enhance their confidence as an effective documenter and an efficient interprofessional communicator.

ACKNOWLEDGEMENTS

This chapter acknowledges The Ottawa Hospital and the Vancouver Coastal Health Authority for their contributions and permissions to reprint their currently established clinical documentation forms as samples for this chapter. Their collaboration is greatly appreciated.

Critical Thinking Case Scenarios

▶ Susan, a second-year nursing student, sat down to complete her narrative documentation. When she reviewed the earlier documentation in her patient's chart, she realizes that her assigned registered nurse has already charted the foley catheter insertion and dressing change that Susan had completed. Susan is upset and not sure what to document now. What should Susan do? Should she still record her assessment and actions for her patient's dressing change and bladder distension?

▶ Chris, a fourth-year nursing student, realized that he recorded in Patient Smith's flow sheet instead of Patient Smyth's. He has fully completed the flow sheet with black ink pen. He is not sure what to do so he asks his classmate, Allison, for advice. What advice should Allison give Chris regarding this documentation error?

▶ Bev, the clinical professor, walks up to one of her students, Susan, who is documenting on the patient's flow sheet. Bev is surprised to see Susan using a bright, glitter, pink gel pen. The flow sheet documentation is bright pink and colourful! What should Bev say to Susan?

▶ John's patient, Mrs. Weightman, a 65-year-old, had a right total knee replacement 3 days ago. At 7 PM, Mrs. Weightman complains of severe pain (6/10) to her right knee. John, RN, offers her prn pain medication but she refuses. Mrs. Weightman states, "I am fine if I don't move." What should John do?

Multiple-Choice Questions

1. The wound care consultant, Sarah, wants an update on Mr. Rioux's leg wound. She has asked Shane, the home care nurse, to fax his flow sheets, progress notes, and wound care plan to her. How should Shane fax Mr. Rioux's information?
   a. Shane photocopies all Mr. Rioux's wound care documentation for the past week and then faxes them to wound consultant fax number listed on the distribution list before he leaves the office to see another patient.
   b. Shane calls Sarah and verifies her fax number. Then, he completes a cover sheet where confidentiality is clearly written. He faxes Mr. Rioux's wound assessment sheet and progress notes. While he waits for the fax activity record to verify full transmission of the fax, he makes a note in Mr. Rioux's chart that he has faxed information to the wound consultant.
   c. Shane tells Sarah that he cannot fax any information because of patient confidentiality.
   d. Shane photocopies all Mr. Rioux's wound care documentation for the past week and he completes a fax cover sheet. He faxes the document to wound consultant fax number listed on the distribution list. The fax activity report shows the transmission failed so Shane leaves the entire fax document on his desk to refax later.

2. Becky's patient had three large bowel movements this morning. Where should she chart this information?
   a. She should record it in the patient's progress notes.
   b. She should not document it.
   c. She should put × 3 on the daily flow sheet in the bowel movement column.
   d. She should record it in the kardex.

3. Mrs. Sam refuses the suppository offered by registered nurse, Austin. She tells Austin that she has a large bowel movement last evening so, "My bowels are just fine, thank you!" This is not recorded anywhere in the patient's chart, what should Austin do?
   a. Austin should trust Mrs. Sam's statement. She may have had a bowel movement without the evening nursing staff being aware. But, he should document this assessment and intervention in the patient's progress notes.
   b. Austin should give Mrs. Sam the suppository to make sure that she has a bowel movement.
   c. Austin should confront Mrs. Sam that none of the nurses recorded any bowel movement yesterday.
   d. Austin should contact the physician to verify if he should give Mrs. Sam the suppository.

4. Brianna is a new staff member at the Winnipeg General Hospital. A senior staff member tells Brianna that she does not have to chart everything on her patient because "this hospital charts by exclusion." How can Brianna verify how she should chart in this new workplace?
   a. Brianna should check the agency policies for documentation guidelines.
   b. Brianna should continue her charting manner as she is responsible for her own documentation and no one else's.
   c. Brianna should follow the staff member's advice and begin charting by exception.
   d. Brianna should ask another colleague or the nursing educator on the unit.

5. When is it appropriate to let another health-care professional document on your behalf?
   a. When both the colleague and you were present for the intervention—You both saw the same thing!
   b. Anytime, the more someone else does, the less you have to do!

c. You should always complete your documentation on your own patients—It is your responsibility to care and document on your patients!

d. When your patient is having an emergency such as stopped breathing, the rapid response team or emergency team will instruct the ICU nurse to become the recorder—You are just following instructions!

Suggested Lab Activities

Here are a few suggested lab activities to enhance your documentation practice:

● Describe your dinner last night, including the food items, placement from each other, and amount.

● Find a classmate who has a cut, sore, or wound. Assess his wound and document its size, shape, depth, colour, odor, and any drainage. Once you have completed your documentation, swamp charting notes and compare each other's narrative of the wound. Whose documentation descriptively matches the wound?

● Write a progress note (narrative format) about your lab professor's appearance and behaviours. Then, review your progress note with a classmate. Whose note is most visibly descriptive? What words best describe your professor?

● After each psychomotor lab, practice your documentation of your nursing skill.

REFERENCES AND SUGGESTED READINGS

Ares v. Venner, [1970] S.C.R. 608. Id. (vLex No.: VLEX-37662931). Retrieved from http://ca.vlex.com/vid/ares-v-venner-37662931

British Columbia Laws. (1996). *Chapter 124: Evidence act. RSBC 1996* (Sect. 51). Retrieved from http://www.bclaws.ca/Recon /document/freeside/—%20E%20—/Evidence%20Act%20%20 RSBC%201996%20%20c.%20124/00_96124_01.xml

Chart smart: The A-to-Z guide to better nursing documentation (2nd ed.). (2007). Philadelphia, PA: Lippincott Williams & Wilkins.

College of Nurses of Ontario. (2002). *Nursing documentation standards*. Toronto, ON: Author.

College of Nurses of Ontario. (2009). *Practice standard: Documentation, revised 2008* (Pub. No. 41001). Retrieved from http://www .cno.org/docs/prac/41001_documentation.pdf

College of Registered Nurses of British Columbia. (2007). *Practice standard for registered nurses and nurse practitioners: Nursing documentation*. Retrieved from http://www.crnbc.ca/downloads /334.pdf

College of Registered Nurses of British Columbia. (2008). *Professional standards for registered nurses and nurse practitioners* (Rev. ed.) Retrieved from http://www.crnbc.ca/downloads/128.pdf

Henneman, E. A. (2009). Patient safety and technology. *AACN Advanced Critical Care, 20*(2), 128–132.

Lippincott manual of nursing practice series: Documentation. (2007). Philadelphia, PA: Lippincott Williams & Wilkins.

Nursing know-how: Charting patient care. (2009). Philadelphia, PA: Lippincott Williams & Wilkins.

Service Ontario Publications. (1993). *Nursing Act, 1991: Ontario regulation 799/93— Professional misconduct.* Retrieved from http:// www.e-laws.gov.on.ca/html/regs/english/elaws_regs_930799 _e.htm

Informatics, E-Technologies, and Nursing

NOREEN CAVAN FRISCH AND
ELIZABETH BORYCKI

As a nursing student living in an age of information and technology, Amy uses various technologies to retrieve information throughout her day. Sometimes, she uses the information to change her activities because she makes judgments about the information she has and thinks about how it will impact her. As a student entering the health-care workforce, she finds her technology use expands for professional reasons. The information she obtains, considers, and records for other professionals will impact her patients. In this chapter, we will follow some of Amy's technology usage as we present information on health-care technologies. We begin by finding Amy early in the morning (7 AM) checking her daily schedule on her computer. Her calendar tells her that she has class at 9 AM, a session in her nursing arts lab at 1 PM, followed by an assignment to go to the long-term care facility, and perform an assessment interview on the patient she will care for tomorrow. At her computer, she also finds an e-mail from her adviser telling her that their 11:30 AM meeting will be cancelled today and that they need to reschedule for tomorrow. Getting in her car to drive to school, she learns from the traffic report that the freeway entrance she normally takes has had an accident so she reroutes her journey to another road. Before she even begins her school day, she's used her home computer to plan her day, her e-mail to check her appointments, and information from the traffic report to drive efficiently so she can get to school on time. We'll check in with Amy throughout this chapter as we think about technology and information in our lives.

CHAPTER OBJECTIVES

By the end of this chapter, you will be able to:

1. Describe the meaning of nursing informatics and the informatics revolution impacting all of nursing practice.
2. Identify how nurses make use of computers for professional purposes.
3. Describe a number of high-tech tools used by nurses to enhance nursing practice.
4. Explain the meaning of EHRs, EMRs, and PHRs and nurses' use of standardized languages to enter nursing data into digital formats.
5. Critically evaluate the controversy in nursing related to use of digital versus narrative documentation.
6. Identify the nursing informatics competencies needed for beginning, intermediate, and advanced practice in informatics.
7. Develop a personal plan for responsible inclusion of informatics and e-health technology into one's own professional practice.

KEY TERMS

Canadian-Health Outcomes for Better Information and Care (C-HOBIC) A major project in Canada to collect data on nurse-sensitive or nurse-related outcomes and use these data to inform patient care.

Canadian Nurses Informatics Association (CNIA) A national organization of nurses that serves to help nurses learn, share, research, and create informatics-related projects and experiences that can help to boost the competencies, theory, and practice of informatics on a national level.

Classification Schemes An assignment of objects into groups based on characteristics that they have in common.

Computer Science The field of expertise that develops computer systems permitting transmission, recording, and retrieval of data.

Data Sets Clusters of core data, used on a regular basis by most professionals in a discipline while delivering patient care.

Electronic Health Record (EHR) A digital repository of individuals' information about their lifetime health statuses and their interactions with the health-care system.

Electronic Medical Record (EMR) Digital health record that can be found in a private practitioner's office or in a clinic.

Electronic Patient Record (EPR)   A digital record used by health professionals involved in a patient's care in a health-care organization (e.g., a hospital or long-term care facility).

Health Informatics   Use of information technology to support the creation and use of health-related data, information, and technology.

Information Literacy   The ability to know when information is needed, being able to find it, and, ultimately, being able to use that information effectively.

International Classification of Nursing Practice (ICNP)   A comprehensive vocabulary for nursing that permits computerized documentation of all aspects of nursing judgments, activities, and outcomes.

NANDA-International   A nursing organization that develops, reviews, and publishes a list of nursing diagnostic labels organized into a hierarchy of domains, classes, and diagnoses.

Nursing Informatics   The confluence of nursing, clinical, information, and management sciences in the development, design, implementation, and evaluation of computer software, hardware, and health-care devices as they are used to support patients and nurses in the hospital, home, and community within the context of nursing and

where nursing science and nursing theory come together with health informatics.

Nursing Informatics Specialist   One who integrates the nursing, clinical, information, and management sciences in the development, design, implementation, and evaluation of computer software, hardware and medical devices as they are used, to support patients and nurses in the hospital, home, and community within the context of nursing practice.

Nursing Interventions Classification (NIC)   A comprehensive list of activities regarded as within the scope and domain of nursing practice.

Nursing Outcomes Classification (NOC)   A comprehensive list of nurse-sensitive outcomes.

Systematized Nomenclature of Medicine Clinical Terms   A clinical terminology that is used in health care for building electronic records.

Taxonomies   Restricted sets of phrases, generally numerated and arranged into a hierarchy.

Translational Vocabularies   Systems that permit data interchange from one vocabulary to another by providing the ability for data entered into a record in one system to be "mapped" or "linked" to data entered through another system.

What Is Nursing Informatics?

Historically, **nursing informatics** described the confluence of disciplinary work where nursing science and theory came together with **computer science**. This definition of nursing informatics was based on the definitions of nursing science and nursing theory (described elsewhere in this text) that refer to the disciplinary knowledge of nursing (science) and the ways in which nurses come to understand and interpret that knowledge (theory). Nursing certainly holds a body of knowledge about health, wellness, illness and recovery, health-care delivery, and nursing activities supportive to patient needs and wants. Nursing theories give us a means to reflect on the situations in which we find ourselves and our patients, providing direction and guidance to us when we need to select a course of action. In contrast, computer science can be thought of as a study of computing systems and computation and defined as the science that developed computer systems permitting transmission, recording, and retrieval of data. The focus of computer science theory has been on understanding computing systems and methods (i.e., methods of computer design, the underlying mathematical algorithms that allow for the processing of information, the development of tools and the methods for testing computation). **Health informatics** has its origins in the field of computer science (Shortliffe & Cimino, 2006).

Over the past few decades in both Canada and globally, we have seen the emergence and development of health informatics as a discipline. Health informatics uses information technology to create and support the use of health related data, information and technology. Health Informatics brings various disciplines together to promote "effective organization, analysis, management, and use

of information in health care in order to facilitate optimal health care delivery" (Travers & Mandelkehr, 2008, p. 127). In this definition, nursing informatics can be considered a subfield of health informatics that draws on and contributes to nursing science and health informatics (Kushniruk, 2011). Therefore, a more modern and contemporary definition of nursing informatics that is reflective of this change in Canada and internationally has emerged. In Canada, nursing informatics is the integration of the nursing, clinical, information, computer, and management sciences in the development, design, implementation, and evaluation of computer software, hardware, and health-care devices as they are used to support patients, nurses, and health-care organizations in the hospital, home, and community settings.

We've all been told that knowledge is doubling at a rapid pace; in fact, Naisbitt reported in his book *Megatrends* that by 2020, knowledge will double every 73 days (Naisbitt, 1991). It is clear that no one can keep up with such vast amounts of new knowledge being reported. In nursing particularly, new evidence is being accumulated every day, and some of this information may be relevant to your work tomorrow. Nursing informatics knowledge is also growing at a rapid pace as the number of nurses who are practicing and conducting research in this field continues to grow. Nurses who work in the field of nursing informatics support the ability to access information because large sets of information are collected in ways that (through the use of computers) you can search, find, sort, and select that information pertinent to your use. In the modern health-care world, it is impossible to imagine a future where nursing informatics competencies will not be required for effective professional practice; yet, we are still at the beginnings of an informatics revolution in our discipline, and we are on the cusp of a new world of nursing. To begin our exploration of this world, we start with background about the development of these fields.

Background: Development of the Fields of Health Care and Nursing Informatics

As early as the 1970s, practitioners who were early adopters of new technologies began to apply the techniques of computer science to health-care practices. Some primary care providers began exploring the use of computers for documentation of patient visits. Some nurses began using computer-generated self-care instructions to give patients information about home management of health conditions. Some hospitals began using technologies to track inventories of medications and equipment on their shelves. Some researchers began developing and testing the first computer-based patient records to be used in hospital settings (Shortliffe & Cimino, 2006). Even though this work was innovative, we find that today health care is behind other fields (industries) in technological and information use. Consider the question in Box 24.1.

What happened that put health care behind banking and other fields in technology use? First, health care is a complicated endeavor. Each patient is unique with his or her own specific health-care issues. Patients may experience disease differently (Shortell & Kaluzny, 2006), and the process of providing health care involves several disciplines, many locations where care is provided (e.g., hospital, home) as well as the involvement of many governmental agencies and services (e.g., federal and provincial governments, regional health authorities). Further, patient information is not only confidential but also very private. The field of health care may have more challenges in creating systems and adapting to change than any other profession. Given the difficulties, the progress that has been made is remarkable.

Nursing Participation in Development Informatics

Nurses have been active in the development of health information systems, but sometimes, their contributions are unknown to many in our discipline. As early as the 1970s, nurses began to explore potential uses of computers and information systems in several ways. In 1974, at the first meeting of the International Medical Informatics Conference (MedInfo) in Stockholm, Sweden, there were five nurses who presented papers. These nurses from Europe and North America discussed topics, such as how to display data in an intensive care unit (ICU), the impact of computers on nurses, the design of nursing protocols for a hospital information system, and issues related to drug administration (Saba, 2001). In 1972, nurses from the United States and Canada met to begin the development of a language system of nursing terms—the initial work that later became the taxonomy of nursing diagnoses completed by the North American Nursing Diagnosis Association (NANDA). The organization's name *North American* was in recognition of the Canadian involvement. (The organization has since renamed itself to **NANDA-International** to recognize the worldwide uptake and participation in its work.) Among other Canadian nurses, Winnifred C. Mills of the Registered Nurse Association of Alberta was active in the initial work and served on the first ever diagnostic review committee for nursing terms. Two nursing authors and pioneers in this field, Maureen Scholes and Barry Barber, were the first to use the term *nursing informatics* in 1980 (Scholes & Barber, 1980). That same year marked the establishment of the first nursing journal in the specialty *Computers in Nursing (CIN)*. Around the same time, the International Medical Informatics Association (IMIA) formally established a nursing working group. This nursing informatics group held its first international open forum in 1982 and has held such forums every 3 years, including one held in Montréal in 2012. In 1989, the International Council of Nurses (ICN) began its work to develop a unified language system for nursing, the **International Classification of Nursing Practice (ICNP)**. To serve as the voice of Canadian nurses in the field, the **Canadian Nurses Informatics Association (CNIA)** was established in 2000, and the *Canadian Journal of Nursing Informatics* was launched in 2005. Canadian nurses have worked with their counterparts around the world to contribute to the advancement of health care using computers and technologies for the betterment of patient and patient care, and together, nurses from around the globe have developed competency standards for practice in our changing world.

BOX 24.1   Technology in Your Life

Consider your use of technology in daily life and work:
Do you
- Use a debit card to buy groceries at the store?
- Pay your bills online?
- Use a computer to schedule an appointment for your car to get an oil change?
- Look at bank statements and your accounts over your computer?
- Get text messages from your cell phone carrier?
- Buy an airline ticket through a computer-based service?
- Call your friends on Skype?
- Retrieve your own health laboratory data via computer?
- Read your health record on your computer?
- Make an appointment with your health-care provider over your computer?
- Receive e-mails from your health-care provider?

If you are like most Canadians, you will have used computers for business, banking, and communication more often and more frequently than you have for your own personal health care. Do you know why? Try to list the barriers to computerized access to health information as opposed to banking information. Discuss with your classmates.

Current Essential Standards

Nursing informatics specialists and educators have projected the knowledge, competencies, and skills needed for modern practice. These can be thought about at the basic level (that which every nurse needs) and the specialist level (those a nursing informatics specialist–prepared at a master level needs; Gugerty & Sensmeier, 2010; Staggers, Gassert, & Curran, 2001). The Canadian Nurses Association (CNA) offers students and practicing nurses the opportunity to develop basic or core nursing informatics competencies. Nursing students can log on to the NurseOne portal and can complete the Health Informatics Training System (HITS) online course. Originally developed in Ireland, the course was customized for the Canadian context and is currently delivered over the World Wide Web (WWW or Web). Through this certification program, nurses can develop basic competencies in health and nursing informatics. Upon completion of the program, nurses will have developed basic knowledge in three core areas of health informatics: IT use in health care, information management in health care, and IT systems use in health care (Canadian Nurses Association [CNA], 2010). As a starting point for the example of the beginning nurse outlined in Box 24.2, you can read an overview of the basic competencies that are covered by the course.

Around the world, nurses are recognizing and working toward the development of basic nursing informatics competencies and their integration into undergraduate nursing programs (Gugerty & Sensmeier, 2010; Staggers et al., 2001). Nurses are working together to identify existing (e.g., ability to use an electronic patient record) and emerging basic nursing informatics competencies (e.g., the use of mobile phones in clinical settings) that a nursing student will need into the future. Nursing informatics competencies will be among the many skill sets that nursing students will need to develop in order to effectively obtain and use information from differing electronic sources to be used for their decision-making involving patients, families, and health-care systems (Gugerty & Sensmeier, 2010; Staggers et al., 2001).

According to the CNA e-health strategies plan, future nurses will be able to

- integrate information and communication technologies (ICTs) into their practice to achieve positive patient outcomes,
- identify the required information and knowledge they need to support their practice,
- better plan to address nursing human resource needs,
- develop new models of nursing practice and health services delivery that will be supported,
- connect nurses to develop patient care solutions,
- improve the quality of nurses' work environments using ICTs, and
- contribute to the global nursing community (CNA, 2006).

In order to meet these competencies, you will need to be able to use certain technological and intellectual tools. Technological tools include computer software (e.g., electronic health records), hardware (e.g., desktop computers, laptop computers, or mobile phones), and medical devices (e.g., intravenous pumps, ventilators) that are used in providing patient care and communicating with other health professionals. The section that follows describes the technological tools you'll need to be able to use in order to meet these competencies.

Technological Tools Required to Meet Informatics Competencies

Nurses need to use computers in several ways along with other devices and systems that support our work. Although the following list is not exhaustive, the discussion gives you an idea of the technologies and tools you will become acquainted with as you progress through nursing education.

Use of Computer Software and Hardware

You probably already use a computer in many aspects of your life. You may use computer hardware such as a desktop computer or a laptop to complete your assignments, a tablet computer (e.g., an iPad or a Kindle) to read a book or journal article in preparation for a class, or a mobile smartphone (e.g., iPhone, Blackberry) to contact friends or family or to check your e-mail. You may even use a smartphone application to self-manage your diet or

---

BOX 24.2 Nursing Informatics Competences

Core Areas
- Basic competency areas

The Basics of Information Technology in Health Care
- Computer hardware
- Computer software
- Networks and health informatics

The Basics of Information Management in Health Care
- Data, information, and knowledge
- Information security, privacy, and confidentiality (i.e., protecting information)

The Basics of Information Technology Systems in Health Care
- Information systems
- Clinical, decision support, and administrative

Source: *Health Informatics Training System (HITS). A training program available through the Healthcare Information Management Systems Society (HIMSS).* Retrieved from http://www.himss.org/Index.asp

your exercise schedule. Some people have discontinued traditional telephones in favour of a mobile phone to be reachable by friends and family anytime and anywhere and have access to the Internet.

Each of these types of hardware has software that can help you organize your life, communicate with others, and carry out activities at school, at home, or at work. You may have used a computer to search the Internet to find the university or college that you now attend, and likely, you did a comparison of your school against some other schools before you decided where to apply. Finding your school of nursing may have been your first professional use of a computer. In the following texts, we'll describe some others.

Finding Nursing Knowledge

As a nursing student, you need to find nursing knowledge and professional information to support your learning. As a nurse, you need to find information to support your practice decisions and to keep your knowledge current and up-to-date in the field of nursing. This means that you need to find nursing knowledge that is professional, scholarly, and current. Professional nursing literature is organized in two ways: There is published literature found in books, professional nursing journals, and trade magazines; and there are published reports, discussion papers, and data from nursing and health-care agencies. You will find printed books in the campus bookstore or the library of the college or university where you are currently studying nursing. Electronic books are found in university libraries as well as on the Internet, book stores, and public libraries. The books and journal articles you find through the library at your college or university or in the library of your regional health authority have been selected by faculty and librarians as valuable sources of information for you. Articles in professional publications are retrievable from professional indexes found in your college or university library through search engines similar to using Internet browsers. These indexes for nursing are the Cumulative Index for Nursing and Allied Health Literature (CINAHL) and MEDLINE. As their titles suggest, CINAHL contains the titles, abstracts, and some of the full texts of nursing articles and those of other health disciplines such as physical and occupational therapy. MEDLINE is a database that has references to journal articles from the life and biomedical sciences and informatics (MEDLINE, 2010). MEDLINE also includes many nursing periodicals, so there is some overlap between these two sources of information. CINAHL is your best first source for nursing information along with the texts recommended to you by your faculty. As a new student, your faculty or your school librarians will give you an introduction to how to search for information online so that you can get access to the materials in these indexes. Do pay attention to these beginning sessions because access to information through these systems will be your key to the knowledge you need for school and beyond.

Amy, our student planning to complete a health assessment of her patient this afternoon, has 30 minutes after class today to go to the library and look up some information that might be helpful. She knows that her patient is an 87-year-old man who has hypertension and diabetes. She wants to find information on the relationship between these two conditions, so she goes to a computer to perform a CINAHL search on the topics. She finds that once she entered the two conditions as search terms, she retrieved a list of 7,172 articles. Knowing that this is way too many, she remembered she had to use the advanced search function to limit her search to something more focused and manageable. So, she entered the advanced search function and used key terms of *diabetes-type 2*, *hypertension*, and *elderly males*, limited the search for the past 5 years and for review articles in core nursing journals. Then, she found only one article related to home monitoring of BP in elderly patients. So Amy went from way too many to not enough to learn from her search. She tried again and searched for the same key terms, but this time in all nursing journals retrieving any journal article. This time, she found a list of 25 articles on topics such as epidemiology of the conditions, diet and risk factors, relationship to obesity, and case management ideas. She then began to read the abstracts online to determine if she wanted to retrieve any of the full articles. Amy's trial-and-error approach helped to make her a more savvy user of CINAHL as one of her new professional tools.

The articles, reports, position statements, and other professional information that are published through an organization may be more difficult for you to find. This body of information is sometimes called *gray literature* because it is not always found in the indexes cited earlier. It will most likely be found online on reliable and valid professional websites offering downloading (e.g., the CNA website has position papers about nursing informatics in Canada). You may be able to find this literature through Internet searches using key words, topics of interest, or through the organization's web page. This body of gray literature may be harder to find than journal articles indexed in CINAHL, and it may also be more difficult to evaluate the accuracy or currency of some of the information. However, if you are searching a web page from a trusted nursing organization, the information should be credible.

To test your ability to find, use your computer to find information about nursing; try the learning activity in Box 24.3. Upon completion of the activity, you will have accomplished the first competency for nursing informatics—the ability to find and retrieve professional nursing knowledge.

In searching for and finding nursing information, you are developing your **information literacy** skills. *Information Literacy* is the term used to describe the ability to know when information is needed, being able to find it, and ultimately being able to effectively use that information. As a nurse, you will be building your information literacy skills

BOX 24.3 Finding Nursing Knowledge

Once you have been oriented to your library system, try out your information literacy skills by doing the following:

1. Select a topic of personal interest (e.g., palliative care) and complete a search on CINAHL for the topic. Then, limit the search to only articles published over the past 5 years and then limit to research articles only. What did you find? (you may also limit to a particular age group of patients as well). Then, complete the same search using MEDLINE. What differences are there between these two search tools?
2. Enter another topic of interest (e.g., HL7) into a major Internet search engine.

What did you find? How would you know if the source was professional, credible, and believable? Discuss this with your faculty and classmates. Begin now to develop abilities to evaluate the usefulness of information retrieved from the Internet.

---

throughout your career. One of the first steps in becoming information literate is knowing what is correct, reliable, and ready to bring into your practice.

Some of the gray literature you find on the Internet may be incorrect or may be misleading (Agency for Healthcare Research and Quality, 1997; Stvilia, Twidale, Smith, & Gasser, 2008). For example, concerns have arisen about the quality, accuracy, and correctness of information found in online resources such as Wikipedia (Agency for Healthcare Research and Quality, 1997; Giles, 2005). The quality of health information on the Internet is considered to be a public health concern as patients may use incorrect or inaccurate information to inform their health-related decision-making. In your role as a nurse, you may at some point teach your patients how to evaluate the quality of the information they find on the Internet. In the past, several tools and rating scales were developed by researchers to help health professionals educate patients about how to identify websites that provide high quality and accurate health information (Eysenbach & Köhler, 2002; Eysenbach, Powell, Kuss, & Sa, 2002; Gagliardi & Jadad, 2002). Upon evaluation, however, very few of these tools could be assessed objectively (Bernstam, Shelton, Walji, & Meric-Bernstam, 2005). When patients and their families ask you to help them understand information they have found on the Internet or direct them to credible and accurate health information resources, your best response may be to consider the source (a governmental or respected health-care agency) and see if the information comes with cited references. Understanding where patients obtain their information, how they use this information, and how you can help them identify credible sources of health information is a role you may have as a nurse.

Finding Patient Care Information

Just as you need to find accurate nursing knowledge, you also need information about your assigned patients. You need to have some information in advance of providing care because

you need to know the current state of the individual's health, the treatments being provided, and the possible risks and projected outcomes of the treatment plan.

Prior to the informatics revolution, all of the patient data we had was written down in a narrative on paper in the form of a patient record or chart (Shortliffe & Cimino, 2006). These records were kept in many institutions, such as hospitals, clinics and doctor's offices, public health agencies, home care agencies, extended-care facilities, and any other agencies providing patient care. Most patients had differing parts of their paper patient records stored in multiple places. Usually, there was no one place where all of the patient's data would be stored. All of this is currently in the process of changing with the establishment and use of the electronic health records or EHRs.

Electronic Health Records

An **electronic health record (EHR)** is a digital repository of a patient's information about his or her lifetime health status and interactions with the health-care system. A patient's information is stored in an EHR in such a way that health professionals who are involved in the patient's health care can use the record to obtain information to support their patient care decisions and activities (Nagle, 2007). Although definitions of the EHR vary, there is agreement that an EHR is a comprehensive digital record of a patient's health-care information and encounters with the health-care system, available in real time, accessible by care providers, and used for the purpose of making health decisions and providing health care. Some authors make a distinction among the EHR, the **electronic medical record (EMR)**, and the **electronic patient record (EPR)** (Nagle, 2007; Thede & Sewell, 2010). When distinctions are made, the EMR refers to the digital record that can be found in a private practitioner's office or in a clinic. In contrast, the EPR is an electronic or digital record that is used by health professionals involved in a patient's care in a health-care organization, such as a hospital or long-term care facility. Unlike the EMR and the EPR, the EHR is a transportable, longitudinal set of data that is used by health-care organizations, physician practices or clinics, and other providers such as nurses. The EHR incorporates only selected information from an individual's interactions with the health-care system over the course of a patient's lifetime. Data contained in an EHR may include laboratory values, digital imaging, pharmaceutical information, transcribed reports, and clinical documentation elements. Data are entered into the EHR according to certain international data standards that permit the data to be coded so that they are machine retrievable as well as being readable by people (Thede & Sewell, 2010). See Table 24.1 for a comparison of these terms.

Given all of the data in an EHR, it quickly becomes a complex record. Figure 24.1 presents a visual picture of the concepts and elements of an EHR. As seen in the figure, information from various units providing care (e.g., nursing, radiology, laboratory) are all collected at the unit level and

TABLE 24.1	Similar Words, Different Meanings: Electronic Health Records, Electronic Medical Records, and Electronic Patient Records		
Term	Electronic Health Record	Electronic Medical Record	Electronic Patient Record
Content	Digital information about an individual's lifetime health status and interaction with the health system	Digital record that records a patient's interactions with a clinic or office providing direct care	Digital record at a health-care organization used by health professionals involved with patient's care at that organization
Accessibility	Individual determines who has access to the EHR and which parts of the record are readable by whom	Health-care providers offering services to the patient at the office or clinic	Health-care professionals working at the institution who have need to know the information in order to provide care

then put together through a computer network so that there is a comprehensive documentation of everything that happened with or for the patient in one place. Advantages to using an EHR include the fact that data can be used to evaluate a patient's condition over time and can also be used to pool data from several patients to evaluate how well a practice, unit, regional health authority, or province is reaching its patient care goals. Ideally, data entered into an EHR can be tagged for simultaneous entry into an EMR, reducing the need for repetitive entry of data in differing forms for different purposes. At the same time, electronic coding provides for sharing of data by multiple care providers (e.g., the history and physical, a consult, a nursing assessment, or a social worker's discharge plan).

The benefits of an EHR to nursing can be substantial. With the use of information systems that support the EHR, patient and caregiver data can be used to help nurses at point of care. Nursing has always been an information-intensive profession, and the EHR provides nurses with information in a manner that can be readily employed to develop plans of care, communicate findings to other health professionals, as well as being used in the analysis of staffing and budgets to efficiently manage health-care resources (CNA, 2001). Data that describes nursing practice can be retrieved from an EHR and used to communicate and evaluate the impact of nursing care on the health of individuals and communities (Coenen, McNeil, Bakken, Bickford, & Warren, 2001). Thus, advances in information management and computer technology have broad implications for nursing.

Use of the Internet for Professional Networking

Most readers will have used the Internet for some kind of social networking or social support. Sites such as Facebook are widely known and used by people to find friends, stay connected with others, and communicate with people who have interests similar to themselves. Further, social networks or web-based clubs that connect people with similar interests have emerged and number in the thousands. People who restore cars, play chess, listen to music, follow dance workshops, or just about any other activity connect with each other through web pages that provide information and also permit people to comment about the information to one another.

Think Joe is a nursing student who has had a Facebook page for several years. He has many friends on this site and communicates information about his interesting activities, sometimes posting pictures of himself and his friends. Now that he is a nursing student, he begins to wonder if his patients and coworkers have access to his more personal information. He also wonders about what to do if a patient or coworker asks to be his friend on Facebook. Lastly, because being in nursing school is his major activity now, he is thinking about what he can and cannot put on his page about his own new experiences. What would you tell Joe about these matters?

There must be a boundary between professional and private life. Our information age activities lead many people to post personal information on the web that in the past would have been kept more private in a journal or shared only with close friends. Social networking sites have changed how many people communicate. Professional boundaries are now much more difficult to achieve than before. Nursing students are best to assume that any information on a website is potentially retrievable by patients and coworkers and not post ideas, descriptions, or photos of themselves depicting any clinical setting. Further, they should not become a friend to a patient in a virtual world, just as they should not socialize a patient outside of the nurse–patient relationship.

Today, there is also a professional use of social technology as nurses connect with each other to exchange information and ideas about their professional practice. Not surprisingly, the CNIA has a networking feature on its website so that members can have conversations with one another about issues they face. We suggest that you access the website of this and other nursing organizations of interest to you and look for the interactive features that membership in the organization will give you. You will find that more and more nursing organizations provide connectivity to online conversations as a means of establishing a membership that is committed, engaged, and exchanging knowledge regularly.

Professional connectivity through the web has been taken to another level as well. There are both nursing and health networks whose purposes are to connect professionals who live in geographically distant settings with one another for the purpose of information exchange, mentorship, knowledge development, and professional support. Different from

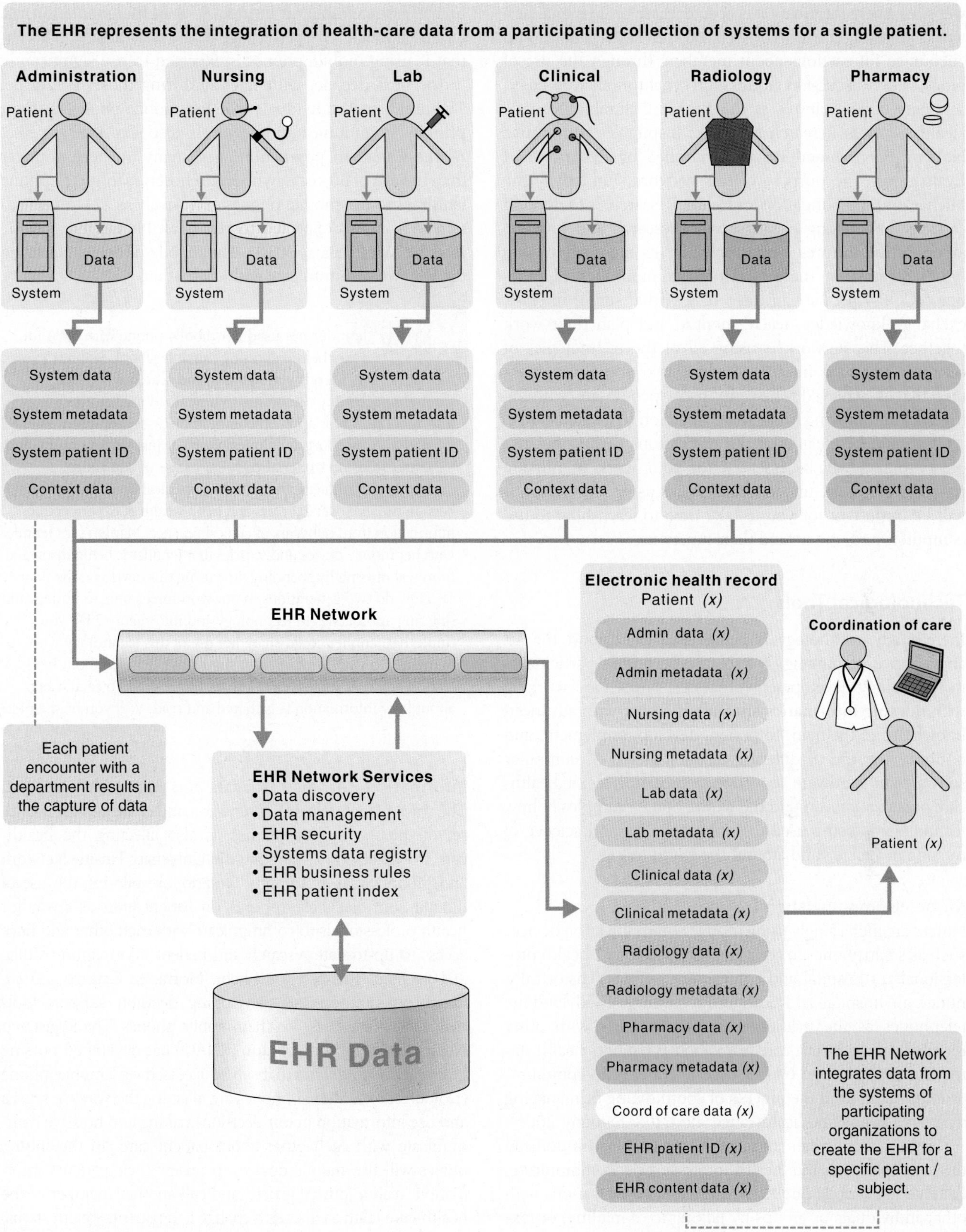

The EHR represents the integration of health-care data from a participating collection of systems for a single patient.

Administration	Nursing	Lab	Clinical	Radiology	Pharmacy
Patient	Patient	Patient	Patient	Patient	Patient
System — Data	System — Data	System — Data	System — Data	System — Data	System — Data
System data	System data	System data	System data	System data	System data
System metadata	System metadata	System metadata	System metadata	System metadata	System metadata
System patient ID	System patient ID	System patient ID	System patient ID	System patient ID	System patient ID
Context data	Context data	Context data	Context data	Context data	Context data

EHR Network

Each patient encounter with a department results in the capture of data

EHR Network Services
- Data discovery
- Data management
- EHR security
- Systems data registry
- EHR business rules
- EHR patient index

EHR Data

Electronic health record
Patient *(x)*

- Admin data *(x)*
- Admin metadata *(x)*
- Nursing data *(x)*
- Nursing metadata *(x)*
- Lab data *(x)*
- Lab metadata *(x)*
- Clinical data *(x)*
- Clinical metadata *(x)*
- Radiology data *(x)*
- Radiology metadata *(x)*
- Pharmacy data *(x)*
- Pharmacy metadata *(x)*
- Coord of care data *(x)*
- EHR patient ID *(x)*
- EHR content data *(x)*

Coordination of care

Patient *(x)*

The EHR Network integrates data from the systems of participating organizations to create the EHR for a specific patient / subject.

Figure 24.1 Concept overview of an EHR.

websites where information is posted, these professional networks are using the tools of Web 2.0 and 3.0 to support and encourage interactions about members through the use of blogs, wikis, discussion groups, and synchronous web-based seminars. One example is the British Columbia Nursing Health Services Research Network: InspireNet (**I**nnovative **N**ursing **S**ervices and **P**ractice **I**nformed by **R**esearch and **E**valuation). The purpose of this network, funded by the Michael Smith Foundation for Health Research, is to develop capacity for nursing health services research and provide, among other features, opportunity for its members to join Action Teams. In these electronic communities of practice (eCOPs) people can meet in a virtual sense, interact, exchange knowledge, teach, mentor, and plan their work together. This network is using all of the technologies of computers and the Internet to create a collaborative advantage that is achieved when groups of people are working together and moving in the same direction to create change.

It should be clear from the discussions earlier that use of computers will be essential for your work in nursing practice. If you are uncomfortable with using computers, it will be important for you to take time to learn how to use computers and understand their functions.

Technological Tools

Increasingly, technology is being used to support the art and science of nursing. Nurses are becoming participants in technology development processes. Nurses are working with **nursing informatics specialists** (those with advanced knowledge in the field) to design, develop, implement, and optimize the use of differing technologies (i.e., computer software and hardware, as well as medical devices) in health-care organizations around the world. Some examples of how technology is being used to support the art and science of nursing in Canada and around the world follow.

Mobile Communication Devices

Nurses are increasingly using mobile communication devices such as smartphones to communicate with other health professionals in hospital and community settings. Historically, nurses in hospital and community settings used landline telephones as the method of communicating with other members of the health-care team about a patient's health status and health needs. Nurses used telephones to communicate information in the process of coordinating or managing a patient's health and health care (Shortell & Kaluzny, 2006).

In the last few years, mobile phones have revolutionized the way patients and health professionals communicate. Patients use mobile phones to engage in conversations with other individuals or groups by talking to, e-mailing, or texting their friends, family, or workplace colleagues. Current Canadian statistics suggests 85% of Canadians use mobile phones in their everyday lives with about 45% of those using smart phones (Interactive Advertising Bureau Canada, 2012). Outside of Canada, mobile phone usage rates are even higher. For example, in Europe, 95% of the population use mobile phones. The percentage of the Canadian population that is using mobile phones is expected to rise significantly in the next decade, with rates mirroring those in Europe. The number of individuals who use mobile phones as their primary communication device is also expected to rise. As the Canadian population ages, many of those younger than the age of 30 years, who have chosen to forgo telephone landlines to use mobile phones exclusively as a communication tool is also expected to rise (Cell Phones Etc., 2007; Internet World Stats, 2010). The mobile phone is changing the way we communicate with each other.

Think Jennifer has used her mobile phone with apps for years before entering nursing school. She retrieves messages, calls friend, plays games, and searches the web throughout the day. She wants to download medication/drug information, access apps on common diseases, and use this information to support her clinical work. It just seems natural and a useful extension of her already savvy use of equipment.

Marilyn is Jennifer's preceptor on a medical floor. Marilyn has been in nursing over 20 years and has a wealth of experience and information from her years of clinical practice. Marilyn sees Jennifer with her mobile device and worries that Jennifer is being distracted from real nursing by spending time using this device on the floor.

How do two generations in our workforce come to understand differing approaches to technology and information? Do you think that Jennifer could share her use of this technology with Marilyn? Do you think Marilyn should ask Jennifer about her technology use? Increasingly, nurses have to talk to each other about how information is gathered and read. Will you be the first?

Information Retrieval Devices and Patient Monitoring

The wave of technological innovation and change in the world, set off by the mobile phones, is also affecting the health-care workplace. For example, the University Health Network and Mount Sinai in Toronto, Ontario, are piloting the use of iPhones and Blackberry phones on patient units as a way for health professionals to communicate with each other and have access to up-to-date research and patient information (Mulla, 2010; Quan, Rossos, Kottachchi, Morra, & Cafazzo, 2010). Other organizations are developing decision support tools that nurses can access via their mobile phones. The Registered Nurses Association of Ontario (RNAO) has developed nursing best practice guidelines that can be accessed via a mobile phone (Doran, 2009). Mobile phones are affecting the way we search and use information in our decision-making and how we communicate with each other about patient care. In the future, nurses will use mobile devices to review their patient's information, read a journal article, and call another member of the health-care team to discuss a change in a patient's health status.

Other mobile devices that a nurse may encounter in the hospital include carts that have a laptop computer mounted on them that are able to send and receive information (i.e., wireless carts or computers on wheels [COWs]). Nurses can move these carts from room to room. The laptop computer on the cart allows the nurse to view the patient's EPR while with the patient and to enter new assessment information into the EPR instead of returning to the nursing station to document (Andersen, Lindgaard, Prgomet, Creswick, & Westbrook, 2009). Medication administration systems have also been added to these wireless carts allowing nurses to use this information to support their decision-making prior to administering a medication and bedside documentation after the medication has been administered (Kushniruk, Borycki, Kuwata, & Watanabe, 2008).

COWs are often used to record assessment and intake data and, in some cases, have a standard assessment format that can be used to obtain new data and update the record.

This afternoon, Amy goes to the long-term care facility to meet Mr. McNeil, her patient. Amy learns that she can use her assessment interview to update the patient's record and is encouraged to do so. She has a series of questions to ask Mr. McNeil about his state of health and how he is managing. She brings the COW into the room, sits down beside him so that they are both in chairs and begins asking her questions. She has to ask a question and either place a tick on a box (e.g., "Are you sleeping well at night?") or write down his answer and then move on to the next question. She finds she is having trouble asking questions, listening, recording, and interacting with Mr. McNeil all at the same time. She has already learned that nurse–patient interactions are the foundation of nursing practice. She starts to think that the COW is getting in the way. Of course, Amy is right. The COW can be a useful tool to record and retrieve information at the bedside, but it can also be a barrier to therapeutic interactions. Amy excuses herself and talks to her preceptor about this. She learned that many nurses will simply talk to their patients and listen carefully to carry on a conversation. Her preceptor emphasized that she should let Mr. McNeil tell his story and advised her to prepare notes to cue herself about the items she really needed to learn about. Then, she was advised to record on the COW occasionally and not to let the recording of information be the focus of her patient encounter, rather the encounter itself should be foregrounded. Amy found this worked and has listed the issue of learning to interact with patients while documenting on the computer as one of her learning goals for the term.

Computer-Equipped Devices

In the next few years, more health-care devices that have been historically used by nurses to monitor a patient's health status (e.g., cardiac monitors), deliver treatments (e.g., intravenous pumps), or sustain life (e.g., the ventilator) will be integrated with the EPR. These devices will automatically record their data about the patient's health status and the activities they are undertaking directly into the EPR. Nurses will need to have an in-depth conceptual understanding of how these devices work—how they monitor a patient's health status and how

they are implementing interventions (e.g., medications) all using the EPR (Martíínez et al., 2009; Rausch & Judd, 2006).

Amy spends 2 hours of her afternoon in the nursing skills lab where she is practicing basic skills such as vital signs, transfer techniques, and performing hygiene. She is proficient in taking vital signs now and has practiced both in the lab and at the long-term care facility. She learned today from her instructor that the new hospital where she will go for her next practicum has "smart beds." These smart beds have pulse oximetry and vital sign monitors in the bed that can be attached to the patients' fingers and arms so that pulse and blood pressure are automatically recorded on the computerized record. She will be able to read the results on a screen in the patient's room. Her instructor points out that the principles of accurate readings and documentation using old and new technologies are the same, but certainly the means of carrying out these principles are different. Amy learns that in a fully electronic smart bed system, she needs to ensure not only that the equipment is used correctly but also that the bed is actually connected to the right patient and right electronic record. Although in the fully electronic system, some of the work is done for Amy, she does have additional considerations to ensure accurate assessment data and records are maintained.

Tools for Informatics Competencies

In the previous sections, you were introduced to informatics competencies and the technological tools you will need for professional practice. For 21st century practice, there is no question that you need to know how to retrieve nursing knowledge, how to obtain information about your patients, and how to use other high-tech tools in the delivery of patient care. Although use of technological and computer tools are critical for effective patient care, they are not sufficient alone. You will need to know what to do with the information you have, learn how to use these tools, and use your nursing judgments when you practice. The purpose of this section is to help you learn about how to use health information technologies and other devices to make meaning of patient data and how to record the important parts of your care encounters in the EHR. The following sections address documentation, communication among nurses, and communication among nurses and other members of the health-care team.

Documentation of Patient Care

Documentation of nursing observations and patient care is a fundamental nursing activity that is addressed in Chapter 23. Although no one goes into nursing solely for record keeping, documentation and communication through the clinical record is one of our most important nursing activities. Complete nursing documentation includes recording of objective and subjective data, our assessment of that data, planning and implementation of care related to the data, and evaluation and communication with other health-care team members. For example, we record an assessment of a patient's mental status, identify that this patient may be at a higher risk for falling related to mental status, develop and implement a plan of care to increase safety, communicate our concern to other nurses and health-care team members on the unit, and then evaluate. We need to document our assessments in a format so others know what we have observed and done, what we judge as plan of care, and what the appropriate nursing actions need to be for the nurse or nurses who work with the patient. There is a large body of knowledge regarding nursing handoffs—the process of turning over the care of a patient from one nurse to another. Because this is outside the scope of this chapter, it is important for you to understand the hazards in the handoff of information (i.e., information passed between nurses and how this information about a patient is critical to providing safe care). The nurses caring for the patient will not be alerted to risks, needed supports, and/or needed treatments for the patient if information is lost. Remember that one major purpose of clinical documentation is that information be available, noticed, and retrievable by the nurse providing the care in the moment. In the following section, we will address documentation in digital formats and focus on what you'll need to know in order to document patient care in electronic formats that can be used by other health-care team members through computers.

Think

Cheryl is a nurse who works on a very busy surgical unit. One day, she received 3 postsurgery admissions to her unit within 1 hour's time. The nurse reporting off to her indicated that one of these patients, Mr. Green, had been given pain medication right before the transfer, and Cheryl acknowledged that she understood the report. On assessment, Cheryl found that Mr. Green seemed quite restless and uncomfortable, and upon looking at the patient's record, Cheryl found no indication of pain medication having been given. Now, Cheryl wonders if she heard the report correctly. She says to herself, "Did the nurse say he had been given pain medication or that he had not?" Cheryl wonders, "Could I have been wrong?"

Cheryl's situation is not uncommon. Errors associated with handoffs happen when information being provided during the handoff is not verified at the time of receiving the patient, in this case, by looking at the record. So what should Cheryl do now?

For safety reasons, Cheryl contacts the nurse and learns that, indeed, the medication had been given and the previous nurse had forgotten to document the administration. Cheryl's actions not only avoid a possible overdose of medication, her knowledge of prior medication also provides important information to her ongoing assessment and support to Mr. Green.

Computer-Coded Documentation

A computerized information system can only understand or take in data that is coded in such a way that the computer knows what the data represents. For example, a health condition is recorded into an EHR through a numeric code associated with the World Health Organization's (WHO) International Classification of Diseases (ICD). The care provider indicates the name of the condition (Type 2 diabetes), and the code for the patient's condition is recorded in the EHR. In the health-care field, the condition of Type 2 diabetes is a condition understood worldwide as having a clear meaning. According to the ICD classification, Type 2 diabetes means "a metabolic disorder characterized by high blood glucose in the context of insulin resistance and relative insulin deficiency" (http://www.icd9data.com/2010/Volume1). The same would be true of other health conditions such as congestive heart failure (CHF) or essential hypertension.

Nursing information is a much more difficult domain for computerization. The ICD language is considered a standardized language and has been accepted by WHO and organizations throughout the world, as the agreed upon definitions of medical conditions. A similar diagnostic system, the *Diagnostic and Statistical Manual* (DSM), exists for psychiatric conditions. In nursing, there are several systems worldwide that have attempted to create a standard so that nursing phenomenon or nursing issues/concerns/diagnoses can be entered electronically and coded digitally. In this way, nursing considerations can be documented in the record in a fashion similar to medical and psychiatric conditions. One reason these systems have been developed is so that data representing nursing assessments, judgments, and care are included in the documentation and prepared in a format readable by the EHR. Doing so provides the ability for nursing data to be maintained electronically in the database of the clinical record, rather than being outside of that database. The implications for nursing are great. Nursing data that are part of the electronic record can be retrieved later to look back on the nursing judgments, care, and outcomes to determine the probable outcomes of nursing practices. They can also be used to answer questions about patient groups. For example, a complete electronic documentation system permits us to ask, "What nursing issues were identified as priority by patients with diabetes and the nurses on a particular unit?" or "In what situations were patients with diabetes also considered to be at risk for falls, in need of individual or group teaching, or in need of patient/family follow-up support after hospital discharge? What did the nurses do in each of these situations? What was the outcome of the patient care provided?" Because these data require use of a standardized nursing language, a nurse using an electronic system to record nursing data must learn the standardized language as well as learning the knowledge, competencies, and skills of providing care. We will discuss some of the issues in nursing related to use of standardized languages in the section that follows. Table 24.2 offers one example of nursing data presented in a narrative (noncomputer codable) fashion and the same data presented through use of a standardized language system that permits coding of that data.

TABLE 24.2	Case Example: Narrative Notes and Standardized Terms

Mrs. Smith is an 80-year-old woman who has fallen in her kitchen and fractured her wrist. She is admitted to your unit tonight and she will need surgery in the morning for her wrist. It is now 2100 hours. She is awake and in pain (she says on a scale of 7 out of 10), her arm and wrist are in a splint. She is to have nothing by mouth (NPO) after midnight and may have liquids now. She has never had surgery before. She has medication ordered for pain control. She is in relatively good health, but she is overweight. Vital signs and blood pressure (BP) are normal. She has a history of dizziness from time to time that has not been worked up, and there is no diagnosis related to her dizziness. Her husband, Mr. Smith, is with her tonight and he seems fairly anxious about her care.

Narrative	Standard Language Use: Codable Terms
Mrs. Smith, 80 y/o female admitted at 2100 hrs. from ED after a fall at home, with DX of Colles fracture left wrist. Splint in place. She reports pain, 7 on a scale of 10; is alert, appears anxious, expressing fear of surgery. Given orientation to unit. Hx of dizziness. Spouse visiting this evening.	Priority concerns: Pain/comfort Fear of surgery (anxiety) Fall risk Need for orientation to unit environment Sleep/rest, need for
Plan: Maintain comfort, institute safety measures, promote sleep, NPO at midnight	Individualized care: Family processes, interrupted Situational crises

Judgments Over Plans of Care/Nursing Actions

Another distinct advantage of collecting data in electronic format and using a fully implemented electronic record for documentation is the ability to build reminders of best practice and decision supports into the record. These are tools that alert the nurse to issues that may have critical relevance to care. For example, when a patient (e.g., the one described in Table 24.2) comes into a unit and has initial assessment data entered including a history of an injury due to a fall, having received pain medication, and currently experiencing dizziness, the computer system would automatically alert the nurse to initiate a *fall protocol* so that actions to prevent a fall while in the hospital could be implemented. The actual fall protocol may differ from one institution to another, but clearly issues of mobility and mobility supports, height of the bed, use of bed rails, call lights, and protection against falls are all essential parts of the patient care plan. The computer alert system serves as an automatic reminder that there are data in the system that indicate the nurse needs to consider this aspect of care. The more sophisticated the system, the better able the system will be in providing alerts that are pertinent. The practicing nurse needs knowledge about how to use such systems, to understand how the alerts work, and the knowledge to interact with the system; that is, to know when the alert does or does not apply to the situation at hand.

Through the eyes of a nurse

Nicole is a first-year student just getting to know her hospital unit. She found that there is a decision alert on the record for her patient reminding her that her patient is not to receive food for 1 hour after taking a specific medication. Nicole does remember this but finds the alert a good backup. Then Nicole hears two experienced nurses talking about the fact that they just tune out alerts as information simply gets in the way of their own work flow. Nicole is witnessing the tension between having alerts that are useful and supportive of care and alerts that are so high in number that they lose their value. She wonders if there is something that could be done differently by the nurses or with the system. Nicole decides it would be good to talk with her instructor and classmates about these alerts and decision supports and to observe the ways in which these are received.

(personal experience of the authors)

Interdisciplinary Use of Computerized Records

The EHR is a communication tool that other members of the health-care team also use to document and communicate information about a patient. Communication may include documenting information about the patient's health status, so that other members of the health-care team are aware of the patient's progress (Shortliffe & Cimino, 2006). Communication may also involve asking other members of the health-care team to perform activities aimed at improving the patient's health status (Kuziemsky et al., 2009). For example, a physician may write an order in the physician order entry component of the EPR. The order would go to the pharmacy, where a pharmacist would review the order and fill the prescription. The nurse would also receive a message via the EPR from the physician order entry system in his or her medication administration system. Here, the nurse would receive the order and review it and later give the medication at the appropriate time. In the meantime, the pharmacist, after reviewing the order and filling the prescription would send the patient's medication to the patient unit so that it would be available for the nurse to administer (Shortliffe & Cimino, 2006). It has been suggested the EPR can be a powerful tool for supporting communication and information exchange between health professionals. However, health professionals must be aware that EPRs should not replace the communication and problem solving that arises when members of the health-care team work together to manage patient health issues (Beuscart-Zéphir, Pelayo, Anceaux, Maxwell, & Guerlinger, 2007).

Issues for Nursing

Worldwide, nurses are reporting that the use of nursing systems in EHRs improve the quality of care and permit documentation of nursing activities that would otherwise be overlooked in settings that focus only on physician-related aspects of care (Scholes & Barber, 1980). Yet, there exist several areas of debate and concern over several issues. First, if a standardized documentation system can adequately record nursing practice; second, which of the several nursing systems available should be used; and third, the legitimate concerns about privacy, use, and access to any compilation of personal data.

Electronic Documentation

As stated earlier, it is not easy for nursing to approach standardization of language, probably because more than other domains of practice, nursing focuses on the individualization of care to meet very specific patient needs. Nursing is a discipline that is holistic, representing the notions of care and caring, nurturing and support, compassion, relational practice, and therapeutic presence. The nurse and the patient together determine all decisions about plans of care and directions of care. Nurses upholding the values of the discipline would never decide for the patient or family what patient needs should be addressed without consulting with the patients and significant others about their viewpoints and priority concerns. Yet, many in nursing perceive these standardized systems represent as more of an intrusion into the integrity of the nurse–patient interaction than a help to it. Some believe that the language used in standardized systems represents an adoption of a paternalistic model of practice and have called for nurses to refuse using such systems. Consider the divergent points of view that appear in the nursing literature about standardized nursing systems in Box 24.4.

These debates in nursing create immense difficulties for our discipline in the 21st century information age. We are currently working in systems that are rapidly moving toward complete electronic documentation of care. Nursing will either move to become an integral part of the electronic record or it will not be included in digitized format. This will have implications for nurses' ability to evaluate trend data, document nursing outcomes, and be evident in systems that will record data in paperless forms. In 2002, Frisch and Kelley stated, "Professional practice requires reflection based on theory and appropriate frameworks, and calls on the

---

BOX 24.4 Two Points of View on Computerized Documentation

Consider the following two quotes from the nursing literature:

Critical care nurses rely heavily on information technology to allow them to focus their energy on the care of the patient rather than the interpretation of voluminous data generated by automated systems. A well-developed information system can maximize the time that nurses spend on direct patient care . . . (Zytkowski, 2003, p. 277)

This [computerized] documentation serves as a general guide for healthcare cost containment and instead of individualizing healthcare services . . . Using . . . clinical support systems which incorporate computer logic and decision-making systems may be harmful to persons. (Milton, 2007, p. 35)

Ask yourself: How can two nursing authors look at the same issues and reach such different conclusions?

Please discuss these ideas with your classmates, faculty, and the nurses with whom you work and think about what you'd recommend as you take in knowledge and gain practice experience throughout your educational program.

---

experienced nurse to use intuition to guide aspects of care. On the other hand documentation of care in a standardized format . . . is required to enter the evolving world of computerized records" (p. 59). In 2012, we are basically still in the same place in nursing, although other disciplines and agencies have moved forward more rapidly to fully embrace the information age. To address this ongoing concern, we will first focus on the issue of choice of standardized language with discussion of what is does and does not record.

Standardization of Nursing Languages

The development of nursing standardized languages or nursing terminologies has been an evolutionary process, taking place over the past 40 years, resulting in several approaches to identify, document, and retrieve nursing information. Early work on nursing languages centered on nurses' realization that *that which is unnamed is unnoticed*. Nurses believed that their work was not understood and therefore, undervalued. Observing that much of what they assessed, thought, did, and evaluated was never written down, nurses embarked on a path to develop language to express nursing and to document nurse's work. Nurses' efforts to develop their standardized languages over the ensuing years have resulted in several creditable systems, all coded for computerized data entry.

Early work in nursing resulted in the development of data sets, classifications, and taxonomies or controlled vocabularies for nursing that could be used to describe and classify patient status, nursing interventions, and patient outcomes (Hardiker, Derek, & Casey, 2000). Other works outside of nursing resulted in systems that permit cross-mapping or the ability to translate information entered and coded in one

TABLE 24.3	Summary of Terms Used in Standardized Languages for Nursing	
Term	**Definitions***	**Examples**
Data set	Clusters of coded data, used on a regular basis by most professionals delivering care	The Nursing Minimum Data Set (NMDS), developed in 1991 (Werley et al.,1991) as a set of items thought to provide descriptions of basic client, nursing, and provider information. This data set includes 16 elements including client data, nursing diagnoses or care concerns, and provider elements (such as provider ID).
Classification system	Groups of terms that are categorized based on common characteristics Criteria for inclusion as a classification are that the terms be clinically useful, clearly defined, have a process for periodic review, and have unique identifiers or codes for entry into an electronic system	The Nursing Interventions Classification (NIC), now in its fourth edition (Bulechek et al., 2008), lists 542 defined nursing interventions. The Nursing Outcomes Classification (NOC), now in its fifth edition (Moorhead et al., 2008), lists 385 defined, measurable nursing outcomes.
Taxonomy	Controlled vocabularies or languages that are a set of phrases, numerated and arranged into a hierarchy	NANDA-I taxonomy of nursing diagnoses, now in its 9th revision (NANDA-I, 2009), lists 137 diagnostic labels with definitions and defining characteristics of each. The taxonomy's hierarchy has three levels: domains, classes, and nursing diagnoses. These levels categorize concepts into four domains (e.g., physiological or psychosocial), present 27 classes (e.g., fluid and electrolyte or communication) and, finally, arrange diagnoses under the appropriate class.
Translational vocabulary	Clinical terminology system used in building health-care records that permits health information entered into a record in one system to be mapped or linked to data entered into a record through another system A translational vocabulary permits data interchange.	Systemized Nomenclature of Medical Clinical Terms (SNOMED-CT). SNOMED is a system used in building electronic records that permits information systems to talk to one another. Thus, data entered into a system using a medical diagnostic system (such as ICD-10), a psychiatric system (e.g., *DSM-IV-TR*), and a nursing system can map information across systems. Similarly, data from one nursing system can be mapped against data from another nursing system.

*Hardiker et al., 2000.

system to information entered and coded into another. These systems are **translational vocabularies**. See Table 24.3 for the definition and use of these terms. Each of these concepts refers to a different type of standardized terms based on level of abstraction/specificity, and each has its use in nursing documentation and care.

Data Sets

Data sets are clusters of core data that are used on a regular basis by most professionals while delivering care within a discipline. As early as 1991, Werley, Devine, Zorn, Ryan, and Westra presented a Nursing Minimum Data Set (NMDS) that was a set of items thought to provide an accurate description of basic patient, nursing, and provider information. The intent was to provide a standardized data format to ensure consistent data entry, accessibility, and retrievability of nursing information. The NMDS was nursing's initial attempt to standardize the collection of essential nursing data and is comparable to traditional forms of documentation (van Bemmel & Musen, 1997). The NMDS has 16 base elements that include patient elements (gender, date of birth), nursing (nursing diagnosis or priority concern), and provider elements (provider identification [ID]). The NMDS remains a formal structure for electronic recording of the minimal elements necessary to document patient care.

Classification Schemes

Classification schemes are described as an assignment of objects into groups based on characteristics that they have in common; for example, origin, composition, structure, and function (Coenen et al., 2001). Classification schemes for nursing provide common terms for the patient care elements such as those recorded in the NMDS. Criteria for inclusion as a classification scheme for nursing are that the terms be clinically useful, clearly defined, having a process for review at periodic intervals, and having unique identifiers or codes for entry into an electronic system. The **Nursing Interventions Classification (NIC)** (Bulechek, Butcher, & Dochterman, 2008) and **Nursing Outcomes Classification (NOC)** (Moorhead, Johnson, Maas, & Swanson, 2008) are examples of classification schemes for nursing (Ball, Hannah, Newbold, & Douglas, 2000). These classifications schemes have been in existence for years, being revised and updated every 4 years, and are currently in their fourth and fifth editions, respectively. There are 542 and 385 terms on these classifications, and although not representing everything possible in nursing practice, they represent a very comprehensive list of nursing activities and nurse-sensitive outcomes.

By means of comparison, other classification schemes that nurses know and use include the ICD, now in its 10th revision (ICD-10), as well as the DSM system (now in its

4th revision [*DSM-IV-TR*]) mentioned earlier in this chapter. The ICD and DSM are more inclusive of their respective domains of practice than the existing nursing classification schemes.

Taxonomies/Controlled Vocabularies

Taxonomies, also considered controlled vocabularies or languages, are a "restricted set of phrases, generally numerated and arranged into a hierarchy" (Hardiker et al., 2000, p. 524). Taxonomic terms are coded to enable clinicians to capture clinical data at the point of care and are amenable for use in an electronic environment. Of the nursing taxonomies in existence, the first developed and the most widely known is the NANDA taxonomy of nursing diagnosis. Originally and published in 1987, this taxonomy has now been through nine revisions and stands as the most complete list of nursing diagnostic labels with definitions in the world. NANDA is now NANDA-International, having evolved to an international nursing organization with members from at least 23 countries. The NANDA-I taxonomy currently has 137 diagnostic labels and has been translated into 17 languages. The taxonomic hierarchy for NANDA-I has three levels: domains, classes, and nursing diagnoses. For example, one domain is *health promotion*, and under this domain are the classes of *health awareness* and *health management*. Another domain is *comfort*, and the associated classes are *physical comfort*, *environmental comfort*, and *social comfort*. Actual nursing diagnostic labels are provided in association with each class. The taxonomy adds *axes* to each diagnosis to provide for a diagnostic statement that includes a depiction of the diagnostic process (the diagnostic concept, the subject of the diagnosis, the location, the patient's age, the time, and the status of the diagnosis [actual, risk, wellness]). Thus, using the NANDA-I taxonomy as an example, it can be seen that a taxonomy is not the same as a classification scheme. A taxonomy has a structure and hierarchy of terms dictated by a framework selected for the system. At present, the NANDA-I taxonomy is used in many nursing information systems throughout the world but is less popular in Canada.

A Unified Nursing Language

The examples of data sets, classifications, and taxonomies for nursing illustrate that each system was developed for one aspect of nursing, but none provide a comprehensive nursing language that could be used in an EHR or that meet the need to describe, define, and document all of nursing's phenomena. The differences inherent in these systems act as a barrier that prevents direct comparison and free exchange of nursing information. Current and future demands on information systems require terminologies to support data reuse and comparisons of data captured and are critical for comparative outcome analysis (Coenen et al., 2001; McCormick et al., 1994). The ICNP was produced to provide such unifying language.

The ICNP was developed through the ICN in the 1990s, partly in response to the need for a unifying language.

Another goal was a response to criticism that the extant nursing languages represented a limited view of nursing and could not be readily translated to suffice for cross-cultural, international use. The first or *alpha* version of the ICNP was released as a standardized vocabulary that would present nursing phenomena of concern: nursing diagnoses, nursing interventions, and nursing outcomes. There have been three revisions to date and the current version (Version 2.0) was released in 2009 (ICN, 2009). This version contains a catalogue of precombined terms that is composed of subsets of diagnoses, actions, and outcomes specific to various practice areas. The ICNP is designed to be used in two ways. The first is as a compositional vocabulary (a list of nursing terms, much like a classification scheme). The second is as a terminology reference, meaning that it can provide a means for cross-mapping terms of existing nursing terminologies to enable comparisons of nursing data across organizations and various health sectors. The ICNP is not a taxonomy nor is it exactly a classification system. It is a comprehensive vocabulary for nursing that permits computerized documentation of all aspects of nursing judgments, activities, and outcomes. The ICNP Version 2.0 makes use of a core data set derived from the nursing minimum data set literature. It includes axes to document the focus of nursing attention, the nursing judgment, and a statement about who the patient is, along with the nursing action, the means of carrying out the nursing action, the location of care, and the time period involved in the nursing encounter (ICN, 2009). These axes are needed for inclusion in EHRs according to international standards of EHRs (International Organization for Standardization [ISO], 2003). ICNP has been endorsed by the CNA as the "most universal, generic, and comprehensive foundational classification system for nursing . . ." (CNA, 2001, p. 14).

Think   Tom is a nursing student and has just completed a full, hour long assessment of one of his patients, Mr. Smith. Tom learns that Mr. Smith is facing surgery soon for prostate cancer and is experiencing a considerable amount of anxiety over both his diagnosis and need for treatment. Mr. Smith has a past history of difficult situations in hospital that contribute to his feelings of anxiety. Tom wants to alert nurses who will care for Mr. Smith that the patient will need their support in dealing with the presurgical procedures. Tom looks at information he has on nursing languages and believes he can relay the information by indicating two major nursing concerns: *need for preoperative teaching* and *fear of upcoming surgery*. Tom worries that use of these word phrases may not provide enough information for the receiving nurses to understand Mr. Smith.

Tom is experiencing first hand the issues in nursing related to how we communicate complex human feelings and human responses to health conditions in shorthand language. If Tom writes these two issues down and you were the nurse to read them, would you understand enough to plan your care of Mr. Smith? Take this opportunity to reflect on how such information might guide your approach to the patient.

Translational Vocabularies

Systematized Nomenclature of Medicine Clinical Terms or simply SNOMED CT is a clinical terminology that is used in health care for building electronic records (e.g., EHRs, EPRs, and EMRs). SNOMED CT helps health information systems communicate with each other (i.e., facilitates electronic health data interchange) (International Health Terminology Standards Development Organization [IHTSDO], 2010). In health care, the ability of one health information system to talk to another system and be understood is referred to as interoperability. ICD, DSM, ICNP, and other nursing terminologies have been mapped to SNOMED CT (Bakken et al., 2002; Hardiker, Casey, Coenen, & Konicek, 2006). When terminologies are mapped to each other (e.g., SNOMED CT to ICNP), translation can occur between the terminologies, and the health information systems that use these differing terminologies. This situation is likely to occur when there are hospital, home care records, and outpatient clinic records, or when there are records from private offices, long-term care facilities, and emergency rooms that all deal with the same patient population. SNOMED CT provides a means for electronic health-care data interchange (IHTSDO, 2010) and has the endorsement of Canada Health Infoway (CHI), a not-for-profit organization that works with all provinces and territories to accelerate the use of EHRs as a Canadian standard. It is important for nurses to understand that SNOMED CT is in the process of incorporating the ICNP and already has other nursing languages included. Thus, an EHR system that is not SNOMED CT compatible may not have the capacity to record nursing-specific data. It must also be noted that not all relationships between the terminologies (i.e., nursing and SNOMED CT) have been fully mapped and further research is needed in this area of nursing informatics (Bakken et al., 2002; Hardiker et al., 2006). Lastly, it should be noted that although there are current efforts to map ICNP to SNOMED CT, it may evolve that ICNP will become the translational vocabulary for all nursing terms.

Challenges

ICNP has the potential to establish a dynamic vocabulary for nursing across Canada because it can provide a coding structure for use in a pan-Canadian EHR (CNA, 2008b). This goal cannot be reached without universal uptake and considerable education of nurses on computer-based systems and computerized cross-mapping of nursing terms.

The ICNP terms are fairly straightforward; however, the volume of concepts required for full documentation of nursing is daunting. At this point, many organizations in Canada have implemented clinical information systems at the basic admission/ discharge/ transfer functionality. Those organizations that are beginning to use electronic clinical documentation are struggling with integrating the systems into mainstream practice. Greater consideration needs to be given to the bigger picture of standard language integration. Although CHI has endorsed ICNP for Canada, the country still needs a cadre of educated nurses who understand the systems and their importance to nursing reach the national goals.

Unlike the other nursing classification and taxonomic systems, the ICNP does not include definitions of all terms. It is the most comprehensive system for labeling nursing phenomena and avoids the challenges of translation of meaning across languages and cultures. The full use of the ICNP will require that Canadian nurses develop consistent and reliable meanings for every term used in the system (or at least for the terms they use). To accomplish this, Canadian nurses could document meanings attributed to terms at local/regional or national levels. They would then follow the lead of nurses in other locations (e.g., Korea, Italy, and Brazil) who have already addressed these definitional issues in their countries (Cho & Park, 2006; da Nóbrega & de Gutierrez, 2000; Sansoni & Giustini, 2006). Another method of attributing meaning would be to use the terms as defined in other extant systems and to cross-map to the ICNP. Without such work, the ability of Canadian nurses to interpret nursing data across health information systems, health-care organizations, and among provinces and territories could be limited. With these additional efforts, the system for Canada can be a most exciting collection of nursing data with ability to review, refine, and impact our work.

Measuring Nursing Outcomes

The ability to collect outcomes data for documentation of the nursing's contribution to patient care is a challenge for nurses. The NOC referred to earlier as a nursing classification system does include many nursing outcomes and provides computer-coding and measurement tools for each outcome. This is an excellent system, but its uptake is dependent on universal use of the system in all areas and specialty practices within the discipline and access to this system on electronic records is limited. There is a Canadian initiative, the **Canadian-Health Outcomes for Better Information and Care (C-HOBIC)**, which is a major project to collect data on nurse-sensitive or nurse-related outcomes and to use these data to inform care. This initiative requires your attention and support as it moves to become an important Canadian undertaking on behalf of nursing.

Canadian-Health Outcomes for Better Information and Care

The C-HOBIC project builds on an Ontario initiative that in 2007 sought to use standard language and assessment tools to record admission and discharge data for patients in acute care areas as well as in continuing or long-term care. The project originated through an agreement between CNA and CHI for use in EHRs. As designed, the objectives of the project are to

- standardize the language concepts used by C-HOBIC to ICNP;
- standardize the language concepts used by C-HOBIC ICNP;

TABLE 24.4	Canadia-Health Outcomes for Better Information and Care: Outcomes and Measures
Outcomes	**Measurement**
Functional status	Self-performance of ADL rated on measures of level of independence
Therapeutic self-care	Readiness for discharge—measures of knowledge of self-care requirements.
Symptom management (pain, nausea, fatigue, dyspnea)	Measures of intensity, duration and frequency of the symptom
Safety (falls, pressure ulcers)	Number of falls in unit of time; Number of pressure ulcers, staging of ulcers
Patient satisfaction with patient care	Satisfaction measures.

ADL, activities of daily living.

- capture patient outcome data related to nursing care across four sectors of the health system: acute care, complex continuing care, long-term care, and home care; and
- store the captured and standardized data in relevant, secure jurisdictional data repositories or databases in preparation for entry into provincial EHRs.

At the time of this writing, the data are being gathered in Manitoba, Prince Edward Island, and Saskatchewan. Each outcome being measured has a definition and measurement parameters so that the outcomes can be referred back to specific nursing inputs or actions. See Table 24.4 for details about the outcomes and measurements. In 2008, the CNA released an important document, *Mapping Canadian Clinical Outcomes in ICNP*, that details the processes applied to definitions and mapping across systems. This effort was the first in the country and likely one of the first is the world that addressed nursing's need to systematically record intake and outcome assessment data and begin to relate that data to nursing activities. Further, because the project maps to the ICNP, it is the first and foremost effort in defining and understanding the use of the ICNP terms in a Canadian context. Although there is still a long way to go to document and retrieve comprehensive data on all aspects of nursing, the C-HOBIC project stands as a very innovative and important initiative for Canadian nursing. There is no question that all nurses should support the inclusion of C-HOBIC data in the EHR systems at their place of work.

Privacy and Ethics

There are significant issues of privacy, confidentiality, access, and right to know when we begin dealing with digitized health-care information. As nurses, our work and guidance in these areas comes from the CNA Code of Ethics (CNA, 2008a)

The Code presents five major principles governing nursing practice (discussed in Chapter 4). Principle No. 5 deals directly with these issues: *Nurses recognize the importance of privacy and confidentiality and safeguard personal, family and community information obtained in the context of a professional relationship.* The specific issues related to privacy, confidentiality, and safeguarding become challenging as we think about the positive opportunity to send health-care information and records instantaneously from one locality to another (e.g., from a rural clinic to an urban emergency department) while ensuring that access to this information is restricted only to those care providers who need this information to make appropriate clinical judgments.

Systems-Level Privacy Issues

The international standards that set out not only what needs to be included in an EHR but also how it will be coded and transmitted to ensure privacy and confidentiality are established through the International Organization for Standardization (ISO) in Geneva (ISO, 2003). Further, there is an international organization called *Health Level Seven* (HL7) that sets standards for functional interoperability and exchange of data across systems. The term *Level Seven* means that the standards set are at the seventh or very highest messaging level. These HL7 standards dictate the protocols used for transmission and exchange and meet the most stringent standards for ensuring privacy is maintained while permitting data exchange across systems. HL7 is becoming the global standard for systems, and Canada has an HL7 Canada Council that participates in this work.

Practice-Level Privacy Issues

At the level of the practicing nurse, there are standard procedures you will learn to ensure that patient privacy is being respected. Computerized records are set up so that some form of authentication is required. This means that there is a verification of the identity of the person logging in. To access the record, there has to be a way for your identity to be established, typically accomplished with a login (User ID) and password. You must never give your password to another person because the password permits only you to access private information in the records. Policies on how often to change passwords vary but are put into place by system administrators charged with overseeing the operations. These policies are based on an accepted understanding that, over time, passwords can become compromised, thus new ones are needed on a regular basis (Thede & Sewell, 2010). Another feature of many electronic records systems is that there is an automatic logout, so that if you leave a computer to carry out patient care and do not manually log yourself out, the system will do that for you. This is done so that others may not enter into the system under your account. We advise that you ask about the automatic logout feature of any system you use.

In addition, most public institutions in Canada have a privacy officer whose role is to oversee policies and practices on behalf of those served. A privacy officer plays an important role, particularly when there are questions or concerns about any specific case. You might inquire about the role of the privacy officer in the places where you begin work.

Amy has completed her basic assessment of Mr. McNeil and returns the next day to provide care. Amy carries a personal digital assistant (PDA) with information she has downloaded that gives her access to health and nursing resources, such as lab value ranges, nursing assessment questions, a medical dictionary, and also a feature where she can record text herself. She begins to record her assessment and developing care plan for Mr. McNeil. Amy has discovered that Mr. McNeil is having difficulties with sleep (not being able to fall asleep at night and awakening several times during the night) and that he is not eating much because "he doesn't care for his food." He is not getting any exercise, although he thinks he might enjoy walking more. As she writes down her thoughts, she questions if she can really carry this information home with her to complete the care plan tonight. She is very correct to be thinking about this. If the data she has on her PDA could be retrieved and Mr. McNeil could be identified as the individual she has written about, she would be violating his right to privacy. Even knowing the patient's age and gender could be enough to identify the individual in some settings. So, Amy realizes she must not record any information that could be traced back to her patient on her PDA. She may record general information, for example, on development of sleep protocols, but she may not record any individual client information on her personal device that she will carry outside of the care facility itself.

Access to What?

Before we leave the issue of privacy and access, consider some other (sometimes difficult) issues about access. Please refer back to Figure 24.1 where we can see several parts of the EHR. Ask yourself: What part of the record does a nurse need to see in order to give safe, effective care? In the figure, nursing is given its own *data silo* along with administration, laboratory, and other areas. Intriguingly, nursing's place is near the top, just under administration. In this visual, nursing also has a place on the electronic health network and in the final EHR. One might ask: Why is nursing separated from the silo termed *clinical*? A paper health record does not have a method to limit access to only one section. Once that paper record is opened, a care provider can view laboratory results, problem lists, nursing notes, physician orders, or any part of the record. In contrast, the EHR is a database that can support multiple distinct views of subsets of the entire data set. Each view may require a different set of privileges for access. Although the EHR may hold complete data from various disciplines, limiting access can be set in ways that prevent the kind of sharing of plans and progress that would otherwise facilitate high-quality interdisciplinary care. Further, if data are not digitized and stored in the EHR in the first place, any discussion about sharing that data is meaningless. If data are included in the EHR but not viewable by one or more disciplines, then the record may lose a significant portion of its value. Consider this example, nurses might need to know

the position of an enterostomy tube for which they have responsibility, but in some implementations, they might not have access to radiology data. Or, if a nurse doesn't have access to laboratory data on international normalized ratio (INR; means of reporting prothrombin time), that nurse's ability to safely administer anticoagulant medications may be impaired. Similarly, nurses and social workers planning for discharge may have legitimate needs to know about the home environments, neighbourhood, local services, and potential risk factors for the patients they serve but could be restricted from access to administrative data that hold such information. There are dual issues of privilege or right to know/need to know and issues of privacy/confidentiality regarding information held in various parts of the EHR database. As a new nurse, likely working in a setting where some of these issues have not yet been fully explored, it is important to know which parts of the record you and the nurses have been given access, which parts are restricted, and for what reasons. In some EHRs, these decisions are being made by software designers, who may not have a clinical background and/or by administrators that may lack a full understanding of the complexities of modern nursing practice. We believe that every implementation plan requires input from at least one nurse cognizant of these matters. It may be instructive for you to ask who the nursing representative is in your setting and have a conversation with that person as you begin to gain access to electronic health-care data in your student role.

Nursing Roles Related to Informatics

As the number of electronic records implemented in hospital, community, clinic, and long-term care settings grows, so will the roles of nurses in informatics. Nurses have an important role in the design, implementation, and evaluation of EHRs and the medical devices that can be used in conjunction with EHRs (e.g., intravenous pumps).

Generalist (User)

As a nurse working in a hospital, clinic, community, or long-term care setting at differing points in your career, you will be asked by health informatics professionals and nursing informatics specialists to participate in evaluations of new software, hardware, and health-care devices before they are purchased or implemented in your work setting. Take these opportunities to participate and get involved. Volunteer for committees that are involved in purchasing differing types of technologies for your work setting. This will give you a chance to find out what types of technologies are being reviewed, and it will allow you to participate in the decision-making process. Review the evidence-based literature that is published to learn about how the technology has impacted other nurses and other health professionals. Participate in the decision-making process (Ball et al., 2000). Think about the impact the technology will have on patient care, your information seeking and decision-making, and communication between you and other nurses as well as other health professionals (Borycki, Lemieux-Charles, Nagle, & Eysenbach, 2009; Kuziemsky et al., 2009). Advocate for opportunities for other nurses to test the technology and determine if it is the right technology for your work setting. Express your thoughts about how technology can support or disrupt nursing practice so the best technology can be purchased by your organization. If your organization is·implementing a new technology such as an EHR or a wireless cart, volunteer to be part of the implementation. Volunteer to be a *super user* (i.e., an individual who has detailed knowledge about the technology) or a technology champion (i.e., an individual who helps others learn about the technology and advocates for new users). As a super user, you can help other nurses who are using the technology for the first time in a real-world setting (after they have completed their training) to effectively use and integrate the technology into the patient care, their work as nurses and with other members of the nursing and health-care team (Walker, Bieber, & Richards, 2006). As a technology champion, you can help nurses to learn about a new technology. You can also advocate for nurses with health informatics professionals when the technology needs to be modified or customized so that it better meets the needs of the nurses using the technology in their daily practice (Hoyt, Sutton, & Yoshihashi, 2007).

Manager

The manager is aware of the ways in which technology can support and disrupt nursing practice. Technologies can help support nurse assessment and decision-making. For example, technologies such as EHRs collect a considerable amount of data. When analyzed, data can be used to support a manager's decision-making, can provide insights into the types of patients that are being cared for on your unit, and can assess effectiveness of nurse interventions currently in use. A technology such as an EHR can be a powerful tool for supporting nursing practice and managerial decision-making because it can provide data that can be used to inform nursing practice changes (Ball et al., 2000; Shortliffe & Cimino, 2006).

Technology, when not designed and/or implemented well, can be disruptive to nurses' work. For example, some researchers have found that poorly designed technology can lead to technology-induced errors (i.e., errors that arise from the use and interactions with technology; Kushniruk, Triola, Borycki, Stein, & Kannry, 2005). Other researchers have found that poorly designed and implemented health-care technologies can lead to a poor fit with the clinical demands of the work setting. These researchers have noted that nurses will bypass or develop work-arounds in an attempt to circumvent the barriers to providing patient care that have been introduced by the new technology (Kushniruk, Borycki, Kuwata, & Kannry, 2006). Be aware that these situations may arise in the workplace. Work with the nurses on your unit to identify those features and functions of the technology that are disruptive to nursing practice and identify the cases in which they affect nursing practice positively and negatively. Describe the issues your nursing staff are experiencing to the IT department and engage in a discussion about how the technology can be modified so that it better supports nurses' work. Speak with your chief nursing officer about your concerns and describe how the technology has affected nursing practice. Work together with the IT department and your chief nursing officer to modify the technology so that it better meets the needs of the nurses on your unit.

Leader—Clinical Nurse Specialist

The clinical nurse specialist (CNS) recognizes the power of technology to act as one more tool that can be used to support nursing practice. When introducing a practice change, the CNS should consider teaching a nurse about the practice change, describing the associated policies and procedures, providing the tools to be able to make the change, and revising the technologies nurses use as a further support to the practice changes. For example, when introducing a new wound care guideline to the unit, CNS should consider educating nurses about the new guideline, introducing new policies and procedures to support the use of the guidelines, and an electronic decision support tool that nurses can use at the bedside to support their decision-making involving the practice change. Use technologies such as the EHR as a source of data that can help the nurses on your unit identify the key health issues that patients have identified. In your department or regional health authority, the CNS uses this information to design and evaluate the introduction of new nursing interventions and to assess their impacts on patient outcomes (Purvis & Brenny-Fitzpatrick, 2010; Shortliffe & Cimino, 2006).

Whether you are a nurse, a nurse manager, or a CNS, understand the technologies that are present in your health-care setting and how they can both help and hinder nursing practice. Think about being active in informatics projects and issues.

Our Current and Future World

Throughout this chapter, we have followed Amy in her day encountering nurses need for information and nurses need to use technologies wisely. We've seen her use technology to plan her day's schedule and retrieve data about health conditions. She has encountered a situation where the technology itself became a barrier to the human interaction so important to patient care. We've also seen that she has encountered new issues of privacy and confidentiality with need to be sure that private information is never carried out of the health-care setting. Lastly, she has encountered a situation related to smart beds where she as the nurse has to be "smarter" than the bed to ensure accuracy of information. In our technologically enabled world, most nursing students will, like Amy, encounter issues of accuracy, quality and safety, relational practice, and ethics that arise because of technologies. Thoughtful and reflective practice is the cornerstone of technology use, and this is something Amy has learned today.

As you continue in your studies and begin your careers, you will encounter challenges that we may not begin to conceptualize today. Your challenge in nursing will be to bring the blend of high tech and high touch into a world where people need care that is compassionate, kind, and effective. Our use of electronic records, home care monitoring systems, and shorthand reports of nursing concerns in standardized languages cannot overtake our need to connect individually with the real people who depend on us for their care. As you complete this chapter, think about this world of home and self-care monitoring, communicating by texting, creating virtual connections between health-care providers and patients. How do you envision relational practice, caring and healing, and person-to-person connection in an electronic and virtual world? We ask you to envision the means to provide such aspects of care in these future environments. You will be the nurses who enter into these worlds, finding the means to keep nursing grounded in its history and values as we move forward in environments unimaginable to our discipline's founders.

SUMMARY

In this chapter, you have been introduced to many issues that are influencing nursing today. There is a complicated world that brings nursing science together with computing science and information science—this is the field we call nursing informatics. There is no way that nurses can function without competencies to find and use professional information, and increasingly, there is no way that nurses can access patient record systems without use of computers. We need to think about computers as tools to assist us in performing our nursing roles, much as we need to use a stethoscope in performing our assessment duties. Computers are our access to information, and as an information-dependent profession, we must use them wisely and efficiently.

In addition to computers, there are other high-tech tools that are coming into our practices. Home monitoring equipment, mobile devices, medication administration systems, EHRs, and other tools provide us the ability to perform our work differently than in previous generations of nursing practice. These are tools that provide *support* to our work; these tools are not *our* work. We recommend learning to use these tools, remaining open to new ideas, and maintaining a critical stance to always ask how the tool assists in provision of care, how it may disrupt or detract from care, and how can we modify the tool to better support nursing practice and patient care.

We've discussed the topics of EHRs and other digitalized health records and how nursing can use standardized terms to enter nursing data into digitalized formats. As nurses entering Canadian systems, it is important for you to know the development of these standardized nursing systems and their relevance today in our move to the ICNP and our desire to adopt the C-HOBIC initiative across the country. We have discussed the benefits and challenges of each of the extant systems.

We've presented the issues prevalent in our discipline regarding a debate over whether nursing can be true to its values of compassionate, individualized care while entering the information age of coded terms, documentation of care plans, and measurement of outcomes. We maintain that it can and that it must. We ask that every new nurse seriously consider the issues of why we have reason to be concerned that nursing will be subsumed into a technological system devoid of human experience. Ask yourself what you and other nurses can and should do about these concerns and develop a personal plan for how you might address them as you enter nursing practice.

Lastly, we discussed the important issues and challenges of privacy, confidentiality, and access privileges in regard to electronic records. Maintaining records in digital format creates wonderful opportunities to share information in real time across geographic boundaries but, at the same time, raises significant issues regarding data security. Every nurse must maintain vigilance authentication, access, and privacy.

We hope that this introduction has captured your interest and that some of you will consider moving on to the specialized work of the nursing informatician!

Critical Thinking Case Scenarios

▶ Nursing student Mary is in a conversation with two nurses on the unit where she is assigned. One nurse expresses concerns over an imminent move to an EHR stating, "We simply haven't got time to be involved, yet they want us to try out a new form for data entry! I don't care what they do!" Then, the other nurse chimes in by saying, "It's just one more phase that we'll be going through, so let's just get on with our work." What should Mary say? If you were Mary, what would you think?

1. What happens to nursing when nurses are too involved to contribute to and critically evaluate the EHR?
2. When nurses truly are too busy, what are the options?
3. Who makes the decisions about clinical records when nurses are too busy to be involved?

▶ James is a nursing student who has come to the hospital unit tonight to obtain information about the patient he is assigned to care for tomorrow morning. He logs into the computerized record when another nurse, who usually works on another floor, comes to his side and says, "I usually don't work here, so can I see that screen so I can get on with my work tonight?" What should James do?

1. Are there any situations where it would be permissible for James to share confidential and private information?
2. What are the principles involved in keeping such information private?

▶ Nancy is a nurse who is using a computerized system for medication administration. The prescribed dose of the medicine seems to be too high for the patient; yet the decision supports do not indicate that there is any concern with the drug dose. What should Nancy do?

1. Can we rely on computerized systems to find errors before we commit them?
2. When do we know if our system is working or is compromised?
3. Who is accountable, legally and morally, when a system fails?

▶ In a conversation with a group of nurses, student Jeanine hears her colleagues stating, "We don't want to use standardized, shorthand languages to document what we do. Our descriptions are much more accurate and important for patient documentation." What should Jeanine say?

1. What are the benefits of rich narrative descriptions?
2. What are the benefits of computer-coded information?
3. Are these mutually exclusive?
4. Why do informaticists describe the narrative records as those which go to the "data cemetery"?

▶ Emily is a nursing student who will be assigned to work in the surgical ICU for the next 2 weeks. Her nursing instructor has asked Emily to do a literature search to find information about the topic of sleep disturbances in the ICU. What should Emily do? How will Emily know if she has obtained current and pertinent information?

1. How would Emily begin her search at your school or hospital?
2. When will Emily know if her search was sufficient for providing care?
3. What should Emily do if she encounters data about sleep hygiene techniques that have not been used on her unit?

Multiple-Choice Study Questions

1. Nursing informatics is:
   a. The intersection of nursing science and theory with computing and information science
   b. Nursing's ability to retrieve information for practice
   c. Individual nurse's ability to search professional literature
   d. The ability to code nursing data on an electronic health record

2. With regard to development of information systems, nurses were:
   a. Not involved in early development.
   b. Active participants since the 1970s
   c. Late adopters of computerized systems
   d. Silent recipients of systems developed by others

3. The ICNP is:
   a. The Institute for the Collaboration of Nurse Practitioners
   b. A taxonomy for nursing diagnoses
   c. A statement of nursing phenomenon of concern
   d. A unified language system that permits coding of nursing terms

4. One of the essential nursing informatics competencies for new graduates is ability to:
   a. Write computer codes for nursing data
   b. Read computer codes for nursing data
   c. Retrieve trended data from existing records
   d. Use computers for documenting nursing data

5. Information literacy in nursing refers to the ability to:
   a. Understand one's own health data
   b. Find creditable and useful information when needed
   c. Use CINAHL to find articles
   d. Find and read gray literature on the Internet

6. An EHR is:
   a. A personal health record kept by the hospital
   b. An individual's record of emergency and clinic visits
   c. A record of patient and health-care agency encounters
   d. A digital record of a patient's encounters with the health system

7. The Nursing Outcomes Classification is:
   a. A comprehensive list of nurse-sensitive outcomes
   b. A translational vocabulary of nursing terms and health conditions
   c. A list of nursing activities
   d. A trended series of expected practices for patient care

8. C-HOBIC is:
   a. An international database for nursing practice
   b. A list of Canadian terms for nursing practice
   c. A translational vocabulary for nursing terms
   d. Project to document outcomes of patient care

9. A nurse using a digital format for recording data must know how to:
   a. Write narrative descriptions of the condition she sees.
   b. Select an inventory of nursing concepts
   c. Adopt a translational vocabulary to nursing ideas
   d. Use a standardized language for nursing

10. Worldwide, nurses are:
    a. Adopting computerization of their work with enthusiasm
    b. Completing analyses of trended data on outcomes of nursing practice
    c. Using the same standardized language to document their care
    d. Entering the information age with both interest and skepticism

11. The standardized nursing language that includes definitions of term as well as defining characteristics is:
  a. ICD-10
  b. ICNP
  c. NANDA-I
  d. *DSM-IV-TR*

12. The advantage of the ICNP as a language for nurses in Canada is:
  a. It is a unified language system.
  b. It was developed by CHI.
  c. It has been translated into both English and French in a Canadian context.
  d. It is included in the SNOMED CT database.

13. To maintain privacy in a computerized system, each nurse must:
  a. Maintain diligence in keeping his or her own passwords protected.
  b. Logout of the system each day.
  c. Tell patient's families that data are kept digitally.
  d. Tell the patient everything that is written down in the record.

14. Access to the EHR for nurses and other health professionals is:
  a. The same as in paper records
  b. Unrestricted by discipline
  c. Determined by administrators developing the computer systems
  d. Dictated by the patients

15. Nursing informatics is a specialty for:
  a. Those with an interest in information science
  b. Nurses prepared at the master's level
  c. Professionals who support nurses in nursing's work
  d. Nurses who wish to share data

REFERENCES AND SUGGESTED READINGS

Agency for Healthcare Research and Quality. (1997). *Quality of health information on the Internet.* Retrieved from http://www.ahrq.gov/qual/hiirpt.htm

Andersen, P., Lindgaard, A. M., Prgomet, M., Creswick, N., & Westbrook, J. I. (2009). Mobile and fixed computer use by doctors and nurses on hospital wards: Multi-method study on the relationships between clinician role, clinical task, and device choice. *Journal of Medical Internet Research, 11*(3), e32.

Bakken, S., Warren, J. J., Lundberg, C., Casey, A., Correia, C., Konicek, D., & Zingo, C. (2002). An evaluation of the usefulness of two terminology models for integrating nursing diagnosis concepts into SNOMED Clinical Terms®. *International Journal of Medical Informatics, 68,* 71–77.

Ball, M. J., Hannah, K. J., Newbold, S. K., & Douglas, J. V. (Eds.). (2000). *Nursing informatics: Where caring and technology meet* (3rd ed.). New York, NY: Springer Publishing.

Bernstam, E. V., Shelton, D. M., Walji, M., & Meric-Bernstam, F. (2005). Instruments to assess the quality of health information on the World Wide Web: What can our patients actually use. *International Journal of Medical Informatics, 74*(1), 13–19.

Beuscart-Zéphir, M. C., Pelayo, S., Anceaux, F., Maxwell, D., & Guerlinger, S. (2007). Cognitive analysis of physicians and nurses cooperation in the medication ordering and administration process. *International Journal of Medical Informatics, 76,* S65–S77.

Borycki, E. M., Lemieux-Charles, L., Nagle, L., & Eysenbach, G. (2009). Evaluating the impact of hybrid electronic-paper environments upon novice nurse information seeking. *Methods of Information in Medicine, 48,* 137–143.

Bulechek, G. M., Butcher, H., & Dochterman, J. M. (2008). *Nursing interventions classification (NIC)* (5th ed.). St. Louis, MO: Mosby.

Canada Health Infoway. (2009). *Building a healthy legacy together: Annual report 2008–2009.* Toronto, ON: Author.

Canada's Health Informatics Association. (2011). *COACH definition of health informatics.* Toronto, ON Author.: Retrieved from http://www.coachorg.com/health_informatics/about_health_informatics.htm

Canadian Nurses Association. (2001). What is nursing informatics? and why is it so important? *Nursing Now: Issues and Trends in Canadian Nursing, 11,* 1–4.

Canadian Nurses Association. (2006). *E-nursing strategy for Canada.* Ottawa, ON: Author.

Canadian Nurses Association. (2008a). *Code of ethics for registered nurses.* Retrieved from http://www.cna-nurses.ca/CNA/documents/pdf/publications/Code_of_Ethics_2008_e.pdf

Canadian Nurses Association. (2008b). *Mapping Canadian clinical outcomes in ICNP.* Retrieved from http://www.cna-aiic.ca/c-hobic/documents/pdf/ICNP_Mapping_2008_e.pdf

Canadian Nurses Association. (2010). Retrieved from https://frontlineinformatics.sslpowered.com/frontlineinformatics.ca/courses_hitscontent.html

Cell Phones Etc. (2007). *Use of mobile phones almost level with landline–Canada statistics.* Retrieved from http://cellphones.ca/news/post002323/

Cho, I., & Park, H. A. (2006). Evaluation of the expressiveness of an ICNP-based nursing data dictionary in a computerized nursing record system. *Journal of the American Medical Informatics Association, 13*(4), 456–464.

Coenen, A., McNeil, B., Bakken, S., Bickford, C., & Warren, J. J. (2001). Toward comparable nursing data: American Nurses Association criteria for data sets, classification systems and nomenclatures. *Computers in Nursing, 19*(6), 240–246.

da Nóbrega, M. M., & de Gutierrez, M. G. (2000). Semantic equivalence of the Nursing Phenomena Classification of ICNP: Alpha version in Brazilian Portuguese. *International Nursing Review, 47,* 19–27.

Doran, D. (2009). The emerging role of PDAs in information use and clinical decision making. *Evidence-Based Nursing, 12,* 35–38.

Eysenbach, G., & Köhler, C. (2002). How do consumers search for an appraise health information on the world wide web? Qualitative study using focus groups, usability tests, and in-depth interviews. *British Medical Journal, 324,* 573–577.

Eysenbach, G., Powell, J., Kuss, O., & Sa, E. R. (2002). Empirical studies assessing the quality of health information for consumers on the world wide web: A systematic review. *Journal of the American Medical Association, 287*(20), 2691–2700.

Frisch, N., & Kelley, J. H. (2002). Nursing diagnosis and nursing theory: Exploration of factors inhibiting and supporting simultaneous use. *Nursing Diagnosis, 3*(2), 53–61.

Gagliardi, A., & Jadad, A. R. (2002). Examination of instruments used to rate quality of health information on the internet: Chronicle of a voyage with an unclear destination. *British Medical Journal, 324,* 569–573.

Giles, J. (2005). Internet encyclopaedias go head to head. *Nature, 438*, 900–901.

Gugerty, B., & Sensmeier, J. (2010). Informatics competencies for nurse across roles and international boundaries. In C. A. Weaver, C. W. Delaney, P. Weber, & R. L. Carr (Eds.), *Nursing and informatics for the 21st century: An international look at practice, education and EHR trends* (2nd ed., pp. 129–144). Chicago, IL: Healthcare Information and Management Systems Society.

Hardiker, N. R., Casey, A., Coenen, A., & Konicek, D. (2006). Mutual enhancement of diverse terminologies. *American Medical Informatics Association Annual Symposium Proceedings Archive*, 319–323.

Hardiker, N. R., Derek, H., & Casey, A. (2000). Standards for nursing terminology. *Journal of the American Medical Informatics Association, 7*(6), 523–528.

Hoyt, R., Sutton, M., & Yoshihashi, A. (2007). *Medical informatics: Practical guide for the healthcare professional.* Retrieved from http://www.mse.mef.unizg.hr/msedb/slike/pisac21/file39p21.pdf

Interactive Advertising Bureau Canada. (2012). *Mobile in Canada: A summary of current facts + trends.* Retrieved from http://www.iabcanada.com/wp-ontent/uploads/2012/04/IABCanada_MobileInCanada_041012_FINAL.pdf

International Council of Nurses. (2009). *ICNP® Version 2.* Geneva, Switzerland: Author.

International Health Terminology Standards Development Organization. (2010). *SNOMED-CT.* Retrieved from http://www.ihtsdo.org/snomed-ct

International Organization for Standardization. (2003). *Health informatics—Integration of a reference terminology model for nursing (ISO 18104).* Geneva, Switzerland: Author.

Internet World Stats. (2010). *Usage and population statistics.* Retrieved from http://www.internetworldstats.com/

Kushniruk, A. (2011). The HIP competency framework: Applications to improve health informatics education and professionalism in Canada and internationally. *Healthcare Information Management and Communications Canada, 24*(4), 28–29.

Kushniruk, A. W., Borycki E., & Kuo, M. H. (2010). Advances in electronic health records in Denmark: From national strategy to effective healthcare system implementation. *Acta Informatica Medica, 18*(2), 99–102.

Kushniruk, A. W., Borycki, E. M., Kuwata, S., & Kannry, J. (2006). Predicting changes in workflow resulting from healthcare information systems: Ensuring the safety of healthcare. *Healthcare Quarterly, 9*, 78–82.

Kushniruk, A. W., Borycki, E. M., Kuwata, S., & Watanabe, H. (2008). Using a low cost simulation approach for assessing the impact of a medication administration workflow. *Studies in Health Technology and Informatics, 136*, 567–572.

Kushniruk, A. W., Triola, M., Borycki, E. M., Stein, B., & Kannry, J. (2005). Technology induced error and usability: The relationship between usability problems and prescription errors when using a handheld application. *International Journal of Medical Informatics, 74*(7–8), 519–526.

Kuziemsky, C. E., Borycki, E. M., Purkis, M. E., Black, F. M., Boyle, M., Cloutier-Fischer, D., . . . Wong, H. (2009). An interdisciplinary team communication framework and its application to healthcare 'e-teams' systems design. *BMC Medical Informatics and Decision Making, 15*, 9–43.

Marin, H. D. F., & Lorenzi, N. M. (2010). International initiatives in nursing informatics. In C. A. Weaver, C. W. Delaney, P. Weber, & R. L. Carr (Eds.), *Nursing informatics for the 21st century: An international look at practice, education and EHR trends* (2nd ed., pp. 45–52). Chicago, IL: Healthcare Information and Management Systems Society.

Martíínez, I., Trigo, J. D., Martínez-Espronceda, M., Escayola, P., Muñoz, P., Serrano, L., & García, J. (2009, September). *Integration proposal through standard-based design of an end-to-end platform for p-Health environments.* Paper presented at

31st Annual International Conference on the IEEE EMBS, Minneapolis, MN.

McCormick, K., Lang, N., Zielstorff, R., Milholland, D. K., Saba, V., & Jacox, A. (1994). Toward standard classification schemes for nursing language: Recommendations of the American Nurses Association Steering Committee on Databases to support clinical nursing practice. *Journal of the American Medical Informatics Association, 1*(6), 421–427.

MEDLINE. (2010). *Fact sheet: MEDLINE.* Retrieved from http://www.nlm.nih.gov/pubs/factsheets/medline.html

Milton, G. L. (2007). Information and human freedom: Nursing implications and ethical decision-making in the 21st century. *Nursing Science Quarterly, 20*(1), 33–36.

Moorhead, S., Johnson, M., Maas, M., & Swanson, E. (2008). *Nursing outcomes classification (NOC)* (4th ed.). St. Louis, MO: Mosby.

Mulla, F. (2010). *Success is not making money, it is making time.* Retrieved from http://faheemmulla.com/blog/?p=314

Müller-Staub, M., Needham, I., Odenbreit, M., Lavin, M. A., & van Achterberg, T. (2007). Improved quality of nursing documentation: Results of a nursing diagnosis, interventions and outcomes implementation study. *International Journal of Nursing Terminologies and Classifications, 18*(1), 5–17.

Nagle, L. M. (2007). Informatics: Emerging concepts and issues. *Nursing Leadership, 20*(1), 30–32.

Nagle, L. M., Marin, H. D. F., & Delaney, C. W. (2010). The Americas: Overview of HER national strategies and significance for nursing. In C. A. Weaver, C. W. Delaney, P. Weber, & R. L. Carr (Eds.), *Nursing informatics for the 21st century: An international look at practice, education, and EHR trends* (2nd ed., pp. 285–293). Chicago, IL: Healthcare Information and Management Systems Society.

Nahm, E. S., Vaydia, V., Ho, D., Scharf, B., & Seagull, J. (2007). Outcomes assessment of clinical information system implementation: A practical guide. *Nursing Outlook, 55*, 282–288.

Naisbitt, J. (1991). *Megatrends 2000: Ten new directions for the 1990's.* New York, NY: Morrow.

North American Nursing Diagnosis Association. (1987). *Taxonomy 1 with complete diagnosis.* St. Louis, MO: Author.

North American Nursing Diagnosis Association International. (2009). *NANDA-I Nursing diagnoses: Definitions and classification 2009–2011.* West Sussex, United Kingdom: Wiley.

Purvis, S., & Brenny-Fitzpatrick, M. (2010). Innovative use of electronic health record reports by clinical nurse specialists. *Clinical Nurse Specialist, 24*(6), 289–294.

Quan, S., Rossos, P. G., Kottachchi, D., Morra, D., & Cafazzo, J. A. (2010). Apples or BlackBerrys? Clinical use and evaluation of the iPhone platform in a BlackBerry-dominated hospital environment. *Electronic Healthcare, 9*(1), 3–8.

Rausch, T. L., & Judd, T. M. (2006, August/September). *The development of an interoperable roadmap for medical devices.* Paper presented at the Proceedings of the 28th IEEE EMBS Annual International Conference, New York, NY.

Saba, V. K. (2001). Nursing informatics: Yesterday, today, and tomorrow. *International Nursing Review, 48*, 177–187.

Sansoni, J., & Giustini, M. (2006). More than terminology: Using ICNP to enhance nursing's visibility in Italy. *International Nursing Review, 53*, 21–27.

Scholes, M., & Barber, B. (1980). Towards nursing informatics. In D. A. D. Lindberg & S. Kaihara (Eds.), *MedInfo 1980* (pp. 70–73). Amsterdam, The Netherlands: North-Holland.

Shortell, S. M., & Kaluzny, A. D. (2006). *Health care management: Organization design and behaviour* (5th ed.). Scarborough, ON: Delmar Thomson Learning.

Shortliffe, E. H., & Cimino, J. J. (2006). *Biomedical informatics: Computer applications in health care and biomedicine.* New York, NY: Springer Verlag.

Staggers, N., Gassert, C. A., & Curran, C. A. (2001). Informatics competencies for nurses at all four levels of practice. *Journal of Nursing Education, 40*, 303–316.

Stvilia, B., Twidale, M. B., Smith, L. C., & Gasser, L. (2008). Information quality work organizations in Wikipedia. *Journal of the American Society for Information Science and Technology, 59*(6), 983–2001.

Thede, L. O., & Sewell J. P. (2010). *Informatics and nursing.* Philadelphia, PA: Lippincott Williams & Wilkins.

Travers, D., & Mandelkehr, L. (2008). The emerging field of health informatics. *North Carolina Medical Journal, 69*(2), 127–131.

U.S. Government. (1995). *High performance computing and communication: Technology for the national information infrastructure.* Washington, DC: Author.

van Bemmel, J. H., & Musen, M. A. (1997). *Handbook of medical informatics.* Houten, The Netherlands: Bohn Stafleu van Loghum.

Walker, J. M., Bieber, E. J., & Richards, R. (2006). *Implementing and electronic health record system.* New York, NY: Springer Publishing.

Werley, H. H., Devine, E. C., Zorn, C. R., Ryan, P., & Westra, B. L. (1991). The nursing minimum data set: Abstraction tool for standardized, comparable, essential data. *The American Journal of Public Health, 81*(4), 421–426.

Zytkowski, M. E. (2003). Nursing informatics: The key to unlocking contemporary nursing practice. *AACN Clinical Issues, 14*(3), 271–281.

Reflection and Reflexivity: On Being a Nurse

JOY L. JOHNSON

Mathew, a senior nursing student, is midway through his 8-hour clinical day shift on a medical unit. It has been a challenging morning. One of his patients is confused and keeps trying to crawl out of bed. The patient's family is very upset with the use of restraints and has reported this to the nursing manager. Another patient is not tolerating his medication and has just vomited his breakfast all over his bed. Mathew dreads going into the room. On top of this, the porter has just arrived to transfer one of his patients for tests, and the patient is nowhere to be found. The porter is impatient and tells Mathew he may not be cut out to be a nurse. Mathew feels frustrated. The nurses he works with seem so much more advanced than him. He is not sure he even likes the work and realizes he is only half way through the morning!

CHAPTER OBJECTIVES

By the end of this chapter, you will be able to:

1. Describe why reflection is a key aspect of nursing practice.
2. Distinguish between reflection in action and reflection on action.
3. Apply reflective questioning to your own practice.
4. Identify key differences between novice and expert nurses.
5. Reflexively consider the assumptions that underlie your practice as a nurse.
6. Describe the key elements of effective or artful nursing practice.

KEY TERMS

Art of Nursing The art of nursing encompasses the capacity to carry out nursing procedures and techniques; developed dexterity or proficiency; the ability to connect with patients; the ability to critically think; and the integration of these principles, procedures, and techniques into one's nursing practice.

Othering Othering is a process that identifies those that are thought to be different from ourselves or the mainstream, and in so doing, reinforces and reproduces positions of power and subordination.

Reflection The process of wondering about a phenomenon and seeking a deeper understanding of it.

Reflection in Action Reflection that occurs in the moment as you are engaged in a particular action. This type of reflection helps us to think about whether we are getting things right.

Reflection on Action Reflection that occurs when we think back on what we have done and consider how what we did contributed to a particular outcome.

Reflexivity The process of critically considering and questioning the assumptions and values that motivate and underlie our nursing practice.

Through the eyes of a nurse

*T*he life of a nursing student is fascinating. You are faced with daily challenges and constantly confronted with new situations that will test your resolve to become a registered nurse. During your studies, you will likely find yourself asking, "Is nursing right for me? Do I have what it takes? Will I know what to do?" You might also find yourself thinking, "Nursing is not what I thought it would be." These reflections are entirely appropriate. Indeed, if you are asking these questions, then you are well on your way to becoming a nurse. In my view, an effective nurse is one who reflects on his practice and asks the hard questions.

(personal reflection of a nurse)

On Reflection, Reflexivity, and the Art of Nursing

The purpose of this chapter is to encourage reflection on questions and concerns that are central to nursing. **Reflection** is a process of wondering about a phenomenon and seeking a deeper understanding. This process is key to becoming an artful and skilled nurse. Artful nursing is complex and includes such things as manual skill, the ability to connect with patients, and the ability to critically think. It is the combination of all of these aspects that makes for an artful nurse (Fig. 25.1).

Although there are many questions that concern us as nurses, this chapter focuses on very broad questions, such as "What inspires nurses to seek a career in nursing?" "What is the nature of nursing?" "What core competencies are embedded in nursing practice?" "How do nursing skills develop over time?" "What are the special ways that nurses manage to care for patients' physical needs?" "What does artful or skillful nursing practice involve?" "How can a nurse develop reflective skills?" "How does reflexivity differ from reflection and how can it be honed?"

In this chapter, we reflect on some of the key factors that can shape one's nursing career. Questions are posed in order to encourage you to reflect on your own nursing practice. Reflection and reflexivity are essential skills for nurses and are explored in the following sections. The art of nursing is covered in depth in the latter portion of the chapter.

Reflection

There are aspects of nursing that cannot be taught. We can teach knowledge and skills; however, nursing students must learn to be nurses through observation, reflection, and practice. For example, we can teach the steps required to change a sterile dressing, but students learn through experience how to handle instruments, make meaningful observations about healing wounds, and respond to patients' questions. A fundamentals textbook provides you with rules, guidelines, and principles for how to perform various procedures. These guidelines and principles are necessary, particularly for the novice nurse, because they provide a foundation for how to proceed. The challenge is that guidelines based on sound scientific evidence are generally founded on what is required. But science and, in turn, guidelines provide directions about what commonly should take place, whereas nurses must deal with individual patients, not general situations. The rules must sometimes be adapted to meet the personal and contextual factors that shape the situation. This is why nurses need to develop and use their skills using reflection. Schön (1983) revolutionized the way we think about professional practice in *The Reflective Practitioner*. He argued that the practice arena is ever changing and increasingly complex. He also maintained that the situations we face in professional practice are not problems to be solved but rather problematic situations characterized by uncertainty, disorder, and indeterminacy. Schön recognized that a professional approach solely based on technical rationality, in which rules are applied to technical problems, is inadequate. Technical rationality is based on the premise that problem solving only requires adherence to a set of rules. An important assumption underlying this approach is that all elements of a situation can be predicted and controlled. Schön maintained that the thinking on one's feet that is required of a professional involves thinking about doing something while we are doing it. In so doing, we adjust our approach as we proceed. Accordingly, a practitioner's reflection in practice can serve as a corrective; we try something, observe the response, and modify our approach if required. Schön made an important distinction between reflection *on* action and reflection *in* action.

Reflection on Action

Reflection on action occurs when we think back on what we have done and consider how what we did contributed to a particular outcome. This type of reflection is valuable because it can help us learn and help us shape our future action.

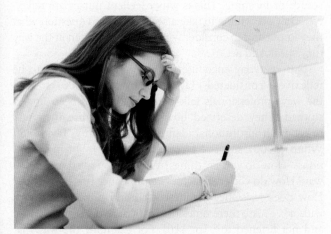

Figure 25.1 Writing, or "journaling," is a valuable exercise for a nurse to learn to be a reflective practitioner.

For example, after an encounter with a patient, you may want to ask yourself, "How did the patient respond to my actions? What could I have done differently?" Asking questions such as these can help us improve our practice. This is why nursing students are frequently asked to keep journals. Your professors and instructors want to understand the ways that you are reflecting on your practice. You can also reflect on action as you observe other nurses providing care and listen to your classmates discuss their clinical encounters. These observations provide valuable learning opportunities when you critically reflect on what you are observing or hearing, and by determining how your reflections can help shape your practice. A reflection on an action you observe might be as simple as, "I will never do that to a patient!" But your learning can be extended by considering what might have motivated the action you observed and why the action you observed was problematic. Reflection is a skill that can be honed, and students should be encouraged to work diligently to develop these skills.

Think Thompson and Thompson (2008) suggested three simple questions that can be used to help one reflect on one's practice:
- *What?* (What happened?—Think about the key details; try to consider multiple perspectives.)
- *So what?* (Reflect on what occurred by thinking about what motivated the actions and how the situation could have been different.)
- *Now what?* (Formulate an action plan by determining how you will approach a similar situation in the future or by identifying the knowledge and skills you need to develop.)

Reflection in Action

Reflection in action occurs in the moment as you are engaged in a particular action. This type of reflection helps us to think about whether we are getting things right. Is the patient responding the way you expect? How can you adjust your approach to obtain a better result? Often, novice nurses just want to get through a situation and rush through the procedure without taking the time to pay attention to how the patient is responding. This is the paradox of nursing: Initially, the skills seem to be the most important thing to master, but eventually, these skills are second nature and do not need to be the focus of attention. As you learn new skills, intentionally practice shifting your focus from the skill at hand to the patient's response. Schön (1983) likened reflection in action to an "on the spot experiment"; you try something and observe its effect.

Reflexivity

Whereas reflection involves asking questions about what we have done or are doing, **reflexivity** moves us deeper into critically considering and questioning the assumptions and values that motivate and underlie our nursing practice. This process pushes us to be aware of our own interests and motivations and, in particular, to consider the power, privilege, and biases that may affect our interactions with

TABLE 25.1	Comparing Reflection and Reflexivity
Reflection	• Considering the key elements of a situation, asking questions about what factors led to particular outcomes • Determining what different types of actions might be taken in the future
Reflexivity	• Considering taken-for-granted assumptions • Asking questions about what might underlie our actions or the practices in a system • Critically determining what personal or system changes might need to be made

our patients. A reflexive approach compels us to interrogate previously taken-for-granted assumptions and to question the broader societal discourses that influence the way we perceive certain situations. See Table 25.1 for a comparison of the concepts of reflection and reflexivity.

Through the eyes of a nurse

I recently encountered a nursing student who was discussing the clinical experiences to which she had been assigned. She indicated that she "loved nursing" but was not enjoying her clinical experience in a particular hospital because it largely involved caring for the elderly and for new immigrants with poor English language skills. She intended no malice in sharing this impression with me, but I left this conversation troubled and hoping that she might find cause to reflect on what she had said.
(personal reflection of a nurse)

The way we act, the things we say, and the way we say them reveal our knowledge; in this way, we might say that in nursing practice, we embody our knowledge in our actions. Much of this knowledge is implicit and is learned through observation or experience. It is problematic, however, to simply act on this tacit knowledge without considering its source or meaning. This is why excellent nurses are reflexive. They are willing to take a second look, to question what they know, and to consider what might be hidden in the way they speak and act.

Our everyday encounters with our patients need to be reflexively considered. Taylor and White (2000) studied the ways professionals talk—an area that has been understudied. They described how professionals use their talk to establish institutional identity and authority. Taylor and White (2000) suggested considering the following questions: "How do you say things? Why do you say them in that way? How do you try to achieve compliance from [patients]? How does resistance manifest itself and how do you deal with it? . . . Are there times that patients' voices are silenced and not listened to?" (p. 116). For example, the way that nurses dispense information to patients often suggests that there is no room for patients to question what is being said.

In subtle ways, the talk of nurses might discount particular patients, especially those with less privilege or power. In developing reflexive practice, you can pay attention to your own professional talk.

Through the eyes of a nurse

*I*n my own practice, I have found myself on occasion making assumptions about a person based on her diagnosis or appearance. For example, I have observed nurses making assumptions about patients based on how they are dressed. One common example is assuming that a patient dressed in a sari (traditional Indian clothing) does not speak English.

(personal reflection of a nurse)

A study focused on South Asian women's interactions with health-care providers found that providers engaged in several othering practices (Johnson et al., 2004). **Othering** is a process that identifies those that are thought to be different from ourselves or the mainstream, and in so doing, reinforces and reproduces positions of power and subordination. The analysis revealed that the health-care providers in the study made overgeneralizations about culture, race, and health-care practices. They made claims such as, "South Asian women do not do breast self-examinations" or "South Asians are the most noncompliant patients I have ever come across." At times, these statements were overtly racist or had strong racist undertones. The health professionals who made these statements were concerned professionals and likely had no awareness of how their talk could serve to marginalize or hurt others. This is why reflexivity is so important. When we make observations about certain "types" of patients or when we express reluctance to care for someone, for whatever reason, it is time to reflect on what is underlying our assumption.

Through the eyes of a nurse

*E*arly in my nursing career, I cared for a patient recovering from surgery who also had a diagnosis of schizophrenia. He was recovering well from his surgery and was going to be discharged home to the group home where he lived. I was to do the discharge teaching. I had met and cared for patients with schizophrenia in my rotations as a nursing student but on reflection had not yet grasped that the diagnosis does not affect intelligence. In performing my discharge teaching with this patient, I oversimplified the instructions and kept asking him if he was following my instructions. The patient had read the discharge information in the pamphlet I provided him and understood what I was doing and told me that he was not "stupid." This is one example where I needed to reconsider the assumptions I was making about the patients I was caring for.

(personal reflection of a nurse)

Think about a time when the way you cared for someone may have unintentionally reflected biases or unfounded assumptions about that person. What can you learn from this reflection?

The Multifaceted Qualities and Skills of the Nurse

It is particularly worthwhile to reflect on what motivated us to enter the nursing profession. We all have our reasons for pursuing a career in nursing. In a recent video entitled, *Reasons for Becoming a Nurse*, the woman on the video emphasized factors such as flexible hours, job opportunities, and good pay. Although all of these reasons might be important, sustaining a career in nursing requires consideration of more than working conditions or benefits. Nursing is demanding, and if you are not committed to the profession for reasons beyond those mentioned in the video, there could be a misfit with your interests, values, skills, and desires—a career in nursing could quickly become unsatisfying.

The ways in which we describe our day and the work we do influence others. In order to shape the next generation of nurses, it can help to share with others the aspects of your nursing practice that you love. Our passion for our work is an important impetus for our own actions and for those of future nurses.

Think Consider what inspired you to become a nurse. What was it about nursing that appealed to you? Was there a particular person who influenced your decision? How do you see yourself inspiring others to consider a career in nursing?

Being a Nurse

A central question that confronts all nurses is, "What does it mean to *be* a nurse?" On the face of this, it might appear to be a simple question, and yet if one ponders the question long enough, the answer seems more and more complex. We can describe what nurses do and their various roles and responsibilities, but considering what it means to be a nurse suggests a more philosophical question. It is a question to return to many times over a career, and it is one that all nurses should consider and reconsider. Making an allowance for the evolving answers to this question can help to ground us as nurses and provide us with direction for action.

We will be asked to do many things as nurses. Demands will be placed on us by patients, families, other professionals, management, industry representatives, governments, professional organizations, and others, and we need to ask ourselves whether what we are being asked to do fits within the scope of nursing. For example, at one time, the nurses in one of the mental health facilities in British Columbia had the regular night shift duty of rolling cigarettes for the patients.

They were likely told this needed to be done and so filled the void. Through hindsight, we realize that what these nurses were doing was likely not an activity that nurses should assume, and it points to the need for all of us to reflect on the nature of nursing. In doing so, we imply questions about the dimensions of nursing practice and what is expected of nurses. Considering the answer to what it means to be a nurse also provides a yardstick against which to measure ourselves.

Beyond Nursing Regulations

As specified by regulatory agencies, the scope of nursing practice is the level of responsibility or health services a nurse is legally authorized to provide, including procedures, actions, and processes. Although nursing regulatory bodies set out the minimum educational requirements, competencies, and standards required for practice, their approach is based on legislation and regulatory frameworks. The scopes of practice change from time to time, and how they are determined results from careful consideration by policy makers, in consultation and negotiation with other stakeholders, including other health professionals and the public. This collaboration ensures that attention has been given to how a change (i.e., in what practitioners can do) would affect the profession seeking the change, other health-care professions, the broader health-care system, and the potential for risk to the public. Although we must practice within the scope of these legal frameworks, we cannot assume that this approach is enough to guide us in our actions. These frameworks are very broad in nature and do not tell us what nurses should do in individual situations nor is it expected that all nurses will be competent to carry out the full scope of practice as specified within these regulatory frameworks. It is the individual registered nurse's responsibility to determine what to do in particular situations and whether they are competent to carry out a particular activity.

The importance of competency surfaces consistently when nurses talk about effective patient care. In a study on the meaning of effective patient care, Hogston (1995) interviewed nurses and found that competence is a key ingredient in the provision of high-quality care. A nurse in Hogston's (1995) study commented, "I tend to think of [quality] as the standard that you would want to receive yourself. . . . " This is an important insight. Although it is worthwhile to reflect on the care we would like to receive should we become ill, we must also consider the unique care requirements that our patients might have. We cannot assume that what works for us will work for our patients or that what works for one patient will work for others.

Competencies Required for Nursing Practice

Benner (1984) was one of the first nurses to describe the competencies embedded in nursing practice. Based on interviews with nurses and observations of nursing practice, she identified seven domains of competencies:

1. The helping role,
2. The teaching or coaching function,
3. The diagnostic monitoring function,
4. Effective management of rapidly changing situations,
5. Administering and monitoring therapeutic interventions and therapeutics,
6. Monitoring and ensuring the quality of health-care practices, and
7. Organizational and work-role competencies.

To demonstrate the competencies associated with each domain, Benner (1984) used exemplars. She suggested that because knowledge is embedded in practice, these stories or exemplars are necessary to demonstrate the competency. As an example, a competency in the domain of the helping role is *providing comfort measures and preserving personhood in the face of pain and extreme breakdown*. Consider how this competency is embedded in the following exemplar in which a nurse described providing care to a patient with diabetes who was blind and gravely ill.

> Expert nurse: And that day, we washed her hair, which hadn't been washed in weeks. We got her up out of bed and sat her up. She just loved to get up off her back. She had been so sick and forced to be on her back; she had a decubitus [pressure ulcer] forming. And any little thing that we did for her—wash her hair, set her up, and take her limbs through range of motion—was just a delight for her. And she let us know that. She told me just how wonderful it was to have people read to her, so I did bring a book in. She had told me about a book she was interested in, and her cousin, who was a student nurse here, and I would take turns reading to her and she just loved that. (Benner, 1984, p. 56)

This exemplar is powerful because it not only demonstrates the relevant competencies (e.g., bathing, skin care, range-of-motion exercises, comfort measures) but also demonstrates that expert nurses do not lose sight of the way that small gestures can make a significant difference in a patient's life.

Through the eyes of a patient

In the recent past, my sister-in-law was diagnosed with leukemia and had a bone marrow transplant. She was hospitalized for close to 3 months, and we visited her almost daily; we often stepped in to perform small tasks, such as giving her back rubs and mouth care. We were concerned about her feet because she was immunocompromised, and there was a concern that she might have been developing a fungal infection in her feet. We decided to give her regular foot care. I will never forget the day a nurse walked in and, on seeing us providing foot care, proclaimed, "Oh, it's spa day!" This declaration saddened me because the nurse could not "read" the situation. She did not understand what her patient required and thus saw the provision of foot care as a luxury rather than as a necessary and routine preventative measure.

(personal reflection of a patient's family member)

From Novice to Expert

As nurses, it is important to reflect on our knowledge, skills and abilities, and how we gain expertise over time. Benner's (1984) book, *From Novice to Expert*, illuminated the results of a study that she conducted about the knowledge embedded in clinical nursing practice. She recognized that nurses accrue practical knowledge over time. She was particularly interested in the "know-how" that nurses develop and noted that this type of knowledge is very different from "know-that" knowledge. A fundamentals textbook provides practical fact-based knowledge. Know-that knowledge can be written about or repeated to others, but know-how can only be developed through practice. For example, you might read about the principles involved in changing a sterile dressing, but the more complete knowledge and understanding of actually changing a dressing can only be developed by practice. Benner recognized this important distinction and described how nurses develop expertise overtime. She identified five stages of expertise (Table 25.2).

It is important to recognize that a novice nurse will necessarily depend on procedures and rules. Fundamental nursing textbooks provide the steps that need to be followed to perform particular skills.

TABLE 25.2	Benner's Five Stages of Expertise
Stage	**Characteristics**
The novice	Lacks experience Uses rules to guide practice Does not necessarily pick up on contextual cues Uses attributes of a situation or measurable parameters to make decisions
The advanced beginner	Has enough real-life experience to understand the meaning of contextual cues Can develop guidelines for action Starts to hone ability to identify relevant aspects of a situation
The competent practitioner	Sees actions in relation to long-term goals or plans Able to outline most important aspects of the situation Uses conscious, deliberate planning Is efficient and organized Knows what to expect in a typical patient's situation Can modify plans when expectations are not met
The proficient practitioner	Perceives situations as a whole Understands long-term implications Knows how to read nuances Decision-making is less laboured Can quickly decide what is required
The expert	Does not always rely on rules to connect the understanding to a situation Has an intuitive grasp Able to quickly zero in on what is required

Source: Benner, P. (1984). *From novice to expert: Excellence and power in clinical nursing practice*. Menlo Park, CA: Addison-Wesley.

Another important insight of Benner (1984) is that expertise is gained not with the passing of time or by merely putting in the hours but rather by reflecting on and refining one's understanding of nursing practice and gaining new knowledge through practice. Nurses who have different levels of expertise analyse situations differently. Whereas a competent nurse might use problem-solving and analytic strategies to decide what a patient needs, the expert nurse might sense what is required, have trouble explaining her specific reasoning, and only retrospectively be able to articulate what course of action was taken. This means that you should not always expect to practice at the same level of proficiency that the registered nurses you observe and work with possess. Your skills will develop over time, with experience and education combined with reflection and reflexivity. To develop expertise, you simultaneously reflect on your practice and develop your reflective skills.

Bodies and Physical Care

Although many professions deal with body parts (ears, eyes, bones), nurses are concerned with the entire body and all of its functions. The relationship between a nurse and a patient is unlike others because it is often formed when a patient is particularly vulnerable. As a nurse, you will see patients in defenseless situations, and you will be expected to assist them with many aspects of body care. It is important to reflect on the proximity and intimacy that you will have with your patients. This relationship is a privilege, and it is an aspect of nursing that is often downplayed or not spoken about directly. Lawler (1991) recognized that care for the body is a topic that is often off limits, so she set out to study the ways that nurses negotiate various norms, values, taboos, beliefs, and ways of behaving with respect to the body. In the context of hospitalization, patients can require assistance with routine tasks such as going to the toilet, showering, or cleaning one's teeth.

Through the eyes of a student

As a nursing student, I recall being concerned about what I would do when I needed to insert a urinary catheter in a male patient. Similarly, I recall fretting that I was not strong enough to be a nurse when I felt faint after seeing (and smelling) a seriously infected leg ulcer. The first bedpans I emptied were a real "wake-up call" to those aspects of nursing that are often not discussed in the classroom or elsewhere.

(personal reflection of a nursing student)

Lawler (1991) recognized that despite the awareness that a patient is not just a body, at times, nurses need to get through a particular procedure by focusing on the routine of that procedure. In her research, she observed the speed and ease with which many nurses approached and made sense of their patients' vulnerability. She recounted the problems nurses face when we care for bodies and the ways patient care can be managed more effectively. In her book, Lawler described so-mological practices that nurses use when providing physical care. Some of the most promising strategies that nurses use to protect their patients when providing physical care follow.

Minifisms

Lawler (1991) coined the term *minifism* to capture the ways that nurses manage potentially problematic, embarrassing, or distressing situations, such as a patient with a bed full of feces or a large pool of blood on the floor. Minifisms involve verbally minimizing the size, severity, or significance of a particular event. These techniques help the nurse to bring a situation under control. An example of a minifism is a statement such as, "Oh dear, a bit of a mess. We will have this cleaned up in no time." This strategy minimizes the patient's embarrassment and also can mask the nurse's shock or displeasure at what must be done. Nurses use mini-fisms to diffuse their own responses to unpleasant situations and to reduce patient stress and anxiety about their vulner-ability and embarrassment. It is an equalizer for the patient in an unfamiliar social setting. Although some might argue that the use of minifisms is inauthentic because they mask the feelings of the nurse, it is worth considering the burden placed on patients when such views are shared.

Through the eyes of a student

I was to change the dressing covering an ulcer on a patient's leg. A nurse was to accompany me to help guide me through the complicated process. I had been told the ulcer was very "mucky." I had never seen any-thing like it though. It was oozing green serous fluid and was black in the middle, and it smelled. The patient was very anxious and wanted to know if the smell bothered me and what I thought about the wound. The nurse sensed my discomfort and stepped in quickly and said, "Oh, we hardly smell a thing, and I can see a little pink (pointing to the wound) here." The patient smiled and seemed to relax.

(personal reflection of a nursing student)

Asking Visitors to Leave

Another important strategy for body care involves guarding the patient's privacy. Lawler (1991) pointed out that asking visitors to leave the room during intimate care not only saves the patient from embarrassment but can also help the nurse minimize his or her own potential embarrassment. Perform-ing body care is often easier when there is no audience.

Discourse Privatization

Lawler (1991) uses discourse to refer to the discussions that nurses have with their patients. It is sometimes very easy to forget that on a day-to-day basis, nurses deal with very private matters. Nurses also protect patients by ensuring that discussions about their patients' bodily functions are

restricted to the patient and nurse. Nurses do this by talk-ing in a quiet voice only to the patient or speaking with the patient away from the hearing of others.

Through the eyes of a patient

I recall visiting my grandfather in the hospital, and the nurse came in, interrupting the conversation, and asked him in a loud voice, "Have your bowels moved?" Grandfather was a very proper man, and this embarrassed him and me.

(personal reflection of a patient's family member)

Managing Nauseating Situations and Body Products

Lawler (1991) noted that there are symbolic systems that govern approaches to body products. Symbolic systems are used when we are unable or unwilling to directly address a phenomenon. For example, many people are reluctant to use or are unaware of the technical terms for feces, urine, penis, vagina, etc. and instead use gestures or nicknames to express themselves.

Body products such as sputum and feces can be diffi-cult for anyone to encounter. Nurses, however, recognize that patients should be protected from the perception that a particular task is difficult or unpleasant. Some of the ways nurses manage are to focus on the details of the task, to take time out by offering a plausible excuse ("I need another towel, back in a minute"), or to focus on the experience of the patient instead of their own concerns.

Lawler's (1991) research shed light on an area of nursing practice that is not often talked about but that is extremely important to the provision of patient care. The strategies she described may provide a useful starting point as you con-sider how you will manage the physical care of patients. In the end, every nurse needs to determine his or her own strategies for managing difficult situations and in protecting patients.

Think What types of strategies do you use to manage potentially difficult or embarrassing situations that involve providing physical care to your patients?

The Art of Nursing: What Does It Mean to Be a Really Great Nurse?

Nurses are not merely technicians; they cannot simply select from a list of interventions and apply them to a patient. There is an art involved in providing excellent care for our patients that encompasses knowledge, judgment, and skill. Early in my career, I was intrigued by the notion of how we know what to do when we practice nursing and was motivated to study the **art of nursing**. I conducted a philosophical study in which I set out to consider the ways that nursing art has been conceptualized by nursing scholars from the time of Florence Nightingale into the modern era (Johnson, 1994). The study brought to light five separate senses of nursing art, each of which is an important ingredient in providing excellent or artful care (summarized in Table 25.3).

The Ability to Find Meaning in Patient Encounters

When a nurse walks into a patient's room, how does he or she decide what to do first? The situations that confront us as nurses are complex and often characterized by uncertainty. There is much to take in, including the patient's physical position, his or her demeanour, extent of colour in the skin, facial expression, the state of the room, the state of the equipment, the emotional comportment of the patient, what the patient is saying, and who else is present. This situation is further complicated when patients cannot express their needs, as is the case with infants or unconscious patients. In these complex contexts, the nurse must grasp the meaning of the situation and determine what is relevant. The process of grasping meaning involves determining the significance of what we see, hear, touch, and smell, including emotions, objects, gestures, and sounds. This ability involves an immediate perceptual capacity—the nurse sees and understands. It is the artful nurse who can sense patterns or have a feel

for what is required. The meanings that the nurse derives are often difficult to express in language; they are tacit and derived from an intuitive capacity. The nurse learns to recognize patterns and therefore makes sense of ambiguous, unstructured situations. An important feature of this aspect of nursing art is that it is holistic. Rather than engaging in incremental, deliberative analysis, the situation is grasped as a whole. This type of capacity can be honed or developed. Over time, a nurse learns to become sensitive to the signals and feelings that he or she is experiencing.

The Ability to Establish a Meaningful Connection With the Patient

Nurses often have a great deal on their minds. They have many tasks to accomplish and many demands placed on them. When we care for a patient and are rushed or impatient, the patient senses our irritability. Similarly, patients know when our minds are elsewhere; they can be made to feel invisible and that their concerns do not matter. An effective connection between a nurse and a patient is an essential element of artful nursing practice. This connection can be fleeting or long term and provides the vehicle through which physical and emotional support is offered. This form of nursing art is expressed in a nurse's actions. The connection cannot be expressed through words; rather, the connection is lived between

TABLE 25.3 Dimensions of the Art of Nursing	
The Five Senses of Nursing Art	**The Artful Nurse**
The ability to grasp meaning in patient encounters	• Determines the significance of what is seen, heard, touched, and smelled • Determines the significance of emotions, objects, gestures, and sounds • Takes in the whole patient • Grasps meaning • Senses patterns • Uses intuitive capacity • Uses a holistic approach
The ability to establish a meaningful connection with the patient	• Creates a quality connection with the patient • Expresses authentic concern, compassion, and care • Is emotionally sensitive to other human beings • Is affirming patients as human beings • Makes a genuine connection • Lets go of other concerns and tasks while caring for the patient • Pays attention to what a patient is saying
The ability to skillfully perform nursing activities	• Develops skills dexterity or proficiency • Integrates principles, procedures, and techniques into practice • Seamlessly integrates principles into action • Develops patient-centered goals
The ability to rationally determine an appropriates course of nursing action	• Has a keen intellect • Is action-oriented and focused on producing particular outcomes • Uses interventions and ends reasoning • Has an action orientation • Has a vision for the patient • Applies logical reasoning
The ability to morally conduct one's practice	• Avoids harm to patients • Strives to benefit the patient • Makes moral choices in the performance of care • Is committed to providing competent care for patients • Sustains excellent practice • Is caring and concerned for others

human beings and is evident in the synchronicity between the nurse and the patient. The nurse's words and behaviour give communicable form to the knowledge of this connection.

The authentic concern, compassion, and care that the nurse expresses are evidence of this nursing art. Scott (2000) identified that an important aspect of good nursing is having an emotional sensitivity to other human beings. This form of nursing art is based on affirming patients as human beings and not treating them as objects. The work of Buber (1958) is often invoked when discussing this form of connection. Buber contrasted two forms of relationships: "I–it" and "I–thou." I–it relationships are subject-to-object relationships and arise from a stance of separation and detachment. It is very easy to slip into this stance when encountering any patient who does not fit the mould of the good patient: those who act out, complain, or do not comply with treatments or directions. The I–thou relationship is one of subject-to-subject relationship and is premised on a notion of connectedness and affirmation of another person's being.

Making a Genuine Connection

An essential element of establishing genuine connections is being sincere and authentic. Rather than playing the role of a nurse, the artful nurse *is* a nurse. It is evident to the patient when we are inauthentic and pretend to show concern or compassion. In turn, this can create a distance between our patients and us. Parse (1992) referred to the preferred type of connection as a genuine or true presence. True presence involves letting go of other concerns and tasks, paying attention to what a patient is saying, and responding based on what you honestly think or feel. When we are truly present, we are not reciting a scripted response, such as "The doctor will take care of that," but instead are focused and engaged.

The Ability to Skillfully Perform Nursing Activities

The ability to hear a heart murmur, distinguish different breath sounds, start an intravenous drip, or insert a nasogastric tube are all important elements of nursing practice. Often, nursing students focus on these skills and are unable to attend to the other elements of nursing art. When focused on doing a sterile dressing, it is easy to forget to pay attention to what is happening to the patient. Skills are important, but alone, they are not enough. The artful nurse has the capacity to carry out nursing procedures and techniques. Skill refers to a developed dexterity or proficiency and is a behavioural ability. Skillful nursing practice involves integrating principles, procedures, and techniques into one's nursing practice. A nurse may know what to do and can recite the steps of a procedure, but the art of nursing involves seamlessly integrating these principles into action.

Skillful nursing practice can be developed over time. This is why students are encouraged to practice procedures in the context of virtual or clinical simulation labs. Learners should actively seek opportunities to use their skills in the real world of the clinical setting. There are certain qualities that we look for in this form of nursing art. These include fluidity of movement, coordination, and efficiency. When

a novice nurse is observed returning to a supply cupboard several times over the course of a procedure and he fumbles with equipment, makes an error in a procedure, or seems to run out of hands, there is evidence that the art of skillfully performing the nursing activity has not been mastered.

For a nursing student, there are many skills to acquire. It is easy to become overly focused on the skills and proficiency and lose sight of the fact that these skills are means to an end. We learn to do particular things to help patients to regain their health. If we lose sight of the particular patient-centered goals, then we are in danger of becoming mere technicians. It is easy to become preoccupied in completing tasks efficiently, but a good nurse does so while paying attention to the patient's other needs.

The Ability to Rationally Determine an Appropriate Course of Nursing Action

Nursing art is not only a matter of intuiting, connecting, and performing skills. An artful nurse must also have a keen intellect and use it. Nurses face complex problems and must reason through what should be done; this form of nursing art is action-oriented and involves producing particular outcomes. For example, when we realize that a patient's blood pressure is rapidly dropping, we must rationally determine what should be done to stabilize the patient (the desired outcome). Thinking through what might be causing the blood pressure to drop (vasodilation, fluid loss) and how to mitigate the effects of the drop in blood pressure (increase the intravenous fluid flow, place the patient flat) are aspects of determining an appropriate course of action. This aspect of nursing art relies heavily on evidence, specifically scientific evidence. Orem (1988) noted that science is a first and necessary condition for nursing art. Nursing research produces knowledge that can help a nurse think through an appropriate action. This form of nursing art is about means and ends reasoning. A nurse must think through the goals he or she has for a patient and determine what means (interventions) could be used to help the patient achieve those goals. This is why nurses create nursing care plans—these plans provide evidence of the goals they have set for their patients and the interventions selected for achieving those goals.

The action orientation of nursing is an important consideration but is often forgotten. Nursing is not simply a matter of blindly following procedures, doling out medications, and getting through a shift with all patients alive and accounted for. Artful nurses have a vision for each of their patients and work toward helping patients realize particular goals. To determine a course of action, the artful nurse applies logical reasoning in determining which scientific principles and theories are applicable to the problems identified in their practice. When nursing instructors inquire about your plans for a patient or ask about why you are taking a particular course of action, they are helping you to hone this skill. This form of nursing art can be judged according to whether an appropriate course of action was selected and ultimately according to whether the identified goals were achieved.

The Ability to Morally Conduct One's Practice

An artful nurse, like any good practitioner, practices in such a way that seeks to avoid harm and to benefit the patient. Because nursing involves human action, and this action affects other humans, it is by nature a moral endeavor. Good nursing and moral nursing practice are synonymous. Nurses may be technically competent and knowledgeable, but if they do not make moral choices in the performance of their care, then they are not artful. This form of nursing art presupposes that one has the necessary skills to practice. Benner (2001) drew on the Aristotelian distinction of *techne*, the knowing required for the making of outcomes, and *phronesis*, the knowing that requires moral agency, discernment, and relationship, and she argued that nursing as a practice requires both these forms of knowing.

A key ingredient in the moral aspect of nursing art is a commitment to providing competent care for patients. This means sustaining excellent practice even when we are tired, facing staffing shortages, or when we receive no acknowledgment for our efforts. The artful nurse is not motivated by self-aggrandizement but instead is motivated by care and concern for others. It is this concern that helps us to pay attention to the necessary details and that guides our caregiving.

Conclusion

This chapter posed several questions. The important message for you is that these are questions that all nurses should ponder from time to time. Being a nurse is multifaceted. As is emphasized throughout this textbook, nursing involves knowing, thinking, being, interacting, and understanding. Nursing care will continue to change and evolve, but these essential elements remain constant. All nurses must commit to lifelong learning. Two essential tools assist you in the process of continuing to learn: reflection and reflexivity. Increasingly, the regulatory colleges or associations of the provinces and territories of Canada include reflective practice–identified strengths, limitations, and learning needs as components of the strategies employed for continued competence. The identification of reflective practice as an expectation of the practicing nurse illustrates the extent to which the concept of reflection has been accepted by the profession of nursing.

Now that Mathew understands that it is unfair to compare himself to expert nurses, he is feeling better. He has the tools to help him to reflect on his challenging day. He realizes he has learned a lot and that he will do things differently next time. He is prepared to deal with the vomit in the bed without embarrassing the patient. He considers what it must be like for the family who has a love one restrained and realizes he could have done a better job of explaining the situation and empathizing with their concerns. He realizes he is a nurse in the making.

Critical Thinking Case Scenario

▶ A psychiatrist was heard to recently state that he found it ironic that one of the easiest tasks for nurses—administering medications—seemed to be something that nurses spent the most time on, whereas one of the most difficult tasks—having meaningful therapeutic interactions with patients—was often left to care aides. One could easily dismiss this comment as an uninformed observation of a physician. But instead, this observation pushes us to consider why this was the case. What assumptions do we make about medication administration? Why is it that we do not readily engage therapeutically with our patients? It is a lack of time or a lack of skill or confidence? Reflexive practice necessitates willingness to question or reconsider aspects of our practice that we often take for granted.

▶ Compare and contrast the following two scenarios. How are the approaches different?

Expert nurse: I walked into Mrs. Nguyen's room and sensed immediately that something was wrong. She was postoperative day 2 and was diaphoretic and pale. I quickly reached for the blood pressure cuff while asking her if she was feeling okay. She was drowsy. Her blood pressure was lower than normal. I turned up the volume of her IV, put the call bell on, and asked the unit clerk to call the resident immediately. I had seen a situation like this before and knew the patient could crash quickly.

Nursing student: I walked into the room and told Mrs. Nguyen that I would be her nursing student for the day. She seemed very drowsy, but it was early in the morning. I proceeded with taking the required vital signs and found them all to be within normal range, although her blood pressure was a bit lower than it had been. I completed my head to toe assessment; all the while, Mrs. Nguyen seemed to become more and more drowsy. I had trouble waking her and decided to go speak to the assigned registered nurse. I thought perhaps the effects of her sleeping pill had not worn off.

Multiple-Choice Questions

1. Which of the following is an aspect of the art of nursing?
   a. Technical proficiency
   b. Ability to forge a personal connection with patients
   c. Critical thinking
   d. All of the above

2. Kayla says, "Indian patients are so stubborn! I feel like I always need to convince them to do anything, even though it's all for their own good." What is Kayla exhibiting here?
   a. Subordinating
   b. Othering
   c. Reflecting
   d. Assuming

3. Joseph is changing the sheets on his patient's bed. As he works, he watches his patient's face for signs of discomfort or nervousness, ready to change his methods, or stop for a moment if necessary. What is Joseph doing?
   a. Othering
   b. Reflection on action
   c. Reflection in action
   d. Technical rationality

4. In the text, three simple questions are suggested to help in reflection on action. Which of the following is NOT one of the questions?
   a. So what?
   b. What?
   c. Who?
   d. Now what?

5. Which of the following did Benner identify as core competencies of nursing practice?
   a. Diagnosing/monitoring
   b. Coaching/teaching
   c. Administering therapies
   d. All of the above

6. On a particularly busy morning, Ginny comes into Mrs. Morgan's room to find her crying; she has accidentally bumped her breakfast tray, pulling her orange juice, oatmeal, and milk all over herself. Ginny says, "No worries! Let me just pop out for some towels and clean sheets and we'll have this taken care of in a moment." Which of the following best describes Ginny's response?
   a. Artfulness
   b. Efficiency
   c. Minifism
   d. Othering

REFERENCES AND SUGGESTED READINGS

Benner, P. (1984). *From novice to expert: Excellence and power in clinical nursing practice*. Menlo Park, CA: Addison-Wesley.

Benner, P. (2001). The roles of embodiment, emotion and life-world for rationality and agency in nursing practice. *Nursing Philosophy, 1,* 5–19.

Buber, M. (1958). *I and thou* (2nd ed.; R. G. Smith, Trans.). New York, NY: Charles Scribner's Sons.

Hogston, R. (1995). Quality nursing care: A qualitative enquiry. *Journal of Advanced Nursing, 21,*116–124.

Johnson, J. L. (1994). A dialectical examination of the art of nursing. *Advances in Nursing Science, 17,* 1–14.

Johnson, J. L., Bottorff, J. L., Browne, A. J., Grewal, S., Hilton, B. A., & Clarke, H. (2004). Othering and being othered in the context of health care service. *Health Communication, 16,*253–271.

Lawler, J. (1991). *Behind the screens: Nursing, somology and the problem of the body*. Harlow, United Kingdom: Churchill Livingstone, Medical Division of Longman Group.

Nelson, S., & Purkis, M. E. (2004). Mandatory reflection: The Canadian reconstitution of the competent nurse. *Nursing Inquiry, 11,* 247–257.

Orem, D. E. (1988). The form of nursing science. *Nursing Science Quarterly, 1,* 75–79.

Parse, R. R. (1992). Human becoming: Parse's theory of nursing. *Nursing Science Quarterly, 5,* 35–42.

Schön, D. A. (1983). *The reflective practitioner: How professionals think in action*. New York, NY: Basic Books.

Scott, A. (2000). Emotion, moral perception, and nursing practice. *Nursing Philosophy, 1,* 123–133.

Taylor, C., & White, S. (2000). *Practising reflexivity in health and welfare: Making knowledge*. Buckingham, United Kingdom: Open University Press.

Thompson, S., & Thompson, N. (2008). *The critically reflective practitioner*. Basingstoke, United Kingdom: Palgrave MacMillan.

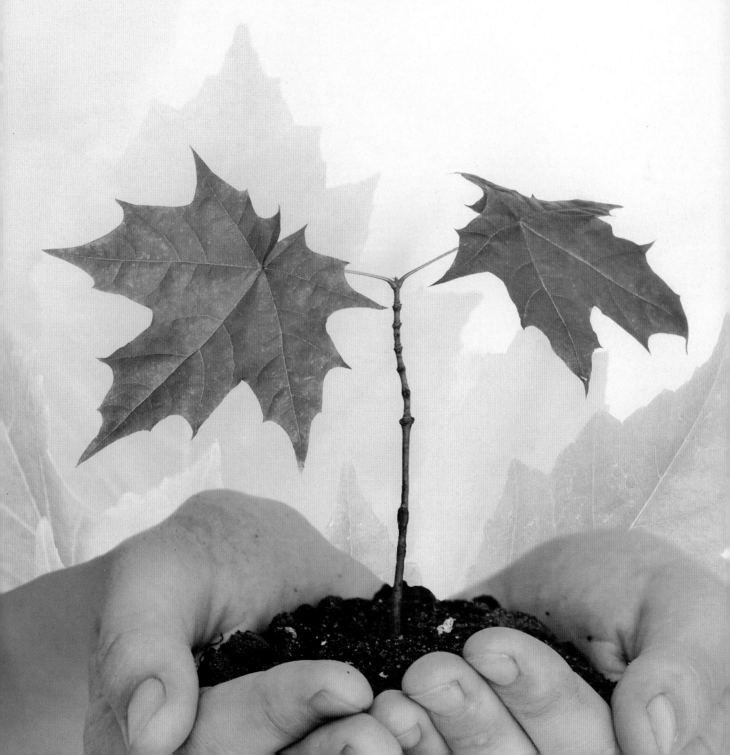

four
Interacting

Communication: At the Heart of Nursing Practice

ANDREA CHUTE

Makenzie is a first-year nursing student in a Bachelor of Science in Nursing program. As part of the program requirements, Makenzie is required to complete a professional communication course. On the first day of class, the professor poses the following question: "If this communication course were offered as an elective, how many of you would take it as part of your nursing program?" Makenzie responds, "We already know how to communicate. We have been communicating all our lives." The professor then poses the following questions for Makenzie and classmates to think about.

What can you tell me about the stages and competencies a nurse is expected to foster within a therapeutic relationship?

How does nonverbal communication influence relationships with patients, families, coworkers, and interprofessional team members?

What strategies would you use to encourage a patient and/or family to disclose personal and health-related information?

How often do you reflect on your ability to communicate, effectively?

CHAPTER OBJECTIVES

By the end of this chapter, you will be able to:

1. Define communication.
2. Describe the five levels of communication.
3. Describe each component within the human communication as transaction model.
4. Describe the purpose of communication within each of the four phases of the nurse–patient therapeutic relationship.
5. Identify the relational practice competencies required to initiate and maintain the therapeutic relationship.
6. Describe how verbal and nonverbal language influences communication.
7. Describe the perception process and how it influences communication.
8. Differentiate between behavioural communications techniques intended to enhance communication and those that block communication.
9. Explain how communication varies with individuals facing physical and emotional challenges.
10. Differentiate between behaviours contributing to incivility and those that create a healthy work environment.
11. Identify the three types of conflict resolution styles.
12. Explain the influence of social media on communication.
13. Discuss the relevance of cultural safety in nursing.

KEY TERMS

Active Listening A communication technique requiring the nurse to be present physically and emotionally by listening attentively to the patient.

Aggressive Communication Any form of communication that is self-focused and disregards the feelings, opinions, and rights of the listener.

Assertiveness Any form of communication that takes into consideration the thoughts, ideas, opinions, and rights of the listener.

Authenticity The ability to be genuine and true to yourself in word, deed, and action.

Bypassing The miscommunication that occurs when a word possesses different meaning for different people.

Channel The medium or pathway through which a message is sent.

Clarification Technique used to ensure a message has been understood.

(continued on page 600)

Closed-Ended Questions   Constrained question requiring a limited response.

Communication   The two-way process of exchanging, acting on, and assigning meaning to messages.

Confidentiality   The assurance given to an individual that his or her personal and private information will not be shared indiscriminately and without consent.

Conflict Resolution   A method and process used in facilitating the peaceful ending of conflict.

Connotative   Subjective meaning of a word.

Cultural Competence   Awareness and understanding of a patient's culture.

Cultural Safety   Concerned with the discourse on culture and health inequities experienced by marginalized populations.

Culture   A set of traditions, norms, attitudes, values, and beliefs that is shared amongst a particular group and passed down from one generation to the other.

Decoding   The process by which the receiver interprets of the meaning of the verbal and nonverbal messages sent by the sender.

Denotative   Literal meaning of a word.

Direct Perception Checking   Being verbally direct in clarifying your interpretation of an individual's behaviour.

Emoticons   Figurative pictures used to convey emotional context created from the arrangement of specific keyboard characters.

Empathy   The ability to imagine how or what someone else might be feeling or experiencing.

Encoding   Process by which the sender translates his or her thoughts, ideas, or emotions into a code in such a way that can be understood by the receiver of the message.

Feedback   The formal or informal, verbal or nonverbal, intentional or unintentional response to a message.

Human Communication as Transaction   Communication that is interactive and occurs simultaneously between the sender and receiver of a message.

Incivility   Rude, insensitive, and disrespectful behaviour demonstrating a lack of regard for others.

Indirect Perception Checking   Seeking additional information by way of nonverbal cues to confirm or refute your interpretation of an individual's behaviour.

Intentionality   Being deliberate in thought, word, and deed.

Interpersonal Communication   The simultaneous exchange of information between two individuals, whereby they mutually influence one another with the goal of creating shared meaning and understanding.

Interprofessional Team   Individuals from various health disciplines possessing diverse knowledge and skills who share goals and collaborate.

Intimate Zone   Comfort area between two individuals that are well acquainted (less than 18 in.).

Intrapersonal Communication   Occurs within each individual and comprises our thought and internal voice.

Message   The intentional or unintentional, verbal or nonverbal or written components of communication.

Mutuality   Amount of shared understanding, meaning, and connectedness.

Noise   The interference that occurs during the process of sending/ Communication other than verbal or written that comprises codes such as kinesics (gestures, posture, and movement), appearance, eye contact, facial expressions, vocalics, and touch encoding and receiving/decoding of messages.

Nonconfrontational Communication   A conflict management/resolution approach in which an individual avoids conflict by engaging in nonconfrontational behavior.

Nonverbal Communication   Communication other than verbal or written that comprises codes such as kinesics (gestures, posture, and movement), appearance, eye contact, facial expressions, vocalics, and touch.

Open-Ended Questions   Questions designed to elicit elaborate response.

Paraphrasing   Communication technique in which the listener repeats in his or her own words what he or she have understood the speaker to say.

Passive-Aggressive Behaviour   A nonconfrontational style of conflict resolution in which an individual chooses to back away, avoid, or give in to another person if he or she sense conflict may result.

Perception   The process of how individuals view themselves, others, and situations.

Perception Checking   Verifying the accuracy of your perceptions.

Personal Zone   Comfort zone in which most conversations occur; between 18 in. and 4 ft.

Probing   Guides the conversation and encourages a patient to expand on or further explore his or her thoughts, ideas, and feelings.

Proxemics   The study of space, personal space, and proximity of individuals to each other.

Public Communication   Communication that occurs at least 12 ft away and is often preferred by presenters in class or at conferences.

Public Zone   Comfort zone in which individuals address others while speaking at conference or lecturing in about 12 ft.

Rapport   An aspect of relationship building whereby individuals share a feeling of mutual trust, affinity, understanding, and connectedness.

Receiver   The individual(s) responsible for listening, observing, and decoding the message by the sender.

Reflective Practice   A problem-solving and learning process involving reviewing, analyzing, and comprehending events, situations, and actions and implementing strategies for positive transformation.

Relational Practice   Practice guided by conscious participation with clients using relational skills that include listening, questioning, empathy, mutuality, reciprocity, self-observation, reflection, and a sensitivity to emotional contexts.

Self-Awareness   The competence to be cognizant and reflective of one's own thoughts, feelings, attitudes, attributes, and actions.

Self-Disclosure   Communication technique of voluntarily sharing information and experiences with others.

Sender   The individual(s) initiating the thought, idea, or emotion and encodes the message in such a way that it will be understood by the receiver.

Sharing Observations   The process of making others aware of what you are observing.

Silence   Remaining quiet yet still being with a patient and nonverbally indicating interest in the hope of encouraging expression of feelings or thoughts.

Small Group Communication   Two to 15 individuals participating in the exchange of thoughts, ideas, and information.

Social Zone   Comfort zone of 4 to 12 ft in which most social and professional relationships occur.

Summary   Condensed version of what an individual has said, shared, or written.

Sympathy   A subjective, nontherapeutic communication technique of overidentifying with a patient's feelings.

Therapeutic Communication   Intentional and purposeful interpersonal communication techniques used by health-care workers, with the goal of enhancing the physical, emotional and spiritual needs of a patient.

Therapeutic Relationships   Constructive relationship between a nurse and a patient, consisting of four progressive phases: pre-orientation, orientation, working, and termination.

Transpersonal Communication   Aspect of communication that pertains to spiritual inquiry.

Trust   Relying on someone without doubt or question.

The Importance of Communication for Nurses

Nursing students are often eager to read, watch, and practice psychomotor or task-related skills, such as dressing changes, and medication administration, including intramuscular injections. When it comes to professional interpersonal communication, some students may not understand the importance of a formal communication course or even a chapter within a nursing textbook dedicated to enhancing therapeutic nurse–patient relationships and interprofessional collaboration. Similar to learning psychomotor skills, the ability to become proficient in professional communication requires skill, knowledge, motivation, self-awareness, practice, reflection, and critical thinking.

Think about your communication style: How often do people misunderstand what you have said? How often have you misunderstood what another person has said to you? At one point or another, we all either have been misunderstood or misunderstood someone. In our personal lives, misunderstandings occur on a daily basis, usually with no serious consequences. In health care, ineffective communication may result in medical or nursing errors, decreased patient outcomes and satisfaction, longer patient stays, and possible disciplinary action against the nurse (Sheldon, 2005). Communicating effectively is a professional competency delineated within provincial and territorial nursing practice standards and is also outlined within the Canadian Nurses Association (CNA) Code of Ethics (2008). Therefore, it is essential for nurses to possess the ability to understand patients as well as be understood by those they care for. It is expected that nurses communicate efficiently, accurately, effectively, and ethically with each other, the patient, and/or family as well as with various interprofessional team members such as physicians, occupational therapists (OT), physical therapists (PT), dieticians, social workers, and pharmacists in order to assess, plan, implement, and evaluate individualized plans of care (Sheldon, 2005).

Communicating effectively improves employability, enhances personal and professional relationships, and improves overall health. Making positive changes to lifelong habits can be difficult and uncomfortable; therefore, to become a more proficient communicator, it is imperative for you to learn to be comfortable being uncomfortable. Before you can make improvements, it is important to examine and reflect on your current ability to communicate. One way to begin is by taking the "How Good Are Your Communication Skills" quiz in Table 26.1.

In addition to examining your current communication ability, the key to achieving effective communication is knowing the definition and levels of communication as well as understanding how the communication process works, all of which will be explored in this chapter.

Through the eyes of a student

*M*eeting a patient for the first time was nerve-wracking. I was so scared. I could not sleep the night before. I had my new scrubs ready, name tag, and bright white shoes, so at least I would look professional, but I also needed to sound professional, and that's the part that worried me. How do I start the conversation? What do I talk about? How do I make the conversation meaningful? What if the patient does not want to talk? What if I don't know what to say? What if I don't know anything about the patient's culture? What if the patient asks questions I cannot answer? What if the patient does not speak English? What if the patient is really sick and needs the nurse, how do I call the nurse? It was apparent that communicating with my friends was not the same as communicating clearly with a patient. This scared me.

(personal reflection of a nursing student)

Communication

Communication can be defined as a process by which information is exchanged between individuals (Berman & Snyder, 2012). This two-way exchange takes many forms such as verbal and nonverbal, written and electronic, and includes alternative mediums, such as dance, music, painting, and sculpture (Berman & Snyder, 2012; Sheldon, 2005). It is through these mediums that individuals assign meaning based on emotional interpretation of what they feel is being communicated.

Human beings are social by nature and as such, have an innate need to communicate our physical, psychological, and spiritual needs with others. Despite which method of communication you choose, it may be viewed as cooperative, uncooperative, effective, or ineffective (Berman & Snyder, 2012; Sheldon, 2005). Nurses engaged in the nurse–patient relationship strive for cooperative and effective communication but sometimes find their communication with patients, families, and interprofessional team members to be met with obstruction, contributing to ineffective communication.

To achieve effective communication, nurses must have a clear purpose for communicating with a patient, possess the ability to adapt their message to others, ensure the message contains appropriate content, and is expressed through one or more channels with the least amount of noise (Beebe, Beebe, & Ivy, 2013). Never stop trying to reach this ideal transaction.

Levels of Communication

In the capacity of a professional, a nurse may use up to five diverse levels of communication: (1) intrapersonal, otherwise referred to as our *self-talk* or *internal thoughts*; (2) transpersonal communication; (3) interpersonal communication,

TABLE 26.1	How Good Are Your Communication Skills?

Instructions:

For each statement, circle the number in the column that best describes you. Please answer questions as you actually are (rather than how you think you should be), and don't worry if some questions seem to score in the 'wrong direction'. When you are finished, calculate your score.

	Not at all	Rarely	Sometimes	Often	Very often
1. I try to anticipate and predict possible causes of confusion, and I deal with them up front.	1	2	3	4	5
2. When I write a memo, email, or other document, I give all of the background information and detail I can to make sure that my message is understood.	1	2	3	4	5
3. If I don't understand something, I tend to keep this to myself and figure it out later.	1	2	3	4	5
4. I'm sometimes surprised to find that people haven't understood what I've said.	1	2	3	4	5
5. I can tend to say what I think, without worrying about how the other person perceives it. I assume that we'll be able to work it out later.	1	2	3	4	5
6. When people talk to me, I try to see their perspectives.	1	2	3	4	5
7. I use email to communicate complex issues with people. It's quick and efficient.	1	2	3	4	5
8. When I finish writing a report, memo, or email, I scan it quickly for typos and so forth, and then send it off right away.	1	2	3	4	5
9. When talking to people, I pay attention to their body language.	1	2	3	4	5
10. I use diagrams and charts to help express my ideas.	1	2	3	4	5
11. Before I communicate, I think about what the person needs to know, and how best to convey it.	1	2	3	4	5
12. When someone's talking to me, I think about what I'm going to say next to make sure I get my point across correctly.	1	2	3	4	5
13. Before I send a message, I think about the best way to communicate it (in person, over the phone, in a newsletter, via memo, and so on).	1	2	3	4	5
14. I try to help people understand the underlying concepts behind the point I am discussing. This reduces misconceptions and increases understanding.	1	2	3	4	5
15. I consider cultural barriers when planning my communications.	1	2	3	4	5

Score Interpretation

Score	Comment
56-75	Excellent! You understand your role as a communicator, both when you send messages, and when you receive them. You anticipate problems, and you choose the right ways of communicating. People respect you for your ability to communicate clearly, and they appreciate your listening skills.
36-55	You're a capable communicator, but you sometimes experience communication problems. Take the time to think about your approach to communication, and focus on receiving messages effectively, as much as sending them. This will help you improve.
15-35	You need to keep working on your communication skills. You are not expressing yourself clearly, and you may not be receiving messages correctly either. The good news is that, by paying attention to communication, you can be much more effective at work, and enjoy much better working relationships!

Reprinted with permission from Mind Tools Ltd. (1996–2013). *How good are your communication skills?* London, United Kingdom: Author.

which occurs between two people; (4) small group communication, occurring amongst 2 to 15 individuals; and (5) public communication (Beebe et al., 2013).

Intrapersonal Communication

Intrapersonal communication is commonly referred to as *self-talk* or the internal and often competing conversations and struggles we have regarding our thoughts, feelings, perceptions, values, beliefs, and attitudes toward another person, situation, or task (Beebe et al., 2013). The attitude you have greatly determines your success or failure in communicating with others, communicating within a given situation, or communicating while completing a task. Attitude drives thinking, and thinking drives behaviour; so if you combine a negative attitude with negative thoughts, chances are you will behave and communicate in an obstructive and ineffective manner. Through self-awareness, you possess the power to stomp out negative intrapersonal attitudes and thoughts. Consciously, choose a positive attitude by thinking, believing, and communicating the positive power of you!

Nurses frequently use intrapersonal communication when critically thinking about a patient's condition and when initiating and working through the nursing process. Observing a patient with signs of diaphoresis, lethargy, and confusion may lead you to think to yourself, "I know the patient is diabetic, I wonder if her blood sugar is low" (Jakubec & Astle, 2014). When in the process of communicating, intrapersonal communication can interfere with the nurse's as well as the patient's ability to be present and actively listening (further discussed in the section on the transactional model).

Transpersonal Communication

The area of **transpersonal communication**, spirituality, or spiritual inquiry is considered by many nurses to be uncomfortable and an area they lack knowledge in. However, engaging in transpersonal communication is a choice and an area where nurses have the opportunity to make a significant difference in the lives of patients experiencing uncertainty (Jakubec & Astle, 2014). Discussions of what spirituality means to the patient, how his or her spirituality helps him or her in difficult circumstances, and its significance within the context of his or her lived experience enable nurses to relate and connect with the patient in a deeper level and require the nurse to employ both therapeutic and relational practice competencies (Doane & Varcoe, 2005; Jakubec & Astle, 2014).

Interpersonal Communication

Interpersonal communication is the simultaneous exchange of information between two individuals, whereby they mutually influence one another with the goal of creating shared meaning and understanding that is necessary when initiating or maintaining relationships (Beebe et al., 2013; Fig. 26.1). Within the context of the nurse–patient relationship, nurses use interpersonal communication skills throughout each phase of the therapeutic relationship and the nursing process. An important aspect of effective interpersonal communication is the nurses' ability to treat each and every person they communicate with as a unique human being, possessing unique talents, qualities, skills, and needs (Beebe et al., 2013).

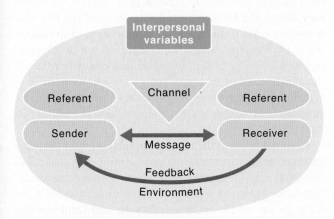

Figure 26.1 Interpersonal communication.

Despite the widespread use of social media channels from Twitter, texting, blogging to e-mailing, face-to-face is still the preferred method of engaging in interpersonal communication (Jakubec & Astle, 2014). Electronic communication is further discussed under social media.

Small Group Communication

Nursing is not an isolated profession. Most nurses will be required to work and communicate within small groups. Nurses engage in **small group communication** during change of shift report, staff meetings, patient care conferences, professional development in-services program, leading patient support, self-help, or teaching groups and when working on committees and research teams (Jakubec & Astle, 2014). Nursing students participate in small group communication in class, study groups, and group presentations. This type of communication is goal-directed and occurs when 2 to 15 individuals participate in the exchange of thoughts, ideas, and information. Professional and personal success depends on how effectively individuals work and communicate in small groups. Groups exist to support individuals in achieving outcomes that would otherwise not be met by working alone (Mitchell, 2014). Therefore, a nurse should possess a sound understanding of the nature, process, and dynamics of small groups (Jakubec & Astle, 2014). The milieu of a small group should offer the comfort and sense of security required for individuals to feel safe to express their opinions, ideas, thoughts, and feelings openly and honestly without fear of disrespect, embarrassment, or humiliation. Furthermore, the dynamics of a group should revolve around the values and principles of respect, inclusivity, open-mindedness, active listening, and being other-oriented (Arnold & Boggs, 2011).

Public Communication

In order to advance our profession, we need to communicate to the public and our peers what it is we do, what we know, what we have learned, where we are going, and how we plan to get there. Nurses are in unique positions to espouse the virtues of health-related issues affecting our profession, communities, and our nation. Nurses who communicate one-on-one or in groups within our communities; teach at universities; present at local, national, and international conferences; address or work with the media; or engage in political advocacy—all contribute to and advance our profession through **public communication** (Jakubec & Astle, 2014). When engaging in public communication, the chance of miscommunication is higher due to the fact that individuals may perceive the message differently if the message itself is abstract or worded abstractly. Therefore, to minimize the chance of miscommunication, pay special attention to the codes of nonverbal communication (see section on nonverbal communication) and use them in a manner that is positive and leaves little room for interpretation (Jakubec & Astle, 2014).

Elements of the Communication Process

The communication process is a cycle that involves a sender, a message, receiver, and a response or feedback. It is an active, two-way, reciprocal process of exchange, where the receiver becomes the sender and the sender becomes a receiver. The process of interpersonal communication is interactive, dynamic, cyclical, and involves interpersonal as well as intrapersonal processes.

Human Communication as Transaction

Human communication as transaction closely resembles human interpersonal communication as the sender and receiver of communication respond to each other simultaneously through verbal and/or nonverbal feedback. Additionally, this model (Fig. 26.2) depicts communication as being relational with individuals sharing accountability and responsibility for their roles, challenges, and achievements within the context of interpersonal communication. Furthermore, the transaction model takes into account the barriers that influence communication. Having a working knowledge of the transaction model enables individuals to explore the many influencing factors that both contribute to and impede effective communication in our everyday personal and professional lives. Although not focused on nursing specifically, this model requires nurses to critically think about and practice the skills related to self-reflection, self-awareness, being other-oriented, and adaptable in order to communicate most effectively within a given situation.

Sender

The **sender** of the message is usually the person(s) initiating communication. However, because communication is a two-way process involving a receiver of information, the

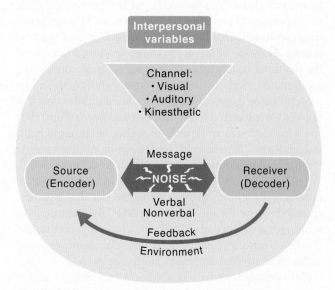

Figure 26.2 Components within the human communication as transaction model.

process is both simultaneous and ongoing. Therefore, individuals engaged in communication share the roles of sender and receiver. It is the responsibility of the sender to **encode** the information, conveying thoughts, ideas, or emotions in such a manner that will be understood by the receiver as well as to verify that the recipient understands the message. Nurses are required to ethically encode their message by taking into account their tone of voice, gestures, choice of words, and arrangement of words. Additionally, they are required to individualize each message to the patient, family member, colleague, and interdisciplinary team member by taking into consideration the age, education, and literacy level, cognitive ability, culture, language, and professional knowledge of the individual(s) they are communicating with (Mitchell, 2014).

Receiver

The **receiver** is the individual(s) responsible for listening, observing, and decoding the message by the sender. **Decoding** refers to the interpretation of the meaning of the verbal and nonverbal messages sent by the sender. For effective communication to occur, the meaning of the decoded message must correspond with the meaning of the encoded message. Ineffective communication occurs when the receiver misinterprets the meaning of the encoded message. Influences contributing to ineffective communication include, but are not limited to, noise, individuals' values, beliefs, attitude, and self-knowledge (Beebe et al., 2013). It is the receiver's responsibility to clarify with the sender if he or she may have misunderstood or misinterpreted the message. Nurses engaged in a collaborative and therapeutic relationship will frequently use clarification as a method to ensure the messages sent and received were interpreted correctly.

Message and Channel

The **message** is the content being communicated through verbal, written, nonverbal gestures, and body language (Beebe et al., 2013). We send messages that are either intentional (smile or a verbal "Hello") or unintentional (turn your back on someone you are speaking with or put your head on your desk in class) (Beebe et al., 2013). What then may distort the message from being received the way that it was intended is the receiver's interpretation of the meaning of the message? Several factors such as use of language, jargon, knowledge of the individual, and emotion influence the effectiveness of messages being sent and received. It is essential that individuals send messages utilizing concrete language and reflects clarity and conciseness (Jakubec & Astle, 2014).

Channel refers to the medium or method used to send a message. Nurses must use the most appropriate channel to effectively convey their message. Face-to-face communication is the preferred channel to use because it enables the nurse to use visual, auditory, olfactory, and tactile senses. Other channels used by nurses are telephones, both landlines and cellular; Internet and fax; audio and video recording; and written documentation. Yet, the most common channels in today's society revolve around social media (text, Skype, e-mail), but ironically, these contribute to a great deal of ineffective communication.

Noise

Within the communication process, noise is a significant factor that interferes with effective communication, yet it is often overlooked. Within the nurse–patient relationship, **noise** is interference that prevents messages from being correctly understood on the part of the nurse, patient, or both. Noise interference may be classified as *physiological* (age, aphasia, pain, hunger, visual or auditory problems, fatigue, illness, and dying/death), *psychological* (biases, anger, embarrassment, task-focused), *environmental/external* (call bells, background conversations, interruptions, equipment malfunctions [phones/faxes/IV pump] and lighting), or *semantic* (language differences, nursing jargon; Adler, Rolls, & Proctor, 2012; Beebe et al., 2013; Devito, Shimoni, & Clark, 2005).

Because noise is always present, nurses must take into account the influence of noise and consciously try to eliminate the number of interfering elements (Table 26.2). Additional elements that can be attributed to misunderstandings and ineffective communication are individual's culture, education level, communication, and listening skills.

Feedback

Feedback occurs once the receiver interprets the meaning of the message and provides a verbal or nonverbal, intentional or unintentional response to the sender (Beebe et al., 2013). This process validates that the message sent was received and understood. Failing to receive appropriate feedback can have detrimental effects on the nurse–patient relationship. In an attempt to elicit as much feedback from patients, nurses are purposeful when choosing the most effective communication strategies for their individual patient.

Communication Categories

Communication categories cover verbal communication, and here, we are referring for the most part to spoken words, nonverbal communications, including facial expression and proxemics, as well as the issue of personal space and its impact on effective communication.

Verbal Communication

As with most words, the term *communication* has both a denotative and a connotative meaning that differs according to the context in which it is used as well as how the individual(s) assigns its meaning. The **denotative** meaning

TABLE 26.2	Types of Noise That Interfere With Communication	
Types of Noise	**Nurse**	**Patient**
Physiological	Pain or discomfort	Pain or discomfort
	Fatigue	Hearing or visually impaired
	Hunger/thirst	Hunger/thirst
Psychological	Stereotypes	Stereotypes
	Biases	Biases
	Emotions	Emotions
	Embarrassment	Embarrassment
	Assumptions	Fear of the unknown
	Intrapersonal communication	Grief
	Stress	Anxiety
	Task focused or preoccupied	Intrapersonal communication
Environmental/	Call bells	Call bells
External	Background conversations	Other patient conversations
	Interruptions	Other patients snoring/moaning
	Equipment malfunctions (phones/faxes/IV pump)	Smells
	Dim lights	Interruptions
	Radio/TV	Bright lights
	Temperature	Radio/TV
	Nonverbal communication	Temperature
		Electronic communication (cell phones/texting/games)
		Nonverbal communication
Semantic	Language barrier	Language barrier
	Nursing jargon/slang	Complex language not understood by the patient
		Culturally specific phrases/slang

Adapted from Adler, R. B., Rolls, J. A., & Proctor, R. F., II. (2012). *Look* (Canadian ed.). Toronto, ON: Nelson; Beebe, S. A., Beebe, S. J., & Ivy, D. K. (2013). *Communication principles for a lifetime* (5th ed.). Toronto, ON: Pearson Allyn & Bacon; Devito, J. A., Shimoni, R., & Clark, D. (2005). *Building interpersonal communication skills* (2nd Canadian ed.). Toronto, ON: Pearson Allyn & Bacon.

of communication is the literal definition as is found in a dictionary (Beebe, Beebe, Redmond, & Geerinck, 2007). The **connotative** meaning of communication is subjective and created from emotional experience. It is often the connotative meaning of words that contribute to ineffective communication. Because we know that words alone do not have meaning, rather individuals assign meanings to words based on their own self-knowledge, miscommunication may occur when two people assign diverse meaning to the same word. This concept is called **bypassing**, and you have most likely experienced bypassing if you have ever responded by saying, "That is not what I meant" (Engleberg & Wynn, 2011). An example of bypassing would be, if Ashley were sitting in a coffee shop with her friend, Joe, and at some point, she asks him to leave. What she means by the word *leave* is for Joe to leave the coffee shop, whereas Joe interprets the word to mean leave the table.

Nurses cannot assume that the patient or interprofessional team members will interpret words correctly and as intended. Should you perceive that bypassing has occurred, simply clarify with the other person as soon as possible. As verbal communication is the main form of communication for nurses, they should be intentional and mindful about what they say, how they say it, and the effect their words may have on another individual.

Nonverbal Communication

Communication is a complex process and is much more than linguistics (Jirwe, Gerrish, & Emami, 2010). As up to 90% of what you say is not verbal, it is essential that nurses are diligent in assessing **nonverbal communication** codes (Grover, 2005). It is not surprising that nonverbal messages are more believable than the spoken word. At each phase of the therapeutic relationship, the nurse is looking for congruence between what the patient is verbally stating and what the patient is exhibiting in terms of nonverbal signals or body language (tone, facial expressions, gestures, and proxemics) in addition to the shared assumptions between the communicants regarding the context and purpose of the exchange (Jirwe et al., 2010). The patient may declare he or she is not in pain, but the nurse observes the patient curled up in the fetal position, limited eye contact, and furrowed brows. This would indicate to the nurse that there is incongruence and requires further follow-up (Taylor, Lillis, LeMone, & Lynn, 2011). Nurses working to enhance cultural safety need to ensure they have an understanding of the cultural variations of nonverbal signals that occur within and between cultures. The communication code related to tone, facial expression, gesture, and proxemics follow.

Eye Contact

The saying, "I was trying to catch their eye," is often heard when an individual is attempting to initiate communication with another person. Eye contact is a nonverbal way of initiating, maintaining, and enhancing honesty, trust, respect, and openness within personal and therapeutic relationships. Most of us value and expect eye contact when communicating with others. Eye contact is somewhat tied to truthfulness, especially in children. Aversion to eye contact may be a nonverbal sign of lying, guilt, avoidance, defensiveness, or anxiety (Taylor et al., 2011). However, not all cultures ascribe to the importance of eye contact in communication. Aboriginal and some Asian populations view eye contact as challenging or an invasion of privacy. Absence of eye contact in some cultures demonstrates respect toward and for positions of status in families and within communities. Keep in mind that the patient's perception of eye contact also influences communication. Patients may perceive that a lack of eye contact on the part of the nurse indicates lack of interest in the therapeutic relationship or that they are not being honest. In performing certain skills, such as dressing and ostomy changes, the patient may look at the nurse's eyes to obtain information. If the nurse's eyes widen or narrow, the patient may perceive something is wrong. Being perceptually aware of cultural expectation, meaning, and context of eye contact is essential for facilitating the therapeutic relationship.

Gestures

When communicating with others, we frequently use nonverbal gestures to compliment/accentuate or substitute verbal messages (Beebe et al., 2013). Being aware that gestures are culture bound and that not all patients will interpret them the same way, nurses should keep this in mind when using this form of nonverbal communication. For example, in North America, the common gesture depicted in Figure 26.3 means *okay*. However, in France, it means *zero* or *worthless*. How patients use gestures might be confusing to a nurse as well, so clarifying the intended meaning of the gestures is recommended.

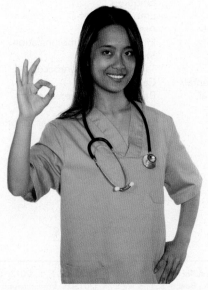

Figure 26.3 Nonverbal gestures. This common hand gesture means different things to different cultures.

Proxemics

Proxemics is a subcategory of nonverbal communication and refers to the spacial zones individuals establish to protect themselves against unwarranted physical closeness and contact (Austin & Boyd, 2010). At some time or another, each of us will work, socialize, and establish relationships based on our unique comfort levels. Typically, we establish spacial territory in our work areas (offices/cubicles or desks) and in our neighbourhoods (fences) that signals to others where our personal space lies. Relationships, culture, and the environment influence the study of space. For example, people from Japan are used to living, working, and relating to others within close spaces/distances (Engleberg & Wynn, 2011). Canadians typically require more space and distance in order to feel comfortable where we live, work, and socialize. However, as space in urban areas within Canada is becoming increasingly scarce, a cultural shift in how we view, identify, and protect our space and distance will likely occur as we live, work, and socialize in closer proximity. Depending on the type of work performed, nurses will usually have experience in all zones. What needs to be kept in the forefront of a nurse's mind is how culture and level of self-awareness (their own and others) influence communication when working with patients in the intimate and personal zones. We always want to do our very best to make each patient comfortable, but that requires an understanding of what that means to the patient and nurse. The tasks, values, and principles when working in each zone are discussed in the following sections (Austin & Boyd, 2010; Jakubec & Astle, 2014).

Intimate Space

Intimate zone is measured at less than 18 in. (<0.5 m). Comfort at this degree of closeness between patient and nurse will be culturally and individually specific. Within intimate space, the nurse will complete personal care, assessments, and procedures; demonstrate empathy; and use therapeutic touch. Working in this space may be uncomfortable and embarrassing to many individuals, the nurse should demonstrate respect by seeking permission and explaining what they or another member of the interprofessional team are planning to do and about how long it will take. Employing cultural safety ideology is essential for working this close with patients (Austin & Boyd, 2010; Jakubec & Astle, 2014).

Personal Space

Personal zone generally measures between 18 in. and 4 ft (0.5 to 1.5 m). This is the realm of space where nurses and interprofessional team members will spend most time sitting, communicating, and teaching the patient (Wilkinson & Treas, 2011). Patients are quite protective of the personal space that exists in and around their bed (otherwise known as the curtain area). If the curtain is closed, announce your presence and seek permission before entering the patient's personal space. Be respectful by seeking permission before going through the bedside table that may contain the patient's personal items (Austin & Boyd, 2010; Jakubec & Astle, 2014).

Social Space

Social zone measures between 4 to 12 ft (1.5 to 3 m) and is usually not effective in advancing the therapeutic relationship. If a nurse were to inquire about the well-being of a patient from his or her room door, as in the case of isolation precautions, the patient may perceive that the nurse is impersonal or too lazy to put on the appropriate personal protective equipment (gown, mask, gloves, and cap). However, in the case of a patient conference, teaching a small class or leading a support group in which individuals are seated around a table, this distance may be quite appropriate (Austin & Boyd, 2010, Jakubec & Astle, 2014; Wilkinson & Treas, 2011).

Public Space

Public zone is measured at distances greater than 12 ft (>3 m). This distance is most effectively used by professors in educational settings, individuals speaking at professional development conferences, or by politicians speaking within communities. The drawback to this space is it affords little opportunity to get to know individuals as the group as a whole is usually addressed (Beebe et al., 2013).

Facial Expressions

The seven universal emotions communicated via facial expressions are sad, happy, surprise, fear, disgust, anger, and contempt (Beebe et al., 2007). Influences on the expression of emotion are both cultural and physiological, and a nurse needs to possess an awareness of both, while focusing on the unique meaning behind the expression as it applies to the patient (Fig. 26.4). Is the patient crying because they are happy, sad, or relieved? Nurses should recognize that the expression of emotion varies within families and cultures. If a patient has passed away and the nurse walks in the room and finds one daughter smiling and one daughter crying, how does emotion and the perception of emotion influence interaction? Would the nurse perceive the daughter that is smiling to be cold and uncaring or relieved that the patient is no longer suffering? Inquiring about the meaning behind the expression of emotion is essential to providing nonjudgmental and compassionate care.

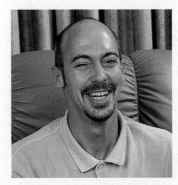

Figure 26.4 Nonverbal message, facial expression. Meaning behind facial expressions is influenced by physiology and culture.

Physical and psychological disorders (stroke, depression, dementia, Parkinson, and schizophrenia), treatments (Botox), effect of some medications (antipsychotics), and developmental disorders (Asperger) for which a patient experiences a flat or blunt affect complicate communication between the nurse and patient.

As we age, we learn to manage our emotions and adapt them according to the event or situation. The culture of technology has also influenced how we express emotions online. **Emoticons** are symbolic pictures intended to add emotional context to informal written and electronic communication. The concern with the use of emoticons is in the deciphering of their meaning. As emoticons evolve and increase in use, the chance for misunderstanding and miscommunication is heightened. Emoticons may be appropriate for social relationships, but you should be cautious when using them to communicate informally with patients, and they should never be used in documentation or interprofessional communication.

Through the eyes of a nurse

I grew up in this community and know a lot of our patients on a personal level. Every morning, I draw a happy face or some other emoticon on the patients white boards in their room. When I go for a break, I draw another emoticon, and when I leave at the end of my shift, I draw two emoticons. One depicting the hope of a good night's rest, and the other illustrating they are in good hands with the next nurse coming on shift. I feel connected with my patients when I use emoticons, especially with the children. Not all patients understand the meaning of each emoticon, but that opportunity alone allows me to engage further with them and demonstrates my caring and compassion. I don't document using emoticons, though. That would be unprofessional and violate standards of practice.

(personal reflection of Kate, a nurse)

Therapeutic Communication

Making meaningful connections with patients and their families is the underpinning of nursing practice. The **therapeutic relationship** between a nurse and a patient is purposeful, goal-directed, time-limited, and always with the intent of advancing the best interests and outcomes of the patient (Registered Nurses Association of Ontario [RNAO], 2006). Although nurses comprise one half of the nurse–patient relationship, the crux of the relationship is not about the nurse; it is always about the patient. Although most nurses place a high value on initiating and maintaining the therapeutic relationship, it is important to keep in mind that nurses placing their needs above those of the

patient run the risk of violating the therapeutic relationship. To communicate in a therapeutic manner requires nurses to communicate with rather than to a patient.

Recognizing the difference between personal and professional therapeutic relationships is essential to nurses. Table 26.3 outlines the differences between personal and professional relationships (College of Registered Nurses of British Columbia [CRNBC], 2006). When nurses seek to advance the therapeutic relationship, they do so by consciously choosing to work through the phases of the relationship by using relational inquiry and the competencies enveloped in **relational practice** (Fig. 26.5). Relational practice uses relational inquiry that is guided by mindful engagement with patients using skills such as listening, questioning, empathy, mutuality, reciprocity, self-observation, reflection, and sensitivity to emotional contexts. Relational practice encompasses the therapeutic nurse–patient relationship as well as interprofessional relationships (College and Association of Registered Nurses of Alberta [CARNA], 2006; Doane & Varcoe, 2005; Fletcher, 1999).

The Nursing Challenge

Given the complexities of both patients and the health-care system, nurses working to establish therapeutic relationships often struggle with the competing demands and expectations of patients/families/interdisciplinary team members and the institution while simultaneously compelled to take the time to hear the patient's story, identifying what the patient needs right now and exploring what this experience means within the context of the patient's life (Doane & Varcoe, 2007). The premise of relational inquiry views therapeutic relationships as unique, meaningful, and responsive. Therefore, a requisite to relational inquiry is the nurse's readiness to move beyond the iceberg effect (Doane, & Varcoe, 2007) of labeling and objectifying patients. For example, the man in room 403, the abdominal pain in room 403, or the lady with the laceration (Doane & Varcoe, 2007). These labels neither create nor enable nurses to establish relational space, to act with intent nor assess the contextual and personal factors such as (a) how the determinants of health currently affect the patient's health and well-being, (b) the patient's readiness to communicate and ability to respond in a meaningful way, and (c) the patient's set of life experiences that may be impeding his or her health and well-being. It is only through this initial and ongoing assessment within each phase of the therapeutic relationship that the nurse is able to view the relationship as relational and unique.

Phases of the Therapeutic Relationship

The therapeutic relationship between nurse and patient is supported through the overlapping phases of pre-interaction (also called *pre-orientation*), orientation, working, and termination (Forchuk & Dorsay, 1995). On a daily basis, we communicate and make connections with friends, acquaintances, and colleagues, mostly through the use of basic, social, and conversational amenities such as taking turns speaking and listening, disclosure, and persuasion. Although the

TABLE 26.3	Differences Between Personal and Professional Relationships	
Characteristic	Professional Relationship (nurse–client)	Personal Relationship (casual, friendship, romantic, sexual)
Behaviour	Regulated by a code of ethics and professional standards.	Guided by personal values and beliefs.
Remuneration	Nurse is paid to provide care to client.	No payment for being in the relationship.
Length of relationship	Limited for the length of the client's need for nursing care.	May last a lifetime.
Location of relationship	Place defined and limited to where nursing care is provided.	Place unlimited; often undefined.
Purpose of relationship	Goal-directed to provide care to client.	Pleasure, interest-directed.
Structure of relationship	Nurse provides care to client.	Spontaneous, unstructured.
Power of balance	Unequal: nurse has more power due to authority, knowledge, influence and access to privileged information about client.	Relatively equal.
Responsibility for relationship	Nurse (not client) responsible for establishing and maintaining professional relationship.	Equal responsibility to establish and maintain.
Preparation for relationship	Nurse requires formal knowledge, preparation, orientation and training.	Does not require formal knowledge, preparation, orientation and training.
Time spent in relationship	Nurse employed under contractual agreement that outlines hours of work for contact between the nurse and client.	Personal choice for how much time is spent in the relationship.

Reprinted with permission from College of Registered Nurses of British Columbia. (2006). *Nurse–client relationships.*
Retrieved from https://crnbc.ca/Standards/Lists/StandardResources/page8/406NurseClientRelationships.pdf

skills used in social relationships may be enough to sustain those relationships, the skills required by nurses within a therapeutic relationship are as unique and complex as the patients themselves. Nurses need to possess the knowledge of and be able to seamlessly integrate behavioural and relational practice skills as they navigate through the phases of the therapeutic relationship. Additionally, nurses should be aware of the complex factors that influence communication and the development of the nurse–patient relationship.

Pre-Orientation Phase

Prior to meeting a patient, nurses attend a shift report and review the Kardex and patient chart. The data needs to be completely objective, but as is the nature of human beings, subjectivity and labeling of patients is often communicated. Nurses and nursing students need to employ critical communication and thinking skills when reviewing patient data, recognizing

that patient conditions and behaviours change throughout the course of the patient's stay or treatment, being mindful to enter the relationship with a nonjudgmental and open attitude. Accepting subjectivity as reported and entering the relationship with preconceived thoughts is disrespectful and unprofessional.

Orientation Phase

Self-knowledge on the part of the nurse is one of the greatest influences when communicating within the orientation phase. The nurse is able to recognize that his or her self-knowledge is shaped by his or her own determinants of health, including nationality, race, culture, gender, economics, and early childhood experiences and development as well as relationships, accomplishments, beliefs, and values (RNAO, 2006) and is different from that of a patient's. Only with this realization is the nurse able to prevent imposing their issues, beliefs, and values on the patient (RNAO, 2006).

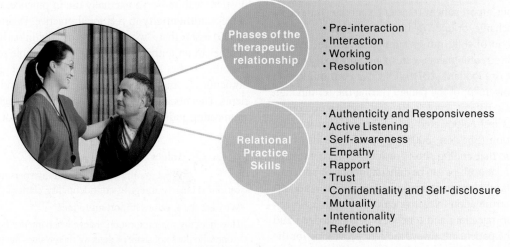

Figure 26. 5 The phases and relational skills that comprise the nurse-patient relationship.

Keeping this in mind, the nurse employs specific communication skills to initiate a relationship with the patient.

An experienced nurse possesses the awareness that the reward of a positive first impression is immeasurable to building rapport, trust, and meaningful communications with patients. Investing the time now by properly introducing yourself, explaining your role and purpose to the patient with a warm and genuine smile by saying, "Good morning, my name is Sarah, I am a first-year nursing student at MacEwan University, and I will be helping you with morning care." Following this, inquire about how the patient would like to be addressed, "May I call you Mike or would you prefer Mr. Snelling?" Furthermore, inquiring about how the patient perceives his or her current health status by employing open-ended, probing, and clarification questions engages the patient to tell his or her story. This basic introduction goes a long way in establishing rapport (see the section on rapport). Although this may not always guarantee a successful relationship, it does provide a positive foundation in moving toward a collaborative working relationship. As the nurse and the patient are getting to know one another, fostering trust and maintaining confidentiality is crucial in this and every phase of the therapeutic relationship.

Working Phase

In this phase, the nurse acknowledges that collaboration is the key to patient success. When engaged in the third phase of the therapeutic relationship, the nurse uses effective communication strategies such as silence, touch, open-ended questions, paraphrasing, shared observation, self-disclosure, and listening (refer to section on effective communication strategies [Goddard, 2010]). Through the use of such skills, the patient is empowered to express and explore his or her feelings, establish goals, and identify realistic strategies (Burger & Goddard, 2010). If the nurse fails to listen to the patient's lived experience or projects his or her self-knowledge and expectations onto the patient, this phase will most likely result in conflict with the nurse having to respond to patient complaints.

Termination

Terminating the nurse–patient relationship may occur at the end of each shift, upon patient transfer to another unit or facility, upon discharge, or upon death. In situations of transfer, discharge, or end of shift, nurses summarize for the patient the patient's care requirements, care plan, and goals met or unmet (Burger & Goddard, 2010). Effective communication and active involvement of the patient during the termination phase enhances patient knowledge and health outcomes, whereas nurses feel empowered and experience an increase in job satisfaction (Sheldon, 2005). However, we also need to acknowledge that ending short- or long-term therapeutic nurse–patient relationships can be difficult for one or both parties. Patients should be encouraged to express their emotions regarding the termination. Negative emotions such as anger, frustration, fear, rejection, and loneliness acknowledged and expressed by the patient are always thought provoking for the nurse. Providing nonjudgmental support and encouragement

will often give patients the motivation empowerment needed to move forward (Sheldon, 2005). Finding emotional closure for the nurse is an undervalued goal and is usually not a part of a nurse's formal education. Nurses can experience feelings of sadness, grief, frustration, anxiety, and dissatisfaction when these relationships end. It is important to be self-aware, acknowledge your feelings, and talk to other colleagues about how you are feeling. You might be surprised to find out others share the same or similar feelings. Seeking out effective coping strategies in this phase will assist you now and in the future.

The relational practice skills shown in Figure 26.5 are fundamental to relational inquiry in establishing therapeutic relationships.

Relational Practice Competencies

Nursing is the caring profession, and our concern for and about others runs deep and can be seen on every unit of every hospital, care centre, clinic, and within our communities. Initiating a meaningful relationship with a patient is a conscious decision nurses make every day. Communicating in an authentic and responsive manner is fundamental to creating relational space and advancing the nurse–patient relationship. These capacities are intertwined, and nurses strive to engage in relationships that extend beyond the physical and spoken word (Hartrick, 1997) where they are equally concerned with saying the right thing as well as mindful about being with the patient. The premise of being responsive is actively listening to the patient describe his or her experience, thoughts, and feelings, and being purposeful in responding to the expressed feelings and thoughts as they become apparent (Hartrick, 1997).

Authenticity

In order for you to make meaningful connections with patients, you need to be true to yourself, actively present, and genuine in how you communicate and interact with patients. Being self-aware, reflecting, and analyzing the congruence between the values, beliefs, and attitudes you verbalize and demonstrate with those you actually use in practice, will help you achieve **authenticity** in relational practice. Doane and Varcoe (2005) assert that, "when a nurse has the initiative to be with another in an authentic way, she or he is able to respond to the other as they are in the moment" (p. 193). However, being authentic is sometimes challenging for nurses and nursing students. Patients are very good at spotting a nurse that is communicating and behaving in a manner that is not authentic.

Think *Values*

What are my values toward interpersonal communication? (Honesty, integrity, confidentiality, clarity . . .)

Why are these values important to me?

How does my communication change when interacting with someone who does not share or perceive these values the same way I do?

Active Listening

Patients often become disillusioned with the health-care team/system when they feel their voice has been silenced or their concerns are not heard or responded to. When engaged in **active listening**, the nurse is present both physically and emotionally, expresses genuine interest, takes the initiative to understand, and provides feedback to ensure the patient feels heard (Browning & Waite, 2010). With the intention of paying attention and listening deeply to the needs of a patient, nurses must become experts at being with the patient. This means that the nurse must first establish a safe environment for the patient to share his or her lived experience. Until the patient feels safe enough to disclose his or her thoughts, feelings, and emotions as well as his or her medical history, nurses have little to listen to. Listening is not the same as hearing. It is an integrative process that can positively enhance patient outcomes and well-being (Browning & Waite, 2010). Listening is at the heart of nursing practice and while most of us would like to think we listen, how many of us truly listen well. You can identify your own barriers and strategies for effective listening in Table 26.4.

Although it is essential for nurses to truly listen to what the patient is saying, it is equally important to listen to what he or she is not saying. This is not always easy to accomplish, but as you practice and gain more experience being with patients, you will begin to pick up on subtle cues such as a change in vocalics referring to the rate, tone, and pitch of speech; shifting position; change in eye contact; avoiding questions; or changing the subject (Shannon, 2011). The skill of listening is complex, nurses need to practice being other-oriented when listening and to realize that while they are listening to gather information to learn the patient's story or to empathize, the patient listens for very different reasons. A patient listens to be heard, acknowledged, and recognized and to feel that he or she is being cared for with compassion. When a nurse considers the reasons for listening, engages in the act of listening, and is able to take into account the needs of others, he or she will truly comprehend that listening is both a process and an outcome (Shannon, 2011).

Additional active listening strategies that the nurse uses may include verbal (asking clarifying questions, paraphrasing and empathizing) and nonverbal skills such as empathy or touch and those depicted by the acronym SURETY (**S**it, **U**ncross, **R**elax, **E**ye contact, **T**ouch, **Y**our intuition; see Box 26.1) in order to facilitate the relational space needed for active listening to occur (Stickley, 2011).

1. Why is it important for me to actively listen to the patient?
2. How am I demonstrating that I actively listen?
3. What strategies can I use to facilitate active listening?
4. What prevents me from actively listening?
5. What are the consequences to the nurse–patient relationship if I fail to actively listen?

Self-Awareness

Nurses who are self-aware focus the therapeutic relationship on meeting the needs of the patient rather than their own needs (Sheldon, 2005). **Self-awareness** is a critical component in establishing therapeutic relationships and relational space. Nurses spend a great deal of time getting to know, to understand, to care for and about their patients. In order for a nurse to truly help a patient within the therapeutic relationship, it is necessary for the nurse to consciously engage in self-awareness by reflecting on his or her inner world of past experiences, thoughts, feelings, needs, fears, strengths, and weaknesses to understand how some or all of these, knowingly and authentically guide their outer world of behaviour and actions (Eckroth-Bucher, 2010).

Through this ongoing and lifelong process, the nurse achieves a high degree of insight and awareness of self and is then able to avoid projecting his or her attitude, values, beliefs, and judgments onto others. When a nurse acknowledges feelings of anxiety or uncertainty in how to communicate with patients in certain situations, the nurse is empowered to manage the anxiety rather than allowing the anxiety to control his or her mind, body, or situation (Jack & Smith, 2007). Reflecting on specific questions such

TABLE 26.4	Listening Barriers and Strategies
Barriers to Listening	**Strategies for Listening**
Self-absorbed/personal agenda	**STOP** talking (same letters in "listen" as there are in "silent").
Information overload	**LOOK** at the nonverbal/body language of both the speaker and listener (fatigue/hunger/distractions).
Focused on the speaker rather than the message	**LISTEN** to the speakers ideas/thoughts for meaning rather than reacting to trigger words.
Noise (physical/psychological/environmental/semantic)	Give undivided attention by eliminating the distractions.
Feeling unwell	Be empathetic.
Multitasking	Practice self-awareness.
Emotions	Use self-talk to manage emotions.

Source: Beebe, S. A., Beebe, S. J., Redmond, M. B., & Geerinck, T. M. (2007). *Interpersonal communication relating to others* (4th Canadian ed.). Toronto, ON: Pearson Allyn & Bacon.

BOX 26.1 SURETY in Achieving Active Listening

Sit at an angle to the patient: This will assist in establishing a nonconfrontational and comfortable environment. This posture indicates to a patient that you are engaged and wanting to listen to his or her story.

Uncross legs and arms: This posture suggests that you are receptive and open to what the patient is relaying. Caution must be taken to refrain from slouching, which may convey an informal and unprofessional attitude. To cross legs and arms (closed posture) may create defensiveness on the part of the nurse and/or patient.

Relax: In some cases, being relaxed (no fidgeting) is easier said than done, but it is important for the nurse to create a relaxed environment and communicate that you are comfortable in the presence of the patient. Learning to convey an appropriate level of comfort may feel unnatural in the beginning, but it is a significant posture that produces surprisingly positive results.

Eye contact: Eyes that specifically avert to the clock or doorway indicate that you are may be bored, uninterested, or have someplace more important to be. Although staring at a patient is

considered intrusive and disrespectful, initiating and maintaining intermittent eye contact is a powerful technique that communicates respect, responsiveness, engagement, and willingness on the part of the nurse to listen to what a patient is saying. It is important to note that the practice of eye contact is not universal but rather varies within and between cultures.

Touch: A nurse using touch for the purposes of fostering the therapeutic relationship does so in such a manner that communicates respect, compassion, understanding, caring, and empathy. The practice of touch requires nurses to be culturally sensitive to the knowledge that what is considered appropriate and therapeutic varies within and between cultures.

Your Intuition: Nurses often rely on their sense of intuition. Although not a science, nurses learn through experience and confidence to trust their intuition, depending on environment, roles, and situations.

Stickley (2011) suggests that all of the SURETY components should be applied through the nurse's sense of intuition.

Adapted from Stickley, T. (2011). From SOLER to SURETY for effective non-verbal communication. *Nurse Education in Practice, 11,* 395–398. doi:10.1016/j.nepr.2011.03.021

as the following will provide the nurse with the strength needed to be proactive rather than reactive in times of uncertainty.

"Why do I feel the way I do?"
"Why do I react to people and situations the way that I do?"
"What needs to change?"
"What strategies are available to me?"
"How will these changes enhance the therapeutic relationship?"

Because self-awareness is a competency for relational practice, the nurse must consciously be aware of his or her own ability to effectively communicate. As a professional, the nurse is responsible and accountable for his or her knowledge, skills, and abilities as he or she relates to interpersonal communication, relational practice, and therapeutic relationships. As a framework for achieving self-awareness in communication competence, the nurse can apply the conscious competence model, sometimes called the *learning matrix*. The matrix suggests that learners are initially unaware of what they don't know. As they gain recognition of what they don't know, they consciously seek to acquire a skill and then consciously use that skill or knowledge. Eventually, when the skill can be completed without thinking, on autopilot, the learner has reached unconscious competence (College of Occupational Therapists of Ontario, 2009). This model consists of four stages as outlined in Box 26.2.

As seen in the following example, this model may be applied to communication competence in nursing. Derek recently acquired his registration as a registered nurse (RN) and obtained his first nursing job. While working day shift, Derek was approached by a patient requesting pain medication. Derek informed the patient that he was not her nurse and that she needed to find her nurse. Staff frequently noted that Derek's style of communication is abrupt,

distant, and primarily task-oriented, meaning that Derek only communicated with his patients when performing a task and even then was not engaged. Due to the number of complaints the charge nurse was receiving regarding Derek's communication, she decided to inform Derek of the effect his communication skills were having on others. Derek

BOX 26.2 Conscious Competence Model

Unconscious Incompetence

The nurse who is unconsciously incompetent is unaware that he or she is communicating in manner that is inconsistent with the expectations outlined in the CNA Code of Ethics, provincial standards of practice, or by their employer's code of conduct.

Conscious Incompetence

A consciously incompetent nurse has been made aware that his or her relational and communication skills fall below expectations. It is at this stage that the nurse may have received disciplinary action and/or be required to attain the knowledge, skills, and attributes related to effective communication.

Unconscious Competence

The unconscious competent nurse continues to practice and implement the relevant knowledge, skills, and attributes to improve how he or she communicates and relates to others. This is not yet an integrated skill.

Conscious Competence

The conscious competent nurse is able to consistently communicate safely, competently, and ethically. Additionally, the nurse possesses the ability to implement and provide rationale for using the most appropriate behavioural and relational communication skills required within various situations.

was unaware (Stage 1: unconscious incompetence) that his communication skills were being perceived in a negative way and, as a new graduate, was feeling overwhelmed by the responsibilities of his position. This is Stage 2: conscious incompetence, as Derek has now been made aware of the need to improve his communication skills. Derek attends monthly in-services program and acquires the relevant knowledge, skills and attributes needed to facilitate effective communication. He puts into practice what he learned but admits that it does not feel natural at times (Stage 3: unconscious competence), but with more time, practice, and feedback, he is confident that one day, he will be proficient in integrating effective communication skills in all situations (Stage 4: conscious competence).

The process of becoming self-aware can at times seem daunting, but it is essential and provides the nurse with a valuable opportunity to acquire deeper understanding of the self, which at the end of the day will ultimately enhance both personal and professional development.

Enhancing Self-Awareness

We can look to three core concepts as a guide to enhancing our self-awareness: listen and watch others, self-disclosure, and seek feedback.

Listen and watch others. We acquire a great deal of information about ourselves when we take the time to listen and observe the behaviour of others. Nursing students often begin the process of self-awareness when they buddy or shadow other nurses and seek constructive feedback. With almost every interpersonal interaction, nurses receive explicit or hidden comments regarding their communication, which can either be ignored or used to increase self-awareness (Devito et al., 2005).

Self-disclosure. Sharing about oneself assists in making connections with others. The more you disclose about yourself, the more likely others will reciprocate and provide feedback as to how they see you.

Seek feedback. Oftentimes, when receiving feedback, we hear only what we want to hear. Truly being aware of how others view you can be a humbling experience. It takes courage, an open mind, and an understanding of intention when seeking feedback from others. When we ask questions such as, "What was your first impression of me?" "How do you feel I did?" and "What do you think my strengths and weaknesses are?" these provide a better understanding of who we are and how others view us. The feedback you receive will depend on your perception, whom you ask, and the relationship you have with that person. For example, colleagues may view Makenzie as quiet, competent, and serious with the ability to do many tasks at once, whereas at the local community center, she is viewed as outgoing, fun, laid back, and resourceful. As a requirement in most provinces/territories, nurses are encouraged to seek feedback from peers as well as participate in yearly performance reviews. Nurses seeking feedback find that it is often an emotional experience, but as long as the feedback remains professional, no boundaries are crossed. It is only when we understand how others view us that we can grow as both nurses and human beings. Box 26.3 provides suggestions for how to present and accept feedback in a constructive manner.

Empathy

A nurse's ability to effectively express **empathy** is one of the most important components in the therapeutic relationship. Empathy is the ability to emotionally and cognitively

---

BOX 26.3 Giving and Receiving of Constructive Feedback

When receiving feedback, consider the following:

- Be open-minded and listen to what the other person is saying.
- If you do not understand the feedback, admit so, and ask questions.
- If you disagree with the feedback, say so in a polite and respectful manner and be willing to discuss the differences.
- Understand and believe that the feedback is given in the spirit of advancement.
- If you become emotional, you have the right to stop the session and continue at another time.
- Reflect on the feedback you received, how it made you feel, how you responded, and what you would do differently next time.
- Use "I" statements.
- Understand the purpose of feedback and that it is meant to be constructive and essential in advancing education, professional development, and patient safety.
- The success in receiving feedback largely depends on your perception of feedback.

When providing feedback,

- Establish a safe environment in which you feel comfortable providing/discussing and the other individual feels comfortable listening/discussing.
- Balance the amount you speak with listening.
- Allow enough time for the individual receiving the feedback to respond.
- Feedback should be specific and to the point.
- Feedback should be focused on issues or competencies rather than of a personal nature.
- Balance the positive and negative feedback.
- Reflect on the feedback you provided, how you provided the feedback, the response you received, how you feel, how you responded, and what you would do differently next time. Understand that the purpose of feedback and that it is meant to be constructive and essential in advancing education professional development and patient safety.
- The success in providing feedback largely depends on your perception of feedback.

understand and communicate the experiences and feelings from another's point of view. The art of empathizing takes practice, patience, creativity, and courage to understand how, why, what the patient experiences, and the unique meaning attributed by the patient. Empathy is a skill that most of us began learning as children when playing with others. We learned that we did not like it when other kids took our toys, hurt our feelings, or pushed us on the playground.

A question often posed by nursing students is how to be empathetic to a patient expressing an unfamiliar emotion or experience. The answer is complex and requires the nursing student to offer a nonjudgmental verbal or nonverbal response.

It also helps to step back and ask, "If this happened to me or someone I care about, how might I feel?" or "What would I be most concerned or fearful about?" Verbal responses from the nurse may include, "I understand how scary this is for you. . . ." or "It must be frustrating for you to have to wait so long. . . ." to convey understanding of the experience and can be used separately or in conjunction with a nonverbal empathic response to further facilitate trust between the nurse and patient.

Rapport

Rapport is the primary influencing factor in the development of trust and understanding within the nurse–patient relationship (Belcher & Jones, 2009). Establishing rapport can be challenging for both new graduates and experienced nurses. Communication, the personalities of the nurse and patient, the nurse's bedside manner, experience, and initiative are fundamental elements in achieving rapport (Belcher & Jones, 2009). Strategies to build rapport with patients can be found in Box 26.4.

The Health Quality Council of Alberta (HQCA) in collaboration with Alberta Health Services (AHS) established the ReLATE|ReSPOND program (Table 26.5) to provide strategies for nurses and other health-care providers to use when establishing rapport with patients. The premise of the program suggests that when used effectively, nurses spend more time successfully engaged in patient care and less time responding to patient issues. The relate aspect of the program addresses the manner in which patients would like nurses to communicate with them and includes both the behavioural

---

BOX 26.4 Strategies for Building Rapport

1. Introduce yourself.
2. Address the patient by his or her preferred name.
3. Explain your role and purpose.
4. Actively listen.
5. Find ways to connect with your patient on a human level. Get to know who he or she really is.
6. Establish trust and comfort by being respectful, genuine, authentic, open-minded, and nonjudgmental.
7. Anticipate the patient's needs and follow-through with what you say you are going to do.
8. Communicate frequently with your patient throughout the shift and let him or her know when you leave and come back from breaks and at the end of shift. Provide the patient the name of the nurse covering for breaks as well as the next nurse assuming his or her care.

---

aspect of communication (clarifying questions) and the relational aspect of communication (respect, listen, empathize, and explain). The respond portion of the program teaches nurses how to effectively and efficiently communicate and attempt to resolve issues by keeping in mind that the patient/family want to feel cared for and about; that their voice has been heard; their issue has been acknowledged; and that they are kept informed as to the status of the issue and resolution.

Trust

For the purposes of this chapter, **trust** is described as an evolutionary process and an attitude in which an individual relies with confidence on another (Belcher & Jones, 2009). Good communication, knowledge, respect, honesty, confidence, self-reliance, and commitment were identified by Washington (1990) and Arnold and Boggs (2011) as being essential elements of trust. Trust is a core value in initiating and maintaining therapeutic relationships.

Nursing is recognized as being one of the most trusted professions; therefore, it is prudent for nurses to keep in mind that the value of trust within therapeutic relationships takes time to develop and if that trust is breached, it may take longer to

---

TABLE 26.5	Relate/Respond		
R	Respect the dignity and privacy of the patient	R	Recognize the complainant's perspective
E	Explain who you are; what you are going to do; identify staff that may be assisting you; how long you will take; what the patient can expect in the future (i.e., lab or diagnostic tests; visit from physician; procedures planned)	E	Establish rapport with complainant
		S	Single out the complainant's real issue
		P	Provide information to the complainant about what you are going to do
L	Listen to what the patient/family is really saying	O	Operationalize the intended plan of care
A	Ask clarifying questions	N	Notify the complainant about progress towards resolving the complaint
T	Try to be flexible and offer alternatives		
E	Empathize with the stress that accompanies illness	D	Discuss the circumstances of the complaint with a supervisor and Document according to organizational policies

Reprinted with permission from Health Quality Council of Alberta. (n.d.). *ReLATE|ReSPOND*. Retrieved from http://www.hqca.ca/index.php?id=216

reestablish, if at all. If patients feel, for whatever reason, that they cannot trust their nurse, they may be left feeling betrayed, anxious, vulnerable, and powerless (Sellman, 2006). Therefore, the idea of care without trust is unfathomable (Sellman, 2007). On an innate level, individuals want and need to trust others, but due to varying circumstances, each of us will learn to internalize this value differently. Belcher and Jones (2009) identify that the personalities of the nurse and patient, friendliness of the nurse, the nurse's willingness to care, in addition to their vested interest in establishing rapport contribute to the development of trusting relationships. When trust is established, patients expect that the nurse will provide care and communicate in a manner that is safe, competent, and ethical (Belcher & Jones, 2009; Canadian Nurses Association [CNA], 2008).

In accordance with the CNA Code of Ethics (CNA, 2008), "Nurses build trustworthy relationships as the foundation of meaningful communication, recognizing that building these relationships involves a conscious effort. Such relationships are critical to understanding people's needs and concerns" (p. 8).

Self-Disclosure and Confidentiality

The intention and expectation of **self-disclosure** within social and personal relationships is very different from that expected within the professional environment of nursing. Self-disclosure on the part of the nurse should occur only if the information is deemed to be therapeutically beneficial for the patient. First-year students often struggle with knowing what is and is not appropriate to share with patients. Disclosing your name, where you attend school, why you chose to enter the nursing profession, interests, and hobbies are social and safe topics that help establish trust and rapport. Disclosing your home address or phone number, financial status or concerns as well as past or current personal relationships would be considered inappropriate and crossing the professional boundary. Should you have doubts about what you should and should not disclose with patients, always consult the CNA Code of Ethics, employer, or regulatory body (CARNA, 2005). The concept of self-disclosure is intertwined with the concepts of trust and **confidentiality**, all of which are requisites for establishing and maintaining therapeutic relationships (Fig. 26.6). Confidentiality is a

moral obligation of nondisclosure and implies that the information a patient chooses to disclose will not be shared without consent (Austin & Boyd, 2010; Berman & Snyder, 2012). Therefore, in order to disclose personal information, the patient first has to trust the nurse, and in order to trust the nurse, the patient must believe that his or her personal information will be kept confidential and only disclosed with pertinent care providers.

Through the eyes of a student

*A*s an in-class exercise, our instructor provided each student with a small piece of paper and an envelope. We were asked to write our first name on the outside of the envelope and then asked to write on the small piece of paper some information about ourselves that we would consider to be personal and confidential and would not want openly shared in class. At this time, the room became quiet, followed by some moaning and reluctance to participate. When the last student had sealed his envelope, we were instructed to pass the envelope to a student seated on the other side of the room and to place the envelope in front of us. The instructor then asked the following questions:

1. What are you feeling?
2. How easy or difficult was it for you to disclose personal and private information?
3. How important is trust and confidentiality right now?
4. What would this be like from a patient's perspective?

As a nursing student, I expect patients to disclose all their personal health and social information, but it was only in the large group discussion did I realize how scared, vulnerable, and anxious some patients must feel disclosing such information. I now realize how quickly I need to create relational space and establish rapport and trust. I also need to communicate why I am collecting the information, what I will be doing with the information, and who has access to it.

What I learned most of all is that I never want a patient to feel the way I did during that exercise. Lesson learned!
(personal reflection of a nursing student)

Mutuality and Intentionality

Mutuality can be defined as finding common ground in others' experiences, goals, values, beliefs, thoughts, and feelings. Nurses use mutuality in acknowledging and honouring the differences that exist in the therapeutic relationship. The outcome of mutuality is a shared sense of understanding, personal responsibility, and satisfaction (Grover, 2005). **Intentionality** is one of the main concepts that motivates, guides, shapes, and affirms the caring value of nursing practice (Purnell, 2002). What motivates nurses to be intentional about demonstrating caring thoughts, attitude, and behaviour is hopefully an intrinsic motivation or desire to

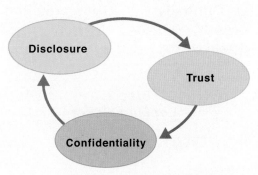

Figure 26.6 Requisite concepts of self-disclosure.

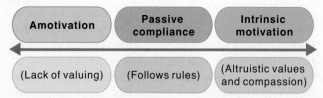

Figure 26.7 Intentionality of caring.

interact, engage with, and know their patient; to improve patient outcomes; and to collaborate with and to help patients understand and clarify the meaning of their health and healing experiences (Hartrick, 1997; Porr & Egan, 2013). The intentionality of caring (Fig. 26.7) runs along a continuum, ranging from a motivation (lack of valuing) in which the nurse chooses not to demonstrate caring behaviours, to intrinsic motivation (altruistic values and compassion), in which the nurse is authentically motivated to demonstrate concern for others and ensures nursing actions are in the best interest of the patient (Porr & Egan, 2013). Think box outlines some questions for you to think about as to whether or not you communicate authentically and with intention.

Think
1. In what ways do you communicate authentically?
2. Are you intentional about what you say and how you say it?
3. How does your communication demonstrate intentionality?

Honouring Complexity and Ambiguity

"Nurses need to learn to acknowledge that complexity and ambiguity are inherent characteristics of every human experience" (Hartrick, 1997, p. 526). Furthermore, it is only when both the patient and nurse expand their capacity to trust; honour uncertainty; and learn to question feelings, thoughts, and meaning of their experience will they begin to comprehend the relevance of the experience and then be able to make meaningful and intentional choices (Hartrick, 1997). Nurses are able to honour complexity and ambiguity by continually assessing, adapting, evaluating, and revising their understanding of the patient's lived experience.

Reflective Practice

Reflective practice is a process of mentally reviewing, analyzing, and comprehending events, situations, and actions that occur in our everyday work and personal lives (Oelofsen, 2012). Although reflective practice often occurs during and after experiential learning, it also encompasses the aesthetic, personal, and ethical ways of knowing (Horton-Deutsch & Sherwood, 2008).

Nurses develop a feeling for what they do, but it cannot always be verbally expressed. Nurses need and desire adequate ways to express themselves and reflective practice provides a mechanism through which they can communicate and justify the importance of their practice and practice knowledge.

The use of reflection ensures nurses are continually learning by assimilating theory into practice and developing self-awareness, all of which contributes to safe, competent, ethical care, and communication. The model of reflective practice by Oelofsen (2012) can be easily integrated into any nursing practice area. The model, as depicted in Figure 26.8, comprises three stages. The first stage is curiosity or the nurse's power of observation, perception, and questioning. In order to comprehend a situation, the types of questions nurses may reflect on include, but are not limited to, the following (Oelofsen, 2012):

- What happened?
- How did I react?
- What was good/bad about the experience?
- What else might be occurring?
- What sense can I make of the situation?
- What was it like from the patient's perspective?
- How did it affect me? How did it affect the team?
- What would I or the team do differently next time?

Stage 2 requires the nurse to take a closer look at some or all of the questions in Step 1. Examining and analyzing a given experience, situation, or event and the effect it had on us enables practitioners the opportunity to step back; slow down their thoughts, feelings, and actions and articulate the experience; and explore the underlying beliefs regarding their own practice (Oelofsen, 2012). However, as we work in collaboration with others, it is necessary for the nurse to embrace the values of being open-minded and other-oriented in order to truly listen to or accept other perspectives on a given situation or experience (Oelofsen, 2012).

The goal of reflective practice is transformation (Stage 3). This model encourages self-awareness and insight, which are key components in the transformation stage, whereby positive changes to behaviour or practice are initiated and sustained.

The process of reflective practice is never ending and should be a regular practice in your development as a nurse.

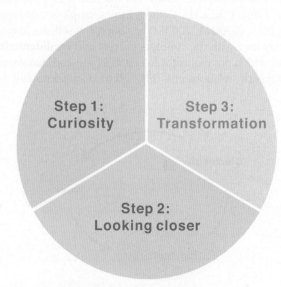

Figure 26.8 Reflective practice model.

In terms of reflecting on your ability to effectively communicate, you should explore the question, "Why do I communicate the way that I do?" as well as identify and explore the assumptions underlying your current attitudes, values, and beliefs pertaining to interpersonal communication (see Think box; Horton-Deusch & Sherwood, 2008).

Think

1. How do I feel my attitude affects my ability to communicate?
2. What are my beliefs and values about interpersonal communication?
3. Why do I feel my beliefs and values are important to me?
4. How do I feel my values impact my ability to communicate?
5. How do I feel when I am communicating with someone who does not share the same values, beliefs, or attitude as I do?
6. How do I differentiate between social and professional communication?

Through critical reflection, individuals develop the emotional intelligence and self-awareness to communicate authentically and with intention.

How Does Perception Influence Communication?

Have you ever wanted to know how others see you or what their first impression of you was? On some level, we may or may not want to know, but nevertheless, it would be interesting to examine our own barriers and strategies to perceptual accuracy (Box 26.5). **Perception** is the process of selecting, organizing, and assigning meaning to the world around us (Adler et al., 2012). In today's world, we are inundated with information from a plethora of sources, making it impossible to remember or even pay attention to all that goes on around us (Adler et al., 2012).

Perception Process

Perception is one influence on interpersonal and therapeutic relationships as well as on relational inquiry and practice. Each of us views people, events, and emotions differently, and how we perceive events and people influences how and what we communicate. What you see depends on how you select, organize, and assign meaning to the details.

Think In 2011, Duval Guillaume Modem, a communications agency located in Antwerp, Belgium, conducted an original experiment involving unsuspecting couples entering a movie theatre filled with 148 burly men sporting various tattoos and dressed in black t-shirts and/or leather jackets. Only two seats were left and situated in the middle of the theatre. If you were to enter this theatre, consider how perception might influence your thinking and subsequent behaviour.

1. What would you be thinking?
2. How would you react?
3. Would you stay or would you leave?
4. What perceptions do you feel the men in the theatre would have if you stayed or left?

BOX 26.5   Self-Assessment of Perceptual Accuracy

Instructions: Respond to each of the following statements with T for "true" if the statement is usually or generally accurate in describing your behaviour and with F for "false" if the statement is usually or generally inaccurate in describing your behaviour. Try to avoid the tendency to give what you feel is the desired response.

1. I base most of my impressions of people on the first few minutes of our meeting. ____
2. I make predictions about people's behaviours that generally prove true. ____
3. I have clear ideas of what people of different national, racial, and religious groups are really like. ____
4. I generally look for lots of cues about a person's attitudes and behaviours rather than his or her physical and psychological characteristics. ____
5. I avoid making assumptions about what is going on in someone else's head on the basis of his or her behaviour. ____
6. I pay special attention to behaviours of people that might contradict my initial impression. ____
7. On the power of my observations of others, I formulate guesses about them (which I am willing to revise) rather than firmly held conclusions. ____

8. I avoid making judgments about others until I learn a great deal about them and see them in various situations. ____
9. After I formulate an initial impression, I check my perceptions. ____

How did you do?

This brief perception test was designed to assist you in self-reflection rather than provide you with a specific score. Questions 1, 2, and 3 refer to tendencies to judge others on the basis of first impressions, self-fulfilling prophecies, and stereotypes. Ideally, you would have responded with false to these because they represent barriers to perceptual accuracy. Questions 4 to 9 suggest specific guidelines for increasing accuracy of people perceptions: looking for various cues, avoiding the tendency to read the minds of others, being especially alert to contradictory cues, formulating hypotheses rather than conclusions, recognizing the diversity in others, and delaying conclusions until more information is acquired. Ideally, you would have answered true to these questions as they represent strategies of increasing perceptual accuracy.

Source: Adapted from Devito, J. A., Shimoni, R., & Clark, D. (2005). *Building interpersonal communication skills* (2nd Canadian ed.). Toronto, ON: Pearson Allyn & Bacon.

Selection and Organization

As previously mentioned, at any given moment, we are inundated with multiple sensory stimuli, and using our five senses helps us to select which stimuli to focus on and which to ignore. A stimulus that catches our attention is often related to our emotions, desires, interests, and memories (Engleberg & Wynn, 2011). Adler et al. (2012) acknowledge that the intensity of stimuli, repetition, and motives (looking to purchase a new truck you are more likely to notice all the trucks in your environment) within our environment contribute to our ability to attend and select certain stimuli or ignore particular cues. For example, if you work with someone you really like, you may be more likely to ignore some negative cues.

After selecting the stimuli, the next step is to organize it in a way that is meaningful to you. This is achieved through classification, figure–ground differentiation, or closure. We tend to organize individuals according to five perceptual constructs: Physical constructs help us classify individuals according to physical attributes, gender, race, age, beautiful or ugly, and thin or fat (Adler et al., 2012). Role constructs classify individuals according to status, social position, occupation, marital status, mother, father, sister, aunt, etc. (Adler et al., 2012). Classification according to social behaviour, such as friendly, helpful, nice, mean, unhelpful, and aloof, is an aspect of the interaction construct (Adler et al., 2012). Psychological constructs classify individuals as being inquisitive, anxious, or timid (Adler et al., 2012), and the last schemata is membership construct in which individuals are classified according to the group(s) they participate in, such as girl guides, scouts, committees, etc. (Adler et al., 2012).

Regardless of the fact that we may not have all the information we need about an individual, we classify according to the stated schemata and continue to apply a label and fill in the rest of the information with our own attitudes, beliefs, and values. The inference we make is either correct or incorrect, and the concern here is in the formation and perpetuation of stereotypes (Beebe et al., 2013). Consider the schemata you use to classify your peers, instructors, patients, and interprofessional team member and then consider how the schemata influences both therapeutic and professional relationships. Within a hospital environment, suppose you saw a female walking past you wearing scrubs. Based on the individual's gender, attire, and work environment, you may infer that the individual is a nurse. Suppose you see another individual wearing scrubs and lab coat and carrying a basket containing needles and blood collection tubes and conclude the person is a lab technician. Taking the observed information allows you to organize it into "nurse" and "lab technician." However, changing the context to a grocery store may or may alter your perception that the individual wearing scrubs may be a nurse but may allow you to consider that the individual could also be a lab technician, dental hygienist, or veterinarian technician (Beebe et al., 2007).

Figure 26.9 demonstrates the principle of figure–ground differentiation as you may notice a stimulus that stands out as a figure against a less noticeable ground, enabling you to choose from two figure–ground relationships (Beebe et al., 2013).

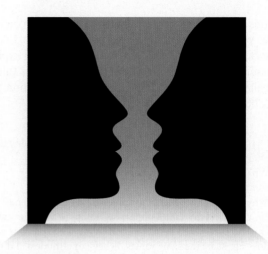

Figure 26.9 Figure–ground differentiation. Do you see two heads or a vase?

Therefore, whether you see a vase or two faces will depend on if you focus on the light or dark aspects of the image.

Interpretation

The interactions between a nurse and patient or nurse and colleague frequently consist of judgments, perceptions, actions, and reactions (Sheldon, 2005). Judgments often occur from perception, which results in a verbal or nonverbal action and reaction. The power of perception greatly influences present and future interactions. Failing to check whether or not the perception of a patient's behaviour is accurate generally leads to an assumption, breakdown in communication, demonstrates disrespectful behaviour, and negatively affects the therapeutic relationship. Listening to the subjective opinion about a patient and his or her condition, attitude, and behaviour perpetuates the cycle of labeling, stereotyping, and contributes to decreased outcomes for the patient.

Through the eyes of a student

I attended morning report on our busy medicine unit, collecting data about my first patient from the Kardex and the taped report from the night nurse. The night nurse said, "Mrs. P. refuses to eat, is difficult to provide care, bites and spits at staff, is miserable, and difficult to work with." I was scared to see this patient but asked my instructor, "What do I do? I don't want to get bit! Did you hear what they said in report about my patient? Why would you assign me that patient when they say she bites, spits, and refuses care?"

My instructor reminded me that the report held both objective and subjective data. To be fair to the patient, I need to review the patient's chart, including the nursing notes. He reminded me that what I hear about patients would influence how I see the patient, which will subsequently influence how I approach and provide care to the patient.

I introduced myself to Mrs. P. in a professional manner and then inquired as to how she was feeling. With a little probing, she said she was in pain and that she did not want any care. I said I would let the nurse know about her pain and would be right back. When I returned to the room, Mrs. P. continued to tell me how she was feeling, not only physically but also emotionally. I pulled up a chair and let her tell her story. I had provided no physical care to that point but she agreed I could come back in 15 minutes to wash her.

Looking back at morning report, I can't believe I almost blew the opportunity of working with Mrs. P by believing what others thought about her. What Mrs. P. needed from me was compassion, caring, and to take the time to listen.

(personal reflection of a nursing student)

Perception Checking

Psychologists Richard Block and Harold Yuker (1992) acknowledge that "perception often is a poor representation of reality. Yet it is important to recognize that a person's behaviour is controlled less by what is actually true, than what the person believes is true. Perceptions may be more important than reality in determining behaviour" (Block & Yuker, 1989, p. 239).

In order to enhance perceptual understanding and to avoid miscommunication, nurses use the behavioural technique of perception checking. The purpose of **perception checking** is to clarify nonverbal behaviour with a verbal statement. There are two ways in which perception checking can be used. Through **indirect perception checking**, individuals passively seek additional nonverbal information (eye contact, body language, tone of voice) that supports or contradicts the interpretation of behaviour (Beebe et al., 2013).

Direct perception checking consists of simply asking the individual or a third party whether your interpretation of the perception is correct (Beebe et al., 2013). Direct perception checking involves the following three steps:

1. A clear description of the behaviour you observed
2. Two possible interpretations of the behaviour
3. Pose a clarifying question.

Box 26.6 provides a few examples of direct perception checking.

BOX 26.6 Indirect Perception Checking

"When you left the table suddenly," (behaviour) "I wasn't sure if you felt sick" (first interpretation) "or just had to use the washroom" (second interpretation). "How are you feeling?" (seeking clarification).

Therapeutic Communication Techniques

Therapeutic communication encourages self-disclosure, increases feelings of self-worth, and promotes self-awareness. Approaches such as open-ended questioning, clarification statements, probing and paraphrasing, sharing your observations, summarizing, and the value of silence are explored. When the nurse uses these behavioural skills correctly, the patient views the nurse as being supportive, caring, and compassionate which in turn leads the patient to feel heard, valued, recognized, and acknowledged.

Open-Ended Questions

Open-ended questions are frequently used when obtaining patient health histories or when the nurse requires an expanded response or explanation from the patient. Asking questions that begin with *what, when, where, why,* and *how* forms open-ended questioning. This type of questioning enables the nurse to introduce an idea or area for discussion and allows the patient to form free and complete responses, (Mitchell, 2014). The intent behind using open-ended questions is to encourage the patient to talk by exploring, clarifying, or describing his or her thoughts and feelings, as these questions require more than a simple yes or no response (Mitchell, 2014). The following scenario provides an example of open-ended questions:

Nurse: *What* did your wife make you for breakfast this morning?
Patient: Sara made me two scrambled eggs, two slices of toast, cup of oatmeal, and coffee.
Nurse: *How* much of each were you able to eat?
Patient: I ate half of the eggs, one slice of plain toast, and most of the coffee. I was not able to eat the oatmeal.
Nurse: *Why* were you not able to eat the oatmeal?
Patient: I started to have pain and felt sick.

Clarification

Nurses will use **clarification** as a way to ensure they have heard the patient correctly and to check or verify information that they feel may be unclear. Restating an unclear message, asking the person to rephrase, or asking for an example are all types of clarification. Clarification is often used with perception checking. Examples of clarifying questions may include the following:

1. "When you said you felt sick this morning, I am not sure I understand what you meant by the word *sick*, please explain."
2. "Before you continue, I just want to make sure that I heard you correctly when you said that you were not able to finish eating your breakfast because you started to feel unwell during breakfast?"

Probing

Probing, also called *focusing*, is a technique used to encourage a patient to expand on or further explore his or her thoughts, ideas, and feelings. Probing is used to guide the direction of the conversation to cover important topics, without interrupting the patient if they are discussing something of importance (Mitchell, 2014). This particular technique is helpful when the discussion fails to move forward. Using the previous scenario, an example of probing would be, "Tell me more about the pain you experienced at breakfast" or "Please continue with what you were saying about having pain this morning. . . ."

Paraphrasing

Paraphrasing is the ability to repeat in your own words the essential thoughts, ideas, and feelings a patient is trying to convey. By using paraphrasing effectively, the patient understands that you are actively listening, engaged, and that you care about him or her. However, in order to paraphrase correctly, the nurse needs to be fully present and actively listening (Box 26.7). In order to effectively paraphrase, practice is essential (Jakubec & Astle, 2014).

Sharing Observations

Sharing observations occurs when a nurse verbally communicates his or her observations regarding how a patient looks, behaves, or sounds (Jakubec & Astle, 2014). Many patients are reluctant to disclose or are unsure of how to verbalize their feelings. When the nurse observes behaviours such as nail biting, clenched hands, scratching, or restlessness, it is important to share those with the patient. It is only when the patient understands that his or her behaviour is noticed by the nurse that the patient feels that he or she can explain the meaning of the behaviour. Statements such as, "I have noticed that every time the doctor enters the room you start biting your bottom lip. . . ." "Your hands are clenched, and you are sweating quite a bit" or "I have not seen you eat anything off your tray this morning" offer the patient the opportunity to verify, correct, or elaborate on the meaning.

Caution needs to be taken on the part of the nurse to ensure that the observations being shared with the patient are objective, void from drawing and stating conclusions or assumptions and remain nonjudgmental (Jakubec & Astle, 2014). Sharing observations with a patient should only be done to enhance trust, honesty, and disclosure and should never be used to embarrass or distress the patient and/or family (Jakubec & Astle, 2014).

Silence

To nurses, **silence** means to be quiet while at the same time nonverbally indicating interest in what the patient is relaying (Austin & Boyd, 2010). Depending on culture and self-knowledge, you may view silence as golden, appropriate, comforting, safe, and affirming, or it may be viewed as awkward, uncomfortable, or inappropriate. In today's environment of social media, we are constantly inundated with electronic communication (discussed further on in the chapter). According to Bunkers (2013), the concept of silence within the technological era has implications to patient's health and well-being. Nurses often struggle with when to be silent, when not to be silent, and when to seek silence. Using silence to facilitate the lived experience of a patient offers integrity, dignity, and respect and provides both the nurse and the patient the opportunity to acquire a different perspective as well as the capacity to "let be and live with complexity and ambiguity" (Doane & Varcoe, 2005; Jacubek & Astle, 2010). However, more often than not, in interpersonal communication, we believe silence as the act of refraining from speaking will actually enhance dialogue (Back, Bauer-Wu, Rushton, & Halifax, 2009).

Silence can have a therapeutic, neutral, or destructive effect on the therapeutic relationship. When asking questions, the normal response time is between 15 and 30 seconds, but consideration must be given to the patient's culture and medical condition. When response time is greater than 30 seconds, inexperienced nurses and nursing students acknowledge that the experience can be awkard. First-year students meeting a patient for the very first time are full of questions, with most of them not pertaining to the patient but rather the experience.

"How do I start the conversation?"
"What if I run out of questions?"
"What do I do if there is prolonged silence?"

Nurses are most familiar with using invitational silence within the nurse–patient relationships. This technique is used with the intention of enhancing the nurses understanding of the patient's lived experience. This typology is focused on the therapeutic benefit of mindfully being with a patient and being comfortable with spontaneous episodes of silence. Noting that, with silence, the nurse possesses the opportunity to assess and obtain additional nonverbal data that can positively influence the nurse–patient relationship (Back et al., 2009).

Nurses understand what compassion means and what it looks like, and they understand what silence is and how it can

---

BOX 26.7   Accurate and Inaccurate Paraphrasing Statements

Patient: The doctor wants me to do cardio exercise every day, but I have been walking around my house and doing daily household chores such as vacuuming, laundry, and making meals, and I am exhausted at the end of the day. I don't know if I can do more than that.

Accurate paraphrasing: You are exhausted from doing daily chores, and you are unsure whether or not you are able to do the additional cardio exercises the doctor is requesting.

Inaccurate paraphrasing: You feel that household chores are a form of cardio exercise?

Patient: No matter what I eat, I have always been slightly overweight, and I am happy with where my weight is now. I feel I am relatively healthy; I just need to cut down on the salt and fast food. I don't think I need to follow the cardiac diet suggested by the doctor.

Effective paraphrasing: I hear you saying that you are healthy and happy, so you don't feel that you need to follow a cardiac diet.

Ineffective paraphrasing: You don't care about your health.

be used to foster relationships. However, the concept of compassionate silence is relatively new to nursing. In order to use compassionate silence for a therapeutic benefit, nurses need to be knowledgeable on the mental capacities of attention, intention, emotional balance in addition to the prosocial mental qualities of empathy, and compassion (Back et al., 2009).

When using compassionate silence with patients of varying cultures, nurses must learn to create meaning by appreciating and honouring the patient's culture by being with, moving in, and around the room in a calm and quiet/silent manner (Back et al., 2009). Silence in varying amounts is needed for personal reflection and self-awareness. Nurses would do well to remember that, "Just as misused silence damages, wise silence heals" (Feldman, 2003, p. 12).

Challenges of Silence

Silence can be intimidating, but the key to being comfortable with silence is first understanding the nature of silence and then reflecting on the uncomfortable situation created by silence. Table 26.6 summarizes the current research as to the typology of silence.

Awkward silence results when nurses are waiting for a response or don't know how to respond to a patient or situation. Most of the time, nurses use silence with no real purpose or benefit to the patient whereby making silence virtually nontherapeutic. When awkward silence occurs, there is the potential for the nurse to transfer his or her feelings of uncertainty onto the patient which then can be interpreted by the patient as judgmental and disapproving (Back et al., 2009).

Summarizing

In situations such as when a nurse is completing a health/admission history or during patient/family conferences, **summarizing** is a helpful technique to concisely recap what the patient, family, or members of the interdisciplinary team have shared. Usually, summarizing occurs upon completion of a history or conference; however, leaving it to the end sometimes prevents the patient or others from clarifying information or asking additional questions. Therefore, summarization is most effective part way through a history or conference. "Before we conclude, I just want to review a few main points of what you have told me . . ." or "To recap, what has been discussed so far . . ." Summarizing is

especially beneficial to a patient in the termination phase of the therapeutic nurse–patient relationship (Jakubec & Astle, 2010).

Patients With Unique Communication Needs

Every nurse has the goal to communicate as effectively as possible with each patient. Patients experiencing temporary or permanent verbal, auditory, visual, cognitive, or linguistic impairments (Fig. 26.10) may be angry, frustrated, anxious or happy, resilient, and accepting of their situation (Johansson, Carlsson, & Sonnander, 2012). The key to communicating with individuals possessing unique communication needs is the nurse's ability to get to know the patient and determine how the patient perceives the impairment before being able to effectively help the patient.

Regardless of how the patient perceives his or her situation, a nurse's comfort, patience, creativity, and adaptability will be challenged. It is also important for nurses to self-monitor their level of frustration in attempting to communicate and refrain from turning and walking away from a patient, which in and of itself may create patient distress, hopelessness, or depression (Hemsley, Balandin, & Worrall, 2012). When communicating with individuals possessing unique communication needs, nurses identify time and work load demands as the main intervening variable preventing effective communication leading to decreased patient satisfaction and increase risk of an adverse event occurring (Hemsley et al., 2011). If the nurse demonstrates compassion and kindness, initiates and makes the time to try various strategies, and is then able to identify the best strategies enabling a connection with the patient, the better the outcome will be for the patient. Having said that, another essential component in the communication process is for the nurse to formally communicate with interprofessional team members the strategies that work best for the patient to use and understand. At the end of the day, nurses frequently employ a wide range of adaptive communication strategies to improve patient outcomes and satisfaction and to prevent adverse events from occurring (Hemsley et al., 2011). Box 26.8 outlines some strategies to consider when communicating with patients possessing unique communication needs (Green, 2012; Jakubec & Astle, 2014; Mitchell, 2014; Webb, 2011).

TABLE 26.6	Typology of Silence
Type of Silence	**Intention of Health-Care Provider**
Awkward	Often occurs spontaneously and is unintentional, although meant to be therapeutic. May conceal distractions, judgements, biases or ambivalence on the part of the health-care worker.
Invitational	Purposeful and intentional in that the health-care worker may utilize an empathic technique in facilitating the patient to reflect on their values, beliefs, feelings and experiences.
Compassionate	The health-care worker recognizes that an impromptu period of silence has occurred during conversation, while completing a task or when entering a patients environment and actively creates meaning and compassion for the patient.

Source: Back, A. L., Bauer-Wu, S. M., Rushton, C. H., & Halifax, J. (2009).Compassionate silence in the patient–clinician encounter: A contemplative approach. *Journal of Palliative Medicine, 12*(12), 1113–1117. doi:10.1089/jpm.2009.0175

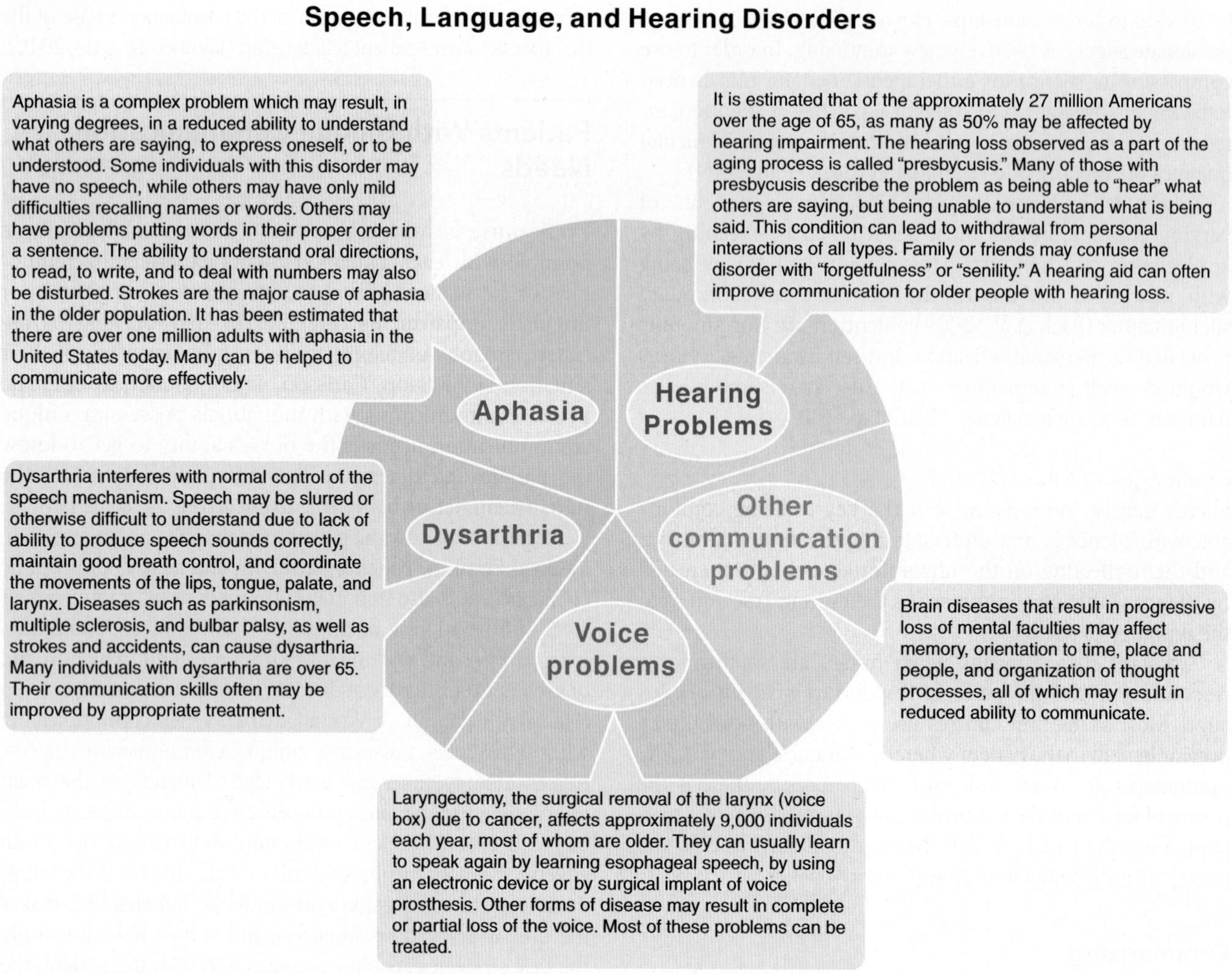

Speech, Language, and Hearing Disorders

Aphasia is a complex problem which may result, in varying degrees, in a reduced ability to understand what others are saying, to express oneself, or to be understood. Some individuals with this disorder may have no speech, while others may have only mild difficulties recalling names or words. Others may have problems putting words in their proper order in a sentence. The ability to understand oral directions, to read, to write, and to deal with numbers may also be disturbed. Strokes are the major cause of aphasia in the older population. It has been estimated that there are over one million adults with aphasia in the United States today. Many can be helped to communicate more effectively.

It is estimated that of the approximately 27 million Americans over the age of 65, as many as 50% may be affected by hearing impairment. The hearing loss observed as a part of the aging process is called "presbycusis." Many of those with presbycusis describe the problem as being able to "hear" what others are saying, but being unable to understand what is being said. This condition can lead to withdrawal from personal interactions of all types. Family or friends may confuse the disorder with "forgetfulness" or "senility." A hearing aid can often improve communication for older people with hearing loss.

Dysarthria interferes with normal control of the speech mechanism. Speech may be slurred or otherwise difficult to understand due to lack of ability to produce speech sounds correctly, maintain good breath control, and coordinate the movements of the lips, tongue, palate, and larynx. Diseases such as parkinsonism, multiple sclerosis, and bulbar palsy, as well as strokes and accidents, can cause dysarthria. Many individuals with dysarthria are over 65. Their communication skills often may be improved by appropriate treatment.

Brain diseases that result in progressive loss of mental faculties may affect memory, orientation to time, place and people, and organization of thought processes, all of which may result in reduced ability to communicate.

Aphasia

Hearing Problems

Dysarthria

Other communication problems

Voice problems

Laryngectomy, the surgical removal of the larynx (voice box) due to cancer, affects approximately 9,000 individuals each year, most of whom are older. They can usually learn to speak again by learning esophageal speech, by using an electronic device or by surgical implant of voice prosthesis. Other forms of disease may result in complete or partial loss of the voice. Most of these problems can be treated.

Figure 26.10 Speech, language, and hearing disorders.

Through the eyes of a student

Contigo (With You)

I was walking out of another patient's room when I came upon Helen in the hallway. Helen was restrained in a wheelchair. She has dementia, and she cannot speak English. She speaks Spanish. Below is a poem I wrote about my interactions with Helen.

I am here. I am here with you. You reached out to me.
I hold you. I hold your hand. You draw me close to you. You cry.
You bury your cheek against my shoulder.
I am not afraid to see, hear, or feel you cry.
I feel you hurting, and I cannot help but hurt with you.
I do not know you. I do not know the laugher you have lived—or the lives you have changed.
Changed. Oh, I am Changed. I am Changed by you.
You speak words that I cannot understand.
It is neither my fault nor yours. It is simply what it is:
I am but one person, but I have learned that one person can hold your hand, listen to you speak; offer you tissues as you weep.

I choose to be this person when I see you. I choose to care for you. I choose to care about you.
I do not suffer, as you suffer. I would never know the depth of what you experience, but I am here for you as best I can be.
I am you. You are me. We are in this moment.
Did I help you forget, if but for a moment, that you are hurting?
You communicate with me, but I cannot understand and so I do not know;
I will never give up on you. I will never turn a blind eye.
You feel alone. I know.
I am here. I am here with you.
If you grasp for me, I will hold you.
If you speak to me, I will listen.
You look at me.
I see you.
You pause to utter: Gracias (Thank You)
I understand.

(Jody Pon, second-year nursing student, MacEwan University)

BOX 26.8 Strategies for Individuals With Unique Communication Needs

Patients With Speaking Challenges
- Introduce yourself.
- Determine if the patient is able to understand what you are trying to communicate. In other words, don't assume the patient that cannot speak also cannot understand.
- Explain what you are doing and how long it will take.
- Face the patient when you are speaking.
- Actively listen, be patient, and refrain from interrupting the patient.
- When asking a question, provide enough time for the patient to respond.
- Rephrase the question if needed but avoid repeating the question because this may lead to patient anxiety and frustration.
- Determine the patient's preferred method of communication and any augmenting and alternative communication devices the patient may be using (gestures, white board, sign language, communication board, pen and paper, or computer technology).
- Be honest and inform the patient should you not understand what he or she is trying to communicate.
- If the patient is elderly, refrain from using **elderspeak** language such as love, dear, sweetie, honey (Williams, K., Kemper, S., & Hummert, M. L., 2004).
- Communicate with respect, caring, compassion, and patience.

Patients Who Are Unresponsive/Dying
- Knock before entering the patient's room.
- Announce your presence if curtain is closed around bed.
- Speak in a normal tone/rate and pitch.
- Explain procedures you are performing.
- Call the patient by his or her preferred name.
- Patients are still able to hear, so use caution in what and how you are speaking.
- Refrain from third-party discussions near the patient (speaking about the patient in the presence of the patient or staff carrying on own discussions and ignoring the patient).
- Use of therapeutic touch may be comforting to the patient.
- Encourage and facilitate family and friends in speaking to the patient.
- Consider the patient's culture and inquire about what should and should not be done in the room (e.g., some Aboriginal persons request nurses to work quietly and slowly in and around the patient so as not to disturb the connection with ancestors).
- Communicate with respect, caring, compassion, and patience.

Patients With Cognitive Challenges
- Introduce yourself.
- Address the patient by his or her preferred name.
- Identify the patient's preferred method of communication.
- Identify and use communication aids deemed to enhance the patient's communication.
- Speak in a normal tone, rate, and pitch.
- Clear and concise verbal communication.
- Gentle and appropriate questioning.

- Monitor the patient's body language and nonverbal cues.
- Refrain from leading questions, "You've been well?" or "You have not been ill, have you?" because patients will often tell us what they think we want to hear; so if you lead a patient in the direction you want (often unintentionally), that will most likely be the response you will get.
- Actively listen by implementing SURETY.
- Use therapeutic touch when you need to gain the patients attention.
- Monitor the environment and keep excess noise to a minimum, especially during interactions.
- Use appropriate augmentative and alternative communication methods.
- Communicate with respect, caring, compassion, and patience.

Patients With Vision Challenges
- Ensure the patient wears glasses/contacts if at bedside.
- Speak in a normal tone, rate, and pitch.
- Introduce yourself.
- Explain what you are doing and how long it will take.
- If vision impairment is severe, let the patient know when you are leaving the room.
- Determine the patient's preferred methods for communication (augmentative and alternative communication methods).
- If communicating in writing, use large font.
- Communicate with respect, caring, compassion, and patience.

Patients With Hearing Challenges
- Ensure the hearing aid is patent and clean and the battery is working.
- Face the patient when speaking.
- If the patient does not wear hearing aids, speak near, or into the unaffected ear (hearing impaired in right ear, you would then speak to the patient on his or her left side).
- Speak in a normal tone and pitch. Refrain from speaking loudly.
- Determine the patients preferred method of communication and any augmenting and alternative communication devices the patient may be using.
- Communicate with respect, caring, compassion, and patience.

Patients With Linguistic Challenges
- Speak in a normal tone, rate, and pitch.
- Introduce yourself.
- Explain as best as you can what you are doing.
- Determine the patients preferred method of communication.
- Learn a few key words or phrases in the patient's language.
- Create or use a communication board in the patient's language.
- Use caution when gesturing. Meanings are often culturally specific.
- Use an interpreter if available. Interpreters may be hired by the facility or you may use staff on the unit or in the facility as well as members of the patient's family.
- Communicate with respect, caring, compassion, and patience.

Nontherapeutic Communication Techniques

Behavioural communication techniques considered to be nontherapeutic are often perceived by the patient as being unsupportive and contribute to the patient feeling devalued, disrespected, and not heard, recognized, or acknowledged. Some of these have been discussed earlier, such as making judgments, interrupting, and inaccurate paraphrasing. The key ineffective approaches to be discussed in this section include giving advice, closed-ended questions, changing the subject, automatic response, false reassurances, expressions of sympathy, and expressing disapproval. Additional contributing factors to ineffective communication include noise, individual values, beliefs, attitude, and self-knowledge.

Giving Advice

Providing patients with subjective opinions such as, "If I were you, . . ." or "What you should do is . . ." is nontherapeutic and imposes the nurse's values, beliefs, and judgments onto the patient, thus violating the nurse–patient relationship. This is an area that can lead patients to become dependent on nurses or blame nurses for undesirable outcomes. When patients are unsure of what to do, it is the nurse's role to assist them in exploring the situation and attempt to resolve the problem autonomously. Therefore, during times when patients are seeking advice or personal opinions, the nurse may choose to respond with, "Tell me what you already know about . . ." or "I want to know what your feelings are toward . . ." because these statements empower the patient to examine his or her own thoughts and feelings, as well as assist in identifying strategies that may be used to achieve the desired outcome. As long as the nurse provides objective data and available resources to the patient, provision of expert advice will remain therapeutic.

Closed-Ended Questions

Questions starting with "Do you," "Have you," or "Are you" usually elicit one-word responses of either yes or no. Generally speaking, asking a **closed-ended question** virtually guarantees that you will have to ask an open-ended question to get the information that you need. Only in emergency situations where the most amount of information is sought in a short period of time are closed-ended questions most effective.

Changing the Subject

At one point or another, we have all done this, whether it was in our personal or professional lives. When a patient is discussing a particular subject matter of importance to them and the nurse changes the subject due to feeling uncomfortable or anxious surrounding the topic of discussion, the patient–nurse relationship has shifted. Not only does it imply that the nurse is not interested in hearing what or how the patient feels but also demonstrates a lack of empathy and mutuality (Jakubec & Astle, 2010) and results with the nurse placing focus on himself or herself rather than on the patient. By changing the subject, the needs of the patient will not be met, and this directly violates the purpose of the therapeutic relationship.

Automatic Responses

Expressions of stereotypes and clichés are examples of automatic responses. In social exchanges, questions such as, "How's it going?" or "How are you?" are thoughtless and generic yet are frequently offered automatic social responses. In a casual social exchange, most of us are expecting to hear "Fine" or "Good," but when someone challenges the response with "I'm not doing very well," it often takes us

by surprise, and we then feel obligated to listen to what the individual has to say or quickly make an excuse to leave.

Automatic responses may come up when working in a particularly busy clinical setting or when the nurse is excessively task-oriented and focused on a procedure rather than on interacting with the patient. Automatic responses then tend to assimilate into one's practice. When a nurse consciously chooses to use automatic responses with patients, the relationship is sure to remain superficial and nontherapeutic. A better response is for the nurse to engage the patient by asking, "Tell me how you slept" or "Tell me about your day." These responses are individualized to the patient and indicate that the nurse is interested in the patient's perspective.

False Reassurance or Reassuring Clichés

The temptation to offer hope and reassurance not founded on facts can interfere with an opportunity for open communication. Communicating with patients using reassuring clichés such as "Everything will be okay" or "Don't worry" or "I'm sure you will feel better in no time" denies and discounts the right of the patient to feel the way he or she is feeling or to think the way he or she does about a certain situation, making the patient feel that his or her perception is incorrect or unimportant. Using false reassurance is also an indication that the nurse is trying to reduce his or her own level of discomfort with the topic area or situation.

Through the eyes of a nurse

As a new graduate working on a busy medical unit, I was approached one evening by a gentleman who was scheduled for open heart surgery the next morning. As I was preparing my medications, he stood by my cart and told me he was scared about the surgery. Being task-focused at the time, I responded with, "You have a good surgeon, I am sure everything will be okay. I will come and talk to you later." Later, never came. The next night I called the cardiac intensive unit to inquire as to the gentleman's condition and was informed that he did not make it through the surgery. That was 22 years ago, and to this day, I can't believe I provided him with such false reassurance and missed an opportunity to connect with him. I have since learned to integrate relational practice into my busy practice, and no matter how busy I am, my focus is always on the needs (physical, social, psychological) of the patient. *(personal reflection of a nurse)*

Sympathy

Sympathy is the subjective sharing of feelings of distress or sorrow. Sympathy can include a feeling of pity for the other person's situation. It is different from empathy, which is the ability to imagine oneself in the situation of another person, feeling with rather than feeling for. Sympathy is a compassionate response toward a patient; however, it is not as effective as empathy. When a nurse indicates that he or she feels sorry for the patient's situation, the automatic response on the part of a patient is to say, "That's okay, it's not your fault," which again changes the dynamics of the nurse–patient relationship by putting the focus on the nurse rather than the patient. Being sympathetic prevents the patient from discussing his or her thoughts and feelings and places him or her in a victim state. Nurses need to be empathetic toward a patient's situation by trying to understand the meaning of the experience from the patient's viewpoint. It is only by being empathetic can the relationship remain therapeutic.

Expressing Approval or Disapproval

In statements that express personal judgment, "I agree with you" or "I don't think you made the right choice," the nurse imposes his or her values, beliefs, attitude, and judgment onto the patient and subsequently violates the therapeutic relationship. Avoid using terms such as *should, ought, good, bad, right,* and *wrong* because they communicate your personal view (Jakubec & Astle, 2014). Voicing approval may seem like positive feedback; however, it implies to the patient that the behaviour is the only acceptable choice. Pejorative statements made by the nurse imply the patient needs to gain your approval and may lead the patient to become angry, which will further block communication. Instead, the nurse should use techniques that encourage the patient to verbalize, elaborate on, or examine his or her own views.

Belittling Feelings

When patients develop the courage to verbalize how they feel and the nurse responds by saying, "You shouldn't feel that way" or "I know exactly how you feel," he or she devalues and dismisses the patients feelings and indicates that what they are feeling is trivial, unimportant, and insignificant. A nurse may never truly know exactly how a patient feels, but he or she can be empathetic by communicating understanding, acceptance, and genuine interest. This can be achieved by having the nurse simply acknowledge the feelings expressed by the patient. For instance, the nurse may respond with "I can only imagine how confusing, difficult, upsetting, frustrating . . . this must be for you."

Defensive Responses

When we feel that others are being critical of or questioning our competence, the natural human tendency is to respond in a defensive manner. However, between the nurse and patient, defensiveness breeds defensiveness, which is neither constructive nor therapeutic. There is always a reason for the patient/family display of anger, the challenge in these situations is in being able to look past the anger and acknowledge, value, and respond in a thoughtful and constructive manner to what the patient has expressed. More often than not, the defensiveness seen in patients is not really what is going on with the patient; rather, it is often an effective way of getting your attention. In order to respond therapeutically to the concerns or criticism, it is important for the nurse to remain calm, actively listen, and employ the relate/respond and assertiveness strategies discussed in this chapter. Uncovering hidden feelings will often result from using these strategies (Jakubec & Astle, 2014).

Nurses should strive to find a balance in using the science of communication, which are the behavioural skills concerned about saying the right thing at the right time, with the art of communication, which is concerned with the relational competencies of being, knowing, doing, and examining the meaning and complexity of the human experience.

Collaborative Interprofessional Communication

In a health-care milieu faced with increasing patient acuity, concerns with patient safety and staff shortages, it is paramount that health-care professionals work collaboratively within interprofessional teams and/or groups to safeguard the provision of quality care and improved health outcomes (Bainbridge, Nasmith, Orchard, & Wood, 2010). An **interprofessional team** is defined as "multiple health disciplines with diverse knowledge and skills who share an integrated set of goals and who utilize interdependent collaboration that involves communication, sharing of knowledge and coordination of services to provide services to patients/clients and their caregiving systems" (RNAO, 2013, para. 1).

The success of effective, collaborative communication centers on being other-oriented, which means understanding the manner in which each profession or discipline perceives communication. Understanding and embracing the differences between nurse and physician communications will go a long way to enhancing interprofessional communication. In general, physicians are taught to verbally communicate and document in a precise, concise, and problem-oriented manner, whereas nurses are taught to communicate narratively and descriptively. These differences may lead physicians to become frustrated, irritated, and impatient waiting for all relevant data to be communicated (Johnson, Martin, & Markle-Elder, 2007; Mitchell, 2014; Pope, Rodzen, & Spross, 2008).

We all share the same goal, and our communication needs to reflect that, whether it is at the bedside, on each unit or clinic, in care conferences, in the community or via the patient care record. Additionally, nurses communicate with "peers and colleagues in order to contribute to professional development" (Wilkinson & Treas, 2011, p. 359) and would be prudent to use techniques such as active listening, relational competencies, effective verbal and nonverbal skills, be respectful of individual proxemics, assertive rather than passive or aggressive communication, and group communication skills of cohesiveness and interaction (trust, honesty, free flow of communication, cooperative, and supportive) to enhance their overall interprofessional and collaborative relationships (Taylor et al., 2011).

The Situation-Background-Assessment-Recommendation Model

Using a framework that requires communication to be concise in relaying pertinent information improves interprofessional communication and patient outcomes (Wilkinson & Treas, 2011). The situation-background-assessment-

BOX 26.9 Situation-Background-Assessment-Recommendation Framework

SBAR report to physician about a critical situation

S

Situation
I am calling about <u><patient's name and location></u>
The patient's code status is <u><code status></u>
The problem I am calling about is _____.
I am afraid the patient is going to arrest.

I have just assessed the patient personally:

Vital signs are: Blood pressure_____/_____, Pulse _____, Respiration _____ and temperature_____

I am concerned about the:
Blood pressure because it is over 200 or less than 100 or 30 mmHg below usual.
Pulse because it is over 140 or less than 50.
Respiration because it is less than 5 or over 40.
Temperature because it is less than 96 or over 104.

B

Background
The patient's mental status is:
Alert and oriented to person place and time.
Confused and cooperative or non-cooperative.
Agitated or combative.
Lethargic but conversant and able to swallow.
Stuporous and not talking clearly and possibly not able to swallow.
Comotose. Eyes closed. Not responding to stimulation.
The skin is:
Warm and dry
Pale
Mottled
Diaphoretic
Extremities are cold
Extremities are warm
The patient   is not or is on oxygen.
The patient has been on _____ (l/min) or (%) oxygen for _____ minutes (hours).
The oximeter is reading _____ %.
The oximeter does not detect a good pulse and is giving erratic readings.

A

Assessment
This is what I think the problem is: <u><say what you think is the problem></u>
The problem seems to be   cardiac infection neurologic respiratory _____.
I am not sure what the problem is but the patient is deteriorating.
The patient seems to be unstable and may get worse, we need to do something.

R

Recommendation
I   suggest or request that you <u><say what you would like to see done></u> .
Transfer the patient to critical care.
Come to see the patient at this time.
Talk to the patient or family about code status.
Ask the on-call family practice resident to see the patient now.
Ask for a consultant to see the patient now.
Are any tests needed:
Do you need any tests like CXR, ABG, EKG, CBC, or BMP?
Others?
If a change in treatment is ordered then ask:
How long do you want vital signs?
How long to you expect the problem to last?
If the patient does not get better when would you want us to call again?

This SBAR tool was developed by Kaiser Permanente. Please feel free to use and reproduce these materials in the spirit of patient safety,
and please retain this footer in the spirit of appropriate recognition.

recommendation (SBAR; Box 26.9) framework supports communication between members of the health-care team. SBAR is an easy-to-remember focused model for framing any conversation about patients, setting expectations about how and what will be communicated among team members. Especially supportive of situations requiring immediate attention and action, SBAR can enhance an environment of teamwork while fostering patient safety.

The SBAR model can be adapted to any health-care setting and is widely used within interprofessional teams (nurse–nurse and nurse–physician) and has been shown to be an effective way to communicate urgent and nonurgent patient and patient safety issues (Canadian Patient Safety Institute, 2011).

Creating a Healthy Work Environment

Civility is at the heart of the healthy working environment with open lines of communication. The acronym CREST reflects the relationship between civility and trust, respect, engagement, and support, all of which are interconnected. Figure 26.11 outlines the elements required to maintain civility in the workplace. Improving interprofessional communication is a priority for many health-care organizations.

Barriers to Professional Communication

Ineffective communication between nurse and physician and nurse to nurse are cited as being the main factors contributing to disruptive work environments (Felblinger, 2008). The most common disruptive behaviour occurring within the interprofessional environment is incivility. Incivility is commonly described as behaviours that are perceived to be rude, distasteful, intimidating, or undesirable, all of which undermine the dignity of another (Clark & Ahten, 2011). Other terms linked with incivility are "lateral violence, horizontal violence, relational aggression, and bullying" (Clark & Ahten, 2011, para. 1). Incivility can be

TABLE 26.7	Behaviours Contributing to Incivility
Personal insults	Treating colleagues as if they
Invading personal space	did not exist
Uninvited physical contact	Inappropriate sexual comments/
Threats and intimidation	advances
• In person	Racial slurs
• Telephone	Offensive ethnic humour
• E-mail	Shaming
• Other social media	Criticizing team members in
channels	front of others
(Twitter/Facebook)	Humiliation
Sarcasm	Rude interruptions
• Jokes	Two-faced attacks
• Teasing	Emotional tirades
Dirty looks	Withholding essential information
Gossiping	Spreading rumours
	Damaging coworkers reputation
	Refusing to work collaboratively
	Failing to share credit for
	collaborative work

Source: Clark, C. M., & Ahten, S. M. (2011). The downward spiral: Incivility in nursing/Interviewer: Laura A. Stokowski. *Medscape Nursing*. Retrieved from http://www.medscape.com/viewarticle/739328; Felblinger, D. M. (2008). Incivility and bullying in the workplace and nurses' shame responses. *Journal of Obstetrics, Gynecologic, and Neonatal Nursing, 37*, 234–242. doi:10.1111/j.1552-6909.2008.00227.x; Porto, G., & Lauve, R. (2006). Disruptive clinician behaviors: A persistent threat to patient safety. *Patient Safety & Quality Healthcare*, 1–11. Retrieved from http://qrshealthcare.com/PDFs/PSQH3%204_Porto%20Preprint-3.pdf; Pfifferling, J. H. (2003). Developing and implementing a policy to deal with disruptive staff members. *Oncology Issues, 18*, 1–5. Retrieved from http://accc-cancer.org/oncology_issues/articles/mayjun03/pfifferling.pdf

seen on a daily basis in every capacity of our lives. Students experience incivility regardless of program or educational institution. We can see it at the grocery store, shopping malls, gas stations, or banks. Incivility is prevalent and, at times, endured in our society, but it is not and should never be acceptable or excused. This is especially true in nursing, where 60% of graduate nurses admit to leaving their first position within 6 months due to some form of incivility (Griffin, 2004). The expression, "Nurses eat their young," is standard lore within our profession (Brown, 2010), and although often said in jest, this expression instils that this is something our profession at one time condoned. However, today, it is an excuse for bullying, harassment, and generally behaving badly.

Behaviours considered to contribute to **incivility** are listed in Table 26.7. Any form of incivility may at some point have a negative effect on the recipient, the culture of the unit, clinic, or organization. Let's not forget the patient, in whom incivility contributes to mortality, compromises patient safety, and decreases quality of life and satisfaction (Felblinger, 2008; Rosenstein & O'Daniel, 2005).

Incivility often occurs when people are stressed, unhappy, and in a hurry. Incivility erodes self-esteem, creates conflict in personal and work-related relationships, increases tension, contaminates the work environment, and may lead to violence (Clark & Ahten, 2011). This can

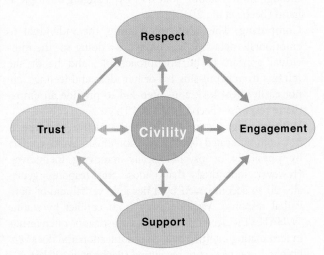

Figure 26.11 CREST.

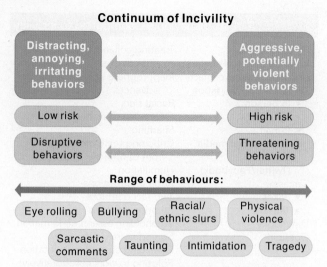

Continuum of Incivility

Figure 26.12 Continuum of incivility. (Redrawn from Clark, C. [2009, revised 2012]. From incivility to civility: Transforming the culture. *Reflections on Nursing Leadership*, 36(3), with permission.)

be seen in the continuum depicted in Figure 26.12 as behaviours associated with incivility range from subtle to threatening and include, but are not limited to, gossiping and sarcasm, verbal, written, or physical intimidation, and threats (Clark & Ahten, 2011).

Transforming the Workplace Environment

As organizations and regional/territorial/national regulatory bodies develop, revise, and implement standards for interprofessional teamwork focusing on optimizing quality outcomes for all persons affiliated with and/or use our health-care system (RNAO, 2012), nurses need to know how to respond to incivility in a safe, healthy, and professional manner.

Effective and open communication is the cure to establishing civility. So, how do we achieve this? Examining how you communicate when faced with inappropriate behaviour, how you respond to inappropriate behaviour, and how you resolve conflict that often results from such behaviour is a first and formidable step.

The fact that nurses work in stressful environments with patients and interprofessional team members having varying backgrounds, cultures, values, beliefs, and attitudes makes conflict a common occurrence. Therefore, when individuals and/or groups experience negative emotional responses such as fear, anger, hurt, anxiety, and frustration to perceived disagreements and intrusions, destructive conflict generally ensues (Pettrey, 2003; RNAO, 2012). However, conflict can be constructive, but some of us learned over time how to respond to conflict in an unhealthy manner. Managing conflict appropriately requires nurses and interprofessional team members to manage perception of the issue, event, or situation (Ellis & Abbott, 2011) and understand their conflict resolution styles so that they may acquire the relevant knowledge, skills, and attributes that foster civility and a healthy work environment.

Conflict Resolution

Interpersonal conflict in our daily personal and professional lives is inevitable and occurs when individuals cannot agree on a way in which their needs can be met (Beebe et al., 2013). What matters most is how you think, feel, and respond to conflict situations. Acknowledging how you perceive conflict and how you feel when in conflict is a part of self-awareness and leads to opportunities for personal and professional growth. **Conflict resolution** is a process and an outcome that involves an understanding of the nature of conflict and implementing the skills, rules, and processes to manage and resolve conflict (Beebe et al., 2013).

Conflict Style

Depending on culture, past experiences, the situation, and perception and level of comfort, there are several behavioural styles to choose from when individuals feel their needs are not being met. Again, understanding that each approach has unique aspects and yield different results may assist you in recognizing whether your approach to conflict resolution is constructive or destructive.

The **nonconfrontational** or nonassertive approach avoids conflict at all cost (Adler et al., 2012; Beebe et al., 2013). Individuals may present with a pattern of avoiding expressing their opinions or feelings, protecting their rights, and identifying and meeting their needs or accommodating by giving in or giving up and putting the other person's needs above their own (Adler et al., 2012; Beebe et al., 2013). The nonconfrontational approach encompasses four responses that may be used by individuals subscribing to this approach to conflict.

1. **Placating:** Avoid conflict as they wish to please others out of a fear of rejection, are uneasy with negative emotions, refrain from becoming upset, and quickly agree with others in an attempt to avoid conflict (Beebe et al., 2013).
2. **Distracting:** Individuals responding in this manner attempt to avoid tense, stressful, or conflict situations through humor (telling jokes) or by changing the topic at hand (Beebe et al., 2013).
3. **Computing:** This response requires the individual to emotionally detach from conflict. By doing so, the individual appears to be unapproachable, and he or she refrains from expressing his or her ideas and feelings, are not easily provoked, and often fail to provide an empathetic response (Beebe et al., 2013).
4. **Withdrawing:** Often, the most destructive response is not communicated effectively. Individuals avoid conflict by physically or psychologically removing themselves. However, individuals that choose this response generally do so accompanied by a negative verbal and/or nonverbal response. Walking away from conflict by stating "WHATEVER" accompanied by a sarcastic tone often results in terminating interpersonal communication and does very little to foster respect or resolution (Beebe et al., 2013).

When using this approach as their primary method of managing conflict, individuals often do not feel heard, recognized, or acknowledged, which in most cases, leads to feelings of resentment. However, the nonconfrontational approach is not always the worst approach to take, especially in situations where the risks outweigh the benefits or you are not truly invested.

The polar opposite of nonconfrontational is the confrontational or **aggressive communication** approach, a style in which individuals express their feelings and opinions and advocate for their needs in a way that demeans or violates the rights of others (Adler et al., 2012; Beebe et al., 2013). Thus, aggressive communicators can be verbally and/or physically abusive. Aggressive responses may be in the form of verbally attacking the character or competence of an individual or other forms of uncivil behaviour, which may include blaming and scapegoating, all of which demonstrates that the individual possesses little insight into the effect his or her behaviour has on others. Individuals that subscribe to this type of conflict resolution style often appear to get what they want. However, in looking long term, the aggressive approach will not achieve cooperation from others.

Interpersonal conflict with patients and families is often highly emotional, and an aggressive response from a patient/family is usually an angry response. This response is generally out of fear for their loved one, a sense of helplessness, or not being heard. Responding in an aggressive manner will only feed further aggression in the other individual. If you can remember that the aggressive response is usually an emotional one and use empathy and the cooperative and assertiveness strategies discussed in this chapter, successful resolution is more likely to occur.

Passive-aggressive behaviour occurs when an individual expresses his or her anger/resentment/hostility in a manner that is incomprehensible (Adler et al., 2012; Beebe et al., 2013) and appears to actually be kind and caring. This type of conflict resolution style is intimidating, counterproductive, and does nothing in attempts to constructively resolve conflict. People that employ this conflict management style appear to get what they want in the short term, but similar to those choosing aggressive behaviour, results in destructive and short-lived personal and working relationships.

The cooperative or **assertiveness** approach is the ability to state what you want, feel, think, or believe in a manner that is open, direct, honest, and nonjudgmental while ensuring your rights as well as the other person's rights are respected (Adler et al., 2012; Beebe et al., 2013; Wilkinson & Treas, 2011). Assertive persons can state their opinions and feelings, advocating for their rights and needs in such a manner that is respectful of the rights of others, valuing themselves, their time, and their emotional, spiritual, and physical well-being. In essence, assertiveness reframes blame, as it demonstrates ownership of thoughts, feelings, and actions in working toward resolution in a much more cooperative and constructive manner by viewing the conflict as something that is issue-focused and can be resolved.

Cooperative and Assertiveness Strategies

Most of us have used each style of conflict resolution at various times throughout our lives, but being assertive on a consistent basis is a learning process that involves self-awareness, courage, conscious effort, and commitment (Cloke & Goldsmith, 2011; Pettrey, 2003; RNAO, 2012). There are several strategies that can assist you in becoming more assertive and taking a cooperative approach in resolving conflict. Employing these strategies, as well as the effective communication strategies discussed in this chapter, enables nurses to be assertive and proactive rather than passive-aggressive and reactive in conflict situations they themselves are involved in, or are at the very least, facilitating (Pettrey, 2003).

1. **Controlling emotions.** The first element in being assertive in resolving conflict is controlling your emotions. Emotional noise prevents individuals from actively listening (Pettrey, 2003). "Our instinctual response is either 'fight,' which may be exhibited as sarcasm or anger, or 'flight,' exhibited as avoidance or silent treatment" (Pettrey, 2003, p. 21), otherwise referred to as "silence or violence" (Pettrey, 2003).

2. **Self-awareness.** Enhancing self-awareness through reflection is key to understanding the reasons underlying the emotional response; in addition to identifying and implementing, realistic strategies can assist in regulating emotions (Pettrey, 2003).

3. **Be other-oriented.** Because there are at least two individuals involved in interpersonal conflict, take into consideration where the other person may be coming from: how he or she may be feeling and look past his or her emotional response (distracter) in order to identify what the real issue is.

4. **Focus on the issue, not personality.** Clearly identify what the issue is. Perception check with the other person to assess if your perception is correct or not. Remain issue-focused and avoid attacking the character or personal traits of the other person. Avoid bringing up personal grievances and maintain a nonjudgmental verbal and nonverbal approach (Beebe et al., 2013).

5. **Use "I" language.** Using "I" language indicates that you own your thoughts and behaviours and that you are taking ownership of the situation or issue (Beebe et al., 2007). Using "I" language removes the defensiveness and helps reframe the issue, situation, or event as well as maintains the self-worth of the other person (Beebe et al., 2007). "Your room is always messy" most likely will not get it cleaned up. Instead, try saying, "When I come home from work, I don't enjoy having to clean up your room. I would appreciate if you would tidy up your room when you come home."

6. **Focus on shared interest.** Emphasize commonalities in interests, values, and expectations (Beebe et al., 2013).

7. **Monitor your nonverbal behaviour.** Seek congruence with your verbal and nonverbal language. Appropriate eye contact and using SURETY indicate genuine interest in the well-being of the other person. Ensure tone of voice and gestures are appropriate and culturally sensitive (Stickley, 2011).

8. **Brainstorm for possible solutions.** Seek workable solutions from each person involved in the conflict.

9. **Apologize.** Take responsibility for your part of the conflict. There are three parts to a correct apology. Say, "I apologize," clearly and concisely articulate what it is that you are taking responsibility for, and say, "What can I do to make this better?"

10. **Present yourself as equal rather than superior.** By asserting the phrase, "Let's work on finding a feasible solution together," will most likely achieve a collaborative environment conducive to resolving conflict (Beebe et al., 2007).

11. **Seek collaboration.** This requires all individuals involved in the conflict to respectfully communicate by expressing a desired interest in achieving a WIN-WIN outcome or goal (CRNBC, 2012).

Challenging Conversations

A challenging or difficult conversation is any conversation that you anticipate or engage in that makes you uncomfortable. Nursing is full of challenging conversations, and avoiding them achieves very little, except procrastination. Most of us feel ill prepared to have these conversations in our personal lives let alone with a patient or colleague. We procrastinate having these conversations out of a fear or lack of confidence and ability. No doubt, prior to these conversations, our intrapersonal thoughts and feelings go to the most negative of reactions and responses. Conversations regarding performance, conflict resolution, death, and dying have one element in common—high emotional context. You can manage challenging conversations by recalling the principles of relational practice, conflict resolution, and effective communication strategies.

Social Media Influence on Communication

Here's a challenge to you: Would you be willing to give up all forms of electronic and social media communication for 12 weeks? Students frequently say that without being able to text, view Facebook, or e-mail, they would experience anxiety, stress, and social isolation. They explain that social media is a part of who they are and how they stay connected with others. There has been much debate about the effect social media has on interpersonal communication. Even the cell phone makers recognize the necessity for face-to-face interpersonal communication. Consider that the iPhone now has *Facetime*. Think about the cultural influence of social media on interpersonal communication. When you go into any public place and see people sitting together, many are using some form of social media, but are they truly communicating with one another?

With the advent of the electronic health-care record and being able to schedule and e-mail appointments, lab, and other diagnostic test results as well as teaching and discharge instructions, nurses need to know when it is and is not appropriate to e-mail private information and should consult the policies pertaining to electronic and social media communication (Berman & Snyder, 2012).

Through the eyes of a nurse

Recently, I observed two nursing students texting to each other while standing side by side. One student was asked why he was texting when he could simply talk to the person standing beside him. The response was that texting was easier and that it "took the emotion out of communication." Both students nodded in agreement. This was unsettling to me as these students are entering a profession that endures a great deal of emotion. What is so wrong with emotional expression? A number of questions were going through my mind. How will these students connect with patients? How will these students provide emotional support to their patients and colleagues? If our profession is based on the value of caring, what effect is social media truly having on our future nurses? On our profession? When I am a patient someday, I want my nurse to look at me when I am speaking. I need and want face-to-face interpersonal contact. I want to look into your eyes and know that you care about me as a patient, as a person. So, my advice for all the future nurses out there is to put the technology away and sit and talk with one another and, most importantly, with your patients and families.

(personal reflection of a nurse)

Professional Standards and Electronic Media

Nurses using Facebook, text messaging, e-mailing, tweeting, and blogging must abide by the standards of professional practice that subsume the virtual world as well as the physical world (CRNBC, 2013a). The act of using the channels associated with social media in and of itself is not the problem. The problem lies with the individual using social media in such a manner that violates professional relationships, integrity, trust, boundaries, privacy, and confidentiality (CRNBC, 2013a). The next time you are communicating via the channels of social media, ask yourself the questions in the Think box.

Think *Social Media*

1. Will my actions affect my reputation as a nurse?
2. Am I sharing photos or information about a patient or situation in the workplace?
3. Would I feel comfortable posting my photos in a public place? If no, then refrain from posting them online.
4. Are my personal comments acceptable for both public and work environments?
5. Does this violate the CNA Code of Ethics or provincial standards of practice?

Recommendations for using social media in a responsible manner are delineated in Table 26.8.

TABLE 26.8	Recommendations for Responsible Use of Social Media
Competence	Build your social media competence. You need to know the technology and have the skills and judgment to use it appropriately and ethically. Know that even if you use the highest privacy settings, others can copy and share your information without your knowledge or permission. Be aware of social media's evolving culture and changing technology. Reflect on your intent and possible consequences of your online behaviour - before you blog, post, or tweet.
Image	Manage your virtual image. Use the same level of professionalism in your online interactions as you do face-to-face. Keep your personal and professional lives separate. Use different accounts for personal and professional activities.
Privacy	Respect your client's privacy and protect your own. Be aware that using social media to seek information about your clients could affect your relationship with the client or create a responsibility for you to act. Set and maintain your privacy settings to limit access to your personal information.
Boundaries	Maintain professional boundaries. Just as with face-to-face relationships, you must set and communicate these boundaries with clients online. Anticipate requests from clients and know how you'll respond. End your professional relationships appropriately. Be ready for and don't accept "friend" requests.
Expectations	Use caution if you identify yourself as a nurse online. If you do so, others may ask for advice, which could lead to a nurse-client relationship. Using a name that hides your identify does not release you from this expectation. Know this and practice accordingly.
Integrity	Protect your and the profession's integrity. Use proper communication channels to discuss, report and resolve workplace issues - not the internet. Refer to colleagues or clients online with the same level of response as you would in the workplace. Before you blog, tweet or share information about your practice, reflect on your intentions and the possible consequences. Understand that "liking" someone's disrespectful comments is not much different than making them yourself.
Policies	Know and follow employer policies on using social media, photography, computers and mobile devices, including personal, at work. If you communicate with clients via social media, work with your employer to develop policies.
Accountability	Make sure you can answer for your actions. Reflect on why, how, and when you use social media and help others do the same. Know that personal use of social media while working could be viewed as client abandonment. If you are unable to discuss your online behaviour with others, consider this a red flag. Use professional judgment to keep your obligations to clients, colleagues, and employers front and center.

Reprinted with permission from College of Registered Nurses of British Columbia. (2013). *Nine recommendations for using social media responsibly.* Vancouver, BC: Author.

The following Think box provides a social media case scenario. After reading the scenario, reflect and critically apply your provincial standards of practice.

Think Anna blogged to stay in touch with her family, friends and former colleagues. She wrote colourfully about her community and work, always careful not to use names. Her former colleagues often commented on her posts, sharing their own stories. They agreed that sometimes patients were unappreciative and managers didn't care.

A comment from a former patient caused Anna to re-read her blog. She saw that her descriptions had details such as when things happened and patient ages, genders and health issues. Anyone who knew Anna, the patient or the agency would know whom she was talking about. In addition, her posts and the comments from her colleagues were disrespectful of patient and workplaces. Seeing that she had crossed a line, Anna deleted her blog.

Eventually, Anna's employer learned of the blog. He said Anna had breached patient privacy and damaged the community's trust in the agency and its employees. In addition, he called her previous employer to tell them about their staff's comments on the blog and their failure to report that Anna was breaching confidentiality. Anna and two other nurses were reported to their regulatory body.

Do you feel Anna should have been reported to her regulatory body? Does reading this case study change how you view social media's influence in a nurse's personal and professional life? Does reading this case study change how you will use social media in the future?

Social media case studies. Retrieved from https://crnbc.ca/Standards /practiceresources/socialmedia/Pages/SocialMediaCases.aspx

Patients and Social Media

In recognizing that social media is about connecting, nurses should examine the possible untoward effects that patients may experience if they don't have, are unable to access, in situations or areas where Wi-Fi is unavailable or where electronic devices are prohibited. The patient may feel disconnected from friends and family and from other patients; nurses should be cognizant of the socioeconomics and individual's determinants of health because not everyone owns, has access to, or possesses the skills and devices to communicate via social media channels (Berman & Snyder, 2012).

Communicating Cultural Safety

As we live and work in multicultural environments, embracing cultural diversity within health care provides a rich milieu in which we have the opportunity to not only create healthy workplaces but also strive to provide care that is respectful of an individual's culture. Patient-centered care requires that nurses to be aware of their own culture, the patient's culture, and how both impact the therapeutic relationship (College of Nurses of Ontario, 2009).

Culture extends beyond nationality and includes attributes, physical characteristics, norms, values, beliefs, language, and communication that a group of individuals identify as their own (Long, 2012). We also need to acknowledge that culture is learned and passed down from one generation to the next and adapts in response to a generation or individual's experiences and environment (Long, 2012). This is an important point, as on occasion, nurses can make the assumption that a younger member of the family is able to communicate or translate for the older family member who is the patient. This may no longer be the case because more and more of the younger generation were born in Canada and are unable to speak the familial language.

Being **culturally competent** implies that nurses are self-aware regarding their thoughts, values, beliefs, and attitudes without letting them have an unjustified influence on those from other cultures. Further, a culturally competent nurse demonstrates an awareness and understanding of the patient's culture, embraces cultural differences, and adapts care that is congruent with the patient's culture (College of Nurses of Ontario, 2009). Nurses who do not feel prepared to practice cultural competent care fail to correctly or sufficiently communicate, assess, evaluate, and adjust the care plan to address the unique cultural needs and preferences of their patient may inadvertently compromise care and treatment (Long, 2012).

Although cultural competence is a significant concept, it can sometimes overlook systemic hindrances, which make it inadequate to fully address health-care disparities (CNA, 2010). A relatively new concept known as **cultural safety**, developed through Australian and New Zealand nursing practitioners, endorses greater equity in health and health care. The primary focus is on the identification, analysis, research, and education of the root causes of health disparities (CNA, 2010). From a global health perspective, cultural safety is both a process and an outcome (CNA, 2010).

Creating an Environment of Cultural Safety

How do we achieve cultural safety in our own working environments? Once again, reflection, self-awareness, and communication are key factors. In order to provide care that respects the culture of a patient, nurses must first reflect on their own culture. How would you describe your culture? We all have one but articulating what culture means to each of us can be an arduous process. Such questions as, "How does your culture influence family celebrations?" "How does your culture influence you when you are ill?" or "What are your beliefs about illness?" makes reflection even more complicated. However, understanding our culture influences how we interact and respond to others. Through reflection, we are able to gain a better sense of self and identify any personal biases or stereotypes that we hold that may ultimately influence the care and treatment we provide (Flowers, 2004). This is the first step toward developing cultural competence and safety (Krainovich-Miller et al., 2008). Cultural safety requires nurses to be nonjudgmental; respectful, supportive, and protective of patient rights, values, and beliefs, and that the care provided is not perceived as demeaning, di-

minishing, or disempowering (Hughes & McKay, 2012). At times, it may be necessary to challenge the status quo in order to advocate for what is important to the patient (Hughes & McKay, 2012). Being open-minded in assessing and analyzing the determinants of health for the patient will go a long way in understanding the unique needs of the patient.

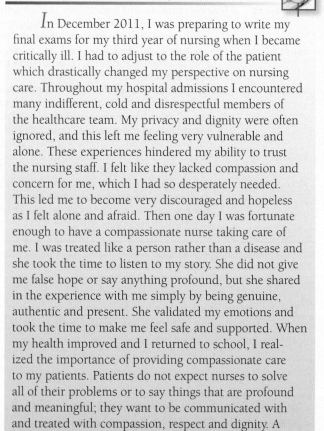

Through the eyes of a student

In December 2011, I was preparing to write my final exams for my third year of nursing when I became critically ill. I had to adjust to the role of the patient which drastically changed my perspective on nursing care. Throughout my hospital admissions I encountered many indifferent, cold and disrespectful members of the healthcare team. My privacy and dignity were often ignored, and this left me feeling very vulnerable and alone. These experiences hindered my ability to trust the nursing staff. I felt like they lacked compassion and concern for me, which I had so desperately needed. This led me to become very discouraged and hopeless as I felt alone and afraid. Then one day I was fortunate enough to have a compassionate nurse taking care of me. I was treated like a person rather than a disease and she took the time to listen to my story. She did not give me false hope or say anything profound, but she shared in the experience with me simply by being genuine, authentic and present. She validated my emotions and took the time to make me feel safe and supported. When my health improved and I returned to school, I realized the importance of providing compassionate care to my patients. Patients do not expect nurses to solve all of their problems or to say things that are profound and meaningful; they want to be communicated with and treated with compassion, respect and dignity. A nurse's simple touch, listening ear, friendly smile and caring heart can help to provide patients with comfort and place them at ease. I understand that nursing is a demanding profession, but I encourage nurses to take the time to recognize, appreciate, empathize and reflect on how difficult it is to be the patient.

(personal reflection of Amanda Dembicki, MacEwan University)

Challenges

When communicating with others from varying age groups, cultural backgrounds, and socioeconomic status, miscommunication can occur (Hughes & McKay, 2012). Strategies for enhancing communication include the use of translators (employees, hired translators, or family members), picture communication boards, and appropriate gestures/pantomime, thus ensuring information translated enhances cultural safety (see Chapter 13 for more on cultural safety.)

Communicating from the heart is rewarding but emotionally exhausting. It takes courage to communicate effectively with others. It also takes courage to acknowledge areas for improvement as well as the willingness to make positive changes that better our lives, the lives of our patients, and interprofessional team members. It is important to remember the courage we and our patients possess and how fundamentally vital it is for nurses to encourage patients in thought, word, and deed to remember the possibilities, to never give up.

Makenzie is now in the last term of her nursing program and is asked to speak with first-year nursing students regarding the importance of communication in nursing. Makenzie begins by reiterating her thoughts regarding the relevance of having to take a communications course when she was in her first year of the program. The thoughts Makenzie shares are congruent with most of the students she is speaking with. Makenzie explains that it was not until she spent time in the clinical setting did she understand the profound difference communication makes to the quality of a patient's life and the quality of her work. Makenzie reinforced with the students that every time they enter a patients room; engage in care, treatments, or procedures; or participate in report and patient conferences, they have the opportunity to use the competencies that foster therapeutic and interprofessional relationships. Communication is more than what you say; it includes your appearance and actions and is influenced by patient's perceptions. Makenzie went on to explain specific behavioural and relational techniques that encourage patients to feel safe enough to disclose their thoughts, ideas, and feelings. Makenzie said she had no idea going into nursing that she would need to be aware of boundaries, maintaining confidentiality, the importance of being self-aware, or that nursing was not just about the science of performing skills. "If that is all we believe, then we do a disservice to our patients and ourselves. Nursing is about applying the science with the skilful art of knowing the patients and obtaining their lived experiences, along with the relational aspect of learning to be comfortable just being with a patient and honouring the uniqueness of that experience. Reflecting on why, how, and what I can do differently to improve my ability to effectively communicate has now become part of my nursing practice. Communication is truly the heart of nursing practice."

Critical Thinking Case Scenarios

▶ Mr. Kirkland was admitted to hospital a week ago and underwent a cholecystectomy. He is postoperative day 3 and tolerating a regular diet. At his morning assessment, Mr. Kirkland asks if he can have six pieces of bacon (three pieces for him and three pieces for his daughter). Mr. Kirkland stated that for years, both he and his daughter have gone out once a month for bacon and eggs. According to the information on his chart, Mr. Kirkland is of Jewish faith. Knowing that the consumption of pork is prohibited in his religion, what critical thinking and communication skills would support the nurse in maintaining cultural competence?

▶ Ben has worked as a charge nurse in a long-term care facility for over 10 years. Recently, Sam, another RN on the unit, approached him in an aggressive manner demanding that he change her patient assignment. Ben attempted to find out why Sam wanted her assignment changed and did not receive a verbal response. Rather, Ben was verbally attacked at morning report and for a week, Ben was the recipient of eye rolls, sarcastic comments, and the silent treatment. How can Ben assertively address Sam and find out why she wants her assignment changed? How can Ben resolve this conflict? How can Ben be assertive in addressing Sam's incivility toward him?

▶ Mrs. Bailey is a 34-year-old single mother of a 3-year-old girl named Izabella. Mrs. Bailey was recently admitted to the palliative care unit with ovarian cancer. One night, she confides in you that she is scared to die, scared for her daughter growing up without a mother, and angry that all this happened to her. She states she never went to church as a child and doesn't know what she believes in but states, "I am a spiritual person." Mrs. Bailey then states that she is overwhelmed as she thought she would have more time to come to grips with her disease and cannot think clearly. What communication skills can you use to help Mrs. Bailey?

▶ Jen is a second-year nursing student and is completing a sterile dressing change. Jen's instructor, David, is there to observe and provide feedback. While setting up the tray, Jen breaks the sterile field, and David informs her of this and asks her to go and get another tray while he stays and talks to her patient. Jen returns with a tray and sets up again. Jen engages very little with her patient during the dressing change, which is unusual for her because she is normally cheerful and cognizant of explaining what is going to happen to her patients. David provides Jen with some minor guidance and reminders throughout the dressing change. When David sits down with Jen to review how things went, Jen breaks down in tears. David is unclear about why Jen is upset and decides to not continue with the session and asks Jen to think about the events of today and they will sit down tomorrow for a discussion. What is your perception about what led Jen to break down? Provide an example of David's perception checking with Jen. How would you use the reflective practice model in reflecting about the interaction between student, patient, and instructor? What feedback strategies would you suggest both David and Jen review?

Multiple-Choice Questions

1. "You mentioned earlier that you are scared, I am not sure what you mean by this. Please, elaborate?" What communication technique is being used?
   a. Paraphrasing
   b. Open-ended questioning
   c. Clarification
   d. Probing

2. Sarah notices that her patient, James, is holding his abdomen and taking small breaths. She asks if James is in pain, and he states, "No." Sarah then informs James of what she is observing. What communication technique is Sarah using?
   a. Sharing observation
   b. Clarification
   c. Closed-ended questioning
   d. Providing information

3. During communication class, the instructor notices that some students are not paying attention or engaged in the lecture. The instructor states there will be a pop quiz and proceeds to administer the quiz. Nathan thinks to himself, "I did not do the readings for this week. I hope the questions are not too hard." What type of communication is Nathan engaged in?
   a. Interpersonal
   b. Transpersonal
   c. Intrapersonal
   d. Impersonal

4. As a student, you are instructing a small group of seniors in wheelchair yoga. Considering proxemics, at which zone is the student in when leading this group?
   a. Personal
   b. Intimate
   c. Public
   d. Social

5. Lucy is caring for Mrs. Dell, an 85-year-old patient with cognitive impairment. What is the best strategy for Lucy to use when communicating with Mrs. Dell?
   a. Make use of a communication board.
   b. Gain Mrs. Dell's attention before conversing.
   c. Ensure you explain in depth what you are doing.
   d. Repeat the question if Mrs. Dell does not immediately respond.

6. Upon reflection, Robin feels he is having difficulty communicating effectively in a collaborative manner with members of the interprofessional team. What strategy should Robin use to improve his ability to communicate effectively within the interprofessional team?
   a. Be respectful of individual proxemics.
   b. Learn the roles of each member of the interdisciplinary team.

   c. Emphasize his accomplishments.
   d. Focus on the task at hand while nonverbally demonstrating that he is listening.

Suggested Lab Activities

Mask-Making Exercise

● This activity occurs in two stages. The first stage is the making of the mask. Using plaster of paris or gypsum, students work in dyads or triads. Placing plastic wrap over the partner's face (nose and mouth holes are mandatory), the student will apply the gypsum (dipped in water and excess moisture removed) strips evenly to their partner's face. Students have the choice of making a whole or half mask. This is usually left up to each student to communicate his or her wishes to his or her partner. Once the gypsum has been applied, let sit for about 5 minutes and then remove and let dry overnight.

Part 2: Students will bring their masks (and any other items they want to adorn their mask with such as feathers, beads, paint, glitter, etc.) back to class and be instructed to depict concepts learned in class. For example, students may be asked to draw their interpretation of self-concept (this one is a trick, as the mask itself is the image of the student), conflict, culture, value, belief, attitude, nonverbal communication, groups, diversity, listening, perception, and interpersonal communication. Once the students have completed their masks, they are asked to explain to each other (in small groups) what their mask means to them.

Power of Perception

● Working in small groups, go to an area where you can sit and observe others (restaurant, mall, library, etc.). Take turns at interpreting the actions/nonverbals/interactions of individuals you are observing. Share your interpretation and then, as a small group, consider other alternative interpretations. Discuss how you came to the interpretation and what influenced your interpretation. Discuss how communication is influenced by perception.

Conflict Resolution

● Using the reflective practice model discussed in this chapter, think of a recent interpersonal conflict you experienced. Write how you would resolve the conflict in a passive manner; an aggressive manner, and, finally, an assertive manner. Indicate the communication skills that are used or not used within each conflict resolution style as well as the impact this recent experience had on you. Given what you now know, what would you do differently?

REFERENCES AND SUGGESTED READINGS

Adler, R. B., Rolls, J. A., & Proctor, R. F., II. (2012). *Look* (Canadian ed.). Toronto, ON: Nelson.

Arnold, E. C., & Boggs, K. (2011). *Interpersonal relationships: Professional communication skills for nurses* (6th ed.). Toronto, ON: Elsevier.

Austin, W., & Boyd, M. A. (2010). *Psychiatric & mental health nursing for Canadian practice* (2nd ed.). Philadelphia, PA: Lippincott Williams & Wilkins.

Back, A. L., Bauer-Wu, S. M., Rushton, C. H., & Halifax, J. (2009). Compassionate silence in the patient–clinician encounter: A contemplative approach. *Journal of Palliative Medicine, 12*(12), 1113–1117. doi:10.1089/jpm.2009.0175

Bainbridge, L., Nasmith, L., Orchard, C., & Wood, V. (2010). Competencies for interprofessional collaboration. *Journal of Physical Therapy Education, 24*(1), 6–11.

Beebe, S. A., Beebe, S. J., & Ivy, D. K. (2013). *Communication principles for a lifetime* (5th ed.). Toronto, ON: Pearson Allyn & Bacon.

Beebe, S. A., Beebe, S. J., Redmond, M. B., & Geerinck, T. M. (2007). *Interpersonal communication relating to others* (4th Canadian ed.). Toronto, ON: Pearson Allyn & Bacon.

Belcher, M., & Jones, L. K. (2009). Graduate nurses' experiences of developing trust in the nurse–patient relationship. *Contemporary Nurse, 31*, 142–152. doi:10.5172/conu.673.31.2.142

Berman, A., & Snyder, S. (2012). *Kozier & Erb's fundamentals of nursing* (9th ed.). Upper Saddle River, NJ: Pearson.

Block, J. R., & Yuker, H. (1992). *Can you believe your eyes?* New York, NY: Brunner/Mazel.

Brown, T. (2010, February 11). When the nurse is a bully. *New York Times*. Retrieved from http://well.blogs.nytimes.com/2010/02/11/when-the-nurse-is-a-bully/

Browning, S., & Waite, R. (2010). The gift of listening: JUST listening strategies. *Nursing Forum, 45*(3), 150–158. doi:10.1111/j.1744-6198.2010.00179.x

Bunkers, S. S. (2013). Silence: A double-edged sword. *Nursing Science Quarterly, 26*(1), 7–11. doi:10.1177/0894318412466739

Burger, J., & Goddard, N. (2010). Communication. In P. A. Potter, A. G. Perry, J. C. Ross-Kerr, & M. J. Wood (Eds.), *Fundamentals of nursing* (Rev. 4th ed., pp. 245–264). Toronto, ON: Elsevier Canada.

Canadian Nurses Association. (2008). *Code of ethics for registered nurses*. Retrieved from http://www.cna-aiic.ca

Canadian Nurses Association. (2010). *Position statement: Promoting cultural competence in nursing*. Retrieved from http://www2.cna-aiic.ca/CNA/documents/pdf/publications/PS114_Cultural_Competence_2010_e.pdf

Canadian Patient Safety Institute. (2011). *Teamwork and communication in healthcare. A literature review*. Retrieved from http://www.patientsafetyinstitute.ca/English/toolsResources/teamworkCommunication/Documents/Canadian%20Framework%20for%20Teamwork%20and%20Communications.pdf

Clark, C. M., & Ahten, S. M. (2011). The downward spiral: Incivility in nursing/Interviewer: Laura A. Stokowski. *Medscape Nursing*. Retrieved from http://www.medscape.com/viewarticle/739328

Cloke, K., & Goldsmith, J. (2011). *Resolving conflicts at work: Ten strategies for everyone on the job* (3rd ed.). San Francisco, CA: John Wiley & Sons, Inc.

College and Association of Registered Nurses of Alberta. (2005). *Professional boundaries and the nurse–client relationship: Keeping it safe and therapeutic guidelines for registered nurses*. Retrieved from http://www.crnns.ca/documents/ProfessionalBoundaries2012.pdf

College and Association of Registered Nurses of Alberta. (2006). *Entry to practice competencies for the registered nurse profession*. Retrieved from http://www.nurses.ab.ca/Carna-Admin/Uploads/Entry-to-Practice%20Competencies.pdf

College of Nurses of Ontario. (2009). *Practice guidelines: Culturally sensitive care*. Retrieved from http://www.cno.org/Global/docs/prac/41040_CulturallySens.pdf

College of Occupational Therapists of Ontario. (2009). *Conscious competence model*. Retrieved from http://www.coto.org/pdf/QA_ConsciousCompetence.pdf

College of Registered Nurses of British Columbia. (2006). *Nurse–client relationships*. Retrieved from https://crnbc.ca/Standards/Lists/StandardResources/406NurseClientRelationships.pdf

College of Registered Nurses of British Columbia (2012) *Professional standards*. Retrieved from https://crnbc.ca/Standards/Lists/StandardResources/128ProfessionalStandards.pdf

College of Registered Nurses of British Columbia. (2013a). *Social media: Professionalism, nurses, and social media*. Retrieved from https://crnbc.ca/Standards/Confidentiality/Pages/SocialMedia.aspx

College of Registered Nurses of British Columbia. (2013b). *Social media cases*. Retrieved from https://crnbc.ca/Standards/practiceresources/socialmedia/Pages/SocialMediaCases.aspx

Devito, J. A., Shimoni, R., & Clark, D. (2005). *Building interpersonal communication skills* (2nd Canadian ed.). Toronto, ON: Pearson Allyn & Bacon.

Doane, G. H., & Varcoe, C. (2005). *Family nursing as relational inquiry: Developing health-promoting practice*. Philadelphia, PA: Lippincott Williams & Wilkins.

Doane, G. H., & Varcoe, C. (2007). Relational practice and nursing obligations. *Advances in Nursing Science, 30*(3), 192–205. doi:10.1097/01.ANS.0000286619.31398.fc

Duval Guillaume Modem. (2011). *Carlsberg stunts with bikers in cinema*. Retrieved from http://www.duvalguillaume.com/news/2011/carlsberg-stunts-with-bikers-in-cinema

Eckroth-Bucher, M. (2010). Self-awareness: A review and analysis of a basic nursing concept. *Advances in Nursing Sciences, 33*(4), 297–309. doi:10.1097/ANS.0b013e3181fb2e4c

Ellis, P., & Abbott, J. (2011). Strategies for managing conflict within the team. *Journal of Renal Nursing, 3*(1), 40–43.

Engleberg, I. N., & Wynn, D. R. (2011). *Think communication*. Boston, MA: Allyn & Bacon.

Felblinger, D. M. (2008). Incivility and bullying in the workplace and nurses' shame responses. *Journal of Obstetrics, Gynecologic, and Neonatal Nursing, 37*, 234–242. doi:10.1111/j.1552-6909.2008.00227.x

Feldman, C. (2003). *Silence: How to find inner peace in a busy world*. Berkeley, CA: Rodmell Press.

Fletcher, J. (1999). *Disappearing acts: Gender, power, and relational practice at work*. Cambridge, MA: MIT Press.

Flowers, D. L. (2004). Culturally competent nursing care: A challenge for the 21st century. *Critical Care Nurse, 24*(4), 48–52.

Forchuk, C., & Dorsay, J. P. (1995). Hildegard Peplau meets family systems nursing: Innovation in theory-based practice. *Journal of Advanced Nursing, 21*, 110–115. Retrieved from http://onlinelibrary.wiley.com/journal/10.1111/(ISSN)1365-2648

Green, D. (2012). Communication and cognitive impairment. *Nursing & Residential Care, 14*(9), 446–449.

Griffin, M. (2004). Teaching cognitive rehearsal as a shield for lateral violence: An intervention for newly licensed nurses. *The Journal of Continuing Education in Nursing, 35*(6), 257–263. Retrieved from http://baylorirvinged.files.wordpress.com/2011/07/lateralviolence1.pdf

Grover, S. (2005). Shaping effective communication skills and therapeutic relationships at work. The foundation of collaboration. *American Association of Occupational Health Nurses, 53*(4), 177–182. Retrieved from http://www.biomed-search.com/nih/Shaping-effective-communication-skills-therapeutic/15853294.html

Hartrick, G. A. (1997). Relational capacity: The foundation for interpersonal nursing practice. *Journal of Advanced Nursing, 26,* 523–528.

Hartrick, G. A. (1999). Transcending behaviorism in communication education. *Journal of Nursing Education, 38,* 17–22.

Hartrick, G. A. (2002). Beyond behavioural skills to human-involved processes: Relational nursing practice and interpretive pedagogy. *Journal of Nursing Education, 41*(9), 400–404.

Health Quality Council of Alberta. (n.d.). *ReLATE|ReSPOND.* Retrieved from http://www.hqca.ca/index.php?id=216

Hemsley, B., Balandin, S., & Worrall, L. (2012). Nursing the patient with complex communication needs: Time as a barrier and a facilitator to successful communication in hospital. *Journal of Advanced Nursing, 68*(1), 116–126. doi:10.1111/j.1365=2648.2011.05722.x

Horton-Deutsch, S., & Sherwood, G. (2008). Reflection: An educational strategy to develop emotionally-competent nurse leaders. *Journal of Nursing Management, 16,* 946–954. doi:10.1111/j.1365-2834.2008.00957.x

Hughes, M., & McKay, L. (2012). Making the links between cultural safety and let's get real. *Nursing New Zealand, 18*(4), 26–28. Retrieved from http://www.nzno.org.nz/services/journalskai_tiaki/kai_tiaki_nursing_new_zealand

Jack, K., & Smith, A. (2007). Promoting self-awareness in nurses to improve nursing practice. *Nursing Standard, 21*(32), 47–52. Retrieved from http://nursingstandard.rcnpublishing.co.uk

Jakubec, S. L., & Astle, B. J. (2014). Communication. In P. A. Potter, A. G. Perry, J. C. Ross-Kerr, M. J. Wood, B. J. Astle, & W. Duggleby (Eds.), *Fundamentals of nursing* (5th ed., pp. 242–261). Toronto, ON: Elsevier Canada.

Jirwe, M., Gerrish, K., & Emami, A. (2010). Student nurses' experiences of communication in cross-cultural care encounters. *Scandinavian Journal of Caring Sciences, 24,* 436–444. doi:10.1111/j.1471-6712.2009.00733.x

Johansson, M. B., Carlsson, M., & Sonnander, K. (2012). Communication difficulties and the use of communication strategies: From the perspective of individuals with aphasia. *International Journal of Language & Communication Disorders, 47,* 144–155. doi:10.1111/j.1460-6984.2011.00089.x

Johnson, C. L., Martin, S. L. D., & Markle-Elder, S. (2007). Stopping verbal abuse in the workplace. *American Journal of Nursing, 107*(4), 32–34.

Krainovich-Miller, B., Yost, J. M., Norman, R. G., Auerhahn, C., Dobal, M., Lowry, M., & Moffa, C. (2008). Measuring cultural awareness of nursing students: A first step toward cultural competency. *Journal of Transcultural Nursing, 19*(3), 250–258. doi:10.1177/1043659608317451

Long, T. B. (2012). Overview of teaching strategies for cultural competence in nursing students. *Journal of Cultural Diversity, 19*(3), 102–108. Retrieved from http://www.tuckerpub.com/jcd.htm

Mitchell, M. G. (2014). Caring and communicating. In B. Kozier, G. Erb, A. Berman, S. J. Snyder, M. Buck, L. Yiu, & L. Stamler (Eds.), *Fundamentals of Canadian nursing* (3rd Canadian ed., pp. 422–454). Upper Saddle River, NJ: Pearson.

Oelofsen, N. (2012). Using reflective practice in frontline nursing. *Nursing Times, 108*(24), 22–24.

Pettrey, L. (2003). Who let the dogs out? Managing conflict with courage and skill. *Critical Care Nursing, 23,* 21–24. Retrieved from http://ccn.aacnjournals.org/

Pope, B. B., Rodzen, L., & Spross, G. (2008). Raising the SBAR: How better communication improves patient outcomes. *Nursing 2012, 38*(3), 41–43.

Porr, C., & Egan, R. (2013). How does the nurse educator measure caring? *International Journal of Nursing Education Scholarship, 10*(1), 1–9. doi:10.1515/ijnes-2012-0011

Purnell, M. J. (2002). Why nurses nurse! Intentionality in nursing. *Holistic Nursing Practice, 16*(4).

Registered Nurses Association of Ontario. (2006). *Establishing therapeutic relationships.* Retrieved from http://rnao.ca/sites/rnao-ca/files/Establishing_Therapeutic_Relationships.pdf

Registered Nurses Association of Ontario. (2007). *Embracing cultural diversity in healthcare.* Retrieved from http://rnao.ca/sites/rnaoca/files/Embracing_Cultural_Diversity_in_Health_Care_-_Developing_Cultural_Competence.pdf

Registered Nurses Association of Ontario. (2012). *Managing conflict in healthcare teams.* Retrieved from http://rnao.ca/bpg/guidelines/managing-conflict-healthcare-teams

Registered Nurses Association of Ontario. (2013). *Interprofessional teamwork in healthcare.* Retrieved from http://rnao.ca/bpg/guidelines/interprofessional-team-work-healthcare

Rosenstein, A. H., & O'Daniel, M. (2005). Disruptive behavior and clinical outcomes: Perceptions of nurses and physicians. *American Journal of Nursing, 105,* 54–64. Retrieved from http://journals.lww.com/ajnonline/pages/default.aspx

Sellman, D. (2006). The importance of being trustworthy. *Nursing Ethics, 13*(2), 105–115. Retrieved from http://online.sagepub.com/search/results?src_selected=selectComplete&submit=yes&journal_set=spnej&productpage=nej&src=selected&fulltext=the+importance+of+being+trustworthy&sendit.x=0&sendit.y=0&sendit=Go

Sellman, D. (2007). Trusting patients, trusting nurses. *Nursing Philosophy, 8*(1), 28–36. doi:10.1111/j.1466-769X.2007.00294.x

Shannon, M. T. (2011). Please hear what I'm not saying. *The Permanente Journal, 15*(2), e114–e117. Retrieved from http://www.thepermanentejournal.org/issues/2011/spring.html

Sheldon, L. (2005). *Communication for nurses: Talking with patients.* Mississauga, ON: Jones & Bartlett.

Stickley, T. (2011). From SOLER to SURETY for effective non-verbal communication. *Nurse Education in Practice, 11,* 395–398. doi:10.1016/j.nepr.2011.03.021

Taylor, C. R., Lillis, C., LeMone, P., & Lynn, P. (2011). *Fundamentals of nursing: The art and science of nursing care* (7th ed.). Philadelphia, PA: Lippincott Williams & Wilkins.

Thomas, C. M., Bertram, E., & Johnson, D. (2009). The SBAR Communication Technique. Teaching Nursing Students Professional Communication Skills. *Nurse Educator, 34*(4), 176–180. doi:10.1097/NNE.0b013e3181aaba54

Washington, G. T. (1990). Trust: A critical element in critical care nursing. *Focus on Critical Care/American Association of Critical-Care Nurses, 17*(5), 418–421.

Webb, L. (2011). *Nursing: Communication skills in practice.* New York, NY: Oxford University Press.

Wilkinson, J. M., & Treas L. S. (2011). *Fundamentals of nursing* (2nd ed.). Philadelphia, PA: F.A. Davis Company.

Williams, K., Kemper, S., & Hummert, M. L. (2004). Enhancing communication with older adults: Overcoming elderspeak. *Journal of Gerontological Nursing, 30*(10), 17–25.

Addressing Developmental Needs Across the Lifespan

KATHRYN ROUSSEAU

J amaal is a first-year nursing student in a baccalaureate program in Ontario. His first clinical placement will be at a long-term care facility in the city. Jamaal confides to his instructor that he has very little experience with the elderly and feels uncomfortable around them. His grandparents do not live in the country, and he has not seen them for many years. He is worried that he will not know how to communicate effectively with his elderly patients or provide them with the care they need.

CHAPTER OBJECTIVES

By the end of this chapter, you will be able to:

1. Identify the major developmental theories that inform nursing care across the lifespan.
2. Describe how growth and development influences approaches to nursing care.
3. Use effective communication skills recognizing lifespan considerations.
4. Conduct health assessment of individuals across the lifespan.
5. Identify common health-care needs associated with each developmental stage.
6. Describe nursing strategies to support healthy development across the lifespan.

KEY TERMS

Accommodation   Alterations made to existing schemas based on new experiences and information (Piaget, 1993).

Ageism   A form of prejudice characterized by discrimination against people based on their age, generally referring to the elderly population.

Aging   Complex biologic process of growing older that is influenced by health status, psychological well-being, and social relationships.

Anticipatory Guidance   A nursing intervention that helps patients and family members understand and prepare for normal developmental changes and identify the risks associated with each developmental stage.

Assimilation   The process of adding new information into our already existing schemas (Piaget, 1993).

Attachment   Connection developed between an infant and his or her mother or main caregiver that is the basis for development of trust.

Average   Midpoint within the broader range of normal.

Baby Boomers   A generation of people born in the post–World War II period from 1947 to 1966.

Development   Continuous process of increased skills and ability to function.

Fontanels   Soft membranous gaps on the infant's skull that allow for growth of the brain during the infant period. These are commonly called "soft spots."

Growth   An increase in physical size and capacity over time.

Life Review   The process of reflecting back on one's life (Erikson, 1980).

Menopause   Period in which women experience a permanent end to their menstrual cycle and the end to fertility.

Midlife Crisis   The experience of dissatisfaction with one's current life that may occur when an individual reevaluates his or her beliefs and values, leading to change in lifestyle behaviours.

Nature Versus Nurture   An expression used to describe the debate between the roles of heredity and environment in human development.

Negativism   Expected behaviour in which a toddler consistently refuses to follow commands or respond to suggestions.

Normal   A range of behaviours or a time span that conforms to expected principles of growth and development.

Puberty   Normal period of development manifested in onset of sexual maturation of the body occurring during the adolescent period.

Regression   A temporary withdrawal to earlier developmental behaviours, usually resulting from a stressful situation.

Sandwich Generation   Adults, usually in the period of middle age, who simultaneously have responsibility for their own children and for their aging parents.

Schema   Term coined by Piaget (1993) to describe the process by which an individual develops cognitive maps to organize and interpret information.

Taking a Lifespan Approach

From conception until death, humans share a common developmental path, but each person travels that path in unique ways. The terms *growth* and *development* are commonly used to describe this process. Each has a distinct meaning, but the two are linked in a close relationship. **Growth** refers to an increase in physical size and capacity. It would include components such as changes in height and weight, increased size and functioning of internal organs, and the increasing complexity of the brain and nervous system. **Development**, on the other hand, is the continuous process of increased skills and ability to function. For example, by the end of the first year, an infant has increased in size and muscle strength so that the developmental milestones of standing upright and beginning to walk can occur.

Both growth and development are affected by genetic and environmental factors. For example, the height of a person at maturity is strongly influenced by the height of the parents. This predetermined endpoint is also affected by outside factors, such as the quality of nutrition received as a child or by medical conditions that can affect growth. The phrase *nature versus nurture* is often used to describe the debate between the roles of heredity and environment in human development. This debate about **nature versus nurture** has continued for centuries over which factor has more influence in the overall development of the individual. However, it is clear that both are influential. Our inborn abilities and traits are shaped in the environment in which we learn and mature.

Principles of Growth and Development

There is a set of principles to describe the patterns of growth and development. These principles explain typical development as an orderly and predictable process. Nevertheless, individuals will demonstrate differences in the timing and the order in which development occurs. Although one girl may show early signs of puberty at the age of 9 years, another might not show any signs until several years later. Both fall within the normal range for pubertal changes, but each has her own pace of growth. The principles of growth and development are outlined in Box 27.1.

It is important to understand the difference between the concepts of normal and average, as used to describe the developmental process. The term **normal** expresses a range of behaviours or a time span that conforms to the principles. **Average**, however, is more specific, locating a midpoint within the range of normal. In the previous example about the onset of puberty, the normal range for early pubertal changes is from approximately age 8 to 13 years; the average age is 10 years (Hockenberry & Wilson, 2007).

Stages of Growth and Development

For purposes of describing the human developmental processes that occur, the lifespan is divided arbitrarily into stages (Table 27.1). Each stage shares particular characteristics that can

---

BOX 27.1   Principles of Growth and Development

1. Growth and development is a continuous process, but the pace is uneven.
2. Growth and development involves interactions of genetics and environment. Development of language, for example, depends on biologic readiness and on social interactions.
3. Development proceeds from the head downward (cephalocaudal) and from the body outward (proximodistal).
4. Development proceeds from simple to complex and from general to specific.
5. The sequence of development is predictable, but the timing and duration will vary with the individual.
6. Sensitive periods exist in which individuals are biologically mature enough to acquire skills that could not be achieved prior to that.

Source: Bee, H., Boyd, D., & Johnson, P. (2009). *Lifespan development* (3rd ed.). Toronto, ON: Pearson; Edelman, C., & Mandle, C. (2010). *Health promotion throughout the life span* (7th ed.). St. Louis, MO: Mosby Elsevier.

---

be described in a way that is distinct from the stage preceding or following it, with transitions that are flexible. Society's ideas shift over time, and research has led to new understanding of the developments that take place in each stage.

In addition, cultural beliefs and practices can influence expected roles and behaviours. A clear example of this has occurred within the adolescent stage, which in the past was described as the period between the ages of 13 and 18 years. However, in Canada, many youth delay the transition to adulthood, spending more time in school before moving on to adult employment (Kroes & Watling, 2009). Therefore, the defined upper range of adolescence in Canada could be said to extend up to the age of 22 years. Conversely, in cultures elsewhere in the world, the adolescent period may be very short because entry into the responsibilities of the adult world occurs much earlier.

Theories of Growth and Development

Freud's Theory of Psychosexual Development

Sigmund Freud made important contributions to our understanding of the human mind. He was the first to explore the concept of the unconscious mind and the way it influences our personalities and behaviours (Bee, Boyd, & Johnson, 2009). Many other viewpoints have emerged since Freud proposed his theories, and some of his ideas are less widely regarded. Nevertheless, his psychosexual theory is still considered important because it was an early and influential stage of development theory, and many other theorists used it as a starting place.

Freud believed that successful movement through the psychosexual stages of childhood could be expected to result in well-adjusted adults. Therefore, the way the basic desires of

TABLE 27.1	Developmental Stages	
Stage	Age Period	Characteristics
Infancy	Birth to 1 year of age Neonatal period: birth to 1 month of age	Period of rapid growth High level of dependence on parent or caregiver
Toddler	1–3 years of age	Rapid development of motor skills and language Period of exploration and limit testing
Preschool/Early childhood	3–6 years of age	Rate of physical growth slows New experiences in the outside world teach social skills.
School age/Middle childhood	6–12 years of age	Increase in cognitive and social skills Becomes more physically agile Peer relationships become more important.
Adolescence	13–19 years of age	Puberty and development of physical and sexual maturity Establishing personal identity and values Risk-taking behaviours may occur as limits are tested.
Young adulthood	20–35 years of age	Establishment of career Development of own lifestyle, including intimate relationships and beginning own family
Middle adulthood	36–65 years of age	Career and family well established but also several lifestyle changes such as children leaving home, aging parents, and planning for retirement
Late adulthood	65 years of age and older Young old: 65–74 years of age Middle old: 75–85 years of age Old old: 85 years of age and older	Time of reflection of personal past and finding satisfaction with life Adaptation to series of losses such as retirement, physical changes of aging, increased dependence on others, and death of spouse

childhood were addressed was critical to how adult personalities developed. He described children as working through five stages of development: oral, anal, phallic, latency, and genital. Each stage centers on the pleasurable sensations from a specific area of the body. Table 27.2 describes the major features of each of the stages.

Piaget's Theory of Cognitive Development

Piaget (1964/1993, 1972/2008) constructed a model to describe cognitive development in childhood. Piaget's theory is based on the idea that an infant is born with innate abilities to build cognitive maps, which he called **schema**. These cognitive maps become more complex and sophisticated in response to stimuli from the external environment as the child experiences the environment, adapting those mental maps as needed. When new information is received that reinforces or adds to previous information, the child incorporates that to the existing schema in a process known as **assimilation**. If new information contradicts what has previously been learned, a process of **accommodation** occurs in which the schema is changed to reflect new knowledge.

Piaget identified four stages of cognitive development: sensorimotor, preoperational, concrete operational, and formal operational. All children pass through the stages in sequence; however, the speed of development can vary from individual to individual. A description of the characteristics of each stage is found in Table 27.2. By the adolescent period, individuals have developed the capacity for complex and coherent thought processes (Piaget, 1972/2008).

Erikson's Psychosocial Stages of Development

Erikson (1980) expanded our understanding of human development with an emphasis on the importance of social interactions. He noted that his theory presented human growth "from the point of view of the conflicts, inner and outer, which the healthy personality weathers, emerging and re-emerging with an increased sense of inner unity, with an increase of good judgment, and an increase in the capacity to do well, according to the standards of those who are significant to him" (Erikson, 1980, p. 52).

Erikson's developmental stages expanded well beyond Piaget to incorporate the entire lifespan, identifying eight stages, from birth to old age. A psychosocial crisis occurring within each stage must be resolved for development of a health personality. Erikson identified both positive and negative outcomes for each stage. The childhood period from birth to adolescence comprises the first five stages. The details for those stages are summarized in Table 27.2. By expanding his theory into the adult period, Erikson introduced the idea that psychological and social development is a lifelong process, occurring in response to the changes that are experienced as we age. A brief summary of the three adult stages is found in Table 27.3.

Moral Development Theories of Kohlberg and Gilligan

Children develop their moral sense through their interactions first within the family and later with other adults and their peers. Lawrence Kohlberg's theory describes the development of principles of justice occurring over time, beginning at

TABLE 27.2 Developmental Stages and Tasks of Infancy, Childhood, and Adolescence

Psychosexual Stage (Freud)	Psychosocial Stage (Erikson)	Cognitive Development (Piaget)
Infancy: Birth to 12 Months *Oral–Sensory* Pleasures center on gratification found in use of mouth and lips. Oral activities include sucking, biting, chewing, and vocalizing.	*Trust vs. mistrust* Basic trust—a sense of the world as a safe place, people as dependable and helpful. Consistent, loving care by nurturing person is essential. Outcomes: hope, faith, confidence, optimism Mistrust—develops when nurturing care is absent, deficient, inconsistent, or rejecting. Outcomes: suspicion, insecurity, pessimism	*Sensorimotor* (age 1½–2 years) Thought derives from sensation and movement. Progress occurs from reflex activity to simple repetitive behaviours. Develops early sense of cause/effect, time, space Concept of object permanence Task: differentiation of self from objects, locating self in physical space
Toddler: 12–36 Months *Anal–Urethral* Interest centers around anal sphincter. Develops ability to withhold or expel fecal material at will Climate surrounding toilet training influences child's personality. Associated traits include possessiveness, retentiveness, aggressiveness, pronounced messiness or tidiness, punctuality, or shame.	*Autonomy vs. shame and doubt* Autonomy—centers around increasing ability to control body, self, and environment; want to "do" for self. Sense of self-reliance and adequacy develops from being permitted to make choices. Outcomes: willpower, self-control Shame and doubt—arises when child is made to feel self-conscious, ashamed, or made dependent in areas in which he or she is capable of taking control. Outcomes: self-consciousness, lack of control	*Sensorimotor* (age 1½–2 years) Uses active experimentation to achieve goals Awareness of cause/effect Awareness of spatial relationships Imitation, domestic mimicry *Preconceptual* (age 2–4 years) Egocentric thought, self as standard of judgment Unable to take viewpoint of others Begin to think and reason conceptually Increasing use of language Thinking is transductive (relating particular to particular).
Preschool (Early Childhood): Age 3–5 Years *Phallic–Locomotion* Interest focused around genital area Recognizes differences between sexes Identification with parent of same sex Oedipal or Electra complexes, penis envy, castration fears	*Initiative vs. guilt* Initiative—sense of confidence that allows child to plan, take action, and test what kind of person he or she can be; reinforced by freedom, opportunity, and encouragement. Outcomes: purpose and direction Guilt—occurs when made to feel bad about initiatives made. Outcomes: guilt, anxiety, fear, dependence	*Preconceptual* (age 4 years) as above *Preoperational or intuitive* (age 4–7 years) Transition to increased symbolic functioning Ability to think in terms of classes, see relationships, deal with number concepts Defines objects in terms of their use Still egocentric, unable to see another's point of view
School Age (Middle Childhood): Age 6–12 Years *Latency* Resolution of phallic conflicts Attention turned from sexuality to tasks of socialization Quiescent period of sexuality	*Industry vs. inferiority* Industry—characterized by sense of confidence and competence in ability to produce, build, and make; needs and wants real achievement. Child learns to compete and cooperate and to use rules. Outcomes: method, competency Inferiority—may feel inadequate if too much or too little is expected of child or if the child feels he or she cannot live up to standards set for him or her. Outcomes: feelings of inadequacy	*Preoperational* (age 7 years) as above *Concrete operational* Development of logical reasoning Thinking is tied to what is observable. Concepts of reversibility, conservation Thinks in terms of numbers, classes, and relations Beginning deductive reasoning Overcoming egocentrism No longer fooled by appearances
Adolescence: Age 13–19 Years *Genital* Period of puberty Beginning of adult sexuality Awakening of sexual pressures and conflicts	*Identity vs. role confusion* Identity—sense of who one is, where one has been, and where one is going; brings together all things learned about self; integrates into a whole that makes sense. Peer relationships and group identity are important. Outcomes: inner consistency, fidelity ("to thine own self be true") Role confusion—confusion about self; inability to form a consistent identity from many roles, aspirations, and identifications. Outcomes: confusion about personal identity	*Formal operational* Capacity to think hypothetically Able to imagine the thoughts of others Able to hold many dimensions in mind at once Attacks problems from angle of all possible combinations of relations and variables Can consider abstract, theoretical, and philosophical matters

References: Bee, H., Boyd, D., & Johnson, P. (2009). *Lifespan development* (3rd ed.). Toronto, ON: Pearson; Dacey, J. S., Travers, J., & Fiore, L. (2009). *Human development across the life span* (7th ed.). New York, NY: McGraw-Hill; Erikson, E. H. (1980). *Identity and the life cycle.* New York, NY: Norton.

TABLE 27.3	Erikson's Psychosocial Stages of Adulthood			
Stage	Developmental Crisis	Description	Positive Outcomes	Negative Outcomes
Young adult (19–35 years)	Intimacy vs. isolation	Intimacy is the ability to form close relationships without losing one's own identity. Isolation is the tendency to separate oneself from love, friendship, and community	Ability to form close personal relationships	Fear of commitment, promiscuity, loneliness
Middle adulthood (36–64 years)	Generativity vs. stagnation	Generativity is interest in establishing and guiding the next generation and the ability to contribute to society in a meaningful way. Stagnation occurs when the person fails to be a productive member of society.	Feeling of accomplishment	Dissatisfaction with life, self-absorption
Late adulthood (65 years and older)	Integrity vs. despair	Integrity involves the ability to come to terms with one's life, to face the end of life, and to find meaning. Despair is a sense of disappointment with one's life in the face of the losses experienced with aging.	Sense of life achievement, wisdom	Regret, depression, living in the past

Source: Bee, H., Boyd, D., & Johnson, P. (2009). *Lifespan development* (3rd ed.). Toronto, ON: Pearson; Dacey, J. S., Travers, J., & Fiore, L. (2009). *Human development across the life span* (7th ed.). New York, NY: McGraw-Hill; Erikson, E. H. (1980). *Identity and the life cycle.* New York, NY: Norton

about the age of 4 years. His theory of moral development is organized in three levels of increased sophistication in moral thinking, with two stages to each level (Dacey, Travers, & Fiore, 2009). Not all individuals proceed to the highest levels of moral development, and only a small number of adults reason at the postconventional level of morality.

Theorist Carol Gilligan objected to the strictly male orientation of Kohlberg's theory, arguing that the moral reasoning of females would develop differently because of their socialization to be caring and more concerned with interpersonal relationships. She described three moral stages based on an ethics of caring, proceeding from an initial period of self-interest to a sense of responsibility for others and finally to a place of harmony that resolves the conflict between the two (Dacey et al., 2009).

Thinking About Growth and Development Across the Lifespan

It is essential for nurses to have a basic understanding of the normal patterns of growth and development at various stages within the life cycle. This knowledge is useful at all steps of the nursing process. In conducting an assessment, it is important to know what the norms will be for the patient's age in order to identify any variations that are occurring. How would it be possible to recognize an elevated blood pressure without an understanding of what is the normal range? In planning and implementing care, a nurse's approach might be modified based on the communication abilities of the patient. As an example, teaching breathing exercises to a 4-year-old will need to involve play activities rather than written instructions.

Growth and Development Across the Lifespan

The Infant Period

The term *infant* may be used generally to describe the period from birth to the age 12 months, although some sources will expand the period to 15, 18, or 24 months. The term *neonate* or *newborn* refers to the first 30 days of life.

Physical Development

The infant period is characterized by rapid growth. An infant's head is disproportionately large and heavy compared to the rest of his or her body. It takes several months before the infant will have good control of his or her head. The baby's ability to control his or her own body movements progresses rapidly, from random movements of arms and legs at birth to purposeful activities such as picking up small objects and beginning to walk unassisted. By the end of the first year of life, an infant will have tripled in weight since birth and will have increased body length by about 50%.

The most dramatic growth occurs in the infant brain, which more than doubles in size during the first year. The bones of the skull are not fused at birth, and two soft spots, known as **fontanels**, are present, allowing for expansion of the skull to accommodate this growth. Neural connections become more extensive and complex, and the neurons become myelinated, permitting the rapid and dramatic developmental achievements of infancy (Estes & Buck, 2008).

The infant's organ systems are immature at birth, and it takes some months for them to stabilize. For example, an infant's regulation of body temperature is underdeveloped and hypothermia can occur rapidly if the infant is not kept warm. The respiratory system is also not fully formed, with fewer alveoli and a reduced ability to produce mucus. Digestive processes are not fully developed, so an infant cannot completely digest some nutrients. Antibodies transferred from the mother at the time of birth bolster an infant's immunity during the first 3 months of life, but after that time period, the infant is more susceptible to infections.

An infant's hearing and sense of touch are both very well developed at birth, and the senses of smell and taste also begin to develop in utero. On the other hand, an infant's vision develops more slowly. At birth, an infant can track bright light but cannot focus on close objects. By 1 year of age, depth and colour perception are present, and visual acuity is about 20/200.

Psychosocial Development

Infants are completely dependent on others to meet their needs, and it is through the care response that basic trust, as described by Erikson, is established (Erikson, 1980). The newborn first develops a deep connection, known as **attachment**, to his or her mother or main caregiver and then later extends the attachment to other close caregiving people in his or her environment (Fig. 27.1). The infant seeks to maintain contact with and elicit care from others through behaviours such as crying, smiling, clinging, raising his or her arms to be picked up, or crawling toward the caregiver. At about the age of 8 months, the infant clearly distinguishes between those with whom he or she has an attachment and others and will begin to "make strange," reacting to strangers by crying and by clinging to his or her parent. By the end of the first year, a child who feels secure will begin to venture outward.

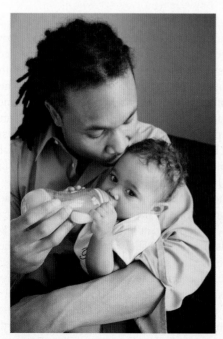

Figure 27.1 A father cuddles his infant daughter, fostering the development of trust.

Cognitive Development

At this life stage, the infant is in Piaget's sensorimotor period, which will last until the preschool age. Cognitive development derives first from sensations of his or her own body and then through interactions with the environment. Inborn reflex activity progresses to simple repetitive behaviours. A newborn may suck on his or her fist when he or she randomly brings it to his or her mouth but a short period later, learns to repeat that sensation by bringing the hand to his or her mouth purposefully. Hand–eye coordination improves as vision develops. The infant is able to identify what behaviours are effective in achieving goals such as getting attention from caregivers and learns to repeat them.

Communication

From birth, infants possess the ability to process sounds and can distinguish between speech sounds and other noises. They also have the ability to communicate their needs. Although their primary mode of communication is crying, they also make other sounds, such as gurgling and fussing, and provide cues through facial expressions and body movements. Mothers rapidly become attuned to the meanings of their babies' sounds and can detect the subtle differences between a hungry cry, a pain cry, and a bored cry. The ability of the mother to recognize the differences and respond appropriately to the crying influences the responsiveness of the infant (Del Vecchio, Walter, & O'Leary, 2009).

The developing infant rapidly gains social skills that enhance communication. By approximately 2 months, a social smile is acquired to respond to the adults in the environments, and shortly thereafter, the baby makes cooing and laughing sounds. By the middle of the first year of life, the infant will develop babbling, making sounds that are not comprehensible to others but clearly have meaning to the infant (Goldstein, Schwade, Briesch, & Syal, 2010). The sequences of babbling sounds develop the tones and phrasing of the spoken language that the infant hears and are part of the learning process in the development of language (Bee et al., 2009).

The Toddler Period

The toddler stage begins when the child takes his or her first steps alone, at 12 to 15 months, and continues until approximately 3 years of age.

Physical Development

The rate of growth slows between the age of 1 and 3 years, but the toddler makes great strides in motor skill development. The toddler's head is still disproportionately large, and the trunk of the body becomes quite long compared to limb length. Toddlers have a typical lumbar lordosis, which gives them a potbellied look. They progress from standing and walking unsteadily to being able to run, manage stairs, kick a ball, and ride tricycles. Manual dexterity also increases, so that the toddler progresses from making simple stacks of blocks to being able to draw recognizable stick figures.

By the age of 3 years, most body systems are relatively mature. The toddler's brain continues to grow and reaches 75% of adult size after 2 years of age. The fontanels of the skull close completely, although the bones remain flexible. Chest size and respiratory capacity increases. A full set of 20 primary teeth have erupted, and the digestive system is sufficiently developed to permit the toddler to eat and digest a range of solid foods. A significant change is the toddler's capability to control his or her bladder and bowels making toilet training feasible. Visual acuity and hand–eye coordination improve.

Psychosocial Development

The toddler begins to assert a desire for independence, and he or she seeks to control his or her own body and his or her environment. According to Erikson (1980), the major task of the period is the quest for autonomy. The toddler shows strong determination to do things for himself or herself, such as feeding or dressing and rejecting the commands or assistance of others. **Negativism**, in which the toddler consistently refuses to follow commands or respond to suggestions, is evident in the frequent use of the word *no* and in the occurrence of temper tantrums.

The toddler's social circle expands to include other adults and playmates. Nevertheless, he or she still is strongly attached to the caregivers and may experience a high degree of separation anxiety when away from them. Toddlers imitate others' behaviours and engage in parallel play with other children (Fig. 27.2).

Cognitive Development

At the beginning of the toddler period, the child is still in Piaget's sensorimotor period during which he or she explores his or her world by touching, tasting, looking, and listening. He or she actively experiments with objects in his or her environment and develops a beginning awareness of cause and effect. As the toddler progresses into the preconceptual period,

he or she begins to think and reason conceptually but not necessarily logically. Egocentric thinking prevails, and the toddler assumes that other people think and feel as he or she does.

Communication

During the toddler phase, the acquisition of language occurs, beginning with single words and rapidly progressing. By the age of 3 years, he or she is able to communicate with a vocabulary of approximately 900 to 1,000 words. Nevertheless, the limits of the language skills mean that toddlers often communicate by other means, such as pointing or crying. The temper tantrums that are typical of the 2-year-old may reflect frustration with the limits of communication (Hockenberry & Wilson, 2007). The focus of the toddler's language is self-centered, used to communicate his or her wants and needs.

The Preschool Period—Early Childhood

During the preschool years, ages 3 to 5 years, the child emerges as a social being. Physical growth is slowing while emotional and intellectual progress is apparent.

Physical Development

The pace of physical growth slows during the preschool period. As body proportions start to change, the preschooler appears slimmer and more graceful. Arms and legs grow so that the head and trunk seem more proportional. The lumbar lordosis of the toddler period disappears, making way for a more erect posture. As gross motor and fine motor skills become well developed, the child can manage such activities as throwing a ball, balancing on one foot, and cutting with scissors.

Organ systems continue to mature. Respiratory and cardiac capacity expands. All primary teeth are present, and by the end of the preschool period, permanent teeth may begin to erupt. The immune system is boosted as it responds to pathogens in the child's environment. All sensory systems are well developed. By the end of the fifth year, visual acuity should be 20/20.

Psychosocial Development

The developmental task of the preschool period is acquiring a sense of initiative. The preschooler develops this through play, which becomes more social and interactive. A child at this age can begin to play cooperatively and manages simple games. Although parents remain the central figures in the preschooler's life, peers become significant as well. At this point, the preschooler learns to control his or her behaviour in social situations.

The preschool child actively seeks out answers, repeatedly asking *why*. The ability to imagine emerges, which greatly enhances his or her understanding of the world but can also lead to unrealistic thinking and fears. He or she will explore his or her abilities, testing the limits of his or her physical skills. The young child engages in sexual curiosity,

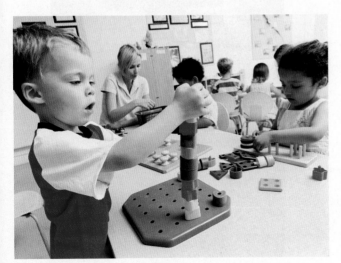

Figure 27.2 The toddler engages in parallel play with other children of the same age.

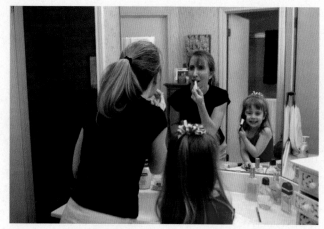

Figure 27.3 The preschool-age girl imitates her mother, while she is putting on makeup, as part of her gender identification.

exploring his or her own genitals and inquisitive about the differences between girls and boys. Gender identification is forming, and the preschooler likes to imitate the same-gender parent (Fig. 27.3). An early sense of right and wrong develops, and following rules becomes important.

Cognitive Development

The preschool child moves from Piaget's preconceptual stage of the sensorimotor period, where thinking is very concrete, to the preoperational period. Thinking becomes more intuitive and imaginative, and the child is able to both relate memories and visualize future events. The child can differentiate between the inner self and the outer world, but egocentrism persists. Magical thinking takes place, in which the child believes he or she has power over what is happening in the world around him or her. The preschool child will be interested in books and begins to understand the concepts of words on the page as symbols for something in the real world.

Communication

At this stage, receptive communication, the ability to understand what is said, greatly exceeds expressive communication. Over the course of the preschool period, the child develops an expanding vocabulary to express themselves. He or she talks almost continuously, asking questions and telling stories. The structure of speech is increasingly complex and should be entirely comprehensible to others. At this stage, the child is likely to be very literal in his or her understanding of the meaning of words. The nurse who tells the 4-year-old he or she is going to get *a shot* might find a rather alarmed child who is expecting a gun to appear.

The School-Age Period—Middle and Late Childhood

The school-age period can be divided into middle childhood (6 to 8 years of age) and late childhood (8 to 12 years of age). The school-age years can also be divided into juvenile and preadolescent periods. The juvenile period begins at approx-

imately age 6 years. Preadolescence (or prepuberty) usually begins at 9 or 10 years of age and ends with the onset of puberty around 11 or 12 years of age.

Physical Development

The school-age child becomes taller and slimmer. Growth tends to occur in spurts, often with an upsurge at the end of this stage at the onset of puberty. Girls enter prepubescence about 2 years earlier than boys. Size differences between the genders are often noticeable at the end of middle childhood. Advanced motor activities, indicating full myelination of nervous system, become noticeable. The child becomes very agile and active, capable of a wide range of gross motor skills, such as skipping, riding a bike, and playing sports (Fig. 27.4). Fine motor skills, such as drawing, model building, and writing, become possible. During this stage, the primary teeth are lost, and all secondary teeth, except for wisdom teeth, erupt by the end of the childhood period. Children may be self-conscious because of missing teeth or the oversized appearance of the permanent teeth when they first emerge.

Psychosocial Development

The middle childhood period is identified by the achievement of a sense of industry. There is eagerness to learn new things and to take on new challenges. At the beginning of the school-age period, the child is generally quite pleasant to be around. Emotions are more stable with fewer outbursts than in the earlier periods. Family relationships remain important, but friendships with peers become more significant. Peer association in the early years of the period

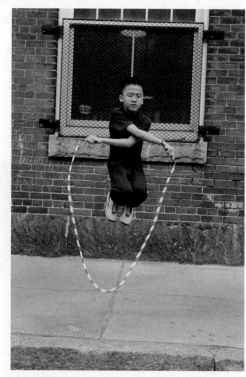

Figure 27.4 School-age children develop increased physical dexterity, which means they can enjoy an activity such as skipping rope.

tends to be same sex, but later on, the school-age child will have friends of both genders. The daily interactions with friends at school and at play provide valuable social lessons, such as following the rules in games, playing fair, and controlling anger. The child gains increasing levels of independence, spending more time away from home, and parents may struggle with the need to let go of their control.

Cognitive Development

The school-age child enters the period of concrete operations in which he or she is able to perform quite complex mental processes (Piaget, 1964/1993, 2008). One important mental task mastered is the concept of conservation, which is the ability to see that the properties of matter are preserved despite different kinds of physical transformation. For example, the child learns that a set volume of liquid stays the same despite the size and shape of the container it is in. The egocentrism of earlier development periods subsides during middle childhood. The school-age child is able to think more conceptually about things and can see the viewpoint of others. Based on the moral development that comes from more flexibility in thinking, he or she begins to value fairness in relationships.

Communication

In middle childhood, there is tremendous expansion of vocabulary and demonstration of correct use of grammar and syntax. By the end of the period, the child understands approximately 50,000 words and speaks in ways that are similar to adults. The application of language becomes socially useful in negotiating relationships with peers and adults. The school-age child delights in the use of words, enjoying word games and rhyming. By developing reading and writing skills, the child learns to communicate in written language. At age 6 years, the child is learning to read. By age 12 years, he or she is reading to learn. Communication can now be used meaningfully in both oral and written forms (Dacey et al., 2009).

The Adolescent Period

The adolescent period approximately spans 13 to 19 years of age. It is characterized by the onset of puberty, the development of physical and sexual maturity, and the establishment of personal identity and values.

Physical Development

Following the stable, slow growth patterns of the preschool- and school-age periods, the physical changes of the adolescent period are quite dramatic. Another period of rapid growth occurs for several years and then continues somewhat more slowly until growth to full adult size is completed. **Puberty** signals the onset of sexual maturation of the body and brings dramatic body changes. Puberty in females begins with the development of secondary sex characteristics, such as growth of pubic hair and breast growth, and is followed by the onset of menstrual periods. Boys experience testicular enlargement,

growth of body hair, and seminal emissions. There is a wide time range for the onset and pace of the pubertal changes, with females entering puberty about 2 years ahead of males. For this reason, adolescents of the same chronological age can differ greatly in size and appearance.

Psychosocial Development

A search for personal identity characterizes the adolescent period of psychosocial development. Initially, the adolescent must incorporate into his or her body image the physical changes that are occurring and cope with the emergence of sexual feelings. Young people who experience the changes of puberty earlier or later than their friends may struggle with feeling different from peers. Similarly, a teenager with a chronic illness may be challenged with trying to fit in. The adolescent period can be tumultuous for both the teenager and his or her parents as he or she strives to establish personal independence while being still dependent on family for most needs. Peer relationships grow in importance, and the nature of friendships change qualitatively as the teenager learns to demonstrate more caring and concern for others (Fig. 27.5). Early experimentation with developing intimate relationships with members of the opposite sex occurs. Older adolescence (17 to 19 years of age) becomes a transition to the adult period, with many young people developing mature relationships and making decisions about future careers.

Through the eyes of a patient

*B*eing a teenager with diabetes started off being a difficult experience for me. I was starting at a brand new high school, and besides the 25 or so kids I had been going to school with for the last several years, no one was going to know that I was diabetic. I wanted to keep it that way. I would go to the bathroom every day at lunch to test my blood sugar and give my insulin. Only a few of my closest friends knew I was diabetic. This all changed when I was 17 and I had a seizure while out for lunch with friends from school. Only one person with me knew I was diabetic and knew what was going on. An ambulance was called and I was fine, but everyone now knew I was diabetic. As I grew and matured through my teenage years, I began to realize that it didn't matter who knew that I was diabetic. It was something that I did not need to hide but something to be proud of. If people didn't like seeing me give needles in public, then it was up to them to turn away. If they were interested in what I was doing, I was more than happy to explain to them what I was doing and answer any questions they may have. I take any opportunity I can get to help educate the general public about many of the misconceptions surrounding diabetes. This is something I started doing a little as a teenager through my final years of high school and I always do now at every opportunity I can get!

(personal reflection of Susan, a patient)

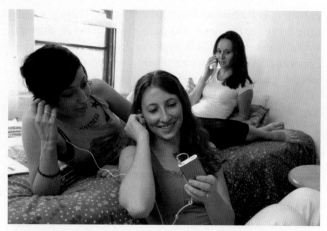

Figure 27.5 Enjoying shared interests with peers is very important during the adolescent period.

Cognitive Development

Around the age of 12 years, the adolescent becomes capable of complex and sophisticated thought processes as the final cognitive stage of formal operations emerges. This stage includes the ability to think abstractly and conceptually, but there will be a wide range of individual achievement of this ability. Abstract reasoning skills may not be highly developed until quite late in the adolescent period. Adolescents may regress to concrete thinking skills in stressful or highly emotional situations. The adolescent becomes more self-absorbed and reflective about his or her own experiences, which leads to more mature moral judgments.

Communication

Adolescents possess a full range of vocabulary with which to express themselves. They learn to use more complex language and to adapt their communication according to the situation. They make use of many avenues to communicate with each other, including text messaging, Internet chat programs, and telephoning as well as face-to-face contacts. On the other hand, the communication with parents often becomes less open and less frequent. Many parents note that their teenage child becomes monosyllabic when addressed.

As part of their forming an identity separate from the adults in their lives, each generation of teenagers develops its own vernacular. The meaning of specific words, phrases, and acronyms make rapid shifts, and the slang of today will be obsolete a few years in the future. Adults would be wise to avoid using slang terminology with the teenager. Whether it is an effort to be up-to-date or to build common bonds, the likelihood of misusing slang is very high.

The Young Adulthood Period

During the young adulthood period (from about age 20 to 35 years), the focus is on the development of his or her own lifestyle. This includes the establishment of a career, the formation of intimate relationships, and beginning a family.

Physical Development

The peak of physical development is reached during the first decade of the young adult period. Physical changes begin to slow down. Maximum height and muscle mass is achieved. Sexual development is completed and reproductive function is at its optimum. Internal organs function at their most effective level and have a reserve capacity that is normally not called on. The brain continues to develop until the mid-20s, with increased myelination and the ongoing addition and pruning of neurons (Simpson, 2008). Most young adults perceive themselves as at the peak of health and do not anticipate health problems.

As the person approaches the age of 30 years, there is already evidence of the body slowing down and becoming less efficient. As spinal disks compress, there is a loss in height, and the amount of fatty tissue in the body increases, creating concerns about weight. Cardiac output, muscle strength, and neurological reaction time decreases. By the end of the young adult period, a person might see himself or herself as potentially vulnerable to health problems.

Psychosocial Development

The young adult period is a critical stage when the individual leaves the security of his or her parents to carve out his or her own place in the world. To achieve Erikson's task of intimacy, the young adult will need to establish a mature, trusting relationship with a significant other in which there can be sharing of hopes and fears (Erikson, 1980). This intimacy may be expressed in a heterosexual or homosexual relationship. The individual makes decisions about the commitments of partnering and marriage and about parenting and raising a family (Fig. 27.6).

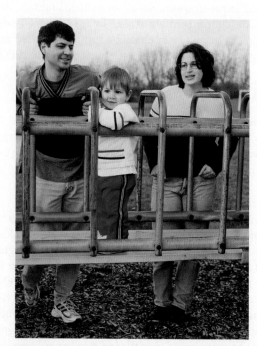

Figure 27.6 As young adults, decisions are made about marriage and family.

Important decisions about careers and work life must be made during this period. In the early 20s, the individual might pursue college or university education to achieve career goals. Moving out of the parents' home might be delayed for economic reasons, and this could potentially impair the ability of the young adult to establish a more mature relationship with his or her family. The phenomenon of young adults who *boomerang*, returning home after moving out, is a common feature of the 21st century (Clark, 2007). However, by the end of the period, the young adult should be established in career and relationship, with long-range plans for the remainder of his or her life.

Cognitive Development

When the cognitive stage of formal operations is achieved during adolescence, the young adult possesses a full range of cognitive skills. The individual develops the ability to focus on practical matters and to cope more easily with the demands of the rapidly changing world.

As the young adult gains knowledge and experience, he or she is increasingly able to consider complex phenomena such as abstract concepts, human relationships, and ethical issues. Piaget (2008) notes that the young adult will become specialized in his or her thinking based on particular aptitudes and interests.

Communication

A young adult with an extensive vocabulary can express thoughts and feelings fully. Being more emotionally stable than in earlier life periods, he or she has the ability to process thoughts and feelings more fully before expressing them. Most young adults are comfortable with using modern technology in a myriad of ways to communicate. When different levels of language are used, the person can tailor vocabulary and tone to match the situation, recognizing, for example, that online chatting with friends calls for a different style of language than a presentation to a committee at work. It is important to note that vocabulary may be very specialized according to the individual's education and interests. An engineer might use highly technical language in work situations but not understand medical terminology.

The Middle Adulthood Period

The middle adulthood period covers a major portion of the human lifespan, from age 36 to 65 years. During this time, the individual's career and family are generally well established, but several significant changes occur, such as children leaving home, retirement, and changes in health status.

Physical Development

Most adults enter the middle adulthood period in good physical shape. Although there is some slowing down of physical function, it is quite gradual. The degree and rate of change is highly individual, dependent on factors such as genetics, lifestyle, and social environment. Some expected physical changes that will occur include loss of muscle mass, slower tissue regeneration, decreased gastrointestinal motility, and reduced kidney function, but many of these will not be noticeable to the individual. Skin changes include loss of elasticity, appearing as sagging and wrinkles, and emergence of age spots. Hair will become thinner and begin to turn gray. Men will notice the onset of male pattern baldness. A change in vision, known as *presbyopia*, results in a decreased ability of the eyes to adjust for close vision. As a result, most people in middle age eventually need reading glasses or bifocal lenses.

For women, the most dramatic change of middle age is the onset of **menopause**, which generally occurs between the age of 40 and 55 years. In addition to the cessation of menstrual periods, the menopausal woman may experience a range of uncomfortable symptoms, such as hot flashes, palpitations, and mood swings. After menopause, women are at risk for loss of bone mass, predisposing them to osteoporosis. Although men do not experience a change corresponding to menopause and can remain fertile into old age, androgen levels gradually decrease, affecting sexual function.

Psychosocial Development

Adults at middle age are drawn to what Erikson termed the *task of generativity*, the experience of which can take several forms. It may be the satisfaction of caring for and nurturing the next generations, or it may be expressed through creativity and contributions to society (Fig. 27.7). Women and men may experience the middle-age period in different ways. Women who have focused for many years on their family responsibilities may find themselves liberated

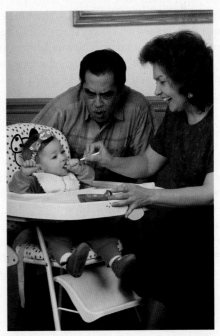

Figure 27.7 Becoming a grandparent is one of the joys of the middle adulthood period.

by the launching of their adult children and may demonstrate more assertiveness and confidence in their careers. Conversely, men who have been career focused begin to think about retirement and restructuring their lives to place more emphasis on their relationships. Adults who weather the challenges of the period can experience great satisfaction with their lives (Bee et al., 2009).

There is great diversity in the social roles of the middle adulthood period that has more to do with individuals' life events than with chronological age. For example, a woman of 45 years of age who has adult children leaving home will have a very different midlife experience than a woman of the same age who had her first child at the age of 40 years and is still dealing with preschoolers at home. Other individuals might find themselves laid off from work in their 40s, changing careers, or returning to school. Often, the middle-aged adult will find himself or herself part of the **sandwich generation**, still assisting adolescent and young adult children while at the same time providing care for aging parents. The new role of grandparenting may begin, and many adults in this period are actively involved in the raising of their grandchildren.

Cognitive Development and Communication

Middle-aged adults maintain full cognitive functioning with no loss of abilities in the areas of abstract thinking, problem solving, learning, or memory. Reaction time slows, and hand–eye coordination declines slightly over the midlife period, which may affect the rate of physical response in some situations such as catching an object falling off a countertop. The middle-aged adult is often very focused on career-related cognitive skills and is most highly motivated to learn when the information is relevant to personal goals.

Middle-aged adults have a mature range of communications skills learned and refined through their life experience. They have been somewhat slower than younger generations to make full use of modern communication technology, such as the Internet, but are rapidly catching up, making use of online resources and e-mail more regularly (Veenhof & Timusk, 2009).

The Older Adult Period

Aging is a complex and varied process affected by many factors, such as health status, family relationships, and psychological well-being. In general terms, the older adult period is considered to begin at the age of 65 years and is divided into three categories: young old (65 to 74 years of age), middle old (75 to 85 years of age), and old old (85 years of age and older). However, these categories are very arbitrary and often may not reflect the self-identification of an individual.

Physical Development

The older adult period is characterized by slow but significant decline in most areas of physical functioning as part of the normal **aging** process. The rate and degree of those

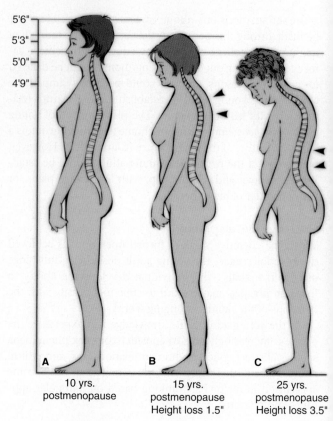

Figure 27.8 Elderly women may develop osteoporosis, which can cause a stooped posture.

changes will vary widely among individuals, and not all changes will be apparent in all elderly patients.

Because of atrophy of intervertebral disks, there will be a loss in stature. This is even more evident if the older adult has lost bone mass due to osteoporosis, and this may be accompanied by a stooped posture (Fig. 27.8). Overall muscle strength and tone is lost. Body joints, particularly knees and hips, experience degenerative changes causing stiffness and restricted range of motion. Reaction time becomes slower, and balance becomes more uncertain, which can increase the risk for falls. As a result, many older people gradually become more cautious about things such as walking down stairs or climbing ladders.

All five senses experience changes associated with aging. There is a loss in visual acuity due to increasing presbyopia and development of opacity of the lens. Less acute sense of taste and smell may affect the older adult's appetite. Some degree of hearing loss can be expected due to normal aging changes and to a lifetime of exposure to noise. Men are more likely to experience a degree of deafness possibly due to noise levels of their work environments. Sensitivity to heat, cold, and pain diminishes due to loss of nerve receptors in the skin, placing the elderly at increased risk for burns.

All organ systems also experience decreased functioning. Pulmonary efficiency is reduced, and the working capacity of the heart diminishes. Blood pressure gradually increases due to changes in the arteries. The elderly patient may have problems with indigestion or constipation because of slowed functioning of the gastrointestinal tract. The older adult may have problems with urinary frequency and urgency because of reduced bladder size. The immune system becomes less effective, increasing the risk of infections, such as influenza or pneumonia.

Psychosocial Development

Erikson (1980) describes the final developmental task of achieving integrity as the process of looking back on life and accepting it, having adapted to the triumphs and disappointments, without significant regret about the choices made. People who are unable to look backward with satisfaction may fail to achieve this task and may experience depression and despair. At the end of life, elderly people generally engage in reflection on their past, doing **life review**. The process of life review is investigated in the accompanying research box.

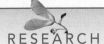

RESEARCH

LIFE REVIEW AS A TOOL FOR PROMOTING WELL-BEING IN THE ELDERLY

Life review is the process of thinking back on one's life and communicating about one's life to another person. Achieving the developmental task of integrity requires acceptance of one's own past and present life. When older adults have the opportunity to reminisce about their life stories, they can find meaning, acceptance, and a sense of control of their lives.

Study

Mastel-Smith, McFarlane, Sierpina, Malecha, and Haile (2007) conducted a study with community-based elderly, testing the usefulness of a life review workshop. The intervention was developed to provide the older adults the opportunity to reflect on, write, and share their life stories. Thirty-three men and women participated in the study and were randomly assigned to an intervention group and to a control group. The intervention used, a Life Story Workshop, involved 2-hour workshops weekly for 10 weeks, during which the participants engaged in the writing and sharing of stories about their lives. Both groups completed the Brief Symptom Inventory subscale, which measures levels of depression before and after the study period.

The study group who participated in the writing program reported significantly fewer depressive symptoms than were reported by those in the control group. The authors concluded that reminiscence and life review activities have the potential to improve the mental health of community-dwelling older adults.

Bohlmeijer, Roemer, Cuijpers, and Smit (2007) conducted a meta-analysis of 15 studies of the usefulness of reminiscence and life review and similarly concluded that "reminiscence in general, but especially life review, are potentially effective methods for the enhancement of psychological well-being in older adults" (p. 291).

Nursing Implications

Nurses who work with the older adults in the community or in long-term care settings can facilitate reminiscence with their patients. Encouraging this reflective process can provide an opportunity for nurses to learn about and appreciate the lives of their patients as well as supporting the older adults' own process of life review. Activities which are useful include writing activities about the past, telling of life stories individually or in groups, or looking through photo albums. Reminiscing may evoke both positive and negative emotions in the patients, so nurses must be prepared to allow for full expression of the feelings and to handle their own emotional responses.

Bohlmeijer, E., Roemer, M., Cuijpers, P., Smit, F. (2007). The effects of reminiscence on psychological well-being in older adults: A meta-analysis. Aging & Mental Health, 11(3), 291–300; Mastel-Smith, B., McFarlane, J., Sierpina, M., Malecha, A., Haile, B. (2007). Improving depressive symptoms in community-dwelling older adults: A psychosocial intervention using life review and writing. Journal of Gerontological Nursing, 33(5), 13–19.

Most older adults will have retired by age 65 years, and their children will have grown and left home. The challenge for the older adult may be to identify meaningful activities they will be able to pursue even in the face of declining physical abilities. Many find outlets in hobbies, traveling, volunteer work, and grandparenting. Over time, the elderly experience a series of losses, such as deaths of family members and friends, or the need to move out of their family home into assisted living facilities. The older adult also adapts to continuing declines in health and ultimately must face the inevitability of death.

Cognitive Development

The changes in sensory function can affect the older adult's cognitive processes, but often, the difficulties are more a matter of speed than of ability. If the elderly person is having difficulty with vision or hearing, the ability to respond quickly and effectively to changes in the environment is affected. Most older adults do not experience cognitive impairment and are able to maintain mental functions such as problem solving and judgment. There is a reduction in the number of neurons in the brain with aging; as a result, processing of some information, such as retrieval of past memories, may be slower.

Many older adults worry about developing dementia, so intermittent problems with memory retrieval or information processing may make them anxious about losing their mental abilities. However, cognitive impairment is not an inevitable result of aging. Health problems, such as high blood pressure, heart disease, or chronic respiratory disease, may interfere with blood flow to the brain, causing some limitations.

Communication

Many older adults maintain the capacity to communicate effectively, but sensory and physical limitation may affect the facility with which they are able to receive and transmit information. Because much of communication is nonverbal, an elderly patient with poor vision may have difficulty interpreting facial expressions or other body language cues. In some elderly people, there are physiological changes in speaking ability, and their voices become weaker or more difficult to understand. A health impairment, such as a stroke, may cause significant communication difficulties such as facial paralysis or aphasia, a total or partial loss of the power to use or understand words.

Consider the case at the beginning of the chapter about Jamaal, who was worried about being able to communicate with an elderly patient. It seems likely that he would not be alone in his concern. Students frequently feel nervous about interacting with older adults. The instructor will help the students develop communication skills in the long-term care setting. Some tips for interacting with an elderly patient:

- Assess the patient's ability to communicate. What eyesight or hearing problems does he or she have? Is his or her speech clear? Is there any evidence that he or she is confused?
- Show respect to the patient. Address him or her by his or her title and last name (e.g., Mr. Watson). Focus on the patient as a person, keeping in mind that this elderly person, now living in a single room in a nursing home, has had a full and interesting life.
- When communicating, create a quiet environment to reduce distracting outside noises.
- Ensure that the patient is wearing any assistive devices such as glasses or hearing aid.
- Sit at the patient's level so he or she can see your face more readily. Face the patient when talking and maintain eye contact. Remember to smile. If the resident is accepting to touch, it is appropriate to use gentle touch, such as placing a hand on his or her arm.
- Use open-ended communication to identify topics that are of interest to the patient. Is the patient interested in talking about current news, particular hobbies or sports, or his or her family?
- Consider using reminiscence as a strategy. Talk about the patient's former work, hobbies, and family. If possible, look at photo albums or other mementos.
- Acknowledge and respect the patient's feelings. Reminiscence may bring back moments of sadness and moments of joy.
- Be patient when listening and be aware of when the elderly person gets tired and wants to rest.

Performing Assessments Across the Lifespan

Knowledge of developmental, physiological, and psychological norms for each stage of development is essential when preparing to interview and examine patients. The nurse's approach needs to be adapted to the developmental needs as well as to the individual preferences of the patient. While conducting the health interview and gathering information about the presenting issue, it is important to be aware of the specific health risks of each age group. Nurses need to base specific screening questions within the health history on this information. Table 27.4 provides an overview of some of the basic screening that should be included for each age group.

Infants and Toddlers

Much of the information that needs to be gathered about an infant's or toddler's health and developmental status will be obtained from the interview with the parent. The parent is the constant in the child's life, can provide valuable information about the child's usual patterns of behaviour, and will be attuned to even small changes that the nurse might not notice. In addition to information about the child's health status, data can be gained about factors that influence the child's life, such as family structure, cultural influences, or environmental factors.

When performing a physical assessment of an infant or toddler, considerable information about the child's physical and emotional state can be gained by simply observing the child. While chatting with the parent, the nurse can note the child's general size, appearance, and mood. By establishing a warm, caring relationship with the parent, the nurse communicates to the infant or toddler that he or she can be trusted. It is helpful to keep the parent involved throughout the examination by having him or her hold the child in his or her lap for portions of the examination or by asking him or her to stand close by where the infant or toddler can see his or her face. The nurse must be flexible in the sequence of the assessment, beginning with the easiest procedures and doing the more invasive portions near the end. Play can be used as a technique to gain the child's cooperation, such as allowing the toddler to listen to a teddy bear's chest with the stethoscope.

Developmental Screening of Infants and Children

Developmental screening is carried out in order to identify early those children who may not be meeting developmental milestones. If a developmental lag is suspected, referral can then be made to specialists for more extensive assessment. Developmental screening tools consist of a checklist of some of the important skills that a child should accomplish by a certain age. These developmental tools are not focused enough to screen for specific disorders such as autism. Specialized tools are available that concentrate on more narrowly defined problems.

Performing screening can also provide reassurance to parents by identifying children who are meeting developmental guidelines and can help parents learn about normal child development. The results should be shared with the parents and should be fully explained. The information can then be used to plan intervention strategies, such as identifying activities to encourage healthy development.

General screening tools check the following areas of development: gross motor skills, fine motor skills, vision, hearing, communication, social-emotional, cognitive, and self-help skills. There are several widely used screening tools available for nurses. Common ones include the Denver Developmental Screening Test II (DDST-II), Ages and Stages Questionnaires (ASQ), and

TABLE 27.4	Health Screening Across the Lifespan
Age Group	**Areas of Assessment and Screening**
Infant	• Weight, length, and head circumference; plot on growth chart and watch trends. • Vision and hearing screening • Mother–infant attachment behaviours; parenting style • Nutrition: breast-feeding or iron-fortified formula feeding and vitamin D supplements; addition of solid foods after age 6 months • Sleep patterns • Teething • Injury prevention: car seat, sleep positioning, crib safety, choking risks (safe toys), smoking in the home, smoke detectors • Immunization history and parent plans for immunization • Developmental milestones; use screening tool such as NDDS. • Family conflict, child abuse
Toddler	• Weight, height, and head circumference (to 18 months); plot on growth chart and watch trends. • Hearing inquiry or screening • Nutrition: breast-feeding or homogenous milk and solid foods (use Canada's Food Guide); weaning to cup • Teething, dental care • Injury prevention: car seat, childproofing of home, poisons, choking hazards, pool safety, smoking in home • Immunizations • Developmental milestones; use screening tool. • Day care participation • Parenting questions, family conflict, child abuse
Early childhood	• Height, length; plot on growth chart and watch trends. • Vision and hearing screening • Nutrition: Canada's Food Guide • Dental care, dentist visits • Injury prevention: car seat/booster, bicycle helmets, water safety • Immunizations • Developmental milestones; use screening tool. • Day care, school readiness • Parenting questions, family conflict, child abuse
School age/Middle childhood	• Height, weight; onset of puberty • Nutrition: Canada's Food Guide, prevention of obesity • Dental care, loss of primary teeth, dentist visits • Injury prevention: bicycle helmets, water safety, sports safety • Immunizations: HPV for females aged 11 and 12 years • School issues • Parenting questions, family conflict, child abuse
Adolescent	• Height, weight, BMI; pubertal changes • Body image • Nutrition: healthy choices, junk food • Immunizations including influenza and HPV vaccine • School issues • Risk behaviours: tobacco, alcohol and drug use, driving • Sexual activity, level of sexual information including birth control, STDs • Dating violence
Young adult	• Height, weight, BMI • Nutrition, exercise • Influenza immunization • Alcohol, tobacco, and drug use • Family planning, birth control methods, STD risks • Cancer screening: Discuss breast or testicular self-examination, sun risks, and Pap smear (female). • Dating or spousal violence
Middle-aged adult	• Height, weight, BMI, waist–hip ratio • Nutrition, exercise • Influenza immunization • Alcohol, tobacco, and drug use • Heart health: blood pressure, cholesterol test • Discuss cancer screening: breast or testicular self-examination, Pap smear and mammogram (female), colorectal screening. • Discuss diabetes screening and risk. • Family violence

(continued on page 652)

TABLE 27.4	Health Screening Across the Lifespan (continued)
Age Group	**Areas of Assessment and Screening**
Older adult	• Height, weight, BMI • Nutrition and exercise pattern • Dentition • Influenza immunization • Discuss cancer screening (as above) • Hearing and vision, use of aids • Review of medications • Mobility assessment: gait, balance, risk for falls, use of aids, bone density tests (women) • Cognitive function: Mini-Mental State Examination, if indicated • Social relationships, family caregivers • Elder abuse • Advance directives

BMI, body mass index; HPV, human papillomavirus; NDSS, Nipissing District Developmental Screen; STD, sexually transmitted disease.

References: Greig, A., Constantin, E., Carsley, S., & Cummings, C. (2010). Preventive health care visits for children and adolescents aged six to 17 years: The Greig Health Record—Executive summary. *Paediatrics & Child Health, 15*(3), 157–162; Rourke, L., Rourke. J., & Leduc, D. (2009). *Rourke baby record.* Retrieved from http://www.rourkebabyrecord.ca; U.S. Preventive Services Task Force. (2009). *Guide to clinical preventative services.* Retrieved from http://www.ahrq.gov/clinic/pocketgd09/

the Nipissing District Developmental Screen (NDDS). Some, such as the Denver II, require the screening to be carried out by a professional with training. Others, such as the NDDS, can be done by the nurse or by the parent. A sample of the NDDS for an 18-month-old child is shown in Figure 27.9.

These developmental screening tools are designed to be used from infancy to age 5 years. At the present time, there are no comprehensive developmental screening tests for use during the middle childhood or adolescent periods. However, there are some tools available to screen for specific problems in the older age groups. The pediatric symptom checklist can be used to identify cognitive, emotional, and behavioural problems, so that appropriate interventions can be initiated.

Preschool- and School-Age Children

As the children get older and their ability to communicate develops, their participation in the health interview process will increase. Parents continue to be an important source of information about the child's health history and status.

Because small children's thought processes are concrete, literal, and egocentric, it is important to use language that is clear, direct, and simple. For example, the nurse can refer to a blood pressure cuff as "hugging the arm tight" as it is pumped up. The nurse can also ask a small child to "point to where it hurts" rather than immediately prodding at the child's body. A school-age child is much more likely to be able to provide accurate information when asked.

Adolescents

The adolescent is in a transitional phase from dependence to independence. In early adolescence, the parents still assume most of the responsibility for their child's health care, but by late adolescence, the teenager is often managing most of

his or her own medical needs. The nurse needs to assess where the adolescent is in the transition phase to determine how much or how little involvement the parent should have in the interview. The setting where the adolescent is being interviewed or examined should be appropriate for adolescent patients. The nurse needs to show a genuine interest in the adolescent from the outset. Establishing a partnership with the teenage patient helps to create a trusting, therapeutic relationship. Chatting for a few minutes in an informal way before the interview begins may be a helpful strategy. The nurse should address the adolescent patient before addressing the parents so that the message is clear that the adolescent's needs and concerns are the primary focus.

The need for privacy during the interview with a teenager is very important. The adolescent may be reluctant to reveal important information if it is possible that the conversations can be overheard. It may be difficult to provide privacy in some settings, such as the hospital unit or the emergency room, but effort should be made to do so. Confidentiality should be discussed, and the limits of confidentiality should be made clear to the adolescent and the family.

Young and Middle-Aged Adults

In assessing the developmental needs of an adult, the nurse needs to recognize that each patient's situation will be unique based on his or her age, life experience, and health status. Most adults will have had previous experiences within the health-care system that will influence their perceptions and attitudes. For example, some may see the nurse or doctor as expert and be passive in their relationship to the health-care team. Others may choose a more active role in making their health-care decisions. The nurse should explore those perceptions and encourage the patient's participation in decision-making. Establishing an open and collaborative

ndds.ca
nipissing district developmental screen®

Child's Name: _____

Birthdate: _____ Today's Date: _____

The Nipissing District Developmental Screen is a checklist designed to help monitor your child's development.

Y   N   BY **EIGHTEEN MONTHS** OF AGE, DOES YOUR CHILD:

O O   1 Identify pictures in a book? *("show me the baby")**

O O   2 Use a variety of familiar gestures?
           (waving, pushing, giving, reaching up)*

O O   3 Follow directions using "on" and "under"?
           ("put the cup on the table")*

O O   4 Make at least four different consonant sounds? *(b, n, d, h, g, w)**

O O   5 Point to at least three different body parts when asked?
           ("where is your nose?")*

O O   6 Say 20 or more words? *(words do not have to be clear)*

O O   7 Hold a cup to drink? **

O O   8 Pick up and eat finger food?

O O   9 Help with dressing by putting out arms and legs? **

O O 10 Walk up a few stairs holding your hand?

O O 11 Walk alone?

O O 12 Squat to pick up a toy and stand back up without falling?

O O 13 Push and pull toys or other objects while walking forward? *A*

O O 14 Stack three or more blocks?

O O 15 Show affection towards people, pets, or toys?

O O 16 Point to show you something?

O O 17 Look at you when you are talking
           or playing together?

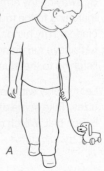

A

18 MONTHS English

* Examples provided are only suggestions.
   You may use similar examples from your family experience.

** Item may not be common to all cultures.

Figure 27.9 Sample of NDDS form and instructions for an 18-month-old. (*continued on page 654*)

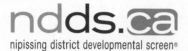
nipissing district developmental screen®

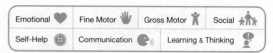

Emotional 💙	Fine Motor ✋	Gross Motor 🧍	Social 👪
Self-Help 🔘	Communication 🔊	Learning & Thinking ❗	

The following **activities for your child** will help you play your part in your child's development.

💚 I feel safe and secure when I know what is expected of me. You can help me with this by following routines and setting limits. Praise my good behaviour.

✋ I like toys that I can pull apart and put back together—large building blocks, containers with lids, or plastic links. Talk to me about what I am doing using words like "push" and "pull".

I'm not too little to play with large crayons. Let's scribble and talk about our art work.

🧍 Don't be afraid to let me see what I can do with my body. I need to practise climbing, swinging, jumping, running, going up and down stairs, and going down slides. Stay close to me so I don't get hurt.

Play some of my favourite music. Encourage me to move to the music by swaying my arms, moving slowly, marching to the music, hopping, clapping my hands, tapping my legs. Let's have fun doing actions while listening to the music.

Let me play with balls of different sizes. Take some of the air out of a beach ball. Watch me kick, throw, and try to catch it.

👪 I want to do things just like you. Let me have toys so I can pretend to have tea parties, dress up, and play mommy or daddy.

I like new toys, so find the local toy lending library or play groups in our community.

🔊 I am learning new words every day. Put pictures of people or objects in a bag and say "1, 2, 3, what do we see?" and pull a picture from the bag.

Pretend to talk to me on the phone or encourage me to call someone.

❗ Help me to notice familiar sounds such as birds chirping, car or truck motors, airplanes, dogs barking, sirens, or splashing water. Imitate the noise you hear and see if I will imitate you. Encourage me by smiling and clapping.

I like simple puzzles with two to four pieces and shape-sorters with simple shapes. Encourage me to match the pieces by taking turns with me.

I enjoy exploring the world, but I need to know that you are close by. I may cry when you leave me with others, so give me a hug and tell me you will be back.

I may get ear infections. Talk to my doctor about signs and symptoms.

Figure 27.9 *(continued)*

relationship with the adult patient will facilitate the assessment. This permits the nurse and patient to jointly explore what health practices and health goals will be addressed.

During the assessment, the nurse needs to attend to any actual health concerns that the patient may have. In addition, it is important to investigate the health practices and health risks of the patient. Young adults generally enjoy good health, but an investigation of their lifestyle behaviours may reveal risks. Information about nutrition, exercise patterns, smoking, and alcohol use should be gathered. Middle-aged adults will be developing awareness of their aging and have concerns about the potential development of health problems as they age, such as hypertension, heart disease, or cancer. Refer to Table 27.4 for specific screening topics for the adult period.

Older Adults

The older adult period is very wide ranging, covering a period of up to 30 years or more, and the elderly are a very diverse group of people. Although some generalizations can be made, it is important to recognize the vast differences that will occur between individuals. The nurse must guard against **ageism**, a way of thinking about the elderly based on negative attitudes and/or stereotypes (Ontario Human Rights Commission, 2010). For example, it should not be assumed than an elderly patient will be hard of hearing or confused.

Conducting assessments of elderly patients may require additional time because of the length of their health history and the complexity associated with their health problems. In some cases, it may help to have a family member present with the consent of the patient, but confidentiality must always be maintained. The nurse should be careful to include the patient in the interaction when a family member is present.

The nurse's assessment of the elderly patient should include comprehensive information about the physical, psychosocial, psychological, and functional aspects. It should include family relationships, social networks, and interests. A thorough appraisal of activities of daily living (ADL) should also be done. Refer to Table 27.4 for screening topics.

Screening Tools for Use With the Elderly

Several screening tools are available that can be used as part of a geriatric assessment. Assessment tools enable the nurse to efficiently assess an elderly patient's current level of function, cognition, and safety. Tools can be chosen to target specific areas of concern. For example, tools are available to assess risk for falls, risk for skin breakdown, ADL, risk for depression, and cognitive function. ADL scales are the most frequently used tools. ADL evaluations can be used to provide an overview of functional status and to determine if the elderly patient has any activity limitations. Use of a standardized tool assists the communication of information among the health-care team and makes monitoring of changes over time more effective. Examples of screening tools available include the Morse Falls Scale (1989), the Folstein Mini-Mental State Examination (1975), and the Katz Basic Activities of Daily Living Scale (1983).

Supporting Health Across the Lifespan

The lifespan approach is a useful way for nurses to be able to explore health promotion needs of their patients and to identify opportunities to provide appropriate information and assistance. A clear understanding of lifespan development allows nurses to target specific issues that are significant for each age group and to develop nursing strategies that fit the developmental needs and capacities of the patient. **Anticipatory guidance** is a nursing tool that helps patients and family members to better understand and prepare for normal developmental changes and identify the risks associated with each developmental stage. In the course of providing meaningful assistance to the patient, the nurse acts in multiple roles: teacher, counselor, advocate, and change agent.

The developmental approach is also important when caring for patients during periods of illness or hospitalization. The age and developmental stage of the patient will affect the ability of the person to cope with the challenge of illness. A preschooler who is having emergency surgery will have trouble understanding what is happening and will need support to deal with the unfamiliar and unpleasant experience. On the other hand, a middle-aged patient having surgery will have a better understanding of what is happening and a wider range of coping skills. For patients who are experiencing a chronic health problem, a nurse should have an understanding of the lifespan issues which may affect the patient's experience of the illness. For example, a young adult who is diagnosed with arthritis may be concerned about how this will affect career and relationship decisions, whereas for an older adult, the concerns may be more about loss of independence.

Infancy

Achievement of Developmental Tasks

The development of trust is achieved through caring parent–infant interactions. When parents attend to the infant's basic needs for food, warmth, comfort, and love, the baby learns that the world is a safe place. When the infant's needs are not appropriately met, a sense of mistrust can develop. Nurses need to be alert to any barriers that may exist to the formation of warm attachment between the parent and infant or in the ability of the parents to properly provide care. Nurses can promote early parent–infant bonding by encouraging parents to touch and care for the infant and to smile and talk to the infant. Teaching the parents how to care for basic needs, such as feeding and bathing, will help them feel confident in their ability to properly care for their baby.

Providing sensory stimulation encourages the infant's cognitive development. Nurses can encourage parents and family members by offering suggestions about appropriate ways to interact with the infant. Examples of stimulating activities can include talking and singing to the baby, placing colourful mobiles in the crib, and providing toys with various textures to experience. Interactive games, such as peekaboo or pat-a-cake, will amuse the infant. Toys that are geared to the infant's age can encourage cognitive development. Initially, toys should be chosen are stimulating to the infant's vision and hearing. As the baby develops increased motor skills, parents can provide toys that the child can safely manipulate, such as plastic rings or blocks.

When caring for an infant who is ill or hospitalized, nurses should implement strategies that support the development of trust. Because parents know their infant best and have learned to respond to the infant's cues, nurses should encourage parents to participate in the baby's care. Grandparents and other caregivers can also be involved, particularly if parents are not able to be present.

Nutrition

An infant needs to consume high-quality nutrients that are readily processed by the immature digestive system. Important nutrients that must be available include water, protein, fat, carbohydrates, vitamins, and iron.

Exclusive breast-feeding for the first 6 months is recommended as ideal. Breast milk provides the essential nutrients the baby needs in a form that is readily digestible. Nurses should actively promote breast-feeding by providing information to mothers about the benefits and giving practical information about how to breast-feed successfully (Fig. 27.10). It is important to identify possible barriers to breast-feeding, such as lack of knowledge, and address concerns.

Infants who are not breast-fed should receive a cow's milk–based formula that is iron fortified. Clear instructions should be given to parents about accurate and safe preparation and storage of formulas. Fruit juice, water, or other beverages should not be given. Parents or caregivers should always hold the infant for bottle feedings and not put the baby to bed with a bottle.

Solid food should not be introduced until the age of 6 months in order to prevent the occurrence of allergies. Solid foods from a spoon should be introduced one at a time at an interval of about 7 days, beginning with small portions of iron-fortified cereals and then vegetables and fruit. A wide range of foods with increasing texture can gradually be offered. Egg whites should not be given to children younger than the age of 1 year because of possible allergic reaction. Honey should also be avoided because it can harbor spores of *Clostridium*

botulinum, which can cause infant botulism (Ontario Society of Nutrition Professionals in Public Health, 2008).

The infant should continue with breast-feeding or formula for the first year of life. The infant should not receive more than 120 ml (4 oz) of juice per day because the sugar content will satisfy the infant's hunger, and he or she may be discouraged from eating more nutrient-dense foods (Ontario Society of Nutrition Professionals in Public Health, 2008). By the age of about 8 months, the infant can be offered breast milk or formula from a cup.

Safety

Because infants are totally dependent on others and are undergoing rapid changes in developmental skills, caregivers must be constantly alert to safety risks in the infant's environment. As the infant's motor skills progress from rolling over to crawling and standing, the range of hazards in the environment increases. Helping parents recognize the developmental changes that will occur can prepare them to identify the risks that their infant will face. Nurses should provide information to parents and other caregivers, such as grandparents, about childproofing of the home. This should include such measures as placing gates across stairwells, storing poisonous substances out of reach, and reducing the temperature of hot water heaters. When traveling with the infant in a motor vehicle, a properly installed rear-facing car seat should always be used (Fig. 27.11). See Table 27.5 for further car seat information.

A major health risk in the first year of life is sudden infant death syndrome (SIDS), the sudden, unexplained death of an infant younger than 1 year of age. By definition, the cause of the death is unknown. Nevertheless, risk factors for the occurrence of SIDS have been identified, including sleep position, co-sleeping, and exposure to tobacco smoke. Several measures to reduce the risks have been identified. Refer to Box 27.2 for information about infant positioning to prevent SIDS.

Sleep Patterns

Initially, infants sleep approximately 18 to 20 hours/day, as demanded by their rapid growth. By the end of the first year, this is usually reduced to about 12 hours/day. This may

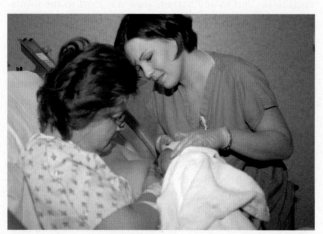

Figure 27.10 A nurse provides education, support, and encouragement to a breast-feeding mother.

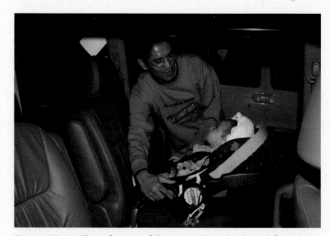

Figure 27.11 The infant is safely secured in a backward-facing car seat in the back seat of the car.

TABLE 27.5   Car Seat Guidelines

Stage	Seat Type	Guidelines
Stage 1	Rear-facing infant seat	Used from birth to approximately 1 year of age, but it is recommended that parents continue to use it for as long as it fits the infant's size. It is important to follow the manufacturer's instructions and guidelines for the weight and height that are allowed. Must always be installed in back seat of car away from front airbags Install according to car seat and auto manufacturer's recommendations.
Stage 2	Forward-facing child seat	Used until child is over 18 kg (40 lb), approximately 4 years of age Installed in back seat of car and anchored by a tether strap Shoulder straps should be at or above the child's shoulders, and chest clip should be level with the child's armpits.
Stage 3	Booster seat	Used until child is 36 kg (80 lb) Should be used in the back seat of the car Must use the correct seat belt system with the booster seat Put the lap belt low and snug across the hips, and always put the shoulder belt over the shoulder and across the chest.
Stage 4	Seat belt use	Can be used when child is over 36 kg (80 lb), approximately 8 years of age If the child is still too small for a seat belt, continue to use a booster seat. Put the lap belt low and snug across the hips and the shoulder belt over the shoulder and across the chest. Never put the shoulder belt under the arm.

Notes:
- All car seats have expiration dates and should not be used beyond that date.
- Car seats should not be used if they have been in an accident.
- All car seats must comply with Canadian standards. Seats purchased outside Canada, do not comply with Canada's regulations.

Reference: Transport Canada. (2013). *Car seats, seat belts and your child*. Retrieved from http://www.tc.gc.ca/eng /roadsafety/safedrivers-childsafety-car-index-873.htm

BOX 27.2   Back to Sleep and Tummy Time

Sudden infant death syndrome (SIDS) refers to the sudden and unexpected death of an apparently healthy infant. In Canada, SIDS is the leading cause of death in the period between 28 days and 1 year. About 90% of SIDS deaths happen before 6 months old. No single specific cause of SIDS has been identified, but several risk factors have been identified, including prone sleeping position, overheating, and exposure to tobacco smoke. More recently, co-sleeping has been identified as an additional factor.

In 1999, the campaign called *Back to Sleep*, using the international slogan, was launched in Canada to encourage parents and caregivers to place infants on their backs in their cribs. Since that time, the incidence of SIDS in Canada has been reduced by more than 50%, although it remains a leading cause of death in infants. The declines in rates are attributed in large part to the educational campaigns.

Nurses should share important information about managing the risk factors for SIDS with parents.

- Position baby on its back on a firm, flat surface to sleep. Instruct other caregivers to do the same.
- Infants should sleep in a crib for the first year of life.
- Provide the baby with a smoke-free environment—both before and after birth.
- Avoid soft mattresses, comforters, stuffed toys, and bumper pads in the baby's crib.
- Have the baby sleep in a crib next to a parent's bed for the first 6 months.
- Breast-feeding may give some protection against SIDS.

- Sleeping with an infant on a sofa is associated with a particularly high risk of sudden unexpected death in infancy.
- Once the infant is old enough to turn over independently, it is alright to allow sleeping prone.

There is now growing evidence that one outcome of this very successful information campaign is the risk for development of positional plagiocephaly, known as *flat head*, caused by the infant lying on the back consistently. It may contribute to some delay in motor development, such as rolling over and crawling, due to lack of time placed on the abdomen. It is now advised that infants have supervised time placed on their stomachs while awake to help with development and prevent flat spots developing.

Nurses should teach the following points to parents:

- Baby should spend some time face-down (tummy time) when awake and being watched by an adult.
- Change the position of the infant's head throughout the day to prevent pressure to the same side. Devices that restrict the movement of the baby's head are not recommended.
- Limit the time the infant is on his or her back in car seats, infant swings, and infant carriers.
- Reverse the head-to-toe position of the infant's crib weekly and change the position of the toys or mobiles.
- Alternate the position the infant is held when feeding, placing in the left arm for one feed and the right arm for the next.
- If the baby is fretful when placed in prone position, build up the tummy time gradually, beginning with a few minutes at a time, three times a day.

References: Miller, L. C., Johnson, A., Duggan, L., & Behm, M. (2009). Consequences of the "back to sleep" program in infants. *Journal of Pediatric Nursing, 26*(4), 364–368. doi:10.1016/j.pedn.2009.10.004; Trifunov, W. (2009). *The practice of bed sharing: A systematic literature and policy review*. Ottawa, ON: Public Health Agency of Canada. Retrieved from http://www.phac-aspc.gc.ca/dca-dea/prenatal/pbs-ppl-eng.php

involve a long period of nighttime sleep plus one or more naps in the daytime. There is, however, no predictable sleeping schedule that each baby will follow. Parents may become frustrated when the infant is awake and fussy in the night and may need reassurance that this problem is temporary.

Nurses can help parents to identify the behavioural cues that indicate that their infant is ready to settle for sleep. Tired signs can include fretfulness, facial grimaces, or rubbing eyes. Nurses can offer helpful suggestions to parents for promoting healthy sleep patterns, such as providing a quiet room for the infant and creating settling-down rituals such as rocking.

Immunizations

Infants are born with a degree of natural immunity, in the form of antibodies from their mothers, but this does not last past the first year. Vaccines are a safe and effective way to prevent various potentially serious diseases. Immunization not only protects the infant or child who receives it but also provides protection from exposure to disease to those people who, for reasons such as allergies, cannot be given vaccines. Vaccines are very safe, and side effects such as redness and soreness at the site of injection are generally minor. In Canada, vaccines to prevent a number of diseases, such as measles, whooping cough, polio, and hepatitis B, are considered routine and are provided free in all provinces and territories. Schedules for immunization have been developed to ensure that maximum possible protection is achieved, starting at the age of 2 months. In Canada, the recommended schedule is developed by the National Advisory Committee on Immunization under the authority of the Public Health Agency of Canada, but publicly funded immunization schedules may vary by province or territory. Refer to Table 27.6 for the recommended childhood immunization schedule.

TABLE 27.6	Recommended Childhood Immunization Schedule
Age of Immunization	**Vaccine**
2 months old	Diphtheria, tetanus, and acellular pertussis + inactivated poliovirus (DTaP/IPV)
4 months old	Haemophilus influenzae type b (Hib)
6 months old	Pneumococcal conjugate (Pneu-C-7)
12 months old	Measles, mumps, rubella (MMR) Meningococcal C conjugate (Men-C)
15 months old	Varicella (chickenpox) (Var) Pneu-C-7
18 months old	DTaP/IPV MMR
4–6 years old	DTaP/IPV
9–13 years old	Hepatitis B (HB)
9–13 years old (female)	Human papillomavirus (HPV)
14–16 years old	Tetanus and diphtheria (Td)
Every 10 years thereafter	Td
Every year (in autumn)	Influenza

References: Ministry of Health and Long-Term Care, Ontario. (2009). *Publicly funded immunization schedules for Ontario—January 2009*. Retrieved from http://www.health.gov.on.ca/english/providers/program/immun/pdf /schedule.pdf; Public Health Agency of Canada. (2010c). *Recommendations from the National Advisory Committee on Immunization (NACI)*. Retrieved from http://www.phac-aspc.gc.ca/im/is-cv/index-eng.php#a

Parents may have questions about the risks associated with immunization. A lot of information, accurate and inaccurate, is widely circulated. Parents worry that vaccines can cause the development of problems such as autism or SIDS. However, researchers have concluded that there is no evidence of a link between vaccines and autism or any other illnesses (Health Canada, 2009). When a parent expresses reluctance about having immunizations given, it is important to explore the reasons behind the reluctance and discuss the issues with the parent clearly, providing accurate information (Public Health Agency of Canada, 2009a).

Toddler Period

Achievement of Developmental Tasks

As toddlers strive to achieve autonomy, they exert their independence by actively exploring their world and by asserting their demands to do things for themselves. In the process of exploring, they investigate every corner of their space, climbing onto, crawling under, touching, tasting, and smelling the objects they encounter. They test their relationship to their parents by pushing the limits of their power. The frequent use of the words *no* and *mine* are their way of expressing their separateness and independence. A parent may find it very frustrating and confusing when the 2-year-old refuses the offer of a favourite toy and then, as soon as it is put away, becomes equally determined to have it. It is important to understand that the negativism is not a personal rejection of the parents' requests. This type of behaviour is just part of the process by which the child is learning to control things in his or her world.

A temper tantrum is a typical response of a toddler who is thwarted in his or her attempts to be independent and does not have the language skills to verbalize frustration or other psychological resources to manage the situation (Hockenberry & Wilson, 2007). He or she may scream, throw himself or herself on the floor, and possibly hit or bite. To help parents cope with temper tantrums, nurses can offer strategies to prevent them and to deal with them. Tantrums can be prevented by maintaining clear consistent limits, by keeping routines simple, and by only providing realistic choices. It is not recommended, for example, to ask a toddler if he or she wants to go to bed, but it is possible to offer a choice of a toy to take to bed. When a tantrum occurs, it is advisable to ignore the behaviour provided there is no risk of injury. Punishment is not useful. Once the tantrum is over, the child can be distracted from the original issue that precipitated the event by offering a different activity.

Because it is important to provide opportunities for the toddler to explore, parents are advised to adjust the environment to fit the child, such as childproofing the kitchen so that the toddler who is investigating the contents of a cupboard will not encounter poisons but will find some pots and pans to bang. Toys can be chosen to challenge the child to develop skills, such as nesting or stacking blocks, riding toys, or durable books.

The toddler's need for more autonomy may come into direct conflict with safely limits, parental rules, or the similar needs of playmates. Parents need to find ways to accommodate and encourage the toddlers' search for autonomy while providing appropriate boundaries to their behaviours. Patience, understanding, and a consistent approach are essential for negotiating this developmental period.

Hospitalization, or other types of separation from caregivers, is a very stressful experience for toddlers. The child may react strongly with screaming and crying and will often reject comforting from any stranger (Hockenberry & Wilson, 2007). Nurses should encourage parents to visit and provide care during the hospitalization. Familiar items from home, such as special blankets or stuffed toys, can be used to provide comforting. Because toddlers are used to being active and exploring environment, they may feel confined and frustrated in hospital. In such stressful situations, **regression**, a temporary withdrawal to earlier developmental behaviours, commonly occurs. For example, the toddler may want the comfort of a bottle after he or she has been weaned to a cup. Nurses can reassure parents that the toddler's behaviour is not abnormal and that usual routines can be resumed once the child is home again.

Nutrition

In the second year of life as the rate of growth slows, the toddler requires a somewhat lower calorie intake. Some toddlers become *picky eaters*, refusing to try new foods or rejecting previously eaten foods. This may result in the risk of nutritional deficiency and cause concern to their parents (Dovey, Staples, Gibson, & Halford, 2008). Parents may find themselves challenged to meet the child's nutritional needs. Toddlers will benefit from having small servings at regular mealtimes supplemented with healthy snacks between meals.

Whole cow's milk can be used to replace or supplement breast milk or to replace formula. The toddler should drink approximately 500 to 750 ml (16 to 25 oz) of milk a day to meet the needs for calcium and phosphorus. Parents should be discouraged from giving large quantities of milk because it will discourage the toddler from eating other foods and may result in iron deficiency (Ontario Society of Nutrition Professionals in Public Health, 2008).

Toddlers are usually very interested in feeding themselves and, when encouraged to do so, rapidly become skillful at managing spoons and cups. Weaning from bottle to cup is generally accomplished early in the toddler period.

Parents should provide a range of healthy and age-appropriate foods for the child, but the child's appetite should determine the amount of food consumed. Parents need to be flexible during this phase to avoid turning mealtime into a battleground. Although the toddler's appetite may be highly variable and the food intake may seem inadequate, most toddlers consume the necessary amount of food for their needs.

Toilet Training

Most children achieve bladder and bowel control between 24 and 48 months of age, and the process from beginning toilet training to independent toileting may take 3 to 6 months. Girls tend to achieve control earlier than boys. Bladder and bowel control do not necessarily occur at the

same time, and nighttime wetting might persist after daytime control is established. For children with physical or mental disabilities, the process may take much longer and requires a lot of patience on the part of caregivers.

Nurses should recommend a child-oriented approach and offer anticipatory guidance to parents about toilet training. The right time for toilet training is not related to the toddler's chronological age but to psychological and physical readiness. Before beginning toilet training, the child should be able to stay dry for several hours, walk to the potty chair, and sit stably on it. He or she should be able to follow simple commands and be able to communicate the need to sit on the toilet or potty chair. When the toddler starts communicating that he or she is wet or soiled and is uncomfortable with that, it is a good time to start.

Parents must also be able and willing to devote time and attention to the ongoing process of toilet training, which may take weeks or months to completely accomplish. All caregivers for the child, including day care workers or grandparents, should be included in the plans so that a consistent routine can be established. The plans also include deciding on the terminology that will be used with the child to refer to urination or bowel movements.

The entire toilet-training experience should be shaped to be a positive experience for the child, a sign of growing up to be a "big boy" or "big girl." The parent should use praise and encouragement, celebrating any successes. Accidents will inevitably occur, and parents should be patient and supportive when they do. Parents may feel frustrated when the process does not go smoothly or quickly, but scolding or punishing the toddler should be avoided.

Safety

As toddlers become more mobile, they begin to explore their environment, which can put them in danger of a new range of injuries, such as falls, poisoning, electrocution, drowning, and burns. Preventing these injuries requires careful preparation and constant vigilance from parents. Parents often do not recognize many of the hazards in the home environment and do not always perceive their own toddler as vulnerable to some obvious risks (Gaines & Schwebel, 2009). Nurses can help parents to properly safeguard their home environment by helping them identify the specific risks that toddlers face and the potential hazards around them. If parents try to view the world from the toddler's level, they will more readily see the hazards, such as lamp cords or sharp edges on coffee tables. It is also advisable to remind parents to watch for the risks in other places they frequently visit, such as grandparents' homes or the child's day care centre.

Toddlers are able to eat a wider range of foods, and this increases the risk of aspiration. Hard, small, round, and stick solid foods can block the airway and can become a significant choking hazard. Examples of hazardous food include popcorn, peanuts, hard candies, and hot dogs cut into rounds. During mealtime, the child should be fed at a pace that allows him or her to chew the food completely. Food items such as hot dogs need to be cut into small irregular-shaped pieces. Because toddlers may still be inclined to put things such as toys in the mouth, small toy parts or items continue to be a choking risk.

Early Childhood Period

Achievement of Developmental Tasks

In developing a sense of initiative, preschool children increase their exploration of the environment. The child needs to expand his or her world through exposure to more social experiences, particularly with other children of his or her own age. Parents can provide this kind of exposure through play groups or preschool settings. Further, parents can encourage the child to learn social skills by using opportunities such as restaurant visits to teach essential social skills. Because children like to imitate adult behaviours at this time, social outings provide a good opportunity to learn basic interpersonal skills.

Preschoolers are able to think more complexly and are often very imaginative. They commonly tell made-up tall tales and may have some difficulty in separating their stories from reality (Piaget, 2008). Parents need to be made aware that this is part of their cognitive development and help them understand the difference between what is real and what is storytelling. Because of their active imagination, preschoolers may develop fears. Common fears include fear of the dark, fear of being left alone, or fear of being hurt. If parents express their own fears, such as a fear of the dentist, these can also be communicated to the child. Involve children in finding ways to cope with their fears. For example, parents can try strategies such as using a nightlight and then exploring the shadows in the room with the child.

For children in the early childhood period, being ill and hospitalized can be a very threatening experience. They have a poor understanding of how their body functions. In addition, they view all experiences egocentrically and therefore think that everything has to do with them, so they may worry about everything they see happening around them. It is important that nurses prepare the child for any unpleasant procedure, such as an injection, by explaining what he or she is going to do and how much it will hurt, using language that the child will understand.

Nutrition

During the early childhood period, the child's appetite will vary from day to day depending on activity level or the occurrence of a growth spurt. The range of foods eaten gradually increases with repeated experiences with new foods, but it may take multiple exposures to a new food before it is accepted. Children may engage in simple food preparation activities to encourage them to try these foods. Parents should be advised that it is important that the child determines the quantity of food eaten because forcing a child to eat may lead to either overeating or aversion to certain foods (Ontario Society of Nutrition Professionals in Public Health, 2008).

Parents should role model good eating habits because at this age, the preschooler emulates the behaviours of the adults in his or her life. Effort should be made to make mealtimes a pleasurable family experience. Focus should be on the interaction over the meal, so diversions such as the television (TV) or toys at the table should be eliminated.

Safety

The preschool-age child has developed greater physical agility and improved ability to listen more to parents' instructions, reducing some of the injury risks common to the infant or toddler period, such as simple falls or choking on small toy parts. Nevertheless, injuries continue to be a significant health hazard for this period, particularly pedestrian and motor vehicle accidents. When the child is learning new physical skills, such as riding a bike, parents need to reinforce instructions about safety. Close supervision is still necessary when children are in the yard or at the playground. At this age, the emphasis should be on educating the child in safe behaviours, such as street safety or helmet use. Parents should be good role models for their children by always using appropriate safety measures themselves.

School Readiness

In Canada, the availability of early childhood education programs varies by province and by local school district. However, all jurisdictions offer some form of pre-elementary education. The Council of Ministers of Education, Canada (CMEC) has released a policy statement entitled *Learn Canada 2020*. The CMEC proposed that children should have access to high-quality early childhood education to prepare them for elementary school (Council of Ministers of Education [CMEC], 2008).

In most districts, pre-kindergarten and kindergarten programs are optional. Parents need to decide if their child will benefit from the programs and if he or she is ready to participate. Box 27.3 lists some criteria for determining if a child is ready to attend a structured school experience.

BOX 27.3 School Readiness Checklist

A child who is beginning school should be able to:

- Understand that when mother or father leaves, he or she will return.
- Tolerate being away from parents or caregivers.
- Play for a short period without an adult's constant assistance.
- Know how to share and to take turns.
- Play well with other children.
- Pay attention for short periods of time.
- Speak well enough to ask for what he or she needs.
- Recognize his or her own name in writing.
- Help put away toys and materials in the classroom.
- Dress and undress self.
- Use the toilet independently.

Reference: Elementary Teachers' Federation of Ontario. (2010). *School readiness*. Retrieved from http://www.etfo.ca/Resources/ForParents/SchoolReadiness/Pages/default.aspx

Nurses can provide advice to parents on how to help their child develop school readiness skills. Establishing regular habits is important, such as having a set bedtime and a routine of picking up and putting away toys. Parents can engage the child in school-related activities such as drawing or colouring and reading books on a regular basis. In the weeks before starting school, the child should have the opportunity to visit the school or the school yard. Parents should always talk in a positive way about the kinds of things that the child will do at school.

Middle Childhood Period

Achievement of Developmental Tasks

In the middle childhood period, parents will need to recognize that there will be changes in the child's relationship to parents and peers. Relationships with peers gain importance and are necessary to the healthy psychosocial development of children. Positive interactions with others of the same age can foster self-esteem and the sense of well-being. Some children may have difficulty making friends and parents can help by exposing them to many opportunities such as trips to the park, sports teams, youth groups, and church groups. Parents cannot control who their child chooses as friends and may sometimes dislike the choices the child makes. Forbidding the friendship is not useful; the parents should instead discuss with their child why he or she has chosen this particular friend, which may provide insight for the parents into the child's social needs.

Parents spend less time with their child in the middle childhood period than in earlier stages and may express concerns about their ability to be a positive influence for the child. Nurses can reassure parents that their impact in the life of the child is still very strong. One important measure parents can take is to be positive role models to their child. Parents need to focus on helping their child become more independent. They can do this by talking with their child about his or her daily experiences and discussing what is important to the child and by encouraging him or her to make good decisions.

Children in this stage are accustomed to be active and busy, so illness and hospitalization makes them feel very bored and restless. Nurses should provide meaningful activities to keep them occupied. Time structuring is a useful strategy, using a clock and sometimes a calendar, to provide them with a schedule that allows them some degree of control of their hospital day. The child should be allowed some decision-making about the timing of necessary treatments and procedures whenever possible. At this age, children have a better understanding of how their body works and benefit from clear descriptions of what is going on and what to expect.

Prevention of Childhood Obesity

Over the last 25 years, Canada has experienced a significant increase in the number of overweight and obese children. Obesity rates among children and youth have soared; 1 in 5 school-age Canadians are now overweight or obese. Childhood obesity is a matter for concern because over time, it increases the risk of developing chronic health problems, such as heart disease, stroke, and Type 2 diabetes (Public Health Agency of Canada, 2010a). The increase in prevalence of childhood obesity may also increase the occurrence of mental health problems. Research suggests that teasing and social stigma are factors leading to low self-esteem in obese children (Wang, Wild, Kipp, Kuhle, & Veugelers, 2009).

Promotion of healthy nutrition and exercise is crucial to the prevention of childhood obesity. Being overweight for children, as in adults, is most directly related to poor eating habits and insufficient physical activity. Evidence suggests that the nutritional and exercise habits of Canada's children are problematic. The percentage of physically inactive school-age children is disturbingly high. In contrast, the percentage of children reporting daily intake of fruits, vegetables, and low-fat milk is low (Boyce, King, & Roche, 2008). The nutritional and exercise habits of children are influenced by multiple factors such as economic status, social environment, genetics, education, and culture (Public Health Agency of Canada, 2010c).

Nurses can help children to develop the lifelong health habits they need to prevent obesity through education of the parents and the children and through advocacy for programs that promote healthy nutrition and exercise. Canada's Food Guide, which promotes a healthy eating pattern based on scientific evidence, is an essential resource for teaching children and parents (Health Canada, 2011a). The child's diet should include a range of healthy foods and limits on the consumption of junk foods. Foods that are high in fat, empty calories, and salt should be restricted.

Parents should be encouraged to model healthy behaviours in their own eating habits. Children are more likely to try new foods and eat various foods if the parents also do. Parents can involve children in selecting healthy snacks and preparing meals at home. Media messages and peers will influence the food choices that the school-age child makes. Nurses can be influential by working with groups of children, discussing the influences of media messages and helping children learn how to make good food choice decisions.

The other important component in preventing childhood obesity is promotion of regular physical activity. In addition to preventing obesity, exercise develops cardiovascular fitness, strength, flexibility, and bone density. Canada's Physical Activity Guides for Children and for Youth recommends 90 minutes of physical exercise daily during childhood, 30 minutes of which should be vigorous activity, such as running or playing soccer. Inactive children can begin with 30 minutes of activity and gradually increase the length of time engaged in being active to achieve this goal (Public Health Agency of Canada, 2010b). Engaging in activity as a family is an effective way to increase the health of all family members and to teach children of the value of exercise. Children will be more likely to be active if they perceive the activity as fun and recreational. When teaching children, it is important to emphasize the short-term benefits rather than the long-term health gains (Lau et al., 2007).

It is important to encourage children to limit the amount of time spent in sedentary pursuits, such as watching television and videos, surfing the Internet, or playing computer games 2 hours a day or less. This will reduce the exposure to food advertising, reduce the intake of junk foods consumed while watching TV, and provide more time for active pursuits (Public Health Agency of Canada, 2010b). A simple strategy to increase a child's activity level is the encouragement of active transportation, which is any form of human-powered transportation such as walking, skateboarding, or cycling. Schools are pivotal settings for support of the development of active lifestyles, so implementation of school-based programs is encouraged.

School Experience

School is a major influence in the child's life in the middle childhood period, meeting social and educational needs. It provides them with opportunities to achieve a sense of industry and to build self-esteem through successful completion of work and projects. Parents need to be alert to stressors in the school environment that may cause emotional damage and affect the child's ability to participate fully, such as learning disorders or bullying.

Bullying continues to be a widespread problem in Canada, with a large proportion of children who identified themselves as involved in bullying, either as the victim, the bully, or both (Boyce et al., 2008). Bullying is harmful to children, contributing to physical and mental health problems and educational difficulties. It is essential to identify those children who are being bullied or are at risk for bullying and to provide support in order to prevent the negative outcomes. Children need to be encouraged to report bullying. Adults, including teachers, nurses, and parents, must convey the message that they will actively work to make the bullying stop.

Injury Prevention

School-age children have developed improved coordination and muscular control. They also have developed the ability to understand risks and make decisions to keep themselves safe. However, during this age period, children are more independent, are exposed to more risks, and may engage in risk-taking behaviours. Children may engage in risky challenges with their peers as a way to gain social acceptance.

Injuries remain the leading cause of death and remain a significant cause of hospitalizations for children in middle childhood. Some injuries, such as head and spinal cord injuries, can result in significant long-term disability (Public Health Agency of Canada, 2009b). Boys are significantly more likely to be injured than girls. Major sources of injury include motor vehicle accidents, bicycle injury, and sports injuries. Bicycle accidents are associated with minor injuries, such as bruises and sprains, and with major injuries, including serious head and spinal cord injuries. Activities, such as skateboarding, in-line skating, and trampoline use,

---

BOX 27.4   Trampoline Safety

Home trampolines are popular with children, and in recent years, they are often seen in the backyards of many families. Unfortunately, they are also dangerous because they can cause serious injuries if they are not used properly.

The increasing availability of low-cost backyard trampolines has resulted to a dramatic increase in the number of injuries from trampoline use. Most injuries occurred in the 5- to 14-year age group. Injuries can occur from falling off of the trampoline or from colliding with another child on the trampoline. However, almost 50% of all trampoline-related injuries were caused by simply jumping on the trampoline. The injuries can be severe, including fractures, dislocations, and spinal injuries. Trampoline injuries accounted for proportionately more hospital admissions than any other kind of sports injury.

The Canadian Paediatric Society in 2007 recommended that trampolines should not be regarded as play equipment and should not be used at home or in outside playgrounds. Healthcare professionals are advised to warn parents of the dangers associated with trampoline use. Nevertheless, the popularity of trampolines continues to increase. When families do use a home trampoline, the following advice should be given to decrease the risk of injuries:

- Make sure the trampoline is correctly assembled and is set up on level ground surrounded by a material, such as sand, that will absorb impact. The trampoline should have padding over the springs, hooks, and frame.
- Children should be closely supervised by an adult when on the trampoline. Safety netting may be used, but it cannot replace appropriate supervision.
- Only one child at a time should use the trampoline.
- Children younger than age 6 years should not be on the trampoline.
- Teach children to always jump in the centre of the trampoline.
- Somersaults and flips should only be done in proper facilities with supervision of a trained instructor.

References: Canadian Paediatric Society. (2007). Trampoline use in homes and playgrounds. *Paediatric Child Health, 12*(6), 501–505; Public Health Agency of Canada. (2009b). *Child and youth injury in review.* Retrieved from http://www.phac-aspc.gc.ca/publicat/cyi-bej/2009/index-eng.php

---

are common sources of head injuries, fractures, and sprains. Refer to Box 27.4 for information about trampoline safety.

Nurses have a role in safety education for children and for parents. Parents may not be fully aware of the risks that exist in the child's environment, especially those related to the child's developmental level. Inspection of sports equipment and use of safety equipment, such as helmets and pads, should be reviewed. Bicycle safety and sports safety are important topics to discuss with groups of children in this age period (Fig. 27.12).

Preadolescence and the Development of Sexual Identity

Toward the end of middle childhood, before the actual onset of puberty, children will begin to show physical and emotional signs of approaching puberty. Girls experience an

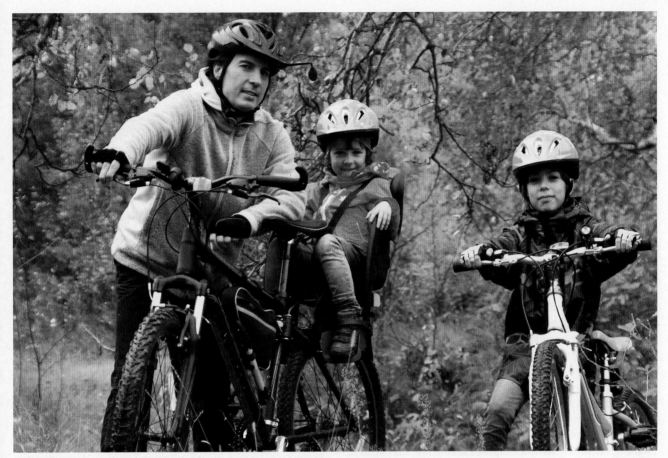

Figure 27.12 A father role models safe behaviour by wearing a helmet while bicycling with his children.

earlier growth spurt, and there will be noticeable differences in size and development between the genders. There are so many developmental and social changes occurring that the preadolescent may experience increased anxiety and moodiness. Children may become self-conscious about their physical appearance, particularly if it occurs earlier or later than their peers. Parents may be unsettled by the changes in their child, particularly mood changes and rebellious behaviours, and react unfavorably, causing an increase in parent–child conflict. Patience, understanding, and open communication on the part of parents will make the transition period easier.

The prepubescent child becomes interested in, yet often shy around, members of the opposite sex. As he or she develops skills in interacting with members of the opposite sex, peer pressure becomes a powerful motivating force in his or her social relationships. Increased curiosity about sexuality may lead to some sexual experimentation such as masturbation or mutual exploration of each other's bodies.

Nurses can help parents and preadolescents cope with this period of great change by providing anticipatory guidance. Understanding the normal process of pubertal development can ease the child's and the parents' anxiety. Education about sex and sexuality should focus on the normal processes that are occurring and address issues about normal sexual feelings. Children's questions should be answered truthfully and in a matter-of-fact way, providing practical information such as explaining how to use a tampon or what a wet dream is. Nurses can promote health sexuality by emphasizing that it is part of each individual's identity and a normal part of growing toward adulthood.

Adolescence

Achievement of Developmental Tasks

Adolescents are involved in the development of their personal identity, which involves a degree of psychological and physical separation from their parents. Teenagers tend to spend less time at home with the rest of the family and are often less likely to openly share information about themselves. Peer groups become very important to the teenager as he or she develops his or her skills in forming and maintaining more mature social and intimate relationships. At the same time that the adolescent is learning to be independent, the parents must learn to let go. Nurses can provide information about normal adolescent development to parents to support them as they adapt to being less of a direct influence on their adolescent child.

Development of a healthy body image is a component of the search for identity in the adolescent period. Body image develops through self-evaluation and is influenced by the messages from parents, friends, and media. The significant physical changes of puberty can magnify body image concerns. Impairments of body image have become widespread among adolescents, particularly females. Poor body image is linked to problems of low self-esteem and can lead to eating disorders (Boyce et al., 2008). Nurses should monitor their teenage patients for possible body image issues and implement interventions to foster a healthy body image. It is important to listen to adolescents talk about their health and determine if their concerns are related to body image. Adolescents may talk about needing to lose weight or ask for dieting advice. Nurses can use these conversations as an opportunity to open discussions around body image. The message that bodies come in many different sizes and shapes and that these differences are normal should be clearly presented. Nurses can also use these opportunities with teenagers to encourage healthy eating and exercise patterns, pointing out that these are more effective in creating a healthy appearance than dieting.

With adolescent patients, nurses should turn their attention away from parents and move toward providing education and support directly to the adolescent. Cognitively, adolescents are capable of understanding information, realizing consequences and thinking introspectively. Nurses need to engage in a collaborative relationship with their adolescent patients, showing respect for their emerging sense of personal identity and their increasing ability to make decisions. A proactive approach that focuses on the strengths and positive attributes of the adolescent rather than always focusing on problems will help in establishing an effective therapeutic relationship with the teenager. By providing accurate information and exploring choices with the adolescent, the nurse can promote decision-making that supports a healthy lifestyle (Duncan et al., 2007).

Adolescents spend much of their time with others of their own age, whether in person, on the phone, or online. Illness and hospitalization separates them from their usual support systems and activities. They dislike being dependent on others and may perceive themselves as being treated like a child, particularly if they are placed on a pediatric unit. Nurses should engage them in a respectful manner, allowing them decision-making opportunities and providing clear information. They need access to enjoyable activities and the means to be in contact with their peers (Fig. 27.13).

Preventing Health Risks

The overall health of adolescents in Canada shows worrisome trends. The Centre for Addiction and Mental Health (CAMH) conducted a survey of adolescents in Ontario, which showed a substantial increase in the number of teenagers who reported poor physical health and a high proportion of overweight or obesity. Injury rates also appear to be increasing. The high percentage of adolescents (30%) who report psychological distress in the form of anxiety or depression also continues to be troubling. Lifestyle patterns, such as large amounts of time spent in sedentary activities and lack of physical activity, were identified as factors contributing to the findings (Paglia-Boak et al., 2010).

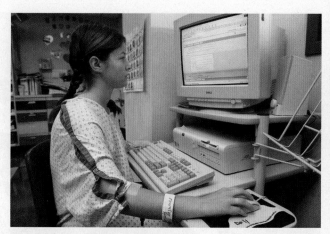

Figure 27.13 Hospitalized adolescents benefit from having access to some of their usual activities.

The main threats to the health of adolescents are preventable risk behaviours. The health-related actions of adolescence predict the likely behaviours for their adult years. Development of unhealthy habits during the teen years means those habits will be more difficult to change in the future. Like their school-age counterparts, the overall health of adolescents is threatened by the problem of obesity related to insufficient exercise and poor nutritional habits. Other preventable risks include unsafe sexual practices, substance abuse, and risk-taking behaviours that lead to injury. Promoting healthy decision-making during the adolescent period will have payoffs for the future. Adolescents need to be encouraged to live healthy, balanced lifestyles and be monitored for unhealthy behaviours (Lau et al., 2007).

Risk-taking is normal behaviour for an adolescent as a means to learn about his or her environment and assert his or her independence. Consequently, simply telling teenagers to avoid all risk behaviours is not a productive health promotion strategy. Instead, adolescents should be helped to develop sound decision-making skills to manage risks in a safe and responsible way (Duncan et al., 2007). For example, rather than lecturing a teenager about drinking alcohol, the nurse can engage him in discussions about the associated risks such as binge drinking or drinking and driving. Parents should continue to be involved in their teenager's life by providing clear guidelines for acceptable behaviour and monitoring the child's activities. Nurses can provide guidance to help parents find the right balance between providing supervision and supporting independence. Encouraging teenagers to participate in youth groups, school teams, and other social organizations also promotes health social attitudes and supports healthy development.

Sexual Health

The emergence of sexual feelings can be confusing and overwhelming, and it is important to acknowledge to adolescents that romantic and sexual feelings are normal. At some point during adolescence, sexual orientation will be identified. Adolescents who are lesbian, gay, or bisexual need assistance to be comfortable with their sexual orientation, including handling such challenges as disclosing it to others. Teenagers need to understand that healthy sexuality is about making their own choices. Nurses can discuss with their teenage patients how to make safe, healthy decisions about being sexually active, reinforcing the idea that the decision to have sex should be well thought out.

Adolescents with knowledge about safe sex practices, including contraception information, are not more likely to be sexually active but will be safer when they choose to be. Adolescents may underestimate the risks of unprotected sex. Knowledge is the key to counteracting this risky notion. The information provided needs to match the learning needs of the teenagers (refer to research review, "Adolescent Sexual Health"). Nurses should address the specific questions raised by their adolescent patients and provide accurate instruction on how to protect themselves and their partners from unwanted pregnancy and sexually transmitted diseases.

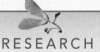

RESEARCH

ADOLESCENT SEXUAL HEALTH

The teen years are a critical time for providing sexual health education and prevention services. The sexual health wants and needs of adolescents have not always been well understood, and the services provided have often been inadequate.

Study

The Toronto Teen Survey set out to develop a comprehensive picture of the sexual knowledge and practices of the diverse population of adolescents in Toronto and identify their sexual health wants and needs. The researchers surveyed 1,216 adolescents, between the ages of 13 and 17 years, using a quantitative survey questionnaire. The sample was deliberately diverse and included a large number of racialized youth and adolescents who often are unheard. The findings from the survey were then discussed with focus groups of service providers, such as public health practitioners, social workers, and clinic personnel.

The findings showed that a large proportion of the teens are sexually active in various ways, including kissing, oral sex, vaginal intercourse, and anal sex. Most teens have not made use of the sexual health-care services offered by clinics, and among those who did, they were generally unhappy with the atmosphere in the clinics. The things that they want from a clinic include privacy and confidentiality, accurate information, and a place where they feel comfortable asking questions. The fear of being judged and the concern that the services were not confidential were the largest barriers to accessing services. The service providers identified systemic barriers in their workplaces to providing effective sexual health services to the youth.

Most teenagers (97%) identified that they had received some form of sexual health education, but a large percentage reported that the major sources of

information are their peers and the media, which often provides inaccurate or distorted information. The level of inaccurate information that teens possess remains high. There is a significant gap between what youth are being taught and what they want to know. Most teens were interested in learning about healthy relationships, sexual pleasure, and HIV/AIDS.

Nursing Implications
Promoting healthy sexual development needs to be more than about preventing disease and pregnancy. Education programs need to address respect for healthy sexuality, an appreciation of pleasure, and communication skills in negotiating with partners as well as the knowledge that supports the teens' ability to protect their sexual health, such as education about STIs, HIV/AIDS, and pregnancy, is important.

Teens need to be participants in the planning of services. Because peers are often the primary source of information, development of peer-based services should be increased. Nurses can work in partnership with their adolescent patients to identify the most useful means to support healthy sexuality.

In a culturally diverse population, as is typical of many communities across Canada, it is important to avoid a "one size fits all" strategy. The specific wants and needs of each adolescent should be assessed, so that the education and counseling that is provided is appropriate and effective.

Flicker, S., Flynn, S., Larkin, J., Travers, R., Guta, A., Pole, J., & Layne, C. (2009). Sexpress: The Toronto teen survey report. Toronto, ON: Planned Parenthood Toronto.

Young Adulthood

Achievement of Developmental Tasks
Healthy development in the young adulthood period is linked to establishment of satisfactory intimate relationships and to the achievement of social goals, such as establishment of a fulfilling career. In recent decades, making the transition to adulthood is taking longer. Establishing a career often takes more years of education, resulting in postponement of plans to marry or cohabit and start a family (Clark, 2007). As a result, at age 35 years, which is often considered the endpoint of young adulthood, many young adults find themselves still heavily involved in meeting the tasks of the young adult period.

For some young people, accomplishing the transition to adulthood produces increased anxiety and stress. The types of stress encountered can include work-related stress, pressures to succeed, financial worries, difficulties balancing family demands and work, or marital conflict. Stress can manifest itself in the form of physical illnesses, emotional disorders, or substance abuse problems. Nurses need to monitor their young adult patients' stress levels and provide information about stress management strategies.

Mental illness, in the form of depression, anxiety, and serious psychiatric disorders such as schizophrenia, is a prominent health issue, affecting about 15% to 25% of adults in the early years of the young adulthood period. Suicide is a leading cause of death for this age group (Kroes & Watling, 2009). Nurses should be alert to signs of depression and suicidal ideation. Some signs to watch for include self-neglect, feelings of hopelessness, anxiety, sleep disorders, and excessive drug or alcohol use. Referral should be made to an appropriate mental health professional when signs are apparent.

Illnesses during the young adulthood period create a disruption in the normal daily activities. Concerns about caring for children or missing work become an additional stressor. Nurses need to be alert to the compelling concerns of the patient and assist him or her in identification of strategies to manage those concerns. To give young adults a sense of control, it is important to keep them informed and involved in all decisions related to their health. Chronic illnesses, such as multiple sclerosis or cancer, are sometimes diagnosed during the young adult period and will produce challenges to the achievement of developmental tasks. Nurses can provide support to these patients as they restructure their lives to accommodate intimate relationships, family decisions, and work demands.

Nutrition and Activity

Because physical growth slows after adolescence, the nutritional needs of the adult period are reduced. This need to reduce the caloric intake may come as a surprise to young adults who find they are gaining weight more easily than in the past. The challenge of health eating may be aggravated by the fact that young adults lead very busy lives and may not take time to prepare healthy foods. They end up choosing convenience foods and fast foods, which are often higher in fat, calories, sugar, and sodium.

When discussing nutrition with patients, nurses can help them identify the less healthy choices and encourage them to track their eating patterns. Developing the habit of reading the nutritional information on packaged foods and restaurant menus is a means to increase awareness of what they are eating. This is the first step in making better nutritional choices (Health Canada, 2011b).

Many young adults feel they do not have enough time for an exercise program and that they cannot afford the costs of a gym membership. Nurses can help them overcome these barriers by reinforcing the need to make regular exercise a priority and by discussing lower cost options such as walking or biking. Young adults need to choose activities that are enjoyable and that they can make time for in their busy schedule.

Sexual Health and Family Planning

Young adults have the maturity to establish fulfilling intimate relationships and enjoy a satisfying sexual life. For nurses, promoting healthy sexuality involves more than teaching how to avoid sexually transmitted infections (STIs) and unintended pregnancies. It also involves helping the young adult develop the ability to sustain good sexual and reproductive health. Young adults should be encouraged to have regular medical checkups and be tested for STIs

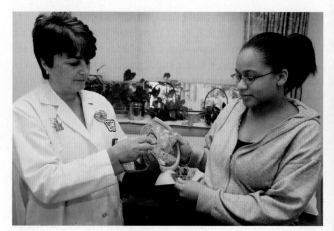

Figure 27.14 The nurse uses a teaching model to help a young woman learn about contraception.

if needed. Women should have regular Pap smears and be taught to perform breast self-examination.

The ready availability of contraception makes it possible for young adults to choose whether or when they wish to have a child. Many young couples are deferring parenthood for career or financial reasons; other couples may choose to remain childless. Nurses can support their decision-making about childbearing by providing information about the wide range of contraception options that are available (Fig. 27.14). Once a couple has decided to begin their family, anticipatory guidance about prepregnancy and prenatal care should be provided along with information about parenting. Many women are postponing childbearing into their 30s and later, and as a consequence, some are encountering difficulties with getting pregnant. Nurses can provide support, reassurance, and information about the management of infertility and the options available to couples if they are not able to conceive.

Middle Adulthood

Developmental Considerations

Middle-aged adults confront the developmental task of being productive and reaching out to the next generation. Those who succeed feel that they are making a contribution in their communities and to the world, whereas some people struggle with feelings of being unproductive and isolated. Because each adult has a long personal history up to this point, there is a great variation in how midlife is experienced. Whereas some middle-aged adults are still raising small children, others may have already launched their families and may be planning retirement. Concerns during midlife are quite broad and center on career issues, conjugal relationships, and raising families.

Most people during middle adulthood feel fulfilled and content with their life course. However, some may experience burnout in their careers, challenges in managing their personal lives, or pessimistic reactions to the idea of aging. A **midlife crisis** may occur, in which they reevaluate their beliefs and values and experience dissatisfaction with the current state of their lives. This crisis might manifest itself in minor ways such as making changes in hair colour or beginning a new exercise regimen. At a more significant level, it can result in marital breakdown, sudden job changes, depression, or substance abuse. Avoiding the midlife crisis requires self-reflection and setting of realistic goals, which may involve revising career decisions or refocusing on personal relationships. An active lifestyle is an effective way to prevent anxiety related to concerns about aging. Encouraging adults to focus on maintaining a healthy lifestyle can give them a feeling of control over some aspects of their lives.

The Sandwich Generation

Many middle-aged adults become part of the sandwich generation in which they find themselves being caregivers for their aging parents while still providing care for their own children and may find themselves providing care for grandchildren as well. The pileup of demands for care of multiple people creates physical, mental, and emotional stress, particularly for middle-aged women (Fig. 27.15). The increased burden may create complicated personal schedules and result in reduced income because of the need to reduce work hours. Research has shown

that these multigenerational caregivers are less likely to engage in health behaviours. They are more likely to choose unhealthy foods, to limit exercise, and to smoke cigarettes (Chassin, Macy, Seo, Presson, & Sherman, 2010). Nurses should monitor middle-aged caregivers for levels of stress and unhealthy coping behaviours and provide recommendations for managing stress and for increasing health-promoting activities.

Health Patterns

Healthy and unhealthy lifestyles and attitudes are important issues for those in middle adulthood. Although the adult years are, for the most part, a time of vigor and good health, health concerns begin to emerge. The most significant health problems of middle adulthood are increased level of risk for cardiovascular disease and for cancer. Chronic conditions, such as arthritis, hypertension, and Type 2 diabetes, may be diagnosed at this time. Self-destructive habits of earlier years, such as tobacco use, excessive alcohol intake, overeating, and lack of exercise, begin to catch up to the person at middle age (Edelman & Mandle, 2010).

Middle-aged adults need to make active attempts to improve their health; they can no longer assume good health as a norm. Nurses can address many of the health needs of this group through health promotion strategies targeted at their specific needs. Nurses can offer education and encouragement in the areas of improving nutrition and increasing exercise. Other useful approaches include smoking cessation programs and counseling in areas of stress and acceptance of aging.

Nutrition and Exercise

Obesity rates in Canada are highest in the midlife period. Efforts to control weight by healthier eating and regular exercise should be undertaken. Poor nutrition and sedentary living are associated with risk factors linked to the most common chronic illnesses.

Regular physical activity can play an important part in the prevention of chronic diseases such as cardiovascular disease and Type 2 diabetes (Fig. 27.16). People who are already physically active are at the lowest risk for developing these chronic diseases; however, the greatest health improvements occur for people who are not fit and then become more active. Nurses can make use of this information to encourage those who are inclined to be sedentary to take steps to increase their exercise levels. Adults can improve their activity level gradually by engaging in healthy activities that they enjoy. Participating in activities with friends and family is also a good way to socialize and stay motivated.

Nurses can recommend dietary guidelines, such as use of Canada's Food Guide or the Dietary Approaches to Stopping Hypertension (DASH) diet, as recommended by the Heart and Stroke Foundation. Research has shown that the DASH plan can reduce the risk of developing high blood pressure and can also lower elevated blood pressure. In addition, the total cholesterol and low-density lipoprotein (LDL) were lower. The DASH diet is similar to Canada's Food Guide but recommends a larger number of servings of fruits and vegetable and

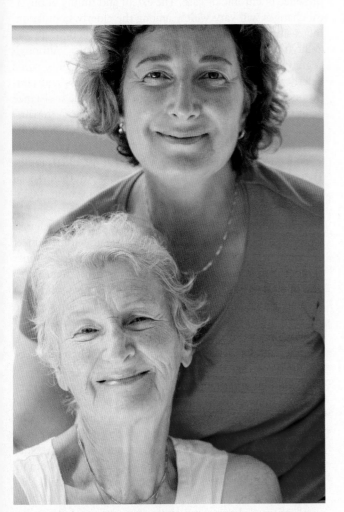

Figure 27.15 A middle-aged woman finds herself in the role of caregiver to her mother.

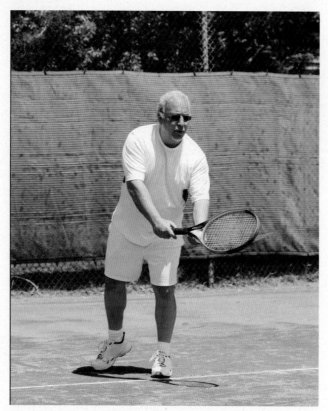

Figure 27.16 Middle-aged adults benefit from regular exercise.

emphasizes lower salt intake (Heart and Stroke Foundation, 2008). As the need for vitamin D increases after age 50 years, all adults older than the age of 50 years should take a daily vitamin D supplement of 10 μg (400 International Units).

Menopause

For most women, menopause occurs between their late 40s and their 50s. Every woman experiences menopause differently. For many, the symptoms are only mildly inconvenient, but some women may experience significant discomfort. Common symptoms include hot flashes, night sweats, general malaise, and changes in sexual response. There are a range of options available for management of menopausal symptoms; the nurse can provide advice and support so women can make decisions that are appropriate to their own needs. Lifestyle changes, including weight loss, regular exercise, and avoidance of triggers such as alcohol or hot drinks, may be helpful to reduce mild symptoms. Use of hormone replacement therapy or of alternative therapies, such as herbal medications, should be discussed with their primary healthcare provider to weigh out the risks and benefits (Society of Obstetricians and Gynecologists of Canada, 2009).

Postmenopause, women experience higher risks for heart disease, diabetes, osteoporosis, and cancer due to loss of the protective effects of estrogen and due to the aging process. Mammogram screening for breast cancer is recommended after the age of 50 years, and all women should have regular physical examinations. Supplements of calcium and vitamin D intake should be used to maintain normal bone density. A regular exercise program that includes weight-bearing exercise is essential to the prevention of bone loss.

Late Adulthood

Experience of Change and Loss

The lives of older adults are characterized by multiple changes and losses, each of them demanding emotional and social adjustments as they occur. Most adults retire at some time in their 60s or earlier, and there is an emerging trend toward later retirement (Statistics Canada, 2011). The adjustment to retirement involves changes in social status and income. After retirement, many people find worthwhile pursuits for the extra time in such activities as traveling or becoming involved in part-time or volunteer work. Retirement or changes in health may result in them giving up their homes and moving into smaller apartments or senior living facilities. Although this may be physically or financially necessary, there are emotional costs to giving up a long-time home and getting rid of prized possessions.

The normal aging process leads to gradual loss of physical strength and health, which may be accelerated by the presence of chronic disease. The extent and timing of physical changes will vary widely among the elderly population. Increasing age brings with it increased limitations in the ability to manage ADL and loss of independence. Although cognitive impairment is not part of normal aging, some elderly will develop problems with forgetfulness and confusion. An older adult may have to rely on the assistance of others for things such as transportation, home repairs, or physical care. Faced with all these changes, older adults must find ways to redefine and maintain their quality of life.

Social isolation can become a problem for older adults. They may progressively lose connections to their social network because of retirement, illness, or relocation. Maintaining ties with other people is important to prevent loneliness. Many communities have services and groups, such as senior centres, which offer a range of programs to help meet the social needs of older adults. An increasingly large number of older people are making use of the Internet as a means to stay in contact with friends and family members who have become geographically dispersed. Using this linkage can improve their connections to their social supports and prevent loneliness (Sum, Mathews, Hughes, & Campbell, 2008).

Older adults' relationship with their children must be redefined, so that they can remain involved in the lives of their children and grandchildren in a meaningful way. They may find themselves in a position of accepting care from the same people they were responsible for in earlier years. The longer the older adult lives, the more people will be lost from his or her life. Siblings and friends die, and commonly, older adults are faced with the loss of a spouse (Fig. 27.17). Coming to terms with the deaths of loved ones may be difficult. Ultimately, they must deal with the prospect of their own death.

All of these changes and losses create sorrow and grieving and can have a negative effect on an elderly person's self-esteem.

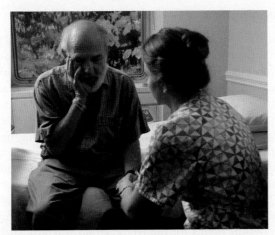

Figure 27.17 An elderly man is experiencing the loss of his wife after 60 years of marriage.

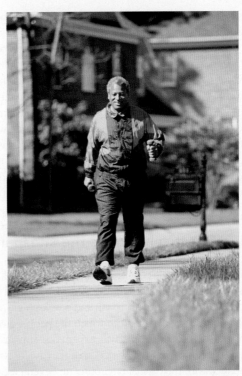

Figure 27.18 An elderly man maintains his health by participating in regular exercise.

Common responses to grief are depression, social withdrawal, and irritability, so nurses should be alert to these symptoms in the elderly person and provide support. To achieve a sense of psychological integrity, older adults must look back at their own lives and come to terms with the changes, losses, successes, and failures. The process of engaging patients in reminiscence or life review, as described earlier in the Research Review, "Life Review as a Tool for Promoting Well-Being in the Elderly," is a useful strategy for nurses to assist their elderly patients with this process.

Whenever older adults experience serious illness, they and their family caregivers may become fearful that recovery will not be complete and that their ability to care for themselves will be diminished. Health crises, such as a stroke or a fracture of the hip, often do result in permanent impairments, creating an increased need for care from others. Nurses can be instrumental in helping the older adults maintain their quality of life in the face of the changes they experience. In some cases, nurses provide the direct physical care to meet basic needs. They can also help by providing referrals to available resources, educating family caregivers and supporting the older adults in making decisions about their future.

Nutrition and Exercise for the Elderly

Older adults are at a higher risk of developing poor nutrition that can affect their overall health unfavorably. Encouraging them to plan nutritious meals and eat healthily can be challenging. Factors associated with aging, such as diminished sense of taste and smell, dental changes, and reduced activity levels, can affect appetitive and caloric needs. Older adults with impaired mobility or financial constraints may not be able to purchase the types of foods necessary to a healthy diet. Living alone often results in reduced motivation for preparing full meals regularly. Canada's Food Guide continues to be a valuable source for dietary advice for the elderly; however, the lower number of servings recommended in each food group should be used because of the reduced caloric needs of the elderly. Smaller, more frequent meals are also recommended. Community programs such as Meals on Wheels that provides well-balanced, low-cost meals are available to seniors.

The physical changes related to normal aging lead to a decline in bone density, strength, flexibility, balance, and overall cardiovascular fitness. If the older adult becomes more inactive, the rate of decline accelerates. Older adults benefit from aerobic exercise, stretching, and weight-bearing activity to maintain their level of function (Fig. 27.18). Canada's Physical Activity Guide to Healthy Active Living for Older Adults recommends 30 to 60 minutes of physical activity daily, which can be done in smaller time increments if prolonged periods of exercise are not well tolerated (Public Health Agency of Canada, 2007). Remaining physically active helps extend health and independence. Nurses can engage older adults in discussions about what types of activity they enjoy and are capable of doing and can encourage them to pursue these activities on a regular basis.

Falls Prevention

Falls are the most common cause of injury and a leading cause of death for the elderly. Approximately one third of people older than the age of 65 years fall once or more each year. Most of these falls occur at home while performing usual daily activities. The chances of falling increase with age due to poor vision, unsteady gait, and poor balance. Chronic illnesses, such as arthritis or Parkinson disease, and medication side effects may increase the level of risk. Older persons may be reluctant to use equipment, such as canes or walkers, which could reduce their risk. Anxiety about ambulating safely and fear of falling can result in older adults reducing their level of activity, which causes further decline in physical well-being and further increase the risk for falls (Scott & Rajabai, 2007).

Nurses should include a falls risk assessment into their patient assessments on a regular basis. A review of medications should be done to identify if any are contributing to possible light-headedness or unsteadiness. A safety review should be conducted during home visits, identifying such hazards as cluttered furniture, loose rugs, locks, or hand rails. Nurses should explore strategies for preventing falls with the older adult. Recommend measures that can be useful in preventing falls include wearing supportive footwear or using safety equipment such as walkers or grab rails. Older adults benefit from regular physical activity to reduce the risk of falls, particularly exercises to promote balance, muscle strength, and endurance are best for reducing falls.

Nursing Effectively Across the Lifespan

The ability to provide effective nursing care across the lifespan requires more than an understanding of developmental theory and information about normal growth and development. An appreciation of the societal context in which the people grow and develop is also needed. People will experience similar developmental trajectories, but the choices that they make will vary in accordance with their social environment. Several aspects of changing Canadian society will be explored to illustrate this.

Demographic Shifts—An Aging Society

Baby boomers, a generation of people born in the post–World War II period from 1947 to 1966, are a large demographic group who, at each developmental stage of their lives, have had a huge societal impact. When this group was in school-age and adolescent periods, large numbers of schools needed to be built; and when they reached the end of the period, many schools experienced the challenges of lower enrollments. As they move toward retirement and old age, there is increasing emphasis on products and services directed at retirees and seniors, such as senior communities. Succeeding generations have been affected by being in the shadow of this momentous demographic bubble.

Current baby boomers will become senior citizens in the next two decades. Canadians are also living longer than ever before, with a life expectancy of more than 80 years of age. Because of this, recent projections for Canada show that the proportion of older adults could be double that of children in the population by the 2030s. This shift in age patterns in Canada will have an impact on many aspects of Canadian society, and one of the most significant will be health and health care. Although most older adults can look forward to years with a good quality of life, not all will enjoy good health. The prevalence of chronic conditions, such as hypertension, Type 2 diabetes, and arthritis, will likely rise. Because seniors account for a proportionately larger part of health service demands, the need for nurses will increase. Nurses will be needed to provide direct supportive and rehabilitative care to this generation. But even more, they will be needed for important roles in health promotion to help support health and prevent illness.

Changing Society—Cultural Diversity

Canada's ethnic and cultural diversity, which has been a feature of the nation from its earliest history, will continue to increase significantly during the next two decades. By 2031, about one fourth of the population will be foreign born. Diversity will grow among those who are Canadian-born, with increased religious diversity within the population as well (Statistics Canada, 2010). Canada has long had a multicultural tradition, which tolerates and respects different cultural values within the framework of Canadian culture.

The achievement of developmental tasks may be manifested differently across cultural groups. In some cases, the physical norms for the ethnic group will vary slightly from the widely used population norms. Different cultural or religious groups may have diverse expectations and behaviours within each of the developmental stages. For example, adolescent rebellion against authority in a traditional Muslim household might be manifested by refusal to wear a hijab; in a family of English Canadians, the rebellion might take the form of underage drinking. Beliefs about infant feeding, disciplinary practices, and attitudes toward the elderly are a few examples of ways in which Canadians can differ. Health practices also have cultural implications, such as breast-feeding attitudes, co-bedding, and dietary practices.

Nurses engaged in promoting healthy growth and development need to make sure they are providing culturally sensitive care. The cultural context must be assessed to identify the values and belief systems of the patients. Any anticipatory guidance plan should take ethnic and religious beliefs into consideration and must be acceptable within the cultural belief system of the people.

Changes in Health-Care Delivery

Toward 2020: Visions for Nursing calls for a change in the way nurses provide care (Villeneuve & MacDonald, 2006). Preventative care across the lifespan will be important in the future support health and prevent injury and disease. A strenuous and coordinated effort must be made to reverse trends related to obesity, poor nutrition, and inadequate exercise. The shift in focus from illness to health will mean the nursing care will become more community based. Nurses will be knowledge brokers and advocates for the people in their care.

Canadians are seeking to be more in charge of their own health care. They want more information and are demanding that health-care professionals be responsive to their needs. Through use of the Internet and other media, they have expanding sources of information that they can access but may experience confusion and overload with the amount of information available. Nurses can facilitate their efforts to be informed and to change their health behaviours by assessing their information needs and providing clear advice on how to meet those needs at all ages across the lifespan.

Critical Thinking Case Scenarios

▶ Rhea, a third-year nursing student, is in clinical placement in a school, working with a Grade 5 class 1 day a week. The teacher has read the recommendations regarding increasing children's physical activity level and asks Rhea to help implement a program in the classroom. What would be suitable activities for children in this age group? What strategies can be used to motivate the students to become more active?

▶ Henry, age 55 years, is housebound because of his multiple sclerosis, and he has begun to use the Internet for e-mailing his family and reading his daily paper. He asks his visiting nurse about using the Internet to find health information. He wants to know where he can find good, accurate information. What guidance should be given to Henry to help him identify reliable information? What are some useful Internet sites that could be suggested?

▶ Maria is 80 years old, and she walks with a cane. At her last checkup, her doctor told her she needed to build more physical activity into her life. How can the nurse motivate her to remain active? What types of activity might be suitable?

Multiple-Choice Questions

1. Matthew, age 6 months, always puts his toy blocks and stuffed animals in his mouth. This reflects which of Piaget's stages of cognitive development?
   a. Sensorimotor
   b. Concrete operations
   c. Reflective motion
   d. Preoperational

2. Marusia, age 16 years, is in 11th grade and is doing well in all her subjects at school. She would be placed in which of Erikson's stage?
   a. Initiative versus guilt
   b. Industry versus authority
   c. Identity versus role confusion
   d. Integrity versus despair

3. Pagna, age 22 months, wants a toy that his sister has and when he can't have it starts to scream and throws himself on the floor. How should his parents handle his tantrum?
   a. Pick him up and give him a quick smack on his bottom to get him to stop.
   b. Ensure that he is safe from injury but otherwise ignore the behaviour.
   c. Put him in his crib and close the door to his room.
   d. Take the toy from the sister and give it to him to calm him down.

4. Ken, 45 years old, who has been single-mindedly climbing the career ladder, suddenly feels that he has no more opportunity for advancement. He also feels that he has neglected his family and has made wrong decisions in charting his life's course. Ken's feelings are probably signs of:
   a. A self-centered personality
   b. An unsuccessful passage through early adulthood
   c. The onset of a psychiatric disorder
   d. A normal developmental crisis of middle age

5. Maria makes regular nursing visits to her elderly patient, Mrs. Harper, in her home. At each visit, Mrs. Harper likes to show the nurse photos of her family and talk about her experiences growing up on a farm and raising her family on the same farm. Maria listens attentively and encourages this because:
   a. Encouraging reminiscence helps her patient's life review.
   b. She can assess her patient's short-term memory.
   c. She grew up on farm and enjoys the farming stories.
   d. This is a therapeutic technique to manage her patient's depression.

6. A nurse is counseling David, age 27 years, about healthy nutrition and exercise patterns. This emphasis on health promotion is intended to modify risk factors related to:
   a. Cirrhosis of the liver
   b. Colon cancer
   c. Coronary artery disease
   d. STIs

Suggested Lab Activities

1. Aging Game

This game is designed to help the nursing student develop a personal understanding of the aging process by experiencing some of the realities and needs of the older adult. Players will gain insight necessary to respect the concerns of daily living that the older adult faces.

Equipment:

- Cotton balls for ears to diminish hearing acuity
- Tongue depressors or tape to splint fingers of dominant hand inside gloves to mock joint stiffness
- Vinyl gloves for hands to decrease the sensation of touch
- Glasses smeared with petroleum jelly to mock vision pattern changes
- Switch shoes on feet to evoke gait pattern changes

Activity:

Students work in pairs. One student dresses to be the older adult and is accompanied by the other student in the role of nurse. They spend 15 to 20 minutes walking in the corridors and on stairs, going to the washroom, and speaking to others they meet in the halls. The students then switch roles and repeat the process.

Discussion:

In groups after the activity, the students should discuss feelings about physical limitations they experienced and social judgments they may have perceived. The groups can engage in discussion of related issues such as financial limitation to purchasing assistive devices and the effect of limitations on ADL.

2. Developmental Assessment of an Infant or Small Child

Students will conduct a developmental assessment of the child using a tool such as the NDDS. Students who have access to an infant or small child (age 2 months to 4 years) are asked to bring the child to a lab session. The child should be well known to the student (own child, sibling, niece or nephew).

Preparation:

Students work in groups of three or four. They identify the age of their participating child and identify and acquire the equipment needed for testing. Creation of a safe and supportive setting for the testing procedure should be discussed.

Activity:

The student who brings the child acts the parent role. The other students conduct the developmental assessment. They should encourage the child, as much as possible, to perform the skill, but "parent" report can be used when necessary to gather the information.

Discussion:

After the activity, the following can be discussed:
- What were the challenges in completing the assessment?
- What techniques were effective in doing the assessment?
- How are the test procedures and results communicated to the parent?
- What would be the next step if some developmental areas were noted to be lagging?

REFERENCES AND SUGGESTED READINGS

Bee, H., Boyd, D., & Johnson, P. (2009). *Lifespan development* (3rd ed.). Toronto, ON: Pearson.

Boyce, W. F., King, M. A., & Roche, J. (2008). *Healthy settings for young people in Canada.* Ottawa, ON: Public Health Agency of Canada. Retrieved from http://www.phac-aspc.gc.ca

Chassin, L., Macy, J. T., Seo, D. C., Presson, C. C., & Sherman, S. J. (2010). The association between membership in the sandwich generation and health behaviors: A longitudinal study. *Journal of Applied Developmental Psychology, 31*(1), 38–46. doi:10.1016/j.appdev.2009.06.001

Clark, W. (2007). Delayed transitions of young adults. *Canadian Social Trends, 84,* 14–22.

Dacey, J. S., Travers, J., & Fiore, L. (2009). *Human development across the lifespan* (7th ed.). New York, NY: McGraw-Hill.

Del Vecchio, T., Walter, A., & O'Leary, S. (2009). Affective and physiological factors predicting maternal response to infant crying. *Infant Behavior and Development, 32*(1), 117–122. doi:10.1016/j.infbeh.2008.10.005

Dovey, T. M., Staples, P. A., Gibson, E. L., & Halford, J. C. G. (2008). Food neophobia and 'picky/fussy' eating in children: A review. *Appetite, 50,* 181–193. doi:10.1016/j.appet.2007.09.009

Duncan, P. M., Garcia, A. C., Frankowski, B. L., Carey, P. A., Kallock, E. A., Dixon, R. D., & Shaw, J. S. (2007). Inspiring healthy adolescent choices: A rationale for and guide to strength promotion in primary care. *Journal of Adolescent Health, 41,* 525–535.

Edelman, C., & Mandle, C. (2010). *Health promotion throughout the life span* (7th ed.). St. Louis, MO: Mosby Elsevier.

Erikson, E. H. (1980). *Identity and the life cycle.* New York, NY: Norton.

Estes, M. E., & Buck, M. (2008). *Health assessment and physical examination.* Toronto, ON: Thompson Nelson.

Gaines, J., & Schwebel, D. (2009). Recognition of home injury risks by novice parents of toddlers. *Accident Analysis & Prevention, 41*(5), 1070–1074. doi:10.1016/j.aap.2009.06.010

Goldstein, M. H., Schwade, J., Briesch, J., & Syal, S. (2010). Learning while babbling: Prelinguistic object-directed vocalizations indicate a readiness to learn. *Infancy, 15*(4), 362–391. doi:10.1111/j.1532-7078.2009.00020.x

Health Canada. (2009). *Misconceptions about vaccine safety.* Retrieved from http://www.hc-sc.gc.ca/hl-vs/iyh-vsv/med/misconception-eng.php

Health Canada. (2011a). *Canada's food guide.* Retrieved from http://www.hc-sc.gc.ca/fn-an/food-guide-aliment/index-eng.php

Health Canada. (2011b). *Eating well with Canada's food guide—A resource for educators and communicators.* Retrieved from http://www.hc-sc.gc.ca/fn-an/food-guide-aliment/educ-comm/resource-ressource-eng.php

Hockenberry, M., & Wilson, D. (2007). *Wong's nursing care of infants and children* (8th ed.). St. Louis, MO: Mosby.

Kroes, G., & Watling, J. (2009). *Healthy transitions to adulthood: Moving to integrated mental health care.* Ottawa, ON: Policy Research Initiative.

Lau, D. C., Douketis, J. D., Morrison, K. M., Hramiak, I. M., Sharma, A. M., & Ur, E. (2007). 2006 Canadian clinical practice guidelines on the management and prevention of obesity in adults and children [Summary]. *Canadian Medical Association Journal, 176*(8), S1–S13.

Paglia-Boak, A., Mann, R. E., Adlaf, E. M., Beitchman, J. H., Wolfe, D., & Rehm, J. (2010). *The mental health and well-being of Ontario students, 1991-2009.* Retrieved from http://www.camh.net/Research/osdus.html

Piaget, J. (1993). Development and learning. In M. Gauvin & M. Cole (Eds.), *Readings on the development of children* (2nd ed.). New York, NY: W. H. Freeman and Company. (Reprinted from *Piaget rediscovered,* pp. 7–20, by R. E. Ripple & V. N. Rockcastle, Eds., 1964, Ithaca, NY: Cornell University Press)

Piaget, J. (2008). Intellectual evolution from adolescence to adulthood. *Human Development, 51,* 40–47. doi:10.1159/000112531 (Original work published 1972)

Scott, V., & Rajabai, F. (2007). *Seniors' falls can be prevented.* Vancouver, BC: BC Injury Research and Prevention Unit and the BC Falls and Injury Prevention Coalition. Retrieved from http://www.injuryresearch.bc.ca

Society of Obstetricians and Gynecologists of Canada. (2009). Menopause and osteoporosis update 2009. *Journal of Obstetrics and Gynaecology Canada, 31*(1), S1–S42.

Sum, S., Mathews, R. M., Hughes, I., & Campbell, A. (2008). Internet use and loneliness in older adults. *Cyberpsychology & Behavior, 11*(2), 208–211. doi:10.1089/cpb.2007.0010

Veenhof, B., & Timusk, P. (2009). Online activities of Canadian boomers and seniors. *Canadian Social Trends, 88,* 25–32.

Villeneuve, M., & MacDonald, J. (2006). *Toward 2020: Visions for nursing.* Ottawa, ON: Canadian Nurses Association.

Wang, F., Wild, T. C., Kipp, W., Kuhle, S., & Veugelers, P. J. (2009). The influence of childhood obesity on the development of self-esteem. *Statistics Canada Health Reports, 20*(2), 21–27.

Fostering a Positive Self-Concept

ELAINE MORDOCH

Jason and Emily are first-year nursing students who are going on their first clinical practicum. Their practicum setting is an assisted living complex in the community where they will be conducting basic nursing assessments and care with various people. In the practice lab, they have been taking vital signs, positioning people for bath care, and learning how to conduct basic health assessments. On the first day of clinical, their instructor asks them to focus on developing rapport with their patients. The goal is to try and understand who their patients are beyond their medical diagnoses. During their clinical conference at the end of the day, Jason and Emily are to report what they have learned and how they have gathered this information. Prior to meeting their patients, they discuss how to go about this, what to do if their patient is not friendly, and how to reach a beginning understanding of the essence of the person. How do you think they should proceed?

CHAPTER OBJECTIVES

By the end of this chapter, you will be able to:

1. Discuss how positive self-concept relates to nursing practice in both the student nurse and the patient.
2. Explain the development of your self-concept during your formative years and the influences on its development.
3. Explore the development of your professional self-concept at this stage of your nursing education.
4. Determine how culture, family, community, and societal forces influence self-concept.
5. Compare the concepts of inclusion and exclusion and how they relate to a positive self-concept.
6. Develop an understanding of how self-concept is affected by illness and disability.
7. Identify ways nurses and nursing students can foster positive self-esteem in their patients.

KEY TERMS

Culture A group of people who identify with each other on the basis of some common purpose, need, or background; a set of learned socially transmitted behaviours and beliefs arising from interactions within the group.

Personhood The uniqueness of each human being, combined with a sense of personal continuity and personal autonomy.

Self-Awareness Being cognizant of one's own beliefs, thoughts, motivations, biases, and physical and emotional limitations and the impact these components may have on others.

Self-Concept The sum of one's beliefs about oneself, which develops over time.

Self-Esteem Attitude about oneself; emotional appraisal of one's worth.

Self-Identity The integration of social and occupational roles and affiliations and self-attributed personality traits, attitudes, and beliefs about political ideology, religion, gender, and sexuality; influences goal-directed behaviour and interpersonal relationships.

Therapeutic Use of Self How nurses use themselves, their personality, and their way of being to assist others to regain health. Nurses must practice ongoing self-awareness, an ability to serve as a role model, and a sense of ethics and responsibility toward their patients' well-being.

World View The way a group of people see their world, their physical and symbolic space, and their place in the world.

Deciding to become a nurse is a life-changing decision. You may have been attracted to a career in nursing after watching exciting television episodes of *ER*, or you were influenced by personal and family experiences with illness. Other reasons for choosing nursing could include being influenced by a positive nurse role model, being told that you "would make a good nurse," or, possibly, by seeing a need in your community that you would like to address. These are only a few of the reasons why people choose nursing as a career.

During your journey to become a nurse, you will be challenged to develop not only an understanding of patients' and their families' behaviours but also your own behaviours, assumptions, and thoughts. Much of this awareness will cause you to reflect on who you are and how you became the person you are at this moment in time; in other words, how your self-concept developed. This chapter will assist you to examine how you became the person you are and how you can use your **personhood**, by which we mean your unique personal qualities, combined with a sense of personal continuity and autonomy, to foster a positive self-concept in patients, families, and communities as well as members of the health-care team with whom you interact in nursing practice.

What Is Self-Concept?

Self-concept is the sum of beliefs about one's self that develops over time: Who am I and what can I become? How we feel about ourselves sometimes may fluctuate in different situations and with different people, but in a healthy person with a positive self-concept, our core beliefs and feelings about ourselves remain intact. For example, consider your position as a nursing student, being challenged with performing new skills in the clinical setting. Most students will experience reasonable doubt and some anxiety about this new experience. This can lead to temporary doubt about one's abilities to perform and to problem-solve ways to be successful. A positive self-concept will allow one to more easily scale new learning experiences. In a helping relationship, a healthy self-concept in the nurse and in the patient is the ideal situation within which to provide care. However, just as new learning experiences challenge students, so can situations arising from illness seriously challenge the self-concepts of patients and their families. No matter where you practice nursing—whether in geriatrics, pediatrics, psychiatry, or surgery—both your and your patient's self-concept will influence the healing process. An essential part of the nursing role is to provide therapeutic care that will nurture a positive self-concept in patients and families. Remember that self-concept is an open dynamic system, and as you develop your identity as a nurse, your professional self-concept will also form (Cunha & Goncalves, 2009). This will help you to maintain professional boundaries in nurse–patient relationships while providing optimal care.

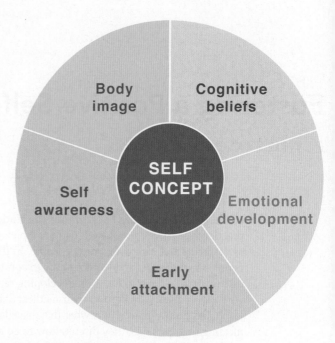

Figure 28.1 Influences on self-concept.

Self-Awareness

Self-concept is influenced by several factors, one of which is **self-awareness**, which is cognizance of one's beliefs, thoughts, motivations, biases, attributes, and limitations and how these aspects of oneself impact others. Cultivating self-awareness is a helpful practice that you can use throughout the development of your nursing practice. Nursing students have various opportunities to think and work on self-awareness. For example, use of the Asian mandala, a circular art form that encourages reflection, has helped student nurses develop understanding of self and their self-concepts in their new role as nurses (Mahar, Iwasiw, & Evans, 2012). The diagram, "Influences on Self-Concept" (Fig. 28.1), illustrates other aspects that impact your self-concept.

Formation of Self-Concept

As a beginning nursing student, it is important for you to start to understand self-concept in both yourself and your patients and their families. Ask yourself the questions in Box 28.1 to

---

BOX 28.1 Student Self-Awareness Exercise

1. Develop a time line of your life to date. Insert the dates of major developmental milestones that you managed well and which promoted your self-concept.
2. Draw a second time line and insert influencing factors that may have placed limits on your developing self-concept.
3. Consider how you managed to overcome these factors. What helped you? What hindered you?
4. Pick one major influencing factor and relate how this might help you to understand the self-concept of someone who is living with a major illness.

help you reflect on the concepts in this chapter. This will help you to promote holistic healing. There is a vast body of knowledge that describes the development of self-concept. For our purposes, we will consider some of the essential key points that will get you started to think about how nurses can nurture self-concepts within themselves, patients and their families, and health-care team members within nursing practice.

The Growth and Developmental Perspective

Self-concept is affected by early attachment to a principal caregiver and how the caregiver meets the foundational emotional and physical needs of the infant and child (Bowlby, 1969). Ongoing experiences throughout the growth and developmental life cycle impact the development of self-concept and are described in Erikson's theory of psychosocial development (Erikson, 1968, 1987; for more on this topic, refer to Chapter 27). The ability to recognize emotions simultaneously develops with the self-concept. Different emotional states of contentment, joy, interest, surprise, distress, sadness, anger, disgust, and fear begin in infancy (Harter, 1996). The reactions of caregivers to these emotions may positively or negatively influence the infant's beginning sense of self. Positive emotions originating in infancy, such as joy and contentment, promote mental and physical well-being. Joy generates confidence and courage, and interest generates engagement with the environment (Izard, 2002).

From the ages of 6 to 12 years, children undergo considerable emotional development, which has the potential to contribute to close relationships with parents and in developing friendships. Positive emotions also act as a buffer for negative life events (Izard, 2002). Children learn self-acceptance, identification and management of feelings, problem solving, and development of interpersonal relationships. As children's analytical abilities increase, they understand more complex emotions such as shame, guilt, and pride and learn to appraise the meaning of a situation (Meerum-Terwogt & Stegge, 2001). How children are able to perform the tasks required of them and fulfill their roles as students, sons, daughters, and friends influences how they see themselves. The successful acquisition of abilities contributes to the formation of a positive self-concept.

Eric Erikson studied the development of humans over the life span and his work highlighted the formation of **self-identity**, particularly in the stages of adolescence. Self-identity may be ongoing and achieved over the life span. You may reflect on your own self-identity and how it has developed and changed over the years. Think back to your adolescence and how you self-identified at that time and how you do so now.

In early adolescence, abstract thought begins to develop. The young adolescent is unable to integrate a self-portrait. This is further reinforced by the fact that others may hold varying opinions of the adolescent. In middle adolescence, cognitive-developmental changes account for shifting self-evaluations, unpredictable behaviours, and mood swings that many adolescents experience (Harter, 1999). Within the later stages of adolescence, self-concept and abstract thinking

are further developed with experiences now being subject to higher levels of thought and analysis. Spurr, Bally, Ogenchuk, and Walker (2012) identified, in a Canadian study with 280 high school students, significant factors that adolescents associated with a sense of their well-being. Factors were social relationships, self-esteem, and self-concept. For those of you who may become pediatric nurses, this evidence can inform your future practice to assess self-concept and self-esteem and work with adolescents to develop a strong sense of self. Young adults face the task of developing intimacy with a confidant and potential life partner, establishing a career path, and taking on the responsibilities of families. The extent to which these tasks are accomplished influences the development of a positive self-concept in mainstream society.

Mature adults and late life adults face the tasks of maintaining a generative productive lifestyle and integrating ego integrity into the last stages of life. Ego integrity, wherein the individual can look on his or her life achievements with satisfaction, is the final testament to a positive self-concept (Erikson, 1968, 1982). However, as you will see in nursing practice, not all late life adults achieve ego integrity. In a nursing study identifying factors influencing suicidal thoughts in late life men, researchers Oliffe, Han, Ogrodniczuk, Philips, and Roy (2011) found that the participants struggled with cumulative losses, had difficulty expressing emotions related to these losses, and were concerned about being labeled as weak for expressing sensitive feelings. In addition, they often felt that they did not live up to the idealized role of male provider. This is an example of the importance of understanding self-concept and the ways it may affect health and well-being. Erikson's theory of psychosocial development highlights the unique developmental stages that occur during the lifespan. Look at Table 28.1 showing Erikson's theory of psychosocial development and reflect on your progression of developmental stages to date.

An Environmental Perspective

Another perspective to consider in the development of self-concept is Uri Bronfenbrenner's classic work on the environmental perspective (Bronfenbrenner, 1994). His ideas help

TABLE 28.1	Erikson's Theory of Psychosocial Development
Stages of Personality Development	**Ego Strength**
Trust vs. mistrust (infant)	Hope
Autonomy vs. self-doubt (toddler)	Will power
Initiative vs. guilt (early childhood)	Purpose
Industry vs. inferiority (school age)	Competence
Identity vs. identity diffusion (teen age)	Fidelity
Intimacy vs. isolation (young adult)	Love
Generativity vs. stagnation (mature adult)	Caring
Ego integrity vs. ego despair (late adult)	Wisdom

If one stage is not completed, it is difficult to complete the tasks of the following stages.
Source: Erikson, E. (1968). *Identity: Youth and crisis*. New York, NY: Norton; Erikson, E. (1982). *The life cycle completed: A review*. New York, NY: Norton.

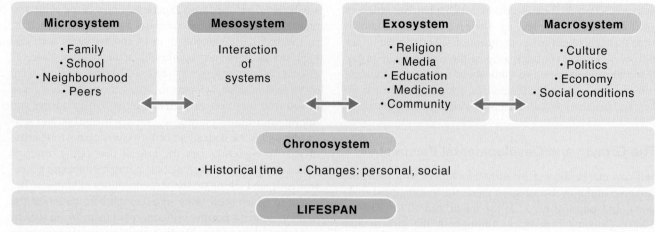

Figure 28.2 Bronfenbrenner's ecological systems approach. (Adapted from Bronfenbrenner & Morris, 2006). The Bioecological Model of Human Development. Bronfenbrenner, U., & Morris, P. A. (2006). The bioecological model of human development. In R. M. Lerner & W. Damon (Eds.), *Handbook of child psychology: Theoretical models of human development* (6th ed., Vol. 1, pp. 793–828). Hoboken, NJ: John Wiley & Sons.

us understand that there is a complex bidirectional interaction between child development and the ecological systems within which the child interacts. Bronfenbrenner classifies these systems as the microsystem, mesosystem, exosystem, macrosystem, and chronosystems. Let's look at the main ideas associated with each system.

The microsystem comprises the child's activities and interactions within the child's immediate surroundings; for example, the family home. The mesosystem refers to connections between this environment and other systems wherein the child interacts, such as day care, church, and school. The exosystem consists of other social systems such as health policy and employment. The macrosystem considers laws, customs, and societal resources. The chronosystem recognizes the historical influences and the passing of time. Bronfenbrenner's (1994) perspective identifies the complexity of the interactions between systems and their influence on child development and self-concept. Bronfenbrenner's work illustrates that how children are able to fulfill their growth and developmental tasks and develop their abilities is also influenced by the context of children's lives within their families, communities, and the larger society.

Knowledge of both Erikson's (1968, 1982) and Bronfenbrenner's (1994) perspectives will help you to understand your personal self-concept development and consider possible influences on the self-concept of your patients and their families. Refer to the diagram of Bronfenbrenner's ecological model in Figure 28.2 and consider how you were and still are influenced by this multisystems approach.

Self-Esteem

Self-esteem is the term used to describe the way you think and feel about yourself. The amount of self-esteem someone has depends on many factors, including parental attitudes and childrearing style and life experiences. Failures, life disappointments, and being mistreated by others may cause some people to feel badly about themselves and experience *low self-esteem*. Having *high self-esteem* means feeling confident, worthy, and positive regarding yourself. You may notice people with high self-esteem project a sense of self-worth, belonging, and security. They may tend to be successful due to their confidence when taking on challenges and risking failure to achieve their personal goals. Refer to Box 28.2 for some of the characteristics of people with high or low self-esteem.

Punishment and abuse, poverty, economic deprivation, failure in school, and even self-criticism are among the factors that affect our feelings of self-worth. Race, religion, the media, culture, and sex all have some influence on how we feel about ourselves. Because development of self-esteem begins in childhood, parents and caregivers help promote

---

BOX 28.2   Personal Characteristics of High and Low Self-Esteem

A person with high self-esteem will be able to
- Act independently
- Assume responsibility
- Take pride in his or her accomplishments
- Tolerate frustration
- Attempt new tasks and challenges
- Handle positive and negative emotions
- Offer assistance to others

A person with low self-esteem will
- Avoid trying new things
- Feel unloved and unwanted
- Blame others for his or her own shortcomings
- Feel or pretend to feel emotionally indifferent
- Be unable to tolerate a normal level of frustration
- Put down his or her own talents and abilities
- Be easily influenced

healthy self-esteem through encouragement and a focus on multiple areas of enjoyment.

Cycle of Encouragement and Discouragement

Let's consider how encouragement and discouragement may influence the development of self-concepts.

Discouragement

If children are met with repeated failures, they become discouraged; lose motivation and confidence; and experience feelings of frustration, anger, fear, and depression. Without sufficient resources or tools to assist them to improve or find attainable goals, children will develop a sense of helplessness and diminished self-concept and worth. Typical reactions of children to repeated failures are aggression, denial, and withdrawal (Harter, 1999). It is not unusual for people facing major health challenges to have similar reactions and feelings. Illness-related events wherein both adults and children experience altered body image, or repeated failure to perform previously ordinary easy tasks, can lead to the same feelings. In addition, Rogers's (1961) theory of incongruence noted that the ideal self and the real self must be congruent for a healthy self-concept. In situations such as illness, the ideal and the real self may be distant leading to a poor self-concept (Rogers, 1961). As a nurse, you can expect to assist patients to work through these negative emotions that can undermine their attempts to deal with losses related to illness. Nurses do their best to understand the underlying meaning of behaviours and emotions. This facilitates fostering and nurturing more healthy responses to restore and build on the patient's self-concept (Benner & Wrubel, 1988).

Encouragement

Self-concept is fostered by realistic encouragement that assists children to develop confidence, have feelings of control of their own lives, take appropriate risks, continue trying, and strive to improve. This fosters belonging, competence, and feelings of self-worth. Adults and children faced with illness and disability require consistent and realistic encouragement to rebuild their confidence and abilities to manage their situations. Nurses use interventions that accept patients wherever they are in their illness experience, guide them to take appropriate risks, and provide opportunities for success in rehabilitation. These actions foster and restore the self-concept of patients and families affected by illness. The messages that we receive from others influence how we see ourselves in relation to others (Hartrick Doane & Varcoe, 2005).

Nursing students themselves may go through cycles of encouragement and discouragement with high stress levels related to the demands of their studies. Sawatsky et al. (2012) studied Canadian university students and found that those students who believed that they were unable to manage their stress were prone to developing depression, whereas those that believed that they could manage were less vulnerable to psychological difficulties. Nursing students when cultivating on-going self-awareness can learn effective ways to manage stress and build self-efficacy in stress management.

Think Anne had been on the medical ward for 6 weeks after suffering a stroke that left her unable to walk without assistance. She has become unsure of herself and unwilling to attempt the suggested physiotherapy exercises. She was often observed sitting in her chair looking out the window with a sad expression on her face. At times, she became irritable with the nurses. She also has Parkinson disease and anxiety. From interactions with Anne and her family, we learned she had always needed reassurance and familiar people around her to try new things. Knowing this, we arranged our patient assignment so that the number of different nurses working with Anne was minimized. This provided consistency in care and allowed Anne to develop trust with familiar nurses. We also arranged for her husband to be present when the physiotherapist visited. Together, we worked to provide a safe and reassuring environment for Anne. Staff and family encouraged her to participate in therapy. Gradually, Anne developed the confidence to learn to walk with her walker.

1. How did the nursing team provide a nurturing environment to restore Anne's self-confidence and self-concept?
2. How do you imagine Anne's self-concept changed after her stroke?
3. What questions would you like to ask Anne and her husband to gather more data on Anne's current self-concept?

Before leaving our discussion of the formation of self-concept, there are two additional points to consider: self-concept in relation to family and self-concept in collective societies.

Self-Concept in Relation to Family

The dominant North American society prizes individualism. It expects and desires that when children become adults, they will separate from their family of origin to establish their own nuclear families. These expectations influence the development of self-concept and also the measures by which individuals judge themselves. Other cultures within Canadian society have differing world views and do not desire that adult children separate from the family. In these cultures, individual identity may be subsumed within the collective of the family (Kirmayer, Tait, & Simpson, 2009). For our purposes, **culture** refers to a group of people who identify with each other on the basis of some common purpose, need, or background. It may also be a set of learned socially transmitted behaviours and beliefs arising from interactions within the group.

A **world view** is the way an individual or a group of people see their physical and symbolic space and their place in the world. How do different world views influence the development of self-concepts in diverse cultural groups likely to be seen in nursing practice? Differences between cultures are often insidiously incorporated into the psyche and self-concept of nurses, patients, and their families.

Self-Concept in Collective Societies

Western world views emphasize the value of individualism. Individuals are expected to advance themselves financially, academically, and socially to the best of their ability with the belief that this will lead to a more advantageous place in society. In other cultures, such as the Aboriginal cultures, the individual grows up with a world view that places value on multiple connections with family, community, and environment. Striving solely for oneself is not highly valued. Although the traditional Aboriginal world view may vary from tribe to tribe, the commonality of ideas of self within a group collective exists. This is an important consideration when nurses work with Aboriginal people whose self-concept is founded on belief systems, which honour the collective group (Kirmayer & Valaskakis, 2009). Nursing students who have some experiences with Aboriginal cultures tend to do better and experience less anxiety than the students who have not had that opportunity. The students who were exposed to some interactions with Aboriginal people more easily developed cultural self-efficacy wherein they felt comfortable working with diverse cultures (Quine, Hadjistavropoulos, & Alberts, 2012).

As a nurse, you will expect diverse cultural groups to have unique world views influencing their group members' self-concepts and actions. For example, in some Asian and Middle Eastern cultures, obligation to the community will take precedence over individual obligation. The individual and the family will be shamed if this obligation is not honoured. Even within cultural groups, diversity of beliefs and norms occurs and must be considered in the complex development of an individual's self-concept (Shebib, 2011). This diversity is part of the fascination of nursing in a multicultural society.

Think Shannon is an urban nursing student who has requested a clinical placement in a northern Manitoba hospital. She is interested in experiencing nursing within a multicultural setting. Shannon is a third-generation Canadian whose ethnic background is Anglo-Saxon. During her first week on the medical unit, she is given a brief orientation to the diverse cultural groups (Cree, Dene, Inuit) that the hospital serves. The following week, she is caring for a 33-year-old Dene man recently diagnosed with insulin-dependent diabetes. Upon entering the room to discuss diet and insulin management, she notices that seven of the man's relatives are sitting in the room. She becomes flustered and announces she will return. Her patient signals that she can stay. Shannon feels conspicuous and is unsure how to proceed.

1. What would you do? What is your rationale for this action?
2. How is Shannon's self-concept affected by her cultural and ethnic background?
3. How is her Dene patient's self-concept likely affected by his cultural and ethnic background?
4. How would you confirm your assumptions?

The Illness Experience and Its Relationship to the Self-Concept

When a healthy individual becomes ill, a major shift occurs in multiple aspects of the individual's life. Illness results in alterations to physical and mental health frequently evidenced by anxiety and depression, acute stress, and trauma reactions (Mate, 2004). Illness may have a significant impact on the individual's level of independence and functioning, cause alterations in appearance, and changed role performance. These changes and accompanying losses understandably affect the self-concept at a time when the integrity of the patient's

being is threatened. Long-standing views of oneself may be challenged and threatened by illness. Disfiguring illness and surgeries will affect the self-concept of patients, making them feel less desirable and confident in their expression of sexuality. Consider how having a heart attack might lead to fear of exertion and thus impede sexual performance or cause avoidance of sexual activity. Mental illnesses, such as schizophrenia, are highly stigmatized and can cause people with the illness to feel isolated and worthless. People living with schizophrenia state that using cannabis helps them to feel more connected with people and increases their sense of belonging and self-worth (Francoeur & Baker, 2010). In situations of physical and mental illness, how would the patient's self-esteem potentially be decreased? How would you approach working with this patient and family? How would your own attitudes and comfort level with sexuality impede or facilitate your intervention?

As a nurse, you will become sensitized to your patients' and their families' role changes resulting from illness and accident. In times of crisis, both families and patients will have altered self-concepts and self-esteem. In fact, our nursing diagnoses recognize these as areas in which nurses can assist. Imagine the feelings and sense of self a young person who develops epilepsy experiences in trying to understand the changes this will make in her life, the elderly person who develops diabetes after being recently widowed, or the family struggling with the loss of personhood in their elderly parent who is in late-stage dementia. Each situation can be a significant challenge to the self-concept of the individuals involved. As a student nurse, there are times when you will feel ineffective in dealing with situations where you feel you can only minimally affect outcomes and your self-concept will be challenged. This is not unusual; in fact, at times, even experienced nurses will have these feelings. All of these experiences in nursing practice in combination with your foundational growth and developmental and life experiences, help you to develop your unique style of therapeutic use of self in your nursing practice. **Therapeutic use of self** is a crucial element in building a helping relationship with the many people and their families with whom you will assist as a nurse.

Finally, it is important for you as a student to develop strategies that will nurture your self-concept and develop your full potential. These strategies will assist you to maintain and build a strong professional self and will assist in building good relationships with other health-care providers. Nurses work within both intra- and interprofessional health-care teams and ongoing self-awareness will facilitate strong inter-collegial relationships.

By the end of their first clinical practicum, Jason and Emily notice changes in their own sense of self-esteem; for example, when they are feeling low in confidence with a new procedure or when one of them had a positive exchange with a patient. They also notice how their own confidence can positively affect the patient's sense of well-being. They have begun learning to recognize examples of low and high self-esteem and to think about how situations can affect feelings about self.

Conclusion

As a student nurse, you have already started to learn about effective communication, assertion, and conflict resolution so that you can be a fully functioning team member. In this chapter, you have discovered that all concepts that link to your self-concept are a foundational part of who you will become as a nurse. Nurturing your self-concept and being aware of how you react in diverse situations, who you are as a person and a nurse, will assist you to manage issues of nurse bullying and horizontal violence and work toward collaborative and respectful relationships (Johnson & Rea, 2009).

Critical Thinking Case Scenarios

▶ Kyle is a student nurse who is in his senior practicum experience on a busy medical unit. His preceptor is a nurse who has been practicing for 4 years. This is her first time in the role of preceptor. About midway through the practicum, Kyle and the preceptor begin to have a tense relationship. This is partially caused by the fact that Kyle feels that the preceptor only sees what is wrong with his work, is constantly criticizing him, and feels that the feedback he is receiving does not acknowledge his efforts. The preceptor is worried her license is "on the line" and perceives the student as defensive.

1. How might the self-concept of the student nurse be influencing his perceptions of the situation?
2. How might the self-concept of the preceptor be influencing her perception of the situation?
3. How might increased self-awareness of both student and preceptor improve the situation?

▶ Sylvia is a 90-year-old woman who is admitted to the hospital for investigation of a suspected transient ischemic attack (TIA). She has been living in the community with home care supports and family assistance. When you approach her and introduce yourself as her student nurse and that you will be caring for her this evening, she replies in an angry voice that she does not need anyone to take care of her, especially a student, and to leave her alone. You feel yourself becoming angry and catch yourself thinking, "Fine, I have enough to do."

1. What accounts for your reaction from your personal life experiences and your position as a student nurse?
2. What is the possible meaning of Sylvia's behaviour and how would you interpret this related to self-concept theory and Erikson's developmental stages?
3. How could this experience influence the development of your professional self-concept?

▶ Louise is a 75-year-old woman who is a retired accountant. She comes to the community clinic where you are a student nurse. She is concerned about recent vision changes. During your interaction with her, you develop an excellent rapport and are feeling satisfied with how the interaction is proceeding. She then tells you she is a lesbian who has recently come out of the closet. You notice a change in your attitude and an anxious feeling arising within you. You attempt to control your nonverbal communication.

1. What accounts for your change in attitude and your anxiety?
2. What response(s) do you consider appropriate in this situation?
3. How might sexual orientation influence the development and maintenance of a healthy self-concept?

Multiple-Choice Questions

1. You are a nurse on the geriatric medical ward. Mr. Jones is hospitalized for an exacerbation of chronic obstructive pulmonary disease (COPD) triggered by a recent relapse from his alcohol recovery program. When you were growing up, your father had problems with alcohol that often led to family quarrels. You notice that your interactions with Mr. Jones are short, and you are feeling anxious completing his care. What does your reaction and behaviour best indicate?
   a. Insufficient knowledge about the patient
   b. Your organizational skills still require development.
   c. You are unable to handle difficult situations.
   d. An expected response related to your past experiences

2. Your patient is a Dene woman from northern Manitoba. Her care plan indicates a diagnosis of low self-esteem. What culturally sensitive approaches would you use to gather data and interact with her?
   a. Gain knowledge of the Dene culture and communication norms.
   b. Gain knowledge of the history of the Dene people.
   c. Use therapeutic touch in your communication with her.
   d. Sit squarely in front of her and make eye contact.
      1. a, b
      2. a, c
      3. c
      4. all of the above

3. You are a nurse on a busy medical unit that uses a team approach to nursing. You notice that the informal team leader in the group often ignores your suggestions. You begin to feel unsure of your ideas. What is the best way to handle this situation?
   a. Ignore the situation and work around it.
   b. Report this immediately to your unit manager.
   c. Reflect on what is happening and your reactions to it.
   d. Consult with a trusted peer about your perceptions.
      1. a, d
      2. b, d
      3. c, d
      4. b

4. A 16-year-old obese girl is in the community nursing clinic for a weight management program. She states that she is a "loser." She tells you that she feels ugly and has no friends. How would you respond in a way that would enhance her self-concept?
  a. "Once you lose some weight, you will think differently."
  b. "You need to join a sports group."
  c. "I never had many friends when I was your age."
  d. "Tell me about one thing that you are proud of and that makes you happy."

5. Chronic illness often challenges the self-esteem and self-concepts of both patients and families. What type of reactions would you expect from a family whose father has recently undergone an operation that resulted in a permanent colostomy?
  a. The patient will cheerfully accept the colostomy.
  b. The family will have no feelings of repulsion related to managing an ostomy.
  c. Family and patient will have a range of emotions when adjusting to the colostomy.
  d. Family and patient will not feel overwhelmed by the change in bodily functions.

6. James is a 10-year-old boy who has presented in the emergency with a broken arm. He is nervous and anxious. His mother tells you he has a stutter and is difficult to understand. When he talks, you notice he is hesitant and seems embarrassed. What would be the best approach for you to take to help James feel better about himself?
  a. Avoid asking him questions and refer to his mother.
  b. Tell him lots of children stutter.
  c. Reassure him that this will get better as he gets older.
  d. Take time to listen to him and find him a special treat, such as a Popsicle.

REFERENCES AND SUGGESTED READINGS

Benner, P. (1984). *From novice to expert: Excellence and power in clinical nursing practice.* Menlo Park, CA: Addison-Wesley.

Benner, P., & Wrubel, J. (1988). Caring comes first. *The American Journal of Nursing, 88*(8), 1072–1075.

Bowlby, J. (1969). *Attachment and loss: Attachment* (Vol. 1). New York, NY: Basic Books.

Bronfenbrenner, U. (1994). Ecological models of human development. In T. Husen & T. N. Postlethaite (Eds.), *International encyclopedia of education* (Vol. 3, 2nd ed., pp. 1643–1647). Oxford, England: Elsevier Sciences.

Cunha, C., & Goncalves, M. (2009). Commentary: Accessing the experience of a dialogical self: Some needs and concerns. *Culture & Psychology, 15*(1), 120–133.

Erikson, E. (1968). *Identity: Youth and crisis.* New York, NY: Norton.

Erikson, E. (1987). *The life cycle completed: A review.* New York, NY: Norton.

Francoeur, N., & Baker, C. (2010). Attraction to cannabis among men with schizophrenia: A phenomenological study. *Canadian Journal of Nursing Research, 42*(1), 132–149.

Harter, S. (1996). Developmental changes in self-understanding across the 5 to 7 year shift. In A. Sameroff & M. Haith (Eds.), *Reason and responsibility: The passage through childhood* (pp. 204–236). Cambridge, United Kingdom: Cambridge University Press.

Harter, S. (1999). *The construction of self: A developmental perspective.* New York, NY: Guildford Press.

Hartrick Doane, G., & Varcoe, C. (2005). *Family nursing as relational inquiry, developing health-promoting practice.* Philadelphia, PA: Lippincott-Williams Wilkins.

Izard, C. E. (2002). Translating emotion theory and research into preventive interventions. *Psychological Bulletin, 128*(5), 796–824.

Johnson, S. L., & Roe, R. L. (2009). Workplace bullying: Concerns for nurse leaders. *Journal of Nursing Administration, 39*(2), 84–90.

Kirmayer, L. J., Simpson, C., & Cargo, M. (2003). Healing traditions: Culture, community and mental health promotion with Canadian Aboriginal peoples. *Australasian Psychiatry, 11*(Suppl. s1).

Kirmayer, L. J., Tait, C. L., & Simpson, C. (2009). The mental health of indigenous people: Transformation of identity and crisis. In L. J. Kirmayer & G. Guthrie Valaskakis (Eds.), *Healing traditions: The mental health of Aboriginal people in Canada* (pp. 3–35). Vancouver, BC: UBC Press.

Kirkmayer, L. J., & Valaskakis, G. G. (2009). *Healing traditions: The mental health of Aboriginal People in Canada.* Vancouver, BC: University of British Columbia Press.

Mahar, D. J., Iwasiw, C. L., & Evans, M. K. (2012). The Mandala: First-year undergraduate nursing students' learning experiences. *International Journal of Nursing Education Scholarship, 9*(1), 1–16.

Mate, G. (2004). *When the body says no: The cost of hidden stress.* Toronto, ON: Random House.

Meerum-Terwogt, M., & Stegge, H. (2001). The development of emotional intelligence. In I. M. Goodyer (Ed.), *The depressed child and adolescent* (2nd ed., pp. 24–45). New York, NY: Cambridge University Press.

Oliffe, J. L., Han, C. S., Ogrodniczuk, J. S., Philips, J. C., & Roy, P. (2011). Suicide from the perspectives of older men who experience depression: A gender analysis. *American Journal of Men's Health, 5*(5), 444–454. doi:10.1177/1557988311408410

Quine, A. S., Hadjistavropoulos, H. D., & Alberts, N. M. (2012). Cultural self-efficacy of Canadian nursing students caring for Aboriginal patients with diabetes. *Journal of Transcultural Nursing, 23*(3), 306–312. doi:10.1177/1043659612441023

Rogers, C. R. (1961). *On becoming a person: A therapist's view of psychotherapy.* Boston, MA: Houghton Mifflin.

Sawatsky, R. G., Ratner, P. A., Richardson, C. G., Washburn, C., Sudmant, W., & Mirwaldt, P. (2012). Stress and depression on students: The medicating role of stress management self-efficacy. *Nursing Research, 61*(1), 13–21.

Shebib, B. (2011). *Choices: Interviewing and counselling skills for Canadians* (4th ed.). Toronto, Canada: Prentice Hall.

Spurr, S., Bally, J., Ogenchuk, M., & Walker, K. (2012). A framework for exploring adolescent wellness. *Pediatric Nursing, 38*(6), 320–326.

Patient Hygiene

CLAIRE TELLIER, HOW LEE, AND JULIE STANTON

Sarah, a first-year nursing student, is scheduled to perform her first bed bath on Mrs. Jones, an 85-year-old female patient with dementia. Despite hours of preparation in lab time, pre-lab readings, and videos, Sarah finds herself nervous and insecure in her ability to perform the bed bath to the satisfaction of her patient and her observing tutor. As Sarah enters the room, she feels nervous because she wants her patient to feel comfortable. Sarah says to her patient, "Good morning Mrs. Jones, my name is Sarah, and I am a nursing student. I will be doing a bed bath this morning, is that alright with you?" Mrs. Jones responds, "Ok, dear." Sarah introduces her tutor, and then she begins to prepare by filling the basin and ensuring a comfortable temperature. In her head, she reviews the steps of the bed bath. She tells Mrs. Jones step-by-step what she will be doing and asks if she has any preferences for her bed bath. As she starts with washing Mrs. Jones's face, Sarah begins to feel more confident. Sarah continues to tell Mrs. Jones what she is doing, checking that everything is to her satisfaction. When Sarah has finished the bed bath, she rubs lotion on Mrs. Jones's back, chest, legs, and arms; she notices that Mrs. Jones is relaxed and enjoying the extra care that she is getting this morning.

CHAPTER OBJECTIVES

By the end of this chapter, you will be able to:

1. Identify strategies to promote patient participation in hygiene practices.
2. Identify the determinants of health and their relation to hygiene practices.
3. Identify common hygiene practices performed by the nurse and/or patient.
4. Apply knowledge of developmental stages to hygiene practices.
5. Identify factors that affect patient's abilities to perform self-care.
6. Incorporate nursing assessment into hygiene practices.
7. Develop an understanding of the process of basic hygiene skills, including bathing, perineal care, care of feet and nails, hair care, shaving, oral care, eye care, ear care, and toileting.
8. Incorporate assessment of the environment into nursing care.

KEY TERMS

Alopecia Loss of hair from the head and/or body.

Bariatric Equipment Devices that are used to help patients who are overweight.

Caries Cavities due to decay of the enamel of teeth.

Cerumen Earwax that forms inside the ear.

Commode A portable toilet, usually with wheels, that can be placed at the bedside of a patient who has limited activity.

Halitosis Mouth odor.

Hygiene Conditions or practices of cleanliness or care of the body that are conducive to health and wellness.

Pannus A large protuberant abdominal skinfold.

Pediculosis An infection with lice.

Perineal Care Routine procedure to cleanse and perform hygiene on the perineum.

Plaque A substance primarily composed of bacteria and saliva that forms on teeth.

Self-Care Refers to a person's ability to perform primary care functions in the following four areas: bathing, feeding, toileting, and dressing; without the help of others.

Tartar Hardened plaque that remains on teeth.

Urinal An external plastic or metal receptacle for collecting urine.

Xerostomia Dry mouth when the oral mucosa becomes drier as saliva production decreases (a common side effect of many medications).

Routine Hygiene Practices

Routine hygiene practices can be performed by either the patient or the nurse, depending on the patient's level of independence. It is common practice for the nurse to encourage the patient to perform self-care as much as possible and provide assistance only as necessary. **Self-care** is personal health-care maintenance, which patients perform independently. There are many factors that affect one's ability to perform self-care, including illness, injury, age, culture, mental health, and cognitive or functional impairment. Self-care includes not just basic bodily hygiene but fitness, eating well, avoiding health hazards (e.g., smoking), and other steps to avoid illness and

promote well-being. See Box 29.1 for information on hygiene and self-care at different points in the lifespan.

In many instances, nurses will assist the patient with self-care deficits by providing hygiene care or support. The ultimate goal of nursing is to provide support for self-care whenever possible, encouraging the patient to build independence and capacity to do for his or her own.

An individual's routine **hygiene** practice is learned from the family but also influenced by culture and social norms. Self-care can change over time due to aging and depending on the individual's life circumstances, among other factors that may affect a person's hygiene practice, such as environment, socioeconomic status, motivation, and energy (Gillaspie-Aviz, 2013). Encouraging patients to be as independent as possible

BOX 29.1   Lifespan Considerations in Hygiene and Self-Care

Newborn and Infant
- The skin of a newborn is easy to damage and is very sensitive.
- Infants do not need to be washed on a daily basis because this may dry out their skin, although a daily hygiene routine should be performed in order to avoid skin rashes and the risk of infection.
- When bathing, ensure that the skinfolds are being washed and look for accumulation of sebum on the scalp to assess for cradle cap.
- Ensure an adequate bath temperature because infants are sensitive to temperature and can easily lose heat from their bodies.
- Oral health needs to be considered at this stage because the infant's first teeth start to erupt half way through infancy.
- Oral hygiene should be performed once a day even prior to the infant's first tooth eruption to prevent early tooth decay.
- When changing an infant diaper, ensure that the infant is never unattended due to the risk of falls.

Toddler and Preschooler
- It is important to maintain hygiene and to educate children on appropriate hygiene habits because these habits are formed early on.
- Proper oral hygiene helps to set good habits and prevent poor oral hygiene later on in life.
- Educate parents to brush their children's teeth at least twice a day to help prevent cavities.

Child and Adolescent
- Body image is very important to consider when assessing adolescent hygiene to help establish good hygiene habits because their bodies are changing.
- Preschool (who attend preschool or child care facilities) and younger school-aged children are susceptible for pediculosis (head lice infestation), which crosses all economic and social boundaries.
- With the hormonal changes that occur during the adolescent years, many developmental changes occur.
- The eccrine and apocrine glands become fully functional, which increases sweating and causes body odor.

- The sebaceous glands become more active, which causes the development of acne.
- To reduce odor and to help prevent or decrease acne, adolescents have to practice hygiene habits more frequently.
- Educating adolescent girls on hygiene practices during their first menarche helps to maintain a healthy reproductive tract.
- It is important to inform adolescent girls of the risk of toxic shock syndrome (TSS) associated with improper use of tampons, although TSS is rare.
- Educating adolescent girls on proper menstrual hygiene will help to prevent TSS.

Adult and Older Adult
- Hygiene care is as important at this stage as the others in order to prevent infection and to help maintain good self-concept and body image.
- Young to middle adult hygiene practices can be affected by factors such as limited functional and cognitive abilities.
- For the older adult, there is an increased risk for infection.
- Special consideration for hygiene care needs to be considered because of the naturally occurring physiological changes of an older adult.
- The older adults' skin loses its ability to moisten, it is thinner, and the skin becomes less elastic; the skin is increasingly fragile and can break down easily.
- The decreased production of saliva may increase the risk of gum disease or cavities; this is known as **xerostomia** or dry mouth.
- Foot care is important for the older adult due to factors such as naturally occurring physiological changes and diseases such as diabetes.
- Certain conditions can lead to poor oral care such as poorly fitting dentures and physiological changes to the gums.
- Sensory deficits and devices need also to be considered at this stage of development because it is more predominant and plays a role in adequate self-care and quality of life.

Source: Baird, S. K., & Briggs, Y. G. (2010). Hygiene. In P. A. Potter, A. G. Perry, J. C. Ross-Kerr, & M. J. Wood (Eds.), *Canadian fundamentals of nursing* (Rev. 4th ed., pp. 829–878). Toronto, ON: Elsevier; Canadian Public Health Association. (2009). *Caring for you and your baby.* Retrieved from http://you-and-your-baby.cpha.ca/_pdf/cyayb_e _final_web.pdf; Frankowski, B. L., & Bocchini, J. A., Jr. (2010). Head lice. *Pediatrics, 126*(2), 392–403; Gillaspie-Aviz, M. (2013). Hygiene and self care. In R. F. Craven, C. J. Hirnle, & S. Jensen (Eds.), *Fundamentals of nursing human health and function* (7th ed., pp. 599–628). Philadelphia, PA: Lippincott Williams & Wilkins; Health Canada. (2011). *It's your health: Menstrual tampons.* Retrieved from http://www.hc-sc.gc.ca/hl-vs/iyh-vsv/prod/tampons-eng.php; London, M. L., Weiland Ladewig, P. A., Ball, J. W., Bindler, R. C., & Cowen, K. J. (2010). *Maternal & child nursing care* (3rd ed.). New Jersey, NY: Pearson.

promotes independence, positive self-esteem, and dignity as well as enables them to maintain as high a level of physical functioning as possible.

Determinants of Health

Health is determined by circumstance and environment, some of which we can control, and others are unchangeable. Many factors combine to affect health, such as where and how we live, what we eat, genetics, the jobs we hold, income and education level, as well as our personal relationships. The determinants of health include:

• the social and economic environment,
• the physical environment, and
• the person's individual characteristics and behaviours.

These determinants—or things that make people healthy or not—include the given factors and many others:

• Income and social status—Higher income and social status are linked to better health. The greater the gap between the richest and poorest people, the greater the differences in health.
• Education—Low education levels are linked with poor health, more stress, and lower self-confidence.
• Physical environment—Safe water and clean air; healthy workplaces; safe houses, communities, and roads all contribute to good health.
• Employment and working conditions—people in employment are healthier, particularly those who have more control over their working conditions.
• Social support networks—Greater support from families, friends, and communities is linked to better health.
• Culture—customs and traditions and the beliefs of the family and community all affect health.
• Genetics—Inheritance plays a part in determining lifespan, healthiness, and the likelihood of developing certain illnesses. Personal behaviour and coping skills—balanced eating, keeping active, smoking, drinking, and how we deal with life's stresses and challenges all affect health.
• Health services—Access and use of services that prevent and treat disease influences health.
• Gender—Men and women suffer from different types of diseases at different ages. (World Health Organization [WHO], 2013a)

Environment

A country's infrastructure has environmental conditions that can affect the population's access to adequate sanitation facilities, clean water, and proper nutrition, especially in rural areas. Globally, increased mortality rates have been linked to inadequate infrastructure, leading to diarrhea (WHO, 2013b).

Environment can also mean the person's living space. Homelessness affects a person's access to basic hygiene facilities. This increases the risk for skin and foot problems and leads to poor oral hygiene. Individuals who are homeless are at greater risk

for skin diseases such as tinea pedis because of inadequate foot hygiene, poor environmental conditions, and limited access to basic hygiene facilities (Howett, Connor, & Downes, 2010). Restrictions within the physical environment, such as the height of a sink or enough space for a wheelchair to maneuver, among other types of disabilities and limitations, can impair an individual's access to adequate hygiene (Gillaspie-Aviz, 2013).

Socioeconomic Status

A person's level of income affects access to necessities such as safe drinking water, hot water, and appropriate facilities (Baird & Briggs, 2010) as well as to health-care services and affordable medications. Access to these resources will affect one's routine self-care practices through the frequency and one's ability to have a preference of hygiene products.

Individual Characteristics and Behaviours

If self-concept and body image are impaired due to depression or mental illness, they may perceive themselves as not worthy to perform self-care (Gillaspie-Aviz, 2013). For example, patients in institutionalized facilities such as long-term care facilities, with no signs of cognitive or physical impairment, but who display symptoms of depression have demonstrated impaired ability to perform activities of daily living (ADL) such as bathing, dressing, and grooming at an independent level (Drageset, Eide, & Ranhoff, 2011).

Cultural Considerations

Culture interplays with social norms that affect self-care practice, preference, and frequency. Cultural practices and beliefs regarding hygiene need to be considered and accepted when assisting with the care of a patient (Baird & Briggs, 2010).

Cognitive and Functional Ability

One's ability to perform self-care at an independent level is dependent on factors such as range of motion, flexibility, mobility, balance, energy, and motivation. The nurse needs to evaluate at what level the patient can participate in his or her own self-care (Baird & Briggs, 2010).

Patient-Centered Nursing Interventions

When providing nursing interventions in hygiene care, it is important to ensure that it is patient-centered and is performed in a timely, equitable, safe, and efficient manner that allows the patient to verbalize his or her personal preferences in order to retain a sense of dignity and autonomy that allows him or her to feel like he or she is a part of the process (Yeo, 2013). While providing hygiene care, consider the specific needs of the patient, including chronic conditions (e.g., diabetes, heart disease), medications, open sores, personal preference, cognitive impairment, and functional impairments. When self-care is altered, and the nurse is providing care, it is an opportunity not only to connect with the patient but also to assess the patient's physical conditions, for instance, bruises, rashes, skin break down, and pressure ulcers (Gillaspie-Aviz, 2013). Every instance of nurse-provided hygiene care is an opportunity to assess the patient. It is important when providing nursing interventions to be aware of the normal function and appearance of the body in order to identify any abnormalities.

General Body and Hair Hygiene

Routine hygiene practices such as bathing and hair washing help to remove dead skin, dirt, and oil. Proper hygiene practices include bathing, hand washing, grooming, dressing, and oral care. These activities help to increase circulation, prevent infection, and maintain the individual's self-concept and body image.

Feet and Nail Care

Foot and nail care are important especially for those with risk factors such as diabetes. The feet and nails are subject to injury or infections, impairing the person's ability to provide self-care (Baird & Briggs, 2010). Regular washing and adequate trimming of the nails is necessary to prevent problems such as ingrown toenails and infections.

Oral Care

Oral hygiene is important in the prevention of oral disease, and the oral cavity should appear moist and pink. Cavities (**caries**) are caused by **plaque** that forms on the teeth; the plaque then combines with existing bacteria in the mouth to cause decay (Gillaspie-Aviz, 2013), a result of inadequate oral care. **Tartar** is formed when the plaque remains on the teeth and then hardens over time (Gillaspie-Aviz, 2013). Evidence has shown that poor oral health can be associated to diseases such as diabetes and heart disease (Canadian Dental Association, 2013a). Poor oral health can affect quality of life because it can alter the way a person speaks, eats, and the overall appearance, ultimately affecting life on all levels, socially, physically, and emotionally (Canadian Dental Association, 2013b).

Risk of Deficit for Self-Care

The nurse identifies factors that may put the patient at risk for a self-care deficit. The following are risk factors that may affect the patient's ability to perform self-care:

- Pain
- Limited mobility
- Neuromuscular impairment
- Changes in cognition or mental status
- Decreased visual acuity or other sensory deficits
- Inability to control bladder or bowel function
- Fatigue or decrease energy level
- Socioeconomic or health determinant–related factors

Physical and mental state assessments can confirm risk factors. If there is incongruence with what the nurse observes and with what the patient states, this should be explored further or taken into account when developing a care plan for the patient.

Providing Care for the Obese Patient

An individual is considered obese if his or her body mass index (BMI) is greater than 30 kg/m^2 and is classified as morbidly obese if his or her weight decreases his or her functional ability. Patients who are obese may have feelings of embarrassment about their weight and be reluctant to ask for assistance with personal care.

Mobility, particularly in small spaces, is difficult for morbidly obese patients. They have skinfolds that are prone to skin breakdown and infection. A large abdominal skinfold, (referred to as the **pannus**), the skin under the breasts, and in the inner thigh area are prone to breakdown and must be assessed, cleansed, and dried thoroughly at least once daily. Any areas of redness or raw-looking skin are reported immediately so that appropriate measures can be taken. Morbidly obese patients may not be able to bend over to perform foot care and have a higher incidence of diabetes and foot problems secondary to their weight. Proper self-cleaning after toileting may also be challenging for these patients, particularly after bowel movements. The nurse may be required to provide assistance with foot and perineal care. Special **bariatric equipment** may be required to hold the increased weight and provide safe care to the patient, such as bariatric beds, wheelchairs, walkers, **commodes**, and mechanical lifts.

Assessing for Alterations in Self-Care

Self-care deficits arise in both community and acute care settings. Deficits can range from short to long term and from simple to complex. Nursing interventions in hygiene care are provided where the nurse identifies a deficit. This is also an opportunity for nursing education in self-care.

Poor Hygiene and Grooming

On visual inspection, hair may be unwashed and uncombed. There may be an odor from the mouth (**halitosis**) or the mouth may have sores or caries, inflamed gums, bleeding or chapped lips, and missing or stained teeth. Clothes may be soiled, disheveled, and inappropriate for the weather or environmental setting. Skin may be dry and dirty, or there may be other skin care issues such as rashes or areas with broken skin. Nail beds may be dirty and broken. The feet may have sores or cracked skin. There may be an unpleasant body odor indicating soiled clothing, or that the patient has not showered or bathed. An odor of urine or feces may indicate difficulty in toileting.

Inability to Demonstrate Self-Care Activities

Difficulties with gross and fine motor coordination may impair the ability to use the bathroom, bathe, dress, and eat. Problems with gross and fine motor skills may be a result of other comorbidities or health issues and are important to document in the patient's health history.

Verbalization of Reluctance to Perform Self-Care

When the patient expresses reluctance or fear to perform self-care activities, physical and mental factors may be present. Physical factors can be related to an existing condition or illness such as pain or fatigue, which leads to inability to perform a self-care activity. Mental factors may be related to mental illness (e.g., depression or schizophrenia), altered cognition, or issues related to self-image and self-esteem.

Health History and Assessment

The nurse gathers subjective and objective data to determine areas that may be problematic for self-care. The nurse asks questions to identify the patient's views toward self-care, feelings about problems and potential solutions, and values and motivation toward changing his or her self-care ability. The nurse maintains therapeutic and nonjudgmental communication techniques and uses open-ended questions to uncover the underlying reasons for and difficulties in performing hygiene and grooming. If family members are present, they can provide perceptions of the patient's self-care ability.

The information provided by the patient is helpful in planning and individualizing patient care, and whenever possible, the patient's hygiene preferences should be taken into account. Keep in mind that due to the scheduled and regimented nature of completing tasks in many health-care facilities, a patient's preferences may not always be met. However, the nurse should try to accommodate patient's preferences if possible.

Normal self-care patterns can be categorized according to the assistance require by the patient. See Table 29.1 for a summary of the levels of care, with Level 0 representing complete independence and Level 4 reflecting complete dependence on others.

TABLE 29.1	Levels of Care	
Level	Description	Example
0	Patient is independent in self-care activities.	Healthy young adult living alone in an apartment
1	Patient uses equipment or devices to perform self-care activities independently.	Older adult who uses a cane for support while walking
2	Patient requires assistance or supervision from another to complete self-care activities.	Adult patient who needs help bathing on the first day after surgery
3	Patient requires assistance or supervision from another and uses devices or equipment.	Older adult who uses a bath chair and needs contact supervision stepping out of the tub
4	Patient completely depends on another to perform self-care activities.	Comatose patient who requires complete care from nursing staff

From Craven, R., Hirnle, C., & Jensen, S. (2013). *Fundamentals of nursing: Human health and function* (7th ed.). Philadelphia, PA: Lippincott Williams & Wilkins.

Dysfunction Identification

The Index of Independence in Activities of Daily Living developed by Katz in 1983 helps with assessment and determining the level of independence in self-care (Table 29.2). This tool provides a comparison of normal self-care with deficits in self-care. Changes to self-care are a normal part of aging and may be altered by illnesses.

TABLE 29.2	Index of Independence in Activities of Daily Living	
ADL	Independent	Dependent
Bathing (sponge, shower, tub)	Patient needs assistance only in bathing a single part (e.g., back or disabled extremity) or bathes self completely.	Patient needs assistance in bathing more than one part of body; needs assistance in getting in or out of tub or does not bathe self.
Dressing	Patient gets clothes from closets and drawers; puts on clothes, outer garments, braces; manages fasteners (act of tying shoes is excluded).	Patient does not dress self or remains partly undressed.
Toileting	Patient gets to toilet, gets on and off toilet, arranges clothes, and cleans organs of excretion (may manage bedpan at night or may not be using mechanical supports).	Patient uses bedpan or commode or needs assistance getting to and using toilet.
Transferring	Patient moves in and out of bed and chair independently (may be using mechanical supports).	Patient needs assistance in moving in or out of bed or chair; does not perform one or more transfers.
Continence	Patient has self-control over urination and defecation.	Patient has partial or total incontinence in urination or defecation; partial or total control by enemas, catheters, or regulated use of urinals or bedpans.
Feeding	Patient gets food from plate into mouth; precutting of meat and preparation of food (e.g., buttering bread) are excluded from evaluation.	Patient needs assistance in feeding; does not eat at all or uses parenteral feeding.

From Craven, R., Hirnle, C., & Jensen, S. (2013). *Fundamentals of nursing: Human health and function* (7th ed.). Philadelphia, PA: Lippincott Williams & Wilkins.

Diagnoses

North American Nursing Diagnosis Association (NANDA) identifies the nursing diagnosis for a patient with a self-care deficit as Self-Care Deficit Syndrome. Related self-care nursing diagnoses and nursing interventions and nursing outcomes can be found in the NANDA and NIC and NOC publications listed in the "References and Suggested Readings" at the end of this chapter.

Providing Hygiene Care to Patients

Patients may feel anxious or embarrassed about requiring assistance with hygiene. It is important to demonstrate respect and sensitivity to patient's preferences, privacy, and modesty. Doors should be closed, and curtains drawn around the patient care area during bathing, dressing, or toileting. Patients may be uncomfortable having these activities provided by a caregiver of the opposite gender; conversely, some care providers might be uncomfortable providing intimate care to a patient of the opposite gender (Inoue, Chapman, & Wynaden, 2006). Patient preferences may be indicated on the care plan in order to assist managers in assigning staff to them appropriately as often as possible.

It is important to promote self-care independence as much as possible in the provision of hygiene care. In order to do this, have necessary supplies and equipment available to assist patients in achieving the highest level of independence possible. Providing a walker to assist a patient in mobilizing to the washroom is an example of a strategy that can be used.

Time spent providing assistance to patients is an opportunity for the nurse to develop a trusting relationship with the patient. Activities such as bathing, shampooing, and brushing a patient's hair can be relaxing and soothing for the patient. Having pleasant conversations during these activities fosters feelings of comfort, well-being, and self-worth. They provide hospitalized or long-term care patients an opportunity to interact with other people.

Specific types of hygienic care are provided at regular intervals to promote patient comfort as well as nurse's planning. Box 29.2 includes common hygiene measures provided.

Bathing and Skin Care

Bathing and skin care are an important part of routine hygiene care. Bathing cleanses the skin of accumulated oil, perspiration, dead skin cells, and certain bacteria. It promotes circulation; warmth dilates superficial arterioles, which brings more blood and nutrients to the skin. In addition, it promotes a sense of well-being for patients, improving morale, appearance, and self-image.

The timing, extent, and type of bath provided to patients depend on multiple factors, including physical abilities, health status, and type of hygiene care required. Timing of routine bathing varies; some patients prefer to bathe early in the day to feel energized and refreshed, whereas evening bathing promotes relaxation. Although it is not always possible to establish routines based on patient's preference, most appreciate the opportunity to wash their hands and faces in the morning and prior to sleep. Bathing frequency is determined by evaluating patient need rather than by adhering to schedules established for staff convenience. Too frequent bathing, especially in older adults, can lead to dry skin contributing to skin breakdown. Patients who are comatose, cognitively impaired, have excessive body excretions or draining wounds, or physically dependent require bathing at least once per day,

---

BOX 29.2   Scheduling Hygiene Care

Early Morning Care
Comfort Measures and Preparation for the Day

- Bedpan, **urinal**, or assistance to bathroom
- Preparation for diagnostic tests or early surgery
- Washing hands and face
- Oral care
- Preparation for breakfast

Morning Care (AM Care)
Hygiene and Grooming

- Bedpan, urinal, or assistance to bathroom
- Bath, shower, or bathing
- Back massage
- Hair care and shaving
- Oral care
- Care for feet and nails
- Dressing
- Bed linen change

- Straightening bedside unit
- Positioning (bed or chair)

Afternoon Care
After Tests, After Lunch, and Before Visitors

- Bedpan, urinal, or assistance to bathroom
- Washing hands and face
- Oral care
- Bed linens and repositioning if needed

Hour-of-Sleep (HS) Care
Comfort Measures and Bedtime

- Bedpan, urinal, or assistance to bathroom
- Washing hands and face
- Oral care
- Back massage
- Bed linens (change soiled linens, fluff pillow, pull out wrinkles)
- Bedclothes
- Straightening unit (place needed night objects within reach)

From Craven, R., Hirnle, C., & Jensen, S. (2013). *Fundamentals of nursing: Human health and function* (7th ed.). Philadelphia, PA: Lippincott Williams & Wilkins.

TABLE 29.3	Therapeutic Baths	
Type	**Purpose**	**Nursing Considerations**
Sitz bath	To cleanse, soothe, and reduce inflammation of perineal or vaginal area after childbirth, vaginal or rectal surgery, or from local irritation of hemorrhoids and fissures	Water temperature depends on the patient's condition and person preference but is usually 40°C to 45°C.
Hot water bath	To relieve muscle spasms and soreness by total immersion	Water temperature should be 45 to 46°C but may be individualized to patient's condition and preference. Remember that older patients, those with sensory deficits, and those with slow or absent reflexes are at risk for burns with hot water. Be alert for vasodilation with resultant orthostatic blood pressure drop and for scalding of skin.
Warm water bath	To cleanse, promote relaxation, and relieve tension	Adjust water temperature to patient's preference.
Cool water bath	To relieve muscle tension or decrease body temperature in febrile patients	Water should be tepid (37°C), not cold. Avoid chilling; shivering may increase body temperature.
Soak	To soften and loosen secretions during dressing changes or to reduce pain and swelling or itching of inflamed or irritated skin	Medications or topical agents may be added to the water. Apply hot, warm, or cold water to an isolated body part.

From Craven, R., Hirnle, C., & Jensen, S. (2013). *Fundamentals of nursing: Human health and function* (7th ed.). Philadelphia, PA: Lippincott Williams & Wilkins.

sometimes more frequently, to assess skin and avoid skin irritation, breakdown, and infection. Bathing provides the nurse with an excellent opportunity to assess the skin for edema, rashes, or areas of redness. Assessment of the patient's psychosocial state, including orientation to time and day, as well as his or her learning needs, for example, related to diabetic foot care, is also possible during provision of hygiene care.

Methods of Bathing

There are multiple methods of assisted bathing, the selection of which is dependent on the patient's conditions and abilities.

- Tub baths
- Stand-up shower
- Sit-down shower with shower chair
- Complete bed bath
- Partial bed bath
- Bag bath
- Partial bath at sink or basin

The nurse considers the patient's abilities when assessing which type of bath to use and select the method that encourages self-care the most effectively. Factors to consider include the patient's energy level, other activities planned for the day, surgical sites or areas of the body needing to be kept dry, preference, and self-care capabilities. Various types of therapeutic baths are listed in Table 29.3.

Certain methods are preferable for patients to perform independently or with limited assistance. By providing required equipment to those patients, the nurse encourages the patients to bathe themselves, providing assistance only for such things as washing their back and feet. Although tub baths provide more effective cleaning and rinsing because the patient is fully submerged, they require greater mobility and agility on the part of the patient. See Skill 29.1 for the steps in assisting patients with a tub bath or shower.

Partial Bed Bath

Partial bed bath includes washing the patient's face, hands, underarms, and perineal region. This type of bed bath may be required for patients with excessive secretions such as sweat or draining wounds or can be used when time does not allow for a full bed bath but the patient requires freshening up. It may also be performed at nighttime to promote a better sleep.

Bag Bath

Disposable bag baths have been introduced in response to concerns regarding infection control and skin drying associated with traditional bathing methods. Improper cleaning of wash basin and tubs promotes growth of Gram-negative organisms. Commercially prepared package baths contain 6 to 10 washcloths remoistened with a combination of water and rinse-free cleanser and are generally stored in a warming unit until needed (Fig. 29.1). A different cloth is used for each part of the patient's body to avoid cross-contamination when washing different body parts. Skin is allowed to air dry when using these products, as towel drying the skin removes the emollient that is left behind. A benefit of bag baths is that they reduce bathing times and increase both patient and nurse satisfaction (Larson et al., 2004).

Working from distal to proximal when washing extremities promotes circulation and venous return. In order to promote skin health and integrity, ensure adequate fluid intake, avoid too frequent bathing with harsh soaps or detergents or water that is too hot, and use of defatting solutions on the skin, such as alcohol. Promote skin moisture with practices, such as applying moisturizer frequently, and encourage patients to do the same.

Bed Bath

Some patients are unable to bathe themselves because they are too weak or even comatose. This may necessitate bathing the patient in bed. See Skill 29.2 for the steps. If time permits and patient desires it, a back rub or massage is generally performed at the end of the bath.

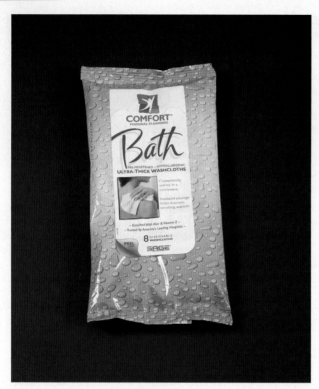

Figure 29.1 Disposable bathing cloths.

Back Massage

A back rub or massage can promote comfort and relaxation, relieve muscle tension, improve sleep, and enhance blood supply to the skin and muscles (Ebersole, Hess, Touhy, Jett, & Scmidt-Luggen, 2008). Positive outcomes related to a back rub include reduction in blood pressure, reduced pain, and decreased anxiety and depression (Zullino, Krenz, Frésard, Cancela, & Khazaal, 2005). Not all patients are comfortable with physical contact; thus, it is important for the nurse to assess the patient's level of comfort with this prior to beginning. It is important to ensure there are no contraindications to back massage. To determine the degree of pressure to use, the nurse observes the patient's verbal and nonverbal response, beginning with light touch and slowly progressing to firmer touch, within the patient's comfort range.

The use of cream or lotion helps the nurse's hands to glide more smoothly over the patient's skin and promotes comfort. Alcohol is not recommended for use during massage because it is drying to the skin and can lead to cracking and skin breakdown in patients with dehydration or older adults.

Patients are positioned appropriately prior to performing a back rub. For patients who can lie in the prone position, this allows the easiest access to the most surface area of the back to the nurse. For immobile patients who cannot lie in this position, a side-lying position can be used. Skill 29.3 demonstrates how to perform a back massage.

Perineal Care

Perineal care is part of a complete bed bath and is performed by the nurse if the patient is unable to do so himself or herself. Performing perineal care may be embarrassing for both the patient

and the nurse, especially when they are of the opposite gender. This is not a reason for the nurse to overlook this important aspect of hygiene care. Providing care using a professional, dignified, and sensible approach can reduce embarrassment and put both parties more at ease (Grant, Giddings, & Beale, 2005).

Due to the fact that perineal tissue is very sensitive, the nurse is cautious to avoid temperature extremes. For patients who cannot be bathed in the tub or shower, pouring water gently over the perineum with the patient sitting on a toilet or bedpan promotes patient comfort and allows for better rinsing.

Patients who are incontinent of urine or feces or have drainage from the perineal area require more frequent cleansing. Patients at greatest risk for infection such as those with indwelling urinary catheters, those recovering from rectal or genital surgery, uncircumcised males, or those who are morbidly obese require more frequent perineal care. Women who are having a menstrual period may require assistance in order to perform appropriate perineal care. While the nurse provides care, there is an opportunity to also provide patient teaching regarding proper perineal and genital care. Patients capable of performing this care independently should always be encouraged to do so. The nurse should always wear gloves when performing perineal care and while handling items that may be contaminated with drainage from the area.

For women, perineal care involves cleansing of the upper inner thighs, the labia majora, and the folds between the labia majora and minora (Fig. 29.2A).

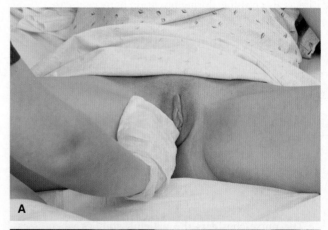

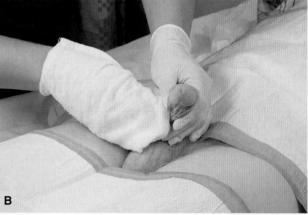

Figure 29.2 Perineal care of female patient (**A**) and male patient (**B**).

Perineal care for men involves cleansing of the upper inner thighs, the penis, and the scrotum. For uncircumcised men, the foreskin of the penis is retracted in order that the glans of the penis can be properly washed. The foreskin is rolled back into place once the skin is clean and dry (Fig. 29.2B). For both men and women, the buttocks and anus are cleansed with the patient lying on his or her side.

Sitz Bath

A sitz bath, or hip bath, can be used to soak a patient's pelvic area in warm water in order to decrease inflammation. This is useful after childbirth or rectal surgery or to decrease inflammation associated with hemorrhoids. By immersing only the pelvic region, heat is applied locally, promoting circulation to the pelvic area without widespread vasodilation, which results when the legs are also immersed. The patient sits in a special chair or tub for 15 to 20 minutes (Fig. 29.3). Portable devices that can be placed in the toilet may be used. These are disposable and circulate warm water through the device from a bag. Water temperature should be maintained between 40° and 43°C to prevent burning the patient.

Care of Feet and Nails

In order to identify health problems, or those at risk for developing foot and nail problems, it is important to assess the appearance of feet and nails. Regular foot and nail care should be incorporated into the patient's regular hygiene

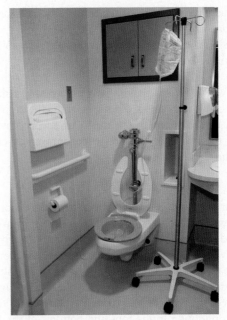

Figure 29.3 Sitz bath.

routine. Table 29.4 describes common foot problems, their causes, and treatment.

Family members or care providers take responsibility for providing thorough, regular foot care to those at high risk if patients are unable to perform this for their own. Patients with visual difficulties, mobility constraints, or cognitive impairment

TABLE 29.4	Common Foot Problems		
Type	Description	Possible Causes	Treatment
Calluses	Flattened thickening of epidermis, often on bottom or side of foot over a bony prominence	Tight shoes or inadequate padding in shoes	Soften by soaking in warm water and abrade with pumice stone.
Corns	Cone-shaped lesion (thickening of epidermis) usually on fourth or fifth toe over toe joint	Pressure from tight shoes	Wear softer, better-fitting shoes or foam protective pads; apply keratolytic agents with salicylic acid to keratinous skin.
Plantar warts	Round or irregular, flattened by pressure, surrounded by cornified epithelium; often painful	Virus, but may be worsened by inadequate circulation or pressure from tight shoes	Remove by curettage, freezing with solid carbon dioxide, or application of salicylic acid.
Bunions (hallux valgus)	Inflammation and thickening of bursa of the great toe joint; enlargement of joint and displacement of toe	Hereditary, degenerative bone and joint disease, and tight shoes or high heels	Surgical intervention may be needed, or patient can achieve symptomatic relief by wearing shoes that are wide at the front.
Ringworm, tinea pedis (athlete's foot)	Redness, scaling, and cracking of skin especially between toes	Fungus, worsened by moist, unventilated environment	Apply antifungal powder or ointment; change socks daily; wear 100% cotton socks to absorb moisture.
Ingrown nails	Inflammation, swelling, and tissue pain at edge of nail	Improper nail trimming, poorly fitting shoes	Prevent by trimming nails straight across and wearing well-fitted shoes. Pain and inflammation are treated with anti-inflammatory agents. Surgical removal of nail may be required.
Foot odor	Excessive foul odor of feet	Possibly from fungal foot infections; exacerbated by hot, moist environment	Decrease excess moisture; use deodorant foot powders, 100% cotton socks, and well-ventilated shoes.

require caregiver or family assistance as well (Canadian Diabetes Association, 2008; Smeltzer & Bare, 2013).

Perfusion can be assessed by evaluating skin colour and temperature. Cold, dusky feet may be a sign of poor circulation. Patients with diabetes mellitus, older adults, and patients with poor circulation have an increased risk of foot problems; and thus, proper foot care and education regarding self-care are essential. The nurse can incorporate teaching into the provision of care to encourage self-care and monitoring for foot problems.

Patients With Diabetes

Particular attention is required when providing foot care to patients with diabetes who are at greater risk for injury due to decreased sensation. Daily inspection and thorough cleansing with warm water and gentle soap is required. Feet should not be soaked in water because this can cause dry skin leading to cracking. Careful attention is paid to thoroughly dry feet, especially between the toes. It is acceptable to apply moisturizing lotion to the tops and bottoms of the feet but never between the toes because excess moisture in this area can lead to infection. Toenails should be trimmed straight across, and their edges filed with an emery board.

Patients With Peripheral Vascular Disease

Patients with peripheral vascular disease are cautioned not to cut nails too short or to cut into calluses. Due to delayed healing times and risk of infection in patients with diabetes and peripheral vascular disease, some institutions have policies in place that prevent nurses from cutting the toenails of these patients. These patients are at increased risk of developing chronic foot ulcers, which heal very slowly and are difficult to treat. It is often challenging to cut the toenails of these patients because they can become thick and distorted, thus increasing the risk of accidental injury. Toenails may be safely filed. Be familiar with your clinical agency's policy prior to providing foot care. Skill 29.4 outlines nursing care of feet and nails.

Patient education is paramount for those with diabetes mellitus or peripheral vascular disease. Research has demonstrated that many patients have not learned or do not practice proper foot and nail care (Canadian Diabetes Association, 2008; Smeltzer & Bare, 2013). It is essential to ensure patients understanding about the direct effect of circulation on the health and integrity of tissues. Review the guidelines for routine foot and nail care from the Canadian Diabetes Association in Box 29.3.

Hair Care

A patient's appearance and sense of well-being can be greatly improved by brushing or combing hair. Patients able to perform this task independently should be given proper equipment and encouraged to do so. Body image is closely related to proper hair care; this includes brushing, combing, and washing hair.

Brushing and Combing

Frequent hair brushing helps keep hair clean by distributing oil along the hair shaft and prevents tangling as well as massaging the scalp and promoting circulation. Patients with long hair who are confined to bed can quickly develop mats and tangles; combing hair daily and tying it back or braiding it helps to minimize this. For patients with scalp incisions or lacerations, blood, topical medications, or dressings can increase tangling. If hair becomes tangled, it is divided into small sections that are brushed first from the ends, working the way up to the roots, and then combed. For patients with tightly curled hair, a wide-toothed comb or pick or firm bristled brush should be used. Combing with the fingers can also loosen tangles. Braids should be undone regularly and the hair combed to ensure appropriate hygiene because braids that are too tight can lead to bald patches. Patient permission should be obtained whenever possible prior to braiding hair. Prior to cutting a patient's hair, the nurse should check his or her institution's policy regarding this practice. Written consent or a doctor's order may be required.

The nurse takes cultural differences into account when caring for patients because these may affect how hair is combed or styled. Consultation with the patient and/or family regarding preferred hairstyle practices is important (Briggs, 2010).

Shampooing

Shampooing hair and scalp removes excess oil, promotes circulation, and provides a relaxing experience for the patient. It provides the nurse with an opportunity to inspect for lice, dandruff, or dermatitis. Ambulatory patients are generally shampooed in a shower or bath chair using hand-held shower nozzles. Those able to sit in a chair may use the sink or a wash basin; however, bending is contraindicated in certain conditions—for example, eye surgery or neck injury. Patients unable to sit up or ambulate can be shampooed in bed using a special trough or tray, which is positioned under the patient's head to catch water and suds, and has a spout for drainage. The nurse ensures the patient is kept warm throughout the process and assesses for fatigue (Skill 29.5). Conditioner may be used to soften hair, decrease tangling, and minimize breakage.

Commercially prepared shampoo caps are available at some institutions, which are kept in a warmer until needed. The cap, containing cleansing solution, is placed on the patient's scalp. Long hair is gathered under the cap. The cap is massaged by either the nurse or the patient to release the cleansing solution and work it into the hair and scalp. No rinsing is required. Hair can either be blow-dried or allowed to air-dry.

Lice

Lice infestation is called **pediculosis**. Pediculosis capitis refers to lice found on the hair of the head, eyebrows, eyelashes, and beard. Pediculosis corporis refers to lice found in body hair, and pediculosis pubis refers to lice found in the hair of the perineal area.

BOX 29.3 Guidelines for Foot Care for Patients With Diabetes Mellitus or Peripheral Vascular Disease

- Inspect feet daily, looking at the tops and soles, heels, and between the toes. A mirror may be required for thorough inspection, or a family member can help.
- Feet should be thoroughly assessed by a health-care professional at least once per year for patients with diabetes mellitus. Those with one or more high-risk foot conditions should be assessed more frequently and referred to a specialist as appropriate.
- Feet should be washed daily with lukewarm water and gentle soap but never soaked. Those with reduced sensation may want to use a bath thermometer to test water temperature and prevent burning. Feel should be thoroughly dried, including between the toes, with a towel.
- Corns or calluses should never be cut, commercial removers should not be used; rather they should be assessed by a physician or podiatrist.
- Apply nonallergenic foot powder if feet perspire heavily.
- Nonallergenic lotion can be gently applied if dryness is noted along the sides of the feet. Excess lotion should be wiped off, and lotion should never be applied between the toes because excess moisture can lead to infection.
- Toenails should be filed straight across and square; scissors, clippers, or other sharp objects should not be used. A podiatrist can be consulted as required.
- Over-the-counter preparations to treat athlete's foot or ingrown toenails should not be used; a physician or podiatrist should be consulted.
- Elastic stockings, knee-high hose, constricting garters, smoking, and crossing the legs while sitting should be avoided because these can impair circulation to the lower extremities.

- Socks or stockings should be changed daily. If feet perspire heavily, change twice daily. Socks should be dry and free of holes or repairs that could cause pressure areas.
- Avoid walking barefoot.
- Shoes should be properly fitted with porous uppers. Soles of shoes should be flexible and nonslip. Shoes should be sturdy, closed in, and not restrict feet. Patients with increased plantar pressure due to erythema or callus should wear shoes that cushion and redistribute pressure. Those with bony deformities, for example, bunions, may require extra wide or deep shoes with cushioned insoles. Shoes should be purchased in the afternoon or evening when feet are larger due to swelling.
- High-heeled, open-toed, or pointed-toe shoes should not be worn.
- New shoes should not be worn for an extended period of time but rather be worn over short periods over several days to be broken in. Observe for signs of skin breakdown or irritation throughout this process.
- Regular exercise improves circulation to the lower extremities. Slow walking and elevation, rotation, flexion, and extension of the feet and ankles also helps. Dangle feet over the side of the bed for 1 minute, then extend both legs and hold them parallel to the bed while lying supine for 1 minute, and then rest for 1 minute.
- Use extra blankets rather than hot water bottles or heating pads.
- Minor cuts should be washed immediately and thoroughly dried using only mild antiseptics such as Neosporin ointment. Iodine or merbromin should be avoided. If cuts or lacerations occur, contact a physician.
- Notify physician or podiatrist of any changes in temperature, colour, or sensation of the feet, or of any abnormal sores, drainage, or pain.

Source: Canadian Diabetes Association. (2008). *2008 Clinical practice guidelines for the prevention and management of diabetes in Canada.* Retrieved from http://www.diabetes.ca/files/cpg2008/cpg-2008.pdf; Canadian Diabetes Association. (2012a). *Foot care: A step towards good health.* Retrieved from http://www.diabetes.ca/diabetes-and-you/healthy-guidelines/foot-care-a-step-toward-good-health/; Canadian Diabetes Association. (2012b). *Skin problems.* Retrieved from http://www.diabetes.ca/diabetes-and-you/living/complications/skin-problems/; Smeltzer, S. C., & Bare, B. (2013). *Brunner & Suddarth's textbook of medical-surgical nursing* (12th ed.). Philadelphia, PA: Lippincott Williams & Wilkins.

Head and pubic lice attach their eggs, called *nits*, to hairs using a sticky substance that makes them difficult to remove. Nits resemble shiny ovals and are visible with good lighting and a magnifying glass. It can be difficult to differentiate between nits and dandruff. Lice live on the skin and bite, causing itching; inflamed bite marks can be seen along the hairline. Body lice suck blood from the skin and live in clothing, which makes them harder to detect. Scratching and hemorrhagic lesions on the skin are indications that body lice may be present.

Permethrin (Nix) is the most common over-the-counter treatment for pediculosis capitis. Generally, this treatment is performed once then repeated a few days later to prevent recurrence. Lindane (Kwell) is the usual treatment for pediculosis corporis or pediculosis pubis and comes in lotion, cream, and shampoo forms. Pubic lice can be difficult to remove due to thicker hair in the area; shampoo should be applied and left on for 12 to 24 hours. Infested clothing should be discarded; linens and clothing used by patients with lice are washed thoroughly in hot water. Furniture, blankets, and carpets can be treated with insecticide. Those with whom affected patients have had intimate or sexual contact should be treated.

If pediculicidal shampoo is prescribed, patients and/or caregivers require instructions on proper use. Neurological side effects may be associated with these shampoos; toxic effects are most likely in the very young or very old and can lead to seizures, dizziness, headaches, paresthesia, and even death. Patients who are HIV positive, those with neurological conditions, neonates, or those weighing less than 50 kg should not use this type of medication (Zurlinden, 2003). Using too much shampoo, too frequent repeating of shampooing, or leaving it on too long are most commonly associated with side effects. Itching is a common side effect of the shampoo, which can cause some patients to overtreat because they incorrectly believe that continued itching means the lice survived the initial treatment (Zurlinden, 2003).

Dandruff

Dandruff refers to generalized scaling of the epidermis of the scalp that is chronic, causes itching, and is associated with flaking white scales. Severe cases can lead involve the auditory canals or eyebrows. In most cases, it can be treated effectively with a keratolytic shampoo; however, severe or persistent cases may require that the patient consult a physician. The nurse should also assess for eczema or scalp dermatitis, which is red, itchy, swollen, and sometimes fluid-filled lumps on the scalp that may ooze and crust (Canadian Dermatology Association, 2013).

Hair Loss

Hair loss and growth are a continuous process. In order to avoid damage to hair, chemical treatments and excessive heat associated with drying on the high setting or electric curling irons should be avoided. To keep hair free of tangles and promote moisture, conditioner should be used.

When male patients reach middle to old age, they may begin to experience male pattern baldness or hair loss. This is thought to be hereditary and can occur earlier in some men. There is currently no known solution other than the use of hair pieces or costly hair transplantation. Certain medications are being developed; however, the long-term outcomes of these are not currently known (Fisk, 2010).

Loss of hair can have significant effects for patient, including altered self-image and sexual identity. Certain conditions can lead to acute hair loss, including stress, high fevers, certain medications, general anesthesia, or childbirth. Hair loss (**alopecia**) is most commonly caused by cancer treatment.

Shaving

Shaving is a simple way to help male patients feel better about their physical appearance, make them more comfortable, and boost their morale. Most men who do not wear beards shave daily. Shaving is easiest after a shower or bath when hair is softened, which reduces cuts and nicks. Alternatively, the hair can be softened with warm towels prior to shaving. Lather the face well with soap or shaving cream, pull the skin taut, and shave with the direction of hair growth to reduce irritation using short, regular strokes (Fig. 29.4). Shaving the patient is a skill that improves with practice.

Patients capable of communication can provide the nurse with instructions about how to shave each area of their face. Dark-skinned patients may have curly facial hair, which can become ingrown if not kept closely shaved. For older men, those with coarser facial hair, or those with decreased energy or fine motor skills, electric razors are easier to use. For patients at risk for bleeding, such as those taking anticoagulants or who have bleeding disorders or thrombocytopenia, electric razors should be used to avoid cuts. When using electric razors, check for frayed cords or other electrical hazards and be familiar with your institution's policy regarding the use of these devices. To maintain appropriate infection control, razors should never be shared between patients.

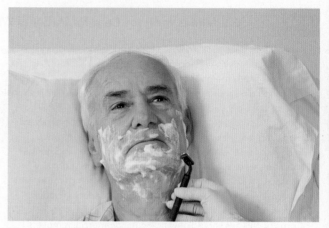

Figure 29.4 Male patient being shaved.

Beards and mustaches need to be trimmed and kept clean of food particles and mucus. Facial hair should be washed during the patient's bath or shower. Never shave off a patient's mustache or beard without obtaining prior consent from the patient. Check your institution's policy regarding this practice because written consent or a physician's order may be required. The nurse considers the cultural and religious preferences or practices of the patient.

For women, shaving the legs and underarms may be considered part of the patient's regular hygiene routine. Shaving is most easily done while bathing or in the shower. Techniques used for women are the same as those used for men.

Oral Care

Oral hygiene is essential for the maintenance of a healthy mouth, teeth, gums, lips, and tongue (Canadian Dental Association, 2013a). Rinsing the mouth soothes dryness and promotes comfort. Brushing teeth removes food, plaque, and bacteria; massages the gums; and relieves discomfort associated with unpleasant tastes and odors. Flossing removes plaque and bacteria from between the teeth, reduces gum inflammation and infection, and helps prevent cavities and periodontal disease. Thorough oral hygiene promotes comfort, enhances well-being, stimulates the appetite, and provides the nurse an opportunity to assess the oral cavity. See Skill 29.6 for guidelines on providing oral care.

Brushing and Flossing

Patients who can brush and floss independently should be encouraged to do so. Water, basins, and other necessary supplies can be provided to patients who are unable to get out of bed. Electric toothbrushes are helpful for those who cannot grip a traditional small-handled toothbrush. Regular toothbrush handles can be enlarged by wrapping with tape, gluing a short piece of plastic tubing around the handle, or piercing a soft rubber ball and pushing the handle through it. Weighted easy-grip handles can be purchased to modify toothbrushes and shaving razors.

Brushing should be encouraged at least four times per day, after meals and before bed. Patients unable to perform oral hygiene this frequently should do it at least once during the day and always before bed. Fluoride toothpaste should be used and all tooth surfaces thoroughly brushed. Soft bristles stimulate gums but will not cause bleeding. Toothbrushes should be replaced every 3 months (Canadian Dental Association, 2013c).

Patients with sensitive gums can use commercially made foam-rubber toothbrushes; however, swabbing does not clean teeth as effectively because plaque accumulates at the base of teeth. These swabs should be used in moderation and only when a proper tooth brushing is not feasible. To moisturize the mouth and improve the texture of the tongue and oral mucosa, a salivary supplement called Moi-Stir is available (Miller, 2009). Rinsing with water, diluted mouthwash, or antiseptic mouthwash can also aid in cleansing and moisturizing the oral cavity.

Some patients are at increased risk for altered mucous membranes, those who are NPO (nothing by mouth), dehydrated, are undergoing chemotherapy or radiation, are malnourished, immunosuppressed, unable to perform oral care independently, have infections in their mouths, or who have undergone oral surgery or trauma. Feeding tubes, nasogastric tubes, and mouth breathing can dry mucous membranes, leading to discomfort and increased risk of skin breakdown. Alcohol-based products such as commercial mouthwashes should be avoided with these patients. Those with drainage or lesions in their mouths or those who are NPO may require oral care as often as every 2 hours. Normal saline rinses can be used to clean the oral cavity effectively upon wakening, after every meal, and at bedtime; every 2 hours if necessary. Mild oral analgesics can also be used for pain control with a physician's order. The patients may have dry lips, which should be moisturized with a water-based lubricant or petroleum jelly. Brushing and flossing are performed gently for these patients in order to prevent bleeding of the gums. They should also be advised to avoid alcohol and stop smoking.

Special Considerations for Patients With Diabetes

Patients with diabetes mellitus are more susceptible to periodontal disease. They should be counseled to visit the dentist every 3 to 4 months, and their oral tissues should be treated gently. These patients need to follow rigid oral hygiene schedules, performing oral care at least four times per day.

Flossing

Encourage or assist patients to floss using waxed or unwaxed floss between all teeth one space at a time. Once-daily flossing is sufficient according to the Canadian Dental Association (2013c). Provide a piece of floss long enough that the patient can use a clean part for each tooth space. Patients receiving chemotherapy or radiation or who take anticoagulants should use unwaxed floss and floss gently near the gumline to avoid bleeding. Applying toothpaste to the teeth before flossing allows fluoride to come into direct contact with the surface of the tooth, which aids in preventing cavities.

Oral Care for the Unconscious Patient

Particular attention must be paid to the provision of oral care in unconscious patients, who require oral care more often, about every 2 hours. These patients are more susceptible to drying of oral mucous membranes caused by thickened salivary secretions because they do not eat or drink, often breathe through their mouths, and are likely to be receiving oxygen therapy. They are unable to swallow the salivary secretions that accumulate in their mouths; these often contain Gram-negative bacteria, which increase their risk for developing nosocomial infections, such as pneumonia, if aspirated into the lungs (Garcia et al., 2009). The use of chlorhexidine mouthwash when providing oral care has been shown to decrease the risk of ventilator-associated pneumonia, reduce the duration of mechanical ventilation, and shorten intensive care unit length of stay (Berry, Davidson, Masters, & Rolls, 2007; Garcia et al., 2009; Munro et al., 2006). The external surfaces of the teeth should be brushed in the usual manner using a soft-bristled brush. Using a padded tongue depressor can help open the teeth to access the interior without risk to the nurse's fingers. Using a toothbrush provides superior cleaning to relying only on foam swabs. In order to prevent aspiration, use only small amounts of liquid and have an oral suction device available.

Denture Care

Patients with dentures should be encouraged to wear them during the day because this improves their ability to eat and talk as well as their appearance, which promotes a positive self-image. As with natural teeth, dentures collect food debris, plaque, and tartar; thus, thorough daily cleansing is imperative. Patients able to perform this independently should be encouraged to do so in order to avoid gingival infection and irritation. Some patients may require assistance with this task. Similar brushing technique is used as for natural teeth. If possible, it is best for the patients to remove their own dentures. If they are unable to do so, the nurse removes the dentures by grasping them with a gauze pad to prevent slipping (Fig. 29.5A).

Bottom dentures are generally easy to remove, but top dentures sometimes need to be moved gently from side to side to break the vacuum seal created by the upper palate. Soft-bristled brushes should be used because hard bristles can damage dentures by causing grooves in them. Dentures should be cleaned with toothpaste and water or with a commercially available denture-cleaning agent (Canadian Dental Association, 2013b) (Fig. 29.5B).

To prevent breakage and warping, dentures should be stored in an enclosed denture cup filled with water labeled with the patient's name. Prior to reinserting dentures, the patient's mouth should be rinsed, and the gums and tongue cleaned with a soft brush. Gently massaging the gums with the brush or a fingertip promotes circulation and serves to toughen the oral mucosa. Patients should not sleep with their dentures in. Patients should be discouraged from removing their dentures and placing them on a tissue or napkin because they can easily be thrown away.

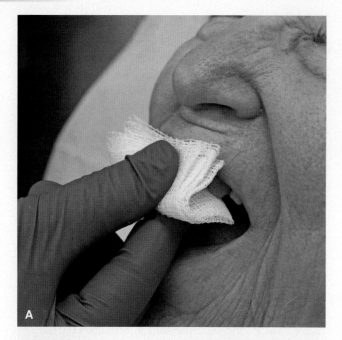

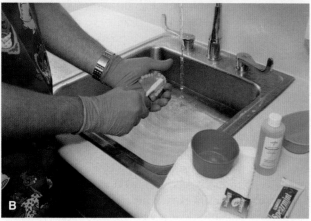

Figure 29.5 **A.** Dentures being removed. **B.** Dentures being cleaned.

Eye Care

Some patients may require assistance with eye care: those who have had eye surgery, injury, infection, or are unconscious. The sclera should be assessed for discoloration, and the conjunctiva evaluated for inflammation and degree of redness. Those with inflammation or excess secretions require assistance cleaning the eye area. This should be done using a washcloth moistened with water, saline, or sterile water. Soap should not be used because it can cause irritation and burning. Direct pressure over the eyeball can cause injury and should be avoided. Eyes should always be cleaned from the inner to outer canthus, using a different part of the cloth for each eye. Generally, eye care should be provided once daily, although unconscious patients may require care more frequently. For these patients, or for those whose eyes do not close completely, an eye patch should be placed over the eye to prevent corneal drying and irritation. Lubricating eyedrops may be provided in accordance with a physician's order.

Eyeglasses and Contact Lenses

Evaluation of visuals aids is an important part of the nurse's assessment. If unable to do so for his or her own due to physical limitation, the nurse will care for the patient's glasses, including documenting where glasses are stored in the patient care record. Glass lenses require daily cleaning and should be washed with warm water; plastic lenses are washed with a special cleaning solution. A lens cloth or soft towel can be used to dry both types of lenses. Glasses should be stored in a safe place within reach of the patient, preferably in his or her case, and labelled with the patient's name to prevent loss.

Some patients have contact lenses, which are small, round, transparent (sometimes coloured) concave disks that fit over the cornea. Several varieties exist, including daily wear, extended wear, and disposable. All types must be removed periodically to protect the eye from ocular infections and corneal ulcers or abrasions, as secretions and foreign substances such as dust can accumulate under the lens as they are worn and irritate the eye. Symptoms such as red conjunctiva, excess tearing, and burning pain are indicative of lens over wear; this can result in distorted vision or infection. Corneal damage can result if contact lenses are left in place too long because they limit the flow of oxygen to the cornea.

After removal of contact lenses, cleaning and disinfecting is required; the method used varies depending on the type of lens. Due to the risk of infection, solutions containing microorganisms such as saliva, tap water, or homemade saline should never be used. Lenses should be rinsed after cleaning with a rinsing and disinfecting solution and stored in rinsing solution. Prior to reinsertion, lenses should be cleaned again with rinsing solution to ensure all particles are removed.

Artificial Eyes

Patients who have had an enucleation (removal of an entire eyeball) will likely have an artificial eye made of either glass or plastic. These may be permanently implanted or removable, which facilitates routine cleaning. Assisting the patient may include help with removal and cleansing of the prosthetic eye. To remove the artificial eye, retract the lower eyelid and apply slight pressure just below the eye to release the suction holding the eye in place. Placing the bulb tip of a small rubber syringe over the artificial eye and squeezing may lift it from its socket. The artificial eye should be cleaned with normal saline and stored in saline or water in a covered, labeled container. The edges of the eye socket and surrounding tissues should be gently cleansed with soft gauze moistened with saline or clean tap water while assessing for redness, swelling, or drainage. The nurse closely monitors for signs of infection as the other eye, or nearby structures such as the sinuses and underlying brain tissue are in close proximity. To reinsert the eye, gently retract the lower lid and slide the eye into the socket, fitting it under the top lid.

Eye Care in the Unconscious Patient

Unconscious patients are at increased risk for corneal ulceration, which can potentially lead to blindness. Because the blink reflex is lost, the patient's eye may remain open and

BOX 29.4 Cerumen/Ear Wax Removal

- Ear wax removal can often be safely performed at home. Patient should never insert objects into the ear to attempt to remove wax.
- Ceruminolytic solutions to dissolve wax in the ear canal are instilled by drops. Solutions include mineral oil, baby oil, glycerin, water, peroxide-based eardrops (e.g., Debrox), hydrogen peroxide, and saline solution.
- Irrigation involves using a syringe to rinse out the ear canal with water or saline, after the wax has been softened or dissolved by a ceruminolytic agent.

become very dry. The nurse prevents this by providing frequent eye care every 2 hours. Liquid tear solution or saline can be administered to prevent drying.

Ear Care

Routine care of healthy ears is minimal. The external ear should be inspected for inflamed tissue, drainage, or discomfort. The auricles should be gently cleaned with a washcloth, removing excessive **cerumen** by using the twisted end of a clean washcloth while pulling down the auricle. Patients should be instructed never to insert any objects (cotton swabs, bobby pins, or toothpicks) into the ear canal for wax removal because these can cause trauma to the ear canal or puncture the tympanic membrane. Cotton-tipped applicators can push wax further into the ear canal causing blockages. Irrigation can be used if necessary; see Box 29.4 for more on cerumen removal.

Accumulation of excess cerumen is more likely in

- People who use hearing aids
- People who put cotton swabs or other items into their ears
- Older people
- People with developmental disabilities

Care of Hearing Aids

Hearing aids are battery-powered devices used to amplify sound. Newer hearing aids are able to reduce background noise interference and contain computer chips that allow for minute adjustments to adapt to each patient's hearing needs. Hearing aids can be used by patients who are hard of hearing (slight to moderate hearing loss) or by those who are deaf (severe or profound hearing loss). See Box 29.5 for types of hearing aids.

Hearing aids are very expensive and should be carefully handled and stored. When the patient is not wearing them, they should be placed in a labeled container, and the nurse should make note in the care record where they are stored, the type of device, how well it is functioning, how the patient cares for it, and any concerns the patient has about it. Care involves careful handling and storage, cleaning of the ear mold, and replacement of dead batteries. Batteries are checked when not worn by the patient by turning the volume to high. If batteries are working, a loud harsh whistling noise will be heard. If no sound is heard, batteries should be replaced.

BOX 29.5 Types of Hearing Aids

- **Behind-the-ear aid:** The most common type; fits over the ear. An ear mold fits into the ear, and the case containing the microphone, amplifier, receiver volume control, batteries, and temporomandibular switch fits behind the ear.

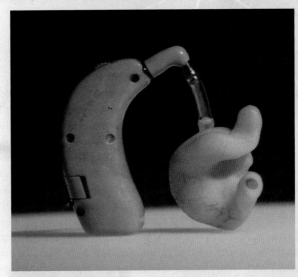

- **In-the-ear aid:** The most compact; has all of the elements located in the ear mold.

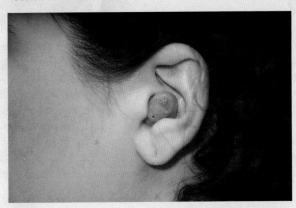

- **Eyeglass aid:** Involves a hearing aid in one or both temples of a pair of eyeglasses. It functions similarly to the behind-the-ear aid, but the components are located in the temples of the glasses.
- **Body-type hearing aid:** Used for the most severe hearing losses. The case looks like a pocket-sized transistor radio and can be clipped into a pocket, undergarment, or harness. The case contains the microphone and amplifier and is connected to a receiver that snaps into an ear mold.

From Craven, R., Hirnle, C., & Jensen, S. (2013). *Fundamentals of nursing: Human health and function* (7th ed.). Philadelphia, PA: Lippincott Williams & Wilkins.

The nurse should turn the hearing aid off prior to placing it in the patient's ear to avoid causing discomfort with sudden loud sounds. Once the aid is fitted into the ear canal, the device can be turned on and the volume adjusted for patient comfort.

Because hearing aids amplify background sounds as well as foreground, patients may have difficulty hearing, especially in noisy environments. For best communication results, always face the patient with a hearing deficit, speaking slowly and clearly when addressing them. If the patient does not understand, try different words rather than a louder voice; enunciating clearly and carefully helps patients to understand. Some patients with hearing impairment can lip-read.

Care of the Unit Environment

Keeping the patient's room as clean and comfortable as possible is an important nursing priority. The room should be safe, comfortable, and free of clutter so that the patient and visitors can move about freely. Temperature and ventilation can be difficult to control from room to room, but noise and odors can be managed to create a more comfortable environment. A neat and tidy room is conducive to healing and promotes a sense of well-being for the patient and his or her families. Ensure equipment is within reach of the patient prior to leaving the room and check if there is anything the patient requires to prevent being called back to the room multiple times. It also provides the patient and family with a sense that the nurse is attentive to their needs.

Beds

Hospital beds can be moved into various positions to promote patient comfort, therapeutic benefit, and safe body mechanics for the nurse (Box 29.6). Many beds have scales built in, so the patient can be weighed even if they are unable to get up. Beds can be raised and lowered to allow nurses to perform tasks without undue back strain (high position) and to allow patients to get in and out of bed more easily and safely (low position). The patient should be provided with instruction on how to adjust the bed independently and cautioned not to raise the bed to a position that might cause him or her harm.

BOX 29.6 Hospital Bed Positions

Flat position: Mattress is completely flat.
Fowler position: The lower part of the bed is raised to the following positions:
  Low Fowler position: Head of bed is elevated to semi-sitting position of 15°–45°. This position also is called semi-Fowler position.
  High Fowler position: Head and trunk are elevated to 80°–90°. This position also is called simply the Fowler position.
Trendelenburg position: The entire bed is tilted with the head downward. This position is not often used because it causes blood pressure to rise and causes hypotension on return to the supine position.
Reverse Trendelenburg position: Entire bed is tilted with feet downward; prevents gastric reflux.

From Craven, R., Hirnle, C., & Jensen, S. (2013). *Fundamentals of nursing: Human health and function* (7th ed.). Philadelphia, PA: Lippincott Williams & Wilkins.

Beds can be adjusted for the following reasons:

- Head of the bed can be elevated to permit eating, improve digestion, reduce reflux, and breathing.
- Head and foot of the bed can be simultaneously elevated to prevent the patient sliding down in bed.
- The foot of the bed can be elevated to elevate legs to reduce swelling.
- The head of the bed can be placed down and the feet up (Trendelenburg position) for certain procedures or to move a heavy patient up in bed.

Special beds are available for patients who, unable turn or move independently, are at increased risk for skin breakdown. Beds and stretchers have side rails to promote patient safety by preventing the patient from falling or getting out of bed independently when he or she is unable to do so safely. Patients can hold onto side rails while moving in bed and getting up and thus promote patient independence. Agency guidelines regarding restrains vary; the nurse must be familiar with institutional policies. In some institutions, having all four rails up is considered restraint.

Footboards provide support to the feet to prevent foot drop and remove some of the weight of bedclothes from the feet and legs. This provides comfort and may relieve pain and improve circulation for patients with swollen legs, feet, or toes. An intravenous (IV) pole may be inserted into the bed frame or may be freestanding beside the bed. There may be hooks suspended from the ceiling from which to hang the IV bag.

Beds contain safety features including locks on the wheels and alarms. Wheels should always be locked when the bed is stationary to avoid accidental movement. Bed alarms should be operational for patients at risk of getting out of bed without assistance.

Bed Making

The nurse inspects linens frequently to ensure they are clean, dry, and wrinkle-free. Patients who are diaphoretic, have draining wounds, or are incontinent may require more frequent linen changes and should be assessed accordingly. Ensuring the patient's bed remains clean, dry, and smooth promotes feelings of well-being for the patient. The nurse should straighten bed linens when they become loose or wrinkled to prevent skin breakdown and check the bed for food debris after meals. Soiled or wet linens should be changed as quickly as possible. See Skill 29.7 for making an occupied bed.

The nurse gathers all necessary linens prior to beginning making the bed. To conserve time and energy, one side of the bed should be made as much as possible prior to moving to the other side. Raising the bed to a comfortable working height and lowering the head of the bed promote good body mechanics for the nurse. The nurse should follow the principles of medical asepsis when changing bed linen by keeping soiled linen away from his or her uniform. Soiled linen should not be shaken, instead rolled up and placed into designated linen bags rather than on the floor. Clean linens must never touch the floor; if this occurs, it should be immediately placed in the laundry.

First-year nursing student Sarah feels elated and satisfied not only with the task she performed for Mrs. Jones but also with the therapeutic relationship and the trust that has been established with her patient. The patient was clearly more relaxed; her hygiene needs met, and now, she is looking forward to more sessions with Sarah. Sarah feels a growing confidence in her abilities in offering hygiene care to and her capacity to form supportive therapeutic relationships with patients.

Conclusion: Key Concepts

- Self-care and hygiene are important in the promotion of health.
- Both children and adults may regress to a lower developmental level during times of stress or illness and require more assistance with self-care.
- Factors that affect self-care include culture, values and beliefs, the environment, patient motivation, emotional status, cognitive abilities, energy levels, acute illness or surgery, pain, and motor deficits.
- Primarily, bathing serves to enhance cleanliness, but its warm water and friction also serve to enhance circulation, and movement during bathing encourages range-of-motion exercises. It also can be relaxing for the patient and promote the development of a therapeutic nurse–patient relationship.
- Care of the eyes, ears, and teeth are important for the maintenance of optimal health. The nurse uses all caution to avoid damaging or losing patients' glasses, contact lenses, hearing aids, or dentures because these items are important to optimal patient functioning as well as expensive to replace.
- To promote comfort and optimize well-being, provide a clean environment and a bed free of wrinkles.

SKILL 29.1 Assisting With the Bath or Shower

Purpose

1. Cleanse the skin, control body odors, and promote self-esteem.
2. Stimulate circulation.
3. Provide an opportunity to assess skin and physical mobility.
4. Provide range-of-motion exercises for joints.
5. Promote relaxation and comfort.

Step

Equipment:
- One or two bath towels
- Bathmat
- One washcloth
- Soap, soap dish, or liquid (non-soap) cleanser
- Personal skin care products (deodorant, powder, lotions, cologne)
- Clean gown or pajamas
- Laundry bag

Assessment:
- Assess patient's ability to perform self-care and amount of assistance he or she needs. Evaluate activity tolerance, cognitive function, musculoskeletal function, and level of comfort to determine type of bath. Note: Encourage the patient to be as independent as possible but not to become excessively fatigued. Pain should not be intensified by the activity.
- Assess the patient's preferences for bathing (i.e., frequency, time of day, type of skin care products).
- Review chart to determine other procedures or therapies the patient is receiving to coordinate scheduling and prevent fatigue.
- Identify patients with special considerations for bathing:
  ○ Older patients: Susceptible to dry skin
  ○ Immobilized patients: Pressure areas on dependent and bony parts; need for range-of-motion exercises to joints
  ○ Patients with altered sensation: Risk for burns from hot water
  ○ Obese or diaphoretic patients: Excessive perspiration or moisture on skin surfaces that rub against each other and provide medium for excoriation and bacterial growth
- Review history for precautions regarding movement or positioning.
- Assess patient's knowledge and practice of hygiene to determine learning needs.

(continued on page 698)

SKILL 29.1 | Assisting With the Bath or Shower (continued)

Procedure

Step	Rationale
Perform hand hygiene.	Reduces microbe transmission
Identify the patient.	Ensures correct patient receives proper assessment or treatment and reduces errors
Close door or bed curtains and explain the procedure to the patient and patient's family.	Ensures patient privacy, increases patient compliance, reduces patient anxiety, and promotes learning
Make sure the tub or shower is clean prior to bathing patient.	Reduces microbe transmission
Prepare bathroom by placing towel or disposable bath mat on door by tub or shower.	Maintains cleanliness and safety for the patient
Accompany or transport patient to the bathroom. Some patients may need to use a shower chair for transportation or support (see Figure 1).	Showering or bathing will be tiring. Transportation and/or sitting in a chair will conserve energy.

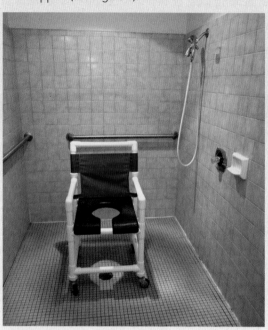

Figure 1

Step	Rationale
Place "occupied" or "in use" sign on door.	The patient needs privacy while bathing. Doors are not usually locked so that the nurse can come in to assist the patient as necessary.
Keep patient covered with a bath blanket until water is ready (see Figure 2).	Keeps the patient warm to prevent chills and ensure privacy/dignity of patient

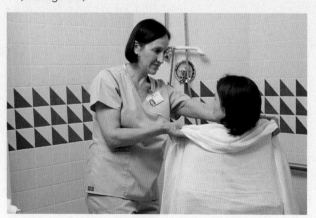

Figure 2

Procedure (continued)

Step

Fill bathtub halfway with warm water (40.6°C). Test water or have patient test water (see Figure 3). If the patient is taking a shower, turn on shower and adjust water temperature.

Rationale

Prevents burns by ensuring temperature is correct for the patient

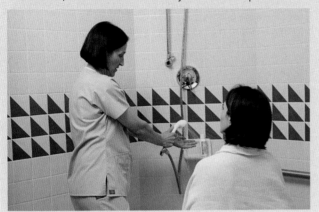

Figure 3

Help patient into shower or tub, providing necessary assistance. Instruct the patient in use of safety bars and call light signal.
Patient may prefer to sit in shower chair to prevent fatigue.
If the patient is unable to shower independently, stay with the patient at all times. (Two nurses may be necessary for some patients.) Use handheld shower to wet patient (see Figure 4). Wash patient with soap and washcloth using long, firm strokes (see Figure 5).

Falls can occur in the shower or tub; provide safety for the patient. Provides for the patient's safety and comfort

Handheld shower allows the nurse to stay dry.

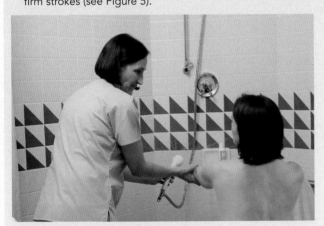

Figure 4

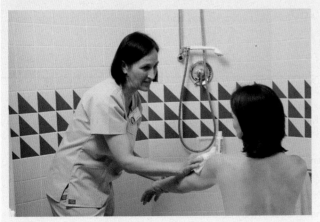

Figure 5

(continued on page 700)

SKILL 29.1   Assisting With the Bath or Shower (continued)

Procedure (continued)

Step	Rationale
If patient is showering or bathing independently, check on patient within 15 minutes. Wash any areas that he or she could not reach.	Prolonged exposure to warm water may cause vasodilation and pooling of blood, which can result in light-headedness and increase fall risk.
Assist with drying (see Figure 6). Help patient out of tub or shower (see Figure 7). If patient is unsteady, drain water before helping patient out of tub.	Prevents falls and maintain patient safety

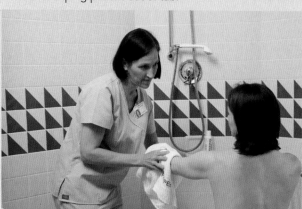

Figure 6

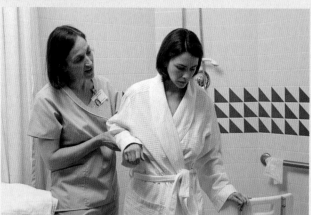

Figure 7

Assist patient with dressing and grooming.	
Help patient to room. Return to bathroom and clean tub or shower according to agency policy. Discard soiled linen. Remove the "occupied/in use" sign on door.	Maintains cleanliness and good infection control practices
Document procedure: 6/1/13: 1000—Weekly bath given, tolerated bath without increased pulse rate or dizziness, no areas of skin breakdown observed. — F. Thomas, RN	Maintains legal record and communicates with health-care team

Lifespan Considerations

Newborn and Infant
- To prevent infection, do not submerge an infant in water until the umbilical cord has fallen off (around 7–10 days of age).

Child
- To prevent drowning, do not leave children younger than 8 years unattended in a bath.
- Supervise the bath so the child washes thoroughly.

Adolescent
- Sebaceous glands become active during puberty. Special cleansing agents may be necessary to treat facial acne. Antiperspirants and more frequent baths will help control body odors.

Older Adult
- Older adults are susceptible to dry skin due to reduced sebaceous gland activity, epidermal thinning, and decreased fluid intake. Use lotions, bath oil, and less soap to reduce the drying effects of aging. Bathing may occur weekly to decrease drying of the skin.
- Check water temperature carefully. Older adults may have decreased sensation and are at risk for burns from hot water.

Home Care Modifications
- Instruct patients at risk for falling to apply lotions and oils after the bath and not put them on in bathtub. Oils can make the bathtub or shower surfaces more slippery.
- Encourage installation of safety devices, such as tub bars, nonskid tub surfaces, and bathroom carpeting to reduce the chance of falls and promote independence.

Collaboration and Delegation
Because unlicensed personnel often assist with showers or bathing, be sure to provide assistants with the following information regarding the patient:
- Any physical limitations or special safety precautions needed
- Amount of help the patient will require
- Any drains, casts, or IVs, along with any precautions or limitations that they will impose during the shower/bath
- Any assessments to report to you (e.g., skin condition under breasts)
- Collaborate with occupational therapy if an occupational therapist (OT) is seeing the patient. Often, OTs want to assess and work with a patient's ability to perform hygiene, so coordination of patient care is important.

SKILL 29.2	Bathing a Patient in Bed

Purpose

Same as Skill 29.1

Step

Equipment:
- Two bath towels
- Two washcloths
- Bath blanket
- Washbasin with warm water (43.3°–46.1°C); test by measuring with bath thermometer or by placing several drops on your inner forearm
- Soap, soap dish, or liquid (nonsoap) cleanser or bag bath packet removed from warmer just before bathing
- Personal skin care products (deodorant, powder, lotions, cologne)
- Clean gown or pajamas
- Laundry bag
- Disposable clean gloves for perineal care

Assessment:
Same as Skill 29. 1.

Procedure

Step	Rationale
Identify the patient.	Ensures correct patient receives proper assessment or treatment and reduces errors
Close door or bed curtains and explain the procedure to the patient and patient's family.	Ensures patient privacy, increases compliance, and reduces anxiety
Help patient use bedpan, urinal, or commode if needed.	The patient will be more comfortable and relaxed after elimination.
Close window and door to decrease drafts.	Provides the patient comfort and minimizes the patient becoming cold
Perform hand hygiene.	Reduces microbe transmission
Raise bed to high position. Lock up side rail on opposite side of bed from your work.	Prevents back strain; prevents the patient from falling out of bed

(continued on page 702)

SKILL 29.2   Bathing a Patient in Bed (continued)

Procedure (continued)

Step	Rationale
Remove top sheet and bedspread and then place bath blanket on patient (see Figure 1). Help the patient move closer to you. If top linen is to be reused, place it on back of chair; otherwise, place it in laundry bag.	A bath blanket provides for patient comfort, warmth, and privacy. Bringing the patient closer to you prevents undue muscle strain and is good back care for the nurse.

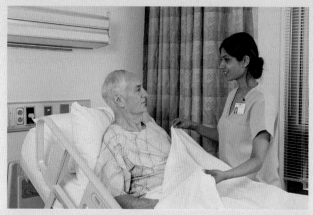

Figure 1

Lay towel across patient's chest (see Figure 2).

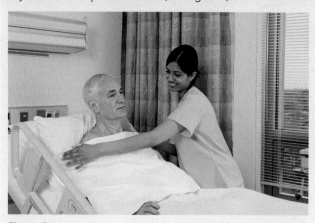

Figure 2

Follow package directions to heat the disposable washcloths in microwave. Remove the cloth from bag bath packet or wet washcloth and fold around your fingers to make a mitt:
- Fold washcloth into thirds (see Figure 3).

Heating per instructions prevents burns.
A mitt retains heat and water better than a loosely held wash-cloth and prevents water from dripping on the patient.

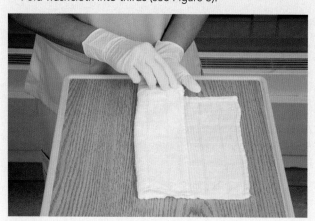

Figure 3

Procedure (continued)

Step	Rationale

Step

- Straighten washcloth to take out wrinkles.
- Fold washcloth over to fit hand.
- Tuck loose ends under edge of washcloth on palm (see Figure 4).

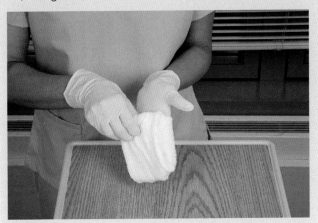

Figure 4

Cleanse eyes with water only, wiping from inner to outer canthus. Use separate corner of mitt for each eye (see Figure 5).

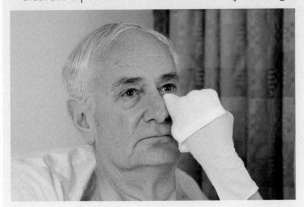

Figure 5

Determine if patient would like soap used on face. Wash face, neck, and ears. Liquid non-detergent cleansing agents are available in some institutions to mix directly into bath water. These products are non-drying and need not be rinsed from the skin.

or

Use a separate cloth to cleanse face.

Rationale

Washing the eye from the inner to outer canthus prevents secretions from entering and irritating nasolacrimal ducts. Using separate corners for each eye prevents contamination and transfer of microorganisms from one eye to the other.

Soap can be drying, especially to the face.

Use separate cloths for the face to prevent transfer of microorganisms from other parts of the body.

(continued on page 704)

SKILL 29.2   Bathing a Patient in Bed (continued)

Procedure (continued)

Step

Fold bath blanket off arm away from you. Place towel lengthwise under arm. Wash, rinse, and dry the arm using long, firm strokes from the fingers toward the axilla (see Figure 6). Wash the axilla. Place folded towel and water basin on patient's bed. Soak patient's hand and then wash and rinse (see Figure 7).

Rationale

Stroking from distal to proximal stimulates circulation and facilitates venous blood return.

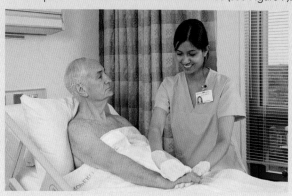

Figure 6

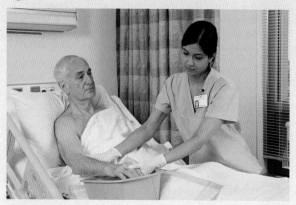

Figure 7
or
Continue to use disposable bag bath cloths as directed on the package, cleansing parts of the body.

Repeat for hand and arm nearest you (see Figure 8).

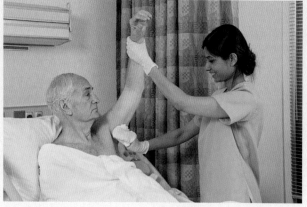

Figure 8

Procedure (continued)

Step	Rationale
Apply deodorant or powder according to patient's preferences. Avoid excessive use of powder or inhalation of powder.	Hygiene products control excess body moisture and odor. Excessive powder can cause caking, which leads to skin irritation; inhalation can cause respiratory difficulty.
Assess bath water temperature and change water if necessary. Side rails should be up.	Changing water ensures that it is warm and comfortable for the patient; side rails prevent falls when nurse leaves the patient to change water
Place bath towel over chest. Fold bath blanket down to below umbilicus.	Keeps the patient warm while preventing unnecessary exposure of body parts
Lift bath towel off chest and bathe chest and abdomen with cloth using long, firm strokes (see Figure 9). Give special attention to skin under the breasts and any other skinfolds if patient is overweight. Rinse and dry well. Apply a light dusting of bath powder under the breasts or between skinfolds.	Toweling and powdering absorb excess moisture and prevent skin maceration and irritation; ensures areas under skinfolds are dry

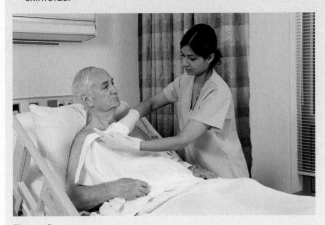

Figure 9

Help patient put on a clean gown (see Figure 10).	Gown prevents exposure of upper body area.

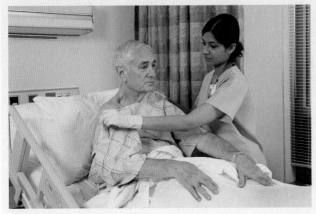

Figure 10

(continued on page 706)

SKILL 29.2   Bathing a Patient in Bed (continued)

Procedure (continued)

Step

Expose leg away from you by folding over bath blanket. Be careful to keep perineum covered.

Lift leg and place bath towel lengthwise under leg. Wash, rinse, and dry leg using long, firm strokes from ankle to thigh (see Figure 11).

Rationale

Preventing unnecessary exposure of body parts maintains the patient's dignity.

Washing from distal to proximal stimulates circulation and facilitates venous blood return.

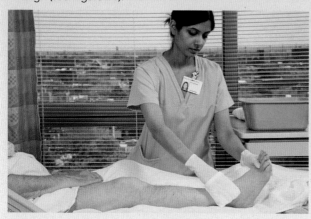

Figure 11

Wash feet. Rinse and dry well. Pay special attention to space between toes (see Figure 12).

Moisture between toes can foster irritation, fungal growth, and skin breakdown.

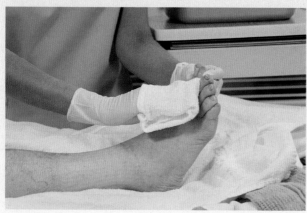

Figure 12

Procedure (continued)

Step	Rationale
Repeat for other leg and foot.	Promotes patient comfort
Assess bath water for warmth. Change water if necessary.	A back rub stimulates circulation and promotes comfort.
Assist patient to side-lying position (see Figure 13). Place bath towel alongside of back and buttocks to protect linen. Wash, rinse, and dry back and buttocks (see Figure 14). Give a back rub with lotion if needed.	

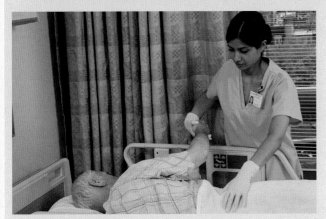

Figure 13

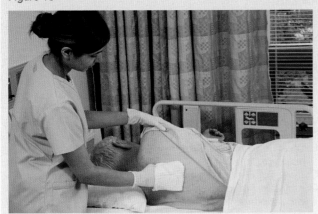

Figure 14

Step	Rationale
Assist patient to supine position. Assess if patient can wash genitals and perineal area independently.	Most patients who are unable to perform perineal care will not ask for assistance with this intimate task, but it is important to keep this area clean to decrease infection risk and prevent odor. This is especially important if the patient has problems with incontinence.
Complete care according to patient's preference. Apply powder, lotion, or cologne. Assist with hair and mouth care. Make bed with clean linen.	Involving the patient promotes self-esteem and self-care efforts.
Clean equipment and return to appropriate storage area. Perform hand hygiene.	Maintains cleanliness
Document procedure:	Maintains legal record and communicates with health-care team
Often noted on a flow sheet, providing information such as complete versus partial bath and the amount of assistance required.	

Home Care Modifications
- Arrange for a hospital bed to help prevent caregiver back strain and assist with turning and moving the patient in bed.
- Commercially available disposable cloths can make bathing easier in the home setting.

Collaboration and Delegation
Same as Skill 29.1.

SKILL 29.3   Massaging the Back

Purpose

1. Stimulate circulation to the skin.
2. Relieve muscle tension.
3. Promote comfort and relaxation.

Step	Rationale
Equipment: • Bath blanket • Bath towel (to absorb excess moisture) • Lotion or powder Assessment: • Assess patient for muscle fatigue, stiffness, complaints of back discomfort, or tension. • Identify patients with impaired physical mobility who may benefit from back massage. • Assess skin for localized areas of redness on the back, shoulders, or hips. • Assess patient's desire for back massage. • Identify conditions that may contraindicate back rub (rib and vertebral fractures, burns, open wounds, or pressure ulcers). • Determine any limitations to positioning for back massage.	Lotion is used to lubricate skin and prevents friction during massage; powder reduces friction and prevents "sticky" feeling on a diaphoretic patient. Powder and lotion are not used together.

Procedure

Step	Rationale
Identify the patient.	Ensures correct patient receives proper assessment or treatment and reduces errors
Close door or bed curtains and explain the procedure to the patient and patient's family.	Ensures patient privacy, increases patient compliance, and reduces patient anxiety
Help patient to side-lying or prone position.	Promotes patient comfort
Expose back, shoulders, upper arms, and sacral area. Cover remainder of body with bath blanket.	Covering areas not being massaged prevents unnecessary exposure and the patient becoming cold while maintaining dignity.
Perform hand hygiene in warm water. Warm lotion by holding container under running warm water.	Warm hands and lotion prevent a startle response and muscle tension from cold lotion and hands.
Pour small amount of lotion into palms.	Lubricating palms decreases friction on the skin during massage.
Inform the patient that you are beginning the massage. Begin massage in sacral area with circular motion. Move hands upward to shoulders, massaging over scapulae in smooth, firm strokes (see Figure 1). Without removing hands from skin, continue in smooth strokes to upper arms and down sides of back to iliac crest. Continue for 3–5 minutes.	Communicate with the patient to avoid startling the patient Continuous, firm pressure promotes relaxation and stimulates circulation.

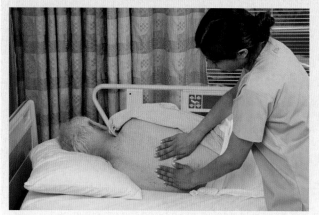

Figure 1

SKILL 29.3	Massaging the Back (continued)

Procedure (continued)

Step	Rationale
While massaging, assess for broken skin areas and whitish or reddened areas that do not disappear. Do not apply pressure over areas of breakdown or redness.	Pressure from massage can traumatize and damage tissues or cause further skin breakdown.
If additional stimulation is desired, nurse can use pétrissage (kneading) over the shoulders and gluteal area and tapotement (tapping) up and down the spine.	
End massage with long, continuous, stroking movements.	Stroking is the most relaxing of the massage movements.
Pat excess lubricant dry with towel. Retie patient's gown and assist to comfortable position.	Promotes patient comfort
Perform hand hygiene.	Reduces microbe transmission
Document procedure:	
Document on a flow sheet that massage was given and the effect of the massage.	Maintains legal record and communicates with health-care team

Collaboration and Delegation
- Encourage unlicensed personnel to provide back massage, especially at bedtime. In some facilities, volunteers are trained to provide back massages for receptive patients. Communicate any positioning restrictions and assessments that they should report.

SKILL 29.4	Performing Foot and Hand Care

Purpose

1. Maintain skin integrity.
2. Provide the patient with comfort and a sense of well-being.
3. Maintain foot function and ability to ambulate.
4. Encourage self-care.

Step

Equipment:
- Waterproof pad
- Washcloths and towels
- Washbasin filled with warm water and soap
- Lotion
- Disposable gloves
- Nail clippers and file
- Cuticle stick

Assessment:
- Observe the patient while mobilizing to assess gait for limping or unusual position. An unnatural gait can be caused by painful feet or bone and muscle disorders.
- Assess the patient's footwear. Socks should always be worn and should be changed daily to absorb excess moisture and prevent fungal infections.
- Identify patients who are at risk for foot or nail problems:
  - Diabetes causes changes in the microvasculature of peripheral tissues. Patients with diabetes have an increased risk for infection from breaks in the skin and may have decreased sensation due to neuropathy.
  - Older patients' ability to perform foot and nail care can be impaired by poor vision, obesity, or musculoskeletal conditions that limit their ability to bend or maintain their balance.
  - Cerebrovascular accidents (CVAs) may cause changes in the patient's gait due to foot drop, muscle weakness, or paralysis.
  - Conditions such as renal failure and congestive heart failure are associated with foot and ankle edema, which interferes with blood flow to tissues and impedes shoes fitting properly.
- Assess the patient's ability to perform self-care.
- Inspect fingers and fingernails, toes, toenails, and feet. Assess the areas between the toes for dryness and cracking.
- Assess the patient's knowledge regarding foot and nail care.
- Review your institution's policy for trimming nails. Some institutions require a physician's order prior to cutting patient's nails, especially if they are high-risk.

(continued on page 710)

SKILL 29.4   Performing Foot and Hand Care (continued)

Procedure

Step	Rationale
Perform hand hygiene.	Reduces transmission of microbes
Identify the patient.	Ensures the correct patient receives the proper assessment or treatment and reduces errors
Provide privacy by closing the door or curtains and explain the procedure to the patient.	Protects patient privacy, increases patient compliance and comfort, and reduces patient anxiety
Assist the patient to transfer to a chair if possible. Elevate the head of the bed for bedridden patients.	Promotes patient comfort
Fill a washbasin with warm water (37.7°–40°C). Place the waterproof pad under the basin. Soak the patient's hands or feet in the basin. Do not soak the feet of patients with diabetes.	Warm water softens nails and nail beds, promotes circulation, and reduces inflammation. In patients with diabetes, soaking increases the risk of burning these patients because peripheral neuropathy affects their sensation.
Place the call bell within reach of the patient. Allow hands or feet to soak for 10–20 minutes.	Softening promotes easier removal of dead epithelial cells and reduces the risk of nails cracking during cutting.
Towel dry the hand or foot that has been soaked. Change the water in the basin for fresh warm water and allow the other extremity to soak while you work on the softened one (see Figure 1).	Soaking the opposite hand or foot while working on the other is an efficient use of time.

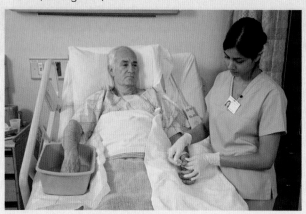

Figure 1

Clean gently under all nails with a cuticle stick. If nails are thick and yellow, the patient may have a fungal infection. Don gloves and eye protection.	Gloves prevent the transmission of infection, and eye protection prevents accidental exposure of the mucous membranes of the eyes.
Cut nails straight across, beginning with the large toe or thumb (see Figure 2). Shape nails gently with a file. File rather than cut the nails of patients with diabetes or circulatory problems.	Trimming straight across prevents the nail from splitting and protects from injury around the nail.

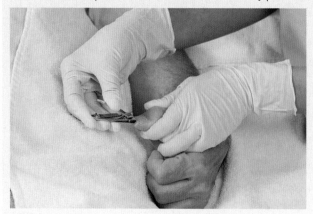

Figure 2

Procedure (continued)

Step	Rationale
Gently push the cuticle of each nail back with a cuticle stick (see Figure 3).	Cuticle care reduces inflammation of the cuticles and the formation of hangnails.

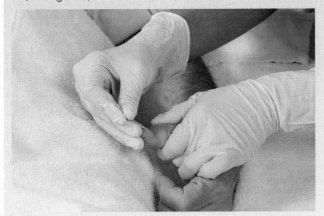

Figure 3

Rinse the foot or hand in warm water.	Removing excess moisture inhibits growth of bacteria and fungus.
Dry thoroughly with a towel, ensuring space between digits is very well dried.	Excess moisture between the toes can lead to maceration and increase fungal growth.
Apply lotion to hands or feet. For patients with diabetes, do not apply lotion between the toes.	
Assist the patient into a comfortable position.	
Remove and dispose of equipment.	Maintains cleanliness and safety
Wash your hands.	Reduces transmission of microbes
Document procedure.	Maintains legal record and communicates with health-care team

Lifespan Considerations

Infant
- Teach parents to care for their infants' nails to prevent infants from scratching themselves. Instruct parents to cut nails straight across using blunt scissors. This is accomplished most easily when the baby is asleep.

Child
- Assess for nail biting, a common concern with school-aged children. This may be a learned behaviour or a symptom of nervousness. Bad-tasting over-the-counter preparations are available to paint on the nails to discourage nail biting. Other measures that can be used include positive reinforcement and rewards.

Older Adult
- Inspect the nails of older adults closely. Older patients often have thick, horny nails due to poor peripheral circulation. Mobility may make nail care a challenge for the elderly.

Collaboration and Delegation
- Refer high-risk patients or those with severely hypertrophied nails to a podiatrist or foot clinic for care. In some institutions, the diabetic nurse or clinician can provide foot care to diabetic or other high-risk patients.

SKILL 29.5   Shampooing the Hair of a Bedridden Patient

Purpose

1. Cleanse the hair and scalp.
2. Promote comfort and improve self-esteem and sense of well-being.
3. Apply medication to scalp and hair as necessary.

Step

Equipment:
- Comb and brush
- Hair dryer (optional)
- Two bath towels, one washcloth
- Shampoo (conditioner, optional)
- Water pitcher
- Plastic shampoo basin
- Washbasin or bucket
- Bath blanket

or

- Disposable shampoo cap (remove from warmer)
- Waterproof pads
- Cotton balls (optional)
- Hydrogen peroxide (optional; used to clean matted blood from hair)

Assessment:
- Assess condition of hair and scalp.
- Determine agency policy about shampooing hair of some patients (e.g., head trauma). Some agencies require a physician's order especially after surgery or trauma involving the head.
- Assess patient's activity level and identify positioning restrictions.
- Assess patient's preference for hair care products. Determine if medicated shampoo has been ordered and is available.

Procedure

Step	Rationale
Perform hand hygiene.	Reduces transmission of microbes
Identify the patient.	Ensures the correct patient receives proper assessment or treatment and reduces chance of errors
Close the door or curtains and explain the procedure to the patient.	Protects patient privacy and improves patient compliance
Place waterproof pads under the patient's head and shoulders and remove pillows.	Ensures bed linens stay clean and dry
Raise the bed to its highest position or a comfortable working height.	Reduces back strain for the nurse
Remove any ties or pins from the hair. Thoroughly but gently brush or comb hair.	Removes tangles and distributes scalp oils to ensure thorough cleansing
Place the bed in a flat position. Place the shampoo basin under the patient's head. Place bath towel around the patient's shoulders and a folded washcloth where the neck rests on the basin.	Shoulder padding protects the patient from getting wet. The washcloths protect the neck from strain and promote comfort.
Fold the bed linens down to the patient's waist. Cover the upper body with a bath blanket.	Keeps the patient warm and protects the patient from water
Place a wastebasket (without the plastic bag) under the spout of the shampoo basin. A chair or table can be used to elevate the wastebasket if necessary.	Water will flow away from the face and head into the wastebasket receptacle.

Procedure (continued)

Step	Rationale

Step

Using a water pitcher, thoroughly wet hair with warm water (approximately 43.3°C) (see Figure 1). Assess water temperature using a thermometer or by placing a small amount of water on your wrist.

Rationale

Wetting the hair in this way protects the face and scalp from getting wet or burned.

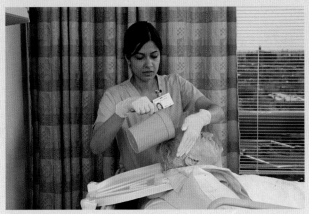

Figure 1

If necessary, use hydrogen peroxide to dissolve matted blood from hair prior to shampooing. The peroxide will feel bubbly and warm; the nurse should reassure the patient that it will not bleach the hair.

Removing blood from hair prior to washing will ensure that the shampoo will reach and cleanse all hair surfaces.

Apply a small amount of shampoo. Massage the scalp with your fingertips while making the shampoo lather. Start at the patient's hairline and work toward the neck (see Figure 2).

Massaging stimulates circulation to the scalp and systematic lathering ensures thorough cleansing.

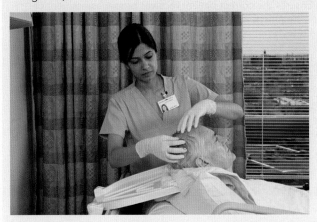

Figure 2

Rinse hair well using warm water. Reapply shampoo and repeat massage.

Rinse hair again thoroughly using warm water. Clean hair should "squeak" when rubbed between the fingers.

Soap residue in hair may cause dryness and irritate hair and scalp.

Apply a small amount of conditioner if the patient desires it. Massage well through the hair, allow to sit for a few minutes, and then rinse well.

Conditioner decreases tangles and makes combing easier, especially with long hair.

(continued on page 714)

SKILL 29.5 | Shampooing the Hair of a Bedridden Patient (continued)

Procedure (continued)

Step	Rationale
Squeeze excess moisture from hair. Wrap bath towel around the hair and gently rub hair and scalp dry (see Figure 3). Use a second towel if necessary.	

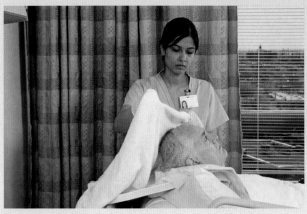

Figure 3

Step	Rationale
Remove equipment and wet towels from the bed. Place a dry towel over the patient's shoulders.	Prevents the patient from getting a chill and promotes comfort
Dry hair with hair dryer if necessary. Comb and style hair.	
Assist patient into a comfortable position.	
Dispose of soiled equipment and linens.	
Alternate Procedure for Using a Dry Shampoo Cap	
Perform hand hygiene.	Reduces transmission of microbes
Identify the patient.	Ensures the correct patient receives proper assessment or treatment and reduces chance of errors
Close the door or curtains and explain the procedure to the patient.	Protects patient privacy and improves patient compliance
Spread towel across the patient's chest and place the shampoo cap on the patient (see Figures 4 and 5).	Provides comfort and prepares the patient for the shampoo

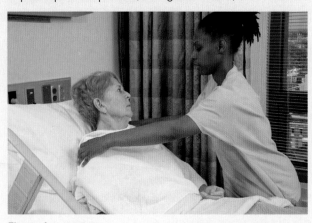

Figure 4

Procedure (continued)

Step	Rationale

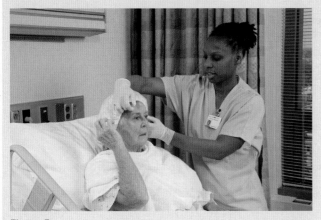

Figure 5

Massage the scalp from the outside of the cap so that dry shampoo is evenly distributed (see Figure 6).

Evenly distributes the shampoo to hair shafts to promote cleaning

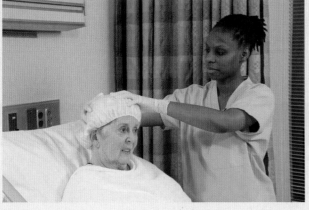

Figure 6

Wait 1–3 minutes for the shampoo to fully saturate the hair.
Remove and discard the shampoo cap.
Use a clean towel to dry the patient's hair.
Comb and style the patient's hair (see Figure 7).

Allows chemical agent to cleanse the hair
Shampoo caps are only used once.
Promotes comfort and prevents the patient getting a chill
Promotes well-being and self-esteem

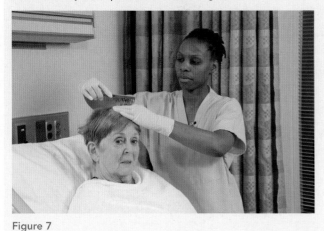

Figure 7

Document procedure.

Maintains a legal record and communicates with other member of health-care team

(continued on page 716)

SKILL 29.5 | Shampooing the Hair of a Bedridden Patient (continued)

Lifespan Considerations

Infant
- Shampooing is usually done during the daily bath to prevent seborrhea (cradle cap), a gray, scaly scalp condition.
- Warm the room and use warmed towels to prevent chilling the baby during the bath.
- Use baby shampoo to decrease eye irritation.

Child
Assess the hair carefully for nits (lice eggs). Pediculosis infestations are common in school-aged children.

Adolescent
- Many adolescents shampoo their hair daily. Offering to shampoo their hair may improve self-esteem and help them feel better.

Older Adult
- Use warm towels to thoroughly dry the hair after shampooing to prevent chilling. Many older adults have decreased amounts of subcutaneous tissue and are easily chilled.
- Older adults may have decreased sensation to heat. Use hair dryers cautiously on a low-heat setting to prevent burning the scalp.

Home Care Considerations
- Ask the family if a relative or friend can help with hair care. Inform the family about helpful equipment, such as disposable shampoo caps, for purchase if showering or bathing is restricted.
- Assist the family with adapting things found in the home (e.g., a dish drainer mat or rolled up plastic garbage bag) for use as a shampoo tray.

Collaboration and Delegation
- Many long-term care facilities and community-based care centres have an in-house beautician who provides hair services for patients. Encourage and make arrangements for such services to promote well-being and enhance self-esteem.

SKILL 29.6 | Providing Oral Care

Purpose

1. Cleanse tooth surfaces to prevent odor and caries.
2. Maintain a hydrated, intact oral mucosa.
3. Promote self-esteem and comfort.

Step	Rationale

Equipment:
• Soft toothbrush (sponge swabs may be used for patients at risk for bleeding)
• Toothpaste
• Cup with water and straw
• Emesis basin
• Washcloth and towel
• Mouthwash (optional; non-alcohol based is preferable)
• Dental floss
• Disposable gloves (if the nurse is providing oral care)
Assessment:
• Inspect lips, buccal membrane, gums, palate, and tongue for lesions or inflammation.
• Assess for caries or halitosis (bad breath).
• Identify patients at risk for oral hygiene complications:
  • Dehydration, NPO status, and nasogastric tubes dry the oral mucosa.
  • Oral airways accumulate secretions and irritate the mucosa.
  • Chemotherapy often results in stomatitis and ulcerations.
  • Anticoagulant therapy or clotting disorders predispose the patient to gum bleeding.
  • Oral surgery or trauma may contraindicate tooth brushing; special rinses may be ordered.
• Determine the patient's ability to assist with the procedure.
• Assess the patient's risk for aspiration.	

Procedure

Step

Perform hand hygiene.
Identify the patient.

Close the door or curtains and explain the procedure to the patient.
Assist the patient to a sitting position. If the patient cannot sit, position him or her in a side-lying position.
Place a towel under the patient's chin.
Moisten the toothbrush with water and apply a small amount of toothpaste (see Figure 1). If the patient is anticoagulated or has a clotting disorder, use a very soft toothbrush or sponge-ended swab to prevent bleeding of gums.

Rationale

Reduces transmission of microbes
Ensures the correct patient received the proper assessment or treatment and reduces errors
Protects patient privacy and promotes patient compliance

High Fowler or side-lying position decreases the risk of choking and aspiration.
Protects the bed linens and patient gown from spills
Limits trauma to the oral mucosa that could cause bleeding

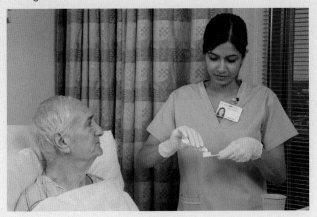

Figure 1

Hand the toothbrush to the patient or don disposable gloves and brush the patient's teeth as follows:
a. Hold the toothbrush at a 45° angle to the gumline (see Figure 2).

Angling the toothbrush allows the brush to reach all tooth surfaces and to penetrate and cleanse under the gumline, where plaque and tartar accumulate.

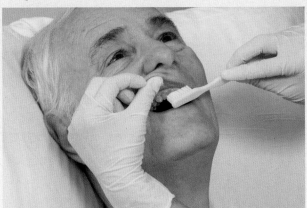

Figure 2

b. Using short, vibrating motions, brush from the gumline to the crown of each tooth. Repeat until both outside and inside of teeth and gums are cleaned.
c. Cleanse biting surfaces by brushing with a back-and-forth stroke.

Bacteria accumulate and grow on the tongue surface.

(continued on page 718)

SKILL 29.6 | Providing Oral Care (continued)

Procedure (continued)

Step

d. Brush the tongue lightly. Avoid stimulating the gag reflex (see Figure 3).

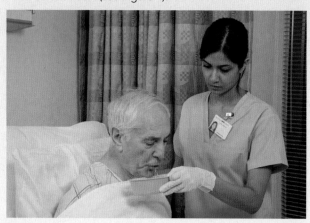

Figure 3

Have patient rinse mouth thoroughly with water and spit into an emesis basin (see Figure 4).

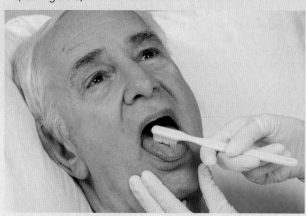

Figure 4

Rationale

Procedure (continued)	
Step	**Rationale**
Remove the emesis basin, set aside, and dry the patient's mouth with a washcloth.	
Floss the patient's teeth (see Figure 5).	Flossing removes particulate matter trapped between the teeth and below the gumline.

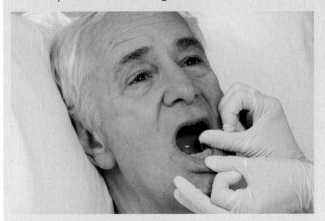

Figure 5

a. Cut a 10-in. piece of dental floss. Wind ends of floss around middle finger of each hand.
b. Using the index fingers to stretch the floss, move the floss up and down around and between the lower teeth. Start at the back lower teeth and work around to the other side.
c. Using the thumb and index finger to stretch the floss, repeat the procedure on the upper teeth.
d. Have the patient rinse his or her mouth thoroughly and spit into the emesis basin.

Remove and dispose of supplies. Help the patient to a comfortable position.	Promotes patient comfort
Remove gloves and perform hand hygiene.	The mouth contains many microorganisms, and hand washing prevents the transmission of infection.

Procedure for the Unconscious Patient

Perform hand hygiene.	Reduces transmission of microbes
Identify the patient.	Ensures the correct patient received the proper assessment or treatment and reduces errors
Close the door or curtains.	Protects patient privacy
Place the patient in a side-lying position.	This position decreases the chance of aspiration.
Place a towel or waterproof pad under the patient's chin.	
Place an emesis basin against the patient's mouth or have a suction catheter positioned to remove secretions from the mouth (see Figure 6).	

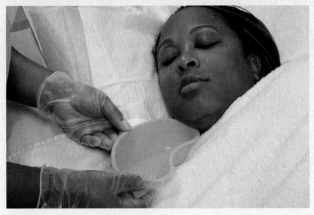

Figure 6

(continued on page 720)

Procedure (continued)

Step

Use a padded tongue blade to gently open the teeth (see Figure 7). Leave it in place between the back molars. Never insert your fingers into the mouth of an unconscious patient.

Rationale

Unconscious patients often respond to oral stimulation by biting down.

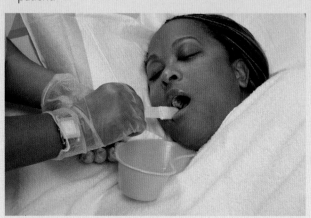

Figure 7

Brush the teeth and gums as directed previously, using a toothbrush or soft sponge-ended swab (see Figures 8 and 9). Cleanse oral cavity using Toothette.

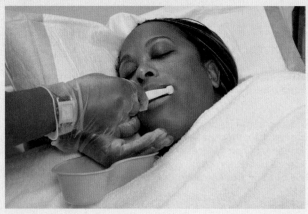

Figure 8

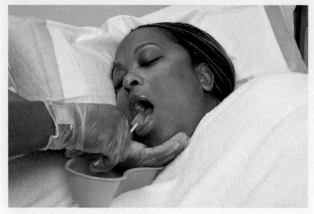

Figure 9

Procedure (continued)	
Step	**Rationale**
Use a small bulb syringe or syringe without a needle to rinse the oral cavity (see Figure 10). Swab or use oral suction to remove any pooled secretions (see Figure 11).	

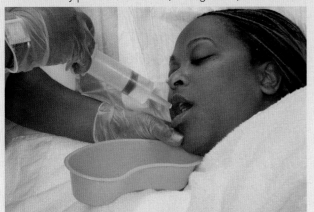

Figure 10

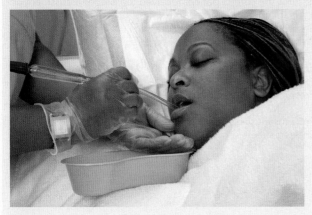

Figure 11

Apply a thin layer of petroleum jelly to lips to prevent drying or cracking.	
Document procedure.	Maintains a legal record and communicates with the health-care team

Lifespan Considerations

Infant
- Use a dry gauze or washcloth to remove accumulated secretions from an infant's gums.
- Use a small, soft-bristled brush after the first teeth have erupted.

Child
- Children younger than 3 or 4 years may not understand what the word *rinse* or *spit* means. Do not offer them water to rinse if they are NPO because they may swallow it.
- In children or teens who wear braces, ensure that all food particles are removed from the wires.

Older Adult
- Many older adults wear full or partial dentures. Be sure dentures are removed and cleaned regularly. Special denture cleansers are available. Brush the gums and any remaining teeth well. Keep dentures in a labeled denture cup to prevent loss or damage.

Home Care Modifications
- When teaching family members who are working with a comatose family member, be sure they can verbalize and demonstrate how to avoid aspirations.

Collaboration and Delegation
- Enlist the aid of OTs to work with patients who are relearning oral care procedures.
- Refer the patient to a dentist if you detect gum disease or caries.

SKILL 29.7   Making an Occupied Bed

Purpose

1. Provide clean linen to a patient who is restricted to his or her bed.
2. Ensure comfort.

Step	Rationale
Equipment: • Top sheet • Bottom sheet • Draw sheet • Blanket (do not change if not soiled) • Pillowcase • Waterproof pads Assessment: • Assess the patient's level of pain; determine when the last analgesic was given, the need for analgesic to ensure that the patient is comfortable. • Determine any position restrictions.	

Procedure

Step	Rationale
Identify the patient.	Ensures the correct patient received the proper assessment or treatment and reduces errors
Close the door and bed curtains.	Ensures patient privacy is maintained
Place equipment on patient's bedside table or chair and not on another patient's bed.	Prevents transmission of microorganisms
Inform the patient and family of the procedure that you will provide at the beginning and throughout.	Ensures that the patient is compliant and informed
Position and lock the side rails up on the opposite side of the bed from which you will be providing care.	Prevents any falls from occurring
Raise the bed to the appropriate height for the nurse.	Prevents muscle strain and injury of the nurse
Remove the top sheet and blanket; do not shake and place it on the bedside table or chair for reuse, unless soiled; and then place in linen bag. Undo the tucked sheets at the foot of the bed (see Figure 1).	Shaking sheets spreads microorganisms.

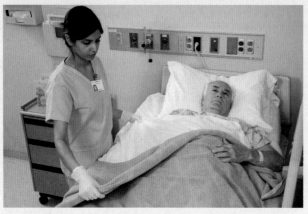

Figure 1

| Leave top sheet or place a bath towel on patient. | Ensures warmth and comfort and promotes privacy |
| Flatten the bed by lowering the head and foot of the bed. Undo the bottom sheet at the head of the bed on your side. | |

Procedure (continued)

Step

Reposition patient to face the opposite side of the nurse. Patient may hold on to the side rail on the opposite side (see Figure 2). Fanfold soiled sheet and tuck underneath the patient's shoulder, back, buttock, and legs (see Figure 3).

Rationale

Fanfold helps to prevent the clean sheets from being soiled.

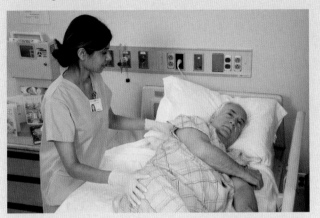

Figure 2

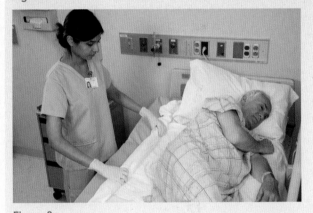

Figure 3

Unfold clean bottom sheet lengthwise. Fold bottom sheet edges over mattress sides and tuck under mattress. If bottom sheet does not have elastic to keep it in place (fitted sheet), perform a mitered corner, by

a. Grasping the edge of the bottom sheet 18 in. from the mattress top
b. Forming a triangle with the sheet by taking the corner of the sheet and laying it flat
c. Tucking the loose end under the mattress, leaving the folded triangle on the top of the mattress
d. Lowering the folded triangle to the side of the mattress and tucking it under

(continued on page 724)

SKILL 29.7 | Making an Occupied Bed (continued)

Procedure (continued)

Step

Once fitted and/or bottom sheet is in place, position the fitted/bottom sheet under the soiled sheet, tucking it under the patient (see Figures 4 and 5).

Rationale

Makes it easier to remove the soiled sheet

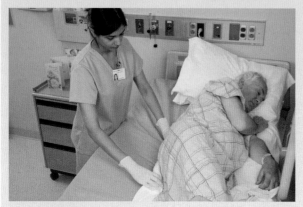

Figure 4

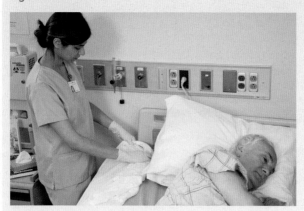

Figure 5

Place the absorbable pad on top of the fitted sheet and center it to the patient, tucking it under the soiled sheets and patient (see Figure 6).

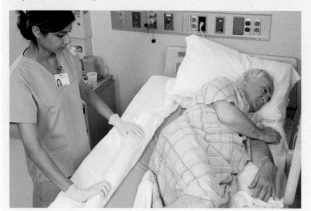

Figure 6

Procedure (continued)	

Step

Secure the side rails on your side. Move to the other side of the bed and lower the rails. Reposition the patient to face the opposite side (see Figure 7).

Rationale

Maintains patient safety

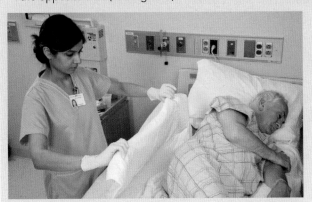

Figure 7

Fold soiled linen into a square and remove it from bed, placing it into the linen bag.

Grasp clean sheet from under the patient (see Figure 8). If using a flat sheet, tuck sheet using mitered corner. If fitted sheet, put over corners of the mattress. Tuck excess sheets tightly under the mattress and flatten absorbable pad, ensuring it is centered to the patient.

Prevents transmission of microorganisms

Secures the linens in place

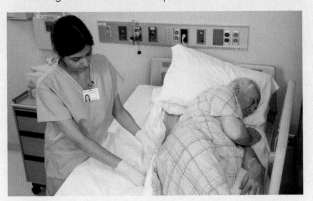

Figure 8

Assist the patient into a comfortable position.

Unfold clean top sheet lengthwise with the crease centered to the patient and unfold the sheet, ensuring that it is smooth. Once the sheet is on top of the patient, remove the towel or soiled top sheet, pulling from underneath the clean top sheet, and place in linen bag.

Maintains patient comfort and safety

Limits the exposure of the patient

(continued on page 726)

SKILL 29.7   Making an Occupied Bed (continued)

Procedure (continued)

Step

Place blanket on top of top sheet; ensure it is evenly covering the bed (see Figure 9). Miter the two bottom corners of the bed and leave the sides untucked (see Figure 10).

Rationale

Mitered corners secure the sheets in place.
Leaving the side untucked ensures comfort to the patient.

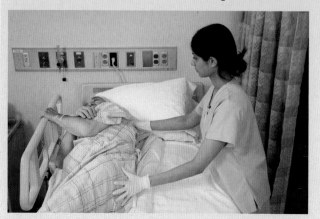

Figure 9

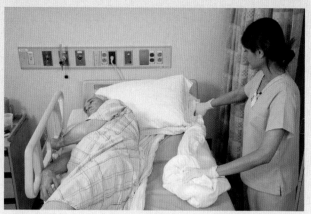

Figure 10

At the foot of the bed, grasp the top covers, pulling slightly to loosen the sheets and form a pleat (see Figure 11).

Ensures patient comfort

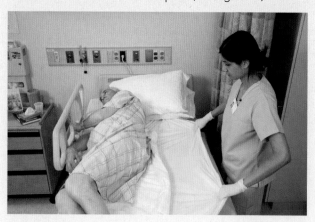

Figure 11

Remove the pillowcase by grasping the seamed end and turning it inside out. Place in linen bag.

Pull clean pillowcase over pillow and tuck one end of pillowcase over the pillow. Adjust pillow so that corners fit the pillowcase. Place pillow centered under the patient's head.

Prevents the transmission of microorganisms

Procedure (continued)

Ensure that that patient is comfortable. Reposition if necessary and arrange bedside table and patient's personal items to be within reach.	Ensures patient safety
Ensure that the call bell is within reach of the patient. Lower the bed to an appropriate and safe height (see Figure 12).	

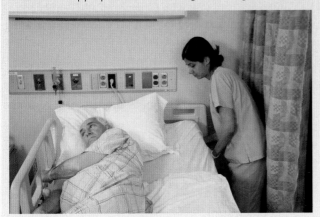

Figure 12
Discard soiled linens, remove gloves, and wash hands. Document procedure.

Prevents the transmission of microorganisms

Collaboration and Delegation
Communicate when help is needed. If repositioning is required be sure to consider patient safety at all times and consider repositioning restrictions.

Critical Thinking Case Scenarios

▶ You are a nurse proving care for Mr. Sigouin, an 85-year-old man who recently experienced a CVA. He has some muscle weakness to his left side and at times as little awareness of his affected side. His wife comes in daily to help her husband with some of his ADL as he requires assistance, and it helps to make her feel a part of his care. She has talked to you about her growing concern with her husband's temperament because he has moments when he is doing his ADL that he becomes extremely frustrated and start to yell.

1. What are some of the factors affecting Mr. Sigouin's ADL?
2. How can you promote independence with his self-care?
3. How would you address Mrs. Sigouin's concern?
4. Develop a care plan for Mr. Sigouin.

▶ Discussing hygiene with a patient can be very personal in nature and requires strong communication and assessment skills. Think about the following three patient/family statements and think specifically about what you would say as the nurse to validate the patient/family's feelings and address their concerns.

• Since my wife had her heart attack, she gets so tired when she tries to take a bath, but she doesn't even want my help.

She's stubborn and won't let anyone help her, and I don't know what to do.
• I don't see the point of bothering with eating or bathing. I have terminal cancer, and I know that I don't have long to live. I just don't see the point of it and want to be left alone in peace.
• I wish my son would come and visit me more often. I could really use his help. I haven't recovered as quickly as I would have liked since my hip surgery, and I'm having trouble getting up to use the bathroom. It's embarrassing to not make it to the toilet in time.

1. What interdisciplinary resources could you use or incorporate into each of these situations to help improve self-care?
2. Are there any specific assessments that you would complete or follow-up questions that you would ask to give you a better understanding of your patient/family?

Multiple-Choice Questions

1. Which of the factors affect one's ability to perform self-care at an independent level the most?
   a. Cognitive and functional ability
   b. Culture and personal preference
   c. Pain, motivation, and energy levels
   d. Socioeconomic status

2. An elderly patient is able to perform self-care with partial assistance, what can the nurse do to empower the patient the most during his self-care?
   a. The nurse can properly communicate the steps of the self-care that she will be performing and continually communicate throughout his self-care.
   b. The nurse can ask the patient what he can do and allow him to do those tasks.
   c. The nurse can ask the patient what he can do himself and ask him to also contribute by indicating what his preferences are for his self-care.
   d. The nurse can give him the basin with a washcloth and ask him to wash his face and his perineal area.

3. A nurse is performing a bed bath on an unconscious patient. What is this patient most at risk for?
   a. Impaired coping
   b. Falls
   c. Skin breakdown
   d. Hygiene self-care deficit

4. Which of the following patients is at the most risk for a self-care deficit?
   a. A surgical patient with pain rated as 5 out of 10
   b. An elderly stroke patient who is alert and oriented with hemiplegia to one side
   c. A patient receiving chemotherapy who has nausea and vomiting
   d. A child who only wants to bathe once a week

5. A nurse is performing an assessment on an elderly patient with Alzheimer dementia. What ADL would she most likely to be able to do independently?
   a. Dressing
   b. Bathing
   c. Toileting
   d. Brushing her hair

6. A home care nurse visits a patient and notices a smell of urine and that the patient uses a cane to mobilize. Which of the following questions would help with your assessment?
   a. Are you able to use the bathroom on your own?
   b. Are you satisfied with your ability to toilet and bathe yourself?

   c. Do you know that you should be cleaning yourself more thoroughly?
   d. Do you feel that you are able to manage your hygiene care independently in your home?

7. A nurse is caring for an elderly patient in the intensive care unit who is mechanically ventilated. The patient has dentures but is not currently wearing them. Which of the following is the most appropriate action?
   a. Rinse the patient's mouth with mouthwash.
   b. Swab out the patient's mouth with a foam swab.
   c. Brush the patient's dentures and put them back into the patient's mouth.
   d. Brush the patient's teeth using small amounts of liquid and an oral suction device.

8. A nurse is providing perineal care to an unconscious female patient. Which of the following is the most important step?
   a. Wash front to back and avoid contamination.
   b. Avoid temperature extremes because the perineal tissue is extremely sensitive.
   c. Include cleansing the folds between the legs and the labia.
   d. Turn the patient on her side to avoid aspiration.

9. Mr. Jones is a diabetic patient. He has an ulcer on his right foot and is being discharged home tomorrow. When providing him with discharge teaching, which of the following is the most important to include?
   a. To soak his feet daily in hot water
   b. To cut his toenails himself and in the shape of a curve
   c. To apply lotion liberally to his feet daily, including between the toes
   d. That he should inspect his feet daily, or have a caregiver do it if he cannot himself

10. You are preparing to provide your patient with hair care. Prior to beginning the procedure, it is MOST important for you to consider:
    a. The patient's preference
    b. The caregiver's preference
    c. The patient's cultural background
    d. The patient's husband's preference

REFERENCES AND SUGGESTED READINGS

Baird, S. K., & Briggs, Y. G. (2010). Hygiene. In P. A. Potter, A. G. Perry, J. C. Ross-Kerr, & M. J. Wood (Eds.), *Canadian fundamentals of nursing* (Rev. 4th ed., pp. 829–878). Toronto, ON: Elsevier.

Berry, A. M., Davidson, P. M., Masters, J., & Rolls, K. (2007). Systematic literature review of oral hygiene practices for intensive care patients receiving mechanical ventilation. *American Journal of Critical Care, 16*, 552–562.

Bulecheck, G. M., Butcher, H. K., McCloskey, J. M., Dochterman, J., & Wagner, C. (2013). *Nursing interventions classification* (NIC; 6th ed.). St Louis, MO: Mosby.

Canadian Dental Association. (2013a). *Oral health: Good for life*. Retrieved from http://www.cda-adc.ca/en/oral_health/cfyt/good_for_life/default.asp

Canadian Dental Association. (2013b). *Your oral health*. Retrieved from www.da-adc.ca/en/oral_health/index.asp

Canadian Dental Association. (2013c). *Flossing & brushing*. Retrieved from http://www.cda-adc.ca/en/oral_health/cfyt/dental_care/flossing_brushing.asp

Canadian Dermatology Association. (2013). *Eczema*. Retrieved from http://www.dermatology.ca/skin-hair-nails/skin/eczema/

Canadian Diabetes Association. (2008). *2008 Clinical practice guidelines for the prevention and management of diabetes in Canada*. Retrieved from http://www.diabetes.ca/files/cpg2008/cpg-2008.pdf

Canadian Heritage. (2012). Cultural diversity: A Canadian perspective. *Canada's Commitment to Cultural Diversity*. Retrieved from http://www.pch.gc.ca/eng/1332871836953/1332872826975

Ciaschini, P., Straus, S., Dolovich, L., Goeree, R., Leung, K., Woods, C., . . . Lee, H. (2009). Community-based intervention to optimise falls risk management: A randomised controlled trial. *Age and Ageing, 38*(6), 724–730. doi:10.1093/ageing/afp176

Drageset, J., Eide, G., & Ranhoff, A. (2011). Depression is associated with poor functioning in activities of daily living among nursing home residents without cognitive impairment. *Journal of Clinical Nursing, 20*(21/22), 3111–3118. doi:10.1111/j.1365-2702.2010.03663.x

Ebersole, P., Hess, P., Touhy, T. A., Jett, K., & Scmidt-Luggen, A. (2008). *Toward healthy aging: Human needs and nursing response* (7th ed.). St. Louis, MO: Mosby.

Fisk, A. (2010). Hygiene. In B. Kozier, G. Erb, A. Berman, S. J. Snyder, S. Raffin-Bouchel, S. Hirst, . . . M. Buck (Eds.), *Fundamentals of Canadian nursing: Concepts, process and practice* (pp. 704–761). Toronto, ON: Pearson Canada.

Garcia, R., Jendresky, L., Colbert, L., Bailey, A., Zaman, A., & Mojumder, M. (2009). Reducing ventilator-associated pneumonia through advanced oral-dental care: A 48-month study. *American Journal of Critical Care, 18*(6), 523–532.

Gillaspie-Aviz, M. (2013). Hygiene and self care. In R. F. Craven, C. J. Hirnle, & S. Jensen (Eds.), *Fundamentals of nursing human health and function* (7th ed., pp. 599–628). Philadelphia, PA: Lippincott Williams & Wilkins.

Grant, B. M., Giddings, L. S., & Beale, J. E. (2005). Vulnerable bodies: Competing discourse of intimate bodily care. *Journal of Nursing Education, 44*(44), 498–504.

Howett, M., Connor, A., & Downes, E. (2010). Nightingale theory and intentional comfort touch in management of tinea pedis in vulnerable populations. *Journal of Holistic Nursing, 28*(4), 244–250. doi:10.1177/0898010110373655

Inoue, M., Chapman, R., & Wynaden, D. (2006). Male nurses' experience providing intimate care for women patients. *Journal of Advanced Nursing, 55*(5), 559–567.

Larson, E. L., Ciliberti, T., Chantler, C., Abraham, J., Lazaro, E. M., Venturanza, M., & Pancholi, P. (2004). Comparison of traditional and disposable bed baths in critically ill patients. *American Journal of Critical Care, 13*, 235–241.

Miller, C. A. (2009). *Nursing for wellness in older adults* (5th ed.). Philadelphia, PA: Lippincott William & Wilkins.

Moorhead, S., Johnson, M., Maas, M. L., & Swanson, E. (2013). *Nursing outcomes classification (NOC): Measurement of health outcomes* (5th ed.). St. Louis, MO: Mosby.

Munro, C. L., Grap, M. M., Elswick, R. K., McKinney, J., Sessler, C., & Hummel, R. S. (2006). Oral health status and development of ventilator associated pneumonia: A descriptive study. *American Journal of Critical Care, 15*, 453–460.

North American Nursing Diagnosis Association International. (2012). *Nursing diagnoses: Definitions and classification, 2012–2014*. Ames, Iowa: Wiley-Blackwell.

Rader, J., Barrick, A., Hoeffer, B., Sloane, P., McKenzie, D., Talerico, K., & Glover, J. (2006). The bathing of older adults with dementia: Easing the unnecessarily unpleasant aspects of assisted bathing. *American Journal of Nursing, 106*(4), 40–49.

Resnick, B. (2004). *Restorative care nursing for older adults*. New York, NY: Springer Publishing.

Sensory Processing Disorder Foundation. (2012). *About sensory processing disorders*. Retrieved from http://www.spdfoundation.net/about-sensory-processing-disorder.html

Smeltzer, S. C., & Bare, B. (2013). *Brunner & Suddarth's textbook of medical-surgical nursing* (12th ed.). Philadelphia, PA: Lippincott Williams & Wilkins.

Smith, M., Darrat, I., & Seidman, M. (2012). Otologic complications of cotton swab use: One institution's experience. *Laryngoscope, 122*(2), 409–411. doi:10.1002/lary.22437

Statistic Canada. (2010). *Pain or discomfort that prevents activities*. Retrieved from http://www.statcan.gc.ca/pub/82-229-x/2009001/status/pdl-eng.htm

Tsai, A., Hsu, H., & Chang, T. (2011). The Mini Nutritional Assessment (MNA) is useful for assessing the risk of malnutrition in adults with intellectual disabilities. *Journal of Clinical Nursing, 20*(23/24), 3295–3303. doi:10.1111/j.1365-2702.2011.03877.x

World Health Organization. (2013a). *The determinants of health*. Retrieved from http://www.who.int/hia/evidence/doh/en/

World Health Organization. (2013b). Water supply, Sanitation, and hygiene development. *Water Sanitation Health*. Retrieved from http://www.who.int/water_sanitation_health/hygiene/en/

Yeo, N. (2013). What really matters: The taste of water and more. *Singapore Nursing Journal, 40*(1), 11–15.

Zullino, D. F., Krenz, S., Frésard, E., Cancela, E., & Khazaal, Y. (2005). Local back massage with an automated massage chair: General muscle and psychophysiologic relaxing properties. *Journal of Alternative and Complementary Medicine, 11*, 1103–1106.

Zurlinden, J. (2003). Drug news: New warnings for Lindane shampoo and lotion. *Nursing Spectrum—Midwest Edition, 40*(6), 10.

Creating Comfort and Managing Pain

JEAN N. HARROWING AND JOAN BRAY

Taylor is in her second clinical rotation as an undergraduate nursing student. She finds Maria, a 29-year-old woman, lying in her hospice bed cuddling and singing softly to her first born child, 3-week-old Sarah. Maria is thinking about the turn her life has taken, away from the hopes she and Ben had 3 years ago when she immigrated to Canada. The couple had met and fallen in love during Ben's mission to her hometown in Central America; they married soon after.

It was at the midpoint of her pregnancy that Maria felt significant and unusual back pain, pelvic heaviness, and bloating. Investigations showed a fast-spreading ovarian cancer. At that moment that she recognized that her life was moving in two directions at once—her anticipation of motherhood shadowed by an invasive tumor robbing her of vital energy and dreams of her future.

At shift report, Taylor heard that the disease has failed to respond favourably to treatment; Maria is not expected to survive more than 6 months. Taylor now finds herself caring for a woman and her family following a very joyous event in their lives, in the midst of very tragic circumstances. She wonders where to begin. She wonders if nursing is going to be the right career for her.

CHAPTER OBJECTIVES

By the end of this chapter, you will be able to:

1. Describe the role of the registered nurse in providing safe and appropriate care to patients and families experiencing terminal illness.
2. Discuss the necessary knowledge, attitudes, and interventions for effective creation of therapeutic presence when working with others in a palliative context.
3. Explain the concepts of pain and comfort and the importance of understanding the patient's interpretation and lived experience of their meaning.
4. Articulate the significance of exploring your personal beliefs and thoughts about living, dying, and death and their impact on your development as a registered nurse.

KEY TERMS

Bereavement Refers to not only the loss of a significant person but also the period of transition for the bereaved individual following that person's death. *Bereavement* is a broad term that encompasses the entire experience of family members and friends in the anticipation, death, and subsequent adjustment to living following the death of a loved one.

Compassion An emotion evoked by the suffering of others, a strength that allows one person to connect with another to acknowledge that suffering, and the desire to ease the accompanying pain.

Compassion Fatigue The distress that accumulates over time after continuous exposure to caregiving situations that are interpreted as traumatic. The effects may be physical, emotional, moral, spiritual, and intellectual.

Complementary and Alternative Therapies A group of diverse medical and health-care systems, practices, and products that are not generally considered part of conventional medicine.

Empathy The ability to truly know another person within a trusting, mutually respectful relationship. Empathy is the most essential ingredient one must have to care for another person.

Grief Sorrow experienced in anticipation of, during, and after a loss. The diverse natural reactions, such as psychological, physical, and social reactions, to the loss of a significant person are characterized by both suffering and growth. Grief is a process that requires time. It is normal to experience grief for many months and years after death.

Holistic Nursing A practice that aims to heal the whole person and draws on nursing knowledge, theories, expertise, and intuition to guide nurses in becoming therapeutic partners with people in their care. This practice recognizes the totality of the human being—the interconnectedness of body, mind, emotion, spirit, social/cultural factors, relationship, context, and environment.

Palliate/Palliative From the Latin *palliare*, meaning to cloak or cover; the term refers to all activities that alleviate the intensity of suffering and symptoms. These activities aim to help patients and their families prepare for and manage life closure and the dying process. The focus of palliative care is to treat all active concerns, prevent new issues from occurring, and promote opportunities for meaningful and valuable experiences, personal and spiritual growth, and self-actualization.

Relational Practice The art and skill of being able to connect with people across differences by joining with them as they are and where they are.

Quality of Life Well-being as defined by the person living with advanced illness. It relates to experiences that are meaningful to the individual. It is the gold standard for palliative care.

Spirituality An existential construct inclusive of all the ways in which a person makes meaning and organizes sense of self around a personal set of beliefs, values, and relationships. It is sometimes understood in terms of transcendence or inspiration. Involvement in a community of faith and practice may be a part of an individual's spirituality.

Suffering A state of distress associated with events that threaten the integrity of a person. It may be accompanied by a perceived lack of options for coping.

Total Pain Suffering related to, and the result of, the person's physical, psychological, social, spiritual, and practical state.

This chapter focuses on the nurse's role in providing comfort and pain management within the context of the transition that occurs while a patient and family receive **palliative** care. It is truly a privilege to be a nurse, working with individuals, families, and communities at the most vulnerable and intimate times of living a life. These moments offer the nurse an extraordinary opportunity to demonstrate the capacity for compassion that is required to support persons on the journey of physical being to nonbeing, through the transition of living to dying to being dead. Although such work is seldom easy, many nurses describe their deep respect for the sacredness of being present with another human being during those final moments as the essence of the person transcends the body and only flesh remains.

Although the emphasis in this chapter is on nursing care for the dying patient and his or her family, the basic principles discussed here can, and should, be applied to any patient regardless of the medical diagnosis. We begin with a "bird's eye view," examining global concepts of providing nursing care to individuals who are facing difficult situations such as terminal illness or spiritual suffering and then "zoom in" to learn about addressing specific challenges such as uncontrolled pain. Although an essential component of expert nursing care is a strong knowledge base, your primary task as a novice nurse is to learn how to engage in **relational practice** with your patients and their families. Without awareness of the person and the context in which she lives life and the ability to meet her where she is, you will not be able to effectively apply your knowledge in a way that respectfully acknowledges her humanity and her care needs. Hence, you will note that this chapter emphasizes thoughtful reflection and the courage to put your own doubts aside as you concentrate on truly listening to what is in the patient's heart as well as observing what is happening to her tissues and organs. Indeed, entire books have been written about all the ideas and interventions that appear in this chapter, and you are encouraged to explore more widely to gain deeper knowledge and broader skills as you simultaneously practice the skills of empathy and **compassion**. Ultimately, the goal is to understand and respond to your patient as a whole person, a fellow human being who is much more than a set of symptoms and body parts. A selection of useful references is provided at the end of this chapter to help you expand your knowledge.

Through the eyes of a nurse

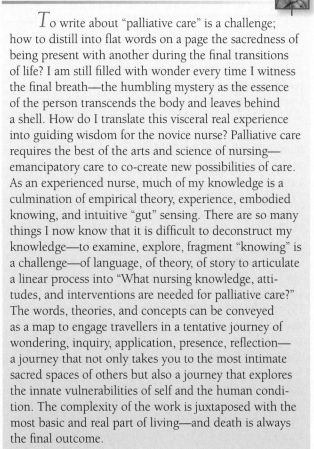

To write about "palliative care" is a challenge; how to distill into flat words on a page the sacredness of being present with another during the final transitions of life? I am still filled with wonder every time I witness the final breath—the humbling mystery as the essence of the person transcends the body and leaves behind a shell. How do I translate this visceral real experience into guiding wisdom for the novice nurse? Palliative care requires the best of the arts and science of nursing—emancipatory care to co-create new possibilities of care. As an experienced nurse, much of my knowledge is a culmination of empirical theory, experience, embodied knowing, and intuitive "gut" sensing. There are so many things I now know that it is difficult to deconstruct my knowledge—to examine, explore, fragment "knowing" is a challenge—of language, of theory, of story to articulate a linear process into "What nursing knowledge, attitudes, and interventions are needed for palliative care?" The words, theories, and concepts can be conveyed as a map to engage travellers in a tentative journey of wondering, inquiry, application, presence, reflection— a journey that not only takes you to the most intimate sacred spaces of others but also a journey that explores the innate vulnerabilities of self and the human condition. The complexity of the work is juxtaposed with the most basic and real part of living—and death is always the final outcome.

(personal reflection of a nurse)

Care, Compassion, and Comfort

As a nursing student, you are learning that registered nurses are committed to providing **holistic** and compassionate care to people in a wide variety of health-related situations. Some of the most critical moments in life happen at times of transition between "what was" and "what will be"; nurses have the unique honour and privilege of being present as people move through those transformations. Our work must be done with great sensitivity, **empathy**, and awareness. Nouwen (1974, pp. 33–34) described empathetic caring in this way:

> The word "care" finds its roots in the Gothic "Kara" which means lament. The basic meaning of care is: to grieve, to experience sorrow, to cry out with. I am very much struck by this background of the word care because we tend to look at caring as an attitude of the strong toward the weak, of the powerful toward the powerless. Still, when we honestly ask ourselves which persons in our lives mean the most to us, we often find that it is those who, instead of giving much advice, solutions, or cures, have chosen rather to share our pain and touch our wounds with a gentle and tender hand.

Through the eyes of a student

I had no idea when I started nursing school that I would be doing palliative care with a woman who is only a few years older than me! I was stunned when I got my patient assignment today from my instructor and saw that I would be caring for Maria, a brand-new mother who wouldn't live to see her baby's first birthday. My great-uncle was in a palliative care program when he died last year, but he was 76, not 29! How could I ever work with a young person? How would I know what to say to her? How could I not feel guilty that I was healthy and she was going to die? What if she cries? My gut reaction was to tell my instructor I couldn't deal with this and to ask for a new assignment. I called him and explained my concerns. He reminded me that Maria was not dead yet and that I might want to think of her as living, not dying. When I thought about this, it made sense. I know that new moms are usually excited and proud of the accomplishment of giving birth, and if I approached Maria with that in mind, I might be able to make a connection with her and not have to worry about saying the "wrong" thing. I decided that if we could base a relationship around her new role as a mom, maybe that would help me be open to hear her story about her cancer and what that was like for her. My instructor also mentioned that there is nothing wrong with being honest about my uncertainty when I talk with Maria—I can tell her that I couldn't imagine what she was going through, but that if she would teach me, I would do my best to help her get what she needs. So, my plan is to prepare for my clinical practice tomorrow by learning about the possible needs of a mother who is adjusting to life with a 3-week-old baby as well as understanding the typical challenges associated with metastatic ovarian cancer. I have an idea that most of my learning will be about courage and compassion, though, and that it will come from real-life experience!

(personal reflection of a nursing student)

Indeed, there are pains that cannot be eliminated and wounds that cannot be fixed; in those cases, providing comfort consists of attending to the individual's complex physical, emotional, social, and spiritual needs within a context of authentic presence and compassion. That choice to engage with people and share the intimacy of the moment requires courage, persistence, and openness; it is not usually a straightforward path to enlightenment and serenity. Often, the nurse must sit quietly and simply pay attention—a challenging task for many of us who believe our hands must be always busy. Indeed, this accompaniment of individuals and families along the final stretch of their life journey may be some of the most difficult work you do as a nurse, but it may also be some of the most rewarding. This therapeutic relationship takes place within a web of teamwork, and you will work in harmony with the patient, family, and other health-care providers. As the most consistent professional directly involved in care, you have the additional responsibility to communicate, advocate, and effectively engage the interdisciplinary team to respond to the dynamic needs of the patient and family.

*T*aylor had all these images in her mind as she summoned the courage to knock on Maria's door for the first time. She took a deep breath, hoping to find the ability to create a space of comfort for both herself and Maria and walked in when Maria answered. The conversation started, "Hi, I am Taylor, I am a second-year nursing student, and I have been assigned to work with you." Maria was at first indifferent to Taylor's presence. With permission, Taylor sat in the chair next to Maria and Sarah and felt her own heart beating as she spoke softly, asking, "How can I support you today?" After some silence, Maria commented, "This has been a good day. At this moment, I feel joy, I still can't believe . . . it is a miracle every time I hold Sarah. I love being a mother! I could sit and hold her all day."

Taylor had been preparing to enter a space filled with sadness and heavy gloom, but Maria's comments made her realize she was a witness to the hope and joy Sarah represented. With appreciation for Maria's perspective, Taylor asked, "What can I do to help you to care for Sarah?"

Nightingale (1860/1969) observed that nursing is based on knowledge; without that knowledge, you cannot call yourself a nurse. Nursing students typically feel a sense of urgency about knowing enough to take care of a patient, as that comprises the visible aspects of your role, the actions that others watch and judge as you interact with people. However, Nightingale emphasized that nursing is more than knowledge of scientific facts and procedures, that nursing requires a certain ethical deportment and the ability to act artfully. Thus, it is important that nurses learn and apply empiric knowledge within a humanistic and equitable context that promotes health for everyone. To accomplish this goal, you will need to cultivate a curiosity for and deliberate pursuit of the theoretical knowledge that will enable you to create a plan relevant to the social, emotional, physical, cultural, and spiritual needs of the people with whom you work.

Healing

Nightingale (1860/1969) also believed that the nurse's role is to create the conditions in which healing can take place. You are curious about how a person can heal when he or she has a terminal illness—these seem to be contradictory concepts. However, as you read about and ponder this notion, you come to understand that the two terms may not be mutually exclusive. Healing can be interpreted as reestablishing integrity or making whole again; it has more to do with the person than the disease (Barnum, 2003). Quinn (2000, p. 42) suggested that healing is a "process of emergence" or coming to know the inner self rather than the disappearance of a set of signs and symptoms. Dossey (2009, p. 21) suggests that healing may or may not occur simultaneously with curing, but that its potential continues until the last breath. Other researchers noted that healing focuses on reconnecting more fully with self and others (McDonough-Means, Kreitzer, & Bell, 2004). Gottlieb (2013, p. 64) says that "healing is not only a noun, but also a verb" that invites the nurse to observe the patient's emotional, spiritual, biologic, and existential status. The nurse can promote healing in the individual by consciously creating a welcoming space in which both can feel secure, listening closely and empathizing, and maintaining hope for the possibility of wellness (Zerwekh, 2006). This may sound challenging and overwhelming, but if you remember that it is your intention to act on your values about and desires to provide care that will be evident to the individual, you will be well on your way to creating that healing environment identified by Nightingale. If you are able to meet Maria where she is in the moment, regardless of where you think she "should" be, you will contribute to her healing (Hartrick Doane & Varcoe, 2005). One way to approach this is to ask yourself not "What can I do?" but "How can I be with this person in this moment in a way that will provide the best possible outcome?" (McKivergin, 2009, p. 725).

What Is Hospice and Hospice Care?

You have probably noticed that much of our modern approach to health care focuses on identifying disease patterns or broken body parts, followed by prescribing a drug or procedure to mend that which is not functioning properly. For many of the health problems we encounter in a lifetime, this approach is satisfactory. An antibiotic to cure an infection, a surgical intervention to replace a damaged joint, counseling sessions to address depression—these interventions are relatively simple and easy to implement to restore or improve an individual's ability to carry on with day-to-day living. However, upon thoughtful reflection, you might realize that almost any disruption in health occurs within a context of contributory factors, threats to normal daily routines, and personal meaning. For example, as a student, you may have experienced a debilitating bout of stomach flu or a cold and the implications for keeping up with your studies as you try to recover from that illness. Perhaps, you were overtired and stressed from late nights of preparing assignments, working at your part-time job, and not eating a balanced diet or getting enough exercise. When you realized you were becoming ill, you may have felt a few moments of anxiety or even panic when you wondered how you could participate in the next day's clinical practice while feeling miserable and exhausted. If you sought medical attention to help you address your situation, your care provider may have carefully listened to your worries about how being sick would affect your ability to keep up with your schoolwork—or your attempts to convey your concerns may have been brushed aside as irrelevant or unimportant. A practitioner who takes into consideration the individual's complete experience and interpretation of personal meaning of an illness and who involves the individual in formulating a set of useful strategies for healing that are relevant and feasible is a practitioner who engages in holistic health care. This approach is particularly significant for someone who is experiencing a life-threatening condition. Most of us do not think much about the notion that our lives will come to an end; if we do, it is only in the abstract, far-distant future that we can imagine such an event. However, the person who has become aware that death will arrive in the next few days, weeks, or months often experiences a tumultuous and confusing array of emotions that may result in physical or behavioural responses that you can observe or inquire about. It is worthwhile for you, the nurse, to explore the personal impact and meaning of the person's unique situation. This means you must have the courage to be present—not always an easy task for a nurse who has been socialized to follow orders, complete tasks, and comply with institutional policy. Also, it is tempting for health-care professionals to believe that "if you have seen one, you've seen them all," but it is critical to teach yourself that you must approach each person as a unique being who understands the world in a unique way. Otherwise, you may try to impose your beliefs and values inappropriately, with the result that the person is not helped, and you are frustrated. When your values collide with those of the individual, you become "a visitor in a foreign country" bound to respectfully honour her integrity by practicing according to her world perspective.

Recall that Taylor has encountered Maria in the hospice setting. Hospice, often called *palliative care*, refers to a philosophical approach to caring for people with the intention of reducing **suffering** (Kastenbaum, 2009) and improving

quality of life (Downing, 2006). Because events at the end of life are often associated with suffering, palliative care is typically understood to be appropriate for persons who are dying. Suffering is linked to distress and pain that cause an individual to experience loss of the meaning and purpose that make life worth living, as defined by that person; suffering threatens the integrity, or intactness, of the whole person. It may have physical, emotional, cognitive, cultural, social, existential, and spiritual aspects and is a profoundly personal and subjective experience (Gregory & English, 1994). Although all human beings will experience suffering at some point in their lives, making it a universal phenomenon, it tends to isolate the individual from family and friends and results in withdrawal into the self as the person tries to sort things out. This can be painful and difficult to witness for the people around the dying person and is a vital consideration for the nurse who wishes to offer holistic care.

Palliative care may be provided in an institutional setting, perhaps a dedicated inpatient unit or as part of a medical unit in an acute care or continuing care environment. It may also be offered through outpatient programs, such as a pain and symptom management clinic, or home care programs. Some comprehensive programs, such as that offered by the Victoria Hospice Society in Victoria, British Columbia (http://www.victoriahospice.org), include **bereavement** counselling, in-home crisis support, and clinical consultation services and educational and research initiatives. Compassionate care of the dying has a long history, going back to ancient times. In recent years, palliative care has come to be understood as a philosophy of, or an approach to, sharing in the care of dying persons and their families rather than a building or location for specialized care provided by a team of medical experts. Palliative care is offered by a highly motivated team of caregivers that may include family members; medical, nursing, and allied health professionals; religious or faith leaders; and volunteers who are committed to help dying people live the remainder of their lives with dignity, quality, and meaning. It is a service based on respect for the dying person's preferences and needs that intends to reduce discomfort, enhance a sense of security and hope, and ease the passage from life to death. It requires acute attention to detail, compassion, and competence.

Unfortunately, not everyone has access to palliative care, despite our advanced knowledge about how to relieve suffering and pain. Our health-care system does not always address the needs of persons who live in poverty, have limited family support or reduced health literacy skills, are aged, perceived as ethno-culturally or racially different, or who suffer from chronic disease; those who also have a terminal illness experience even greater challenges in accessing appropriate end-of-life resources and services (Lewis, DiGiacomo, Currow, & Davidson, 2011; McGibbon & Etowa, 2009; Walshe, Todd, Caress, & Chew-Graham, 2009). Even in a country such as Canada, where you live often dictates the kind of care you are likely to receive (Collier, 2011). Most of the 58 million people in the world who die every year live in low-income countries, which have the scarcest resources; many of these people die unsupported, isolated, and in unspeakable agony because a public health strategy for palliative care does not exist (Stjernswärd, Foley, & Ferris, 2007). Thus, in addition to the provision of direct care to people, it is essential that as a nurse, you engage in the research and policy development process that will positively influence access to comprehensive services for the global community (Canadian Nurses Association, 2008b; Krakauer, Wenk, Buitrago, Jenkins, & Scholten, 2010). Such work will contribute to the achievement of social justice, one of the fundamental principles of the code of ethics (Canadian Nurses Association, 2008a) to which we are held accountable as registered nurses.

Now that she has worked with Maria for several shifts, Taylor is curious about her patient's experience of pain. Maria is taking a small oral dose (4 mg) of extended-release hydromorphone twice daily, and she has never requested additional analgesia for breakthrough pain. Although Taylor has not heard Maria complain directly about pain, she has observed several behaviours (e.g., gently massaging her abdomen as she lay in bed, grimacing when she picked up Sarah) that make her wonder about the presence and intensity of discomfort. Taylor has found an assessment tool that seems to provide the opportunity to gather comprehensive knowledge about pain. She will ask Maria if there is a time this afternoon when they can discuss the topic.

What Is Pain?

Through the eyes of a patient

I have end-stage bowel cancer, and I am going to die soon. I have known this for a while now. It still seems surreal sometimes; at other times, it sits like a rock in my belly, pulling my soul into the earth. As I watch my young daughters bounce around the hospital room when they come with my wife to visit, I know I cannot leave them yet, even though I am so tired of the winter, the pain, and the sense that I am a burden. I feel selfish, but I want to stay just long enough to see . . . to see what? What is realistic to hope for? I want to be here to hold my grandchildren, but I know that is not going to happen. Maybe, I can live just long enough to watch my girls' delight as spring blooms, as they notice the baby robins in the backyard, as they breathlessly ask when we can pull the wading pool out of the garage so they can go "swimming." Can I hang on that long?

Yesterday, the evening nurse came in to ask me about my pain. I told her it was about a 4 on the now-familiar 0 to 10 scale. She responded with alarm, stating that was unacceptable, why didn't I call her to report this, and as she spoke, she began moving toward my portable pain pump. "Whoa!!" I said to her, "what are you doing?" She told me she was going to increase the dosage of my morphine. I told her I didn't want it increased. She looked at me in astonishment and said, "What do you mean? I can relieve your pain by bumping up the infusion, the doctor has already written that order." I quietly told her that I didn't want her to get rid of my pain. She opened her mouth to speak; then she closed it and sat down in the chair and just waited quietly. I finally explained it to her. "As long as I have pain, I know I am still alive." She slowly nodded, and said, "I never thought of it that way. That makes sense, though." She thanked me and told me she would make it a habit to always ask the patient about their pain management goals rather than expect that everyone would naturally want to be pain-free. She thanked me again for forcing her to question her assumptions. I felt good that I had maybe made a difference to her way of being a nurse.

(personal reflection of a patient)

Although many people have tried to define pain, perhaps the most accurate, accepted, and easiest to remember is the definition offered by Margo McCaffery, a registered nurse who has studied and taught about the subject for many years. McCaffery (1968, p. 95) said that "pain is whatever the experiencing person says it is, existing whenever he says it does." In other words, no one can judge the existence and intensity of pain except the person who has it. This is a crucial point because many of us are quick to evaluate the presence, quality, and severity of someone's reports of pain based on factors that have nothing to do with the pain. For example, consider your own response when someone who is laughing and interacting with friends states that she is experiencing severe pain and needs an analgesic. Do you believe her, or do you question her trustworthiness? If a person is asleep, would you assume his pain is minimal? Some people have a mental image of how a person in pain should look or behave; sleeping or laughing are not generally characteristics that fit that expectation. Indeed, researchers have shown that nurses are more likely to offer adequate pain medication to a person who grimaces and reports severe pain than they are to treat someone who smiles while reporting severe pain (McCaffery, Herr, & Pasero, 2011, p. 21). Similarly, people from minority racial or cultural groups are less likely to receive adequate pain control (Lasch, 2000). However, there is a great deal of scientific evidence that supports the accuracy and reliability of the patient's report of pain; therefore, nurses must first of all be aware of their biases and tendencies to judge people rather than to show empathy. Secondly, they must accept and respect the individual's report of pain as they decide how best to intervene. In this way, the individual and nurse are more likely to enter into a trusting and therapeutic relationship.

Based on your knowledge of metastatic cancer, you might anticipate that Maria will experience pain as a result of the tumor that is invading her internal organs. She might respond to your inquiry by confirming escalating pain that interferes with caring for her daughter. What other information do you need to gather before you suggest some possible strategies to Maria? A good pain assessment takes into account a wide array of factors; you will likely find it helpful to follow a systematic process to make sure you cover all the key aspects. You will want to know about the location, intensity, quality, patterns, onset, duration, rhythms, and variations in the pain as well as factors that cause or increase it and the interventions that relieve it. McCaffery et al. (2011) offer several widely used tools to assess and document pain; these authors invite you to duplicate their tools and scales and use them in clinical practice. For other examples of pain assessment tools, see the references at the end of this chapter. When conducting your assessment, it is helpful to remember that the stronger your relationship with the person, the more comfortable he will feel in sharing the very personal story of his pain experience. Furthermore, if the individual is confident that you will do your utmost to help, you are more likely to gather relevant information. Thus, it is critical that you engage in an authentic, respectful relationship with the person. That relationship is complemented by your sense of salience and your capacity for clinical reasoning and clinical imagination (Benner, Sutphen, Leonard, & Day, 2010, p. 15). In other words, you identify and interpret the relevant components of Maria's story of pain and engage in a process of clinical reasoning to negotiate an effective resolution, guided by your vision of future possibilities.

It is important to understand that pain comprises not only a physical component but is manifest in other ways as well. Dame Cicely Saunders, educated as a nurse, social worker, and finally as a physician who founded St. Christopher's Hospice in London, England in 1967, suggested the term "**total pain**" to describe multidimensional causes and effects of pain (Saunders, 1976). She believed that to assess and treat pain, one must consider the emotional, spiritual, and social components of the pain experience. Furthermore, there is often more than one pain, especially if the person has a complex disease such as cancer. Several different pathological processes may occur simultaneously, resulting in different sensations and requiring different treatments. Additionally, factors such as fear or anxiety often accompany pain, and there is evidence that suggests they may help a person cope with the pain, or they may make the pain worse (McCaffery et al., 2011). Hence, there is a need for careful and detailed assessment in order to arrive at appropriate treatment options.

Once you learn about the person's pain and its patterns, you will be in a position to observe, assess, and anticipate her needs. You might consider asking her to document her response to the treatment plan using a pain diary. Using the person's goals, ask her to note the time and dose of the drug or strategy as well as its effectiveness in meeting the desired outcomes. You will quickly notice what strategies are working well and where changes need to be made to better meet the goals. Such a diary will also help you plan your nursing care activities. For example, if the person reports increased pain associated with his morning bath, you will plan to offer an analgesic prior to the next bath to take advantage of the maximal efficacy of the drug. In this way, you will build the person's confidence, enhance his quality of life, and perhaps restore some of his hope for a meaningful future. You must not underestimate your ability to make profound contributions to a person's life by your simple but careful attention to significant details!

Adequate relief of pain requires extensive knowledge of a wide range of treatment modalities. Although pharmacologic management plays a major role, there are many other options available for consideration. The gate control theory (Melzack & Wall, 1965) includes the notion that the perception of pain may be altered by stimulating other sensory pathways that interfere with the transmission of pain messages to the brain. Use of this theory to guide your practice will lead you to try interventions such as distraction techniques (e.g., music or funny movies), acupressure, massage, or application of heat or cold to reduce or minimize discomfort.

Pharmacologic Pain Management

There are three main groups of analgesics commonly used to treat most types of pain: nonopioids, opioids, and adjuvant drugs. This section offers a basic introduction to the uses and characteristics of each group.

Nonopioids

Acetaminophen and nonsteroidal anti-inflammatory drugs (NSAIDs) comprise this group of analgesics. These drugs are used to control mild to moderate pain (analgesic) and fever (antipyretic); the NSAIDs are also anti-inflammatory. Drugs in this group represent the first step on the World Health Organization (WHO) Analgesic Ladder (WHO, 1996) and are often used as multipurpose interventions to deal with both chronic and acute pain that originates from bone, joint, or soft tissue injury or inflammation. It is essential to give the lowest effective dose for the shortest time needed, to avoid problems associated with long-term use. There is a wide range of choice available in this category, so if the side effects of one drug are unacceptable, others can be tried. Although these drugs are generally considered safe, they are limited in their ability to treat severe pain.

Opioids

The second step of the WHO Analgesic Ladder recommends the use of opioid analgesics for persistent pain that does not respond adequately to nonopioid use alone. Morphine is the prototype, or gold standard, to which other opioids are compared (Pasero, Quinn, Portenoy, McCaffery, & Rizos, 2011).

The major concern with these medications is the potential for life-threatening respiratory depression; therefore, as the nurse, you must monitor the individual receiving the drug very closely for signs of excessive sedation. If pain relief is not achieved initially, the dose will be increased gradually (titrated) under close supervision.

Although opioids are very effective for many types of moderate to severe pain, there are several misconceptions about their use that often act as a barrier. For example, many people, including health-care professionals, worry about the potential for addiction, a chronic neurologic and biologic disease characterized by continued craving for the drug's effects other than pain relief. Addiction is very rare in persons suffering from terminal conditions (Pasero & Portenoy, 2011), and concerns about it should not preclude the consideration of opioids for people in intractable pain. Similarly, some people believe that opioids should not be used in early stages for fear that they "won't work" later on. However, a useful property of these analgesics is that there is no maximum dose for most of them, so the dose can be titrated as needed as long as the response (safety and side effects) remains acceptable. Furthermore, there are times when the side effects of the drug are desirable—for example, a person who is gasping for breath because of pulmonary edema secondary to lung cancer will often benefit from oral or nebulized administration of morphine to ease the awful sensation of being unable to breathe (Pasero, Quinn, et al., 2011). It is imperative to understand the pharmacokinetics of the medications, so that you can make use of their properties to enhance comfort and quality of life.

There are several opioid-induced adverse effects, in addition to the sedation and respiratory depression already mentioned, that you must anticipate or prevent. Constipation and nausea are common and may be distressful enough that the person terminates use of the analgesic prematurely. This is an unfortunate situation because the removal of opioids as a treatment option severely limits the chances of managing the pain. Thus, it is essential that you educate care providers and the individual about potential side effects and ways to prevent them rather than allowing these issues to arise. Other less common but equally distressing problems associated with opioids include pruritus (itching), myoclonus (jerking or twitching), and mental confusion or delirium. If at all possible, you must prevent these effects from occurring; if that is not feasible, it is critical that you anticipate, monitor frequently, and be prepared to treat adverse effects immediately. As a member of the interdisciplinary team, you will collaborate with your colleagues (e.g., pharmacist, physician) to determine most appropriate intervention. Your goal is to provide competent care that facilitates comfort, confidence, and quality of life.

Adjuvants

An adjuvant, or nontraditional, analgesic is a drug that is normally used for a non-pain indication but which can provide analgesia for some painful conditions (Pasero, Polomano,

Portenoy, & McCaffery, 2011). Clinical experience with these medications has been mainly with neuropathic (nerve) pain and chronic (persistent) non-cancer conditions such as fibromyalgia and bone pain as well as other non-pain symptoms. However, ongoing research is revealing new roles for these drugs; thus, it is vital that you stay up-to-date with current evidence. Classes of drugs included in this category are antidepressants, corticosteroids, cannabinoids, anticonvulsants, local anesthetics, and anticholinergics. Some of them relieve pain by themselves, whereas others are used in combination with opioids or nonopioids—it depends on the condition being treated. As a nurse, you need to understand the underlying mechanisms of pain and analgesia, as well as the pharmacotherapeutic action of specific drugs, to know what nontraditional medications might be helpful to ease the discomfort of a particular condition.

The use of adjuvant medications to relieve pain is not always easily implemented. At times, it requires significant trial and error because there is insufficient evidence and experience about the effectiveness and efficacy of nontraditional analgesics on some conditions. Dosing regimens vary, so it is prudent for the interdisciplinary team to consider a strategy whereby the patient begins with low initial doses and titrates gradually to optimize therapeutic benefits and balance analgesia with adverse effects.

Pain assessment and management comprise a complex set of skills that can take years to develop. However, regardless of your level of expertise, the process always begins with your ability to engage in a therapeutic relationship with the suffering individual, your authentic intention to provide empathetic care, your commitment to explore the details of the person's experience, and your capacity to advocate for the well-being of both the individual and family members. There are times when reaching the person's goals will require you to advocate in a way that resists bureaucracy and challenges the notion that "we always do it this way." Society tends to doubt people who say they are in pain and admire those who suffer in silence. As advocates, we must demonstrate our trust of the individual's reports of pain and express compassion when he or she openly expresses that pain. In those situations, it is critical that you are familiar with current evidence and can build a reasonable and solid case for trying something different from the usual approach that will provide a safe and meaningful way to achieve pain control for the person. Remember, you are accountable to the individual, first and foremost. This is a sacred responsibility rooted in the ethical practice of registered nurses (Canadian Nurses Association, 2008b).

Complementary and Alternative Therapies

Over recent decades, life expectancies have lengthened, chronic illnesses have become more prevalent, and society has become better informed about the limitations of conventional or biomedical interventions. Increasingly, people have sought alternatives in an attempt to "fill the gaps" left by orthodox treatments. As contemporary nursing practice continues to encompass more holistic principles, it is important to explore the types of healing modalities that attract interest as well as the role of the nurse in supporting and guiding the client to make informed and safe decisions. Complementary approaches comprise a very wide range of therapies that belong to one of five domains (College and Association of Registered Nurses of Alberta, 2011):

1. Biologically based practices and products supplement the diet and include substances such as herbal medicines, probiotics, and vitamins;
2. Mind and body medicine employs approaches that enhance the influence of the mind on the body's functioning, and include meditation, acupuncture, guided imagery, and yoga;
3. Manipulative and body-base practices, such as spinal manipulation and massage therapy, focus on the structures and systems of the body;
4. Energy medicine promotes healing through manipulation of energy fields using techniques such as qi gong, healing touch, and Reiki; and
5. Whole medicine systems comprise practices based on evidence accumulated over long periods of time, such as Ayurvedic and traditional Chinese medicine.

You can see that there is a strong focus on connections and interactions within the mind-body-spirit entity. Such approaches are used by people at all stages and conditions of life to treat or prevent many different types of health concerns, including chronic illnesses that do not always respond well to conventional Western or biomedical treatments. An expanding body of scientific evidence is accumulating as more research funds and efforts are devoted to examining the usefulness and safety of such treatments; an excellent source for current information is the National Center for Complementary and Alternative Medicine (http://nccam.nih.gov/). Over time, use of complementary therapies is becoming more accepted by practitioners of biomedical medicine and clients alike, a fact that is reflected in improved coverage by many health insurance plans. Many people use both conventional and complementary approaches to achieve relief from symptoms and to enhance their sense of well-being.

Complementary and alternative therapies may be particularly useful at the end of life, when the focus shifts from cure of disease to quality of remaining life. Many people use or indicate interest in using such approaches in the hospice setting (Mansky & Wallerstedt, 2006; Nelson, 2006; Rahim-Jamal et al., 2011; Running, Shreffler-Grant, & Andrews, 2008) to relieve symptoms, boost the immune system, and control side effects. Furthermore, researchers often show that clients report psycho-spiritual, physical, and social benefits (e.g., Leow, Drury, & Poon, 2010; Selman, Williams, & Simms, 2012) following implementation of such treatments, although there also are authors who challenge those claims (Downey et al., 2009). Although the jury is still out regarding statistically significant evidence, it is necessary that you have the conversation with your client; it is likely that some kind of complementary treatment has been or is being used. The client may not recognize or refer to the treatment as a complementary or alternative therapy, so you will need to consider carefully how you ask your questions. You may wish to determine the client's interest in exploring options that might increase comfort and provide information on which she can make an informed decision about safety and efficacy. Some interventions you may be able to provide yourself (e.g., music, guided imagery, relaxation), and others require training and certification (e.g., therapeutic touch, acupuncture). If you are interested in specialization training leading to practice as a holistic nurse, please visit the Canadian Holistic Nurses Association (http://www.chna.ca/).

Principles of Pain Management

There are some important basic principles to keep in mind when you are working with a person who lives with pain. As you know, pain can be overwhelming; an efficient and effective process to address it will bring comfort to the individual and will enhance his or her confidence in your ability and willingness to acknowledge and meet his or her needs. The principles that can guide your practice are the following:

1. Always remember the notion of "total pain" and be prepared to investigate, treat, and evaluate all dimensions and manifestations of pain.
2. Include the person, family, and other caregivers in the pain treatment plan. Be guided by the person's goals for pain relief and educate yourself and the team appropriately.
3. Do a thorough assessment of the pain and do it as quickly as possible.
4. Initiate treatment of the pain as rapidly as you can, even if the only tools you can access immediately are acetaminophen and a foot massage. Consider untreated pain to be a medical emergency.
5. Use a stepped approach to analgesia that responds to the severity of the pain. Become familiar with the use and titration of palliative medications and complementary interventions.
6. Choose the simplest approach before moving to more complicated or invasive techniques (e.g., give medication orally whenever possible).
7. Constant pain requires around-the-clock administration of analgesics to maintain therapeutic levels of analgesia. Access to additional analgesia for breakthrough pain is critical and must be built into the treatment plan.
8. Ensure the person has as much control as possible over the administration of analgesia techniques, including the decision to use breakthrough doses when pain suddenly escalates.
9. Anticipate and treat other symptoms, such as nausea and constipation, aggressively.
10. Never give up hope of achieving pain relief to the extent desired by the person. Keep trying different approaches, if necessary, and remain flexible.

Maria agrees to speak with Taylor after lunch about her pain. Before Taylor has a chance to ask any questions, Maria lies back against her pillows, stares at the ceiling, and begins to recite the areas in her body that hurt. Taylor listens carefully and is startled to see tears sliding silently down Maria's face as she talks about pain that has gradually escalated over the past few days. Taylor doesn't want to interrupt, so she wordlessly takes Maria's hand. When Maria pauses, Taylor asks about the impact of the pain on Maria's life.

Other Symptoms

Pain is not the only symptom that may accompany life-threatening illness. Many other problems can disrupt the quality of life of the individual. It is beyond the scope of this text to discuss all of the possible concerns and their treatment, but a few of the more common ones are described. You are encouraged to be vigilant and thoughtful in your care, so that you identify and address symptoms before they overwhelm the individual. Anticipate the emergence of symptoms, question their etiology, and insist that they be treated. This process often involves careful detective work to determine the underlying problem and persistent advocacy to convince health-care colleagues to engage in the comprehensive assessment necessary to adequately remedy the situation to the individual's satisfaction. Furthermore, it is not unusual to find that the treatment of one symptom leads to the emergence of another. Your nursing care must be meticulous and thorough.

Some of the more common physical, emotional, and spiritual problems, in addition to pain, that affect individuals at the end of life include the following:

- nausea, vomiting
- constipation
- dyspnea
- fatigue
- anxiety, depression
- pruritus
- hiccoughs
- diarrhea
- existential distress
- loneliness, isolation
- problems related to decreased mobility (e.g., skin breakdown, joint pain, compromised organ function).

The list is long and incomplete and is beyond the scope of this text to discuss in detail. There are many excellent resources that provide extensive explanations of etiology, diagnosis, and clinical management (see end of chapter). Several symptoms are addressed briefly in the following sections to give you a sense of their complexity, the importance of pattern recognition and clinical judgment, and the need for team effort to overcome the distress that may result. Remember that the individual makes the ultimate decision about whether to treat or not and what side effects are acceptable. Adverse effects that for other people may be minor irritants might be major obstacles for the dying individual. Despite your own personal beliefs or opinions, you must focus on ensuring the individual has access to the best information, support for his decision, the opportunity to change his mind, and your command of best efforts to help him achieve his goals.

Nausea and Vomiting

There are numerous reasons why an individual may experience nausea and vomiting during the course of a terminal illness. Anxiety and fear; chemicals produced by a tumor; gastric irritation from drugs; metabolic alterations such as hypercalcemia resulting from the disease process; radiation therapy; constipation caused by opioids; the presence of ascites; coughing; vertigo; hepatomegaly; and increased intracranial pressure—these are a few of the factors that may cause or accompany these symptoms. Understanding the root cause can be very complex. For example, nausea may cause pain, or pain may cause nausea. You will want to gather a detailed history and do a careful physical examination to determine how best to diagnose and treat the problem. You must be very knowledgeable about all body systems and metabolic processes as well as the mechanisms of various treatments to successfully address the problem.

It is essential that you consider simple or less invasive measures first. If anxiety and fear contribute to nausea, spending time listening to and authentically validating the individual's concerns, or requesting the attendance of a chaplain may be the most effective intervention. If smells or tastes trigger nausea, you need to eliminate those from the environment. Offering sour or bland foods may be effective. Techniques that promote relaxation or distraction often are useful.

You will also want to rule out the most common causes before proceeding to more complicated explanations for the symptoms. For example, constipation often leads to nausea and should be one of your primary considerations. Constipation should always be anticipated and prevented with prophylactic use of stool softeners and/or oral or rectal stimulants, along with careful attention to establishment of a regular bowel routine. Sometimes, nausea is antibiotic-induced; if so, you may need to consult with the physician and pharmacist about a change of medication or its administration. If nausea is caused by mechanical pressure, such as an expanding tumor in the brain, treatment may include shrinking the mass through radiation therapy or use of corticosteroid drugs. There are many types of antiemetic drugs that work on different factors and pathways, and you may need to combine two or more agents to successfully address the problem. As well, you may need to include adjuvant drugs such as anxiolytics for their antiemetic properties. It is evident that nausea and vomiting are not simple and straightforward issues and that they require your utmost diligence to overcome in collaboration with members of your interdisciplinary team.

Involving the individual and family members in your plan is critical. Careful explanations and excellent education will facilitate successful interventions. Awareness of the potential adverse side effects of medications such as xerostomia, sedation, and blurred vision will allow the individual to make an informed decision about using the drug. Offering nonpharmacologic recommendations such as maintaining exquisite oral hygiene and using ginger candy or tea to minimize nausea (Vogel, Wilson, & Melvin, 2004) may permit a measure of control and comfort for the individual. Your best attempts to include the individual and his or her caregivers in choosing, assessing, and adjusting interventions for maximum benefit will also provide dividends in the creation of a trusting and therapeutic relationship.

Constipation

Constipation is a common and very distressing symptom with many possible causes including the presence of a tumor mass in the intestine, use of opioids and other drugs, spinal cord compression, metabolic disorders such as hypercalcemia and hyperkalemia, anxiety or depression, sedentary lifestyle, dehydration, and chronic diseases such as diabetes and amyotrophic lateral sclerosis that have a neurologic or endocrine effect. You will need to listen carefully to the individual's story as you take a detailed history and perform a physical examination and then compile the salient cues to arrive at a nursing diagnosis. Managing constipation might require that you manually disimpact the individual, offer nonpharmacologic treatment such as increasing fluid and fibre intake in conjunction with physical activity, or administer medications to increase bulk or soften the stool, and/or lubricate or stimulate the bowel. An individual who takes opioid drugs will almost always require stool softeners at the same time to prevent constipation; the doses may be much higher than you are accustomed to providing to people who are not using opioids for analgesia. Generally, you will continue to increase the dose slowly until the individual achieves the desired effect. A person who is taking 300 mg of morphine daily may need 10 or more tablets of a stool softener such as Senekot-S to maintain regular bowel function. As you might imagine, it is crucial that you educate the individual and family, and perhaps your colleagues as well, in the effective use of such agents.

Dyspnea

The sensation of being unable to breathe properly is very distressing to the individual and his or her caregivers. It is very common in people with terminal cancer and, as with other symptoms, has a host of possible causes. Anxiety, infections, heart failure, anemia, bronchoconstriction as a result of tumor mass, and even the toxic effects of cancer therapy may all result in the feeling of suffocation or being out of breath. Your assessment is likely to reveal rapid (tachypnea) or deep (hyperpnea) respirations, low oxygen or high carbon dioxide levels, and restlessness or agitation. Treatment will depend on the cause but may include blood transfusion, oxygen therapy, administration of medications to promote diuresis or heart function, chest physiotherapy to release and move secretions, elevation of the head of the bed, relaxation techniques, nebulized or systemic administration of morphine, elimination of allergens or smoke from the environment, and a fan to gently circulate air. Educating the individual and family about strategies to reduce oxygen demand and use of nonpharmacologic therapies will help them choose the most appropriate techniques to minimize this symptom.

Interdisciplinary Teamwork

By now, you will recognize that there are many interrelated and overlapping symptoms that contribute to the impact of the illness experience for the individual and his or her caregivers. Whether associated with the disease process or its treatment, all symptoms have the potential to be distressing at best and life-threatening at worst. Furthermore, their presence and treatment are factors in the memories that are being created for the surviving family members that will not easily be forgotten. It must be a priority for you to anticipate, recognize, study, document, and alleviate those symptoms as swiftly and expertly as possible. It is unlikely that you have or that any one health-care professional has the complete set of skills, knowledge, and capacity necessary to adequately address all the symptoms and side effects that manifest throughout the course of the illness. Therefore, it is critical that you work as part of an interdisciplinary team collective to identify and achieve the goals of the individual and family who ultimately direct the activities of the team.

You will recall from your pathophysiology studies that the human body is an amazing and complex organism with many backup mechanisms to ensure competent execution of the many processes required to sustain life. However, at some point, disease can overwhelm one or more of those systems, and they fail in their efforts to function effectively. As well, treatment aimed at overcoming the disease or its symptoms can adversely affect the performance of organs and systems. A simple example is the use of antibiotics to treat infection; the normal bacteria in the gut are often destroyed by these drugs, causing diarrhea. Another example is the use of opioid drugs to control pain, with the unintended side effects of debilitating constipation and nausea or vomiting. In both cases, the secondary effects of essential treatment can be devastating for the individual and may lead to the need for invasive or uncomfortable interventions. Hence, it is critical that you understand and anticipate these possible side effects and prevent them whenever possible. It is beyond the scope of this chapter to go into detail about all of the possible trajectories, challenges, and knowledge that you might experience in your care of patients. Therefore, you must explore helpful resources and engage in interdisciplinary discussions with your team. Ultimately, you are charged with the responsibility of finding the appropriate answers to facilitate the best experience possible for your patient and the family.

Comforting and Supporting the Family

He cannot bring up her fear.
She is afraid of being alone.
He cannot see that she is not angry at him.
They chase one another in ordinary circles.
They love each other.
(Larsen, 2002, p. 84)

When you provide palliative care, you almost always are caring for a family as well as an individual. That family comprises whoever the person says it does; it may be a group of people connected by genetic or marital ties, or it may include people who depend on one another for emotional, physical, economic, and/or other types of support. It is important for you to explore and understand the structure and functioning of all members of the family (just as you do with the human body), so that you can identify appropriate interventions to help the family cope with the stress of losing a member. A useful first step is to construct a genogram or ecomap so that you can visualize and document relationships and patterns of interaction (Wright & Leahey, 2009). You will need to carefully observe body language, communication styles, and behaviours as you spend time with the family. Be aware that although you may see behaviours that seem unhealthy or dysfunctional to you, you must interpret their role and purpose in the context of the family with which you are working before you label them as problematic. Your goal is to strengthen the capacity and integrity of the whole family while at the same time accommodating the exceptional needs of the ill person. Therefore, you must assess and appreciate how the family is making sense of the situation and what is required to support the difficult process of becoming an entity that no longer includes the physical presence of the sick individual. To accomplish this, you will commit yourself to being a witness to suffering, a seeker of understanding, and a guide through transition.

Family members often take on much of the responsibility of caring for a dying loved one in the final weeks, months, or sometimes years of life. This can be both gratifying and costly, as it brings the satisfaction of being able to contribute to quality of life, but it may also be exhausting for the caregiver—physically, emotionally, economically, and spiritually. In addition to managing daily care and environmental needs for the ill individual, the caregiver must also prepare himself or herself for the death. It is very likely that family members will each experience personal suffering; in addition, they may come to recognize their own assets and strengths as they adapt to and function in an unimaginably challenging situation. As you develop your relationship with the family, it is important that you observe, acknowledge, and validate the experiences of each member and offer support with the intention of restoring wellness.

Nursing Interventions

One of the first lessons for many nurses concerns the family member's need to have some degree of influence in what often feels like an unpredictable, chaotic situation. Consequently, you may be startled to receive an angry or hostile response to your friendly greeting to the patient's visiting family member. Before you respond defensively, it is helpful to consider the situation from that person's perspective. For example, if you walk into Maria's room at the beginning of your shift only to be confronted by an angry Ben who blames you for the significant weight loss he notices in his wife, you need to take a breath and consider what Ben is feeling. Daily, he watches Maria shrink before his eyes, and he, who promised to protect and care for her always, is completely helpless to meet that obligation. Nothing he can do will prevent her health from deteriorating, nothing will postpone her death. He is exhausted physically and spiritually. Are you surprised that he would express his anger by lashing out at you? Are you going to take it personally, or will you respond with compassion and understanding for his anguish? You might acknowledge his pain and helplessness by saying, "Ben, it must be terrible to watch Maria losing weight. I have noticed over the past few days that her appetite is changing; she doesn't seem to be as hungry. Is there anything you can think of that she might enjoy eating or drinking?" Depending on his response, you might look for an opportunity to gently discuss and normalize the diminished oral intake that typically accompanies the process of dying. By raising the topic with Ben, you will be able to explore the meaning of Maria's behaviour and the extent to which he has integrated it into his own life.

Through the eyes of a nurse

When I think about providing comfort, I visualize the integration of mind, body, and spirit. There are no "simple tasks" in nursing because meeting the most basic of the "essential ordinary" requires me to engage with the whole of the human condition. Karl Rahner (as cited in Perry, 2009, p. 17) wrote that we often take for granted ordinary everyday activities of living such as eating, sitting down, sleeping, and bathing until "something turns up which restricts or prohibits us from doing them." Two key ways in which nurses attend to the essential ordinary include attention to little things and keeping the promise to never abandon (Perry, 2009). Florence Nightingale understood and promoted the importance of the essential ordinary: cleanliness, ventilation, nourishment, and rest. It is in attention to the small, intimate interactions of personal care—warming the towels, placing the water jug close at hand, following the person's lead in the way things are done—that the nurse conveys compassion and respect for the individual. Even though the nature of nursing care has changed with increasingly complex technology, greater acuity, and shorter hospital stays, it is still the basic caring, the essential ordinary, that means so much to people who are ill or dying (Iliffe, 2002).
(personal reflection of a nurse)

Story

We construct meaning in our lives through the process of the grand narrative of living a life. How we construct the stories of our existence brings forth our interpretation of the past, our hopes for the future, and our engagement with the present. The significance we give to events, characters, and the progression of plot lines gives texture to our constructed reality. The aspects of human experience that capture our attention or stories, both oral and written, give our lives definition and substance and serve as a way of creating evidence of our existence. In creating the story, we are transformed; the process of assigning language or giving voice is our attempt to define our world.

As nurses, we live in the realm of co-created narratives. The same character may be involved in several stories. As Maria's story slowly emerges, it converges with the story Taylor is creating. The mere presence of one story shapes the plot and reveals what is possible—to support or constrain the imagined future, to enhance or diminish the present, and to respect or ignore the influence of past. Listening for the narrative (Hartrick Doane & Varcoe, 2005) offers a sense of person and family as influenced by culture, social structure, dominate ideology, and language. Story transforms both the storyteller and the storykeeper. The telling and retelling of the story helps to define and redefine personhood and the significance of events. Story gives a different dimension to time and space; past, present, and future are embedded in the narrative. As Taylor's story is created, think about how it converges with Maria's story, with Ben's story, and with Sarah's story. Think about how Taylor enters the intertwined stories of Maria's family at a time when the future has just been changed in extraordinary ways. As Chinn and Kramer (2011, p. 142) say,

The person and the family face a period of tension and uncertainty during which the new imaged future is a dreaded future that was never imagined before. As a nurse, you begin with small everyday acts of nursing care. With each nursing interaction, you begin to create with the patient and family a new plot that cannot be fully anticipated in advance. On the basis of your experience and background as a nurse, you are able to help the patient and family image a new future. It is perhaps not the ultimately desired future, but it may be one that they can begin to embrace. Some elements of the new future involve small everyday things, such as learning to function with only one arm. Other elements of the new future are more complicated. . . .

In this situation, it is a future without the physical presence of Maria—wife and mother. You can imagine how difficult it must be for Ben to think about that future. For Taylor, a separate story is being constructed. She is trying to make sense of being a nurse—this may not be what she expected, and she has to find a way to understand the experience and make it a part of her own reality. She may feel she has to tell the story to determine its meaning and significance, so she calls her friend or meets with her instructor. In so doing, she is mindful of the responsibilities associated with confidentiality and the boundaries imposed by the code of ethics (Canadian Nurses Association, 2008a). As Taylor reconstructs the storyline, she has freedom to exaggerate, fictionalize, emphasize, and reshape the actual experience to reveal possibilities and visions for the future. You might think this is dishonest, but in reality, we all tell stories in this way. It allows us to imagine and explore other avenues for interpreting and responding to the situation that we can then apply to similar experiences in the future (Chinn & Kramer, 2011).

Comfort

The essential ordinary discussed earlier referred to activities of daily living—the patterns and rhythms of each day, the basic human needs. Although these activities may bring to mind Maslow's hierarchy of needs, we propose that living a life is not a process neatly divided into distinct layers of boxes decreasing in size and culminating in a perfect triangle as a way of giving definition to human needs. In a palliative care situation, you may wish to reconsider your notion of basic needs. For example, are basic needs restricted to toileting, hydration, and mobility? Or might the need to ponder the greater spiritual aspects of life have more immediate significance? The client might be focused on her **spirituality**, her thoughts about the meaning and purpose of her existence. As you observe that process in another person, you may find yourself asking questions about your own life, such as, "What do I believe will happen after my death? Has my life made a difference? How do I, as a nurse, know what is important at any moment in time?"

Maria and Ben had many dreams for Sarah and many hopes for their future as a loving family. Taylor is beginning to see that the story of Maria and Ben is a complex, many-layered one, and she wonders how a nurse would best provide care. She also questions her own concerns and uncertainties about life and death and wonders how they will influence her ability to care for someone like Maria and what will happen to her in the process.

A hallmark of nursing continues to be the expectation of providing comfort. What exactly is comfort? What is the experience of being comforted? What are the values, beliefs, and ethics of comfort? How does a nurse offer comfort? The word *comfort* comes from *confortare*, which means to strengthen greatly. There are many different perspectives and ideas about comfort, depending on whether you are offering or receiving it, but one that might be helpful to the nurse was proposed by Kolcaba (2003, p. 251): Comfort is concerned with meeting needs for relief, ease, and transcendence by nursing modalities in the four dimensions of human experience (physical, psycho-spiritual, sociocultural, and environmental). This understanding of comfort is based on a view of the world as an interconnected whole and nursing as a relational encounter between people. Thus, providing comfort engages you as a nurse meeting the person in that sacred space where you recognize needs and have the intention, capacity, and desire to respond. According to Kolcaba, your interventions may include standard actions to maintain physiological stability and control pain; coaching activities to provide reassurance and instill hope; and food for the soul, those special acts that make a person feel cared for and strengthened. You have many options for providing comfort to Maria; her guidance and your presence will contribute to nursing care that will enable her to address her unique story.

Through the eyes of a nurse

The privilege of nursing involves the responsibility to engage with those significant transitions of life . . . birth and death. In a small community, the nurse can be called upon to attend both events in a single shift. That anticipation of the first breath and anticipation of the final one are opportunities to honour the sacred by our presence. The following story is recounted by a nurse as she reflected on the diversity and challenge of her night shift at a rural Canadian hospital. "I remember that the maternity unit entrance was framed by lovely tall windows. Just outside the large swinging doors was a single patient room with two women in it and the family waiting room.

As I rushed by, hurrying to a couple that had just delivered their baby and another that was about to give birth, my sense of connection to the space of the room with the two women grew. While getting tea and toast for the new family, I quickly brought tea to the woman who was soothing, encouraging, and coaxing her dying friend. I will never forget watching her wipe her dying friend's face telling her, 'Remember when we came here—wasn't that crazy times ehhh, remember your dog, remember . . .?' On another trip past their door, the friend beckoned me in. A minute later, her dying companion turned, looked skyward, smiled, and died. Afterward, as I left the room, I stood for a breath—the moment was filled with grace—the intersecting wards were still and quiet, only the motionless wheelchairs and IV poles stood as totems, watching. It was three or four in the morning. The other nurses were working together in another room to complete a burn dressing. I turned towards maternity, knowing soon the sky would lighten and the trees outside would slowly reveal themselves from their black blanket. The swinging door opened, and the about-to-be grandmother told me it was time. I entered their sacred space to assist as their baby revealed himself. Death and birth are the same."

(personal reflection of Jeddie Russell, RN, BScN, MAdEd)

Grief and Bereavement

"To walk through grief is a heroic journey. No other challenge in life approaches it" (Tappouni, 2013, p. xvii). Loss and death are everyday occurrences, yet the effects last a lifetime. Nurses frequently witness the raw emotions that slam into patients and their families as they realize the magnitude of the situation. Wilson (2000) shares the story of the life and death of his teenage son, revealing the brutal, physical, and overpowering onslaught of sensations that threatened to tear him apart. Family members often plead with the nurse to explain how they are to cope with and survive the depths of sorrow that appear to stretch endlessly into the future. As a nurse, you must have the courage to be present with family members in these most awful moments, to witness their profound loss, and to honour the life that is gone. The survivors need to know that the process will take much time and hard work, as they struggle to find ways to accommodate the loss into their lives. It often surprises people to know that they cannot "get over" loss; that it will change their lives in ways they cannot begin to imagine. The process is a long and winding journey that must be travelled in solitude because no two individuals have identical experiences and relationships with the person who has died. There is no time limit to grief, yet we live in a world that sometimes fails to acknowledge that fact. Consider the length of bereavement or compassionate leave

allowed by many employers—often less than a week—and the expectations of friends and family who may lose patience with manifestations of the person who experienced the loss, or the harried family physician whose 15-minute appointment does not allow for the messiness that often characterizes grief. It is important that you remind the family that they must work through the process at their own speed and in their own time and that they must resist any pressures, self-imposed or otherwise, to avoid or rush through grief.

You might have heard of Elisabeth Kübler-Ross, a Swiss American psychiatrist who pioneered the study of death and dying in the 1960s. Her well-known book, *On Death and Dying*, was published in 1969 and describes the emotions and challenges that dying and bereaved people might experience. Although she has been criticized for her presentation of dying as a process that comprises five distinct stages, careful readers will note that she emphasized it is not a standard one-size-fits-all event. Individuals may not move through the stages in a particular order or may remain in each stage for varied amounts of time. Human responses and emotions are not always predictable nor are they necessarily symptoms of disease—they must be interpreted as a way of "re-learning the world" (Attig, 1996) and one's place in it—a normal, healthy, albeit difficult, lengthy, and challenging transition. The nurse must be prepared to support each person's personal journey and to normalize the wide and sometimes wild range of responses.

Many other authors have written about loss, **grief**, and bereavement. Kastenbaum (2009) distinguishes among several categories of grief, including anticipatory (grieving before the death happens), disenfranchised (the hidden grief that may not be readily resolved because it is not recognized by others, as when a woman experiences a miscarriage), and complicated (grief that is so debilitating and enduring that the individual appears to be headed for catastrophe). Psychiatrist Colin Murray Parkes (2006) observes that love and loss are two sides of the same coin and discusses patterns of grief in the context of different types of emotional attachments (e.g., secure, anxious, ambivalent, and avoidant) between individuals. Rando (1984, 2000) is a clinical psychologist and thanatologist (specialist in death and dying issues) who has published many books on specific forms of grief, such as that experienced by parents when a child dies, and complicated and anticipatory mourning as well as guidelines for caregiver interventions. Rando (1984, p. 115) also notes there is truth to the saying "once bereaved, always bereaved"—the grief will be there in some form for the rest of a person's life. Thus, it is important that we gently help family members to understand that the pain and sorrow can only be accommodated into but never eliminated from their lives as they seek insight into the meaning of the loss.

As a registered nurse, supporting a bereaved person requires empathy, that ability to sense the patient's world "as if it were your own but without ever losing the 'as if' quality" (Rogers, 1992, p. 829). We all come to the care-giving context with our personal experiences regarding loss that must be recognized and their impact acknowledged before we can engage in therapeutic relationships with others. Moreover, many of us spend little time considering our lives as finite entities, preferring to avoid contemplation of the end of our existence on the planet. However, taking the time to reflect on your life and losses and responding to yourself with empathy and compassion will enable you to do the same for your patients. When you invest your emotions and energy in another person, you will confront loss when the relationship ends, so you must expect to deal with grief from time to time over the span of your nursing career. It is important to develop a set of strategies to help you cope with your feelings to ensure your own health and well-being.

Assiduous attention to self-care is essential to protect against **compassion fatigue** and to create a personal work environment that will lead instead to compassion satisfaction (Harrowing, 2011). It is possible to find inspiration and a sense of revitalization, even in situations that are extraordinarily sad. Nurturing an appreciative, positive approach is an important step, as is engaging in meaningful relationships with patients (Perry, 2008), to achieving fulfillment in your work (Burtson & Stichler, 2010). You might focus on your efforts to relieve suffering and find contentment as you ease the patient's distress. It is always advisable to identify a mentor, perhaps an experienced nurse whose work you admire and who can listen to your ideas and offer his or her own experiences of learning to find meaning. Finding a balance between work and play is also a critical component—taking time to participate in activities that are relaxing and enjoyable, to be with supportive people who validate your humanity, and to recognize indications that you need to remove yourself from damaging or traumatic situations are all suggestions that will help you in your journey; you can probably think of other ways to cope with stress that have been effective in the past. Ultimately, your efforts will help you remain healthy while providing thoughtful, comprehensive, holistic care to your patient and family.

RESEARCH

NURSES' MORAL EXPERIENCES AND DECISION-MAKING

Nurses engage in a complex decision-making process when determining the best course of action in a crisis situation. There are many factors to be considered in a short period of time as the nurse attempts to honour the goals and wishes of everyone involved. The situation may become a moral dilemma and result in moral distress for the nurse, reflecting the myriad of tensions and rewards inherent in the event.

Study

Six nurses who worked in a Canadian pediatric hospice facility participated in a qualitative study designed to help us understand the moral experiences they encountered related to the administration of as-needed antiseizure medications to their patients. The nurses, with between 2 and 30 years of work experience, were asked to share stories about the experience of making decisions about giving these medications to children who had been admitted to the hospice to allow their families a period of temporary respite. When children were brought to the hospice, their parents explained the nature of the seizures as well as the protocol used for determining if, when, and how the drugs were to be administered. The nurses were asked about the goals they were trying to attain in making decisions about giving the drugs, their satisfaction or dissatisfaction with the decisions, and the factors that influenced the time and method of drug administration. The researchers listened to their stories and identified themes that were commonly mentioned and that explained how the participants interpreted their experiences.

The nurses noted that although they needed a strong clinical knowledge base about seizures and their pharmaceutical treatment, their decisions also had to accommodate the family's wishes and experience. The parents generally had been dealing with the seizures at home and had worked out an effective response. For example, sometimes they allowed the seizure to proceed, knowing that it was self-limiting and would cause little harm to the child; the preference was often to avoid sedating the child (a common side effect of the antiseizure drugs) if possible. On the other hand, the nurses were well aware that seizures can lead to respiratory arrest and even death. Thus, their decisions were critical. The overarching theme they described to the researchers had to do with *not on my watch*, meaning they were very concerned with making the right decision to ensure no adverse effects were sustained while maintaining quality of life for the child. It was indeed a balancing act of knowing the child and parents and being willing to engage in the uncertainty of changing seizure patterns. To accomplish their goals, the nurses had to be prepared to bear witness as the child endured the suffering associated with seizures, constantly on the alert for changes in the child's behaviour, connected with the parents, and skilled enough to "do what is right." The participants found that they were very aware of time as they observed and comforted the child during a seizure, and they often experienced distress both as they witnessed the seizure and as they struggled to make the appropriate decision. They also spent time reflecting on the decision in order to come to terms with it.

Nursing Implications

This research study speaks clearly of the importance of story—both the nurses' stories and those of their patients and families—and how stories intersect as we carry out our responsibilities. The study also demonstrates the complexity of the work done by nurses and how, even after many years of experience, we may struggle to make the best decision possible. Nurses need strong clinical knowledge, but also essential to excellent care is the ability to open a safe space for dialogue and trust, as nurses and families enter into a sacred partnership to ensure the best possible care for the patient. Even when nurses are unhappy with their decisions, the choice to bear witness and accompany the patient in his or her journey is highly valued by families. The process of decision-making is a moral experience for nurses because it always occurs within a context of relationship and uncertainty. Finally, making and acting on decisions involves ethical questioning and sometimes distress, but it also leads to self-understanding for nurses.

Rashotte, J., King, J., Thomas, M., & Cragg, B. (2011). Nurses' moral experience of administering prn anti-seizure medications in pediatric palliative care. Canadian Journal of Nursing Research, 43(3), 58–77.

Palliative Care in the Community

As important as it is to develop expertise in individual and family care to address end-of-life concerns, it is also vital that nurses examine and participate in the palliative care needs of communities and the country. In Canada, palliative care programs began with the expansion of cancer care programs in the 1970s and were designed to meet local needs. Special palliative care units were developed in hospitals, first in Winnipeg at St. Boniface General Hospital in 1974, followed soon after by a unit at the Royal Victoria Hospital in Montreal. Later, programs were implemented by volunteer-based hospice societies. In the 1980s, services became more widely available in communities through home care programs. Palliative care service guidelines were published by Health and Welfare Canada, and the University of Ottawa established the first institute for research and education in palliative care. The Canadian Palliative Care Association was formed in 1991; 10 years later, its name changed to the Canadian Hospice Palliative Care Association (CHPCA) in recognition of the interchangeable use of the terms *hospice* and *palliative* in this country (CHPCA, 2011). In 2003, the Government of Canada introduced the Compassionate Care Benefit, which allows Canadians who are caring for dying family members the opportunity to temporarily leave their jobs with support from the federal Employment Insurance program (Service Canada, 2011). It was clear that many Canadians were becoming aware of the importance of developing and expanding hospice palliative care services to meet the growing need to recognize the complex concerns of people facing the end of life.

Over the past three decades, many advancements have led to improvements in care for Canadians who face terminal illness and chronic pain. However, much remains to be done.

We are part of an aging society; we are living longer than ever before but with more complex health conditions. The vast majority of us will need palliative care services to ease the journey through the dying process. However, as Senator Sharon Carstairs (2010, p. 3) indicated in her important report, at least 70% of Canadians do not have access to equitable palliative care services. People who live in rural or remote areas, for example, may have to travel long distances to obtain care (CHPCA, 2010). The option of dying at home is not possible for many First Nations elders; instead, they may live their final days in unfamiliar urban hospitals far from family networks (Parliamentary Committee on Palliative and Compassionate Care [PCPCC], 2011). Although the Compassionate Care Benefit is a step in the right direction, it is limited in its scope and may not fully address the needs of family caregivers. On the other hand, there are good examples of integrated, multidisciplinary programs in this country that reflect excellent, evidence-informed practices such as use of common assessment tools, collaborative care plans, seamless and consistent care across settings, and support for family caregivers prior to and following the death of their loved one (CHPCA, 2010). Increasingly, access to hospice palliative care and pain management services is seen as a basic human right, fundamental to the quality of life of all citizens. As a nurse committed to advocacy and social justice for all persons, it becomes your responsibility to recognize, learn about, and promote change at all levels to ensure equitable access for all Canadians—indeed all citizens on the planet—to primary health care that meets needs throughout the lifespan (PCPCC, 2011; Sepúlveda, Marlin, Yoshida, & Ullrich, 2002). A good starting point is to explore the models that offer gold standard care in Canada, such as the New Brunswick Extra-Mural Program, the Niagara West Shared Care Model for Palliative Care, Victoria Hospice, and the Edmonton Regional Palliative Care Program (for website addresses, see "Web Resources" at thePoint). These programs are among the well-established and highly respected programs in this country that offer invaluable resources and information based on extensive evidence and experience in improving the transition from life to death for countless families.

Maria, with Ben's support, has asked to be discharged so that they can go home and be a family for as long as possible. With the guidance of her instructor, Taylor arranges a meeting of Ben, Maria, the social worker, and the home care nurse. Together, they identify the family's needs and organize the appropriate services. As well, Ben's mother is able to come and stay with the family for a few weeks. When the family is at last ready to leave the hospital, Taylor accompanies them to the door and with tears in her eyes thanks Maria for allowing her to be part of her care.

Six weeks later, Taylor receives a message from the home care nurse saying that Maria died peacefully at home the previous day. Taylor attends the memorial service where she takes a moment to tell Ben how sorry she is for his bereavement. He replies that he is so grateful that Maria was able to be at home and that it was the hardest thing he has ever experienced. He hugs Sarah tightly and thanks Taylor for her help. Taylor thinks about how much she has learned in the past 2 months—about life, nursing, and herself. She muses about the words of Hartrick Doane and Varcoe (2005, p. 110) who said that nursing is about respecting the "human experiences of mystery, diversity, and paradox." She realizes that she has indeed chosen the right career after all.

Critical Thinking Case Scenarios

Suzanne

▶ Suzanne is a 54-year-old school teacher who has been admitted for treatment of multiple myeloma, a malignant disease of plasma cells diagnosed 2 years ago. She is described by her husband and children as very outgoing and people-oriented, with great hopes to overcome her cancer so that she can continue to enjoy her three grandchildren. She has been undergoing aggressive chemotherapy but now has developed some of the common side effects: overwhelming fatigue, constant nausea, mucositis, and diarrhea. She has a central venous line in place for parenteral nutrition and intravenous antibiotics because any food she ingests she immediately vomits. As a result of her neutropenia, she has been placed in reverse isolation to protect her from infection. Suzanne asks many questions about her condition and prognosis, but her chart reveals little information other than lab values and blood work results. She looks to you like she is dying, but there is no record of any frank discussion with her and her family about her wishes. You wonder if this situation represents a conflict between cure-oriented treatment and care-oriented treatment.

How might you go about discovering the answer to this question? What strategies can you use to develop an authentic relationship with this family? How can you find out what the patient's priorities are? What impact will you bring to the relationship? What skills and knowledge do you need to acquire in order to be able to be therapeutic for this family? What beliefs and assumptions do you hold that will influence your care? How will you document your assessments and interventions?

Dave

▶ Dave is 38 years old, the father of 12-year-old twins, and has severe pain as a result of bone metastases from advanced prostate cancer. He is very reluctant to take opioid medications because he wants to remain alert and able to participate in his children's activities. He also does not want the drugs in the house because of the danger to the children.

How might you approach this situation? What personal beliefs and assumptions do you need to acknowledge before you listen to Dave's story? How can you support him in his journey?

Multiple-Choice Questions

1. A patient who has been chatting with visitors tells you that her pain intensity is 5 on a 0 to 10 scale. How should you document this finding?
   a. By recording a rating that is lower than the one reported by the patient.
   b. By recording a rating of 5.
   c. By recording that the patient doesn't appear to be in pain.
   d. By recording that the patient doesn't understand how to use the pain rating scale.

2. The best way for nurses to approach their patients' experiences of sadness and grief is to:
   a. Look for solutions that will fix the problem.
   b. Ask someone with more skills to take over.
   c. Accept that it is just the way things are.
   d. Trust in people's capacity to deal with difficulty.

3. An important strategy to inform your nursing care is to:
   a. Learn the patterns and rhythms of the patient's experience.
   b. Review the chart for new orders several times each day.
   c. Carry and refer frequently to an approved drug guide.
   d. Teach patients the reason for their symptoms.

4. Palliative hospice care services in Canada are:
   a. Available to every citizen.
   b. Only provided in acute care and cancer treatment centres.
   c. Not easily accessed by people living in remote areas.
   d. Only available for older adults.

5. One strategy to fulfill your professional obligation to promote social justice is to:
   a. Ensure the patient has good pain management.
   b. Advocate for universal access to palliative care services.
   c. Participate in nursing union activities.
   d. Volunteer for the social committee at your worksite.

Suggested Lab Activities

My Story

● Loss, grief, and bereavement are universal experiences we have all encountered in life. Through the process of exploring our stories, we gain an understanding of the significance of our journey in recreating meaning in our life after a significant loss. Try this reflective story activity to consider your own narrative around grief and its implications for your life and your nursing career. It may help to consider loss in its broadest sense; you may not have experienced the death of someone close to you, but you have likely gone through a transition (e.g., leaving behind childhood, graduation from high school, moving away from home for the first time, divorce) that included feelings of sadness or sorrow.

1. Writing the story

- Find a quiet space where you will not be interrupted during the documentation of your story.
- Imagine, recreate, and document your story of loss, grief, and bereavement. The story will be documented in the first person ("I"), thus situating "self" in the details of the story.
- Write the story: Capture the details. These may include the following components:
  - Context—describe the physical setting, relevant factors influencing the situation, and overall purpose of interactions;
  - Characters—who was involved in the story;
  - Convey the atmosphere, feelings, attitudes, and emotional tone of the story;
  - Plotline—how did the story unfold?

2. Reflective wonderings

- How did/does this story influence your life?
- What have you come to appreciate about the process of grief?
- What personal/family rituals, beliefs, or traditions were involved in this story?
- How did this loss challenge all dimensions of your being? Consider physical, mental, emotional, and spiritual aspects.
- How did the presence or absence of others influence your journey? What was helpful? What actions/interactions with others did you find supportive?
- As a registered nurse, how do you envision being a "therapeutic presence" when interacting with others?

⬤ Find a partner and read the following poem aloud, as indicated.

Come With Me (adapted from Crowe, 1996)
Both:
    Listen to these words I whisper
    Press your lips to mine.
    Keep me in your arms
    Forever entwined.

One:
    Come with me, I'll show you the way
    Will you follow me into the night?
    Come with me, relinquish this day
    And the angels will hasten our flight.
Other:
    I will not follow you into the dark
    Who knows what morning we'll find.
    Stay with me, never depart
    How can you leave your true love behind?
One:
    Come with me, you promised to be
    My companion through all of our days.
    Come with me, it's easy, you'll see
    How you just let the light slip away.
Other:
    I have been faithful through heartache and tears
    True, in the way that I know.
    Stay with me, I'm troubled, I'm weary
    But I am not ready to go.
Both:
    Listen to these words I whisper
    Press your lips to mine.
    Keep me in your arms
    Forever entwined.
One:
    Come with me, darkness is falling
    I've stepped from the circle of time.
    Come with me, though voices are calling
    I weep for to leave you behind.
Other:
    For so many years I have walked by your side,
    Your hand was pressed in my own.
    Sail away, slip out with the tide
    For someday both our hearts will be home.

Discuss possible scenarios: Who is speaking to whom, and what are the tensions in their conversation? What message does each person convey? What emotions is each experiencing? What happens in the end? What do you think happens next? What is the most important thing you can contribute as a nurse and human being if you witness such a conversation?

REFERENCES AND SUGGESTED READINGS

American Holistic Nursing Association. (2012). *What is holistic nursing?* Retrieved from http://www.ahna.org/AboutUs/Whatis HolisticNursing/tabid/1165/Default.aspx

Attig, T. (1996). *How we grieve: Relearning the world.* New York, NY: Oxford.

Barnum, B. S. (2003). *Spirituality in nursing: From traditional to new age* (2nd ed.). New York, NY: Springer.

Benner, P., Sutphen, M., Leonard, V., & Day, L. (2010). *Educating nurses: A call for radical transformation.* Stanford, CA: Jossey-Bass.

Burtson, P. L., & Stichler, J. F. (2010). Nursing work environment and nurse caring: Relationship among motivational factors. *Journal of Advanced Nursing, 66*(8), 1819–1831. doi:10.1111/j.1365-2648.2010.05336.x

Canadian Hospice Palliative Care Association. (2010). *Policy brief on hospice palliative care: Quality end-of-life care? It depends on where you live . . . and where you die.* Ottawa, ON: Author.

Canadian Hospice Palliative Care Association. (2011). *Canadian Hospice Palliative Care Association.* Retrieved from http://www.chpca.net/Home

Canadian Nurses Association. (2008a). *Code of ethics for registered nurses.* Ottawa, ON: Author.

Canadian Nurses Association. (2008b). *Providing nursing care at the end of life.* Ottawa, ON: Author.

Carstairs, S. (2010). *Raising the bar: A roadmap for the future of palliative care in Canada.* Ottawa, ON: The Senate of Canada.

Chinn, P. L., & Kramer, M. K. (2011). *Integrated theory and knowledge development in nursing* (8th ed.). St. Louis, MO: Elsevier.

Christ, G. H., Bonanno, G., Malkinson, R., & Rubin, S. (2003). Bereavement experiences after the death of a child. In M. J. Field & R. E. Behrman (Eds.), *When children die: Improving palliative and end-of-life care for children and their families* (pp. 553–579). Washington, DC: National Academies Press.

College and Association of Registered Nurses of Alberta. (2011). *Complementary and/or alternative therapy and natural health products: Standards for registered nurses.* Edmonton, AB: Author.

Collier, R. (2011). Access to palliative care varies widely across Canada. *Canadian Medical Association Journal, 183*(2), E87–E88.

Crowe, S. (Writer). (1996). Come with me [Audio]. In S. Crowe, D. Hok, & A. Schuld (Producer), *The door to the river.* Sofia, Bulgaria: Corvus Records.

Dossey, B. M. (2009). Integral and holistic nursing: Local to global. In B. M. Dossey & L. Keegan (Eds.), *Holistic nursing: A handbook for practice* (5th ed., pp. 3–46). Sudbury, MA: Jones and Bartlett.

Downey, L., Diehr, P., Standish, L. J., Patrick, D. L., Kozak, L., Fisher, D., . . . Lafferty, W. E. (2009). Might massage or guided meditation provide "means to a better end"? Primary outcomes from an efficacy trial with patients at the end of life. *Journal of Palliative Care, 25*(2), 100–108.

Downing, G. M. (Ed.). (2006). *Companion booklet: Medical care of the dying* (4th ed.). Victoria, BC: Victoria Hospice Society.

Ferris, F. D., Balfour, H. M., Bowen, K., Farley, J., Hardwick, M., Lamontagne, C., . . . West, P. J. (2002). *A model to guide hospice palliative care: Based on national principles and norms of practice.* Ottawa, ON: Canadian Hospice Palliative Care Association.

Gottlieb, L. N. (2013). *Strengths-based nursing care: Health and healing for person and family.* New York, NY: Springer.

Gregory, D. M., & English, J. C. (1994). The myth of control: Suffering in palliative care. *Journal of Palliative Care, 10*(2), 18–22.

Harrowing, J. N. (2011). Compassion practice by Ugandan nurses who provide HIV care. *Online Journal of Issues in Nursing, 16*(1), 5. doi:10.3912/OJIN.Vol16No01Man05

Hartrick Doane, G., & Varcoe, C. (2005). *Family nursing as relational practice: Developing health-promoting practice.* Philadelphia, PA: Lippincott Williams & Wilkins.

Iliffe, J. (2002). Heeding the words of Florence. *Australian Nursing Journal, 9*(10), 1.

Kastenbaum, R. J. (2009). *Death, society, and human experience* (10th ed.). Boston, MA: Allyn & Bacon.

Kolcaba, K. (2003). *Comfort theory and practice.* New York, NY: Springer.

Krakauer, E. L., Wenk, R., Buitrago, R., Jenkins, P., & Scholten, W. (2010). Opioid inaccessibility and its human consequences: Reports from the field. *Journal of Pain and Palliative Care Pharmacotherapy, 24*(3), 239–243. doi:10.3109/15360288.2010.501852

Kübler-Ross, E. (1969). *On death and dying.* New York, NY: Simon & Schuster.

Larsen, L. (2002). *Facing the final mystery.* Malibu, CA: Blue Sky Press.

Lasch, K. E. (2000). Culture, pain, and culturally sensitive pain care. *Pain Management Nursing, 1*(Suppl. 1), 16–22.

Leow, Q. H. M., Drury, V. B., & Poon, W. H. (2010). A qualitative exploration of patients' experiences of music therapy in an inpatient hospice in Singapore. *International Journal of Palliative Nursing, 16*(7), 344–350.

Lewis, J. M., DiGiacomo, M., Currow, D. C., & Davidson, P. M. (2011). Dying in the margins: Understanding palliative care and socioeconomic deprivation in the developed world. *Journal of Pain and Symptom Management, 42*(1), 105–118. doi:10.1016/j.jpainsymman.2010.10.265

Mansky, P. J., & Wallerstedt, D. B. (2006). Complementary medicine in palliative care and cancer symptom management. *Cancer Journal, 12*(5), 425–431.

McCaffery, M. (1968). *Nursing practice theories related to cognition, bodily pain, and man-environment interactions.* Los Angeles, CA: University of California.

McCaffery, M., Herr, K., & Pasero, C. (2011). Assessment. In C. Pasero & M. McCaffery (Eds.), *Pain assessment and pharmacologic management* (pp. 13–176). St. Louis, MO: Mosby.

McDonough-Means, S. I., Kreitzer, M. J., & Bell, I. R. (2004). Fostering a healing presence and investigating its mediators. *Journal of Alternative and Complementary Medicine, 10*(Suppl. 1), S25–S41.

McGibbon, E. A., & Etowa, J. B. (2009). *Anti-racist health care practice.* Toronto, ON: Canadian Scholars' Press.

McKivergin, M. (2009). The nurse as an instrument of healing. In B. M. Dossey & L. Keegan (Eds.), *Holistic nursing: A handbook for practice* (5th ed., pp. 721–737). Sudbury, MA: Jones and Bartlett.

Melzack, R., & Wall, P. D. (1965). Pain mechanisms: A new theory. *Science, 150*(3699), 971–979.

National Center for Complementary and Alternative Medicine. (2011). *What is complementary and alternative medicine?* Retrieved from http://nccam.nih.gov/sites/nccam.nih.gov/files/D347_05-25-2012.pdf

Nelson, J. P. (2006). Being in tune with life: Complementary therapy use and well-being in residential hospice residents. *Journal of Holistic Nursing, 24*(3), 152–161. doi:10.1177/0898010105282524

Nightingale, F. (1969). *Notes on nursing: What it is and what it is not.* New York, NY: Dover. (Original work published 1860).

Nouwen, H. J. M. (1974). *Out of solitude: Three meditations on the Christian life.* Notre Dame, IN: Ava Maria Press.

Parliamentary Committee on Palliative and Compassionate Care. (2011). *Not to be forgotten: Care of vulnerable Canadians.* Ottawa, ON: Author.

Parkes, C. (2006). *Love and loss: The roots of grief and its complications.* New York, NY: Routledge.

Pasero, C., Polomano, R. C., Portenoy, R. K., & McCaffery, M. (2011). Adjuvant analgesics. In C. Pasero & M. McCaffery (Eds.), *Pain assessment and pharmacologic management* (pp. 623–818). St. Louis, MO: Mosby.

Pasero, C., & Portenoy, R. K. (2011). Neurophysiology of pain and analgesia and the pathophysiology of neuropathic pain. In C. Pasero & M. McCaffery (Eds.), *Pain assessment and pharmacologic management* (pp. 1–12). St. Louis, MO: Mosby.

Pasero, C., Quinn, T. E., Portenoy, R. K., McCaffery, M., & Rizos, A. (2011). Opioid analgesics. In C. Pasero & M. McCaffery (Eds.), *Pain assessment and pharmacologic management* (pp. 277–622). St. Louis, MO: Mosby.

Pereira, J. (2008). *The Pallium palliative pocketbook: A peer-reviewed, referenced resource.* Edmonton, AB: The Pallium Project.

Perry, B. (2008). Why exemplary oncology nurses seem to avoid compassion fatigue. *Canadian Oncology Nursing Journal, 18*(2), 87–99.

Perry, B. (2009). Conveying compassion through attention to the essential ordinary. *Nursing Older People, 21*(6), 14–21.

Quinn, J. F. (2000). Transpersonal human caring and healing. In B. M. Dossey, L. Keegan, L. G. Kolkmeier, & C. E. Guzzetta (Eds.), *Holistic health promotion: A guide for practice* (3rd ed., pp. 37–48). Gaithersburg, MD: Aspen.

Rahim-Jamal, S., Sarte, A., Kozak, J., Bodell, K., Barroetavena, M. C., Gallagher, R., & Leis, A. (2011). Hospice residents' interest in complementary and alternative medicine (CAM) at end of life: A pilot study in hospice residences in British Columbia. *Journal of Palliative Care, 27*(2), 134–140.

Rahner, K. (1965). *Everyday things.* London, United Kingdom: Sheed & Ward.

Rando, T. A. (1984). *Grief, death, and dying: Clinical interventions for caregivers*. Champaign, IL: Research Press.

Rando, T. A. (Ed.). (2000). *Clinical dimensions of anticipatory mourning: Theory and practice in working with the dying, their loved ones, and their caregivers*. Champaign, IL: Research Press.

Rogers, C. (1992). The necessary and sufficient conditions of therapeutic personality change. *Journal of Consulting and Clinical Psychology, 60*(6), 827–832.

Running, A., Shreffler-Grant, J., & Andrews, W. (2008). A survey of hospices' use of complementary therapy. *Journal of Hospice & Palliative Nursing, 10*(5), 304–312. doi:10.1097/01.NJH.0000319177.25294.e5

Saunders, C. (1976). *Care of the dying*. London, United Kingdom: Nursing Times.

Selman, L. E., Williams, J., & Simms, V. (2012). A mixed-methods evaluation of complementary therapy services in palliative care: Yoga and dance therapy. *European Journal of Cancer Care, 21*(1), 87–97. doi:10.1111/j.1365-2354.2011.01285.x

Sepúlveda, C., Marlin, A., Yoshida, T., & Ullrich, A. (2002). Palliative care: The World Health Organization's global perspective. *Journal of Pain and Symptom Management, 24*(2), 91–96. doi:10.1016/s0885-3924(02)00440-2

Service Canada. (2011). *Employment Insurance (EI) compassionate care benefits*. Retrieved from http://www.servicecanada.gc.ca/eng/ei/types/compassionate_care.shtml

Stjernswärd, J., Foley, K. M., & Ferris, F. D. (2007). The public health strategy for palliative care. *Journal of Pain and Symptom Management, 33*(5), 486–493. doi:10.1016/j.jpainsymman.2007.02.016

Stroebe, M. S., Hansson, R. O., Stroebe, W., & Schut, H. (2001). Concepts and issues in contemporary research on bereavement. In M. S. Stroebe, R. O. Hansson, W. Stroebe, & H. Schut (Eds.), *Handbook of bereavement research: Consequences, coping, and caring* (pp. 671–703). Washington, DC: American Psychological Association.

Stroebe, M. S., & Schut, H. (1999). The dual process model of coping with bereavement: Rationale and description. *Death Studies, 23*, 197–224.

Tappouni, T. (2013). *The gifts of grief: Finding light in the darkness of loss*. San Antonio, TX: Hierophant.

Vogel, W. H., Wilson, M. A., & Melvin, M. S. (2004). *Advanced practice oncology & palliative care guidelines*. Philadelphia, PA: Lippincott Williams & Wilkins.

Walshe, C., Todd, C., Caress, A., & Chew-Graham, C. (2009). Patterns of access to community palliative care services: A literature review. *Journal of Pain & Symptom Management, 37*(5), 884–912. doi:10.1016/j.jpainsymman.2008.05.004

Wilson, A. (2000). The continent of cancer. *Canadian Medical Association Journal, 163*(12), 1620–1621.

World Health Organization. (1996). *Cancer pain relief*. Geneva, Switzerland: Author.

Wright, L. M., & Leahey, M. (2009). *Nurses and families: A guide to family assessment and intervention* (5th ed.). Philadelphia, PA: F. A. Davis.

Zerwekh, J. V. (2006). *Nursing care at the end of life: Palliative care for patients and families*. Philadelphia, PA: F. A. Davis.

Balancing Activity and Rest

SARAH KOSTIUK AND SHERRY ARVIDSON

Mackenna, a fourth-year nursing student working at the public health clinic, meets her patient, Mr. Jones, who is 28 years of age and is married with two young children. Mackenna discovered that Mr. Jones has recently started a job as a geologist at different oil sites, and his new job requires him to work from 3:00 PM until midnight every night for a week, followed by a stretch of 5 days off. Mr. Jones is not used to working such late hours because his previous job for the past 3 years was from 9 AM to 5 PM. During the visit, Mackenna notices that Mr. Jones has dark circles under his eyes, increased yawning, and slow responses. When Mackenna asks Mr. Jones how he was finding his new job, Mr. Jones replies that he was still trying to find a way to balance his life. Mackenna continues the visit by assessing Mr. Jones's quality of sleep. Mr. Jones discloses that he finds it difficult to sleep after he gets home from his shift. Mackenna identifies that since Mr. Jones began his new job, he has not been going for his regular morning jogs and has been eating more unhealthy foods. Mr. Jones reports that he has no energy and finds he has to drink a lot of caffeine to stay awake. He says he spends most of his free time watching television or going on the computer. Mr. Jones wonders: What factors are causing him to feel the way he does? If there is anything he can do to better balance his activity with rest? What are the consequences of sitting on the couch too long and not exercising?

CHAPTER OBJECTIVES

By the end of this chapter, you will be able to:

1. Explain the importance of balancing activity with rest.
2. Identify the stages of sleep and the related activity in each stage.
3. Discuss the issues that could result from a lack of rest.
4. Differentiate among the various sleep disorders and their related causes.
5. Describe factors that affect sleep.
6. Gain a beginning understanding of interventions to assist a patient to improve the quality of sleep.
7. Develop an understanding of nurse-assisted movements.
8. Develop a basic understanding of the benefits of activity and exercise.
9. Describe healthy age-related activity and exercise.
10. Gain an awareness of positioning in regard to patient care.

KEY TERMS

Active Range of Motion   When a person performs a range of motion activities without needing assistance.

Activities of Daily Living (ADL)   Everyday endeavors that people do to meet their basic needs, such as going to the bathroom, performing hygiene, being able to dress, and eating.

Activity   The process of movement.

Aerobic Exercise   Planned, structured, and focused activities that last over 10 minutes and increase a person's breathing and heart rate.

Body Alignment   The action of keeping the body in a state of normal position.

Body Mechanics   Using proper assistive devices, body movements, and body positioning to prevent injuries.

Circadian Rhythms   The human body's physical, mental, and behavioural changes that occur in a 24-hour cycle that generally follows the light and darkness cycles.

Dorsal Recumbent Position   Bed is flat, keeping the patient's head in a straight line with his or her entire body.

Duration   The time spent to complete an activity.

Electroencephalogram (EEG)   An instrument used to measure, analyze, and record brain wave activity.

Ergonomics   Education about keeping the proper postural position during movement and lifting so that the body maintains a normal body alignment to avoid injury.

Fowler Position   The head of the bed is at 45° angle above the horizon of the bed.

Frequency   The number of times an activity is performed.

Gait   The speed, stride width, stride step, stride length, and stride movement that occur as a person walks.

High Fowler Position   The angle of the head of the bed is at a 90° angle above the horizon of the bed.

Hypersomnia   Excessive daytime sleepiness.

Immobility   Inability to move a part or all of the body to some degree.

Insomnia   Difficulty initiating sleep, or maintaining sleep, or waking too early and not being able to get back to sleep.

Intensity   The effort needed to perform an activity.

Lateral Position   When a person is lying on his or her hip with the shoulder, arm of the lying side forward, leg of lying side straight.

Lithotomy Position   The head of the bed is flat with the foot of the bed increased so that the patient's legs are bent in bed.

Narcolepsy   A neurological disorder that affects the control of sleep and wakefulness, characterized by extreme sleepiness or falling asleep during the day.

Nonrapid Eye Movement (NREM) Sleep   Consists of discrete stages of a reduction in physiological activity.

Parasomnias   Lack of progression from one sleep state to the next; may result in bizarre behaviours.

Passive Range of Motion   When a patient requires assistance to perform different range of movement with respect to the body's joints.

Postural tone   A person's unconscious, patterned, muscle tension that extends across the body axis.

Prone Position   Lying on stomach with the arms to the side and head turned to the side.

Range of Motion (ROM)   The movement of a joint within its normal limits.

Rapid Eye Movement (REM) Sleep   An active period of sleep marked by intense brain activity.

Rest   Not participating in strenuous activity that is either mental or physical.

Restless Leg Syndrome   A sleep disorder characterized by uncomfortable sensations and an irresistible urge to move the legs to relieve the sensation; can lead to sleep deprivation and increased stress levels; commonly seen in older adults.

Reverse Trendelenburg Position   Bed is flat and tilted so that the head is above the feet.

Sedentary Behaviours   Actions that require very little physical energy to perform, such as watching a movie or playing a video game.

Semi-Fowler Position   The head of the bed is at 30° angle above the horizon of the bed.

Shift Work   Work schedules that are not within typical 9 AM to 5 PM daytime work hours.

Sims Position   When a person is lying close to a prone position but has a slightly lateral position and is lying on the side of his or her shoulder and hip while the other shoulder and hip are slightly forward.

Sleep   Expected regular period of decreased awareness to the external stimuli.

Sleep Apnea   Irregular breathing that causes multiple awakenings.

Sleep Architecture   Having the right combination of REM and NREM sleep.

Sleep Deprivation   Lack of sufficient restorative sleep over a cumulative period so as to cause physical or psychiatric symptoms and affect routine performances of tasks. When the body does not regularly get adequate sleep (between 7 and 9 hours), deprivation may manifest with frequent sleepiness, nodding off, difficulty concentrating, lapses in memory, poor performance, and mood changes. Shift workers are often the hardest hit.

Sleep Hygiene   Personal sleep habits.

Supine Position   When a person is lying on his or her back side with his or her feet in a neural position and arms to the side of the body.

Trendelenburg Position   Bed is flat, but it is tilted so that feet of a person are higher than the head and trunk.

Turning and Repositioning   The action of moving a person from one position into a new position to shift the pressure off different pressure points on the body.

Activity, Rest, and Sleep in Balance—Introduction

Balancing activity and rest is important for healthy body functions. Adequate rest is essential for wellness. Sleep is essential for a person's health, body function, and healing. The amount of activity and rest that an individual requires depends on various factors such as age, physiological state, and individual needs.

Regular physical activity and exercise are recognized as essential aspects of health promotion and chronic disease prevention (Kokkinos, 2012).

This chapter explores the phenomenon of sleep and the importance of activity by discussing the stages of sleep, the importance of sleep and rest, the effects of inadequate sleep, sleep disorders, inhibitors of sleep, healthy sleep hygiene tips nurses can teach patients as well as practice, the importance of participating in activity, the aspects of normal movements, the potential consequences associated with a lack of mobility, and the care needed for patients with decreased mobility.

Rest

Rest is being in a state of relaxation, such as ceasing from motion, closing ones' eyes, eliminating stressors, and refraining from thinking about anything particular (Polanía, Paulus, & Nitsche, 2012). Rest can mean leisure; it can include not only relaxation techniques (such as meditation, biofeedback, and deep breathing), but it also includes exercise such as walking, yoga, or Tai Chi. Some people use massage to improve their restful state. Methods that are used to relax people are structured to decrease the arousal system and are selected based on whether the targeted treatment in need is physiological or cognitive in nature (Saddichha, 2010). *Rest* is a term that is sometimes used synonymously with *sleep* because when a person is asleep, he or she is generally not engaging in physical activities. Both sleep and rest are important to maintaining a person's wellness because they allow the body to enter into a state of lower activity where it can work to restore itself. A major part of balancing activity and rest is getting adequate sleep.

Sleep

An important aspect of sleep is that a person rests when he or she is asleep. **Sleep** is a natural and changeable state of consciousness with a temporary interruption in perceptual, sensory, and voluntary motor activity that occurs at regular intervals with alternating periods of wakefulness (Liberalesso et al., 2012). The period of sleep is when our body secretes many important hormones that affect growth, regulate energy,

TABLE 31.1	Recommended Amount of Sleep Throughout the Lifespan
Age	**Recommended Amount of Sleep**
Infants	17 hours
Children	10 hours
Teenagers	10 hours
Adults	8 hours
Older adults	8 hours

Adapted from National Heart Lung and Blood Institute. (2011). *Your guide to a healthy sleep.* Bethesda, MD: U.S. Department of Health and Human Services; Public Health Service; National Institute of Health; and National Heart, Lung, and Blood Institute. Retrieved from http://www.nhlbi.nih.gov/health/public/sleep/healthy_sleep.pdf

BOX 31.1	Sleep Hygiene Activities That Enhance Sleep

- Bedtime routine
- Regular exercise
- Eating right
- Relaxation techniques
- Comfortable sleep environment

Adapted with permission from University of Maryland Medical Center. (2010). *Sleep disorders center: Sleep hygiene: Helpful hints to help you sleep.* Retrieved from http://www.umm.edu/sleep/sleep_hyg.htm

and control metabolic and endocrine functions (National Heart, Lung, and Blood Institute [NHLBI], 2011). Sleep is reported to be associated with reduced heart rate, blood pressure, respiratory rate, oxygen consumption, anxiety, arousal, and overall basal metabolic levels leading to a hypometabolic state (Nagendra, Maruthai, & Kutty, 2012).

A typical pattern of sleep and activity in humans within a 24-hour period is a 12- to 16-hour cycle of wakefulness with the remainder of the time spent at rest (University of Maryland Medical Center [UMMC], 2010a). Most people need about 6 to 9 hours of sleep every night, and anything less can adversely affect their health (Cartwright, Dang-Vu, Ellenbogen, & Foulkes, 2012; National Institute of Neurological Disorders and Stroke [NINDS], 2007) (Table 31.1). Some people find that 20-minute naps assist them to battle daytime sleepiness and feel more alert, whereas others who find it makes harder for them to sleep at night, and it enhances their daytime drowsiness (NHLBI, 2011).

Sleep hygiene refers to the habits that a person participates in that affects the quality and quantity of sleep; for instance, healthy sleep hygiene practices might include regular times for sleeping and waking, avoiding television or computer use an hour before bed, not napping during the day, and avoiding alcoholic beverages (Table 31.2).

For decades, researchers around the world have studied the phenomenon of sleep. It is suggested that patterns of sleep have changed over the past decades with patterns of sleep changing

TABLE 31.2	Habits to Avoid to Enhance Sleep
Habit	**Time of Day to Avoid**
Caffeine	For up to 4 hours before bed
Vigorous exercise	Approximately 2–3 hours before bed
Spicy or heavy food	During bedtime snacks
Stressful activities	Right before bed
Alcohol	Around 4 hours before bed
Naps	In the late afternoon
Taking certain medications	Just prior to sleep

Adapted with permission from University of Maryland Medical Center. (2010). *Sleep disorders center: Sleep hygiene: Helpful hints to help you sleep.* Retrieved from http://www.umm.edu/sleep/sleep_hyg.htm

over our lifespans (Cartwright et al., 2012). Sleep is believed to occur in different stages of a sleep cycle (Cartwright et al., 2012; NHLBI, 2011). The purpose of sleep has been debated throughout history and is still definitively unknown. Some believe that the purpose for sleep is to enhance memory, muscles healing, immune systems, daytime alertness, mood, and regulate hormones (Cartwright et al., 2012; NHLBI, 2011). A person's quality of sleep can be affected by other disturbances, such as insomnia or hypersomnia (Cartwright et al., 2012). Additionally, several lifestyle factors and sleep habits can also affect the quality of a person's sleep, such as caffeine intake, or environmental conditions (UMMC, 2010a). Researchers have identified several sleep habits, or sleep hygiene tips, that are able to assist people in enhancing their sleep. For example, a person may sleep better if he or she avoids engaging in certain activities before bedtime (UMMC, 2010c) (Box 31.1).

Activity and Exercise

Activity is just as important as sleep to our health and well-being. **Activity** is known as a process of doing something. Being active possesses many benefits for a person's health; for instance, physical activity promotes metabolism, increases a person's spirit, and maintains the function of the heart (Ontario Ministry of Health and Long-Term Care [MOHLTC], 2011c). If a person does not move or is inactive, it can lead to several health issues. Lack of activity, just as lack of sleep, can result in reduced mental acuity, mood alteration, and weight gain, among many other health issues discussed in greater detail in this chapter, including the issues, care, and impact that limited mobility or immobility has on patient care.

What Is Sleep?

Feeling the need to sleep becomes overwhelming if you put off going to sleep because of the regulation of two substances in your body: adenosine and melatonin (NHLBI, 2011). When a person is awake, adenosine builds up in the blood, and while a person sleeps, the body breaks down the adenosine (NHLBI, 2011). It is believed that the buildup of adenosine level signals us to sleep and that a lack of sleep alters the regulation of the adenosine levels, which may result in sleeping longer and at odd times (NHLBI, 2011). Melatonin is the other substance

BOX 31.2 Physiological Changes in Nonrapid Eye Movement

- Blood pressure decreases.
- Heart rate decreases.
- Peripheral blood vessels dilate.
- Cardiac output decreases.
- Muscles relax.
- Basal metabolic rate decreases.
- Growth hormone levels increase.
- Intracranial pressure decreases.
- Respirations fall.
- Body temperature decreases.
- Diminished eye movement

BOX 31.3 Physiological Changes in Rapid Eye Movement

- Increased brain stimulation
- Voluntary muscle relaxation
- Irregular heart rate
- Irregular respirations
- Fluctuations on blood pressure
- Impaired temperature regulation

that helps regulate our sleep patterns. The natural hormone melatonin is what is believed to cause a person to feel drowsy at night (NHLBI, 2011). Light and darkness are other cues that communicate to our bodies that it is time for rest (NHLBI, 2011). Our bodies send out messages to make us feel awake or sleepy at certain times during a 24-hour period.

Stages of Sleep

Sleep is considered to occur in stages, and each of these discrete stages has different characteristics which are regulated by distinct neural centers (NHLBI, 2011). Sleep pattern stages are revealed through the use of an **electroencephalogram (EEG)**. Our brains still remain very active when we sleep. Sleep is believed to consist of two discrete stages known as nonrapid eye movement (NREM) and rapid eye movement (REM) (Sharma & Kavuru, 2010). **Nonrapid eye movement**

(NREM) sleep is characterized by a reduction in physiological activity of brain waves and is believe to be further broken down in the N1, N2, N3 stages of sleep (Sharma & Kavuru, 2010). As a person moves through the NREM sleep stages, he or she progressively become characterized by more cortical neuron activity and a stable autonomic function as well have an increased arousal threshold (NHLBI, 2011). As sleep moves from the NREM stage to the REM stage, it becomes more pronounced, and our breathing, heart rate, and blood pressure decreases (Harvard University, 2009; NHLBI, 2011) (Box 31.2). **Rapid eye movement (REM) sleep** is an active period of sleep characterized by intense brain activity with increased shallow breathing, REM, increased heart rate, and temporary muscle paralysis (NHLBI, 2011) (Box 31.3). It is during our NREM sleep that our bodies are believed to undergo repair and restoration (UMMC, 2010a). After being in a REM sleep, we move back into a NREM sleep. In a night, a person experiences repeated cycles of the stages of sleep that last about 90 minutes (Waterhouse, Fukuda, & Morita, 2012).

Researchers at National Heart, Lung, and Blood Institute (NHLBI, 2011) identified four stages of sleep (Table 31.3).

TABLE 31.3	Stages of Sleep	
Stages of Sleep	**Corresponding Activity**	**Physiological Changes**
Stage 1	Brain waves and muscle activity slows. Muscle jerking may be present. May experience feeling of falling Light sleep that only lasts a few minutes Can be easily awakened 75%–80% of sleep during the night is NREM (NHLBI, 2011).	Person feels drowsy and relaxed. Eyes rolls from side to side. Slight decrease in heart rate and respirations.
Stage 2	Eye movement stops. Brain waves become slower. Alternating muscle tone and relaxation Lasts 10–15 minutes but constitutes 44%–55% of total sleep (NHLBI, 2011) Person requires more stimulation to awaken.	Continual slowing of body processes. Eyes have limited movement. Body temperature drops.
Stages 3 and 4	Presence of slow delta waves fluctuating in intensity Sleep is deeper without eye movement. Decreased muscle activity Deepest stages of sleep Difficult to arouse	Blood pressure decreases. Breathing rate decreases. Body temperature drops. No disturbance to sensory stimuli. Skeletal muscles are very relaxed. Reflexes are diminished. Snoring may occur.

Adapted from National Heart Lung and Blood Institute. (2011). *Your guide to a healthy sleep.* Bethesda, MD: U.S. Department of Health and Human Services; Public Health Service; National Institute of Health; and National Heart, Lung, and Blood Institute.

Stage 1 is a presleep phase, the time of drowsiness, or transition from being awake to falling asleep. Brain waves and muscle activity begin to slow down, muscle jerking may be present, and a feeling of falling may be experienced (NHLBI, 2011). This stage lasts a few minutes to a half hour. If a person has difficulty falling asleep, this period can last an hour or longer.

Stage 2 is a period of light sleep during which eye movement stops, brain waves become slower, there are occasional shifts in periods of muscle tone mixed with periods of muscle relaxation, and a person's heart rate and body temperature decrease (NHLBI, 2011; NINDS, 2007). A person is relatively easily roused in this stage. This stage lasts about 10 to 20 minutes.

Stage 3 and 4 are characterized by the presence of slow delta brain waves alternating with faster and slower brain waves, a drop in blood pressure, slowed breathing, and a lower body temperature as the body becomes immobile (NHLBI, 2011). Sleep in this stage is deeper with no eye movement, decreased muscle activity, and maintained muscle functioning, and it is the stage in which bedwetting, night terrors, or sleepwalking may occur (NHLBI, 2011). The person is difficult to arouse during this stage of sleep.

Each stage plays an essential role to promote healthy body function and to have the right balance to obtain a restorative sleep that will promote processes such as learning, memory, mood, and concentration.

Sleep Architecture

Sleep architecture refers to the right proportion of REM and NREM sleep stages for adequate rest and supporting wellness. An important note to remember is the quantity of sleep is just as crucial as the quality of sleep. Keeping track of your sleep patterns, nutritional intake, and exercise schedule can identify measures to improve or secure a good night's rest. A sleep diary will help you to track sleep patterns and lead you to interventions to promote a healthy well-being (Box 31.4). Lifestyle and behavioral interventions that can help promote sleep include lifestyle changes, physical activity, maintaining a sleep schedule, relaxation techniques, and cognitive behavioral therapy.

Issues Resulting From a Lack of Sleep

Sleeping for less than 6 hours in duration increases a person's risk for developing chronic diseases, such as stroke and cancer (Ruesten, Weikert, Fietze, & Boeing, 2012). **Sleep deprivation** means that person has poor quality sleep and/or short duration of sleep (Lo & Lee, 2012). If an adult gets less than 8 hours of quality sleep, he or she is at risk of sleep deprivation (Tewari, Soliz, Billota, Garg, & Singh, 2011). *Microsleeps* are another mark of sleep deprivation. Microsleeps are a phenomenon characterized by a gradual reduction in the level control to stay awake, along with a continuous decrease in psychomotor performances, reduced reaction times, lowered perception of risks, and severely decreased attention span (Sena et al., 2012). In many cases,

---

BOX 31.4   Sleep Diary

Sleep Diary	Month/Day/Year

Time I went to bed

Time I woke up this morning

Number of hours slept last night

Number of awakenings during my sleep at night

How long I took to fall asleep last night

Sleep aid medications taken at night time

How awake did I feel when I got up this morning:

   1—Wide awake

   2—Awake but a little tired

   3—Sleepy

Number of caffeinated drinks and time I had them today

Number of alcoholic drinks and time when consumed today

Naptimes and length of naps today

Exercise times and lengths of time exercising

How sleepy did I feel during the day today:

   1—So sleepy struggled to stay awake during much of the day

   2—Somewhat tired

   3—Fairly alert

   4—Wide awake

---

people are not aware that they are experiencing microsleeps. When people became increasingly sleepy, they have a decreased ability to perform tasks (Czisch et al., 2012). Sleep deprivation is extremely common in contemporary society and is considered to be a frequent cause of behavioral disorders, mood disturbances, decreased alertness, and lowered cognitive performance (Liberalesso et al., 2012).

It is not uncommon for people to be sleep deprived to some degree. Sleep deprivation can cause physiological and cognitive changes, such as decreased memory, slowed thought processes, increased irritability, decreased job performance, and impaired emotional control (Harvard University, 2009; Tewari et al., 2011). Challenges with sleep are particularly common in patients with mental health disorders, diabetes, and cardiovascular disease (Saddichha, 2010). Another medical condition that is well known to disrupt sleep is gastroesophageal reflux disease (GERD) (Lindam, Jansson, Nordensted, Pedersen, & Lagergren, 2012). People with GERD generally are awoken or cannot sleep from the symptoms of the disease, such as experiencing pain behind the breastbone, tasting bitter acidic fluids, or having heartburn because the disease causes a regurgitation of stomach acid into their esophagus and mouth (Lindam et al., 2012). Prolonged lack of sleep is also stressful to immune and endocrine systems, increasing a person's risk of critical illnesses such as obesity, diabetes, and hypertension (NHLBI, 2011).

For example, people with sleep apnea are known to be at an increased risk of hypertension and sudden death from cardiac causes during the night (Canadian Sleep Society [CSS], 2007; NHLBI, 2011). Although the exact purpose of sleep is still at debate, it is clear that sleep is an important aspect of our overall health and well-being.

Through the eyes of a student

As a first-year nursing student, rest and sleep have become particularly important to me. When I make getting an adequate amount of sleep a priority, I see vast improvements with my focus, performance in clinical, and ability to study for exams. To ensure I get enough rest mentally, I also make a point of working rest into my daytime schedule, where I take a break from schoolwork and only focus on my personal life.

(personal reflection of J. Cran, nursing student, February 8, 2012)

Sleep Disorders

Conditions that interfere with sleep (excluding environmental factors) can be identified as sleep disorders. There are some classic symptoms of sleep disorders, such as twitting as a person falls asleep (NHLBI, 2011) (Box 31.5). Classes of sleep disorders are categorized by sleep disturbances, parasomnias, and sleep pattern disruptions associated with mental illness. Other factors that interfere with sleep include inadequate sleep hygiene, effects of drugs and alcohol, and dietary changes. Sleep disturbances include disorders such as insomnia, narcolepsy, hypersomnia, sleep apnea, restless leg syndrome, and parasomnia.

Insomnia

Insomnia refers to an inadequate quantity or quality of sleep that interferes with normal daytime functioning (Harvard University, 2009; Hayward, Jordan, & Croft, 2012). A person may experience insomnia if he or she has difficulty falling asleep or staying asleep or experience early awakening (Harvard University,

---

BOX 31.5 Common Signs of a Sleep Disorder

- It takes more than 30 minutes to fall asleep at night with frequent awakenings and then have difficulty falling back to sleep.
- Waking up too early in the morning
- Feeling tired and fatigued despite spending 8 hours of sleep at night
- Feeling sleepy during the day and fall asleep quickly if an opportunity presents
- Loud snoring, gasping, or making choking sounds while sleeping
- Creeping, tingling, and burning sensations in your feet
- Dreamlike experiences trying to fall asleep
- Jerking movements to limbs
- Regular intake of stimulants during the day to stay awake

2009; Hayward et al., 2012). In some cases, insomnia can be situational and last only a few days, or it can be chronic where it lasts longer than a month (UMMC, 2010b). The causes of insomnia may relate to psychological conditions including depression, stress, and feeling overwhelmed (NHLBI, 2011). Medical illness and neurological conditions including breathing conditions, stomach upset, cardiac disorders, hot flashes, arthritis, increased frequency of elimination, stroke, Parkinson disease, and dementia may have an impact on getting a restful sleep (Harvard University, 2009; Saddichha, 2010).

If the patient's current sleep hygiene techniques are not effective, treating insomnia may require implementing healthy sleep habits or pharmaceutical medication (Harvard University, 2009; Hayward et al., 2012). For instance, some patients may take melatonin (a hormone that is produced by the pineal gland) as a dietary supplement because in low doses, it may help people to feel sleepy (NHLBI, 2011).

Hypersomnia

Hypersomnia is another sleep disorder characterized by excessive prolonged sleepiness and difficulties waking from sleep (NINDS, 2008; Shah, Bang, & Bhagat, 2010). It is believed that the causes of hypersomnia can be narcolepsy, idiopathic hypersomnia, sleep apnea, pain disorders, and mood disorders (Proctor & Bianchi, 2012). Idiopathic hypersomnia differs from narcolepsy because the sleep with idiopathic hypersomnia is not as irresistible and is less refreshing (Knudsen & Culebras, 2011). Symptoms of hypersomnia include irritability, difficulties concentrating, excessive sleepiness, slowed responses, and decreased energy (NINDS, 2008; Knudsen & Culebras, 2011). Treatment may consist of treating the underlying causes, practicing healthy sleep hygiene, or taking medications such as stimulants to increase alertness (NINDS, 2008; Proctor & Bianchi, 2012). Depending on the individual causes of hypersomnia, a treatment plan will be tailored toward each situation. Obtaining a complete and accurate history of the individual with hypersomnia is vital toward the success of the treatments.

Narcolepsy

Narcolepsy is a neurological disorder that causes people to fall asleep at any given time of day when they want to be awake (CSS, 2007; UMMC, 2010b). In people with narcolepsy, sleep begins immediately with REM sleep, and fragments of REM occur involuntarily throughout the waking hours (NHLBI, 2011). It is believed that genetic and environmental factors are contributors to this disorder (Ajayi, Kinagi, & Haslett, 2012; CSS, 2007). In some cases, people may experience symptoms of cataplexy, sleep paralysis, and hypnotic hallucinations. Cataplexy is a sudden loss of muscle control that generally occurs when a person has intense emotional disturbances (CSS, 2007; UMMC, 2010b). Sleep paralysis is loss of mobility, speech, or ability to breathe when a person awakes or is falling asleep (CSS, 2007; NHLBI, 2011). Hypnotic hallucinations are strong and bizarre sensations similar to dreaming just as a person awakes or goes to sleep (UMMC, 2010b). Narcolepsy can be frightening and not knowing when one might fall asleep can have serious consequences to overall quality of life.

Researchers believe that narcolepsy may be caused by a deficiency of hypocretin in the brain because the chemical is known to prevent cataplexy and improve wakefulness (Ajayi et al., 2012; CSS, 2007). At this point, there is no cure for narcolepsy; however, symptoms can be alleviated to the point of near-normal functioning in many patients. Treatment for narcolepsy may include an evaluation by the sleep clinic. Keeping a sleep diary as well as a record of symptoms and their severity will help to track the frequency and intensity experienced by the patient (Harvard University, 2009; Saddichha, 2010). Treatments that are used to alleviate symptoms of narcolepsy include using stimulants to improve alertness and diminish daytime excessive sleepiness, scheduling daytime naps, regular exercise, and education (Ajayi et al., 2012). Behavioral modification is also an essential treatment that is often used to treat patients with narcolepsy (UMMC, 2010b). Because the symptoms may vary among each individual affected with narcolepsy, it is important to remember to treat every person affected according to the symptoms he or she experiences.

Sleep Apnea

One of the most common sleep disorders is sleep apnea. **Sleep apnea** can be defined as prolonged and repetitive cessations of airflow causing sleep arousal and occasional oxygen desaturation (Adegunsoye & Ramachandran, 2012). With sleep apnea, breathing stops while sleeping. Obstructive sleep apnea is a common chronic form of sleep apnea in which a person's airways are completely or partially obstructed, causing episodes of apnea or hypopnea, respectively (Adegunsoye & Ramachandran, 2012). Obstructive sleep apnea occurs when a person's tongue, tonsils, or soft palate in the back of the mouth prevent airflow from reaching the area of the throat. Contributing factors of obstructive sleep apnea may include being overweight; having a narrow airway; and excessive amounts of tissue including the tongue, tonsils, and soft palate (Veasey, 2012). There are some factors that put a person at risk for sleep apnea (Box 31.6). The most common underlying pathophysiology of obstructive sleep apnea is a partial or complete collapse of the upper airway during sleep states that lead to momentary interruptions in ventilation (Zhang & Veasey, 2013). When a person stops breathing from sleep apnea, the brain quickly realizes and makes the needed efforts to breathe, such as waking the

person up (UMMC, 2010b). Not everyone who snores has sleep apnea, but a lot of people who have sleep apnea are known to snore. In some instances, a partner may not even know his or her partner has sleep apnea issues (UMMC, 2010b). A person with apnea who has disrupted sleep may have the same symptoms that are seen in person with a lack of sleep, such as decreased concentration, fatigue, and daytime sleepiness (Adegunsoye & Ramachandran, 2012).

Treatment for sleep apnea may involve continuous positive airway pressure (CPAP) machine, which involves a mask being place over the person's nose or nose and mouth when he or she sleeps in order to maintain a pressure that will keep the person's airways open (UMMC, 2010b). For the cases of positional obstructive sleep apnea, treatment involves repositioning the patient in a semi-upright position (UMMC, 2010b). Other treatments for sleep apnea are avoiding sedatives, surgically removing the tissue blocking the airway, losing any excessive weight, and using a dental device at night to keep a person's jaw in a certain position to help alleviate breathing obstructions (UMMC, 2010b). The choice of treatment will depend on the individual's preference and situation.

Restless Leg Syndrome

When a person experiences tingling, pain, burning, cramping, and crawling sensations in the lower legs or feet, which worsen with rest, this is known as **restless leg syndrome** (UMMC, 2010b), also called Willis-Ekbom Disease (WED). Restless leg syndrome is a chronic sensorimotor disorder, but its exact pathophysiology is not entirely understood (Mitchell, 2010). Cases of restless leg syndrome are considered to be either a primary or secondary forms caused by both delineating genetic and idiopathic contributions and the involvement of other underlying pathologies, respectively (Mitchell, 2010). Secondary forms of this disorder are treating by addressing the underlying causes or associated medical conditions (Mitchell, 2010). Factors noted to be associated with restless leg syndrome include family history, pregnancy, low iron or folate levels or anemia, kidney failure, diabetes, rheumatoid arthritis, peripheral neuropathy, and excessive caffeine consumption (NHLBI, 2011). People with restless leg syndrome may find it difficult to relax and fall asleep because the tingling, pain, and cramping become very unsettling (CSS, 2008; Garcia-Borreguero et al., 2011). The severity of symptoms range from mild to intolerable. The unpleasant sensations may even awaken individuals with restless leg syndrome from their sleep. People with the disorder may feel an urge to walk or move to relieve the sensation in their legs. Walking is one way that people with restless leg syndrome are able to relieve the unpleasant sensations (UMMC, 2010b).

Treatments for restless leg syndrome depend on the cause and may include behavioural and pharmacological approaches (CSS, 2008; Garcia-Borreguero et al., 2011). Making lifestyle changes such as eating a healthy diet, reducing caffeine intake, eliminating alcohol consumption, and practicing sleep hygiene are some strategies to lessen the severity and impact on patients living with restless leg syndrome.

BOX 31.6 Factors Making People Prone to Sleep Apnea

- Family history
- Relaxed throat and tongue while asleep
- Enlarged tonsils and adenoids
- Being overweight
- Anatomy—small airway in the mouth and throat areas
- Congestion due to allergies narrowing the airway

Stretching and yoga have also been used to help manage the symptoms of restless leg disorder (UMMC, 2010b). If a patient has iron deficiency anemia, iron supplements, vitamin B$_{12}$, or folate may provide relief. Some people may even use anti-Parkinson medications, antiseizure, or pain medications to treat the symptoms (UMMC, 2010b). Not every person will be treated the same way for the disorder; it is important to tailor the treatment to fit the person's situation.

Through the eyes of a patient

Sometimes, my feet bother me during the night, and at times, they even feel as if ants are crawling on the soles of my feet. The unpleasant restless feelings in my feet have been occurring for years, and no one seems to be able to fully explain what is happening. I am now taking iron for a low blood count and have to get my blood tested every 6 months to a year. To manage the undesirable sensations, I massage my feet and rub them with lotion. The sensations have interfered with my sleep because I can only rest for a short period of time, and then I need to move my feet around or get up and walk at night to stop the feelings in my feet.

(personal reflection of S. Mosiuk, patient, February 2, 2012)

How does Mr. Jones know if he is getting enough sleep? What can he do to better track his sleep patterns?

Sleep architecture is a mixed balance between NREM and REM. If you are functioning without any signs of drowsiness, feelings of fatigue, or emotional instability, then you are on the right track of balancing sleep with your individual activities of daily living. Mr. Jones could keep a sleep diary to better track his sleep pattern.

Through the eyes of a nurse

It is important to balance activity with sleep because if you don't, your body catches up, and you are likely to become ill and feel stressed with life's demands. At times, I feel the need to take a nap after working for 5 days in a row, but I have to limit the naptime or else my entire night is spent staring at the walls. Learning to adjust the amount of sleep one needs is essential to function with an open mind.

(personal reflection of K. Arvidson, nurse, February 3, 2012)

Parasomnia

Not all sleep disorders involve difficulty falling or staying asleep; some people experience parasomnia sleep disorders. **Parasomnias** can be defined as an unintentional motor or a subjective phenomenon that occurs during the transition from sleep to wake states, or when a person is aroused from sleep (Shah et al., 2010). With parasomnia sleep disorders, a person's walking, talking, and body functions are not suppressed as they should be during the sleep (NHLBI, 2011). Parasomnias sleep disorders are commonly seen in children who generally outgrow it, people who are excessively tired, people who have neurological disorders, or people who are taking certain medications (NHLBI, 2011). Some of the parasomnia sleep disorders include sleepwalking, night terrors, and bedwetting (NHLBI, 2011). A person with parasomnia sleep disorders may sit up in bed and start talking aloud while he or she is asleep. People who sleepwalk might look at you, talk to you, and even perform tasks (UMMC, 2010b). It is important to take precautions to keep the person with parasomnia safe from harm. For instance, some families keep the windows and doors locked so that sleepwalkers cannot leave the house when an episode occurs (UMMC, 2010b).

Inhibitors of Sleep

Several factors exist that can inhibit a person's ability to sleep or remain asleep (see Table 31.2). A person with sleep disturbances needs help to identify if there are factors that he or she can change. A nurse can assist a patient in uncovering the factors that are altering his or her sleep. Some of the factors that a person can alter to obtain a better sleep are consuming less caffeine, avoiding alcohol and drugs, eliminating environmental intrusions, minimizing stress, eliminating certain medication, avoiding shift work, and controlling pain from health issues.

Effects of Caffeine

Many people in Western society turn toward caffeine to battle unwanted sleepiness, especially in the daytime. Caffeine can be consumed in the form of coffee, chocolate, teas, and some soft drinks (NHLBI, 2011). Energy drinks can contain significant levels of caffeine (Campbell et al., 2013; Rainbow Rehabilitation Centers, 2008). Caffeine works by inhibiting adenosine's sleep signal because it binds the adenosine to neuron receptors (Cartwright et al., 2012; NHLBI, 2011). Caffeine can remain active in the body for hours after it is consumed and should avoided within 4 to 6 hours before bed because it decreases a person's quality of sleep (UMMC, 2010c). In Canada, research indicates that adults ingest 60% of their daily caffeine intake from coffee; about 30% from tea; and 10% comes from cola beverages, chocolate products, and medicines (*Its Your Health: Caffeine*, 2010). Research shows that in Canada, children younger than 5 years old consume about 55% off caffeine from cola drinks, about 30% from tea, and about 14% from chocolate (*Its Your Health: Caffeine*, 2010).

Several potential health issues can result in people who consume more than the recommended daily dose of caffeine, such as sleep disturbances, irregular heart rates, and irritability (*Its Your Health: Caffeine,* 2010). Nurses can teach patients the importance of avoiding taking any caffeine before bedtime to help improve the quality of their sleep. It is important that nurses remind patients of the different items that contain caffeine, the daily limit of caffeine, and the different types of noncaffeinated or decaffeinated items that they can consume around bedtime instead.

Effects of Alcohol and Drugs

Alcohol and drugs are among other substances that are capable of affecting a person's quality of sleep and rest. Alcohol is a commonly ingested legal drug. A recent survey of Canadians 15 years and older shows that 78.0% of Canadians reported drinking in the past year (Health Canada, 2012). Many people report resorting to using alcohol to assist them in falling asleep (NHLBI, 2011). Although alcohol may help some people fall asleep initially, the quality of sleep may be affected because alcohol has stimulant effects as the levels in the blood begin to lower (UMMC, 2010c). Over time, the use of alcohol can affect a person's sleep by further exacerbating sleep disorders, such as apnea and snoring (NHLBI, 2011). Comparably, the use of illegal drugs can also affect a person's sleep by either inhibiting the ability to sleep or to stay awake. For example, the uses of methamphetamines, amphetamines, and cocaine can cause difficulties sleeping (National Institute on Drug Abuse [NIDA], 2011). Drugs such as heroin, morphine, and marijuana have been known to cause drowsiness and difficulties staying awake (NIDA, 2011). Nicotine is also a drug that is a stimulant and can inhibit the ability to sleep. Nicotine initially acts as a stimulant by enhancing the release of neurotransmitters accelerating many body reactions causing an increase in the level of excitement (Ratsch, Steadman, & Bogossian, 2010). If a patient uses any of these substances, a nurse can teach about the effects of using these drugs on sleep patterns.

Effects of the Environment

A person's sleep is potentially affected by the environment in which he or she is attempting to sleep or rest. A comfortable, dry, warm, quiet, dark, well-ventilated place is identified as the ideal environment to promote sleep (Harvard University, 2009; UMMC, 2010c). A person is less likely to relax and thus fall asleep in a room that is lit-up, loud, unsafe, too hot, too cold, wet, or uncomfortable. To illustrate, if a person shares a room or bed with another person who snores, wakes frequently in the night, or retires to bed later, he or she can experience difficulties sleeping. Some partners sleep in different rooms because their partner's snoring disrupts their sleep (NHLBI, 2011). Regular disruptions to a person's sleep may eventually lead to health problems and delayed healing. It is important for nurses to help a patient to find and create an environment in which a patient feels comfortable enough to sleep the entire night uninterrupted. A nurse can adjust a patient's environment by dimming the lighting, closing the door

to help eliminate noise, and ensuring the patient is warm. One study on patients in intensive care found that earplugs and eye masks resulted in the patients getting more REM time, they were less aroused, and they had an increase in their nocturnal melatonin levels (Hu, Jiang, Zeng, Chen, & Zhang, 2010).

Effects of Stress

Stress and sleep act as counterparts because stress increases arousal and sleep decreases stress (Hasson & Gustavsson, 2010). Beyond the environment and certain substances, high stress levels have also been identified in the literature as being a factor that is capable of inhibiting a person's quality of sleep (Hurst, 2008; UMMC, 2010c). People who are stressed or anxious will have troubles sleeping if they are unable to control thoughts, images, and emotions that are worrying them (Saddichha, 2010). When a person is stressed, he or she tends to find it hard to settle down and relax to go to sleep. The cause may be that during times of high stress the human body releases more cortisol, causing us to become more aroused and less able to relax (NHLBI, 2011). Some may find they cannot sleep because they are thinking about things they have done or need to do. If a patient is experiencing difficulties sleeping due to stress, a nurse should assist a patient to identify ways in which the patient can cope with stress, such as exercising regularly, reassessing the patient's responsibility, or participating in relaxation techniques. Some have found taking time to address their worries before bed helps them deal with their stress so that they can sleep (UMMC, 2010c). Before going to bed, some people find it helpful to write down their stressors and make a plan to deal with them or instead to focus on the accomplishments of the day.

Effects of Medications

A few common medications that have been identified to cause issues with sleep are β-blockers, α-blockers, antidepressants, and nicotine (Harvard University, 2010). Other medications that are known to affect sleep are antiarrhythmic medications, steroids, prednisone, some asthma medications, diuretics, and thyroid medications (Harvard University, 2010). Medications that have amphetamine and antidepressants are known to inhibit a person's REM sleep (Cartwright et al., 2012). Because some of the patient's medications may contain substances that disrupt sleep, it is important that a nurse teaches the patient which medications may impact sleep patterns and about the importance of scheduling these medications to be taken at a time that they will not interfere with sleep. For example, for patients taking diuretics, it is better if they take them earlier in the day so that they are not awakened by the need to urinate. Some medications used to help a person sleep are generally referred to as sleeping pills (Box 31.7). Most over-the-counter (OTC) sleeping pills contain antihistamines that are capable of making a person feel sleepy but can result in a hangover effect the next morning (Health Canada, *Seniors, Sleeping Pills and Tranquillizers* [Brochure], 2011). In general,

BOX 31.7 Downside of Sleeping Pills, Over-the-Counter Sleep Aids, and Medications

- Side effects: mild to severe feeling of being hung over, drowsy, and confused
- Drug tolerance: over a period of time, may need to take more pills to help sleep
- Drug dependence: eventually can be unable to sleep without them
- Withdrawal symptoms: Symptoms such as nausea, sweating, and shaking can occur if a person stops taking the medication abruptly.
- Drug interactions: life-threatening interactions with other medications
- Rebound insomnia: Insomnia can become worse if a person stops taking the pills after using them for a long period of time.
- Untreated disorder: The pills may mask the underlying disorder and prevent proper treatment from occurring.

Adapted from Saddichha, S. (2010). Diagnosis and treatment of chronic insomnia. *Annals of Indian Academy of Neurology, 13*(2), 94–102.

sleep medications are most effective when used sparingly for short-term situations. Sometimes, sleep aids are used at the beginning of treatment for insomnia, especially if the sleep deprivation has been severe. Sleeping pills should be used with caution to avoid dependence and tolerance (Health Canada, *Seniors, Sleeping Pills and Tranquillizers* [Brochure], 2011). It is best to try a range of sleep therapies that do not require medication before resorting to use medication to help with sleep.

Effects of Shift Work

Another factor that is known to affect a person's sleep is work schedule. Many jobs including health-care professionals such as nurses and doctors require their employees to work non-traditional hours that are outside of the regular 9 AM to 5 PM work hours. **Shift work** is the term used to describe non-traditional work hours where a person may work a full shift during evenings, weekends, or nights (Hurst, 2008; Zencirci & Arslan, 2011). Shift work has been known to cause several health issues if a person does not get the recommended amount of sleep in a 24-hour period (NHLBI, 2011). Zencirci and Arslan (2011) conducted a study on 483 nurses who worked shift work and found that most of the participants of the study had difficulties sleeping after they worked night shifts, and they had sleep problems for the past month. Another study found a continuous decline in nurses' quality of sleep beginning from their last semester of nursing education and over the last 3 years into their working life (Hasson & Gustavsson, 2010). The study found that the greatest decline in sleep quality occurred during the time the nurses were transitioning from a student to working in the nursing profession (Hasson & Gustavsson, 2010). The cause is related to our body's **circadian rhythms**, which are physical, mental,

and behavioural changes that follow a roughly 24-hour cycle, responding primarily to light and darkness. Circadian sleep rhythm is our biologic clock that is regulated by our brain and hormones (Tewari et al., 2011). It is believed that our brains receive light inputs from our retina to signal us to wake and the pineal gland secretion of melatonin at night to signal sleep (Tewari et al., 2011). Our daily sleep and wake cycle help to regulate our hormones and physiological processes, and shift work disrupts these patterns and behaviours, leading to an increased risk of developing cardiovascular disorders, metabolic disorders, gastrointestinal disorders, some cancers, and mental disorders (Gamble et al., 2011).

When we make changes to our normal rhythms, our bodies may experience difficulties falling asleep at irregular times. It is important for patients and nurses who follow a shift work schedule to practice healthy sleep hygiene to ensure that they obtain an adequate amount of sleep in a 24-hour period to maintain their health.

Think *Effects of Shift Work*

Nurses on your unit work 12-hour rotating shifts, which are a combination of days and nights. Shifts are regularly scheduled so that nurses never work more than three night or day shifts in a row. The shifts are also scheduled so that nurses have time off before having turnaround from working night shift to working day shift. Some nurses think that they can handle a short turnaround time from nights to day shifts, and some believe that they can handle working more than three nights in a row. One night that you are working, you find out that one of your fellow nurses on shift has worked the last five nights in a row because he picked up two overtime shifts. Do you think that this could be a problem?

The shifts are scheduled this way to help prevent nurses from experiencing the effects of shift work. Our bodies have a circadian rhyme that signals our bodies to want to sleep at night and be awake in the day. When we do not follow the normal pattern of our circadian rhyme, then our bodies can experience alterations in its normal functioning.

Through the eyes of a nurse

I have been working shift work as a registered nurse for the past 7 years. Learning how to sleep to prepare for my clinical shifts was a difficult journey. I tried taking advice that was given to me by my final preceptor back when I was a student, which was to allow myself to sleep in as long as I could after getting off my first night shift. Her advice enables me to stay alert on night shifts until approximately 3 AM, and then I become drowsy. To combat my drowsiness, I go for a break around 3 AM and refuel with food. I now find that I sleep better between night shifts and that I feel better on the second night in a row that I work the night shift.

(personal reflection of J. Cherwinski, nurse, 2012)

Effects of Pain or Discomfort

Health issues or pain may also affect a person's sleep. When a person is in pain, it is hard for him or her to feel relaxed and sleep. Some illnesses that cause pain that can disrupt a person's sleep include arthritis, premenstrual syndrome, heartburn, and acid reflux disorders (UMMC, 2010c). Pain that disrupts sleep may also result from an acute episode such as surgery or an injury. Pain can increase the number of times a person awakes from sleep, breaking the NREM and REM cycles and diminishing the quality of the person's sleep (NHLBI, 2011). If a patient is experiencing sleep disturbances due to pain or discomfort, the nurse can teach the patient and provide interventions to address the factors disrupting the patient's sleep. Some interventions include administering pain medications, repositioning the patient, and teaching relaxation techniques.

Through the eyes of a nurse

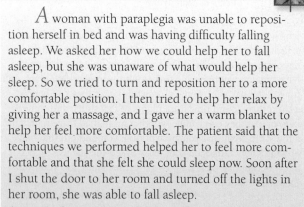

A woman with paraplegia was unable to reposition herself in bed and was having difficulty falling asleep. We asked her how we could help her to fall asleep, but she was unaware of what would help her sleep. So we tried to turn and reposition her to a more comfortable position. I then tried to help her relax by giving her a massage, and I gave her a warm blanket to help her feel more comfortable. The patient said that the techniques we performed helped her to feel more comfortable and that she felt she could sleep now. Soon after I shut the door to her room and turned off the lights in her room, she was able to fall asleep.

(*personal reflection of C. Kostiuk, nurse, January 20, 2012*)

Healthy Sleep Hygiene Practices

Several habits can help a person to obtain a better sleep quality. A nurse can help by creating an environment adequate for the patient's sleep needs. It is also helpful for a nurse to monitor and address the patient needs to improve the sleep pattern of the individual and promote a pattern of sleep that is adequate for performing the normal functioning of daily living activities. Both nurses and their patients can enhance their sleep by forming and practicing healthy sleep hygiene habits (see Box 31.1). Simply, sleep hygiene is the health practices, environmental factors, or routines that may be beneficial to sleep (Jan et al., 2010). Sleep hygiene practices can include the sleep environment, sleep schedule, and bedtime activities (Jan et al., 2010). A few sleep hygiene practices that can promote sleep include developing a sleep routine, exercising regularly, practicing healthy eating patterns, adapting the environment, and using relaxation practices.

Developing a Sleep Routine

One of the habits often cited to enhance sleeping is developing a healthy bedtime routine. A regular healthy bedtime routine can be as simple as consistently going to bed and waking at the same time every day even on days off or when on vacation (Jan et al., 2010). Other techniques that are suggested for creating a healthy sleep routine are reading before bed, having a hot bath, and engaging in relaxation techniques (Harvard University, 2009; NHLBI, 2011). Other tips include avoiding talking on the phone, watching television, using computers, exercising, eating a big snack, or smoking right before bedtime because they can disrupt a person's sleep (Saddichha, 2010). The purpose of developing a healthy bedtime routine is to create a signal that will tell the body to relax in preparation for sleep and when to awake (NHLBI, 2011). Nurses can work with patients to find daily routines to promote sleep that fit their preferences and lifestyles. For instance, a patient may develop a healthy sleep routine that consists of first changing into sleep attire, brushing the teeth, followed by reading a magazine in bed until the patient falls asleep.

Healthy Eating Patterns

Developing healthy eating patterns can promote a healthy sleep patterns. For instance, it is recommended that people avoid eating heavy meals before bedtime in order to enhance their quality of sleep (NHLBI, 2011). It is believed that foods that are of plant origin have a positive effect on a person's sleep duration, such foods as vegetables, fruits, milk, starchy foods, readymade cereals, and olive oil (Moreira et al., 2010). Conversely, foods that are high in fat and sugar have a negative effect on a person's sleep duration such as fast food, sugar sweetened beverages, and pastry (Moreira et al., 2010). Some foods that contain tryptophan can help promote sleep (Rainbow Rehabilitation Centers, 2008; UMMC, 2010c). Foods that are heavy or spicy should be avoided before bedtime because they can inhibit sleep (UMMC, 2010c).

People should also avoid drinking too many fluids before bed because it can cause waking frequently to urinate (NHLBI, 2011). An appropriate bedtime snack would be a glass of milk or a bowl of cereal.

Forming healthy eating patterns also involves being mindful of how we eat throughout the day. A study conducted on nurses revealed that regular breakfast eaters had lower stress levels, experienced less cognitive failures, and had fewer accidents at work (Chaplin & Smith, 2011). On the other hand, people who did not eat regular breakfasts and people who snacked on crisps, chocolate, and biscuits had higher stress, increased cognitive failures, and increased injuries outside of work (Chaplin & Smith, 2011). Literature also suggest that people should avoid ingesting foods that are high in caffeine because they can give you a sudden rush of energy but then soon make you feel drowsy again (NHLBI, 2011). Breakfast cereal and toast have been found to increase a person's alertness (Chaplin & Smith, 2011). To avoid drowsiness after meals, a person may want to eat light meals that are not high in caffeine or sugar, such as soups, vegetable plates, or salads. The Canadian Centre for Occupational Health and Safety (2012) recommended workers avoid eating candy bars and drinking pop for quick energy because the energy dissipates quickly, and instead, they suggest eating crackers with cheese or nuts because both of which provide some protein for longer energy. Nurses can teach patients about healthy eating practices that can enhance patients' sleep.

Adapting the Environment

Environmental factors can also affect the quantity and quality of sleep. Some patients may need to alter to their sleep environment in order to improve their sleep; for example, choosing or creating a dark cozy environment, away from noise (Harvard University, 2009; NHLBI, 2011). In order to make a sleep environment conducive to sleep, persons can consider dark blinds to block out light, making their beds comfortable with a good mattress, and wearing eye covers to block out light. Another intervention that a person can do is to generate white noise, which is sound that will block out noise that will hinder the sleep (Jan et al., 2010). A nurse can suggest that the patient having trouble sleeping in the hospital due to noise use earplugs or create white noise with a fan to help the patient sleep. One way that a nurse can make a person's bed more comfortable is to get the patient a warm blanket or an extra pillow. Some behaviors that a person should avoid in the bedroom because it cause disruption to a person's ability to sleep are watching television, using computers, smoking, or watching the clock (Saddichha, 2010). Shift workers that need to sleep in the day, such as nurses, may find altering their sleep environment particularly important to promote their sleep. Conversely, to battle unwanted sleepiness, a nurse or patient can also adjust the environment by opening up blinds, turning on lights, and performing activities to promote wakefulness. Adjusting the environment assists in balancing a person's sleep and activity so that they occur during the appropriate times.

Using Relaxation Practices

It is a good habit for people to practice techniques that relax their mind because it can help them to feel content and at peace and better prepared for sleep. One type of relaxation practice is meditation. Meditative practices are believed to integrate the brain functions and regulate different physiological mechanisms to result in a state of mental and physical well-being (Nagendra et al., 2012). Meditation causes the body to experience regulatory changes at various behavioural levels that favor sleep (Nagendra et al., 2012), which makes people feel rested. Relaxation techniques can help to reduce arousal, such as imagery training to stop intrusive thoughts and racing mind (Saddichha, 2010). Also helpful to relaxation are breathing techniques, such as having a person breathe in and out slowly (Saddichha, 2010).

A few techniques that are helpful to promote sleep include relaxation stretches, imagery, cognitive therapy, and deep breathing ("Overcoming Insomnia," 2011). Progressive relaxation is a technique that requires a person to listen to relaxing audio sounds (UMMC, 2013), including the sounds of the ocean or rain. Some people find spiritual practices such as meditation, yoga, mantra, and prayer very calming and relaxing (Merkur, 2012). A nurse should work to uncover any mind and spiritual practices that a patient may already use or may develop to use as a healthy sleep hygiene practice. It may be beneficial for patients to try out different relaxation practices to find the ones that work best for them.

Exercising Regularly

Developing a regular exercise routine has many benefits for wellness and is identified as a support to healthy sleep hygiene. Regular daily exercise of 30 to 60 minutes is believed to improve a person's quality of sleep (Harvard University, 2009; UMMC, 2010c). Men and women who exercised regularly sleep better at nighttime (Hurst, 2008; NHLBI, 2011). However, when strenuous activities are done within 3 hours of bedtime, it can actually stimulate the person to become more awake (NHLBI, 2011). It is recommended that a person schedule more strenuous exercise for earlier in the day to promote improved daytime energy (NHLBI, 2011). Shift workers may want to schedule exercise during their night shifts because exercise is known to give you more energy (MOHLTC, 2011a). Nurses can teach patients about the benefits of participating in regular daily physical activity and the importance of avoiding strenuous activity before bed. Together, the nurse and the patient can develop a daily exercise schedule that fits the patient's life, such as going for a 30-minute morning walk every day, having a daily game of golf, or joining a daily 30-minute exercise class. It is important to find an activity that fits the patient's life or he or she may be less likely to commit to the exercise routine.

Activity and Exercise

Activity and exercise are important for all ages, for a range of daily events. Activity can be referred to as a regular process of doing something, such as grocery shopping, sweeping, or gardening (Koeneman, Verheijden, Chinapaw, & Hopman-Rock, 2011). Being active has many benefits for a person's health; for instance, physical activity promotes healthy metabolism, increases a person's spirit, and maintains the function of the heart (MOHLTC, 2011c). In order for people to participate in daily activities, it takes body movements, coordination, and balance. Exercise is more than simply moving to perform daily functions; it is planned, scheduled, and purposeful. People can benefit greatly from exercise, but too much exercise can be harmful.

The following section outlines the benefits for people who participate in adequate activities and exercise, along with some interventions that help patients with mobility challenges.

Normal Movement

The human body has the ability to perform several different movements. An upright bipedal walk is one of the most common motor functions that adults perform (Ivanenko, Wright, George, & Gurfinkel, 2013). Other movements that a human can perform are sitting, standing, lifting, pulling, and pushing (Ghosh, Bagchi, Sen, & Bandyopadhyay, 2011). When people are doing normal movement, they need to practice ergonomics to avoid injuries. **Ergonomics** is the education of maintaining a proper posture and body alignment during normal movements in an effort to avoid injuries (Ghosh et al., 2011). Several factors are important to ergonomics for maintaining a person's safety, health, comfort, and efficiency while they perform actions at work and in everyday life (Ghosh et al., 2011). Some of the factors include body posture, body movements, plus environmental factors such as noise, vibrations, illumination, climate, chemical substances, operation, and work organization (Ghosh et al., 2011). Using improper ergonomics can lead to injuries. Nurses should practice proper ergonomics because their jobs put them at high risk for work injuries with all the standing, walking, pushing, pulling, and turning they have to perform several times a shift. The implementation of ergonomics have had significant effects on increasing production, decreasing medical costs, reducing psychological pressure, increasing job satisfaction, and increasing efficiency (Juibari, Sanagu, & Farrokhi, 2010). It is important that nurses not only teach their patients about ergonomics but that they also practice proper ergonomics in their patient care.

Posture Alignment

The human body can better avoid injury when it keeps a normal posture alignment because an impaired posture leads to fatigue, skeletal asymmetry, and pain as the muscles strain in order to maintain abnormal posture, leading to spasms and pain (Zagyapan, Iyem, Kurkcuoglu, Pelin, & Tekindal, 2012). In a standing position a normal human posture, or stance, is slightly tilted forward so that the centre of the body projects forward of the ankle joint (Mignardot, Olivier, Promayon, & Nougier, 2013). In other words, a stable posture standing includes a person's head over the shoulders, shoulders in line with the hips, hips in line above the knees, and the knees in line with the ankles (Fig. 31.1). The actions of twisting, bending, and overreaching force a person into a non-neutral position that can increase the overall discomfort and pain in a person's back, neck, and shoulders (Ghosh et al., 2010). The basis of a human posture during sitting or standing is the **postural tone** of the skeletal muscles (Ivanenko et al., 2013). Postural tone is known as a person's unconscious, low-scale, long-lasting muscle tension that is spread over the body alignment in a particular pattern (Ivanenko et al., 2013). Certain diseases can lead to abnormal postures, such as scoliosis, cerebral palsy, and Parkinson. Obesity, pregnancy, atrophy, and fractures can also alter a person's posture. Maintaining a static posture, such as sitting or standing for a long period of time, increases

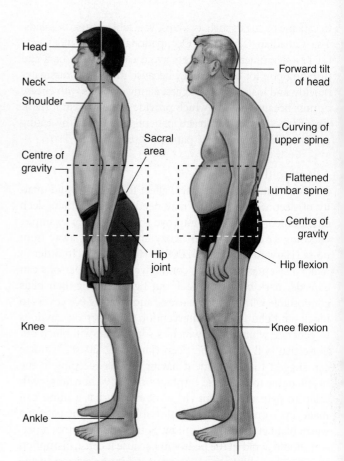

Figure 31.1 Body alignment and centre of gravity.

the demand on the musculoskeletal system's muscles, ligaments, and other soft tissues (Ghosh et al., 2010). Overtime, a static posture can cause discomfort in the back, neck, and shoulders (Ghosh et al., 2010). Prolonged sitting can cause compression of the discs in the spine because sitting alters the normal curvature of the spine, which puts pressure on these discs (Ghosh et al., 2010). People need to realize the importance of the body's posture during motion to better keep the body in balance and help prevent injuries (Zeng & Zhao, 2011). Nurses need to remember to keep a proper body alignment during movement and at their work stations to prevent injuries. Additionally, a nurse should assist a patient to set up the environment so the patient can maintain a proper body alignment and avoid injury.

Joint Mobility

Another important aspect to maintaining health is keeping the joint flexible and functioning through its full and fluid range of motion (Fig. 31.2). **Range of motion (ROM)** refers to moving a joint within its normal full range (Arthritis Consumer Experts, 2011). Two types of ROM activities exist to help maintain joint mobility, which are active range of motion and passive range of motion. **Active range of motion** occurs when a person performs the ROM activities on his or her own (Thomson Reuters, 2011a). **Passive range of motion** takes place with the help of another person, who

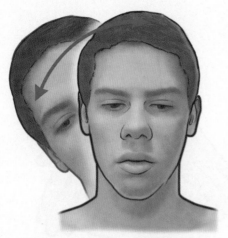

Neck and cervical spine: lateral flexion.

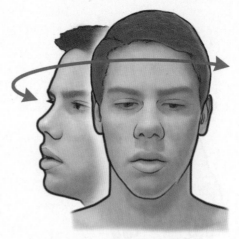

Neck and cervical spine: rotation.

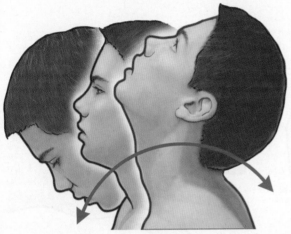

Neck and cervical spine: flexion, extension, and hyperextension.

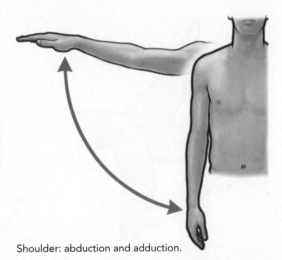

Shoulder: abduction and adduction.

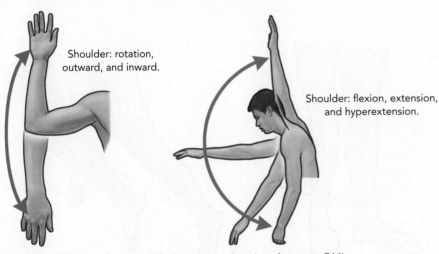

Shoulder: rotation, outward, and inward.

Shoulder: flexion, extension, and hyperextension.

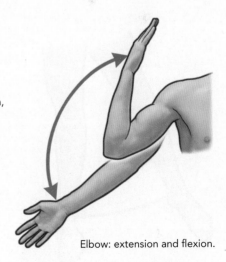

Elbow: extension and flexion.

Figure 31.2 Range-of-motion (ROM) exercises. *(continued on page 764)*

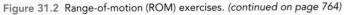

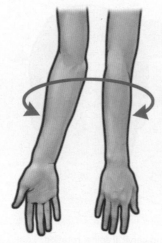

Forearm: supination and pronation.

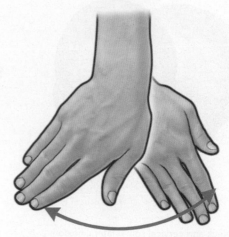

Wrist: ulnar flexion (adduction) and radial flexion (abduction).

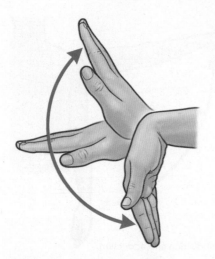

Wrist: flexion, extension, and hyperextension.

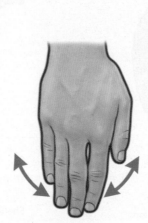

Fingers: adduction and abduction.

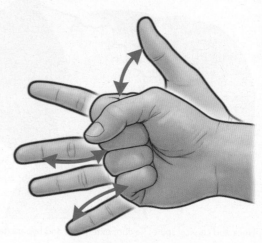

Fingers: flexion and extension.

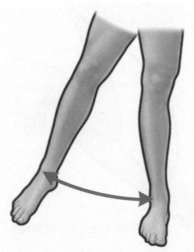

Hip: adduction and abduction.

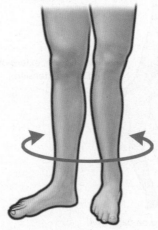

Hip: rotation, outward, and inward.

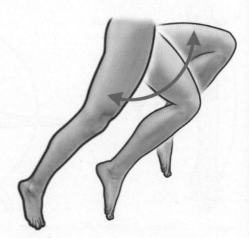

Hip: flexion, extension, and hyperextension.

Figure 31.2 *(continued)*

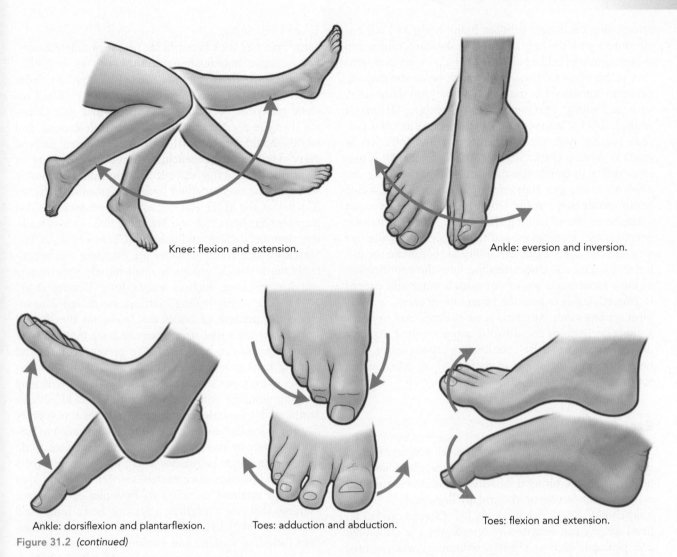

Knee: flexion and extension.

Ankle: eversion and inversion.

Ankle: dorsiflexion and plantarflexion.

Toes: adduction and abduction.

Toes: flexion and extension.

Figure 31.2 *(continued)*

performs the joint's movement while the patient is in a prone or neutral and relaxed state, until the point of slight resistance is felt in the limb (Thomson Reuters, 2011a). This might be done by a nurse, masseuse, physical therapist, chiropractor, or other practitioner. Performing ROM activities daily will support continued independence and well-being, plus it can enhance the performance of everyday activities. It is imperative that a nurse or patient performs ROM activities that fit the patient's situation to avoid injury. Engaging in activities that promote ROM can help keep blood and oxygen flowing to tissues and joints, maintaining flexibility and avoiding stiffening or immobility (Thomson Reuters, 2011a). Immobility can lead to fluid stasis and shortening of the muscles resulting in limited movement of the joint that causes pain. A person's joint flexibility may decrease with age, injury, and certain diseases that affect the musculoskeletal system.

Balance

In order for people to perform actions such as sitting or walking, they need to be able to balance. A human being's balance is controlled by the human vestibular system, which has a structure that simultaneously and accurately detects variables from our senses, which are then interpreted by the central and peripheral neural systems (Zeng & Zhao, 2011). Humans are able to identify their positions using their eyes, ears, the vestibular system, joints, and skin (Zeng & Zhao, 2011). Balance is regulated by the continuously adjusting the body's center of pressure and the body's center of mass (Mignardot et al., 2013). Adjustments in a person's balance are made accordingly using the feedback mechanism coordinated by the central and peripheral neural systems (Zeng & Zhao, 2011). Alterations to a person's balance can lead to inability to perform daily actions and puts them at risk for falls.

Coordinated Movement

In order to do actions in our daily lives and at work, we have to coordinate movements. It takes coordination to do actions such as grasping, reaching, pointing, upright standing, walking, chewing, and speech production (Zelic, Mottet, & Lagarde, 2012). Coordinating movements requires our joints to participate in multisensory information exchanges between brain, body, and our environment with the help of our sight, hearing, touch, and proprioception (Zelic et al., 2012). If a person's multisensory information exchange is blocked, he or she may experience limitations in the ability to perform daily tasks, such as walking, opening a door, or reaching (Huang & Ahmed, 2011). Walking takes the coordination of a person's posture with the lower extremity and lower trunk joints in motion (Park, Schöner, & Scholz, 2012). A person's ability to coordinate these muscles for walking can affect his or her gait. **Gait** refers to a person's speed, stride width, stride step, stride length, and stride movement when he or she is walking (Hass et al., 2012). Diseases, genetics, age, medication, and trauma are among the factors that can affect a person's ability to coordinate the different movements. Understanding how the coordination of these movements works can assist a nurse and patient to plan strategies to help the patient move about and perform actions safely. At times, some patients may need assistance to perform coordinating actions, to use assistive devices to perform these coordinating actions safely, or to help them gain the ability to perform these coordinating actions.

Exercise

Exercise is a subcategory of physical activity that is planned, organized, repetitive, and focused to improve health, whereas physical activity includes unstructured activities that can occur in our daily lives, such as household chores (Koeneman et al., 2011). *Exercise* can be defined as physical activities or sports that are structured and planned, such as jogging, swimming, water sports, ball games, hiking, and dancing (Mak, Ho, Lo, McManus, & Lam, 2011). Participating in physical activity has many benefits such as increased mood and energy levels (MOHLTC, 2011a). Based on excerpts from "Physical Activity of Canadian Adults: Accelerometer Results from the 2007 to 2009 Canadian Health Measures Survey," the results of the Canadian Health Measures Survey (CHMS) indicate that only 5% of adults participate in the recommended 30 minutes of activity a day 5 days a week (Colley et al., 2011). When we exercise, our blood flow increases, and certain hormones that are beneficial to our health are released into our bloodstream. When a person exercises, endorphins within the body are released, promoting a feeling of well-being (MOHLTC, 2011b). Physical activity is also known to lower our blood pressure, blood sugars, and cholesterol levels, as well as it helps prevent diabetes, hypertension, stroke, and heart disease (MOHLTC, 2011c). Exercise is recommended to help prevent osteoarthritis, dementia, depression, and cancer (MOHLTC, 2011c). Activity benefits people who are physically challenged because it prevents as well as controls the secondary conditions and loss of mobility (Rosenberg, Bombardier, Hoffman, & Belza, 2011).

Types of Exercise

Some exercises are a better fit for people of different ages. For example, muscle-strengthening, such as weightlifting programs, are usually not needed for children. Some exercises that are used appropriately with children include basketball, dancing, tag, cycling, and stair climbing (Berry et al., 2012). Older children, adolescents, and adults should try to participate in a planned exercise every day. There are benefits to regularly engaging in planned exercises that include **aerobic exercise**, muscle strengthening exercises, and bone strengthening exercises (Cooney et al., 2011). Aerobic activities are exercises that increase your heart rate and breathing rate, such as walking, running, cycling, and dancing (Cooney et al., 2011). Muscle-strengthening activities are exercises that repetitively work muscle groups to elicit muscle hypertrophy and strengthening, such as weightlifting (Cooney et al., 2011). Bone strengthening exercises are designed to increase the strength of bones that make up the skeletal system. Exercises that strengthen the bone increase peak bone mass and can be beneficial to prevent diseases and enhance bone growth (Bergmann et al., 2011). A few examples of exercises that are associated with strengthening bone are jumping and running (Bergmann et al., 2011). Adults should exercise for at least 30 minutes almost every day of the week (Cooney et al, 2011). People need to participate safely in exercises. Some people may want to do high energy, high endurance exercises, whereas others should do low endurance exercises. Jogging, tennis, spin classes, or rhythmic exercises are examples of endurance exercises that can strengthen a person's heart, lungs, and circulation (MOHLTC, 2011c). Lower endurance exercises including walking and swimming can also promote healthy heart, lungs, and circulation (MOHLTC, 2011c). Older adults may prefer to do lower endurance exercises. Flexibility exercises such as yoga, tai chi, and stretches are also excellent activities to do regularly because they can increase a person's ROM and balance (MOHLTC, 2011c). It is important to tailor the exercise activities to meet a person's individual needs to avoid injury.

Strength-Building Exercise

It is important to build muscle strength, which can be done with weight training, climbing stairs, and push-ups (MOHLTC, 2011c). There are three main types of muscle contractions that can be done during exercise to help strength muscles: isometric, isotonic, and isokinetic. Isometric exercises refer to activities in which a person contracts a muscle, but there is not muscle shortening (Natural Standard, 2012). An example of isometric exercise is holding your body in one position and pushing against the wall with your arms without actually bending a joint or otherwise moving. Isotonic exercises refer to activities in which a person contracts a muscle with muscle shortening (Natural Standard, 2012). Doing bicep curls would be an example of an isotonic exercise. Isokinetic exercises require the person to contract the muscles in combination with shortening the muscles at a constant controlled rate (Natural Standard, 2012). A person is engaging in isokinetic exercises when he or she is using weight machines at the gym. Nurses can work with patients to perform and develop daily activities in which they can strengthen their muscles, increase their flexibility, and enhance their endurance.

Postexercise Recovery

Just as important as teaching about exercise, nurses can teach patients about avoiding overexerting themselves and taking regular periods of rest. Exercise may lead to some muscle soreness initially, but it should go away. For instance, when people engage in high-intensity exercise, they often experience muscle soreness and decreased performance that eventually goes away (Arent, Senso, Golem, & McKeever, 2010). Exercise should not be painful, although there may be a feeling of exertion or burning in the muscle group being used. If a person experiences pain while exercising, he or she should immediately stop. Prolonged postworkout pain may be an indication of strain and overexertion. Resting postexercise is just as important as exercising. It is important for people postexercise to take sufficient rest before their next workout to allow for recovery, stretch to help the muscles recover faster, have a cool-down period versus stopping exercise abruptly, follow a balanced diet, and drink adequate fluid replacement (Lateef, 2010).

One way to pace the level of activity is to monitor the intensity, duration, and frequency of the exercises. **Intensity** refers to the amount of effort that is required to perform the activity (Groeneveldt et al., 2013; Kokkinos, 2012), such as vigorous or light aerobics. The **duration** speaks to how long a person performs an activity (Groeneveldt et al., 2013), which would include monitoring the amount of running time, such as running for 30 minutes or 20 minutes. **Frequency** speaks to the number of times that a person engages in the activity (Groeneveldt et al., 2013) such as running three times a week. A patient should start slow and build up an exercise routine as tolerated to avoid injury.

Benefits of Exercise

People benefit from exercise for several reasons. Regular exercise has a positive impact on cognition and brain function, such as motor skills and motor memory (Roig, Skriver, Lundbye-Jensen, Kiens, & Nielsen, 2012). Exercise training has been shown to be an effective nonpharmacological way of reducing physical difficulties in older people and even the risk of falls (Bocalini, Serra, Rica, & Santos, 2010). Additionally, literature suggested that regular physical activity aids in preventing cardiovascular diseases, preventing some cancers, reducing body weight, increasing mood, preventing diabetes, and increasing a person's life expectancy (McNaughton, Crawford, Ball & Salmon, 2012).

Factors Affecting Body Alignment and Activity

Our bodies have to work against the force of gravity to balance and smooth out the bended parts of our bodies with the ground (Hundozi-Hysenaj, Hysenaj, Hysenaj, & Shalaj, 2012). This phenomenon of opposing active and passive forces occurs within each body part's physiological limits (Hundozi-Hysenaj et al., 2012). If people do not stay within their normal body alignment during activity, then injuries, pain, and muscle spasms can occur (Zagyapan et al., 2012). Some common injuries that can occur if a person does not stay within his or her normal body alignment during activity are muscle sprains, torn tendons, and broken bones. Some people have diseases, injuries, or deformities that result in an unbalanced body alignment, such as osteoporosis, thoracic kyphosis, or lumbar lordosis (Wang et al., 2012). Other diseases that cause issues with posture alignment are stroke, Parkinson disease, cerebral palsy, and spinal cord injury (Fregly, Boninger, & Reinkensmeyer, 2012). When a person has muscular misbalance of spine that alters the posture, such as spina bifida, it affects everyday activities (Hundozi-Hysenaj et al., 2012). Obese patients can have issues with maintaining postural stability during a standing position (Mignardot et al., 2012). Treatment for eliminating the factors affecting the posture alignment depends on and must be tailored to the underlying cause.

Growth and Development

Activity plays a big part in a person's growth and development. The size and shape of a person's skeleton may be influenced by genetics, but it is also affected by the mechanical loading that occurs with physical activity (National Institute of Arthritis and Musculoskeletal and Skin Diseases, 2011). Weight-bearing and intense impact activities create the greatest benefit on a person's growth (National Institute of Arthritis and Musculoskeletal and Skin Diseases, 2011). However, high-impact activities can be harmful to people who are frail. For instance, osteoporosis is a disease in which bone density is decreased, leaving bones vulnerable to fracture (National Institute of Health Osteoporosis and Related Bone Diseases, 2012), and therefore, high-impact activities may be more harmful.

Nutrition

If people are not taking in enough nutrients, it can greatly affect their ability to participate in activities and exercise. For instance, if people exercise too much and are not eating enough, they are at high risk for developing several serious problems that could affect their health, they may lose the ability to remain active, and they may sustain an injury (National Institute of Health Osteoporosis and Related Bone Diseases, 2012). It is important for nurses to understand the modifiable determinants of nutrition that apply to their patients, the physical activity behaviors of their patients, and to take into account the specific life-stage context of their patients because it can assist the nurses in developing appropriate interventions that will promote health and prevent chronic disease (McNaughton et al., 2012). Similarly, it is also imperative that a person's socioeconomic position is taken into account when assessing and planning nutrition and physical activity behaviors (McNaughton et al., 2012), or the interventions may not be successful. Literature recommends eating diets that are high in vegetables and fruits because they have a strong association with a reduced risk of several chronic diseases (Boeing et al., 2012). Nurses can emulate and teach patients about the importance of eating a diet balanced between the food groups. The main food groups are vegetables, fruits, dairy products, meats, and grains (Moore, Singer, Qureshi, Bradlee, & Daniels, 2012). A few ways that a nurse can help promote good nutrition with the patients are to encourage them to eat healthy foods, encourage them to drink enough water, make mealtimes pleasant, offer them choices for meals, and record their food and fluid intake (Burke, 2011).

Personal Values and Attitudes

Like nutrition, motivation plays a vital role in participation of activity and exercise (Teixeira, Carraça, Markland, Silva, & Ryan, 2012). People may be unmotivated to exercise because of low interest, they perceive they lack the competence for the task, or they do not see it as highly important (Teixeira et al., 2012). Some people feel they are too busy to exercise because they are trying to juggle several roles at once, such as working, going to school, and raising families. People may also believe that there are no exercises that they enjoy doing. Some people may not be aware of the effects that not exercising can have on them or even think they are immune to the effects of not exercising. A nurse needs to interview the patient and find out what his or her perceptions are about exercising and health. Once the nurse understands the patient's personal values, he or she can implement interventions to address the underlying issues, such as implementing patient education. It is important for a nurse to work with patients to schedule regular appropriate exercise.

External Factors

There are some external factors to think about with regard to exercise. For instance, exercising in cold air can be hard on the lungs. Inspired air in normal temperature is warmed up to body temperature before entering the lungs by the upper airway's heat exchange system; however, because people breathe from their mouth instead of their nose, this system is compromised during exercise in cold weather (Turmel, Bougault, & Boulet, 2012). People should try to avoid exercising in cold weather or dress appropriately if they are. It is a good idea to have an alternative plan for exercising if the weather is too cold, such as doing a workout tape at home. Con-

versely, exercising in the heat is commonly thought to cause dehydration (Murray & Costa, 2012). Thus, people need to think about the environment when considering what exercise is appropriate. Some things to consider with the environment when exercising are the lighting in the exercise area, the maintenance of the exercise equipment, and access to the exercise building. Whether the exercising environment is the neighborhood, a gym, or the home environment, it needs to be appropriate for the person to stay active (Rosenberg et al., 2011). For instance, a person may not want to exercise outside if he or she does not feel the neighborhood is safe so he or she may want to purchase a gym membership or a treadmill for his or her home to stay active. Nurses need to consider the patient's environment when they are planning exercise regimes.

Physical and Mental Health

Some people may not exercise because they feel that they do not have the energy to exercise. For some people, exercising is hard or painful because of their physical condition. Some of the conditions that are known to affect a person's ability to move are frailty, arthritis, multiple sclerosis, diabetes complications, amputation, or stroke (Rosenberg et al., 2011). Pain and fatigue are two common reasons that people with physical conditions have fluctuations in physical activity patterns (Rosenberg et al., 2011). A nurse should find a time to exercise the patient when the patient has more energy and is not exhausted or someone could get injured. In addition, patients may want to take a pain medication before exercising to stop pain from hindering their physical activities.

Effects of Inactivity/Immobility

Even though the benefits of activity and exercise are known to many, there are still people who are inactive or have limited mobility. Being inactive is a personal choice for some, and they engage in sedentary behaviours. **Sedentary behaviours** are actions that require little physical energy, such as watching television and using a computer (Rutten, Savelberg, Biddle, & Kremers, 2013). When a person is unable to move in his or her own environment or move objects in his or her environment unassisted, it is referred to as having **immobility** (Cowan et al., 2012). People who have impaired mobility can suffer from deconditioning, muscle weakness, and infections (Zomorodi, Topley, & McAnaw, 2012). A person who is immobile is at risk for several health issues, such as pressure sores or ulcers (Best, Desharnais, Boily, Miller, & Camp, 2012). Prolonged immobility is known to cause muscle weakness conversely, respiratory complications, and a risk of thrombosis (Makhabah, Martino, & Ambrosino, 2013). The treatment for patients who have decreased mobility generally includes regular repositioning, skin protectors such as sheep skin sheets, and daily assessments for complications (Mistiaen et al., 2010). In some cases, people may have immobility issues that affect their ability to perform typical self-care activities, called **activities of daily living (ADL)**, which include eating, bathing, grooming, feeding, and toileting activities (Kumar & Jim, 2010). Nurses can help patients with immobility maintain their ADL by providing encouragement, using assistive devices for the patients to perform their own ADL, or performing some of the ADL for the patients if they are unable to. Wheelchairs, walking aids, and prosthetic limbs are a few aids that can assist people with impaired mobility (Cowan et al., 2012).

Body Mechanics for Nurses

Patients with decreased mobility may need assistance moving themselves and objects. When a nurse is moving objects or patients, there are certain movements can help maintain a proper posture or **body alignment**. A proper body alignment requires keeping a centerline of gravity, spinal alignment, and/or keeping a good base of support. To maintain a centerline of gravity and good base, a nurse should have his or her head above his or her shoulders, shoulders above and in line with hips, hips in line and above his or her knees, and knees in line and above his or her feet (see Fig. 31.1). Factors such as lifting a heavy load, having improper body flexion, using improper body rotation, and having an unbalanced weight load can cause a nurse to get injured at work (Tinubu, Mbada, Oyeyemi, & Fabunmi, 2010). When lifting an object, the nurse must adjust to the additional weight by positioning the additional weight so it is moved within its centre of gravity. Similarly, if a nurse is pivoting, then he or she needs to ensure he or she turns, keeping shoulders, hips, and feet in the same direction as he or she moves. Our arm muscles are designed to pull better than they push; nurses and patients should pull objects rather than push objects to avoid injuries.

Nurses are required to perform physically demanding tasks on daily basis, such as turning or repositioning patients. The physical demanding tasks put nurses at risk for injuries by placing strain on their muscles and joints. To avoid injuries, nurses need to use proper assistive devices, movements, and postures of **body mechanics**. Proper body mechanics help to keep the nurse from injury; it also helps to ensure the nurse moves the patient or object safely. A nurse should always ensure that patients keep a proper body posture and use proper body mechanics when they are moving. Nurses can take certain steps when moving patients and objects to keep proper body mechanics (Skill 31.1).

Some of the assistive devices that are available for proper body mechanics are (a) slider sheets to help move patients in bed, (b) ceiling lifts to move patients, (c) beds that rise up to a nurse's core level when moving a patient, and (d) slider boards to move patients. Nurses should ensure they are trained on how to use assistive moving devices properly and when to use the different assistive moving devices to avoid work-related injuries from occurring (ECRI Institute, 2011). Therefore, it is essential that a nurse has the required agency training to use these assistive devices according to the policies and regulations.

Positioning Patients

For patients at rest, a good body alignment may entail placing them in a position in which the movable parts of their body are aligned without any stress on their muscles or skeleton (Kader et al., 2011; Registered Nurses' Association of Ontario, 2007). Nurses need to be aware of the beneficial ways to position a patient's body so that he or she is in proper alignment and is comfortable. Assistive devices can help to position patients in bed so they keep proper body alignment, such as foam wedges (Kader et al., 2011). Foot paddings are also used to help prevent a patient's foot muscles from becoming weak (ECRI Institute, 2011). There are several positions that patient can be placed in to keep proper body alignment, such as the supine position, prone position, side-lying position, and Sims position (Fig. 31.3). A nurse can place a patient in **supine position**, which requires a patient to lie on his or her back (Burke, 2011), with feet in a neural position and arms at the side. When a nurse is positioning a patient on the patient's back, he or she can place a pillow behind the patient's shoulder, head, weaker arm, or hip to promote comfort (Kader, et al., 2011). Another position that can be used is **prone position**, where the patient lies on his or her stomach with arms at the side, and head turned to the side (Burke, 2011). A person can also be placed so that he or she is lying on the right or left hip in a **lateral position** (Burke, 2011). When a patient is on lying on his or her side, a nurse may want to place one or two pillows under the patient's head, leg of the side not being laid on, the weaker shoulder, and back, while keeping the lying side leg straight (Kader et al., 2011). **Sims position** is another position that could be used, where the person is lying in a half prone and half lateral position (Burke, 2011). To help maintain the position of a patient while sitting up in a chair, a nurse may want ensure the individual is seated at the centre of the chair, with arms placed forward onto pillows on the patient's lap or wheelchair table; while in this position, the patient's feet should be placed flat on floor or on wheelchair footrests with knees bent directly above the feet (Kader et al., 2011). Some of the common devices used for positioning patients are pillows, wedges, slings, and trochanter rolls (Kader et al., 2011). Nurses need to always ensure that a patient is safe at rest and during transfer. During patient transfers to a chair, the patient's weaker side should always be supported, and if appropriate, it may be useful to install a bar at the beside of the patient so the patient can use it with the stronger arm to push himself or herself up to the standing position (Kader et al., 2011). To transfer patients, a nurse can use sliding sheets, transfer belts, ceiling lifts, or band slings to help the nurse maintain proper body alignment of himself or herself and the patient to prevent injuries; as well, these help to protect the patients from sheering injuries or other injuries that can occur during the transfer (Best et al., 2012).

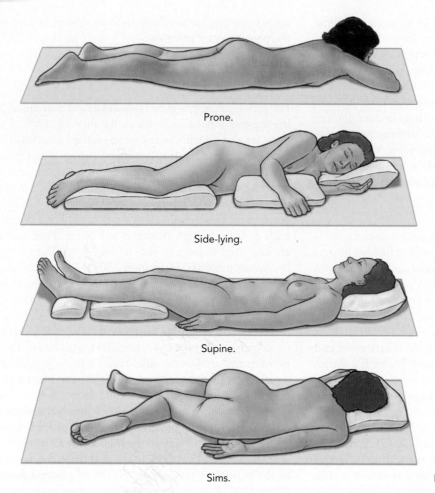

Prone.

Side-lying.

Supine.

Sims.

Figure 31.3 Patient positioning.

Commonly Used Bed Positions

A patient's bed can be moved to different positions in an effort to improve care. For instance, the head of bed and legs of a bed can altered to be higher or lower to enhance patient care. The elevation of the bed's head is often referred to as the angle of the head of the bed and is expressed in degrees of elevation above horizontal (Niël-Weise et al., 2011). Depending on the position of the head and legs of the bed, there are different positions the bed can be in to promote care. Some of the main positions are prone, semi-Fowler, Fowler, dorsal recumbent, lithotomy, and Trendelenburg position (Fig. 31.4). The **dorsal recumbent position** is where the entire bed is flat so that the patient's back is in line with his or her head and in a straight line with the rest of the body (ECRI Institute, 2011). In the **Trendelenburg position**, the bed is flat, but it is tilted so that the patient's head and trunk are lower than the feet (ECRI Institute, 2011). A **lithotomy position** calls for the head of the bed to be flat and the foot of the bed raised so that the patient is in the supine position with legs bent (ECRI Institute, 2011). **Reverse Trendelenburg position** is when the bed is flat but tilted so that the feet are lower than the head (ECRI Institute, 2011). **Semi-Fowler position** is when the head of the bed is at a 30° angle above the rest of the bed

(Burke, 2011). A **Fowler position** is when the head of the bed is in the upright position (Burke, 2011) at a 45° angle above the horizon of the bed. And **high Fowler position** is when the angle of the head of bed is 90° from the rest of the bed (Burke, 2011).

Assisting Patients With Mobility

Some patients may have a decreased ability or a complete loss of ability to move about in their environment. A nurse needs to be able to identify and address a patient's needs for maneuvering in the environment. Several aids and interventions can assist a nurse to help a client safely mobilize.

Ambulating Patients

Functional limitations can lead to the inability to perform particular actions, tasks, and activities such as rolling, getting out of bed, transferring, walking, climbing, bending, lifting, and carrying (Kumar & Jim, 2010). Nurses and caregivers assist patients with these limitations to ambulate. Critically ill patients who have decreased mobility need assistance from the nurse to be turned side to side, pulled up in bed, or transferred from bed to a stretcher for a test

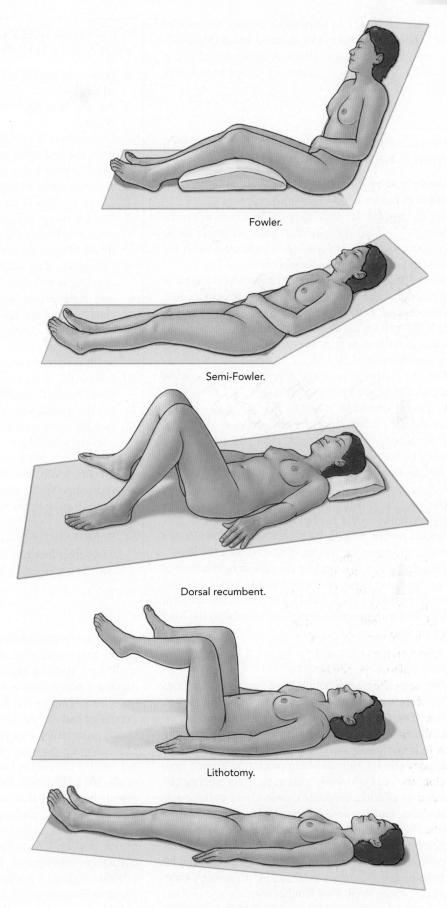

Fowler.

Semi-Fowler.

Dorsal recumbent.

Lithotomy.

Trendelenburg.

Figure 31.4 Bed positioning.

(Zomorodi et al., 2012). In some cases, a nurse will have to prompt residents to perform a sit-to-stand action (Slaughter, Estabrooks, Jones, & Wagg, 2011). A nurse should follow safe guidelines for getting a patient out of bed to ambulate (Nursing Guideline 31.1).

NURSING GUIDELINE 31.1: GETTING PATIENTS FROM BED TO STANDING POSITION

1. Have the patient roll to the side and keep his or her arms in front of him or her.
2. With the arm that is on the opposite side from where the patient is lying, ask the patient to place his or her hands flat against the surface of the bed by in front of his or her trunk area with the arm slightly bent.
3. Have the patient place the other arm in a position that his or her elbow is slightly bent and against the surface of the bed.
4. In one motion, have the patient push the trunk of his or her body up with the elbow and hand that is against the surface of the bed, as he or she carefully swings his or her legs over the side of the bed.
5. Allow the patient to sit at the edge of the bed for a few minutes before attempting to stand.
6. The patient should be sitting so that his or her head is over the ears facing forward, with ears over shoulders, the shoulders in line and over the hips. The patient's legs should be shoulder width apart with the knees in line and above the feet. The feet need to be flat on the ground and pointing forward.
7. Make sure the patient has on footwear with a good grip. Apply a transfer belt if needed.
8. Have the patient move his or her feet up and down on the floor to make sure the feet are in contact with the floor.
9. When the patient is ready, give the patient instructions to place his or her hands on the bed beside him or her, and "on the count of 1, 2, 3, stand." The patient should push off the bed with his or her hands and stand with the head looking up.

Mechanical Aids

Assistive devices exist for training and functional activities with patients who have limited function (Kumar & Jim, 2010). For example, prosthesis such as artificial limbs, orthotic splints, and supportive braces are useful in assisting people to perform activities (Kumar & Jim, 2010). Slings or harness can prevent pain and help protect an injured limb (Kader et al., 2011). Mobility aids such as locomotive devices such as wheelchairs, prone crawlers, and walking aids such as canes, crutches and walkers are also used in to assist people with activities (Kumar & Jim, 2010) (See Skills 31.2). Transferring residents can require the aid of a second healthcare professional to assist or even the use of a mechanical lift or a transfer belt (Slaughter et al., 2011) (Nursing Guideline 31.2). Nurses need to be familiar with the use of these devices and their agency policies for using the devices safely.

NURSING GUIDELINE 31.2: MOVING A PATIENT WITH A LIFT TO A WHEELCHAIR

1. Gather the needed equipment, such as the lift swing and wheelchair.
2. Put the wheelchair close to the bed and put on the brakes.
3. Ensure there is a clear path for transferring the patient.
4. Raise the bed up to you and your coworker's core area, which is your lower trunk area.
5. Tell the patient what you are doing.
6. Check equipment for defects or appropriateness.
7. Use a turning technique to put the lift sling under the patient by having the patient turn on the one side to put the lift sling underneath him or her.
8. Put the lift sling underneath the patient so that half of the sling is rolled up; place the rolled-up end along the side of the patient and the other end leave folded out.
9. Have the patient turn back down and then onto the opposite side. Gently grab the rolled-up end and spread out the sling evenly. The sling should now be underneath the patient and covering both sides of the body.
10. Follow the designated policy and correctly attach the sling's hooks to the lift.
11. Lift the patient with the lift.
12. Steadily move patient in the lift until he or she is directly over the wheelchair.
13. Slowly, one nurse will lower the patient down with the lift while the other nurse guides the patient to right spot in the wheelchair. Ensure the patient is far enough back in the wheelchair to keep a proper body alignment.
14. Unhook the sling and place the patient's feet on the wheelchair footrest. Attach any necessary safety devices, such as a wheelchair belt.

Turn and Reposition

Turning and repositioning are important interventions that nurses may implement with patients who have mobility challenges. **Turning and repositioning** refers the process of moving a person into a new position to prevent complications from lying in one position too long (Lyder & Ayello, 2008; Pattanshetty & Gaude, 2010). When a person is left in one position for long periods of time, he or she is at risk of developing pressure ulcers over the bony prominences because the circulation becomes decreased to that area (Best et al., 2012; Thomson Reuters, 2011b). Some of the bony prominence areas that are prone to developing pressure ulcers if there is a prolonged mechanical load on them are the hips, elbows, shoulders, buttocks, heels, or knees. Lying in one position for too long may also cause problems with circulation, constipation, and breathing (Thomson Reuters, 2011b). Turning a patient regularly also helps to improve his or her breathing (Pattanshetty & Gaude, 2010). A nurse should change the positioning of a patient, such as from lying on the back to lying on the side, once every 2 hours (Burke, 2011; Pattanshetty & Gaude, 2010). The use of positioning cushions, elbow pads, booties, pressure shifting mattresses, and mattresses over surfaces can help prevent pressure ulcers in patients with decreased mobility (Burke, 2011). Some patients may not be able to go into certain positions based on their condition or circumstance; therefore, a nurse must ensure the patient is safe to be in the positions.

For patients who can turn or shift on their own, it is important for the nurse to remind and teach the importance of shifting their weight frequently to prevent pressure ulcers. The use of positioning pillows, rolls, padding, and pressure-shifting mattresses are aids known to reduce complications of immobility (ECRI Institute, 2011).

RESEARCH
TRUNK RELEASE MANEUVER

Study
Placing elderly patients in a high Fowler position is a very common practice in health-care settings because it is known to aid in digestion and breathing. Recently, however, high Fowler is being perceived to cause discomfort and risk of pressure ulcers because of a believed increase pressure magnitude on the sacral and gluteal areas of the body and possible shearing force. The study aimed to evaluate the effect of a low-tech and time-efficient Trunk Release Maneuver (TRM) on the sacral and gluteal pressure, trunk displacement, and the perceived discomfort in older adults. The TRM is a standardized practice in which the patient's trunk is pulled forward and away from the surface of the bed without lifting the backsides with either a positioning sling or a slider sheet. The study used a randomized controlled trial method on a sample of adults living in the community who were 60 years of age and older. There was an intervention group of 59 participants who received the TRM, whereas the control group of 58 participants used the standard high Fowler position. The study's results did not show the intervention had an effect on perceived discomfort; however, the researchers believe this result occurred because pain can be hard to measure. The results showed the TRM intervention was effective for releasing the pressure of the participants in the sacral and gluteal regions. It also showed that the intervention can relieve the contact between the skin and the surface of the support in the trunk area.

Nursing Implications
Treatments for pressure ulcers can cause a significant financial burden on the Canadian health-care system. The populations of people at risk of pressure ulcers are older adults who often have limited mobility and activity tolerance that causes them to be in bed most of the time. These patients do most of their daily activities in bed, such as eating, bathing, socializing, and sleeping in their bed. The TRM may be able to help prevent them for developing pressure ulcers. It is a simple practice for repositioning that can easily be implemented by nurses within the health-care system.

Best, K. L., Desharnais, G., Boily, J., Miller, W. C., & Camp, P. G. (2012). The effect of a trunk release maneuver on Peak Pressure Index, trunk displacement and perceived discomfort in older adults seated in a high Fowler's position: A randomized controlled trial. BMC Geriatrics, 12, 72.

Develop Daily Activities of Exercise

It is clear that nurses should encourage physical activity to promote the health and well-being for their clients. Nurses do this in part by helping develop an activity plan that fits the patients' levels of capacity, activity, and life context. In order to help patients develop daily activities, nurses need to properly assess and identify patient needs. To illustrate, if a patient has a disability that inhibits him or her from jogging, then the nurse needs to find another activity for the person that will provide similar benefits. In addition, a nurse needs to be able to identify and address a patient's lack of mobility. If a patient is unable to move in bed, then a nurse needs to be aware of the techniques to safely move and position a patient while maintaining a proper body alignment for himself or herself and the patient. Several aids and methods can assist a nurse in positioning and moving a patient safely.

Assessing Activity and Rest

It is important for a nurse to assess the patient's activity and rest. Therefore, it is important that a nurse conducts health histories and physical examinations to provide individuals with information and guidance for illness prevention and the maintenance of a healthy lifestyle. One of the ways a nurse can assess a patient's rest is with a sleep diary (Saddichha, 2010) (see Box 31.5). Information could also be gained by asking patients when they go to sleep at night, if they wake at night, when they wake up, if they take daytime naps, and if they are tired in the day. A nurse should also ask about the patients' use of sleep aids and medical history for disorders that put them at a higher risk for sleep disorders (Saddichha, 2010). Another tool that can assist in assessing a patient's sleep is an Epworth Sleepiness Scale (ESS), which is a questionnaire that measures daytime sleepiness (Tewari et al., 2011). The Pittsburgh Sleep Quality Index (PSQI) is another tool to assess a person's quality of sleep that is composed of self-rated questions and questions rated by the bed partner or roommate (Tewari et al., 2011).

To assess a patient's level of activity, a nurse can ask specific question geared toward activities, nutrition, and exercise. For instance, one question to ask a patient is how much time he or she spends on activities and exercise, such as walking, bicycling, gardening, housekeeping, and sports (Buffart et al., 2012). It is also important to ask the patient about the intensity, frequency, and length of time spent doing these activities (Buffart et al., 2012). Knowing if a patient rests between activities is also important to a patient's care. It is important to assess the patient's tolerance of the activities and exercise, he or she engages in (Buffart et al., 2012); you can ask the patient if he or she is fatigued, sore, or energized after exercising. A physical assessment may also help to determine joint mobility, muscle strength, balance, body alignment, coordination, and flexibility. Sociodemographic factors and clinical factors are also important for understanding activity and exercise needs (Buffart et al., 2012). For example, it is important to know if they work; their eating habits, age, and gender; if they have access to a gym; or if they smoke. Furthermore, a nurse will want to assess if the patient has any limitations with his or her mobility or if he or she uses assistive device, such as a cane.

Diagnosing

Once the nurse has gathered information about the patient's activity, rest, sleep, and exercise habits, he or she can develop nursing diagnoses to help direct the patient's plan for care. Some of the North American Nursing Diagnosis Association International (NANDA-I) identified nursing diagnoses that are relevant and applicable to activity and rest include the following:

- Activity Intolerance (specific level)
- Activity Intolerance, risk for
- Activity Planning, ineffective
- Disuse Syndrome, risk for
- Diversional Activity, deficient
- Fatigue
- Insomnia
- Lifestyle, sedentary
- Mobility, impaired bed
- Mobility, impaired wheelchair
- Sleep, readiness for enhanced
- Sleep Deprivation
- Sleep Pattern, disturbed
- Transfer Ability, impaired
- Walking, impaired. (Doenges, Moorhouse, & Murr, 2012, p. 40)

Planning

During the planning stage, it is important for a nurse to involve the patient and other health-care members. If a nurse does not involve the patient in the plan, then the plan may not be successful because it will not be tailored to the patient's personal needs. Goals and interventions should also be made with the patient during the planning stage so that they are appropriate, realistic, and achievable in regard to the patient's sleep, rest, activity, exercise, or mobility. An end result may be to maintain or improve an aspect of the patient's activity and rest. Planning then should include addressing any obstacle that prevents the patient's success and planning interventions that can help reach the patient's goal for rest or activity. For example, to address potential obstacles, a nurse may want to develop an alternative plan that if the patient cannot walk outside, then the patient could go walk on the treadmill. Another example of planning to address obstacles is having a plan that the patient stays in bed and countdown from 10 if the nurse finds the patient having issues falling asleep. Any time a nurse is planning with the patient about the patient's rest and activity, he or she must ensure that the plan does not over exert the patient and is within the patient's limits, or injuries can occur. Remember, it is better to start with smaller steps and slowly increase the goals to improve the patient's performance.

Implementing

Nurses should support and assist the patient as needed in implementing their planned interventions. Implementing the interventions should be done safely and in line with best practice. As the nurse and patient are implementing the plan, they should be observing the effectiveness of the interventions, and adjustments should be made if needed. Regular documentation of the interventions implemented and the methods used is essential. Just as important is the need to document any interventions that were not done as well as a reason. To illustrate the importance, a patient may not participate in range of motion activities because he or she is undergoing a diagnostic test. This is different than if the patient did not participate because he or she is in pain. Documenting the implementation will help to evaluate and reassess the care plan.

Evaluating

A nurse should consider several factors in regard to evaluating a patient's mobility, activity, rest, and exercise. Any observations that the nurse makes during the patient's engagement in daily activities, sleep, rest, exercises, or movements should be documented and included in the evaluation of the patient's care. For instance, it is important for a nurse to evaluate the quality, length, and duration of the patient's sleep. The patient can possibly use a sleep diary to evaluate sleep quality. It should be noted if the patient feels tired or drowsy during the day or need naps. Knowing a patient's sleep quality is important for planning his or her activities. If a patient is sleepy, then you would not want to plan strenuous activities or he or she can be at risk for injury. One of the aspects to determine is how the patient tolerated activity, mobility, or exercise, such as if he or she is fatigued, comfortable, dizzy, stiff, or feeling weak. Additionally, a nurse should determine if the patient suffered any injuries when engaged in these tasks. A nurse can assess for injuries by looking at the skin for any cuts, redness, or swelling. A patient should never be forced to perform activities or do exercises if he or she feels dizzy or fatigued because it can put him or her at risk for injuries. It is important for a nurse and patient to evaluate the outcomes of patient's mobility, rest, activity, and exercise plan; goals; and intervention so that they determine if they need to make alterations to better optimize the patient's health from a holistic standpoint.

Conclusion

People need to ensure they get the recommended amount of sleep and balance their activity and rest. Although sleep is still a phenomenon whose purpose remains debated, it appears to be a regular important part of our lives. It is apparent that there are several effects that sleep has on a person's health and well-being. Several factors exist that can hinder quality of sleep that people should try to eliminate or address. A person can enhance sleep and rest by practicing healthy sleep hygiene techniques. Nurses need to ensure that they promote healthy sleep patterns for their patients. In addition to rest, exercise and activity are important to maintain and promote good health. A lack of mobility or inability to exercise can have effects on the human body and overall health. While moving and exercising, it is important to keep proper body alignment to avoid injuries. If a patient or nurse is moving someone or something, he or she should keep proper body alignment and avoid stretching, twisting, or pulling to prevent injuries and maintain his or

her health. A nurse should be aware of the different positions and aids to help maintain a body alignment. At times, certain patient may have a limited ability to move about in the environment or even completely lose the ability to move about in the environment. If a patient is unable to move in the environment, then a nurse should be able to implement actions to help the patient safely move and evaluate the outcomes to optimize the patient's health. Sleep, rest, activity, exercise, and mobility are important to people's health and well-being.

Mackenna and Mr. Jones worked together to develop a plan to improve his sleep and adjust to his new job that requires shift work. Some of the interventions they developed to improve Mr. Jones's quality of sleep include avoiding caffeine and heavy meals close to bedtime. Also, developing a bedtime routine, having light snacks high in carbohydrates, creating a sleep environment, and relaxing his mind and spirit before bedtime will be helpful to enhance Mr. Jones's sleep. In addition, they developed daily physical activity and exercise plans. It is important that Mackenna works with Mr. Jones to develop a plan that fits his life, schedule, limits, and needs. Mackenna also encouraged Mr. Jones to see his doctor if the problem persists or worsens.

SKILL 31.1 Steps for Implementing Proper Body Mechanics

Steps for Proper Body Mechanics	Description
Assess before taking actions.	Before moving a patient or object, assess and make sure there is a clear safe path to move the object or patient in. Assess a patient's mental, physical, and emotional states before moving him or her. Determine if assistance or assistive devices are needed to move a patient.
Use your large muscles and core muscles for moving, lifting, and transferring.	Ensure you have a good grip on what you are moving; keep your elbows bent by your side and close to your centre trunk. Your hips should be in line with your knees, and your knees should be bent with your legs slightly apart. As you move, use your core stomach and thigh muscles and not your back muscles as you move the object.
Move the object at the correct level.	Move the object by keeping it close to your centre trunk area and keep the normal body alignment. Avoid twisting, stretching, and pulling. Bend at the knees to pick up objects at core level and don't lift with your back. Pivoting should be with your heels or toes, and your knees slightly bent with your face pointing in the same direction that you are moving and the object close to your body. Adjust a bed height to core level, which is around your waist level when dealing with patients in bed.

SKILL 31.2 Mechanical Aids

Cane	A patient's cane should be as high off the ground to meet the patient's crease in the wrist when standing. When a patient uses the cane, he or she should keep his or her elbow slightly bent in the hand that is opposite to the affected side. As the patient walks, the affected leg should move in line with the cane. To begin, the patient should position the cane a slightly ahead and step off the affected leg.
Walker	Make sure the patient has the walker touching the ground when he or she uses it. When a patient uses the walker, he or she should grip the handles with his or her hands and slide the walker ahead of him or her and then step in toward the walker. Patients should not walk all the way into the walker when he or she steps into it.
Crutches	A patient's crutches should reach just below the armpit, 1.5 in. when standing. The patient's elbows should be slightly bent when he or she places hands on the handgrips. When the patient uses the crutches, he or she should place the top of the crutches 1.5 in. below the armpit and held tightly by his or her side using the handgrips. To begin, the patient should slightly lean forward and put the crutches slightly ahead of him or her and move in toward him or her.

Critical Thinking Case Scenarios

▶ Mrs. Hall is a registered nurse on a surgical ward and cares for patients after they have general surgeries. It is important that Mrs. Hall gets enough sleep before her shifts because her job requires critical thinking and constant movement. The night before Mrs. Hall was to do a series of day shifts, her child became ill throughout the night and she ended up only getting 4 hours of sleep. The next day at work, Mrs. Hall noticed that she had difficulties carrying out the medication calculations and remembering the formulas for the calculations.

What are some effects that a lack of sleep can have on memory and thinking? Why is it important to balance activity and rest? What are some safety issues that might result from a lack of adequate sleep with Mrs. Hall? What are some alternative measures that Mrs. Hall could take that would allow her to get adequate sleep and function safely at work?

▶ A young wife is worried because she says her husband stops breathing for short periods at night whenever he sleeps on his back. She says she notices it is worse after he drinks alcohol. Her husband is a heavier man and has been known to be a loud snorer. She wonders what is happening to him at night when he stops breathing. How can you explain what is occurring? What would you advise her and her husband to do and why?

▶ Mr. Lemon is 22 years old, single, and has been experiencing episodes of sleepless nights. Mr. Lemon has recently been diagnosed with diabetes mellitus. The reason for his admission to the hospital is unstable blood sugars. Mr. Lemon has been up all night because of frequent urination. How can the nurse promote a balance between activity and rest for Mr. Lemon? What are some areas the nurse could explore with Mr. Lemon to help achieve this balance?

▶ Mr. Thompson, 53 years of age, has been experiencing minimal sleep at night, is restless, and has a burning sensation on the soles of his feet. Mr. Thompson has tried several remedies including medications to help him sleep. Mr. Thompson has also been taking medications for a recent cold and nasal congestion. He reads or watches TV in bed hoping that it will help him relax and fall asleep. Mr. Thompson enjoys a glass or two of wine before bed and often will drink a cup of tea hoping that the warmth will relax and promote a restful night. What contributing factors may be preventing Mr. Thompson from getting a good night's sleep?

Multiple-Choice Questions

1. A nurse is packing his meal for his night shift and contemplates what to choose to help him stay awake for his entire night shift. What foods and beverages could he choose to enhance alertness?
   a. Deep fried chicken wings and dip
   b. Leftover steak and mashed potatoes
   c. Fresh vegetables and dip
   d. Double chocolate chip muffins

2. Which of the following is a psychological symptom associated with poor sleep?
   a. Moodiness
   b. Happiness
   c. Loneliness
   d. Terror

3. A nursing student is having difficulty sleeping at night. Which of the following would be an example of a poor sleep hygiene practice?
   a. Going to bed and waking at the same time every day
   b. Choosing to not watching a scary movie before bed
   c. Practicing mantra
   d. Eating pizza during late night study sessions.

4. If young man is using cocaine, how can it affect his sleep?
   a. He may experience insomnia.
   b. He may experience daytime drowsiness.
   c. There will likely be no effect on his sleep.
   d. He may develop narcolepsy.

5. If a nurse is trying to avoid ingesting substances that contain caffeine on his night shift, which of the following should he have?
   a. Chai tea
   b. Milk
   c. Soft drink
   d. Energy bars

6. A nurse performing ROM exercises for a patient with immobility knows to perform the exercises until:
   a. Maximum resistance of the joint is felt.
   b. Slight resistance of the joint is felt.
   c. The patient yells to stop.
   d. The patient states he is experiencing pain.

7. Mrs. Henry is an 84-year-old with a recent admission to the hospital for shortness of breath. She is wondering why she is experiencing mild muscle and joint stiffness in her legs prior to discharge. Mrs. Henry has been on bed rest for a large portion of her stay in the hospital until all diagnostic test results were negative. Your best answer for this response would be:
   a. Immobility can lead to fluid buildup, resulting in limited movement of the joint.
   b. Mrs. Henry may have a blood clot in her legs.
   c. Mrs. Henry is 84 years of age, and she is entitled to rest.
   d. Immobility causes a decrease in the amount of synovial fluid in joints.

8. With restless leg syndrome, patients often experience unusual sensations in their feet and legs that prevent them from achieving adequate and quality sleep. Identify which of the following is an intervention to assist in promoting a restful sleep with patients experiencing restless leg syndrome.
   a. Drinking caffeine before bed
   b. Acupuncture therapy

c. Stress reduction
d. Cold baths

9. Pearl is a 24-year-old teacher assigned to teach a new grade for the academic school year. While shopping for new school clothes, Pearl slipped and fell. She now has a wound on her arm, for which she comes in daily to get dressed. While in the emergency department, she reports feeling tired and stressed because she has new responsibilities as a teacher and has been experiencing difficulties sleeping at night and staying awake during the day. She wants to do well in her teaching position but feels anxious and is worried that things will not work out this year. Identify which of the following is a nursing intervention to help Pearl with a healthy sleeping pattern.
   a. Ask her how much television she watches.
   b. Tell Pearl to try to lie in bed and think about her day before sleeping.
   c. Encourage Pearl to keep a sleep diary which will track the hours slept, amount of time awake at night, exercise throughout the day, and types of beverage intake.
   d. Tell her to eat a heavy meal before bed so that she feels sleepy.

10. What are the three types of muscle contractions that can strengthen muscles?
   a. Isometric, tonic, endurance
   b. Isotonic, velocity, endurance
   c. Isokinestic, frequency, isotonic
   d. Isokinetic, isotonic, and isometric

11. An example of an isokinetic activity is:
   a. Running
   b. Walking
   c. Using weight machines
   d. Swimming

12. The benefits of a regular exercise plan includes the following, except:
   a. Increased muscle tone
   b. Enhanced general well-being
   c. Decreased circulation
   d. Decreased muscle building

13. While performing passive ROM exercises with an individual, the nurse needs to remember to:
   a. Exercise the extremity to the point of pain and then stop.
   b. Support the extremity when the client expresses signs or symptoms of discomfort.
   c. Exercise the extremity to the point where resistance is felt.
   d. Massage the area where pain is felt on the extremity.

Suggested Lab Activities

Practice Relaxation Training of Deep Breathing

1. Sit in a cross-legged position with your hands gently folded on your lap.
2. Maintain a straight sitting posture.
3. Close your eyes and concentrate on your breathing.
4. Take a deep breath in through your nose and hold it for 2 seconds.
5. After holding your deep breath in for 2 seconds, slowly release your breath through your mouth.
6. Repeat this process 10 times.

Practice Guided Imagery

● Have one person lying on a mat in a comfortable position with his or her eyes closed while another person reads the following scene. The person who is on the mat should feel relaxed and sleepy while and after the scene is read.

● Scene: Imagine yourself on warm summer day walking along the ocean shoreline with not another person in sight. A gentle warm breeze is blowing through your hair and making small waves splashing along the ocean shoreline. As you walk along the peaceful shoreline, you feel the soft sand between your toes. You stop to notice that ocean water is a beautiful fresh turquoise blue and you decide to take a deep breath in, and you smell the fresh smell of the ocean air. While you are standing there breathing in the fresh air, you hear above the light breeze the sounds of birds singing in the air. You look to the sky and notice two birds flying gracefully above you so you decide to lie down in the soft white sand and take in the beauty of the moment. As you are lying in the soft white sand, you feel the warm comforting sun against your skin as if it is a soft warm blanket. You feel so comfortable and relaxed you decide to close your eyes and take a rest in the serenity of the scenery.

Develop a Bedtime Routine

● Identify your typical pattern before bedtime. Write down what you do before retiring to bed in the form of a list. Look at the list and see if you can identify any healthy and unhealthy sleep habits in your routine. If you have unhealthy sleep habits, think of healthy sleep hygiene practices that you can do instead. Now, replace your unhealthy habits with the new healthy sleep habits in the list. If you could not identify any unhealthy sleep habits and had only healthy sleep habits, see if there are other healthy sleep hygiene practices that you want to change or add. Once you have adapted your list, you should have a new bedtime routine that you could implement to enhance your sleep.

Practice Range of Motion

● With another person acting as a patient, practice performing the ROM movements as illustrated in Figure 31.1, once as active ROM and once as passive ROM. Be sure to support the joints for passive ROM, and give appropriate instructions and support for active ROM.

Practice Repositioning in Bed

● With another person acting as a patient who is unable to turn on his or her own, practice repositioning a person in the different positions, such as a prone, semi-Fowler, Fowler, side-lying, dorsal, dorsal recumbent, Sims position, lithotomy, knee-chest, and Trendelenburg. Discuss how the "patient" felt in the positions, the benefits of the positions, and the difficulties moving the patient into these positions. Discuss the steps for the nurse and the patient so that they both keep proper body mechanics during the process of turning and repositioning.

REFERENCES AND SUGGESTING READINGS

Adegunsoye, A., & Ramachandran, S. (2012). Etiopathogenetic mechanisms of pulmonary hypertension in sleep-related breathing disorders. *Pulmonary Medicine.* Advance online publication. doi:10.1155/2012/273591

Ajayi, S., Kinagi, R., & Haslett, E. (2012). Obstetric management of a patient with narcolepsy and cataplexy: A case report. *Case Reports in Obstetrics Gynecology.* Advance online publication. doi:10.1155/2012/982039

An, H. M., Baek, E. H., Jang, S., Lee, D. K., Kim, M. J., Kim, J. R., . . . Ha, N. J. (2010). Efficacy of lactic acid bacteria (LAB) supplement in management of constipation among nursing home residents. *Nutrition Journal, 9*, 5. doi:10.1186/1475-2891-9-5

Arent, S. M., Senso, M., Golem, D. L., & McKeever, K. H. (2010). The effects of theaflavin-enriched black tea extract on muscle soreness, oxidative stress, inflammation, and endocrine responses to acute anaerobic interval training: A randomized, double-blind, crossover study. *Journal of International Society of Sports Nutrition, 7*, 11. doi:10.1186/1550-2783-7-11

Arthritis Consumer Experts. (2011, June). Exercise and good nutrition: Essentials for a complete arthritis treatment plan. *JointHealth Monthly*, 1–4. Retrieved from http://jointhealth.org/pdfs/JointHealth-monthly-2011-June.pdf

Bergmann, P., Body, J., Boonen, S., Boutsen, Y., Devogelaer, J., Goemaere, S., . . . Rozenberg, S. (2011). Loading and skeletal development and maintenance. *Journal of Osteoporosis.* doi:10.4061/2011/786752

Berry, D., McMurray, R., Schwartz, T., Skelly, A., Sanchez, M., Neal, M., & Hall, G. (2012). Rationale, design, methodology and sample characteristics for the family partners for health study: A cluster randomized controlled study. *BMC Public Health, 12*(250). doi:10.1186/1471-2458-12-250

Best, K. L., Desharnais, G., Boily, J., Miller, W. C., & Camp, P. G. (2012). The effect of a trunk release maneuver on Peak Pressure Index, trunk displacement and perceived discomfort in older adults seated in a high Fowler's position: A randomized controlled trial. *BMC Geriatrics, 12*, 72.

Bocalini, D. S., Serra, A. J., Rica, R. L., & Santos, L. D. (2010). Repercussions of training and detraining by water-based exercise on functional fitness and quality of life: A short-term follow-up in healthy older women. *Clinics (Sao Paulo), 65*(12), 1305–1309.

Boeing, H., Bechthold, A., Bub, A., Ellinger, S., Haller, D., Kroke, A., . . . Watzl, B. (2012). Critical review: Vegetables and fruit in the prevention of chronic diseases. *European Journal of Nutrition, 51*(6), 637–663.

Buffart, L. M., Thong, M. S., Schep, G., Chinapaw, M. J., Brug, J., & Poll-Franse, L. V. (2012). Self-reported physical activity: Its correlates and relationship with health-related quality of life in a large cohort of colorectal cancer survivors. *PLoS One, 7*(5). doi:10.1371/journal.pone.0036164

Burke, A. (2011). *Preventing pressure ulcers.* Retrieved from http://www.nursingassistanteducation.com/site/courses/eng/nae-ppu-eng.ph

Campbell, B., Wilborn, C., Bounty, P. L., Taylor, L., Nelson, M., Greenwood, M., . . . Kreider, R. B. (2013). International Society of Sports Nutrition position stand: Energy drinks. *Journal of International Society of Sports Nutrition, 10*(1). doi:10.1186/1550-2783-10-1

Canadian Centre for Occupational Health and Safety. (2012). *Rotational shiftwork.* Retrieved from http://www.ccohs.ca/oshanswers/ergonomics/shiftwrk.html

Canadian Sleep Society. (2007). *Narcolepsy and cataplexy.* Retrieved from http://canadiansleepsociety.com

Canadian Sleep Society. (2008). *Restless leg syndrome (RLS) and periodic limb movement disorder (PLM-D) during sleep.* Retrieved from http://canadiansleepsociety.com/MainSite/pdf/brochure/CSS_Brochure_RLS.pdf

Cartwright, R. D., Dang-Vu, T., Ellenbogen, J. M., & Foulkes, D. (2012). Sleep. *Encyclopædia Britannica.* Retrieved from http://www.britannica.com/EBchecked/topic/548545/sleep

Celis-Morales, C. A., Perez-Bravo, F., Ibañes, L., Salas, C., Bailey, M. E., & Gill, J. M. (2012). Objective vs. self-reported physical activity and sedentary time: Effects of measurement method on relationships with risk biomarkers. *PLoS One, 7*(5), e36345. doi:10.1371/journal.pone.0036345

Chaplin, K., & Smith, A. P. (2011). Breakfast and snacks: Associations with cognitive failures, minor injuries, accidents and stress. *Nutrients, 3*(5), 515–538. doi:10.3390/nu3050515

Colley, R. C., Garriguet, D., Janssen, I., Craig, C. L., Clarke, J., & Tremblay, M. S. (2011). Physical activity of Canadian adults: Accelerometer results from the 2007 to 2009 Canadian health measures survey (Catalogue number 82-003-XWE2011001). *Health Reports, 22*(1). Retrieved from http://www.statcan.gc.ca/pub/82-003-x/2011001/article/11397-eng.htm

Cooney, J., Law, R.-J., Matschke, V., Lemmey, A. B., Moore, J. P., Ahmad, Y., . . . Thom, J. M. (2011). Benefits of exercise in rheumatoid arthritis. *Journal of Aging Research, 2011.* doi:10.4061/2011/681640

Cowan, R. E., Fregly, B. J., Boninger, M. L., Chan, L., Rodgers, M. M., & Reinkensmeyer, D. J. (2012). Recent trends in assistive technology for mobility. *Journal of NeuroEngineering Rehabilitation, 9*, 20. doi:10.1186/1743-0003-9-20

Czisch, M., Wehrle, R., Harsay, H. A., Wetter, T. C., Holsboer, F., Sämann, P. G., & Drummond, S. P. (2012). On the need of objective vigilance monitoring: Effects of sleep loss on target detection and task-negative activity using combined EEG/fMRI. *Frontier Neurology, 3*, 67. doi:10.3389/fneur.2012.00067

Doenges, M. E., Moorhouse, M. F., & Murr, A. C. (2012). *Nurse's pocket guide: Diagnoses, prioritized interventions, and rationales* (12th ed.). Philadelphia, PA: F. A. Davis.

ECRI Institute. (2011, January). Patient positioning [Risk analysis]. *Healthcare Risk Control: Surgery and Anesthesia, 6*, 4.

Epstein, L. H., Roemmich, J. N., Cavanaugh, M. D., & Paluch, R. A. (2011). The motivation to be sedentary predicts weight change when sedentary behaviors are reduced. *International*

Journal of Behavioral Nutrition and Physical Activity, 8, 13. doi:10.1186/1479-5868-8-13

Fregly, B. J., Boninger, M. L., & Reinkensmeyer, D. J. (2012). Personalized neuromusculoskeletal modeling to improve treatment of mobility impairments: A perspective from European research sites. *Journal of NeuroEngineering Rehabilitation, 9*, 18. doi:10.1186/1743-0003-9-18

Gamble, K. L., Motsinger-Reif, A. A., Hida, A., Borsetti, H. M., Servick, S. V., Ciarleglio, C. M., . . . Johnson, C. H. (2011). Shift work in nurses: Contribution of phenotypes and genotypes to adaptation. *PLoS One, 6*(4), e18395. doi:10.1371/journal.pone.0018395

Garcia-Borreguero, D., Stillman, P., Benes, H., Buschmann, H., Chaudhuri, K. R., Gonzales Rodríguez, V. M., . . . Zucconi, M. (2011). Algorithms for the diagnosis and treatment of restless legs syndrome in primary care. *BMC Neurology, 11*, 28. doi:10.1186/1471-2377-11-28

Ghosh, S., Bagchi, A., Sen, D., & Bandyopadhyay, P. (2011). Ergonomics: A bridge between fundamentals and applied research. *Indian Journal Occupational Environment Medicine, 15*(1), 14–17. doi:10.4103/0019-5278.83000

Ghosh, T., Das, B., & Gangopadhyay, S. (2010). Work-related musculoskeletal disorder: An occupational disorder of the goldsmiths in India. *Indian Journal of Community Medicine, 35*(2), 321–325. doi:10.4103/0970-0218.66890

Groeneveldt, L., Mein, G., Garrod, R., Jewell, A., Van-Someren, K., Stephens, R., . . . Yong, K. (2013). A mixed exercise training programme is feasible and safe and may improve quality of life and muscle strength in multiple myeloma survivors. *BMC Cancer, 13*, 31. doi:10.1186/1471-2407-13-31

Harvard University. (2009). *Insomnia: Restoring restful sleep.* Retrieved from http://www.health.harvard.edu/newsweek/insomnia-restoring-restful-sleep.htm

Harvard University. (2010). *Medications that can affect sleep.* Retrieved from https://www.health.harvard.edu/newsletters/Harvard_Womens_Health_Watch/2010/July/medications-that-can-affect-sleep

Hass, C. J., Malczak, P., Nocera, J., Stegemöller, E. L., Wagle Shukala, A., Malaty, I., . . . McFarland, N. (2012). Quantitative normative gait data in a large cohort of ambulatory persons with Parkinson's disease. *PLoS One, 7*(8), e42337. doi:10.1371/journal.pone.0042337

Hasson, D., & Gustavsson, P. (2010). Declining sleep quality among nurses: A population-based four-year longitudinal study on the transition from nursing education to working life. *PLoS One, 5*(12), e14265. doi:10.1371/journal.pone.0014265

Hayward, R. A., Jordan, K. P., & Croft, P. (2012). The relationship of primary health care use with persistence of insomnia: A prospective cohort study. *BMC Family Practice, 13*, 8. doi:10.1186/1471-2296-13-8

Health Canada. (2010). *It's your health: Caffeine.* Retrieved from http://www.hc-sc.gc.ca/fn-an/securit/addit/caf/food-caf-aliments-eng.php (Original work published 2006)

Health Canada. (2011). *Seniors, sleeping pills and tranquillizers* [Brochure]. Retrieved from http://www.phac-aspc.gc.ca/seniors-aines/publications/public/medication/sleep-dormir/pills-somniferes/index-eng.php

Health Canada. (2012). *Canadian alcohol and drug use monitoring survey: Summary of results for 2011.* Retrieved from http://www.hc-sc.gc.ca/hc-ps/drugs-drogues/stat/_2011/summary-sommaire-eng.php#a7

Horsted, F., West, J., & Grainge, M. J. (2012). Risk of venous thromboembolism in patients with cancer: A systematic review and meta-analysis. *PLoS One, 9*(7), e1001275. doi:10.1371/journal.pmed.1001275

Hu, R.-F., Jiang, X.-Y., Zeng, Y.-M., Chen, X.-Y., & Zhang, Y.-H. (2010). Effects of earplugs and eye masks on nocturnal sleep, melatonin and cortisol in a simulated intensive care unit environment. *Critical Care, 14*(2), R66. doi:10.1186/cc8965

Huang, H. J., & Ahmed, A. A. (2011). Tradeoff between stability and maneuverability during whole-body movements. *PLoS One, 6*(7), e21815. doi:10.1371/journal.pone.0021815

Hundozi-Hysenaj, H., Hysenaj, V., Hysenaj, V., & Shalaj, I. (2012). Postural disharmony in relation to the back pain and physiotherapeutic rehabilitation. *Acta Informatica Medica, 20*(2), 103–105. doi:10.5455/aim.2012.20.103-105

Hurst, M. (2008). Who gets any sleep these days? Sleep patterns of Canadians (Catalogue Number 11-008-XWE2008001). *Canadian Social Trends,* (85). Retrieved from http://www.statcan.gc.ca/pub/11-008-x/2008001/article/10553-eng.htm

Ivanenko, Y. P., Wright, W. G., George, R. J., & Gurfinkel, V. S. (2013). Trunk orientation, stability, and quadrupedalism. *Frontier Neurology, 4*, 20. doi:10.3389/fneur.2013.00020

Jain, A. K. (2011). The rational treatment of fractures: Use the evidence with caution. *Indian Journal of Orthopaedics, 45*(2), 101–102. doi:10.4103/0019-5413.77125

Jan, J. E., Asante, K. O., Conry, J. L., Fast, D. K., Bax, M. C., Ipsiroglu, O. S., . . . Wasdell, M. B. (2010). Sleep health issues for children with FASD: Clinical considerations. *International Journal of Pediatrics.* Advance online publication. doi:10.1155/2010/639048

Juibari, L., Sanagu, A., & Farrokhi, N. (2010). The relationship between knowledge of ergonomic science and the occupational health among nursing staff affiliated to Golestan University of Medical Sciences. *Iranian Journal of Nursing and Midwifery Research, 15*(4), 185–189.

Kader, E., Korner-Bitensky, N., Sitcoff, E., Goulamhoussen, L., Laroui, R., Liu, S., . . . Tang, S. (2011). *Positioning.* Retrieved from http://www.strokengine.ca

Khan, F., Amatya, B., & Turner-Stokes, L. (2011). Symptomatic therapy and rehabilitation in primary progressive multiple sclerosis. *Neurology Research International.* Advance online publication. doi:10.1155/2011/740505

Knudsen, R. P., & Culebras, A. (2011). Hypersomnolence. In S. Gilman (Ed.), *MedLink neurology.* San Diego, CA: MedLink Corporation. Retrieved from http://www.medlink.com

Koeneman, M. A., Verheijden, M. W., Chinapaw, M. J., & Hopman-Rock, M. (2011). Determinants of physical activity and exercise in healthy older adults: A systematic review. *International Journal of Behavioral Nutrition and Physical Activity, 8*, 142. doi:10.1186/1479-5868-8-142

Kokkinos, P. (2012). Physical activity, health benefits, and mortality risk. *ISRN Cardiology.* doi:10.5402/2012/718789

Kumar, S. P., & Jim, A. (2010). Physical therapy in palliative care: From symptom control to quality of life: A critical review. *Indian Journal of Palliative Care, 16*(3), 138–146. doi:10.4103/0973-1075.73670

Lateef, F. (2010). Post exercise ice water immersion: Is it a form of active recovery? *Journal of Emergencies, Trauma, and Shock, 3*(3), 302. doi:10.4103/0974-2700.66570

Liberalesso, P. B., D'Andrea, K. F., Cordeiro, M. L., Zeigelboim, B. S., Marques, J. M., & Jurkiewicz, A. L. (2012). Effects of sleep deprivation on central auditory processing. *BMC Neuroscience, 13*, 83. doi:10.1186/1471-2202-13-83

Lindam, A., Jansson, C., Nordensted, H., Pedersen, N. L., & Lagergren, J. (2012). A population-based study of gastroesophageal reflux disease and sleep problems in elderly twins. *PLoS One, 7*(10), e48602. doi:10.1371/journal.pone.0048602

Lo, C. M., & Lee, P. H. (2012). Prevalence and impacts of poor sleep on quality of life and associated factors of good sleepers in a sample of older Chinese adults. *Health and Quality of Life Outcomes, 10*, 72. doi:10.1186/1477-7525-10-72

Lyder, C. H., & Ayello, E. A. (2008). Pressure ulcers: Patient safety issues. In R. G. Hughes (Ed.), *Patient safety and quality: An evidence-based handbook for nurses* (Vol. 1, pp. 267–299). Rockville, MD: Agency for Healthcare Research and Quality. Retrieved from http://www.ncbi.nlm.nih.gov/books/NBK2650/

Mak, K.-K., Ho, S.-Y., Lo, W.-S., McManus, A. M., & Lam, T.-H. (2011). Prevalence of exercise and non-exercise physical activity in Chinese adolescents. *International Journal of Behavioral Nutrition and Physical Activity*, 8, 3. doi:10.1186/1479-5868-8-3

Mak, M. K., Pang, M. Y., & Mok, V. (2012). Gait difficulty, postural instability, and muscle weakness are associated with fear of falling in people with Parkinson's disease. *Parkinson's Disease*. Advance online publication. doi:10.1155/2012/901721

Makhabah, D. N., Martino, F., & Ambrosino, N. (2013). Perioperative physiotherapy. *Multidisciplinary Respiratory Medicine*, 8(1), 4. doi:10.1186/2049-6958-8-4

McNaughton, S. A., Crawford, D., Ball, K., & Salmon, J. (2012). Understanding determinants of nutrition, physical activity and quality of life among older adults: The Wellbeing, Eating and Exercise for a Long Life (WELL) study. *Health Quality of Life Outcomes*, 10, 109. doi:10.1186/1477-7525-10-109

Merkur, D. (2012). Meditation. *Encyclopædia Britannica*. Retrieved from http://www.britannica.com/EBchecked/topic/372609/meditation

Mignardot, J.-B., Olivier, I., Promayon, E., & Nougier, V. (2012). Obesity impact on the attentional cost for controlling posture. *PLoS One*, 5(12), e14387. doi:10.1371/journal.pone.0014387

Mignardot, J.-B., Olivier, I., Promayon, E., & Nougier, V. (2013). Origins of balance disorders during a daily living movement in obese: Can biomechanical factors explain everything? *PLoS One*, 8(4), e60491. doi:10.1371/journal.pone.0060491

Mistiaen, P., Ament, A., Francke, A. L., Achterberg, W., Halfens, R., Huizinga, J., & Post, H. (2010). An economic appraisal of the Australian Medical Sheepskin for the prevention of sacral pressure ulcers from a nursing home perspective. *BioMed Central Health Service Research*, 10, 226. doi:10.1186/1472-6963-10-226

Mitchell, U. H. (2010). Use of near-infrared light to reduce symptoms associated with restless legs syndrome in a woman: A case report. *Journal of Medical Case Reports*, 4, 286. doi:10.1186/1752-1947-4-286

Moore, L. L., Singer, M. R., Qureshi, M. M., Bradlee, M. L., & Daniels, S. R. (2012). Food group intake and micronutrient adequacy in adolescent girls. *Nutrients*, 4(11), 1692–1708. doi:10.3390/nu4111692

Moreira, P., Santos, S., Padrão, P., Cordeiro, T., Bessa, M., Valente, H., . . . Moreira, A. (2010). Food patterns according to sociodemographics, physical activity, sleeping and obesity in Portuguese children. *International Journal of Environmental Research and Public Health*, 7(3), 1121–1138. doi:10.3390/ijerph7031121

Murray, A., & Costa, R. J. (2012). Born to run. Studying the limits of human performance. *BioMed Central*, 10, 76. doi:10.1186/1741-7015-10-76

Nagendra, R. P., Maruthai, N., & Kutty, B. M. (2012). Meditation and its regulatory role on sleep. *Frontiers in Neurology*, 3, 54. doi:10.3389/fneur.2012.00054

National Heart, Lung, and Blood Institute. (2011). *Your guide to healthy sleep*. Retrieved from http://www.nhlbi.nih.gov/health/public/sleep/healthy_sleep.pdf

National Institute of Arthritis and Musculoskeletal and Skin Diseases. (2011). *Childhood exercise leads to sustained improvements in bone mass*. Retrieved from http://www.niams.nih.gov/News_and_Events/Spotlight_on_Research/2011/child_exercise_bone.asp

National Institute of Health Osteoporosis and Related Bone Diseases. (2012). *Exercise and bone health for women: The skeletal risk of overtraining*. Retrieved from http://www.niams.nih.gov/Health_Info/Bone/Bone_Health/Exercise/fitness_bonehealth.asp

National Institute of Neurological Disorders and Stroke. (2007). *Brain basics: Understanding sleep*. Retrieved from http://www.ninds.nih.gov/disorders/brain_basics/understanding_sleep.htm

National Institute of Neurological Disorders and Stroke. (2008). *NINDS hypersomnia information page*. Retrieved from http://www.ninds.nih.gov/disorders/hypersomnia/hypersomnia.htm

National Institute on Drug Abuse. (2011). *Commonly abused drugs chart*. Retrieved from http://www.drugabuse.gov/drugs-abuse/commonly-abused-drugs/commonly-abused-drugs-chart

Natural Standard. (2012). *Isometric muscle training*. Retrieved from http://www.naturalstandard.com/databases/hw/generic-isometricmuscletraining.asp

Niël-Weise, B. S., Gastmeier, P., Kola, A., Vonberg, R. P., Wille, J. C., & Broek, P. J. (2011). An evidence-based recommendation on bed head elevation for mechanically ventilated patients. *Critical Care*, 15(2), R111. doi:10.1186/cc10135

Ontario Ministry of Health and Long-Term Care. (2011a). *Physical activity challenges and solutions*. Retrieved from http://www.mhp.gov.on.ca/en/healthy-ontario/active-living/challenges.asp

Ontario Ministry of Health and Long-Term Care. (2011b). *Why be active?* Retrieved from http://www.mhp.gov.on.ca/en/healthy-ontario/active-living/being-active.asp

Ontario Ministry of Health and Long-Term Care. (2011c). *Why exercise is vital to health*. Retrieved from http://www.mhp.gov.on.ca/en/active-living/exercise.asp

Overcoming Insomnia. (2011, February). *Harvard Mental Health Letter*. Retrieved from http://www.health.harvard.edu/newsletters/Harvard_Mental_Health_Letter/2011/February/overcoming-insomnia

Park, E., Schöner, G., & Scholz, J. P. (2012). Functional synergies underlying control of upright posture during changes in head orientation. *PLoS One*, 7(8), e41583. doi:10.1371/journal.pone.0041583

Pattanshetty, R. B., & Gaude, G. S. (2010). Effect of multimodality chest physiotherapy in prevention of ventilator-associated pneumonia: A randomized clinical trial. *Indian Journal of Critical Care Medicine*, 14(2), 70–76. doi:10.4103/0972-5229.68218

Polanía, R., Paulus, W., & Nitsche, M. (2012). Reorganizing the intrinsic functional architecture of the human primary motor cortex during rest with non-invasive cortical stimulation. *PLOS One*, 7(1), e30971. doi:10.1371/journal.pone.0030971

Proctor, A., & Bianchi, M. T. (2012). Clinical pharmacology in sleep medicine. *ISRN Pharmacology*. Advance online publication. doi:10.5402/2012/914168

Rainbow Rehabilitation Centers. (2008). Sleep disorders & nutrition. *Nutritional News*. Retrieved from http://www.rainbowrehab.com/RainbowVisions/article_downloads/articles/Art-NUT-SleepNutrition.pdf

Ratsch, A., Steadman, K. J., & Bogossian, F. (2010). The pituri story: A review of the historical literature surrounding traditional Australian Aboriginal use of nicotine in Central Australia. *Journal Ethnobiology and Ethnomedicine*, 6, 26. doi:10.1186/1746-4269-6-26

Registered Nurses' Association of Ontario. (2007). *Positioning techniques in long-term care: Self-directed learning package for health care providers*. Toronto, ON: Author.

Roig, M., Skriver, K., Lundbye-Jensen, J., Kiens, B., & Nielsen, J. B. (2012). A single bout of exercise improves motor memory. *PLoS One*, 7(9), e44594. doi:10.1371/journal.pone.0044594

Rosenberg, D. E., Bombardier, C. H., Hoffman, J. M., & Belza, B. (2011). Physical activity among persons aging with mobility disabilities: Shaping a research agenda. *Journal of Aging Research*. Retrieved from http://www.ncbi.nlm.nih.gov/pmc/articles/PMC3124953/

Ruesten, A. V., Weikert, C., Fietze, I., & Boeing, H. (2012). Association of sleep duration with chronic diseases in the European Prospective Investigation into Cancer and Nutrition (EPIC)-Potsdam study. *PLoS One*, 7(1), e30972. doi:10.1371/journal.pone.0030972

Rutten, G. M., Savelberg, H. H., Biddle, S. J., & Kremers, A. S. (2013). Interrupting long periods of sitting: Good STUFF. *International Journal of Behavioral Nutrition and Physical Activity*, 10, 1. doi:10.1186/1479-5868-10-1

Saddichha, S. (2010). Diagnosis and treatment of chronic insomnia. *Annals Indian Academy Neurology, 13*(2), 94–102. doi:10.4103/0972-2327.64628

Sanchez, N. F., Stierman, B., Saab, S., Mahajan, D., Yeung, H., & Francois, A. F. (2012). Physical activity reduces risk for colon polyps in a multiethnic colorectal cancer screening population. *BMC Research Notes, 5,* 312. doi:10.1186/1756-0500-5-312

Seene, T., & Kaasik, P. (2012). Role of exercise therapy in prevention of decline in aging muscle function: Glucocorticoid myopathy and unloading. *Journal of Aging Research.* Advance online publication. doi:10.1155/2012/172492

Sena, P., Attianese, P., Carbone, F., Pellegrino, A., Pinto, A., & Villecco, F. (2012). A fuzzy model to interpret data of drive performances from patients with sleep deprivation. *Computational and Mathematical Methods in Medicine.* Advance online publication. doi:10.1155/2012/868410

Shah, N., Bang, A., & Bhagat, A. (2010). Indian research on sleep disorders. *Indian Journal of Psychiatry, 52*(Suppl. 1), S255–S259. doi:10.4103/0019-5545.69242

Sharma, S., & Kavuru, M. (2010). Sleep and metabolism: An overview. *International Journal of Endocrinology.* Advance online publication. doi:10.1155/2010/270832

Slaughter, S. E., Estabrooks, C. A., Jones, A., & Wagg, A. S. (2011). Mobility of Vulnerable Elders (MOVE): Study protocol to evaluate the implementation and outcomes of a mobility intervention in long-term care facilities. *BioMed Central Geriatrics, 11,* 84. doi:10.1186/1471-2318-11-84

Swartz, A. M., Squires, L., & Strath, S. J. (2011). Energy expenditure of interruptions to sedentary behavior. *International Journal of Behavioral Nutrition and Physical Activity, 8,* 69. doi:10.1186/1479-5868-8-69

Teixeira, P. J., Carraça, E. V., Markland, D., Silva, M. N., & Ryan, R. M. (2012). Exercise, physical activity, and self-determination theory: A systematic review. *International Journal of Behavioral Nutrition and Physical Activity, 9,* 78. doi:10.1186/1479-5868-9-78

Tewari, A., Soliz, J., Billota, F., Garg, S., & Singh, H. (2011). Does our sleep debt affect patients' safety? *Indian Journal of Anaesthesia, 55*(1), 12–17. doi:10.4103/0019-5049.76572

Thomson Reuters. (2011a). *Passive range of motion exercises: What are passive range of motion exercises?* Retrieved from http://www.drugs.com/cg/passive-range-of-motion-exercises.html

Thomson Reuters. (2011b). *How to turn a person in bed.* Retrieved from http://www.drugs.com/cg/how-to-turn-a-person-in-bed.html

Tinubu, B., Mbada, C. E., Oyeyemi, A., & Fabunmi, A. (2010). Work-related musculoskeletal disorders among nurses in Ibadan, South-west Nigeria: a cross-sectional survey. *BMC Musculoskeletal Disorders, 11*(12). doi:10.1186/1471-2474-11-12

Turmel, J., Bougault, V., & Boulet, L.-P. (2012). Seasonal variations of cough reflex sensitivity in elite athletes training in cold air environment. *Cough, 8,* 2. doi:10.1186/1745-9974-8-2

Tzeng, H.-M. (2010). Perspectives of staff nurses of the reasons for and the nature of patient-initiated call lights: An exploratory survey study in four USA hospitals. *BioMed Central Health Services Research, 10,* 52. doi:10.1186/1472-6963-10-52

University of Maryland Medical Center. (2010a). *Sleep disorders center: Normal sleep.* Retrieved from http://www.umm.edu/sleep/normal_sleep.htm

University of Maryland Medical Center. (2010b). *Sleep disorders center: Sleep disorders.* Retrieved from http://www.umm.edu/sleep/sleep_dis_main.htm

University of Maryland Medical Center. (2010c). *Sleep disorders center: Sleep hygiene: Helpful hints to help you sleep.* Retrieved from http://www.umm.edu/sleep/sleep_hyg.htm

University of Maryland Medical Center. (2013). *Sleep Disorders Center: Relaxation techniques.* Retrieved from http://www.umm.edu/sleep/relax_tech.htm

Veasey, S. C. (2012). Piecing together phenotypes of brain injury and dysfunction in obstructive sleep apnea. *Frontier Neurology, 3,* 139. doi:10.3389/fneur.2012.00139

Waidyatilaka, I., Lanerolle, P., Wickremasinghe, R., Atukorala, S., Somasundaram, N., & Silva, A. D. (2013). Sedentary behaviour and physical activity in South Asian women: Time to review current recommendations? *PLoS One, 8*(3), e58328. doi:10.1371/journal.pone.0058328

Wang, H.-J., Giambini, H., Zhang, W.-J., Ye, G.-H., Zhao, C., An, K.-N., . . . Chen, C. (2012). A modified sagittal spine postural classification and its relationship to deformities and spinal mobility in a Chinese osteoporotic population. *PLoS One, 7*(6), e38560. doi:10.1371/journal.pone.0038560

Waterhouse, J., Fukuda, Y., & Morita, T. (2012). Daily rhythms of the sleep-wake cycle. *Journal of Physiological Anthropology, 31*(1), 5. doi:10.1186/1880-6805-31-5

Wijndaele, K., Brage, S., Besson, H., Khaw, K.-T., Sharp, S. J., Luben, R., . . . Ekelund, U. (2011). Television viewing and incident cardiovascular disease: Prospective associations and mediation analysis in the EPIC Norfolk Study. *PLoS One, 6*(5), e20058. doi:10.1371/journal.pone.0020058

Zagyapan, R., Iyem, C., Kurkcuoglu, A., Pelin, C., & Tekindal, M. A. (2012). The relationship between balance, muscles, and anthropomorphic features in young adults. *Anatomy Research International.* Advance online publication. doi:10.1155/2012/146063

Zelic, G., Mottet, D., & Lagarde, J. (2012). Behavioral impact of unisensory and multisensory audio-tactile events: Pros and cons for interlimb coordination in juggling. *PLoS One, 7*(2), e32308. doi:10.1371/journal.pone.0032308

Zencirci, A. D., & Arslan, S. (2011). Morning-evening type and burnout level as factors influencing sleep quality of shift nurses: A questionnaire study. *Croatian Medical Journal, 52*(4), 527–537. Retrieved from http://www.ncbi.nlm.nih.gov/pmc/articles/PMC3160700/?tool=pmcentrez

Zeng, H., & Zhao, Y. (2011). Sensing movement: Microsensors for body motion measurement. *Sensors (Basel), 11*(1), 638–660. doi:10.3390/s110100638

Zhang, J., & Veasey, S. (2013). Making sense of oxidative stress in obstructive sleep apnea: Mediator or distracter? *Frontiers in Neurology, 3,* 179. doi:10.3389/fneur.2012.00179

Zomorodi, M., Topley, D., & McAnaw, M. (2012). Developing a mobility protocol for early mobilization of patients in a surgical/trauma ICU. *Critical Care Research and Practice.* Advance online publication. doi:10.1155/2012/964547

Oxygenation

chapter
32

DEBBIE RICKEARD AND KATHLEEN S. RODGER

Jason, a first-year nursing student, has his first patient assignment in the nursing home. He is excited and nervous to meet his patient. Jason has learned that his patient is Mr. Pipe, a 70-year-old male. Mr. Pipe's medical history includes high blood pressure (hypertension), a 40-year pack per day smoking history, and recent diagnosis of emphysema. The patient has been admitted with fever, chills, and cough with increased clear sputum production. As Jason enters the room, he observes Mr. Pipe sitting up in bed, with the head of the bed elevated to 45°, and breathing very quickly (tachypnea). His respirations appear laboured, and his colour appears pale. Mr. Pipe tries to talk with Jason but is unable to speak in full sentences because he needs to pause to catch his breath. Jason is unsure how to proceed with his patient's assessments at this time.

CHAPTER OBJECTIVES

By the end of this chapter, you will be able to:

1. Describe the structures and functions of the respiratory system.
2. Understand the physiological processes related to gas diffusion, ventilation, and perfusion.
3. Identify common conditions associated with the respiratory system.
4. Understand and describe the effects of hypoxemia.
5. Identify and describe age-related considerations with respiratory function.
6. Identify and describe assessment of the respiratory system and its role in oxygenation.
7. Identify and describe lifestyle and environmental factors associated with respiratory conditions.
8. Identify and explain common health alterations in respiratory function.
9. Identify nursing diagnoses related to oxygenation based on information gathered from patient assessments.
10. Identify common diagnostic tests associated with the respiratory system.
11. Successfully complete the associated chapter case study.

KEY TERMS

Alveoli Microscopic air sacs contained within the lungs where gases are exchanged.

Asthma A chronic inflammatory respiratory disease marked by periodic attacks of wheezing, shortness of breath, a tight feeling in the chest, and a cough that may produce mucous. It is caused by an allergic reaction, certain drugs or irritants, exercise, or emotional stress.

Atelectasis A collapse of some or all of the alveoli in the lungs. This is often related to a disease process or hypo-inflation of lung tissue.

Atrioventricular (AV) Node Part of the electrical system in the heart that transmits electrical impulses located between the right atrium and right ventricle.

Autoregulation The continual adjustment or self-regulation of a biochemical or physiological system to maintain a stable state.

Bradypnea Respirations that are a slow rate. In an adult patient, bradypnea is a respiratory rate less than 12 breaths/min.

Bronchoconstriction Narrowing of the bronchial airways.

Bronchodilators Medications prescribed to help open the bronchial tubes (airways) of the lungs, allowing more air to flow through them.

Bronchospasm Intermittent narrowing or closure of bronchial airways often triggered by exposure to allergens or in acute asthma attacks.

Carbon Dioxide (CO_2) A colourless gas, heavier than air, that is eliminated during expiration as a part of the respiratory cycle. If CO_2 accumulates in the body, the pH of the blood decreases.

Cardiac Cycle The sequence of events beginning with the depolarization of the electrical pathway in the heart, resulting in contraction of the myocardium and the ejection of blood through the ventricles.

Chronic Bronchitis Inflammation of the mucous membrane of the bronchial tree. It is characterized by hypertrophy and hyperplasia of seromucous glands and goblet cells that line the bronchi which results in a productive cough.

Chronic Obstructive Pulmonary Disease A condition characterized by progressive, debilitative pulmonary symptoms involving increased resistance to air movement, prolongation of the expiratory phase of respiration, and loss of elasticity of the lung tissue.

Cough A sudden, noisy expulsion of air from the lungs, with or without expectoration.

Crackles   An adventitious lung sound heard on auscultation of the chest, produced by air passing over retained airway secretions or the sudden opening of collapsed airways.

Diastole   Relaxation phase of the myocardium during the cardiac cycle that allows for filling of the ventricular chambers prior to the onset of cardiac muscle contraction.

Diffusion   The tendency of molecules of a substance (gas, liquid, or solid) to move from a region of high concentration to one of lower concentration.

Dyspnea   Difficulty breathing or shortness of breath.

Emphysema   A lung disorder where the alveolar walls are affected resulting in a loss of elasticity of the lungs.

Expiration   The act of expelling air from the lungs.

Huff Coughing   A forced expiratory technique performed by the patient as a series of quick, short exhalations. This promotes bronchial hygiene by increasing the expectoration of respiratory excretions.

Hypoxemia   Insufficient oxygenation of the arterial blood.

Hypoxia   Lack of adequate oxygen at the tissue level.

Incentive Spirometer   A device used to increase air movement in and out of the lungs. Incentive spirometers are given to patients to produce maximum effort during deep breathing and prevent atelectasis.

Inspiration   The act of drawing air into the lungs.

Orthopnea   Laboured breathing that occurs when the patient is lying flat.

Oxygen   A colourless, odourless gas present in the atmosphere essential to respiration and life.

PaO$_2$ The partial pressure of oxygen present in arterial blood.

Parenchyma of the lung   Any form of lung tissue including bronchioles, bronchi, blood vessels, interstitium, and alveoli.

Perfusion   The circulation of blood through organs and tissues to supply nutrients and oxygen.

Pleural Effusion   An excess of fluid that accumulates in the pleural space.

Pleural Space   The potential space between the two pleura (visceral and parietal) of the lungs. The thin space between the two pleural layers is known as the *pleural cavity*; it contains a small amount of pleural fluid.

Pneumonia   Inflammation of the lungs, usually due to infection with bacteria or viruses or other pathogenic organisms.

SaO$_2$ The percentage of saturated oxygen present in the blood measured by pulse oximetry. Frequently considered part of vital sign assessment, SaO$_2$ is an indicator of adequate oxygenation. In adults, this measurement is usually 100% with normal ranges above a minimum of 92%.

Stridor   A harsh, high-pitched respiratory sound, often due to airway obstruction.

Surfactant   A surface agent produced in the alveoli of the lungs that decreases the surface tension of the fluid lining the alveoli, permitting expansion.

Tachypnea   A rapid rate of respiration. In an adult patient, tachypnea would be respiratory rates exceeding 20 breaths/min.

Tidal Volume   The volume of air that is passed in and out of the lungs during a single inspiratory/expiratory cycle.

Tracheostomy   The surgical opening of the trachea to provide a secure and open airway.

Ventilation   The movement of air in and out of the lungs.

Wheezes   A continuous musical sound heard predominantly during expiration that is caused by narrowing of the lumen of a respiratory passage.

Understanding the Respiratory System

The respiratory system delivers **oxygen** (the gaseous element required to release energy) to the bloodstream and removes excess carbon dioxide from the body. To achieve this process, there needs to be ventilation, diffusion (the movement of gases between alveoli in the lungs and the bloodstream), and **perfusion** (the movement of blood into and out of the capillary beds surrounding the alveoli of the lungs to the organs and tissues of the body). Patients with compromised oxygenation status need careful assessment and priority clinical care to achieve an adequate level of oxygenation.

Respiratory System Structures

The respiratory system includes airways and lungs (called the *pulmonary system*), bony thorax, and respiratory muscles; see the diagram in Figure 32.1.

The airways of the respiratory system consist of an upper and lower part. The upper airway warms, filters, and humidifies inhaled air and before it travels to the lower airway and includes the nasopharynx, oropharynx, laryngopharynx, and larynx. These structures are lined with a ciliated mucosa having a very rich vascular supply. The mucosal lining warms and humidifies inspired air and removes foreign particles from the air as it passes into the lungs.

The larynx connects the upper and lower airways and houses the vocal cords. The laryngeal box is formed of three large cartilages: the epiglottis, thyroid, and cricoid.

The lower respiratory airways include both conducting airways and the acinus. The conducting airways include the trachea, right and left mainstem bronchi, secondary bronchi, and bronchioles. The gas exchange units called the *acinus* include the respiratory bronchioles and the alveoli.

The thorax boundaries are the sternum, 12 ribs, and 12 thoracic vertebrae. Muscles of respiration include the diaphragm and intercostals, whereas the accessory muscles include the abdominal, sternocleidomastoid, and the pectoral muscles. The right lung has three lobes, whereas the left lung has two lobes, due to the proximity of the heart.

The lungs are lined by the visceral pleura, but the chest wall is lined by the parietal pleura. In between these two layers is the **pleural space**, which has a negative pressure that prevents the lungs from separating from the chest wall. The lungs contain the **alveoli** saclike dilations (about 500 million in the lungs), which are the key structures in gas exchange. The great alveolar or septal cells, also called *pneumocyte II cells*, manufacture **surfactant**, which acts to lower the surface tension of the alveoli and prevent collapse of the alveoli, which is referred to as **atelectasis**.

Gas exchange takes place across the alveolar-capillary membrane. This membrane is thin and has an immense surface area that promotes the alveolar ducts, diffusion of oxygen from the alveoli into the blood and carbon dioxide out of the blood and into the alveoli to be exhaled.

Respiration

Respiration refers to the mechanical process of breathing; that is, inhaling oxygen and exhaling **carbon dioxide (CO_2)**. In contrast, **ventilation** refers to the adequacy of respiration or breathing. Ventilation is the flow of mixture of gases into and out of lungs and is regulated by respiratory control

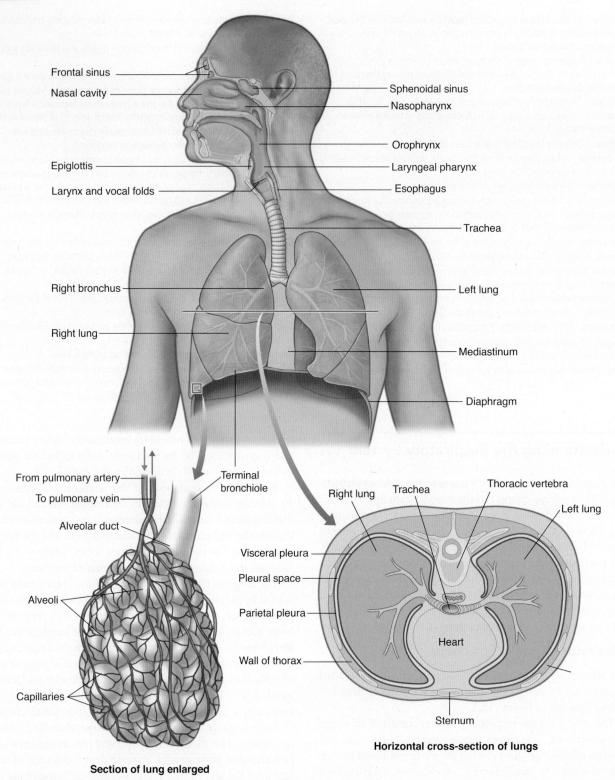

Frontal sinus

Nasal cavity

Epiglottis

Larynx and vocal folds

Sphenoidal sinus

Nasopharynx

Orophrynx

Laryngeal pharynx

Esophagus

Right bronchus

Right lung

Trachea

Left lung

Mediastinum

Diaphragm

From pulmonary artery

To pulmonary vein

Alveolar duct

Alveoli

Capillaries

Terminal bronchiole

Right lung

Trachea

Thoracic vertebra

Left lung

Visceral pleura

Pleural space

Parietal pleura

Wall of thorax

Heart

Sternum

Horizontal cross-section of lungs

Section of lung enlarged

Figure 32.1 Respiratory system.

centres in the pons and medulla oblongata, which are located in the brainstem. The rate and depth of ventilation are constantly adjusted in response to changes in concentrations of hydrogen ion (pH) and CO_2 in the blood. For example, if a patient has an increase in the CO_2 in the blood or a decrease in pH in the body's fluids, the respiratory control centre signals the body to stimulate faster and deeper ventilation.

A decrease in blood oxygen concentration (hypoxemia) will also stimulate ventilation but to a lesser degree.

Inhalation of air is initiated when the diaphragm contracts, pulling downward and thereby increasing the size of the thoracic space. At the same time, the external muscles contract which elevate and separate the ribs and move the sternum forward. The effect of increasing the space inside the thorax is to decrease the intrathoracic pressure, allowing the atmospheric air to fill the lungs.

Stretch receptors in the lung tissue send signals back to the brain to cause cessation of inhalation, preventing over distension of the lungs. Exhalation occurs when the respiratory muscles relax, thereby reducing the size of the intrathoracic space, increasing the intrathoracic pressure, and forcing air to exit the lungs. Under normal circumstances, exhalation is a passive process.

When the movement of air is impeded, the patient may have to use additional muscles to increase the ventilatory effort. These accessory muscles of ventilation include the sternocleidomastoid, abdominal, and internal intercostal muscles. When accessory muscles are required for breathing, the work of breathing is said to be increased.

 ### Alveolar Gas Exchange

The exchange of oxygen from the alveoli into the pulmonary capillary blood is called *external respiration*. Oxygen diffuses across the alveolar membrane in response to a concentration gradient. The oxygen moves from higher concentrations (the alveoli) to lower concentrations (the pulmonary capillary blood). At the same time, CO_2 diffuses from the blood to the alveolar space, also in response to a concentration gradient (Fig. 32.2).

Oxygen Transport and Perfusion

Once the diffusion of oxygen across the alveolar-capillary membrane occurs, the oxygen molecules are dissolved in the blood plasma. Three factors influence the capacity of the blood to carry oxygen: the amount of dissolved oxygen in the plasma, the hemoglobin level, and the tendency of the hemoglobin to bind with oxygen. Only 1% to 5% of the total oxygen is carried in the plasma. The oxygen-carrying capacity of the blood is greatly enhanced by the presence of hemoglobin in the red blood cells (erythrocytes).

The amount of oxygen carried in a sample of blood is measured in two ways. Oxygen dissolved in plasma is expressed as the partial pressure of oxygen (PaO_2). The normal PaO_2 in arterial blood is 80 to 100 mmHg. The vast majority of oxygen in the blood is carried bound to the hemoglobin molecule. The amount of oxygen bound to hemoglobin is expressed as the percentage of hemoglobin that is saturated with oxygen (referred to as SaO_2), with 100% being fully saturated. Normal saturation of arterial blood (SaO_2) is about 96% to 98%.

Circulation

Once bound to hemoglobin, the oxygen is delivered to the cells of the body for tissue perfusion by the process of circulation. Circulation of the blood is the function of the heart and blood vessels. The heart is a muscular pump that is divided into four chambers: the right and left atria and the right and left ventricles (Fig. 32.3). Valves allow for unidirectional blood flow through the chambers.

A single cycle of atrial and ventricular contraction and relaxation is referred to as a **cardiac cycle**, which is a both mechanical and electrical event. The electrical activity of the heart involves the generation and transmission of electrical current by specialized cells known as the *cardiac conduction system* (Fig. 32.4). A small mass of cells in the right atrium, the sinoatrial node or the SA node, is the intrinsic pacemaker of the heart. The impulses of the SA node travel along specialized internodal pathways to spread throughout the atria resulting in the mechanical contraction of the atria. The electrical impulse is then transmitted down to the ventricles through the **atrioventricular node (AV) node**, which lies in the lower part of the right atrium. From the AV node, it spreads to the bundles of His, right and left bundle branches, and the Purkinje fibres.

This results in the mechanical contraction of the ventricles. The sequential contraction and relaxation of the atria and ventricles is an essential factor in the cyclical filling and emptying of the chambers, which produce circulation. This cycle occurs approximately 6 to 100 times per minute, depending on the patient's age, gender, and condition.

The process of chamber filling is referred to as **diastole**, and the process of emptying is systole (Fig. 32.5). Right atrial diastole occurs as the right atrium fills from the blood that returns to the heart from the superior and inferior vena cava. Left atrial diastole occurs as the left atrium fills from the blood that returns to the heart from the pulmonary veins. As the pressure rises in the atria, the valves that separate the atrium and ventricles (tricuspid on the right side and mitral on the left side) open, permitting the blood to begin flowing into the ventricles. This is called *passive filling* and accounts for approximately 70% of the total cardiac output. Ventricular filling is further augmented by the contraction of the atrium (atrial systole). This further ventricular filling is called the *atrial kick*. It accounts for approximately another 30% of the total cardiac output.

Filling of the ventricles causes the intraventricular pressure to rise. When the intraventricular pressure exceeds the pressure in the atria, the AV valves close. The ventricular muscle then begins to contract, further increasing the

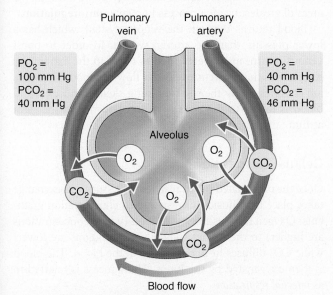

Figure 32.2 Gas exchange in the pulmonary capillary.

Pulmonary vein

Pulmonary artery

PO_2 = 100 mm Hg
PCO_2 = 40 mm Hg

PO_2 = 40 mm Hg
PCO_2 = 46 mm Hg

Alveolus

O_2 O_2 O_2 CO_2 CO_2 CO_2

Blood flow

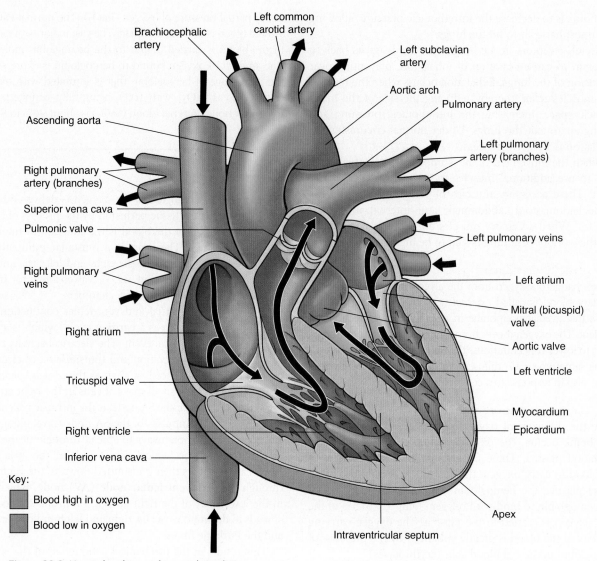

Figure 32.3 Heart chambers, valves, and circulation.

pressure until it is sufficient to force the semilunar valves open (pulmonic on the right and aortic on the left). As contraction of the ventricular walls proceeds, blood is forced out of the ventricles and into the circulation (ventricular systole).

Blood leaving the right ventricle is pumped into the pulmonary artery, which quickly branches into the right and left pulmonary arteries. They further divide down to the pulmonary capillary beds that surround the alveoli. It is at this point that alveolar-capillary gas exchanges take place. From the pulmonary capillaries, the oxygenated blood flows into the pulmonary veins and to the left atrium to the left ventricle. The left ventricle pumps the oxygenated blood to the rest of the body through the aortic valve and aorta.

The aorta divides into many branches that reach out to every organ in the body (Fig. 32.6). Blood flow through the arterial system is driven by the pressure generated during ventricular systole and is influenced by the volume and thickness of the blood as well as the resistance within the arterial system. Blood flow to specific organs and tissues may be increased or reduced by the relaxation or contraction of

precapillary sphincters that regulates flow of blood. This mechanism allows for redistribution of blood flow to the areas of greatest need, a process known as **autoregulation**.

Blood returns through the venous system, which has a lower pressure than the arterial system. In order to boost venous return, many veins such as those in the extremities have valves that prevent backward flow of blood. The veins are compressed by their surrounding skeletal muscles, and blood is forced to the vena cava and returned to the right atrium.

Cellular Respiration

Once the oxygenated blood reaches the tissues, gas exchange takes place by diffusion in response to concentration gradients. Oxygen diffuses from the blood (where concentrations are higher) to the tissues (where concentrations are lower) while CO_2 diffuses from the tissues to the blood. The blood is then oxygenated by the lungs. This process is referred to as *internal respiration*.

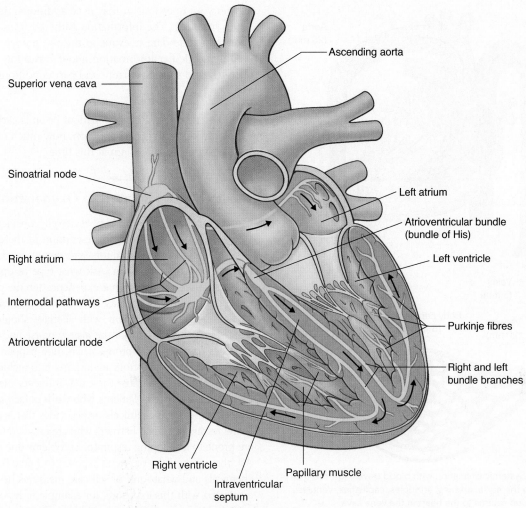

Figure 32.4 The electrical conduction system of the heart.

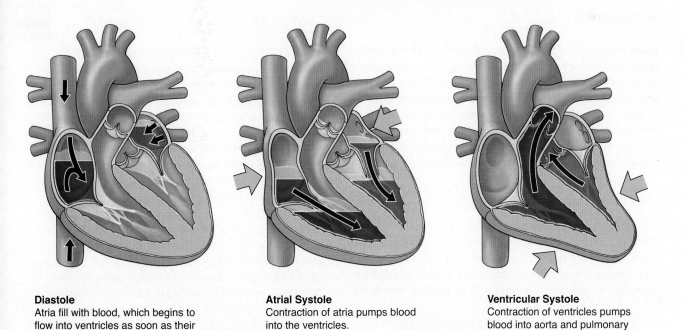

Diastole
Atria fill with blood, which begins to flow into ventricles as soon as their walls relax.

Atrial Systole
Contraction of atria pumps blood into the ventricles.

Ventricular Systole
Contraction of ventricles pumps blood into aorta and pulmonary arteries.

Figure 32.5 Pumping action of the heart.

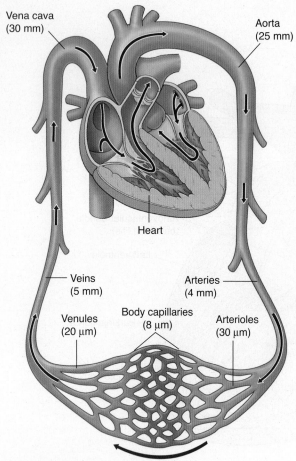

Vena cava
(30 mm)

Aorta
(25 mm)

Heart

Veins
(5 mm)

Arteries
(4 mm)

Venules
(20 μm)

Body capillaries
(8 μm)

Arterioles
(30 μm)

Figure 32.6 Systemic circulation with blood travelling from the heart through the aorta, arteries, arterioles, capillaries, venules, and veins. Blood returns to the heart in the vena cava.

Assessment

Assessment entails taking a focused health history, noting symptoms, history of respiratory illness, history of smoking or drug abuse, level of pain and fatigue, and treatments or medications used to date. The physical assessment includes inspection of the respiratory system, paying attention to rate, depth, and regularity of breathing; as well as palpation, percussion, and auscultation of breath sounds, taking into consideration the age and current condition of the patient.

Health History

An accurate health history is obtained from the patient, including a review of all body systems and focused attention to the respiratory system. The patient may be seeking health care due to a respiratory concern, but a complete physical examination of the patient should also be done to review the function of all body systems.

Use your discretion when carrying out the physical assessment, keeping in mind that the patient may be in acute respiratory distress and fatigued. If the patient is experiencing **dyspnea**, he or she may be unable to speak or

answer your questions or may need additional time to pause while speaking. The information gathered from the history should include data relevant to the respiratory system, including particular information about breathing difficulties, allergies, and specific current and past conditions.

Remember Mr. Pipe, the patient Jason is caring for? Given Mr Pipe's physical condition, how much of the health history should Jason obtain at this time?

Health History Related to Oxygenation

Current health history should be reviewed, considering present symptoms and the onset and description of these symptoms along with a focused respiratory assessment, according to the patient's presenting concern. Ask what type of upper respiratory conditions the patient has experienced in the past, including common illnesses such as colds, sore throats, allergies, and sinus concerns. The patient with allergies should be asked what specific triggers make the allergy worse and what he or she does to relieve symptoms when they happen. Questions about environmental factors are important to include in assessment of the patient, because these may influence the function of the respiratory system. Patients who work in factories or farms may be exposed to chemicals or pesticides that act as irritants to the respiratory tract. Farmers who are exposed to grain dust are prone to developing respiratory problems due to irritation. Ask the patient if he or she is exposed to home or workplace chemicals and what kind of self-care measures he or she uses associated with this exposure; for example, if he or she wears a mask. Medication history should be reviewed, paying special attention to medications that are used for respiratory disorders.

Through the eyes of a nurse

A 70-year-old female patient was admitted to our emergency department. She was brought in by family because she was acting tired and had been gradually been feeling less well, although there was no significant history of any medical problems.

On admission into emergency, she was sleepy and difficult to arouse. ABGs showed a very high level of CO_2, and her PaO_2 was quite decreased. Her respirations were markedly slow. Diagnostic tests, including blood work and chest x-rays, did not show anything unusual. Eventually, the patient deteriorated to the point that she required intubation and mechanical ventilation to maintain gas exchange.

This case was strange, given that the patient had no medical history of any health problems. A CT scan was performed which showed the patient had a tumor in her brain, pressing on her medulla, which controls the autonomic function of respiration.

This case showed me how the signs and symptoms the patient presents with may not always have an obvious cause, and it may turn out to be something that you did not expect.

The way that I assessed and treated the patient was based on her symptoms, and the observations about her decreased respiratory rate along with the blood gas results led us to believe there was more to investigate with this patient.

(personal reflection of a nurse)

Common Respiratory Symptoms

Wheezing

Wheezing is a high-pitched musical noise that is produced as a result of air movement through a narrowed airway. It is often heard on inspiration but may also be heard on expiration. Wheezing is often associated with asthma but can be associated with airway obstruction.

Cough

A **cough** is an abrupt discharge of air from the lungs to clear the trachea bronchi and lungs from some type of irritant. If the patient reports a cough, it's important for the nurse to ask about the quality of the cough (congested, harsh, dry) because some illnesses have a characteristic cough. For example, a cough that is continuous throughout the day and night usually indicates a respiratory infection. A cough that occurs only in the morning may be due to sinusitis; coughing clears the airways from discharge that has accumulated during sleep. Ask if the patient is expectorating any sputum, and if so, how often this is occurring. Ask if the sputum is blood tinged or has any detectable odor. A complete symptom analysis is essential to help guide diagnosis and treatment for the patient (see Chapter 20 on Health Assessment).

Dyspnea

Dyspnea is often due to underlying heart disease, or pulmonary diseases such as chronic obstructive pulmonary disease or asthma, but can also occur with acute conditions including respiratory infections such as pneumonia or pulmonary emboli. Dyspnea, the subjective feeling of uncomfortable or difficult breathing, is a clinical sign of hypoxia. A patient with shortness of breath may feel fatigued from the effort of breathing and may not be able to fully participate in routine activities of daily living.

Note that Mr. Pipe is currently having dyspnea. What do you think is the cause of Mr. Pipe's dyspnea?

History of Respiratory Illness

Patients who have challenges with oxygenation often have a history of difficulty with respiratory infections or other conditions. Many respiratory conditions are chronic and progressively debilitative in nature. Patients may have a history of lower respiratory tract illnesses such as asthma, chronic obstructive pulmonary disease, and **pneumonia** (inflammation of the lungs usually due to infection) or infectious lung disease such as tuberculosis. Respiratory symptoms may be caused by other diseases, such as congestive heart failure, **pleural effusion**, anemia, or certain cancers; therefore, the history of those illnesses is important to obtain. Ask the patient if there is a history of respiratory disease in his or her family.

Cigarette Smoking

Cigarette smoking is a common risk factor in many respiratory and cardiovascular illnesses as well as cancers. Identify if the patient currently smokes, how much he or she smoke, the number of packs per day (PPD), and the number of years he or she has smoked. The Canadian Tobacco Use Monitoring Survey (CTUMS) results from June 2010 identified that 18% of the Canadian population age 15 years and older were current smokers. In view of disease prevention, these statistics have important implications for health teaching for individual patient as well as populations. Box 32.1 reviews evidence-based practice for smoking cessation from the Registered Nurses Association of Ontario (RNAO).

Think The patient in emergency department (ED) was gasping for breath and coughing. The family member reported that the patient smoked two packs of cigarettes a day for at least 30 years. A chest x-ray revealed loss of lung tissue consistent with severe chronic obstructive lung disease and acute pneumonia. Best practice guidelines identify the important role that nurses and the health-care team have in motivating and supporting patients to stop smoking in a sensitive, nonjudgmental manner. The evidence suggests that if health-care providers implement smoking cessation interventions, it would reduce the number of smokers and decrease the related tobacco diseases.

Substance Abuse and Exposures

The person who chronically abuses alcohol or drugs often has poor nutritional intake, which can lead to anemia, the result being decreased oxygen-carrying capacity, further leading to other illnesses that affect the respiratory system. Excessive intake of alcohol or other drugs can depress the respiratory centre, which in turn reduces the rate and depth of respiration

---

BOX 32.1 Evidence-Based Practice for Smoking Cessation

RNAO has developed evidence-based best practice guidelines around smoking cessation. The aim of the guidelines is to have nurses create opportunities to encourage smoking cessation through brief counseling and minimal interventions with patients. For example, while obtaining a health history from a patient who smokes cigarettes, part of the interaction should include documenting amount of tobacco used and assessing the patient's readiness to quit smoking.

Other helpful interventions may include the following:

- Referral to the Canadian Cancer Society's Smokers' Helpline 1-877-513-5333 or http://www.smokershelpline.ca
- Offer support and self-help resources, such as booklets.
- Inform about or refer to a community stop smoking clinic or service.
- Refer to other health-care provider.

and reduces the amount of inhaled oxygen. Chronic substance abuse from inhaling crack cocaine or fumes can cause direct damage to the tissues of the lungs that can lead to permanent lung damage and reduced lung capacity.

Pain

The patient's subjective experience of pain and discomfort is an important clue to diagnoses and treatment. Inquire if the patient is experiencing any chest pain when breathing. Is the pain sharp or dull? Does it occur on **inspiration** (inhalation) or **expiration** (exhalation)? Does the pain radiate? What does it feels like? Pain on inspiration can indicate infection such as pneumonia. It is important to ask when the pain started, if it is getting better or worse, or if any measures have been taken to relieve it (heat, cold, medication, rest, etc.).

Fatigue

Fatigue can be an indication of inadequate oxygenation. Ask if the patient has been experiencing fatigue or having interrupted sleep patterns from breathing difficulties. Does the patient have difficulty lying flat or require more than one pillow to be comfortable in sleep? Specifically inquire about fatigue when performing usual activities of daily living.

Treatment of Symptoms

Inquire if the patient has done anything to treat his or her symptoms, such as medications. It's important to review what medications the patient takes on an ongoing/regular basis, including prescribed and natural remedies, as well as over-the-counter preparations. Patients who take medications regularly should be screened for medication toxicity as many medications (e.g., theophylline) can quickly rise to toxic levels.

Respiratory Physical Assessment

Assessment of the respiratory system requires knowledge of anatomy and surface landmarks, underlying structures, and the ventilatory and respiratory functions of the lungs. The techniques of inspection, palpation, percussion, and auscultation are used during this assessment. See Chapter 20 for a complete overview of physical assessment. Consider age-related variations to assessment findings and planning care by review of Boxes 32.2 and 32.3.

BOX 32.2 **Age-Related Changes: Newborn and Pediatric Variations Respiratory Assessment**

- One of the greatest adaptations, the transition from in utero to newborn extra uterine life is moving from lungs filled with fluid to lungs that quickly fill with air.
- The newborns' chests are small, and their airways are short.
- Aspiration is a risk during the immediate newborn stage.
- Newborns have a rapid respiratory rate (30 to 60 breaths/min), use abdominal muscles to aid respiration, and are obligate nose breathers.

BOX 32.3 **Age-Related Changes: Older Adults Respiratory Assessment**

The cardiac and respiratory systems undergo changes throughout the aging process. These changes are associated with atherosclerotic plaque formation in the arterial system, which will affect the perfusion of lung tissue, and thus, its ability to exchange gases.

Due to the effects of osteoporosis, the thoracic cage typically becomes rounder and barrel shaped. Kyphosis (an outward curvature of the thoracic spine) may also occur, causing the person to tilt his or her head forward or back to compensate.

Chest expansion may become reduced, but it should remain symmetrical. Over time, gas exchange declines from diminishing chest expansion, leading to lower oxygen saturation levels.

The trachea and bronchi become enlarged from calcification of the airways. The alveoli enlarge, decreasing the surface area available for gas exchange. The number of functional cilia is reduced, causing a decrease in the effectiveness of the cough mechanism, placing the older adult at greater risk of respiratory infections.

Alterations in Respiratory Function (Oxygenation)

Conditions and illnesses that affect ventilation or oxygen transport cause alterations in respiratory function. Some common respiratory health challenges include infectious lung disease, airway obstruction, chronic obstructive pulmonary disease, and asthma, along with discussions of some fundamental nursing principles.

Hypoxia

Hypoxia refers to a state of insufficient oxygen levels in the blood, caused primarily by hypoventilation, hyperventilation, or airway obstruction. The PaO_2 falls to a low level, which causes signs and symptoms of **hypoxemia** such as tachycardia, **tachypnea**, shallow or laboured breathing, restlessness, and/or confusion. Due to dyspnea, the patient may have trouble forming words. Other manifestations of hypoxia may occur such as cardiac decompensation, and/or eventually respiratory failure, especially if the underlying cause of the hypoxia is not addressed. Hypoxia may accompany any of these health challenges: pneumonia, chronic obstructive pulmonary disease, asthma, and airway obstruction.

Pneumonia

Pneumonia is an infection of the lung **parenchyma** caused by a microorganism such as bacteria and viruses as well as fungal or tubercular agents. The upper airways in healthy adults are defended by protective defense mechanisms such as filtration of air, cough reflex, alveolar macrophage action, and the action of cilia in the upper airways to remove harmful organisms. When defense mechanisms are reduced or incompetent, microorganisms can enter and attach to vulnerable tissue,

TABLE 32.1	Types of Pneumonia
Types of Pneumonia	Transmittal
Community acquired	Acquired from external environment, prevalent in community; commonly streptococcal
Hospital acquired	Causative organism originates and spread within hospital setting; commonly pseudomonas
Aspiration	Caused from abnormal entry of microorganisms and secretions into lower airways in compromised patients
	Damage to lung can occur from toxins associated with aspirated material (gastrointestinal [GI] contents).
Opportunistic	Causative organism may be associated with other body illnesses, common in patients with COPD or who are immunosuppressed from radiation or chemotherapy for example.

causing infection to develop. Organisms that enter the lungs and cause pneumonia reach the lung by three main methods:

- Aspiration from the nasopharynx or oropharynx
- Inhalation of microbes present in the air
- Hematogenous spread (via the bloodstream) from an infection somewhere else in the body

No matter the causative agent, pneumonia causes congestion and spread of organisms throughout the lung tissues. Alveoli become filled with exudate, thus reducing the surface available for gas exchange, resulting in signs of hypoxia in the patient. Bronchopneumonia means that the pneumonia is diffusely spread throughout the lungs and bronchi. Lobar pneumonia is more localized in one or more lobes of the lung. Lobar and bronchopneumonia can be differentiated on a chest x-ray. Several types of pneumonia are listed in Table 32.1.

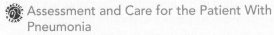 Assessment and Care for the Patient With Pneumonia

The patient with pneumonia requires diligent respiratory assessment (including auscultation of lung fields). Regular evaluation of respiratory status (improvement or decline) is a key nursing action in caring for patients with pneumonia (Nursing Guidelines 32.1).

NURSING GUIDELINES 32.1: AUSCULTATION

When you are auscultating the patient's lungs, practice the following:

- Ask the patient to breathe deeply through his or her mouth.
- Listen at all locations.
- Listen to the full inhalation and exhalation at each location.
- Take your time and concentrate—learning to recognize breath sounds takes time and practice.

The increased respiratory effort that accompanies pneumonia consumes energy and is drying to the oral mucous membranes. Providing adequate oral and or intravenous (IV) fluid intake and encouraging oral hygiene are important in the care of the patient with pneumonia. Providing small, nourishing frequent meals helps to replace calories that are easily lost during the work of breathing and fighting infection.

Therapeutic positioning helps to promote oxygenation and drainage of respiratory secretions. Incentive spirometry, and deep breathing and coughing exercises help to promote chest expansion and improve oxygenation.

Patients with pneumonia are usually treated with anti-infective drug therapy, unless the pneumonia is viral in origin, in which case anti-infective drugs are not effective, because they are designed to treat bacterial or fungal infection. Regular and timely administration of anti-infective agents is necessary to completely eradicate the causative organism. Health teaching for the patient related to medication purpose and directions is important to ensure compliance with treatment. Patients must take the full course of the prescribed anti-infective medications to ensure successful recovery from pneumonia. Patients will sometimes stop taking anti-infective medication if they are feeling better, making them more at risk for recurrence. This commonly happens when patients are discharged home on anti-infective therapy.

Oxygen Therapy

Oxygen therapy is used as a supportive measure when oxygenation levels are not sufficient. Thus, regular monitoring of SaO_2 levels, respiratory rate, vital signs, and assessment of the patient's colour and indicators of respiratory effort are necessary. Oxygen should be administered based on need, saturation levels, and physician or respiratory therapist prescriptions. If the patient with pneumonia has thick tenacious oral secretions and is coughing, humidification of oxygen is recommended to loosen secretions and encourage expectoration.

Patients should be taught deep breathing and coughing techniques to encourage oxygenation and may require pillows to support the chest and/or abdomen to ensure they are able to cough effectively to clear secretions. Patients may experience pain while coughing, and analgesics for pain management may be helpful. Fever may be present and should be monitored closely and treated with antipyretic medication (e.g., acetaminophen) and fluids.

Promotion and supervision of proper nutrition is important. This includes provision of small frequent meals according to food preferences to maintain energy requirements, adequate protein intake to promote healing, and considerable fluid intake (orally or parenterally) to support hydration and liquefy secretions.

The patient with pneumonia is often fatigued from the work of breathing (and resultant hypoxia) as well as the infection itself. The nurse should recommend limiting activity while promoting rest, comfort, and quiet. Positioning the patient in high Fowler position allows for appropriate chest expansion and oxygenation and relieves dyspnea.

Airway Obstruction

Airway obstruction can be either complete or partial and may be due to aspiration of food or a foreign body, laryngeal edema following extubation, central nervous system (CNS) depression, or severe allergic reactions. Symptoms may include **stridor**, a harsh, high-pitched respiratory sound; as well as panic levels of fear and anxiety, restlessness, rapid or absent respiration, choking, chest retractions, or wheezing (partial); and use of accessory muscles for respiration. Airway obstruction is a medical emergency and requires prompt attention to regain a patent airway. The nurse must be alert to the risk for patients who are at greatest risk such as those with cancer of the larynx and those with existing **tracheostomy**.

Diagnostics for the Patient With Airway Obstruction

The patient with complete or partial airway obstruction should have oxygen saturations monitored closely and may have blood examined for hemoglobin levels and white blood cell counts. Depending on the cause of airway obstruction, monitoring the white blood cell count is important to prevent infection. If the cause of airway obstruction is not apparent, chest x-rays, pulmonary function tests, and bronchoscopy may be performed.

Assessment and Care for the Patient With Airway Obstruction

Close monitoring of the patient's airway is critical. Partial obstruction of the airway may quickly progress to complete obstruction. The nurse must observe for signs of worsening obstruction such as stridor, use of accessory muscles for breathing, suprasternal, and intercostal in drawing. In the case of complete airway obstruction, the physician may perform a tracheotomy to establish a functional airway.

Chronic Obstructive Pulmonary Disease

Chronic obstructive pulmonary disease, commonly referred to as COPD, refers to airway disorders that are obstructive in nature, meaning that gas exchange in the lungs is decreased because the flow of air is trapped, and the ability to exhale becomes difficult, prolonging the expiratory period. The two main airway diseases that are categorized as COPD are emphysema and chronic bronchitis. Often, these two conditions are present together.

Exposure to tobacco smoke is one of the primary causes of COPD; dyspnea is the prevailing symptom. Although primarily a lung disease, as COPD advances, it can cause skeletal muscle dysfunction, right-sided heart failure, polycythemia, mental depression, and altered nutrition.

Emphysema and Chronic Bronchitis

Emphysema is a condition where the alveoli become abnormally enlarged and, over time, are destroyed along with the surrounding capillary beds. Airways are narrow and nonelastic, impairing gas exchange. **Chronic bronchitis** is an obstructive pulmonary disease of the larger airways, demonstrated by a chronic productive cough that is present for at least 3 months per year for 2 years in succession.

With emphysema or chronic bronchitis, air becomes trapped in diseased airways and lung tissue, leading to dyspnea, an altered ventilation-perfusion ratio, and an overall state of hypoventilation and impaired gas exchange. Patients may experience cough, excessive sputum production, and dyspnea.

Early symptoms include a cough that often occurs in the morning upon rising and dyspnea upon exertion, which makes every day routine activities increasingly difficult. A typical patient with COPD had a barrel-shaped chest, which occurs due to the air trapping in the lungs, distending the chest wall. As COPD progresses into advanced stages, patients experience weight loss and anorexia due to the high metabolic demands associated with the work of breathing.

Assessment and Care for the Patient With Chronic Obstructive Pulmonary Disease

Acute exacerbations of COPD are common. Typically, patients with COPD contract an infection such as a cold or virus, which can quickly develop into pneumonia. During an acute exacerbation, the nurse should assess breath sounds, respiratory rate, and effort and administer oxygen if indicated. Persons with COPD may require O_2 at higher flow rates, especially when their conditions are advanced. Refer to Nursing Guidelines 32.2 for administrating oxygen to patients with COPD.

Asthma

Asthma is a chronic inflammation of the airways that causes varying degrees of obstruction leading to recurrent episodes of wheezing, coughing, chest tightness, and dyspnea. Asthma may be triggered by environmental allergens or infectious agents. Symptoms arise from stimulation of the immune system in genetically predisposed individuals, which causes **bronchoconstriction**, and narrowing of the smaller airway passages of the lungs.

The key features of asthma are airway inflammation and hyperresponsiveness. Bronchoconstriction occurs in carrying degrees in accordance with the degree of airway inflammation. **Bronchospasm** is an early symptom of an asthma attack, indicating the action of the inflammatory response in the lung tissue. As inflammation increases, so does the immune response, which causes release of inflammatory mediators including histamine, bradykinin, leukotrienes, and others. The combination of these effects leads to bronchoconstriction, which can over time become severe, resulting in airflow obstruction.

**NURSING GUIDELINES 32.2:
ADMINISTERING OXYGEN TO PATIENTS WITH CHRONIC OBSTRUCTIVE PULMONARY DISEASE**

- Be aware of patient's past and present oxygen requirements such as home oxygen.
- Titrate oxygen to the lowest effective dose according to oxygen saturation levels and physical symptoms.
- Perform ongoing physical and cognitive assessment of the patient.

Asthma symptoms range from mild to severe. A mild attack can produce wheezing, cough, and use of accessory muscles to support breathing. An attack that escalates may include tachycardia; diaphoresis; and increasing accessory muscle use with rapid, laboured breathing. A prolonged attack can lead to physical exhaustion, diminished breath sounds, and inadequate SaO_2, which may require mechanical ventilation in severe cases.

An important characteristic of asthma is the episodic and unpredictable nature of the disease, which can be influenced by cold, heat, stressful events, exercise, allergens, and/or infections. The morbidity associated with asthma is dramatic, and efforts are directed toward accurate assessment of severity, adequate and timely medical treatment as well as compliance with treatment guidelines and patient education.

Asthma is treated with inhaled glucocorticoid medications, anti-inflammatory agents, bronchodilators, and anti-allergic agents. Each patient should be evaluated for knowledge of his or her symptoms and be given health teaching about medication use and prevention of future attacks.

Assessment and Care for the Patient With Asthma

Patients with an acute exacerbation of asthma require close monitoring of their oxygen saturation levels and may require administration of oxygen. Monitor breath sounds and administer bronchodilator medications, following up with reassessment after administration of bronchodilator medications is crucial. Encourage fluid intake to optimize fluid balance and liquefy secretions to aid removal.

Providing a calm and reassuring approach to the patient is helpful to reduce anxiety and facilitate relaxation. Evaluate the patient's current knowledge of asthma treatment and reinforce information, such as asthma treatment action plan, awareness of triggers, and the patient's understanding of his or her prescribed medications and use. Having the patient demonstrate the use of inhaler devices is useful in determining proper technique and ensuring compliance. See Nursing Guidelines 32.3 for asthma action plans.

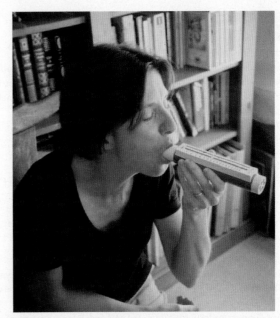

Figure 32.7 Peak flow metres measure the highest volume of airflow during a forced expiration.

Figure 32.7 illustrates the use of a flow meter. The zones used in the asthma action plan are shown in Figure 32.8. Box 32.4 reviews common diagnostic tests related to oxygenation.

Nursing Diagnosis

Care of the patient experiencing oxygenation issues need to be prioritized based on maintaining a patent airway, breathing, and circulation. Table 32.2 lists the primary nursing diagnoses related to maintaining airway, breathing, and circulation.

NURSING GUIDELINES 32.3: ASTHMA ACTION PLANS

Asthma action plans help patients identify how effectively their asthma is controlled.

Each zone indicates action to be taken if symptoms worsen.

- The green zone indicates symptoms are controlled and require no immediate action.
- The yellow zone indicates symptoms are uncontrolled and require medical attention.
- The red zone indicates asthma is dangerously uncontrolled and immediate medical attention is required.

Asthma action plans are available through pharmacies or from the Canadian Lung Association (http://www.lung.ca/_resources/asthma_action_plan.pdf).

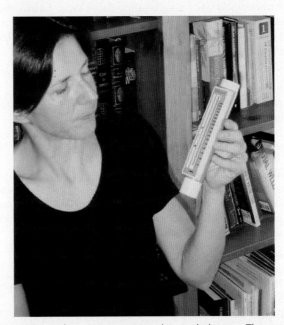

Figure 32.8 Volume is measure in colour-coded zones: The green zone signifies 80% to 100% of personal best; yellow, 60% to 80%; and red, less than 60%. If peak falls below the red zone, the patient should take the appropriate actions prescribed by his or her health care provider.

BOX 32.4 Diagnostic Tests

Arterial Blood Gas and pH Analysis

These examine arterial blood to determine the pressure exerted by oxygen and CO_2 in the blood and the blood pH. This test measures the adequacy of oxygenation, ventilation, and perfusion. Normal results are as follows: pH (7.35 to 7.45), PCO_2 (35 to 45 mmHg), PO_2 (80 to 100 mmHg), HCO_3^- (22–26 mEq/L), and base excess or deficit (−2 to +2 mmol/L).

Preparation
- Explain to the patient that this test requires an arterial puncture and collection of a blood specimen.
- The radial, brachial, or femoral arteries are usually the sites of choice.
- Perform Allen test to ensure adequate ulnar blood flow when using radial artery.

Aftercare
- Record supplemental oxygen or respirator settings on laboratory slip.
- The arterial specimen is immediately placed on ice and taken to the laboratory.
- Apply pressure for 5 to 10 minutes and watch for evidence of bleeding. If patient is taking anticoagulants, pressure must be applied for a longer interval.

Cytologic Study

This involves a microscopic examination of sputum and the cells it contains. It is done primarily to detect cells that may be malignant, determine organisms causing infection, and identify blood or pus in the sputum.

Preparation
- Collect the specimen, if possible, in the morning before breakfast. The test usually involves 3 successive days of sputum collection. About 1 tsp of sputum is needed for a specimen.
- Instruct the patient that saliva is not a satisfactory specimen.
- Patient should take a deep breath and then expel the air with a deep cough.
- Expectorate the specimen into a sterile specimen container with the appropriate preservative, if indicated.
- Close the container with a tight-fitting lid.

Aftercare
- Advise the patient to inform the nurse when the specimen has been obtained.
- Label and package the specimen and send it to the laboratory as soon as possible.

Endoscopic Studies

These involve direct visualization of a body cavity. A bronchoscope is used to examine the larynx, bronchi, and trachea. Bronchoscopy is used to view lesions, obtain a biopsy, improve drainage, remove foreign substances, evaluate trauma, and drain abscesses.

Preparation
- Verify that an informed consent was obtained.
- The patient should be nothing by mouth (NPO) for 6 to 8 hours before the test.
- An analgesic, sedative, and/or anticholinergic may be administered before the test.
- Local anesthetic is sprayed into the throat.

Aftercare
- Withhold food and fluids until the gag reflex returns.
- Check vital signs according to the protocol.
- Observe carefully for signs of respiratory impairment. Emergency resuscitation equipment should be available.
- Warm saline gargles may relieve throat irritation once the gag reflex has returned.

Skin Tests

These determine antigen–antibody reactions. In intradermal tests, antigens (to which the patient may have previously been exposed) are injected into the superficial layer of the skin with a needle and syringe to evaluate immune response.

Preparation
- Check patient's history for hypersensitivity to any of the test antigens. If positive, notify the physician before performing test.
- Cleanse the test area with alcohol and allow it to dry.

Aftercare
- Instruct the patient to have the test results read at the appropriate time.
- After reading the results, document the reaction, noting the amount of erythema or induration. Record the test, time, date, method, and site of administration on the patient record.

Radiography

Radiography is an x-ray examination of the lungs and the thoracic cavity. Radiographic examinations of the lungs are done to help diagnose pulmonary diseases and to determine the progress or development of disease.

Preparation
- Instruct patient to remove clothing to the waist and put on gown. All metal jewelry should be removed.
- The patient will be required to take a deep breath and hold it during the radiograph.

Aftercare
- No special care is required after chest radiograph.

Lung Scan

Lung scan is the recording on a photographic plate of the emissions of radioactive waves from a substance injected into a vein as it circulates through the lung. A *perfusion scan* (Q scan) is done to measure integrity of pulmonary blood vessels and evaluate blood flow abnormalities (e.g., pulmonary emboli). A *ventilation scan* (V scan) is done to detect ventilation abnormalities (especially in patients with emphysema). Both scans used together provide greater and more accurate diagnostic information than either test used solely.

Preparation
- Verify that an informed consent was obtained, if required by agency.
- Explain that no fasting is required.
- Patient should be told to remove jewelry from the chest area.

Aftercare
- No special care is required after the lung scan.
- Reassure patient that no radiation precautions are necessary.

Adapted from Fischbach, F., & Dunning, M. (2009). *A manual of laboratory and diagnostic tests* (8th ed.). Philadelphia, of medical-surgical nursing (12th ed.). Philadelphia, PA: Lippincott Williams & Wilkins; Fischbach, F., & Dunning, M. (2006). *Common laboratory and diagnostic tests* (4th ed.). Philadelphia, PA: Lippincott Williams & Wilkins.

TABLE 32.2 Nursing Diagnosis and Defining Characteristics

Nursing Diagnosis	Defining Characteristics

Ineffective Airway Clearance related to
• Airway obstruction
  – Obstruction of the airway by the tongue
  – Obstruction of the airway by secretion
  – Upper airway obstruction caused by edema of the larynx or glottis
  – Obstruction of the trachea or a bronchus by foreign body aspiration
  – Partial occlusion of the bronchi and bronchioles by infection, inflammation, or spasm or occlusion or compression by a tumor mass
  – Occlusion of the more distal airways by changes that may occur with COPD
	– Reporting of shortness of breath or feeling as though suffocating
	– Difficulty speaking or completing sentences
	– Cough
	  ▪ Effective or ineffective
	  ▪ Productive or nonproductive
	– Diminished breath sounds over the peripheral lung fields
	– Adventitious breath sounds such as **crackles** or **wheezes**
	– Complete obstruction of a large-sized airway may result in a loss of breath sounds over the affected area.

Ineffective Breathing Patterns related to
• Airway or tracheobronchial obstruction
• Thoracic or abdominal pain
  – Avoids taking deep breaths or coughing due to surgical pain.
  – CNS depression
  – Anesthetics
  – Narcotics
  – Lesions affecting the brainstem
  – Neuromuscular impairment
  – Guillain-Barré syndrome
  – Myasthenia gravis
  – Alterations of thoracic structures
  – Scoliosis
  – Kyphosis
  – Chest wall injury
  – Fractured ribs
	– Dyspnea
	– Cough tachypnea
	– Diminished chest excursion
	– Asymmetric chest excursion
	– Breath sound changes
	– Increased $PaCO_2$
	– Decreased PaO_2

Impaired Gas Exchange related to – Inadequate alveolar ventilation – Hypoventilation – Decreased inspired oxygen – High altitudes – Alveolar-capillary membrane changes – Congestive heart failure – Decreased hemoglobin – Anemia – Ventilation-perfusion mismatch – Pulmonary embolus – Emphysema	– Tachycardia – Tachypnea – Cyanosis (late sign) – Neurologic changes: restless, confusion, anxious – Decreased exercise capacity, fatigue – Breath sound changes – Decreased PaO_2, decreased SaO_2 – Elevation of arterial lactate levels
Risk for Aspiration related to – Decreased level of consciousness – Impaired gag or cough reflex – Increased intra-abdominal pressure – Impaired swallowing – Facial/oral/neck surgery or trauma	– Dyspnea – Cough – Tachypnea – Tachycardia – Fever – Breath sound changes – Arterial blood gases (ABGs) changes: hypoxemia with hypocapnia

Interventions to Promote Airway Clearance

Interventions to promote airway clearance focus on clearing the airway secretions, relieving bronchial spasm, and, when necessary, using an artificial airway. There are many interventions to promote an open or patent airway obstructed by mucus or a foreign body. These may be an interdisciplinary if there are concerns about the appropriateness of the intervention or if the obstruction does not respond to treatment.

The need for specific interventions to promote bronchial hygiene and a clear airway is based on physical assessment, results of diagnostic tests such as an x-ray, and additional sources of informal as indicated. Hypoxemia will result if the patient does not have a clear airway and gas exchange cannot take place. Box 32.5 lists the signs and symptoms that may be observed with hypoxemia. Any one or combination

BOX 32.5 Signs and Symptoms of Hypoxemia

Symptoms may include the following:
Cyanosis (late sign)
Dyspnea
Tachypnea
Decreased level of consciousness
Increased work of breathing
Loss of protective airway (conscious sedation)
Agitation
Confusion
Disorientation
Tachycardia/bradycardia
Promotion of airway clearance

BOX 32.6 Pursed-Lip Breathing Technique

1. Instruct patient to relax his or her neck and shoulder muscles.
2. Then instruct patient to breathe in (inhale) slowly through his or her nose (smell the coffee) for two counts, keeping his or her mouth closed.
3. Following inhalation, instruct the patient to pucker or "purse" his or her lips as if you were going to whistle or gently flicker the flame of a candle.
4. Instruct patient to breathe out (exhale) slowly and gently through pursed lips (blow out the candles) while counting to four.

of the following therapies is used: patient positioning, deep breathing and coughing, hydration, chest physiotherapy, and medications. Prior to any of these procedures, the patient requires teaching of the purpose of the intervention and what to expect.

Patient Positioning

Frequent position changes and ambulation promote oxygenation and respiration; the patient is positioned for maximum chest expansion. The semi-Fowler or high Fowler positions allow for patients who are immobile to maximize their chest expansion. **Orthopnea** is the laboured breathing that occurs when a patient is lying flat.

The orthopneic position is a variation of the high Fowler position and is used for patients who have difficulty breathing. The head of the bed is at a 90° angle (high Fowler). The bedside table is then place across the bed and one or two pillows are placed on top of the table. The patient leans forward with his or her arms on or bedside the pillows (Fig. 32.9A).

Patients with advanced lung disease will often assume a tripod position. In this position, patients are leaning forward, with their hands on their knees to help ease breathing when breathing difficulties occur (Fig. 32.9B). This provides a position that optimizes respiratory mechanics.

Deep Breathing and Coughing

The nurse can promote airway clearance and respiratory function by encouraging a patient to deep breathe and cough to remove secretions. Taking in deep breaths facilitates the opening of the alveoli, improving gas exchange. Coughing helps to mobilize secretions. Deep breathing and coughing is important for patients who have limited mobility or on bed rest. It is indicated for patients with such respiratory conditions as chronic obstructive lung disease, postabdominal or thoracic surgery, and pneumonia.

Pursed-lip breathing is commonly employed to help a patient develop control over his or her breathing, slow his or her pace of breathing, and make it more effective (Box 32.6). By using pursed lips, a resistance to the air flowing out of

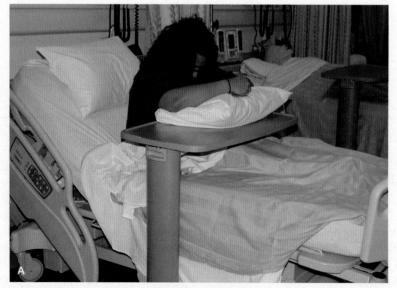
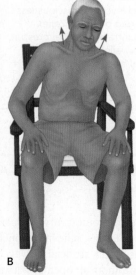

Figure 32.9 **A.** Orthopneic position. **B.** Tripod position

the lungs is created. This prolongs exhalation and prevents airway collapse by maintaining positive airway pressure.

Coughing should be controlled using a **huff coughing** technique. The patient is instructed to cough twice as the first cough loosens the secretions and the second cough will assist with expelling the secretions. Huff coughing has the patient leaning forward, and when he or she exhales, he or she makes a sharp "huff" sound. The force helps to clear the airways. Deep breathing and coughing can be fatiguing. The patient is encouraged to rest in between these exercises and avoid prolong episodes of coughing. Although deep breathing and coughing is effective, some patients require assistance or a motivator to do the task effectively.

Incentive Spirometer

Incentive spirometer is a device that assists patients with deep breathing by providing visual feedback about the depth of their breaths. There are two types of spirometers: flow-oriented and volume-oriented. The flow-oriented incentive spirometer has one or more plastic chambers with freely moveable coloured balls (Fig. 32.10A). As the patient inhales slowly, the balls are elevated to a premarked area. The goal is to keep the balls elevated for as long as possible to ensure maximal sustained inhalation. Even if the slow inspiration does not elevate the balls, this pattern may achieve greater lung expansion. Box 32.7 lists contraindications and complications with incentive spirometer.

Volume-oriented incentive spirometer has a bellow that the patient must raise to a predetermined volume by inhaling slowly (Fig. 32.10B). With this type of spirometer, a known inspiratory volume can be achieved and measured with each breath.

The incentive spirometer supports the patient's efforts to maintain or improve pulmonary ventilation. It will loosen secretions, prevent atelectasis, and facilitate gas exchange. The patient is encouraged to use the incentive spirometer at least four times every hour, taking 10 breaths each time. After each set of 10 deep breaths, the patient should

---

BOX 32.7   Incentive Spirometer Contraindications and Complications

Contraindications
- Patient is uncooperative, or patient is unable to understand or demonstrate proper use of the device.
- Patients unable to deep breathe effectively (e.g., with vital capacity [VC] less than about 10 ml/kg or inspiratory capacity [IC] less than about one third of predicted).
- The presence of an open tracheal stoma is not a contraindication but requires adaptation of the spirometer.

Complications
- Ineffective unless closely supervised or performed as ordered
- Inappropriate as sole treatment for major lung collapse or consolidation
- Hyperventilation
- Barotrauma (emphysematous lungs)
- Discomfort secondary to inadequate pain control
- Hypoxia secondary to interruption of prescribed oxygen therapy if face mask or shield is being used
- Exacerbation of bronchospasm
- Fatigue

---

practice coughing to be sure the lungs are clear. If they have an incision, it should be supported when coughing by placing a pillow firmly against it. See Box 32.7 for contraindication and complications related to using an incentive spirometer.

Monitor Hydration

In a dry environment or if the patient becomes dehydrated, the normally thin secretions thicken and are more difficult to expectorate. Unless contraindicated by other illnesses such as congestive heart failure or renal failure, increased fluid intake often keeps secretions thin and prevents stagnation of mucus, which can lead to airway

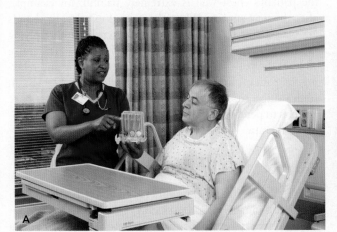
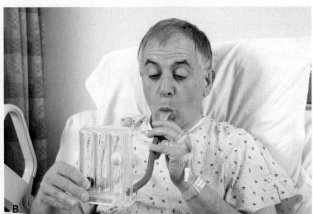

Figure 32.10   A. Flow-oriented incentive spirometer. **B.** Patient using incentive spirometer.

infection, airway obstruction, shortness of breath, increased work of breathing, and abnormal gas exchange. In dry environments, humidifiers add water vapor to inspired room air or can be used with oxygen devices to provide moistened air to the patient. Using a humidifier with an oxygen device prevents drying of the mucous membranes. The moistening of inspired air assists to loosen secretions for expectoration.

Chest Physiotherapy

Postural drainage, positioning, and chest percussion and vibration are all methods of chest physiotherapy. Together, these techniques mobilize and eliminate secretions, assist with expanding lung tissue, and promote more efficient use of respiratory muscles. This is especially important in a patient who has limited mobility or is bedridden. Chest physiotherapy helps to prevent atelectasis or pneumonia.

These various techniques may be used in sequence in different lung drainage positions and are preceded by bronchodilator therapy and followed by deep breathing and coughing. Chest physiotherapy includes changing of the patient's position from supine to upright, which affects gas exchange. If the patient has a unilateral (one side) lung disease, for example, pneumonia on the right lung, positioning the patient with the healthy lung down improves oxygenation and will decrease shunting when the good lung is in the dependent position. Positioning the patient with the diseased lung down may result in hypoxemia.

Chest Percussion and Vibration

Chest percussion and vibration are performed to dislodge secretions in the patient's airways. Contraindications for chest percussion and vibration are listed in Box 32.8. To perform

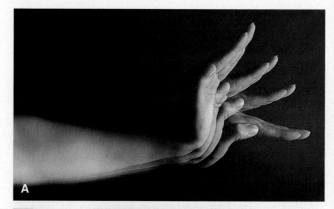
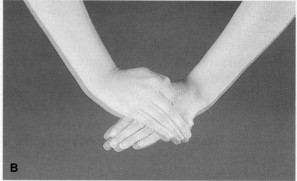

Figure 32.11 A. The cupping position and function of the hand on manual percussion of lung area. **B.** The position and action of the hands necessary to use vibration to loosen respiratory secretion in the lungs.

percussion, the patient is asked to breathe slowly and deeply using the diaphragm to promote a relaxed breathing pattern. The nurse uses cupped hands with fingers flexed and thumbs pressed in tightly (Fig. 32.11A). The hands in this position are rhythmically tapped against the patient's anterior and posterior chest, about 1 to 2 minutes for each segment. When done correctly, percussion should create a hollow or a clapping sound.

Vibration is done while the patient exhales through pursed lips. Vibration will be used instead of percussion if the patient's chest wall is extremely painful; for example, after thoracic surgery. While the patient exhales, the hands are placed side by side with fingers extended and applying the flat of the palm over the affected chest area. The nurse vibrates the patient's chest by quickly contracting and relaxing the patient's arm and shoulder muscles (Fig. 32.11B). In some critical care units, they use specialized beds that have options to percuss, vibrate, or provide continuous lateral rotation therapy.

Postural Drainage

To be effective, chest physiotherapy should be done with postural drainage, which uses gravity to encourage peripheral pulmonary secretions to empty into the major bronchi

---

BOX 32.8 Contraindications for Chest Physiotherapy

Contraindications for Postural Drainage
- Head injury
- Inability to cough
- Obesity
- Recent eye surgery or injury
- Recent meal or during tube feeding

Contraindications to Percussion/Vibration
- Fractured ribs or an unstable chest wall
- Untreated pneumothorax
- Acute asthma or bronchospasm
- Cervical cord injury
- Tuberculosis
- Osteoporosis
- Active pulmonary bleeding or pulmonary embolus

Postural Drainage Positions

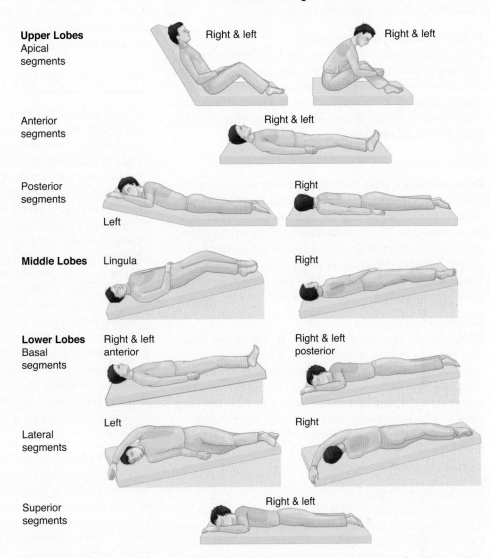

Upper Lobes
Apical segments — Right & left / Right & left

Anterior segments — Right & left

Posterior segments — Left / Right

Middle Lobes — Lingula / Right

Lower Lobes
Basal segments — Right & left anterior / Right & left posterior

Lateral segments — Left / Right

Superior segments — Right & left

Figure 32.12 Various postural drainage positions are used to mobilize secretions from specific lobes and segments of the lung.

or trachea (Fig. 32.12). Secretions drain best with the patient positioned upright so that the bronchi are perpendicular to the floor. Lower and middle lobe bronchi usually empty best with the patient in the head-down position while the upper lobe bronchi in the head-up position. Postural drainage is not indicated for all patients.

Medications

Many respiratory disorders interfere with airway clearance, breathing patterns, and gas exchange. Medications are often used in the management of these disorders. Types of drugs commonly used are anti-inflammatory agents and bronchodilators.

Anti-Inflammatory Agents

Anti-inflammatory agents play an important role in the treatment of respiratory disorders such as asthma or exacerbation of the obstructive lung disease. They are used to reduce the inflammation of the airways. Anti-inflammatory agents include corticosteroids, mast cell stabilizers, and leukotriene receptor antagonists.

Corticosteroids

These agents are the most effective anti-inflammatory agents used to reverse airflow obstruction. They work by suppressing the body's immune system and reducing the inflammation. Corticosteroids can be given orally, by IV, or by inhaler. Hydrocortisone (Solu Cortef), prednisone (Apo-Prednisone), and methylprednisolone (Solu Medrol) may be given intravenously. Prednisone (Apo-Prednisone) is also available by oral route.

Mast Cell Stabilizers

Mast cell stabilizers prevent the release of inflammatory substances that are released with exposure to allergens or other stimuli. These drugs are used prophylactically to prevent airway narrowing after an exposure to an allergen. Sodium cromoglycate (Intal) is taken by inhalation.

Leukotriene Receptor Antagonists

Leukotriene receptor antagonists block inflammatory mediators that cause bronchoconstriction, mucous secretion, and airway swelling. They are used in the management of exercise-induced bronchospasm, asthma, and allergic rhinitis. Montelukast (Singulair) and zafirlukast (Accolate) are given by oral administration.

Bronchodilators

Bronchodilators relax bronchial smooth muscles which dilate the airways. If both bronchodilators and anti-inflammatory drugs are ordered by inhaler, the bronchodilator is given first. The bronchodilator will open the airway, allowing more bronchioles exposed to the anti-inflammatory inhaler. Bronchodilators can be divided into three categories. These are $\beta2$-adrenergic agonists, anticholinergic agents, and methylxanthines.

β2-Adrenergic Agonists

$\beta2$-Adrenergic agonists stimulate the $\beta2$-adrenergic receptors, resulting in bronchodilation. The $\beta1$-adrenergic receptors in the heart may also be stimulated and lead to increased heart rate, hyperactivity, and tremors. These agents are available both orally and by inhaler. Inhaled therapy has been shown to produce comparable bronchodilation and fewer systemic adverse effects. Salbutamol (Ventolin), terbutaline (Bricanyl), and fenoterol (Berotec) are commonly used short-acting $\beta2$-adrenergic agonists.

Anticholinergic Agents

Anticholinergic agents block the action of acetylcholine in the bronchial smooth muscle preventing bronchoconstriction. Ipratropium (Atrovent) and tiotropium (Spiriva) are given by inhalation for maintenance therapy of bronchoconstriction associated with obstructive lung disease.

Administering Oxygen Therapy

The primary indication for oxygen therapy is hypoxemia. Oxygen uptake in the pulmonary capillary beds that surround the alveoli can be improved by increasing the concentration of oxygen in the alveolar air; increasing the partial pressure of oxygen in the alveoli (PaO_2) increases the driving pressure for gas **diffusion** across the alveolar-capillary membrane. The amount of oxygen required depends on the pathophysiological mechanisms affecting the patient's oxygenation status. Once oxygen therapy has been initiated, the patient's respiratory status needs to be continuously assessed. The percentage of oxygen in the inspired air is called the *fraction of inspired oxygen*, or FiO_2, and is expressed as a percentage. Normal atmospheric air has an FiO_2 of 21%. Supplemental oxygen

delivery systems are able to increase the FiO_2 from 24% to 100%. Oxygen, as in the administration of any drug, when administered correctly may be lifesaving, but it is not without complications.

Through the eyes of a patient

*I*t was midafternoon, and I began to feel like I was not getting enough air. I seemed to be breathing more quickly like I was walking fast but I was lying in bed. I had oxygen on and just could not figure out what the problem was with my breathing. One of the nurses came in and asked how I was doing. I told her about my breathing. She said the oxygen would help and left the room.

About 15 minutes later, another nurse came into my room. She asked how I was doing. I told her my breathing was getting more difficult, and I felt like I was sweating by this time. She quickly checked my oxygen level and my oxygen equipment. She noted that although the oxygen prongs were in my nose, somehow the tubing became disconnected and I was not getting any oxygen. The nurse reconnected the tubing and soon, I began to have easier time breathing. She said my oxygen levels were going up. I am thankful that she took the time to check not only that the tubing was in my nose but that the equipment was hooked up properly and working.

(personal reflection of a patient)

Inappropriate dose and failure to monitor treatment can have serious consequences. Although we need oxygen, too much can result in oxygen toxicity. Patients who have pulmonary disease associated with CO_2 retention may become insensitive to CO_2 levels to drive their respiratory rates (Box 32.9). Vigilant monitoring to detect and correct adverse effects swiftly is essential.

Oxygen is supplied in several different ways. In the acute care setting (hospitals) or in long-term care facilities (nursing homes), it is usually piped into wall outlets at the

BOX 32.9 Response to Oxygen Therapy

Carefully monitor your patient's response to oxygen. Recall that the two chemoreceptors in the respiratory centre that control the drive to breathe respond to CO_2 and oxygen. A $PaCO_2$ accumulation in the blood triggers the respiratory drive in healthy people. In a patient with COPD, he or she develops a tolerance for a high $PaCO_2$ level over time, and as a result, the patient's respiratory centre may lose its sensitivity to the chronically elevated $PaCO_2$. Consequently, giving oxygen to this patient could depress the respiratory rate, leading to bradypnea and/or respiratory arrest. Therefore, if oxygen is required by the patient, it is given at the lowest rate needed to oxygenate the patient, as identified by the patient's clinical condition and ABGs.

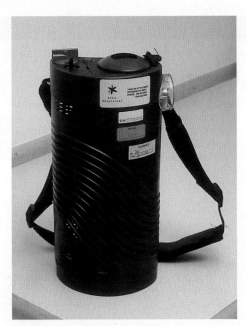

Figure 32.13 Portable oxygen tank.

The Flow Meter

To use an oxygen wall outlet, the nurse needs to attach the flow meter (Fig. 32.14). The flow meter is set to off, and then pressure applied. If there is no humidification bottle being attached, an oxygen nipple (also called a *Christmas tree*) is attached to the base of the flow meter. For the patient who requires humidification of his or her oxygen, a humidifier bottle can be attached to the base of the flow meter.

After the prescribed oxygen tubing and delivery device is attached to the oxygen nipple or the humidification bottle,

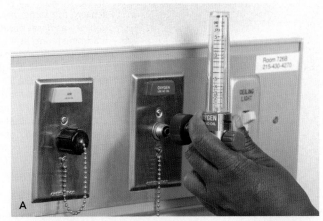

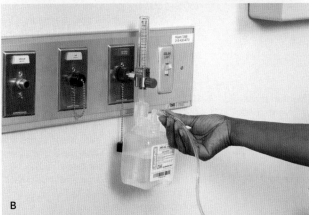

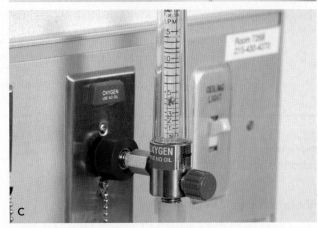

Figure 32.14 **A.** Flow meter inserted into oxygen wall outlet. **B.** Humidification bottle and oxygen tubing attached to flow meter. **C.** Setting the oxygen rate on the flow meter.

patient's bedside, readily available for use at all times. Tanks or cylinders of oxygen that are under pressure are available either when there are no wall outlets or used when a patient on oxygen therapy is being transferred to another area (Fig. 32.13).

Following safety precautions is imperative with oxygen therapy (Box 32.10). Oxygen is a nonflammable, nonexplosive gas. It does not burn; however, it does support combustion, meaning that many materials will ignite more readily in an oxygen-enriched environment.

BOX 32.10 Safety Considerations With Oxygen Therapy

Highly concentrated sources of oxygen promote rapid combustion. Oxygen itself is not flammable, but the addition of concentrated oxygen to a fire greatly increases its intensity and can aid the combustion of materials (e.g., metals) that are relatively inert under normal conditions.

Use "No Smoking, Oxygen in Use" signs to warn visitors not to smoke near the patient.

No open flame or products that are combustible should be permitted when oxygen is in use. These include petroleum jelly, oils, and aerosol sprays.

A spark from a cigarette, electric razor, or other electrical device could easily ignite oxygen-saturated hair or bedclothes around the patient. Explosion-proof plugs should be used for vaporizers and humidifier attachments.

Care must be taken with oxygen equipment used in the hospital. Cylinders should be kept in carts or have collars for safe storage. If not stored in a cart, smaller canisters may be laid on the floor. Knocking cylinders together can cause sparks, so bumping them should be avoided.

TABLE 32.3   Oxygen Delivery Devices and Guidelines for Use

Delivery Device	Oxygen Concentration Administered	Administration Guidelines	Advantages	Disadvantages
Nasal cannula	Low flow 1–6 L/min (24%–44% FiO_2) 1 L/min = 24% 2 L/min = 28% 3 L/min = 32% 4 L/min = 36% 5 L/min = 40% 6 L/min = 44%	– Ensure patency of nostrils with penlight; position prongs in nostrils. – Position the cannula tubing behind the ears and under the chin, sliding the adjuster upward under the chin to secure. – This device can be used with mouth breathers and still achieve the same oxygen delivery as nasal breathers. – If administering at 4 L/min or longer, add humidification.	Easy to apply, disposable, low cost; usually well tolerated by the patient	The cannula can be easily dislodged; causes dryness which can lead to bleeding; and deviated septum can block flow of oxygen.
Simple mask	6–10 L/min (40%–60% FiO_2)	– Ensure the mask is tight fitting on the patient. – Place the mask over the patient's nose, mouth, and chin, and then mold metal edge to the bridge of the nose. – Minimum oxygen flow rate needs to be 6 L or CO_2 will build up in the mask.	Easy to apply; disposable; inexpensive	Poor compliance by patients as the mask is uncomfortable, suffocating to them. The mask must be removed for eating, and nasal cannula may need to be applied to provide supplemental oxygenation. In unconscious patient who vomits, he or she may aspirate his or her emesis as mask blocks vomitus.
Nonrebreathing mask— reservoir mask	6–10 L/min (60%–100%)	Delivers the highest percentage of oxygen without intubation and mechanical ventilation; same as simple mask plus: – Make sure one-way valves are secure and functioning. – Monitor for buildup of CO_2 if valves are not functioning.	Same as simple mask High FiO_2	Same as simple mask; potential suffocation hazard
Venturi mask— venti mask	4–10 L/min (24%–55% concentration of oxygen)	Same as simple mask plus: – Ensure that the proper device is used and the oxygen flow rate is set at the amount specified to deliver the ordered FiO_2.	Same as simple mask Allows for precise concentration administration	Same as simple mask; potential suffocation hazard
Face tent	4–8 L/min (30%–50% concentration of oxygen)	Same as simple mask	Used when masks are poorly tolerated by the patient	Frequently inspect facial skin for dampness or chafing. The face needs to be kept dry.
Oxygen tent	Tent delivers approximately 30% concentration of oxygen	The tent needs to be filled with oxygen first. This is done by setting the flow meter at 15 L/min for approximately 5 minutes. Then, it is adjusted to the ordered rate (10–15 L/min)	Used for the pediatric population; the child may be able to tolerate oxygen provided by an oxygen tent.	The tent needs to be cooled because it can become very warm. The child needs to be covered with a gown or blanket to prevent chilling and dampness for the condensation that builds in the tent.

the flow meter is turned to the ordered level of oxygen, indicated by the line in the middle of the ball.

Methods of Delivery

Oxygen therapy can be delivered by many different devices. Table 32.3 describes the various oxygen devices. Common problems with these devices include system leaks and obstructions, device displacement, and skin irritation. These devices are classified as either low-flow or high-flow systems. Figure 32.15 illustrates various types of oxygen devices. Administration of oxygen is outlined in Skill 32.1.

Low-Flow Systems

A low-flow oxygen delivery system provides supplemental oxygen at less than or equal to 8 L/min. These devices result

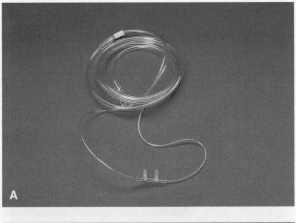
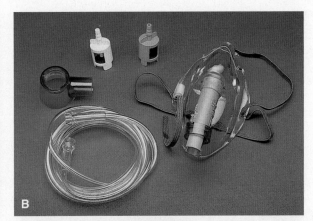
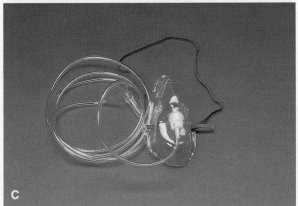
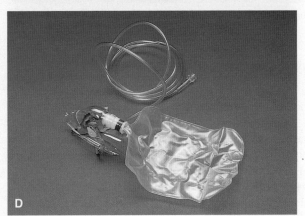

Figure 32.15 Oxygen devices.

in variable FiO_2 as the inspired oxygen is mixed with room air. The patient's ventilation pattern will also affect the FiO_2. As the patient's respiratory pattern changes, the inspired oxygen concentration varies because of differing amounts of room air gas that is mixing with the constant flow of oxygen from the device. Low-flow systems include nasal cannula, simple oxygen mask, partial rebreathing mask with reservoir bag, and nonrebreathing mask with reservoir bag.

Think

To Use or Not Use the Prongs

Often, patients require oxygen per nasal prongs throughout the day. When patients go to the bathroom, they remove their oxygen and the tubing with the nasal prongs ends up on the floor. When patients return to bed, they are short of breath. They retrieve the nasal prongs and put them into their nares.

Some may think that the patient using the nasal prongs that have been on the floor is not a problem. Some may feel that because the patient only has to walk a short distance to the bathroom that being without the oxygen would be okay.

There are two distinct problems in this situation that often occurs in a hospital unit. One is the contamination of the nasal prongs from being on the floor. This is an infection control issue. When nasal prongs are removed, they should be placed in a bag to keep them clean for the patient. A bigger problem is that that patient has not been provided extension tubing to ensure that he or she is able to reach the bathroom and still be supplied with his or her oxygen source.

Reservoir Systems

A reservoir system is a device to collect and store oxygen between breaths. The patient is able to draw from the reservoir of oxygen to meet his or her inspiratory volume needs. Although the reservoir system can deliver a higher FiO_2 than a low-flow system, there is still a mixing of the inspired oxygen with room air. Reservoir systems include simple face masks, partial rebreathing masks, and nonrebreathing masks.

With a high-flow system, the FiO_2 of oxygen delivered to the patient is exact. It is not affected by the patient's ventilatory pattern. A high-flow system includes the Venturi mask, also known as the *venti mask*.

Oxygen Therapy for a Patient With a Tracheostomy

A patient with a tracheostomy requires constant humidification to the airway with a tracheostomy collar. The tracheostomy bypasses the normal filtering and humidification process of the nose and mouth. This collar is curved and has straps that adjust to fit around the patient's neck (Fig. 32.16). The two ports include an exhalation port that must remain patent at all times, the other port connects to the oxygen source, with the flow rate set at 10 L/min. The tubing is connected to a humidification device to provide humidified air to the lower airways via the tracheostomy tube opening.

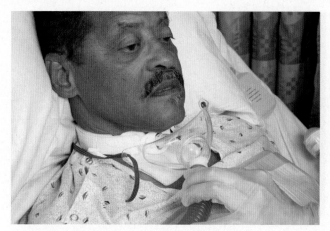

Figure 32.16 Tracheostomy Shield for Oxygenation

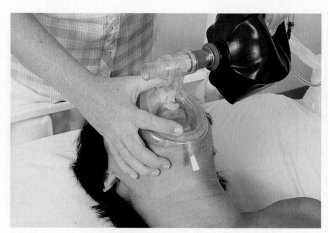

Figure 32.17 Self-inflating bag-valve-device (Ambu Bag)

Oxygen Toxicity

The most detrimental effect of breathing a high concentration of oxygen is the development of oxygen toxicity. It can occur in any patient breathing oxygen concentrations of greater than 50% for more than 24 hours. Patients most likely to develop oxygen toxicity are those who require high oxygen concentrations for extended periods.

Hyperoxia, or the administration of high oxygen concentrations, produces free radicals. These radicals are responsible for the initial damage to the alveolar-capillary membrane. Oxygen free radicals are toxic metabolites of oxygen metabolism. The end result is damage to the lung tissue and vasculature, resulting in the initiation of a critical lung issue referred to as *adult respiratory distress syndrome* (ARDS). In Box 32.11 are the clinical manifestations of oxygen toxicity and guidelines for prevention.

Manual Ventilation

Manual resuscitation is typically used in an emergency situation such as respiratory or cardiopulmonary arrest. A self-inflating bag-valve device commonly referred to as

an *Ambu bag* (Fig. 32.17) may be attached to a face mask, endotracheal tube, or a tracheostomy to allow manual delivery of oxygen to the patient. The Ambu bag's tubing is connected to the nipple or Christmas tree adapter on the oxygen flow meter. The mask must be tightly fitted around the patient's nose and mouth. Effective bag-valve device ventilation requires adequate training and frequent practice.

The volume of air that passes in and out of the lungs with a single inspiratory/expiratory cycle is referred to as **tidal volume**. The force of squeezing the bag determines the amount of tidal volume the patient will receive. When using an Ambu bag, the nurse should squeeze the bag to deliver enough volume to produce a chest rise. This is generally 6 to 7 ml/kg over 1 minute. Giving the patient more tidal volume will increase the risk of gastric distention.

When delivering breaths with this device, it is important to allow time for complete exhalation to prevent air trapping, which may cause hypotension, and increase the risk for barotrauma, especially in those patients with obstructive airway disease.

BOX 32.11   Oxygen Toxicity

Clinical Manifestations Associated With Oxygen Toxicity
- Substernal chest pain exaggerated with deep breathing
- Dyspnea
- Nasal stuffiness
- Sore throat
- Eye and ear discomforts
- Damage to type II alveolar cells responsible for the production of surfactant

Guidelines to Prevent Oxygen Toxicity
- Limit use of 100% oxygen to brief periods.
- As early as possible, reduce FiO$_2$ to lowest possible level to maintain oxygenation.

Mechanical Ventilation

Mechanical ventilation uses a ventilator machine to move oxygen into the patient's lungs. Ventilators are classified as either negative pressure ventilators or positive pressure ventilators. Indications for mechanical ventilation may include acute respiratory failure such as pneumonia or pulmonary embolism, respiratory centre depression such as stroke or brain trauma, and neuromuscular disturbances such as spinal cord injury or Guillain-Barré syndrome.

Negative pressure ventilators include the iron lung, the cuirass, and the body wrap. These types of ventilators pull the thorax outward and allow the air to flow into the lungs (Fig. 32.18). They work on a similar principle to how we take spontaneous breaths.

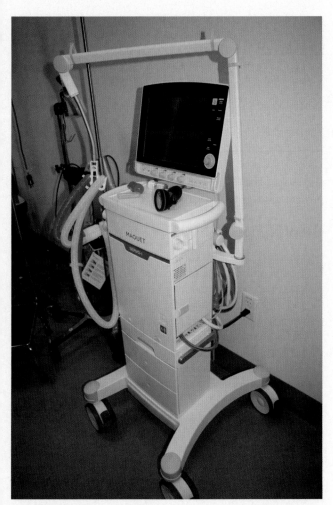

Figure 32.18 Positive pressure ventilator.

Positive pressure ventilators are categorized as volume or pressure ventilators and have various modes. These types of ventilators exert a positive pressure on the airway that forces the air into the lungs.

Caring for a patient who requires mechanical ventilation requires extensive training. Detailed information regarding nursing interventions and specific ventilator settings is a topic covered in critical care and advanced practice courses.

Noninvasive Positive Pressure Ventilation

Noninvasive positive pressure ventilation (NPPV) refers to positive pressure ventilation delivered through a noninvasive measures (nasal mask, facemask, or nasal plugs) rather than an invasive measure, such as an endotracheal tube or tracheostomy. The modes of ventilation for NPPV most commonly used are continuous positive airway pressure (CPAP) or bilevel positive airway pressure (BiPAP).

CPAP provides constant low-flow pressure into the airways to hold the airways open and mobilize secretions. BiPAP delivers a different pressure during inspiration and expiration. NPPV may be used for such conditions as sleep apnea, hypercapnic acidosis, cardiogenic pulmonary edema, and hypoxemic respiratory failure.

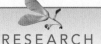

RESEARCH

OBSTRUCTIVE SLEEP APNEA

Obstructive sleep apnea (OSA) affects many Canadians. Although it can be easily diagnosed and treated, the problem is most people aren't aware they have it. Sleep apnea is an involuntary cessation of breathing during sleep.

There are three types of sleep apnea: obstructive, central, and mixed. OSA occurs when the patient's breathing efforts are intact, but air movement is blocked by a temporary obstruction. Central sleep apnea is characterized by the absence of any breathing effort and is associated with brain disease rather than airway blockage. Mixed sleep apnea combines characteristics of both central and OSA types. OSA is the most common.

Most people with OSA are obese individuals. As they gain weight and their necks become thicker, the result is excess tissue in the back of the throat that narrows the airway and limits the amount of air that can pass through. OSA is increasingly being recognized as an important risk factor in cardiovascular and cerebrovascular diseases.

Study

In a recent prospective longitudinal cohort study, 105 patients who presented with a ST-segment elevation myocardial infarction (STEMI) underwent an overnight sleep study during their admission. The study found that 42% of the patients who presented with a STEMI had severe OSA and 61 (58%) nonsevere OSA. After adjusting for age and body mass index, severe OSA remains an independent predictor of adverse events at 18 months follow-up.

The present study is the first report on the association of untreated severe OSA with long-term clinical outcomes in patients admitted for STEMI. They demonstrate that the adverse event rate in patients with severe OSA is 5 times as high as in those without severe OSA.

Implications to Practice

The physiological impact of disrupted breathing and sleep patterns and how, over time, physical changes occur in the body that specifically affect the heart and either exacerbate existing heart disease or contribute to new-onset heart disease.

From this study and others on OSA, there are major implications for nursing. Asking patients about their breathing and sleep patterns at night is important in assessing patients who may be experiencing OSA. It is concerning that a common modifiable risk factor for cardiac disease (sleep apnea) remains largely underdiagnosed and undertreated in clinical practice. Valid OSA assessment is an important part of a nursing comprehensive assessment of modifiable risk factors for patients.

Lee, C. H., Khoo, S. M., Chan, M. Y., Wong, H. B., Low, A. F., Phua, Q. H., . . . Yeo, T. C. (2011). *Severe obstructive sleep apnea and outcomes following myocardial infarction.* Journal of Clinical Sleep Medicine, 7(6), 616–621.

Oxygen Saturation Monitoring With Pulse Oximetry

Pulse oximetry is a simple procedure used to noninvasively monitor arterial oxygen saturation. Performed either intermittently or continuously, based on the patient's need or situation, it can provide an early and immediate warning of impending hypoxemia. Oxygen saturation is an indicator of the percentage of hemoglobin saturated with oxygen. The reading is obtained from a pulse oximeter device that uses a light sensor that contains two sources of light (red and infrared) absorbed by hemoglobin and transmitted through tissues to a photodetector. Pulse oximetry was covered in Chapter 21, Measuring Vital Signs.

Through the eyes of a student

When I entered my patient's room, he told me he was having some difficulty breathing but not any worse than other mornings. I started my assessment with his vital signs. As I was taking the patient's blood pressure and heart rate, his shortness of breath seemed to be increasing. I felt it was important to get the pulse oximetry reading. I found a nurse using the equipment and explained my patient's assessment findings. The nurse immediately brought the pulse oximeter to my patient's room. The reading was 85%. The physician was called and oxygen therapy was ordered. Assessing my patient's change in status and the need for obtaining further information impacted my patient's outcome.

(personal reflection of a nursing student)

Artificial Airways

An artificial airway is inserted to establish and maintain a patent airway. Assessing a patient's airway and maintaining a patent airway requires attentive patient care. Four common types of airways include oropharyngeal, nasopharyngeal, endotracheal, and tracheostomy. The selection of the appropriate artificial airway is important not only to maintain the

TABLE 32.4	Oral and Nasopharyngeal Airway Sizes	
Size of Patient	Size of Oral Airway	Size of Nasopharyngeal Airway
Large adult	5	8–9
Medium adult	4	7–8
Small adult	3	6–7

airway but also to maximize therapeutic interventions and prevent damage to the patient's own airway.

Oropharyngeal Airway

Oropharyngeal airways (oral airways) are usually made of a hard-curved disposable plastic. The airway is only placed in patients who are unconscious, as the device will stimulate the gag reflex, and increase the risk of vomiting and aspiration in a semiconscious or conscious patient.

Oral airways are manufactured in various lengths and widths for adults, children, and infants; sizing depends on the age and size of the patient (Table 32.4). If the airway is too small, it can cause airway obstruction, or if too large, the tongue may be displaced against the oropharynx. Oral airways are used to facilitate suctioning of the pharynx and prevent patients from biting their tongues. In the intubated patient, the oral airway acts as a bite block, preventing the patient from biting and occluding the endotracheal tube.

One way to select the appropriate size is to measure the airway by placing the flange alongside the patient's lips and the oral airway tip alongside the angle of the jaw (Fig. 32.19). Improper insertion can results in tooth damage or laceration to the roof of the mouth, lips, or tongue. It is important to remember that an oral airway should never be placed in a patient who is actively having a seizure.

Nasopharyngeal Airway

Nasopharyngeal airways have three parts: the flange, cannula, and bevel tip (Fig. 32.20). The flange is often referred to as the trumpet for its wide trumpetlike end that prevents

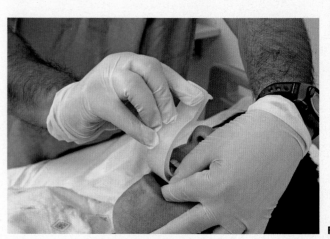

A

Figure 32.19 Measuring the oropharyngeal airway **(A)** and insertion **(B)**.

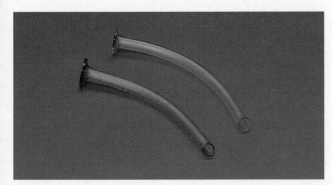

Figure 32.20 Nasopharyngeal airways.

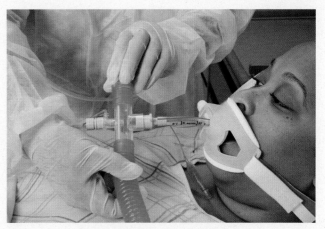

Figure 32.22 ET tube attached to ventilator tubing.

further slippage into the airway. The hollow shaft of the cannula permits airflow into the hypopharynx. The tip is the distal opening of the tube.

The external diameter of the nasopharyngeal airway should be slightly smaller than the patient's external nares opening. The length of the nasopharyngeal airway is determined by measuring the distance between the naris and the tragus of the ear. Nasopharyngeal airway sizing is shown in Table 32.4. An improper size may result in increased airway resistance and mucosal trauma. If the airway is too small, there will be limited airway flow. A too large airway may result in gastric distention, gagging, and vomiting.

Nasopharyngeal airways are used to facilitate tracheobronchial secretions by directing the catheter to the hypopharynx. This can be used in a conscious patient who requires frequent suctioning to clear secretions. The nasopharyngeal airway decreases mucosal trauma during the suctioning.

Endotracheal Tube

Endotracheal (ET) tubes are used to maintain a patent airway or to facilitate mechanical ventilation (Fig. 32.21). ET tubes bypass the upper airway structures altogether; they may be inserted via the nose or mouth. Because ET tubes prevent effective coughing, they necessitate periodic removal of pulmonary secretions with suctioning.

ET intubation can be done either nasally or orally. Nasal intubation is contraindicated in patients with facial trauma or suspected fractures at the base of the skull or postcranial surgeries. Nasal intubation is associated with increased risk for sinusitis and the development of ventilator-associated pneumonia (VAP). Figure 32.22 illustrates the intubated patient attached to the ventilator.

Because ET tubes bypass the filtration and humidification normally provided by the nose and oropharynx, care must be taken to humidify the inspired air and to prevent introduction of pathogenic organisms into the lung.

Oral care must be provided every 2 to 4 hours to the patient who is intubated. Patients who are intubated, especially for more than 24 hours, have an increased risk for VAP. It is thought that VAP is related to aspiration of gastric or oral secretions and bacteria related to dental plaque. Evidence-based research on VAP is outlined in Box 32.12. A special ET tube called a *subglottic endotracheal tube* to prevent VAP is illustrated in Figure 32.23.

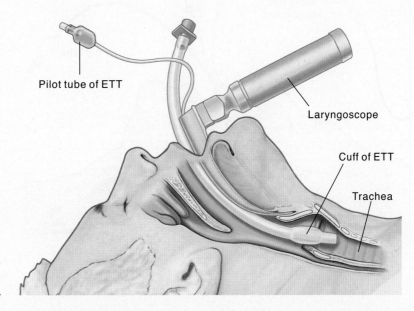

Pilot tube of ETT

Laryngoscope

Cuff of ETT

Trachea

Figure 32.21 ET tube.

BOX 32.12 Evidence-Based Bundles to Reduce Risks for Ventilator-Associated Pneumonia

Background

Ventilator-associated pneumonia (VAP) is defined as an airway infection that develops more than 48 hours after the patient is intubated. Reducing mortality due to VAP requires an organized process that guarantees early recognition of pneumonia and consistent application of the best evidence-based practices.

The ventilator bundle is a series of interventions related to ventilator care that, when implemented together, will achieve significantly better outcomes than when implemented individually.

The key components of the ventilator bundle are as follows:

- Elevation of the head of the bed
- Daily sedation vacations and assessment of readiness to extubate
- Peptic ulcer disease prophylaxis
- Deep venous thrombosis prophylaxis
- Daily oral care with chlorhexidine
- ET tubes that are designed to provide subglottic suction

A. Elevation of the Head of the Bed

The recommended elevation is 30° to 45°. Elevating the head of the bed is an integral part of the ventilator bundle. It is not completely clear whether raising the head of the bed decreases the risk of aspiration of gastrointestinal contents or secretions from the oral or nasal cavities. Elevating the head of the bed unless contraindicated also improves the patient's ventilatory efforts and decreases atelectasis.

B. Daily Sedation Vacations With Assessment of Readiness to Extubate

Reducing the sedation decreases the amount of time spent on mechanical ventilation and, therefore, the risk of VAP. When patients are under less sedation, it becomes easier to wean them from the ventilator. Patients are more awake to cough, deep breathe, and mobilize secretions when they are extubated.

Sedation vacations are not without risks, however. Patients who are not sedated as deeply will have an increased potential for self-extubation. Therefore, the maneuver must be conducted in a careful fashion.

C. Peptic Ulcer Disease Prophylaxis

Patients who are critically ill can have a higher incidence of stress ulcers due to the physiological and psychological stress that they are under. Aspiration of the acidic gastric contents may result in a worsening pneumonia or pneumonitis.

D. Deep Venous Thrombosis Prophylaxis

Applying deep vein thrombosis (DVT) prophylaxis to all sedentary patients is very important. The risk of venous thromboembolism is reduced if prophylaxis is consistently applied.

E. Daily Oral Care With Chlorhexidine

Dental plaque biofilms are colonized by respiratory pathogens in mechanically ventilated patients. Dental plaque develops in patients who are mechanically ventilated because of the lack of mechanical chewing and the absence of saliva, which minimizes the development of biofilm on the teeth. Dental plaque can be a significant reservoir for potential respiratory pathogens that cause VAP. Chlorhexidine antiseptic has long been approved as an inhibitor of dental plaque formation and gingivitis.

F. Subglottic Suction

By microaspiration along the cuff, contaminated secretions can pass into the lower respiratory tract and can become a potential cause of lower airway infection including VAP. ET tubes modified to permit continuous subglottic suctioning have been shown to decrease the incidence of VAP.

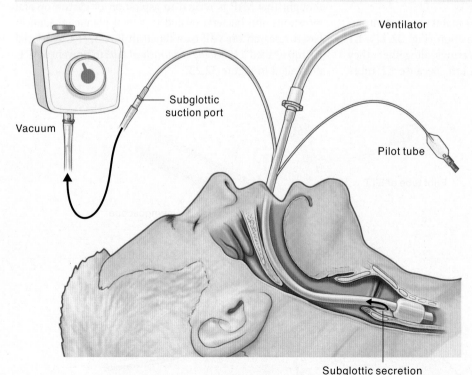

Figure 32.23 Subglottic ET tube suction.

Ventilator

Subglottic suction port

Vacuum

Pilot tube

Subglottic secretion

Tracheostomy Tubes

Tracheostomy refers to a surgical procedure an incision is made below the cricoid cartilage through the second to fourth tracheal rings. *Tracheostomy* refers to the opening (or stoma) made by the incision. The tracheostomy tube is the artificial airway that is inserted to keep the stoma open. A stoma that is less than 48 hours old has not fully formed a tract. If the tracheostomy tube is dislodged, the stoma may close and the patient will not have an open airway. For this reason, when providing tracheostomy care on a patient with a fresh tracheostomy, the nurse should have assistance.

A tracheostomy tube is different from an ET tube in that it has an outer cannula, a flange, and an inner cannula. The outer cannula forms the body of the tracheostomy tube. The flange is attached to the outer cannula and assists in stabilizing the tube in the trachea. The inner cannula, which can be removed for easy cleaning, inserts inside the outer cannula. During insertion, an obturator replaces the inner cannula. Its smooth surface minimizes tracheal trauma. When the tracheostomy tube is inserted, the obturator is removed and replaced by the inner cannula that is then locked into place. A same-size tracheostomy tube should be available at the bedside for emergency replacement in case of accidental dislodgement of the tube. Figure 32.24 illustrates the parts of the uncuffed tracheostomy tube.

A tracheostomy tube may have a cuff, which is a balloon inflated with air to maintain a seal around the tube. A cuffed tube is appropriate for patients who need mechanic ventilation or for whom aspiration is a risk. The cuff limits aspiration of oral and gastric secretions. Children's trachea are small enough that they generally do not require a cuffed tube. Figure 32.25 illustrates the cuffed tracheostomy tube.

A fenestrated tracheostomy tube allows a patient to speak. The tube has an opening in the curvature of the posterior wall of the cannula. The matching fenestrated inner cannula is inserted into the outer cannula (Fig. 32.26). The patient can communicate when he or she occludes (cover or close) the tracheostomy tube opening with his or her finger or with the use of a speaking valve called a *Passy-Muir valve* (Fig. 32.27).

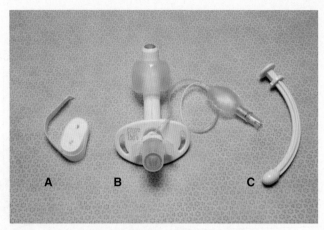

Figure 32.25 Cuffed tracheostomy tube.

Increased Risk of Infection

A tracheostomy tube is a foreign to the body, and the body responds by increasing secretion production. The tracheostomy bypasses the upper airway and its protective and hydrating mechanisms. This puts the patient with a tracheostomy at increased risk for infection. The secretions become thick, which increases the risk for occlusion of the inner cannula. Tracheostomy patients should receive humidified air or oxygen and scheduled tracheostomy care as per the organization's policy, or more frequently as required by the patient. Skill 32.2 outlines the steps for tracheostomy care.

Interventions to Promote Airway Clearance

Administration of supplemental oxygen provides a sufficient concentration of inspired oxygen to permit full use of the oxygen-carrying capacity of the arterial blood to ensure adequate tissue perfusion. At the same time, interventions are required to promote airway clearance. These interventions focus on clearing the airways of secretions, relieving

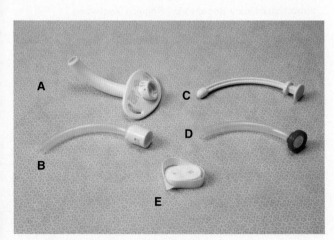

Figure 32.24 Uncuffed tracheostomy tube.

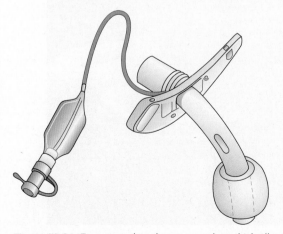

Figure 32.26 Fenestrated tracheostomy tube, which allows the patient to talk.

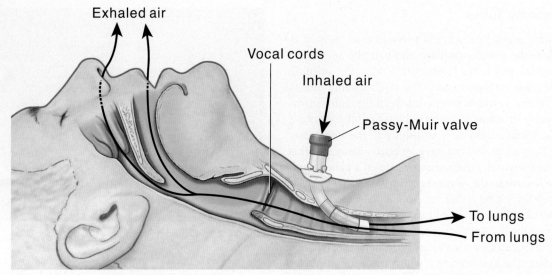

Figure 32.27 Speaking valve (Passy-Muir valve).

bronchospasm, and, when necessary, bypassing the natural airway structures with an artificial airway.

The Yankauer

The Yankauer (tonsillar tip), suction device made of rigid plastic, can be used for oral pharyngeal suctioning (Fig. 32.28). The Yankauer is angled to facilitate removal of pharyngeal secretions through the mouth, particularly useful in removing copious amounts of secretions such as emesis. The Yankauer is only an oral suction catheter and because of its size is not used to suction the nares. The steps for using a Yankauer suctioning catheter are outlined in Skill 32.3.

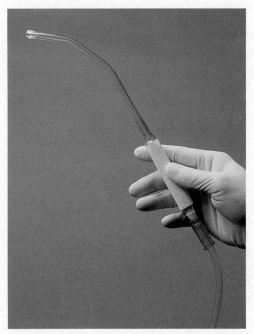

Figure 32.28 Yankauer suction catheter to clear oral cavity of excess secretions.

Nasopharyngeal and Oropharyngeal Suctioning

Nasopharyngeal and oropharyngeal suctioning maintains a patent airway by removing secretions from the pharynx (or throat) and the trachea. This procedure helps maintain a patent airway to promote optimal exchange of oxygen and CO_2 and to prevent pneumonia that results from pooling of secretions. The clinical indications and complications of suctioning are listed in Box 32.13. Suctioning is paramount for the removal of secretions and maintaining a patent airway; however, it is not without potential complications and should only be done when needed and never longer than 10 to 15 seconds in duration.

Nasopharyngeal and oropharyngeal suctioning is used when suctioning with a Yankauer device is ineffective or when the lower airway requires removal of secretions. This type of suctioning involves inserting a suction catheter into

BOX 32.13 Indications and Complications of Suctioning

Indications That a Patient May Require Suctioning
- Visual observation of secretions in the airway
- Determination of the presence of secretions by chest auscultation
- Coughing
- Deterioration of the patient's oxygenation as noted by his or her oxygen saturation level

Complications of Suctioning
- Hypoxemia
- Cardiac arrhythmias
- Vagal nerve stimulation resulting in bradycardia and hypotension
- Increased intracranial pressure
- Trauma to the mucosal membrane resulting in bleeding
- Nosocomial infection

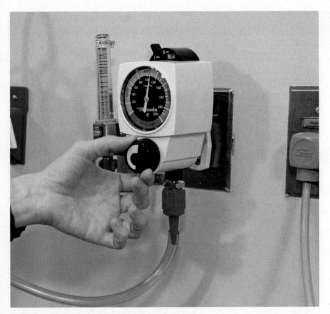

Figure 32.29 Adjusting wall suction.

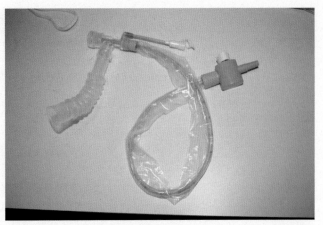

Figure 32.30 In-line suction catheter (Closed suctioning system)

the nares to the pharynx or through the mouth into the trachea. Negative pressure is then applied to suction out the secretions (Fig. 32.29). See Table 32.5 for choosing the appropriate size of suction catheter and amount of suction based on the patient's age.

The major differences between pharyngeal and tracheal suctioning are the depth suctioned and the potential for complications. Pharyngeal suctioning only removes secretions from the back of the throat and requires clean technique (see Chapter 20). Tracheal suctioning extends into the lower airway and necessitates aseptic technique. Skill 32.4 outlines the steps for performing nasopharyngeal and oropharyngeal suctioning.

Endotracheal Tube Suctioning

A patient who is intubated will require suctioning of the ET tube only when clinically indicated. Suctioning of the ET tube is generally performed by the closed-suction method

(also called *in-line suctioning*) (Fig. 32.30). The closed-suction technique allows for the maintenance of oxygenation and ventilation. This technique decreases the risk for spreading of tracheal secretion with suction-induced coughing. Normal saline is used to clear the suction tubing. The steps for closed suctioning technique are outlined in Skill 32.5.

Tracheostomy Tube Suctioning

Suctioning of the tracheostomy tube can be performed with the closed in-line suction method described in Skill 32.5. This method is primarily used when the patient is on a ventilator. A second method is the open-suction technique. As with an ET tube, the patient should only be suctioned when it is clinically indicated. Adequate hydration and humidification is necessary for the patient to assist with keeping the secretions thinned. Instillation of a bolus of normal saline solution into the tracheostomy or ET tube does not thin secretions. It contributes to lower airway contamination, irritation of the bronchial tree, and decreased oxygenation.

Now that Jason has learned about oxygenation, the various assessments, and modes of treatment, he feels more confident in caring for Mr. Pipe. Jason recognizes that he needs to establish interventions that will maintain a patent airway, improve the patient's ease and comfort in breathing, as well as maintain ventilation and oxygenation. Priority nursing diagnoses that Jason has established include Ineffective Breathing Pattern, Impaired Gas Exchange, and Ineffective Airway Clearance. From the readings, Jason realizes that his nursing interventions will include respiratory assessment; implementing measures to clear secretions, such as incentive spirometer; initiating oxygen therapy per physician's orders; administering medications as ordered; and maintaining a healthy breathing pattern through pursed-lip breathing. Jason is excited to learn more about the care of a patient with oxygenation condition and put his knowledge into practice.

TABLE 32.5	Suction Catheters and Vacuum Setting
Age	Size of Catheter (French)
Infants	5–8
Children	8–10
Adult	12–18
Vacuum Setting	**Wall Suction**
Infants	50–95 mmHg
Children	95–110 mmHg
Adults	100–120 mmHg

SKILL 32.1   Oxygen Administration

Reviewing Pertinent Information

Step	Rationale
Assess patient's respiratory status including pulse oximetry or ABGs if available.	Important to know why the patient is to receive supplemental oxygen
Verify written order for oxygen therapy, including methods of delivery and flow rate.	Oxygen is a drug, and its use must be ordered by a physician. Oxygen delivered by nasal cannula, mask, or venture mask is expressed in litres per minute (L/min).

Preparing for Implementation

Step	Rationale
Wash hands.	Prevents the spread of microorganisms to the supplies being used and handled and prevents further spread to the patient
Gather supplies needed: • Gloves • Supplemental oxygen device • Oxygen flow meter to attach to wall oxygen outlet or portable oxygen tank • Oxygen humidifier, if required	Important to get organized prior to administering oxygen to the patient Organization can save valuable time for the patient requiring oxygen and prevent deterioration in the patient's condition.
Prepare the equipment: • Check functioning of oxygen wall outlet or portable tank.	Wall outlets are sealed by heavy steel valves that prevent the escape of oxygen from the system. If you hear hissing from the valve, the flow meter is not fully engaged. Ensuring the portable tank is functioning and is filled with oxygen is important to prevent a loss of oxygen delivery to the patient.
• If humidification is used, remove the cover from the humidifier bottle to expose the adapter that connects the bottle to the flow meter. Attach the bottle to the flow meter by screwing the plastic nut on the adapter to the threaded outlet of the flow meter.	If long-term oxygen therapy is anticipated, if the flow is 6 L/min or higher, or if drying of the respiratory mucosa and/or thick secretions are present, humidification of oxygen is indicated. Short-term and/or low-flow oxygen use, such as during a clinical procedure, may not require humidification.
• Attach oxygen tubing to the port on the humidifier bottle or the "Christmas tree" end of the nipple adapter. Turn on oxygen flow by turning the thumbscrew (wall outlet) or knob (tank).	Establishes proper functioning of equipment. If humidifier bottle is used, bubbling of oxygen through the bottle will be noted. In addition, verify flow by feeling for the flow of air from the oxygen tubing.
Prepare the patient: • Verify the correct patient with two identifiers.	Prior to performing a procedure, the nurse should ensure the correct identification of the patient for the intended intervention to reduce error.
• Explain to the patient and family the reason for supplemental oxygenation.	This communication evaluates and reinforces teaching. Patients who are more knowledgeable about the process are usually more comfortable asking questions.
• Instruct patient and family that oxygen increases the risk of fire. Even though smoking is not allowed in any organization, the importance of no combustibles around oxygen is important. Check that all electrical equipment in use in the room has been inspected for electrical safety.	Teaching can provide the necessary understanding that will foster more effective outcomes through patient participation. Explanation reduces anxiety. Oxygen, although not itself flammable, makes fires burn more readily than they otherwise would, so strict safety must be enforced. Faulty electrical equipment may produce sparks that could ignite materials nearby.
• Assess the patient for obstruction of the nasal passages by observing breathing patterns and inspecting nasal passages with a penlight. Notify physician if significant obstruction is present.	If nasal passages are obstructed, oxygen delivery by nasal cannula will be ineffective, and another route should be chosen.

Administering Oxygen

Step	Rationale
1. Put on gloves. – Gloves need to be applied when checking patency of nasal passages.	Gloves will protect the patient from surface organisms from the nurse's hands and will protect the nurse from possible body secretions that may come into contact with the nurse's hands during the administration procedure.
2. Adjust flow rate to the prescribed amount.	As for any drug, correct dosing of oxygen is essential. Both insufficient and excessive amounts can be harmful to the patient.
3. Apply supplemental oxygen device on the patient. If applying oxygen per nasal prongs, point the curves of prongs toward the floor of the nostril.	Directs the flow of oxygen into the nasal cavity where it will mix with inspired room air
4. If applying nasal cannula, loop the cannula tubing over the patient's ears; adjust the fit of the tubing by sliding the adjust cuff upward to hold the cannula in place. If applying supplemental oxygen with a strap, adjust the strap around the patient's head. The strap should fit securely around the middle of the head.	The strapping of the supplemental oxygen device should be secured but not so tight to cause skin breakdown behind or above the ears or at the back of the scalp.
5. Assess the patient's nares, face, ears, and scalp every 4 hours for signs of skin irritation or breakdown. At the same time, inspect the nasal prongs or mask device for the presence of secretions that may need to be wiped down.	Pressure from the tubing, cannula or mask, may cause skin breakdown. Accumulation of secretions can impair the flow of oxygen.

Engaging in Evaluation

Step	Rationale
1. Observe for decreased anxiety, improved level of consciousness, decreased fatigue, absence of dizziness, improved vital signs, and oxygen saturation.	Provides assessment of effectiveness of interventions
2. Monitor ABG levels or oxygen saturation using pulse oximetry.	Documents patient's level of oxygenation
3. Observe patient's nares and nasal mucous membranes and check back of ears or back of head for skin breakdown.	Oxygen therapy can cause drying of nasal mucosa and skin breakdown where the delivery device comes in contact with the face, ears, and back of head.

Documenting Effectively

Step	Rationale
Document in a timely manner and include the following: – Date and time – Patient and family education – Respiratory and vital signs assessment before and after supplemental oxygen	Documentation is the key communicative method between health-care professionals.

SKILL 32.2   Tracheostomy Care

Preparing for Tracheostomy Care

Step	Rationale
1. Observe signs that tracheostomy care needs to be performed; signs may include loose or soiled dressing or wet ties from excessive secretions.	Soiled or moist dressings may be a medium for microorganisms.
	Loose dressings are unsafe because the tracheostomy tube may become dislodged.
2. Suction tracheostomy.	Suctioning clears tracheostomy tube of secretions and prevents clogging of the tube when removing inner cannula.
3. Remove old dressing and dispose of soiled dressing material and used catheter.	Disposing of soiled dressing and suction catheter in waste receptacle reduces spread of microorganisms.
4. Organize equipment for tracheostomy dressing, cannula, and tie change:	Organization of equipment in advance ensures efficient procedure.

4. Organize equipment for tracheostomy dressing, cannula, and tie change:
Hydrogen peroxide
Sterile normal saline
Three to four sterile 4 × 4 gauze sponges
Two long-handled cotton swabs
Fresh sterile tracheostomy dressing
Two sterile basins
Small sterile brush
Twill tape approximately 60–75 cm long
Sterile gloves
Sterile inner cannula, correctly sized to patient
Scissors
- Open sterile tracheostomy kit using sterile technique to develop sterile field.
- Open three sterile 4 × 4 gauze sponges and place within tracheostomy kit field.
- Open sterile basin(s) and place on sterile field; add hydrogen peroxide to one, saline to the other using sterile pouring technique.
- Dampen one 4 × 4 with sterile hydrogen peroxide, dampen one 4 × 4 with sterile saline, and leave one 4 × 4 dry.
- Cut ties on diagonal and lay aside on clean area.
- Open two long-handled cotton swabs and dampen one with saline and the other with hydrogen peroxide.
   Open sterile brush and place onto sterile field.
   Open sterile disposable or nondisposable inner cannula and place on sterile field.

Apply sterile gloves.
Remove oxygen source, keeping it close by.

Tracheostomy suctioning is a sterile procedure.
Oxygen will need to be removed in order to perform tracheostomy change, but oxygen should be kept in close proximity to patient to ensure adequate oxygenation during procedure.

Stabilize tracheostomy tube at all times during procedure.

To prevent discomfort to patient or accidental dislodgement

Disposable cannula removal and reinsertion:
- Touching only the outer aspect of the tracheostomy, withdraw old inner cannula and dispose in receptacle.
- Replace with new cannula.
- Ensure cannula locks in place.
- Using hydrogen peroxide–soaked swabs and one 4 × 4 gauze, clean around the outer cannula and surrounding skin, working outward in a circular motion, extending to ~5–10 cm around stoma.

Hydrogen peroxide cleanses the secretions from the stoma site and prevents microbial growth.

- Repeat earlier process using saline-soaked cotton swabs and 4 × 4 gauze.

Rinses skin surface of hydrogen peroxide

- Using dry 4 × 4 gauze, dry outer surfaces of tracheostomy and surrounding skin.

Drying prevents growth of microorganisms.

- Reapply oxygen source.

To ensure adequate oxygenation is maintained

Reviewing Pertinent Information

Step	Rationale
Nondisposable cannula reinsertion:	
• Place tracheostomy collar or oxygen source near to outer cannula.	To ensure adequate oxygenation is maintained
• Touching only the outer aspect of the tracheostomy, withdraw old inner cannula and drop into hydrogen peroxide basin.	This action initiates the cleansing process.
• Maintain oxygen source during cleansing of inner cannula.	To ensure adequate oxygenation is maintained
• Quickly clean inner cannula with scrub brush with peroxide solution; rinse with normal saline (using nondominant hand to pour saline).	Scrubbing action provides mechanical force to aid cleansing of debris and microorganisms.
• Replace inner cannula ensuring it is locked in place.	Ensures safety and security
• Reapply oxygen source.	
Resecure tracheostomy with ties (applies to both disposable and nondisposable procedures).	Ensures tracheostomy is secured/prevents dislodgement
• If two persons are present, have one secure the tracheostomy tube while the other threads the ties through the faceplate of the tracheostomy.	It is easier and safer to have an assistant because this avoids accidental dislodgement and expedites the process.
• If another person is not available, thread ties through the faceplate of the tracheostomy while maintaining a firm grasp of the tracheostomy tube.	
• Do not remove old tracheostomy ties until new ones are secured.	Ensures tracheostomy is secured/prevents dislodgement
Discard gloves and other wastes.	Reduces transmission of microorganisms
Cap and date saline and hydrogen peroxide containers as per institutional policy.	Recapping prevents contamination and maintains sterility. Saline should be used within 24 hours of opening.
Position patient and provide comfort or perform any additional hygienic care.	Promotes comfort and hygiene to support health
Assess respiratory status, comparing to previous baseline	Identifies any untoward assessment findings which may signal further nursing action(s) Verifies adequate placement of cannula and stability of tracheostomy
Assess skin condition around tracheostomy tube and ties.	Identifies any areas of skin breakdown; confirms patient's comfort

SKILL 32.3 Performing Oral Pharyngeal (Yankauer) Suctioning

Reviewing Pertinent Information

Step	Rationale
Observe for signs and symptoms associated with upper airway obstruction that may require oral pharyngeal suctioning: gurgling, drooling, excessive oral secretions, vomitus in mouth, and coughing without clearing airway.	Physical signs and symptoms may indicate need to perform this procedure. Worsening status may result in total airway obstruction and hypoxia. The risk of aspiration of gastric contents and airway obstruction is increased in patients with vomiting, delayed gastric emptying, impaired cough, or gag reflex.

Preparing for Implementation

Step	Rationale
Wash hands.	Prevents the spread of microorganisms to the supplies being used and handled, and prevents further spread to the patient.
Gather supplies needed: • Gloves • Yankauer catheter • Sterile water and cup • Suction equipment	Important to get organized prior to initiating the procedure as this may need to be done emergently
Prepare the equipment: • Pour sterile water into the cup.	For cleansing catheter after suctioning
• Turn suction device on; set regulator to appropriate negative pressure.	Elevated pressure settings increase risk of trauma to the oral mucosa.
• Check the suction by suctioning up the water through the Yankauer.	Ensures equipment functions and lubricates the Yankauer
Prepare the patient: • Verify the correct patient with two identifiers.	Prior to performing a procedure, the nurse should ensure the correct identification of the patient for the intended intervention to reduce error.
• Explain to the patient and family how the procedure will clear airway secretions.	This communication evaluates and reinforces teaching. Patients who are more knowledgeable about the process are usually more comfortable asking questions.
• Explain that the patient may cough, gag, or sneeze during or after the procedure.	Teaching can provide the understanding that will foster more effective outcomes through patient participation.
• Practice splinting of surgical incision if necessary.	Splinting the incision during coughing decreases movement and subsequent pain during this activity.
• Position patient with towel or drape across his or her chest.	Protects patient's gown and linens from contamination by secretions
• If patient is vomiting or choking, place in lateral side-lying position to perform the suctioning.	Position decreases risk of aspiration.

Preparing for Suctioning

Step	Rationale
1. Put on gloves.	Gloves will protect the patient from surface organisms from the nurse's hands and will protect the nurse from possible body secretions that may come into contact with the nurse's hands during the administration procedure.
2. Remove oxygen mask if present. Nasal cannula may remain in place. Keep oxygen near patient's face. Be prepared to quickly reapply the supplemental oxygen if respiratory distress develops.	Allows access to mouth
3. Insert Yankauer suction catheter into mouth along the gum line to pharynx. Move catheter around mouth until secretions are cleared. Encourage patient to cough. If patient has other tubing in place such as a nasogastric tube or feeding tube, be careful not to dislodge the tubing.	Catheter provides continuous suction. Take care not to allow suction tip to invaginate oral mucosal surfaces. Coughing moves secretions from lower airway into mouth and upper airway.

Preparing for Suctioning (continued)

Step	Rationale
4. Rinse catheter with water in cup or basin until tubing is clear of secretions. Turn off suction unless procedure needs to be repeated.	Rinsing catheter reduces probability of transmission of micro-organisms. Cleaning the tubing enhances delivery of the set suction pressure.
5 Patient's face may need to be washed if secretions are on skin.	Prevents skin breakdown
6. Reassess respiratory status. Repeat procedure, if indicated.	Necessary to continue or cease intervention or to choose another intervention
7. Discard remainder of water. Discard disposable cup into appropriate receptacle.	Reduces transmission of microorganisms Moist environments encourage microorganism's growth.
8. Place catheter in a non-airtight container. It should be stored in an area where it will not come in contact with secretions or excretions or contaminate clean supplies.	Closure in an airtight container promotes bacterial growth.
9. Remove gloves and wash hands.	Reduces transmission of microorganisms to other patients; clean equipment should not be handled with contaminated gloves.

Engaging in Evaluation

Step	Rationale
Compare assessment findings before and after procedure. Auscultate chest and airways for adventitious sounds.	Identifies physiological response to the suction procedure

Documenting Effectively

Step	Rationale
Document in a timely manner and include the following: • Date and time • Amount, consistency, and colour of secretions • How patient tolerated procedure • Evaluation of procedure • Teaching to patient and family	Documentation is the key communicative method between health-care professionals. Documenting the amount, consistency, and colour of secretions, nursing care, and expected and unexpected outcomes provides baseline for future assessments.

SKILL 32.4　Nasopharyngeal and Oropharyngeal Suctioning

Reviewing Pertinent Information

Step	Rationale
Assess signs and symptoms of upper and lower airway obstruction requiring suctioning including wheezes, crackles, or gurgling on inspiration or expiration; restlessness; ineffective coughing; tachypnea; hypertension or hypotension; cyanosis; decreased level of consciousness; and excess nasal secretions, drooling, gastric secretions, or vomitus in the mouth.	Suctioning is an uncomfortable and traumatic procedure and should be used only when required through patient assessment.
Check patient's chart for low platelet count, use of anticoagulants, and recent history of epistaxis or nasal trauma.	Suctioning can be traumatic to the mucosal membranes, and excessive bleeding can occur with certain conditions.
Determine factors that normally influence upper or lower airway functioning such as the following: • Fluid status • Lack of humidity • Infection	Fluid overload may increase amount of secretions, whereas dehydration promotes thicker secretions. Dry environment can thicken secretions and make them more difficult to expectorate. Respiratory infections are prone to increased secretions that are thicker and sometimes more difficult to expectorate.

(continued on page 818)

SKILL 32.4 Nasopharyngeal and Oropharyngeal Suctioning (continued)

Preparing for Suctioning

Step	Rationale
Wash hands.	Prevents the spread of microorganisms to the supplies being used and handled and prevents further spread to the patient
Gather supplies needed:	Important to have equipment organized
• Suction source	
• Extension tubing connected to suction device	
• Sterile suction kit	
• Sterile water-soluble lubricant	
• Small bottle of sterile water or normal saline if not included in kit	Important for protection from splattering from a vigorous productive cough
• Gown, mask, goggles, or face shield	
Prepare the equipment:	The patient's mouth may require suctioning prior to insertion of the oral airway.
• Ensure that suction is working.	
Prepare the patient by	
• Checking patient identifying information using a two-step method; checking the patient armband and then asking the patient to verify name	Double-checking patient identification decreases potential for error greatly.
• Explaining the procedure to the patient and family (if patient's condition allows)	Explanations decrease patient and family anxiety. This process identifies knowledge deficits regarding the patient's condition, the procedure, and risk and benefits of the procedure.

Nasopharyngeal and Oropharyngeal Suctioning

Step	Rationale
1. Put on gloves.	Gloves will protect the patient from surface organisms from the nurse's hands and will protect the nurse from possible body secretions that may come into contact with the nurse's hands during the administration procedure.
2. Choose the most appropriate route (nasopharyngeal or oropharyngeal) for the patient. If nasopharyngeal approach is used, consider insertion of nasopharyngeal airway.	The oropharyngeal approach is easier but requires that the patient cooperates. The nasopharyngeal route can be more effective for reaching the posterior oropharynx but is contraindicated in patients with deviated nasal septum, nasal polyps, or tendency toward excessive bleeding.
3. Position patient in a high Fowler position or semi-Fowler position.	Maximizes lung expansion and effective coughing
4. Connect extension tubing to suction device and adjust suction control to between 110 and 120 mmHg.	Excessive negative pressure can cause tissue trauma, whereas insufficient pressure will be ineffective.
5. Put on gown, mask, and goggles or face shield as indicated.	Protects from splattering with body fluids
6. Using sterile technique, open the suction kit. Consider the inside wrapper of the kit to be sterile and spread the wrapper out carefully to create a small sterile field.	Produces an area in which to lace sterile items
7. Open a packet of sterile water-soluble lubricant and squeeze out the contents of the packet onto the sterile field.	Lubricant will be used to further lubricate the catheter tip if the nasopharyngeal route is used.
8. If sterile water or saline is not included in the kit, pour about 100 ml of solution into the sterile container provided in the kit.	This solution will be used to lubricate and rinse the catheter to clear secretions.
9. Put on sterile gloves using sterile gloving technique.	The gloves should be kept sterile to avoid introducing pathogens into the patient's airway.
10. Designate one hand as sterile and the other as clean to touch nonsterile items.	Usually, the dominant hand is the sterile hand, whereas the nondominant hand is clean. This prevents contamination of sterile supplies while allowing you to hand unsterile items.
11. Using your sterile hand, pick up the suction catheter. Grasp the plastic connector end between your thumb and forefinger and coil the tip around your remaining fingers.	Prevents accidental contamination of the catheter tip

Nasopharyngeal and Oropharyngeal Suctioning (continued)

Step	Rationale
12. Pick up the extension tubing with your clean hand and connect the suction catheter to the extension tubing.	The extension tubing is not sterile.
13. Position your clean hand with the thumb over the catheter's suctions port.	Suction is activated by occluding this port with the thumb. Releasing the port deactivates the suction.
14. Dip the catheter into the sterile solution and activate the suction. Observe as the solution is drawn into the catheter.	Test the suction device as well as lubricate the interior of the catheter to enhance the clearance of secretions.
15. For oropharyngeal suctioning, ask the patient to open his or her mouth. Without activating the suction, gently insert the catheter and advance until you reach the pool of secretions or until the patient coughs.	To minimize trauma, do not apply suction while the catheter is being advanced.
16. For nasopharyngeal suctioning, estimate the distance from the tip of patient's nose to the earlobe and grasp the catheter between your thumb and forefinger at a point equal to this distance from the catheter tip.	Ensures placement of the catheter tip in the oropharynx and not in the trachea
17. Insert the catheter into the naris or the nasopharyngeal airway if in place with the suction control port uncovered. Slight rotation of the catheter may be used. Advance the catheter to the point marked by your thumb and forefinger.	Guides the catheter toward the posterior oropharynx along the floor of the nasal cavity
18. If resistance is met, do not force the catheter. Withdraw it and attempt insertion via the opposite naris.	Forceful insertion may cause tissue damage.
19. Apply suction intermittently by occluding the suction control port with your thumb; at the same time, slowly rotate the catheter by rolling it between your thumb and fingers while slowly withdrawing. Apply suction for no longer than 15 seconds at a time. Repeat steps 18 and 19 as required with brief rest period in between.	Prolonged suction applied to a single area of tissue can cause damage. Suctioning longer than 15 seconds can lead to hypoxemia.
20. Withdraw the catheter by looping it around fingers as the catheter is removed.	Allows control over the catheter and prevents secretions from splattering
21. Dip catheter into the sterile solution and apply suction.	Clears the extension tubing of secretions that would promote bacterial growth.
22. Disconnect the catheter from the extension tubing. Holding the coiled catheter in the gloved hand, remove the glove by pulling it over the catheter. Discard catheter and gloves in appropriate containers.	Contains the catheter and secretions in the glove for disposal
23. Wash hands.	Prevents the transmission of pathogens

Engaging in Evaluation

Step	Rationale
Reassess patient's respiratory status and verify airway patency.	Validates the effectiveness of the suctioning procedure

Documenting Effectively

Step	Rationale
Documents the procedure in a timely manner and include the following: • Amount, colour, and odor of secretions • Patient's tolerance of suctioning procedure • Respiratory assessment and vital signs pre- and postprocedure. • Patient and family education	Documentation is the key communicative method between health-care professionals. Documenting cardiopulmonary status, patient care, and expected and unexpected outcomes provides baseline for future assessments.

SKILL 32.5   Endotracheal Suctioning

Reviewing Pertinent Information

Step	Rationale
Assess signs and symptoms of upper and lower airway obstruction requiring suctioning including wheezes, crackles, or gurgling on inspiration or expiration; restlessness; ineffective coughing; tachypnea; hypertension or hypotension; cyanosis; decreased level of consciousness; and excess nasal secretions, drooling, gastric secretions, or vomitus in the mouth.	Suctioning is an uncomfortable and traumatic procedure and should be used only when required through patient assessment.
Check patient's chart for low platelet count, use of anticoagulants, and recent history of epistaxis or nasal trauma.	Suctioning can be traumatic to the mucosal membranes and excessive bleeding can occur with certain conditions.
Determine factors that normally influence upper or lower airway functioning such as the following: • Fluid status • Lack of humidity • Infection	Fluid overload may increase amount of secretions, whereas dehydration promotes thicker secretions. Dry environment can thicken secretions and make them more difficult to expectorate. Respiratory infections are prone to increased secretions that are thicker and sometimes more difficult to expectorate.

Preparing for Suctioning

Step	Rationale
Wash hands.	Prevents the spread of microorganisms to the supplies being used and handled and prevents further spread to the patient
Gather supplies needed: • Closed suction setup • Sterile saline solution lavage containers • Suction catheter for oral and nasal suctioning • Source of suction • Connecting tube • Nonsterile gloves • Gown, mask, goggles, or face shield	Important to have equipment organized Important for protection from splattering from a vigorous productive cough
Prepare the equipment: • Ensure that suction is working.	This ensures that the suction equipment is working properly before hand and is ready to suction the patient as required.
Prepare the patient by • Checking patient identifying information using a two-step method; checking the patient armband and then asking the patient to verify name. • Explaining the procedure to the patient and family (if patient's condition allows)	Double-checking patient identification decreases potential for error greatly. Explanations decrease patient and family anxiety. This process identifies knowledge deficits regarding the patient's condition, the procedure, and risk and benefits of the procedure.

Endotracheal Suctioning Closed Method

Step	Rationale
1. Put on gloves.	Gloves will protect the patient from surface organisms from the nurse's hands and will protect the nurse from possible body secretions that may come into contact with the nurse's hands during the administration procedure.
2. Position patient in a high Fowler position or semi-Fowler position.	Maximizes lung expansion and effective coughing
3. Turn on suction and set vacuum regulator to 100–120 mmHg.	The amount of suction applied should be only enough to remove secretions effectively. High negative pressure settings may increase tracheal mucosal damage.
4. Connect the suction tubing to the closed system suction port and unlock the thumb valve.	The suction port is kept locked between suctioning.
5. Hyperoxygenate the patient for at least 30 seconds by either • Using the suction hyperoxygenation button on the ventilator • Increasing the ventilator's FiO$_2$ to 100% • Disconnecting the ventilator from the ET tube and attach the self-inflating manual resuscitation bag-valve device to the tube (Ambu bag)	Hyperoxygenation with 100% oxygen is used to prevent hypoxemia during the suctioning procedure. This usually takes five to six breaths over 30 seconds.
6. With the control vent of the suction catheter open, gently but quickly insert the catheter with the dominant hand into the ET tube until resistance is met or patient is coughing.	Suction should not be applied as the catheter is being inserted. This limits tissue trauma and minimizes the decrease in oxygen levels.

Endotracheal Suctioning Closed Method (continued)

7. Push thumb valve down with dominant thumb to apply continuous suction. Secure ET tube with nondominant hand and completely withdraw the catheter for less than 10 seconds into the sterile catheter sleeve. Stop withdrawal when the black marker ring appears inside the sleeve and release the thumb valve. Do not pull too far or you will stretch the sleeve.

Decreases in arterial oxygen levels during suction can be minimized with brief suction periods

8. Hyperoxygenate for 30 seconds before each pass of catheter. Repeat steps 6 and 7.

The number of passes to suction the ET tube should be based on amount of secretions and the patient's response to the suctioning procedure.

9. When the lower airway is cleared from secretions, oropharyngeal and/or nasopharyngeal suctioning can be performed with a separate catheter or Yankauer.

Suctioning the oropharyngeal area if secretions are present promotes patient comfort and oral hygiene.

10. Be sure that the black marker ring is visible in the sleeve. Instill sterile saline into the side port of the in-line suction catheter. Apply continuous suction while instilling the solution to clear the tubing. Ensure that the suction catheter tubing is pulled back so that the solution is not instilled into the patient's trachea.

The suction tubing needs to be cleared to reduce transmission of microorganisms.

Instilling normal saline into the patient's trachea can result in bronchospasm, tracheal irritation, and extreme coughing.

11. Put the thumb valve on the catheter in the lock position.

Prevents accidental engagement of the suction

12. Wash hands.

Prevents the transmission of pathogens

Tracheostomy Suctioning

Step	Rationale
• Gather equipment: • Suction catheter • Sterile saline • Clean towel • Sterile basin • Sterile gloves in appropriate size • Oxygen source • Ambu bag • Suctioning kit suction device set to appropriate pressure for tracheal suctioning (100–120 mmHg for adults)	Organization of equipment in advance ensures efficient procedure.
Put on one disposable clean glove on dominant hand. Attach suction catheter to suction apparatus. Dispose of both suction catheter and glove before proceeding.	Verifies function of suction apparatus
Set proper setting on suction apparatus.	
Ensure patient is in comfortable position—for conscious patient, position in semi-Fowler position with clean towel draped across chest. For unconscious patient, place in side-lying position.	Ensures patient comfort and eases access for nurse
Obtain baseline respiratory assessment of patient.	Provides baseline assessment and reevaluation postprocedure
Apply safety eyewear.	Prevents contamination
Open suctioning kit; fill sterile basin with small amount of sterile saline.	Creates sterile field from which to work
Open suction catheter package using sterile technique. Place suction catheter on the sterile field.	Allows for easier access of catheter once dominant hand is covered in sterile glove
Open package of sterile gloves; apply sterile gloves, being mindful that nondominant hand will not remain sterile.	Dominant hand will be performing procedure involving sterile contact with patient. Nondominant hand will be used to maneuver nonsterile equipment (e.g., oxygenation devices)
Check that suction equipment is functional by suctioning a small amount of water into the suction catheter.	Ensures catheter is working and lubricates catheter and tubing; lubrication facilitates movement of secretions through catheter.
Open tracheostomy adapter if patient is mechanically ventilated.	Allows for access of artificial airway Promotes optimal oxygenation
Using dominant hand, grasp catheter firmly and insert catheter in to trachea during inhalation (have patient take deep breath during insertion if possible).	Suctioning during insertion can cause irritation of the tracheal mucosa.
Without applying suction, insert the catheter into tracheostomy using dominant thumb and forefinger as a guide until opposition is met, or patient coughs, and then withdraw 1 cm. Rotate catheter.	When opposition is met, you have probably touched the tracheal wall, so withdrawing the catheter reduces that stimulus, making it less irritating to the patient.
Apply intermittent suction to catheter by depressing thumb over opening of catheter for up to 10–15 seconds.	Intermittent suction is less caustic to tracheal mucosa. Suctioning longer than 10 seconds can be associated with cardiopulmonary distress.

(continued on page 822)

SKILL 32.5   Endotracheal Suctioning (continued)

Tracheostomy Suctioning (continued)

Rotate catheter as it is withdrawn.	Rotation of catheter minimizes trauma to mucosa.
Assess patient's tolerance of suctioning procedure.	Determines how patient is coping with the procedure; repeated suctioning can induce hypoxia or arrhythmias.
Flush catheter with saline.	Flushing clears catheter and lubricates it for the next insertion.
Hyperoxygenate patient for at least 30 seconds. If patient on a ventilator, use the ventilator for hyperventilation and hyperoxygenation. If patient on a oxygen delivery device, increase the litre flow to deliver 100% oxygen. A ambu bag may also be used to hyperoxygenate the patient.	Tracheostomy suctioning may compromise the patient's oxygenation status.
Allow a rest interval of 30 seconds to 1 minute if additional suctioning is needed. No more than three suctioning passes should be done at one time.	Suctioning in intervals provides time for reoxygenation of airways.
Reapply oxygen source and have patient take a few deep breaths if possible.	Allows for optimal oxygenation following suctioning procedure
Suction patient's oropharynx following the last pass of tracheal suctioning. Do not reinsert catheter once oropharynx has been suctioned.	Suctioning the mouth clears secretions that the patient may be unable to clear on his or her own. Oropharynx contains multiple microorganisms; thus, it is suctioned last to prevent contamination.
Once suctioning is complete, detach suction catheter from connective tubing. Rotate catheter into dominant gloved hand and then remove glove with catheter remaining tucked inside glove.	Retaining catheter inside glove reduces transmission of microorganisms. Contaminated items should not touch clean surfaces.

Engaging in Evaluation

Step	Rationale
Reassess patient's respiratory status and verify airway patency.	Validates the effectiveness of the suctioning procedure

Documenting Effectively

Step	Rationale
Document in a timely manner and include the following: • Amount, colour, and odour of secretions • Patient's tolerance of suctioning procedure • Respiratory assessment and vital signs pre- and postprocedure. • Patient and family education	Documentation is the key communicative method between health-care professionals. Documenting the amount, colour and odour of secretions, patient care, and expected and unexpected outcomes provides baseline for future assessments.

Critical Thinking Case Scenarios

▶ A patient went into respiratory arrest, and a code blue call went out. The patient was intubated, recovered, but subsequently rearrested. The second attempt to resuscitate failed, and the patient died. When staff was cleaning up, they noticed that the tubing from the Ambu bag had been connected to the wall outlet and regulator pictured here. Was the Ambu bag connected to an oxygen outlet? Based on this type of outlet, what was the concentration of oxygen that the patient was receiving? How would this impact the patient's outcome?

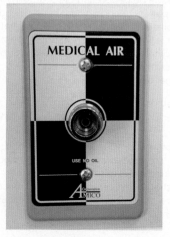

Medical air outlet.

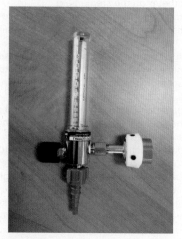

Regulator.

▶ A patient who is on continuous oxygen through nasal prongs tells the nurse that her nose is dry. In further assessment, the nurse sees that the patient had put petroleum jelly (Vaseline) in her nose. Do you think this could be a problem with the petroleum jelly and the use of oxygen? What nursing interventions could the nurse implement for the patient's dry nasal mucosal membranes? What health teaching points should the nurse make with the patient regarding oxygen safety?

▶ A patient returns from the operating room following a surgical procedure that required a general anesthetic. In the postanesthetic care unit, the patient is alert and oriented but having a great deal of pain. The ordered pain medication (analgesic) is given. Ten minutes later, the patient is not responding to the nurse, and the respiratory rate is less than 6 breaths/min. The nurse calls for help. What should the nurse do initially to maintain a patent airway? What interventions should the nurse initiate to ensure that the patient is being oxygenated?

▶ You are a nursing student in a clinical learning experience on a medicine unit. You are assisting the registered nurse with morning care and go into Mr. Jones's room to begin his morning care. You notice that Mr. Jones is having difficulty breathing, his respirations are rapid and laboured, and his colour is greyish. He is unable to speak clearly due to his laboured breathing. You notice his oxygen tubing and mask have fallen onto the floor. What will you do first to help Mr. Jones?

▶ You are working as a nursing student on a surgery unit. Mrs. Helmsby, a 48-year-old patient, returned from the operating room 4 hours ago. She is very sleepy. While you monitor her vital signs, you notice her respiratory rate is 10 breaths/min, and her skin colour is pale. Her oxygen saturation level is 89%. Her oxygen is running via nasal cannula at 3 L/min. What will you do first to help Mrs. Helmsby?

Multiple-Choice Questions

1. A pulse oximetry monitor indicates a sudden change in the patient's SaO$_2$ from 95% to 85%. The *first action* the nurse should take is to:
   a. Order stat ABGs.
   b. Notify the physician of the change.
   c. Check the position of the probe on the finger or earlobe.
   d. Start oxygen administration by nasal cannula at 2 L/min.

2. What intervention before suctioning will decrease hypoxia during suctioning?
   a. Use the Ambu bag with 100% oxygen.
   b. Lubricate suction catheter.

c. Suction for only 25 to 30 seconds
d. Use a small catheter to suction.

3. Normally, ventilation is regulated by the central chemoreceptors response to levels of:
   a. O$_2$
   b. CO$_2$
   c. PCO$_2$
   d. pH

4. What assessment data indicates the need for suctioning a patient with a tracheostomy tube?
   a. Difficulty breathing, tachypnea, change in the level of consciousness
   b. Difficulty breathing, slow respiratory rate, pink skin colour
   c. Restlessness, bradycardia, decreased respiratory rate
   d. Restlessness, bradycardia, increased respiratory rate

5. Which part of the tracheostomy tube is removed by the nurse for cleaning?
   a. Outer cannula
   b. Cuffed cannula
   c. Inner cannula
   d. Uncuffed cannula

6. A patient has undergone abdominal surgery. The surgeon has ordered incentive spirometry. Which of the following nursing actions will most help the patient use the incentive spirometer?
   a. Keep a loose seal around the mouthpiece to prevent pressure buildup in the alveoli.
   b. Use the "huff" cough before the patient uses the spirometer.
   c. Cough after each breath on the spirometer.
   d. Sit as upright as possible and splint the abdominal incision.

7. A patient attends the clinic for a respiratory assessment related to his chronic asthma. The nurse understands that the most important teaching point for this patient is:
   a. Hand washing
   b. Nutrition education
   c. Proper medication use
   d. Maintaining airway patency

8. Which of the following statements is true about vesicular breath sounds?
   a. They are most notable in the peripheral lung fields and are best heard over the base of the lung.
   b. They are most notable on expiration and sound like air blowing through a pipe.
   c. They are best heard during expiration and sound high pitched.
   d. They are heard throughout the respiratory cycle.

9. Priority *nursing assessments* for a patient with pneumonia would include:

 a. Blood pressure and pulse measurement
 b. Respiratory rate and oxygen saturation measurement
 c. ABGs
 d. Chest x-ray

10. Mr. Smith, who has a history of COPD, is admitted to the patient unit with dyspnea. The nurse understands that a priority nursing diagnosis for Mr Smith will be:

 a. Impaired Gas Exchange
 b. Decreased Cardiac Output
 c. Ineffective Airway Clearance
 d. Knowledge Deficit

Suggested Lab Activities

● When in a health-care facility, observe how many patients are on various types of oxygen therapy. Determine why the patient is on that specific type of oxygen therapy. Discuss your findings with your fellow students.

● Look at this website on lung sounds: http://www.med.ucla.edu/wilkes/lungintro.htm. Identify when a patient may have the adventitious lung sounds.

● Review the guidelines set by the RNAO for smoking cessation at http://rnao.ca/search/node/smoking%2520cessation. Discuss smoking cessation based on these guidelines with family members, fellow student, or any population of smoker such as high school students. Reflect on these discussions by thinking how you felt initiating the discussion, how you felt the discussion went, and what would you have done differently.

● In your community and province, identify environmental factors that may influence the development of lung conditions. Identify what lung conditions that the population is at risk for based on these environmental factors. What can be done to reduce these environmental factors?

SUGGESTED READINGS

Brophy, K., & Collins A. (2010). Clinical drug therapy for Canadian practice (2nd ed.). Philadelphia, PA: Lippincott Williams and Wilkins.

Canadian Nurses Association. (2006). *Towards 2020: Visions for nursing.* Retrieved from http://www2.cna-aiic.ca/CNA/documents/pdf/publications/Toward-2020-e.pdf

Casey, G. (2011). Pulse oximetry—What are we really measuring? *Nursing New Zealand, 17*(3), 24–29.

Critical care nursing made incredibly easy. (2012). Philadelphia, PA: Lippincott Williams & Wilkins.

Day, R. A. (2012). Thorax and lungs assessment. In T. C. Stephen, D. L. Skillen, R. A. Day, & S. Jensen (Eds.), *Canadian Jensen's nursing health assessment: A best practice approach* (pp. 452–492). Philadelphia, PA: Lippincott Williams & Wilkins.

Hennefer, D., & Lawson, E. (2009). Pharmacology—A systems approach: Respiratory system. *British Journal of Healthcare Assistants, 3*(3), 148–151.

Hudak, B. M., Gallo, B. M., & Morton, P. G. (Eds.). (2013). *Critical care nursing: A holistic approach* (10th ed.). Philadelphia, PA: Lippincott Williams & Wilkins.

Lewis, S. L., Heitkemper, M. L., Dirksen, S. R., O'Brien. P., & Bucher, L. (2010). In M. Barry, S. Goldsworthy, & D. Goodridge (Canadian Eds.), *Medical-surgical nursing in Canada. Assessment and management of clinical problems.* Toronto, ON: Elsevier.

Leyshon, J. (2011). Improving inhaler technique in patients with asthma. *Nursing Standard, 26*(9), 49–56.

McCance, K. L., & Huether, S. E. (2010). *Pathophysiology* (6th ed.). Philadelphia, PA: Mosby.

Sole, M., Penoyer, D. A., Bennett, M., Bertrand, J., & Talbert, S. (2011). Oropharyngeal secretion volume in intubated patients: the importance of oral suctioning. *American Journal of Critical Care, 20*(6), e141–e145. doi:10.4037/ajcc2011178

Speroni, K., Lucas, J., Dugan, L., O'Meara-Lett, M., Putman, M., Daniel, M., & Atherton, M. (2011). Comparative effectiveness of standard endotracheal tubes vs. endotracheal tubes with continuous subglottic suctioning on ventilator-associated pneumonia rates. *Nursing Economic$, 29*(1), 15–37.

Standring, D., & Oddie, D. (2011). Prevention of ventilator-associated pneumonia. *British Journal of Cardiac Nursing, 6*(6), 286–290.

Stoller, J. K. (2011). An overview of home oxygen delivery devices and prescribing practices. *Canadian Journal of Respiratory Therapy, 47*(4), 22–27.

Taylor, C., Lillis, C., LeMone, P., & Lynn, P. (2011). *Fundamentals of nursing: The art and science of nursing care.* Retrieved from http://wk-trusted-auth.ipublishcentral.com/services/trustedauth/reader/isbn/9780781793834?partnerKey=w1WcOVItAWsvkr2CoOOemMyBXE6EFM%2fyNbWMX%2bGkk7o%3d&userID=tpXyJvungLd2PjSzAUc5GtlYfesSi5DXQg%2fk%2b1mh4LU8VtN5byac%2bnz38i49b3oiVMor6ezAWtayx8beLL9Qxw%3d%3d

Urden, L. D., Stacy, K. M., & Lough, M. E. (2010). *Critical care nursing: Diagnosis and management* (6th ed.). St. Louis, MO: Mosby/Elsevier.

Vincent, J., Dalton, & Cianferoni, S. (2010). Diagnosis, management and prevention of ventilator-associated pneumonia: An update. *Drugs, 70*(15), 1927–1944. doi:10.2165/11538080-000000000-00000

Wiegand, D. (2010). *AACN procedure manual for critical care.* Philadelphia, PA: W. B. Saunders.

Supporting Fluid and Electrolyte Balance

DEBBIE FRASER AND WILLIAM DIEHL-JONES

Bill is a third-year nursing student doing his clinical rotation in pediatric emergency. Connor is a 3-year-old boy who is brought into the emergency ward with a chief complaint of diarrhea and vomiting, which his mother states began 3 days ago. During Bill's assessment, he notes that Connor appears listless, with dry mucous membranes and poor skin turgor. His mother also states that her son appears to have lost approximately 0.5 kg since the onset of the current illness. Bill begins to think about the effects of the sustained fluid loss and how it may be impacting Connor's fluid and electrolyte balance. What fluid shifts might be occurring? Which electrolytes might be of chief concern?

CHAPTER OBJECTIVES

By the end of this chapter, you will be able to:

1. Identify the fluid and electrolyte composition of the intracellular and extracellular fluid compartments.
2. Outline the methods by which fluid and electrolytes move between various body compartments.
3. Discuss the role of the kidney, lungs, and endocrine glands in maintaining the body's normal fluid, electrolyte, and acid–base balance.
4. Describe the effects of age, gender, and body composition on fluid and electrolyte balance.
5. Explain the steps in assessing a patient's hydration status.
6. Discuss the regulation of sodium, potassium, calcium, phosphate, and magnesium in the human body.
7. Identify the etiology, signs and symptoms, and nursing intervention for imbalances in sodium, potassium, calcium, phosphate, and magnesium.
8. Distinguish between metabolic and respiratory acidosis and alkalosis.
9. Analyze acid–base imbalances.
10. Outline the types of fluids that are administered parenterally.
11. Discuss the potential complications of intravenous therapy.
12. Develop a plan of care for a patient requiring intravenous fluids.

KEY TERMS

Acidemia Refers to the state of low blood pH.

Acidosis Refers to an increase in acidity (a decrease in pH) in body fluids (usually plasma). A distinction between acidemia and acidosis is that acidosis is used to describe the physiological processes leading to a low blood pH. For example, "respiratory acidosis" implies that the cause of the lower blood pH is due to a respiratory problem (e.g., hypoventilation).

Active Transport The movement of a molecule against a concentration gradient. This process requires a transporter and energy, usually adenosine triphosphate.

Adenosine Triphosphate (ATP) A molecule that transfers energy through the cleavage of phosphate bonds. ATP is required for active transport.

Alkalemia Refers to the state of high blood pH.

Alkalosis In contrast to its counterpart (acidosis), this refers to a decrease in acidity (an increase in pH) in body fluids (usually plasma). Similarly, alkalosis is used to describe the physiological processes leading to a high blood pH.

Anions Any negatively charged ion (e.g., Cl^-).

Atrial Natriuretic Peptide (ANP) A peptide hormone released by the atrial myocardium. ANP is a powerful vasodilator and reduces water and Na^+ loads in the circulatory system.

Brain Natriuretic Peptide (BNP) A peptide hormone secreted by the ventricular myocardium in response to excessive stretching of myocardial cells. BNP binds to ANP receptors. Its effects are weaker than ANP but longer lasting, making it a good indicator for diagnosing heart failure.

(continued on page 826)

Bundles Groups of care practices that, together, decrease the risk of central line infections.

Cations Any positively charged ion (e.g., Na^+).

Central Venous Access Device (CVAD) Intravenous devices such as peripherally inserted central catheter lines, percutaneous central venous catheters, tunneled central venous catheters, and port devices that allow direct access to large central veins.

Colloid A substance evenly dispersed through another medium. In physiological terms, colloid is primarily composed of dissolved proteins or other organic molecules. There is some debate over whether colloid or crystalloid solutions should be used in particular intravenous (IV) therapies.

Colloid Oncotic Pressure Pressure created by protein molecules such as albumin.

Concentration Gradient A gradual change in solute concentration between two regions. In physiological terms, this usually refers to the difference in electrolyte concentration across the cell membrane.

Crystalloid Aqueous suspensions of mineral salts. The term *crystalloid* is derived from the fact that salts typically form crystals when not in an aqueous medium. Typically, crystalloids are smaller than colloids and can pass through a semipermeable membrane.

Crystalloid Oncotic Pressure Pressure created by electrolytes such as sodium.

Dehydration Refers to a deficit in body water. This can be the result of either excessive fluid loss or inadequate fluid intake.

Diffusion Refers to the movement of a solute from a high concentration of that solute to a region of lower concentration (down the solute's concentration gradient).

Drop Factor Refers to the number of drops per millilitre of solution. The drop factor is determined by the size of the opening in an IV infusion apparatus.

Electrolytes Charged molecules (positive or negative) in a solution.

Extracellular Fluid (ECF) Refers to fluid found outside of the cell, specifically in the intravascular space within the blood vessels, between the cells in the interstitial space, and in the transcellular spaces.

Filtration Separation of molecules based on size, usually driven by hydrostatic pressure.

Hydrostatic Pressure The force created by the pumping action of the heart and the effects of gravity.

Hypertonic A condition in which a specified fluid has a higher osmotic pressure compared to another fluid. This differs from *hyperosmotic* in that it is a descriptive term that implies how a cell or tissue will believe in solution. For example, a red blood cell in a hypertonic solution will shrink as a result of the osmotic flow of water out of the cell.

Hypotonic A condition in which a specified fluid has a lower osmotic pressure compared to another fluid. This differs from *hypoosmotic* in that it is a descriptive term that implies how a cell or tissue will behave in solution. For example, a red blood cell in a hypotonic fluid will swell or even lyse (burst) as a result of the osmotic flow of water into the cell.

Hypovolemia The state in which there is decrease in fluid volume, typically of blood plasma.

Insensible Water Losses Water losses (e.g., evaporation of sweat or exhalation of water vapour) about which an individual is unaware.

Ionized The process of converting a molecule or substance into ions, usually by removing one or more electrons

Isotonic A condition in which a specified fluid has the same osmotic pressure compared to another fluid. This is essentially a numerical term. A cell exposed to an isotonic fluid will neither shrink nor swell. Normal saline (0.9% NaCl, or 300 mmol/L) is both isoosmotic and isotonic. A glucose solution that is 300 mmol is also isoosmotic with respect to a cell, but it is not isotonic.

Milliequivalents An expression of the chemical combining power of an electrolyte in a solution. One equivalent (Eq) is the weight in grams of an element that combines with 1 g of H^+ ions. When cations (e.g., Na^+) and anions (e.g., Cl^-) combine, they do so according to charge, not weight. One mole of a univalent cation is equal to 1 Eq because it can replace H^+ to combine with 1 Eq of Cl^-. The clinical usefulness of milliequivalents is that they are a better method of measuring the concentration of ions in serum than milligrams. For example, if you wanted to balance the number of male and female patients in a hospital ward, it would be more accurate to have 10 males and 10 females, rather than trying to balance by weight.

Oncotic Pressure Osmotic pressure exerted by proteins and other organic molecules. Also referred to as *colloid osmotic pressure* (see definition of *colloid*).

Osmolality The number of particles or solutes contained in fluids in the body by weight, which is the number of milliosmoles (mOsm) per kilogram of solution.

Osmolarity A measure of the number of solute particles in a fluid, defined as the number of osmoles (Osm) solute per litre (L) of solvent.

Osmosis Refers to the movement of water through a semipermeable membrane. This always occurs from a low concentration of solute to a high concentration of solute.

Osmotic Pressure The amount of pressure required to stop net osmotic flow of water across a semipermeable membrane. Generally, osmotic water flow occurs in a direction toward the side of a membrane where there is a higher concentration of solute or dissolved particles.

pH A measure of the acidity of a solution. Mathematically, it can be calculated as $pH = -\log_{10}[H^+]$.

Peripherally Inserted Central Catheter (PICC) Line A specially designed catheter that is inserted into a peripheral vein and advanced until the tip rests in the superior or inferior vena cava.

Plasma Osmolality The number of solute particles in 1 kg of plasma. Osmolality is a major determinant of total body water. Plasma osmolality is 280 to 300 mmol/kg.

Sensible Water Losses Measurable water losses via urine and feces (of which an individual can said to be "aware").

Solute Any substance dissolved in another substance. In clinical terms, this refers to a molecule such as glucose (the solute) dissolved in plasma (the solvent).

Solvent In clinical applications, a fluid such as water into which a solute is dissolve, for example, D5W refers to an IV solution of water (the solvent) into which has been dissolved 5% dextrose.

Specific gravity Measures the density of a liquid, in this case urine, compared to sterile water, which has a specific gravity of 1.00. The value is a reflection of the number of solutes in the urine.

Third Spacing Refers to the movement of body fluids (usually blood or plasma) into a compartment that is not usually perfused with fluids. For example, third spacing occurs in the abdominal cavity where it is referred to as *ascites*.

Tonicity The effect of a solution's osmolality on cell size. Cell size changes as water moves across cell membranes in response to changes in osmolality.

Total Parenteral Nutrition (TPN) An IV solution containing glucose, proteins, fats, minerals, and vitamins.

The balance of water and electrolytes is fundamental to life and health. Maintaining this balance is a complex process dependent on communication and interaction between several body systems. Fluid and electrolyte and acid–base regulation is affected by age and gender, body type, activity, and intake and is altered in time of illness. As a nurse, it's important to understand the normal process of fluid and electrolyte and acid–base regulation in order to anticipate problems and assist patients in optimizing their health.

Composition of Body Fluids

Approximately 60% of a person's body weight is composed of water; although this can vary according to age, gender, and body composition, the noteworthy point is that a very large proportion of body mass is composed of water, which in turn is a medium for a complex mixture of electrolytes (charged atoms and molecules), proteins, lipids, and, depending on the body fluid compartment, cells. Body fat has less water than lean tissue. In women, who tend to have more body fat than men, 55% of their body mass is water. Total body water (TBW) also changes from infancy to adulthood; newborns are 75% to 80% water, whereas a 1-year-old is about 65% water (Fig. 33.1). Water is vital for health

BOX 33.1	Functions of Water

- Building block for body cells and tissues
- **Solvent** for solutes such as proteins and electrolytes
- Involved in breakdown of carbohydrates, fats, and proteins
- Transports nutrients to the cells and waste products to the kidney
- Participates in thermoregulation by limiting changes in body temperature
- Acts as a lubricant and shock absorber

and has several functions in the body. These are outlined in Box 33.1.

The distribution of body water is divided into two compartments: the intracellular space or fluid in the cells (ICF), which accounts for 40% of TBW, and the extracellular space or fluid outside the cells, which has 20% of TBW (Fig. 33.2). **Extracellular fluid (ECF)** is found in three areas of the body: the intravascular space within the blood vessels, between the cells in the interstitial space, and in the transcellular spaces. Transcellular fluids include cerebrospinal fluid, intraocular fluid, and fluids found in the pleural and pericardial spaces and the gastrointestinal (GI) tract.

The ECF and ICF are separated by semipermeable membranes that allow water to move freely between the compartments. The fluid in each of these compartments is tightly regulated, particularly between the intracellular and extracellular compartments. Not only relative quantities in these compartments have to be controlled; the balance of specific electrolytes and other dissolved particles is essential for optimal health. In cases such as Connor's, from the opening scenario, there has been a loss of both fluid and specific electrolytes (most likely due to an infectious condition known as *gastroenteritis*). Furthermore, there have been fluid and electrolyte losses and shifts between compartments. How his body attempts to compensate for these shifts and the specific

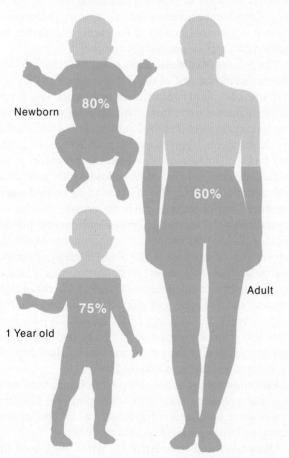

Figure 33.1 Changes in body water composition over the lifespan.

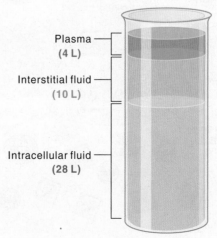

Figure 33.2 Distribution of body water.

nursing interventions that will be required to return normal physiological homeostasis is part of our continuing discussions throughout this chapter.

Movement of Fluids and Solutes

Several mechanisms affect the movement of molecules and water across cell membranes. These include diffusion, active transport, osmosis, and filtration. Some substances such as the waste product urea move by simple **diffusion** from areas of high urea concentration to areas of low urea concentration. When such concentration difference exists, it is known as a **concentration gradient**. The plasma membrane of tissue cells typically generates a barrier to the free exchange of many solutes or dissolved molecules in plasma. In some cases, carrier molecules use energy in the form of **adenosine triphosphate (ATP)** to move particles across a membrane, a process known as **active transport**. Active transport requires ATP to move substances from an area of low concentration of that substance to one of a higher concentration. The sodium-potassium pump (or Na^+-K^+-ATPase) is an example of a pump that uses ATP to maintain a higher concentration of potassium inside cells and a high concentration of sodium outside the cells (Fig. 33.3).

Other mechanism for transporting molecules across the cell membrane include ion channels, facilitative transporters, and water pores. Ion channels are essentially proteins that span the plasma membrane. They have openings of specific pore sizes that are relatively selective for specific ions. For example, a sodium channel allows sodium ions to cross the membrane but not potassium ions. When there is net movement of an ion through a channel (or primarily one-way movement), the main force that favors that movement is a concentration

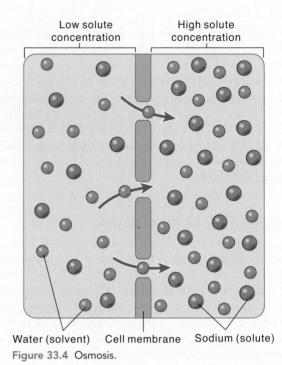

Water (solvent)   Cell membrane   Sodium (solute)
Figure 33.4 Osmosis.

gradient. Molecules such as glucose use facilitative transporters, and as with ions, such movement is driven by concentration gradients. Finally, special proteins called *aquaporins* form channels for water to cross the cell membrane. In the presence of antidiuretic hormone (ADH), these water channels are inserted in the renal tubules of the kidney to enhance water reabsorption and are hormonally controlled.

The process of **osmosis** refers to the movement of water, whether from one side of the cell membrane to another or from one body fluid compartment to another. This involves the movement of water from compartments where there is a low concentration of dissolved substances known as **solutes** to compartments where there are more solutes (Fig. 33.4). Two types of solutes generate **osmotic pressure**: proteins such as albumin, referred to as **colloid** which generate colloid osmotic pressure, also referred to as **colloid oncotic pressure**, and electrolytes such as sodium, referred to as **crystalloids** which generate **crystalloid oncotic pressure**. Because blood contains more protein than interstitial fluid, colloid osmotic pressure in the blood is greater than in the interstitial fluid. In contrast, crystalline osmotic pressure is equal between compartments because each compartment contains equal numbers of electrolytes. The movement of water between the ICF and ECF depends on both hydrostatic and osmotic pressure. In the body, **hydrostatic pressure** is generated by the weight and force of fluid created by the pumping of the heart and by gravity.

Filtration results in the movement of fluid from an area of higher pressure to one with lower pressure. The formation of urine or filtrate in the tubules of the kidney is one example of the movement of fluid by filtration.

Osmolality and **osmolarity** are terms often used interchangeably, although there is a subtle difference between

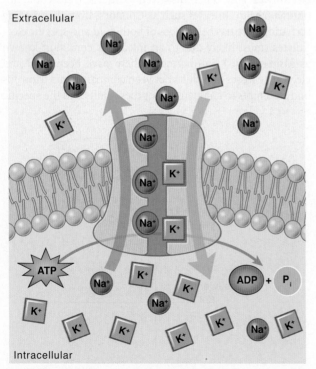

Figure 33.3 Active transport: sodium-potassium pump.

Hyponatremia:
Na+ less than 130 mEq/L

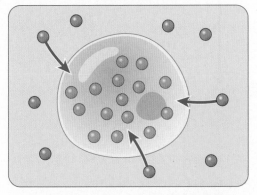

Cell swells as water is pulled in from ECF—
low solute-to-water ratio

Hypernatremia:
Na+ greater than 150 mEq/L

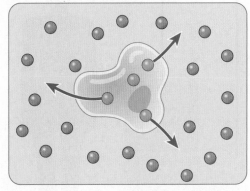

Cell shrinks as water is pulled out into ECF —
high solute-to-solvent ratio

Figure 33.5 Effect of extracellular sodium level on cell size. Blue spheres represent water molecules.

the two. *Osmolality* refers to the number of particles or solutes contained in fluids in the body by weight, which is the number of milliosmoles (mOsm) per kilogram of solution. Normal **plasma osmolality** is 270 to 300 mOsm/kg. Osmolarity is the concentration of solutes in fluid measured by volume; that is, the number of mOsm/L. Osmolality reflects the ability of the solution in a fluid compartment to generate osmotic pressure and to affect the movement of water. **Tonicity** is the term used to describe the effect that a solution has on cell size, describing that portion of the particles in a solution that actually affect cell size by causing water to move into or out of cells. When body fluids in two compartments are similar in osmolality, they are said to be **isotonic**. Isotonic solutions don't pull water in either direction (there is no net movement into one compartment versus another). When one solution has sufficient solutes to generate an osmolality greater than 300 mOsm/kg, it is said to be **hypertonic**; a solution with an osmolality of less than 270 mOsm/kg is **hypotonic**. Some of the particles that make up a solution's osmolality also move freely back and forth across cell membranes and therefore do not contribute to water movement or change cell size (Fig. 33.5). One very important point to remember is that a solution may be isosmotic but not isotonic. For example, a 300 mOsm/L solution of glucose has the same osmolality as that of ICFs. However, the glucose solution is not isotonic when compared to the cell. This is because glucose is very quickly metabolized or stored in the body, and the osmolality of the infusion will essentially be reduced to 0. The relevance of this fact is that certain intravenous (IV) fluids that we may give to a patient (e.g., most solutions containing glucose) will essentially be hypotonic with respect to the cell.

Regulation of Water Balance

Most water in our body comes from the fluids and food that we eat and drink each day. In addition, about 300 ml of water is generated each day through the breakdown of

carbohydrates, fats, and proteins (Whitmire, 2008). Water is excreted from the body through urine and feces (termed **sensible water losses**) and through evaporation from the skin and respiratory tract (**insensible water losses**). Figure 33.6 demonstrates the normal balance of daily intake and output. Insensible water losses increase when the ambient air temperature increases, with exercise, and with conditions such as fever or burns.

The kidney is the major regulator of both water and sodium balance in the body. Each day, the kidney filters about 180 L of plasma and produces 1,500 ml of urine or about 40 to 80 ml/hour of urine. Urine production depends on an adequate delivery of blood to the kidney and on delivery of filtrate from the glomerulus of the kidney to the loop of Henle, where water and electrolytes are reabsorbed. Urine production and hence water balance is also influenced by several hormones and regulatory mechanisms. The body's goal in regulating water volumes is to ensure that there is enough circulating blood volume to bring oxygen and nutrients to the tissues and to remove waste products from the cells. Because water follows sodium (think osmosis), if the kidney changes the amount of sodium it excretes or reabsorbs, water excretion and absorption will also change. It is mainly the regulation of sodium that is altered to maintain water balance in the body. However, plasma proteins—most notably albumin—are also important. Albumin (produced in the liver) has several important functions, including acting as a carrier for substances in blood and by acting as an osmotic agent that keeps fluid in the blood vascular space. Inadequate albumin, whether through liver disease or through loss as a result of kidney disease (albumin is not normally filtered by the kidney) will result in excessive fluid accumulating in the interstitial spaces, a condition known as *edema*.

Several mechanisms, including hormones, the nervous system, and blood vessels work in combination to maintain normal fluid balance. Receptors in kidneys and in other

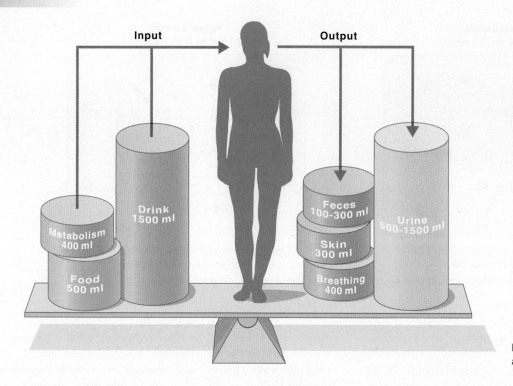

Input   **Output**

Metabolism 400 ml

Food 500 ml

Drink 1500 ml

Feces 100–300 ml

Skin 300 ml

Breathing 400 ml

Urine 500–1500 ml

Figure 33.6   Normal daily intake and output.

parts of the body respond to changes in blood volume (and therefore blood pressure) and/or Na^+ concentration by activating or suppressing three important hormone mechanisms: the secretion of arginine vasopressin (AVP) from the posterior pituitary gland; the renin-angiotensin-aldosterone system (RAAS), which originate in the kidneys; and the lining of the heart, which produces **atrial natriuretic peptide (ANP)** and **brain natriuretic peptide (BNP)**. ANP and BNP are produced when the cells in the myocardium become stretched such as might occur with fluid overload and act as diuretics to reduce fluid volume.

An increase of only 1% to 4% in plasma osmolality stimulates the release of AVP from the posterior pituitary gland. AVP targets cells in the kidney, stimulating the reabsorption of water. Other regulatory mechanisms become activated by a decrease in plasma volume of approximately 4% to 15% (Haskal, 2007). In this case, arterial baroreceptors become activated, and induce the sensation of thirst in specific areas of the brain (Agrawal, Agarwal, Joshi & Ghosh, 2008). Excess fluid volume has the opposite effect, suppressing both thirst and the release of AVP and the RAAS.

Activation of RAAS starts with either a decrease in blood volume or a decrease in Na^+. This stimulates the release of the enzyme renin from a part of the kidney called the *juxtaglomerular apparatus*. From there, renin converts another molecule in blood (angiotensinogen) into angiotensin I, which is converted by still another blood enzyme (angiotensin-converting enzyme or ACE) into angiotensin II. This hormone has several functions. Angiotensin II causes vasoconstriction, which works to increase circulating blood volume. It also stimulates aldosterone secretion from the adrenal cortex. Aldosterone increases sodium reabsorption

and potassium excretion in the distal tubule of the kidney. When this occurs, the body reclaims more Na^+. Equally importantly, water follows Na^+ via osmosis out of the renal tubules and back into plasma. In this way, both water and Na^+ deficits can be corrected.

The third mechanism involves the heart. Fluid overload also activates baroreceptors in the atria, which release ANP and BNP, substances that increase excretion of sodium and water. Together, these diverse organs and factors regulate water and electrolyte balance in body fluids.

Disorders of Fluid Balance

Normally, the body's regulatory mechanisms maintain the balance of fluid and electrolytes within a normal range. When healthy people feel thirsty, they drink; however, when they are ill, the sensation of thirst may be suppressed or ignored. During times of increased demand or illness, the normal balance of either fluids, electrolytes, or both can be lost.

Hypovolemia

An excessive loss of ECF and electrolytes results in low circulating blood volume or **hypovolemia**. Hypovolemia occurs when both water and electrolytes are lost in normal proportions and occurs in patients with acute blood loss, severe burns, or fluid shifts into the interstitial tissue from conditions such as fever and sweating, infection, or shock. Hypovolemia can also occur when the vascular space is increased such as when drugs are used that cause vasodilation. The patient may not show any symptoms until 10% to 20% of his or her blood volume has been lost. Signs and symptoms of hypovolemia include dizziness, decreased blood pressure, tachycardia, weak pulses, and poor perfusion. Treatment of hypovolemia is directed at restoring the intravascular blood volume with fluid replacement. The type of fluid used will depend on the source of the fluid loss. If hypovolemia is caused by hemorrhage, then a blood transfusion may be required.

Dehydration

Unlike hypovolemia where both water and electrolytes are lost in equal proportions, **dehydration** involves a deficit of water alone. Dehydration occurs in situations where water intake is less than water loss, such as when exercising or sweating excessively or with GI losses from vomiting or diarrhea. It may also occur in patients who cannot access water, such as those with mobility or communication issues, those that are restrained, or have altered thirst sensation. The elderly people are at particular risk for dehydration because of decreased intake and increased fluid losses. Compounding these risk factors, elderly persons have a relative resistance to the effects of AVP and have diminished aldosterone levels. In addition, issues with cognitive impairment, mobility, vision, and swallowing may influence fluid intake. At the other end of the life spectrum, infants are also vulnerable to dehydration because they have an increased surface area for insensible water loss and a limited ability to concentrate their urine and excrete solutes. They also have a high metabolic rate with a limited ability to express thirst.

Symptoms of dehydration occur with as little as 2% loss in body water and include thirst, decreased appetite, weakness, headache, dizziness, tachycardia, incoherent speech, dry mucous membranes, weight loss, decreased urine output, concentrated urine, and decreased blood pressure. Dehydration increases the risk of falls, kidney stones, and urinary tract infections in the elderly (Jequier & Constant, 2010). Treatment of dehydration centers on replacing water either through oral intake of administration of IV fluids.

Thinking back to Connor in the opening scenario, it will be important for Bill to carefully assess Connor for the signs of dehydration discussed in this section.

Hypervolemia

Too much fluid in the ECF compartment, and, in particular, in the intravascular space, results when the kidneys cannot excrete enough sodium and water to maintain fluid balance. This can occur in patients with renal or heart failure, cirrhosis of the liver (which results in inadequate albumin production), or when too much IV fluid is given. It can also occur in situations where large amounts of fluid shift from the interstitial or intracellular space to the ECF. Symptoms of hypervolemia include edema, increased blood pressure, tachypnea, shortness of breath, weight gain, distended neck veins, and wet breath sounds.

Third Spacing

Fluid balance between the intravascular and interstitial spaces is maintained by fluid volumes, hydrostatic pressure, and **oncotic pressure**. Lymphatic drainage and capillary permeability also play a role. When this balance is disrupted, excess fluid moves from the blood vessels into the interstitial space, resulting in edema, as described previously. An extension of this process is **third spacing**, which involves the movement of fluid into compartments that are not normally part of the exchange between ECF and ICF. An example of one such compartment is the abdomen; when fluid seeps into the abdominal compartment, a condition known as *ascites* develops. This is diagnosable by the nurse as a fluid wave across the abdomen when one side is tapped gently (Fig. 33.7).

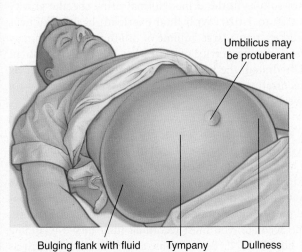
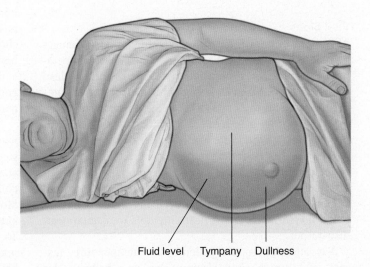

Umbilicus may be protuberant

Bulging flank with fluid   Tympany   Dullness

Fluid level   Tympany   Dullness

Figure 33.7 Ascites.

Because the abdominal cavity is not normally part of the fluid exchange, it becomes difficult for that fluid to return to the ECF compartment. Third spacing is the result of imbalances in either blood hydrostatic pressure or oncotic pressure and typically begins with fluid overload, which often is the result of either overzealous fluid replacement or renal dysfunction. Furthermore, hydrostatic pressure is altered by conditions such as heart failure, which increases venous pressure, causing fluid to back up into the interstitial space and, if the fluid imbalance is severe enough, it can become third spaced. Colloid oncotic pressure is decreased when albumin levels are low. Recall that albumin is important in osmotic balance and is in fact the most important source of oncotic pressure. Other causes of this spacing include increased capillary permeability as the result of burns, tissue trauma, hypoxia, sepsis, and anaphylaxis. Lymph obstruction commonly occurs when lymph nodes are removed during surgery for cancer and results in localized edema.

Assessing Fluid Balance

A careful nursing assessment is a key step in determining a patient's hydration status and assisting the patient in improving his or her health. Begin by asking the patient if he or she feels thirsty. Inquiring about fluid and food intake for the past 24 hours will give you a sense of how much water the patient has taken in. Ask your patient if he or she is passing normal amounts of urine and stool. Ask about the colour of the urine by comparing it to water (dilute urine), straw (normal), and tea (concentrated or containing blood). Ask if the patient has been vomiting or has diarrhea and ask about exercise, intense sweating, or prolonged periods of sun and heat exposure. Remember to ask about any medical illnesses, surgeries, and any other signs or symptoms of illness. Questions about a family history of kidney or GI conditions may provide clues to the patient's current condition.

Vital Signs

Alterations in intravascular fluid volume produce changes in vital signs. Begin by measuring your patient's temperature. Fever increases insensible water losses and can lead to dehydration. Manually assess your patient's pulse, noting the rate and rhythm as well as the pulse's characteristics. Tachycardia may result from either hypervolemia or hypovolemia as the heart works harder to supply oxygen to the tissues. A bounding pulse may reflect an increase in vascular volume, whereas a weak thready pulse may result from dehydration. Blood pressure is also affected by fluid volume. With progressing hypovolemia or dehydration, blood pressure falls as the heart attempts to maintain cardiac output.

Pay attention to the patient's skin temperature, texture, and turgor. Cold clammy skin is a hallmark for several medical conditions including dehydration and hypovolemia. As the patient tries to compensate for low vascular volume, vasoconstriction occurs and results in extremities that are cool to touch. Sweaty skin suggests the presence of increased fluid losses, which can impact intravascular volume.

Tissue turgor reflects tissue hydration in healthy children and young adults. It is less reliable in the elderly where decreased skin elasticity occurs as part of the aging process. To assess tissue turgor, grasp the skin over a bony prominence. Pinch the skin gently and hold for a few seconds. As you let go, note how long it takes to flatten out. A pinch that is slow to flatten is a sign of dehydration. The presence of edema is assessed by applying pressure over the shin, ankle, or back of the hand for 3 to 5 seconds and releasing. An indentation that persists for longer than 20 to 30 seconds is seen in patients with pitting edema. Edema can be graded according to its severity (Fig. 33.8).

Capillary refill time (CRT) is a reflection of tissue perfusion. Decreased intravascular volume can result in delayed CRT. To assess CRT, apply firm pressure on the back of the patient's hand for about 5 seconds and release. Note how long it takes for the perfusion to return once the pressure is released. A delay of longer than 2 seconds is abnormal. CRT may not be accurate if the patient has pitting edema or fever. Fever causes dilation of blood vessels shortening CRT (Scales & Pilsworth, 2008).

Listen to your patient's lungs for the presence of adventitious sounds. Patients with fluid overload may have fluid in the alveoli resulting in crackles on auscultation.

Urine Testing

In addition to asking about or observing the colour of the patient's urine, the concentration of urine can be tested by measuring the **specific gravity** or urine osmolality. Specific gravity measures the density of a liquid, in this case urine, compared to sterile water, which has a specific gravity of 1.00. The value is a reflection of the number of solutes in the urine. Normal urine specific gravity is 1.010 to 1.020. With fluid overload, healthy kidneys should excrete a large volume of dilute urine, which may have a specific gravity of close to 1.00. When a patient is dehydrated, the healthy kidney will conserve water by concentrating the urine bringing the specific gravity up above 1.020.

A hospitalized patient with fluid balance disturbances may require additional monitoring. Measuring the patient's weight each day is a useful tool in determining fluid gains and losses. This is especially important in infants and young children as well as in people with congestive heart failure. Monitoring fluid intake and urine output can also provide precise information about hour-to-hour fluid balance. To be accurate, you must record all fluid intake including oral liquids, food, IV infusions, and fluid boluses such as blood transfusions or medications. Noting the fluid volumes

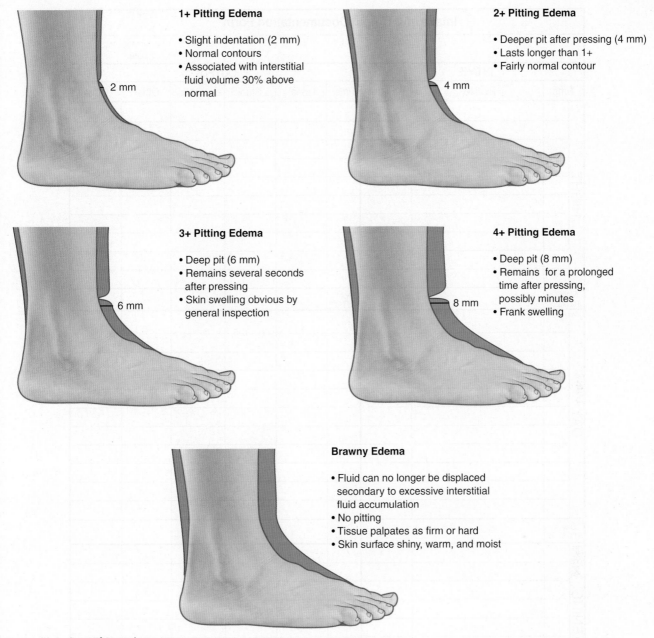

1+ Pitting Edema

- Slight indentation (2 mm)
- Normal contours
- Associated with interstitial fluid volume 30% above normal

2 mm

2+ Pitting Edema

- Deeper pit after pressing (4 mm)
- Lasts longer than 1+
- Fairly normal contour

4 mm

3+ Pitting Edema

- Deep pit (6 mm)
- Remains several seconds after pressing
- Skin swelling obvious by general inspection

6 mm

4+ Pitting Edema

- Deep pit (8 mm)
- Remains for a prolonged time after pressing, possibly minutes
- Frank swelling

8 mm

Brawny Edema

- Fluid can no longer be displaced secondary to excessive interstitial fluid accumulation
- No pitting
- Tissue palpates as firm or hard
- Skin surface shiny, warm, and moist

Figure 33.8 Quantifying edema.

of commonly used cups and glasses will make this process easier. Compare the patient's prescribed fluid intake to actual intake at regular intervals to ensure that the desired intake is achieved.

Measure and record all fluid losses so that you can balance these losses against fluid intake to reflect ongoing changes in overall fluid status. Common sources of fluid loss include drainage from blood loss, nasogastric and chest tubes, colostomy bags, liquid stool, and urine. Estimate any losses such as vomiting so that fluid balance calculations can be as accurate as possible. Most hospitals have a standardized form for recording both intake and output (Fig. 33.9).

Assessing dehydration in children is especially important because they are more vulnerable to fluid losses and cardiovascular collapse. The Canadian Paediatric Society (CPS) has developed guidelines for oral rehydration that are based on an accurate assessment of the degree of dehydration present. Table 33.1 presents the CPS dehydration assessment score.

This scoring system can be used on Connor, our 3-year-old with vomiting and diarrhea, to determine his level of dehydration. Once Bill determines whether Connor has mild, moderate, or severe dehydration, then a plan for fluid replacement can be established.

Intake and Output Documentation Form

					Bed		Date	

	INTAKE			OUTPUT				
Time	PO/NG	Amount	Time	Urine	Stool	Emesis/Gastric	Other	Other
NIGHT								
Night TOTAL			Night TOTAL					
DAY								
Day TOTAL			Day TOTAL					
EVENING								
Evening TOTAL			Evening TOTAL					

Figure 33.9 Example of an intake–output form.

TABLE 33.1	Assessing Dehydration in Children*	
Mild (<5%)	**Moderate (5%–10%)**	**Severe (>10%)**
Slightly decreased urine output	Decreased urine output	Markedly decreased or absent urine output
Slightly increased thirst	Moderately increased thirst	Greatly increased thirst
Slightly dry mucous membrane	Dry mucous membrane	Very dry mucous membrane
Slightly elevated heart rate	Elevated heart rate	Greatly elevated heart rate
	Decreased skin turgor	Decreased skin turgor
	Sunken eyes	Very sunken eyes
	Sunken anterior fontanel	Very sunken anterior fontanel
		Lethargy
		Cold extremities
		Hypotension
		Coma

*Some of these signs may not be present.

Source: Canadian Paediatric Society Nutrition Committee. (2006). Oral rehydration therapy and early refeeding in the management of childhood gastroenteritis. *Paediatrics & Child Health, 11*(8), 528.

Electrolytes

Body fluids contain several dissolved particles. Some particles break apart into simpler molecules that carry an electrical charge (Fig. 33.10). These electrically charged molecules or ions are known as **electrolytes**. Electrolytes with a positive charge such as sodium (Na^+), potassium (K^+), calcium (Ca^{++}), and magnesium (Mg^{++}) are known as **cations**, whereas those with a negative charge such as chloride (Cl^-) and bicarbonate (HCO_3^-) are known as **anions**. The concentration of these electrolytes differs in different body compartments, but in a healthy person, the number of cations in each compartment is balanced by equal numbers of anions (Fig. 33.11).

Sodium

With a normal concentration of 135 to 145 mmol/L, sodium is the most abundant electrolyte in the ECF. Because water follows sodium, sodium plays an important role in regulating water balance in the body and is the main determinant of plasma osmolality. As sodium levels increase in either the ICF or ECF compartments, water will follow the flow of sodium as it is drawn by osmosis. The net flow of water stops when osmolality equalizes. In addition to

	ICF (mmol/L)	ECF (mmol/L)
Na^+	10–14	135–145
K^+	140–150	3.5–5.0
Cl^-	3–4	98–106
Ca^{++}	<0.25	2.1–2.6
HCO_3^-	7–10	0.8–1.45
Mg^{++}	Variable	0.75–1.25
P_i	75	0.8–1.45

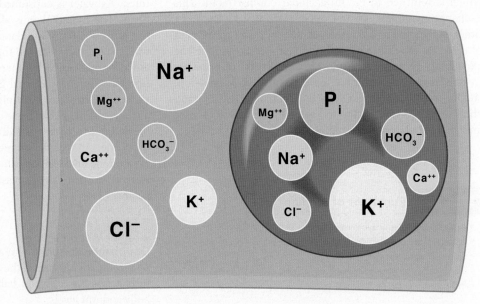

Figure 33.10 Distribution of electrolytes in fluid compartments.

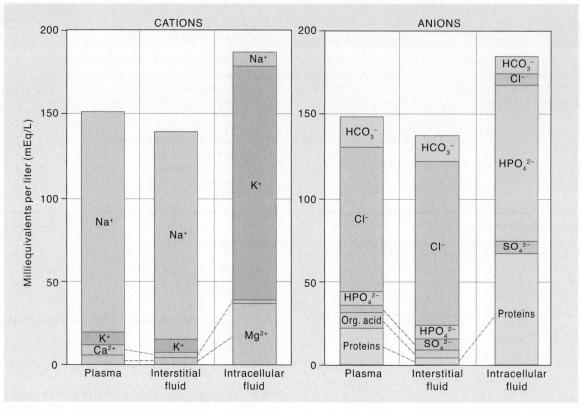

Figure 33.11 Normal electrolyte distribution.

maintaining plasma osmolality and water balance, sodium plays an important role in balancing intracellular and extracellular electrolyte levels (Box 33.2). Together with potassium, the primary intracellular cation, the sodium–potassium pump uses ATP or energy to move sodium out of the cells and into the ECF in exchange for potassium, which is returned to the intracellular compartment. This exchange maintains sodium outside the cell at levels 14 times higher than that inside of the cell. The movement of these cations, coupled with ion channels, results in the excitability of nerve cells and the conduction of impulses in muscle and nerve fibres. As a positively charged ion, sodium readily combines with bicarbonate ($HCO3^-$) and chloride (Cl^-). This helps to maintain normal acid–base and charge balance in the blood.

BOX 33.2 Functions of Sodium

- Activates cellular enzyme reactions
- Assists in the conduction of nerve impulses
- Controls water movement
- Contributes to acid–base balance
- Promotes muscle contractility

Regulation of Sodium

Sodium is a common ingredient in our food and beverages and is easily absorbed from the small intestine. Excess sodium is excreted by the kidneys. The basic process is as follows: When sodium levels in the blood increase, osmolality increases, and osmoreceptors in the hypothalamus stimulate thirst. As water is consumed, normal plasma osmolality returns. The hypothalamus also stimulates AVP release from the posterior pituitary gland, which, in turn, causes more water to be reabsorbed in the kidney. Normal sodium levels are also maintained by alterations in aldosterone, a steroid hormone from the adrenal gland. When the adrenal cortex produces aldosterone (a mineralocorticoid) in response to angiotensin II, aldosterone acts on distal tubular cells of the kidney to reabsorb sodium, chloride, and water from the urine. As plasma sodium levels drop, the secretion of aldosterone and AVP are suppressed and water excretion returns to normal (see discussion under "Regulation of Water Balance").

Sodium Imbalances

Disturbances in sodium balance are quite common in hospitalized patients and in the elderly patients. Often, the disturbance is one of water balance rather than with the total body sodium levels.

Hyponatremia

When plasma sodium levels drop below 135 mmol/L, hyponatremia results (Crawford & Harris, 2011b). One of the more common electrolyte imbalances, hyponatremia occurs in up to 30% of hospitalized patients (Agrawal et al., 2008). Hyponatremia is more common in elderly patients and is thought to result from impaired renal sodium conservation (Whitmire, 2008). Low levels of sodium in the blood are found in three situations: an excessive level of TBW with a normal amount of body sodium, a high level of body sodium with a higher level of body water, and a low level of sodium with a normal level of body water (Box 33.3). Hypotonic hyponatremia is the most common type of hyponatremia and usually results from the ingestion of large amounts of hypotonic fluid—for example, following surgery; in marathon runners (see "Through the Eyes of a Patient"); or with some drugs including ecstasy, carbamazepine, theophylline, and diuretics (Reddy & Mooradian, 2009). Hypertonic hyponatremia is uncommon but can occur when a patient's blood sugar is high. Glucose increases the osmolality of the blood by drawing water from the cells and into the blood, resulting in dilution of the sodium in the blood.

Through the eyes of a patient

*T*owards the end of a scorching hot marathon race in Regina, I began to feel dizzy and to experience difficulties with my vision. I remember crossing the finishing line then collapsing in the heat. I didn't know what was happening to me, and I was scared and felt like I was dying. Then, everything went black.

When I woke up, I had ice packs under my arms, electrodes attached to my chest, and an IV line inserted just above my wrist. I was in the medical aid tent. I remember asking if I was having a heart attack. The nurse who was beside me said, "No," and that I had gotten overheated and needed some fluids in my blood. Concerned, I asked him what was wrong with my blood. He said that my sugar levels were low and so was my sodium. He told me I was getting saline to help fix the sodium problem as well as sugar. He also said he was keeping a close watch on me, and that I should be feeling better in a while. Having the nurse explain this to me really helped me to remain calm. And true enough, an hour later I felt much better.

Later, I asked the nurse what might have caused my low sodium, and he said it was quite likely it was because I had drunk too much water on the marathon course, and this diluted the sodium in my blood, even though I was sweating a lot. He also told me that the condition was called hyponatremia. I found this puzzling; I had tried to drink enough water so that I wouldn't get dehydrated but didn't know that I could drink too much water. When I talked to a more experienced runner, she said that next time, I should drink only according my thirst, and that next time, I should choose a sports drink that has sugar and electrolytes in it. I have since made this my practice, and I have never again needed the medical aid tent!

(personal reflection of a patient)

Syndrome of Inappropriate Antidiuretic Hormone

Syndrome of inappropriate antidiuretic hormone (SIADH) causes hyponatremia as a result of the loss of the normal regulation of AVP, leading to water retention and concentrated urine. SIADH occurs in patients with pneumonia, emphysema, meningitis, and with CNS injuries or tumors. SIADH can also be triggered by drugs including carbamazepine, selective serotonin reuptake inhibitors (SSRIs), and theophylline (Goh, 2004).

Symptoms of Hyponatremia

The symptoms of hyponatremia depend on the blood level and on how quickly the sodium levels have dropped. Chronic hyponatremia is better tolerated than an acute drop in plasma sodium. Because of the important role that sodium plays in regulating the movement of water in the body, low sodium levels cause fluid shifts that can result in cerebral edema. Signs and symptoms of cerebral edema include headaches, lethargy, confusion, difficulty with walking and balance, nausea, and vomiting. Seizures and coma can occur when sodium levels drop below 120 mmol/L (Goh, 2004). Treatment of hypovolemia depends on the cause. Fluid restriction is used when excessive fluid volumes cause hyponatremia. Diuretics may also be used to reduce fluid volumes. If body fluid volumes are low or normal, IV sodium can be given to correct the hyponatremia.

BOX 33.3 Classification of Hyponatremia

Hypotonic hyponatremia: Normal or increased water intake with impaired renal function or excessive water intake with normal renal function

Isotonic hyponatremia: ECF volume is expanded with fluid that doesn't contain sodium.

Hypertonic hyponatremia: An increase in osmolarity in the ECF causes fluid to move into the ECF (i.e., hyperglycemia).

Hypovolemic hyponatremia: Low ECF volume caused by sodium and water loss from the kidneys or other body fluids; causes include thiazide diuretics, vomiting, diarrhea, excessive sweating, or third-space losses.

Dilutional or hypervolemic hyponatremia: Excessive water in the ECF; for example, congestive heart failure

RESEARCH

CALCULATING SODIUM REPLACEMENT IN CHILDREN

The most common electrolyte imbalance in hospitalized children is hyponatremia. This is a dangerous condition in which neurologic disturbances, seizure, and even death are often manifested secondary to low plasma Na^+ concentrations.

Hyponatremia can be the result of either a deficit of Na^+ or a positive balance of electrolyte-free water (EFW). The latter is the most likely scenario, although there has been much debate about the actual cause(s). Hatherill (2004) maintained that it is the total volumes of parenteral maintenance solutions (PMS) infused that are at fault, and that formulae for estimating pediatric fluid requirements are too generous and result in excessive volumes being infused, thereby causing dilutional hyponatremia. Taylor and Durward (2004) also took issue with traditional formulae for estimating PMS requirements, although these authors were of the opinion that the chief problem is that fluid requirements are based on a healthy pediatric population. Furthermore, they suggested that isotonic PMS such as normal saline are safer given that they are more effective at maintaining tonicity (see "Keyterms") and thus help to balance fluids between the ICF and ECF. Taylor and Durward (2004) posited that the use of hypotonic IV fluids (e.g., 0.45% saline or D5W) contribute to hyponatremia in hospitalized children, particularly after surgery.

Until recently, no clear answer has been forthcoming, mainly due to the ethical dilemmas inherent in doing any randomized controlled clinical trials with children. However, new research in this area has helped to resolve the debate (Choong et al., 2011). In a randomized controlled trial conducted in Hamilton, Ontario, surgical patients between 6 months and 16 years of age with a postoperative stay of more than 24 hours were enrolled in a blinded study to test whether hypotonic PMS or isotonic PMS were associated with hyponatremia. The primary outcome measure was acute hyponatremia, whereas the secondary outcome measures were severe hyponatremia, hypernatremia, adverse events associated with low Na^+, and ADH levels. To ensure the safety of all study participants, an independent medical safety officer reviewed all plasma sodium levels and informed the treating physician whether children were approaching any predefined safety thresholds.

The results strongly suggest that the risk of postoperative hyponatremia in children is significantly higher with hypotonic PMS compared to isotonic PMS. Choong et al. (2011) therefore suggest that isotonic saline is a safer empiric choice for postoperative children, although they stress the point that ". . . there is no 'ideal' PMS for all children. As with any drug, responses to intravenous fluid therapy should be monitored, and clinicians' decisions with respect to the most appropriate PMS to use should be individualized and goal-directed" (Choong et al., 2011, p. 863).

Choong, K., Arora, S., Cheng, J., Farrokhyar, F., Reddy, D., Thabane, L., & Walton, J. M. (2011). *Hypotonic versus isotonic maintenance fluids after surgery for children: A randomized controlled trial.* Pediatrics, 128, 857–866.

Hatherill, M. (2004). *Rubbing salt in the wound. The case against isotonic parenteral maintenance solution.* Archives of Disease in Childhood, 89, 414–418.

Taylor, D., & Durward, A. (2004). *Pouring salt on troubled waters. The case for isotonic parenteral maintenance solution.* Archives of Disease in Childhood, 89, 411–414.

Hypernatremia

Hypernatremia is defined as plasma sodium levels of greater than 145 mmol/L. Hypernatremia results from inadequate water intake, excessive water loss, impaired thirst, or excessive sodium administration (Box 33.4). In humans, the thirst mechanism is very sensitive, so hypernatremia is rare in conscious patients with access to water. In most healthy people, the body compensates for water loss by reducing urine output and by stimulating thirst, as described previously. Hypernatremia does occur in about 1% of hospitalized patients, usually those who are critically ill. The thirst sensation decreases with aging; therefore, the elderly patients are more susceptible to hypernatremia. Renal fluid loss may occur if the kidney is unable to concentrate the urine in response to increasing plasma osmolality. Signs of hypernatremia include flushed skin, dry tongue, hyperthermia, increased thirst, decreased urine output, restlessness or lethargy, brisk reflexes, neuromuscular irritability, or coma. Treatment consists of increased oral water intake if tolerated or the administration of hypotonic IV fluid.

Potassium

Potassium (K^+) is the major cation in the ICF. Normal plasma potassium is 3.5 to 5 mmol/L with a ratio of ICF–ECF potassium of 30:1. Potassium is not stored in the body and must be consumed daily. Unlike sodium, the concentration of potassium doesn't change very much in response to changes

---

BOX 33.4 Causes of Hypernatremia

Inadequate water intake
Decreased consciousness
Unable to communicate thirst
Unable to access water
Lesion in thirst centre
Increased insensible water losses
Renal losses (diabetes insipidus, hyperglycemia causing diuresis)
Burns, vomiting, diarrhea
Cushing disease
Seawater intake
Hypertonic feedings
Hyperaldosteronism

BOX 33.5 Functions of Potassium

- Maintains cellular osmolality and electrical neutrality
- Plays an important role in protein and glycogen synthesis
- Assists in the conduction of nerve impulses
- Contributes to acid–base regulation
- Allows normal cardiac, skeletal, and smooth muscle function

in TBW. Potassium plays a major role in cardiac contractility as well as in skeletal and smooth muscle function. Box 33.5 lists the functions of potassium. The body is acutely sensitive to potassium disturbances, and it must be monitored carefully.

Regulation of Potassium

Potassium moves into the urine by passively traveling down the concentration gradient from a higher concentration of potassium in the blood to a lower concentration in the urine. Some potassium is also excreted in feces and sweat. Reabsorption of potassium occurs is an active process (requiring energy) and is affected by the sodium-potassium pump and by the body's acid–base balance. Normally, in the distal tubule of the kidney, hydrogen or potassium is excreted in exchange for sodium. When the blood pH is low (acidosis) and the body is trying to excrete hydrogen, then potassium is retained, resulting in hyperkalemia. When the pH of the blood is high (alkalosis), potassium is excreted and hydrogen is retained, leading to a low blood level of potassium (hypokalemia). The kidney is efficient at excreting excess potassium but not as good at conserving potassium when levels are low. Insulin secretion promotes movement of potassium from the ECF to the ICF, thereby resulting in low plasma potassium levels. The most common causes of potassium balance disturbances are outlined in Table 33.2.

Potassium Imbalances

Changes in plasma potassium result from changes in the overall amount of potassium in the body or from shifts of potassium out of the cells and into the ECF.

TABLE 33.2 Common Causes of Potassium Balance Disturbances

Causes of Hypokalemia	Causes of Hyperkalemia
Loss of body fluids (diuretics, vomiting, diarrhea, excessive sweating, gastric drainage)*	Excessive potassium intake
	Renal failure*
	Major tissue injuries
Congestive heart failure	Infection
Stress	Acidosis
Hyperaldosteronism	Hemolysis
Alkalosis	Addison disease
Excessive ingestion of licorice	Hyperaldosteronism
	Medications (e.g., potassium-sparing diuretics, ACE inhibitors, NSAIDs)

NSAIDs, nonsteroidal anti-inflammatory drugs.

*Most common cause.

Hypokalemia

Hypokalemia is one of the most common electrolyte disturbances occurring in about 20% of hospitalized patients (Unwin, Luft, & Shirley, 2011). It is usually mild with levels between 3 and 3.5 mmol/L. Moderate hypokalemia is defined by levels of 2.5 to 3 mmol/L, and severe hypokalemia occurs when levels drop below 2.5 mmol/L. Hypokalemia is more common in patients with infections, those on dialysis, and those taking psychiatric medications. Alcoholism, HIV infection, and eating disorders also increase the risk of hypokalemia. Severe or chronic diarrhea is the most common nonrenal cause of hypokalemia. Insulin increases the cellular uptake of potassium as does higher than normal blood pH.

Signs of hypokalemia are usually seen when plasma potassium drops below 3.0 mmol/L and include weakness, muscle cramps, arrhythmias, rapid weak and irregular pulse, decreased reflexes, flatulence, vomiting, abdominal distension, and paralytic ileus. Treatment of hypokalemia is aimed at finding and fixing the underlying cause. A high-potassium diet may be recommended for mild hypokalemia. Good sources of potassium include whole grains, greens, potatoes, beans, oranges, and bananas. Oral potassium supplements can also be given. Severe hypokalemia may require IV potassium; however, IV potassium is extremely dangerous and is never given IV push. It is only given by infusion pump, and its use is governed by institution policies and safety checks.

Hyperkalemia

Hyperkalemia is defined as plasma potassium levels of greater than 5 mmol/L. Hyperkalemia is unlikely to develop when the kidneys are functioning normally. Pseudohyperkalemia (falsely elevated plasma potassium levels) can result from errors in collection of the blood such as bruising or squeezing the sample site or using a tourniquet that is too tight. The most common sign of hyperkalemia is a change in the electrocardiogram (EKG) (Fig. 33.12). Other signs and symptoms include muscle weakness, speech problems, nausea, diarrhea, and intestinal cramping (Crawford & Harris, 2011b).

Treatment of hyperkalemia includes identifying and treating the underlying cause. Mild cases of hyperkalemia can be managed with a low-potassium diet. If hyperkalemia is more severe, a cation exchange resin can be administered rectally. Dialysis may be needed in severe cases.

Calcium

Calcium is another of the body's major cations. It plays a major role in the transmission of electrical impulses both in muscle and in the nervous system. Calcium levels inside cells are also very critical because this ion is involved in regulating muscle contraction and can have a profound impact on heart activity. The functions of calcium are outlined in Box 33.6. Ninety-eight percent of calcium in the body is stored in the bones and teeth with the remainder found in the ECF and to a much smaller extent in the cells. Forty-five percent of the calcium in the ECF is bound to plasma proteins such as albumin, and 5% is bound to other ions

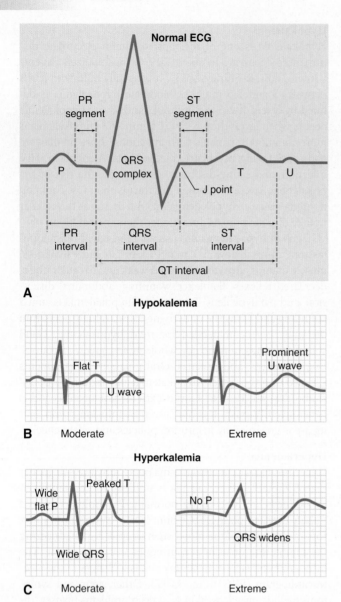

Normal ECG

PR segment

ST segment

QRS complex

P

J point

T

U

PR interval

QRS interval

ST interval

QT interval

A

Hypokalemia

Flat T

U wave

Prominent U wave

B Moderate   Extreme

Hyperkalemia

Wide flat P

Peaked T

No P

Wide QRS

QRS widens

C Moderate   Extreme

Figure 33.12 ECG changes seen in Potassium imbalances.

such as phosphate. The remaining 50% of calcium in the ECF is in its free form, also known as **ionized** calcium. Normally, when plasma calcium is measured in a laboratory, it is the total amount of calcium in the plasma that is reported. Under some circumstances such as when a patient is critically ill or has a low albumin level, then an ionized calcium may be ordered. Normal total plasma calcium is 2.20 to

---

2.56 mmol/L, whereas normal ionized calcium levels are 1.0 to 1.4 mmol/L. Under the influence of vitamin D, calcium is absorbed from the GI tract and excreted by the kidneys.

Regulation of Calcium

Calcium balance is maintained by a complex interaction of hormones that influence movement of calcium in and out of the bones and also control both absorption and excretion (Fig. 33.13). The three hormones which regulate calcium balance are parathyroid hormone (PTH); calcitonin; and calcitriol (1,25[OH]$_2$D), the active form of vitamin D. When calcium levels in the blood drop, PTH is released by the parathyroid glands, which causes more calcium to be released from the bones and reabsorbed by the kidney. PTH also converts vitamin D into calcitriol, which in turn increases calcium absorption from the small intestine and promotes release of calcium from the bones. When plasma calcium levels are high, PTH secretion is inhibited, and calcitonin is released from the thyroid gland. Calcitonin inhibits the release of calcium from the bones and also reduces renal reabsorption of calcium. The acid–base balance in the blood also affects the amount of ionized or free calcium in the blood. When the blood becomes more alkalotic, calcium binds more readily to albumin decreasing the amount of available calcium in the blood. When the blood becomes more acidotic, ionized calcium levels increase (Crawford & Harris, 2012).

Calcium Imbalances

Although calcium levels are normally tightly controlled, hypocalcemia and hypercalcemia occur with illness or hormone imbalances. Because of the critical role that calcium plays in muscle and nervous system function, imbalances can have a major impact on well-being. It is important to remember that calcium and magnesium levels are interrelated with low magnesium levels, leading to hypocalcemia. Conversely, phosphate and calcium have a reciprocal relationship. Low levels of phosphate lead to hypercalcemia, and rapid correction of hypophosphatemia can lead to hypocalcemia.

Hypocalcemia

Hypocalcemia is common in hospitalized patients and is defined as a total plasma level of less than 2.1 mmol/L. Various conditions can lead to hypocalcemia including inadequate intake of calcium or vitamin D, low levels of magnesium that decreases PTH secretion, hypoparathyroidism, malabsorption from the GI tract (celiac disease), high levels of phosphorous, pancreatitis, and renal failure, leading to excessive renal excretion.

Signs and symptoms depend on the plasma level of calcium and on how quickly hypocalcemia develops. Mild hypocalcemia may be asymptomatic and only detected with blood screening. Symptoms are usually related to the heart, nerves, and muscles. Muscle cramps and tremors are common as is tingling and numbness in the extremities. Hoarseness and shortness of breath may result from bronchospasms and laryngospasms. Acute hypocalcemia may present with congestive heart failure, arrhythmias, and seizures, whereas symptoms of long-term low calcium levels include brittle

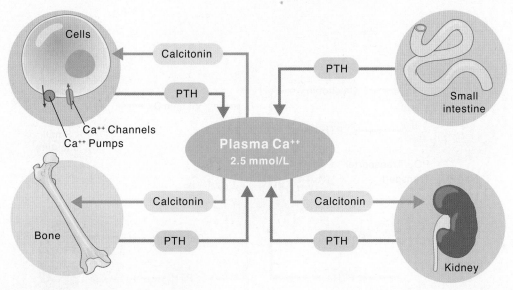

Figure 33.13 Plasma calcium regulation.

nails, dry and itchy skin, cataracts, and poor oral health (Beach, 2010).

Patients with hypocalcemia will require a workup to determine the underlying cause. Mild cases of hypocalcemia can be treated with a diet high in calcium and vitamin D. Oral calcium supplements can also be given. More severe cases of hypocalcemia will require IV supplementation and close observation. When caring for a patient with significant hypocalcemia, you will need to implement seizure precautions and safety measures to prevent falls, which may result from a seizure or loss of consciousness. Close monitoring of vital signs and observation for cardiac arrhythmias is also an important part of nursing care.

Hypercalcemia

Hypercalcemia is less common than hypocalcemia but can be life-threatening if levels are significantly elevated. Hypercalcemia can be classified as mild, moderate, or severe, depending on the plasma calcium levels. Mild hypercalcemia is defined as elevations in total plasma calcium of 2.5 to 3 mmol/L or an ionized calcium of 1.4 to 2 mmol/L. Moderate disease occurs with levels of 3 to 3.5 total calcium or 2 to 2.5 mmol/L ionized calcium. Severe hypercalcemia occurs with a total calcium level of greater than 3.5 mmol/L or an ionized level that exceeds 2.5 (Agraharkar, 2010).

The most common cause of hypercalcemia is hyperparathyroidism. Other causes include malignancies, hyperthyroidism, prolonged immobility, multiple fractures, hypophosphatemia, excessive vitamin D intake, and the use of thiazide diuretics.

Signs and symptoms of hypercalcemia will depend on plasma calcium levels. Mild elevations may be asymptomatic. Early signs of elevated calcium include fatigue, and as levels increase, patients may complain of anxiety, depression, muscle weakness, and confusion. Severe elevations result in sleepiness and loss of consciousness. Cardiac arrhythmias and hypertension may develop, and GI findings include nausea, vomiting, and constipation. Kidney stones, peptic ulcers, or pancreatitis may occur in patients with prolonged hypercalcemia.

Management of hypercalcemia depends on the severity and the underlying cause. Urgent treatment includes the use of IV fluids to dilute plasma calcium and promote diuresis. Diuretics may be used to blood sodium and calcium reabsorption in the kidneys. Weight-bearing exercise should be encouraged to promote bone absorption of calcium. Diet restrictions may be appropriate depending on the cause of the hypercalcemia.

Phosphate

Phosphate is primarily an intracellular anion with much higher concentrations in the ICF compared to the ECF. Phosphate enters the cells through facilitated transport. Like calcium, most of the body's phosphate is stored in the bones and as part of the extracellular matrix. It is responsible for bone structure, storage, and transfer of energy (ATP) and is an acid–base buffer. Box 33.7 outlines the functions of phosphate. The normal plasma phosphate range is 0.8 to 1.6 mmol/L. Normal phosphate levels are higher in children than in adults and are also increased in pregnancy. Phosphate absorption from the GI tract is determined by dietary intake and the plasma concentration of phosphate and vitamin D levels. Excess phosphate is excreted in the urine with the kidney, playing the major role in regulating phosphate balance.

BOX 33.7 Functions of Phosphate

- Acts as an acid–base buffer
- Essential for cell membrane integrity, bone and teeth strength
- Part of ATP and 2,3-Diphosphoglycerate (2,3-DPG), which is essential for oxygen delivery to the tissues
- Plays a role in carbohydrate, fat, and protein metabolism
- Required for normal nerve and muscle function
- Plays a role in phagocytosis and platelet function

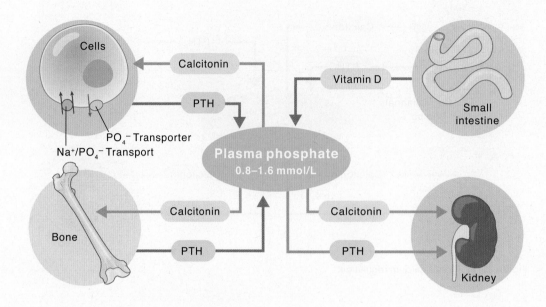

Figure 33.14 Regulation of plasma phosphate levels.

Regulation of Phosphate

The regulation of phosphate is not completely understood, but it is closely tied to calcium levels. When plasma calcium levels are low, PTH is released and increases release of both calcium and phosphate from the bone. PTH decreases the reabsorption of phosphate in the urine, resulting in a net drop in plasma phosphate. Low dietary intake of phosphate and low levels of PTH result in increased reabsorption of phosphate from the urine. High vitamin D levels also enhance phosphate reabsorption (Fig. 33.14). High levels of phosphate in the blood decrease the conversion of vitamin D to calcitriol and result in increased secretion of PTH resulting in more urinary excretion of phosphate. Calcitonin encourages the transport of phosphate into the bones and the cells.

An increase in blood pH causes phosphate to shift from the ECF to the ICF, creating a drop in plasma phosphate levels. Conversely, a lower blood pH causes more phosphate to enter the ECF, elevating blood levels.

Phosphate Imbalances

Imbalances in phosphate levels usually result from altered intestinal absorption, renal disease, bone resorption, or redistribution between the cells and the intravascular space. Because of the close relationship between phosphate and calcium, investigations to determine the underlying cause of phosphate imbalances should include an evaluation of calcium, vitamin D, and PTH levels.

Hypophosphatemia

Hypophosphatemia occurs when plasma phosphate levels drop below 0.8 mmol/L. Causes of low plasma phosphate levels include increased insulin, especially after refeeding a malnourished patient, overuse of antacids containing aluminum or magnesium, chronic diarrhea, hyperparathyroidism,

vitamin D deficiency, acute renal failure, alcoholism, and large burns. Because phosphate is present in so many foods, inadequate intake is rarely the cause of low phosphate levels.

Mild hypophosphatemia is usually asymptomatic. Signs and symptoms of more significant hypophosphatemia include bone pain; weakness; fatigue; confusion; numbness and tingling; congestive heart failure; respiratory failure; trouble swallowing; and chronic low phosphate levels leading to kidney stones, rickets, and osteopenia. Management of low phosphate levels is dependent on the underlying cause and the severity of the condition. Treatment of mild to moderate hypophosphatemia includes a diet high in phosphate-rich foods such as dairy products, meat, and legumes. Oral supplements can also be taken. Vitamin D supplements are indicated if vitamin D deficiency is present. More severe cases of hypophosphatemia require correction with IV phosphate supplements.

Hyperphosphatemia

When plasma phosphate levels exceed 1.6 mmol/L, the patient is said to have hyperphosphatemia. Plasma calcium levels are usually low in the presence of high plasma phosphate levels. Hypoparathyroidism is the most common cause of hyperphosphatemia because PTH normally decreases renal reabsorption of phosphate. Chronic renal failure and too much vitamin D can both cause phosphate levels in the blood to increase. Excessive intake can cause hyperphosphatemia, but this is unusual if the kidneys are working normally. Most patients are asymptomatic; those with symptoms usually have signs of hypocalcemia, including muscle twitching and cramping, numbness and tingling around the mouth, itchy skin, and bone and muscle pain.

Chronic hyperphosphatemia such as that seen with patients in renal failure can lead to calcifications (calcium and phosphate complexes), which can be deposited in the skin,

---

BOX 33.8 Functions of Magnesium

- Plays a role in the formation of ATP
- Plays a role in carbohydrate, fat, and protein metabolism
- Necessary for PTH secretion and normal serum calcium levels
- Acts as a vasodilator
- Aids in the function of the sodium-potassium pump
- Is a cofactor in more than 300 enzyme reactions (Crawford & Harris, 2011a)

---

joints, tendons, eyes, and blood vessels. Treatment begins with identification of the underlying cause. Management includes a low-phosphate diet and the administration of phosphate binders such as magnesium-containing antacids. In severe cases, IV fluids containing sodium can be used to dilute the concentration of phosphate in the blood.

Magnesium

After potassium, magnesium is the second most abundant intracellular cation. Most magnesium (about 60%) is stored in the bones with the remaining 40% in the cells, muscle, and in the ECF. Only 1% to 2% of total body magnesium is found in the ECF, 1/3 of that is bound to albumin, and the remaining 2/3 is free or ionized. The normal plasma magnesium level is 0.8 to 1.2 mmol/L. Ionized magnesium is important in maintaining normal neuromuscular activity. Box 33.8 outlines the functions of magnesium. Magnesium is found in foods such as grains, legumes, green vegetables, dairy products, dried fruit, and fish. It is absorbed in the GI tract and excreted by the kidney. Renal regulation of magnesium levels is poorly understood. Magnesium movement in the kidney occurs by passive diffusion, and reabsorption is influenced by both plasma magnesium and plasma calcium levels. Several hormones play a role in magnesium regulation including PTH, calcitonin, glucagon, and AVP, but the mechanisms of action of these hormones is not yet clear.

Magnesium Imbalances

Magnesium stores in the bones are not readily depleted when plasma magnesium levels drop. Likewise, an increase in plasma magnesium does not stimulate bone storage; therefore, the normal kidney function is essential for magnesium balance.

Hypomagnesemia

Hypomagnesemia (level less than 0.8 mmol/L) occurs in up to 12% of hospitalized patients and in a much higher percentage of those requiring intensive care. GI causes of hypomagnesemia include chronic diarrhea, malnutrition, and chronic alcoholism. Increased renal losses may occur with diuretic use or in renal failure. Diabetic ketoacidosis (DKA), hypokalemia, and hypoalbuminemia can also cause low plasma magnesium levels. Low magnesium levels block the release of calcium from the cells and also decrease PTH secretion leading to hypocalcemia.

Because hypomagnesemia and hypocalcemia (or hypokalemia) often coexist, symptoms of hypomagnesemia mimic those of both these imbalances and include muscle weakness or tremors, difficulty with balance, exaggerated deep tendon reflexes, and seizures. Changes in cardiac rhythm may be seen, including a wide QRS complex and flattened T waves. Alterations in mood, depression, and anxiety may occur, as might confusion and hallucinations. Management of hypomagnesemia is based on identifying and treating the underlying cause. Oral magnesium supplements can be used in asymptomatic patients or those with mild hypomagnesemia. A diet high in magnesium-containing foods should also be encouraged. Those patients with severe hypomagnesemia will need IV replacement fluid containing magnesium. Careful monitoring is required during therapy.

Hypermagnesemia

High magnesium levels (>1.2 mmol/L) are less common than low magnesium levels. In people with healthy kidneys, excessive intake is usually eliminated by the kidneys. Renal failure is the primary cause of hypermagnesemia. In some individuals, especially those with renal impairment, ingestion of laxatives or antacids containing magnesium may elevate blood levels. Magnesium-containing drugs are contraindicated in renal failure. Administration of IV magnesium is sometimes given to pregnant women with preeclampsia and can result in elevated levels of magnesium and neuromuscular symptoms. Mild elevations in plasma magnesium usually don't produce symptoms. More significant increases result in symptoms such as nausea and vomiting, low blood pressure, decreased deep tendon reflexes, lethargy, and respiratory depression. Muscle weakness is common and can progress to paralysis. Hypermagnesemia can be prevented by avoiding magnesium-containing drugs in patients with renal failure. IV solutions containing magnesium should be discontinued if symptoms of hypermagnesemia develop. Dialysis may be needed to treat severe symptoms. Common fluid and electrolyte imbalances are summarized in Table 33.3.

Acid–Base Physiology

The body's biochemical and cellular reactions are designed to function best under balanced conditions referred to as *homeostasis*. Metabolic processes within the body produce waste products in the form of acids, which must be balanced by the production of buffers or bases in order to maintain an optimal acid–base balance or **pH**. pH is an expression of the concentration of hydrogen ions (H^+) in a solution. pH is based on a negative logarithmic scale; therefore, the more hydrogen ions in a solution, the lower the pH will be and the more acidic the solution is. On the pH scale, 7 represents a neutral solution, measures between 0 and 7 are said to be acid, and numbers between 7 and 14 are alkaline. Pure water has a neutral pH of 7, whereas gastric or stomach secretions have a pH of 1 to 1.3 and pancreatic secretions have a pH of close to 10.

An acid is any substance that can release hydrogen ions, whereas a base is any substance that can accept or bind with a hydrogen ion. For example, hydrochloric or stomach acid donates a hydrogen ion as follows: $HCl \rightarrow H^+ + Cl^-$, whereas bicarbonate accepts a hydrogen ion: $HCO_3^- + H^+ \rightarrow H_2CO_3$.

TABLE 33.3	Major Fluid and Electrolyte Imbalances	
Imbalance	**Contributing Factors**	**Signs/Symptoms and Laboratory Findings**
Fluid volume deficit (hypovolemia and dehydration)	Loss of water and electrolytes, due to fever, excess sweating, burns, blood loss, and third-space fluid shifts; and decreased intake, as in anorexia, nausea, and inability to gain access to fluid. Diabetes insipidus and uncontrolled diabetes mellitus also contribute to a depletion of ECF volume.	Acute weight loss, ↓ skin turgor, oliguria, concentrated urine, weak rapid pulse, capillary filling time prolonged, ↓ blood pressure, flattened neck veins, dizziness, weakness, thirst and confusion, ↑ pulse, muscle cramps, and sunken eyes *Labs indicate:* ↑ hemoglobin and hematocrit, ↑ serum and urine osmolality and specific gravity, ↓ urine sodium, ↑ urea and creatinine, and ↑ urine specific gravity and osmolality
Fluid volume excess (hypervolemia)	Compromised regulatory mechanisms, such as renal failure, heart failure, and cirrhosis; overzealous administration of sodium-containing fluids; and fluid shifts (i.e., treatment of burns)	Acute weight gain, peripheral edema and ascites, distended jugular veins, wet breath sounds, shortness of breath, ↑ blood pressure, bounding pulse and cough, and ↑ respiratory rate *Labs indicate:* ↓ hemoglobin and hematocrit, ↓ serum and urine osmolality, and ↓ urine sodium and specific gravity
Sodium deficit (hyponatremia) Serum sodium <135 mmol/L	Loss of sodium, as in use of diuretics, loss of GI fluids, renal disease, and adrenal insufficiency. Gain of water, as in excessive administration of D5W and water supplements for patients receiving hypotonic tube feedings; disease states associated with SIADH such as head trauma; and medications associated with water retention (ecstasy, theophylline, and certain tranquilizers). Hyperglycemia and heart failure cause a loss of sodium.	Anorexia, nausea and vomiting, headache, lethargy, dizziness, confusion, muscle cramps and weakness, muscular twitching, seizures, weight gain, edema *Labs indicate:* ↓ serum and urine sodium, and ↓ urine specific gravity and osmolality
Sodium excess (hypernatremia) Serum sodium >145 mmol/L	Water deprivation in patients unable to drink at will, hypertonic tube feedings without adequate water supplements, heatstroke, and burns; and excess sodium bicarbonate and sodium chloride administration	Thirst, elevated body temperature, swollen dry tongue and sticky mucous membranes, hallucinations, lethargy, restlessness, irritability, focal or grand mal seizures, pulmonary edema, hyperreflexia, twitching, nausea, vomiting, and anorexia *Labs indicate:* ↑ serum sodium, ↓ urine sodium, ↑ urine specific gravity and osmolality, ↓ CVP
Potassium deficit (hypokalemia) Serum potassium <3.5 mmol/L	Diarrhea, vomiting, gastric suction, corticosteroid administration, dialysis, eating disorders, osmotic diuresis, alkalosis, starvation, diuretics, and infections	Fatigue, anorexia, nausea and vomiting, muscle weakness or cramps, polyuria, decreased bowel motility, arrhythmias, paresthesias, leg cramps, ileus, abdominal distention, and hypoactive reflexes *ECG:* flattened T waves, prominent U waves, ST depression, and prolonged PR interval
Potassium excess (hyperkalemia) Serum potassium >5.0 mmol/L	Pseudohyperkalemia, oliguric renal failure, metabolic acidosis, Addison disease, crush injury, burns, stored bank blood transfusions, and rapid IV administration of potassium	Muscle weakness, arrhythmias, flaccid paralysis, paresthesias, intestinal colic, cramps, abdominal distention, irritability, and anxiety *ECG:* tall tented T waves, prolonged PR interval and QRS duration, absent P waves, and ST depression
Calcium deficit (hypocalcemia) Serum calcium <2.1 mmol/L	Hypoparathyroidism (may follow thyroid surgery or radical neck dissection), malabsorption, pancreatitis, alkalosis, vitamin D deficiency, peritonitis, chronic diarrhea, ↑ PO_4, fistulas, burns, and alcoholism	Numbness, tingling of fingers, toes, and cir-cumoral region; seizures, hyperactive deep tendon reflexes, irritability, bronchospasm, anxiety, impaired clotting time, and ↓ BP *ECG:* prolonged QT interval and lengthened ST *Labs indicate:* ↓ Mg^{++}

Imbalance	Contributing Factors	Signs/Symptoms and Laboratory Findings
Calcium excess (hypercalcemia) Serum calcium >2.5 mmol/L	Hyperparathyroidism, malignant neoplastic disease, prolonged immobilization, overuse of calcium supplements, vitamin D excess, acidosis, and thiazide diuretic use	Muscular weakness, constipation, anorexia, nausea and vomiting, polyuria and polydipsia, hypoactive deep tendon reflexes, lethargy, and bone pain *ECG:* shortened ST segment and QT interval, bradycardia, and heart blocks
Magnesium deficit (hypomagnesemia) Serum magnesium <0.8 mmol/L	Chronic alcoholism, hyperparathyroidism, malabsorptive disorders, DKA, refeeding after starvation, chronic laxative use, diarrhea, heart failure, decreased serum K^+ and Ca^{++}, and certain pharmacologic agents (e.g., gentamicin)	Neuromuscular irritability, insomnia, mood changes, anorexia, vomiting, increased tendon reflexes, and ↑ BP *ECG:* PVCs, flat or inverted T waves, depressed ST segment, prolonged PR interval, and widened QRS
Magnesium excess (hypermagnesemia) Serum magnesium >1.2 mmol/L	Renal failure (particularly when magnesium-containing medications are administered), adrenal insufficiency, excessive IV magnesium administration, DKA, and hypothyroidism	Flushing, nausea and vomiting, low blood pressure, muscle weakness, drowsiness, hypoactive reflexes, depressed respirations, and coma *ECG:* tachycardia → bradycardia, prolonged PR interval and QRS, and peaked T waves
Phosphorus deficit (hypophosphatemia) Serum phosphorus <0.8 mmol/L	Refeeding after starvation; alcohol withdrawal; DKA; respiratory and metabolic alkalosis; ↓ magnesium; ↓ potassium; hyperparathyroidism; vomiting; diarrhea; hyperventilation; and vitamin D deficiency associated with malabsorptive disorders, burns, acid–base disorders, parenteral nutrition, and diuretic and antacid use	Paresthesias, muscle weakness, bone pain and tenderness, chest pain, confusion, cardiomyopathy, and seizures
Phosphorus excess (hyperphosphatemia) Serum phosphorus >1.6 mmol/L	Acute and chronic renal failure, excessive intake of phosphorus, vitamin D excess, respiratory and metabolic acidosis, hypoparathyroidism, and volume depletion	Muscle twitching; tachycardia; anorexia; nausea and vomiting; muscle weakness; signs and symptoms of hypocalcemia; hyperactive reflexes; and soft tissue calcifications in lungs, heart, kidneys, and cornea

↑, increased; ↓, decreased; →, ; BP, blood pressure; CVP, central venous pressure; ECG, electrocardiogram; PO_4, phosphate; PVCs, premature ventricular contraction; DKA, diabetic ketoacidosis.

Adapted from Smeltzer, S. C., Bare, B. G., Hinkle, J. L., & Cheever, K. H. (2010). *Brunner and Suddarth's textbook of medical-surgical nursing* (12th ed.). Philadelphia, PA: Lippincott Williams & Wilkins.

The normal pH of human blood is 7.35 to 7.45. Disease processes can alter the pH of the blood and, if not corrected, can alter cellular function and ultimately cause death. The most common acid in the body is carbonic acid, formed from carbon dioxide and water: $H_2O + CO_2 \rightarrow H_2CO_3$, whereas bicarbonate ($HCO_3^-$) is the most common base. The ratio of bicarbonate to carbonic acid in the ECF is normal 20:1 (Fig. 33.15). This ratio is important in maintaining a normal pH. A blood pH of less than 7.35, termed **acidemia**, can result from an excess production of hydrogen ions or a loss of bicarbonate. **Alkalemia**, or a pH greater than 7.45, occurs when there is excess bicarbonate or a lack of hydrogen ions.

There are three major systems that contribute to acid–base regulation: the lungs, the kidneys, and the buffer systems.

The Lungs

Carbon dioxide is produced as a byproduct of many cellular reactions and combines with water to make carbonic acid. By regulating the amount of carbon dioxide excreted, the lungs regulate carbonic acid levels. Increased carbon CO_2 levels in the blood trigger chemoreceptors in the medulla, which in turn stimulate the lungs to increase the rate and depth of respirations and more carbon dioxide is exhaled. In healthy lungs, this process can rapidly decrease the amount of carbonic acid in the body and return the pH to normal levels. If CO_2 levels decrease, the process is reversed, the rate and depth of respirations decreases, and more carbonic acid is formed to keep the pH within the desired level.

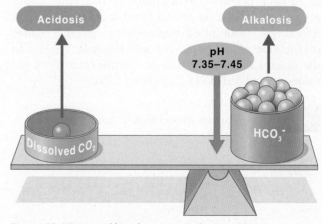

Figure 33.15 Normal bicarbonate to carbonic acid ratio.

The Kidneys

The kidneys are responsible for regulating the body's bicarbonate levels. In response to changing pH levels, the kidney alters the amount of hydrogen that is excreted and the amount of bicarbonate that is formed or excreted. When the plasma pH is low (acidosis), the kidneys excrete hydrogen ions and form and retain more bicarbonate ions: $H_2CO_2 \rightarrow$ excreted H^+ + retained HCO_3^-.

In the presence of alkalosis, H^+ is retained and less bicarbonate is formed or retained. This process occurs over a period of hours rather than the minutes it takes for the lungs to restore normal pH levels. In elderly patients or those with impaired renal function, bicarbonate adjustments can take several days (Pruitt, 2010).

Buffer Systems

A buffer is similar to a sponge that can soak up and release free hydrogen ions. The carbonic acid–bicarbonate system described previously is the body's most important buffer and acts in the following way: $H_2O + CO_3 \leftrightarrow H_2CO_3 \leftrightarrow H^+ + HCO_3^-$. Note that this reaction can go either to the left or to the right, dependent on whether the body is gaining or losing hydrogen ions. Carbonic anhydrase is the enzyme that permits the conversion of water and carbon dioxide into carbonic acid. This buffering system is useful as a transport mechanism for carbon dioxide; it also explains the relationship between carbon dioxide levels in the body and the pH of body fluids, as is discussed on the next section.

Other buffer systems include hemoglobin and plasma proteins, which can bind with hydrogen ions both in the plasma and in red blood cells, and the phosphate buffer system. The phosphate buffer system is active in ICF, especially in the renal tubules.

Acid–Base Disorders

Several disease processes can result in a disturbance in the body's acid–base balance. In addition to data obtained from the patient's history and physical assessment, an arterial blood gas is performed to determine the type of imbalance present. Analysis of an arterial blood sample will provide information about blood oxygen levels and the relative contribution of the respiratory and metabolic systems to the patient's acid–base imbalance. Normal adult blood gas values are outlined in Box 33.9 (Pruitt, 2010).

BOX 33.9   Normal Blood Gas Values

pH	7.35–7.45
PaO_2	80–100 mmHg
$PaCO_2$	35–45 mmHg
HCO_3^-	22–26 mmol/L
SaO_2	95%–100%

Acid–base abnormalities occur when the carbonic acid to bicarbonate ratio is altered. When the primary cause of the disturbance is respiratory, the result is respiratory **acidosis** or **alkalosis**. When the bicarbonate balance is altered, the result is metabolic acidosis or alkalosis. In many cases, combined metabolic and respiratory disturbance can occur. A pH of less than 7.35 indicates acidosis, whereas a pH of greater than 7.45 is alkalosis. The amount of oxygen and carbon dioxide dissolved in arterial blood is measured, and their partial pressure (P) or tension is reported as PaO_2 and $PaCO_2$ with the "a" indicating an arterial sample.

A PaO_2 of less than 80 indicates that less oxygen is being transported in the blood, whereas a high PaO_2 reflects an elevated blood oxygen level. Most oxygen (about 97%) in the blood is bound to hemoglobin in the red blood cells. Oxygen saturation measures the percentage of hemoglobin that is saturated with oxygen. Normally, at least 95% of the hemoglobin in the blood is saturated with oxygen.

$PaCO_2$ is a measure of the activity of the respiratory system. An elevated $PaCO_2$ occurs when the lungs are unable to adequately excrete or "blow off" carbon dioxide. This may occur if CO_2 produced in the body cannot reach the gas exchange membrane of the alveoli because of problems with lung perfusion, if the gas exchange membrane is not functioning because of damage or disease processes, or if the patient's respiratory depth or rate is inadequate to match the rate of carbon dioxide production. When CO_2 levels in the blood increase, more carbonic acid will be produced, leading to a decrease in pH and the development of respiratory acidosis. Conversely, a low $PaCO_2$ occurs when excess amounts of CO_2 are excreted from the lungs, usually as a result of an elevated respiratory rate. The resulting decrease in carbonic acid in the blood leads to respiratory alkalosis.

Tip: increased $CO_2 \rightarrow$ increased $H_2CO_3 \rightarrow$ decreased pH; decreased $CO_2 \rightarrow$ decreased $H_2CO_3 \rightarrow$ increased pH

The bicarbonate level (HCO_3^-) reflects the metabolic or nonrespiratory contribution to acid–base balance. Recall that the kidneys regulate bicarbonate levels by altering the formation and retention of bicarbonate ions. A shortage of bicarbonate ions leaves more H^+ unbuffered, resulting in a lower pH or metabolic acidosis, whereas excess bicarbonate leads to metabolic alkalosis.

Tip: increased $HCO_3 \rightarrow$ increased pH; decreased $HCO_3 \rightarrow$ decreased pH

Low levels of bicarbonate (metabolic acidosis) result from conditions such as renal failure, DKA starvation, or diarrhea. Metabolic alkalosis results from the loss of gastric acid seen in prolonged vomiting or nasogastric tube drainage.

Because cellular function is optimal at normal pH levels, the body will attempt to compensate for dysfunction in either the metabolic or respiratory system by altering the function of the opposite system. The lungs will compensate for a metabolic disturbance by increasing or decreasing the rate and depth of respirations until a normal pH is restored. Remember that, in the case of healthy lungs, this can be done in a matter of minutes to hours.

When the disturbance originates with the lungs, the kidneys attempt to compensate by altering the excretion of bicarbonate, retaining more bicarbonate to compensate for respiratory acidosis and excreting more bicarbonate to compensate for respiratory alkalosis. When the body is unable to compensate for a disturbance, correction may be required. *Correction* refers to the use of interventions such as mechanical ventilation or pharmacologic buffers to restore a normal pH.

Intravenous Therapy

IV therapy, used to administer fluids, electrolytes, drugs, and blood products, is common in hospitalized patients. It is estimated that over 90% of hospitalized patients require IV therapy. Most IV solutions are administered by inserting a needle into a vein (venipuncture) and threading a plastic catheter into a peripheral vein. The plastic catheter is left in the vein for the duration of the required IV therapy. If prolonged IV access is required, the IV site is changed according to institution policy or if the catheter becomes dislodged from the vein. In most institutions, nurses are responsible for establishing IV access and administering the appropriate IV solution, monitoring the IV site at regular intervals, tracking the patient's intake, and discontinuing therapy when it is no longer needed. In addition, nurses must also assess the patient on an ongoing basis for signs of the effectiveness of the therapy and for any adverse effects that may result from IV therapy.

The selection of both the IV site and the solution to be infused depends on the purpose of the IV, anticipated duration of therapy, and on patient factors such as age. Let's begin by looking at the indications for IV therapy.

Indications for Intravenous Therapy

Patients who are unable to eat or drink properly may need IV therapy to maintain fluid and electrolyte balance. Others may have a preexisting fluid or electrolyte imbalance that needs to be corrected or may need medications that can only be administered parenterally. Finally, some patients will require the administration of blood products or parenteral nutrition.

Intravenous Solutions

IV solutions contain water combined with dextrose or electrolytes. There are several standard IV solutions containing a combination of water and dextrose, or dextrose and saline, or saline. Plain water is never given intravenously because it moves too quickly into the ICF and would cause cells to swell and burst. IV solutions may be hypotonic, isotonic, or hypertonic. Isotonic solutions such as normal saline have an osmolality similar to that of plasma. Because the osmolality is close to that of plasma, it expands the ECF but does not cause red blood cells to change size. Hypotonic solutions such as half-strength saline can be used to replace fluid in the cells because the solution contains fewer solutes than plasma and will move into the cells to equalize the osmolality between the ECF and ICF. Hypertonic solutions contain more solutes than plasma and draw water into the ECF. This fluid shift can cause cells to shrink and must be used with caution. Solutions containing dextrose deserve special mention because although they may initially have a higher osmolality than plasma, glucose is quickly metabolized, leaving an isotonic or even hypotonic solution. Table 33.4 outlines the most common IV solutions.

Various electrolytes can be added to IV solutions to restore electrolyte imbalances. It is important to consider the final osmolality of any IV solution with additives. Solutions with higher concentrations of solutes may need to be administered into a vein with a large volume of blood capable of diluting the IV solution. Central veins such as the superior or inferior vena cava are more suited for hypertonic solutions but must be accessed through special catheters such as a **peripherally inserted central**

TABLE 33.4	Common Intravenous Solutions
D5W	Used to supply water in a dehydrated patient and in the treatment of hypernatremia; contains 50 g of glucose per litre Osmolality is 252 mOsm/L. Initially, an isotonic solution; glucose is rapidly metabolized leaving a hypotonic solution.
10% Dextrose in water (D10W)	Is initially hypertonic but, as glucose is metabolized, becomes hypotonic; contains 100 g of glucose per litre and supplies 340 cal/L; supplies water and calories
0.9% NaCl	An isotonic solution (308 mOsm/L) often used as a volume expander; contains 154 mmol/L of sodium; provides no calories and contains too much sodium and chloride to be used as a maintenance solution; only solution that can be given with blood products
0.45% NaCl (½ normal saline)	A hypotonic solution (154 mOsm/L) containing small amounts of sodium and chloride; used to replace fluid volume in patients with hypernatremia
Lactated Ringer	An isotonic solution containing sodium chloride, potassium, calcium, and bicarbonate in concentrations similar to plasma; used to treat hypovolemia and mild metabolic acidosis; may be used as a volume expander; cannot be used with renal failure because it contains potassium
5% Dextrose in 0.45% NaCl	A hypertonic solution that can be used to treat hypovolemia or to maintain fluid intake
5% Dextrose in 0.9% NaCl	Supplies calories and sodium; can be used to treat hypovolemia

catheter (PICC) line or through a central line inserted via a cutdown procedure.

For patients who are unable to eat, IV solutions can be used to provide calories and nutrients. **Total parenteral nutrition (TPN)** is a specially formulated solution that contains glucose, protein, fats, minerals, and vitamins. Although it is possible to administer some TPN formulations in a peripheral vein, the higher concentration of solutes in most TPN solutions require that they be given through a catheter inserted into a large or central vein.

Blood products including whole blood, packed red blood cells, platelets, albumin, plasma, and cryoprecipitate are given by IV.

Various medications are administered by IV. The IV route may be desirable because it allows the medication to enter the circulation quickly. This also makes the IV route more hazardous because of the speed in which adverse reactions can occur. Medications given by IV may be given by continuous infusion or by a bolus infusion given into the IV line. When giving drugs by the IV route, it is important to follow recognized drug administration guidelines or the manufacturer's recommendations regarding drug dilution and speed of administration. Prior to giving any medication, you must follow the standard safety checks to determine that the patient has been correctly identified and has no history of allergic reactions to medications, that the drug is the correct one,

the dose is correct, the route of administration is correct, and that the time for administration is correct.

Choosing an Intravenous Site

Several factors need to be considered when choosing an IV site. Patient factors such as age, weight, and health condition may render some sites more appropriate than others. For example, the hands and feet may be a poor choice in a patient with edema. Patients who have had axillary nodes removed should not have a venipuncture in that arm. An IV should never be started near an intended surgical site. The ability to secure an IV site is a consideration in young children or in someone with delirium or dementia. The veins of the arms are generally good sites for an IV infusion (Fig. 33.16). Choose the nondominant arm if possible so that the patient can continue to use his or her dominant hand. An IV started in the antecubital vein is difficult to secure and should not be a first choice. The vessels on the back of the hand are suitable for IV lines in children and adults; however, for the elderly patients, these vessels may be too fragile. Vessels in the legs are not normally used for IV lines in adult patients because of the risk of venous stagnation. In infants, vessels on the top of the foot are used when other options are limited.

The type of IV solution to be infused should also be considered in selecting an IV site. Hypertonic solutions, those

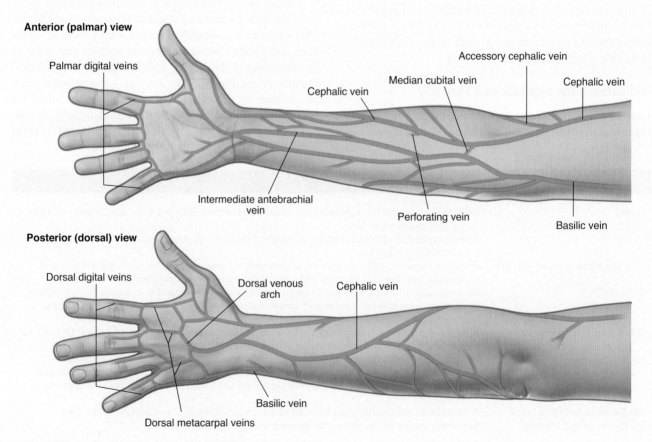

Figure 33.16 Site selection for peripheral IV line.

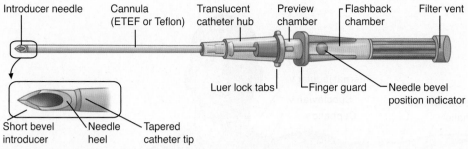

Figure 33.17 Catheters and cannulas for IV therapy.

that are administered rapidly and those containing medications or electrolytes (e.g., calcium) that are irritating to the veins, dictate the need for a large vein; in some cases, a CVAD.

As a general rule, the smallest, shortest catheter inserted into the largest available vein will result in the fewest complications. Of course, not all solutions can be administered through a small cannula.

> ### Think *How Many Pokes?*
>
> You are assisting a senior nurse in starting an IV infusion in an elderly patient. After the third unsuccessful attempt, the nurse is unable to establish the IV. The patient is crying and clearly uncomfortable. Do you think that this nurse should try a fourth time to start the IV?
>
> Some hospital units or wards have established policies guiding the number of attempts an individual should make at starting an IV before asking someone else to try. Some nurses feel that after two or, at most three attempts, someone else should be called to start the IV. This is especially true in populations where IV access can be more challenging such as in children or the elderly. It is important to remember that even the most skilled health-care providers can have difficulty in establishing an IV and that this is not a reflection of their overall skills or abilities.

Types of Intravenous Catheters

There are various catheters and cannulas available to provide IV therapy (Fig. 33.17). The choice of device depends on the purpose of the IV; the patient's age, size, and physical condition; the type of solution to be infused; and the preference of the operator.

The type of catheter or cannula available varies from institution to institution. Peripheral venous catheters are suitable for most short-term infusions, provided the concentration of the IV fluid is not too hypertonic for infusion into the smaller peripheral veins. When a patient requires IV therapy for a longer period of time, if the required IV solution is hypertonic or if the peripheral veins are fragile or damaged, access to a larger vein may be required. In that case, a **central venous access device (CVAD)**

could be inserted. The tip of a central line is positioned in a larger vein, usually the superior or inferior vena cava where the increased blood flow can more rapidly disperse and dilute hypertonic solutions. The risk of infiltration is lower in central lines, which are less likely to move outside the blood vessel.

Peripheral Venous Catheters

The most common type of peripheral venous line is an over-the-needle catheter with a soft plastic sheet over a metal needle. These catheters, come in sizes from 16 to 24 gauge and lengths of 25 to 45 mm (Dougherty, 2008). Keep in mind that the lower the gauge, the larger the size of the catheter and therefore the faster the fluid will flow through the catheter. Larger gauge catheters are more likely to damage the vein than smaller catheters. Once the needle enters the vein, it is removed, leaving the plastic sheath or cannula in the vein. In adults, peripheral IV insertion sites are usually rotated every 72 to 96 hours to avoid injury to the vein (Scales, 2008). Because IV access in children are more difficult to obtain and do not last as long as those in an adult, they are usually left in place until they are no longer needed or until a complication develops.

Central Venous Access Devices

CVADs are becoming more common in both hospital and community settings. In addition to providing access for IV therapy, some CVADs can also be used for blood sampling and pressure monitoring. Various CVADs are available including PICC lines, percutaneous central venous catheters, tunneled central venous catheters, and port devices. An x-ray is required to confirm the placement of a CVAD.

Peripherally Inserted Central Catheter Lines

Central venous catheters can be inserted into a peripheral vein and advanced until the tip reaches a central vein (Fig. 33.18). These catheters are referred to as *peripherally inserted central catheters (PICCs) lines*. PICC lines are inserted by physicians or registered nurses with specialized training and typically remain in place for several weeks unless complications develop. Nursing care of a patient with a PICC line

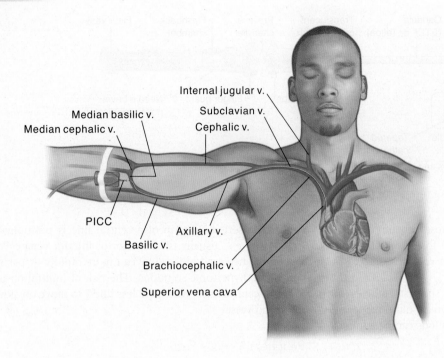

Internal jugular v.
Median basilic v.
Subclavian v.
Median cephalic v.
Cephalic v.
PICC
Axillary v.
Basilic v.
Brachiocephalic v.
Superior vena cava

Figure 33.18 Placement of PICC.

includes monitoring the condition of the insertion site and the line. Sterile dressing changes are done if the dressing is loose or soiled and according to institutional policy. Nursing Guideline 33.1 outlines steps in the care of a patient with a PICC line.

NURSING GUIDELINE 33.1: NURSING CARE OF THE PATIENT WITH A PERIPHERALLY INSERTED CENTRAL CATHETER LINE

- Assess the insertion site and extremity below the site according to institution policy.
- Solution and tubing changes are performed as indicated by institution policy. These are usually done with sterile technique.
- Keep the external portion of the catheter coiled under dressing and secure to avoid any traction on the tubing.
- Access the line only as needed using sterile technique and according to institution policy.
- When flushing the line, use saline or saline with heparin according to medical orders.
- Use sterile technique to change dressings as outlined in institution policy and if loose or solid.
- Avoid venipuncture and blood pressure measurement in involved arm.
- Document:
  - Appearance of site and extremity
  - Date of dressing and line change
  - Insertion distance marking at insertion site, if available
  - Complications, if any

Adapted from Taylor, C. R., Lillis, C., LeMone, P., & Lynn, P. (2011). *Fundamentals of nursing: The art and science of nursing care* (7th ed., p. 1708). Philadelphia, PA: Lippincott Williams & Wilkins.

Percutaneous and Tunneled Central Catheters

Percutaneous central catheters are usually inserted into the internal jugular, subclavian, or femoral vein. Tunnelled catheters are inserted into the subcutaneous tissue 3 to 6 in. from the entry into the vein. It is initially sutured into place. A cuff around the tunnelled portion of the catheter helps to stabilize the catheter. These catheters provide access for hypertonic solutions or for longer term use such as for TPN or medications.

Central lines must be monitored carefully. Because they remain in place for longer periods of time, there is an increased risk of bloodstream infections. Dressing and tubing changes must be done with careful attention to sterile technique.

Implanted Ports

Ports have a catheter, which is inserted into the internal jugular or subclavian vein. The catheter is attached to a reservoir, which is inserted under the skin in the upper chest. No part of the system is visible outside the body. Medications such as antibiotics or chemotherapy can be injected into the reservoir, or an IV infusion can be administered into the reservoir. Ports are designed for long-term intermittent infusions such as chemotherapy or antibiotic administration.

Starting an Intravenous Infusion

Like medications, IV solutions must be checked carefully prior to initiating an infusion. Check to ensure that the correct solution has been prepared for the correct patient. Compare the label on the IV bag to the patient's prescription and compare the name and identifying information on the patients chart to the patient's identification band.

Examine the IV solution to ensure that is not discoloured and does not have undissolved particles. Because of the added risks associated with infusing blood products, most institutions have additional safety procedures that must be undertaken before initiating a transfusion of blood products. Depending on the solution and the type of line being used, an in-line filter may be added to further reduce the risk of contamination. The steps for starting an IV infusion are outlined in Skill 33.1.

Through the eyes of a nurse

I remember as a student nurse how excited I was at the prospect of starting my first IV line in a patient. Beforehand, I had reviewed the mechanics of setting up the IV: checking who and what the IV was for, preparing the line itself, landmarking and preparing the actual site, proper technique for insertion, looking for flashback and removing the stylet, and securing the IV. To my immense pride, the first attempt worked! However, in the months to follow, I wasn't always so successful, and I often watched in frustration and awe as more experienced nurses were able to establish IV access in "difficult" patients.

In time, as one becomes an experienced nurse, it is possible to appreciate both the science and the art behind IV therapy. It is not simply the mechanical skill that confers competence; an understanding of the rationale behind IV therapy is just as important. And then there is that elusive "skill" which cannot always be explained, but which the more experienced nurses seemed to have. Moreover, the expert also needs to "see" the patient, which is a critical part of both the nurse–patient relationship and of assessing the effects of the medication being administered. As my mechanical skills developed, the other more advanced competencies started coming as well.

(personal reflection of a nurse)

Changing the Intravenous Solution

As a nurse, you will be responsible for changing the IV solution when the bag is empty or when the IV order changes. The IV bag is usually changed at least every 24 hours. The frequency of the IV tubing change is dictated by institution policy. Any time an IV line is opened, aseptic technique must be used to reduce the risk of infection. Follow your hospital protocol to minimize the risk of errors and complications.

Nursing Care of the Patient Receiving Intravenous Therapy

In addition to the assessments listed in Skill 33.1, nurses are also responsible for determining and maintaining the proper flow rate and ensuring that the patient is safe and

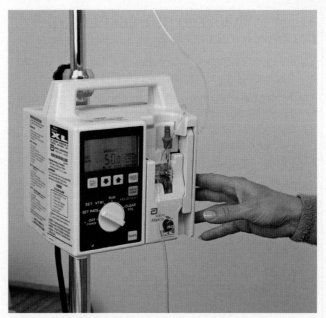

Figure 33.19 Programmable IV pump.

comfortable while receiving IV therapy. The physician or nurse practitioner orders the IV infusion as an hourly rate or as a specified volume of fluid given over a certain time period; for example, 30 ml over 3 hours. The volume of fluid is divided by the time to determine an hourly rate of infusion. For infusions given with a programmable pump, the total volume to be infused and the hourly IV are entered into the pump (Fig. 33.19). When using a free flow or gravity system, the drip rate must be calculated and then adjusted to ensure that the patient receives the correct amount of fluid.

The IV **drop factor** (drops per millilitre of solution) varies according to the infusion apparatus and is different for products manufactured by different companies. Macrodrop infusion sets typically have a drop factor of 10, 15, or 20 drops/ml, whereas microdrop systems have a drop factor of 60. Once you know the drop factor for the IV apparatus, then a formula can be used to calculate the appropriate drop rate (Nursing Guideline 33.2).

Hourly time intervals can be marked on the IV bag and used to check that the fluid is infused at the appropriate rate. The IV should be checked at least every hour to ensure that the correct volume is infusing. Infusion rates can be altered by various factors such as a position change, clots or obstructions in the cannula, compression of the IV tubing, and changes in the patient's blood pressure. For pediatric patients, a volume control device (Buretrol or Soluset for example) is used to reduce the risk of giving too much fluid (Fig. 33.20).

Managing a Saline Lock

In some situations, a patient may require intermittent IV access for administration of medications or fluids. In this case, the IV can be converted to heparin or saline lock. Nursing Guideline 33.3 provides information on changing an IV to an intermittent access device.

NURSING GUIDELINE 33.2: REGULATING INTRAVENOUS FLOW RATE

Follow agency's guidelines to determine if infusion should be administered by electronic pump or by gravity.

- Check physician's order for IV solution.
- Check patency of IV line and needle.
- Verify drop factor (number of drops in 1 mL) of the equipment in use.
- Calculate the flow rate.

EXAMPLE—Administer 1,000 mL D$_5$W over 10 hours (set delivers 60 gtt/1 mL).

a. Standard formula

$$\text{gtt/min} = \frac{\text{volume (mL)} \times \text{drop factor (gtt/mL)}}{\text{time (in minutes)}}$$

$$\text{gtt/min} = \frac{1,000 \text{ mL} \times 60}{600 \text{ (60 min} \times 10 \text{ h)}}$$

$$= \frac{60,000}{600}$$

$$= 100 \text{ gtt/min}$$

b. Short formula using milliliters per hour

$$\text{gtt/min} = \frac{\text{milliliters per hour} \times \text{drop factor (gtt/mL)}}{\text{time (60 min)}}$$

Find milliliters per hour by dividing 1,000 mL by 10 hours:

$$\frac{1,000}{10} = 100 \text{ mL/hr}$$

$$\text{gtt/min} = \frac{100 \text{ mL} \times 60}{60 \text{ min}}$$

$$= \frac{6,000}{60}$$

$$= 100 \text{ gtt/min}$$

From Taylor, C. R., Lillis, C., LeMone, P., & Lynn, P. (2011). Fluid, electrolyte, and acid-base balance. In C. R. Taylor, C. Lilis, P. LeMone, & P. Lynn (Eds.), *Fundamentals of nursing: The art and science of nursing care* (7th ed., p. 1414). Philadelphia, PA: Lippincott Williams & Wilkins.

Discontinuing an Intravenous Infusion

When the required fluids have been administered and the patient is eating and drinking well, IV therapy is discontinued. It may also be discontinued if complications develop. To discontinue an IV, begin by obtaining a small sterile gauze and tape or a small occlusive dressing. Put on nonsterile gloves because you may come into contact with the patient's blood. Turn off the infusion pump and close the roller clamp to occlude the tubing. Gently remove the dressing over the IV insertion site, taking care not to dislodge the catheter. Place a sterile gauze over the insertion site and withdraw the catheter. Place gentle pressure over the site until any bleeding has stopped. Cover the site with a small dressing. Check the catheter to ensure that it was intact on removal. Document the time that therapy was stopped, the condition of the catheter insertion site, and the total amount of fluid that was

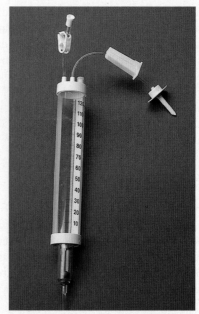

Figure 33.20 Volume control set.

infused. Note any complications of therapy and any nursing interventions taken.

Removal of the Peripherally Inserted Central Catheter Line

The removal of a PICC line is governed by agency policies. A member of the PICC insertion team or a nurse with specialized training may be responsible for PICC line removal. When a central or PICC line is removed, special precautions

NURSING GUIDELINE 33.3: CONVERTING AN INTRAVENOUS TO AN INTERMITTENT ACCESS DEVICE

- Gather your supplies.
  - Extension tubing (short plastic tubing with a cap or injection port)
  - Tape and label
  - Nonlatex gloves
- Wash your hands and put on gloves.
- Close the roller clamp on the existing IV tubing.
- Label the extension tubing with the date and time and your initials.
- Flush the extension tubing with saline or saline with heparin.
- Using clean technique, disconnect the IV tubing and connect the extension set.
- Flush the extension set with saline or saline with heparin according to the patient's medical orders or institution policy.
- Observe the IV site and assess the patient's comfort and tolerance of the procedure.
- Document the procedure, including the following:
  - Date and time therapy initiated
  - Type and amount of flush
  - Condition of the insertion site
  - Patient's response to procedure

TABLE 33.5 Complications of Intravenous Therapy

Complication/Cause	Signs and Symptoms	Nursing Considerations
Infiltration: the escape of fluid into the subcutaneous tissue Dislodged needle Penetrated vessel wall	Swelling, pallor, coldness, or pain around the infusion site; significant decrease in the flow rate	Check the infusion site several times per shift for symptoms. Discontinue the infusion if symptoms occur. Restart the infusion at a different site. Limit the movement of the extremity with the IV.
Sepsis: microorganisms invade the bloodstream through the catheter insertion site. Poor insertion technique Multilumen catheters Long-term catheter insertion Frequent dressing changes Immunocompromised patient	Red and tender insertion site Fever, malaise, other vital sign changes	Assess catheter site daily. Notify physician immediately for any sign of infection. Follow agency protocol for culture of drainage. Use scrupulous aseptic technique when starting an infusion.
Phlebitis: an inflammation of a vein Mechanical trauma from needle or catheter Chemical trauma from solution Septic (due to contamination) Thrombus: a blood clot Tissue trauma from needle or catheter	Local, acute tenderness; redness, warmth, and slight edema of the vein above the insertion site Symptoms similar to phlebitis; IV fluid flow may cease if clot obstructs needle.	Discontinue the infusion immediately. Apply warm, moist compresses to the affected site. Avoid further use of the vein Restart the infusion in another vein. Stop the infusion immediately. Apply warm compresses as ordered by the physician. Restart the IV at another site. Do not rub or massage the affected area.
Electrolyte imbalances	Depending on type of electrolyte solution	Notify the physician immediately. Monitor vital signs. Carefully monitor the rate of fluid flow. Check the rate frequently for accuracy. Collect blood work as ordered.
Fluid overload: the condition caused when too large a volume of fluid infuses into the circulatory system	Engorged neck veins, increased blood pressure, and difficulty in breathing (dyspnea)	If symptoms develop, slow the rate of infusion. Notify the physician immediately. Monitor vital signs. Carefully monitor the rate of fluid flow. Check the rate frequently for accuracy.
Air embolus: air in the circulatory system Break in the IV system above the heart level allowing air in the circulatory system as a bolus	Respiratory distress Increased heart rate Cyanosis Decreased blood pressure Change in level of consciousness	Pinch off catheter or secure system to prevent entry of air. Place patient on left side in Trendelenburg position. Call for immediate assistance. Monitor vital signs and pulse oximetry.

Adapted from Taylor, C. R., Lillis, C., LeMone, P., & Lynn, P. (2011). Fluid, electrolyte, and acid–base balance. In C. R. Taylor, C. Lilis, P. LeMone, & P. Lynn (Eds.), *Fundamentals of nursing: The art and science of nursing care* (7th ed., pp. 1414–1489). Philadelphia, PA: Lippincott Williams & Wilkins.

are used to ensure that the catheter is intact and that no air enters the blood vessel. The patient is usually placed flat on the bed or in Trendelenburg position and asked to perform a Valsalva maneuver while the line is removed. Gentle traction is placed on the catheter avoiding tugging or twisting. If resistance is encountered, the procedure is stopped and a physician or nurse practitioner is notified. Once the catheter is removed, an occlusive dressing is placed over the site and left in place for 48 to 72 hours.

Complications of Intravenous Therapy

IV therapy requires careful monitoring both to assess the effectiveness of therapy and also to watch for complications. It is important that you monitor your patient at regular intervals and carefully document your findings. Common complications include infiltration, phlebitis, infection, fluid overload, and electrolyte imbalances. Air embolism and

catheter breakage are less common and occur mainly with central lines rather than with peripheral IV lines. Table 33.5 summarizes the common IV complications.

Infiltration

Infiltration occurs when IV fluid leaks into the interstitial tissue, often as a result of the catheter tip slipping through the wall of the vein. Signs of infiltration include pain and swelling at the insertion site. The IV will likely infuse more slowly. Some IV solutions such as TPN or those containing calcium are very irritating to the vein and can cause serious tissue damage if the infiltration is not recognized quickly. Infiltrations can be graded according to symptoms and severity (Table 33.6).

Phlebitis

The presence of an IV catheter is irritating to the vein and can cause an inflammation (phlebitis). If a blood clot forms in the vein, the resulting inflammation is labeled

TABLE 33.6	Millam Scale of Intravenous Infiltrations
Stage	**Symptoms**
Stage I	Painful IV site, no erythema, no swelling
Stage II	Painful IV site, slight swelling (0%–20%), no blanching, good pulse below infiltration site, brisk capillary refill below infiltration site
Stage III	Painful IV site, marked swelling (30%–50%), blanching, skin cool to touch, good pulse below infiltration site, brisk capillary refill below infiltration site
Stage IV	Painful IV site, very marked swelling (>50%), blanching, skin cool to touch, decreased or absent pulse,* capillary refill >4 seconds,* skin breakdown or necrosis*

*The presence of any of the marked conditions constitutes a stage IV infiltration.

From Millam, D. A. (1988). Managing complications of IV therapy. *Nursing, 18*(3), 34–43.

thrombophlebitis. Redness and warmth over the insertion site or the vessel proximal to the IV site are signs of phlebitis. Discomfort is also present. Phlebitis is more likely to develop as the length of time the IV is in place increases. Other risk factors include polyvinyl chloride catheters, small vein size, and IV placement in the lower extremities. The IV site should be assessed according to unit protocol for phlebitis, using a standardized grading scale (Box 33.10).

Infection

When IV sites are routinely changed, the risk of infection is lessened. CVADs are more likely to become infected than peripheral IV lines because they remain in place longer. The patient who is immunocompromised is also at increased risk of infection. Many agencies have adopted a standardized approach to central line care known as a **bundle**. Bundles are simply groups of practices that, together, are more likely to decrease line infections. Hand hygiene, sterile two-person line changes, and limiting the number of times a line can be opened are examples of practices thought to decrease central line infections.

Fluid Overload

Rapid administration of IV fluids can exceed the kidney's ability to handle the fluid volume leading to a state of fluid overload. Patients with congestive heart failure, those with renal disease, infants, and the elderly are especially vulnerable. Signs of fluid overload include increased blood pressure, respiratory distress, crackles in the lung fields, edema, and increased weight. The risk of fluid overload is decreased with careful monitoring of the rate and quantity of fluid administered.

Electrolyte Imbalances

Excessive administration of fluid can lead to dilutional hyponatremia. Administration of 0.9% saline or infusions containing electrolytes can lead to high levels of these electrolytes.

BOX 33.10 Infiltration Scale

Grade and document infiltration according to the most severe presenting indicator.

Grade	Clinical Criteria
0	No symptoms
1	Skin blanched
	Edema <1 in. in any direction
	Cool to touch
	With or without pain
2	Skin blanched
	Edema 1–6 in. in any direction
	Cool to touch
	With or without pain
3	Skin blanched, translucent
	Gross edema >6 in. in any direction
	Cool to touch
	Mild to moderate pain
	Possible numbness
4	Skin blanched, translucent
	Skin tight, leaking
	Skin discoloured, bruised, swollen
	Gross edema >6 in. in any direction
	Deep pitting tissue edema
	Circulatory impairment
	Moderate to severe pain
	Infiltration of any amount of blood product, irritant, or vesicant

Adapted from Infusion Nurses Society. (2006). Infusion nursing standards of practice. *Journal of Infusion Nursing, 29*(1S), S60.

The nurse should monitor lab results and assess the patient frequently for signs and symptoms of electrolyte disturbances.

Remember Connor, the 3-year-old boy in the emergency ward with nausea and vomiting? Connor was assessed as having moderate dehydration (see Table 33.1). His urine was dark yellow and the specific gravity was 1.025. Blood work was done that showed a serum sodium level of 142 and a serum potassium of 3.7 mmol/L. Connor was kept in the emergency room for 6 hours and during that time received oral rehydration therapy (ORT) of 100 ml/kg. Flavored ORT popsicles were given first followed by small amounts of flavored ORT liquid. After 4 hours, Connor had not experienced any further vomiting and was playing happily with his toy cars. Connor's mother was instructed to continue to replace any fluid losses with equal amounts of pediatric oral rehydration drinks or popsicles and that Connor should resume his normal diet. Connor's mother was further taught to monitor Connor for signs of dehydration and to return to the emergency department if Connor became dehydrated or could not tolerate oral therapy (Leung et al., 2006).

SKILL 33.1	Establishing an Intravenous Line

Review Pertinent Information

Step	Rationale
Verify order for IV therapy, check solution label against the order, and identify patient. Check for allergies (i.e., latex, iodine).	Serious errors can be avoided by careful checking. Checking for allergies reduces risk of allergic reaction.

Preparing Intravenous Line Start

Step	Rationale
Wash hands.	Prevents the spread of microorganisms to the supplies being used and handled and prevents further spread to the patient
Gather supplies needed: • Gloves • IV solution • Tourniquet • IV catheter or cannula • IV administration set • Needleless connector (if needed) • IV infusion pump (if using) • Alcohol swabs or equivalent • Tape or transparent dressing • Label for the site	Important to get organized prior to beginning the procedure; organization can save time and reduce the potential for errors. The use of IV pumps, fluid administration sets, and needleless connectors is dictated by the type of IV infusion, the age of the patient, and institutional policy.
Prepare the equipment by: • Inserting the fluid administration set into the labeled IV solution • Priming the tubing by filling it with the IV solution • Closing the roller clamp until the IV has been established • Inserting the IV tubing into the infusion pump (if being used) and programming the pump according to the patient's IV order • Labeling the tubing with the date and time and your initials	 The tubing should be free of air in order to reduce the risk of air embolism. Closing the roller clamp will prevent the loss of any IV fluid. If an infusion pump is being used, it should be programmed in order to ensure that it is ready to use when the IV has been established. The IV bag and tubing should be labeled with the date and time they were opened in order to ensure that solutions and tubing is changed at the interval dictated by institution policy or manufacturers' recommendations.
Prepare the patient by: • Checking patient's identifying information using a two-step method; checking the patient's armband and then asking the patient to verify name • Checking the IV solution order against the armband • Explaining the purpose of the IV and the process of establishing catheter • Adjusting the bed or chair height and creating privacy; position patient's arm below heart level to encourage capillary filling. Place protective pad on bed under patient's arm. • Completing any necessary preadministration assessments • Providing patient teaching about the infusion and needed follow-up	Double-checking patient identification decreases potential for error greatly. Explaining the purpose of the IV and what will occur fosters patient collaboration and increases patient comfort. Proper positioning will increase likelihood of success and provide comfort for patient. Teaching can provide the necessary understanding that will foster more effective outcomes through patient participation.

Establishing the Intravenous Line

Step	Rationale
Wash hands and put on nonlatex gloves.	Gloves will protect the patient from surface organisms from the nurse's hands and will protect the nurse from possible body secretions that may come into contact with the nurse's hands during the administration procedure. Use of nonlatex gloves reducing the patient's exposure to a potential allergen

(continued on page 856)

SKILL 33.1 Establishing an Intravenous Line (continued)

Establishing the Intravenous Line (continued)

Step	Rationale
Select site for the IV. Use distal veins of the hands and arms first.	Selection of the site should be based on the purpose of the IV, the age of the patient, and the patient's condition.
	Careful site selection will increase likelihood of successful venipuncture and preservation of vein. Using distal sites first preserves sites proximal to the previously cannulated site for subsequent venipunctures. Veins of feet and lower extremity should be avoided due to risk of thrombophlebitis. (In consultation with the physician, the saphenous vein of the ankle or dorsum of the foot may occasionally be used.)
Choose IV cannula or catheter.	Length and gauge of cannula should be appropriate for both site and purpose of infusion. The shortest gauge and length needed to deliver prescribed therapy should be used. Inspect the needle or cannula to make sure there are no imperfections.
Apply a tourniquet 4–6 in. above the site and identify a suitable vein (see Figure 1).	This will distend the veins and allow them to be visualized.

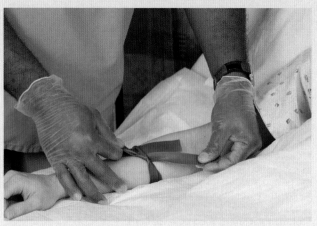

Figure 1 Applying the tourniquet. (Source: Taylor et al., 2011)

Palpate for a pulse distal to the tourniquet. Ask patient to open and close fist several times or position patient's arm in a dependent position to distend a vein.	The tourniquet should never be tight enough to occlude arterial flow. If a radial pulse cannot be palpated distal to the tourniquet, it is too tight. A new tourniquet should be used for each patient to prevent the transmission of microorganisms. A clenched fist encourages the vein to protrude. Positioning the arm below the level of the patient's heart promotes capillary filling. Warm packs applied for 10–20 minutes prior to venipuncture can promote vasodilation. Bedside ultrasound-guided visualization of vein location and assessment of venous pathway and flow using ultrasonic waves may also be used.
Prepare site by scrubbing with chlorhexidine gluconate or povidone-iodine swabs for 2–3 minutes in circular motion, moving outward from injection site. Allow to dry.	Strict asepsis and careful site preparation are essential to prevent infection.
a. If the site selected is excessively hairy, clip hair. (Check agency's policy and procedure about this practice.)	Hair removal should be performed with scissors or electric clippers. Shaving should not be done with a razor because of the potential for microabrasions that increase the risk of infection.
Note: Isopropyl alcohol 70% is an alternative solution that may be used.	Depilatories should not be used due to the potential for dermal allergic reactions and/or irritation.
With hand not holding the venous access device, steady patient's arm and use finger or thumb to pull skin taut over vessel.	Applying traction to the vein helps to stabilize it.
Hold needle bevel up and at 5° to 25° angle, depending on the depth of the vein; pierce skin to reach but not penetrate vein.	Bevel-down technique is necessary for small veins to prevent extravasation. One-step method of catheter insertion directly into vein with immediate thrust through the skin is excellent for large veins but may cause a hematoma if used in small veins.
Decrease angle of needle further until nearly parallel with skin and then enter vein either directly above or from the side in one quick motion.	Two-stage procedure decreases chance of thrusting needle through posterior wall of vein as skin is entered. No attempt should be made to reinsert the stylet because of risk of severing or puncturing the catheter.

Establishing the Intravenous Line (continued)

Step	Rationale
If backflow of blood is visible, straighten angle and advance needle. Additional steps for catheter inserted over needle are as follows:	Backflow may not occur if vein is small; this position decreases chance of puncturing posterior wall of vein.
a. Advance needle 0.6 cm (1/4–1/2 in.) after successful venipuncture.	a. Advancing the needle slightly makes certain the plastic catheter has entered the vein.
b. Hold needle hub and slide catheter over the needle into the vein. Never reinsert needle into a plastic catheter or pull the catheter back into the needle.	b. Reinsertion of the needle or pulling the catheter back can sever the catheter, causing catheter embolism.
c. Remove needle while pressing lightly on the skin over the catheter tip; hold catheter hub in place.	c. Slight pressure prevents bleeding before tubing is attached.
d. Never reinsert a stylet back into a catheter.	d. The stylet can shear off a piece of the plastic if reinserted.
e. Never reuse the same catheter.	e. Reusing the same catheter can cause infection.
Release tourniquet and attach infusion tubing; open clamp enough to allow drip.	Releasing the tourniquet restores blood flow and avoids potential ischemic damage to the area distal to the IV insertion site.
Cover the insertion site with a transparent dressing, bandage, or sterile gauze according to hospital policy and procedure. Tape in place with nonallergenic tape but do not encircle extremity. Tape a small loop of IV tubing onto dressing (see Figure 2).	Transparent dressings allow assessment of the insertion site for phlebitis, infiltration, and infection without removing the dressing. Tape applied around extremity can act as a tourniquet and impede blood flow and infusion of fluid. The loop decreases the chance of inadvertent cannula removal if the tubing is pulled.

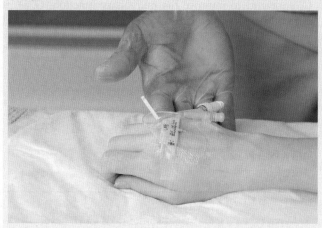

Figure 2 Applying the dressing. (Source: Taylor et al., 2011)

Step	Rationale
A padded, appropriate-length arm board may be applied to an area of flexion (neurovascular checks should be performed frequently).	This secures cannula placement and allows correct flow rate (neurovascular checks assess nerve, muscle, and vascular function to be sure function is not affected by immobilization).
Calculate infusion rate and regulate flow of infusion. See Nursing Guideline 33-2.	Infusion must be regulated carefully to prevent overinfusion or underinfusion. Calculation of the IV rate is essential for the safe delivery of fluids. Safe administration requires knowledge of the volume of fluid to be infused, total infusion time, and calibration of the administration set (found on the IV tubing package; 10, 12, 15, or 60 drops to deliver 1 ml of fluid).
Discard needles, stylets, or guidewires into a puncture-resistant needle container that meets institutional requirements. Remove gloves and perform hand hygiene.	Proper disposal of sharps decreases risk of needlesticks.

Engaging in Evaluation

Step	Rationale
Document patient response to IV start	How was the procedure for the patient? Was the patient able to cope with the procedure or was it painful?
Document effect of intervention	
Effect of intervention (e.g., Is the IV fluid flowing appropriately? Is the IV site free from bleeding, swelling, or discolouration?)	Monitoring for therapeutic effects will assist in ensuring the IV is working for the patient.
Monitor on an ongoing basis for signs of IV complications (infiltration, infection, bleeding, fluid overload, electrolyte imbalances).	An interstitial IV has the potential to cause serious injury or below the insertion site. Skin infections may develop at the site of IV insertion. Administration of fluid and electrolytes may result in overload or imbalances.

(continued on page 858)

SKILL 33.1	Establishing an Intravenous Line (continued)

Documenting Effectively

Step	Rationale
Document in a timely manner and include the following: • Date and time therapy initiated • Type and amount of solution additives and dosages • Flow rate • Gauge, length, and type of vascular access device • Catheter insertion site and type of dressing applied • Patient response to procedure • Patient teaching and name and title of the health-care provider who inserted the catheter	Documentation is the key communicative method between health-care professionals. The more complete the documentation, the better other health-care team members are able to assess and monitor the IV.

Adapted from Smeltzer, S. C., Hinkle, J. L., & Cheever, K. H. (2010). Fluid and electrolyte: Balance and disturbance. In S. C. Smeltzer, B. G. Bare, J. L. Hinkle, & K. H. Cheever (Eds.), *Brunner and Suddarth's textbook of medical and surgical nursing* (12th ed., p. 263). Philadelphia, PA: Lippincott Williams & Wilkins.

Critical Thinking Case Scenarios

Hypernatremia Case Study

▶ Mrs. Henry is an 86-year-old woman who lives alone in a seniors' complex. Her daughter brought Mrs. Henry to an urgent care clinic after she noticed that Mrs. Henry was becoming increasingly agitated and that her breathing was sounding laboured. On examination, you noticed that Mrs. Henry has a fever (39.5°C) and that her other vital signs are as follows: heart rate = 110 beats/min; blood pressure = 98/64 mmHg; respiratory rate = 24 breaths/min and laboured. Auscultation revealed that there was reduced air entry bilaterally and that crackles were audible. A sputum sample comes back from the lab as negative, but her plasma Na^+ concentration is 148 mmol/L.

1. Is your patient's Na^+ high, low, or within normal limits?
2. What are some plausible explanations for how Mrs. Henry's plasma Na^+ became altered? Could her age and social context be related to the altered electrolyte status?
3. How might her Na^+ levels explain her signs and symptoms?

Anion Gap Case Study

▶ J. D. is a 21-year-old male with Type 1 diabetes. He is admitted to the emergency room unconscious, and you detect a "fruity" odor on his breath. His chemistry panel comes back showing a high blood sugar (14 mmol/L), plasma K^+ is 3.2 mmol/L and an anion gap of $^+14$.

1. Define *anion gap*.
2. What does the anion gap in this case signify? Why is K^+ so low?
3. What is the normal treatment for DKA?
4. Why do you think J. D. is presenting with DKA at this time?

Acid–Base Case Study

▶ G. D. is a 62-year-old male who was diagnosed with emphysema 2 years ago. He has a 32-year history of cigarette smoking (which he continues to do) and is on medication (Combivent) to improve his pulmonary function. G. D. is currently on the medical ward for assessment and clinical workup. His blood gases currently are as follows:

Arterial Blood Gases	G. D.'s Values	Normal Range	Units
pH	7.28	7.35–7.45	
pCO_2	50.8	35–45	mmHg
pO_2	77.2	≥80	mmHg
Hemoglobin saturation	90%	≥95%	
HCO_3^-	24.7	22–26	mmol/L

1. What type of acid–base disorder does G. D. have?
2. What is the likely cause of this disorder?
3. Why is G. D.'s bicarbonate below normal?

Multiple-Choice Questions

1. The normal proportion of TBW in an adult is approximately:
   a. 50%
   b. 60%
   c. 75%
   d. 80%

2. The dominant extracellular cation and anion are:
   a. Sodium and bicarbonate
   b. Potassium and chloride
   c. Potassium and phosphate
   d. Sodium and chloride

3. If serum sodium is 145 mOsm/L, what is the best estimate of overall serum osmolarity?
   a. 72.5 mOsm/L
   b. 145 mOsm/L
   c. 300 mOsm/L
   d. 345 mOsm/L

4. The recommended replacement for extracellular volume fluid loss due to dehydration is:
   a. Isotonic (normal) saline solution
   b. D5W
   c. Lactated Ringer
   d. One-half normal saline solution plus 20 mmol potassium chloride per litre

5. Lactated Ringer is an isotonic, crystalloid solution that contains several electrolytes. If 800 ml are infused, what will be the net gain into the extravascular compartment?
   a. 100 ml
   b. 200 ml
   c. 400 ml
   d. 600 ml

6. The most common electrolyte disturbance in hospitalized children is:
   a. Hypernatremia
   b. Hyponatremia
   c. Hypokalemia
   d. Hyperchloremia

Suggested Lab Activities

● Keep track of your fluid intake for the next 24 hours. How does your intake compare to the average presented in Figure 33.6 in this chapter? How do you think your output compares? What changes might you make to improve your body's fluid balance?

● What is the recommended daily salt intake for the average adult? Look on the Internet to determine what the average daily salt intake is for an adult in North America. Go to the supermarket and check the ingredient list for four or five popular frozen packed meals. How does the salt content of those meals compare to the recommended daily salt intake?

● Think about methods you can use to ease the pain and discomfort associated with venipuncture. What nonpharmacologic measures might you use? What topical preparations are available to numb the skin? How would you modify your approach for a child? For someone who is disoriented?

● When in a health-care facility, examine the policy for infusing blood products. What steps have been put in place to ensure patient safety during a blood transfusion?

REFERENCES AND SUGGESTED READINGS

Agraharkar, M. (2010). Hypercalcemia. *Medscape*. Retrieved from http://www.emedicine.medscape.com/article/240681-overview

Agrawal, V., Agarwal, M., Joshi, S. R., & Ghosh, A. K. (2008). Hyponatremia and hypernatremia: Disorders of water balance. *Journal of the Association of Physicians of India, 56,* 956–964.

Ayers, P., & Warrington, L. (2008). Diagnosis and treatment of simple acid-base disorders. *Nutrition in Clinical Practice, 23*(2), 122–127.

Beach, C. B. (2010). Hypocalcemia in emergency medicine clinical presentation. *Medscape*. Retrieved from http://www.emedicine.medscape.com/article/767260-clinical#a0216

Brown, B., & Ellerman, B. (2006). Understanding blood gas interpretation. *Newborn and Infant Reviews, 6*(2), 57–62.

Crawford, A., & Harris, H. (2011a). Balancing act: Hypomagnesemia and hypermagnesemia. *Nursing 2011, 41*(8), 52–55.

Crawford, A., & Harris, H. (2011b). Balancing act: Sodium and potassium. *Nursing 2011, 41*(7), 44–50.

Crawford, A., & Harris, H. (2011c). I.V. fluids: What nurses need to know. *Nursing 2011, 41*(5), 30–38.

Crawford, A., & Harris, H. (2012). Balancing act: Calcium and phosphorus. *Nursing 2012, 42*(1), 36–42.

Dougherty, L. (2008). Peripheral cannulation. *Nursing Standard, 22*(52), 49–56.

Gabriel, J. (2008a). Infusion therapy part one: Minimizing the risks. *Nursing Standard, 22*(31), 51–56.

Gabriel, J. (2008b). Infusion therapy part two: Prevention and management of complications. *Nursing Standard, 22*(32), 41–48.

Goh, K. P. (2004). Management of hypernatremia. *American Family Physician, 69,* 2387–2394.

Haskal, R. (2007). Current issues for nurse practitioners: Hyponatremia. *Journal of the American Academy of Nurse Practitioners, 19,* 563–579.

Holcomb, S. S. (2008). Third-spacing: When body fluid shifts. *Nursing 2008, 38*(7), 50–53.

Jequier, E., & Constant, F. (2010). Water as an essential nutrient: The physiologic basis of hydration. *European Journal of Clinical Nutrition, 64,* 115–123.

Lavery, I., & Ingram, P. (2008). Safe practice in intravenous medicines administration. *Nursing Standard, 22*(46), 44–47.

Leung, A., Prince, T., & Canadian Paediatric Society, Nutrition and Gastroenterology Committee. (2006). Oral rehydration therapy and early refeeding in the management of childhood gastroenteritis. *Paediatrics and Child Health, 11*(8), 527–531.

Nitu, M., Montgomery, G., & Eigen, H. (2011). Acid-base disorders. *Pediatrics in Review, 32*(6), 240–250.

Palmer, B. F. (2008). Approach to fluid and electrolyte disorders and acid-base problems. *Primary Care Clinics in Office Practice, 35,* 195–213.

Pruitt, B. (2010). Interpreting ABGs. *Nursing 2010, 40*(7), 35–36.

Reddy, P., & Mooradian, A. D. (2009). Diagnosis and management of hyponatremia in hospitalized patients. *International Journal of Clinical Practice, 63*(10), 1494–1508.

Reynolds, R. M., Padfield, P. L., & Seckl, J. R. (2006). Disorders of sodium balance. *British Medical Journal, 332,* 702–705.

Rhoda, K. M., Porter, M. J., & Quintini, C. (2011). Fluid and electrolyte management: Putting a plan in motion. *Journal of Parenteral and Enteral Nutrition, 35,* 675–685.

Scales, K. (2008). Intravenous therapy: A guide to good practice. *British Journal of Nursing, 17*(19), S4–S12.

Scales, K., & Pilsworth, J. (2008). The importance of fluid balance in clinical practice. *Nursing Standard, 22*(47), 50–57.

Shoulders-Odom, B. (2000).Using an algorithm to interpret arterial blood gases. *Dimensions of Critical Care Nursing, 19*(1), 36–41.

Sweeney, J. (2010). Managing hypernatremia. *Nursing 2010, 40*(9), 63.

Taylor, C. R., Lillis, C., LeMone, P., & Lynn, P. (2011). Fluid, electrolyte, and acid–base balance. In C. R. Taylor, C. Lilis, P. LeMone, & P. Lynn (Eds.), *Fundamentals of nursing: The art and science of nursing care* (7th ed., pp. 1414–1489). Philadelphia, PA: Lippincott Williams & Wilkins.

Unwin, R. J., Luft, F. C., & Shirley, D. G. (2011). Pathophysiology and management of hypokalemia: A clinical perspective. *Nature Reviews. Nephrology, 7,* 75–84.

Whitmire, S. J. (2008). Nutrition-focused evaluation and management of dysnatremias. *Nutrition in Clinical Practice, 23*(2), 108–121.

Ensuring Nutrition

CHRISTINE WELLINGTON AND LINDA PATRICK

P amela (a second-year nursing student) is just beginning her first day of clinical placement in a nursing home and has been assigned to a unit with individuals who have mild dementia. Pamela notices that two of the patients have not eaten anything from their breakfast and lunch trays. She believes this is not a good situation, but she has observed that the dietary staff simply removed the uneaten meals without showing any concern. Pamela is wondering what she should do. Should she discuss this with the busy, overworked nursing staff or leave the situation to the attention of the dietary staff who may report the uneaten meals to the food service supervisor?

CHAPTER OBJECTIVES

By the end of this chapter, you will be able to:

1. Integrate knowledge, assessments, and skills related to nutrition into your daily practice.
2. Calculate energy requirements for an individual and list at least three methods that can be used to assess the body's composition.
3. Interact with health-care professionals and engage with patients in the teaching and promotion of healthy diet choices.
4. Describe the nutrients in foods and the roles they play in the body.
5. Explain the importance of nutrition in the life cycle for promoting health as well as reducing the incidence of certain diseases, such as diabetes and heart disease.
6. Think critically about the principles of diet therapy and the management of common nutrition problems.

KEY TERMS

Body Mass Index (BMI) A measurement representing the ratio of a person's body weight to height. This is an indicator of overweight, obesity, or underweight that is calculated: weight in kilograms divided by height in meters squared (kg/m^2).

Calorie A unit of energy defined as the amount of heat required to raise the temperature of 1 kg of water by 1°C.

Dietary Reference Intake (DRI) A general term that includes the four specific types of nutrient recommendations (adequate intake [AI], estimated average requirement [EAR], recommended dietary allowance [RDA], and tolerable upper intake level [UL]). DRIs are used for nutrient recommendations for Canada's healthy population.

Enteral Nutrition (EN) A method of supplying nutrients through the body's feeding tract with a feeding tube.

Glycemic Index (GI) A ranking of foods according to their potential for raising blood glucose relative to a standard food. The standard food is white bread or glucose. Foods with low GI may help to control blood glucose level, control appetite, and control cholesterol level.

High-Density Lipoprotein (HDL) Lipoproteins that remove cholesterol from the tissues and bring the cholesterol to the liver for it to be disposed. HDLs contain a large amount of protein.

Ideal Body Weight (IBW) Also called *desirable body weight*, is the weight that we expect an individual to weigh based on his or her age, height, and sex.

Joule (J) A unit of energy defined as the force of 1 N traveling a distance of 1 m. The calorie to joule conversion ratio is 1 kcal = 4.2 kJ.

Kilocalorie Because a calorie is only a very small amount of energy, the energy content of foods is most often listed in units of 1,000 calories (cal) or 1 kilocalories (kcal).

Low-Density Lipoprotein (LDL) Lipoproteins that transport lipids from the liver to other tissues in the body. LDLs contain a large amount of cholesterol.

Malnutrition Any condition caused by excess (overnutrition) or deficient (undernutrition) food energy or nutrient intake or an imbalance of nutrients.

Monounsaturated Fats A fatty acid that contains one point of unsaturation.

Parenteral Nutrition (PN) A method of supplying nutrients through an intravenous, bypassing the usual process of eating and digestion.

Trans fat Type of unsaturated fat (monounsaturated or polyunsaturated). Trans fats occur naturally, in small amounts, in meat and dairy products. Manufacturers create trans fats by partially hydrogenating plant oils. Partial hydrogenation changes a fat's molecular structure. Trans fats are not needed in the body and are not beneficial for an individual's health.

Healthy Lifestyles and Nutrition

Proper nutrition combined with regular physical activity can prevent some diseases and reduce the risk for developing others as well as increase feelings of well-being. For example, proper nutrition can play a role in reducing both anxiety and depression. It is important that nurses can identify nutrition issues so they can work both singly and collaboratively with registered dietitians and other members of the health team to improve the nutritional health of Canadians. Most, if not all, baccalaureate programs now include a course on nutrition. Whether you encounter patients in the hospital setting, or clients in community agencies or in their homes, nutrition will be an important part of your nursing practice. It is also important for nurses to take care of their own nutritional needs because inadequate nutrition can affect work performance.

As a nursing student, Pamela wondered why she needed to know about the nutritional status of her patients when there were dietitians and other health-care team members who played a key role in ensuring nutrition at the hospital. After discussing this with her clinical instructor, she learned that assessing nutritional status is the combined responsibility of the health-care team including the registered nurse. It is also important to include the patient and the patient's family in nutritional plans to ensure that the patient receives adequate nutrition. In Pamela's nursing theory class, she learned that the quality of nutrition affects a patient's speed of recovery from disease and how quickly he or she regains daily functional abilities. Pamela now knows that she needs to be aware that many diseases are related to nutrition, including heart and respiratory diseases, specific cancers, and diabetes.

Through the eyes of a nurse

I always make sure that I eat breakfast before starting my morning shift and take my breaks at work and eat a nutritious lunch. I bring snacks or lunch even when working the midnight shift. I learned the hard way about skipping meals when working by experiencing low blood sugar on a day when I did not eat any food before or during the shift. I started feeling light-headed, and I nearly passed out. I could tell that my thinking was not clear, and I almost gave the wrong medication to a patient because I could not concentrate. Thank goodness, I was able to realize what was happening to me before I made a medication error and caused harm to a patient.

(personal reflection of a nurse)

 Energy Requirements

In this section, we explore the basic science of nutrition, reviewing some of the concepts you are also learning in physiology. Specifically, this section focuses on the major nutrients, including carbohydrates, lipids, proteins, vitamins, and minerals, and the principles of diet evaluation, nutritional assessment, weight control, and energy balance.

Energy is defined as the capacity to do work. You need to recall some physics here; don't worry, we are more interested in having you understand energy in an applied rather than a theoretical way. Energy is measured in several ways and reported using different units of measure such as joules, watts, ergs, and calories. The **calorie** is the most commonly reported food energy value in North America. In Canada, the International System of Units is used, and food energy is often reported in joules. A calorie (cal) is a unit of energy defined as the amount of heat required to raise the temperature of 1 kg of water by 1°C. Because a calorie is only a very small amount of energy, the energy content of foods is most often listed in units of 1,000 calories or **kilocalories** (kcal). A **joule (J)** is a unit of energy defined as the force of 1 N traveling a distance of 1 m. The calorie to joule conversion ratio is 1 kcal = 4.2 kJ. Food scientists measure food energy in calories, which is units of heat measurement. Units of weight—grams—measure food and nutrient quantities.

In the human body, the energy from food comes from three basic sources: protein, fat, and carbohydrate. Each of these sources must be converted into adenosine triphosphate (ATP). ATP is the common currency of energy for virtually all cells of the body. If you remember biology, glycolysis is a sequence of reactions where glucose is converted to pyruvate, which produces ATP.

Fat is the most energy-rich nutrient, containing 37.6 kjoules/g (9 kcal/g). Carbohydrate and protein each contain 16.7 kjoules/g (4 kcal/g). The energy ratio that is of most interest for this chapter is that the intake of 3,500 extra calories of food will add 0.454 kg or 1 lb (remember that 1 kg = 2.2 lb) of fat to your body. Many of your patients will want to know the relationship between calories and weight loss. People on weight-reducing diets know they must expend 3,500 kcal to lose 1 lb of fat. Ideally, it is best to add or subtract 500 kcal a day to either gain or lose 1 lb of fat a week. If exercise is involved, more calories can be burned to assist with the weight loss process.

Calculating Your Patient's Energy Requirements

In the majority of inpatient health-care facilities, a dietitian will usually be responsible for calculating your patients' energy (caloric) needs. However, you could use some of the following methods for determining your patient's basic energy requirements in those situations when a dietitian is unavailable.

One simple method for estimating an adult's energy needs:

Adult males: kilogram of body weight × 24 = calories per day
Adult females: kilogram of body weight × 22 = calories per day

(Remember to divide by 2.2 when converting pounds to kilogram.)

TABLE 34.1	Physical Activity Coefficients			
	Sedentary	Low Active	Active	Very Active
	Examples of activities—daily living activities (household chores)	Examples of activities—daily living activities and 30–60 minutes of moderate activity (e.g., walking)	Examples of activities—daily living activities and at least 60 minutes of moderate activity	Examples of activities—daily living activities and at least 60 minutes of moderate activity and 60 minutes of vigorous activity or 120 minutes of moderate activity
Boys ages 3–18 years	1.0	1.13	1.26	1.42
Girls ages 3–18 years	1.0	1.16	1.31	1.56
Men 19+ years	1.0	1.11	1.25	1.48
Women 19+ years	1.0	1.12	1.27	1.45

Source: Health Canada. (2010). *Dietary reference intakes tables*. Retrieved from http://www.hc-sc.gc.ca/fn-an /nutrition/reference/table/index-eng.php#eeer

As an example, a woman who weighs 70 kg (about 154 lbs) needs 1,540 cal/day. If she wants to lose weight to reach 59 kg (about 130 lb), she needs to reduce her calorie intake to about 1,300 cal/day (without taking extra exercise into account).

Estimated Energy Requirement

The estimated energy requirement (EER) is the intake that is needed to maintain the energy balance for a healthy individual. Health Canada (2010b) has published *Dietary Reference Intake Tables* that can be accessed for quick numbers. This formula takes into account the person's age, sex, weight, height, and physical activity (PA) level. See Table 34.1 for calculating physical activity coefficients.

The common formula used for healthy adults is

Estimated Energy Requirement (kcal/day) = Total Energy Expenditure

Men $EER = 662 - (9.53 \times age\ [y]) + PA \times \{(15.91 \times weight\ [kg]) + (539.6 \times height\ [m])\}$

Women $EER = 354 - (6.91 \times age\ [y]) + PA \times \{(9.36 \times weight\ [kg]) + (726 \times height\ [m])\}$

Take a moment to calculate your own EER.

Body Weight Standards

Ideal body weight (IBW), also called *desirable body weight*, is the weight that we expect an individual to weigh based on age, height, and sex (Fig. 34.1). There are several methods used to determine IBW. The simplest formula is to use height as the baseline:

Adult males:

For the height of 152.4 cm (5 ft), that person should weigh 45.5 kg (100 lb). For every 2.54 cm (1 inch) above 152.4 cm (5 ft), add 2.72 kg (6 lb).

Thus, a Caucasian man of 180.34 cm (5 in. 11 ft) should ideally weigh 61.82 kg (166 lb).

Adult females:

For the height of 152.4 cm (5 ft), that person should weigh 45.5 kg (100 lb). For every 2.54 cm (1 inch) above 152.4 cm (5 ft), add 2.27 kg (5 lb).

Thus, a Caucasian woman of 160.02 cm (3 ft, 5 in.) should ideally weigh 52.31 kg (115 lb).

This method is not very accurate and does not apply to people who are very short or very tall.

The Body Mass Index

Most individuals working in today's health-care system now use the **body mass index (BMI)**, a measurement representing the ratio of a person's body weight to his or her height.

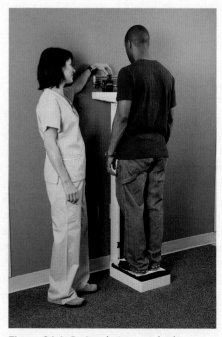

Figure 34.1 Patient being weighed.

This is an indicator of overweight, obesity, or underweight that is calculated as weight in kilograms divided by height in metres squared (kg/m²). It should not be used for visible minority populations, pregnant and breast-feeding women, and athletes (muscle weighs more than fat, thus producing an inaccurate number) as the values for BMI have been developed primarily on Caucasian men and, to a lesser extent, women. Overweight and obesity are based on the BMI. BMI is highly correlated with body fat and is widely used to indicate health risks.

One point to consider is that BMI does not differentiate between males and females. Discussion point: Is it a concern that BMI does not differentiate between males and females?

Calculating BMI using kilograms and metres:
Weight in kilograms ÷ Height in metres
Hints: Remember that 2.2 lb = 1 kg and 39.37 in. = 1 m.
Calculating BMI using pounds and inches:
Weight in pounds ÷ Height in inches × 704.5

There are many calculators or charts available that can quickly give you BMI numbers. The Health Canada (2012a) website is a useful source for charts on BMI.

BMI is classified into six categories, each representing a different level of risk; refer to Table 34.2 for a breakout of these categories.

Overweight and obesity are known risk factors for

- Diabetes
- Coronary heart disease
- High blood cholesterol
- Stroke
- Hypertension
- Gallbladder disease
- Osteoarthritis (degeneration of cartilage and bone of joints)
- Sleep apnea and other breathing problems
- Some forms of cancer (breast, colorectal, endometrial, and kidney)

Obesity is also associated with

- Complications of pregnancy
- Menstrual irregularities
- Hirsutism (presence of excess body and facial hair)
- Stress incontinence (urine leakage caused by weak pelvic floor muscles)
- Psychological disorders, such as depression
- Increased surgical risk
- Increased mortality

A recent variant on BMI combines BMI with waist size to offer a more accurate picture of a person's risk for developing health conditions. For example, and in addition to the BMI category, a waist size of more than 35 in. or 88 cm for women, or more than 40 in. or 102 cm for men, places one at risk for developing health (cardiovascular) conditions.

Waist–Hip Ratio

The waist–hip ratio is a measure of truncal fatness. To calculate waist–hip ratio, measure the waist at the smallest part. Measure the hips at the widest part.

Waist–Hip Ratio = Waist Circumference ÷ Hip Circumference

You have a lower risk of developing certain medical conditions if your waist–hip ratio is less than 0.8 for women and 1.0 for men.

Healthy Waists

The Heart and Stroke Foundation of Canada (2009) is focusing on healthy waist measurements. Fat in the abdominal area can increase a person's risk of developing Type 2 diabetes, hypertension, heart disease, and stroke. Refer to Table 34.3 to view the healthy waist measurement recommendations according to ethnicity.

Apple-Shaped Versus Pear-Shaped Body

Individuals with apple-shaped bodies store their fat around the chest and abdominal area, which contains many important organs, including the heart. This body type has a higher risk of developing high blood pressure, high blood cholesterol, Type 2 diabetes, gallbladder disease, heart disease, and stroke. Individuals with pear-shaped bodies store fat around their hips and thighs. For more information on

TABLE 34.2	Health Risk Classification According to Body Mass Index	
Classification	BMI Category (kg/m²)	Risk of Developing Health Problems
Underweight	<18.5	Increased
Normal weight	18.5–24.9	Least
Overweight	25.0–29.9	Increased
Obese class I	30.0–34.9	High
Obese class II	35.0–39.9	Very high
Obese class III	≥40.0	Extremely high

For persons 65 years and older, the "normal" range may begin slightly above BMI 18.5 and extend into the "overweight" range.
Source: Health Canada. (2003). *Canadian guidelines for body weight classification in adults.* Ottawa, ON: Minister of Public Works and Government Services Canada.

TABLE 34.3	Healthy Waists	
Ethnicity	Male	Female
European/Caucasian, sub-Saharan Africans, Eastern Mediterranean, Middle Eastern	102 cm (40 in.)	88 cm (35 in.)
South Asian, Malaysian, Asian, Chinese, Japanese, Ethnic South and Central Americans	90 cm (35 in.)	80 cm (32 in.)

Source: Heart and Stroke Foundation of Canada. (2009). Healthy waists. Retrieved from http://www.heartandstroke.com/site/c.iklQLcMWJtE/b.3876195/

body shape and its impact on health, the Heart and Stroke Foundation of Canada (2009) website offers good information on this topic.

The Nutrients in Foods and Their Role in the Body

Nutrients are classified into the following six classes: carbohydrate, fat, protein, vitamins, minerals, and water (Table 34.4). Carbohydrate, protein, and fat are energy-yielding nutrients that are converted into the energy that your body uses for fuel. Vitamins, minerals, and water do not produce energy, but they are involved in many other important functions of the body.

Carbohydrates

The human brain and the nervous system operate with carbohydrates as their main energy source. Carbohydrates (CHO) are compounds composed of carbon, hydrogen, and oxygen and are a major source of energy. The minimum amount of carbohydrate needed per day for healthy brain function is 130 g (one slice of bread is equal to approximately 15 g of carbohydrate.). A healthy Canadian adult should consume between 45% and 65% of their total daily calories from carbohydrates. Most carbohydrates come from plant-based foods. Milk is the only animal-sourced food that contains a significant amount of carbohydrate. Carbohydrates are divided into two categories: simple and complex.

Simple Carbohydrates

Simple carbohydrates are often called *simple sugars*. Food sources of simple carbohydrates (categories are monosaccharides and disaccharides) include honey, sugar, corn syrup, and naturally occurring sugar found in fruit, some vegetables, and milk. When you consume simple carbohydrates, they can be used as energy or stored by the body very quickly because they are absorbed directly into the bloodstream during digestion. When you eat disaccharides, they must be split apart into monosaccharides before entering the bloodstream.

TABLE 34.4	The Six Classes of Nutrients
Carbohydrates	Macronutrient Organic—contains carbon
Fat	Macronutrient Organic
Protein	Macronutrient Organic
Water	Macronutrient
Vitamins	Micronutrient Organic
Minerals	Micronutrient

BOX 34.1 Lactose Intolerance

The most common carbohydrate malabsorption is lactose malabsorption. Lactose is a disaccharide composed of the following monosaccharides: galactose and glucose.

Lactose is found only in milk and milk products but is a common additive to foods (e.g., certain brands of salt and vinegar chips) and medications (Matthews, 2005).

The amount of lactase (the intestinal enzyme that splits the disaccharide lactose to monosaccharides during digestion) available in the body is highest at birth and decreases with age.

Secondary lactase deficiency can occur as a result of the following:

• Disease or infection
• Injury to the small intestine
• Surgery
• Malnutrition

When there is inadequate lactase available for digestion, lactose will travel to the large intestine undigested and unabsorbed. Bacteria in the large intestine will cause the lactose to undergo fermentation, which creates increased gas and abdominal cramping. Undigested lactose pulls additional water into the large intestine, contributing to bloating, distention, increased flatulence, abdominal cramping, and, for some individuals, diarrhea.

When milk and milk products are avoided because of lactase deficiency, there is risk of inadequate intake for calcium, riboflavin, and vitamin D.

Lactase deficiency is seen in the following populations: Asian, Latino, African, African American, and American Indians

---

Remember learning in your high school science class that monosaccharides are single sugars? The three monosaccharides are glucose, fructose, and galactose. Disaccharides are linked pairs of the single monosaccharides. All three have glucose as part of their makeup. They are lactose (milk sugar), maltose (two glucose units), and sucrose (table sugar). The most common carbohydrate malabsorption is often referred to as lactose intolerance (Box 34.1).

In our chapter opening scenario, Pamela, our nursing student, identified that missing meals could lead to problems, so she decided to talk to the unit manager about the two patients who did not consume any of their breakfast and lunch. The unit manager suggested that she talk to the patients and explore with them why they did not eat their food.

The first patient Pamela spoke to was Mr. J., who appeared to be relatively coherent and friendly as well. He told Pamela why he didn't eat. He told her that for breakfast, he was given cereal with milk, a glass of milk, and orange juice. He was given a bowl of cream of broccoli soup with macaroni and cheese for lunch. He told her that every time he has milk or a milk product, he gets a bloated stomach, suffers from intestinal gas, and often develops diarrhea within a short time after eating. Pamela found out that he was newly admitted to this nursing home and had not spoken to anyone about this problem. Pamela noted that there was no information on the chart from family members about this issue either.

Pamela went to the unit manager and explained the reason Mr. J. chose not to eat his meal. She documented this issue in his chart and left a message for the food service staff to adjust his menu for the time being and then she made a referral to the dietitian to review his dietary restrictions.

Complex Carbohydrates

Complex carbohydrates are mostly composed of polysaccharides, which are long strands of glucose units. Foods in this group include starch and fibre. Grains such as wheat, rice, and corn are the major source of starches. Fibre is found in plants including legumes, fruit, vegetables, and the outer part of the cereal grain. Starch, most fibres, and the body's stores of glycogen are polysaccharides. Our body must break these long chains into the monosaccharide glucose so that we can use this fuel for energy. In the human body, carbohydrate, which is not immediately metabolized, may be stored as glycogen in the muscles and liver as an easily accessible source of energy. We can digest most starches, although some starch in plants is not digestible and this is called *resistant starch*. Resistant starch (starch that escapes digestion in the small intestine) may be important as a protector against colon cancer. When we try to digest this resistant starch, butyrate, which is a fatty acid, is produced, and this may protect us against colon cancer. Foods that are high in resistant starch include legumes (beans, peas, and lentils), raw potatoes, and unripe bananas.

A healthy diet should include plenty of fibre. Fibre is the part of plant foods that your body cannot digest. Research shows that a diet high in fibre may reduce the risk of colorectal cancer. Eating plenty of fibre may also help you maintain a healthy body weight, which reduces the risk of several cancers. Fibre is divided into two main classes: soluble and insoluble.

Soluble Fibre

Soluble fibres dissolve in water. They form gels that are viscous (a sticky, gummy, or gel-like consistency that flows fairly slowly), and they are digested by the bacteria in the colon. Foods high in soluble fibre include barley, legumes, fruit (apple), oats, and vegetables. This includes pectins and gums. This type of fibre is often associated with lower risk for certain diseases; for example, it may protect against heart disease by possibly reducing the absorption of cholesterol. It may also help those individuals living with diabetes by delaying gastric emptying, which causes a slower influx of glucose into the bloodstream, therefore decreasing the postprandial (after eating a meal) blood sugar.

Insoluble Fibre

This type of fibre does not dissolve in water and does not form gels. It is less fermented in the colon. Foods high in insoluble fibre include cellulose, hemicellulose, outer layers of whole grains (e.g., bran), the strings in celery, the skins of vegetables, and fruit. This type of fibre helps with elimination of waste products.

Daily Fibre Requirements

It is recommended that healthy adults consume between 25 and 35 g of fibre a day. Many people do not seem to be aware of this requirement because according to a recent report by the Heart and Stroke Foundation (2012), Canadian adults are consuming only half that amount. A sample high-fibre menu is shown next.

SAMPLE MENU:

Breakfast
2 slices of whole wheat bread (4 g fibre)
1 tbsp honey
½ cup applesauce (1.5 g fibre)

Morning Snack
4 whole wheat crackers (1.7 g fibre)
1 oz cheese

Lunch
2 oz canned tuna
2 6-in. corn tortillas (3.2 g fibre)
½ cup blackberries (3.8 g fibre)

Afternoon Snack
2 oz oat bran muffin (2.7 g fibre)
1 pear (5.1 g fibre)

Supper
3 oz baked chicken
1 medium-baked sweet potato (4.8 g fibre)
½ cup broccoli (2.5 g fibre)
½ cup corn (2.1 g fibre)

Total fibre = 31.4 g

According to Health Canada (2010b) guidelines, 2 g of fibre per serving is considered a source of fibre, 4 g per serving is considered a high source of fibre, and 6 g of fibre per serving is considered a very high source of fibre. It is important that health professionals recommend that to remain healthy, individuals choose higher fibre foods more often. Think about how much fibre you are consuming each day. Would you be able to consume the foods listed in the sample menu? Dietitians encourage individuals to consume their fibre from food sources rather than supplements.

Glycemic Index

The **glycemic index (GI)** ranks carbohydrates according to their effect on our blood glucose levels in comparison to a standard food (glucose or white bread). Meals containing high glycemic foods can cause the blood glucose to rise to high levels in comparison to meals that have low glycemic foods, even though both meals could be equal in terms of the number of calories and nutrients they contain. A high glycemic meal causes a much higher insulin output, which can lead

BOX 34.2 Glycemic Index of Foods

FOOD	GLYCEMIC INDEX
Examples of High GI Foods: 70 or More	
Bread—white	70
Russet potato baked without fat	78
Rice—instant	87
Cereal (Corn Flakes, Rice Krispies)	92, 82
Donut, cake type	76
Examples of Medium GI Foods: 56–69	
Rice, basmati	58
Black bean soup	64
Blueberry muffin	59
Shredded wheat spoon size	58
Examples of Low GI Foods: 55 or less	
Fruits: apple, pear	38, 38
Vegetables: yam, carrots	37, 47
Whole grains (oatmeal, barley)	49, 25
Legumes: chickpeas, lentils	28, 29

Sources: Brand-Miller, J., Wolever, T., Colagiuri, S., & Foster-Powell, K. (1999). *The glucose revolution*. New York, NY: Marlowe & Company; Atkinson, F. S., Foster-Powell, K., & Brand-Miller, J. C. (2008). International tables of glycemic index and glycemic load values: 2008. *Diabetes Care, 12*, 2281–2283.

to an increase in the storage of glycogen and fat in the body. Choosing carbohydrates with a low GI (which produce only small fluctuations in blood glucose and insulin levels) helps our long-term health by reducing the risk of heart disease and diabetes and is the key to maintaining weight loss (Box 34.2).

Carbohydrates and Blood Sugar

Carbohydrates affect blood glucose when they are broken down into sugar during the digestive process. Managing carbohydrate intake by counting the grams of carbohydrate and evenly distributing them throughout the day will help regulate blood sugar levels in those individuals with diabetes. For people with diabetes, a registered dietitian will usually be consulted in managing their diets. The dietitian will calculate the daily amount of carbohydrate for individuals that will meet their specific needs. Carbohydrate is the key nutrient that affects the postprandial glycemic response. Usually, individuals consume between 45 and 60 g of carbohydrate at a meal and 15 and 30 g of carbohydrate at snack time. Counting grams of carbohydrate provides flexibility and helps people increase their confidence in managing diabetes.

Fat

You've likely heard many negative things about fat. It seems that almost every food product on the grocery shelves is available as low fat or fat free, and many people talk about cutting back on their fat intake. In this section, we note the importance of fat and its role in the human body. There are three classifications of fat: triglycerides (about 95% of lipids in food and in the body are triglycerides), phospholipids (lecithin is one example), and sterols (cholesterol being the most common sterol). Fats differ in chain length and degree of saturation (saturated and unsaturated). See Table 34.5 for types and sources of fats.

TABLE 34.5 Types and Sources of Fats

Type of Fat	Foods	Important Points to Remember
Monounsaturated fat	Olive oil, canola oil, some soft nonhydrogenated margarines—read label carefully, peanut oil, avocados, nuts (almonds, cashews, pecans)	Good or healthy fats because they can lower your bad (LDL) cholesterol
Polyunsaturated fat	Corn oil, cottonseed oil, safflower oil, soybean oil, sunflower oil, walnuts, pumpkin or sunflower seeds	Polyunsaturated fats are also healthy fats.
Essential polyunsaturated fat Omega-3	Omega-3 fats are found in fatty fish such as salmon, mackerel, albacore tuna, trout, herring and sardines, and omega eggs. Some plant foods contain omega-3 fatty acids: tofu and some soybean products, walnuts, flaxseed, and canola oil.	These fats also help lower blood cholesterol. Omega-6 and omega-3 are important structural components of cell membranes. When incorporated into phospholipids, they affect cell membrane properties such as fluidity, flexibility, permeability, and the activity of membrane bound enzymes. Omega-3 fats help prevent stickiness and clotting of blood.
Omega-6 (linoleic acid is the main omega-6 fatty acid in foods)	Omega-6 fats are found in safflower, soybean, sunflower and corn oils, in some soft nonhydrogenated margarines, and nuts and seeds such as almonds, pecans, Brazil nuts, sunflower seeds, and sesame seeds.	
Saturated fat	Animal foods: fatty meats, poultry with skin, lard, high-fat milks, cheese, and yogurts; some baked goods and fried foods can contain high levels of saturated fats. It is important to read labels. Plant foods: coconut and palm oils	Saturated fats raise the level of cholesterol in your blood. High levels of blood cholesterol increase your risk of heart disease and stroke.
Trans fat	Created when hydrogen is added to vegetable oils (turn a liquid oil into a hard fat) Shortening	Trans fat can increase the bad LDL cholesterol. Trans fat can reduce the level of good cholesterol HDL.

Fat has many roles in the body.

- It is the body's major storage form of energy. A pound of body fat is equal to 3,500 cal of energy.
- Fat is part of the cell membrane of cells in the body.
- Fat deposits insulate the body and cushion the vital organs.
- The fat-soluble vitamins (A, D, E, and K) require fat for their absorption.
- Fat slows down the rate at which the stomach empties and therefore gives you a feeling of satiety (feeling full).
- Fat is a concentrated source of calories and provides 37.6 kjoules/g (9 kcal/g). Triglycerides are composed of three fatty acids that are attached to glycerol.

In a healthy diet, fat should only make up about 20% to 35% of a person's total daily calorie intake. It is important to limit saturated fat to less than 10% of calories and to limit **trans fat** to less than 1% of calories of a person's daily intake (EatRight Ontario, 2011). Trans fatty acids are a type of unsaturated fat. Trans fats occur naturally, in small amounts, in meat and dairy products. Manufacturers create trans fats by partially hydrogenating plant oils. Partial hydrogenation changes a fat's molecular structure. Trans fats are not needed in the body and are not beneficial for an individual's health.

For quick information to provide to your patients, use the following ideal guideline recommendations: Females should aim to consume no more than approximately 60 to 65 g of fat a day, whereas men should consume no more than approximately 90 g of fat a day. These values are ideal, although some sources quote lower recommendations: women—between 45 and 75 g of fat a day and men—between 60 and 105 g of fat a day.

Saturated Fatty Acids

Saturated fats increase blood levels of **low-density lipoprotein (LDL)**. Lipoproteins transport lipids from the liver to other tissues in the body. LDLs contain a large amount of cholesterol and are commonly known as bad cholesterol. LDL cholesterol is a risk factor for heart disease. Some examples of foods with saturated fats include butter, hard margarine, fatty cuts of meat, high-fat dairy products, and palm oil. It is important to limit your intake of saturated fat in order to optimize your health. Current daily consumption guidelines recommend consuming less than 10% of calories from fat in the form of saturated fat (Heart and Stroke Foundation, 2011).

Trans Fatty Acids

Trans fatty acids, also called *trans fats*, increase blood levels of LDL cholesterol. Trans fat can decrease the levels of beneficial cholesterol, or **high-density lipoprotein (HDL)**. HDL removes cholesterol from the tissues and brings the cholesterol to the liver for it to be disposed. HDLs contain a large amount of protein. Foods made with hydrogenated or partially hydrogenated vegetable oil are high in trans fatty acids. They are also present at low levels in dairy products, beef, and lamb. It is important to limit the intake of trans fats because

research shows they are strongly related to plaque buildup in arteries and contribute to high cholesterol levels and heart disease. Many school boards in Canada will not allow the sale of food items on the school premises if they contain trans fat. The focus on reducing trans fatty acid intake has food manufacturers looking for new methods for processing foods to decrease or even eliminate trans fat in their products. Current guidelines recommend consuming less than 1% of trans fat a day (Heart and Stroke Foundation, 2010).

Unsaturated Fatty Acids

Did you know that the leading cause of death in industrialized countries is coronary heart disease? Studies conducted over the past several decades have demonstrated that when monounsaturated or polyunsaturated fats replace the saturated and trans fat in our meal plans, it is good for our heart health. These fats help to lower blood cholesterol if used in place of saturated fats. The more unsaturated a fat, the more liquid it is at room temperature.

Monounsaturated Fats

Monounsaturated fats include olive oil, peanut oil, and canola oil. Dark-coloured olive oils contain phytochemicals, which are also good for the body. It is recommended that Canadians substitute monounsaturated fats and polyunsaturated fats for saturated fats in the diet because both lower LDL cholesterol levels in the blood. When reading labels, choose a product that has 2 g of fat or less of saturated fat per tablespoon. It is also recommended to replace saturated fats and trans fats with unsaturated fats from vegetables, legumes, and nuts.

Essential Polyunsaturated Fatty Acids

Certain essential fatty acids are needed in the body, but the body cannot make them in sufficient amounts. Essential fatty acids include linoleic acid (unsaturated omega-6 fatty acid) and linolenic acid (omega-3 fatty acid). Essential fatty acids have many important functions in the body: muscle relaxation and contraction, blood vessel clotting formation, regulation of blood lipids, and immune response. A deficiency of essential fatty acids in the diet will adversely affect reproduction and the functions of the skin, kidney, and liver.

Linoleic acid, also called omega-6, can be found in nuts and seeds. It is also found in vegetable oils (soybean, cottonseed, corn, sunflower, and safflower). Linolenic acid is an omega-3 fatty acid. Eicosapentaenoic acid (EPA) and docosahexaenoic acid (DHA), which are part of the omega-3 fatty acids, are found in the oils of certain fish. A diet that includes fatty fish in two to three meals each week can provide a healthy amount of omega-3 fatty acids. A balanced diet that includes grains, nuts (walnuts), seeds (flaxseeds), oils (canola), and leafy green vegetables will supply all of the essential fatty acids. Salmon, sardines, herring, mackerel, and other cold water fatty fish contain omega-3 fatty acid. Dietitians of Canada (2011) suggests that persons with heart disease who are not consuming enough dietary sources of omega-3 fatty acids should discuss the possible use of supplements with their physician or dietitian.

Through the eyes of a nurse

*A*s a nurse, I had the opportunity to work in a community health centre, and I participated in health promotion programs with the dietitian. I learned that a healthy heart class is a great program to offer to your patients. Nurses working in clinics with patients and families can also be effective educators in providing patient education for coronary risk reduction and dietary fat intake. Once the initial information has been provided to the patient, a referral for a formal dietary consultation appointment with the dietitian is necessary for improving understanding, fostering commitment to a healthy heart diet, and achieving lipid control. *(personal reflection of a nurse)*

Protein

Proteins are made up of amino acids (nitrogen-containing molecules that combine to form proteins). There are approximately 20 different amino acids. Nine of these amino acids are considered essential; they must be consumed in the diet because the body cannot synthesize them. In contrast, the other 11 nonessential amino acids can be synthesized in the body. In people who have metabolic disorders, amino acids classified as nonessential may become essential, in which case, they are referred to as conditionally essential amino acids. For example, people who have phenylketonuria (PKU) cannot make tyrosine from phenylalanine. If there is not enough phenylalanine or the body cannot convert phenylalanine from tyrosine, then tyrosine becomes conditionally essential in a person's diet (see Box 34.3 for more information on PKU).

BOX 34.3 Phenylketonuria

As a nurse, you may work with newborn babies. All babies are routinely tested for PKU at birth. PKU is a genetic disorder of metabolism that is inherited. People with PKU (an autosomal recessive disorder where the gene coding for the enzyme phenylalanine hydroxylase is defective and leads to the inability to convert the amino acid phenylalanine to tyrosine) cannot process a portion of the protein called phenylalanine (Phe), which is in almost all food that we eat, except fats and sugars. If the Phe cannot be digested, it builds up in the body and can damage the brain, permanently affecting mental functioning. Treatment includes a lifelong special diet to regulate the amount of Phe consumed and avoidance of foods that are very high in protein, such as milk, meat, eggs, and nuts. There is a special commercial infant formula available for PKU babies. It has 95% of the phenylalanine removed from its protein source, providing just enough phenylalanine for basic needs. With a special diet, children who have PKU develop normally but are encouraged to stay on a diet that helps control the amount of Phe and preserve brain health and to control hyperactivity and aggressive behaviour. Regular blood tests determine the adequacy of the amounts.

When a food contains all of the essential amino acids, it is considered to be a complete protein source. If a food does not contain all the essential amino acids, then it is considered to be an incomplete protein. There are foods that may be eaten separately that offer incomplete proteins but when they are combined, they contain adequate amounts of all the essential amino acids. This is called mutual supplementation or protein complementation. The amino acids missing in one food are supplied in the other food with protein complementation. Rice and beans are a common example of protein complementation. Rice contains low amounts of certain essential amino acids while other essential amino acids are found in greater amounts in dry beans—combined they make a complete source. It is good to consume both types of foods to insure that all of the essential amino acids are consumed on a daily basis (Melina & Davis, 2003).

Recommendations for Protein Intake

The recommended protein intake for a healthy Canadian adult is between 10% and 35% of total daily calories. A quick formula to remember is that a healthy adult requires 0.8 g of protein per kilogram of body weight. See Box 34.4 for the metabolic functions of protein.

Nitrogen Balance

Nitrogen balance is the amount of nitrogen consumed compared to the amount of nitrogen excreted over a specific period of time. Studies have shown that in a healthy individual, the amount of protein taken into the body is equal to the amount of protein excreted from the body. A person with an injury excretes more nitrogen than is ingested and therefore is in negative nitrogen balance. A pregnant woman or a growing child consumes more protein than is excreted and is therefore in a positive nitrogen balance.

Malnutrition

Protein–energy malnutrition (PEM) occurs when an individual consumes too little protein and energy. It is the most common form of **malnutrition** in the world today. Two other types of protein deficiencies are marasmus and kwashiorkor,

BOX 34.4 The Metabolic Functions of Proteins

- Proteins are considered the building blocks of the body. They are needed for growth and repair of tissue.
- They are also part of body structure (collagen and muscle—fibrous protein).
- Proteins transport materials throughout the body.
- Proteins come in many different forms: enzymes, antibodies, hormones, transportation, oxygen carriers, filaments of hair, part of the nails, tendons, ligaments, and so forth.
- Protein can be used for energy if there is insufficient fat and carbohydrate coming from the diet. Unlike carbohydrate and fat, excess protein cannot be stored for future use.
- Proteins work as a defense for the body; that is, the immune system.

but they are not commonly seen in North America. Marasmus, a PEM that results from inadequate intakes of protein, energy, and other nutrients, is the calorie deficiency disease. It is malnutrition that includes emaciation and occurs mainly in young children because of very limited calorie and protein intake. Kwashiorkor is a form of PEM that is seen often in developing countries in infants and toddlers that are fed a cereal diet that provides adequate energy but inadequate protein. It is a disease related to protein malnutrition. This is more commonly seen in young children who have been weaned from protein-rich breast milk at the birth of a sibling and live on a protein-poor carbohydrate food source.

Malnutrition among older adults living at home is a serious nutrition problem that can lead to disease and frailty; minor ailments can become major health problems. The Mini-Nutritional Assessment (MNA) tool can be used to assess the risk of malnutrition (Soini, Routasalo, & Lagström, 2004). Please note that more information on malnutrition are presented later in the chapter.

Wound Healing

Protein depletion can affect the rate and quality of wound healing. There is an increase in demand for protein by the body in the presence of a wound, and the protein requirement further increases with sepsis (a systematic inflammatory response syndrome or SIRS). Protein is required for the inflammatory process, the immune response, and the development of granulation tissue. The main protein synthesized during the healing process is collagen, and the strength of the collagen determines wound strength. If a patient has a low protein intake even for a short period of time, this can result in a significant delay in wound healing. Low protein intake has also been shown to affect remodeling of the wound (Brown & Phelps Maloy, 2005).

Nurses and dietitians have key roles in a multidisciplinary health team, and nurses need an effective referral system to call in a registered dietitian for treatment advice for those patients who are not in positive nitrogen balance and not consuming enough calories (Anderson, 2005). Nurses also need to assess protein-related nutrition risk indicators such as the following:

Low albumin (<3.5 mg/dl)
Low body weight (<85% IBW)
5% to 10% significant weight loss over 1 month
Low serum transferrin (<170 mg/dl)

Vitamins

Vitamins are organic compounds that are needed in small amounts. Most vitamins are not synthesized in the body so they must be acquired from dietary sources. Vitamin insufficiency can cause health problems.

Vitamins are classified according to their solubility. The fat-soluble vitamins are vitamins A, D, E, and K. The water-soluble vitamins are ascorbic acid (vitamin C), thiamin, riboflavin, niacin, pyridoxine, biotin, pantothenic acid, folate, and cobalamin. See Table 34.6 for a list of the main dietary sources of vitamins.

Unique Considerations for Vitamin D

Vitamin D is unique in that the body can synthesize it with the help of sunlight. During the winter months when sunlight is reduced, people will often need to take vitamin D supplements. Additionally, because of concerns about skin cancer, many people are wearing sunscreens to block ultraviolet (UV) light. Researchers have found that wearing sunscreen continuously can reduce the amount of vitamin D a person is able to synthesize. For example, sunscreens with a sun protection factor of 8 or more appear to block vitamin D–producing UV rays. Consequently, vitamin D supplementation is now necessary during both warm and cold months. Health Canada recommends that in addition to following Canada's Food Guide, all adults over the age of 50 should take a daily vitamin D supplement of 10 micrograms (mcg) or 400 IU (Health Canada, 2010g).

Current research has shown that vitamin D_3 might be more than three times as effective as vitamin D_2 in raising serum 25(OH)D concentrations and maintaining those levels for a longer time (Houghton & Vieth, 2006). As such, many pharmaceutical companies are reformulating their supplements to contain vitamin D_3 instead of vitamin D_2.

Vitamin D for Infants and Children

Breast milk is the optimal food for infants. It is recommended that all breast-fed, full-term infants in Canada receive a daily vitamin D supplement of 10 mcg (400 International Unit) (Health Canada, 2010d). After 1 year, all children should have a daily intake of 15 mcg (600 International Units) of vitamin D (Health Canada, 2010g). Supplementation should begin at birth and continue until the infant's diet includes at least 10 mcg (400 International Unit) per day of vitamin D from other dietary sources, or until the breast-fed infant reaches 1 year of age (Health Canada, 2010d).

Infants born to mothers who are vitamin D deficient are at increased risk for developing a vitamin D deficiency. A vitamin D supplement is recommended because sunlight is the main source of vitamin D for humans. Exposure to sun is not recommended for long periods of time for infants, who are at a higher risk for overexposure to sunlight. Their skin is thin and they are more sensitive to UV rays. Vitamin D deficiency causes rickets in children.

Vitamin D status may also play a role in the protection against the development of other diseases. For example, vitamin D may be involved in the "inhibition of proliferation of a number of malignant cells including breast and prostate cancer cells and protection against certain immune mediated disorders including multiple sclerosis" (Raghuwanshi, Joshi, & Christakos, 2008, p. 338). The dietary reference intake for vitamin D has recently changed (Health Canada, 2010g). See Table 34.7 for the new dietary reference intake recommendations for vitamin D.

(text continues on page 872)

TABLE 34.6 Main Dietary Sources of Vitamins and Their Role

Vitamin	Source	Function	Deficiency	Toxicity
Vitamin A (antioxidant—as beta carotene)	Fortified milk and margarine, butter, liver Beta-carotene: spinach, dark leafy green vegetables, broccoli, apricots, peaches, cantaloupe, squash, carrots, sweet potato, pumpkin	Vision, growth and repair of body tissues, maintenance of mucous membrane, reproduction, bone and tooth formation, immune system, hormone synthesis	Night blindness, impaired bone growth, changes in skin texture—bumps on the skin	Birth defects, nausea, diarrhea, blurred vision, bone pain
Vitamin D	The body can make vitamin D from the sun. Fortified milk, eggs, liver, and fish	Calcium and phosphorus metabolism and absorption	Osteomalacia in adults Rickets in children Joint pain, soft bones	Deposits of calcium in organs, mental retardation, and abnormal bone growth
Vitamin E (antioxidant)	Vegetable oils, liver, egg yolk, nuts, and seeds.	Protects red blood cells	Anemia, red blood cell breakage	May increase bleeding
Vitamin K	Bacteria make it in the digestive tract. Leafy green vegetables	Blood clotting proteins, calcium metabolism	Hemorrhaging	Interferes with anticlotting medications
Thiamin	Pork, meat, liver, fish, poultry, whole grain and enriched breads and cereals, legumes	Coenzyme for conversion of pyruvate to acetyl coenzyme A (acetyl CoA), which enters the Krebs cycle to produce energy	Beriberi, mental confusion, anorexia, and weight loss	None known
Riboflavin	Milk, leafy green vegetables, liver, whole grain and enriched breads and cereals	Coenzymes helping to form $FMNH_2$ and $FADH_2$ FMN and FAD are coenzymes that catalyze the oxidation of fatty acids in glucose metabolism. FMN is needed for the conversion of pyridoxine (B_6) to pyridoxal phosphate. FAD is required for the biosynthesis of niacin from the amino acid tryptophan.	Photophobia; tearing; burning and itching of the eyes; soreness and burning of lips, mouth, and tongue Advanced symptoms—cheilosis (fissure of the lips) and angular stomatitis (cracks in the skin at the corners of the mouth)	None known
Niacin	Meat, poultry, fish, whole grain and enriched breads and cereals, legumes	Coenzymes NAD and NADPH are involved with hundreds of enzymes involved in the metabolism of carbohydrates, fatty acids, and amino acids.	Muscle weakness, anorexia, indigestion, and skin eruptions Pellagra, which is the 4 Ds (dermatitis, dementia, diarrhea, and death), tremors and sore tongue (beef tongue)	Doses of 1–2 g three times per day can affect the liver, histamine release that causes flushing may cause problems in those individuals with asthma or peptic ulcer disease
Pantothenic acid	In many foods (cereal, rice, mushrooms, corn, yogurt, potatoes, chicken, milk, banana)	Coenzyme in energy metabolism. CoA is important in the formation of acetyl CoA, which is involved in TCA cycle to release energy.	Impairments in lipid synthesis and energy production Deficiencies are rare because it is widespread in foods.	None known
Pyridoxine (vitamin B_6)	Cereal, potato, banana, rice, chicken, pork chop, baked beans, beef, tuna, whole wheat bread	Coenzyme for many enzymes involved in metabolism of amino acids, neurotransmitters, glycogen, heme and steroids	Weakness, sleeplessness, peripheral neuropathies, cheilosis, glossitis, stomatitis, and impaired cell-mediated immunity	Sensory neuropathy marked by changes in gait and peripheral sensation
Biotin	In many foods (peanuts, almonds, soy protein, eggs, yogurt, nonfat milk, and sweet potatoes)	Coenzyme in energy metabolism, fat synthesis, and glycogen formation Linked to folic acid, pantothenic acid, and vitamin B_{12}	Caused by feeding raw egg white, inflammatory bowel diseases or achlorhydria Biotin is linked to the metabolic roles of folic acid, pantothenic acid, and vitamin B_{12}.	None known

TABLE 34.6	Main Dietary Sources of Vitamins and Their Role (continued)			
Vitamin	Source	Function	Deficiency	Toxicity
Folate	Liver, mushrooms, green leafy vegetables, lean beef, potatoes, whole wheat bread, orange juice, and dried beans	Enzyme cosubstrate in many synthesis reactions in the metabolism of amino acids, formation of red and white blood cells in bone marrow	Impaired biosynthesis of DNA and RNA, thus reducing cell division Megaloblastic, macrocytic anemia	May affect zinc
Cobalamin (vitamin B_{12})	Animal products, meat, fish, liver, poultry, milk, fortified foods	Red blood cell formation, nerve cells Megaloblastic anemia	Macrocytic anemia, smooth red tongue, fatigue, nerve degeneration	None known
Ascorbic acid (vitamin C; antioxidant)	Orange juice, grapefruit juice, lemons, limes, tomato juice, kiwi	Involved in synthesis of collagen and carnitine; acts as a reducing agent to keep iron in its ferrous state; needed for proper lung function, decreases severity of colds, essential for the oxidation of phenylalanine and tyrosine, the conversion of folate to tetrahydrofolic acid, and neurotransmitter serotonin and the formation of norepinephrine from dopamine	Scurvy Impaired wound healing; edema; hemorrhages and weakness in bone, cartilage, teeth, and connective tissues; bleeding gums; rheumatic pains in legs; skin lesions; and psychological changes— hysteria, hypochondria, depression	Gastrointestinal upset and diarrhea and may form renal oxalate stones

FAD, Flavin Adenine Dinucleotide; FMN, Flavin Mononucleotide; NAD, Nicotinamide Adenine Dinucleotide; NADPH, Nicotinamide Adenine Dinucleotide Phosphate; TCA, Tricarboxylic acid cycle.

TABLE 34.7	Dietary Reference Intake for Vitamin D and Calcium	
DRI for Vitamin D Age Group	Recommended Dietary Allowance (RDA) per Day	Tolerable Upper Intake Level (UL) per Day
Infants 0–6 months	400 International Unit (10 mcg)*	1,000 International Unit (25 mcg)
Infants 7–12 months	400 International Unit (10 mcg)*	1,500 International Unit (38 mcg)
Children 1–3 years	600 International Unit (15 mcg)	2,500 International Unit (63 mcg)
Children 4–8 years	600 International Unit (15 mcg)	3,000 International Unit (75 mcg)
Children and adults 9–70 years	600 International Unit (15 mcg)	4,000 International Unit (100 mcg)
Adults >70 years	800 International Unit (20 mcg)	4,000 International Unit (100 mcg)
Pregnancy and lactation	600 International Unit (15 mcg)	4,000 International Unit (100 mcg)

DRI for Calcium Age Group	Recommended Dietary Allowance (RDA) per Day	Tolerable Upper Intake Level (UL) per Day
Infants 0–6 months	200 mg*	1,000 mg
Infants 7–12 months	260 mg*	1,500 mg
Children 1–3 years	700 mg	2,500 mg
Children 4–8 years	1,000 mg	2,500 mg
Children 9–18 years	1,300 mg	3,000 mg
Adults 19–50 years	1,000 mg	2,500 mg
Adults 51–70 years		
Men	1,000 mg	2,000 mg
Women	1,200 mg	2,000 mg
Adults >70 years	1,200 mg	2,000 mg
Pregnancy and lactation		
14–18 years	1,300 mg	3,000 mg
19–50 years	1,000 mg	2,500 mg

*AI rather than RDAs.
The IOM report states that there are no additional health benefits associated with vitamin D intakes above the level of the new RDA.
Total vitamin D intake should remain below the level of the new UL to avoid possible adverse effects.
The IOM report states that there are no additional health benefits associated with calcium intakes above the level of the new RDA.
Total calcium intake should remain below the level of the new UL to avoid possible adverse effects.
Source: Health Canada. (2010). *Vitamin D and calcium: Updated dietary reference intakes.* Retrieved from http://www.hc-sc.gc.ca/fn-an/nutrition/reference/table/ref_vitam_tbl-eng.php

Important Facts About Folate

Folate (a B vitamin that acts as part of a coenzyme that is needed in the manufacture of new cells) plays an important role in the first few weeks of pregnancy. The folate that is added to foods and supplements is folic acid. This nutrient has been added to wheat flour in Canada in the past few years because many women in childbearing years do not consume enough folate. It is important to know that too much folate can mask a vitamin B_{12} deficiency. "Because many pregnancies are unplanned, all women who could become pregnant should take a daily multivitamin containing 400 mcg (0.4 mg) of folic acid. At a minimum, start taking your supplement 3 months before you get pregnant" (Health Canada, 2013, "Key Messages On Folate," para. 3).

Important Facts About Vitamin B_{12}

There are several reasons why a person may become deficient in vitamin B_{12}, including inadequate absorption (the most common cause of vitamin B_{12} deficiency) and inadequate consumption. See Box 34.5 for the causes of inadequate absorption.

In many older adults, absorption of vitamin B_{12} may be inadequate because stomach acidity is decreased. Decreased stomach acidity reduces the body's ability to remove vitamin B_{12} from the protein in meat. Inadequate consumption can result in vitamin B_{12} deficiency, which develops in people who do not consume any animal products (e.g., vegans) unless they take supplements.

The Changing Evidence on Vitamins and Minerals

Information regarding vitamins and minerals is changing. Studies in the last few years have shown that some vitamins and minerals may have other roles beyond those functions that have been associated with deficiency diseases. For example, it is known that vitamin D is needed for healthy bones and is protective against bone diseases (rickets/osteomalacia), but there is some new evidence to show that vitamin D also protects against certain types of cancers (Gorham et al., 2005).

It is also known that deficiencies in multiple nutrients besides calcium have been associated with the development of osteoporosis (Nieves, 2005). In the past, professionals only looked at the role of calcium with osteoporosis. Currently, researchers are looking at all the nutrients that

BOX 34.5 Causes of Inadequate Absorption

- Overgrowth of bacteria in part of the small intestine
- Malabsorption disorders
- Inflammatory bowel disease (Crohn disease and ulcerative colitis)
- Surgery that removes the part of the small intestine where vitamin B_{12} is absorbed
- Drugs such as antacids and metformin
- Lack of intrinsic factor
- Decreased stomach acidity (common among older people)

support mineralization: calcium, phosphorus, magnesium, and vitamin D. Zinc and vitamin K are involved in increasing concentrations of calcium and phosphorus locally in order to facilitate precipitation at appropriate sites for mineralization.

It is important to connect with a registered dietitian who can continuously update your knowledge base on vitamins. Many patients take vitamin and mineral supplements that can interact with medications. For example, calcium supplements should not be taken with thyroid medication or tetracycline. Calcium supplements should also not be taken at mealtimes because it can interfere with iron absorption. Patients could end up with a vitamin/mineral deficiency or might inactivate their medications if they are not instructed properly. Thus, communication between health-care professionals is essential for effective patient care.

Minerals

Minerals are inorganic substances that are not broken down during digestion and absorption. They are not destroyed by heat or light and have a role in many body processes. They are naturally occurring inorganic compounds that can be divided into two categories: macrominerals, which are essential minerals and occur in large amounts in the body and are needed in the diet on a daily basis in large quantities, and microminerals, which are essential minerals that are only needed in small amounts (the total amount found in the human body is less than 5 g). See Table 34.8 for the main dietary sources of minerals.

Important Facts About Calcium

The nutrient bioavailability (the amount of a nutrient our bodies can absorb and use) of calcium depends on our age and our need for calcium. Infants and children normally absorb around 60% of the calcium they consume in their diet because their requirements for calcium are high at this time of life. Pregnant and breast-feeding women only absorb around 50% of the calcium they consume, whereas healthy adults absorb even less, taking in only 30% of their dietary calcium. Although older adults have a significant need for calcium, metabolic changes related to aging lower the level of calcium absorption in the small intestine of older adults. When our calcium needs are high, the body normally increases the absorption from the small intestine.

It is important to know that our bodies cannot absorb more than 500 mg of calcium at one time. Even if a supplement contains 1000 mg of calcium, the amount that a person can absorb at any one time is less. Consequently, in order to maximize daily calcium intake it is important to advise patients to spread out their calcium intake throughout the day. Refer to Box 34.6 for information about calcium supplements.

The absorption of calcium in the body can be affected by several things. The presence of other compounds in foods along with calcium can inhibit its absorption. For example, phytates and oxalates (compounds present in plant foods)

TABLE 34.8 Main Dietary Sources of Minerals and Their Role

Mineral	Source	Function	Deficiency	Toxicity
Macrominerals				
Calcium	Cow's milk and dairy products; dark leafy green vegetables (kale, turnip greens, broccoli) Salmon with bones, tofu processed in calcium sulphate, almonds	Most of the calcium is found in the bones, and the bones support and protect the body's soft tissues. Required for nerve transmission, muscle contraction, cell membranes, and helps with maintenance of blood pressure and is necessary for blood clotting	Low bone mass which could contribute to osteomalacia and may play a role in colon cancer and hypertension	Calcification of soft tissues; interference of absorption of iron, zinc, and manganese
Phosphorus	Protein sources: meat, poultry, fish, eggs, milk and milk products, nuts, legumes, cereals, and grains	Phosphate is needed for DNA and RNA. ATP contains phosphate bonds. Phosphorus is part of every cell membrane in the body.	Not very common; neurological, muscular, skeletal, and renal changes will occur.	A low dietary calcium/phosphorus ratio can result in faster bone turnover, which may result in a reduction of bone density.
Magnesium	Magnesium is in many foods: seeds, nuts, legumes, dark green vegetables, milk, and cereal grains.	Cofactor for more than 300 enzymes; needed for synthesis of fatty acids and proteins and the glycolytic pathway Neuromuscular transmission requires magnesium.	Rare; when deficiency occurs, there are tremors, muscle spasms, nausea, and vomiting.	Can inhibit bone calcification
Microminerals				
Iron	Liver, oysters, fish, lean meat and poultry, dried beans, egg yolks, dried fruits, dark molasses, and whole grains	Red blood cells, blood and respiratory transport of oxygen and carbon dioxide, immune function, and cognitive performance	Most common nutrition deficiency Anemia	Oxidation of LDL cholesterol, arterial vessel damage
Zinc	Meat, fish, poultry, milk and milk products, oysters, liver, whole grain cereals, dry beans	Part of 300 enzymes; structural role of several proteins and functions as a signal in brain cells, immune function.	Short stature, hypogonadism, mild anemia	Interferes with copper absorption; gastrointestinal irritation and vomiting
Fluoride	Drinking water with fluoride added; seafood	Tooth enamel	Does not cause a disease	Discoloration of teeth
Copper	Animal products (not milk), shellfish, muscle meats, chocolate, nuts, cereal grains, dried fruits	Part of many enzymes	Anemia, neutropenia, and skeletal abnormalities	Toxicity occurs from supplements.
Ultra trace minerals				
Iodine	Seafood (clams, sardine, saltwater fish), iodized salt	Goiter	Thyroid disease or disorder	
Selenium (antioxidant)	Anything grown in ground, but the selenium content of soil must be adequate; Brazil nuts, seafood, liver, meat, and poultry	Exists in several proteins	Keshan disease	Skin and nail changes, tooth decay
Chromium	Brewer's yeast, oysters, potatoes, seafood, whole grains, cheese, chicken, meat, and bran	Potentiates insulin action Carbohydrate, lipid, and protein metabolism	Insulin resistance and lipid abnormalities	Skin lesions

occur naturally in calcium-containing foods such as seeds, nuts, spinach, rhubarb, and Swiss chard. The phytates and oxalates bind to some of the calcium and do not allow the calcium to be absorbed in the small intestine. If a person takes calcium at the same time as he or she takes iron, zinc, magnesium, or phosphorus, these minerals may interact with each other, which can affect the absorption and the body's utilization of all of them. A high intake of insoluble fibre can bind calcium in the intestine and decrease its absorption. If a person consumes tea with food or with a calcium supplement, tannins in tea can also bind with calcium in the intestine and decrease its absorption. In contrast, the absorption of calcium may be increased in the presence of lactose or vitamin D. The dietary reference intake for calcium has recently changed. See Table 34.7 for the dietary reference intake recommendations for calcium intake.

Important Facts About Iron

Iron is an essential nutrient. It is a part of many proteins and enzymes and is essential for the regulation of cell growth and differentiation. Human bodies store iron in two forms: ferritin (major intracellular store of iron that carries bound iron from the brush border to the basolateral membrane of the absorbing cell) and hemosiderin (a complex, insoluble form of storage iron). The most common places where iron is stored in the body are in the liver, bone marrow, intestinal mucosa, and spleen.

Absorption of iron is higher when a person's iron stores are low. Iron absorption is better when a person has a good amount of stomach acid. There are two types of iron found in food: heme iron and nonheme iron. Heme iron is part of hemoglobin and myoglobin and is found in animal-based foods (meat, fish, and poultry), whereas nonheme iron is found in both animal and plant-based foods. Heme iron has a better absorption rate (may be as high as 25%) in the digestive system than nonheme iron (only around 5%).

Iron absorption is increased by meat protein factor (MPF). The mechanism by which MPF increases the absorption of nonheme iron in other foods is unknown.

Vitamin C (ascorbic acid) increases the absorption of nonheme iron as well.

Dietary factors can decrease the absorption of iron, including the consumption of phytates (legumes, rice, and whole grains), carbonates, phosphates, polyphenols (tannins in tea and coffee, oregano, and red wine), vegetable protein (soybean), and calcium. Iron in egg yolk is not absorbed well because of the presence of phosvitin. For more information about iron deficiency, refer to Table 34.9.

Water

Water is the most important nutrient in the human body because it is part of every cell, tissue, and organ, contributing about 60% to 70% of a person's body weight. Water is often called the fluid of life because every cell in the body needs water to be able to function properly, and every process in the body occurs in a water medium. Water plays an important role in maintaining body temperature. Water is part of three compartments in the body including the intracellular, the extracellular, and the vascular system. A healthy person needs to have a proper fluid balance. Too little water (dehydration) or too much water in the body (water intoxication—occurs when water intake is in excess of the body's ability to excrete it) can both have serious health impacts. So how much fluid should we drink in a day? The amount most often recommended is known as the "8 × 8" guideline: Eight glasses of 8 oz of liquid per day, not including caffeinated and alcoholic beverages (Negoianu & Goldfarb, 2008). However, Negoianu and Goldfarb (2008) report that there is no scientific evidence, not one study, and no single outcome to support the 8 × 8 guideline. Nevertheless, we do know that too little fluid can lead to dehydration and too much fluid can lead to water intoxification. For more reading on

TABLE 34.9	Information About Iron Deficiency
Iron deficiency	Most common nutrient deficiency in the world
	Infants, young children, adolescent girls, premenopausal women, and pregnant women are at a high risk for developing iron deficiency.
Stage 1	Decrease in iron stores, resulting in reduced levels of ferritin; often physical symptoms are not seen because hemoglobin levels are not affected.
Stage 2	Decrease in the transport of iron; transferrin is decreased; the production of heme starts to decrease leading to symptoms of reduced work capacity.
Iron deficiency anemia	The production of red blood cells decreases and hemoglobin levels are low.
Stage 3	Impaired work performance, general fatigue, depressed immune system, impaired cognitive and nerve function, paleness, impaired memory occur.

TABLE 34.10		Dietary Reference Intake for Water	
Age in Years (Males)	Water (L/day)	Age in Years (Females)	Water (L/day)
0–0.5	0.7	0–0.5	0.7
0.5–1	0.8	0.5–1	0.8
1–3	1.3	1–3	1.3
4–8	1.7	4–8	1.7
9–13	2.4	9–13	2.1
14–18	3.3	14–18	2.3
19–30	3.7	19–30	2.7
31–50	3.7	31–50	2.7
>50	3.7	>50	2.7

this topic, go to the website for the *Journal of the American Society of Nephrology* for the article by Negoianu and Goldfarb (2008). For information on the dietary reference intake for water, see Table 34.10.

Dehydration

Dehydration (depletion of body fluid that occurs when fluid excretion is greater than fluid intake) is a serious and potentially life-threatening situation that can develop if water intake is interrupted. Healthy adults can usually only survive up to 10 days without water intake, whereas children can only survive for at most 5 days. Despite its importance, most individuals do not drink enough water on a daily basis to maintain healthy levels of hydration. Water is regularly lost from the body within a 24-hour period. It is mainly lost through urine but is also lost in sweat and water vapor through the breathing mechanism. It must constantly be replaced or dehydration will occur.

Dehydration can lead to renal problems and constipation. Dehydration may also decrease the ability of the mucosal membranes in the upper respiratory tract to effectively block bacteria and airborne particles, making an individual susceptible to infection. Children, older adults, individuals with learning disabilities, and those who have had their colons surgically removed (because of bowel disease) should be particularly encouraged to drink fluids to maintain their health.

Causes of dehydration include the following:

- Alcohol
- Caffeine
- Suntanning
- Improper intake of fluids
- Smoking
- Diarrhea
- Vomiting
- Illness
- Infection

Fluid Retention

Edema is a condition where fluid builds up in the tissue spaces of the body, producing fluid imbalance and swelling. Some common causes of fluid retention are hot weather, burns, and medications. Edema can also be a symptom of serious conditions such as chronic lung disease, liver disease, heart failure, peripheral vascular disorders, and kidney disease. Treatment may include a mild fluid restriction, a change in medication, a low sodium diet, and ongoing medical supervision.

If you cannot remember the dietary reference intake for fluid intake, here is an easy formula to use for daily water consumption recommendations:

1 ml of water for every kilocalories consumed for adults
1.5 ml of water for every kilocalories consumed for infants
Sources of water include both beverages and solid food.

For more information on the physical findings in association with dehydration, refer to Table 34.11. The Health Canada website (Health Canada, 2011b) offers a detailed description of the definitions and physical findings associated with dehydration as well as the clinical practice guidelines for treatment.

Through the eyes of a nurse

*E*ncouraging my patients to drink fluids is a nursing responsibility that I take very seriously in my practice (often a common diet prescription seen in the chart is "push fluids"). Preventing dehydration is an important part of the preventative care for my patients, which can, in some circumstances, save their lives. As a nurse, I know that it is important to communicate with the dietary department and the dietitian to make sure ample fluids are provided for my patients. Also, you must make sure that your patients can reach their container of fluids and can take a drink independently.

(personal reflection of a nurse)

Nutrient Recommendations

Nutrient recommendations are guides used as standards for measuring the energy and nutrient intakes for individuals. Dietitians use these recommendations to assess intakes, and with this information, they can provide information on the amounts of food and nutrients patients need to consume. The nutrient recommendations for energy, macronutrients, vitamins, minerals, and water have been established by Canadian and American scientists through a review process overseen by the U.S. National Academies, which is an independent, nongovernmental body; and they are published as **dietary reference intake (DRI)**, a general term that includes the four specific types of nutrient recommendations: adequate intake (AI), estimated average requirement (EAR), recommended dietary allowance (RDA), and

TABLE 34.11	Physical Findings in Association With Degree of Dehydration		
Clinical Sign	Mild Dehydration	Moderate Dehydration*	Severe Dehydration*
Fluid loss (% of body weight)	<6%	6%–10%	>10%
Radial pulse	Normal	Rapid, weak	Very rapid, feeble
Respiration	Normal	Deep	Deep, rapid
Systolic blood pressure	Normal	Low	Very low or undetectable
Skin turgor	Retracts rapidly	Retracts slowly, arms and legs feel cool to touch	Retracts very slowly, cold and clammy to touch or hot, dry skin
Mouth	Dry, sticky saliva	Dry	
Eyes	Normal	Sunken, possibly no tearing	Very sunken
Mentation	Alert	Restless, light-headed	Drowsy, light-headed, and continues for 2 minutes after standing, confusion, comatose
Urine output	Normal or reduced with dark yellow colour	Scant, dark brown colour	Oliguria
Voice	Normal	Hoarse	Inaudible
Thirst	Increased	Even more increased thirst	
Muscle	Normal	Cramps	

*Moderate: must be addressed quickly because it can progress to rapid deterioration requiring complex clinical intervention.
   Severe: requires immediate attention (can lead to delirium, coma, and death).

tolerable upper intake level (UL). DRIs are used for nutrient recommendations for both Canada and the United States. The Canadian governing bodies for health and medicine have accepted these standards.

DRIs are dietary standards for healthy people. EAR is a value that is estimated to meet the requirements of half the healthy individuals of a group. RDA is the amount of a nutrient needed to meet the requirements of most of the healthy population (97% to 98%). AI is the recommended daily intake level looking at observed or experimental determinations of approximate nutrient intake by a group of healthy individuals. UL is the highest daily intake amount of a nutrient that should not risk adverse health effects for almost all individuals in the general population. Canadians can use the daily values from the food label to assist in making good choices among the wide variety of foods available in the supermarket. You will find more information on Canada's guidelines for healthy eating in Box 34.7.

BOX 34.7 Canada's Guidelines for Healthy Eating

- Enjoy a variety of foods.
- Emphasize cereals, breads, other grain products, vegetables, and fruits.
- Choose low-fat dairy products, lean meats, and foods prepared with little or no fat.
- Achieve and maintain a healthy body weight by enjoying regular physical activity and healthy eating.
- Limit salt, alcohol, and caffeine.

Eating Well With Canada's Food Guide

Eating Well with Canada's Food Guide (Fig. 34.2) helps Canadians plan healthy meals when they include foods from the four food groups:

- Vegetables and fruit
- Grain products
- Milk and alternates
- Meat and Alternates

These food guide sources provide advice for specific ages: children, women of childbearing years, and men and women over the age of fifty.

Physical Activity Guide

Nutritional needs are directly impacted by the amount of physical activity. The physical activity guide published by the Public Health Agency of Canada was created to help Canadians make good choices for exercise. Exercise will help prevent disease and improve overall health. It reduces stress, strengthens the heart and lungs, increases energy levels, and helps maintain and achieve a healthy body weight. (See Web Resources on thePoint for a link to the Public Health Agency site and the guidelines.)

Food Labels

Educated consumers can make healthier food choices when they understand the meaning of the information on food labels. Health Canada regulates the labeling of food

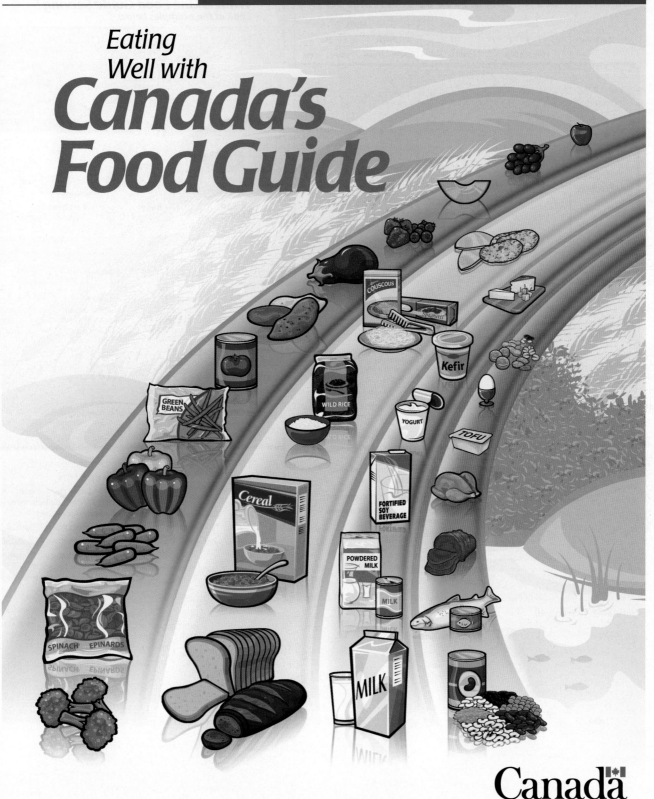

Figure 34.2 Canada's Food Guide and Serving Suggestions. (Reproduced with permission from Health Canada. (n.d.). *Recommended number of food guide servings per day.* Retrieved from http://www.hc-sc.gc.ca/fn-an/food-guide-aliment/index-eng.php *(continued on page 878)*

Recommended Number of *Food Guide Servings* per Day

	Children			Teens		Adults			
Age in Years	2-3	4-8	9-13	14-18		19-50		51+	
Sex	Girls and Boys			Females	Males	Females	Males	Females	Males
Vegetables and Fruit	4	5	6	7	8	7-8	8-10	7	7
Grain Products	3	4	6	6	7	6-7	8	6	7
Milk and Alternatives	2	2	3-4	3-4	3-4	2	2	3	3
Meat and Alternatives	1	1	1-2	2	3	2	3	2	3

The chart above shows how many Food Guide Servings you need from each of the four food groups every day.

Having the amount and type of food recommended and following the tips in *Canada's Food Guide* will help:

- Meet your needs for vitamins, minerals and other nutrients.
- Reduce your risk of obesity, type 2 diabetes, heart disease, certain types of cancer and osteoporosis.
- Contribute to your overall health and vitality.

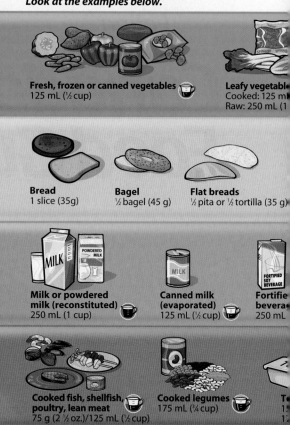

What is One Food Guide Serving?
Look at the examples below.

Fresh, frozen or canned vegetables
125 mL (½ cup)

Leafy vegetable
Cooked: 125 m
Raw: 250 mL (1

Bread
1 slice (35g)

Bagel
½ bagel (45 g)

Flat breads
½ pita or ½ tortilla (35 g)

Milk or powdered milk (reconstituted)
250 mL (1 cup)

Canned milk (evaporated)
125 mL (½ cup)

**Fortifie
bevera**
250 mL

Cooked fish, shellfish, poultry, lean meat
75 g (2 ½ oz.)/125 mL (½ cup)

Cooked legumes
175 mL (¾ cup)

**T
1
1**

Oils and Fats
- Include a small amount – 30 to
  each day. This includes oil usec
  and mayonnaise.
- Use vegetable oils such as canc
- Choose soft margarines that ar
- Limit butter, hard margarine, la

Figure 34.2 (*continued*)

Make each Food Guide Serving count...
wherever you are – at home, at school, at work or when eating out!

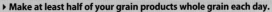

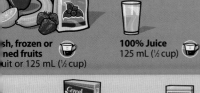

‣ **Eat at least one dark green and one orange vegetable each day.**
- Go for dark green vegetables such as broccoli, romaine lettuce and spinach.
- Go for orange vegetables such as carrots, sweet potatoes and winter squash.

‣ **Choose vegetables and fruit prepared with little or no added fat, sugar or salt.**
- Enjoy vegetables steamed, baked or stir-fried instead of deep-fried.

‣ **Have vegetables and fruit more often than juice.**

sh, frozen or
ned fruits
uit or 125 mL (½ cup)

100% Juice
125 mL (½ cup)

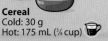
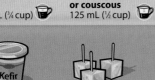

Cereal
Cold: 30 g
Hot: 175 mL (¾ cup)

Cooked pasta
or couscous
125 mL (½ cup)

‣ **Make at least half of your grain products whole grain each day.**
- Eat a variety of whole grains such as barley, brown rice, oats, quinoa and wild rice.
- Enjoy whole grain breads, oatmeal or whole wheat pasta.

‣ **Choose grain products that are lower in fat, sugar or salt.**
- Compare the Nutrition Facts table on labels to make wise choices.
- Enjoy the true taste of grain products. When adding sauces or spreads, use small amounts.

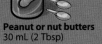

Yogurt
75 g
¾ cup)

Kefir
175 g
(¾ cup)

Cheese
50 g (1 ½ oz.)

‣ **Drink skim, 1%, or 2% milk each day.**
- Have 500 mL (2 cups) of milk every day for adequate vitamin D.
- Drink fortified soy beverages if you do not drink milk.

‣ **Select lower fat milk alternatives.**
- Compare the Nutrition Facts table on yogurts or cheeses to make wise choices.

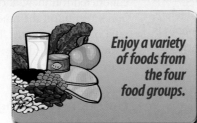
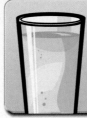

gs
ggs

Peanut or nut butters
30 mL (2 Tbsp)

Shelled nuts
and seeds
60 mL (¼ cup)

‣ **Have meat alternatives such as beans, lentils and tofu often.**

‣ **Eat at least two Food Guide Servings of fish each week.***
- Choose fish such as char, herring, mackerel, salmon, sardines and trout.

‣ **Select lean meat and alternatives prepared with little or no added fat or salt.**
- Trim the visible fat from meats. Remove the skin on poultry.
- Use cooking methods such as roasting, baking or poaching that require little or no added fat.
- If you eat luncheon meats, sausages or prepackaged meats, choose those lower in salt (sodium) and fat.

f unsaturated fat
sings, margarine

rans fats.

Enjoy a variety of foods from the four food groups.

Satisfy your thirst with water!

Drink water regularly. It's a calorie-free way to quench your thirst. Drink more water in hot weather or when you are very active.

* Health Canada provides advice for limiting exposure to mercury from certain types of fish. Refer to www.healthcanada.gc.ca for the latest information.

Whole Wheat Pita			
Nutrition Facts			
Per 1 pita (60 g)			
Amount		% Daily Value	
Calories **170**			
Fat **2 g**		**3%**	
Saturated Fat **0.2 g** + Trans Fat **0 g**		**2%**	
Cholesterol **0 mg**			
Sodium **320 mg**		**14%**	
Carbohydrate **35 mg**		**12%**	
Fibre **5 g**		**20%**	
Sugars **1 g**			
Protein **6 g**			
Vitamin A	**0%**	Vitamin C	**0%**
Calcium	**2%**	Iron	**15%**

Figure 34.3 Food label.

products in Canada with the Food and Drugs Act, which makes nutrition labeling mandatory on most food labels (Fig. 34.3).

The ingredient list is where ingredients must be listed in descending order by weight. The nutrition facts table is where calories and 13 core nutrients are listed with amounts for one serving of that particular food item. Nutrient content claims are based on standardized serving sizes. Health claims are defined by Health Canada, which are currently limited to five health claims. Since 2003, certain health claims have been allowed between diet and health benefits for selected relationships (Health Canada, 2007b; Box 34.8).

BOX 34.8 Health Claims

Since 2003, health benefit claims have been allowed on the following relationships:

- Between a healthy diet low in sodium and high in potassium and reduced risk of high blood pressure
- Between a healthy diet with adequate calcium and vitamin D and reduced risk of osteoporosis
- Between a healthy diet low in saturated and trans fat and reduced risk of heart disease
- Between a healthy diet rich in vegetables and fruit and reduced risk of some types of cancers
- Between nonfermentable carbohydrates in gums and hard candies and reduction in dental caries

The nutrition facts table shows

- Serving size and servings in the package
- Calories, calories from fat, and calories from saturated and trans fats per serving
- Percent daily values: how much a serving of food contributes to your overall intake of the various nutrients listed on each label. The daily value of 2,000 cal is based on recommendations for a healthy adult diet.

For more information on nutrition throughout the life cycle, refer to Box 34.9.

Nutrition Screening and Assessment

How will you apply the knowledge you have about nutrition, nutrition status, and healthy eating in your professional practice? This next section shows you the skills and tools that you need to provide nutrition care. Let's begin by discussing how you will assess the nutritional status of your patients.

Nutrition screening and assessment are important parts of the nutrition care process, which involves the assessment of the person's nutritional status, nutrition diagnosis, medical nutrition therapy, and monitoring and evaluation of therapy. It is important to assess the nutrition adequacy for each patient. An individual's nutrient intake is influenced by several considerations including income level, eating behaviour, emotional status, culture, disease states, ability to consume food, ability to chew food, ability to digest food and, finally, the ability to absorb food. A nutrition assessment should be conducted routinely, and this necessitates the use of a nutrition screening at the time of the patient's admission to a hospital or nursing home. The nutritional assessment includes a nutritional-based physical exam that is tailored for each individual patient.

Nutrition Screening

A nutrition screening process is used to identify those individuals who are malnourished or at risk from malnourishment. The findings from an initial screen will determine whether further assessment is needed. All qualified health-care professionals should be able to complete a nutrition screening process by employing a nutrition screening tool (Fig. 34.4).

Nutrition Assessment

A nutrition assessment is a comprehensive evaluation that is conducted by a registered dietitian. The assessment will provide information that will identify those individuals who require nutrition support therapy; it will enable health-care professionals to improve or maintain a person's nutrition status; it will identify the appropriate medical nutrition therapy; and finally, it allows health-care professionals to monitor the effectiveness of the nutrition intervention (Box 34.10).

(text continues on page 888)

BOX 34.9 Nutrition Throughout the Life Cycle—Key Points to Consider

Preconception

Women with less than 17% body fat will often not menstruate.

Women with less than 22% body fat often do not ovulate.

Overweight women (greater than 120% IBW) will often have problems getting pregnant because the ratio of testosterone to estrogen is out of balance.

Consume adequate amounts of folate at least 1 month before conception. A multivitamin that has 400 mcg of folic acid is sufficient. It is important to not consume greater than 1,000 mcg since this large amount can mask a vitamin B_{12} deficiency.

Conception

Caffeine consumption may affect fetal outcome.

Ideally, women should avoid intake of alcohol when they are trying to become pregnant.

Pregnancy

Fetal growth and the pregnancy require that mom include extra nutrients based on the DRIs.

The following nutrients are increased during pregnancy: water, energy in the second and third trimesters, carbohydrate, total fibre, linoleic acid, linolenic acid, protein, thiamin, riboflavin, niacin, biotin, pantothenic acid, vitamin B_6, folate, vitamin B_{12}, choline, vitamin C, vitamin A, magnesium, iron, zinc, iodine, selenium, copper, manganese, chromium, and molybdenum.

Refer to the DRI chart in any nutrition textbook or consult with an RD for more details.

First trimester: same caloric intake as a nonpregnant female

Second trimester: Mom needs to consume an additional 340–360 kcal/day.

Third trimester: Mom needs to increase calories another 112 kcal/day.

Folic acid requirements increase during pregnancy. The RDA is 600 mcg/day.

Iron: RDA for iron during pregnancy is 27 mg/day.

Gastrointestinal tract changes, and nausea, vomiting, constipation, or heartburn can occur.

Nutrient needs increase with special attention to protein, iron, iodine, folate, and calcium and vitamin D.

Nausea and vomiting in pregnancy: Separate liquids and solids by at least 1 hour. Have plain foods; often, cold foods work best (cold chicken, fruit, uncooked vegetables, plain grains). Avoid strong smelling foods and consume small, frequent meals.

Heartburn: Consume several small feedings; wear loose fitting clothes.

Infants

Breast-fed infants need additional vitamin D supplementation by 2 months of age and iron.

If an infant is not exclusively or is partially breast-fed, then commercial formulas are the most acceptable alternative to breast milk for the healthy full-term infant.

It is recommended that families introduce nutrient-rich complementary foods at 6 months to meet the increasing nutritional requirements and developmental needs. New recommendations suggest that to prevent iron deficiency; iron-containing foods are recommended as the first foods.

In the first year of life, the baby grows faster than any other time in his or her lifespan. Growth directly relates to nutrition status. Babies only need a small amount of food, but they need more than twice as much of most nutrients. The earlier research provides great information to help you guide your new parents in feeding their babies.

Childhood

Children ages between 1 and 3 years are at high risk for developing iron deficiency anemia.

Calcium, zinc, and vitamin D are important.

Nutrition concerns for childhood are overweight/obesity and underweight, failure to thrive, iron deficiency, dental caries, allergies, and attention deficit hyperactivity disorder (ADHD), which is a common behavioural disorder that affects approximately 8% of school-age children.

Children will eat well with Canada's Food Guide recommendations.

Adolescence

Calcium needs are greater, iron requirements are also increased for the building of bone mass and the increase in red blood cell volume.

In females, iron is needed to support iron lost during menses.

Zinc is important for sexual maturation.

Nutrition concerns are irregular meals and snacking, fast foods and convenience foods, dieting and body image, and the requirement for increased nutrients for the pregnant teen.

Pregnant Teens

Many teens begin pregnancy with a deficiency in vitamins A and D, folate, iron, calcium, and zinc.

It is recommended that pregnant teenagers follow the Canada's Food Guide pattern for their age and eat an extra two to three Food Guide Servings each day.

Pregnant teens need more food to meet their increased energy requirements during pregnancy.

Other nutrients (e.g., zinc) are needed in greater amounts by pregnant teens than by other teenagers (Health Canada, 2010e).

Pregnant teens can meet the increased nutrient needs (e.g., zinc) by taking a daily multivitamin.

Adult Years

Adults require less energy as they get older.

Vitamin D and calcium are important. Canada's Food Guide to Healthy Eating recommends that all individuals older than the age of 50 years should take a daily vitamin D supplement of 10 mcg (400 International Unit).

Nutrition concerns for men are heart disease, prostate cancer, and lung cancer. Alcohol is also a concern. The Nutrition Recommendations for Canadians state that "the Canadian diet should include no more than 5% of total energy as alcohol, or two drinks daily, whichever is less." The more alcohol an individual consumes, the food intake and adequate nutrients decreases. Alcohol provides "empty calories." Alcohol abuse also affects the body's metabolism of nutrients and intestinal cells do not absorb thiamine, folate, and vitamin B_6 well (Canadian Centre on Substance Abuse, 2013).

Aging

Nutrition concerns: sensory loss, oral health, gastrointestinal changes, cardiovascular disease, neurologic function, depression, ulcers, eyesight changes, and decreased immune system

Protein needs are the same for older adults as for young adults.

Vitamin A absorption increases age and therefore the requirement decreases.

It is important to consume enough vitamin B_{12}, B_6, and folate because they may assist in preventing some loss of mental ability.

Dehydration is a major risk for older adults. The thirst mechanism is not as efficient, and the kidneys become less efficient in drawing back water before it is lost in the urine.

Zinc deficiency is common in older adults, which can decrease the appetite and sense of taste.

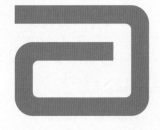

Determine Your Nutritional Health

The warning signs of poor nutritional health are often overlooked. Use this checklist to find out if you or someone you know is at nutritional risk.

Read the statements below. Circle the number in the yes column for those that apply to you or someone you know. For each yes answer, score the number in the box. Total your nutritional score.

	YES
I have an illness or condition that made me change the kind and/or amount of food I eat	2
I eat fewer than 2 meals per day	3
I eat few fruits or vegetables or milk products	2
I have 3 or more drinks of beer, liquor or wine almost every day	2
I have tooth or mouth problems that make it hard for me to eat	2
I don't always have enough money to buy the food I need	4
I eat alone most of the time	1
I take 3 or more different prescribed or over-the-counter drugs a day	1
Without wanting to, I have lost or gained 10 pounds in the last 6 months	2
I am not always physically able to shop, cook and/or feed myself	2
TOTAL	

Total your nutritional score. If it's —

0–2   **Good!** Recheck your nutritional score in 6 months.

3–5   **You are at moderate nutritional risk.** See what can be done to improve your eating habits and lifestyle. Your office on aging, senior nutrition program, senior citizens center or health department can help. Recheck your nutritional score in 3 months.

6 OR MORE   **You are at high nutritional risk.** Bring this checklist the next time you see your doctor, dietitian or other qualified health or social service professional. Talk with them about any problems you may have. Ask for help to improve your nutritional health.

These materials developed and distributed by the Nutritional Screening Initiative, a project of:

AMERICAN ACADEMY
OF FAMILY PHYSICIANS

THE AMERICAN
DIETETIC ASSOCIATION

NATIONAL COUNCIL
ON THE AGING, INC.

Remember that warning signs suggest risk, but do not represent diagnosis of any condition. Turn the page to learn more about the Warning Signs of poor nutritional health.

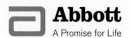

Figure 34.4 Determine Your Nutritional Health checklist. (Reproduced with permission from Abbott Laboratories. (2008). *Determine your nutritional health.* Retrieved from http://www.abbottnutrition.ca/static/cms_workspace/en_CA/content/document/ENS339A08.pdf) *(continued)*

> ## The nutrition checklist is based on the warning signs described below. Use the word DETERMINE to remind you of the warning signs.

DISEASE

Any disease, Illness or chronic condition which causes you to change the way you eat or makes it hard for you to eat, puts your nutritional health at risk. Four out of five adults have chronic diseases that are affected by diet. Confusion or memory loss that keeps getting worse is estimated to affect one out of five or more of older adults. This can make it hard to remember what, when or if you've eaten. Feeling sad or depressed, which happens to about one in eight older adults, can cause big changes in appetite, digestion, energy level, weight and well-being.

EATING POORLY

Eating too little and eating too much both lead to poor health. Eating the same foods day after day or not eating fruit, vegetables, and milk products daily will also cause poor nutritional health. One in five adults skip meals daily. Only 13% of adults eat the minimum amount of fruit and vegetables needed. One in four older adults drink too much alcohol. Many health problems become worse if you drink more than one or two alcoholic beverages per day.

TOOTH LOSS/MOUTH PAIN

A healthy mouth, teeth and gums are needed to eat. Missing, loose or rotten teeth or dentures which don't fit well or cause mouth sores make it hard to eat.

ECONOMIC HARDSHIP

As many as 40% of older Americans have incomes of less than $6,000 per year. Having less—or choosing to spend less—than $25–$30 per week for food makes it very hard to get the foods you need to stay healthy.

REDUCED SOCIAL CONTACT

One-third of all older people live alone. Being with people daily has a positive effect on morale, well-being and eating.

MULTIPLE MEDICINES

Many older Americans must take medicine for health problems. Almost half of older Americans take multiple medicines daily. Growing old may change the way you respond to drugs. The more medicines you take, the greater the chance for side effects such as increased or decreased appetite, change in taste, constipation, weakness, drowsiness, diarrhea, nausea and others. Vitamins or minerals, when taken in large doses, act like drugs and can cause harm. Alert your doctor of everything you take.

INVOLUNTARY WEIGHT LOSS/GAIN

Losing or gaining a lot of weight when you are not trying to do so is an important warning sign that must not be ignored. Being overweight or underweight also increases your chance of poor health.

NEEDS ASSISTANCE IN SELF CARE

Although most older people are able to eat, one out of every five have trouble walking, shopping, buying and cooking food, especially as they get older.

ELDER YEARS ABOVE AGE 80

Most older people lead full and productive lives. But as age increases, risk of frailty and health problems increase. Checking your nutritional health regularly makes good sense.

www.AbbottNutrition.ca
Printed in Canada
© Abbott Laboratories, Limited
ENS/339A08-Feb. 2008

The Nutrition Screening Initiative
2626 Pennsylvania Avenue, NW, Suite 3001, Washington, DC 20037

The Nutrition Screening Initiative is funded in part by a grant from
Ross Laboratories, a division of Abbott Laboratories

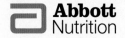

Figure 34.4 (*continued*)

BOX 34.10 Nutritional Assessment

Level 1 Screen

- The Level 1 Screen provides a simple method for identifying individuals who should be referred for more comprehensive nutrition or medical evaluation as well as those who would benefit from other health or community services without the need for a physician's intervention.
- Social services and healthcare professionals in a variety of community and healthcare settings can use the Level 1 Screen.
- It is divided into two categories:

   1. Includes individuals with documented significant weight loss changes or those who are found to have BMI above 27 or below 22.
   2. Includes individuals without quantifiable nutritional deficits, weight loss or abnormal BMI.

Body Mass Index (BMI)

Measure height to the nearest inch and weight to the nearest pound. Record the values below and mark them on the Body Mass Index (BMI) scale to the right. Then use a straight edge (ruler) to connect the two points and circle the spot where this straight line crosses the centre line (body mass index). Record the number below.

Healthy older adults should have a BMI between 24 and 27.

Height (in): _____
Weight (lbs): _____
Body Mass Index: _____
(Number from center column)

Check any boxes that are true for the individual:

[ ] Has lost or gained 10 pounds (or more) in the past
    6 months.
[ ] Body mass index <24
[ ] Body mass index >27

For the remaining sections, please ask the individual which of the statements (if any) is true for him or her and place a check by each that applies.

Eating Habits

[ ] Does not have enough food to eat each day
[ ] Usually eats alone
[ ] Does not eat anything on one or more days each month
[ ] Has poor appetite
[ ] Is on a special diet
[ ] Eats vegetables two or fewer times daily
[ ] Eats milk or milk products once or not at all daily
[ ] Eats fruit or drinks fruit juice once or not at all daily
[ ] Eats breads, cereals, pasta, rice, or other grains five or fewer
    times daily

[ ] Has difficulty chewing or swallowing
[ ] Has more than one alcoholic drink per day (if woman); more
    than two drinks per day (if man)
[ ] Has pain in mouth, teeth, or gums

A physician should be contacted if the individual has gained or lost 10 pounds unexpectedly or without intending to during the past 6 months. A physician should also be notified if the individual's body mass index is above 27 or below 24.

Living Environment

[ ] Lives on an income of less than $6,000 per year
    (per individual in the household)
[ ] Lives alone
[ ] Is housebound
[ ] Is concerned about home security
[ ] Lives in a home with inadequate heating or cooling
[ ] Does not have a stove and/or refrigerator
[ ] Is unable or prefers not to spend money on food
    (<$25–30 per person spent on food each week)

Functional Status

Usually or always needs assistance with (check each that apply):
[ ] Bathing
[ ] Dressing
[ ] Grooming
[ ] Toileting
[ ] Eating
[ ] Walking or moving about
[ ] Traveling (outside the home)
[ ] Preparing food
[ ] Shopping for food or other necessities

If you have checked one or more statements on this screen, the individual you have interviewed may be at **risk** for poor nutritional status. Please refer this individual to the appropriate healthcare or social service professional in your area. For example, a dietitian should be contacted for problems with selecting, preparing, or eating a healthy diet, or a dentist if the individual experiences pain or difficulty when chewing or swallowing. Those individuals whose income, lifestyle, or functional status may endanger their nutritional and overall health should be referred to available community services: home-delivered meals, congregate meal programs, transportation services, counseling services (alcohol abuse, depression, bereavement, etc.), home healthcare agencies, day care programs, etc.

A repeat of this screen is recommended at least once each year—sooner if the individual has a major change in his or her health, income, immediate family (e.g., spouse dies), or functional status.

Nomogram for Body Mass Index

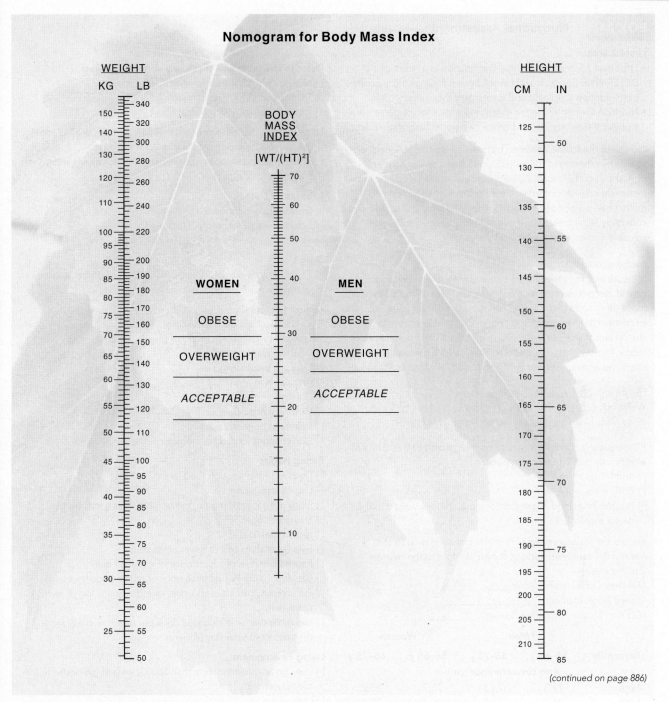

(continued on page 886)

Reprinted with permission by the Nutrition Screening Initiative, a project of the American Academy of Family Physicians, the American Dietetic Association and the National Council on the Aging, Inc., and funded in part by a grant from Ross Products Division, Abbott Laboratories.
Source: http://www.geroeducation.org/HyperText_module/Weight_Loss/html/level_1_screen_body_weight.htm

BOX 34.10 Nutritional Assessment (continued)

Level 2 Screen

- The Level 2 Screen as an initial examination or a result of DETERMINE Checklist and Level 1 Screen findings, incorporates both nutrition screening and assessment measures.
- Nutrition assessment in the elderly includes a focused interview, a physical examination, and review of pertinent laboratory data.

Complete the following screen by interviewing the patient directly and/or by referring to the patient chart. If you do not routinely perform all of the described tests or ask all of the listed questions, please do consider including them, but do not be concerned if the entire screen is not completed. Conducting a minimal screen and collecting serial measurements on older patients can be extremely valuable in monitoring nutritional status.

Anthropometrics

Measure height to the nearest inch and weight to the nearest pound. Record the values below and mark them on the Body Mass Index (BMI) scale to the right. Then use a straight edge (paper, ruler) to connect the two points and circle the spot where this straight line crosses the center fine (body mass index). Record the number below; healthy older adults should have a BMI between 24 and 27; check the appropriate box to flag an abnormally high or low value.

Height (in): _____
Weight (lbs): _____
Body Mass Index: _____ (weight/height)

Please place a check by any statement regarding BMI and recent weight loss that is true for the patient.
[ ] Body mass index <24
[ ] Body mass index >27
[ ] Has lost or gained 10 pounds (or more) of body weight in the past 6 months

Record the measurement of mid-arm circumference to the nearest 0.1 centimeter and of triceps skinfold to the nearest 2 millimeters.
Mid-Arm Circumference (cm): _____
Triceps Skinfold (mm): _____
Mid-Arm Muscle Circumference (cm): _____

Percentile	Men		Women	
	55–65 y	65–75 y	55–65 y	65–75 y
Arm circumference (cm)				
10th	27.3	26.3	25.7	25.2
50th	31.7	30.7	30.3	29.9
95th	36.9	35.5	38.5	37.3
Arm muscle circumference (cm)				
10th	24.5	23.5	19.6	19.5
50th	27.8	26.8	22.5	22.5
95th	32.0	30.6	28.0	27.9
Triceps skinfold (mm)				
10th	6	6	16	14
50th	11	11	25	24
95th	22	22	38	36

From: Frisancho AR. New norms of upper limb fat and muscle areas for assessment of nutritional status. Am J Clin Nutr 1981; 34:2540–2545. c1981 American Society for Clinical Nutrition.

Refer to the table and check any abnormal values:
[ ] Mid-arm muscle circumference <10th percentile
[ ] Triceps skinfold <10th percentile
[ ] Triceps skinfold >95th percentile

Note: mid-arm circumference (cm) − {0.314 × triceps skinfold (mm)} = mid-arm muscle circumference (cm)
For the remaining sections, please place a check by any statements that are true for the patient.

Laboratory Data
[ ] Serum albumin below 3.5 g/dl
[ ] Serum cholesterol below 160 mg/dl
[ ] Serum cholesterol above 240 mg/dl

Drug Use
[ ] Three or more prescription drugs, OTC medications, and/or vitamin/mineral supplements daily

Clinical Features
Presence of (check each that apply):
[ ] Problems with mouth, teeth, or gums
[ ] Difficulty chewing
[ ] Difficulty swallowing
[ ] Angular stomatitis
[ ] Glossitis
[ ] History of bone pain
[ ] History of bone fractures
[ ] Skin changes (dry, loose, nonspecific lesions, edema)

Eating Habits
[ ] Does not have enough food to eat each day
[ ] Usually eats alone
[ ] Does not eat anything on one or more days each month
[ ] Has poor appetite
[ ] Is on a special diet
[ ] Eats vegetables two or fewer times daily
[ ] Eats milk or milk products once or not at all daily
[ ] Eats fruit or drinks fruit juice once or not at all daily
[ ] Eats breads, cereals, pasta, rice, or other grains five or fewer times daily
[ ] Has more than one alcoholic drink per day (if woman); more than two drinks per day (if man)

Living Environment
[ ] Lives on an income of less than $6000 per year (per individual in the household)
[ ] Lives alone
[ ] Is housebound
[ ] Is concerned about home security
[ ] Lives in a home with inadequate heating or cooling
[ ] Does not have a stove and/or refrigerator
[ ] Is unable or prefers not to spend money on food (<$25–30 per person spent on food each week)

Functional Status
Usually or always needs assistance with (check each that apply):
[ ] Bathing
[ ] Dressing
[ ] Grooming
[ ] Toileting
[ ] Eating

[ ] Walking or moving about
[ ] Traveling (outside the home)
[ ] Preparing food
[ ] Shopping for food or other necessities

Mental/Cognitive Status
[ ] Clinical evidence of impairment, e.g., Folstein <26
[ ] Clinical evidence of depressive illness, e.g., Beck Depression
   Inventory >15, Geriatric Depression Scale>5

Patients in whom you have identified one or more **major indicators** of poor nutritional status require immediate medical attention; if **minor indicators** are found, ensure that they are known to a health professional or to the patient's own physician. Patients who display **risk factors** of poor nutritional status should be referred to the appropriate health care or social service professional (dietitian, nurse, dentist, case manager, etc.).

Nomogram for Body Mass Index

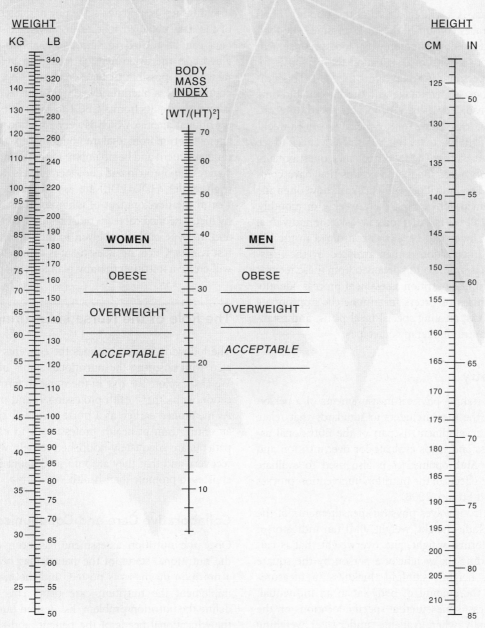

Reprinted with permission by the Nutrition Screening Initiative, a project of the American Academy of Family Physicians, the American Dietetic Association and the National Council on the Aging, Inc., and funded in part by a grant from Ross Products Division, Abbott Laboratories.

Source: http://www.geroeducation.org/HyperText_module/Weight_Loss/html/level_1_screen_body_weight.htm

Patient histories of diet, medical, social, and medication information are all part of the nutrition assessment, but the focal point is the diet history combined with anthropometry, physical assessment, and biochemical analysis. The diet history looks at the person's usual patterns of food intake and food selection. There are several tools used for taking a diet history including a daily food diary, a food frequency questionnaire, and a 24 hour recall.

Taking a Dietary History

A daily food diary is a written record of the amounts of all foods and beverages consumed during a set time. The food record will include information on when food is consumed, place where food is consumed, situation the person is in, and mood that person is in when eating the food. The individual records dietary food intake with the amount and time of day it was consumed. Usually, people are asked to record their intake for at least 3 days (one of the days being a weekend day). You might like to try this yourself as a check to see how healthy your diet is. The food frequency questionnaire is a chart that organizes foods into groups that have common nutrients. The individual will check off how often the foods are consumed; for example daily, weekly, or monthly. The 24-hour recall list is a method that asks the individual to remember all foods and beverages consumed in the last 24 hours. This information is then analyzed by the registered dietitian. The information obtained from these records is used to assist in the nutrition assessment process, identify nutrient deficiencies or excess, determine the appropriate nutrition diagnosis, creating special meal plans, and establishing desired nutrition therapy outcomes.

Anthropometry

Anthropometry (taking physical measurements of a person and comparing the measurements to standards that relate to growth and development) is part of the nutritional assessment process and helps evaluate for overnutrition and undernutrition. Anthropometrics is also used to evaluate and monitor the effects of the nutrition intervention process (Mahan & Escott-Stump, 2008).

Anthropometry involves physical measurements of the patient that includes height, weight, BMI (an indicator of underweight, normal weight, and overweight that is calculated by dividing the weight of a person by the square of the person's height), skinfold thickness (a measurement to assess the amount of body fat in an individual; skinfold thickness is measured at specific locations on the body), and, finally, when available, underwater weighing and bioelectrical impedance analysis (composition analysis using the principle that relative to water, lean tissue has a higher electrical conductivity and lower impedance than fatty tissue; electrodes are attached at several points on the body and a small electrical current is passed through the body). The skinfold thickness measure must be conducted carefully because its validity depends on the accuracy of the measuring technique and the skill of the individual undertaking it. Head circumference and length are measurements conducted in the pediatric population. Anthropometry includes the interpretation of the height, weight, and head circumference measurements by comparing them to standard measurements.

Biochemical Analysis

Several biochemical tests measure nutritional status. The urinalysis test is used as a screening or diagnostic tool. Much of the data obtained reflects urinary tract status but some data can be related to various metabolic disorders (e.g., glucose in the urine may be related to high carbohydrate intake and possible diabetes mellitus). A complete blood count (CBC) is often reviewed by dietitians. As an example, laboratory results from a CBC can assist in the screening for nutritional anemia which is very common (iron deficiency anemia: serum iron, total iron binding capacity [TIBC], ferritin, hematocrit and hemoglobin, B_{12} deficiency or folate deficiency). Lipoprotein and cholesterol levels (total cholesterol, triglycerides, HDL, LDL) are assessed because they play a role in the development of atherosclerosis and are affected by diet. The medical team must realize that the disease itself and the type of therapy given to the patient may affect the test results. Once the assessment is completed, the dietitian will create a nutrition therapy plan for each patient.

The Role of the Nurse in Ensuring Nutrition

The following section outlines the concepts that are associated with ensuring the nutritional status of your patients. We also explore the role of the nurse in terms of communication with other health professionals and patient teaching. As mentioned earlier, as a nurse, you will be working with an entire team of health professionals to ensure that your patients are adequately nourished to help with their illness recovery and that they are informed about healthy lifestyle choices to promote their health.

Collaborative Care and Communication

Once the nutrition assessment has been completed and the nutritional status of the patient has been determined, a nutrition diagnosis is posted, and the medical team can implement the nutrition care plan. This care plan will define the nutrition problem, list desired outcomes, include the educational needs of the patient, and show a plan for monitoring and evaluation. It is important that the healthcare professionals work together to improve the nutritional health of the patient.

There are two primary ways by which we communicate a nutrition assessment: through the patient's record or chart and through a verbal report. In addition, you may also record a patient's fluid intake on a fluid balance record on a feeding record if the patient is receiving enteral or parenteral feedings (discussed later in this chapter), and you may also write your findings in the nurses' notes or interdisciplinary chart. If your agency uses electronic charting, you will be entering your findings directly into an electronic record. Because your daily work will involve working with different levels of health-care workers, you will want to report changes in your patient's nutritional status at unit rounds, end-of-shift reports, and care plan meetings. A serious patient safety issue arises when important information is not handed off to others who will take care of the patient on the next shift or the next day. Effective communication to ensure continuity of care is an essential component of safe and efficient nursing practice.

Patient Teaching

Teaching patients about healthy food choices is a very important role for nurses in various community and hospital settings. For example, instruction in healthy eating takes place in all of the following situations: prenatal nutrition classes, diabetes education, counseling patients in cardiac rehab postmyocardial infarction situations, and dealing with patients who want to lose weight to achieve a healthy BMI or reduce the amount of unhealthy saturated fats in their diet. In many cases, registered nurses teach these classes in partnership with a dietitian. In all these examples, the nurse as part of the teaching team can take advantage of the teachable moment when the patient is most ready to hear the information that is highly relevant to his or her current situation. The timing of the teaching is very important, and you will soon learn as you move from beginning nurse to expert nurse how to identify when a patient is most ready to accept the information about diet that you want to share. It is not unusual for people to need to hear the same information more than once before they are able to integrate permanent changes into their life. If you have a patient in the hospital whom you are teaching about a dietary change and she is not the person who prepares the meals at home, then you should include whoever prepares the patient's meals in the teaching that you do. The same principle will apply if you are teaching children about healthy food choices; you need to design a class that includes a parent or caregiver (Fig. 34.5).

Your teaching sessions, if they are in a hospital setting, will need a few special considerations. One is that you schedule the teaching at a time when the patient is able to listen, with her pain controlled, and that you provide for privacy. Allow the patient time to ask questions and don't try to give him or her too much information at one time. It is also helpful if you can provide written information to support your teaching; the patient can then take home this information and use it as a resource. In some settings, the nurse educator can provide the patient with a telephone number that he or she can call if he or she has questions once home, or if he or she forgets something that he or she was told. Finally, document

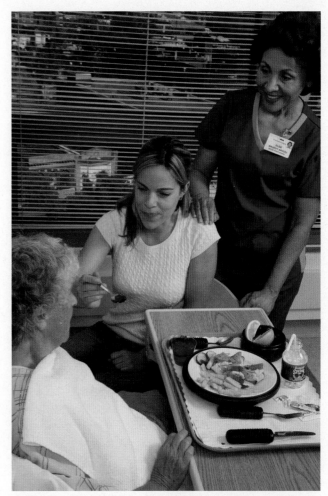

Figure 34.5 Nurse interacting with patient and family member at mealtime.

the details of your teaching sessions in the patient record and report that you did teaching at the team report. Teaching is most effective when nurses can build upon each other's teaching sessions.

Putting It All Together: Understanding Nutrition in the Context of Patient Care

Now that you have some knowledge about food science basics and how to assess the nutrition status of your patients, it is time to apply this knowledge to your nursing practice decisions. Assessment of the nutritional status of your patients will inform numerous clinical decisions that you will make on an ongoing basis. As a member of the health-care team, you will carry out skills that may be uncomfortable for the patient but necessary to ensure that he or she received adequate nutrition if he or she cannot take food or fluids by mouth. As examples, your patients may have experienced a stroke and not be able to swallow food or may have had surgery on the mouth or throat. In the case of premature infants, sucking may be too exhausting for them, so they are fed through a feeding tube inserted down their nose. Whatever the reason, as a nursing student, you will move from observer to participant with the skills for administering enteral and parenteral feedings. If you refer to Chapter 22 on medications, you will recall that medications are also administered via nasogastric tubes and jejunostomy tubes.

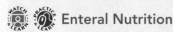

Enteral Nutrition

Enteral nutrition (EN) is a method of supplying nutrients through the body's feeding tract with a feeding tube. EN is a method used for those patients who are at risk for or are undernourished and have a minimal functioning intestine. They are unable to take in their total daily calories and protein in a typical oral form. Use of this mode of feeding is determined through the nutritional assessment (Hernandez, Torres, & Jimenez, 2006) (Fig. 34.6).

It is important to use the screening process to quickly and accurately identify those individuals who are malnourished as well as those who are at risk for developing nutrition-related complications. Nutrition-related complications include the following:

- Infection of wounds
- Slow healing process of wounds
- Longer periods in hospital
- Respiratory infections

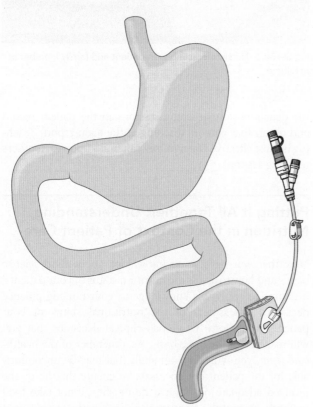

Figure 34.6 Jejunal tube (J tube) feed. Enteral nutrition refers to all types of feeding—gastric (inserts into stomach) and duodenal tube feed (inserts into duodenum). This is just one example of a feeding tube for EN.

Indicators that dietitians and nurses use in the screening process include the following:

- Changes in weight
- Changes in oral food and fluid intake
- Past medical/surgical history

Patients Who Require Enteral Nutrition

EN is used in those patients where a functional gastrointestinal tract can be accessed, but their oral food and fluid intake is not enough to meet their daily estimated energy needs (Skill 34.1). It is important to have at least 1 m of functional gastrointestinal tract when considering EN. The expected length of therapy, risk of aspiration, and the patient's clinical status determine enteral access.

Instead of regular foods, patients are fed special enteral formulas that are available in several forms, including a standard format (nutrients are equal to those consumed by healthy individuals), elemental format (predigested or hydrolyzed macronutrient content), or specialized format (products specifically designed for disease states). Standard formulas are used in most patients. It is important to familiarize yourself with where the formulas as stored and if they have an expiry date. Formulas are usually unrefrigerated until opened and then stored in the fridge to prevent bacterial contamination. You should always check to see how long an enteral feeding can be used once it is opened (read the guidelines on the formula package), but the usual time is 24 to 48 hours and after that leftover formula should be thrown away.

The most common tube feedings provide 1 cal/ml, others provide 1.5 cal/ml, and some formulas will even provide 2 cal/ml. A dietitian will calculate the number of calories needed per feed.

Small bowel feeding may be chosen over gastric feeding. Often, over time, there is a potential for decreased feeding tolerance with gastric feeding, which means there can be an increased risk for pulmonary aspiration of feedings. Aspiration is the leading cause of pneumonia in the intensive care unit (d'Escrivan & Guery, 2005).

The decision about which enteral formula to give to a patient must be made by the dietitian and the rest of the medical team by looking at the underlying clinical situation, the patient's nutrition requirements, and whether the patient's gastrointestinal tract is functioning adequately.

Enteral Delivery Method

After determining the need for EN, the delivery method and formula strength is determined next (Box 34.11).

- Bolus or intermittent is often used for gastric feedings and given to ambulatory patients.
- Continuous is the method commonly used for those patients who cannot tolerate intermittent feeding and often for critically ill patients.
- The cyclic method is often used in the home care setting with the feedings given either in the day or night. This method is a variation of the continuous drip method where

BOX 34.11 Enteral Nutrition

Naso/oroenteric Access

This is the most common method of enteral access because it is the simplest and least expensive method of feeding. Feedings can be administered by bolus, intermittent, or continuous infusions.

Bolus: Bolus feeding is essentially providing the equivalent of a meal, consisting entirely of formula. It requires the infusion of a set amount of formula given either by syringe, or it can be gravity controlled at specific times during the day. The infusion time is brief—it may take several minutes or last up to 20 minutes. Bolus feedings are very convenient for caregivers because feedings are administered only at specific times and larger amounts are given at each sitting.

Intermittent feeding: Intermittent feedings are given at various times in the 24-hour period. Infusion of the formula is either gravity controlled or pump assisted. Infusion time is often 20–60 minutes per feed. This method is used in ambulatory patients.

Continuous feeding: This feedings are infused by an enteral pump. Continuous feedings are given over a 24-hour period at lower volumes per hour.

Long Term (>4 Weeks)

Percutaneous feeding tube

- PEG (gastric): Percutaneous endoscopic gastrostomy tube is generally placed into a patient's stomach as a means of feeding them when they are unable to eat.
- J/PEG (gastric/jejunal)

Gastrostomy tube is the most common method used for long-term feeding.

Source: Charney, P., & Malone, A. (2008). *ADA pocket guide to nutritional assessment* (2nd ed.). Chicago, IL: American Dietetic Association.

the patient is given a constant rate of formula over an 8- to 16-hour period. The head of the bed must be raised to a 45° angle to avoid aspiration.

- Formula dilution is not routinely recommended. Dilution is used if the patient's total fluid requirements are not met through other means.

Transition from EN to oral food intake:

- An assessment must be made to determine a patient's ability to swallow and chew.
- Switch from predigested formula to formulas with intact protein.
- Assess patient for any future dietary modifications once food is introduced (allergies, textures, diseases, and food preferences).

- Dietitian to begin oral diet slowly with restricted lactose if dairy has not been included in the diet for some time.
- Food and beverage intake must be monitored.
- Once the patient consumes approximately half of his or her nutrition needs, then switch to nighttime cycle feedings.
- Enteral feedings are often discontinued when the patient is consuming approximately ¾ of his or her nutrition needs along with consuming 1 L of fluid for at least 3 days.
- Keep monitoring food intake until 100% of needs are met consistently.

Successful EN requires regular monitoring and assessment by the medical team. It is important to identify complications that might occur. See Box 34.12 for a nursing checklist for the patient receiving EN.

BOX 34.12 Checklist for Nursing Care for Patients Receiving Tube Feeding

- Before every tube feeding or every 8 hours, it is important to confirm that the tube is in the correct location.
- Make sure the head of the bed is at a 30° minimum during the administration of the feed and for a half hour postfeed.
- Change the feeding tubing and container every 24 hours unless using a closed system (follow manufacturer's instructions and check the nurse's notes/Kardex for the date and time to be changed).
- Make sure formula is fresh and changed regularly.
- Flush feeding tube with 30 ml of warm water regularly—follow facility guidelines.
- Do not mix medications with the feeding formula.
- Check body weight twice a week.
- Monitor daily intake and output.
- Monitor stool frequency, consistency.
- Look for abdominal distension or patient discomfort.
- Look for edema.

- Monitor hydration status daily. Fluid needs change regularly so this involves looking at electrolytes, protein content of the feeding, changes in stool, pulmonary and renal status, and temperature regulation.
- Monitor gastric residual volume. This assessment can help to identify patients at high risk for aspiration and aspiration-related pneumonia. This test is used to determine whether the patient has been able to empty his or her stomach contents postfeeding.
- Monitor daily electrolytes, creatinine, blood urea nitrogen (BUN), magnesium, phosphorus, and calcium.
- Monitor glucose daily in persons without diabetes until glucose level is stable and monitor at least every 6 hours or according to physician's orders for those individuals living with diabetes.
- Monitor albumin, prealbumin, and transferrin.
- Monitor nitrogen balance weekly.
- Monitor diarrhea because diarrhea is common in tube-fed patients. Sometimes, fibre may need to be added, an antidiarrheal agent is given, or the patient is switched to a new formula.

Nurse's Notes on Enteral Feeding

Enteral feeding is a complex process. The given information provides basic guidelines geared to introduce you to the concept of enteral feeding. As you progress in your education, more knowledge will be introduced. Once you have the opportunity to participate in a patient's EN care process, connect with the registered dietitian who will be able to add more valuable information to improve your skills and increase your knowledge.

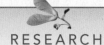

RESEARCH

IMPROVING FEEDING TUBE PLACEMENT TECHNIQUES

In a critical care setting in a U.S. hospital, registered nurses (RNs) and registered dietitians (RDs) work together in teams to place small bowel feeding tubes (SBFT) at the bedside (Gray et al., 2007). These teams verify placement of the tubes by using an electromagnetic tube placement device (ETPD). This method of verifying feeding tube placement has been described as an improvement over traditional feeding tube placement techniques. It is important to note that the feeding tubes are placed in the small bowel distal to the pylorus to avoid gastric stasis. In other words, the feedings are delivered below the level of the stomach to decrease the chances that the patient will aspirate (if the patient vomits, he or she could choke). This is especially important for patients who have their breathing assisted with a ventilator.

Critical care patients often require nutritional support via EN. Early initiation of EN is associated with decreased mortality, decreased complications associated with infection, increased patient safety, and earlier discharge from the hospital. Blind feeding tube insertion by the RN or RD followed by verifying tube placement with x-ray was the traditional approach used. Blind insertion can lead to serious complications when the feeding tube is misplaced. Additionally, if the hospital does not use portable x-ray machines in the intensive care unit (ICU), then it is an additional risk to the patients to transport them from the ICU to the radiology department for an x-ray.

To lower the incidence of serious consequences associated with blind insertion and traditional methods for feeding tube placement, the hospital obtained an ETPD. This device tracks "the approximate location of the SBFT tip during tube placement" (Gray et al., 2007, p. 436). The purpose of the study was to determine if the ETPD improved patient safety outcomes for tube insertion at the bedside. Additional outcomes of interest were success rate of accurate placement of tubes, costs associated with each approach, and timeliness of feeding initiation between the blind technique and the ETPD technique. Remember improved patient outcomes are associated with the initiation of feedings as soon as possible.

The study included two groups of patients or those that had blind insertion and those with ETPD insertion. The study by Gray et al. (2007) followed a detailed protocol to ensure patient safety including specialty training for the nurses and dietitians who inserted the feeding tubes.

As you become more proficient in reading research, you may want to review this study for the detailed protocol that was used. The researchers did report that the ETPD method prevented serious consequences from incorrect tube placement with two patients because of immediate real-time feedback that informed the nurse or dietitian to stop insertion and remove the tube. Findings of the study included a decrease by 50% in the number of x-rays needed to confirm tube placement in the study group. X-rays themselves are associated with a degree of risk for the patient. The SBFT also resulted in earlier feedings due to a shorter turnaround time between when the physician wrote the order and when the first feeding could be given. The researchers in this study found that there was a benefit to RNs and RDs working together (their work complemented each other) to insert the feeding tubes in their critically ill patients. If the patient became unstable, the nurses were able to identify, treat, and stabilize the patient "more readily than the RD" (Gray et al., 2007, p. 442).

The small number of participants was a key limitation of this study, but future studies could replicate this research and use a variety of different patients and settings. Research seeks to improve health-care practices by testing new approaches with a goal to improve patient outcomes while not compromising patient safety. New techniques that improve on a traditional process, inform practice, improve patient outcomes, save money, improve efficiency, and build on interdisciplinary teams are worthy of our attention.

Gray, R., Tynan, C., Reed, L., Hasse, J., Kramlich, M., Roberts, S., . . . Neylon, J. (2007). Bedside electromagnetic-guided feeding tube placement: an improvement over traditional placement technique? Nutrition in Clinical Practice, 22, 436–444.

Parenteral Nutrition

Parenteral nutrition (PN) bypasses the usual digestion in the stomach and bowel using a special liquid food mixture given into the blood through an intravenous (IV) catheter (Skill 34.2). The mixture contains proteins, carbohydrates (sugars), fats, vitamins, and minerals. PN was once called total parenteral nutrition (TPN), or hyperalimentation. PN should be considered for all patients who are malnourished or at risk of malnutrition and have a nonfunctioning or inaccessible gastrointestinal tract, preventing enteral feeding (Fig. 34.7).

Nutrition Screening for Parenteral Nutrition

The screening process is needed first to identify patients who are malnourished or are at risk for developing nutrition complications. Indicators that dietitians and nurses use in the screening process include the following:

- Changes in weight
- Changes in oral food and fluid intake
- Past medical/surgical history
- Food allergies or following a special diet

PN is used for those individuals who are malnourished and are not candidates for EN. Once initiated, PN should be

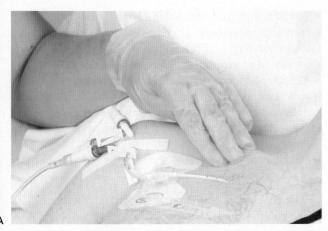

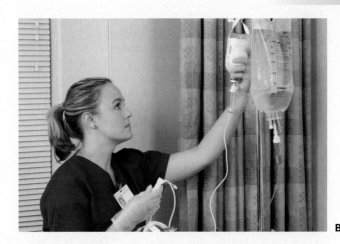

Figure 34.7 PN: hyperalimentation.

administered for at least 7 to 14 days. There is a high risk of infection and this method of feeding is very expensive.

Sites for Venous Access

PN solutions can be delivered through peripheral or central veins, depending on the specific osmolarity of the solution. Peripheral venous access is used with low-osmolarity solutions that are less than 900 mOsm. Peripheral cannulas are often put in at the bedside by a nurse and have a low risk of complications. Thrombophlebitis or inflammation of the vein is the most common complication, which is often caused by infusion of hyperosmolar solutions. Hyperosmolality refers to the osmolality of a solution that is greater than 350 mOsm/kg. Osmolality is the concentration of osmotically active particles per litre. Osmolality of a formula is affected by the concentration of amino acids, carbohydrate, and electrolytes. Normal body fluids are approximately 300 mOsm/L. High osmolality produces an osmotic effect in the stomach and small intestine. Hyperosmolality pulls water into the gastrointestinal tract to dilute the formula concentration. This incoming water into the gastrointestinal tract can cause diarrhea, nausea, and distention. Isotonic formulas do not cause this problem. The high osmolality of PN is damaging to veins, and the nurse will need to assist in peripheral line changes on a regular basis. Temporary central venous catheters are the most common device used in hospital settings. Solutions that use dextrose have a high osmolarity of greater than 900 mOsm and need large diameter, high-flow veins. Veins used most often for central peripheral access are the jugular and the subclavian. There is a greater risk of complications, and it is important to use gowns, sterile gloves, and sterile drape during the insertion placement procedure.

Care of Access Device

The goal is to avoid infections directly at the exit site as well as catheter-related bloodstream infections. Noninfectious complications include catheter occlusion, breakage, and tube dislodgment. Protocols need to be established for hand hygiene, skin antisepsis, catheter site dressings, catheter cap change, and hub care and also catheter patency. Refer to Box 34.13 for a list of complications related to parenteral access devices.

Nutritional Complications of Parenteral Nutrition

Hyperglycemia is high levels of blood glucose levels caused by too little insulin. Symptoms that may be observed: increased thirst, weight loss, tired, frequent urination often occurs, and overfeeding should be prevented. It is important to limit the carbohydrate dose, look for other sources of dextrose (e.g., other medications), and look for changes in medication—for example, corticosteroids affect glycemia. Corticosteroids stimulate gluconeogenesis (the formation of glucose from noncarbohydrate molecules—glycerol and the carbon skeletons of amino acids) in both liver and peripheral tissues. It is possible that corticosteroid treatment may induce hyperglycemia, and therefore, you will want to monitor capillary blood glucose (Skill 34.3) an hour after starting PN, again halfway through PN, and 1 hour post-PN feeding.

Refeeding syndrome results when there is a very quick infusion of substrates, especially carbohydrate, into the plasma. This causes insulin to be released rapidly, and there is a shift of electrolytes into the intracellular space as the glucose moves into the cells for oxidation. There is a decrease in salt and water excretion, and low serum levels of potassium, magnesium, and phosphorus are the result. It occurs after starvation and when a carbohydrate source is introduced back into the diet. Carbohydrate metabolism resumes as glucose becomes

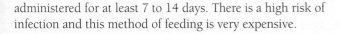

BOX 34.13   Complications of Parenteral Access Devices

- Catheter misplacement
- Nerve injury of the brachial plexus at the time of needle insertion
- Pneumothorax (abnormal presence of air in the pleural cavity resulting in the collapse of the lung)
- Hemothorax (accumulation of blood in the pleural cavity which is the space between the lungs and the walls of the chest) or hydrothorax (accumulation of serous fluid in one or both pleural cavities)
- Air embolism
- Occlusion
- Venous thrombosis
- Dislodgment

BOX 34.14 Monitoring the Patient on Parenteral Nutrition

- CBC differential—weekly in the stable patient
- Prothrombin time (PT) and partial thromboplastin time (PTT) tests weekly in stable patient
- BUN, creatinine—daily for 3 days with initiation of PN and then twice a week in stable patient
- Electrolytes—daily for the first 3 days of starting PN and then twice a week in stable patient
- Serum glucose—monitor every 4 hours until the results are consistently between 5.5 and 8.3 mmol/L.
- Serum triglycerides—to be measured after first bag and then weekly
- Liver function test, bilirubin, prealbumin and C-reactive protein (CRP)—measure on monthly basis.
- Physical assessment—weekly
- Weight—daily
- Fluid balance—daily
- Nitrogen balance—as needed

the major energy source, which then increases insulin production. Refeeding syndrome can be serious and can involve cardiac, respiratory, and neurologic failure. Abnormal glucose metabolism occurs because of the release of glucocorticoids; the body's electrolytes become imbalanced (magnesium, phosphate, and potassium), and thiamin deficiency and fluid and sodium retention can occur. Cholecystitis (inflammation of the gallbladder) can occur, but it is rare.

Liver disease involves the elevation of liver enzymes and is common in the first 2 weeks of PN. PN-associated liver disease is a very serious complication of long-term PN therapy. Unfortunately, it is often recognized too late, when liver injury is irreversible. Therefore, it is important to monitor liver enzymes early on in the treatment and regularly thereafter.

Metabolic bone disease is a decrease in bone mineralization from low vitamin D levels along with hypercalciuria (urinary excretion of calcium greater than 250 mg [6.25 mmol/L] a day or 4 mg [0.1 mmol/kg/day] for individuals who follow an unrestricted diet). It is important to make sure your patient is receiving enough vitamin D. The RD will monitor the vitamin D intake. For more on monitoring the patient on PN, see Box 34.14.

Nutrition Formulae for Parenteral Nutrition

PN is a complex therapy. There are commercially available standard solutions available from the hospital pharmacy, which are composed of all the essential amino acids and some of the nonessential amino acids, carbohydrates, lipid emulsions, electrolytes, vitamins and minerals, and additives. The pharmacist will provide instructions for storage.

The typical parenteral solution will contain

- Dextrose
- Amino acids
- Fat—using essential fats linoleic and linolenic acids
- Electrolytes (calcium, magnesium, phosphorus, sodium, potassium, acetate, and chloride)

- Vitamins and trace minerals (thiamin; riboflavin; niacin; folic acid; pantothenic acid; pyridoxine; cyanocobalamin; biotin; ascorbic acid; vitamins A, D, E, and K; chromium; copper; iron; manganese; selenium; and zinc)
- Additives—glutamine (amino acid occurring in proteins; important in protein metabolism and for immune function) and carnitine (a molecule found in the muscle and liver cells that transports fatty acids across the mitochondrial membrane)
- Osmolarity—This refers to the osmoles of solute per litre of solution (mOsm/L).

The concern of osmolarity is important when one is infusing a high-osmolarity formula through a peripheral vein. Phlebitis and irritation can occur. Osmolarity is not a concern when using central peripheral nutrition.

PN can be administered to individuals of all ages including infants, children, and adults. People can survive on PN for a long period of time. It is discontinued when the intestinal tract is able to handle the digestive process and the person can begin to eat normally again.

Now that Pamela has mastered the fundamental skills and knowledge required to ensure that her patients receive adequate nutrition, she feels confident in reporting to the nurse manager that her two patients did not eat their meals for reasons other than just not being hungry. Her observations prompted her to verbally report the situation to the charge nurse and to document her findings in the patient chart on the fluid balance sheet and in the nurses' notes. A note was made to report and put into the care plan that her two patients required assistance with their meals, to set up their trays, and to be assessed at the next mealtime by a nurse to see if they need further assistance to eat from their trays.

Conclusion

This chapter has introduced you to the basics of food science and the role of nurses in ensuring adequate nutrition for health and healing. You have learned that nurses are members of a team of health professionals with a responsibility for assessing the nutrition status of their patients and for intervening in situations when patients cannot independently take in nourishment because of alterations in their physical and/or mental health. See Box 34.15 for a diet therapy chart of common diseases. Teaching patients about healthy eating requires a commitment by nurses to continuous learning beyond graduation by attending conferences, reading the latest research findings, and being knowledgeable about clinical practice guidelines and best practice guidelines. Your knowledge and skills will continually evolve as you gain experience and learn more about promoting and maintaining healthy nutrition for your patients. An RD can also serve as an excellent resource and help you to understand the latest advancements in nutrition science.

BOX 34.15 Diet Therapy for Common Disorders

Anemia

Megaloblastic

Vitamin B_{12} or folic acid deficiency

Treatment for B_{12} deficiency:

High-protein diet, green leafy vegetables, meats, eggs, milk, and milk products

Treatment for folic acid deficiency:

Fresh fruit (mostly berries), orange juice, dark leafy green vegetables (e.g., spinach, asparagus, broccoli), dried beans and peas, fortified ready-to-eat cereals

Microcytic

Iron deficiency

Treatment:

High-iron foods (liver, beef, dried fruits, green leafy vegetables); ascorbic acid–containing foods increase absorption of dietary iron (citrus foods)

If supplements are prescribed, take iron in the evening with a small snack.

Diarrhea

Treatment:

Replace fluids and electrolytes.

Consume a clear fluid diet (broth, clear diluted juices, popsicles).

Stimulate the gastrointestinal tract by the slow introduction of solid food (plain cereals dry, plain bread, chicken, canned fruits).

Low-residue, low-fat, lactose-free nutrition therapy initially

Avoid caffeine-containing products, alcohol, and high-fibre and gas-producing foods, such as nuts, beans, corn, broccoli, cauliflower, or cabbage.

Sugar alcohols, lactose, fructose, and large amounts of sucrose may make diarrhea worse.

Modest amounts of pectin, fructooligosaccharides (FOS), inulin, oats, and banana flakes may help to control or treat diarrhea.

Diarrhea in Infants and Children

Infants and children are easily dehydrated by large fluid losses.

Replacement of fluid and electrolytes must be started immediately.

Oral rehydration is less invasive and less expensive than IV rehydration.

Diverticulosis

Treatment:

High-fibre diet promotes soft, bulky stools.

Increase the fibre slowly to avoid bloating and gas.

Adequate fluid intake is important (2–3 L/day).

Introduce probiotic foods such as yogurt or kefir to the daily diet.

Kefir is a cultured food that contains beneficial bacteria along with minerals, B vitamins, and amino acids. It is thinner than yogurt and many individuals consume it as a beverage.

Diverticulitis

Treatment:

Initially, rest the bowel and start the patient on clear liquids.

Slowly begin restricted fibre/low-residue nutrition therapy until inflammation and bleeding are no longer a risk.

Elemental nutrition or in some situations, total PN may be needed for the beginning of treatment and then one can slowly return to a high-fibre diet.

Initially, start with a low-fat diet because colonic smooth muscle contractions intensify after a high-fat meal and can cause stomach upset feelings.

Continue to increase fibre slowly after an acute episode is resolved.

Increase the fluid intake once fibre intake increases.

Add a probiotic food such as yogurt or kefir to the daily diet.

Foods such as nuts, popcorn hulls, sunflower seeds, pumpkin seeds, and sesame seeds may need to be limited in some individuals.

Tomato, zucchini, cucumbers, strawberries, and raspberries may not be a problem for most individuals.

(Mahan & Escott-Stump, 2008)

Diabetes Mellitus

Treatment:

Weight management

Exercise

Balance of intake from all food groups (Beyond the Basics Meal Plan: Grains and Starches, Fruits, Milk and Alternates, Other Choices, Vegetables, Meat and Alternates, Fats and Extras)

Encourage consumption of low GI foods.

Check blood fasting glucose and 2 hours postconsumption at various times of the day. (Practice Guidelines 228)

Diabetes Practice Guidelines for Canadians are available online (Canadian Diabetes Association, 2008a, 2012a, 2012b).

Gallbladder Disease

Treatment:

Low-fat diet with small, frequent feedings

Moderate amounts of low-fat protein foods

Coronary Heart Disease

Treatment:

Achieve and maintain a healthy body weight.

Physical activity

Mild sodium restriction

Low saturated and trans fat intake

Increased fruits and vegetable intake (antioxidants)

Increased soluble and insoluble fibre

Consume oily fish twice a week.

Minimize intake of beverages and foods with added sugars.

Alcohol in moderation; moderate alcohol consumption is considered to be up to two standard alcoholic drinks (44 ml spirits, 148 ml wine, or 355 ml beer) per day for men and up to one drink per day for women.

Alcohol and Health in Canada: A Summary of Evidence and Guidelines for Low-Risk Drinking is available online at http://www.ccsa.ca/2011%20CCSA%20Documents/2011-Summary-of-Evidence-and-Guidelines-for-Low-Risk%20Drinking-en.pdf

Gastroesophageal Reflux Disease (GERD)

Treatment:

Encourage weight loss.

Consume low-fat foods.

Avoid alcohol, coffee, black pepper, chocolate, and mint.

(continued on page 896)

BOX 34.15   Diet Therapy for Common Disorders (continued)

Consume small amounts of food, avoid lying down after eating, and sleep with the head of the bed elevated at a 45° angle.
Wear loose fitting clothes.

Hiatal Hernia

Treatment:

Eat small amounts of food at a time.
Avoid alcohol.
Avoid lying down after eating.
Weight reduction

Hypertension

Treatment:

Weight reduction
Moderate physical activity—30 minutes of walking most days of the week.
The Dietary Approaches to Stop Hypertension (DASH) diet
Increase fruit and vegetable consumption.
Sodium restriction (2,300 mg per day)
Consume two to three low-fat dairy products each day.
Increase consumption of whole grains.
Consume smaller portions of lean meats.
Decrease alcohol consumption.
The DASH DIET can be accessed online.
DASH DIET: Your Guide to Lowering Your Blood Pressure With DASH at http://www.nhlbi.nih.gov/health/public/heart/hbp/dash/new_dash.pdf

Lactose Intolerance

Treatment:

Eliminating or restricting the food intake of lactose (dairy foods, lactose added to products)
Those individuals who avoid dairy products should take a calcium and vitamin D supplement.
Lactase enzyme (Lactaid) and milk products treated with lactase enzyme may be beneficial.

Ulcer

Treatment:

Eat three regular meals a day in small portions.
Avoid pepper and chili pepper, chocolate, tea, coffee, and decaffeinated coffee.
Citrus fruits and juices may cause gastric reflux in some individuals.
Avoid alcohol in concentrated forms.
Eat slowly in a calm environment.
Introduce probiotics into the daily meal plan. Probiotics are live microorganisms and they are available in both supplement form and as components of foods and beverages. Probiotics have been shown to boost the immune system and inhibit the growth of harmful bacteria. Yogurt is the most common source of probiotics. Yogurt container must state that probiotics have been added. The terms "live cultures" and "probiotics" are not the same. Live cultures are specific microorganisms added to foods to create the fermentation process, live cultures are also referred to as "starter cultures" (Sanders, 2008; World Gastroenterology Organisation, 2008).

SKILL 34.1   Inserting a Nasogastric Tube for Enteral Feeding

Reviewing Pertinent Information

Step	Rationale
Review the patient's chart for the physician's order about the tube to be inserted (type and size) and the type of feeding that will be administered.	It is your professional responsibility as the RN prior to inserting the nasogastric tube to check the physician's order and to be fully informed about the patient prior to performing the skill.
Note: Other reasons for inserting a nasogastric tube include administration of medications, to establish a means for suctioning stomach contents, to remove stomach contents for gastric analysis in the lab, or to lavage (wash) the stomach in the case of overdose or poisoning.	
Assessment of your patient prior to tube insertion will include the following:	
• Check the chart for a history of nasal injury from surgery or a deviated septum.	Knowing the patient's history and the physical condition of his or her nose will assist in your decision-making about tube insertion. The nares may be blocked or irritated, and you may determine that you cannot insert the tube safely. Use a flashlight or penlight for a better assessment.
• Assess the patient's nose and check for patency of the nares. Use the nostril with the best air flow.	Nasoenteral tubes are contraindicated in patients with recent nasal surgery or trauma that includes nosebleeds.
• Check the patient's gag reflex.	If the patient does not have a gag reflex, he or she may be at risk for choking/aspiration. Checking the gag reflex will also tell you if the patient can swallow the tube.
• Check for a history of recent nasal surgery or nosebleeds and if the patient is on anticoagulant medication.	Patients who are confused or have an impaired level of consciousness may be more at risk for aspiration.
• Explain the procedure to the patient and assess his or her mental status or ability to cooperate with the procedure (as appropriate).	

Preparing for Administration (continued)

Step	Rationale
Wash hands.	Prevents the spread of microorganisms to the supplies being used and handled, and prevents the further spread of microorganisms to the patient
Gather supplies needed:	The patient might have a latex allergy.
• The tube ordered by the physician—large or small bore tube (nonlatex preferred)	The safety and the comfort of the patient are improved when you are organized before starting the procedure.
• Stethoscope	
• 60-ml catheter-tip or Luer Lock syringe	
• Tube fixation device or hypoallergenic tape (check agency policy)—2.5 cm wide	
• pH indicator strip (scale 0.0 to 14.0)	
• Water-soluble lubricant	
• Glass of water and a straw	
• Emesis or K basin	
• Safety pin and rubber band	
• Towel or disposable pad	
• Facial tissues or face cloth	
• Disposable gloves	
• Suction equipment	
• Penlight or flashlight	
• Tongue blade—tongue depressor	
• Clamp or plug (optional)	
Assist the patient to a sitting position—high Fowler's, if possible.	It will be easier for the patient to swallow in a sitting position.
Support the patient's head with a pillow.	Gravity will help the tube insertion in a sitting position.
Place the towel or disposable pad across the patient's chest.	The patient may gag and vomit, so it is best to be prepared and have the K basin close by too.
Have the patient hold some tissue if he or she is able to do so.	

Performing the Skill

Step	Rationale
Introduce yourself to the patient if you have not already done this earlier.	Important for ensuring the patient's safety and fostering a relationship of respect and trust with the patient.
Verify the patient's identity.	It will be more comfortable for the patient if he or she can swallow the tube and feel that he or she has some control during the procedure.
Explain what you are going to do and why it is necessary.	Raising a hand or a finger is a common signal to pause with the tube insertion.
Explain to the patient how to help and identify a signal to indicate to the need to have you pause.	
Wash your hands.	
Use other infection prevention and control procedures (e.g., clean gloves).	Prevents the spread of microorganisms to the patient
Close the door and/or curtains.	Provides for privacy
Determine how far to insert the tube (see Figure 1).	This length approximates the distance from the nose to the stomach and is different for each patient.

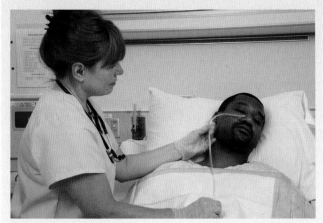

Figure 1

(continued on page 898)

SKILL 34.1   Inserting a Nasogastric Tube for Enteral Feeding (continued)

Performing the Skill

Step	Rationale
Using the tube, mark off the distance from the tip of the patient's nose to the tip of his or her earlobe and then from the tip of the earlobe to the tip of his or her xiphoid. Mark this length with a piece of adhesive tape.	To remember the length measured above
Put on gloves.	Gloves will protect the patient from surface organisms from the nurse's hands and will protect the nurse's hands from possible body secretions that may come into contact with the nurse's hands during tube insertion.
Lubricate the tip of the tube with the water-soluble lubricant or water to make insertion easier.	Lubrication will make the insertion of the tube easier and more comfortable for the patient and minimize trauma to the nostrils and throat during insertion. Water-soluble liquid is safer in case the tube enters the lungs during insertion because it dissolves; petroleum jelly is oil-based and does not dissolve, making it a safety risk for respiratory complications.
Insert the tube into the nostril with the curve in the tubing pointing toward the patient	Tube insertion will be easier if you follow the natural curve in the patient's nose and throat.
Ask the patient to hyperextend neck.	Hyperextension of the neck lessens the curvature of the nasopharyngeal junction.
Gently advance the tube.	This action avoids the turbinates (projections) along the lateral wall.
Direct the tube to the floor of the nostril and toward the ear.	Forcing the tube can cause harm to the patient.
If the tube meets resistance, pull it out, add more lubricant, and insert it into the other nostril.	Tilting the head forward helps the tube go into the posterior pharynx and esophagus. Swallowing moves the epiglottis over the opening into the larynx, which is where you don't want the tube to go.
Once the tube is in the throat, the patient may have the urge to vomit and gag. Ask the patient to tilt his or her head forward and swallow some water using the straw.	You want this procedure to be as comfortable as possible for the patient and for the tube to go into the stomach.
Stop advancing the tube until the patient stops gagging and then advance the tube. Pass the tube 5 to 1 cm each time the patient swallows until you reach the marking on the tube that you made.	
You may need to use the flashlight and look inside the patient's throat if the tube does not advance as it could be coiled in the throat (see Figure 2).	

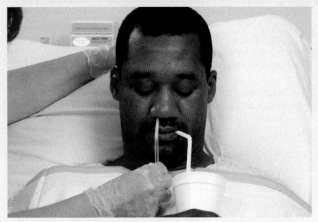

Figure 2

Performing the Skill (continued)

Step

Check placement of tube.
- pH
- Aspiration of stomach contents (see Figure 3)

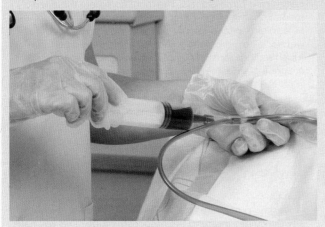

Figure 3

- X-ray
- Place a stethoscope over the patient's epigastrium and inject 10 to 30 ml of air into the tube while listening for bubbling—air through fluid sound (see Figure 4).

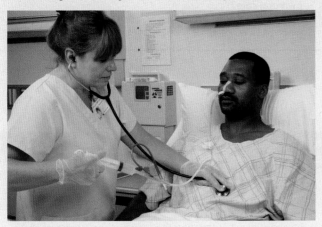

Figure 4

Once the tube is confirmed to be in the stomach, tape the tube to the bridge of the patient's nose.

Secure the tube to the patient's gown.

Attach the tube to suction or feeding apparatus—whatever was ordered.

Use the elastic band and the safety pin to secure the tube to the patient's gown.

Rationale

Gastric contents are usually pH 1 to 5. If your findings indicate a higher pH, the tube may be in the intestinal tract or in the lung. Aspirated stomach contents could be analyzed for the presence of bilirubin to determine correct placement.

An x-ray verifying placement depends on agency policy and a physician's order.

Injecting air is not the most reliable method to check tube placement and may not be in the agency's policies, but it is still one of the methods used.

Keep a small alcohol wipe hand to clean the patient's nose if they have been sweating during tube insertion. The tape will stick better.

This method of taping and securing of the tube is intended to prevent discomfort to the edge of the nostril. Taping to the gown of the patient prevents the tube from dangling and pulling on the nares.

(continued on page 900)

SKILL 34.1   Inserting a Nasogastric Tube for Enteral Feeding (continued)

Documenting Effectively

Step

Document relevant information as per agency policy, but usually, this will include the following:

- The size and type of tube inserted and the date and time of tube insertion
- Colour and amount of gastric contents
- Process used to verify tube placement
- How did the patient tolerate the procedure
- What did you attach the tube to—suction or feeding apparatus
- Plans for follow-up of care for patient with a nasogastric tube, which will include a plan for changing the tube, changing the tape that holds the tube in place, mouth care
- Accurate measurement of patient fluids, either tube feedings, irrigations, or gastric contents.

Rationale

Documentation is the key method of communication among health-care professionals. The more complete the documentation, the better other health-care team members are able to understand exactly what and how the procedure went and how the patient should be monitored and the tube feedings (or suctioning) delivered. All of these steps ensure a greater measure of patient safety.

Engaging in Ongoing Evaluation

Step

Include in the care plan appropriate follow-up and monitor the patient for the following:

- Comfort
- Tolerance of the nasogastric tube
- Continued correct placement of the tube in the stomach
- Patient's understanding of restrictions with having either a tube feeding or continuous suctioning attached
- Colour and amount of gastric contents if suction is attached or if stomach contents are aspirated to check tube placement before a tube feeding

Rationale

How was the procedure for the patient? Did you encounter any difficulties inserting the nasogastric tube? Did you have to stop inserting the tube into one nostril and try the other? How is the patient tolerating the restrictions to their mobility? Are there any tender spots inside the nares?

How is the patient tolerating the tube? Nauseated? How often is he or she receiving oral care? Can he or she do his or her own oral care?

Keep an accurate record of fluid balance, including type, amount, and colour of gastric contents.

SKILL 34.2   Nutrition Administration via Nasogastric or Gastrostomy Tube

Reviewing Pertinent Information

Step

Review the patient's chart and the nursing care plan.

- Check for food allergies.
- Check for other allergies (latex).
- Check the type, amount, rate, route, and how often the feedings or medications are administered.
- Check to see if the patient has experienced any difficulties with a previous feeding.

Rationale

The patient may have an allergy to an ingredient in the formula. The record may also indicate if the patient is having difficulty tolerating the feedings for other reasons; for example, lactose intolerance.

The record may indicate other problems with previous feedings that the physician needs to be notified about; for example, abdominal distention, cramping, or constipation.

Preparing for Administration

Step

Prepare the patient for a tube feeding by assessing the following before administering a tube feeding.

- Check for the presence of bowel sounds, abdominal distention, tenderness, and time of last bowel movement.

Tube placement and patency

Rationale

Formulas with high osmolarity can cause an electrolyte imbalance, causing diarrhea or constipation, intestinal cramping, gastric distention, and loss of fluid. Tube feedings are best tolerated if they are administered at room temperature and delivered slowly.

Feeding tubes can become displaced or clogged. Occlusion of a feeding tube even for a short period of time must be avoided. Clogging can be prevented by flushing the feeding tube with fluid (water) before and after feedings.

Administering a feeding if the tube is not in the stomach can cause aspiration of the feedings.

Preparing for Administration (continued)

Step	Rationale
Gather supplies needed: • Measuring container • Infusion pump (optional) • Water • Formula (as ordered) • pH test strip or meter • K basin • Clean gloves • 60-ml catheter tip syringe • Stethoscope • Gavage tubing	Important to be organized prior to entering the patient's room
Assist the patient to a sitting position by adjusting the bed to at least 60° high Fowler or having him or her sit in a chair as if he or she was going to eat in preparation for a meal.	To prevent aspiration of fluid into the lungs by improving the gravitational flow of the tube feeding fluid Note: If the patient cannot sit up, then a right side-lying position is an alternative position for the feeding.
Introduce yourself to the patient and verify identity by checking the armband and asking to verify his or her name.	Important for ensuring the patient's safety and fostering a relationship of respect and trust with the patient
Wash hands and follow other appropriate infection control measures.	Prevents the spread of microorganisms to the supplies being used and handled, and prevents further spread to the patient
Close room door or curtains around the patient's bed.	Ensures privacy and prevents embarrassment
Confirm placement of tube in the patient's stomach by withdrawing a sample of stomach contents.	The contents of the stomach have a pH of between 1 and 3. The presence of gastric fluid confirms the tube is placed in the stomach.
Check pH level and/or using the 60-ml syringe by attaching it to the tube inject 10 ml of air while listening with your stethoscope over the epigastrium.	Air can be heard entering the stomach. Note: This is not always a reliable method of checking tube placement when the tube has a small bore opening.
Aspirate stomach contents (gastric residuals) and measure in the measuring container.	This is a process for evaluating if gastric emptying is adequate or delayed. If there is 100 ml or more of the previous feeding still sitting in the stomach, call the physician before giving the next feeding.
Put the aspirated stomach contents back through the tube into the stomach.	Gastric contents or residuals are rich in electrolytes. Maintaining electrolyte balance is important.

Administering the Gastric Feeding

Step	Rationale
Prepare the formula at room temperature according to the physician's orders, ensuring the correct amount and strength.	Patient's tolerance will be increased if the strength of the formula is increased gradually. The patient will be less likely to develop diarrhea and gastric intolerance. Room temperature feedings are less likely to cause cramping and discomfort. Formula that is too hot can burn the stomach. Note: Tube feedings bypass the oral and esophageal mucosa that either heat up food or cool down food in normal swallowing.
Continuous feeding is a feeding that continues over a 24-hour period either by gravity drip or feeding pump. Cyclical/intermittent feedings are stopped in between feedings for a 4- to 16-hour period. See Figure 1, a nurse administering intermittent feeding.	Tube feedings can be intermittent/cyclical or continuous. An advantage to a continuous feeding is that it allows for the lowest possible hourly feed rate to meet nutrient requirements. It may also result in better blood glucose levels and increased tolerance given the lower rate. Daytime-only feedings may reduce the risk of aspiration. Tube feedings usually infuse over 3 hours (check agency policy). If a feeding is given too quickly, the patient may be uncomfortable and vomit (risking aspiration) or have cramping. An infusion pump allows for more control by being able to more accurately adjust the rate of infusion for the feeding.

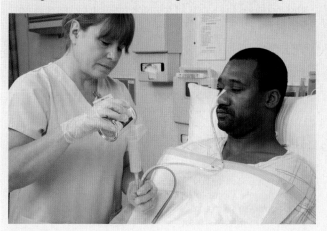

Figure 1

(continued on page 902)

| SKILL 34.2 | Nutrition Administration via Nasogastric or Gastrostomy Tube (continued) |

Administering the Gastric Feeding

Step	Rationale
Connect the gavage tubing to the gastric tube. Hang the tube feeding bag on an IV pole. Pour the desired amount of formula. Connect the tubing to the infusion pump (see Figure 2).	

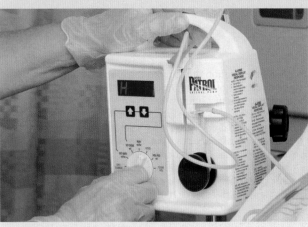

Figure 2

Step	Rationale
Check agency policy for the infusion rate. Set the rate for the infusion. Check gastric residuals every 4 to 6 hours for a continuous feeding. Then, flush the tubing with 30 to 60 ml of water (see Figure 3).	Checking the residuals confirms tube placement has been maintained and that adequate amounts of the tube feeding are being absorbed.

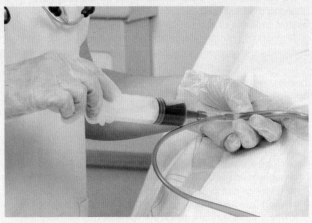

Figure 3

Step	Rationale
Have the patient remain in a sitting position (high Fowler or slightly elevated side-lying position.	Promotes digestion of the feeding, increases patient comfort and increases the safety of the tube feeding by decreasing risk of aspiration.

Engaging in Evaluation

Step	Rationale
Check agency policy for how often tubing should be changed. After discontinuing a feeding, wash any reusable equipment with soap and water. Wash hands.	Clean equipment decreases the chance of contaminating a future feeding with spoiled formula left in the tubing. Prevents the spread of microorganisms

Documenting Effectively

Step	Rationale
Document as per agency policy in a timely manner: • Date and time of feeding • Type of feeding administered • Patient response (tolerance) to the feeding • Other pertinent observations	Documentation is the key communication among health-care professionals. Complete documentation provides for the safe administration of gastric feedings for the patient and the prevention of errors.

SKILL 34.3   Measuring Blood Glucose With a Capillary Blood Specimen

Reviewing Pertinent Information

Step	Rationale
Check the chart and determine: • The purpose for the blood glucose testing • How often the testing is done • When the testing is done • What sites are most often used • How are the sites rotated Assess the following: • The patient's understanding of the procedure • The skin at the puncture site • Check for colour, warmth, and capillary refill. • Check to see if the patient is taking anticoagulant medication.	Important to know why the patient/client is having blood glucose levels monitored Frequent finger pricking for capillary blood samples can cause pain at the site, and over time, the patient may experience decreased sensation in the finger tips. Newer glucometers can use blood samples from the forearm in addition to fingertips. Check the patient's fingertips for signs of trauma and infection. Also, check for adequate blood flow to the puncture site. Choose a different site if you are concerned and report as well as document your findings. If the patient is on anticoagulant medication, she may bleed more excessively from the puncture site.

Preparing for Administration

Step	Rationale
Gather supplies needed: • Blood glucose meter (glucometer) (see Figure 1)	Equipment is specific to the agency and nursing unit you are working on. Become familiar with the policies and procedures at your agency. In home care settings, the patient might use his or her own glucose meter and strips. Alcohol swabs are not used in all settings due to the drying effect they have on skin and the possibility that the alcohol will affect the accuracy of the test. Some agencies have the patient wash hands with soapy water and dry thoroughly instead of using alcohol swabs.

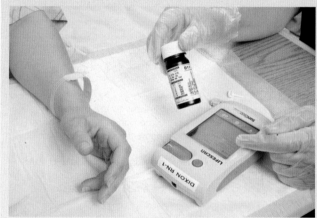

Figure 1

• Blood glucose reagent strips
• Warm cloth or warming device (optional and may not be needed)
• Small piece of gauze
• Antiseptic swab

Step	Rationale
Prepare the equipment: • Calibrate the meter and run a control sample according to the manufacturer's instructions. Prepare the patient: • Introduce yourself. • Check the patient's identity. • Explain the procedure. • Provide for privacy. • Have the patient wash her hands. • Choose a vascular puncture site.	Increases the accuracy of the blood glucose test result. Each manufacturer has instructions for calibrating their blood glucose monitors. Double-checking the patient's identity decreases the chance of an error. Explaining the purpose of the procedure fosters patient collaboration. Cleansing the puncture site decreases the chance of infection. Common sites are the side of an adult's finger, forearm, or the earlobe. Both actions improve blood flow to the extremity.

(continued on page 904)

SKILL 34.3 Measuring Blood Glucose With a Capillary Blood Specimen Feeding (continued)

Preparing for Administration

Step	Rationale
• Prepare site (finger) with a warm cloth if needed or hold the finger in a dependent position (see Figure 2).	

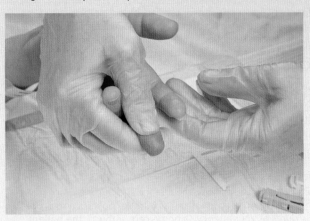

Figure 2
Wash hands.

Prevents the spread of microorganisms to the supplies being used and handled and prevents the further spread of microorganisms to the patient

Performing the Skill

Step	Rationale
Obtain the blood specimen:	Prevents the spread of microorganisms to the patient.
• Put on gloves.	The lancet is designed to pierce the skin at a specific depth that can be adjusted on some injectors (some patients have tougher skin to penetrate)
• Place the lancet in the injector.	
• Place the injector against the site.	Squeezing the site too harshly may damage tissue and interfere with the accuracy of the blood glucose reading.
• Release the needle.	
• Wait for a small bubble of blood to form at the site.	Pressure will help to decrease the amount of bleeding from the puncture site.
• Hold the reagent strip up to the bubble of blood until an adequate amount registers and begins the test on the monitor (see Figure 3).	

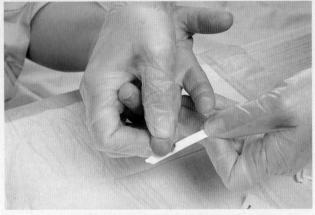

Figure 3

• Have the patient apply pressure to the skin puncture site with gauze.

Performing the Skill (continued)

Step	Rationale
Measure the blood glucose: • The machine will count down the prescribed time and then display a result.	Familiarize yourself with what to expect from the blood glucose monitor at your agency (see Figure 4).

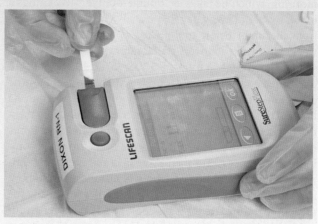

Figure 4

Step	Rationale
Discard the strip in a biohazard container. Discard the lancet in the sharps container.	Agency policy/universal precautions The strip and the lancet have blood on them.

Engaging in Evaluation

Step	Rationale
Compare the blood glucose reading with the normal blood glucose level. Check the puncture site.	To make sure that the bleeding has stopped

Documenting Effectively

Step	Rationale
Report abnormal results to the appropriate member of the health-care team. Record the blood glucose reading on the patient's chart according to agency policy.	Inform the nurse giving medications if this blood glucose reading is going to be used to give medication such as insulin. Documentation is the key communication among health-care professionals.

Critical Thinking Case Scenarios

▶ MB is a 19-year-old white female university nursing student who is health conscious and does not consume animal products. She is 1.63 metres (5 ft 4 in.) and weighs 46 kg (102 lb). Her diet includes tofu, legumes, soy milk, and fruits and vegetables. She eats organic grains with each meal. She does not take any herbal or vitamin/mineral supplements, and she is not on any medications. She does not smoke and abstains from consuming alcohol. Lately, MB has been feeling extra tired. For example, although in the past she usually walked an hour every day, she has not had the energy to do so in the last month. In fact, she has been experiencing shortness of breath walking up the three flights of stairs to her residence room. Her friends have told her that she is looking pale. In the morning while MB is putting on her make-up, she has noticed that her hair is not as shiny, and her gums are pale. MB is wondering why she is not feeling well and why her feeling of fatigue is getting progressively worse. MB has booked an appointment with the student health services nurse practitioner because she is worried something might be seriously wrong with her. If you were the nurse practitioner assessing MB, what would you look at to assist in determining her condition?

▶ RW is a 42-year-old male who has been married for 18 years and has two children ages 12 and 8 years. He works as an English teacher in a high school that is a 45-minute commute from where he lives. He works hard preparing lessons and grading as well as volunteering at the school and finds it very hard to find time for regular exercise. RW loves to cook and spends his weekends creating and cooking new recipes for his family to try. He has found that he has gained weight since the birth of his first child. His father died of a heart attack at age 47 years, and his two older brothers have had heart attacks. Everyone in his family has been diagnosed as having elevated cholesterol levels. RW is 1.8 metres (5 ft 11 in.) in height and weighs 114 kg (252 lb). When he first got married, he weighed 79 kg (178 lb). He does not eat breakfast as he does not have the time. At work, he drinks coffee throughout the morning, which he takes as "double-double." RW brings a lunch to school every day that usually consists of leftovers from the night before and a slice of bread. He brings in weekend dessert leftovers on Mondays and Tuesdays. His school lunch time is from 11:50 AM to 12:40 PM, and MB does not eat again until 8 PM because he volunteers for the chess and literature clubs after school before commuting home. His wife feeds the kids dinner early and takes them to after-school activities, and they usually don't get home until later evening. When RW comes home from his commute, he changes, and then takes his time preparing dinner for himself and his wife. He will taste test throughout the cooking process and has two glasses of wine during the meal preparation. He loves his cooking and feels very hungry by the time supper is ready. He loves creating sauces for his creative dishes. He likes adding all types of cheese for the flavor. He does not always have vegetables for supper. Most nights, he and his wife finish off their meal with a glass of Grand Marnier and a dish of pistachio ice cream. The serving sizes vary each meal depending on the type of meal prepared. Excessive amounts of each food item are common. RW has just gone in for his annual medical checkup. Predict what tests his primary health-care provider is likely to order and what recommendations RW is likely to receive.

▶ Mrs. W is a 75-year-old widowed woman living alone. She weighs 80 kg (175 lb) and is 1.55 metres (5 ft 1 in.) tall, and she has a long history of indigestion. She gets a stomachache after all meals, but it gets worse in the evening. To relieve her discomfort, Mrs. W self-medicates by taking a heavily advertised brand of over-the-counter chewable antacid after each meal and before going to bed at night. Mrs. W worked as a cook for her entire career and was in the habit of testing her food while cooking. She struggled financially all of her life. Mrs. W has gained weight steadily for the last several years with a recent gain after retirement and when her husband passed away 2 years ago. She recalls that her weight was 50 kg (110 lb) on her wedding day. When she retired at 66 years of age, she weighed 67 kg (148 lb), and now she weighs 79 kg (175 lb). She is lonely, and to keep busy, she cooks for her son and daughter-in-law's family 5 days a week. Lately, they have noticed that she is not able to modify recipes as well as in the past and is not balancing all the food groups each meal. Last night for supper, she served rice, potatoes, peas, bread, and butter. She suffers from arthritis and has been taking aspirin for the pain because she does not have any drug coverage. She takes ramipril for hypertension and is taking Lasix for her swollen feet. She has been suffering from chest pains and burning and decided that she needed to see a physician. She told her physician that the food was "coming back up." Her physician ordered several tests

that indicated that she had gastritis without ulceration and decreased esophageal motility with reflux esophagitis. She was advised to stop aspirin and the over-the-counter antacid. She was prescribed Zantac.

Multiple Choice Study Questions

1. How many categories do nutrients fall into?
   a. Two
   b. Three
   c. Four
   d. Six
   e. Eight

2. Which of the following foods has the greatest effect on lowering cholesterol?
   a. Apples
   b. Chicken
   c. Oat bran
   d. Celery
   e. None of the above

3. Vitamin D deficiency in adults is known as:
   a. Pellagra
   b. Sickle cell anemia
   c. Rickets
   d. Osteomalacia
   e. Beriberi

4. Which of the following decreases iron absorption?
   a. Tea
   b. Phytates
   c. Niacin
   d. Both a and b
   e. Both b and c

5. The percentage of calories from fat in the diet should be no more than _____ % with less than _____ % from saturated fat and less than _____ % from trans fat.
   a. 30, 1, 10
   b. 30, 10, 1
   c. 35, 1, 10
   d. 35, 10, 1
   e. 35, 10, 1

6. The absorption of this nutrient increases with aging:
   a. Riboflavin
   b. Vitamin D
   c. Vitamin A
   d. Thiamin
   e. Niacin

7. What vitamin is available in diets containing meat but not in plant-based diets?
   a. Vitamin A
   b. Vitamin D

c. Vitamin B_1

d. Vitamin B_{12}

e. Vitamin B_2

8. High levels of dietary fibre may protect the individual from:
   a. Colon cancer
   b. Rectal cancer
   c. Urinary tract infection
   d. Both a and b
   e. Both b and c

9. One teaspoon of salt is equal to _____ mg of sodium.
   a. 2,000
   b. 2,300
   c. 2,500
   d. 2,600

10. A BMI of 25.0 to 29.9 in an adult would indicate:
    a. Normal weight
    b. Overweight
    c. Underweight
    d. Obesity

Suggested Lab Activity

Vitamin and Mineral Test

● This test simulates stomach acidity.

Take white vinegar and water and mix it 50/50.

Put a small amount of the vinegar water solution in several glasses.

Add one vitamin supplement in each glass and set a timer for 30 minutes.

Some supplements will not break down at all which means that one may eventually find them whole in the stool!

REFERENCES AND SUGGESTED READINGS

Abbott Laboratories. (2008). *Determine you nutritional health checklist.* Retrieved from http://www.abbottnutrition.ca/static/cms_workplace/en_CA/content/document/ENS339A08.pdf

American Society of Parenteral and Enteral Nutrition. (2009). *Definition of terms.* Retrieved from http://www.nutritioncare.org/lcontent.aspx?id=546

Anderson, B. (2005). Nutrition and wound healing: The necessity of assessment. *British Journal of Nursing, 14*(19), S30, S32, S34.

Biology Online. (2010). *ATP.* Retrieved from http://www.biology-online.org/dictionary/Atp

Brown, P., & Phelps Maloy, J. (2005). *Quick reference to wound care.* Burlington, MA: Jones and Bartlett Learning.

Canadian Centre on Substance Abuse. (2013). *Canada's low-risk alcohol drinking guidelines.* Retrieved from http://www.ccsa.ca/2012%20CCSA%20Documents/2012-Canada-Low-Risk-Alcohol-Drinking-Guidelines-Brochure-en.pdf

Canadian Diabetes Association. (2008a). Canadian Diabetes Association 2008 clinical practice guidelines for the prevention and management of diabetes in Canada. *Canadian Journal of Diabetes, 32*(Suppl. 1). Retrieved from http://www.diabetes.ca/files/cpg2008/cpg-2008.pdf

Canadian Diabetes Association. (2008b). *The glycemic index.* Retrieved from http://www.diabetes.ca/files/GlycemicIndex_08.pdf

Canadian Diabetes Association. (2012a). *Beyond the basics.* Retrieved from http://www.diabetes.ca/for-professionals/resources/nutrition/beyond-basics/

Canadian Diabetes Association. (2012b). *Self-monitoring of blood glucose in people.* Retrieved from http://www.diabetes.ca/for-professionals/resources/self-monitoring-of-blood-glucose/

Canadian Food Inspection Agency. (2008). *Labelling of trans fatty acids.* Retrieved from http://www.inspection.gc.ca/english/fssa/labeti/inform/transe.shtml

d'Escrivan, T., & Guery, B. (2005). Prevention and treatment of aspiration pneumonia in intensive care units. *Treatments in Respiratory Medicine, 4*(5), 317–324.

Dietitians of Canada. (2009). *Dietary fat: The food, the bad and the ugly.* Retrieved from http://dietitians.ca/news/frm_resource/imageserver.asp?id=841&document_type=document&popup=true

Dietitians of Canada. (2011). *Eating guidelines for omega 3 fats.* Retrieved from: http://www.dietitians.ca/Nutrition-Resources-A-Z/Factsheets/Fats/Eating-Guidelines-for-Omega-3-Fats.aspx

Dietitians of Canada. (2012a). *Dietary fats.* Retrieved from http://www.dietitians.ca/Dietitians-Views/Dietary-Fats.aspx.

Dietitians of Canada. (2012b). *EATracker.* Retrieved from http://www.eatracker.ca/background.aspx

Dietitians of Canada. (2012c). *Healthy eating is in store for you.* Retrieved from http://www.healthyeatingisinstore.ca/

EatRight Ontario. (2011). *Facts on fats.* Retrieved from http://www.eatrightontario.ca/en/Articles/Heart-Health/Facts-on-Fats

EatRight Ontario. (2012a). *A healthy waist is good for your health.* Retrieved from http://www.eatrightontario.ca/en/Articles/Heart-Health/A-healthy-waist-is-good-for-your-health!.aspx

EatRight Ontario. (2012b). *Tips and facts: Tips on fats.* Retrieved from http://www.eatrightontario.ca/en/viewdocument.aspx?id=57

Egg Farmers of Canada. (2012). *FAQ: Fat.* Retrieved from http://www.eggs.ca/allabouteggs/FAQ_Fat.aspx

Exercise is Medicine. (2008). *Exercise is Medicine.* Retrieved from http://exerciseismedicine.org

Gorham, E. D., Garland, C. F., Garland, F. C., Grant, W. B., Mohr, S. B., Lipkin, M., . . . Holick, M. F. (2005). Vitamin D and prevention of colorectal cancer. *The Journal of Steroid Biochemistry and Molecular Biology, 97*(1–2), 179–194.

Health Canada. (2004). *Vitamin D supplementation for breast-fed infants—2004 Health Canada recommendation.* Retrieved from http://www.hc-sc.gc.ca/fn-an/nutrition/infant-nourisson/vita_d_supp-eng.php

Health Canada. (2007a). *Canada's food guide: Vitamin D for people over 50: Background.* Retrieved from http://www.hc-sc.gc.ca/fn-an/food-guide-aliment/context/vita_d-eng.php

Health Canada. (2007b). *Status of disease risk reduction claims in Canada.* Retrieved from http://www.hc-sc.gc.ca/fn-an/label-etiquet/claims-reclam/permitted_claims-allegations_autorisees-eng.php

Health Canada. (2008). *Trans fats: It's your health.* Retrieved from http://www.hc-sc.gc.ca/hl-vs/iyh-vsv/food-aliment/trans-eng.php

Health Canada. (2010a). *Clinical practice guidelines for nurses in primary care.* Retrieved from http://www.hc-sc.gc.ca/fniah-spnia/services/nurs-infirm/clini/index-eng.php

Health Canada. (2010b). *Dietary reference intakes tables.* Retrieved from http://www.hc-sc.gc.ca/fn-an/nutrition/reference/table/index-eng.php#eeer

Health Canada. (2010c). *Equations to estimate energy requirement.* Retrieved from http://www.hc-sc.gc.ca/fn-an/nutrition/reference/table/index-eng.php

Health Canada. (2010d). *Nutrition for healthy term infants: Recommendations from birth to six months.* Retrieved from http://www.hc-sc.gc.ca/fn-an/nutrition/infant-nourrisson/recom/index-eng.php#a6

Health Canada. (2010e). *Prenatal nutrition guidelines for health professionals—Background on Canada's food guide.* Retrieved from http://www.hc-sc.gc.ca/fn-an/pubs/nutrition/guide-prenatal-eng.php

Health Canada. (2010f). *Prenatal nutrition guidelines for health professionals—Folate contributes to a healthy pregnancy.* Retrieved from http://www.hc-sc.gc.ca/fn-an/pubs/nutrition/folate-eng.php

Health Canada. (2010g). *Vitamin D and calcium: Updated dietary reference intakes.* Retrieved from http://www.hc-sc.gc.ca/fn-an/nutrition/vitamin/vita-d-eng.php

Health Canada. (2011a). *Eating well with Canada's food guide.* Retrieved from http://www.hc-sc.gc.ca/fn-an/food-guide-aliment/index-eng.php

Health Canada. (2011b). *Extreme heat events guidelines: Technical guide for health care workers.* Retrieved from http://www.hc-sc.gc.ca/ewh-semt/pubs/climat/workers-guide-travailleurs/index-eng.php

Health Canada. (2011c). *Food and nutrition: Dietary reference intakes.* Retrieved from http://www.hc-sc.gc.ca/fn-an/nutrition/reference/index-eng.php

Health Canada. (2012a). *Body mass index (BMI) nomogram.* Retrieved from http://www.hc-sc.gc.ca/fn-an/nutrition/weights-poids/guide-ld-adult/bmi_chart_java-graph_imc_java-eng.php

Health Canada. (2012b). *Food and nutrition: Consultation—Nutrition for healthy term infants: Recommendations from birth to six months—DRAFT.* Retrieved from http://www.hc-sc.gc.ca/fn-an/consult/infant-nourrisson/recommendations/index-eng.php

Health Canada. (2013). *Prenatal nutrition guidelines for health professionals—Folate contributes to a healthy pregnancy.* Retrieved from http://www.hc-sc.gc.ca/fn-an/pubs/nutrition/folate-eng.php

Health Canada. (n.d.). *Nutrition for healthy term infants—Statement of the joint working group: Canadian Paediatric Society, Dietitians of Canada and Health Canada.* Retrieved from http://www.hc-sc.gc.ca/fn-an/pubs/infant-nourrisson/nut_infant_nourrisson_term-eng.php

Heart and Stroke Foundation. (2010). *Eliminating trans fats.* Retrieved from http://www.heartandstroke.com/site/c.ikIQLcMWJtE/b.3479251/k.5271/Eliminating_trans_fat.htm

Heart and Stroke Foundation. (2011). *Dietary fats, oils and cholesterol.* Retrieved from http://www.heartandstroke.on.ca/site/c.pvI3IeNWJwE/b.3581947/k.D7AE/Healthy_Living__Dietary_fats_oils_and__cholesterol.htm

Heart and Stroke Foundation. (2012). *Health check—Nutrition facts table.* Retrieved from http://www.heartandstroke.com/site/pp.aspx?c=ikIQLcMWJtE&b=4391511&printmode=1

Heart and Stroke Foundation of Canada. (2009). *Healthy waists.* Retrieved from http://www.heartandstroke.com/site/c.ikIQLcMWJtE/b.3876195/

Hernandez, J. A., Torres, N. P., & Jimenez, A. M. (2006). Clinical use of enteral nutrition. *Nutrición Hospitalaria, 21*(Suppl. 2), 85–87.

Houghton, L. A., & Vieth, R. (2006). The case against ergocalciferol (vitamin D2) as a vitamin supplement. *The American Journal of Clinical Nutrition, 84,* 694–697.

Kalergis, M., De Grandpre, E., & Andersons, E. (2005). The role of the glycemic index in the prevention and management of diabetes: A review and discussion. *Canadian Journal of Diabetes, 29*(1), 27–38.

Mahan, L. K., & Escott-Stump, S. (2008). *Krause's food & nutrition therapy* (12th ed.). Philadelphia, PA: Saunders.

Matthews, S. B., Waud, J. P., Roberts, A. G., & Campbell, A. K. (2005). Systemic lactose intolerance: A new perspective on an old problem. *Postgraduate Medical Journal, 81,* 167–173.

Melina, V., & Davis, B. (2003). *The new becoming vegetarian: The essential guide to a healthy vegetarian diet* (2nd ed.). Summertown, TN: Book Publishing Company.

National Cancer Institute. (2012). *NCI dictionary of cancer terms: Gluconeogenesis.* Retrieved from http://www.cancer.gov/dictionary?cdrid=44111

National Heart Lung and Blood Institute. (2006). *Your guide to lowering your blood pressure with DASH.* Retrieved from http://www.nhlbi.nih.gov/health/public/heart/hbp/dash/new_dash.pdf

National Institute for Health and Clinical Excellence. (2006). *Nutrition support in Adults: Oral nutrition support, enteral tube feeding and parenteral nutrition.* Retrieved from http://www.nice.org.uk/guidance/index.jsp?action=byID&r=true&o=10978

Negoianu, D., & Goldfarb, S. (2008). Just add water. *Journal of the American Society of Nephrology, 19*(6), 1041–1043.

Nieves, J. W. (2005). "Osteoporosis: The role of micronutrients." *American Journal of Clinical Nutrition, 81*(5), 1232S–1239S.

Public Health Agency of Canada. (2011). *Physical activity guide.* Retrieved from http://www.phac-aspc.gc.ca/hp-ps/hl-mvs/pa-ap/index-eng.php

Raghuwanshi, A., Joshi, S. S., & Christakos, S. (2008). Vitamin D and multiple sclerosis. *Journal of Cell Biochemistry, 105*(2), 338–343.

Sanders, M. E. (2008). Use of probiotics and yogurts in maintenance of health. *Journal of Clinical Gastroenterology, 42*(S2), S71–S74.

Soeters, P. B., & Schols, A. M. (2009). Advances in understanding and assessing malnutrition. *Current Opinion in Clinical Nutrition & Metabolic Care, 12*(5), 487–494.

Soini, H., Routasalo, P., & Lagström, H. (2004). Characteristics of the mini-nutritional assessment in elderly home-care patients. *European Journal of Clinical Nutrition, 58*(1), 64–70.

The Engineering Toolbox. (n.d.). *Units of heat—BTU, calorie and joule.* Retrieved from http://www.engineeringtoolbox.com/heat-units-d_664.html

Weight-control Information Network. (2012). *Overweight and obesity statistics.* Retrieved from http://www.win.niddk.nih.gov/statistics/

World Gastroenterology Organisation. (2008). *Probiotics and prebiotics.* Retrieved from http://www.worldgastroenterology.org/assets/downloads/en/pdf/guidelines/19_probiotics_prebiotics.pdf

Supporting Elimination

AMANDA MCEWEN, SARAH LOPEZ, AND
LINDA PATRICK

Jaswinder is beginning the second semester of her first year in a Bachelor of Science in Nursing program in Southwestern Ontario. Her upcoming clinical rotation is at a senior's residence and she is concerned about some of the things she has been teased about by her friends who are not in nursing. Specifically, she is thinking about assisting people with their bowel and bladder needs and especially how she will react to smells. What if she makes the person she is trying to help feel badly about needing a bedpan, or may need to change adult diapers? She wonders how nurses do this work and how she should prepare for her clinical day.

CHAPTER OBJECTIVES

By the end of this chapter, you will be able to:

1. Describe the structure and function of both urinary elimination and bowel elimination.
2. Apply knowledge of anatomy and physiology to assessment and care of patients with alterations in bladder and bowel elimination.
3. Identify common factors that influence elimination patterns including lifespan considerations.
4. Explain the most common alterations in both urinary and bladder elimination.
5. Discuss common diagnostic tests for both urinary and bowel elimination.
6. Promote bowel and bladder health through effective health teaching.
7. Explore risk factors for developing altered urinary and bowel function with patients during health teaching.
8. Use strategies to promote comfort and decrease patient stress during assessment of urinary and bowel functions.

KEY TERMS

Constipation Bowel movements are irregular with feces that may be hard and painful to pass.

Defecation Evacuation or removal of feces from the body through the anus.

Dialysis A process that removes waste and excess fluid from the blood. It is a substitute for people with impaired kidney function (renal failure). The two main types are hemodialysis and peritoneal dialysis.

Diuresis Excessive urine production.

Diuretic Refers to any substance that promotes the production of urine.

Dysuria Difficult urination.

Enuresis The passing of urine while sleeping; often referred to as *bed-wetting*.

Fecal Impaction Hardened and dry feces in the folds of the rectum, resulting from prolonged retention and accumulation of fecal material.

Feces The waste products produced and eliminated from the digestive tract. May also be referred to as *stool*.

Hematuria Blood in the urine.

Hemorrhoids Enlarged and distended veins in the rectum that can be internal or may protrude outside the anus.

Hydronephrosis Water in the kidneys/distention of the kidney pelvis.

Kock Pouch (pronounced "coke") A continent ileal bladder conduit. A portion of ileum is used to form a urine reservoir. Patients can control the passage of urine using intermittent catheterization of this internal reservoir.

Micturition Another term for urination.

Meatus A term used to describe an opening or a natural body passage.

Neurogenic Bladder Absence of bladder control due to a condition that may occur with the brain, the spinal cord, or a nerve condition.

Nocturia Waking up to empty the bladder at night, interrupting sleep patterns.

Occult (Hidden) Blood Blood that is only detected by microscopic examination. A fecal occult blood test looks for blood in feces.

Oliguria Decreased production and elimination of urine.

(continued on page 910)

Peristalsis   A series of muscle contractions that occur in the digestive tract to move gastric contents through to elimination. Peristaltic muscle contractions also move urine from the kidneys into the bladder.

Pyuria   The presence of pus in the urine. Pus is made up of white blood cells and most often indicates the presence of infection.

Reflux   Backflow of urine. Urine moves up the ureters toward the kidney instead of moving down the ureters into the bladder.

Stoma   An opening that is surgically created to reroute a body pathway to the outside of the body.

Urinary Diversion   A surgically created alternate route for urine flow. A nephrostomy refers to urine that is diverted through a surgically created alternate route from the kidney to a stoma.

Urinary Tract Infection (UTI)   An infection in any part of the urinary system (kidneys, ureters, bladder, and urethra). Most infections involve the lower urinary tract—the bladder and the urethra.

Valsalva maneuver   a voluntary contraction of abdominal muscles while holding one's breath causing an increase in intra-abdominal pressure.

Eliminating urine from the bladder and **feces** from the rectum is something you have done every day since birth, but you may not have thought about either in the way that you now need to do as part of your nursing studies. The following section provides a brief overview of elimination processes, and your learning will be enhanced if you refer to anatomy and physiology and health assessment textbooks as resources. We will begin by reviewing urinary function and the organs involved in this process.

Anatomy and Physiology of the Urinary System

In order to eliminate urine, our bodies depend on the function of the kidneys, ureters, bladder, and urethra. Kidneys perform the job of removing waste products from the blood, forming urine. Ureters transport urine from the kidneys to the bladder, where it is contained until you feel the urge to urinate, typically when the bladder is becoming full. The urine leaves the body through the urethra. In order for this process to successfully occur, all organs must be intact and functioning properly. As we take a closer look at each organ involved, this chapter will provide an overview of the urinary and digestive tracts but cannot replace the depth and breadth of knowledge contained in your science textbooks.

Kidneys

There are two kidneys in the body, located between the level of the 12th (last) thoracic vertebra and just above the 3rd lumbar vertebra, on the posterior abdominal wall, one on each side of the vertebral column. Each kidney is encased in a fibrous capsule and cushioned with fat (adipose tissue). As we briefly discuss each of these structures, keep in mind that fluid is filtered in order and refer often to the structures of the urinary system shown in Figure 35.1.

Waste is produced as a by-product of metabolism and collected in the blood for transport to each kidney by a renal (kidney) artery branching from the abdominal aorta. Approximately one fifth (about 1,200 ml) of the body's cardiac output circulates through the kidneys every minute (Patton & Thibodeau, 2010). The nephron is the functional unit of the kidney. Each kidney has more than 1 million nephrons and each nephron consists of two main sections: the renal corpuscle and the renal tubule. Within each nephron (see Fig. 35.2),

three mechanisms work together to process blood plasma and form urine: filtration, tubular reabsorption, and tubular secretion. The renal corpuscle makes up the first area of the nephron and includes Bowman capsule. Bowman capsule (see Fig 35.3) surrounds a group of small blood vessels (capillaries) called the *glomerulus*. Bowman capsule is where urine formation and filtration of blood starts. Because the capillaries of the glomerulus are porous, they permit filtration of water, glucose, urea, creatinine, and other components in the blood into the Bowman capsule. This fluid is called the *glomerular filtrate*. Proteins and red blood cells, however, are too large to be filtered and stay in the capillary. As a result, if large proteins are detected in the urine (proteinuria), it is a sign of glomerular injury.

Next, from Bowman capsule, the glomerular filtrate enters the renal tubule. The renal tubule consists of the proximal convoluted tubule, loop of Henle, and distal convoluted tubule. The collecting duct is made up of the renal tubules of several nephrons. Approximately 65% of the reabsorption and secretion occurring in the tubular system occurs in the proximal tubule (Porth & Pooler, 2010). Substances vital for nutrition (including lactate, amino acids, glucose, and water-soluble vitamins) are almost completely reabsorbed here, whereas electrolytes (sodium, chloride, potassium, etc.) and bicarbonate are 65% to 90% reabsorbed. As this process occurs, a concentration gradient is created, allowing for the osmotic reabsorption of water and urea. Besides reabsorption, cells in the proximal tubule secrete organic cations and anions (including the end products of metabolism, such as urate).

The loop of Henle is involved with controlling the concentration of urine and is divided into three portions: (1) thin descending, (2) thin ascending, and (3) thick ascending. The thin descending segment is highly permeable to water, and water flows out of the urine filtrate as it moves down the segment. Conversely, the ascending limb is impermeable to water. So, as solutes are reabsorbed (and water is unable to follow and remains in the filtrate), the tubular filtrate becomes more dilute. This allows free water to be excreted from the body. The thick portion of the loop of Henle is also impermeable to water and contains a sodium-potassium-chloride cotransport system. Approximately one quarter of the filtered load of sodium, potassium, and chloride gets reabsorbed in this segment, resulting in the passive reabsorption of calcium and magnesium (Porth & Pooler, 2010). This is the site of action for the loop diuretics, such as furosemide (Lasix). In the tubules, other substances (ammonia, creatinine, uric acid, and other metabolites) are secreted into the filtrate to rid them from the body.

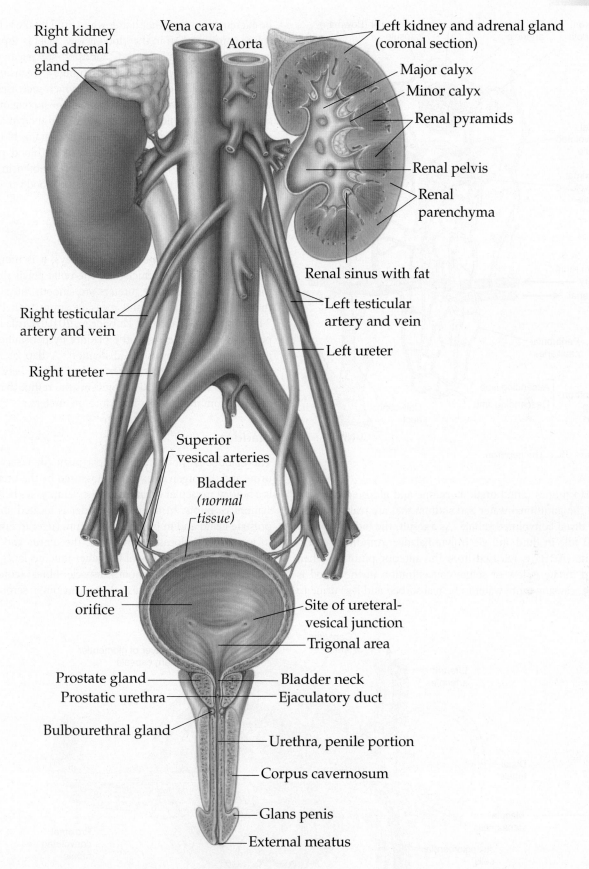

Kidneys and Urinary Tract

Figure 35.1 Urinary tract.

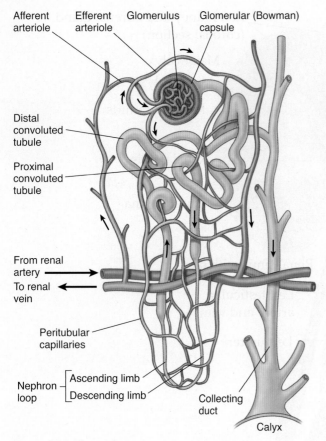

Afferent arteriole

Efferent arteriole

Glomerulus

Glomerular (Bowman) capsule

Distal convoluted tubule

Proximal convoluted tubule

From renal artery

To renal vein

Peritubular capillaries

Nephron loop [Ascending limb / Descending limb]

Collecting duct

Calyx

Figure 35.2 The nephron.

be excreted. On the other hand, when fluid intake is high, or solute concentration in the blood is low, ADH is suppressed and more urine is excreted. Aldosterone, released from the adrenal cortex, also affects the tubule by causing more sodium and water to be reabsorbed, which increases blood volume and decreases urine output. The juxtaglomerular apparatus (or complex) (located where the afferent arteriole passes by the distal convoluted tubule) maintains blood flow by secreting an enzyme called *renin* when blood pressure drops. Renin triggers the production of angiotensin, which causes vasoconstriction (narrowing of the blood vessels) and results in the blood pressure rising.

Ureters

Once the urine is formed in the kidneys, it is transported through the collecting ducts into the renal pelvis then into the ureters. In the adult, ureters are smooth muscle tubes that act as passageways and measure approximately 28 to 34 cm in length (Patton & Thibodeau, 2010). Urine is transported from the ureters to the bladder by peristaltic movements stimulated by urine distention. A flap of mucous membrane acts as a valve, covering the juncture between the ureters and the bladder. This prevents the **reflux** (backflow) of urine from the bladder back into the ureters.

Bladder

The bladder is the storage compartment (or reservoir) for urine and the organ of excretion (assisted by the urethra). It is a hollow, muscular organ that, when empty, lies behind the symphysis pubis. In men, the bladder is located above the prostate gland and in front of the rectum (refer to Fig. 35.1). In women, it is located in front of the uterus and vagina. The bladder wall consists of the inner mucous layer, a layer of connective tissue, smooth muscle fibres (collectively known as the *detrusor muscle*), and an outer serous layer.

Hormones (antidiuretic hormone and aldosterone) control the additional water and sodium that are reabsorbed in the distal convoluted tubule. As a result, the kidneys play a vital role in fluid and electrolyte balance. Antidiuretic hormone (ADH) is released from the anterior pituitary when fluid intake is low or solute concentration in the blood is high, causing more water to be reabsorbed and less urine to

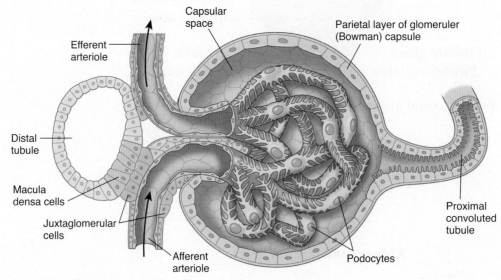

Efferent arteriole

Capsular space

Parietal layer of glomeruler (Bowman) capsule

Distal tubule

Macula densa cells

Juxtaglomerular cells

Afferent arteriole

Podocytes

Proximal convoluted tubule

Figure 35.3 The Bowman capsule.

As the bladder fills with urine, the detrusor muscle allows it to expand and contract during voiding (releasing urine outside the body). The bladder is capable of significant distention and normally holds approximately 500 ml of urine. At the base of the bladder, a triangular area called the *trigone* contains an opening at each of its three angles. Two are for the ureters, whereas one is for the urethra. The internal urethral sphincter is located at the base of the bladder where it connects with the urethra. The sphincter is under voluntary control and prevents the escape of urine from the bladder.

Urethra

Urine passes from the bladder through the urethra to the urinary **meatus** (opening) and outside the body (referred to as *voiding*, *urination*, or **micturition**). Bacteria are washed through the urethra by the turbulent flow of urine, preventing infection. Women, however, are more prone to bacterial infections of the bladder due to the urethra being short, along with the close proximity of the urinary meatus (located between the labia minora, above the vagina, and below the clitoris) to the vagina and anus. In men, the urethra is longer (about 20 cm) and serves as a passageway for both urine and semen. The urinary meatus is located at the distal end or tip of the penis.

The mechanism for voiding starts with involuntary contractions of the detrusor muscle in bladder wall. As the volume of urine increases, the pressure of urine against the inside of the bladder increases and these involuntary contractions develop and strengthen (by a parasympathetic reflex). At the same time, this reflex results in relaxation of the internal urethral sphincter muscles. Together, this can force urine out of the bladder and through the urethra. Urine can flow from the bladder when the external sphincter relaxes. This voluntary control of urination requires the proper functioning of the nerves supplying the pelvic floor, the projection tracts of the central nervous system (CNS), and motor areas of the brain (Patton & Thibodeau, 2010). The pelvic floor muscles support the pelvic organs or the uterus (in women), the bladder, the small intestine, and the rectum.

Urinary Function

It takes a coordinated effort between your brain, bladder, and urethra to release urine from your bladder in a controlled manner. This is a learned skill that cannot occur until the human body is physically, emotionally, and mentally ready. Most people learn to consciously control contraction of the external urethral sphincter muscle to prevent voiding until a suitable time. A child between the ages of 2 and 5 years must be able to recognize the urge to void, control the urge until he or she is in a bathroom, and physically be able to sit on a toilet and then release urine.

In an adult, the bladder may be able to hold up to 500 ml of urine at one time and may need to void five to seven times per day. This depends on fluid intake and on the types of fluids consumed. Typically, once the bladder fills to approximately 250 to 400 ml of urine, signals in the sensory impulses are sent to the sacral spinal cord that are relayed to the pontine micturition centre. If the time and place are appropriate, the impulses are sent back to begin detrusor muscle contraction and urethral sphincter relaxation and the bladder empties. On other occasions, when the time and place are not appropriate, the person suppresses the urge or voluntarily inhibits detrusor contraction. Repeated ignoring of the urge to urinate can increase the pressure so much that the bladder reaches capacity and the sphincter muscle releases regardless.

On the other hand, stressful situations can cause a strong urge to urinate. People can suppress urination (voluntarily) due to perceived time constraints. For instance, nurses often ignore the urge to urinate until they are able to take a break. This can increase the person's risk of a urinary tract infection.

Factors Affecting Voiding

Many factors affect the volume and characteristics of urine production. Factors affecting urination include disease processes, medications, and surgical procedures that interfere with healthy urinary function. An alteration in urinary function can create considerable emotional stress for the patient; therefore, the nurse should be vigilant with assessment skills and prepared to incorporate knowledge of the factors that influence urination into patient teaching.

Developmental Factors

The normal ranges for daily urine output change as we develop and grow from infancy to adulthood and old age. The normal expected range for daily urine output for infants is between 500 and 600 ml; for toddlers, it is between 500 and 800 ml per day; and by school age, children void between 600 and 1,200 ml per day. Older children reach adult capacity of 1,500 ml per day by the age of 14 years. Newborns void as many as 30 to 40 times a day, but small amounts of about 15 to 30 ml at a time. Refer to Table 35.1 for more details about lifespan considerations.

Nutrition and Fluid Intake

The optimal daily amount of fluid intake is between 1,500 and 2,000 ml. The amount of fluid required by the body will fluctuate with excessive loss of body fluids during activity, a fever, or from perspiration. The preferred fluid to drink is water, which helps to flush out the microorganisms that can cause infection or renal calculi (stone) formation. Muscle tone of the urinary tract including the bladder and ureters is further promoted with fluid distending and stretching the muscle. Excessive amounts of caffeine (found in cola,

TABLE 35.1	Lifespan Considerations for Urinary Elimination			
	Newborn and Infant	Toddler and Preschooler	School-Age Child and Adolescent	Adult and Older Adult
Normal daily ranges for urine output	500–600 ml	500–800 ml	Increases from 1,000 to 1,500 ml a day as the child grows and matures	1,500 ml per day
Developmental Considerations for Urinary Function				
Urinary function	Unable to control urine release; lack voluntary control. Frequent small voiding. UTIs are more frequent in female infants than male infants. Congenital malformations of the urinary tract or nervous system may interfere with normal urine elimination.	Voluntary urinary continence is usually achieved between 2.5 and 3 years. Perception of a full bladder is possible and the child is able to verbalize the need to urinate. Also requires physical maturity and fine motor control to remove clothing and to be able to sit on the toilet or potty chair	Urinary elimination patterns include the ability to control urinary function both during the day and night. Some school-age children may experience the involuntary release of urine when they are sleeping. This is called **enuresis**.	The aging process of the cardiovascular system decreases the efficiency of the kidney. Voiding during the night (nocturia) especially in males with an enlarged prostate. Women may experience similar problems of frequent urination due to weakening of the pelvic muscles.

For more information on bed-wetting, visit http://emedicine.medscape.com/article/1014762-overview

tea, and coffee) can stimulate the production of urine and contribute to dehydration. Glucose found in fruit juices and sodium found in carbonated beverages (soda) should be limited as they contribute to urinary changes when consumed in excessive amounts.

Urinary elimination can be affected by diet. With the consumption of foods with a high water content (e.g., fruits, Jello, vegetables, soup), the volume of urine will be greater than if intake of these foods is limited. When ingesting large quantities of salty foods without also increasing water intake, urine will be concentrated, as output will decrease (fluid retention) to maintain the normal concentration of electrolytes. Conversely, consuming large quantities of foods with caffeine (a **diuretic**), may increase urine output. Several factors influence the effects of caffeine on individuals. Some individuals can be more sensitive to the diuretic effects of caffeine, whereas others may build up a tolerance to caffeine and experience minimal or no diuretic effects. This is an important consideration for patients who are experiencing challenges with urinary elimination. Alcohol will increase urine output because it inhibits the production of ADH.

Medications

Urine production may be altered by certain medications. Medications classified as diuretics (sometimes called *water pills*) are used to increase urine output (**diuresis**). Some commonly used diuretics include hydrochlorothiazide,

furosemide, and spironolactone. They each work in a slightly different way, but overall, they lower salt and water in the body, treating edema and lowering blood pressure. Conversely, some medications used to treat other health problems cause urinary retention as a side effect. These include medications with anticholinergic effects, antihistamines, and tricyclic antidepressants. Narcotics can lower the glomerular filtration rate and interfere with the sensation of bladder fullness.

Undergoing Diagnostic Examination and Surgery

Preparation for diagnostic testing and surgery may include fluid restriction, which commonly lowers urine output by decreasing production. Volume depletion can also be caused by blood and fluid loss during surgery. Patients should be able to void within 10 hours after surgery, but there are many other ways that surgery affects this. Spinal anaesthetics can decrease a person's awareness of the need to void and impair the sensory and motor impulses controlling micturition. As a result, the patient will be unable to initiate voiding until after the anaesthesia has worn off. ADH may be released with the stress of surgery, causing decreased urinary output. Being unable to stand up postoperatively and relying on using a bedpan or urinal while supine interferes with normal urinary patterns. Various medications cause urinary retention. Surgery that involves the urinary system, reproductive organs, or intestines can predispose a patient to urinary retention. Trauma to the affected tissues causes edema, which may obstruct urine flow. As a result, any surgery on the urinary tract should involve use of a retention catheter.

Psychological and Psychosocial Factors Affecting Urination

Urinary elimination is typically voluntary. As a result, voiding can be affected by simply thinking about it. If you hear someone talking about needing to void, you may also feel this need; if you hear running water, the feeling may be more intense. In addition, certain conditions (such as position, privacy, and sufficient time) can also stimulate the micturition reflex. Pouring warm water over a patient's inner thigh or perineal area may stimulate voiding, whereas positioning him or her on a cold bedpan may temporarily impede voiding. When a person is anxious (including situations with inadequate privacy or a sense of insufficient time) and cannot relax the abdominal and perineal muscles and external urethral sphincter, then voiding is inhibited. In particular, women have culturally been taught to require more privacy for urinating. Women's public restrooms always have private stalls, but men's public restrooms have open rows of urinals for urinating and fewer available private stalls. People have different personal needs for privacy while voiding. Refer to Skill 35.1, "Assisting the Patient Using a Bedpan."

Putting patients on and off a bedpan requires the mastery of skills to prevent injury (yours and theirs) and promote comfort while respecting privacy. Before going into the clinical setting for the first time, Jaswinder had the opportunity to learn and to practice techniques for safely toileting patients in the clinical skills lab. Practicing these new skills on a peer or a mannequin was not only beneficial for Jaswinder's future patients but also increased both her competence and her self-confidence.

Through the eyes of a nurse

It doesn't take years of practice to notice that patients may be embarrassed to void into a urinal or a bedpan. I advise nursing students to be extra attentive to providing them with privacy and respect and plenty of time in which to try to relax. Pulling the curtains around their bed and closing the door to their room will help put them at ease.

(personal reflection of a nurse)

Body Fluid Loss

The body compensates for the loss of body fluids that can occur with diarrhea, vomiting, excessive diaphoresis (caused by exercise or fever), excess drainage from wound(s), extensive burns, or loss of blood during surgery or from trauma. The kidneys compensate by increasing water reabsorption from the glomerular filtrate to maintain the correct osmolarity (concentration of solutes) of the extracellular fluid (ECF), resulting in decreased urine output. If urine output falls to less than 30 ml/hour, decreased blood flow to the kidneys and other vital organs must be suspected and reported to the physician.

Muscle Tone

Poor abdominal and pelvic floor muscle tone can impair bladder contraction and external urethral sphincter control. This can be caused by prolonged immobility, obesity, stretching of muscles during childbirth, multiple pregnancies, muscle atrophy from menopause (decreased estrogen), chronic constipation, and trauma causing muscle damage. Use of an indwelling urinary catheter causes loss of bladder tone (because it continuously empties the bladder) and can damage urethral sphincters. As a result, when a catheter is removed, the patient may have trouble regaining control of voiding.

Pathological Conditions

Illnesses or health alterations can affect urine formation and excretion. Conditions affecting the kidneys can impede the ability of the nephrons to make urine. Elevated amounts of blood cells or protein can be present in the urine. In renal failure, the kidneys can stop producing urine or produce very little. Heart failure, shock, and hypertension can all affect blood flow to the kidneys, which then limits urine production.

Altered Urinary Function

Urinary function can be impacted by multiple factors; some may be temporary such as not drinking enough fluids causing mild dehydration, but other factors can be of longer duration and may require interventions to correct or manage. Refer to Table 35.2, "Altered Urinary Production and Elimination."

Neurogenic Bladder

Impaired neurological function, including neurological injury after a spinal cord injury or stroke, can interfere with urinary elimination. In a **neurogenic bladder**, the patient cannot tell when the bladder is full and lacks urinary sphincter control. Trauma, hemorrhage, or a tumour affecting the frontal lobes of the brain, the area of the brain that controls voluntary voiding, can lead to incontinence. If injury occurs to the spinal cord at or above the sacral region, the micturition reflex and control of urination will

TABLE 35.2	Altered Urinary Production and Elimination	
Term	**Definition**	**Altered Function and Symptoms**
Dysuria	Pain when voiding	The pain may feel like a burning or stinging sensation. The pain can be caused by inflammation of the bladder or urethra caused by infection or trauma.
Urgency	The feeling associated with having to empty your bladder immediately	Inflammation or infection can create the feeling of impending micturition or the involuntary release or urine. Psychological distress can also cause this reaction.
Frequency	Voiding more often than normal and not related to increased fluid intake	Associated with bladder infections or pressure on the bladder from pregnancy. Patients with a bladder infection will most often complain of both urgency and frequency.
Nocturia	Waking up from sleeping to urinate	Causes can include increased fluid intake, drinking alcohol, increased caffeine intake, and not voiding prior to bedtime. Pregnancy in women and an enlarged prostate in men can cause sleep to be interrupted by the need to void.
Polyuria	An increase in urine production and elimination not associated with taking in increased fluids	The amount of urine produced to be considered polyuria is output greater than 2,500–3,000 ml in a 24-hour period. Medications, caffeine, and alcohol can cause polyuria, as well as medical conditions; that is, diabetes insipidus and diabetes mellitus.
Oliguria	Decreased production of urine	Output of less than 500 ml in 24 hours. Decreased production of urine can be caused by not taking in enough fluid, but also the loss of bodily fluids from hemorrhage, diarrhea, burns, excessive vomiting, and sweating (diaphoresis).
Pyuria	Pus in the urine	Pus is formed by the end products of the body's response to inflammation. The urine will appear cloudy and often will have a strong unpleasant odor. Patients with UTIs will have pyuria caused by the presence of microorganisms and white blood cells in their urine.
Hematuria	Blood in the urine	Very worrisome to patients who may see blood (called gross) in their urine. Blood that cannot be seen visibly is called occult blood and requires microscopic examination to be seen. Causes of hematuria may include trauma, infection, tumours, and surgery.

be affected. Reflex voiding (reflex neurogenic bladder) may result, which means that as soon as the bladder is stretched to a certain level, it will contract without the patient's control, and urine will be lost (urinary incontinence). See Table 35.3 for a summary of the different types of urinary incontinence.

Obstructions

Some conditions can obstruct urine flow from the kidneys to the urethra. Urinary stone(s) can block a ureter and restrict urine flow from the kidney to the bladder. Prostate enlargement, which commonly affects older men, can partially compress or block the urethra, which makes it more difficult to void and empty the bladder. Structural abnormalities in the urinary tract and tumours are other possible causes of urinary obstruction. Urinary catheters or tubes inserted to help drain urine can become kinked or plugged and block urine flow. **Hydronephrosis** is a complication of urinary obstruction. It occurs due to the increased resistance that a block in normal urine flow causes. If untreated, this can cause atrophy and necrosis (death) of renal cells and could result in permanent kidney damage.

Renal Therapy

In the event of permanent renal damage and the death of renal cells, it may be necessary for patients to undergo **dialysis** either temporarily for acute renal failure or for chronic renal failure they may require regular peritoneal or hemodialysis. See Table 35.4 for more details.

Urinary Tract Infections

Urinary tract infections (UTIs) are often caused by microorganisms normally found in the gastrointestinal (GI) tract. This includes the Enterobacteriaceae group of bacteria (*Escherichia coli*, *Proteus*, *Klebsiella*, etc.). Because these microorganisms usually gain access to the urinary system through the urethral meatus, infections of the lower urinary tract are most common (including urethritis [infection of the urethra] and cystitis [infection of the bladder]). Upper UTIs are less common and include infections of the ureters (ureteritis) and the kidney pelvis or tubule system. Because kidney damage and renal failure may occur, upper UTIs are more serious than lower UTIs.

Except at the urethral meatus, the urinary tract is sterile. In the healthy person, voiding tends to flush away bacteria. Infection results when microorganisms from the perineal skin or anus enter the urethra through the urinary meatus. Women are more susceptible to lower UTIs due to the short length of the female urethral meatus and the close proximity of the vagina and anus to the urinary meatus. Prostatic secretions that have antibacterial properties and a longer urethra mean men are less likely to get lower UTIs.

TABLE 35.3	Types of Urinary Incontinence	
Type	**Description**	**Symptoms and Causes**
Functional	Unpredictable and involuntary loss of urine, yet patient has an intact urinary and nervous system	Patient has the urge to void but is unable to reach the bathroom before having a loss of urine. The patient with cognitive deficits may have forgotten what to do. Caused by a change in environment: cognitive, sensory, or motor deficits (e.g., severe arthritis; Alzheimer disease; Parkinson disease; and in the hospital setting, side rails up and call bell out of reach can contribute to functional incontinence)
Overflow	Voluntary or involuntary loss of a small amount of urine that occurs when a person cannot fully empty the bladder. This causes overflow, which can leak out unexpectedly. The person may or may not sense his or her full bladder.	Symptoms can vary from dribbling a few drops of urine to loss of larger amounts with frequency and urgency. Causes include enlarged prostate (in men), blockages of the urethra (from tumours, scar tissue, urinary stones, or swelling from infection), injury to nerves that affect the bladder, medications (including some anticonvulsants and antidepressants), and nerve damage (from diabetes, alcoholism, multiple sclerosis, Parkinson disease, or spina bifida)
Reflex	Involuntary loss of a small or large volume of urine that happens when a specific bladder volume is reached (at somewhat predictable intervals). The person is unable to sense the bladder is full and empties when a certain degree of stretch has occurred.	No awareness of filling bladder, no urge to void, and bladder spasm contraction inhibited Seen in patients with neurological impairment, such as stroke, brain tumour, or spinal cord lesion
Stress	Sudden and involuntary loss of small amounts of urine (less than 50 ml) that occurs during a sudden increase in intra-abdominal pressure	Urinary frequency and urgency; urine loss with increased intra-abdominal pressure Activities that increase intra-abdominal pressure include sneezing, laughing, coughing, lifting, and jumping. Other associated factors include weak pelvic floor muscles (caused by stretching that occurs with childbirth), damage to the bladder neck, obesity, full uterus in third trimester, postmenopausal low estrogen levels, and side effects of medications.
Urge	Strong sense of urgency to void followed by involuntary loss of urine	Urinary urgency, frequency, nocturia, dysuria, and bladder spasms or contractions are often associated. Some patients may experience temporary urge incontinence after removal of an indwelling catheter. Other associated causes include UTIs, stroke, Parkinson disease, Alzheimer disease, bladder irritants, injury, or nervous system damage (such as experienced with multiple sclerosis). Without a known cause, urge incontinence is also referred to as *overactive bladder*.
Total	Involuntary, continuous, and unpredictable urine loss from a nondistended bladder	Sometimes designated when the observed incontinence does not fit other categories Associated factors include a neurological lesion in the brain or spinal cord, injury to the genitourinary area or spinal cord from surgery or trauma, and congenital malformation of the urinary tract or spinal cord.
Mixed	The person experiences the symptoms of more than one type of urinary incontinence, such as stress plus urge incontinence.	

A person's risk for UTIs increases with improper wiping after a bowel movement and after sexual intercourse (which brings microorganisms in contact with the urinary meatus). Refer to Box 35.1 for more health teaching tips to prevent UTIs.

Any diagnostic or therapeutic intervention that places an object in the urethra or bladder, including urinary catheterization, also increases the incidence of UTIs. The biggest factor contributing to the risk of developing a catheter-associated urinary tract infection (CAUTI) is the length of time the catheter remains in situ (Bernard, Hunter, & Moore, 2012). To reduce this risk, nurses must always critically think about the indicated need for catheterization and the length of their use when initiating and maintaining a catheter. If the catheter is no longer needed, advocate on behalf of the patient to the physician to obtain an order for removal (Bernar et al., 2012). Refer to the following research box about the effectiveness of using ultrasound bladder scanners to reduce UTIs.

Think Should an indwelling catheter be left in place for the convenience of not having to get a patient up to void? Should catheters inserted to collect urine samples in the emergency department be removed immediately after obtaining the sample? On the other hand, if the catheter is left in place until further orders are received from the physician, it could save the patient unnecessary stress and discomfort from another catheter insertion.

TABLE 35.4   Renal Replacement Therapies

There are several life-threatening situations that require renal replacement strategies. These situations may be caused by renal failure, end-stage renal disease, or severe abnormalities with electrolytes or fluid management.

Hemodialysis	Peritoneal Dialysis	Organ Transplant
A hemodialysis machine with an artificial kidney (semipermeable filtering membrane) removes excess fluid and waste products from blood. Requires that a patient be "hooked-up" to a machine several times per week. The patient has a specially placed vascular access device called a graft or a fistula that can be accessed through a hemodialysis catheter. The patient is attached to the dialysis machine for several hours at a time. Dialysate fluid is pumped through one side of the filter or artificial kidney. The patient's blood passes on the other side of the membrane. This process involves diffusion, osmosis, and ultrafiltration to pull the excess fluid and waste products across the membrane into the dialysate fluid and then down the drain. The patient's blood is returned to his or her body minus the waste products. Patients require constant monitoring by nurses with specialized skills during the process. Complications can include blood clotting and alterations in vital signs especially if the process is administered too quickly. The vascular access sites need to be monitored for patency.	Peritoneal dialysis does not involve a machine but also uses a semipermeable membrane (the peritoneum). Excess fluid and waste are removed from the blood using osmosis and diffusion similar to the process of hemodialysis. In peritoneal dialysis, the sterile electrolyte dialysate fluid is instilled into the peritoneal cavity by gravity through a surgically placed port or catheter. The patient is not as restricted in his or her physical movements with peritoneal dialysis. The dialysate is left in the cavity for a prescribed period of time and then allowed to drain out by gravity. The fluid brings with it the waste products that crossed the membrane into the dialysate. People can go about their normal activities while the dialysate sits in the peritoneal cavity. They can even perform their own exchanges at home, during the day or overnight. Complications of peritoneal dialysis can include site infection and peritonitis.	In some cases, it is necessary to replace a patient's diseased kidney. The organs used are from either living or cadaver donors. The donor kidney must be a compatible blood and tissue type to reduce the incidence of rejection. A transplant can provide a patient with psychological as well as physical freedom from required dialysis treatments but require special medications (immunosuppressives) for life to prevent rejection. A successful transplant may offer a return to normal kidney function.

BOX 35.1   Health Teaching: Preventing Urinary Tract Infections

To flush bacteria out of the urinary system, ensure you drink eight 250 ml glasses of water daily and avoid or limit bladder irritants such as alcohol and caffeine.

Void often (every 2 to 4 hours) to flush out bacteria and prevent organisms from ascending from the urethra to the bladder.

Girls and women must always wipe the perineal area from front to back after voiding or having a bowel movement.

Do not wait to void; urinate when the need arises.

Void after sexual intercourse.

Keep the perineal area clean and dry, but avoid the use of bubble bath, powder, sprays, or harsh soaps. By being irritants, they can cause inflammation to the urethra and encourage bacterial infection.

Do not douche.

Wear cotton underwear and avoid tight-fitting clothing to limit perineal moisture by improving ventilation.

If UTIs are reoccurring, encourage patients to take showers instead of baths, because bacteria present in the bathwater can enter the urethra.

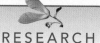

RESEARCH

THE EFFECTIVENESS OF THE ULTRASOUND BLADDER SCANNER IN REDUCING URINARY TRACT INFECTION: A META-ANALYSIS

Background
Urinary retention is defined as being unable to empty the bladder, even if it is full. This can be an acute or chronic problem and is a common postoperative complication. The association between urinary catheterization and UTI has been well documented in the literature. As a result, avoiding unnecessary catheterizations is paramount. The purpose of this study was to synthesize the literature concerning the effectiveness of the ultrasound bladder scanner (see Fig. 35.4) in reducing the risk of CAUTI.

The Study
A meta-analysis study design was used which means that the findings of multiple independent studies were combined and statistically analyzed for a precise estimate of the effect of the treatment. In this study, the treatment was using an ultrasound bladder scanner to measure urinary retention, bladder volume, and decision making about whether or not the patient required a catheter.

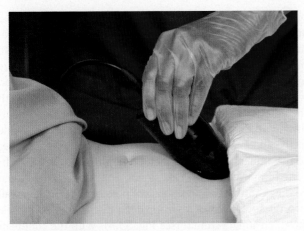

Figure 35.4 Bladder scanner.

Conclusions

The ultrasound bladder scanner was demonstrated to help monitor and evaluate urinary volume and reduced unnecessary urinary catheter use among immediate postoperative patients aged 18 years or older.

Implications for Nursing Students

This meta-analysis demonstrates that the systematic perioperative use of the ultrasound bladder scanner can increase the rate of appropriate catheterizations and reduced patient discomfort, hospital costs, and lengths of hospital stays associated with CAUTI. As a nursing student, you should refer to agency policies for the use of bladder scanners to assess the need for a catheter.

Palese, A., Buchini, S., Deroma, L., & Barbone, F. (2010). The effectiveness of the ultrasound bladder scanner in reducing urinary tract infections: A meta-analysis. Journal of Clinical Nursing, 19, 2970–2979.

Urinary elimination is affected during a UTI in several ways. These include more frequent and painful voiding and a sense of urgency (a feeling of being unable to delay the urge to urinate). The urine may contain pus (pyuria) and blood (hematuria). Renal failure may result if the infection travels to the kidney.

Managing Urinary Incontinence

Urinary incontinence occurs when urine is released from the bladder involuntarily. Regardless of the cause, incontinence is a significant issue for the patients and their families. Incontinence contributes to anxiety and embarrassment for patients who are not prepared for an unexpected loss of urine. Fear of incontinence or bed-wetting can contribute to the limiting of social activities and avoidance of travel. Products are commercially available for daily wear including pads and protective underwear, and patients should be told about measures to protect their clothing during your health teaching. The financial burden associated with the purchase of incontinence products may impact on a patient's activities of daily living, and long-term incontinence may affect the ability of a family to provide care at home.

Through the eyes of a patient

I don't want to wet my pants like a baby, but since my stroke, I have had trouble knowing when I need to go to the bathroom. The pee just comes and I feel bad having to wear the pad in my underwear and that my wife has to help me change when it gets wet. The homecare nurse who visited me today gave me hope when she talked about bladder retraining. I am willing to try anything to stop having this wetting problem. *(personal reflection of a patient)*

Patients in hospital and long-term care facilities may have incontinence pads on their beds or, for male patients, a condom catheter may be applied during the night. It is important for all patients who are incontinent to receive regular skin care and changing of wet products and clothing to prevent chafing, excoriation, and odors. Bladder training is used to reintroduce a more predictable pattern of voiding for patients who have bladder incontinence. Refer to Box 35.2 for more details.

BOX 35.2 Management of Urinary Incontinence

The goal of continence (bladder) training is to decrease how frequently urinary incontinence occurs. A continence training program may include the following nursing interventions:

- Bladder training—requires the patient to postpone voiding, resist the sensation of urgency, and follow a schedule to time voiding instead of according to the urge to void. To correct frequent voiding, ease urgency, and stabilize the bladder, the patient's goal is to gradually extend the time between urination. As a result, bladder training can be used for patients with urge incontinence and bladder instability. In the beginning, the patient can be encouraged to urinate every 2 to 3 hours (except while asleep), and then extend to every 4 to 6 hours. Vital to bladder training, the nurse can teach the patient to practice deep, slow breathing to inhibit the premature urge-to-void sensation.
- Habit training (timed voiding/scheduled toileting)—aims to keep patients dry by having them urinate at regular intervals. As opposed to bladder training, with habit training, the patient voids when the urge arises. This method can be useful for children experiencing urinary dysfunction.
- Prompted voiding—used in addition to habit training. The patient is prompted, or encouraged, to try to void and reminded when to void. This method can be useful for patients with physical or cognitive impairments that require reminders (Registered Nurses' Association of Ontario [RNAO], 2005). The three primary behaviours caregivers use with this intervention are monitoring, prompting, and praising. The caregiver monitors by asking the person, at regular intervals, if he or she needs to use the toilet and be assisted, where necessary, to void at regular intervals (specific to each patient's own schedule as determined by a 3-day record of voiding) (RNAO, 2005). The person is prompted to regularly use the toilet and encouraged to void in between prompted voiding sessions. Positive feedback is given for maintaining bladder control.

Urinary Diversion

A **urinary diversion** is a surgical procedure that changes the normal pathway of urine elimination. This surgically creates a new path for urine flow from the kidneys to a location other than the bladder. The diversion can be temporary, to promote healing after trauma, or for severe chronic UTI. With removal of the bladder (cystectomy) to treat cancer, urinary diversions can be permanent. There are two main types of urinary diversions available: incontinent and continent. Incontinent diversions affect normal elimination because the person no longer has control of urination. A continent diversion alternately gives patients control over the passage of urine.

An example of an incontinent diversion requires the use of an external ostomy appliance to contain the urine, rerouting of ureters from a damaged or diseased urinary system to a **stoma**, an opening surgically created on the patient's abdomen, using a portion of the intestine (urostomy). The two main types of urostomy include ileal conduit (ureters are implanted into a surgically created ileal pouch and closed with sutures, while a stoma in the abdomen is created with the other end of the removed segment of ileum) and ureterostomy (one or both ureters is brought directly to the side of the abdomen, forming small stomas). Some other types of incontinent diversions include **nephrostomy** (urine diverted from the kidney to a stoma) and vesicostomy (when voiding through the urethra is not possible; the bladder wall is surgically attached to an opening in the skin below the navel, creating a stoma) (see Fig. 35.5). With the continent diversion, **Kock** (pronounced *coke*) **pouch** (also known as an *ileal bladder conduit*), a portion of the ileum is used to

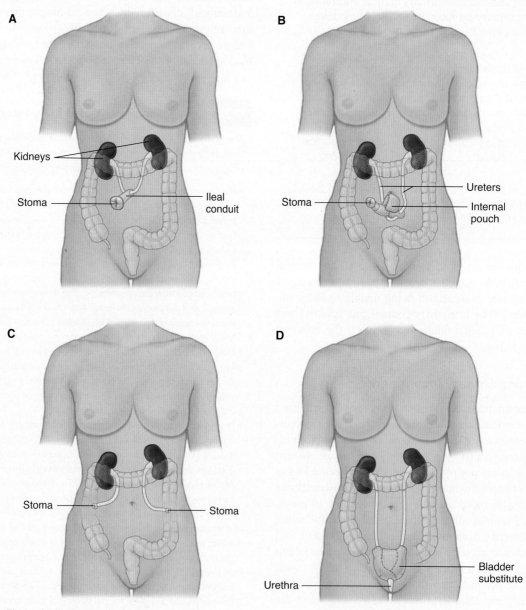

Figure 35.5 Urinary stoma.

create a reservoir for the urine. Nipple valves are surgically created that close as the pouch fills with urine, preventing leakage and backflow of urine toward the kidneys. To empty the pouch, the patient inserts a clean catheter every 4 hours and wears a small dressing between catheterizations to protect the stoma and clothing. Another type of continent diversion is a neobladder (new bladder), which replaces a damaged or diseased bladder with a piece of ileum. This new bladder is sutured to the functioning urethra and patients can control voiding.

When caring for a patient with any urinary diversion, the nurse must accurately assess intake and output, noting any changes in urine clarity, colour, or odour, and frequently monitor the condition of the stoma and surrounding skin. Local irritation and skin breakdown will occur when urine is in contact with the skin for long periods. Further, a urinary diversion threatens the patient's body image. With the help of an enterostomal therapist (a nurse with special training to care for patients with stomas), the patient must be empowered to learn to manage his or her artificial device and realize he or she can wear normal clothing, travel, take part in physical activity, and have sexual relations.

Assessment

A nursing history and assessment of urinary elimination will include asking specific questions about normal elimination patterns. It is important to establish a baseline of normal function and be able to assess for any changes or concerns that the patient may have. Questions will establish the last time the patient voided, the estimated amount at each voiding, colour, presence of any odour, and whether or not the patient wakes at night to void or experiences any discomfort upon voiding.

Jaswinder was assigned to admit a new patient to the unit. She knew from her health assessment class that it was important to use words or terms that patients were comfortable with to assess urinary function. Jaswinder felt a little uneasy at first because her patient looked puzzled when she asked about normal urination habits, so she used the words *peeing* and *passing water* instead. Her patient responded to *peeing* and Jaswinder was able to collect the information she was seeking.

Risk Factor Assessment

Identifying any potential risk factors for an alteration in normal urinary elimination will be accomplished by completing a thorough nursing history. Refer back to the factors affecting urination earlier in this chapter. Assess any recent surgeries, pregnancy, mobility issues, sensory issues such as sight and hearing, physical problems with ambulation that would impact on ambulating to the bathroom, and any acute or chronic medical conditions that could alter urinary function.

Physical Assessment

A comprehensive urinary tract physical assessment usually includes percussion of the kidneys to detect areas of tenderness and palpation and percussion of the bladder are done. Based on individual patient need, according to current concerns and history, the urethral meatus is inspected for discharge, swelling, and inflammation. The nurse must assess the skin for colour, tissue turgor, and edema. The perineum should be inspected for irritation and excoriation if dribbling, incontinence, or dysuria is noted in the patient history.

Assessing Urine

Normal urine is made up of 96% water and 4% solutes (organic and inorganic). The organic solutes include urea (the main organic solute), ammonia, creatinine, and uric acid. Inorganic solutes include sodium, chloride, sulphate, phosphorus, magnesium, and potassium, with sodium chloride being the most abundant inorganic salt. See Table 35.5 for characteristics of normal versus abnormal urine and urinalysis parameters.

Measurement and Assessment of Urine Output

Urine output is collected, measured, and assessed by nurses as part of monitoring fluid balance. As mentioned earlier, adults usually void between 1,500 and 2,000 ml of urine in a 24-hour period. A deviation from the normal amount of urine voided can be an indication of a serious underlying problem such as dehydration, renal failure, renal disease, bleeding, or medication side effects. Urine is collected for lab tests to assess kidney function; that is, a 24-hour creatinine clearance. Creatine is an important part of muscle and creatinine is its breakdown product. It is excreted by the kidneys. As a result, comparing the amount of creatinine in urine to the amount in blood is a good indicator of kidney function.

Testing Urine

It is often the nurse's responsibility to collect urine samples for various tests. The type of test and reason it is being done will determine how the urine is collected (Table 35.6). These include clean voided specimen collection for urinalysis, midstream or clean-catch for urine culture, and timed urine specimens collected for various tests related to the patient's specific illness. All specimens must be labeled with the patient's name and date and time of collection according to agency protocol. Some simple urine tests are done by nurses directly on the nursing units and may include testing for specific gravity, pH, and components not normally

TABLE 35.5	Characteristics of Normal Versus Abnormal Urine and Urinalysis Parameters		
Characteristics	Normal	Abnormal	Significance
Amount (adult)	1,200–1,500 ml (in 24 hours)	Less than 1,200 ml Greater than 1,500 ml A large volume of urine greater than intake	Urine output should be approximately equal to intake. Output less than 30 ml/hour may signify decreased blood flow to the kidneys and should be reported right away.
Colour	Straw, amber	Dark amber Dark orange Red or dark brown	Nearly colourless: increased fluid intake; dark colour: decreased fluid intake Pink, red, dark/rusty brown: red blood cells in urine (hematuria) Menstrual bleeding can also colour urine (but don't confuse with hematuria).
Clarity/turbidity	Transparent/ clear	Hazy, cloudy, smoky Mucus plugs, viscid, thick	Hazy, cloudy, smoky: urine specimen allowed to stand at room temperature. High protein concentrations in patients with renal disease can appear foamy or cloudy. Bacteria, pus, white blood cells, or contaminants such as sperm, prostatic fluid, or vaginal drainage can cause cloudy urine.
Odour	Faint aromatic	Offensive	The more concentrated the urine, the stronger it smells. Stagnant urine, common in patients who are repeatedly incontinent, has an ammonia odour. Some foods, such as asparagus, cause a musty odour; infected urine can have a foul odour; urine high in glucose smells sweet or fruity (acetone or acetoacetic acid are by-products of incomplete fat metabolism that occur with diabetes mellitus or starvation).
pH	Range: 4.5–8 Normal: 6	Less than 4.5 Greater than 8	<6: diet high in meat or some fruits (cranberries); metabolic acidosis (starvation, diabetes mellitus); respiratory acidosis (emphysema) >6: diet high in vegetables and citrus fruits; UTIs; respiratory alkalosis (hyperventilation); metabolic alkalosis (prolonged diuretic therapy, vomiting)
Specific gravity	Range: 1.015–1.025	Less than 1.015 Greater than 1.025	Increased fluid intake; diuretic therapy, renal diseases, diabetes insipidus Decreased fluid intake; excess fluid loss (fever, vomiting, and diarrhea); ADH secretion (stress, trauma)
Protein	None to trace	Present	Present in severe stress, pregnancy-induced hypertension, and renal disease
Glucose	None	Present	Indicates high blood glucose levels; may signify undiagnosed or uncontrolled diabetes mellitus
Ketones	None	Present	The end product of the breakdown of fatty acids; may be present in diabetes mellitus, ketoacidosis, starvation, or in patients who have ingested excessive amounts of acetyl-salicylic acid (Aspirin)
Microscopic exam Red blood cells	0–3	Greater than 3	UTI, trauma to urinary tract, kidney disease, anticoagulant therapy
White blood cells	0–5	Greater than 5	UTI
Bacteria/yeast	None to few	Present	Few: contamination from perineum Many: UTI
Casts (clumping of protein substances)	None to occasional	Present	Many: possible renal diseases

present in urine including ketones, protein, occult blood, and glucose. Nurses in health-care facilities and in home care settings may use commercially prepared kits including paper test strips or dipsticks and reagents that cause a colour change and a chart for comparison.

Urine Culture

Urine is collected for culture and sensitivity when an infection needs to be ruled out and when knowledge is required for prescribing an appropriate antibiotic in the presence of a UTI.

Midstream or Clean-Catch Urine Specimen

Midstream or clean-catch urine are collected when a urine culture is ordered. This is done to identify microorganisms that cause UTIs. Careful collection is necessary to reduce contamination from skin bacteria. A sterile specimen container with a lid is used for the collection of the sample. Many agencies use clean-catch kits for this purpose. Some patients are able to collect the specimen independently with guidance and direction from the nurse. Skill 35.2 explains how to perform a clean-catch or midstream urine collection.

TABLE 35.6	Urine Collection
Test	**Considerations**
Random/clean voided	Collected when a routine urinalysis is ordered
	Collected from a normal void
	Many patients are able to collect the sample independently with clear instruction from the nurse.
	Although the sample is not sterile, it must be kept clean from feces, toilet tissue, and other contaminants.
	A clean specimen cup must be used.
Midstream/clean-catch	Collected when a urine culture and sensitivity is ordered
	A patient may be able to collect the specimen with guidance and/or supervision.
	Care must be taken to ensure the sample is free from contamination from microorganisms.
	A sterile specimen cup is used.
	If the patient has an indwelling catheter, a sterile specimen may be collected through the specimen port found on the collection tubing. Ensure that fresh uncontaminated urine is collected by clamping the collection tubing below the port. Wipe the port with an aseptic swab and then insert a sterile syringe or needleless system if present; withdraw 3–5 ml of urine (per agency policy) and transfer to a sterile container.
Timed urine	Urine is collected over a specified time period; often, this may range from 1 to 2 hours to 24 hours.
	The patient collects all urine produced within the specified period in a small container or hat and then transfers it to a larger collection container, which is often refrigerated or contains preservatives to prevent bacteria growth.
	The timed period begins after the patient urinates; this initial urine is not part of the collection, it ends with a final void at the end of the specified time.
	If one urine is missed during this period, the entire collection is inaccurate and must be restarted.
	This collection is not sterile but must be kept clean of feces and toilet tissue.
	Always check agency policy for specific instructions.

Diagnostic Examinations

There are several visualization procedures available to evaluate urinary function. These include both direct and indirect techniques and are subdivided into noninvasive and invasive radiographic techniques.

Noninvasive Procedures

Noninvasive examinations include intravenous pyelogram (x-ray), renal scan, computerized axial tomography (CT), and ultrasound.

Abdominal Roentgenogram

Abdominal roentgenogram is commonly used to assess the gross anatomy of the urinary tract, giving information on size, symmetry, location, and shape of the kidneys; ureters; and structure of the bladder. It is also called a plain film, KUB (kidneys, ureters, and bladder), or flat plate of the abdomen. Calcifications (stones) or tumours in these organs can be visualized as well as assessment for fractures of surrounding supportive structures such as ribs. Additional diagnostic studies may be required to rule out urinary tract abnormalities. The nurse caring for a patient undergoing a roentgenogram explains the procedure and helps alleviate anxiety. This test is painless and does not require any special bowel preparation unless the physician states otherwise.

Intravenous Pyelogram

The intravenous pyelogram (IVP) (also called an excretory urogram) is an x-ray procedure used to visualize the entire urinary system. It provides a view of the collecting ducts, renal pelvis, ureters, bladder, and urethra. For this test, the patient receives an intravenous (IV) injection of radiopaque (contrast) dye. X-ray views are taken during the IVP at specific intervals as the dye concentrates. A radiograph is taken right after the patient voids to ensure the bladder is emptied fully. The evening before the test, the patient can consume only clear liquids or a light meal and nothing by mouth (NPO) after midnight (sometimes clear liquids are allowed). A bowel preparation to clear the colon of feces is needed because the kidneys and ureters lie behind the intestines. Before the test, the nurse assesses volume status and maintenance prior to this procedure. Other nursing implications include recognizing patients with renal insufficiency who are at an increased risk for altered renal function due to the dye and older patients who are more prone to the nephrotoxic effects due the loss of fluid during bowel preparation. Additional nursing implications include ensuring signed informed consent was obtained, assessing patient for an iodine/IVP dye allergy, explaining injection of the dye may normally cause facial flushing or a feeling of warmth or dizziness, and explaining what's involved during the test. If the radiology department employs nurses, during the test, the nurse would be responsible for assessing the IV site for signs of allergic reaction to the dye (such as respiratory distress, hives, and a drop in blood pressure). After the test, nursing implications include ensuring the patient receives usual diet, encourage fluid intake to lessen dehydration caused by the bowel prep and to aid excretion of the nephrotoxic dye, monitor intake and outputs and report alterations, and watch for a delayed allergic reaction.

Renal Ultrasound

Renal ultrasound uses high frequency, inaudible, reflected sound waves to visualize the kidneys. The velocity of the sound waves varies based on the density of the tissue. Ultrasound is performed with the patient in a prone position but can be done in a sitting position. This painless test is often used to identify renal structures and abnormalities of the kidneys or lower urinary tract. It is also used to assist with percutaneous biopsy. Abnormalities including cysts or tumours in the kidney are easily identified using ultrasonography. A Doppler can be used with the transducer to examine blood flow through the kidneys. The nurse explains the test to the patient and may possibly encourage the patient to drink fluids to distend the bladder. No specific follow-up care is needed after.

Computerized Axial Tomography

Computerized axial tomography (CT) is a computerized x-ray that obtains detailed images of structures within one plane of the body. Internal structures are photographed in thin cross sections that the computer manipulates into a recognizable image on the television monitor. Abnormal pathological conditions including tumours, masses, obstructions, and lymph node enlargement can be visualized using this procedure. Although a noninvasive procedure overall, oral or IV contrast material may be required to enhance the images. If IV contrast is used, a bowel-cleansing oral solution or an enema may also be used, especially if organs in the abdominal cavity will be examined. The nursing implications for this procedure are the same as those listed for the IVP examination. However, the nurse needs to explain that the patient will be placed in a large machine, which could cause feelings of claustrophobia.

Invasive Procedures

Invasive procedures used to visualize components of the urinary system include cystoscopy, angiography, and urodynamic testing.

Cystoscopy

During a cystoscopy (an endoscopic procedure), a lighted flexible instrument called a *cystoscope* is inserted through the urethra to directly visualize the bladder, ureteral orifices, and urethra. This allows the physician to look for stones, tumours, or structural abnormalities. Small stones can be removed or tissue biopsies taken using specialized instruments passed through the cystoscope. The patient must sign a consent form before this procedure. After the procedure, the nurse assesses for urinary retention, hematuria, dysuria, bladder spasms, and any signs or symptoms of a UTI. A retention catheter may remain in situ for a short time after the procedure is over.

Renal Angiogram

A renal angiogram is an invasive radiographical procedure used to evaluate the renal arterial system, most commonly used to detect narrowing or occlusion of the main renal artery or its branches. This procedure can also be used to evaluate masses, such as cysts or neoplasms, to determine changes in blood flow. A catheter is inserted into one of the femoral arteries and advanced to the level of the renal arteries. Then radiopaque contrast dye is injected through the catheter while a series of x-ray images are rapidly taken. There are several nursing implications prior to this test, including ensuring signed informed consent was obtained, assessing for an iodine allergy (because this predicts an allergy to the dye used), ensuring the patient did not eat or drink anything after midnight, explaining the test involves x-rays at intervals after the injection of the dye, and that facial flushing and feeling dizzy and warm are normal responses during injection of the dye. After the test is completed, the nurse is responsible for monitoring vital signs, ensuring the patient maintains bed rest, checking pulse and circulation in the affected extremity, and that the patient keeps the leg straight. The nurse observes for bleeding, increased tenderness, and hematoma formation at the insertion site for 24 hours; maintains a pressure dressing over the site (per agency policy); observes for a possible delayed reaction to the contrast material; monitors intake and outputs; reports abnormalities in urine output to the physician; and encourages fluids to help flush out the dye (to minimize nephrotoxic effects).

Urodynamics

Urodynamic testing includes various studies (uroflowmetry, cystometrogram, and urethral pressure profile) to measure the transport, storage, and elimination of urine in the lower urinary tract. A cystometrogram (CMG) determines the level of function of the detrusor muscle and rules out causes of incontinence. For this particular test, a catheter is inserted, residual volume is measured and emptied, and the bladder is then incrementally filled with sterile saline or carbon dioxide gas. At each increment, pressure is measured, and the patient is asked to report his or her perceptions of bladder fullness, urge to void, and ability to inhibit voiding. There is no special preparation required for urodynamic testing and these studies are usually not painful. However, intermittent discomfort may be experienced. Prior to the test, the nurse explains the procedure and the need for the patient to report sensations as they occur. The nurse should instruct the patient to report sweating, pain, bladder fullness, nausea, or a strong urge to void that occur after the test is completed.

Health Teaching and Promoting Healthy Urinary Elimination

Promoting optimal health and functioning of the urinary tract provides a valuable opportunity for health teaching. All patients should be reminded of the importance of adequate fluid intake, measures to prevent infections of the urinary tract, preserving optimal muscle function in the perineum, and reducing the risk of injury.

Managing Urinary Incontinence

Urinary incontinence is not a normal part of aging and is often treatable. There are many independent nursing interventions to help patients with urinary incontinence, such as

(1) a continence training program (that may include bladder training, prompted voiding, pelvic floor muscle [Kegel] exercises, habit training, and positive reinforcement); (2) meticulous skin care; and (3) for male patients, application of a condom catheter (external drainage device). Refer back to Box 35.2 for management of urinary incontinence.

Kegel Exercises

Exercises that strengthen the floor of the pelvis are called *Kegel exercises*. Pregnancy, childbirth, being overweight, aging, and surgery are all risk factors for mild to severe incontinence related to the weakening of the pelvic floor muscles. Warning signs that the pelvic floor is weakening can begin with leaking a few drops of urine when you sneeze, cough, or laugh really hard. Refer to Box 35.3 for health teaching tips on how to instruct the patient to do Kegel exercises for mild or stress incontinence.

Applying an External Condom Catheter

External or condom catheters are applied and connected to a urinary drainage system in males with incontinence. The condom appliance is preferred over a retention catheter because the risk of UTI is less. Consider the length of time the condom is required and when the patient is experiencing incontinence; some patients may only require it at night. Special care may be required to protect the foreskin and to ensure it is securely attached if it is to be used for more than a few days. Manufacturer's instructions should be closely followed. Skill 35.3 describes how to apply a drainage condom.

Urinary Catheterization

Urinary catheterization of the bladder requires introducing a latex or plastic tube through the urethra into the bladder. The catheter creates a continuous flow of urine in patients who are unable to control urination or who have an obstruction.

BOX 35.3 Instructions for Kegel Exercises

Kegel exercises can strengthen the pelvic floor muscles, but it takes patience, practice, and time for the full benefits to be realized for mild bladder incontinence. There are some tips that you can share with patients to help them do the Kegel exercises correctly.

- Begin by identifying the pelvic floor muscles. Suggest that the patients practice stopping urination in midstream. If they are able to accomplish this, then they have identified the right muscles. Inform them to not make it a habit to stop urine midstream as this can have a negative effect of eventually weakening the bladder muscles and contribute to UTIs due to incomplete emptying of the bladder.
- Instruct patients to lie on their back and tighten or contract their pelvic floor muscles. They should hold the contraction for 5 seconds, relax for 5 seconds and do this routine five times in a row. A goal is to work up to 10-second intervals.
- Remind patients that the exercises will require focus and to breathe during the exercises.
- The goal is to do the exercise routine of 10-second intervals multiple times a day. Some people learn to do the exercises when they are standing up and can discreetly do them while waiting in line at the grocery store and no one knows that they are doing them. Try it!

It also allows for accurate monitoring of urinary output. There are risks associated with catheterization that include UTI and urethral trauma; for this reason, catheterization is often considered as the last choice of care. Less invasive procedures should be considered first.

There are two different types of catheter insertion: indwelling retention catheters and intermittent catheterization. Intermittent catheterization involves inserting a straight, single-use catheter tube (see Fig. 35.6) into the bladder

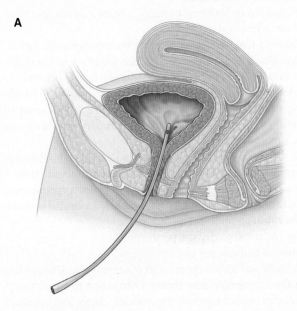
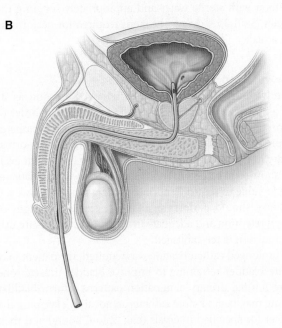

Figure 35.6 Catheter tube.

A

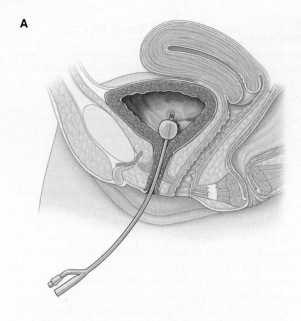

B

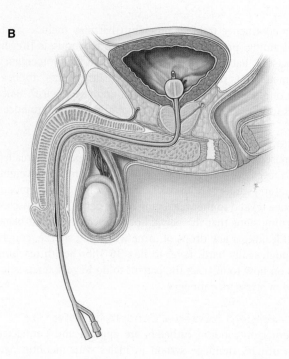

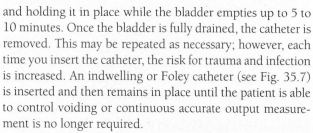

Figure 35.7 Foley catheter.

and holding it in place while the bladder empties up to 5 to 10 minutes. Once the bladder is fully drained, the catheter is removed. This may be repeated as necessary; however, each time you insert the catheter, the risk for trauma and infection is increased. An indwelling or Foley catheter (see Fig. 35.7) is inserted and then remains in place until the patient is able to control voiding or continuous accurate output measurement is no longer required.

Urethral catheterization is performed under the order of a health-care provider. It is important to use strict aseptic technique to reduce the risk of infection. Insertion of both indwelling and intermittent catheters requires the same steps, except an indwelling catheter also involves inflating a balloon with sterile water and appropriately securing the catheter. Skill 35.4 details the steps required for performing both a male and female catheterization.

Removal of an Indwelling Catheter

An indwelling catheter should be removed as soon as its purpose has been achieved; this often requires the order of the primary care provider. Timely removal of the catheter will prevent CAUTI as well as promote the return of normal urinary function. Although urethral swelling may occur even after short-term catheterization (such as a few days), patients are often able to return to normal voiding quickly. However, the nurse should perform regular assessments for signs of urinary retention and adequate urinary output to ensure urinary function is reestablished.

If prolonged catheterization was required, the patient may require bladder retraining to improve bladder muscle tone before normal urinary elimination patterns return. Bladder training may begin before catheter removal by clamping the catheter for specified intervals (e.g., 2 to 4 hours) and then

removing the clamp to simulate normal bladder distention and emptying.

To remove an indwelling urinary catheter:

- Gather the required supplies: a receptacle for disposal, a towel, disposable gloves, and a sterile syringe large enough to deflate the balloon (see the end of the catheter for the size of the balloon in use).
- Enter the patient's room and introduce yourself, identify the patient using institution policy, and explain the procedure and purpose. Wash your hands and use appropriate infection control practices.
- Assist the patient into a supine position, similar to the position for catheterization.
- If required by order or protocol, obtain a sterile specimen prior to removal.
- Carefully remove the tape securing the catheter to the patient. Don gloves and then place the clean towel across the thighs of a male patient or between the legs of a female patient.
- Attach the syringe to the port and withdraw the fluid filling the balloon. If unable to remove the full amount of fluid, notify the charge nurse or primary care provider before proceeding.
- Never pull the catheter while the balloon is still inflated or partially inflated as this may cause injury to the urethra.
- Once all fluid is removed from the balloon, gently pull back on the catheter and withdraw it from the urethra; place it in an appropriate receptacle.
- Use the towel to dry the perineum.
- Remove and discard gloves.
- Measure and record the amount of urine in the drainage bag in the appropriate flow sheets. Ensure that documentation includes time of removal; the amount, clarity, and colour of urine; and the information provided to the patient.

- After the removal, monitor and record the time and amount of the first void as well as total output for 24 hours following removal, per institution policy. Compare output to intake to ensure appropriate bladder function is resumed.
- Assess for abnormal voiding patterns that may suggest urinary retention is occurring (e.g., an output of less than 100 ml per void). If urinary retention is suspected, observe postvoid residual using a bladder scanner and perform straight catheterization as required per institution policy.

Bladder Irrigation

Bladder irrigation is performed with a physician's order, usually to flush or wash out the bladder. Other times, it is used to apply a medication to the bladder lining. Irrigating a catheter may be done to restore or maintain catheter patency; for example, to clear blood clots that may be blocking the tubing. There are two main techniques for bladder or catheter irrigation: closed and open. The closed method is preferred because it is less likely than the open method to cause a UTI. Closed irrigations may be continuous or intermittent and, generally, a three-way catheter is used. To restore catheter patency, the less preferred open method may be used. Because the risk of UTI is higher as the connection between the indwelling catheter and drainage tubing is broken, strict precautions must be used to maintain the sterility of the catheter interior and drainage tubing connector. A double-lumen indwelling catheter is used for open bladder or catheter irrigation. The open method may be necessary to clear mucus or blood clots or to change the catheter. Skill 35.5 details how to perform bladder irrigations.

Anatomy and Physiology of Fecal Elimination

Elimination of the waste products of digestion is an essential bodily function. Let's quickly review the process of digestion.

Digestion begins as food and fluids enter the mouth, mixing with salivary enzymes. This bolus of food then travels down the pharynx, through the esophagus to the stomach, where it is further broken down by acids in the stomach. Next, the food enters the small intestine, which is separated into three sections: the duodenum, the jejunum, and the ileum. The small intestine measures about 2.5 cm in diameter and 6 m in length (Patton & Thibodeau, 2010). Approximately 3 to 10 hours later, the digested products (referred to as *chyme*) enter the large intestine, which includes the cecum, colon, rectum, and anus (see Fig. 35.8).

Large Intestine

The ileocecal valve lies between the small and large intestines (at the junction of the ileum and cecum). The valve functions to slow the movement of semi-digested food in the large intestine (allowing more time for absorption of nutrients) and to prevent the backflow of fecal contents. The large intestine

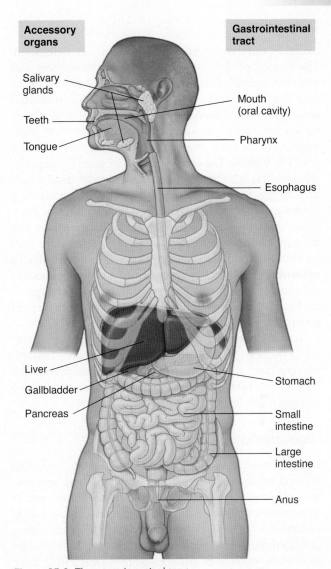

Figure 35.8 The gastrointestinal tract.

extends from the ileocecal valve to the anus, measuring approximately 1.5 m in the adult (Patton & Thibodeau, 2010).

The colon, which makes up most of the large intestine, is composed of four parts: the ascending, transverse, descending, and sigmoid colons. The colon functions to absorb water and nutrients, provide mucosal protection of the intestinal wall, and eliminate feces. Most waste products are eliminated within 48 hours of ingestion, although the colon can contain foods you have consumed in the previous 4 days.

Rectum and Anal Canal

The rectum is the final portion of the GI tract. The average length of the adult rectum is 10 to 15 cm. It is made up of folds of tissue that extend vertically and across the rectum. Within each vertical fold is an artery and vein. The most distal portion of the rectum is the anal canal, which is approximately 3 cm long. The lower anal canal and anal opening are composed of the internal and external sphincter muscles that are involved in defecation.

Defecation

Normally, there are no feces in the rectum until **defecation**. The process of defecation involves both involuntary and voluntary control. Defecation starts when gas (flatus) or the fecal mass distends the walls of the rectum. This stimulates sensory nerves and nerve impulses cause the internal sphincter to relax. This allows more feces to enter the rectum while impulses to the brain create awareness of the need to have a bowel movement. The external sphincter starts to relax, too, although this is controlled by adults and toilet-trained children. If it is not the right time to defecate yet, constricting the levator ani muscles delays defecation by closing the anus. When the time is right, the external sphincter relaxes and pressure can be used to expel feces. This can be done with an increase in intra-abdominal pressure, called a **Valsalva maneuver**; however, this voluntary contraction of abdominal muscles while holding one's breath can cause changes in the heart rate and rhythm. As a result, it is contraindicated in patients experiencing heart problems.

Typical bowel elimination patterns vary from one individual to the next. This can mean that the frequency of defecation can range normally from one or two bowel movements daily to one every few days. It's important when assessing patients to ask them what their typical pattern is.

Characteristics of Normal Feces

Feces are made up of 75% water and 25% solids, including bacteria, undigested fibre, fat, inorganic material, and protein. The major undigested fibre is cellulose. The amount of fibre in one's diet affects the amount of feces produced daily. Normally, feces are soft but formed. When chyme passes quickly through the large intestine, then there is no time for most of the water to be absorbed and the feces will be more fluid, containing as much as 95% water. Feces that contain less water, perhaps from a lower than normal fluid intake, may be hard and difficult to expel. Brown is the normal colour of feces, mainly due to the presence of bilirubin (a red pigment in bile) derivatives and from the bacterial action of the large intestine's normal flora, such as *Escherichia coli*. The odour of feces is caused by the action of microorganisms on the chyme. Approximately 7 to 10 L of flatus (gas) is usually formed in an adult's large intestine every 24 hours. Some gases are swallowed with food and drinks taken by mouth, some are formed through bacterial action on the chyme in the large intestine, and other gas diffuses into the GI tract from the blood. Flatus includes the following gases: carbon dioxide, oxygen, methane, nitrogen, and hydrogen.

Factors Affecting Bowel Elimination

Several factors affect defecation, including fluid intake and output, diet, psychological factors, medications, diagnostic procedures, surgery and anaesthesia, habits, pathological conditions, and pain.

Development

Elimination patterns vary over the lifespan due to many factors, including diet, toilet training, and aging.

Newborns and Infants

The first fecal material passed by a newborn is meconium, an odourless, sticky, black, and tarry feces normally passed up to 24 hours after birth. Transitional feces are generally greenish yellow, loose, and containing mucus; they follow meconium for about a week. Breast-fed infants have bright, mustard yellow feces; whereas formula-fed infants have dark yellow or tan-coloured feces that are more formed. Infants may pass feces after each feeding because the intestine is immature and doesn't absorb water well. So, the feces are liquid, soft, and frequent. As the intestine matures, bacterial flora increases, and after solid foods are started, the feces become firmer and less frequent.

Toddlers

Toddlers start to gain some control of defecation around 1.5 to 2 years of age. The nervous and muscular systems have sufficiently developed to allow bowel control. Generally, once the child becomes aware of the discomfort of a soiled diaper and the sensation indicating the need for a bowel movement, a desire to control daytime bowel movements and use the toilet starts.

School-Age Children and Adolescents

School-age children and adolescents have similar bowel habits to adults. Defecation patterns vary in consistency, quantity, and frequency. Some school-age children experience functional **constipation**, which is the voluntary delay of defecation because of an activity, such as play. Conversely, *encopresis* is the term used to describe the passage or leakage of feces among children past the age of toilet training (usually after age 4 years). Involuntary encopresis is often associated with constipation when liquid feces are expelled, but the hardened and dry feces remains in the rectum. A developmental or emotional problem may be indicated by voluntary soiling.

Older Adults

A common bowel management problem among older adults is constipation. Reduced activity levels, inadequate fluid and fibre intake, and muscle weakness contribute to this. In addition, older adults secrete less mucus in the large intestine. To maintain their normal pattern and prevent constipation, people should get adequate exercise, consume adequate fibre, and drink six to eight glasses of fluid daily.

Older adult patients often believe that regularity means having a bowel movement every day; they should be advised that normal bowel patterns vary significantly from person to person. These patients often seek over-the-counter preparations to relieve what they improperly think is constipation. Consistent use of laxatives inhibits defecation and may actually cause constipation because the user eventually will need larger or stronger doses as the effect decreases with continual use. Continuous laxative use can also be dangerous as they interfere with electrolyte balance and decrease the absorption of some vitamins. It's important for the nurse to evaluate any reports of constipation carefully, and any change in bowel habits that has persisted over several weeks with or without associated weight loss, pain, or fever should be evaluated by a physician.

Diet and Fluid Intake

It is necessary to consume enough bulk (fibre and cellulose) to provide fecal volume. The recommended daily intake of dietary fibre is 25 to 38 g (Dietitians of Canada, 2012). There are two types of dietary fibre—soluble and insoluble—and it is important to consume enough of each type among a variety of foods daily. You can use Canada's Food Guide (downloadable from Health Canada's website) to plan snacks and meals. Their fact sheet provides tips on how to add more fibre-rich foods in your diet. There are different kinds of fibre found in foods such as vegetables, fruit, legumes (peas, beans, lentils), and whole grains and cereals. Soluble fibre is found in some fruits, vegetables, and legumes and can help control blood glucose and cholesterol levels. Insoluble fibre comes from some fruits, vegetables, whole grains, and wheat bran. It helps keep the bowels regular and may protect against colon cancer. Constipation may be improved with a diet that is high in fibre, but this should be done gradually and with an increase in fluid intake to minimize bloating, gas, and diarrhea (Dietitians of Canada, 2012). Foods that cause gas include cabbage, onions, beans, bananas, cauliflower, and apples, whereas cheese, pasta, eggs, and lean meat can cause constipation. Bran, prunes, figs, chocolate, and alcohol are laxative-producing foods. Spicy foods can also produce diarrhea and flatus for some people and excess sugar can also result in diarrhea. Low-residue foods (including rice, eggs, and lean meats) move more slowly through the intestines, but increasing fluid intake with these foods can increase motility.

Eating at irregular times can impair regular defecation, whereas people who eat at the same times every day usually have a regular pattern of peristalsis and bowel movements.

Lactose intolerance causes the difficulty or inability to digest milk and milk products. Lactose is a simple sugar found in milk that is normally broken down by the enzyme lactase. This food intolerance may cause diarrhea, abdominal cramps, gas, bloating, and nausea.

Physical Activity

Being immobile slows **peristalsis**, whereas physical activity promotes peristalsis. Early ambulation is important as soon as possible after surgery or as illness begins to resolve to prevent constipation. Maintaining tone of muscles used to defecate is also important; weak abdominal and pelvic floor muscles make it difficult to increase intra-abdominal pressure necessary during defecation and control the external sphincter. Immobility, lack of exercise, or neurological disease impairing nerve transmission may cause weakened or lost muscle tone. Walking just 15 to 20 minutes daily can aid fecal elimination. If patients are confined to bed, it is important that they perform exercises such as single leg lifts, pelvic tilts, and low trunk rotation (after approval and consultation with the appropriate health-care team members).

Pregnancy

The size of the fetus increases as the pregnancy advances, which puts pressure on the rectum. Passage of feces is impaired by a temporary obstruction caused by the fetus. During the third trimester, peristalsis is slowed, which often causes constipation. Hemorrhoids can be caused by frequent straining during defecation or delivery of the baby. These can sometimes be permanent.

Medications

Some medications can interfere with normal bowel elimination. These include drugs that have an anticholinergic effect (such as specific antihypertensives, analgesics, and antidepressants), iron supplements, opioids, antihistamines, antiparkinsonism medications, and antacids with aluminum that are commonly known to cause constipation.

Pain

Normally, defecating does not cause pain. However, several conditions, such as hemorrhoids, rectal fistulas, and abdominal and rectal surgeries, cause discomfort. The patient may suppress the urge to defecate to avoid pain, which may result in constipation. Constipation is a possible side effect of taking opioid analgesics to relieve pain.

Diagnostic Examinations

Before diagnostic procedures involving visualization of the GI tract, the patient is often restricted from consuming food or fluid. The patient may be given an enema to empty the bowel prior to the exam. This usually interferes with normal bowel elimination until eating has been resumed.

Anaesthesia and Surgery

Peristalsis can be temporarily slowed or stopped by general anaesthetics used during surgery that block parasympathetic impulses to the muscles of the colon. However, local or regional anaesthesia has little to no effect on bowel activity.

Surgery involving directly manipulating the bowel stops peristalsis temporarily. This is called paralytic ileus and usually lasts approximately 24 to 48 hours. If the patient is unable to eat after surgery or remains inactive, this may be further prolonged. Assessing bowel sounds that reflect intestinal motility is important for the nurse to do after surgery. See Chapter 20 for more information on assessing bowel sounds.

Personal Habits

The habit of defecating at a regular time can be started with early bowel training. After breakfast, when the gastrocolic reflex causes large peristaltic waves in the large intestine, many people defecate. If this urge is ignored, the colon absorbs more water out of the feces, hardening it and making it harder to pass. When the conditioned normal defecation reflexes are ignored, these conditioned reflexes are weakened. If this becomes routine, the urge to defecate is ultimately lost. The pressures of time or work may cause people to ignore these urges. Patients in the hospital may suppress the urge to defecate due to the embarrassment, lack of privacy, or because defecation is too uncomfortable.

Ignoring the urge to defecate can cause **hemorrhoids** or swollen and enlarged veins in the folds of the rectum. Hemorrhoids can be very painful, may cause rectal itching, and if severe, may require surgery.

Body Position

The normal position used during defecation is squatting. The design of modern toilets facilitates this posture. This allows the person to properly lean forward, exert intra-abdominal pressure, and tighten the thigh muscles. When a patient is immobilized in bed, especially if in the supine position, he cannot contract the muscles used during defecation. To assist the patient to defecate when using a bedpan, raise the head of the bed to allow a more normal sitting position (refer to Skill 35.1).

Psychological Factors

Anxiety or anger can increase peristaltic activity for some people, resulting in diarrhea. Conversely, slower intestinal motility may result in people who are depressed, causing constipation. How people respond to these emotions depends on differences in the response of the enteric nervous system to vagal stimulation by the brain.

Pathological Conditions

Acquired brain injuries and spinal cord injuries can impair the sensory stimulation needed for defecation. Impaired physical mobility may limit the patient's ability to get assistance or reach a toilet, which may result in fecal incontinence or constipation. Fecal incontinence can also be the result of poorly functioning sphincters.

Bowel Elimination Problems

Common bowel elimination problems may result from emotional stress, physiological changes in the GI tract, disorders affecting defecation, or surgical alteration. These include constipation, impaction, diarrhea, incontinence, and flatulence.

Constipation

Constipation is a decrease in the frequency of bowel movements; the passing of hard, dry feces; and possibly difficult and painful defecation. Constipation usually occurs when there is slow motility in the bowel and if the feces stay in the large intestine too long. Everyone has their own unique pattern of bowel movements influenced by their age; level of activity; fluid intake; diet, including the amount of fibre they eat; stress levels; and perhaps medications they may be taking. It is important when you are collecting a health history to inquire what your patient's normal bowel habits are to establish a baseline to refer back to. As part of your assessment, ask about the use of laxatives, as overuse can contribute to chronic constipation. Feces may appear dry, small, and hard when the patient is constipated and will contribute to fecal impaction if the feces become stuck in the intestine.

As long as there is no associated pain or bloating, a bowel movement pattern of every 4 or more days may be considered normal. For an elderly patient, a bowel movement every 2 to 3 days, without bloating, bleeding, or pain, may be a normal elimination pattern. The nurse should be concerned if the patient's personal pattern changes.

Constipation is a significant health hazard, with straining causing problems to patients who have undergone recent gynecological, rectal, or abdominal surgery. Having difficulty passing feces can cause sutures to separate and the wound to reopen. Patients with cardiovascular disease, glaucoma, and increased intracranial pressure should prevent constipation and avoid using the Valsalva maneuver by exhaling through the mouth during straining.

Fecal Impaction

Fecal impaction occurs when feces accumulates in the rectum and is stuck. Impaction can occur when constipation is not relieved and there is no bowel movement for 3 to 5 days or more. Debilitated, unconscious, or confused patients are those at highest risk for impaction. The barium given for radiological exams of the GI tract can lead to fecal impaction, so measures (such as laxatives) are usually taken to ensure its removal following the test.

The patient may pass liquid or semiliquid feces (which have gone around the impacted or stuck feces) and complain of discomfort but not feel the urge to defecate and continues to complain of feeling full. Patients experiencing fecal impaction may experience abdominal distention, nausea, loss of appetite, and vomiting. Fecal impaction is uncomfortable and needs to be attended to quickly. If the nurse suspects an impaction, a gentle digital examination can be performed to assess the rectum and palpate the impacted mass. It is important to be careful and gentle because stimulating the vagus nerve in the rectal wall can cause the patient's heart rate to drop. However, although digital manipulation and manual removal may be necessary and falls within the nursing scope of practice, some agency policies require a physician's order. Other interventions may include oil retention and cleansing enemas, suppositories, or stool softeners. (See discussion of digital removal of a fecal impaction later in the chapter.)

Diarrhea

Increased GI motility results in **diarrhea** (watery feces) and can be accompanied by stomach pains, mucus, and flatulence. Diarrhea occurs when intestinal contents pass through the intestines too quickly to allow for fluid and nutrient absorption. Increased mucus secretion results from irritation within the colon; feces become more watery, making it difficult or impossible to control the urge to defecate. Diarrhea and the threat of bowel incontinence are sources of embarrassment and concern for the patient. Cramping is often associated with diarrhea; the patient may pass blood, and nausea and vomiting can also occur.

The causes of diarrhea are numerous and most often are the result of irritants that cause inflammation of the digestive tract and irritate the intestinal mucosa. Irritants may include certain foods, food allergies, alcohol, high bacteria levels, or unclean food or contaminated water. Diarrhea is a side effect of many medications, especially antibiotics, because they can disrupt the balance of healthy microbes in the GI tract.

You may have heard about *Clostridium difficile* or *C. difficile*. Our intestinal tract needs normal flora for a healthy mucous lining, and a healthy level of intestinal flora inhibits the growth of *C. difficile*, a spore-producing, Gram-positive, anaerobic bacillus. In patients with a compromised immune system or low levels of healthy flora, *C. difficile* can flourish and release toxins that cause diarrhea.

In infants, it can be difficult to assess diarrhea. A baby bottle-fed formula may have one firm feces every other day, but a breast-fed baby may have five to eight small, soft feces daily. As a result, it is important to note a sudden increase in the number of feces or thinner consistency (increase in fluid content) or if the feces tend to be greenish.

Complications

Serious fluid and electrolyte or acid–base imbalances can result from excess loss of fluid from the colon. Those at highest risk for associated complications are infants, small children, and older adults (see Chapter 33). Another potential complication is skin breakdown; intestinal contents are irritating and cause excoriation to the skin of the perineum and buttocks as diarrheal feces are repeatedly passed. Meticulous skin care and containment of fecal drainage are essential. Zinc oxide or other ointments can be used and the skin should be kept clean and dry. A fecal collector pouch can be used. Prolonged diarrhea will cause fatigue, malaise, weakness, and emaciation. Treating diarrhea involves removing the causes, slowing peristalsis, and providing supportive measures to restore and maintain fluid and electrolyte balance.

Fecal Incontinence

Bowel or **fecal incontinence** is the loss of the ability to voluntarily control passage of feces and gas through the anal sphincter. This may occur irregularly or at specific times, such as following meals. Conditions that impair control or function of the anal sphincter or its nerve supply or that create frequent, watery, large-volume feces can cause incontinence. People who experience fecal incontinence may be emotionally distressed and withdraw from social situations, confining themselves within their homes or hospital rooms to minimize embarrassment. It may harm a patient's body image and be embarrassing and degrading for the patient to have to rely on the nurse for this basic need. People experiencing incontinence may prefer to wear easily washable night garments instead of street clothes. Similarly to diarrhea, meticulous skin care is needed to protect the skin from the irritating and acidic incontinent feces; use of a rectal pouch is an option. Surgical procedures such as repair of the sphincter and fecal diversion or colostomy are used to treat fecal incontinence.

Flatulence

The bowel wall stretches and distends as gas accumulates (**flatulence**) in the intestines. This flatus (air or gas) is primarily caused by the action of bacteria on the chyme in the colon, gas that diffuses into the intestine from the bloodstream, or swallowed air. Drinking carbonated beverages, chewing gum, sucking on candies, smoking, anxiety, drinking from straws, and eating and drinking too quickly can all increase the amount of air swallowed. Intestinal gas is a common cause of abdominal fullness, cramping, and pain and normally escapes from the mouth (belching or eructation) or anus (passing flatus). However, when intestinal motility is slowed, by general anaesthetics, opioid analgesics, abdominal surgery, or immobilization, flatulence can become quite severe, causing abdominal distention and sharp pains. The patient may describe abdominal distention as a feeling of discomfort and fullness. The distended abdomen will appear convexly shaped or protuberant (more than slightly rounded) on inspection. Insertion of a rectal tube or return flow enema may be needed to remove excessive gas. Many high-fibre foods, and notably cabbage, legumes, and onions, often cause increased flatus. As a result, gas-producing foods may best be avoided and increasing dietary fibre should be done gradually. Flatus can also be prevented with movement (ambulation/exercise) to stimulate peristalsis and help the gas escape or get reabsorbed.

Assessment

To assess fecal elimination, the nurse obtains subjective data from the patient, with a nursing history and objective data from physical examination of the patient's abdomen, rectum, and anus. The nurse also inspects the feces and reviews any relevant diagnostic test results.

Nursing History

Although it can be embarrassing for the patient and new nursing student, it is important to gather information about the patient's current bowel elimination pattern. This can include information the nurse obtains from the chart, the patient, or significant others about the patient's normal pattern of elimination; usual characteristics of feces, changes to the patient's normal pattern (bowel elimination patterns vary largely from person to person), any medications, preexisting conditions, or other factors that impact elimination; the presence of an ostomy; and when the patient's last bowel movement was.

Physical Examination

A physical examination of the abdomen includes inspection, auscultation, percussion, and palpation, in this order. Auscultation of bowel sounds must occur prior to palpation, because palpation can stimulate peristalsis. The nurse inspects the area around the anus (perianal area) for any abnormalities, including the presence of hemorrhoids, inflammation, discolourations, or lesions. Refer to Chapter 20 on health assessment and your health assessment textbook for additional information.

Inspection of Feces

The nurse inspects the consistency, colour, shape, odour, and amount of the patient's feces. The feces are examined for the presence of abnormal components such as mucus, parasites, blood, pus, and large quantities of fat or foreign objects.

Diagnostic Studies

There are direct and indirect visualization techniques used to assess the GI tract. In addition, laboratory tests identify abnormal components.

Visualization Techniques

Direct visualization techniques allow the actual viewing of the GI tract. This includes the anal canal (anoscopy), rectum (proctoscopy), rectum and sigmoid colon (proctosigmoidoscopy/sigmoidoscopy), and the large intestine (colonoscopy). X-ray (roentgenography) is used for indirect visualization of the GI tract and can detect obstructions, tumours, ulcers, inflammatory disease, strictures, or such structural changes as a hiatal hernia. Barium, a radiopaque substance, enhances the radiographs. The patient will drink barium sulphate to visualize the upper GI tract or small bowel, or to examine the lower GI tract, the nurse will administer a barium enema. Fluoroscopic examination allows the examiner to watch the flow of barium continuously.

Diagnostic examinations used to visualize GI structures usually require that portions of the bowel be empty of feces. This may involve the use of cathartics and an enema given until the expelled contents are clear. In addition, patients are instructed not to eat or drink anything after midnight (NPO) of the day prior to the examination.

Laboratory Tests

Laboratory tests of fecal contents can identify tumours, infection, and blood.

Collecting Feces Specimens

The nurse is responsible for properly collecting and labeling feces specimens in the appropriate containers and transporting them to the laboratory on time. Instructions to patients include the following: try not to contaminate the feces with urine or menstrual discharge by voiding prior; use a clean bedpan or bedside commode; do not place toilet tissue in the bedpan after defecating; and notify the nurse immediately after defecating, especially if the specimen needs to be sent to the laboratory in a timely manner. When transferring the feces sample to the appropriate specimen container, it is important to wear disposable gloves and follow aseptic technique. It is important to follow the specific instructions for each test, often on the specimen container, to ensure the specimen is obtained properly, including the proper amount and whether it has to be sent immediately to the lab or refrigerated to avoid bacteriological changes. If unsure of the specific instructions, ask laboratory staff.

Testing Feces for Occult Blood

Testing feces for **occult (hidden) blood** (referred to as the *guaiac test*) is used to detect blood from the GI tract present in the feces but not visible to the eye (microscopic amounts). Tumours, ulcers, and inflammatory disease can cause GI bleeding. The nurse can perform this test in the clinical area or it can be sent to the laboratory. The patient can also perform this test at home. The Hemoccult test is the most common guaiac test and involves using a chemical reagent to detect the peroxidase enzyme that is present in the hemoglobin molecule, thereby identifying occult blood. The patient or nurse uses a tongue depressor to transfer a small amount of feces on a card or slide and closes the card. The card is flipped over and reagent is dropped onto the smear on the back. A colour change is observed: blue means blood is present (guaiac positive); any other colour indicates a negative test result. Prior to obtaining a feces sample for this test, the patient must avoid certain foods and medications or the results will be inaccurate. If the patient has recently eaten red meat, radishes, turnips, horseradish, or melons or taken medications that irritate the gastric mucosa (such as acetylsalicylic acid/aspirin or other nonsteroidal anti-inflammatories, steroids, iron preparation, or an anticoagulant), false-positive results may occur. If the patient takes or consumes vitamin C (from food sources or supplements) up to 3 days prior to the test, false-negative results may occur even if bleeding is present.

Nursing Interventions to Promote Regular Defecation

Promoting regular elimination of feces requires adequate amounts of fluids and fibre in the diet as well as opportunities to defecate when the urge occurs, proper positioning, adequate exercise, and privacy.

Medications Affecting Bowel Elimination

Medications may be needed to help induce a bowel movement, relieve flatulence, or control diarrhea by slowing motility.

Laxatives and Cathartics

Patients may need the help of cathartics and laxatives to help empty the bowel to relieve constipation or impaction or as preparation for GI tests and abdominal surgery. Cathartics have a strong, purging effect and include such medications as castor oil, bisacodyl (Dulcolax), and cascara. In comparison, laxatives are milder, producing frequent soft or liquid feces.

These medications are available in oral and suppository forms. Although the oral route is commonly used, suppository cathartics are more effective because they directly stimulate the rectal mucosa. An example of a suppository is bisacodyl that can act within 30 minutes and often causes a strong sudden urge to defecate among older adults. See Table 35.7 for a description of the different types of laxatives.

Older adults in particular often use laxatives improperly. The repeated self-administration of laxatives can lead to chronic constipation by weakening the bowel's natural response to being distended by feces. It is important to encourage a more natural approach to regular defecation by increasing dietary fibre, adequate fluid intake, etc.

TABLE 35.7	Types of Laxatives	
Type	**How They Work**	**Important Information**
	Saline	
Magnesium citrate Magnesium hydroxide (Phillips' Milk of Magnesia) Sodium phosphates (Fleet Enema)	Draw water into the intestines, increasing pressure, which stimulates peristalsis	May be fast acting Prolonged use may affect fluid and electrolyte levels (especially in people with cardiac and renal diseases). Do not use phosphate salts for patients on fluid restriction.
	Irritant/Stimulant	
Senna (Senokot) Bisacodyl (Dulcolax) Castor oil	Irritate the intestinal mucosa or stimulate the nerve endings of the intestinal wall Alter secretion of water and electrolytes	May cause malabsorption, weight loss, and discolour urine May cause severe cramping Prolonged use may cause fluid and electrolyte imbalances.
	Bulk-Producing	
Methylcellulose (Citrucel) Psyllium (Metamucil) Wheat dextrin (Benefiber)	Absorb water (high-fibre content); stimulate peristalsis by adding bulk and stretching intestinal wall	Safe for long-term use Sufficient fluid intake necessary to avoid obstruction May take 12 hours to 3 days to work
	Lubricant	
Mineral oil	Reduces absorption of fecal water in the colon; coats and lubricates feces for easier passage	Oral use long-term may cause lipid pneumonia if aspirated into lungs. Can increase risk for fat emboli when taken with emollients Affects absorption of fat-soluble vitamins
	Surfactants/Stool Softener	
Docusate/Senna (Peri-Colace) Docusate sodium (Colace) Docusate calcium (Surfak)	Docusate—stool softener Senna—mild irritant Detergent that lowers surface tension of feces and allows fat and water to penetrate, softening feces	Slow-acting Not for treatment of chronic constipation; used to prevent constipation
	Osmotic	
Glycerin suppository	Hyperosmotic action (draws water into the bowel); local irritant	Prolonged use may cause fluid and electrolyte imbalances. Replace fluid loss.
Lactulose	Produces osmotic effect in bowel, retaining fluid, causing distention and stimulating peristalsis	
Polyethylene glycol	Nonabsorbable; acts as osmotic agent causing water to be retained in feces	
Sodium sulfate, magnesium sulfate, potassium sulfate	Hyperosmotic action (draws water into the bowel)	
Sorbitol 70%	Produces osmotic effect in bowel, retaining fluid, causing distention and stimulating peristalsis	

Adapted from Lexi-Comp Online. (2014). *Laxatives, classification and properties.* Hudson, OH: Lexi-Comp.

Antiflatulent Medications

Antiflatulent medications (e.g., simethicone) do not decrease flatus production, but they do help facilitate passage through the mouth (belching) or anus. Often, these agents contain an antacid to help neutralize stomach acid and relieve discomfort. Suppositories may help by increasing intestinal motility.

Antidiarrheal Medications

Antidiarrheal medications (e.g., loperamide) slow intestinal motility or absorb extra fluid in the intestine. It is important to determine the cause of the diarrhea, because treating with an antidiarrheal when the cause is a toxin, poison, or infection may cause the diarrhea to persist even longer. Long-term use of antidiarrheal medication available without a prescription (over-the-counter) may lead to dependence. Opiates are effective for treating diarrhea, but also may be habit forming and should be used cautiously.

Administering Enemas

An **enema** is fluid that is placed into the rectum and works by distending the intestine and sometimes also irritates the intestinal mucosa, causing peristalsis to increase, which expels both feces and flatus. Enemas are given to administer medication, prepare the patient for diagnostic tests such as colonoscopies, and before bowel surgery. Some enemas deliver medication, but the most common enemas that you will administer are to relieve gas, constipation, or fecal impaction. The physician may order a cleansing enema to be delivered "high" or "low." This refers to the height of the enema solution bag. Enema solution that is held higher delivers the enema solution with more pressure. The high enema is intended to cleanse the entire colon. There are several types of enemas. See Table 35.8 for common enema solutions and refer to Skill 35.6 for administration of an enema.

Digital Removal of Fecal Impaction

Fecal impaction acts like a plug, blocking feces from moving through to the anus and defecation. The impacted feces may need to be physically removed using a lubricated gloved finger. This procedure can be embarrassing for the patient so you will need to provide privacy, use a calm matter-of-fact approach, and be organized by taking all the equipment that you will need to the room. Equipment necessary for

TABLE 35.8	Common Enema Solutions	
Cleansing Enemas	**Type of Solution**	**Special Considerations**
Cleansing enemas are given to completely evacuate the contents of the colon. A large amount of fluid or the irritation caused by the solution stimulates peristalsis.	Tap water—hypotonic solution with a lower osmotic pressure than the fluids in the interstitial spaces that surround the bowel. Fluid administered stimulates defecation before moving into the interstitial spaces around the bowel.	Should not be repeated due to the risk of water toxicity or circulatory overload if water is absorbed from the colon into the interstitial spaces from the bowel lumen
Most commonly ordered for constipation	Normal saline—safest solution with the same osmotic pressure as the fluids surrounding the bowel in the interstitial spaces	Children should only receive normal saline enemas due to the risk of fluid imbalance.
Each solution has a different osmotic effect on the colon.	Stimulates peristalsis Soapsuds—promote irritation of the lining of the bowel to stimulate peristalsis	Only pure castile soap is safe to use. It is a liquid soap and comes in little packets that are on the units with enema kits.
	Commercially prepared fleet enemas are a hypertonic solution. The hypertonic solution works by pulling fluid into the bowel from the interstitial spaces that surround the bowel. The additional fluid drawn into the colon enlarges or distends the bowel lumen and promotes the passage of feces.	Fleet enemas can be irritating. Patients who cannot tolerate large volumes of fluid may be able to tolerate a fleet enema better. Should not be administered to young patients or patients who are dehydrated Following the administration of the enema, the patient should change from the left side lying or lateral position to the dorsal recumbent position and then to the right lateral position to ensure that the enema fluid moves around the entire colon.
Oil retention enemas	The oil acts as a lubricant in the bowel. The feces absorb the oil and become softer. This process takes time so the patient is expected to retain the enema for up to several hours.	The challenge for administering this type of enema is that it has to be held by the patient in the rectum for up to several hours and may be uncomfortable.
Medicated enemas	Medication is sometimes administered in an enema.	An example of a medicated enema is an enema that contains an antibiotic. Medicated enemas may be ordered prior to bowel surgery to reduce the amount of bacteria in the bowel.

this procedure includes (1) multiple disposable gloves and a gown for yourself, (2) packets of water-soluble lubricant, (3) protection for the bed and floor, and (4) a bedpan and a commode chair close by if you are able to transfer the patient safely. You should instruct the patient to turn to a side-lying position, insert a gloved and lubricated index finger into the rectum, and use a gentle sweeping motion to remove the hardened feces. Be gentle as the bowel can be easily perforated. Once the impacted feces are removed, the patient may then be able to pass a normal bowel movement on a bedpan or the commode chair that you have nearby. Take special precautions to provide for the patient's safety throughout the procedure and provide hygiene care afterward. This intervention can be stressful for the patient and he or she will appreciate the room being well ventilated and the soiled pads with feces being removed as quickly as possible.

Bowel Training Programs

Patients who are recovering from a neurological impairment (e.g., a head injury, stroke, or paralysis) may require a bowel training program (Craven, Hirnle, & Jensen, 2013) to manage their bowel elimination. The goals of bowel retraining are (1) to maintain the consistency of the feces for easier passage and (2) to develop a routine where the patient can defecate at the same time each day using the same techniques to control the pattern of elimination. The patient will take stool softeners, a bulk-producing agent, and use suppositories in preparation for a routine that usually takes place after breakfast each day. A common routine would include taking the prescribed medications, followed by toileting and digital stimulation of the anal opening at the same time every morning (Craven et al., 2013). Strategies to facilitate bowel retraining include pelvic floor exercises, biofeedback techniques, encouragement, reassurance, and abdominal massage.

Jaswinder has prepared herself to care for patients with fecal incontinence by ensuring that she takes all the necessary supplies to the bedside. By being organized, efficient, and using a matter-of-fact approach, she will minimize the stress experienced by herself and her patient.

Bowel Diversion Ostomies

An opening created in the abdominal wall to eliminate feces or urine is called an *ostomy*. There are many types of ostomies, including urinary diversions discussed earlier in the chapter. There are two main types of ostomy used to divert and drain feces: ileostomy and colostomy. An **ileostomy** is an opening into the small bowel (ileum) and a **colostomy** opens into the large bowel (colon). Ostomies used to divert the bowel can be differentiated by whether they are temporary or permanent, their anatomical location, and the construction of the opening (*stoma*). Temporary colostomies may be created for inflammatory conditions to allow the diseased portion of bowel to heal. A permanent colostomy creates a way to expel feces when the rectum or anus cannot function. This may be due to a birth defect or bowel cancer. The portion of the bowel that is diseased may or may not be removed.

The expected output from an ostomy depends on the location. Because the large bowel absorbs water from feces, an ostomy further along the bowel is more formed. An ileostomy produces liquid feces, is constant, and cannot be regulated. Digestive enzymes make the output even more irritating to peristomal skin. For ileostomies, odour is minimal due to fewer bacteria, when compared to colostomies.

Types of Stomas

The types of surgical stomas include single, divided, loop, or double-barreled colostomies. A permanent single (end or terminal) stoma is created by bringing one end of bowel through an opening on the anterior abdominal wall. A divided stoma has two separated edges of bowel brought out onto the abdomen. The proximal, digestive end is the colostomy, whereas the distal end continues to secrete mucus (commonly referred to as a *mucous fistula*). A loop stoma has two ends: the proximal (active) end and the distal (inactive) end. This is usually done as an emergency procedure; it is bulky and harder to manage than a single colostomy. A double-barreled colostomy has proximal and distal loops sutured together with both ends brought up onto the abdomen (see Fig. 35.9).

Ostomy Management

To assist the patient with a fecal diversion, you will need to provide physical care, instruction, and psychological support. See if your agency has a specially trained enterostomal therapy nurse you can collaborate with to provide the proper support and care. There are often multiple community resources available, including national organizations that have local chapters such as the United Ostomy Association of Canada that can provide information and practical and emotional support.

Skin and Stoma Care

All patients who have ostomies require proper skin and stoma care. Fecal contents from a colostomy or ileostomy are irritating to the skin surrounding the stoma. As a result, the peristomal skin should be assessed each time the appliance is changed and any skin breakdown or irritation addressed immediately. The skin should be kept clean by washing and drying thoroughly.

A properly selected ostomy appliance collects feces, controls odour, protects the skin, and is comfortable and inconspicuous. A skin barrier and pouch make up the appliance,

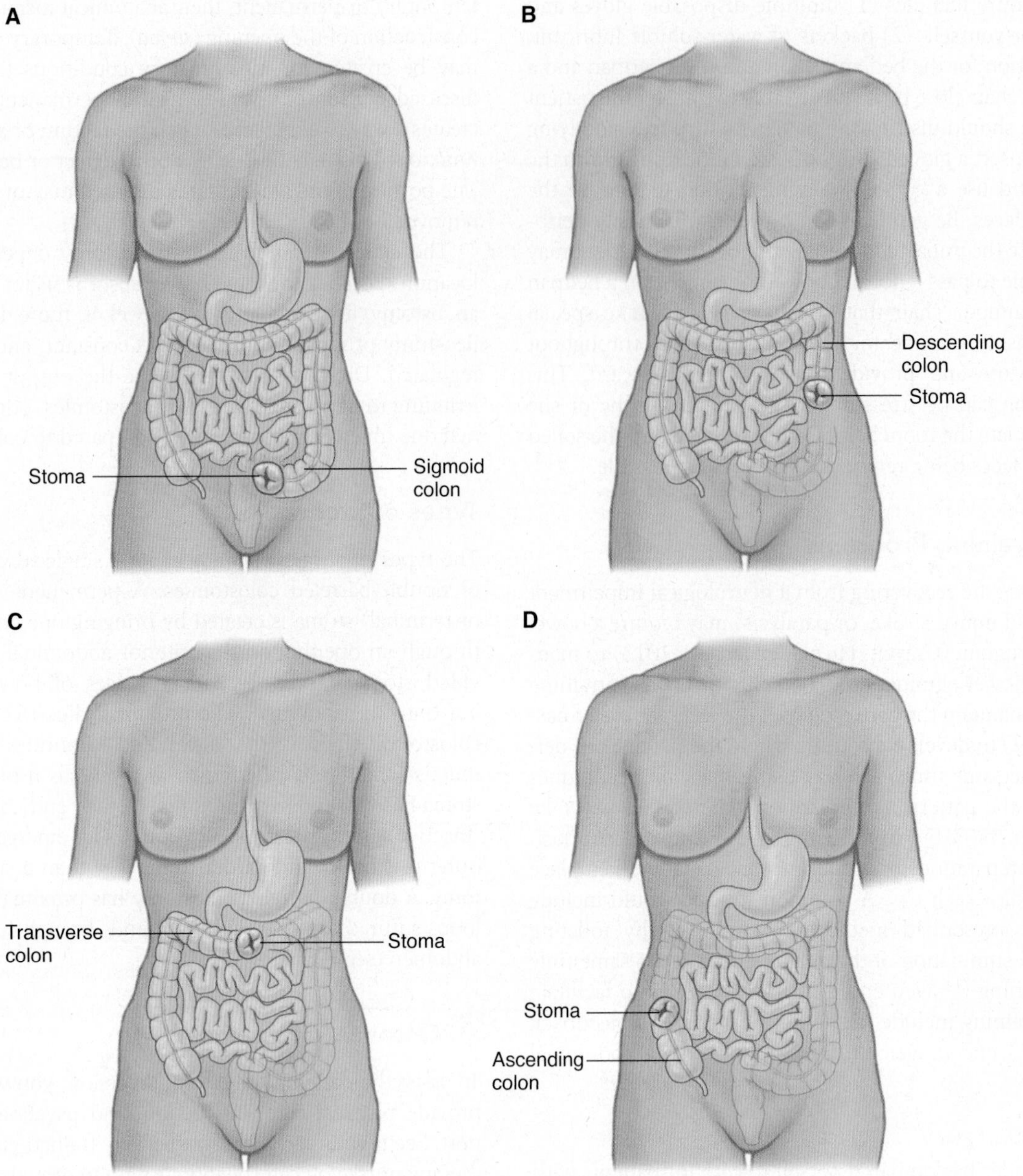

A

Stoma — ⊙ — Sigmoid colon

B

Descending colon

Stoma

C

Transverse colon — Stoma

D

Stoma

Ascending colon

Figure 35.9 Different types of ostomies.

but some patients may prefer to use an adjustable ostomy belt to help hold the pouch firmly in place. There are one-piece ostomy appliances that have the skin barrier already attached to the pouch or two-piece appliances that have a separate skin barrier with flange that connects to a pouch with flange. When using a two-piece appliance, the pouch can be removed for emptying or changing without disrupting the skin barrier. Available skin barriers include pastes, liquid films, and powders. There are also closed and drainable pouches. Unlike a closed pouch, a drainable pouch has a removable clip or integrated closure at the end. Closed are appropriate for a patient who has a regular stoma discharge that only requires emptying once or twice daily, whereas drainable pouches are usually used by patients who need to empty the pouch more than twice daily (refer to Skill 35.7).

To protect the patient's self-esteem, help him or her with odour control. Ambulatory patients should be taught and encouraged to empty the ostomy in the bathroom, avoiding bedside odours. Other important considerations for controlling odour include choosing the appropriate appliance, ensuring it remains intact, and rinsing it thoroughly every time it is emptied. Other methods to control odours include placing a deodorizer in the pouch or selecting a pouch with a charcoal filter.

Follow agency protocol to determine how often to change an intact ostomy appliance. The maximum is 7 days. If feces from the stoma leak onto the peristomal skin or cannot be completely rinsed away, the appliance must be changed. Although the patient may prefer to change his or her appliance daily or whenever soiled, this is not recommended. Frequent changes can cause skin damage and are an unnecessary expense, unless the patient complains of pain or discomfort or has already experienced skin breakdown. Some people choose to remove the entire appliance twice weekly to clean and inspect the skin. For more information on ostomy care and maintenance, including how to change an ostomy appliance, see Skill 35.7.

Irrigating a Colostomy

A colostomy irrigation is a form of stoma management for patients with a sigmoid or descending colostomy. It is similar to an enema. It is unnecessary for ileostomies because the feces are usually liquid. Colostomy irrigation is used to distend the bowel enough that it stimulates peristalsis, which causes evacuation and also eliminates gas and odour. Irrigation should be performed at the same time of day and with the same frequency. It becomes unnecessary to wear a colostomy pouch when a regular pattern of evacuation is achieved (although some patients prefer to wear a smaller pouch over the stoma in case of fecal spillage). Because irrigation allows regaining of some control of fecal elimination, patients may find this helps with the emotional adjustment of living with a colostomy. However, many patients find the procedure to be unpleasant and it can take 45 to 60 minutes to perform. Some patients may choose instead to use rigid dietary regulation. Using irrigation to control evacuation also requires some control of the diet, including the avoidance of foods with a laxative effect.

The amount of fluid needed to stimulate varies from patient to patient. For most, a relatively small amount (300 to 500 ml)

is enough, but for others, up to 1,000 ml may be necessary. The fluid is instilled into the colon through the stoma, and because it has no sphincter, the fluid often returns as it is instilled. This may be reduced with the use of a cone on the irrigating catheter that helps keep the fluid in the bowel during the process. Some potential complications of colostomy irrigation include bowel perforation, peristomal hernias, and electrolyte imbalance (when irrigating large volumes of fluid). These problems are more common among patients who have been using irrigation for several years. The risk for bowel perforation is reduced by ensuring the proper specific equipment is used and by irrigating gently. An enema set should never be used to irrigate a colostomy.

Jaswinder is feeling more confident in assisting her patients with their bowel and bladder needs. Most patients are able to use the toilet with minimal assistance, but others require her help to measure output, apply ostomy devices, ambulate while walking with a urinary catheter inserted, and to use toilet aids such as a commode or an elevated toilet seat. Jaswinder is quite surprised that there are so many skills to learn so that she can safely assist her patients to meet their elimination needs. She is very pleased that she is able to practice skills in the nursing lab before doing them with real patients. Her personal fears about the odours associated with fecal incontinence interfering with her ability to provide care have been lessened by using a matter-of-fact approach to meeting the needs of her patients.

SKILL 35.1 | Assisting the Patient Using a Bedpan

Purpose

- Allows a patient restricted to bed rest to defecate in a receptacle
- Maintains continence despite limited mobility
- Male patients use a bedpan for feces and a urinal for urine
- Female patients use a bedpan for both feces and urine
- See Figure 1 and Figure 2

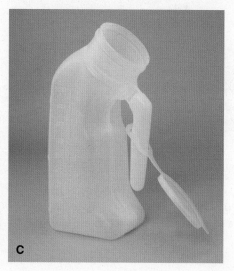

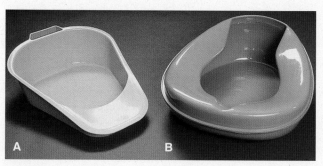

Figure 1

(continued on page 938)

SKILL 35.1   Assisting the Patient Using a Bedpan (continued)

Purpose

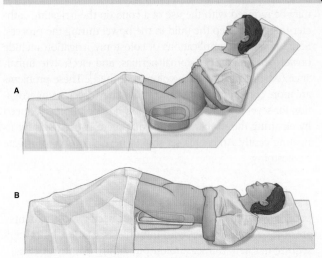

Figure 2

Step	Rationale
• Thoroughly wash hands and use appropriate protective equipment.	• Prevents the spread of infection.
• Provide patient privacy.	• Use of a bedpan is uncomfortable and often embarrassing; providing privacy will help the patient.
• Elevate the side rail on the opposite side of the bed.	• A safety measure to prevent the patient from falling.
• Adjust the height of the bed to a level appropriate to prevent back strain.	• Risk of injury to the nurse is decreased by the use of proper body mechanics.
• Encourage the patient to assist by flexing his or her knees, directing his or her weight to the back of the heels and raising the buttocks. A trapeze bar may be used if available.	• When able, encourage the patient to be active in self-care.
• Assist the patient in lifting by placing one hand under the lower back while resting your elbow on the mattress, using your forearm as a lever.	• The risk of injury to the nurse is decreased by the use of proper lifting techniques; it also provides a sense of security to the patient.
• Position a regular bedpan so that the patient's buttocks rest on the smooth, rounded rim. If using a fracture pan, place it with the flat, lower end under the patient's buttocks (see Figure 3).	• Patient comfort is increased and spillage is avoided with proper placement of the bedpan.

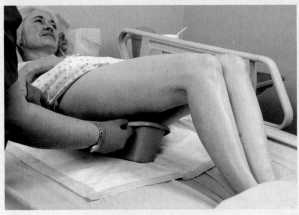

Figure 3

• If the patient is unable to assist with the placement of the bedpan, a second nurse is required to assist in the positioning.

Additional assistance decreases the risk of back injury to the nurse.

Purpose (continued)

Step	Rationale
• Turn the patient onto his or her side and place the bedpan against the buttocks then roll the patient back onto the bedpan (see Figure 4).	• Moving the patient onto his or her side and then back allows for proper placement of the bedpan without the patient having to lift.

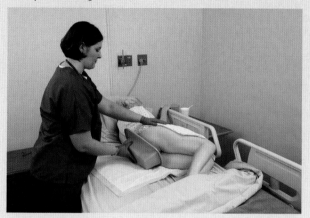

Figure 4

• If permitted, elevate the patient's bed to a semi-Fowler position, providing a more normal lower back position. If elevation is not permitted, provide the patient lower back support with pillows.	• Using pillows or elevating the bed provides for patient comfort and decreases the risk of hyperextension of the back.
• Cover the patient with a bed sheet.	• Assists in maintaining patient dignity and comfort.
• Provide the patient with toilet tissue and place the call bell within his or her reach and, if permitted, leave the patient alone.	• Privacy may make it easier for the patient to have a bowel movement. Encouraging the patient to wipe himself or herself if able promotes self-care.
• Respond to the patient promptly; only allow a maximum of 15 minutes on the bedpan unless the patient is able to remove it independently.	• Pressure ulcers can be caused by excessive time spent on a bedpan.
• Wear gloves when removing the bedpan. Hold the bedpan steady and cover the bedpan and carefully place on a nearby chair with a disposable pad on it. Return the patient to a comfortable position.	• Prevents spilling of bedpan contents, reduces contamination of patient surfaces (the chair), and promotes patient comfort and dignity.
• If assistance is required, wipe the perineum with several layers of toilet tissue; for a female, ensure to wipe from the urethra toward the anus. If specimen collection is required, discard the soiled tissue in a waterproof receptacle other than the bedpan.	• Proper cleansing prevents transfer of microorganisms into the urinary meatus.
• If the patient is dependent, wash the perineal area with soap and water and dry the area thoroughly.	• Proper cleansing helps to prevent excoriation caused by feces left on the skin.
• Offer all patients warm water, soap, a washcloth, and towel for hand washing. Empty and clean the bedpan and then return it to the bedside.	• Assists in preventing infection and increasing patient comfort.
• Remove and dispose of your gloves and wash hands.	• Prevents cross-contamination.
• Appropriately document the odour, colour, amount, and consistency of the urine and feces as well as the condition of the perineum.	• Proper documentation is necessary to track changes in bowel patterns and to help prevent related complication (e.g., constipation).

SKILL 35.2	Specimen Collection—Collecting a Midstream Urine (Clean-Catch)

Purpose

Tests for the presence of microorganisms, the type of organism(s), and the antibodies that the organisms are sensitive.

Step	Rationale
Check the chart and determine: • The purpose for the test.	Important to know why the patient needs a urine sample collected, as this will determine the procedure used to collect the specimen.
Assess: • The patient's understanding of the procedure. • The following: when did the patient last void, the patient's ability to urinate on request. • Physical and intellectual ability to collect the specimen independently.	An alert patient may be instructed to collect the clean-catch sample on his or her own with clear directions.
Prepare the equipment by: • Gathering clean gloves, antiseptic towelettes, sterile cotton balls or 5 × 5 gauze pads, sterile specimen container, specimen label, and laboratory requisition form. • If the patient is not able to ambulate, also obtain a urine receptacle and a basin of warm water, soap, a washcloth, and a towel.	Protective equipment not only ensures the safety of the nurse but is also important to decrease the risk of contamination of the specimen.
Prepare the patient by: • Identifying the patient using patient identifiers such as patient number or date of birth. • Explaining the need for a urine specimen, purpose of the test, and the method that will be used for collection. • Providing clear directions to a patient alert and capable of collecting the sample independently.	
Wash hands and use gloves and other necessary protective equipment.	Reduces the risk of transmission of microorganisms to both patient and nurse.

Performing the Skill

Step	Rationale
If the patient is ambulatory and able to independently collect the sample, instruct him or her on cleansing. • Wash and dry the genitals and perineum with soap and water. • Using antiseptic towelettes, clean the urinary meatus. Female patients (see Figure 1)	• Reduces bacteria that may contaminate the specimen.

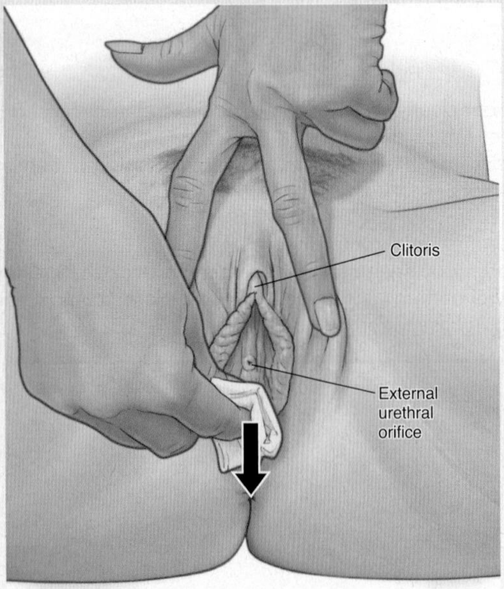

Clitoris

External urethral orifice

Figure 1

• Using each towelette only once, clean the perineum wiping from front to back.	• Wiping from front to back will clean from the area of least to greatest contamination.

Performing the Skill (continued)	
Step	**Rationale**

Step

Male patients (see Figure 2)

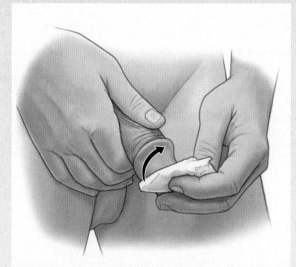

Figure 2

- If uncircumcised, gently retract the foreskin to expose the urinary meatus.
- Use a circular motion to clean the urinary meatus and the distal portion of the penis. Using each towelette only once, clean several centimeters down the shaft of the penis.

If the patient is unable to ambulate or collect the specimen independently, assist him or her to an upright position on a clean commode or bedpan.
- Put on clean gloves
- Clean the urinary meatus and perineal area as outlined earlier.

Collect the specimen from the patient or instruct a capable patient on how to collect it.
- Instruct the patient to begin voiding.

- While ensuring not to touch the container to the perineum or penis, place the specimen container into the midstream of urine.
- Collect the urine into the container.

- Tightly place the cap on the container while touching only the cap and the outside of the container.
- Clean the outside of the container with appropriate disinfectant if necessary.

Label and transport the specimen.
- Ensure the appropriate label is attached to the specimen container and not the lid.
- Ensure the order entry has been input correctly and that the laboratory requisition is correct.
- Place the specimen and requisition in a plastic bag and arrange for immediate transport to the laboratory.

Document
- In the patient's chart, record the time of collection and any observations made such as the colour, odour, and consistency of the sample.
- Ensure to include on the lab slip if the patient is taking antibiotics or is menstruating.

Rationale

- This method cleans from the area of least contamination to the greatest.

- Assisting the patient to a normal anatomical position will facilitate comfort and urination.

- The first few millimetres of urine expelled clears bacteria in the distal urethra and urinary meatus.
- Avoids contaminating the inside of the specimen container as well as the sample.

- Prevents contamination and spilling.

- Prevents transfer of microorganisms to others handling the specimen.

- Accurate labeling and information decreases errors and facilitates timely diagnosis and treatment.

- Immediately starting bacterial cultures prior to the growth of any contaminate organisms decreases the risk of false results.

SKILL 35.3   Applying an External Condom Catheter

Purpose

To collect urine using an external drainage system, allowing for less contact between the urine and skin due to incontinence.

Step	Rationale
Check the chart and determine: • The order and assess the patient's urinary pattern. Assess: • The patient's ability to cooperate with the application and use of the condom catheter. • The integrity of the skin around the penis and perineal area.	• To ensure the condom catheter is the required intervention. • To determine the type and degree of teaching required and if this is the most appropriate continence management for the patient. • Ensure no swelling or excoriation is present, contraindicating the use of the condom catheter. Also provides baseline information for comparison of future assessments.
Prepare the equipment by: • Gathering clean gloves, condom catheter sheath, urinary or leg drainage bag, a drape, basin of warm water and soap, washcloths and towel, and elastic tape/Velcro strap. • Assembling the selected drainage bag for attachment to the condom catheter. • Rolling the condom outward onto itself for easier application. Prepare the patient by: • Introducing yourself to the patient; identify the patient using appropriate identifiers. • Explaining the procedure as well as how he can assist and cooperate. • Positioning the patient in a supine or sitting position, ensuring for comfort. • Raising the bed to a height comfortable for the nurse. Wash hands and apply clean gloves.	 • The patient will tolerate the procedure better if comfortable; a supine position facilitates cleaning of the penis and application of the catheter. • Raising the bed supports good body mechanics. Reduces the transmission of microorganisms and protects the nurse from contact with bodily fluids.

Performing the Skill

Step	Rationale
• Protect patient privacy by closing the door or drawing the curtains. • Drape the patient allowing for privacy, exposing only the penis. • Clean the genitals with warm soapy water, retracting the foreskin if the patient is uncircumcised, ensuring to return the foreskin to the normal position. Dry well. • If the patient becomes erect at any time during the procedure • Some condom catheter kits may include skin preparation wipes and double-sided adhesive tape. Use the preparation and apply the tape in a spiral manner 1 in. from the base of the penis.	• Reduces patient embarrassment. • Minimizes microorganisms that may cause infection. Returning the foreskin to the normal position prevents swelling and constriction once the catheter is in place. • Using a spiral formation when applying the adhesive promotes circulation, preventing edema.

Performing the Skill (continued)

Step

Place the rolled condom at the end of the penis; smoothly unroll it over the penis, leaving 2.5–5 cm between the end of the penis and the connecting tube (see Figure 1).

Rationale

- The extra space prevents irritation and pressure at the tip of the penis and allows for proper drainage of urine.

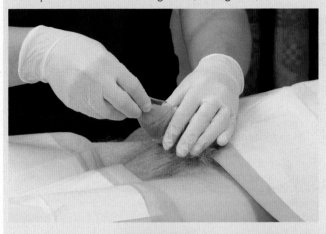

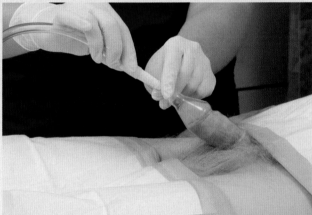

Figure 1

- Gently press the condom against the adhesive strip provided. If no strip or special tape was provided, use a piece of elastic tape or Velcro around the base of the penis in a spiral manner.
- Attach the drainage bag tubing securely to the catheter tubing. Ensure the tip of the penis is not in contact with the condom and that the condom is not twisted.
- Remove gloves and wash hands.
- Ensure the tubing lies over the patient's leg and not under.
- Attach the drainage bag to the side of the bed, instructing the patient to keep the bag below the level of the condom and to avoid looping or kinking the tubing.
- If the patient is ambulatory, attach the drainage bag to the patients leg.
- Thirty minutes following the procedure, assess the penis for swelling or discolouration. If the patient has voided, assess urine flow. Document the findings.
- The condom should be changed and skin care provided.

Document

- Use narrative notes when necessary in addition to forms and checklists.
- Include the time, application of the condom, and important observations.

- Regular tape is not used because it is not flexible and may inhibit blood flow.

- If the condom is twisted or the tip of the penis is blocking the tubing, the flow of urine may be obstructed.

- Promotes urine flow into the drainage bag.
- Keeping the drainage bag below the condom level reduces the occurrence of reflux onto the penis and the introduction of microorganisms.
- Attaching the drainage bag to the leg helps to control movement of the tubing, preventing the material from twisting.
- Swelling or discolouration indicates the condom is too tight. Urine in the tube is present if flow is not obstructed.

SKILL 35.4 Urethral Urinary Catheterization

Purpose

- To complete emptying of the bladder preoperatively
- To monitor urinary output in critically ill patients
- To relieve discomfort related to bladder distention
- To assess residual urine following incomplete bladder emptying
- To obtain a sterile sample
- To provide for intermittent or continuous drainage and/or irrigation
- To keep urine from contacting perineal incisions following surgery
- Incontinence management

Step	Rationale
Check the chart and determine: • The physician's order. • The purpose of the test. Assess: • The required method of catheterization; indwelling or straight and size of catheter. • The patient's ability to cooperate, remain still, and lie in a supine position for the procedure. • When the patient last voided or was catheterized. • Percuss the bladder to check for fullness or distention. • If possible, complete a bladder scan.	It is important to determine why the test has been ordered to allow for appropriate follow-up and assessment. • A straight catheter should be used for temporary decompression/emptying, sample collection, or to assess residual. • An indwelling catheter should be used for ongoing bladder emptying and output measurement/collection. • To determine the amount of urine present in the bladder and the necessity of the catheterization.
Prepare the equipment by: • Gathering an appropriate-sized catheter with an extra one on hand and a catheterization kit including sterilized gloves, waterproof drapes, antiseptic, forceps, lubricant, urine receptacle, specimen container, and disposable clean gloves. • An indwelling catheter also requires a prefilled syringe, a collection bag, and tubing. Prepare the patient by: • Verifying the patient's identity using appropriate identifiers. • Explaining the need for the procedure and how the patient can cooperate. • Assisting the patient into the appropriate position Female: supine with knees flexed, feet spread about 50 cm apart, and hips slightly externally rotated, if possible. Male: supine, thighs slightly abducted or apart. • Providing for privacy. • Establishing adequate lighting, using a lamp if necessary. • Performing routine perineal care.	The use of sterile equipment decreases the risk of infection transmission.
Perform hand hygiene.	Reduces the risk of transmission of disease to patient and nurse.

Performing the Skill

Step	Rationale
• Stand on the appropriate side of the patient's bed; if you are right-handed, stand on the right side of the patient, stand on the left side if you are left-handed. • If inserting an indwelling catheter, open the drainage bag and place it within reach. • If your agency uses Xylocaine gel, apply clean gloves and apply 10–15 ml of Xylocaine gel into the urethra of the male patient. Wait at least 5 minutes before proceeding. • Open the catheterization kit while ensuring the container and contents remain sterile. • Place a waterproof drape under the buttocks (female) or penis (male), making sure not to contaminate the centre of the drape with your hands. • Put on sterile gloves. • Organize the supplies on the sterile field. Open the sterile catheter package; if necessary, saturate cotton balls with sterile antiseptic. Open lubricant package. If collecting a sample, remove the lid from the specimen container and loosely place it on top; place nearby.	One hand will be needed to hold the catheter and it will be difficult to open the package with only one available hand. Xylocaine may be used to decrease discomfort in the male patient. Waiting at least 5 minutes allows the medication to take effect. Maintaining the sterile field decreases the risk of infection transmission.

Performing the Skill (continued)

Step

- Attach the prefilled syringe to the indwelling catheter hub and test the balloon.
- Lubricate the catheter 2.5–5 cm for a female and 5–15 cm for a male and place it within the collection container.
- Place the fenestrated drape over the perineum, exposing the urinary meatus.
- Place the sterile tray and contents onto the sterile drape. Open specimen container.
- Cleanse the meatus. The nondominant hand becomes contaminated once you touch the patient and must remain in position throughout the procedure.

Female: Using your nondominant hand to spread the labia, firmly and gently maintain a position that exposes the urethra. Using the provided antiseptic sticks or saturated cotton ball and forceps, cleanse the area, wiping in a downward direction from the clitoris toward the anus. Using a new cotton ball/stick for each area, wipe along the far labial fold, near labial fold, and then directly over the meatus. Take care not to contaminate your sterile dominant hand while cleansing.

Male: Using your nondominant hand, grasp the penis just below the glans, retracting the foreskin if necessary. Hold the penis upright firmly with gentle tension. Use the antiseptic stick or a saturated cotton ball and forceps to cleanse the penis. In a circular motion starting at the meatus, wipe out around the glans. Repeat this three more times using a new stick/cotton ball each time. Use care not to contaminate your dominant sterile hand. Ensure that the foreskin does not return over the meatus and that the penis is not dropped.

- Insert the catheter.

Firmly grasp the catheter 8–10 cm away from the tip. While the patient takes a slow deep breath, insert the catheter as the patient exhales. Resistance may be felt as the catheter passes through the sphincters. You may gently twist the catheter or apply slight pressure until the sphincters relax. **Do not use force.**

Once urine flow is detected, continue to advance the catheter 5 cm farther.

If the catheter contacts the labia or is accidentally placed in the vagina, it is contaminated and you must use a new sterile catheter. If the catheter is placed in the vagina, leave it in place while attempting to insert the new catheter to avoid confusing the vaginal opening with the urethral meatus.

- Using your nondominant hand, hold the catheter. For male patients, lay the penis onto the drape. Use caution to ensure the catheter does not pull out.
- Inflate the retention balloon with required volume.

While continuing to support the catheter, hold the inflation valve with your nondominant hand. Inflate the balloon with the syringe using your dominant hand.

If the patient reports discomfort, immediately withdraw the instilled fluid, advance the catheter farther, and attempt to inflate the balloon again.

Gently pull on the catheter until resistance is felt. Reduce or reposition the foreskin as required.

- If necessary, collect a urine specimen. Allow 20–30 ml of urine to fill the sterile cup by holding end of catheter over the cup without touching the tip to the jar.
- Allow the straight catheter to continue draining. If required, attach the drainage end of the indwelling catheter to the collecting tubing and bag.

Rationale

Assesses the function of the balloon and allows for replacement before use if necessary.
Increases patient comfort and eases insertion.

Maintains sterility of work environment.

Allows for easy access of supplies during catheter insertion; maintains aseptic technique.

Provides visualization of the meatus.
Cleansing reduces the number of microorganisms present.
Using a new antiseptic wipe on each area reduces cross-contamination.

Lifting the penis perpendicular to the body helps to straighten the urethra.

Further advancement of the catheter ensures it is fully in the bladder. Some agency policies and procedures state that for male patients, advancement to the Y bifurcation of the catheter is necessary.

Discomfort may indicate that the catheter is not placed correctly in the bladder; further advancement is required.

Ensures that the balloon is inflated and placed in the trigone of the bladder (see Fig. 35.8).
Retraction and constriction of the foreskin behind the glans penis (paraphimosis) may occur secondary to catheterization if foreskin is not reduced.

Allows for a sterile collection.

(continued on page 946)

SKILL 35.4   Urethral Urinary Catheterization (continued)

Performing the Skill

- Allow the bladder to completely drain, remembering that only 750–1,000 ml of urine should be drained from the bladder at one time. Review agency policy for further instructions if this should occur; often, clamping of the tubing for some time is indicated.

  Prevents unnecessary trauma to the urethra.

- Once urine flow has stopped, remove the straight catheter. If the catheter is indwelling, use tape or a manufactured catheter—securing device to secure the tubing to the patient. For females, secure it to the inner thigh and the upper thigh or abdomen for males, allowing enough slack for movement. Secure the collecting tubing to the bed linens and hang the bag below the bladder level. Ensure that no tubing falls below the top of the collection bag. (See Figure 1.)

  Maintains comfort.

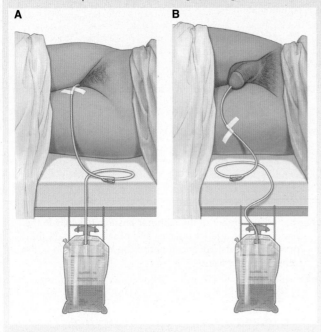

A   **B**

Figure 1

- Cleanse the area of any remaining antiseptic and assist the patient into a comfortable position.
- Using proper receptacles, dispose of the used supplies. Perform hand hygiene.

  Reduces transmission of microorganisms.

Document
- Record within the bedside chart in the appropriate column the time, characteristics, and amount of urine.
- Within narrative notes, record the catheter size and results.

SKILL 35.5 Bladder Irrigation

Purpose

- Maintaining patency of a urinary catheter and tubing (closed continuous irrigation)
- To dislodge a blockage in a urinary catheter or tubing (open intermittent irrigation)

Step	Rationale
Check the patient's chart to determine:	
• The purpose for the procedure.	Allows for anticipation of necessary observations (e.g., blood or mucus in urine).
• The amount and type of irrigant.	An order is required to initiate irrigation. The type and amount of solution may vary per patient or may be left to nurses' discretion or agency policy.
Assess:	
• The type of urinary catheter and drainage system currently in place.	Single (for open intermittent irrigation), double (one lumen to inflate balloon, one for urine outflow), or triple lumen (one lumen to inflate balloon, one to instill irrigation solution, one to allow outflow of urine) catheter.
	Continuous or intermittent irrigation.
• The colour of urine and presence of sediment, mucus, or clots.	Determines if urine is draining freely from bladder.
• Palpate the bladder.	Indicates if patient is having bleeding or sloughing off tissue and may determine if necessary to increase irrigation rates or frequency.
• Empty the drainage bag; measure and record the amount prior to discarding.	To assess for bladder distention.
	Determines baseline for prior urine output measures. An empty drainage bag allows for accurate measurement of urinary output following irrigation.
• Assess for the presence of bladder spasms and discomfort.	May indicate a need for bladder irrigation.
Prepare the equipment by:	
• Gathering two pairs of clean gloves, drainage tubing and bag (if retention catheter not in place), antiseptic swabs, sterile graduated container, sterile irrigation tubing, clamp for catheter tubing, sterile irrigation solution warmed or at room temperature (labeled clearly), infusion tubing, IV pole, and towel.	The use of sterile equipment when appropriate decreases the risk of infection transmission.
Prepare the patient by:	
• Introducing yourself to the patient; identify the patient using appropriate identifiers.	
• Assessing his or her knowledge regarding the purpose of bladder irrigations.	Determines the need for further teaching.
• Providing privacy by pulling bed curtains closed; carefully fold back covers, exposing catheter only. Cover patient's upper body with towel if desired.	Promotes patient comfort and provides easy access to the catheter.
• Positioning patient in a dorsal recumbent or supine position.	Promotes flow of irrigation solution into the bladder.
• Raising the bed to a height comfortable for the nurse.	
Wash hands and apply clean gloves.	

(continued on page 948)

SKILL 35.5   Bladder Irrigation (continued)

Performing the Skill

Step

Rationale

Closed intermittent irrigation (see Figure 1)

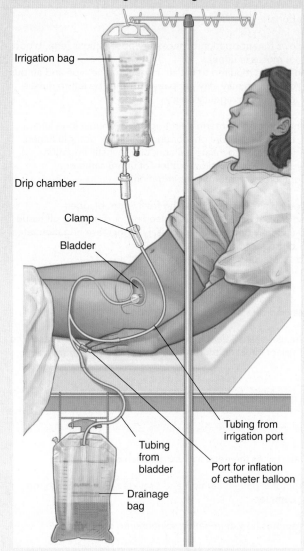

Irrigation bag

Drip chamber

Clamp

Bladder

Tubing from
irrigation port

Tubing
from
bladder

Port for inflation
of catheter balloon

Drainage
bag

Figure 1

- Determine if solution is to remain in bladder, known as "instillation."
- Clamp indwelling retention catheter tubing just below the specimen port if instillation is ordered.
- Draw warm sterile solution into a syringe using an aseptic technique.
- Apply gloves and cleanse injection port with antiseptic swab.
- Insert hub of syringe through port at 30° angle toward the bladder using a blunt or needleless syringe system.
- Slowly inject fluid into catheter and bladder.

- Withdraw the syringe and remove the clamp. Allow the solution to drain into the drainage bag.
- If an instillation is ordered, keep the catheter clamped, allowing the solution to remain in the bladder for the specified time.
- If a triple lumen catheter is in place, a similar irrigation may be performed using irrigation solution and irrigation tubing connected to the irrigation port of the catheter.

Closing the flow clamp allows the solution to be retained in the bladder and in contact with bladder walls.
Avoid cold solution for irrigant or instillation as it may result in bladder spasm and discomfort.
Aseptic technique ensures sterility of irrigation fluid.
Reduces transmission of infection.
Ensures the hub enters the lumen of catheter and flow is directed toward the bladder.
Continuous, slow insertion dislodges sediment and clots without causing trauma to the bladder wall.
Allows it to drain by gravity.

Allows for closed system irrigation.

Performing the Skill (continued)	
Step	**Rationale**
• Assess the drainage for colour, amount, and clarity. The amount of drainage should be equal to the amount of irrigant inserted in addition to expected urinary output. **Closed continuous irrigation**	
• Apply gloves; using aseptic technique, clamp the tubing and insert sterile spike of irrigation tubing into bag of sterile irrigating solution.	Prevents entrance of microorganisms.
• Hang bag of solution on IV pole. Open clamp, allowing solution to flow through tubing, ensuring the end of the tubing remains sterile. Close the clamp.	Removes air from tubing.
• Wipe irrigation port of triple lumen catheter with antiseptic swabs and then securely attach irrigation tubing.	Allows closed system to remain sterile.
• Calculate the drip rate and adjust clamp on irrigation tubing as required. Ensure that clamp on drainage tubing is open, tubing is patent, and no kinks are present. Note the volume of drainage in the drainage bag.	Ensures an even, continuous irrigation of the catheter system. Prevents collection of solution in the bladder, which can cause bladder distention and injury.
• Once procedure is complete, dispose of soiled supplies, remove gloves, and perform hand hygiene.	Prevents the spread of infection.
• Calculate the amount of irrigation fluid and subtract from total output.	Allows for accurate calculation of urinary output.
• Assess and document the characteristics of the output: viscosity; colour; and presence of sediments, clots, or blood. **Document**	Assesses the results of the irrigation.
• In appropriate spaces within the chart, document the procedure, type, and amount of irrigation solution as well as output amount and description.	

SKILL 35.6 Administration of an Enema

Purpose

Used to assist in cleansing, retention, carminative, or return flow.

Step	**Rationale**
Check the chart and determine: • The purpose and goal of the enema administration. • Review the physician's order.	• It is important to understand why the patient requires an enema in order to assess the effectiveness of it. • Assists in determining which solution to prepare and the number of enemas to administer.
Assess: • The patient for last bowel movement; amount, colour, and consistency of the feces; hemorrhoids; mobility; external sphincter control; and abdominal pain.	• Helps to determine need for the enema and influences the assistance required following the procedure.
• For the presence of increased intracranial pressure, glaucoma, or recent rectal or prostate surgery.	• These conditions contradict the administration of enemas.
• The presence of abdominal distention and auscultate for bowel sounds.	• Assists in establishing a baseline for assessing the effectiveness of the enema.
• The patient's level of understanding regarding the purpose and administration of an enema.	• Assists in preparation and teaching.
Prepare the equipment by: • Gathering water-resistant absorbent bed pads, a bath blanket, bedpan, commode or access to toilet, clean gloves, water-soluble lubricant, and paper towel/tissue. **Large-volume enema** • Solution container with tubing of correct size and clamp. • Correct solution, amount, and temperature (37.7°–40°C for adult patients). **Small-volume enema** • Packaged container of enema solution with lubricated tip.	

(continued on page 950)

SKILL 35.6   Administration of an Enema (continued)

Step	Rationale
Prepare the patient by:	
• Identifying the patient using appropriate type and number of identifier per agency protocol.	• Ensures you are administering the enema to the correct patient.
• Explaining the procedure and answering any questions the patient has.	• Understanding increases patient cooperation and reduces anxiety.
• Arranging appropriate equipment at the bedside.	• Ensures preparation and ease of procedure.
• Providing privacy by pulling curtain around bed or closing door.	• Reduces patient embarrassment.
• Raising bed to comfortable working height, raising side rail on patient's left.	• Promotes good body mechanics and patient safety.
• Assisting patient into left side-lying (Sims) position with right knee flexed.	• Allows enema solution to flow downward by gravity along the natural curve of the sigmoid colon and rectum, thus improving retention of solution.
Wash hands and apply clean gloves and any other necessary equipment.	Reduces the transmission of microorganisms and protects the nurse from contact with bodily fluids.

Performing the Skill

Step	Rationale
• Place the waterproof pad under the hips and buttocks.	• Prevents the linen from being soiled.
• Cover the patient with a bath towel, exposing only the rectal area.	• Allows for patient privacy and comfort.
• Lubricate approximately 5 cm of the rectal tube or tip if not pre-lubricated.	• Facilitates insertion of the enema through the sphincters, minimizing trauma.
• With patient in left lateral position, lift the upper buttock.	• Allows for proper visualization of the anus.
• Slowly and smoothly insert the tube into the rectum while directing it toward the umbilicus. (See Figure 1.)	• Decreases spasm of the sphincter and follows the normal shape of the rectum.

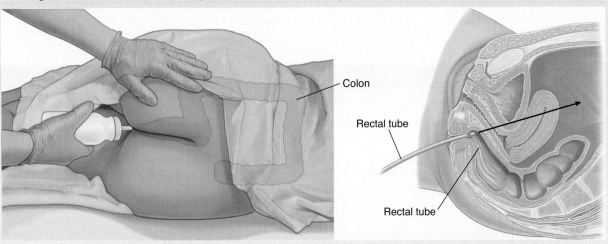

Colon

Rectal tube

Rectal tube

Figure 1

• Fully insert the tube 7–10 cm into the rectum.	• Places the tip of the tube past the anal sphincter and into the rectum.
• Do not force the tube or solution if resistance is met and a small amount of solution does not allow the tube to be advanced.	
• Slowly squeeze the bottle, ensuring that the container is no more than 30 cm higher than the rectum.	• The flow and pressure (force) is increased when the container is held higher.
• Slowly administer the solution; if pain or fullness is experienced by the patient, stop the flow for 30 seconds and then restart at a slower flow.	• Slow administration of the solution and momentarily stopping the flow reduces the risk of intestinal spasm and premature explosion of the solution.
• If a plastic prefilled container is used, roll it up as the fluid is instilled.	
• Following inserting all of the fluid, or when the patient states he or she feels the urge to defecate, remove the enema from the anus.	• This urge usually indicates an adequate amount of fluid has been inserted.
• As you remove the enema, place it into a disposable towel.	• The required time will be noted and may vary depending on the type of enema administered.

Performing the Skill (continued)

Step	Rationale
• Encourage the patient to remain lying, which will assist him or her in retaining the enema solution for the required time. • Assist the patient to sit on the bedpan, commode, or toilet. • Encourage the patient to not flush the toilet or to use a bedpan or commode. Document • In the appropriate place in the patient's chart, record the type and volume of solution. • Describe the results of the enema; include the amount, colour, and consistency of feces. • Record the effectiveness in patient's relief from abdominal distention and flatulence. • Include any difficulties or abnormalities encountered during the procedure.	A sitting position facilitates defecating. • This allows the nurse to observe the feces and collect a specimen as required.

SKILL 35.7 Ostomy Maintenance and Care

Purpose

- To care for and assess the peristomal skin.
- Collection and assessment of amount and output of effluent.
- To promote patient comfort and self-esteem by minimizing odours.

Step	Rationale
Check the patient and chart to determine: • The kind of ostomy and placement on the abdomen. • Orders regarding the care of the ostomy. Assess: • *Stoma colour:* should appear red, similar to the mucosal lining colour of the inner cheek. • *Stoma size and shape:* many stomas will slightly protrude from the abdomen. When new, the stoma may appear swollen; this will decrease over the first 2–3 weeks but may take up to 6 weeks. • *Stomal bleeding:* slight bleeding with initial touching is normal. • *Condition of peristomal skin:* note redness or irritation to the area within 5–12.5 cm surrounding the stoma. Expect transient redness following the removal of adhesive. • *Feces type and amount:* assess the colour, amount, odour, and consistency of feces. • *Symptoms:* reports of burning under the skin barrier can indicate breakdown of tissue. Abdominal distention and discomfort should be noted. • Any learning needs of the patient and his or her family members regarding ostomy self-care. • The patient's emotional well-being, with special consideration for coping and body image changes. Determine the need for the appliance change: • Assess the used appliance for feces leakage. • Ask the patient if he or she is experiencing pain at or around the stoma site. • Assess how full the pouch is. Leakage or discomfort at or around the stoma indicates the need for an appliance change. Consider the most appropriate time to change the appliance: • Avoid times near meals or visitors. • Avoid times that immediately follow meals or medication administration that may stimulate bowel evacuation.	• Important to confirm which is the functioning stoma. • Assists in anticipating supplies needed for the procedure. • Impaired circulation can be indicated by a very pale or darker coloured stoma with a bluish or purplish hue. • If the swelling does not decrease, it can indicate a problem, such as a blockage. • Bleeding at other times or increased amounts should be reported because it can indicate a concern. • Redness can indicate infection of other complications. • Report abnormalities including pus or blood that can indicate complications. • The presence of feces can cause irritation to the peristomal skin. • Burning pain may indicate breakdown underneath the pouch. • If the pouch is overly full, the weight of the bag can cause the bag to loosen, resulting in leaking of feces. • The odour may affect appetite and cause embarrassment to the patient. • Change the ostomy when drainage is least likely to occur.

(continued on page 952)

SKILL 35.7   Ostomy Maintenance and Care (continued)

Step	Rationale
Prepare the equipment by: Gathering: • Disposable gloves • Bedpan • Plastic waterproof bag (for disposable pouches) • Cleaning supplies: tissues, warm water, mild soap (optional), washcloth or cotton balls, and towel • Gauze or tissue pad • Skin barrier (paste, powder, water, or liquid skin sealant) • Measuring guide for stoma • Scissors and pen or pencil • New appliance with optional belt • Tail closure clamp • Pouch deodorant (optional)	
Prepare the patient by: • Introducing yourself and verifying patient identity using agency-required identifiers. • Explaining what you are going to do, why it is necessary, and what he or she can do to help. • Changing of the ostomy appliance should not be painful but may cause distress to the patient. • Providing for privacy, preferably in the bathroom. • Assisting the patient to a comfortable position: lying in bed or standing in the bathroom. Unfasten the belt if one is in use. Perform hand hygiene and apply clean gloves.	• Necessary to ensure patient safety. • Including the patient in the care of the ostomy promotes self-esteem and independence. • Display support and acceptance while changing the appliance quickly and competently. • The bathroom is where patient will provide self-care at home. • A standing or lying position will assist in avoiding wrinkles and facilitate a smoother application.

Performing the Skill

Step	Rationale
• Empty the contents of the pouch into a bedpan or toilet. • If a clamp is being used, do not throw it away; it can be reused. • Assess the feces, noting the consistency, colour, and amount. • While holding the patient's skin tautly, slowly remove the skin barrier, peeling it off beginning at the top and moving downward (see Figure 1).	• Emptying the pouch prior to removal prevents spilling of feces. • Holding the skin tautly prevents skin abrasions and minimizes discomfort.

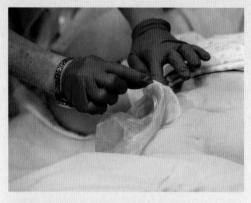

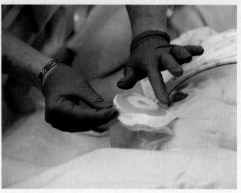

Figure 1

Performing the Skill (continued)

Step	**Rationale**

Step
- Dispose of the pouch in a plastic bag.
- Clean and dry the stoma and peristomal skin (see Figure 2).

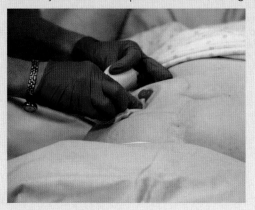

Figure 2

- Use toilet tissue to remove excess feces.
- Use a washcloth with warm water and mild soap (optional) to clean the skin and stoma.
- If soap is used, ensure that it is fragrance and moisturizer free.
- Thoroughly dry the area by gently patting with a towel.
- Assess the stoma for bleeding, colour, size, and shape.
- Assess the peristomal skin for irritation, ulceration, and redness.
- Place a piece of gauze or tissue over the stoma; change as needed (see Figure 3).

Rationale
- Soap may be discouraged because it can cause irritation to the area.
- The adhesives in the skin barrier may be affected by this.

- Avoid excess rubbing because it can abrade the skin.

- Used to absorb leakage from the stoma while appliance is changed.

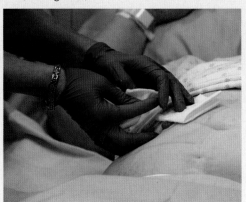

Figure 3

(continued on page 954)

SKILL 35.7   Ostomy Maintenance and Care (continued)

Performing the Skill

Step

- Prepare and apply the peristomal seal/skin barrier.
- Use the guide to size and measure the stoma (see Figure 4).

Rationale

- Minimizes the risk of feces contacting peristomal skin and allows room for the stoma to slightly expand while functioning.

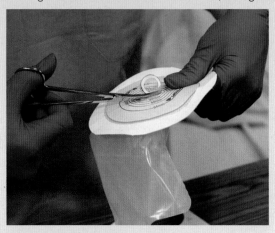

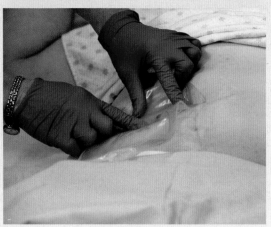

Figure 4

- Trace a circle the same size as the stoma on the back of the skin barrier.
- Make an opening in the skin barrier by cutting out the traced stoma. Ensure that the opening is a maximum of 0.3–0.4 cm larger than the stoma.
- Expose the sticky adhesive by removing the backing of the skin barrier. The backing can be saved to be used as a pattern in the future.
- Remove the gauze/tissue from over the stoma.

- The adhesive in the skin barrier is activated by the heat and pressure.

For a one-piece pouching system: centre the skin barrier and gently press for 30 seconds onto the patient's skin.

For a two-piece pouching system: centre the skin barrier over the stoma while gently pressing it into the skin for 30 seconds. Snap the pouch onto the skin barrier flange or wafer. For drainable pouches, close the pouch following the manufacturer's directions.

Document

- In the appropriate space within the patients chart, record any necessary assessments and interventions. Include change in stoma size, colour that may indicate impairment of circulation, and the presence of peristomal skin irritation. Record the amount and type of drainage, patient's toleration of the procedure, and the skills the patient learned during the procedure.
- Use any applicable forms or checklists provided by the agency and supplement with narrative charting where required.

Critical Thinking Case Scenarios

▶ Older adults or seniors living at home are at risk for health hazards such as falls in the bathroom. Falls may result in painful injuries and permanent disabilities that threaten the independence of the senior who wishes to continue living at home. Nurses working in community settings are key advocates for seniors and through their holistic assessments can make the home a safer environment.

1. What potential hazards exist in the bathroom?
2. Describe the physical assessment required to determine the safety needs of the patient living at home.
3. What environmental assessment is required to reduce the risk for injury for the patient in the bathroom?
4. Discuss the types of bathroom assistive devices available.

▶ Jaswinder is assigned to provide nursing care to a postoperative patient. The patient has an indwelling catheter and is being monitored for input and output. The patient is NPO but has an IV running at 125 ml/hour. Jaswinder assesses the patient's urine output every hour for the first 4 hours. She becomes concerned when there is little urine to measure during one of the postoperative checks.

1. What assessment of the patient should Jaswinder do upon discovering the decreased urine output?
2. Consider that the decreased urine output is due to a kinking of the catheter tube. Describe the actions that Jaswinder should take to rectify the problem and prevent it from happening again.
3. Consider that the decreased or absent urine output is not due to a physical anomaly with the catheter tubing but due to a physical anomaly with the patient. What actions should Jaswinder take to meet the needs of her postoperative patient?

▶ Dorothy is a 70-year-old woman who has just learned that she has a tumour in her bowel. Surgery is planned to remove the cancerous tumour by removing a section of her colon but will also require a postsurgical colostomy. Dorothy is very upset about the colostomy and the impact that it will have on her life.

1. Describe the role of the nurse in meeting Dorothy's emotional needs prior to her undergoing surgery.
2. What knowledge and skills will Dorothy need to care for her colostomy in both the postoperative period and longer term?
3. Describe the assessment of the stoma postoperatively.
4. What is the role of the discharge nurse when preparing Dorothy to go home with a new colostomy?

Multiple-Choice Questions

1. Urine excretion relies on functioning kidneys and:
   a. Ureters
   b. Bladder
   c. Urethra
   d. All of the above

2. The mechanism for the transport of urine into the bladder by the ureters is by:
   a. Dialysis
   b. Peristaltic movements
   c. Vasoconstriction
   d. None of the above

3. The production of ADH is inhibited by:
   a. Tea
   b. Chocolate
   c. Alcohol
   d. Cola drinks

4. Patients should be able to void within _____ hours after surgery.
   a. 2
   b. 6
   c. 10
   d. 24

5. The risk of developing a UTI increases with:
   a. Suppression of the urge to void
   b. Sitting in a wet bathing suit
   c. Using bubble bath and perfumed products
   d. All of the above

6. If urine output falls to less than ___ ml/hour, decreased blood flow to the kidneys and other vital organs must be suspected and reported to the physician.
   a. 10
   b. 30
   c. 60
   d. 120

7. Some conditions can obstruct urine flow from the kidneys to the urethra. These include:
   a. Kidney stones
   b. Enlarged prostate
   c. Tumour
   d. All of the above

8. When caring for a patient with any urinary diversion, the nurse must accurately assess:
   a. Intake and output
   b. Urine clarity
   c. The stoma and surrounding skin
   d. All of the above

9. Feces is made up of:
   a. 75% solids and 25% water
   b. 50% solids and 50% water
   c. 25% solids and 75% water
   d. 100% water

10. Constipation is a common bowel management problem in older adults. The following may contribute to constipation:
    a. Decreased fluid intake
    b. Muscle weakness
    c. Less mucus in the intestinal mucosa
    d. All of the above

11. Excess vagal stimulation during digital rectal examination or forceful digital removal of impacted feces can precipitate:
    a. Damage to the rectal mucosa
    b. Altered cardiac rhythm
    c. Both of the above

REFERENCES AND SUGGESTED READINGS

Bernard, M. S., Hunter, K. F., & Moore, K. N. (2012). A review of strategies to decrease the duration of indwelling urethral catheters and potentially reduce the incidence of catheter-associated urinary tract infections. *Urologic Nursing, 32*(1), 29–37.

Craven, R., Hirnle, C., & Jensen, S. (2013). *Fundamentals of nursing: Human health and function* (7th ed.). Philadelphia, PA: Wolters Kluwer Health/Lippincott Williams & Wilkins.

Dietitians of Canada. (2012). *Healthy eating guidelines for increasing your fibre intake. Why this diet is important.* Retrieved from http://www.dietitians.ca/Nutrition-Resources-A-Z/Factsheets/Fibre/Increasing-Your-Fibre-Intake.aspx

Registered Nurses' Association of Ontario. (2005). *Promoting continence using prompted voiding* (Rev. ed.). Toronto, ON: Author.

Robson, Wm. L. (2013). *Enuresis.* Retrieved from http://emedicine.medscape.com/article/1014762-overview

Patton, K. A., & Thibodeau, G. A. (2010). *Anatomy & physiology* (7th ed.). St. Louis, MO: Mosby Elsevier.

Porth, C. M., & Pooler, C. (2010). Structure and function of the kidney. In R. A. Hannon, C. Pooler, & C. M. Porth (Eds.), *Porth pathophysiology: Concepts of altered health states* (1st Canadian ed., pp. 710–728). Philadelphia, PA: Wolters Kluwer Health/Lippincott Williams & Wilkins.

Skin Care

chapter

36

GLENN DONNELLY, ELIZABETH L. DOMM, AND
BONNIE RAISBECK

Jane Smith is a nursing student in a Canadian university. Today, she is attending student orientation and notices there is a Canadian Cancer Society booth, where volunteer registered nurses offer to assess exposed skin with a camera to determine skin damage from sun exposure. You will meet Jane throughout this chapter as you learn about skin integrity.

CHAPTER OBJECTIVES

By the end of this chapter, you will be able to:

1. Understand the structure and function of the skin.
2. Develop knowledge and skills for assessing the integumentary system.
3. Recognize deviations from normal healthy skin, hair, and nails.
4. Understand the prevention of pressure ulcers.
5. Acquire essential knowledge of nursing interventions to manage pressure ulcers.
6. Develop knowledge of purpose and principles of dressings for skin wounds and wound care.
7. Incorporate health promotion concepts into all aspects of skin care.

KEY TERMS

Actinic Keratosis Single or multiple discrete, dry, rough, and scaly occurrences on sun-exposed skin.

Angioma Soft, red papule caused by a dilated venule.

Apocrine Glands Sweat glands found mainly in the axilla, groin, areolae of the breasts, and bearded regions in the face of adult males. They do not begin to function until puberty, release a milky or yellowish sweat that contains lipids and proteins, and do not play a role in thermoregulation.

Coccygeal Relating to or near the coccyx.

Collagen Strong insoluble protein fibre layer; main component of connective tissue.

Cyanosis A bluish coloration of the skin due to the tissues near the skin surface being low on oxygen.

Dermatitis Inflammation of skin (a rash). There are several different types of dermatitis.

Diaphoresis Excessive perspiration.

Ecchymosis Subcutaneous purpura or hematoma, purple discoloration of skin caused by blood in the subcutaneous tissue. Commonly, but erroneously, called a bruise. Bruises are caused by trauma whereas ecchymoses, a type of purpura, are not caused by trauma.

Eccrine glands Sweat glands.

Epidermal (Langerhans) Dendritic Cells Immune cells whose main function is to process antigen material and present it on the surface of the skin to other cells of the immune system.

Epidermis Outer layer of skin. Together with the dermis forms the cutis. Underneath is the subcutis.

Erythema Diffused redness of the skin. It occurs with any skin injury, infection, or inflammation. Disappears with pressure on the skin (blanching).

Eschar Coagulated crust on surface of wound.

Fissure Elongated opening in the skin.

Greater Trochanter Large bony prominence at the head of the femur.

Hemangioma Bright red nodular plaque usually found in newborn infants.

Hirsutism Excessive hair growth in women on those parts of the body where hair does not normally occur or is minimal, in a male pattern of body hair.

Integument Refers to skin, the largest organ of the body, and to the body system.

Ischial Tuberosity Anatomical area of pelvis between the ischial spine and ischial ramus.

Jaundice Abnormal yellowing of skin, mucous membranes, and white of eyes, caused by hyperbilirubinemia (increased levels of bilirubin in the blood).

Keratin Tough fibrous protein of hair, nails, and integumentary surface.

Keratinocytes Epidermal cell responsible for synthesizing keratin.

Lichenification Thickening and hardening of the skin as a result of irritation.

(continued on page 958)

Lipoma Benign tumor of adipose tissue.

Melanin Yellow-brown pigment produced by melanocytes. It gives colour to hair and skin. Exposure to sunlight stimulates melanin production and it protects skin from ultraviolet rays.

Melanocytes A specialized cell of the skin that produces melanin.

Melanoma Cancer of pigmented epithelial cells. These cells predominantly occur in skin, but are also found in other parts of the body, including the bowel and the eye. Melanoma can originate in any part of the body that contains melanocytes. Melanoma is less common than other skin cancers. However, it is much more dangerous if it is not found early.

Necrosis Devitalized or dead tissue.

Nevi A small pigmented benign tumor, commonly known as a *birthmark*, on the skin.

Osteomyelitis Acute or chronic infection of the bone.

Pallor Lack of colour, paleness.

Palpebral Conjunctivae Lining of the inside of the eyelids.

Papule Superficial solid lesion.

Petechiae Small purplish hemorrhagic spots on the skin.

Prepping Solution Liquid barrier applied to skin.

Prevalence The number of cases of a disease present in a specific population.

Punctate Tiny spots or punctures.

Purpura Red or purple spot(s) on the body (also called *petechiae*), caused by minor broken capillary blood vessels that occur in groups or patches.

Pustule Small raised skin lesion filled with pus.

Scapula Bony structure that connects the humerus and the clavicle or the shoulder blade.

Sebaceous Glands Specialized glands that produce sebum, a waxy substance on hair.

Serosanguineous Pertaining to both blood cells and serum.

Shear Physical change caused by the stress of two parallel layers of skin rubbing on each other.

Slough Nonviable slimy gray or yellow tissue on surface of wound.

Stratum Basale Deepest layer of skin, which has cells that can reproduce themselves.

Stratum Corneum Tough outer layer of epidermis whose cells are full of keratin.

Stratum Germinativum Combined stratum basale and stratum spinosum.

Stratum Granulosum Thin layer of cells in epidermis.

Stratum Lucidum Clear layer between stratum granulosum and stratum corneum.

Stratum Spinosum Layer of epidermis rich in RNA for protein synthesis in production of keratin.

Telangiectasis Tiny blood vessels that become widened and form patterns on the skin. Can develop anywhere on the body but are commonly seen on the face around the nose, cheeks, and chin.

Thrombocytopenia Decrease of platelets in the blood.

Ultraviolet Rays Sunlight rays that are not visible and emit electromagnetic radiation.

Vitiligo Acquired condition that results in loss of pigment in areas of the skin.

Structure and Function of the Skin

The integumentary system is the organ system that protects the body from various kinds of damage, such as loss of water or abrasion from outside. It is the largest of the body's organ systems and is composed of the skin and its appendages (including hair and nails).

The skin, or **integument**, serves many important functions to maintain health and protect internal body structures. The human integumentary system is composed of the skin, nails, hair, sweat glands, and sebaceous glands. Skin is subjected to many environmental stresses: trauma, chemicals, pollutants, pathogens, and damaging **ultraviolet rays**. Skin renews itself on a regular basis and serves as a visual indicator of health. Changes in skin colour may reflect disorders or disease. Skin changes or lesions may be normal aspects of aging or may indicate a serious problem.

Composition of the Integument

The skin is composed of two layers—the highly differentiated **epidermis** and the inner supportive dermis. Beneath these layers is the subcutaneous layer of adipose tissue. The deepest epidermal layer is known as the **stratum basale** or **stratum germinativum** (refer to Fig. 36.1). This layer forms new skin cells. The most abundant cell type is the **keratinocyte**, and each time a keratinocytic stem cell divides, a daughter cell is pushed toward the external surface. The main ingredient of these cells is **keratin**, a protein that is the primary component of the epidermis and hair. **Melanocytes** are also interspersed along this layer, producing the pigment melanin that gives brown tones to the skin and hair. The amount of melanin a person produces varies according to genetic, hormonal, and environmental influences. Tactile cells (Merkel cells) are also found in this layer. These cells are sensitive to touch and when compressed release chemicals that stimulate sensory nerve endings, providing information about objects touching the skin.

Stratum spinosum is known as the *spiny layer*. Each time a keratinocyte stem cell divides, a daughter cell is pushed toward the surface from the stratum basale. Once this new cell enters the stratum spinosum, it begins to differentiate into a nondividing highly specialized keratinocyte. In addition to keratinocytes, this layer also contains **epidermal dendritic (Langerhans) cells**. These cells fight infection in the epidermis. Their phagocytic activity initiates an immune response to protect the body against pathogens that have penetrated the superficial epidermal layers as well as epidermal cancer cells.

Keratinization is the process that occurs in the **stratum granulosum**. The keratinocytes fill up with the protein keratin. This causes the cell's nucleus and organelles to disintegrate, and cell death occurs. The process is not complete

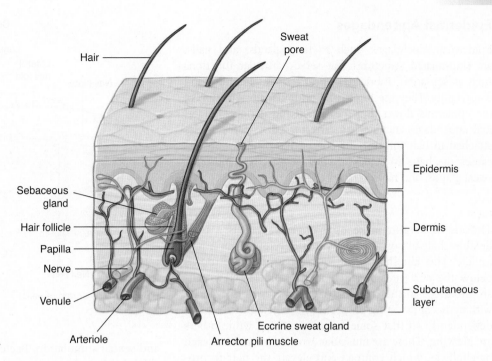

Figure 36.1 Diagram of skin.

until the cells reach the more superficial epidermal layers. A fully keratinized cell is dead because it does not have a nucleus or organelles, but it is structurally strong because of the keratin. **Stratum lucidum** or clear layer is a thin, translucent layer superficial to the stratum granulosum. This layer is only found in the thick skin within the palms of the hands and soles of the feet.

Epidermis

The epidermis is the outer, thinner layer. It provides protection from microbes, chemicals, and excessive water loss. The **stratum corneum** is the outermost layer of the epidermis. This layer consists of about 20 to 30 layers of dead, scaly, interlocking keratinized (cornified) cells and can be compared to the structure of a brick wall. The corneocytes (flattened dead skin cells) are the bricks, and these are secured by a mortar of lipids. Cells are constantly being shed and replaced with new cells from below. Stability of the epidermis is enhanced by the corneocytes ability to retain water. This allows them to swell and remain tightly packed. Desmosomes function like protein rivets. In healthy skin, the essential water level is maintained by the presence of natural moisturizing factor (NMF) and lipids. The skin has a range of functions designed to protect the skin from excessive water loss. Water loss through the skin is minimized by the secretion of sebum onto the skin surface from the sebaceous glands.

Skin is normally mildly acidic with a pH between 5 and 5.5. This provides protection from microbes. The normally dry stratum corneum presents a thickened surface unsuitable for growth of many microorganisms. Secretions from exocrine glands also help prevent growth of microorganisms. If skin structures are damaged, these protective mechanisms are disrupted, leading to impaired skin barrier function and potential breakdown.

Dermis

The dermis, the layer between the epidermis and subcutaneous tissues, ranges in thickness from 0.5 to 3.0 mm. It is composed of connective tissue and contains mainly **collagen** fibres (the main component of connective tissue), although both elastic and reticular fibres are found within the dermis. Dendritic cells are also found in this layer, and these cells provide an immune function, similar to those found in the epidermis. Other components of the dermis are blood vessels, sweat glands, sebaceous glands, hair follicles, nail roots, sensory nerve endings, and *arrector pili*. The dermis contains two major regions: a superficial papillary layer and a deeper reticular layer.

The **collagen** fibres and elastic fibres of the dermis contribute to the physical characteristics of the skin. Collagen fibres impart tensile strength, and elastic fibres allow stretch and recoil during normal movement. Both flexibility and thickness of the dermis are diminished by effects of exposure to ultraviolet light and aging.

The dermis contains sensory nerve fibres that monitor stimuli in both the dermis and epidermis. Touch receptors detect pressure, vibration, and cold and initiate sensory input to the brain. This innervation allows awareness of surroundings and enables us to differentiate among different kinds of sensory signals. Motor nerve fibres control both blood flow and gland secretions. Because the epidermis is avascular, the dermis must supply nutrients to the living cells in the epidermis as well as the dermis. These blood vessels have an important role in body temperature and blood pressure regulation.

Epidermal Appendages

Epidermal appendages, such as hair, glands, and nails, are skin-related structures that serve particular functions such as sensation, lubrication, heat loss or retention, and contractility. They are formed by a tubular invagination of the epidermis down into the underlying dermis. Epidermal appendages include hair, arrector pili (small muscles attached to hair follicles; the contraction of these muscles causes the hairs to stand on end), sebaceous glands, the sweat glands, and nails.

Hair

Threads of keratin make up hair. Each hair is a thin, flexible shaft of cornified cells that develops from a hair follicle. The hair shaft is the visible part, and the root is below the surface embedded in the follicle. New cells are produced in the bulb matrix. Hair growth is cyclical, with active and resting phases. Each follicle functions independently so that some hairs are resting while others are growing. There are muscular arrector pili around each hair follicle, which contract and elevate the hair to produce goose bumps during exposure to cold or in emotional states.

People have three types of hair—lanugo, vellus, and terminal. Lanugo hairs are present in utero but are gone by early childhood. Vellus hair is the downy hair that covers most of the body, particularly in women and children, whereas terminal hair grows on the scalp and eyebrows. After puberty in both male and females, terminal hair is found on the axillae and pubic area. Males also have hair growth on the face and chest. Melanocytes within the hair shaft determine colour. Variations in hair colour, density, and distribution pattern vary considerably according to age, gender, race, and genetics.

Sebaceous Glands

Sebaceous glands provide lubrication, producing the protective lipid-rich substance *sebum*. Sebum (an oily substance that keeps hair and skin supple) is secreted through the hair follicles to lubricate the skin and hair. It forms an emulsion with water that retards moisture loss from the skin. Sebaceous glands are most abundant in the scalp, forehead, face, and chin but are distributed everywhere in the body except the palms and soles.

Sweat Glands

Evaporation of sweat reduces body temperature. There are two types of sweat glands: eccrine and apocrine. **Eccrine glands** open directly onto the skin surface and produce the dilute saline solution called *sweat*. Eccrine glands are distributed throughout the body. **Apocrine glands** open into the hair follicles, becoming active during puberty. They are located mainly in the axillae, anogenital area, nipples, and navel where they produce a thick milky secretion that coincides with emotional

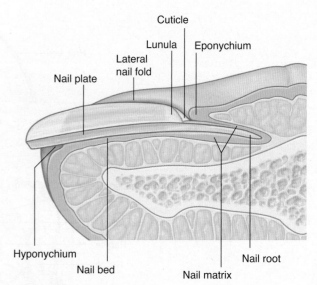

Figure 36.2 Diagram of nails.

and sexual stimulation. Bacterial flora that resides on the skin surface mixes with apocrine secretions to produce a characteristic musky and sometimes strong or unpleasant body odor. Decreased functioning of the apocrine glands occurs with aging.

Nails

Nails are hard plates of keratin on the dorsal edges of the fingers and toes. They serve to protect the distal tips of the fingers and toes from damage during activities such as walking, jumping, catching objects, working with the hands, etc. (Fig. 36.2).

Functions of the Skin

The primary function of skin is protection. The skin protects the body from microbial invasion and protects internal body structures from minor physical trauma and foreign substances. Other functions of the skin include the following:

- Retention of fluid and electrolytes
- Sensory input from the environment through nerve endings and sensory receptors; this enables the body to adapt through temperature regulation or changing position.
- Production of vitamin D_3
- Excretion of sweat, urea, and lactic acid
- Expression of emotion
- Temperature regulation
- Immune function
- Repair of surface wounds
- Provides valuable clues to internal disorders by mirroring systemic disease
- Provides identifying traits such as hair colour, skin colour, and presence of tattoos

Skin Assessment

Techniques used in assessment of the skin include health history, inspection, and palpation. The examiner may detect unusual skin odors as well. Body odors may be related to factors such as poor hygiene or excessive perspiration (hyperhidrosis). The examiner may assess the entire skin surface at one time or, more commonly, each aspect of the skin as the head-to-toe assessment is completed (Table 36.1).

The registered nurse (RN) at the Canadian Cancer Society booth greets Jane Smith, who is next in line for a skin assessment. What questions about Jane's health history related to sun exposure would the RN ask Jane?

TABLE 36.1	Health History Questions

The nurse should ask questions related to following:

Current Health

Chronic illnesses	Diabetes, liver disease, renal disease, autoimmune disorders, etc., which can cause skin changes such as rash, pruritus, or skin lesions
Medications	Side effects from some medications include rashes, hives, photosensitivity, acne, thinning of the skin, etc.
Health-care practices related to the skin	Use of sunscreen Protection from sun exposure Hygiene practices Use of lotions, cosmetics, etc. Use of sunscreen Changes in skin, hair, and nails It is better to ask about changes rather than problems because patients may not recognize that a change could indicate a problem if troublesome symptoms are not present.
Family history *This helps determine predisposition to skin disorders. Some skin disorders have familial or genetic links*	Skin cancer Autoimmune disorders such as lupus erythematosus
Medical history	Skin diseases Skin or nail infections Trauma

Focused Assessment

Commonly reported skin and nail problems include pruritus (itch); pain or discomfort; rash; wounds or lesions; and changes in skin colour, texture, or appearance of nails or hair. Each symptom must be fully evaluated, which includes asking about onset, location, duration, characteristics, severity, provocative (provoking a reaction) or palliative (relieving) factors, related symptoms, medication use, treatment, and patient's perception of the problem.

The memory device using the letters PQRSTU can be used to analyze symptoms. For example, in the patient presenting with a rash:

P (provocative/palliative): Does anything make the rash better or worse? Have you treated the rash with anything? What medications are you taking? Did you notice the rash before you took the medication or after?

Q (quality): What does it look like? (flat? raised?) Has it changed from when you first noticed it? Is there any discomfort or itching associated with it?

R (region/radiation): Where is the rash located? Has it spread from the original area?

S (severity): How bad is it (itching or discomfort) on a scale of 1 to 10? Is it getting better, worse, or staying the same?

T (timing/onset/frequency/duration): Onset—When did the rash start? Duration—How long has the rash been present? Frequency—How often does it occur (if it is a recurrent symptom)? Have you had a similar rash in the past?

U (understanding): Do you have any allergies to foods, plants, skin/hair products, soaps, etc.? Does anyone else in your family have a similar rash? Are there any associated symptoms such as pain in the joints, fatigue, and fever?

Inspection

Inspect the skin for general colour and uniformity of colour. Skin colour normally ranges from whitish pink, to olive tones, to deep brown. Colour should be consistent over the

---

NURSING GUIDELINES 36.1: PHYSICAL EXAMINATION: ROUTINE TECHNIQUES

Inspect the skin for general colour, localized variations in skin colour, and lesions (palpate lesions if present).

Palpate the skin for temperature, moisture, texture, mobility, turgor, edema, and thickness.

Inspect and palpate the scalp and hair for surface characteristics, distribution, colour, quantity, pest inhabitants, texture, and hygiene.

Inspect facial and body hair for distribution, colour, quantity, pest inhabitants, and hygiene.

Inspect and palpate the nails for shape, contour, consistency, colour, thickness, and hygiene.

Equipment needed: good light source (natural light preferable), millimeter ruler, magnifying lens, and gloves (for use if open lesions are present)

entire body with the exception of vascular areas (cheeks, upper chest, and genitalia). These areas may have a pinkish or reddish purple tone.

Generalized Colour Changes

Note any colour alteration over the entire body such as pallor, erythema, cyanosis, or jaundice. **Pallor** is when the reddish-pink skin tone from oxygenated hemoglobin is lost; the skin takes on the colour of connective tissue, which is mostly white in Caucasians. Pallor is seen in states of anxiety or fear because of peripheral vasoconstriction from sympathetic nervous system stimulation. Heart disease, hypoglycemia, exposure to cold, presence of edema, etc. can also cause skin pallor.

In dark-skinned people, the lack of the underlying red skin tone looks different from light-skinned people. Pallor in brown-skinned individuals presents as a more yellowish-brown skin colour than usual; black-skinned individuals will appear ashen or grey. The mucous membranes, lips, and nail beds are good places to observe generalized pallor. When assessing for anemia, a reduction in circulating red blood cells, nail beds, and the **palpebral conjunctiva** (which lines the eye lids) are preferred sites.

Abnormal Findings

Abnormal skin colour may indicate local or systemic disease. Common abnormal findings include cyanosis, pallor, erythema, and jaundice. Other abnormal findings are ecchymoses (bruises), **petechiae**, **purpura**, rash, etc.

Erythema is an intense redness of the skin from excess blood in the dilated superficial capillaries. Erythema is an expected sign with fever and local inflammation. It is an abnormal finding when it is associated with polycythemia, venous stasis, and carbon monoxide poisoning.

Cyanosis is a bluish, mottled discoloration of the skin that signifies decreased perfusion, indicating that the tissues are not being adequately perfused with oxygenated blood. It occurs with shock, heart failure, and congenital heart disease.

Jaundice is exhibited by yellow skin, indicating elevated bilirubin levels in the blood. It is initially noted in the junction of the hard and soft palates in the mouth and in the sclera (white of the eye). In the eye, the yellow of jaundice extends to the edge of the iris. As levels of serum bilirubin rise, jaundice is evident in the skin over the rest of the body. It occurs with hepatitis, cirrhosis of the liver, sickle-cell disease, transfusion reactions, and hemolytic disease of the newborn.

Localized Variations in Skin Colour

Most individuals have localized variations in skin pigmentation. Some normal and abnormal variations of skin pigmentation are described in Table 36.2.

Skin Temperature

Use the dorsal aspect of your hands to evaluate skin temperature. The skin should be warm, and temperature should be consistent for the entire body with the exception of the hands

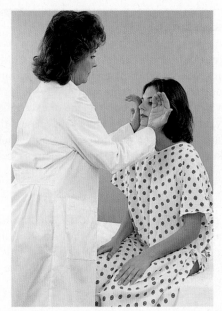

Figure 36.3 Using dorsal aspects of hand to assess bilateral areas of skin.

and feet, which may be cooler if the environment is cool. Compare the two feet and two hands for uniformity (Fig. 36.3).

Abnormal findings include generalized cool skin, which may be associated with shock or hypothermia. A localized area of cool skin may be an indication of poor peripheral perfusion. Generalized hot skin indicates hyperthermia. This may be related to fever, hyperthyroidism (increased metabolic rate), or exercise. Localized areas of hot skin may be related to infection, sunburn, or traumatic injury.

Skin Moisture

Skin is normally dry to the touch. Increased perspiration is a normal finding associated with strenuous activity, increased environmental temperature, and anxiety. Observe the oral mucous membranes for dryness. Normally, the mucous membranes look smooth and moist.

Excessive sweating (**diaphoresis**) is an abnormal finding in the absence of increased environmental temperatures or strenuous activity. Moist skin may indicate hyperthermia, anxiety, pain, or shock. It may also be associated with metabolic conditions such as hyperthyroidism. With dehydration, mucous membranes look dry and the lips look parched and cracked.

Skin Texture

Skin should feel smooth, soft, and intact, with an even surface. Normal exceptions include thickened areas over the hands, feet, elbows, and knees. Excessive dryness, flaking, scaling, or cracking of the skin may be related to environmental or occupational conditions but may be signs of systemic disease or nutritional deficiency. Inspect for areas of maceration (softened skin related to extended periods of wetness), discoloration, or rashes, especially under skinfolds.

TABLE 36.2	Localized Variations in Skin Colour

Normal Variations of Skin Pigmentation

Pigmented nevi (moles)

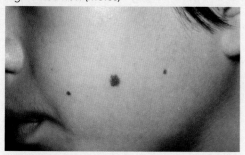

(Stephen, Skillen, Day, & Jensen, 2012)

Moles are considered a normal finding, and most adults have between 10 and 40 moles scattered over the body. They are most commonly found on sun-exposed body surfaces (chest, back, arms, legs, and face). They are usually uniformly tan to dark brown, typically less than 5 mm in size, and may be raised or flat. They may be round or oval with a clearly defined border.

Freckles

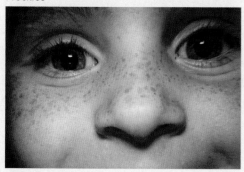

(Stephen et al., 2012)

Small, flat pigmented macules that usually appear on sun-exposed areas

Patch

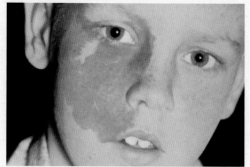

(Stephen et al., 2012)

An area of darker pigmented skin that is usually brown or tan and is often present at birth; some of these patches fade, but many do not change over time.

Striae

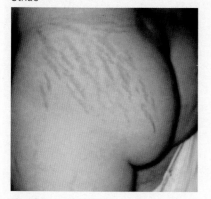

(Stephen et al., 2012)

Silver or pink stretch marks secondary to weight gain or pregnancy

(continued on page 964)

TABLE 36.2 Localized Variations in Skin Colour (continued)

Normal Variations of Skin Pigmentation

Scar

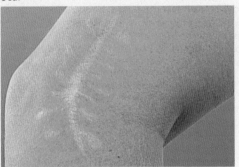

(Stephen et al., 2012)

Narrow line related to an injury or surgery

Tattoo

A common intentional form of body modification made by inserting indelible ink into the dermis layer of the skin to change the pigment.

Abnormal Findings

Skin cancer

Basal cell carcinoma, squamous cell carcinoma, melanoma

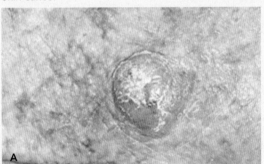
A

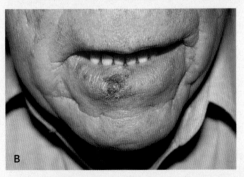
B

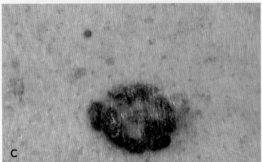
C

(Stephen et al., 2012)

Normal Variations of Skin Pigmentation

Actinic keratosis

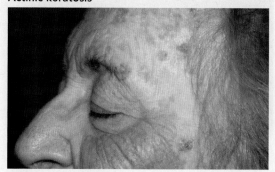

(Stephen et al., 2012)

Actinic (sun) damage that is a precursor of squamous cell carcinoma

Vitiligo

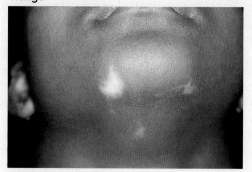

(Stephen et al., 2012)

Patches of unpigmented skin, more common in dark-skinned people and thought to be an autoimmune disorder

Localized areas of hyperpigmentation

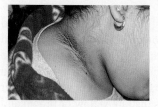

(Stephen et al., 2012)

May be associated with diabetes (acanthosis nigricans) or other endocrine disorders and autoimmune disorders such as systemic lupus erythematosus

---

In hyperthyroidism, the skin feels smoother and softer. In hypothyroidism, the skin feels rough, dry, and flaky.

Mobility and Turgor

Mobility is the skin's ease of rising. Turgor is its ability to return to place promptly after release, assessing dehydration. Skin mobility and turgor are assessed by picking up and slightly pinching the skin on the forearm or under the clavicle on the anterior chest (Fig. 36.4). The skin should move easily when lifted and return to place immediately when released. Tenting is when the pinched skin retains shape for a few seconds before flattening out. Especially in older people, skin that requires more than 2 to 5 seconds to return to a flat position may be dehydrated.

Conditions that reduce skin mobility include edema, excessive scarring, and some connective tissue disorders (e.g., scleroderma). Poor skin turgor is noted if tenting is

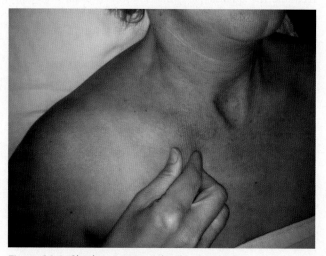

Figure 36.4 Checking turgor under the clavicle.

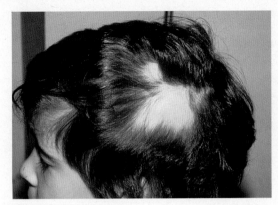

Figure 36.5 Alopecia.

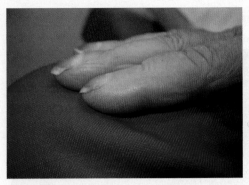

Figure 36.7 Nail clubbing

observed. Decreased turgor is seen in dehydration and extreme weight loss.

Thickness

Thickness of the skin varies according to age and body area. Skin is thickest over the palms of hands and soles of feet and thinnest over the eyelids. A callus is an area of excessive thickening of the skin associated with friction or pressure over a particular surface area. Calluses are commonly found on hands and feet. Very thin, shiny skin occurs with arterial insufficiency.

The Scalp and Hair

The scalp is normally smooth to palpation and shows no evidence of flaking, scaling, redness, or open lesions. The hair is normally shiny and soft, and the texture may range from fine to coarse. Note the quantity and distribution of the hair, and note any areas of hair loss and balding patterns. If areas of isolated hair loss exist, note whether the hair shaft has broken off or whether it is absent. Men may show a gradual, symmetric hair loss on the scalp due to genetic disposition and elevated androgen levels. Women also experience hair loss with aging (Fig. 36.5).

Facial and Body Hair

Examine the quantity and distribution of facial and body hair. Fine vellus hair covers the body, whereas coarser terminal hairs grow at the eyebrows, eyelashes, and scalp.

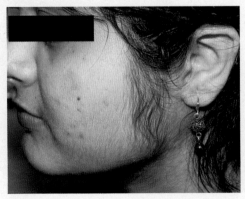

Figure 36.6 Hirsutism.

Male and female distribution patterns differ. In the genital area, the female pattern is an inverted triangle; the male pattern is an upright triangle.

Dull, coarse, and brittle hair may be seen with nutritional deficiencies, hypothyroidism, and exposure to chemicals in hair products. Hyperthyroidism makes the hair texture fine. In **hirsutism**, a female presents with a male pattern of hair distribution on the face and chest, indicating endocrine abnormalities, but this may be related to genetic factors (Fig. 36.6). Parasitic infection with lice will be seen in the presence of nits (eggs) found on the scalp at the base of the hair shaft. Adult lice are very difficult to observe unless the person is heavily infested because they hide easily in the hair.

The Nails

Inspect the edges of the nails; they should be smooth and rounded. The nail surface should be flat in the centre and slightly curved downward at the edges. The skin adjacent to the nail should be intact and not reddened. In light-skinned individuals, nails are pink and blanch with pressure. Darker skinned individuals have nails that are yellow or brown and vertical lines may appear. Note the angle of the nail base; it should be approximately 160°.

Jagged nails may indicate nervous habits or inattention to grooming. Dirty nails may indicate poor hygiene or may be related to occupation. Smokers may have nicotine stained nails. Clubbing of nails occurs with congenital heart disease and chronic obstructive pulmonary disease. Early clubbing is indicated by an angle of 180° and a spongy nail base (Fig. 36.7).

Lesions

Primary, secondary, and vascular skin lesions appear in response to some change in the external or internal environment (Table 36.3). Nurses are responsible for describing lesions in terms of location (e.g., back, face); distribution (i.e., generalized over the entire body or localized); configuration (pattern); as well as colour, shape, borders (or edges), size, texture, consistency (firm or soft), and other characteristics (fluid-filled or solid, exudate, flat, raised, or sunken) (Table 36.4).

(text continues on page 978)

TABLE 36.3	Types of Skin Lesions
Primary Skin Lesions	

Macule

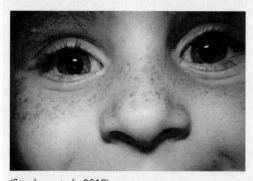

(Stephen et al., 2012)

Flat, circumscribed area that is a change in colour of the skin; 1 mm to 1 cm in size
Examples: freckles, measles, petechiae, flat moles (nevi)

Larger than 1-cm macule

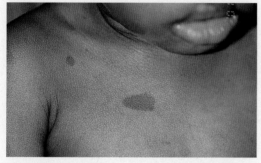

(Stephen et al., 2012)

May have irregular shape
Examples: port wine birthmark, vitiligo, café au lait spots, congenital dermal melanocytosis

Papule

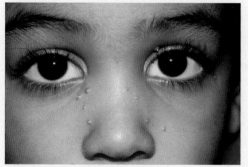

(Stephen et al., 2012)

Circumscribed, solid, elevation of the skin, less than 1 cm
Examples: pimples, warts, elevated moles, cherry **angioma**, skin tags

Pustule

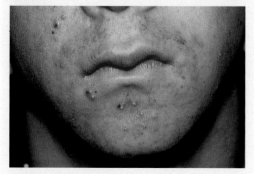

(Stephen et al., 2012)

Vesicle or bulla filled with pus
Examples: impetigo, herpes simplex, acne

(continued on page 968)

| TABLE 36.3 | Types of Skin Lesions (continued) |

Primary Skin Lesions

Plaque

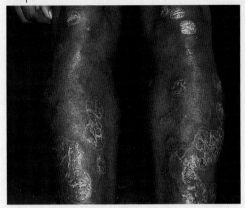

(Stephen et al., 2012)

Elevated, firm, rough lesion greater than 1 cm in diameter
Examples: psoriasis, seborrheic and actinic keratosis, eczema

Wheal

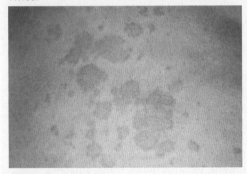

(Stephen et al., 2012)

Elevated, irregularly shaped area of fluid under the skin
Examples: hives, insect bites

Nodule

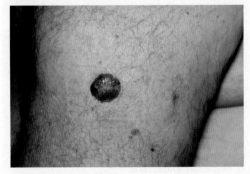

(Stephen et al., 2012)

Elevated, firm, circumscribed lesion extending deeper into the
dermis than a papule; size ranges from 0.5 to 2 cm
Examples: **lipomas**, melanoma, hemangioma, neurofibroma

Primary Skin Lesions (continued)

Tumor

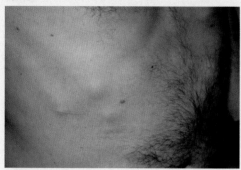

(Stephen et al., 2012)

Elevated, solid lesion extending deeply into the dermis; may have an irregular border and are larger than 2 cm
Examples: lipoma, hemangioma, malignant melanoma

Vesicle

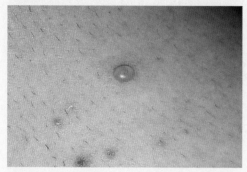

(Stephen et al., 2012)

Elevated, circumscribed, superficial mass filled with serous fluid or blood; less than 0.5 cm
Examples: varicella, herpes zoster, impetigo, eczema

Bulla

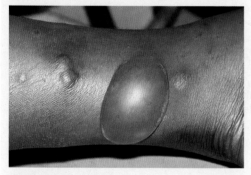

(Stephen et al., 2012)

Vesicle larger than 0.5 cm
Examples: blister, impetigo, drug reaction

Cyst

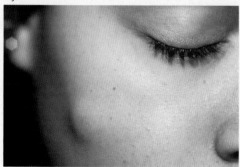

(Stephen et al., 2012)

Elevated, circumscribed, encapsulated, fluid-filled or semisolid mass; a cyst may occur in dermis or subcutaneous layer.
Examples: sebaceous and epidermal cysts, chalazion of the eyelid, cystic acne

(continued on page 970)

TABLE 36.3   Types of Skin Lesions (continued)

Secondary Skin Lesions

Scale

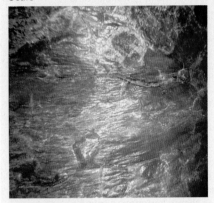

(Stephen et al., 2012)

Shedding, flaky, keratinized cells; may be irregular, thick or thin, dry or greasy; vary in size
Examples: seborrheic dermatitis, eczema

Lichenification

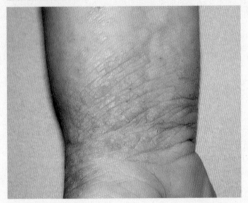

(Stephen et al., 2012)

Rough, thickened, hardened area of epidermis secondary to chronic irritation such as rubbing, itching, or skin irritation
Example: chronic dermatitis

Keloid

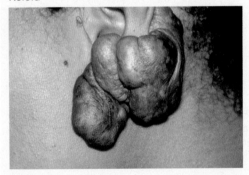

(Stephen et al., 2012)

Elevated, irregular, area of excess scar tissue extending beyond the border of the initial injury; keloids appear at a higher incidence in blacks.

Secondary Skin Lesions (continued)

Scar

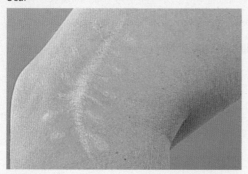

(Stephen et al., 2012)

Flat, irregular area of connective tissue that forms after a lesion or wound has healed; colour of new scars is red or purple; older scars may be silvery or white.
Example: healed surgical wound, acne

Excoriation

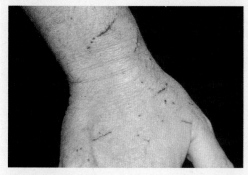

(Stephen et al., 2012)

Linear erosion of the epidermis
Examples: scratches, chemical burns, scabies

Fissure

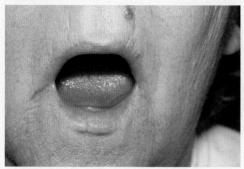

(Stephen et al., 2012)

Linear crack with sharp edges extending into the dermis
Examples: cracks in the hands or feet (athlete's foot)

Crust

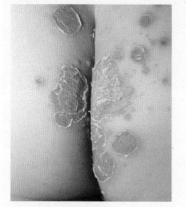

(Stephen et al., 2012)

Dried drainage or blood left on the skin surface when vesicles or pustules burst; vary in colour from tan, to red, to black
Example: scab on abrasion, impetigo, eczema

(continued on page 972)

TABLE 36.3	Types of Skin Lesions (continued)

Secondary Skin Lesions

Erosion

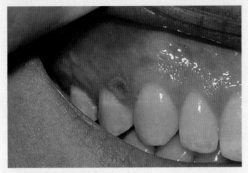

(Stephen et al., 2012)

Shallow depression in the epidermis, moist, follows rupture of vesicle or bulla

Examples: varicella, candidiasis, herpes simplex

Ulcer

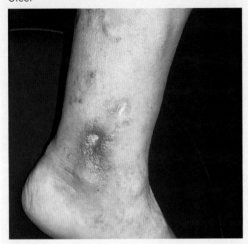

(Stephen et al., 2012)

Deep, irregularly shaped area of epidermis and dermis loss; an ulcer may extend into the subcutaneous tissue, vary in size, may bleed, and may leave scar.

Examples: decubitus ulcers, stasis ulcers, chancres

Atrophy

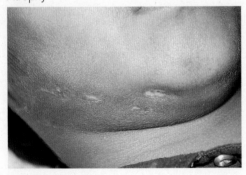

(Stephen et al., 2012)

Thinning of the skin surface resulting from loss of collagen and elastin; skin appears translucent, dry, and paper-like.

Example: Aged skin, striae

Vascular Lesions

Bruise (ecchymosis/contusion)

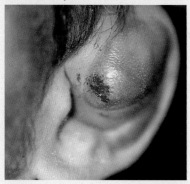

(Stephen, Skillen, Day, & Jensen, 2012)

A large patch of capillary bleeding into skin; colour changes with time from reddish-blue to yellow-brown. In dark-skinned individuals, a recent bruise is a deep, dark, purple patch. Bruises occur from trauma and bleeding disorders.

Hematoma

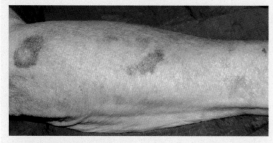

(Stephen et al., 2012)

A bruise that can be palpated

Petechiae

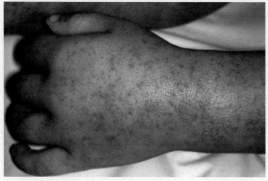

(Stephen et al., 2012)

Pinpoint (1–3 mm) round, discrete lesions as a result of bleeding under the skin; commonly appear in clusters and may look like a rash; usually flat to the touch and do not blanch with pressure; may be red, purple, or brown in colour

(continued on page 974)

TABLE 36.3   Types of Skin Lesions (continued)

Vascular Lesions

Purpura

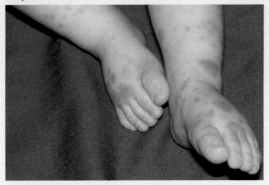

(Stephen et al., 2012)

Confluent patch of petechiae and **ecchymosis** >3 mm; red to purple; seen in **thrombocytopenia** and in older adults as skin becomes more fragile

Hemangiomas

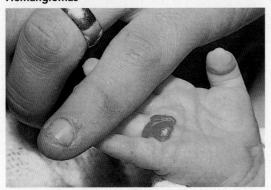

(Stephen et al., 2012)

Caused by a benign proliferation of blood vessels

Telangiectasis (spider veins)

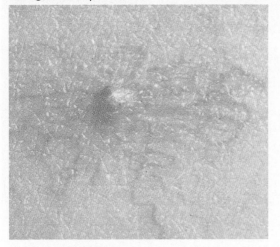

(Stephen et al., 2012)

Caused by vascular dilatation visible on the skin surface; examples are spider angiomas and venous lake.

TABLE 36.4	Shapes and Patterns of Lesions

Shapes of Lesions

Punctate	Small, marked with points or dots (petechiae)

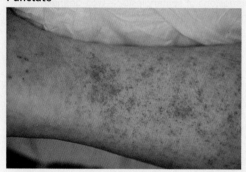

(Jensen)

Annular	Ringlike, circular Example: tinea corporis (ring worm)

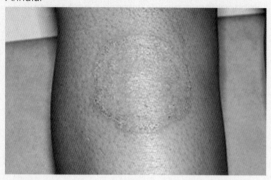

(Jensen)

Iris	Bull's eye (Lyme disease, erythema nodosum)

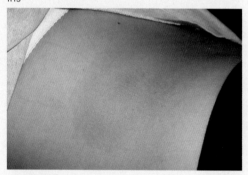

(Jensen)

Serpinous/gyrate	Curving, snakelike

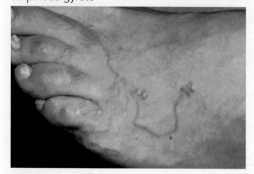

(Jensen)

(continued on page 976)

TABLE 36.4 **Shapes and Patterns of Lesions** (continued)

Patterns of Lesions

Single/discrete

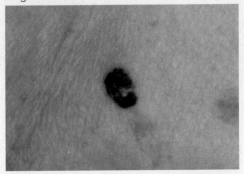

(Jensen)

Separate from other lesions or solitary lesion—well-defined borders (malignant melanoma, insect bite)

Grouped/clustered

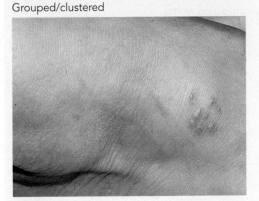

(Jensen)

Lesions that clump together in groups (impetigo, herpes simplex)

Polycyclic

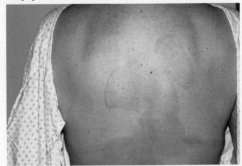

(Jensen)

Annular lesions that come in contact with one another as they spread (tinea corporis/ringworm)

Confluent

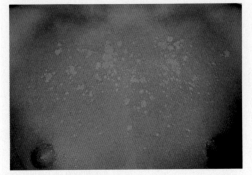

(Jensen)

Lesions that merge together over a large area (urticarial/hives)

Patterns of Lesions (continued)

Linear

Lesions that form a line (poison ivy, contact dermatitis)

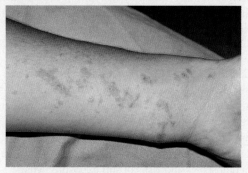

(Jensen)

Asymmetrical

Distributed solely on one side of the body (contact dermatitis)

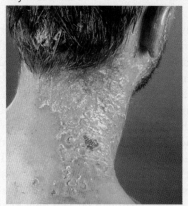

(Jensen)

Zosteriform

Lesions following a nerve (herpes zoster)

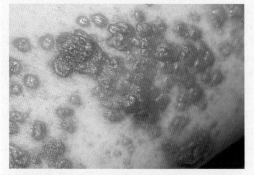

(Jensen)

Generalized

Lesions scattered over the entire body (psoriasis, herpes varicella)

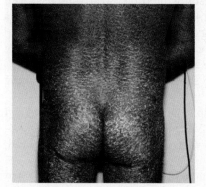

(Jensen)

Skin Cancer

Skin cancer is the most common type of cancer. In 2012, there were an estimated 81,300 cases of nonmelanoma skin cancer and 5,800 cases of melanoma in Canada. This accounts for almost half of all cancers. The number of skin cancer–related deaths was approximately 1,290 in 2012; 320 deaths were related to nonmelanoma and 970 related to melanoma (Canadian Cancer Society, 2012).

Melanoma, the most serious type of skin cancer, develops in the cells (melanocytes) that produce **melanin**—the pigment that gives skin its colour. Melanoma can also form in the eyes and, rarely, in internal organs, such as the intestines.

Most skin cancers are the nonmelanoma type, including basal and squamous cell skin cancers. Most nonmelanoma cancers are basal cell carcinomas. These can damage deeper tissues, such as muscles and bones, although it almost never spreads to other parts of the body. Squamous cell carcinoma is less common, often starting in skin that has been injured or diseased. It sometimes spreads to other parts of the body. There are other types of skin cancer that are not melanoma, but these are much less common. They include Merkel cell carcinoma and several kinds of sarcomas.

Skin Cancer Treatment

Both nonmelanoma and melanoma skin cancer can be successfully treated with early detection and treatment. Recognizing symptoms and going for regular checkups are the best ways to detect skin cancer. Nurses should teach patients about what skin changes to look for and to check their skin regularly, including in areas that are hard to see such as the scalp, soles of the feet, and backs of the legs.

Approximately one third of melanomas occur in existing **nevi** (commonly called *birthmarks*, *beauty marks*, or *moles*). Melanoma frequently occurs on the lower legs and back in women and on the trunk, head, and back in men. The tumors are often dark brown or black. Patients should be taught of the characteristics of normal moles and to consult a healthcare professional immediately if their moles or lesions show any of the clinical signs of melanoma (Fig. 36.8). They should also be taught about sun safety, risk factors for skin cancer, skin self-examination, and the dangers of tanning beds.

Normal moles have the following characteristics:

- Solid tan, brown, black, or flesh colour
- Smaller than 6 mm in diameter (size of a pencil eraser)
- Well-defined edges
- Usually round or oval in shape with flat or dome-like surface
- Emergence before 30 years of age

Sun Safety

The sun generates three forms of ultraviolet radiation: ultraviolet A (UVA), ultraviolet B (UVB), and ultraviolet C (UVC). UVA and UVB are the only rays that reach the earth's surface.

UVA light is commonly called *tanning rays*, and UVB light is commonly called *burning rays*. However, UVA rays can cause burning as well as tanning, and they also inhibit the immune system. Both UVA and UVB rays are believed to cause skin cancer, so there is no such thing as a healthy suntan.

Jane tells the RN at the Canadian Cancer Society booth that her friend, Troy, is a 25-year-old man who is working as a landscaper. Jane is concerned that Troy is getting too much sun exposure as he works 12 to 14 hours a day outdoors in the direct sun. Jane states Troy is resistant to any advice to use sunscreen or chemical sunblock. Given your knowledge of developmental stages and risks of sun exposure, what strategies would you recommend that Jane use when counselling Troy about the dangers of excessive sun exposure?

Sunscreens are lotions that contain materials that absorb or block UVA and UVB rays. They can help protect the skin if used correctly. They must be applied liberally over all exposed body surfaces. A sunscreen must also have a high enough sun protection factor (SPF). SPF is a number determined experimentally by exposing subjects to a light spectrum. The amount of light that induces redness in sunscreen-protected skin, divided by the amount of light that induces redness in unprotected skin, equals the SPF. A sunscreen with an SPF of 15 will delay the onset of sunburn in a person who would otherwise burn in 15 minutes to 150 minutes. Dermatologists recommend using a sunscreen with an SPF of at least 30. This blocks 97% of the sun's rays. Other types of sun protection include wearing a hat with a brim, wraparound sunglasses, and clothing to protect exposed skin.

The intensity of UV rays is greatest during the middle of the day, and exposure to the sun between 10 AM and 4 PM increases potentially damaging effects. Reflection of UV waves off snow, concrete, sand, and water doubles exposure. Help patients to understand the following:

- Avoid direct exposure to the sun between 10 AM and 4 PM or anytime the UV index is 3 or higher.
- Stay in the shade as much as possible, under umbrellas, awnings, or trees.
- Cover skin with loose-fitting, lightweight, tightly woven clothing.
- If exposure to the sun is probable, wear sunscreen with SPF of at least 30. It should be reapplied every 2 to 3 hours and after swimming or perspiring.
- Sunscreen should be applied 20 minutes prior to exposure in order to enhance absorption into the skin.
- Lip balm with SPF should be applied repeatedly during sun exposure.
- Sunglasses that wrap around the eyes should be worn and have at least 99% UVA and UVB protection.
- Wear a hat with a wide brim to protect the face, head, neck, and ears.
- Take these precautions all year round (Canadian Skin Cancer Foundation, 2012).

Melanoma is a less common but most dangerous form of skin cancer since it can spread in the body.

MELANOMA SKIN CANCER
KNOW THE SIGNS, SAVE A LIFE

ABCDEs of Melanoma

A ASYMMETRY
The shape on one side is different than the other side.

B BORDER
The border or visible edge is irregular, ragged and imprecise.

C COLOUR
There is a colour variation with brown, black, red, grey or white within the lesion.

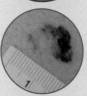

D DIAMETER
Growth is typical of melanoma. It is usually more than 6 mm although it can be less.

E EVOLUTION
Look for change in colour, size, shape or symptom such as itching, tenderness or bleeding.

Photos provided by Dr Joël Claveau

5 steps to SKIN CANCER SELF-EXAM

1 Using a mirror in a well lit room, check the front of your body - face, neck, shoulders, arms, chest, abdomen, thighs and lower legs.

2 Turn sideways, raise your arms and look carefully at the right and left sides of your body, including the underarm area.

3 With a hand-held mirror, check your upper back, neck and scalp. Next, examine your lower back, buttocks, backs of thighs and calves.

4 Examine your forearms, palms, back of the hands, fingernails and in between each finger.

5 Finally, check your feet - the tops, soles, toenails, toes and spaces in between.

PROTECT YOURSELF!
The best ways to protect yourself are to:
• Find out your risk factors
• Learn the early signs, the ABCDEs of melanoma
• Protect yourself from the sun from spring to fall and avoid sunbeds
• Check your skin once a month
• Take action if you see any suspicious spots

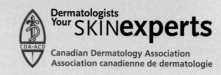

Dermatologists Your SKINexperts
Canadian Dermatology Association
Association canadienne de dermatologie

For further information, visit www.dermatology.ca

Figure 36.8 ABCDE of melanoma.

- Chronic UV exposure without protection or overexposure to artificial light from a tanning bed
- Persons with fair skin, hair, and eyes have less melanin and less protection from UV rays.
- Severe and frequent childhood sunburns
- Prior diagnosis of melanoma
- First-degree relative (e.g., a parent) with melanoma
- Multiple moles or dysplastic nevi
- Recreational lifestyle or occupation that leads to greater sun exposure
- Weakened immune system
- Occupational exposure to coal tar, pitch, creosote, arsenic compounds, or radium
- Spontaneous mutation in a gene (*BRAF*) has been identified that is responsible for 70% of the cases of melanoma.

Risk Factors for Skin Cancer

UV radiation is the most important focus area for both preventing skin cancer and determining risk. Exposure to UV radiation has been shown to cause all types of skin cancer, particularly melanoma. Refer to Box 36.1 for a list of risk factors for melanoma. Patients should be taught of the steps for self-examination listed in Box 36.2.

Dangers of Tanning Beds

In light of a growing body of evidence linking indoor tanning and skin cancer, the Canadian Skin Cancer Foundation strongly recommends avoiding the use of tanning beds. The World Health Organization designated tanning beds "carcinogenic to humans" in 2009 (Box 36.3). First exposure to tanning beds before age 25 years increases the risk of melanoma by 75%. Use of a tanning bed even once is associated with increased risk of melanoma by 15%. Tanning beds have UV doses well above the midday sun—as much as 14 times higher UVA and 4 times higher UVB (Canadian Skin Cancer Foundation, 2012).

BOX 36.2   **Skin Self-Examination**

Patients should be taught to examine their skin on a monthly basis and follow these steps:

1. Get fully undressed and stand in front of a full-length mirror.
2. Carefully look at the entire body, using a handheld mirror to look at areas difficult to see such as the soles of the feet and back.
3. Use a comb or blow-dryer when examining the scalp and examine in a systematic way, section by section.
4. Report any suspicious lesion to a health-care provider.

BOX 36.3   **Skin Cancer**

- One in six Canadians born in the 1990s will develop skin cancer.
- Melanoma is the number one cancer killer of women aged 25 to 30 years.
- The risk of melanoma is 75% greater for people who use tanning beds before the age of 25 years.

Canadian Skin Cancer Foundation, 2012.

Jane asks the RN at the Canadian Cancer Society booth about concerns she has about working at a tanning salon, as Jane has seen an advertisement for a part-time tanning salon attendant. What would the RN tell Jane about ethical implications of a nursing student working at a tanning salon?

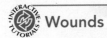

Wounds

Wounds are injuries to the body, the skin in particular, causing a breach of the layers of skin. Wounds are categorized as acute, chronic, and palliative, which relates to the way they develop, their duration, and also the health of the patient. An acute wound is expected to follow the pattern and time frame of wound healing from primary intention. A chronic wound may arise from an acute episode. A pressure ulcer arises from an acute episode of unrelieved pressure. It may take weeks to heal. It becomes chronic because of the length of time it takes to heal as well as the mechanism of healing. Wounds that arise from underlying disease are chronic and generally are hard to heal. Palliative wounds are those that never heal either because of the underlying disease or because people are at the end of life (Grocott, 2012) (Fig. 36.9).

Pressure Ulcers

A pressure ulcer is a localized injury to the skin and/or underlying tissue, usually over a bony prominence, as a result of pressure, or pressure that can occur with **shear** or friction (National Pressure Ulcer Advisory Panel [NPUAP] & European Pressure Ulcer Advisory Panel [EPUAP], 2009, as cited in NPUAP, 2013).

Pressure ulcers are caused by pressure, shear, or friction of the body on an immovable surface, which restricts in blood flow to the skin, leading to tissue damage and cell death. Many pressure ulcers should be avoidable with adequate risk assessment, pressure relieving equipment, and regular turning. Hospital-acquired pressure ulceration represents a major failure in systems to secure patient safety and quality care (Hurd & Posnett, 2009).

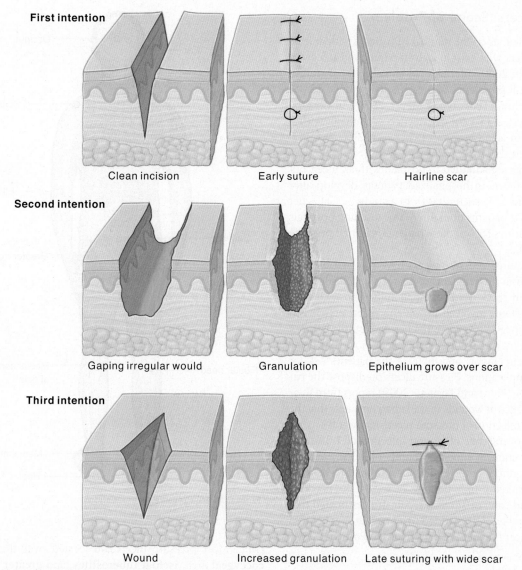

First intention

Clean incision   Early suture   Hairline scar

Second intention

Gaping irregular would   Granulation   Epithelium grows over scar

Third intention

Wound   Increased granulation   Late suturing with wide scar

Figure 36.9 Types of wounds.

RESEARCH

POINT PREVALENCE OF WOUNDS IN A SAMPLE OF ACUTE HOSPITALS IN CANADA

This research was conducted to provide new evidence on wound prevalence and the potential resource impact of nonhealing wounds in the acute care sector by summarizing results from wound audits carried out by 13 acute care hospitals in Canada in 2006 and 2007. Audits were carried out in each hospital by the same team of independent advanced practice nurses using standard data collection forms. The results reported here were derived from the summary reports for each hospital. A total of 3,099 patients were surveyed (median 259 per hospital). In the sample hospitals, the mean prevalence of patients with wounds was 41.2%. Most wounds were pressure ulcers (56.2%) or surgical wounds (31.1%). The mean prevalence of pressure ulcers was 22.9%. Most pressure ulcers (79.3%) were hospital-acquired, and 26.5% were severe (Stage III or IV). The rate of surgical infection was 6.3%. Forty-five percent of patients had dressings changed at least daily, and the mean dressing time was 10.5 minutes.

Nursing Implications

Wounds are a common and potentially expensive occurrence in acute care hospitals. Any wound has the potential to develop complications, which compromise patient safety and increase hospital costs. Ensuring consistent, best-practice wound management programs should be a key priority for hospital managers.

Hurd, T., & Posnett, J. (2009). Point prevalence of wounds in a sample of acute hospitals in Canada. International Wound Journal, 6(4), 287–293.

Pressure Ulcers: Scope of Problem

Prevalence is defined as the number of patients with at least one pressure ulcer who exist in a given population at a given point in time. In 2009, international cross-sectional studies found the overall prevalence of pressure ulcers to be 12.3% (VanGilder, Amlung, Harrison, & Meyer, 2009). In Canada, estimates suggested that the prevalence of patients with a pressure ulcer in acute hospitals is between 24% and 26% (Hurd & Posnett, 2009).

Some patients are admitted to hospital with an ulcer, but most pressure ulcers in hospitalized patients develop after admission (Hurd & Posnett, 2009). In a study by Gallagher et al. (2008), 672 patients from three large teaching hospitals had pressure ulcers; 75% of these patients acquired pressure ulcers in hospital.

Hospital-acquired pressure ulcers have received increasing attention from government, regulatory, and health-care organizations. In 2003, nearly one-half million hospital stays in the United States involved a pressure ulcer, which is a 63% increase since 1993 (Bry, Buescher, & Sandrik, 2012).

Pressure ulcers add to the patient's length of stay, delay the patient's recuperation, and increase the patient's risk for developing complications. Pressure ulcers predispose the patient to infection. Hurd and Posnett (2009) report from their study of prevalence of wounds in Canadian hospitals that the average rate of infection of pressure ulcers is about 8% compared with an overall rate of wound infection of 7.3%, and the rate of infection in surgical wounds of 6.3%. Pressure ulcers often require that the patient be admitted to hospital for lengthy periods of time because of sepsis, the need for complex wound care, or surgical repair. It is estimated that the average number of days added to a hospital stay because of a pressure ulcer is about 8.2 days (Hurd & Posnett, 2009).

Etiology

Pressure ulcers are ischemic lesions of the skin and underlying structures caused by constant pressure that impairs the flow of blood and lymph. They are most likely to develop over bony prominences but can occur on any part of the body that is subjected to external pressure, friction, or shearing forces (Simandl, 2010).

Mechanism of Development

Factors contributing to the development of pressure ulcers include (1) pressure, (2) shearing forces, (3) friction, and (4) moisture. External pressures that exceed capillary pressure disrupt blood supply in the capillary beds. When the pressure between a bony prominence and support surface exceeds normal capillary filling pressure, capillary blood flow is obstructed (Simandl, 2010). Prolonged pressure leads to accumulation of metabolic waste products, which lead to cellular **necrosis**.

The weight of the body puts pressure on the tissues covering bony prominences whether a person is sitting or

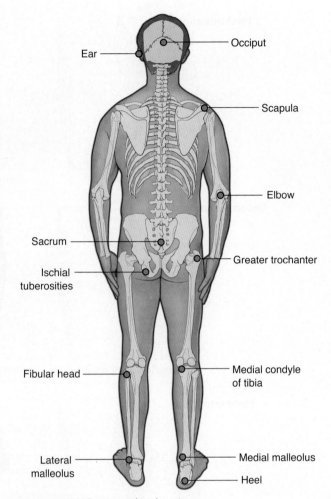

Figure 36.10 Pressure ulcer locations.

lying. Most pressure ulcers are located over the sacrum, **coccygeal** area, **ischial tuberosities**, and **greater trochanters** (Maklebust, 2005). Pressure over a bony prominence is transmitted from the surface to the underlying dense bone, sandwiching all of the tissue between. Therefore, the greatest pressure occurs at the surface of the bone and dissipates outward in a cone-like manner toward the surface of the skin. As a result, extensive underlying tissue damage can be present when a small superficial skin lesion is first noticed (Simandl, 2010) (Fig. 36.10).

Risk Factors

Changes in sensory perception, level of skin moisture, nutrition and hydration status, mobility and circulatory status, as well as fecal and urine incontinence and the presence of shear and friction forces are risk factors for the development of pressure ulcers (Simandl, 2010, p. 1518). These factors place elderly people who have conditions that result in immobility and physiological changes to the skin at risk. In Canada, separations from hospital of elderly people were 5 times more than all other adults in 2009 to 2010 (Canadian Institute of Health Information, 2011).

Causes of Pressure Ulcers

Pressure damage tends to be greatest over bony prominences, where soft tissue can become trapped between the underlying bone and the source of the pressure. Pressure greater than 32 millimeters of mercury (mmHg) obstructs blood supply, preventing oxygen, and nutrients from reaching tissues. The accumulation of metabolic wastes from obstructed blood supply results in the production of free radicals. Free radicals are highly reactive compounds that are known to be highly destructive to body tissues (Martini, 2012). Lying on a standard hospital mattress can induce pressure of 50 to 94 mmHg on the heels, sacrum, and **scapula**. Sitting on a hard surface can result in a local pressure of 300 to 500 mmHg, depending on weight and surface area (Jaul, 2010).

Shearing forces, friction, and moisture are also causes of pressure ulcers. Shearing forces such as those that happen when sliding a patient up in bed stretch and traumatize blood vessels in the underlying tissue. Friction can rub off the outer layers of skin, which then can be accentuated by pressure or shearing, creating an ulcer. Moisture softens the skin to the point that it predisposes the skin to ulceration (Youell & Wright, 2010) (Fig. 36.11).

Assessment

Risk assessment, which is critical in clinical practice, aims to identify susceptible patients and institute appropriate interventions to prevent pressure ulcers. Identification of patients at risk can be accomplished by using one of the several tools available. In Canada, the Braden Scale for Predicting Pressure Sore Risk is commonly used. It is reported to be the most widely used and tested of all risk assessment scales. This scale consists of six subscales used by nurses to assess risk factors that are associated with pressure ulcer development (Cowan, Stechmiller, Rowe, & Kairalla, 2012) (Fig. 36.12).

Using the Braden Scale, nurses can assess six broad categories, including sensory perception, moisture, activity, mobility, nutrition, and friction and shear. Total scores range from 6 to 23, with the lower scores indicating a lower level of functioning and inversely a higher risk of developing a pressure ulcer. A score of 18 or below indicates a risk for developing a pressure ulcer (Fleck, 2012).

Pressure Ulcer Classification System

A common international definition and classification system has been developed and approved for use by the National Pressure Ulcer Advisory Panel (NPUAP) (United States) and the European Pressure Ulcer Advisory Panel (EPUAP) (2009). A four category system has been developed, with additional categories to be used in the United States of America.

Previously, pressure ulcers were graded using Stage I to Stage IV; however the term has recently been changed to "Categories" because "Stages" implies a progression, and that is not always the case. Both terms are used in the following system (Fig. 36.13).

Category/Stage I: Non-Blanchable Redness of Intact Skin

This category includes intact skin with non-blanchable erythema of a localized area, usually over a bony prominence. Discolouration of the skin, warmth, edema, hardness, or pain may also be present. Darkly pigmented skin may not have visible blanching. The area may be more painful, firmer or softer, or warmer or cooler than adjacent tissue. Category I may be difficult to detect in individuals with dark skin tones.

Category/Stage II: Partial Thickness Skin Loss or Blister

Partial thickness loss of dermis is present when there is a shallow open ulcer with a red/pink wound bed without **slough**. It may also present as an intact or open/ruptured serum-filled or **serosanguineous** fluid–filled blister. It presents as a shiny or dry shallow ulcer without slough or bruising. This category should not be used to describe skin tears, blisters from burn injuries, tape burns, incontinence-associated **dermatitis**, maceration, or excoriation.

Category/Stage III: Full-Thickness Skin Loss (Fat Visible)

With full-thickness tissue loss, subcutaneous fat may be visible, but bone, tendons, or muscles are not exposed. Some slough maybe present and may include tunneling under neighboring tissue. The depth of Category III pressure ulcer varies by anatomical location. Shallow ulcers can occur on the bridge of the nose, ear, occipital area, and malleolus where there is no (adipose) subcutaneous tissue. In contrast, areas of significant adiposity, for example, the buttocks, can develop extremely deep Category III pressure ulcers. Bone or tendon is not visible or directly palpable.

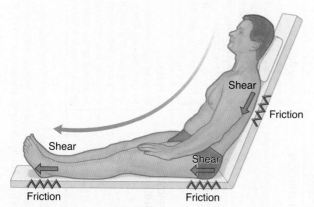

Figure 36.11 Shearing diagram.

BRADEN SCALE FOR PREDICTING PRESSURE SORE RISK

Patient's Name _____ Evaluator's Name _____ Date of Assessment _____

SENSORY PERCEPTION ability to respond meaning-fully to pressure-related discomfort	**1. Completely Limited** Unresponsive (does not moan, flinch, or grasp) to painful stimuli, due to diminished level of con-sciousness or sedation. OR limited ability to feel pain over most of body	**2. Very Limited** Responds only to painful stimuli. Cannot communicate discomfort except by moaning or restlessness OR has a sensory impairment which limits the ability to feel pain or discomfort over ½ of body.	**3. Slightly Limited** Responds to verbal commands, but cannot always communicate discomfort or the need to be turned. OR has some sensory impairment which limits ability to feel pain or discomfort in 1 or 2 extremities.	**4. No Impairment** Responds to verbal commands. Has no sensory deficit which would limit ability to feel or voice pain or discomfort.
MOISTURE degree to which skin is exposed to moisture	**1. Constantly Moist** Skin is kept moist almost constantly by perspiration, urine, etc. Dampness is detected every time patient is moved or turned.	**2. Very Moist** Skin is often, but not always moist. Linen must be changed at least once a shift.	**3. Occasionally Moist:** Skin is occasionally moist, requiring an extra linen change approximately once a day.	**4. Rarely Moist** Skin is usually dry, linen only requires changing at routine intervals.
ACTIVITY degree of physical activity	**1. Bedfast** Confined to bed.	**2. Chairfast** Ability to walk severely limited or non-existent. Cannot bear own weight and/or must be assisted into chair or wheelchair.	**3. Walks Occasionally** Walks occasionally during day, but for very short distances, with or without assistance. Spends majority of each shift in bed or chair	**4. Walks Frequently** Walks outside room at least twice a day and inside room at least once every two hours during working hours.
MOBILITY ability to change and control body position	**1. Completely Immobile** Does not make even slight changes in body or extremity position without assistance	**2. Very Limited** Makes occasional slight changes in body or extremity position but unable to make frequent or significant changes independently.	**3. Slightly Limited** Makes frequent though slight changes in body or extremity position independently.	**4. No Limitation** Makes major and frequent changes in position without assistance.
NUTRITION usual food intake pattern	**1. Very Poor** Never eats a complete meal. Rarely eats more than ⅓ a of any food offered. Eats 2 servings or less of protein (meat or dairy products) per day. Takes fluids poorly. Does not take a liquid dietary supplement OR is NPO and/or maintained on clear liquids or IV's for more than 5 days.	**2. Probably Inadequate** Rarely eats a complete meal and generally eats only about ½ of any food offered. Protein intake includes only 3 servings of meat or dairy products per day. Occasionally will take a dietary supplement. OR receives less than optimum amount of liquid diet or tube feeding	**3. Adequate** Eats over half of most meals. Eats a total of 4 servings of protein (meat, dairy products per day. Occasionally will refuse a meal, but will usually take a supplement when offered OR is on a tube feeding or TPN regimen which probably meets most of nutritional needs	**4. Excellent** Eats most of every meal. Never refuses a meal. Usually eats a total of 4 or more servings of meat and dairy products. Occasionally eats between meals. Does not require supplementation.
FRICTION & SHEAR	**1. Problem** Requires moderate to maximum assis-tance in moving. Complete lifting without sliding against sheets is impossible. Frequently slides down in bed or chair, requiring frequent repositioning with maxi-mum assistance. Spasticity, contractures or agitation leads to almost constant friction	**2. Potential Problem** Moves feebly or requires minimum assistance. During a move skin prob-ably slides to some extent against sheets, chair, restraints or other devices. Maintains relatively good position in chair or bed most of the time but occasionally slides down.	**3. No Apparent Problem** Moves in bed and in chair independently and has sufficient muscle strength to lift up completely during move. Maintains good position in bed or chair.	

Total Score _____

Figure 36.12 Diagram of Braden Risk Assessment Tool. (Permission granted to use tool from Barbara Braden & Nancy Bergstrom, 1988. Reprinted with permission.

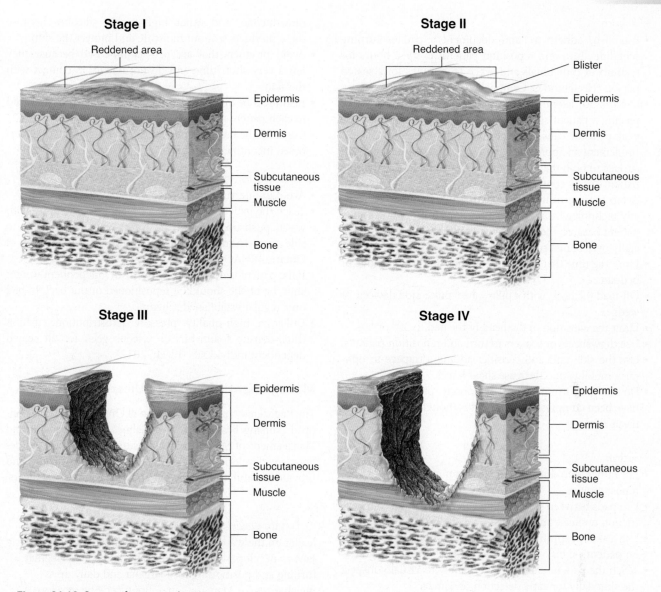

Figure 36.13 Stages of pressure ulcers.

Category/Stage IV: Full-Thickness Tissue Loss (Muscle/Bone Visible)

This category is when there is full-thickness tissue loss with exposed bone, tendon, or muscle. Slough or **eschar** may be present and often include undermining and tunneling. The depth of a Category IV pressure ulcer varies by anatomical location. The bridge of the nose, outer ear, occipital area, and the malleolus of the tibia and fibula do not have adipose or subcutaneous tissue, and these ulcers can be shallow. Category IV ulcers can extend into muscle and/or supporting structures such as fascia, tendon, or joint capsule. This exposure makes **osteomyelitis** or osteitis likely to occur. Exposed bone and muscle is visible or directly palpable (NPUAP & EPUAP, 2009).

The system for use in the United States includes a category titled, "Unclassified: Full-Thickness or Tissue Loss Depth Unknown." This category refers to wounds that cannot be measured because of depth and covering with slough tissue.

Jane Smith is caring for Margaret, an 84-year-old patient who develops a pressure ulcer on her left buttock. It is assessed as Stage II. What are some of the key observations and actions Jane will make to prevent or slow a Stage I pressure ulcer from progressing to a Stage II? Now that the patient has a Stage II pressure ulcer, what are the critical nursing interventions that must be done to heal the ulcer and prevent it from progressing?

Preventing Pressure Ulcers

Pressure ulcer prevention encompasses alleviating the possible causative factors. Preventative strategies should address pressure, shear, friction, moisture, and redistribution of pressure.

Pressure

- Establish, adhere to, and document a patient turning schedule. Turn and reposition patients every 2 hours for recumbent individuals and every 15 minutes for a seated person (Houghton & Campbell, 2013).
- Use the 30° lateral position in a supine patient instead of placing a patient side-lying at 90°. This may decrease the peak pressure caused by the greater trochanter.
- Implement an appropriate pressure-redistribution support surface to both the seated and recumbent surfaces that the patient's body contacts.
- Avoid the use of invalid rings, "donuts," rubber rings, or any technology that has a cutout for cushioning a seated patient because these can actually increase pressures especially over bony prominences.
- Limit the time that the patient spends on the commode or bedpan.
- Off-load the heels with a pillow, heel protection devices, or wedge.
- Limit the elevation of the head of the bed to 30° or less.
- Use drawsheets or soakers to turn and reposition patients.
- Use the side rails and consider adding a trapeze to optimize mobility and decrease shear forces.
- Do not perform massage over bony prominences that have been compressed because it is thought this can cause tissue damage.

Friction

- Lift rather than drag the patient when moving or repositioning.
- Use pads between surfaces that rub together and to relieve friction on heels and elbows.
- Use a skin **prepping solution** or sealant before using tape on patient's skin.
- Teach the patient and his or her family to visually inspect the skin daily for early detection of damage.
- Encourage proper hydration and nutrition.
- Institute an active or passive range-of-motion routine.
- Apply transparent dressings or skin sealants to protect the epidermis.

Moisture

- Apply high-quality moisturizers to the skin to increase skin's water content and thus pliability and strength. Apply moisturizers anytime water comes in contact with the skin, especially after the bath or shower within the 3-minute window of opportunity.
- Protect the skin from body fluids and drainage by absorption.
- Decrease baths and address a patient's need for skin cleansing individually by body region.
- Use moisturizing, soap-free cleansers with a neutral or slightly acidic pH.
- Apply barrier creams that remain in contact with the skin despite cleaning to offer protection from incontinence episodes. Good examples of ingredients include zinc oxide, dimethicone, and other high-quality silicones because these products seal out moisture and protect the skin.
- Avoid products that are petrolatum-based because they last a very short time and do not remain in contact with the skin.
- Institute a bowel and bladder program that is customized to each patient and can be documented.
- Consider the use of some of the newer high-tech polymer-based incontinent products.

Redistribution of Pressure

- Avoid uninterrupted sitting.
- Teach the patient to perform a weight shift (stand up with assist, push-up, bend at the waist, or shift from side to side every 15 minutes) (Registered Nurses' Association of Ontario [RNAO], 2007).
- If the patient is not able to perform an independent weight shift, he or she should be repositioned or put back in bed on a regular established schedule.
- Utilize a high-quality pressure redistribution cushion (high-density foam, air, or viscous gels) for all seated dependent individuals (Fleck, 2012).

Management of Pressure Ulcers

The Registered Nurses Association of Ontario (RNAO) developed Nursing Best Practice Guidelines for Assessment and Management of Stage I to IV Pressure Ulcers. These guidelines are developed using the best evidence available and provide a useful tool to prevent and manage pressure ulcers.

Mary Blevins is an experienced RN who is the team leader on the ward where Margaret is a patient. Mary assists Jane to develop a nursing care plan that includes regular turning and positioning for Margaret and daily dressing changes for Margaret's pressure ulcer. She develops a turning schedule that forms part of the documentation for this patient and enlists the help of her nursing team in implementing this regular turning schedule and dressing changes.

Initial identification of a pressure ulcer requires a complete history and focused physical assessment. This should include the following:

- A psychosocial assessment, including quality of life from the patient's perspective, mental status, social support, culture, resources, stressors, sexuality, alcohol, and drug abuse
- Optimum nutrition facilitates wound healing, maintains immune competence, and decreases the risk of infection. A nutritional assessment is important including consultation with a nutritionist.
- Pain should be assessed routinely and regularly using validated pain assessment tools, including location, frequency, and intensity of pain to determine the presence of underlying disease.

- Assess all patients with existing pressure ulcers to determine their risk for developing additional pressure ulcers. All patients at risk should be place on a high-specification foam mattress rather than standard hospital management.
- Vascular assessment including palpable pedal pulses, capillary refill, ankle/brachial pressure index is recommended (RNAO, 2007).

Consistency in the process for describing pressure ulcers facilitates communication amongst the health-care team. Pressure ulcer treatment requires consistent objective assessments and documentation for proper treatment. Documentation and other forms of communication must reflect valid, reliable data on pressure ulcers and action taken for prevention and treatment (Li & Korniewicz, 2013). Initial assessment of the pressure ulcers should include category or stage, location, surface area, odor, sinus tracts, exudates, appearance of wound bed, and condition of surrounding skin (RNAO, 2007).

Category/Stage I ulcers are managed best by relief of pressure and barrier cream, whereas Category/Stage II with skin loss usually is managed with transparent films because they retain moisture and prevent friction. Category/Stage III should be dressed with synthetic dressings rather than gauze because synthetic dressings cause less pain with less frequent dressing changes. These include hydrocolloids and foam dressings. Surgical repair of Category/Stage III ulcers may include closure, skin grafting, and flaps, depending on the patient's needs. Category/Stage III ulcers can also be treated using electrical stimulation, wound vacuum assisted wound closure, or heat therapy (Doyle & Kowalak, 2009).

Wound bed preparation includes cleaning, debridement, and dressings. Saline or potable water may be used to cleanse most pressure ulcers; solutions with surfactants and/or antimicrobials may be used for wounds with debris or infection. Necrotic or devitalized tissue should be removed to alter the wound healing environment by reducing the bacterial concentration and decreasing the risk of spreading infection. Debridement can be accomplished by removal of necrotic tissue or by the use autolytic solutions and dressings (RNAO, 2007).

Recommendations and supporting evidence is available for a myriad of dressings, including hydrocolloid, transparent film, hydrogel, alginate, foam, polymeric membrane, silver-impregnated, honey-impregnated, iodine-impregnated, gauze, silicon-coated, collagen matrix, and composite dressings for treatment of pressure ulcers (NPUAP & EPUAP, 2009). In cases where anaerobic infection is suspected, occlusive dressings are not recommended (RNAO, 2007).

Infected pressure ulcers do not heal. Prevention, early diagnosis, and effective treatment of infection are critical components for pressure ulcer healing. Early identification of patients at high risk for pressure ulcer infection and early recognition of colonization and local infection with ulcer pain, pocketing, friable granulation tissue, and increased drainage are necessary. Topical antimicrobial agents can be used directly on the infected area of the ulcer, and systemic antibiotics are needed for systemic infections such as cellulitis, osteomyelitis, or sepsis (NPUAP & EPUAP, 2009). There is some evidence to suggest that Chinese herbal medicine ointment is an effective strategy for treating pressure ulcers. Various different herbs are used in these ointments (Zhang et al., 2013).

Unavoidable Pressure Ulcers

Prevention of pressure ulcers is a critical nursing intervention. In the past, it was believed that pressure ulcers are secondary to poor nursing care. It is now recognized that some pressure ulcers are not avoidable. Unavoidable pressure ulcers are those that the patient develops even though the care providers in a facility did perform the critical elements of evaluating the patient's condition and pressure ulcer risk assessment; defined and implemented interventions that are consistent with the patient's needs, goals, and standards of practice; and monitored and evaluated the impact of interventions and revised them as appropriate (Fleck, 2012).

Wound Healing

Successful wound healing requires a cascade of events and a series of physiological responses before resulting in durable tissue repair. Healing by primary intention occurs with wounds where there is minimal tissue loss and edges are neatly approximated, such as surgical wounds or paper cuts (Wagner & Hardin-Pierce, 2014). Wound healing by primary intention occurs in three phases:

1. Initial (3 to 5 days): approximation of incision edges; migration of epithelial cells; clot serves as meshwork
2. Granulation (5 days to 4 weeks): migration of fibroblasts; secretion of collagen; abundance of capillary buds; wound fragile
3. Scar contracture (7 days to several months): remodeling of collagen; strengthening of scar (Source: Wagner & Hardin Pierce, 2014)

Wounds that heal by secondary intention are usually large wounds characterized by irregular wound margins, significant tissue loss, damage, or bacterial infection (Wagner & Hardin-Pierce, 2014). Signs of wound infection include redness, swelling, localized warmth, purulent drainage, and wound tenderness/pain. The person may also have a fever, swollen lymph glands, or red streaks emanating from the wound to surrounding integumentary tissue. A primary incision may become inflamed and infected, resulting in wound reopening and wound healing by secondary intention as the body attempts to close gaping wound edges. All phases of wound healing are prolonged; however, the same activities as healing by primary intention take place and may result in more scar tissue. The nurse must be diligent in noting changes in wound characteristics, such as amount and odor of exudates, inflammation, wound margins, and debris. Systemically, fever and elevation of white blood cell counts indicate wound infections (Wagner & Hardin-Pierce, 2014).

Wound healing by tertiary intention involves wound closure by primary and secondary intention. The wound is left open until the wound bed is free of debris and infection, and then it is closed to heal by primary intention (Wagner & Hardin-Pierce, 2014). Psychologically, an individual may experience several emotions during wound healing. Health professionals will be alert to recognize the emotional and physical effects of wound care and provide support (Wagner & Hardin-Pierce, 2014).

Wound Cleansing

Wound cleansing is the process of using fluids to reduce the bacterial count and to remove dead tissue, waste products, and other agents that have the potential to delay wound healing. Saline can be used to cleanse most pressure ulcers, or solutions with surfactants or antimicrobials are used for ulcers with debris or infection (NPUAP & EPUAP, 2009). Cleansing solutions should be nontoxic, remain effective in the presence of organic material, reduce the number of microorganisms, not cause sensitivity reactions, be available, and cost-effective (Main, 2008). Saline is recommended because it is an isotonic solution that does not interfere with the normal healing process; however, potable tap water, cooled boiled water, and distilled water have been used in some settings (Fernandez & Griffiths, 2012). Authors of a systematic review conclude that there is no good clinical trial evidence to support the use of any particular wound cleansing solution (Moore & Cowman, 2013).

Antiseptic agents, such as alcohol, peroxide, and iodine, have long been used to cleanse wounds primarily because they are effective against both transient and resident flora on the skin and reduce microbial counts either by mechanical removal, chemical action, or both (Atiyeh, Dibo, & Hayek, 2009). Povidine and hydrogen peroxide have been shown to reduce proliferation of normal human fibroblasts pivotal to wound healing, whereas silver-containing compounds and chlorhexidine have not shown the same effect at lower doses (Thomas et al., 2009).

Current wound cleansing practice is to either scrub or irrigate wounds with normal saline, as it is an isotonic solution and does not interfere with normal wound healing. Tap water is sometimes used in the community (Atiyeh et al., 2009). Antiseptic solutions may be used in exceptional circumstances, and caution is advised as the toxicity might outweigh benefits (Main, 2008).

Margaret is turned using the schedule on her nursing care plan. The nurses have been meticulous in assuring that this schedule is adhered to and documented. Nevertheless, Margaret develops a pressure ulcer on her left buttock in which the partial loss of the outer layers of the skin with an open ulcer that is pink-red and has some slough in it. It is assessed as a Stage II ulcer. Mary Blevins, RN, team leader, consults with Jane Smith and recommends that she cover the ulcer with gauze dressing while she makes a referral to the ostomy nurse. The ostomy nurse sees Margaret within an hour. She recommends that her turning schedule be maintained, using a 30° lateral turn rather than a side-lying position. She also recommends heel protectors and placing a pillow underneath Margaret's lower legs to reduce heel pressure on the bed. For Margaret's wound, the ostomy nurse recommends a transparent semipermeable film dressing, which should be left in place until it leaks or for at least 3 to 5 days.

Dressings

The purposes of wound dressings are to protect wounds from contamination and trauma, to absorb exudates, to provide compression to reduce bleeding and swelling, and to supply medications (RNAO, 2007). Recommendations and supporting evidence are available for the use of a myriad of dressings for wounds and pressure ulcers. Selection of a dressing is dependent on a thorough assessment of the wound and the overall status of the patient. Expected patient outcomes include achievement of a clean and healing wound, protection of the wound bed from bacteria and trauma, prevention of wound deterioration, containment of odor and exudates and reduction of pain or preparation of wounds as the patient moves to another setting (Baranoski & Ayello, 2012). The choice of dressing is dependent on factors affecting wound healing. These factors may include presence of devitalized tissue, the wound infection, and moisture balance (Tinne, 2011).

Clean lacerations and surgical wounds, in which the edges are brought together and approximated with sutures or staples, are covered with a dressing to prevent exogenous contamination, immobilize the surgical site, and help to minimize pain. Traditionally, several layers of absorbent gauze and pads designed to wick away drainage have been used. If a dressing is not absorbent, drainage and blood will pool around the sutures or staples, become a medium for bacterial growth, and can lead to abscess formation. A sterile nonadherent strip or ointment can be placed over the incision line to prevent trauma during dressing removal. Initial dressings are usually left in place for 48 to 72 hours. Earlier changes are indicated if the dressing becomes saturated with drainage. If the dressing is moist on the outermost layer, it loses its capability to act as a barrier and must be reinforced with a sterile dressing or changed. Sterile technique is used to change these dressings (Berg, Fleischer, Kuss, Unversagt, & Langer, 2011).

Think Nurses with specialized training in ostomy and wound care are an excellent resource. How would you make a referral to them? What information would you provide them and what questions would you have of them?

Transparent films, hydrocolloid, and hydrogel dressings are recommended as an alternative to gauze. Studies have shown that although the epidermal resurfacing is enhanced with such dressings, the long-term effect is not known. Early reports indicate that the rate of infections is higher in the incision with these three types of dressings, and more research is needed to develop guidelines for use (Cuzzell, 1997; Jones, 2011). Transparent occlusive films provide a good environment for clean with minimal drainage. Hydrocolloids and hydrogel dressings combine the benefits of occlusion and absorbency; they are particularly useful in burn treatment (Barbel & Efron, 2010) (Table 36.5).

Hydrocolloid dressings provide an occlusive, moist environment conducive to wound healing. They provide the advantages of occlusive, reduced frequency of dressing changes, and better absorption. They have a film that controls evaporation, and the semipermeable film facilitates the exchange of oxygen and water vapor. The wound is protected from contamination by exogenous bacteria, and the hydrocolloid layer absorbs exudates (Kim, Lee, Seo, & Rhie, 2013). Similarly, hydrogel dressings have high water content and allow a high rate of evaporation without compromising wound hydration (Barbel & Efron, 2010). Hydrogel dressings are reported to have good biocompatibility (Biazar et al., 2012).

Calcium alginate dressings are used when there is skin loss, open surgical wounds with medium to heavy exudate, and on full-thickness chronic wounds. In the presence of wound exudate, alginates turn into a soluble solution through an ion exchange process (Barbel & Efron, 2010). The soft-woven, seaweed-derived fibres absorb exudate and act as an autolytic agent (Tinne, 2011).

Foams are available in several forms. They generally have several layers of polyurethane foam and may come as a cavity dressing. They are suitable for use in open, draining wounds. Foam dressings are highly absorbent and nonadherent and maintain a moist wound bed. They can be used on wounds with either minimal or copious amounts of drainage (Tinne, 2011).

A wide variety of silver-impregnated wound dressing have become available in recent years. Silver has broad-spectrum antimicrobial efficacy. There is considerable support for use of silver-impregnated dressings because research has confirmed its positive effects (Leaper, 2012); however, closely controlled cell biology studies have demonstrated significant evidence of cytotoxicity (Du Toit & Page, 2009). The silver impregnated into the dressings is known to kill bacteria by deactivating metabolic pathways and genetic machinery and by weakening bacterial cells walls (Kotz, Fisher, McCluskey, Hartwell, & Dharma, 2009).

TABLE 36.5	Dressing Types		
Dressing Type	**Material Used**	**Advantages**	**Disadvantages**
Gauze	Cotton fibres	Inexpensive Accessible	Sheds fibres Traumatic removal Lateral bacteria migration
Semipermeable film/ membranes	Nonporous plasticized polyvinyl polymer	Maintains moist environment Prevents bacterial migration	Does not prevent wound maceration
Calcium alginate	Polymer extract from seaweed	Absorbs excess moisture Prevents maceration Hemostatic capability	Not suitable for dry wounds Requires moisture to prevent traumatic removal
Hydrogel	Cross-linked polymers such as starch and cellulose	Can provide moisture and absorb moderate amount of exudate	Can cause maceration in wounds with heavy exudates
Hydrocolloid	Gelatin, pectin, and polysaccharides	Provides moist hypoxic wound environment	Does not prevent maceration
Foam	Polyurethane	Moist interface Absorbable	Not suitable for dry wounds
Scaffold material	Cadaver dermis or collagen or silicone	Biocompatible	Localized production of lactic acid may affect wound healing
Honey dressing	Medicinal honey	Antimicrobial, antifungal, anti-inflammatory, deodorizing	Requires frequent changes
Iodine dressing	Povidine	Antiseptic	Cytotoxic
Silver dressing	Silver	Antibacterial, antimicrobial	Systemic toxicity
Charcoal	Charcoal	Odor-absorbing	
Composite	Multilayered	Absorbent, autolytic	

Source: Daunton, C., Kothari, S., Smith L., & Steel, D. (2012). A history of material and practices for wound management. *Wound Practice & Research, 20*(4), 174–186; Newton, H. (2013). An introduction to wound healing and dressings. *British Journal of Healthcare Management, 19*(6), 270–274; Registered Nurses' Association of Ontario. (2007). *Nursing best practice guideline. Assessment & management of stage I to IV pressure ulcers.* Toronto, ON: Author.

Dressings impregnated with honey have the potential to promote new tissue regeneration. Based on a scientifically robust study by Du Toit and Page (2009), there is support for the continued use of honey-impregnated dressings by wound care practitioners. The study established that honey-impregnated dressings could modestly stimulate epidermal and dermal cells in vitro. These researchers go on to say that practitioners have highlighted its antimicrobial potential.

Dressings impregnated with iodine are used in some clinical settings, mainly as a disinfectant agent. Iodine- and iodine derivative–impregnated dressings have an absorptive and debriding quality. Higher concentrations of iodine (greater than 0.1% to 20%) are known to be cytotoxic; however, at more dilute amounts, some evidence to suggests that it is not damaging human fibroblasts (Cooper, 2007). Iodine products have not been used by some clinicians because of the perception that iodine is associated with toxicity when used topically. The toxicity of iodine to cells in culture is dose-dependent. Iodine-containing products are ideal to reduce the bacterial count; they are inexpensive but have unknown resistance and systemic toxicity. They also can be used to reduce the need for systemic antibiotics (Leaper & Durani, 2008). In a systematic review of 27 randomized controlled trials, iodine was found not to lead to a reduction or prolongation of wound-healing time compared with other wound dressings or agents. In individual trials, iodine was found to be significantly superior to other antiseptic agents (Vermeulen, Westerbos, & Ubbink, 2010).

Charcoal-impregnated dressing have been use to absorb odor from necrotic tissue (Lee, Anand, Rajendran, & Walker, 2007). Charcoal has the ability to absorb the small gas molecules that are responsible for malodor, and these are attracted to the surface of the charcoal dressing and held there (Hampton, 2006). Charcoal dressings have also been found to absorb bacteria, local toxins, and wound degradation products, thereby promoting wound healing (Kerihuel, 2010).

Medicated dressings have been used as a drug delivery system. Drugs such as Bacitracin, Polysporin, and framycetin (Soframycin) have been used in dressings to control and eradicate infections (Woo, 2011). Zinc- and benzoyl peroxide–impregnated dressings have been shown to promote epithelisation (Barbel & Efron, 2010).

Skin substitutes, such as dressings with scaffolding material, are used when there is loss of a large amount of skin from either an acute or chronic wound. They are manufactured by tissue engineering and combine several different substances with living cells to provide functional skin substitutes. They have an advantage of being readily available and don't require a painful harvest of donor skin. In addition, they promote healing either by stimulating host cytokine generation or by providing cells that may also produce growth factors locally (Barbel & Efron, 2010).

Proper choice of dressings can help facilitate removal of necrotic tissue in dehisced surgical wounds, traumatic injury wounds, and chronic ulcer wounds. Unlike a closed surgical wound, these wounds are often left open to heal by second intention. They are characterized by surface colonization with microorganisms and take much longer to heal. Black wounds represent devitalized necrotic tissue, which should be debrided to control infection and promote healing. Dressings that are moisture-retentive are generally contraindicated on black wound beds because bacterial proliferation is increased. Yellow wounds produce a cream-coloured or grey necrotic slough, which may be accompanied by purulent exudates. Yellow wounds should be covered with moisture retentive dressings, such as hydrocolloids, and alginates may be used to enhance debridement through autolysis in these types of wounds. Dressings to support autolysis trap bacteria that release proteolytic enzymes and liquefy the necrotic tissue beneath occlusive dressings. Red-coloured wounds indicate presence of viable tissue and should be covered with a dressing that retains some moisture (Houghton & Campbell, 2013).

Mechanical debridement can be achieved with wet to dry gauze dressings. Dressings are soaked with saline and placed next to the wound surface. The entire wound is covered with dry gauze pads. As the saline soaked gauze dries, it causes the contact layer to shrink and traps necrotic debris. When the dried dressing is removed the nonviable tissue can be more easily lifted from the wound (Strohal, 2013).

Think Margaret's pressure ulcer progresses to Stage III. Jane Smith is changing her dressing. When she removes the occlusive transparent film on the pressure ulcer, she notices two circular areas about 20 mm in diameter that are black. What factors would a nursing student take into account in assessing the wound? What type of dressing would be best suited to use for this wound? What is your rationale for using the type you have chosen?

Change a Simple Dressing

Nurses apply or change simple dressings to patients' wounds to protect the wound and surrounding skin, to promote healing, and to reduce wound contamination and infection (Baranoski & Ayello, 2012).

Before changing a simple dressing,

1. Assess the need to apply or change a dressing by assessing the patient's skin integrity and wound if the edges of the wound are approximated, if an existing dressing is intact or exudates are present, and if there is a health-care practitioner's order and/or nursing plan of care for dressing changes and wound care. Assess the patient's response to the wound. For example, is the patient anxious, guarding the wound, and expressing or displaying signs of pain

(Bell & McCarthy, 2010). Your assessments provide clues for nursing diagnosis and rationale for applying or changing the dressing to maintain skin integrity and wound care for this person.

2. Nursing diagnosis follows from your assessment of the current status and condition of the patient's skin and existing dressings. Possible nursing diagnoses may include Risk for Infection, Impaired Skin Integrity, Impaired Tissue Integrity, Disturbed Body Image, Anxiety, Acute Pain, Delayed Wound Healing, or Delayed Recovery of skin integrity after surgery or injury (Lynn, 2011).

3. Identify preferred outcome and plan to apply or change dressing. Preferred outcomes may be a clean wound with a dry sterile dressing or removal of a contaminated dressing with application of a sterile dry or moist dressing, removal of trauma, debris, or exudates from the wound bed and application of a sterile wound dressing, or dressing changes that causes the patient the least amount of discomfort or pain (Wilkins & Unverdorben, 2013). Patients may demonstrate understanding for reasons for wound care and dressing changes, and nurses assess for wound healing progression with dressing changes.

Complex Wound Dressing

A complex wound dressing is required for wounds healing with secondary or tertiary intention or when several wounds in any stage of healing are dressed at the same time; for example, when a person has multiple sites of surgery, burns, or trauma. Health-care providers often specifically order complex dressings, including what actions to take prior to, during, and after dressing changes. Complex wounds include some pressure ulcers, burn injuries, and wounds where skin integrity is compromised with extensive abrasions, blisters, penetrating injuries, or infection. A complex wound can require negative pressure wound therapy to bring the edges of a wound together in close approximation or to apply suction to drain exudate from an open wound or fistula. Detailed dressing change procedures required for complex wounds are outlined in health-care orders and in detailed nursing care plans, which a nurse checks before starting a dressing change and may update after changing a dressing.

Principles for changing complex dressings are consistent with changing simple dressings: a nurse gathers supplies, introduces self and identifies patient, accommodates patient's request for analgesic prior to dressing changes, provides for privacy during dressing change, and dons personal protective equipment and performs hand hygiene. The dressing closest to the patient's head (proximal dressing) is changed first, and area is cleaned from centre to periphery of wound, then dried, and treatment applied. New dressing sets may be used for each separate wound, or wounds in close proximity may be cleaned with a common dressing set, if the wounds are in close proximity and not infected. The nurse

uses aseptic technique to clean wounds, and sterile wound dressings are applied to each wound. Complex dressings may require the "cut and fit" of a specifically ordered wound dressing; this is done after the wound is exposed, examined, and cleaned and wound treatment applied, and with the nurse wearing new sterile gloves.

Removing Sutures or Staples

A suture is a thread used to sew wound edges together. Sutures used beneath the skin surface are often made of absorbable material, and sutures used to close wounds at skin surfaces are made from several nonabsorbent materials. Sutures are classified as interrupted, where each stitch is tied and knotted individually, and continuous, where one thread is used to close the wound and tied at the beginning and end of the wound.

A primary care provider orders the removal of sutures or staples, and according to agency policy, physicians or nurses may remove sutures or staples as ordered. Sutures are removed after the wound is cleaned and dried using sterile technique, with special suture scissors that have a short curved cutting tip and a blunt edge that will not cut the patient's skin, or with a suture remover, which resembles a short, curved, blunt-edged blade designed for cutting suture threads (Fig. 36.14).

Staples (or clips) are removed with a specially designed staple remover, with handles and a tip that squeezes the centre of the staple to dislodge and remove it from the patient's skin.

Jane feels she has learned a lot over the past few months about skin care. Particularly in caring for Margaret, she has benefited from the experience of Mary Blevins and the ostomy specialist and has increased confidence in her ability to care for her patients with pressure ulcers and other skin and wound issues.

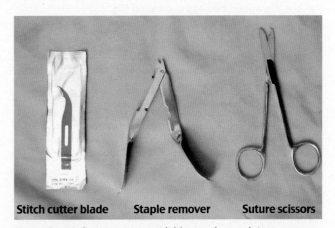

| Stitch cutter blade | Staple remover | Suture scissors |

Figure 36.14 Suture scissors with blunt and curved tips, a suture removal blade in a sterile package, and a staple removal instrument. (Photograph is property of Elizabeth Domm, RN, PhD, used with permission.)

SKILL 36.1 Changing a Dressing on a Wound

Nursing Action	Rationale for Action
Review health-care practitioner's order and nursing care plan for dressing change.	Nursing actions supported by verifying correct patient and planned nursing action
Gather necessary supplies for dressing change. Bring supplies to patient's bedside. Check with the patient to ascertain when the dressing change can be done. Clean area on bedside table or stand; dry area and place dressing supplies in prepared area that is conveniently located close to area where you will change dressing.	Gathering supplies promotes efficiency of time management and organization of nursing actions. Checking with the patient adds to your assessment of the patient's response to the dressing change and demonstrates respect for the patient's preference. Cleaning an area to place supplies aids sanitation and integrity of supplies. Place supplies in a safe, accessible location where you do not have to stretch, twist, or turn your back when changing the dressing.
Perform hand hygiene in view of the patient and put on personal protective equipment as required.	To prevent the spread of microbial contaminants
Identify yourself to the patient and identify the patient. Explain that you are there to change the patient's dressing. Reassess need for prescribed medications or patient positioning for comfort during dressing change. Administer appropriate prescribed medication; allow time for medication to be effective.	Respects the patient's right to know who the caregivers are, right to accept, reschedule, or refuse care; may help to alleviate patient anxiety and/or pain that accompanies dressing change; promote nurse–patient collaboration; and ensures that the right patient receives the right dressing change to prevent error
Close curtains around patient's bed or close door to room. Adjust bed height to be a comfortable working height for the nurse changing the dressing. Position patient just prior to changing the dressing, and cover patient with a bath blanket for non-wound areas that are exposed.	Ensures patient privacy for dressing change; allows access to wound while restricting some movement of air currents over exposed skin Bed at proper height (perhaps elbow height for nurse) helps to promote good body mechanics and prevent muscle strain.
Place a waste receptacle or bag at a convenient place to receive waste during the procedure. Place a waterproof barrier under the wound site.	Dressings that are removed and gauze used to cleanse and dry wound will be placed in waste receptacle. A waterproof pad will prevent wetting of bed linens with wound cleansers or exudates.
Assess visible dressing for presence of wound drains, tubes, or pins securing the dressing to the wound before removing the dressing. Put on clean disposable gloves and loosen tape on the old dressings. If dressings adhere to wound, loosen dressings by moistening dressings with sterile saline solution.	To ensure drains, tubes, or pins are not removed with dressing and to prevent discomfort from tape removal and tension from removal of adherent dressings on healing wound beds
Carefully remove dressing after loosening dressing from the wound by lifting the gauze first from the side so you can see the wound bed as the dressing lifts.	Careful removal of the dressing is more comfortable for the patient and avoids undue disturbance of a newly epithelized wound bed. Lifting the edge of the dressing so you can see beneath the old dressing aids visualization of areas still adherent to the dressing.
Assess the dressing that was removed from the wound for amount, type, colour, consistency, and odor of drainage.	Nursing assessment of wound drainage is documented.
Dispose of old dressing in waste receptacle. Remove gloves and dispose of these in waste receptacle.	Prevents spread of microbial contaminants
Inspect the patient's wound for appearance, drainage, approximation of wound edges, size of wound and check for odor of drainage. Check if drains, tubes, sutures, staples, or wound closure strips are intact.	Nursing assessment of wound is documented.

Nursing Action	Rationale for Action
Using sterile technique, prepare a sterile field with the dressing bundle on the table. Add sterile supplies to the sterile field, if necessary (see Figure 1).	Supplies are within reach, and sterility is maintained of dressing materials.

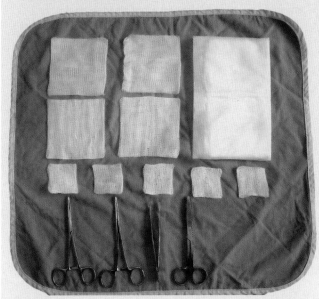

Figure 1A Photograph of opened sterile dressing set, with instruments, gauze, and abdominal dressing. (Property of Elizabeth Domm, RN, PhD, used with permission)

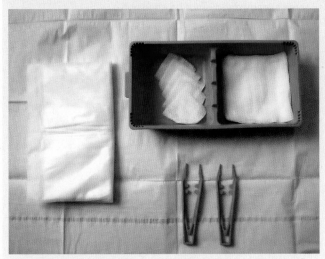

Figure 1B Photograph of single use dressing set. (Property of Elizabeth Domm, RN, PhD, used with permission)

Open the sterile cleaning solution. Depending on the size of the wound, the cleaning solution may be poured onto individual gauze sponges or into a sterile bowl.	
Don sterile gloves.	Sterility is maintained.

(continued on page 994)

SKILL 36.1   Changing a Dressing on a Wound (continued)

Nursing Action	Rationale for Action
Clean the wound with sterile swab that has been moistened with sterile saline solution, from top to bottom and from the centre to the outside, using a clean gauze sponge with cleansing solution for each swipe and then placing that gauze sponge in the waste receptacle (see Figure 2).	Ensures cleaning is carried out from least contaminated to most contaminated; and using new gauze for each wipe ensures area already cleaned is not cleaned again.

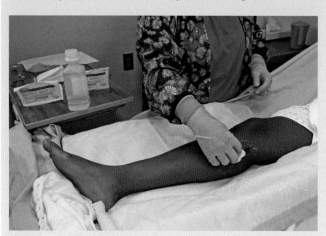

Figure 2 Cleaning wound with dampened gauze. (Source: Lynn, P. [2011]. *Taylor's clinical nursing skills: A nursing process approach* [3rd ed.]. Philadelphia, PA: Lippincott Williams & Wilkins).

Nursing Action	Rationale for Action
Dry the wound using a dry gauze sponge in the same manner: top to bottom and centre to the outside.	Ensures drying is carried out from least contaminated to most contaminated; and using new gauze for each wipe ensures area already dried is not brushed again.
Apply ointment or other wound treatment prescribed to go under the dressing (see Figure 3).	Ointments or wound treatments may be prescribed to inhibit microbial growth or aid wound healing.

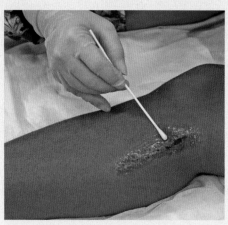

Figure 3 Applying antimicrobial ointment to wound with cotton applicator. (Source: Lynn, P. [2011]. *Taylor's clinical nursing skills: A nursing process approach* [3rd ed.]. Philadelphia, PA: Lippincott Williams & Wilkins).

Nursing Action	Rationale for Action
Cleansing around a drain: If a drain is adjacent to the wound, clean around the wound from centre (cleanest) area to area furthest from drain insertion point, after cleaning and drying the main incision. With gauze sponges, dry after area around drain is cleaned, disposing of each gauze sponge after one cleaning swipe.	Ensures cleaning and drying of area around drain from least contaminated to most contaminated; and using a new gauze for each wipe ensures area already cleaned is not cleaned or dried twice.

Nursing Action	Rationale for Action
Wound cultures: A nurse notices drainage or exudates when a soiled dressing is removed from a wound. After cleaning a wound, the nurse may collect a sample of drainage or exudates for would culture. General instructions to collect a wound culture: After the wound has been cleaned using sterile normal saline, a sterile swab from a culturette tube is moistened with sterile normal saline to more readily absorb organisms and pressed to the wound in the area closest to the wound bed to ensure wound flora rather than skin contaminants are captured. The person collecting the culture sample may press around the wound and gently turn the swab to collect as much tissue or fluid as possible. The swab is then placed into either an aerobic or anaerobic culture tube or both, depending on the type of organism suspected, and transported to the laboratory for culture.	Never collect a sample of wound exudates from old drainage in order to avoid gathering contaminants that have grown in the exudates. There has been debate about the value of collecting wound cultures to aid in diagnosis of wound infection, as false-positive culture results can confound the diagnosis (Spear, 2012).
Apply a dry sterile dressing over the wound. Use forceps to place sterile gauze if preferred (see Figure 4).	Primary dressing goes on over ointment or wound treatment as ordered. This gauze and second dressing layer serves as sterile wick to absorb wound drainage or exudates and wound covering barrier.

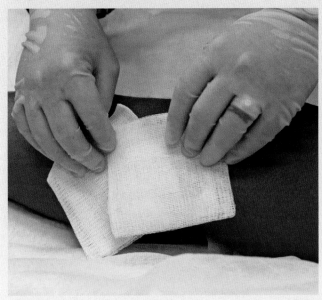

Figure 4 Applying a dry dressing to site. (Source: Lynn, P. [2011]. *Taylor's clinical nursing skills: A nursing process approach* [3rd ed.]. Philadelphia, PA: Lippincott Williams & Wilkins)

Nursing Action	Rationale for Action
Apply second layer of sterile dressing over first layer (this layer may be gauze or absorbant surgical dressing material).	
Remove and discard gloves in waste receptacle. Apply tape or circular roll of gauze to hold dressings to wound.	Disposal of gloves prevents contaminants from spreading. Applying tape is easier without gloves, after wound is covered.
Label the dressing with date and time of dressing change.	Provides communication about dressing change according to plan of care
Remove all remaining supplies, waste receptacle, and cleaning solution. Reposition patient to a comfortable position and return patient's bed to former height.	Provides safety and comfort to patient's environment when supplies are removed and patient's bed is returned to previous height

(continued on page 996)

SKILL 36.1	Changing a Dressing on a Wound (continued)

Nursing Action	Rationale for Action
Remove personal protective equipment and perform hand hygiene.	Reduces the risk of infection
Check and record all wound dressings at least once per shift for all patients.	Assessment of findings and changes in patient condition and vigilance to detect wound complications

1. Evaluate expected outcome of dressing change, which may include the dressing is clean, dry and intact, free of contamination; patient tolerated dressing change well, without expressed discomfort or pain; and the patient's wound appearance is consistent with wound healing.
2. Document the location of the wound, dressing removed, and any characteristics of exudates on the old dressing. Document your assessment of the wound, for instance, the wound edges are approximated, presence of sutures, staples, drains, or tubes. Make a note of redness, swelling, tenderness, edema, or drainage from wound. Document what solution was used to cleanse the wound, such as sterile normal saline, and any application of wound treatment or ointment to wound, and what dressing was applied to the wound. Make a note of any pertinent patient or family reaction to the dressing change, including patient's expression of pain and effectiveness of medication or positioning for the dressing change, and patient education that you offered at the time of the dressing change, such as to tell a nurse if the dressing becomes loose or saturated with drainage (see Figure 5).

8/27/13	1700hr. Dressing removed from lower right leg incision after patient requested and received analgesic 30 minutes prior to dressing change. Moderate serosanguinous drainage noted on lower 1 cm. of dressing, no odor to drainage. Incision edges well approximated with 12 staples in situ. Area cleansed with sterile normal saline, dried and ointment applied as per order. Skin around incision is flesh colored. Skin wound redressed with sterile gauze and a surgical pad, and secured with 1 inch tape. Patient reports adequate pain control after analgesic, states pain is 3 on scale of 1-10 during dressing change. --M.B. RN.

Figure 5 Sample documentation for a dressing change.

SKILL 36.2 Suture and Staple Removal

Assessment and Actions	Rationale for Action
Assessment: Assess order for suture or staple removal, including if all or alternate sutures or staples are to be removed.	To confirm that there is a primary care providers' order to remove sutures or staples from patient's wound
Assess patient, plan and provide privacy, intervene to expose, and clean wound using sterile technique.	
Evaluate appearance of wound, approximation of wound edges, inflammation, or presence of drainage.	It may be contraindicated to remove sutures or staples if wound edges are poorly approximated, inflamed, or there is drainage present.
	Wound is inspected to ascertain the way the wound was sutured before attempting to remove sutures; this will help the nurse detect where suture threads can be grasped with forceps and where to cut a thread to avoid pulling threads beneath the surface of the patient's incision. Principle is to start at the end of the wound closest to the patient's head as this area is proximal.
To remove plain interrupted sutures:	
Using forceps, grasp the knot of the suture on one side of the healed wound, gently lift the knot, and snip the thread of the suture just below the knot, or close to the skin on the side opposite the knot.	Suture is cut below the knot, close to the skin surface to avoid pulling thread that was above the skin surface through the tissue below the skin surface.
Discard the thread and inspect the area where the suture was removed.	The patient may state he or she feels the thread tug or slide through the tissue below the healed incision, so monitor the patient's response as you monitor the wound.
If the wound gapes open after the suture is removed, attach a Steri-Strip across the skin right next to the place where the suture was removed, pulling the edges of the skin together.	To provide additional support and hold wound edges close together
Nurses may remove every second suture along the length of the incision and then return and remove the remaining sutures.	Removing alternate sutures may prevent the wound from gaping open when all sutures are sequentially removed if wound healing is not complete.
Discard the thread and assess the skin surface. Repeat procedure for the length of the patient's incision.	
To remove staples, first check the health-care provider's order. Gather dressing set, sterile normal saline, and staple remover. Cleanse and dry wound using sterile technique; assess characteristics of wound including approximation of wound edges, drainage, or inflammation.	Sterile technique is used to cleanse wound prior to staple removal.
Gently position the foot end of the staple remover under the staple, with the tip above the staple. Compress the handles of the staple remover to free the ends of the staple from the patient's skin, and when the ends of the staple are free, lift the staple and discard.	
Assess the patient's incision and if the patient experienced a "tug" or pain with staple removal.	
Remove alternate staples and assess the incision after each staple removal.	Removing alternate staples may prevent the wound from gaping open should all staples be removed sequentially if wound is not healed.
Clean and dry the incision line after staple removal.	

Critical Thinking Case Scenarios

▶ John West, RN, has a 75-year-old patient named M. K. on his case load. She has a chronic Category III ulcer on her heel that has not shown any progress in the past 3 months. He notices that she has a smoking history of 40 pack years and has not followed her diet instructions. She has refused to be admitted to the hospital because she feels the doctors and nurses don't understand her. What would you include in your health teaching for M. K. to prevent further ulcer development? What interventions would you implement to manage her existing pressure ulcer? What modifications to the management of Category III ulcers would you have to make for M. K.? What other health team members could you involve in her care?

▶ You are the nurse assigned to help a patient who is unconscious with hygiene and mobility. The patient care plan indicates that the person requires complete care and a lift for transfers. Identify how you will prepare to move this patient while preventing skin tears and breakdown, friction shearing, and pressure sores.

▶ A nurse is working at a health information fair and a fair-skinned mother of two young children asks for information on sun safety. What important research findings about skin cancer should the nurse ensure that she relays to this young woman?

Multiple-Choice Questions

1. A nurse is teaching a patient about functions of human skin and tells the patient that intact skin functions as a barrier to:
   a. Invasion by infectious organisms
   b. Sensation
   c. Formation of vitamin D
   d. Pressure ulcers

2. In which way does a nurse play a key role in maintaining a patient's skin integrity?
   a. Waiting for a physician's order before assisting a patient to care for his or her skin
   b. Waiting for the patient to ask about skin care before discussing skin care practices
   c. Never asking a patient about skin care practices
   d. Identifying risks for skin breakdown

3. Which group of patients are at increased risk of developing skin breakdown?
   a. Clients who turn over in bed without prompting
   b. Clients who are undernourished
   c. Clients who ambulate independently
   d. Clients who are 10 kg above their desired weight

4. The nurse notes purple, pinpoint, round, flat lesions approximately 2 mm in diameter scattered over a patient's torso. He would correctly describe the lesions as:
   a. Purpura
   b. Ecchymosis
   c. Petechiae
   d. Hematomas

5. A nurse is teaching a patient about sun safety. Which of the following pieces of information is incorrect?
   a. "Stay out of the sun when the UV index is 7 or higher."
   b. "If you must be in the sun, wear sunscreen with SPF of at least 30."
   c. "Sunscreen should be applied at least 20 minutes prior to exposure."
   d. "Precautions should be taken all year round, including winter."

6. A patient is concerned about skin cancer and asks what he should watch for. The nurse correctly tells him to:
   a. Perform skin self-assessment every 2 months.
   b. Have a physician examine his skin annually.
   c. Report any changes in lesions to a physician or nurse following the ABCDE rule.
   d. Have a family member examine his skin monthly.

7. A patient has erythematous, raised lesions that merge together over her chest and upper arms. When describing this pattern, the nurse would document that the lesions are:
   a. Linear
   b. Symmetrical
   c. Discrete
   d. Confluent

8. Cells that perform the immune function in the skin are:
   a. Keratinocytes
   b. Corneocytes
   c. Dendritic cells
   d. Melanocytes

9. A patient on prolonged bed rest has developed a pressure ulcer. The wound shows no signs of healing even though the client has received skin care and has been turned every 2 hours. Which factor is most likely responsible for the failure to heal?
   a. Inadequate vitamin D intake
   b. Inadequate protein intake
   c. Inadequate massaging of the affected area
   d. Low calcium level

10. A patient on bed rest is assessed using the Braden Scale for Predicting Pressure Sore Risk. The patients score is 17; this score indicates that:
    a. The patient has a Category I pressure sore.
    b. The patient is at risk for developing a pressure sore.
    c. There is no risk of developing a pressure sore.
    d. The patient should be reassessed weekly.

11. A patient sitting in a wheelchair who is unable to move his body needs to be repositioned every:
    a. 2 hours
    b. 15 minutes
    c. Hour
    d. Prn

12. Patients who are at high risk for developing a pressure ulcer should:
    a. Have a nursing care plan that includes a turning schedule
    b. Have a rubber ring placed under their buttocks
    c. Have regular massage over bony prominences that the patient lies on
    d. Be placed in a high Fowler's position rather than in a wheelchair.

Suggested Lab Activities

● Have students practice focused skin assessments on each other, followed by written documentation.

● Have students describe and document photographs of pressure ulcers at various categories of development and locations.

REFERENCES AND SUGGESTED READINGS

Atiyeh, B. S., Dibo, S. A., & Hayek, S. N. (2009). Wound cleansing, topical antiseptics and wound healing. *International Wound Journal, 6*, 420–430.

Baranoski, S., & Ayello, E. A. (2012). Wound dressings: An evolving art and science. *Advances in Skin & Wound Care, 25*(2), 87–92. Retrieved from http://www.woundcarejournal.com

Barbel, A., & Efron, D. (2010). Treatment of wounds. In C. Brunicardi, D. Anderson, T. Billiar, D. Dunn, J. Hunter, J. Mathews, & R. Pollock (Eds.), *Schwartz's principles of surgery*. New York, NY: McGraw-Hill.

Bell, C., & McCarthy, G. (2010). The assessment and treatment of wound pain at dressing change. *British Journal of Nursing, 19*(11), S4–S10.

Berg, A., Fleischer, S., Kuss, O., Unversagt, S., & Langer, G. (2011). Timing of dressing removal in the healing of surgical wounds by primary intention: Quantitative systematic review protocol. *Journal of Advanced Nursing, 68*(2), 264–270.

Biazar, E., Roveimiab, Z., Shahhossieni, G., Khataminezhad, M., Zafari, M., & Majdi, A. (2012). Biocompatibiility evaluation of a new hydrogel dressing based on polyvinylpyrrolidone/polyethylene glycol. *Journal of Biomedicine and Biotechnology.* Advance online publication. doi:10.1155/2012/343989. Retrieved from http://www.ncbi.nlm.nih.gov/pmc/articles/PMC3155791/

Bry, K. E., Buescher, D., & Sandrik, M. (2012). Never say never: A descriptive study of hospital-acquired pressure ulcers in a hospital setting. *Journal of Wound, Ostomy & Continence Nurses Society, 39*(3), 274–281.

Canadian Cancer Society. (2012). *Canadian cancer statistics 2012.* Toronto, ON: Author. Retrieved from http://cancer.ca/~/media/CCS/Canada%20wide/Files%20List/English%20files%20heading/PDF%20-%20Policy%20-%20Canadian%20Cancer%20Statistics%20-%20English/Canadian%20Cancer%20Statistics%202012%20-%20English.ashx

Canadian Cancer Society. (2013a). *Know your skin.* Retrieved from http://www.cancer.ca/BritishColumbiaYukon/Prevention/SunandUV/UsingSunSense/Earlydetectionofskincancer.aspx?sc_lang=en&r=1

Canadian Cancer Society. (2013b). *Vitamin D.* Retrieved from http://www.cancer.ca/Canada-wide/Prevention/VitaminD.aspx?sc_lang=en

Canadian Institute of Health Information. (2011). *Health care in Canada 2011: A focus on seniors and aging.* Retrieved from https://secure.cihi.ca/free_products/HCIC_2011_seniors_report_en.pdf

Canadian Institute for Health Information. (2013). *Compromised wounds in Canada.* Retrieved from http://www.cihi.ca/CIHI-ext-portal/internet/EN/Home/home/cihi000001

Canadian Skin Cancer Foundation. (2012). *Malignant melanoma.* Retrieved from http://www.canadianskincancerfoundation.com/malignant-melanoma.html

Canadian Skin Cancer Foundation. (2013a). *Artificial tanning beds.* Retrieved from http://www.canadianskincancerfoundation.com/tanning-beds.html

Canadian Skin Cancer Foundation. (2013b). *Early detection.* Retrieved from http://www.canadianskincancerfoundation.com/

Cooper, R. A. (2007). Iodine revisited. *International Wound Journal, 4*(2), 124–137.

Cowan, L. J., Stechmiller, J. K., Rowe, M., & Kairalla, J. A. (2012). Enhancing Braden pressure ulcer risk assessment in acutely ill adult veterans. *Wound Repair & Regeneration, 20*, 137–148.

Cuzzell, J. (1997). Choosing a wound dressing. *Geriatric Nursing, 18*(6), 260–265.

Day, R. A., Paul, P., Williams, B., Smeltzer, S. A., & Bare, B. (2010). *Brunner and Suddarth's textbook of Canadian medical surgical nursing* (2nd ed.). Philadelphia, PA: Lippincott Williams & Wilkins.

Doyle, R., & Kowalak, J. (2009). Pressure ulcer care. In *Lippincott's visual encyclopedia of clinical skills* (pp. 427–439). Philadelphia, PA: Lippincott Williams & Wilkins.

Du Toit, D. F., & Page, B. J. (2009). An in vitro evaluation of the cell toxicity of honey and silver dressings. *Journal of Wound Care, 18*(9), 383–389.

European Pressure Ulcer Advisory Panel and National Pressure Ulcer Advisory Panel. (2009). *Treatment of pressure ulcers: Quick reference guide.* Washington, DC: National Pressure Ulcer Advisory Panel.

Fernandez, R., & Griffiths, R. (2012). Water for wound cleansing. *Cochrane Database of Systematic Reviews, 2*, CD003861.

Fleck, C. (2012). Pressure ulcers. *Journal of Legal Nurse Consulting, 23*(1), 4–12.

Gallagher, R., Barry, P., Hartigan, I., McCluskey, P., O'Connor, K., & O'Connor, M. (2008). Prevalence of pressure ulcers in three university teaching hospital in Ireland. *Journal of Tissue Viability, 17*, 103–109.

Gould, D. (2012). Skin flora: Implications for nursing. *Nursing Standard, 26*(33), 48–56.

Green, L. (2011). Emollient therapy for dry and inflammatory skin conditions. *Nursing Standard, 26*(1), 39–46.

Grocott, P. (2012). Managing wounds. In I. Bullock, J. Macleod Clark, & J. Rycroft-Malone (Eds.), *Adult nursing practice: Using evidence in care.* Oxford, United Kingdom: Oxford University Press.

Hampton, S. (2006). Malodourous fungating wounds: How dressings alleviate symptoms. *Wound Care, 13*(6), S31–S38.

Houghton, P. E., & Campbell, K. E. (2013). *Canadian best practice guidelines for the prevention and management of pressure ulcers in people with spinal cord injuries: A resource handbook for clinicians.* Retrieved from http://www.onf.org

Hurd, T., & Posnett, J. (2009). Point prevalence of wounds in a sample of acute hospitals in Canada. *International Wound Journal, 6*(4), 287–293.

Jaul, E. (2010). Assessment and management of pressure ulcers in the elderly: Current strategies. *Drugs Aging, 27*(4), 311–325.

Jones, T. (2011). Wound care. In K. Stone & R. Humphries (Eds.), *Current diagnosis and treatment emergency medicine.* New York, NY: McGraw-Hill.

Kerihuel, J. C. (2010). Effect of activated charcoal dressings on healing outcomes of chronic wounds. *Journal of Wound Care, 19*(5), 208–215.

Kim, S. W., Lee, J. H., Seo, B. F., & Rhie, J. W. (2013). Prospective RCT comparing two hydrocolloid dressings in acute trauma wounds in South Korea. *Journal of Wound Care, 22*(4), 210–213.

Kotz, P., Fisher, J., McCluskey, P., Hartwell, S. D., & Dharma, H. (2009). Use of a new silver barrier dressing, ALLEVYN Ag in exuding chronic wounds. *International Wound Journal, 6*, 186–194.

Leaper, D. (2012). Appropriate use of silver dressings in wounds: International consensus document. *International Wound Journal, 9*(5), 461–464.

Leaper, D. J., & Durani, P. (2008). Topical antimicrobial therapy of chronic wounds healing by secondary intention using iodine products. *International Wound Journal, 5*(2), 361–368.

Lee, G., Anand, S., Rajendran, S., & Walker, I. (2007). Efficacy of commercial dressings in managing malodorous wounds. *British Journal of Nursing, 16*(6), S14–S20.

Li, D., & Korniewicz, M. (2013). Determination of the effectiveness of the electronic health records to document pressure ulcers. *MedSurg Nursing, 22*(1), 17–25.

Lynn, P. (2011). *Taylor's clinical nursing skills: A nursing process approach* (3rd ed.). Philadelphia, PA: Lippincott Williams & Wilkins.

Main, R. C. (2008). Should chlorhexidine gluconate be used in wound cleansing? *Journal of Wound Care, 17*, 112–114.

Maklebust, J. (2005). Pressure ulcers: The great insult. *Nursing Clinics of North America, 40*, 365–389.

Martini, F. (2012). *Fundamentals of anatomy & physiology* (9th ed.). Upper Saddle River, NJ: Pearson.

Massa, J. (2010). Improving efficiency, reducing infection, and enhancing experience. *British Journal of Nursing, 19*(22), 1408–1414.

McKinley, M., O'Loughlin, V., & Bidle, T. (2013). *Anatomy & physiology: An integrative approach*. New York, NY: McGraw-Hill.

Moore, Z. E., & Cowman, S. (2013). Wound cleansing for pressure ulcers. *Cochrane Database of Systematic Reviews, 3*, CD004983.

National Pressure Ulcer Advisory Panel. (2013). *Educational and clinical resources—NPUAP pressure ulcer stages/categories.* Washington, DC: Author. Retrieved from http://www.npuap.org/resources/educational-and-clinical-resources/npuap-pressure-ulcer-stagescategories/

National Pressure Ulcer Advisory Panel & European Pressure Ulcer Advisory Panel. (2009). *International Guideline: Pressure Ulcer Treatment Technical Report.* Retrieved from http://www.npuap.org/wp-content/uploads/2012/03/Final-2009-Treatment-Technical-Report1.pdf

Registered Nurses' Association of Ontario. (2007). *Nursing best practice guideline. Assessment and management of stage 1 to 1V pressure ulcers.* Toronto, ON: Author.

Rupp, M. E., Cavalieri, J., Lyden, E., Kucera, J., Martin, M. A., Fitzgerald, T., . . . VanSchooneveld, T. C. (2012). Effect of hospital-wide chlorhexidine patient bathing on healthcare-associated infections. *Infection Control & Hospital Epidemiology, 33*(11), 1094–1100.

Schofield, J. K., Grindlay, D., & Williams, H. C. (2009). Skin conditions in the UK: A health care needs assessment. *Center of Evidence Based Dermatology.* Retrieved from www.nottingham.ac.uk/SCS/Divisions?EvidenceBasedDermatology/index.aspx

Simandl, G. (2010). Disorders of skin integrity and function. In R. Hannon, C. Pooler, & C. Porth (Eds.), *Porth pathophysiology: Concepts of altered health states* (1st Canadian ed., p. 1448–1528). Philadelphia, PA: Lippincott Williams & Wilkins.

Spear, M. (2012). Best techniques for obtaining wound cultures. *Plastic Surgical Nursing, 32*(1), 34–36.

Stephen, T., Skillen, D., Day, R., & Jensen S. (2012). *Canadian Jensen's nursing health assessment.* Philadelphia, PA: Lippincott Williams & Wilkins.

Strohal, R., Apelqvist, J., Dissemond, J., O'Brien, J., Piaggesi, A., Rimdeika, R., & Young, T. (2013). EWMA document: Debridement. *Journal of Wound Care, 22*(Suppl. 1), S1–S52.

Thomas, G. W., Rael, L. T., Bar-Or, R., Shimonkevitz, R., Mains, C., Slone, D., . . . Bar-Or, D. (2009). Mechanisms of delayed wound healing by commonly used antiseptics. *Journal of Trauma, 66*, 82–91.

Tinne, N. (2011). Wound management. In L. Dougherty & S. Lister (Eds.) *The Royal Marsden Hospital Manual of Clinical Nursing Procedures.* (8th ed., pp. 1166–1201). West Sussex, United Kingdom: John Wiley & Sons.

VanGilder, C., Amlung, S., Harrison, P., & Meyer, S. (2009). Results of a 2008–2009 International Pressure Ulcer Survey and a 3-year acute care unit-specific analysis. *Ostomy Wound Management, 55*, 39–45.

Vermeulen, H., Westerbos, S. J., & Ubbink, D. T. (2010). Benefit and harm of iodine in wound care: A systematic review. *Journal of Hospital Infection, 76*(3), 191–199.

Wagner, K. D., & Hardin-Pierce, M. G. (2014). *High acuity nursing* (6th ed.). Boston, MA: Pearson.

Wilkins, R. G., & Unverdorben, M. (2013). Wound cleaning and wound healing: A concise review. *Advances in Skin & Wound Care, 26*(4), 160–163. Retrieved from http://www.woundcarejournal.com

Woo, T. (2011). Drug affecting the integumentary system. In T. Woo, & A. Wynne (Eds.), *Pharmacotherapeutics for nurse practitioner prescribers* (pp. 679–739). Philadelphia, PA: F. A. Davis.

Youell, L., & Wright, C. (2010). Principles and practices of rehabilitation. In R. Day, P. Paul, B. Williams, S. Smeltzer, & B. Bare (Eds.), *Brunner and Suddarth's textbook of Canadian medical surgical nursing* (2nd ed., pp. 183–217). Philadelphia, PA: Lippincott Williams & Wilkins.

Zhang, Q. H., Sun, Z. R., Yue, J. H., Ren, X., Qiu, L. B., Lv, X. L., & Du, W. (2013). Traditional Chinese medicine for pressure ulcer: A meta-analysis. *International Wound Journal, 10*(2), 221–231.

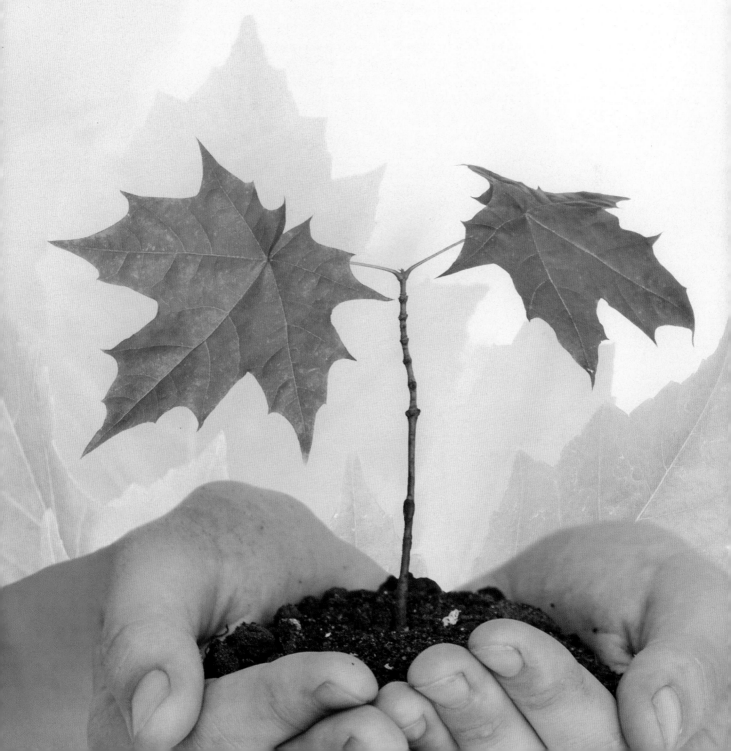

five

Understanding

Immigrant Canadians

KATHRYN A. EDMUNDS AND
JOAN SAMUELS-DENNIS

Kyla is a second-year nursing student in her first clinical rotation in an acute care setting. She is assigned to care for Mrs. Gupta, a 64-year-old woman from India, who has been in Canada for 1 year. Mrs. Gupta had an appendectomy the day before and has had an uneventful recovery so far. However, her English skills are limited, and this is the first time she has been a patient in a Canadian hospital. Her son, who immigrated to Canada with his wife and three children 7 years ago, sponsored Mrs. Gupta to Canada. The application to sponsor Mrs. Gupta as a family relative took 5 years to process. Mrs. Gupta is still getting used to her new life in a new country and the changes she sees in her son and his family as they have adapted to Canada. Kyla was born in Canada and wonders how she will assess and establish a relationship with and care for Mrs. Gupta given the language barrier and their different life experiences.

CHAPTER OBJECTIVES

By the end of this chapter, you will be able to:

1. Describe the history and context of Canadian immigration, diversity, and multiculturalism.
2. Define and differentiate the terms *immigrant, refugee, newcomer, permanent* and *temporary resident,* and *migrant.*
3. Identify current patterns of migration to Canadian and the implications for nursing care.
4. Critically analyze the short- and long-term factors that influence migrants' health.
5. Demonstrate awareness of the nursing skills needed to build relationships and provide care to those affected by migration.
6. Evaluate structural and systemic factors, such as determinants of health, that shape nursing practice with these populations.
7. Identify future trends in migration and global health.
8. Articulate and reflect on nursing's responsibilities for migrants to Canada currently and in the future.

KEY TERMS

Diversity Differences among people reflecting many traits such as gender, country of origin, and religion.

Ethnicity Groups that have a shared identity based on heritage, language, beliefs, and values.

Immigrant Someone who is accepted in another country for the purpose of establishing permanent residence.

Migrant A person who has moved from his or her country or region of origin either temporarily or permanently.

Multiculturalism A societal value that encourages ethno-cultural diversity and emphasizes the freedom of all people to preserve, enhance, and share their cultural heritage.

Newcomer A permanent resident who has been in Canada for 5 years or less before the next census.

Race Artificially created categorizations of people based on skin colour or other biologic characteristics.

Racialization The assignment of value or status to artificially created racial categories that consequently results in inequities at social, economic, and political levels.

Refugee Someone who requests the protection and safety of another country based on the fear of persecution in his or her country of origin.

Social Determinants of Health The familial, contextual, and socio-environmental factors that exert major influences, both positive and negative, on the health of populations.

Transnationalism The ongoing ties and relationships migrants maintain with their countries of origin and form in their sites of relocation.

Undocumented Migrant A person living in another country without authorized and valid migration status.

Visible Minority People living in Canada who are non-Caucasian in race or non-white in colour and who are not Aboriginal.

Introduction

In the 2011 census, 20.6% of the Canadian population reported they were foreign-born, the second highest proportion in the world after Australia (Statistics Canada, 2013). We are home to people from around the globe and the first country in the world to have explicit federal legislation supporting multiculturalism. Perhaps, you immigrated to Canada, or family members from previous generations did so. Many of us have personal and family stories related to migration, stories of hardship and success, of starting over, and change.

In this chapter, you will learn about caring for migrants to Canada in your nursing practice. This requires comprehending the past and current contexts of Canadian immigration as well as the population implications of migration patterns. You need to know some foundational definitions, such as immigrants and refugees, and foundational concepts such as multiculturalism and diversity. We discuss some of the changes to people's health status after migration and the health-care and settlement services that are available to them. We discuss the integration of your knowledge and thinking as you consider factors that commonly influence the health of migrants and how to comprehensively assess and care for your patients. Some of these factors are linked to personal or group risk factors and the stresses and hopes of migration, but many are linked to the social determinants of health as experienced and lived by those who were not born in Canada. We explore the importance of self-reflection and questioning assumptions while developing relationships that span the differences with our patients, colleagues, and in our communities, always remembering that we are all different in some ways as we are similar in others. Finally, we expand our understanding of the projections in global trends in migration and health, including projected changes to the Canadian population. What will these changes mean for nurses and our expectations of expert and comprehensive nursing care for all our patients? We examine the challenges and opportunities for nurses and the implications for nursing research, education, practice, and policy.

The Context of Migration to Canada

People migrate in order "to enjoy the political and economic freedoms and social opportunities that host societies offer, to fulfill themselves, to maximize their abilities, and to improve living conditions for themselves and their family" (Gravel et al., 2010, p. 707). One of the primary reasons countries accept immigrants is to address shortages in various labour sectors and skill levels (Asanin & Wilson, 2008). The federal, provincial, and territorial governments of Canada encourage both permanent and temporary migration and share jurisdiction for policies, programs, and requirements (Citizenship and Immigration Canada [CIC], 2012a).

For numerous reasons including our standard of living, our reputation as a safe haven, and our openness to multiculturalism, Canada is seen as a desirable destination country for those wanting to migrate internationally, and we are a major migrant-receiving nation.

Categories of Migrants

There are very different options, opportunities, routes, and preconditions for people wishing to migrate to Canada. This necessitates discussion of the various terms used to describe or categorize people who relocate internationally. Often, some of these terms are used interchangeably, but they have specific meanings and implications, especially regarding legal rights and access to health and settlement services. You may be used to thinking about the term **immigrant** as a general descriptor for all those who come to Canada. However, within this chapter, we use the term *immigrants* for people who arrive already accepted as permanent residents or who are eligible for permanent residency (Health Canada, 2010). To be a permanent resident means people have the right to settle, remain in Canada, and eventually apply for citizenship. For more definitions on the status for various migrants, look at Box 37.1. Permanent residents include those who meet the criteria and have the skills that Canada needs to be considered in the economic class and their immediate families; family members of people already settled; and **refugees** who have been sponsored into Canada by the federal government or private organizations, such as religious institutions. Refugee status and request for asylum can also be claimed by people who enter Canada needing protection and fearing a return to their home country. While they are waiting for their hearing to determine if their claim will be accepted or denied, they are considered temporary residents. Other categories of temporary residents include foreign workers and international students.

Undocumented migrant refers to those people who are not authorized to be in Canada; for example, family members who come as visitors and stay beyond 6 months, people whose refugee claims have been denied, temporary workers or international students who remain after their visas have expired, and people who have entered the country illegally. Therefore, in this chapter, the term **migrant** will be used to apply to all people who have migrated to Canada regardless of means of arrival, length of stay, or immigration status. *Migrant* and *migration* are more inclusive terms than *immigrant* and *immigration* (Acevedo-Garcia & Almeida, 2012).

Patterns of Migration

In the early 1900s, large numbers of immigrants from the United Kingdom, Europe, and the United States were encouraged, through the offer of free land, to settle in Western Canada (CIC, 2012b). The peak year was 1913, when 400,000 immigrants arrived. Immigration levels then fluctuated, falling during World War I and II and increasing

BOX 37.1 Definitions of Migrants to Canada

Permanent Resident: A person who has been granted permanent resident status in Canada has all of the rights guaranteed under the Canadian Charter of Rights and Freedoms except the right to vote. The three primary CIC categories of permanent residents are:

Economic immigrants
People selected for their skills and ability to contribute to Canada's economy; includes skilled workers, business immigrants, provincial or territorial nominees, and the Canadian experience class; includes the principal applicant and, where applicable, the accompanying spouse and/or dependants

Family class immigrant
People sponsored by a Canadian citizen or a permanent resident living in Canada who is 18 years of age or older; includes spouses, partners, parents, grandparents, and certain other relatives but excludes fiancés

Refugees
Includes government-assisted refugees, privately sponsored refugees, and refugee dependants

Temporary Residents: People lawfully in Canada with valid documentation on a temporary basis, or individuals who seek asylum and remain in the country pending the outcome of their claim. The three primary CIC categories of temporary residents are:

Temporary foreign workers
People who are in Canada principally to work; they are classified based on skill level and skill type

Foreign students
People who are in Canada principally to study

Humanitarian population
Primarily refugee claimants who request refugee protection upon or after arrival in Canada; a refugee claimant whose claim is accepted may make an application for permanent residence. This category also includes other foreign nationals allowed to remain in Canada on humanitarian or compassionate grounds

Source: Citizenship and Immigration Canada. (2012b). *Canada facts and figures 2011. Immigration overview: Permanent and temporary residents.* Ottawa, ON: Author. Retrieved from http://www.cic.gc.ca/english/pdf/research-stats/facts2011.pdf; Health Canada. (2010). Migration health: Embracing a determinants of health approach. *Health Policy Research Bulletin,* (17), 1–52.

following those conflicts. Canada's immigration policy was discriminatory, favouring applicants who were white, and particularly in the case of the United Kingdom, from countries considered to have close historical and cultural ties. Reflecting the changes legislated by the Canadian Bill of Rights in 1960, federal immigration policy was changed in

1962 to eliminate discrimination based on race, religion, and national origin (CIC, 2012b). A point system was introduced in 1967, which took into account age, education, language skill, and economic characteristics (Health Canada, 2010).

The ranking of source countries has changed over time, as illustrated in Table 37.1. The top countries with

Order	1981 Census	1991 Census	1996 Census	2001 Census	2006 Census	2011 Census
1	United Kingdom	Hong Kong	Hong Kong	People's Republic of China	People's Republic of China	Philippines
2	Vietnam	Poland	People's Republic of China	India	India	People's Republic of China
3	United States of America	People's Republic of China	India	Philippines	Philippines	India
4	India	India	Philippines	Pakistan	Pakistan	United States of America
5	Philippines	Philippines	Sri Lanka	Hong Kong	United States of America	Iran
6	Jamaica	United Kingdom	Poland	Iran	South Korea	United Kingdom
7	Hong Kong	Vietnam	Taiwan	Taiwan	Romania	Haiti
8	Portugal	United States of America	Vietnam	United States of America	Iran	Pakistan
9	Taiwan	Lebanon	United States of America	South Korea	United Kingdom	France
10	People's Republic of China	Portugal	United Kingdom	Sri Lanka	Columbia	United Arab Emirates

TABLE 37.1 Top 10 Countries of Birth of Recent Immigrants, 1981 to 2011

Sources: Statistics Canada (2007). *Immigration in Canada: A portrait of the foreign-born population, 2006 census.* Ottawa, ON: Author; Citizenship and Immigration Canada. (2012b). *Canada facts and figures 2011. Immigration overview: Permanent and temporary residents.* Ottawa, ON: Author. Retrieved from http://www.cic.gc.ca/english/pdf/research-stats/facts2011.pdf

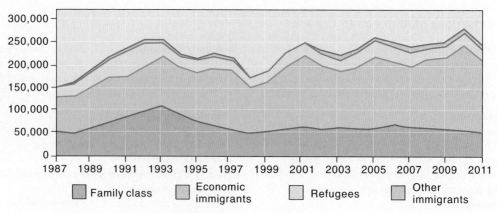

Figure 37.1 Canada—Permanent residents by category, 1987 to 2011.

immigration to Canada are now South Asia and China. With the change in source countries has come an increase in the **visible minority** population, which in Canada refers to people who are non-Caucasian in race or non-white in colour, and does not include Aboriginal peoples. In 2006, 16.2% of the Canadian population identified themselves as a member of a visible minority group; in 2011, that number had increased to 19.1% (Statistics Canada, 2013). Recent immigrants are younger than the Canadian-born population and more highly educated. Currently, 3 out of 4 immigrants to Canada settle in the provinces of British Columbia, Ontario, and Québec. The proportion of immigrants settling in Ontario and British Columbia has decreased over the past 10 years while increasing in the other provinces of Canada (Statistics Canada, 2012a). Québec sets its own immigration requirements, which include commitment to living in a francophone society (Blad & Couton, 2009). This is a mechanism to preserve and promote French as the prevailing language in that province and has implications for the source countries of migration. In Québec, there is a higher proportion of immigrants from French-speaking countries in Africa and the Middle East when compared to the rest of Canada (39% vs. 24%; CIC, 2012b).

As you can observe in Figure 37.1, since 2001, immigration levels have been consistently around 250,000 people per year, although the numbers of economic immigrants (see Box 37.1) has increased proportionally. During 2013, the current federal government plans to maintain yearly admissions of between 240,000 and 265,000 permanent residents. These numbers are unlikely to substantially decrease in the future as sustained levels of immigration are required to maintain or increase our country's population and to support the federal objectives of economic immigration, family reunification, and humanitarian commitments for accepting refugees (CIC, 2012a).

Figure 37.2 shows the sharp increase in the numbers of temporary foreign workers and international students in the past 15 years. In 2011, there were close to 700,000 temporary residents living in Canada, and these numbers are likely to continue to increase. In addition to permanent residents, high-income countries, such as Canada, admit temporary migrants to address shortages in labour sectors. Temporary foreign workers are a labour source that is flexible related to employers' needs and for those in the federal "low-skilled" job classification categories, relatively inexpensive. High-skilled temporary workers can apply to have their spouses and dependents accompany them to Canada; low-skilled workers are required to migrate independently, leaving their families behind. Once temporary workers have reached the end of their time-limited contracts, they must return to their countries of origin. Most Canadians are unaware of the large numbers of temporary workers in Canada and the health-care needs they may have.

Many international students and their families value Canadian postsecondary education. Some international students are eligible to apply for postgraduation work permits after completing their education and can seek work in Canada for up to 3 years (CIC, 2012a). Universities and colleges value international students for their contributions and enrichment to academic life through increased diversity of viewpoints and experiences. However, a key reason colleges and universities recruit international students is economic as international students pay higher tuition than Canadian residents and provide a source of income for academic institutions.

Canadian Diversity and Multiculturalism

Diversity is a broad and inclusive term that encompasses attributes such as gender, age, language, visible and invisible disabilities, national origin, and group affiliations. It is important to avoid limiting our thinking about diversity to one or two characteristics. We are all diverse in many ways, some of which are constant (e.g., your ethnic group), whereas some change (e.g., age), providing many points of connection with others. In Canada, diversity is often con-

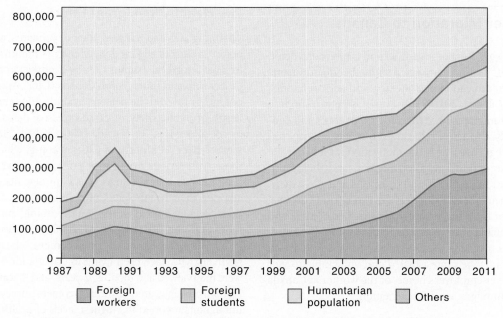

Figure 37.2 Canada—Temporary residents present on December 1st by yearly status, 1987 to 2011.

sidered to be synonymous with **ethnicity**. *Ethnicity*, which refers to groups who share a common social and cultural identity based on heritage, language, and often religion, is just one example of diversity. More than 200 ethnic origins were reported in the 2011 census (Statistics Canada, 2013). Those who reported multiple ethnicities increased to 42.1% of the population, as people could self-identify their ethnicity based on the countries of origin of themselves and their families and could also self-identify their ethnicity as Canadian.

Ethnicity is frequently used as a code word for **race**—socially created categories of people based on the differences of some biologic characteristics, most often skin colour (Benedict, 2013). We are more comfortable talking about ethnic groups than racial groups, which reflect the contested meanings associated with this term. The assumption that the concept of race arises from neutral, objective, biologic differences is incorrect. "This 'genetic' view has been refuted by a growing body of evidence across biological and social sciences that demonstrates that while race makes reference to physiological traits, it is nevertheless a categorization scheme that is social in both its origin and maintenance" (Health Canada, 2010, p. 27). **Racialization** is the social process that constructs racial categories in ways that label behaviour as having racial origins. This is done in order to maintain the prevailing social order and the associated inequities of opportunity (Browne et al., 2009). Experiences of discrimination are common for visible minority populations in Canada and have direct and indirect effects on health (Fuller-Thomson, Noack, & George, 2011).

Multiculturalism refers to the cultural and ethnic diversity in Canada, where the preservation and sharing of that diversity is encouraged and supported. There are historical roots to the multiculturalism we have today. In 1867, Canadian Confederation was a bicultural agreement affirming both French and English heritage. Canada was officially portrayed as two founding nations, albeit with white European origins. Confederation was not inclusive because the First Nations were not acknowledged as a founding population. However, the base was laid to explicitly incorporate differing cultures, languages, and histories within this country in a way that recognized and sustained diversity. In 1971, Canada was the first state in the world to have a multiculturalism policy, and in 1988, the Multiculturalism Act became law. The values reflected in multiculturalism have undergone critique and change in the past decades, from an emphasis on cultural preservation to more nuanced understandings of the dynamics of the cultural pluralism in Canadian society. This has included the relevance of and need for discussion and action related to issues of equity and social justice (Srivastava, 2007).

Migration, ethnicity, and culture are all dynamic, fluid processes of identification and change, although labelling by culture and/or ethnicity tends to dominate the discussion about diversity and multiculturalism. Like racialization, these labels often serve as the dominant explanations for how or why members of certain groups behave and what they believe. These explanations maintain assumptions; are used to justify or rationalize decisions about the provision of health-care services; and contribute to people's experiences of health, social, and economic difficulties (Browne et al., 2009). Ask yourself some critical reasoning questions about racialization: What does it accomplish and whose purposes are being served?

Health After Migration to Canada

Migration is always a major transition and can be considered a determinant of health, intertwined with other determinants such as gender, education and literacy, and socioeconomic status (Health Canada, 2010). However, it is easy to suppose that all or most migrants have the same experiences and concerns. Certainly, the act of relocation to a new country has some similar challenges, as is the motivation for a better life and to improve opportunities for migrants and their families. Yet, migration pathways and prospects and the experiences of health and health-care services can be quite diverse; for example, for the refugee family who has fled conflict and is settled in Canada after years in a refugee camp, the entrepreneur who is investing in a Canadian business, the live-in caregiver who may be quite isolated and vulnerable to violence in his or her employer's home, or the worker in Canada without valid immigration documentation.

Transformative Processes of Migration

Everyone who migrates experiences change, out of which comes transformation in relationships and ways of living and being for all involved, including the host country (Isaacs, 2010). The transition is not easy, and there is often a gap between migrants' expectations of life in Canada and the realities. Conditions such as lack of social support and low-waged insecure employment exacerbate feelings of isolation and stress (Anderson et al., 2010). When there is greater congruence between immigrant groups and their new home, such as a common language and a preexisting community of similar background, the transition to settlement tends to be less challenging. When there are lower levels of congruence, such as differences in skin colour or religion, immigrants experience increased levels of social stress and feelings of anger and depression (Reitmanova & Gustafson, 2009).

The inevitable adjustments that are required after migration can affect individuals and families differently. For example, children who quickly adapt to school or a wife who is employed for the first time can experience resilience and strength in the acquisition of new skills and successful integration into their new society. These situations can also be a source of stress if the changes are perceived as threatening values or roles that some family members want to preserve. Migrants are also well aware of issues of power, marginalization, and stereotyping. It is the process of making sense of their lives in a new country and integrating elements from their previous and current experiences that has the potential for constructive synthesis (Simich, Maiter, & Ochocka, 2009). What helps promote positive migration outcomes is the identification and reinforcement of preexisting strengths and resiliencies, the identification and alteration of barriers that are harmful, and strong formal and informal networks of support. As stated by Anderson et al. (2010), "research with immigrants and refugees gives vivid accounts of narratives of hardships yet illustrates that with sufficient opportunity and support, immigrants and refugees [can] succeed and achieve well-being in Canada" (p. 108).

The Healthy Immigrant Effect

All immigrants and refugees, their dependants, and most temporary residents staying longer than 6 months are required to have a medical examination by a physician authorized by Citizenship and Immigration Canada (CIC). Applications may not be approved if the person's health could "endanger public health or public safety, or cause excessive demands on health or social services" in Canada (CIC, 2012d, Health grounds section, para. 1). In light of CIC screening, which disqualifies those with serious health problems, and better premigration health habits of non-refugees, new immigrants entering Canada rate their health status more highly than the Canadian-born. This is known as the healthy immigrant effect (Maximova & Krahn, 2010; Newbold, 2009). In a survey conducted by Statistics Canada and CIC, **newcomers**, who are permanent residents who have been living in Canada for 5 years or less, were interviewed at 6 months, 2 years, and 4 years after arrival. Not surprisingly, among the newcomers surveyed, economic immigrants reported the highest levels of health, and refugees the lowest (Newbold, 2009). The self-reported health status of all newcomers significantly declines during the first few years after migration and becomes the same as Canadian levels by 10 years postmigration (Maximova & Krahn, 2010). Although the reasons for this are many, current research suggests that the stresses arising from settlement and structural barriers, such as difficulties finding work or poor working conditions play a significant part as well (Newbold, 2009). Limitations in proficiency in either of Canada's official languages were also strongly linked to declines in health for both women and men (Ng, Pottie, & Spitzer, 2011). It is important to note that problems gaining access to health-care services occurred frequently, and 20% of those surveyed had experienced discrimination (Fuller-Thomson et al., 2011). Women reported greater declines in health compared to men, "not only due to the intersecting oppressions related to race, gender and immigrant status, but also to the additional caring responsibilities they have to take on after immigration, particularly among married women with children" (Fuller-Thomson et al., 2011, p. 278).

Resources Available to Migrants

There are various health and settlement resources available to migrants in Canada. However, the availability and fit of services may differ across provinces, territories, and regions, and access to these services can be dependent on immigration status. If it can be difficult for health-care providers to be aware of all the services and the accompanying criteria, think about how confusing it often is for new migrants. Wherever you practice as a nurse, you will need to be aware of a number of community resources. A list of some relevant web resources and links can be found at thePoint.

Health-Care Services

All permanent residents are eligible for publicly funded health insurance, as are temporary foreign workers and international students. However, some provinces or territories may have a waiting period until coverage begins. In those cases, interim private health-care insurance needs to be purchased shortly after arrival. Remember that refugees who have been sponsored into Canada enter as permanent residents and while they are waiting for provincial coverage to begin, have comprehensive health coverage through the Interim Federal Health Program (IFHP) (CIC, 2012c). Coverage for extended health benefits (for both migrants and Canadian citizens), such as dental care, prescription medications and eyeglasses, and visits to optometrists, varies by province or territory. As you can imagine, financial costs for primary and extended health care can be a significant barrier for many migrants. Other common barriers include geographical distances to providers and services, especially for those who rely on public transport; a lack of physicians, particularly female physicians, who are preferred by many migrant women; and language differences whereby one is misunderstood or does not understand instructions (Asanin & Wilson, 2008).

Think *Health Coverage for Refugees*

Which migrants are deserving of publicly funded health care? Who should decide? In 2012, changes were made to the IFHP for refugees. Some refugee claimants, who are in Canada as temporary residents waiting for their claim to be approved or denied, are now eligible only for basic health-care services and then only if their disease poses a threat to public health. Should all refugee claimants be eligible for comprehensive health-care coverage through the IFHP? What about refugee claimants whose applications are denied yet remain in Canada? What will be your responsibility as a nurse to provide care to migrants who may not have health-care coverage?

Addressing barriers by improving the accessibility, suitability, and inclusiveness of health services is necessary to maintain or improve the health of migrants. This often requires innovation in service delivery. Researchers (Guruge, Hunter, Barker, McNally, & Magalhaes, 2010) interviewed immigrant women in Toronto regarding their experiences using a mobile health clinic. These transportable and self-contained clinics provide flexible sites for health care. Not only was the mobile clinic more accessible in terms of location, hours of service, and languages spoken, the care received was perceived as more holistic than mainstream services and sensitive to the premigration and postmigration contexts of the women's lives.

Settlement Services

A primary resource for migrants is the CIC website, which provides information for potential and current permanent and temporary residents and has some interactive components to tailor information to individual needs. Through its settlement program, CIC helps immigrants and refugees with their adjustment and orientation to life in Canada. Their free services include classes in French and English; assistance with forms and applications for finding housing and work; and linking people with resources

in their provinces, territories, and local communities (CIC, 2012a). Spouses and dependents of economic immigrants as well as refugees and family class immigrants are not required to be proficient in one of Canada's two official languages, as a result, more than one quarter of all immigrants do not speak French or English (Health Canada, 2010). This has implications for health because language skills in French or English are particularly important in reducing isolation. Formal and informal support at many levels, such as government-provided settlement programs linking Canadian volunteers with new refugee families, are critical for successful integration. Higher numbers of settlement services used in the first year after arrival have been found to mitigate declines in health status among refugees (Maximova & Krahn, 2010). However, only immigrants and refugees (those people who are or will become permanent residents) are eligible for government-funded settlement services. Few services exist for temporary workers or undocumented migrants. In order to address the health and health promotion needs of all migrants to Canada, short- and long-term support needs to be more inclusive and comprehensive.

Providing Nursing Care

There are clear expectations of nurses in Canada regarding our responsibilities to and beyond individual patients. The Canadian Nurses Association (CNA) Code of Ethics states that "nurses recognize and respect the intrinsic worth of each person . . . [and] . . . support the family, group, population or community receiving care in maintaining their dignity and integrity" (Canadian Nurses Association [CNA], 2008, p. 13). This means recognizing diverse values and understandings of health within social and economic contexts when nursing care is provided. There are also increasing expectations that nurses have an explicit responsibility in identifying, planning, and participating in actions to create a more socially just and healthy society (Browne et al., 2009; Isaacs, 2010). A primary way to engage in social justice is to advocate, which means "actively supporting a right and good cause; supporting others in speaking for themselves or speaking on behalf of those who cannot speak for themselves" (CNA, 2008, p. 22). Advocacy for social justice is expected of nurses in our Code of Ethics in order to address unfairness in the accessibility and distribution of health-care resources and services. It is a professional responsibility that nurses will have the knowledge and skills not only to work with diverse patients but also to work in interprofessional collaboration within our health-care systems for change (CNA, 2011).

Nurses most often advocate on a one-to-one basis; for example, making sure individual patients are aware of relevant resources and facilitating delivery of those resources when patients have difficulties gaining access to services, such as receiving home care after discharge from hospitals. This work is very important and makes an enormous difference in our patients' lives, especially for those who are unfamiliar with our health-care systems. But this is just a part of what we must do to correct unfairness. The most effective advocacy and change for positive health outcomes for many in our country will only take place when we take action across all levels: with individuals, families, communities, institutions, and nationally and internationally (Browne et al., 2009; Doane & Varcoe, 2007) .

Health Priorities of Migrants

The health priorities of migrants can best be understood within the broad context of the **social determinants of health** (SDoH). The World Health Organization (WHO) defines the SDoH as "the conditions in which people are born, grow, live, work and age, including the health system" (World Health Organization [WHO], 2013). The SDoH are one of the key elements of Canada's framework for enhancing the health of our population. Based on past research, expert opinion, and the input of community representatives, the SDoH represent multiple social factors that have been found to be most significant in determining the health outcomes of Canadians (Public Health Agency of Canada, 2011).

In Figure 37.3, the SDoH are organized within three levels, providing a way to understand how each determinant is contextually related to the other. The familial and biologic con-

text is at the centre of the figure reflecting the SDoH of genetic endowment, health practices and coping skills, and child development. The structural context reflects the importance of income, the identities of gender and culture that we hold in Canadian society and the status associated with those identities. The socioeconomic and political context attends to the structuring of our communities and the availability of the community-specific resources needed to support our health. The three levels are interdependent, but current research suggests the SDoH reflecting the socioeconomic and political context has the greatest influence on health and well-being. As for all Canadians, the health priorities and experiences of migrants are inherently linked to the SDoH. In the next section of this chapter, we address several health priorities for this population and examine how the SDoH influence each priority. Keep in mind that these examples will only apply to some, because there are always variations in our lived experiences, and for migrants, many of the issues addressed relate to the opportunities and challenges that accompany different migration pathways and settlement and integration. In addressing the health priorities in the following section, we highlight the impact of the structural, socioeconomic, and political contexts on everyday experiences.

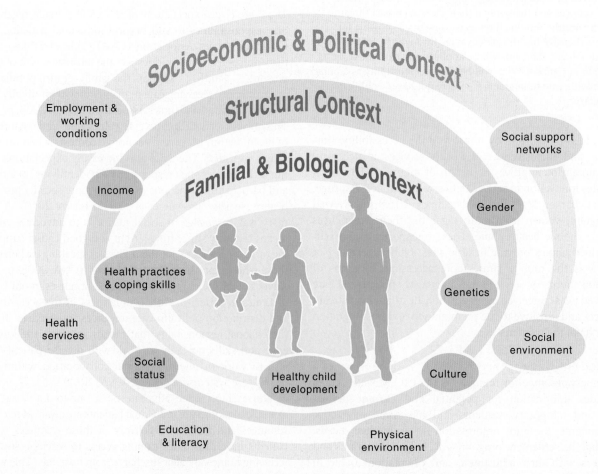

Figure 37.3 SDoH. Source: Samuels-Dennis, J. A., George, A., & Laurio, C. (Eds.). (2013). *Community assessment and advocacy projects: Partnerships for change.* Toronto, ON: Nelson Education.

Employment, Poverty, and Health

Successful resettling in a new country involves establishing economic and social ties that foster independence and self-sufficiency, family and community networks, and developing the language and cultural competencies that make social and employment participation possible (Beiser, 2009). However, research "has demonstrated a strong association between health, income and employment, and between downward mobility and health—factors that affect immigrants who tend to be underpaid and underemployed in Canada" (Health Canada, 2010, p. 29). Among the most recent cohort of immigrants, it takes approximately 7 to 10 years to achieve social and economic stability. Difficulties in finding employment at levels relative to that of their home country are connected to systemic barriers such as licensing for professionals. Structural oppression in the form of racism and social exclusion often perpetuates unemployment, underemployment, and employment that is insecure and unsafe (Health Canada, 2010). When employment is obtained, migrants earn less than their Canadian-born counterparts, even when holding the same position in similar work environments. Although these experiences are not always unique to migrants, it is not surprising then that one third of all refugee families live in poverty during the first 10 years of resettlement (Beiser, 2009).

Factors that intersect to undermine immigrant mental health include lack of family and social support, unemployment and low income, unwelcoming social and physical environments, and the underuse of mental health services (Reitmanova & Gustafson, 2009). In a study by Dean and Wilson (2009), unemployed or underemployed skilled immigrants living in Mississauga, ON, directly related their mental health stressors to low incomes, loss of premigration employment skills, loss of social status, and pressures within their families. The participants also identified that their physical health was affected by the high stress levels and arduous working conditions in their current jobs. Although most refugees experience improved mental health upon arrival to Canada, it has been demonstrated that the trauma associated with forced migration or spending time in a refugee camp and holding a higher status position (i.e., managerial/professional position) prior to migration is highly associated with declines in mental well-being (Maximova & Krahn, 2010).

Through the eyes of a patient

Not too long ago, I lived a comfortable life in Saudi Arabia. We had a large well-kept home; servants who cooked, cleaned, and took care of the children; and a good family business. I was fortunate to have a loving husband and 10 children all of whom I cherished, but two of which I was especially proud. After becoming increasing concerned for our safety, our family made plans to permanently leave Saudi and seek asylum in Canada. We journeyed to India (my husband's home country) with the intent to move on quickly to Canada. In India, my husband and my two dearest children were separated from the rest of us. I have been in Canada now 12 months. . . . I feel as though my world has turned upside down. My husband used to take care of us, but he is not here. Even in all of my sadness, I have to be strong for my children. I don't feel safe, and I don't know who to trust. The social assistance worker says that a nurse will be coming to help me and my family. . . . In Saudi, nurses work in hospitals, how can a hospital nurse help me now?

(personal reflection of Zahara, 53 years old)

Through the eyes of a nurse

In 2004, I was a public health nurse (PHN) with a program called Families First. I received a service referral for a refugee family who was facing many challenges but whose primary concern was locating affordable housing. The family was large, a mother with eight children, who had been separated from other family members. After working with a very skilled interpreter to identify the family's needs, I worked with the family over several months to address their need for housing, childhood education, income, family cohesion, and mental health. Assistance was offered in locating a rental home in a neighbourhood that when compared to their home in Saudi Arabia was satisfactory. The family was referred to several agencies that could support them in furnishing their newly rented home. The oldest child (20 years old) was connected to an English language training centre. One year later, she could proficiently communicate in English and actually became the family liaison. The family was also assisted with becoming aware of the cultural norms for childhood education, and all children were enrolled in school. Looking back, a significant amount of time was dedicated to helping the family settle, but these tasks were very important to establishing a helping–trusting relationship. It was only after establishing this trusting relationship that "Mom" could speak to me about the severe isolation and depression she was experiencing. It is the smallest things that matter. Trust is built by helping someone read a newspaper or in helping them to make a phone call. When trust is established, it is at that time that you can begin to have a conversation about the things that most deeply impact the life and health of the person.

(personal reflection of Babitha, PHN for 5 years)

Unfair treatment of migrants, such as insufficient health and safety protections and violations of employment and labour standards, can give rise to situations of dangerous and precarious employment. In their study of Quebec workers with musculoskeletal injuries, Gravel et al. (2010) found that immigrant workers who had applied for compensation experienced more barriers and problems with the provincial compensation system compared to nonimmigrant workers. Employers challenged immigrant workers' claims more frequently, their diagnoses were less specific, and difficulties continued when they sought reinstatement to their previous jobs.

Employment Environment

Attention also needs to be paid to work environments and the structures and systems under which temporary workers are employed (Edmunds, Berman, Basok, Ford-Gilboe, & Forchuk, 2011). Jobs in agriculture and live-in caregiving represent two occupations that are often undertaken by migrant workers. Research has shown that these groups, when compared to the general population, are at greater risk for workplace injuries or accidents (Preibisch & Hennebry, 2011). Among agricultural workers, potential workplace hazards include chemical exposure, falls, and musculoskeletal injury. Among caregivers, live-in arrangements leave some women vulnerable to long work hours and physical, sexual, emotional, and economic abuse. For both groups discrimination, stress, isolation, and loneliness have the potential to significantly impact their mental health and well-being (Preibisch & Hennebry, 2011).

Within this context, it is both ethical and necessary to take action related to the immediate mental and physical health concerns of migrants as well as the larger sociopolitical SDoH that directly affect health. Such actions would require critical reflection on some important questions. For example, why are migrant men and women more likely to be underemployed in the Canadian workforce? Why do they receive lower pay for doing the same job as their Canadian-born counterparts? Why does this population have fewer chances for advancement, even when their educational level is similar to, or exceeds, the education of those born in Canada? Clearly, there is a need for holistic health and social service programs that attend to the prevention of mental and physical health concerns. An effective prevention strategy will ensure that needed resources and supportive networks are in place to facilitate the retraining and successful entrance of migrants into the labour market. Additionally, diversity strategies aimed at discrimination and other forms of oppression are essential to promoting the integration of migrants into the workforce. These strategies, in turn, will facilitate faster access to good paying jobs, adequate and safe housing, and dramatically reduce the stressors associated with day-to-day survival (Anderson et al., 2010).

Maternal Health and Health Services

Providing appropriate maternal health care to immigrants and refugees is critical to the well-being of the community. In their article, entitled "'They Can't Understand It': Maternity Health and Care Needs of Immigrant Muslim Women in St. John's,

Newfoundland," Reitmanova and Gustafson (2008) explored the needs and barriers to accessing maternity health services from the perspectives of immigrant Muslim women living in St. John's. The article was timely for two reasons: First, few studies have addressed this issue from the perspective of immigrant women in Canada, and second, because of the growing population of Muslim families in Newfoundland and Labrador.

> [Muslim] women reported experiencing discrimination, insensitivity and lack of knowledge about their religious and cultural practices. . . . There were also significant gaps between existing maternity health services and women's needs for emotional support, and culturally/linguistically appropriate information. This gap was further complicated by the functional and cultural adjustments associated with immigration. (Reitmanova & Gustafson, 2008, p. 101)

This research highlights the nurse's obligation to understand the ways in which our health-care system can marginalize members of diverse populations and the varied ways in which we as individuals and professionals limit access to the knowledge and resources needed to promote health. We need to act on the opportunity to expand current approaches to health service delivery, so that they are more inclusive and responsive to the health needs of new migrants. As student nurses, part of your role is to ensure that your practice, which was originally designed to meet the needs of Canadian-born woman, shifts to readily accommodate the needs of our diverse migrant population. You will be practicing within a health-care system that makes certain assumptions about what services and resources are important to provide, under which circumstances, and to whom. As nurses, you will be participating in making decisions regarding service and resource allocation. Nurses frequently support patients navigating through the health-care system, and we are strong and vocal advocates for our patients. However, questions you need to carefully consider include "How am I perpetuating some of the assumptions of my institution and community?" and "How am I participating in judging my patients?" You will witness inequities in the provision of health-care services and resources, and sometimes, the context of constraints, such as lack of funding or strict eligibility requirements, will mean that your decisions will perpetuate unfairness.

Diabetes and Ethnicity

It is anticipated that the prevalence of diabetes in Canada will increase from 11.6% of the population in 2010 to 13.9% in 2030, a shift from approximately 4.1 to 4.9 million people. Within Canada, the increase in the numbers of persons with diabetes will be highest in Alberta, British Columbia, Ontario, and the territories, among people who are between 55 and 69 years of age and those older than 80 years old (Ohinmaa, Jacobs, Simpson, & Johnson, 2004). The prevalence of diabetes will also be affected by the aging of migrants from global regions with high rates of this disease. Diabetes prevention will become an important component of the nurse's role particularly among migrants from certain regions. Migrants from the Middle East experience significantly higher rates of diabetes when compared to long-term residents of Ontario (Creatore et al., 2010). People migrating to Ontario from South Asia, Latin America and the Caribbean, and sub-Saharan Africa are 2 to 3 times more likely than migrants from Western Europe and United States to develop diabetes, regardless of age, sex, time since arrival, and income (Creatore et al., 2010). It has been suggested that the high rates of diabetes among specific migrant groups is related to genetics as well as several socioenvironmental factors associated with immigration including acculturation, stress, social isolation, poverty, and food insecurity (Creatore et al., 2010).

Cervical Cancer

Over their lifetime, 1 in 150 Canadian women are expected to develop cervical cancer, and 1 in 423 will die from the disease (Public Health Agency of Canada, 2013). The incidence of cervical cancer can be significantly decreased if abnormal cervical cells are identified early. However, research conducted over the past two decades has repeatedly shown new immigrants (<3 years in Canada) are less likely to have regular Papanicolaou (Pap) tests as a means of screening for cervical cancer (Latif, 2010; McDonald & Kennedy, 2007). Although immigrants develop cervical cancer at rates comparable to those born in Canada, failure to complete regular Pap tests delays detection and increases the risk of the cancer being invasive at the time of discovery (Khadilkar & Chen, 2013). Acculturation appears to be the single most important factor in determining rates of screening. That is, as immigrant women become aware of and are able to adopt Canadian norms relevant to cervical health, they become engaged in the practice of cervical screening (Khadilkar & Chen, 2013). As many migrants are arriving from countries that traditionally do not offer cervical screening, nurses will have an important role providing education about cervical cancer and appropriate measures for lifelong well-being as well as identifying and modifying barriers to receiving care. This may include creating environments that attend to cultural discomfort with sharing private information and concerns about receiving care from male health-care professionals.

RESEARCH
PROMOTING CANCER SCREENING WITH VIETNAMESE CANADIAN WOMEN

After migration to high-income Western countries, Vietnamese women have a significant increase in breast cancer risk and incidence compared to women in

their countries of origin. Vietnamese women have the highest rates of cervical cancer in the United States and for migrants living in Australia, significantly higher rates compared to the native-born. Increased rates of cancer may in part be due to the low participation rates in cancer screening and prevention programs such as the Pap test.

Study

In this paper, the factors that influenced Vietnamese women's participation in breast and cervical cancer screening were explored from the perspectives of Vietnamese health-care providers through individual in-depth interviews. Four male physicians and two female community health nurses were asked about their experiences of providing care to Vietnamese Canadian women including their perceptions regarding barriers the women experienced in engaging in clinical breast examinations (CBE), breast self-examination (BSE), and mammogram and Pap screening practices; information, health-care programs, and services that would best benefit Vietnamese Canadian women; and participants' perceptions of best strategies to promote breast and cervical cancer screening among the target population.

Conclusion

Male physicians identified that they were uncomfortable, or felt their patients were uncomfortable during breast and cervical examinations in light of cultural valuing of the privacy of the body and reluctance to discuss reproductive or sexual matters between men and women. Traditional hierarchical relationships between physicians and patients with reluctance by patients to directly ask for health-care information, coupled with a high patient/physician ratio was also a challenge. The low socioeconomic status of the Vietnamese Canadian women meant they were frequently changing addresses and/or phone numbers and were employed in jobs where visiting health-care providers often meant lost income. Community health nurses identified limitations in institutional support, such as a lack of interpreters, and budget constraints as significant barriers for both the providers and the women.

Implications for Nursing Students

The study provides a unique perspective on the individual- and system-level factors that influence Vietnamese women's participation in cancer screening programs. Although aware of the difficulties the women experienced, health-care providers felt that barriers could be overcome with funded and consistent promotion of the benefits of cancer screening. Engaging with this population also requires understanding of how the SDoH have shaped women's health-care practices.

Donnelly, T. T. (2008). Challenges in providing breast and cervical cancer screening services to Vietnamese Canadian women: The healthcare providers' perspective. Nursing Inquiry, 15(2), 158–168.

Practice Settings and Roles of Nurses Working With Migrants

Nurses play a vital part in the successful adjustment and adaptation of migrants. You will encounter migrants in every setting in which you practice, including hospitals, clinics, community health services such as public health and home care, and in community health centres and agencies, especially those geared to the settlement and integration of newcomers. As with all your patients, an important component of your practice is being aware of appropriate federal, provincial, territorial, and community services and resources. You may also be practicing nursing through indirect involvement with patients. For example, settlement and literacy organizations often have limited staff and time for resource development. The teaching and learning principles that you will use as you progress through your nursing program will give you a foundation on which you can collaborate to develop much-needed resources, such as health classes or health curricula for English or French language classes, at the same time strengthening programs implemented by community partners (Taylor et al., 2009).

Assessment

A necessary part of the nursing process is assessment, which involves describing and recording the evidence we gather. Particularly, as we assess the health of diverse populations, we must remain aware of the ways in which assessments can act to reinforce stereotypes that marginalize individuals and groups. As nurses, we are always interpreting or filtering the information we gather through a system of values and beliefs that are informed by our professional and personal life experiences. That we are nurses working within various healthcare systems also shapes what we perceive as important, our purposes for how we label it, what outcomes are desirable, and the conclusions we draw for our nursing diagnoses. When we describe, we are always creating and maintaining categories of difference (Allen, 2006).

Take for example the act of performing auscultations to assess a patient's lung sounds. You begin this task by recalling your knowledge and skills relevant to physical assessment and the well-established categories of lung sounds, such as wheezes or rhonchi. In completing your assessment, you have described and drawn a conclusion that supports the difference between a patient with normal lung sounds and a patient with abnormal sounds. The conclusions you draw and nursing interventions you may consider are based on those categories of difference. In this example, it may be challenging to detect how or why we should approach assessment, or the act of describing, in a somewhat different and more complex manner. And what is usually overlooked is a conscious awareness of the power of the person conducting the assessment. Those who have

the authority to describe and then make decisions based on those descriptions are always located within systems of power.

Through the eyes of a student

I was assigned to care for a woman from Egypt who was hospitalized for decubitus ulcers; she was in her mid-40s and had lost her mobility and vision due to multiple sclerosis. Her family, including her husband, sister, and children, had immigrated to Canada 15 years ago and were providing all her care at home. My patient was fluent in Arabic, French, and English, and she had been a physician in Egypt, so she was very knowledgeable and asked many questions. I was a bit intimidated at first because of her medical background and because she did not want me to provide any of her physical care. My patient's sister was at the bedside and was her "eyes," describing me and the other staff who came in and out of the room and what we were doing. I knew it was important that I assess my patient and build a trusting relationship, but I sensed she had put many walls up. I asked if she would allow me to assist while her sister bathed her in order to do a visual assessment. I respected the needs of my patient by facilitating the request to have a female family member care for her, promptly answering questions and assisting with her needs once she trusted me. She told me many stories of what it was like living in Egypt and how her family kept certain traditions that were important to them.

This experience really allowed the theoretical knowledge of comprehensively caring for patients to sink in. I had always thought that I was doing a good job at facilitating the needs of others, but until I had this experience, I was unaware of how truly important it was to understand the backgrounds, values, and beliefs of patients. It seemed all this patient had was her culture and her cultural memories, maybe partly because she had lost so much independence since coming to Canada as her illness had progressed. It was difficult to leave her because she had taught me so much for my future nursing practice, that nursing is not only about the physiological, emotional, and psychosocial needs, it's the way of life that someone has that contributes to all of these needs and is the matrix that shapes the person from their core. When we understand a patient's perspective and life history and respect their beliefs, they often allow us the privilege to be part of their world. It turned out that learning about dressing changes and treating the ulcers was the least of what I needed to do as a student nurse; establishing a relationship was the most important part in order to provide care.

(personal reflection of Aidan, a second-year nursing student)

Through the eyes of a nurse

I usually have four to five patients with high acuity levels and complex needs, and it often feels like there never enough time to provide the kind of nursing care I would like for my patients. Sometimes, it is hard not to feel like patients and families expect too much and don't realize or don't understand all the different procedures that nurses carry out and the multiple responsibilities we have during our shifts. Immigrant patients may be used to very different health-care systems and differing roles of nurses. My student's patient would push the buzzer frequently, and I must admit I rolled my eyes at times when the buzzer went off (again) and the student could see me. That's not the kind of nurse I want to be, and I realized that I needed to find ways to reduce my frustration. Talking with the student helped me understand more about the patient's life before and after she immigrated, the changes she and her family had gone through, and her need to ask many questions. I was very grateful that my student had taken the time to establish a therapeutic relationship and had the time to attend to the patient's needs. I don't have the same amount of time to spend with all my patients, but this experience reminded me to look beyond the procedures and the buzzers and see the whole person.

(personal reflection of Susan, RN, a staff nurse)

Importance of a Holistic Assessment

Most of our assessments focus on individuals. Yet, when we do consider group characteristics, especially for those who are identified as being somehow different, we often assume that certain values and behaviours are universal for that group and do not check with the individual patient. This action on our part ignores both the diversity that occurs within any group and that, as individuals, families, and communities, we are embedded in social and political contexts that shape our daily lives and health (Yang, 2010). The assessment questions in Box 37.2 are tailored to migrants. Rather than being used to describe migrants as

---

BOX 37.2 Assessment Questions

- Tell me about how you came to Canada.
- What was life like for you (and your family) when you first arrived?
- What is life like for you now?
- What has helped you settle in Canada?
- What life challenges are you attempting to manage right now?
- Which of your personal strengths have helped you adjust to life in Canada?
- How would you describe your health right now?
- What helps you to remain healthy?
- What prevents you from being healthy?
- Where do you go for health-care services? What have those experiences been like for you?
- Whom do you rely on or turn to for support?

---

normal or non-normal, the intent of the questions is to discover life stories and past and current challenges and strengths. It should be noted that aside from the questions about migration, these types of questions exploring the contexts and meanings of health could and should be asked of all your patients.

Language and Working With Interpreters

The term *mother tongue* "refers to the first language learned at home in childhood and still understood by the individual at the time of the census" (Statistics Canada, 2012b, p. 1). More than 200 mother tongues were identified in the 2011 census. Immigrant languages, those languages other than English, French, or Aboriginal languages, were the mother tongue for 20.6% of the Canadian population. Of the immigrant-language population, 56% identified their mother tongue as one of the Asian languages, whereas 40% identified a mother tongue of European origin. Asian languages are spoken in the Indian subcontinent, East Asia, and Southeast Asia and include the Chinese languages (Statistics Canada, 2012b).

*K*yla's parents were immigrants from the Philippines, and she remembers hearing them talk about the adjustments they had to make after they arrived in Canada. She also remembers trips to the Philippines with her family and how excited she was to visit with her grandparents and other relatives, but she realized that her extended family's lives in the Philippines were different from her life in Canada. Kyla feels she has some insight into Mrs. Gupta's situation but knows she needs to assess Mrs. Gupta as an individual within the context of her life before and after migration. Mrs. Gupta's son is present when Kyla starts her afternoon shift. He interprets for his mother when Kyla enters the room. Kyla appreciates this but isn't sure if it is appropriate.

Language expresses more than information; it conveys context, meaning, and nuances that can become lost in translation. Interactions with patients become more complicated when there are language barriers, and interpreters are needed. There can be many variations in the interpretation services offered by health-care organizations, ranging from on-site professional interpreters to interpretation services conducted by telephone, and informal interpretation by family members or staff of the institution (Srivastava, 2007). As a student nurse, you need to be aware of the policies regarding the use of interpreters and the resources available in your clinical settings as well as the policies of your school or faculty of nursing. Box 37.3 has some useful approaches.

Building Relationships Within Diversity

We have previously discussed that diversity can occur in many ways. This next section reflects on building relationships with diverse patients, colleagues, and groups of people

BOX 37.3   Strategies for Working Effectively With Interpreters

- Gain the patient's consent to use an interpreter.
- Attempt to identify factors that may influence the interaction, such as differences in dialect, religion, political affiliation, gender, age, and social status.
- Family members, especially spouses or children, should not be asked to interpret.
- Discuss with the interpreter the importance of repeating everything that is spoken by the patient and the nurse.
- Explain to the patient and the interpreter the importance of confidentiality. The interpreter must not disclose patient information to anyone.
- Talk to the patient, not to the interpreter. This reinforces that the communication is between the provider and the patient, assisted by the interpreter.
- Speak in simple terms. Avoid complex terms, jargon, or slang.
- Give the information to the interpreter in short sentences and ask the interpreter to relay the information after each sentence.
- If during an interpretation you sense that more is taking place than what is being relayed to you, ask the interpreter to explain what is being said.
- Ask the interpreter to explain to the patient any discussion between the interpreter and the nurse.
- Write down key points, directions, appointment times, and any other material that has numbers or can easily be confused or forgotten.
- Ask the patient to repeat, in his or her own words, the information you have given.
- Interpreters are part of the process and context of the interaction. They may have valuable insights into where the patient "is coming from."
- After the encounter, ask the interpreter to share his or her perceptions, especially if there was anything about the interaction that made it difficult to interpret.

Adapted from College of Nurses of Ontario. (2009). *Practice guideline: Culturally sensitive care.* Retrieved from http://www.cno.org/Global/docs/prac/41040_CulturallySens.pdf

within contexts of personal expertise, professional authority, and institutional power. The thoughtfulness and skills that nurses require for personal reflexivity in order to develop strong and positive connections with patients is no less important in the workplace and in our communities.

Questioning Assumptions and the Importance of Self-Reflection

As you prepare to practice nursing and interact with migrant patients, you need to be aware of the values and assumptions that shape not only your understanding of migrant populations but also the ways in which you interact with migrants at a fundamental level. This process of critically thinking through your varied assumptions and then shifting your nursing practice to one that is less harmful is called

self-reflexivity. Srivastava (2007) describes self-reflexivity as a process of critical self-examination, in which we are challenged to question our own understanding of reality and our beliefs of who we are; what it means to be a nurse; and our assumptions about individual patients, groups, and communities. Reflection and reflexivity are both important. However, reflection usually occurs "after the fact," whereas reflexivity can occur during interactions and involves explicit attention to structures and systems as well as the personal (refer back to Chapter 25 for a detailed discussion).

Our values, beliefs, and assumptions are often hidden and unexamined but can perpetuate nursing actions that may limit our effectiveness in establishing authentic and therapeutic relationships with members of migrant groups. An important component of self-reflexivity is recognizing how we describe ourselves and the groups with which we identify. Our sense of identity is dynamic and fluid, and we all identify with multiple and different groups at different points in our lives. For example, you may be a student nurse, so you are starting to take on that professional identity, but you also have a gender identity, and you may identify with certain ethnic or migrant groups. The list may be extensive, but it is important to remember that the sometimes simplistic ways in which others label us (or assign identity) may not be how we understand or label ourselves.

So why is self-reflexivity important? Recognition of our assumptions, values, and beliefs (both personal and professional) and the values and beliefs of our institutions and communities is the necessary first step in working toward responses that are inclusive and accepting of diversity and working for change at all levels. Reflexivity prompts us to consider the many factors that influence and shape what we do and whose purposes or agendas are being served. In some instances, the purposes of an educational or health institution such as a hospital may not be in the best interest of the patient or you as a nurse. Holding a community forum to assess the service needs of a community may be a fairly benign and acceptable practice reflecting the valuing of community engagement and public participation, but how does this practice influence inclusivity or exclusivity among members of a migrant population where community forums are unfamiliar and a less acceptable means of consultation? As an example, we might look closely at the criteria for providing certain resources and health services that reflect the cultural and economic realities of Canadian institutions. Reflexivity allows us to question the values and assumptions that underlie such realities and decisions.

Reflexivity also allows us to counter the assumption that nurses and other health-care professionals are neutral or objective in our interactions with patients. None of us are neutral and cannot be separated from the values, perceptions, fears, and strengths that we bring to our encounters with all people. Just as our patients are situated in the systems and structures that influence their lives, nurses (and all health professionals) are also shaped by the contexts of their personal and professional values and the values, assumptions, and policies of their institutions. Box 37.4 provides some

BOX 37.4 Questions for Self-Reflexivity

Reflections About My Personal Self

- What are my assumptions about the life experiences of immigrants, refugees, and temporary residents who arrive in Canada?
- How have my life experiences and/or family history of migration influenced my assumptions and beliefs about migrants?
- How do I assess difference and diversity? For example, is it based on markers of visible difference (from myself) such as ethnicity, skin colour, dress, or language? What are the implications of this? Can difference/diversity be invisible?
- How would I describe myself to others? With which groups do I identify? Why? How does this shape my values and expectations of how people should act?

Reflections About Myself as a Nursing Student

- What assumptions am I making about the health of migrants and the nursing care they need?
- Do I think that all immigrant families are "needy" or will have trouble coping?
- What are my assumptions about the services and resources provided in Canada for migrants? How do these services and resources promote health? Should migrant patients be grateful?
- How do I feel and act toward patients who have different or similar values and behaviours than mine?

- What is my role as a nursing student working with migrants? Is it different/similar than for other patients? Why?
- How do the identities that nurses and patients assign to themselves and to others influence nurse–patient interactions and relationships?
- How do my assessments of patients and the conclusions I draw influence the nursing care I provide? How do nurse–patient power relations shape nursing diagnoses? Is this different and/or similar for migrants?
- How do I resolve disagreement and conflict with peers, teachers, patients, and staff in clinical settings? How do I act inclusively?

Reflections About Context

- How do the institutions in which you will have clinical placements assess, manage, or promote difference and diversity?
- What services and resources are provided to migrants? Why? What are the priorities? How do these services reflect the underlying values of the institutions?
- Should other services and resources be in place? What can you do about this?
- How is power reflected in working with migrants? Who has power and privilege to make decisions? Whose voice counts?
- How do disparities and inequities in the SDoH influence experiences of health and illness in the communities in which migrants live and health-care institutions are located?

---

important questions to consider as you engage in the reflexive process, a process that you will develop and continually hone throughout your nursing career.

Building Relationships With Diverse Patients

Being a nurse requires the art and application of your knowledge, skills, and expertise. The skills and expertise needed to establish caring relationships, understand meanings of health, and advocate for equitable services are not limited to migrants. Because of our formal training and education, nurses may consider themselves to be experts in the nurse–patient relationship. However, we should always recognize that patients are the experts regarding their experiences of health and illness. Also, remember that members of diverse populations are often more aware than professionals of the consequences and implications of the SDoH such as poverty, lost social networks, and systemic and structural constraints, such as restrictive immigration policies or temporary employment contracts. After all, they are the ones situated in and experiencing those consequences.

We need to consider how we judge the values, beliefs, and behaviours of patients from diverse populations. It is often the case that when a patient's behaviour is different from what we, as professionals, have judged to be appropriate, we assign the label of "noncompliance." To label patients as noncompliant harms relationships and reflects our values about who has the power to judge behaviours

and to make the right (or best) health-care decisions for others. It demeans patients (and ourselves) and usually indicates that we have not taken the time to fully explore the patient's level of understanding, the meaning they ascribe to the health-care concern, and factors such as lack of access to providers and services or costs the patient cannot afford.

Building Diversity With Colleagues

Diversity in the Canadian population, including the nursing workforce, will continue to increase. A workforce composed of nurses who are open-minded, inclusive, and respectful of all colleagues is essential for a healthy professional community. In a recent publication, Samuels-Dennis, York, and Barrett (2012) document the migration trends of Jamaican nurses into the Canadian health-care system beginning in the late 1940s up to the present. Their work highlights how this migrant group has helped to transform our health-care system. Although many positive influences were highlighted, the integration of Jamaican nurses into the nursing profession was not without its challenges. Jamaican nurses (first and second generation) often recalled experiences shaped by racism, discrimination, hierarchical oppression, and the constant assumption that they were not good enough. Several nurses discussed concerns that Jamaican nurses tended to remain predominantly in front line or general nursing positions, which often meant caring for the patients with the most challenging illnesses.

They also faced barriers gaining the skills and experiences needed for professional advancement. Some nurses currently practicing in hospital settings expressed concerns that their nursing colleagues and physicians overlooked or ignored their professional opinions but did not do the same for other nurses.

Cultural safety, as discussed in Chapter 13, is not just something we aspire to achieve with individuals, migrant communities, and our colleagues sometime in the future. We must not forget that diversities within and across our workplaces and communities are very much grounded in past and current histories of migration and settlement within contexts of power and oppression. Yet, these differences of experiences and collective beliefs and values also enhance the richness of our neighbourhoods, worksites, and our country by providing opportunities for new insights, perspectives, and change.

Attending to Communities of Migrants

As nurses, our relationships with patients are important to us. For many nurses, this is the most important and meaningful aspect of nursing. Currently, there is a great deal of emphasis on the acquisition of skills an individual nurse needs to work with individual patients, and as student nurses, that is a large part of your education. However, this focus on individual encounters, especially when the patient is identified or described as different because of migration not only obscures the broader SDoH and contexts in which that patient is living but also often conceals the social norms and practices that permit oppression, such as those based on race and gender (Racher & Annis, 2012).

Responding to the needs of migrant communities requires that we view health and the resources needed to support health from a broad perspective, regardless of the settings where patients come for care. Although we still focus on the individuals for whom we are providing care, we also need to focus on the communities in which they live. The WHO (1998) defines a *healthy community* as "one that is continually creating and improving those physical and social environments and expanding those community resources which enable people to mutually support each other in performing all the functions of life and in developing their maximum potential" (p. 13). This definition refers to a process rather than a status. A healthy community does not necessarily have the highest health status but is on a journey continually striving to be healthier. Valuing the health of diverse populations requires us to think about the physical, social, and political factors that influence the health of migrants, who are themselves diverse. It means that as a profession, we are able to partner with migrant patients and communities to build new ways to achieve social change and community well-being.

Building partnerships with migrant communities that are grounded in mutual respect and trust is essential to understanding and appreciating their struggles and beginning the social change process. Box 37.5 highlights seven principles for working with diverse populations as we partner with them to promote their health. Racher and Annis (2012) originally developed the principles during several years of working with groups, organizations, and communities. They noted that because each community is unique, the intent is not to be prescriptive but to offer strategies for reflective practice that attend to the needs of migrant communities.

BOX 37.5 Touchstones for Working With Diverse Communities

- *Reframing diversity and migration as benefits* and understanding that the multiple and varied contributions to our communities and society counteract negative stereotypes.
- *Creating spaces for voices to be heard and groups to be represented* produces opportunities to break down resistance and facilitate social change. Nurses have both the opportunity and responsibility to take action in creating such spaces.
- *Understanding concepts of health, health practices, and health promotion used by different groups* expands the knowledge of nurses. Sharing knowledge creates a foundation for new ideas and the evolution of strategies to achieve and sustain health.
- *Nurses have the responsibility to facilitate partnerships* in order to develop needed programs, confront exclusionary practices and marginalization, and advocate for full participation by all residents of Canada.

- *Effective nursing practice requires the ability to differentiate* between (a) facilitating discussion between people with diverse perspectives to reach a single outcome and (b) facilitating respectful acceptance of multiple and different perspectives within an inclusive framework, which may result in options for outcomes.
- *Examining the assumptions of organizations* within the health care and other systems offers the opportunity for change and growth. Recognizing discrimination, exclusion, or unequal power relations within institutions is an important step toward change. Self-assessment by organizations builds organizational commitment to be inclusive, open, and progressive in meeting the needs of patients. Nurses are advocates and resources for this work.
- *Effective, committed nurses examine their openness, humility, and interpersonal skills*; grow as lifelong learners and reflective practitioners; and critically determine how they choose "to be" in their relationships with diverse individuals, groups, and communities.

Adapted from Racher, F. E., & Annis, R. C. (2012). Honouring culture and diversity in community practice. In A. R. Vollman, E. T. Anderson, & J. McFarlane (Eds.), Canadian community as partner: *Theory & multidisciplinary practice* (3rd ed., pp. 154–176). Philadelphia, PA: Lippincott Williams & Wilkins.

The Future of Migration

The number of global migrants will continue to increase through both international and internal relocation. International migrants now number 214 million people and are projected to increase to 450 million people by 2050 (International Organization for Migration, 2010). There have been significant increases in the numbers of female migrants, temporary foreign workers, undocumented migrants, and refugees. Occurring much more frequently than international migration, to date, approximately 740 million people have migrated internally within their countries of origin (International Organization for Migration, 2010). As with international migrants, an important reason for internal migration is to seek work, such as people from Newfoundland and the Maritime provinces of Canada who obtain employment in Alberta's Oil Sands or the millions of rural residents of China who are migrating to the factories and construction jobs in the major cities of that country. Growth in all forms of migration is related to our increasing global population; changes in economic opportunities related to globalization; high youth unemployment worldwide; and displacement and forced migration through conflict, natural disasters, and climate change.

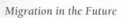 *Think* *Migration in the Future*

In the next few decades, international migration will become more common and more complex as a result of shifting demographics, environmental changes, global political and economic pressures, and technological changes, such as the use of social media. These changes bring both opportunities and challenges. How does environmental or climate change affect migration and health? What are some examples? The use of social media can be an effective communication mechanism for promoting social and political change. How could social networks be used to promote health? Would there be any disadvantages to using social networks for this purpose? How could global pressures for increased migration threaten the human rights and health of migrants?

Changes to the Canadian Population

Over the next few decades, the composition of the Canadian population will continue to change, reflecting the shift in migration to Canada from non-European countries (Fig. 37.4), sustained immigration levels, and low birth rates among the nonimmigrant population. The proportion of foreign-born residents in Canada is projected to increase to between 25% and 28% of the total population or at least 1 person out of

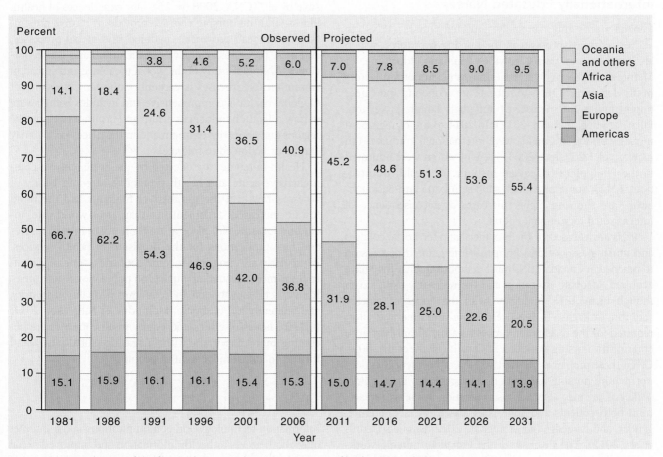

Figure 37.4 Distribution of the foreign-born population by continent of birth, 1981 to 2031.

4 by 2031 (Statistics Canada, 2010). Almost three quarters of the foreign-born in Canada will belong to a visible minority group. It is also predicted that by 2031, between 29% and 32% of all Canadians could be a member of a visible minority group, with South Asians and Chinese remaining the largest visible minority communities. Persons whose mother tongue was neither English nor French accounted for less than 10% of Canada's population in 1981. By 2006, that proportion had risen to 20%, and projections indicate that in 2031, the first language for 3 out of 10 Canadians could be neither English nor French (Statistics Canada, 2010).

Toronto, Vancouver, and Montréal, which are and will continue to be Canada's three largest metropolitan areas, will be home for more than 71% of all visible minority persons in the future (Statistics Canada, 2010). As the number of Canadians who identify with multiple ethnicities continues to increase, dialogue about the meanings and practices of multiculturalism will continue to shift from a past focus on valuing a single ethnic heritage to a more complex and pluralistic understanding. As a nation and as a profession, we need to continually reflect on what we expect of migrants to Canada. Is it possible to have too much integration? Is it possible to have too little? The answers to these questions will vary, but they will offer nurses some direction for the care we provide.

Internationally Educated Nurses

Canada needs internationally educated nurses (IENs) to address current shortages in the nursing workforce, which are predicted to persist (Blythe, Baumann, Rheaume, & McIntosh, 2009). As with other migrants, important factors in the decisions of IENs to relocate are economic and career opportunities for themselves and their families (Newton, Pillay, & Higginbottom, 2012). In 2011, 8.6% of registered nurses working in Canada were international graduates (an increase of 1.2% since 2003), 30% of whom were educated in the Philippines (Canadian Institute for Health Information, 2012). Some provinces, such as Alberta and Saskatchewan, are showing higher increases as a consequence of international recruitment efforts.

IENs are assessed by the provincial and territorial colleges and nursing associations. Prior to being granted permission to practice in Canada, IENs must demonstrate that they have acquired adequate education and the necessary skills. Even though many IENs immigrate with the hopes of quickly acquiring a license to practice nursing, the time and effort required for the registration process is a significant barrier to entering the nursing workforce in Canada (Blythe et al., 2009). Given these problems, IENs may seek employment that does not require nursing registration, a process that is called *deskilling*. They may also face discrimination in the workplace, from both patients and colleagues, based on race, culture, gender, and language (Newton et al., 2012; Samuels-Dennis et al., 2012). The diversity of the Canadian nursing workforce will continue to be shaped by nurses who are educated

internationally. Members of the nursing workforce must be willing to identify and cooperate with one another to address barriers to equity. Additionally, we must build practice environments in which the professional and personal contributions of nurses from diverse and migrant populations are valued and welcomed (Sochan & Singh, 2007).

Think *Internationally Educated Nurses*

The CNA and the International Council of Nurses recognize the right of individual nurses to migrate yet acknowledge that there may be negative effects on the quality of health care in countries where many nurses leave. Is it ethical to recruit IENs from countries with limited resources for educating nurses and providing nursing care? What would the ethical recruitment of IENs look like? What professional and personal challenges are IENs likely to face when they immigrate to Canada? As a profession, what should our role be when assisting IENs after migration? Other than the recruitment of IENs, how might Canada resolve our nursing shortage?

Global Health and Migration

Global health is "the optimal well-being of all humans from the individual and the collective perspective. Health is considered a fundamental right and should be equally accessible by all" (CNA, 2008, p. 25). Our experiences of health, illness, and the nursing care we provide or receive are embedded in local, provincial, national, and global processes, and these processes at all levels shape health and health outcomes. Although study of the global incidence and spread of communicable diseases is certainly important, the concept of global health is comprehensive and includes being aware of how migration influences health and health services in the regions and countries of origin and in the places people may choose or be forced to migrate.

Health outcomes are affected by the availability of comprehensive acute and health promotive care and equity of access. Growth in the numbers of migrants and the trend toward increased settlement in urban areas worldwide, including Canada, will place a strain on urban infrastructures and has implications for the provision of health services. Particularly affecting low-income countries, "one of globalization's most substantial impacts on population health arises from its tendency to increase economic inequality, insecurity, and vulnerability" (Labonte, Mohindra, & Schrecker, 2011, p. 270). Issues of ethics and equity in all countries are becoming more important with increasing globalization and the transnational movement of people.

Use of Technology

Information technology and communication via the Internet offers both access to health information and improved social support systems for migrants. The Internet, which has a vast array of health information from both formal and informal sources, is often available in the user's language of origin. During past waves of migration and prior to modern technological advances, many migrants would have considered relocation a permanent "before" and "after" experience of loss, opportunity, and settlement in a new country. **Transnationalism** refers to significant changes in the ways in which migration is experienced. Currently, and in the future, the maintenance and development of connections with families, networks, and communities across borders will be enhanced and more fluid (Isaacs, 2010). The sense of displacement and lost social networks, experienced by all migrants, are now somewhat tempered by technological resources such as Skype, Google video chat, and cell phones. These advances make it possible for migrants to maintain ongoing and frequent contact with friends and relatives in their countries of origin.

However, when taking into account the actual benefits of technology, it is necessary to recognize that the role one ascribes to technology is directly dependent on context. That is, exposure to technology is both dependent on development within countries and the socioeconomic status of the migrant in their country of origin. Current immigration criteria ensure that those coming to Canada as permanent residents are highly skilled and highly educated. In high-income countries, this likely means prior experience with the Internet and technological resources. However, in other countries, poor or restricted access to the Internet and computers may be the norm. It is important to assess each person for his or her experience in using technology to promote his or her health. Also remember that someone holding a high socioeconomic status in his or her country of origin, even if it is a low-income country, may be more versed in using technologies than someone arriving from a high-income country but of low socioeconomic status.

Public Health

Increases in global migration pose some challenges for public health, such as the heightened potential for the worldwide spread of communicable diseases related to rising levels of tourism, trade, and ease of international travel. Diseases such as HIV/AIDS, Ebola, SARS, tuberculosis, and cholera are now able to spread quickly across geographical distances (Labonte et al., 2011). As you now know, most migrants arrive in Canada healthier than long-term residents of this country and undergo medical screening before entry. However, the perception that migrants can be carriers of disease that put those in the new country at risk still exists (Gushulak, 2007), as illustrated during the H1N1 influenza outbreak in 2009. When temporary agricultural workers, who are usually defined as being from racial groups, were subject to increased screening and media attention that portrayed them as potentially dangerous vectors of H1N1 from their countries of origin and therefore a health threat to Canadians. This focus not only draws our attention away from other global vectors but also maintains our awareness

on individuals or groups who are different from us and the ways in which we may perceive them as a threat rather than the larger structures and systems that affect migrants' health in their home countries and here in Canada (Preibisch & Hennebry, 2011).

The Future of Nursing: Challenges and Opportunities

Challenges and opportunities exist together and create a synergy for reflection, discussion, and action. What can we learn from migrants? Anyone who migrates is changed by that experience, in both anticipated and unanticipated ways. However, what is often minimized, if not forgotten, is that migrants influence and change their new countries as well. As nurses, this means going beyond the ways in which models of cultural competence are often used in our health-care systems, where the cultures of those who are seen as outside the mainstream are viewed as static, unchanging, and homogeneous. What can you learn from your patients? What contributions do migrants bring to your personal and professional relationships with them and to Canada?

The ability of people to access health information from numerous sources will continue to increase, as will the use of complementary and alternative medicine (CNA, 2008). Given the federal government priorities for skilled and professional workers, increasing numbers of migrants will enter Canada with higher levels of formal education than in the past, and they may be more comfortable challenging our assumptions about the Canadian health-care system and the availability of services (Isaacs, 2010).

Working for Change at All Levels

Throughout this chapter, you have been asked to consider the contexts and structures that shape the lives of migrants in Canada. By doing this, we (the authors) hope you are more aware of the complexity of migrants' lives and the need for solutions that address our structures and systems, solutions that ultimately benefit all Canadians (Isaacs, 2010). In the future, nurses will need to respond to increasing rates of population change. This means becoming more knowledgeable regarding the implications for health and nursing care and much more flexible and proactive in initiating and shaping change in our health-care systems through formal and informal partnerships. Change at systemic levels also means addressing public and government accountability, a process that "must include not only an evaluation of the quality and accessibility of services, but also an evaluation of measures in place to promote safe and inviting environments for full participation" (Caxaj & Berman, 2010, p. E28).

As mentioned earlier, the terms *culture* or *ethnicity* are often used as code words for *race*. Racialization is a powerful way to exclude people from full participation in public life. Ensuring that all migrants feel included in Canadian society means having honest discussions about the processes of racialization and further taking action where racialization works to disadvantage others. These discussions and actions are vital and, with the increasing visible minority population, will continue to be needed in the future. Additionally, all nurses need to be aware of how structural, legislative, funding, and policy decisions affect migrants to Canada and be prepared to take responsibility for participating in the dialogue and needed actions (Yang, 2010).

Nursing Research

Past research pertaining to migrants has focused on infectious diseases and conditions of being "at risk" (Gushulak, 2007). Current research often focuses on individual or group health behaviours and outcomes; however, there is lack of research regarding integrating the contextual layers of migration including the SDoH, barriers to health care, and experiences of discrimination (Acevedo-Garcia & Almeida, 2012). Like the narrowness of the nurse focusing only on the individual patient and not taking into account systemic and structural issues, research that focuses on individual behaviour does not give us the complete picture (Yang, 2010).

There is a significant gap in research related to the short- and long-term strengths, resiliencies, and coping skills of all migrants, including those without documentation, and a lack of research focused on gender and on stages throughout the lifespan (Health Canada, 2010; Salehi, 2010). The mental health of migrants is another area that has been understudied, particularly among youth and women, and based on type of migration status and level of education (Dean & Wilson, 2009; Reitmanova & Gustafson, 2009). Migrants, particularly refugees, may find their lives drastically changed because of forces beyond their control, such as war and natural disasters. However, they are not "passive pawns of fate" (Beiser, 2009). We need to know much more about the personal and collective resources used to adjust and adapt in a new country and how can we support resiliency as well as identify what gets in the way.

Research about certain conditions, diseases, or issues will always be needed. However, a balanced approach recognizing strengths within conditions of concern is essential. People who have migrated are not victims. Like any other population in Canada, they need our thoughtful and evidence-informed support and research conducted with their full collaboration, not research about subjects (Salehi, 2010). Some research, such as that related to complementary and alternative medicine, not only has relevance to the migrant population but for the wider Canadian population as well (Roth & Kobayashi, 2008).

Nursing Education

All nurses are expected to have an understanding of the SDoH and the skills to advance social justice and equity (CNA, 2008), although often these concepts are most explicitly taught and experienced in community health theory and clinical courses. Cohen and Gregory (2009) list the following enabling factors in order to promote understanding and the experiential learning of these concepts: The nursing curriculum needs to a focus on these concepts early and throughout the program in all courses; when appropriate, use non-nurse preceptors and mentors, who, especially in the community, often have a holistic and broad viewpoint; and have structured opportunities for students to integrate theory and practice and be supported in critical and reflective thinking. In some clinical settings, students themselves may have an influence on the staff nurses that broaden their perspectives and approaches.

As students and as nurses, you will be providing care to people from many parts of the world. Nursing education needs to go further than providing international experiences, which are usually available for relatively few students. Opportunities are needed for all students to become engaged in and knowledgeable of the role of nurses in an increasingly global and connected world (Mill, Astle, Ogilvie, & Gastaldo, 2010). Similar to becoming proficient in working with the concepts of SDoH, social justice, and equity, awareness of and proficiency working with global health issues is an essential part of nursing care. These enabling factors and comprehensive approaches (Cohen & Gregory, 2009) are relevant for understanding global health. Researchers (Mill et al., 2010) include the need for endorsement by those in faculty and university leadership roles. Opportunities and expectations for interprofessional education and practice are also increasing (CNA, 2011).

Educational institutions, including schools and faculties of nursing, do not function outside of political and social contexts nor are they neutral. Change requires recognizing assumptions and practices that support dominant interests and actively "resisting the political and cultural isolation characteristic of professional education" (Allen, 2006, p. 72). Change requires engagement and courage. Nursing students in Canada have and will become more diverse. Think about your nursing class. Do nursing students who are members of a visible minority group or are migrants themselves feel accepted and understood? Are the backgrounds, experiences, and qualifications of all applicants and students valued equally?

Practice and Policy: Putting It All Together

Nursing practice is the convergence of your professional education, the expertise you will develop, and research, which is needed to not only inform your nursing practice with migrants to Canada but also to have the evidence to influence policy and program development at different levels. There is strong and consistent support in the nursing and health literature for the closer integration of research, education, practice, and policy, always taking into consideration local, national, and international contexts (Beiser, 2009; Browne et al., 2009; Yang, 2010). Again, a focus on individual behaviour misses the larger influences on patients' lives, arising both from their countries of origin and in Canada and lessens our potential for facilitating positive change. As with nursing theories, which help us make sense of a ways of providing care and guide us to better practice decisions, we are more effective when we consider structure, context, and systems in collaboration with others.

We need to pay attention to diverse and multiple voices in education, research, and practice, valuing that people have many kinds of resources and knowledge and recognizing the power relations that occur when someone is accorded the authority and status of a "professional" (Allen, 2006). We need to be aware of how we are reacting to our patients, the assumptions behind our reactions, and how we are being changed or being resistant to change. With increasing global connections available for health information and care, nurses need to know how to support diverse health practices within the context of their professional knowledge (Isaacs, 2010). Keep in mind, though, that when it comes to evidence-informed research or policies, the question that always needs to be asked is, "Who is defining what is considered to be and valued as evidence?" All too often, the recipients of policies have not been consulted, or they have barriers to being included arising from language, lack of transportation, or hours of work.

Conclusion

As chapter authors, we represent two important trends in Canadian immigration. One of us (Joan) is an immigrant herself, coming to Toronto at the age of 10 years from Jamaica at a time when the countries of origin for migration to Canada were changing, and the visible minority population was quickly increasing. The other author (Kathryn) is a third-generation immigrant whose grandparents came from England to Saskatchewan in the early 20th century as part of the federal government's drive to settle the prairies with white Europeans. We share family histories of what it is like to leave your home and start anew while maintaining ties with geographically distant relatives. We also share our identities and values as nurses and nurse educators and our backgrounds in public health nursing. Of course, we have also had many differing individual experiences.

You may have been surprised that this chapter did not contain specific information about specific ethnic, cultural, or migrant groups. What happens all too often in health care is that when descriptions of different groups are given, they become entrenched and focused on the individual while ignoring aspects of patients' lives that may have far

more influence on their health, namely, the SDoH. Instead, we decided to concentrate on the context of migration to Canada, the importance of questioning your assumptions, recognizing the power relations inherent in the act of describing, conducting holistic assessments with every patient, and your professional responsibilities to work for change. You will find general background information about cultural and migration histories relevant and necessary in your practice, so that you have a deeper understanding of how and why people have made the decision to come to Canada. In order to provide comprehensive and meaningful care to your patients, you will need to learn what is important to them, what they understand about their health, and the structures and systems influencing their lives.

Being responsive to diversity means recognizing the variety and complexity of migration pathways, the multiplicity of premigration and postmigration experiences, and differing accessibility to health care once in Canada. Being responsive to diversity also means that even though nursing care is often provided by an individual nurse to an individual patient, it includes identifying barriers within our systems of care and then working to change policies and institutions so there is increased awareness and flexibility to respond to various needs, beliefs, and life contexts, change that has the potential to improve the health of all those residing in Canada.

Kyla has had the experience of other Canadians assuming she is an immigrant because of her name and skin colour. As a student nurse, she sometimes feels that people assume she "knows about immigrants" because she is from an "ethnic" group. She did not know how to approach Mrs. Gupta at first, especially given the language barrier. Kyla checked the policy of her clinical site regarding interpreters, which stated that, when possible, family members should not be acting in this role during nursing and medical assessments and interventions. An on-site interpreter designated by the institution was available and came to Mrs. Gupta's room. Kyla thanked Mrs. Gupta's son for his assistance and then asked for privacy while she assessed her patient. As Kyla assessed Mrs. Gupta's postoperative recovery, she was also able to ask about any other concerns her patient might have. Through the interpreter, Mrs. Gupta said that although she was thankful to be with her son and his family, adjustment to life in Canada had been more difficult than she anticipated. The interpreter was able to provide some information about relevant community resources that could provide some support. By relating to Mrs. Gupta as an individual within the larger context of her family, her community, and life in Canada, Kyla was able to establish a rapport, more fully appreciate the complexity of her patient's experiences, and conduct a holistic nursing assessment.

Critical Thinking Case Scenarios

▶ In your practice as a registered nurse (RN) in the emergency department of a large urban hospital, you are assigned to a 40-year-old female patient who is a recently arrived refugee and is experiencing dizziness and palpitations. You assess her physical symptoms. What else should you be assessing and why?

▶ Mr. Martinez is a 37-year-old, Spanish-speaking migrant worker from central Mexico. On his brother's recommendation, he came to Chatham, Ontario, seeking employment and soon began working 10 to 12 hours a day in local tomato farm. He has no medical history, takes no medications, and is generally fit. He does not speak English and has limited literacy in Spanish, only completing a sixth-grade education. His wife and five children remain in Mexico. His daughter has a chronic illness that uses much of the family's economic resources. Some months after arrival, Mr. Martinez developed palpitations and shortness of breath. His brother brought him to the emergency department of a rural community hospital. His chest radiograph confirmed moderate congestive heart failure and cardiomegaly. His medical condition was stabilized, and he was discharged on a β-blocker, furosemide, and warfarin. The attending physician, Dr. Graham, instructed him not to return to work until he met with a primary care physician and his conditions had significantly improved. Unable to work, Mr. Martinez grew frightened by the uncertainty of his health and the financial difficulties of his family in Mexico. Keeping in mind the various contextual factors that determine health, what specific familial/biologic, structural, and socioeconomic and political factors are most likely to impact Mr. Martinez's health?

Multiple-Choice Questions

1. Match each of the key terms below to the appropriate definitions.
   a. _____ Immigrant
   b. _____ Refugee
   c. _____ Visible minority
   d. _____ Diversity

   I. Defined by the Employment Equity Act as persons, other than Aboriginal peoples, who are non-Caucasian in race or non-white in colour.
   II. Groups that have a shared identity based on heritage, language, beliefs, and values.
   III. A person who has moved from his or her country or region of origin either temporarily or permanently.
   IV. The variation between people in many traits such as gender, age, national origin, beliefs, and values.
   V. A person who fears returning to his or her home country and who seeks the protection of another country.
   VI. An ongoing relationship with the country of origin for migrants residing in a new host society.
   VII. A person who moves into another country for the purpose of settling.

2. The CNA Code of Ethics states that nurses must "recognize and respect the intrinsic worth of each person . . . [and] . . . support the family, group, population or community receiving care in maintaining their dignity and integrity" (CNA, 2008, p. 13). Which of the following nursing activities is most supported by this statement?
   a. The nurse attends conferences and workshop that promote cultural and religious sensitivity.
   b. The nurse conducts research that uncovers the ways in which racialized groups are treated unjustly.
   c. The nurse sits on a committee that assesses and addresses the settlement needs and concerns of refugees and newcomers.
   d. As part of a community planning group that celebrates diversity through an annual health fair, the nurse ensures that cultural artifacts from all ethnic groups living the community are included at the fair.

3. Given what we know about the "healthy immigrant effect," in the first 10 years postmigration, which SDoH is most significant to this population's mental health and well-being?
   a. Employment
   b. Education and literacy
   c. Social networks
   d. Genetic endowment/biology

4. By 2030, it is anticipated that diabetes prevention will become an important component of the nurse's role, particularly as we account for current immigration trends. It is estimated that immigrants from South Asia, Latin America, the Caribbean, and sub-Saharan Africa are 2 to 3 times more likely than immigrants from Western Europe and the United States to develop diabetes even after controlling for age, sex, time since arrival, income level, and immigration-related variables. Which of the following does NOT account for this observed increased in risk for diabetes among migrant populations from these regions?
   a. Genetics
   b. Sex
   c. Acculturation
   d. Health services

5. A nursing student is a member of a university committee charged with planning a day to celebrate Canadian diversity. One suggestion is to have foods representing the diverse ethnic groups within the student body. Some committee members express disagreement stating "cultural foods" would perpetuate stereotyping of certain groups. The student nurse realizes that:
   a. The committee needs to reach unanimous agreement on all suggestions in order to have a successful event.
   b. Values and beliefs regarding positive expressions of multiculturalism are diverse.
   c. The solution would be to promote the total integration of all cultures through assimilation.
   d. Issues of perception and how people are portrayed are not inherent in multiculturalism.

6. A student nurse is working with a migrant family that is experiencing unemployment and risk for homelessness. The family connects with others from their country of origin who offer them food, money to pay the rent, and friendship. Which statement best describes the family's situation?

   a. The family's social networks are strengths in a situation currently shared by many Canadians.

   b. The family is not at risk for poor health because their strong social networks will keep them healthy.

   c. Unemployment and poverty are normal for the newly migrated family and could be considered a rite of passage.

   d. Once family members find employment, they will successfully adapt to Canadian life.

7. A nursing student conducting an assessment of an immigrant family should be demonstrating:

   a. The ability to assess how the family's values and beliefs differ from his or her own.

   b. A thorough and in-depth understanding of the family's health practices.

   c. Comprehensive and complete knowledge about services that support immigrant groups in the community.

   d. Awareness of the intersections of the family's values and migration experience and the SDoH throughout the assessment.

REFERENCES AND SUGGESTED READINGS

Acevedo-Garcia, D., & Almeida, J. (2012). Special issue introduction: Place, migration and health. *Social Science & Medicine (1982)*, 75(12), 2055–2059.

Allen, D. G. (2006). Whiteness and difference in nursing. *Nursing Philosophy: An International Journal for Healthcare Professionals*, 7(2), 65–78.

Anderson, J. M., Reimer, J., Khan, K. B., Simich, L., Neufeld, A., Stewart, M., & Makwarimba, E. (2010). Narratives of "dissonance" and "repositioning" through the lens of critical humanism: Exploring the influences on immigrants' and refugees' health and well-being. *Advances in Nursing Science*, 33(2), 101–112.

Asanin, J., & Wilson, K. (2008). "I spent nine years looking for a doctor": Exploring access to health care among immigrants in Mississauga, Ontario, Canada. *Social Science & Medicine*, 66(6), 1271–1283.

Beiser, M. (2009). Resettling refugees and safeguarding their mental health: Lessons learned from the Canadian refugee resettlement project. *Transcultural Psychiatry*, 46(4), 539–583.

Benedict, R. (2013). Race: What it is not. In L. Back & J. Solomos (Eds.), *Theories of race and racism* (2nd ed., pp. 113–118). New York: NY: Routledge.

Blad, C., & Couton, P. (2009). The rise of an intercultural nation: Immigration, diversity and nationhood in Quebec. *Journal of Ethnic and Migration Studies*, 35(4), 645–667.

Blythe, J., Baumann, A., Rheaume, A., & McIntosh, K. (2009). Nurse migration to Canada: Pathways and pitfalls of workforce integration. *Official Journal of the Transcultural Nursing Society*, 20(2), 202–210.

Browne, A. J., Varcoe, C., Smye, V., Reimer-Kirkham, S., Lynam, M. J., & Wong, S. (2009). Cultural safety and the challenges of translating critically oriented knowledge in practice. *Nursing Philosophy: An International Journal for Healthcare Professionals*, 10(3), 167–179.

Canadian Institute for Health Information. (2012). *Regulated nurses: Canadian trends, 2007 to 2011*. Ottawa, ON: Author.

Canadian Multiculturalism Act, Policy U.S.C. c. 24 (4th Supp.) (1988).

Canadian Nurses Association. (2008). *Code of ethics for registered nurses* (2008 centennial edition). Ottawa, ON: Author.

Canadian Nurses Association. (2011). *Position statement: Interprofessional collaboration*. Retrieved from http://www2.cna-aiic.ca/CNA/documents/pdf/publications/PS117_Interprofessional_Collaboration_2011_e.pdf

Caxaj, C. S., & Berman, H. (2010). Belonging among newcomer youths: Intersecting experiences of inclusion and exclusion. *Advances in Nursing Science*, 33(4), E17–E30.

Citizenship and Immigration Canada. (2012a). *Annual report to parliament on immigration 2012* (No. Ci1-2011E-PDF). Ottawa, ON: Distribution Services Citizenship and Immigration Canada.

Citizenship and Immigration Canada. (2012b). *Canada facts and figures 2011. Immigration overview: Permanent and temporary residents*. Ottawa, ON: Author. Retrieved from http://www.cic.gc.ca/english/pdf/research-stats/facts2011.pdf

Citizenship and Immigration Canada. (2012c). *Health care in Canada*. Retrieved from http://www.cic.gc.ca/english/newcomers/after-health.asp

Citizenship and Immigration Canada. (2012d). *Reasons for inadmissibility*. Retrieved from http://www.cic.gc.ca/english/information/inadmissibility/who.asp

Cohen, B. E., & Gregory, D. (2009). Community health clinical education in Canada: Part 2—Developing competencies to address social justice, equity, and the social determinants of health. *International Journal of Nursing Education Scholarship*, 6. doi:10.2202/1548-923X.1638

Creatore, M. I., Moineddin, R., Booth, G., Manuel, D. H., DesMeules, M., McDermott, S., & Glazier, R. H. (2010). Age- and sex-related prevalence of diabetes mellitus among immigrants to Ontario, Canada. *Canadian Medical Association Journal*, 182(8), 781–789.

Dean, J. A., & Wilson, K. (2009). 'Education? it is irrelevant to my job now. It makes me very depressed . . .': Exploring the health impacts of under/unemployment among highly skilled recent immigrants in Canada. *Ethnicity & Health*, 14(2), 185–204.

Doane, G. H., & Varcoe, C. (2007). Relational practice and nursing obligations. *Advances in Nursing Science*, 30(3), 192–205.

Edmunds, K., Berman, H., Basok, T., Ford-Gilboe, M., & Forchuk, C. (2011). The health of women temporary agricultural workers in Canada: A critical review of the literature. *The Canadian Journal of Nursing Research = Revue Canadienne De Recherche En Sciences Infirmieres*, 43(4), 68–91.

Fuller-Thomson, E., Noack, A. M., & George, U. (2011). Health decline among recent immigrants to Canada: Findings from a nationally-representative longitudinal survey. *Canadian Journal of Public Health*, 102(4), 273–280.

Gravel, S., Vissandjee, B., Lippel, K., Brodeur, J-M., Patry, L., & Champagne, F. (2010). Ethics and the compensation of immigrant workers for work-related injuries and illnesses. *Journal of Immigrant and Minority Health*, 12, 707–714. doi:10.1007/s10903-008-9208-5.

Guruge, S., Hunter, J., Barker, K., McNally, M. J., & Magalhaes, L. (2010). Immigrant women's experiences of receiving care in a mobile health clinic. *Journal of Advanced Nursing*, 66(2), 350–359.

Gushulak, B. (2007). Healthier on arrival? Further insight into the "healthy immigrant effect." *Canadian Medical Association Journal*, *176*(10), 1439–1440.

Health Canada. (2010). Migration health: Embracing a determinants of health approach. *Health Policy Research Bulletin*, (17), 1–52.

International Organization for Migration. (2010). *World Migration Report 2010: The future of migration: Building for capacities for change* (No. 2013). Geneva, Switzerland: Author.

Isaacs, S. (2010). Transnational cultural ecologies: Evolving challenges for nurses in Canada. *Journal of Transcultural Nursing*, *21*(1), 15–22.

Khadilkar, A., & Chen, Y. (2013). Rate of cervical cancer screening associated with immigration status and number of years since immigration in Ontario, Canada. *Journal of Immigrant and Minority Health/Center for Minority Public Health*, *15*(2), 244–248.

Labonte, R., Mohindra, K., & Schrecker, T. (2011). The growing impact of globalization for health and public health practice. *Annual Review of Public Health*, *32*, 263–283.

Latif, E. (2010). Recent immigrants and the use of cervical cancer screening test in Canada. *Journal of Immigrant and Minority Health*, *12*(1), 1–17.

Maximova, K., & Krahn, H. (2010). Health status of refugees settled in Alberta: Changes since arrival. *Canadian Journal of Public Health. Revue Canadienne De Sante Publique*, *101*(4), 322–326.

McDonald, J. T., & Kennedy, S. (2007). Cervical cancer screening by immigrant and minority women in Canada. *Journal of Immigrant and Minority Health/Center for Minority Public Health*, *9*(4), 323–334.

Mill, J., Astle, B. J., Ogilvie, L., & Gastaldo, D. (2010). Linking global citizenship, undergraduate nursing education, and professional nursing: Curricular innovation in the 21st century. *Advances in Nursing Science*, *33*(3), E1–E11.

Newbold, B. (2009). The short-term health of Canada's new immigrant arrivals: Evidence from LSIC. *Ethnicity & Health*, *14*(3), 315–336.

Newton, S., Pillay, J., & Higginbottom, G. (2012). The migration and transitioning experiences of internationally educated nurses: A global perspective. *Journal of Nursing Management*, *20*(4), 534–550.

Ng, E., Pottie, K., & Spitzer, D. (2011). *Official language proficiency and self-reported health among immigrants to Canada* (No. 82-003-X). Ottawa, ON: Statistics Canada.

Ohinmaa, A., Jacobs, P., Simpson, S., & Johnson, J. A. (2004). The projection of prevalence and cost of diabetes in Canada: 2000 to 2016. *Canadian Journal of Diabetes*, *28*, 116–123.

Preibisch, K., & Hennebry, J. (2011). Temporary migration, chronic effects: The health of international migrant workers in Canada. *Canadian Medical Association Journal*, *183*(9), 1033–1038.

Public Health Agency of Canada. (2011). *What determines health?* Retrieved from http://www.phac-aspc.gc.ca/ph-sp/determinants/#determinants

Public Health Agency of Canada. (2013). *Cervical cancer.* Retrieved from http://www.phac-aspc.gc.ca/cd-mc/cancer/cervical_cancer-cancer_du_col_uterus-eng.php

Racher, F. E., & Annis, R. C. (2012). Honouring culture and diversity in community practice. In A. R. Vollman, E. T. Anderson, & J. McFarlane (Eds.), *Canadian community as partner: Theory & multidisciplinary practice* (3rd ed., pp. 154–176). Philadelphia, PA: Lippincott Williams & Wilkins.

Reitmanova, S., & Gustafson, D. L. (2008). "They can't understand it": Maternity health and care needs of immigrant Muslim women in St. John's, Newfoundland. *Maternal and Child Health Journal*, *12*(1), 101–111.

Reitmanova, S., & Gustafson, D. L. (2009). Mental health needs of visible minority immigrants in a small urban center: Recommendations for policy makers and service providers. *Journal of Immigrant and Minority Health*, *11*(1), 46–56.

Roth, M. A., & Kobayashi, K. M. (2008). The use of complementary and alternative medicine among Chinese Canadians: Results from a national survey. *Journal of Immigrant and Minority Health/Center for Minority Public Health*, *10*(6), 517–528.

Salehi, R. (2010). Intersection of health, immigration, and youth: A systematic literature review. *Journal of Immigrant and Minority Health*, *12*(5), 788–797.

Samuels-Dennis, J. A., York, M., & Barrett, D. (2012). The transformational influences of Jamaican nurses on the Canadian health care system. In A. Davis & C. E. James (Eds.), *Jamaica in the Canadian experience: A multiculturalizing presence*. Toronto, ON: Fernwood Publishing.

Simich, L., Maiter, S., & Ochocka, J. (2009). From social liminality to cultural negotiation: Transformative processes in immigrant mental wellbeing. *Anthropology & Medicine*, *16*(3), 253–266.

Sochan, A., & Singh, M. D. (2007). Acculturation and socialization: Voices of internationally educated nurses in Ontario. *International Nursing Review*, *54*(2), 130–136.

Srivastava, R. (Ed.). (2007). *The health care professional's guide to clinical cultural competence*. Toronto, ON: Mosby Elsevier Health Sciences.

Statistics Canada. (2010). *Projections of the diversity of the Canadian population: 2006-2013* (No. 91-551-X). Ottawa, ON: Author.

Statistics Canada. (2012a). *Canada year book 2012: Ethnic diversity and immigration* (No. 91-551-X). Ottawa, ON: Author.

Statistics Canada. (2012b). *Immigrant languages in Canada* (Government No. 98-314-X2011003). Ottawa, ON: Author.

Statistics Canada. (2013). *Immigration and ethnocultural diversity in Canada: National household survey 2011* (Government No. 99-010-X2011001). Ottawa, ON: Author.

Taylor, V., Teh, C., Lam, W., Acorda, E., Li, L., Coronado, G., . . . Hislop, G. (2009). Evaluation of a hepatitis B educational ESL curriculum for Chinese immigrants. *Canadian Journal of Public Health*, *100*(6), 463–466.

World Health Organization. (1998). *Health promotion glossary* (No. WHO/HPR/HEP/98.1). Geneva, Switzerland: Author.

World Health Organization. (2013). *Social determinants of health.* Retrieved from http://www.who.int/social_determinants/en/

Yang, J. S. (2010). Contextualizing immigrant access to health resources. *Journal of Immigrant and Minority Health*, *12*(3), 340–353.

chapter

38

Vulnerable Populations and Nursing: Vulnerability as a Health Equity Concern

BERNADETTE M. PAULY AND COLLEEN VARCOE

$\mathcal{S}$asha is a third-year nursing student. She is doing her clinical placement at a community agency where most clients are homeless or living in unstable housing situations. Many of the people at the agency have unmet health-care needs for wound care, foot problems, chronic respiratory problems, dental care, and infectious diseases. She wonders what could be done to improve access to health care as many of the people she has met do not have a doctor or primary source of health care. As she learns more about people's lives, she begins to question the source of these health-care problems and the role that housing, food, and income play in contributing to the poor health status of the people who come to the agency. She also reflects on the nursing role in addressing both unmet health needs and working to change the conditions that are contributing to the poor health of the individuals, families, and communities affected.

CHAPTER OBJECTIVES

By the end of this chapter, you will be able to:

1. Define vulnerability.
2. Identify the factors that contribute to vulnerability and poor health.
3. Discuss vulnerability in relation to health inequities.
4. Critically assess factors that produce vulnerability for particular populations.
5. Gain an understanding of the social processes that are pathways to poor health.
6. Discuss the difference between inequities in access to health care and inequities in health outcomes.
7. Describe the role of nurses in facilitating access to health care and addressing health inequities for vulnerable populations in various settings.
8. Discuss the political advocacy role of nurses in reducing vulnerability to poor health and improving the health of vulnerable populations.

KEY TERMS

Access to Health Care Refers to the availability and appropriateness of health-care services to meet the needs of those seeking such services.

At Risk A term truncated from attempts to identify specific risks; for example, *at risk of poverty* or *at risk of infection*. This truncated form is often used without designating the particular risks, with the consequence that the risk is implied to reside within the group being designated. For example, at risk youth are implied as embodying the risk, rather than specifying that youth are at risk of homelessness, violence, or poverty.

Determinants of Inequities Those social processes such as stigmatization and discrimination that impact access to the social determinants of health. Social processes such as stigmatization and discrimination impact people differentially depending on their social position.

Disadvantaged Populations Refers to subgroups in the population defined on the basis of shared characteristics associated with increased risk for poor health outcomes; for example, poor health associated with poverty, homelessness, or substance use.

Health Disparities In some countries, such as the United Kingdom, a term used interchangeably with *health inequities*; in the United States, a term generally used to refer to differences in health between people of different ethnic backgrounds, highlighting the impact of racism on health.

Health Equity Refers to fair conditions in society that allow each person to reach his or her potential for health.

Health Inequalities Differences in health among groups in the population that may be either positive or negative.

Health Inequities Those differences in health that are deemed unfair or unjust because they are a product of social processes that can potentially be changed. Health inequities can be distinguished from health inequalities in that health inequities are differences that are judged to be unfair.

Intersectionality Perspective Approach focusing on the multiple social circumstances that shape the lives of individuals and thereby their chances to be healthy.

(continued on page 1028)

Marginalization   Process in which people who are relatively different from the dominant norm are moved to the periphery of society because of their identities, associations, experiences, or environments.

Primary Health Care   The delivery of health care at the most local level of a country's health system. It is essential health care made accessible at an affordable cost with methods that are practical, scientifically sound and socially acceptable.

Social Determinants of Health   The conditions in society that impact the health of the population. This includes factors such as housing, income, social support, employment, education, and access to health care.

Social Exclusion   "Social exclusion is an expression of unequal relations or power among groups in society, which then determine unequal access to economic, social, political and cultural resources" (Galabuzi, 2009). Social exclusion encompasses the structures and processes that shape inequality and access to resources that determine both participation in society and shape health outcomes. Social exclusion may be based on many intersecting forms of discrimination along the lines of class, gender, sexual orientation ability, age, religion, and ethnicity (Benoit & Shumka, 2009).

Social Gradient   Term for the hierarchy that differences in health status follow. The lower one is on the socioeconomic gradient, the poorer the health. This means that health varies on a continuum from better to worse, dependent on income and resources.

Social Justice   A societal situation in which power and decision-making are equally shared and distributed so that all have equal chances in life.

Vulnerability   Being in need, susceptible to injury, and at higher risk of harm than the rest of the population.

Vulnerable Populations   In Canada, groups identified as vulnerable to health inequities as a result of social exclusion include such groups as women, the poor, Aboriginal people, immigrants, elderly people, children living in disadvantaged circumstances, and people experiencing disabilities. *Disadvantaged* and *vulnerable populations* are sometimes used interchangeably.

What Does Vulnerability Mean?

Vulnerability suggests that individuals or groups are in need, at risk of or susceptible to harm because of their exposure to particular social conditions puts them at greater risk of harm than others in the population (Frohlich & Potvin, 2008; Mechanic & Tanner, 2007). The risk of poor health is shaped by living conditions, and the risk of poor health is different for individuals and groups of people at various times in their life and in relation to their social position. **At risk** is a term truncated from attempts to identify specific risks; for example, *at risk of poverty* or *at risk of infection*. This truncated form is often used without designating the particular risks, with the consequence that the risk is implied to reside within the group being designated. For example, at risk youth are implied as embodying the risk, rather than specifying that youth are at risk of homelessness, violence, or poverty. For example, if you are working and studying very hard to become a registered nurse, you may be staying up late to study especially if you have to work to support yourself through school or have responsibilities for the care of others. Lack of sleep, irregular meals, lack of exercise, and stress may make you vulnerable to becoming ill. Vulnerability means that there is a potential for harm to occur. People may become ill after experiencing a period of stress. As well, vulnerability to poor health may accumulate over one's lifetime. For example, lack of adequate nutrition and experiencing abuse in childhood can have cumulative effects and negatively affect one's health in adulthood and access to resources for health such as education and employment (Raphael, 2009a).

Conditions That Shape Vulnerability

Understanding the conditions that shape vulnerability to poor health are important to the care that nurses provide in both acute care and community health settings. In acute care, all patients for whom you provide nursing care can be considered vulnerable. They are vulnerable because they are ill, undergoing treatment or surgery, and may be unable to fully care for themselves. As well, being in hospital increases vulnerability because patients are in unfamiliar situations and away from their families and friends. Some people may be more vulnerable in hospital because they have multiple health problems, preexisting disabilities, or underlying chronic illnesses that may exacerbate the impact of hospitalization on health and/or their ability to recover. Age, gender, and ethnicity play an important role in shaping vulnerability when in hospital. For example, people who are elderly and very ill with compromised immunity may be susceptible to hospital-acquired infections. People who are racialized (identified as "different" or "other" by race) are disadvantaged by implicit and explicit bias on the part of health-care providers and by structural biases in policies and infrastructure (Browne et al., 2011; Green et al., 2007; Smedley, 2012).

In community and public health settings, nurses are concerned with overall population health and with vulnerability to poor health associated with living conditions, such as poverty, unsafe and inadequate housing, and inadequate food. Stigma, previous trauma, violence, or abuse are also part of the conditions that contribute to vulnerability to poor health and are of concern in public health. An important focus of public health nursing work is reducing vulnerability to poor health early in life to reduce or ameliorate the negative cumulative effects of social conditions and processes that impact families' and children's opportunities for health and access to health-care resources that impact future health outcomes.

Individual Vulnerability or Social Conditions?

Vulnerability can be understood as both an individual problem and/or a product of social conditions. Viewing vulnerability only as a problem of individuals overlooks the conditions that create vulnerability to illness and poor health. For example, you may be studying late because you did not prioritize your homework or you had difficulty understanding the assignment and were nervous about asking for help. These are individual explanations. What if you had a disabled family member who required care; a family member who became ill during the exam period; what if you needed to work full-time in order to support your children while attending school; or could not afford a computer and can only study after your roommate is finished doing her homework? Maybe the assignments and exams were scheduled too closely together or there were simply too many course requirements. These possibilities suggest that conditions outside of your control are shaping your ability to study. In a society that highly values individual success and achievement, there is a tendency to focus on individual explanations rather than structural or systemic understandings that produce vulnerability to poor health. To take our example a bit further, student health is rarely considered a systemic or structural problem, except in relation to some specific health concerns such as sexual assault, substance use, suicide, or sexually transmitted infections. Even those problems are often understood only as a consequence of individual choices, not as products of systemic circumstances, including student debt, student poverty, stress related to socially enforced performance expectations, gender norms, and so on.

Individual- and Disease-Focused Vulnerability

Vulnerability in nursing and health care has often been seen through the lens of individual vulnerability to particular social conditions or diseases. According to Raphael, "an individual perspective limits analysis of health risks to individual biomedical and behavioural risk factors for disease" (Raphael, 2009c, p. 21). In an individual-focused approach to vulnerability, health-care activities primarily focus on screening for diseases such as blood pressure or cholesterol screening, treatment for diagnosed disease conditions, and the modification of individual lifestyle factors such as physical activity, diet, and stress management (Raphael, 2009c). Such approaches do not account for the distal factors that impact health behaviours such as poverty, housing, and stigma (Link & Phelan, 1995; Phelan, Link, & Tehranifar, 2010). As a result, lifestyle approaches have not typically worked with low-income groups because of unaddressed factors such as precarious employment or inability to get employment, long work hours, and lack of affordable transportation, all of which impede participation in health education or a healthier lifestyle. Further, lifestyle approaches often focus on educational strategies and overlook underlying determinants of health. For example, education regarding the importance of making nutritious food choices is not useful if people cannot afford nutritious food.

An individual approach to vulnerability contributes to viewing poor health as a problem or failing of the person. However, such individualistic thinking is often applied unevenly, with certain groups of individuals more likely to be blamed for poor health. For example, those who are poor or using drugs are often seen to be at fault for their health problems, whereas those with wealth are less likely to be blamed for the obesity or chronic stress associated with overwork. Individualizing poor health reflects a neoliberal (individualistic) view of the world in which people are seen as responsible for the choices they make in spite of the social conditions in which they live or their access to resources. Individuals are seen as responsible for making poor choices, and the route to achieving good health is to make better or different choices, particularly lifestyle choices. This is sometimes referred to a cultural behavioural explanation of factors that mediate health (Raphael, 2009a). A cultural behavioural explanation often confuses culture as a collective phenomenon with culture as a personal characteristic. Consequently, groups of people, sometimes designated by ethnicity, are attributed certain characteristics (e.g., laziness, volatility, competitiveness) that are seen to influence health. Understood in this way, cultural behaviourist explanations are aligned with individualist explanations (see Chapter 13).

An individual approach tends to focus on individuals as the source of vulnerability rather than the living conditions that contribute to poor health or the social political and economic conditions that shape health inequities (those differences in health that are unfair or unjust and amenable to change; Dahlgren & Whitehead, 2006). Through the media, we are bombarded by messages to exercise more, eat more fruits and vegetables, stop smoking, and drink in moderation. However, what if we do not have access to fresh fruits and vegetables because we live in a remote community and the growing season is short? What if local water rights are such that we can no longer grow our own vegetables? What if there is poor urban transit and unable to afford a car, we are restricted to purchasing food at a high priced poorly stocked neighbourhood store? What if we do not feel safe to go out walking or running in our neighbourhoods? What if we have a chronic condition that limits physical activity? What if alcohol and tobacco are readily available, actively marketed, and routinely part of the social pressure to conform?

Social Determinants

Living conditions or the social and material circumstances of a person's life have been found to have a greater impact on health than individual choices and lifestyle factors (Raphael, 2009c). There are several explanations that provide an understanding of how social and material conditions impact health through various processes. Materialist, neomaterialist, life course, and psychosocial explanations can help us to understand the pathways through which the **social determinants of health** operate (Raphael, 2009a, 2009c).

Materialist explanations focus on how the social determinants of health, such as housing, employment, income, social support, education, and so on, influence health (Raphael, 2009c). A safe secure home, food security, employment, and income to meet basic needs and access to education are needed to adopt healthy behaviours and better health (Jones, 2008). In addition, having control over one's life and having a safe and supportive network of friends and family are part of the essential foundations for good health (World Health Organization, Commission on the Social Determinants of

Health, 2008). Lack of these key determinants increases vulnerability to poor health. Where we work and live are important to our health (World Health Organization, Commission on the Social Determinants of Health, 2008). Our social circumstances and environments shape the choices we make. People in deprived living circumstances experience increased illness and shorter life expectancies than others in the population, even in a country as wealthy as Canada. If these differences are unfair, potentially avoidable, and we can do something about them, then they are considered health inequities (Whitehead & Dahlgren, 2006). A neo-materialist approach focuses on the dynamics that result in an unequal distribution of resources that impact living and working conditions. For example, the introduction of private, for-profit health care means that people with sufficient financial resources are able to access what in some cases may be necessary health care. Lack of affordable housing in Canada has contributed to homelessness and early death for people impacted by homelessness and inadequate housing (Hwang, Wilkins, Tjepkema, O'Campo, & Dunn, 2009). A life course approach highlights the cumulative impact of social and economic conditions on health throughout the lifespan. For example, there is an increased rate of diabetes among Aboriginal populations because of changes in traditional diets that have followed expropriation of land and destruction of sea- and land-based food sources in combination with racism and poverty that affect health over the life course (Frohlich, Ross, & Richmond, 2006; Veenstra, 2009).

Psychosocial explanations focus on the stress associated with uneven distribution of resources in society (Raphael, 2009c). In particular, the social comparison model suggests that one's health is determined by social position and that one's perceptions and the stress associated with different social positioning is responsible for health differences (Raphael, 2009c; Wilkinson & Pickett, 2010). The social comparison model suggests that in societies in which there are significant inequities, stress is high because individuals compare themselves to others (Raphael, 2009c). Repeatedly, researchers have found that both health and health behaviours such as smoking, physical activity, diet, and alcohol use vary by socioeconomic status (Dunn, 2010). It is not only material deprivation that creates vulnerability to poor health but also the stress associated with having very limited resources in a society where there are large differences between rich and poor (Wilkinson & Pickett, 2010). Stress acts directly, through the development of unhealthy behaviours, as well as indirectly, where unhealthy behaviours may be ways to cope with stress. Not surprisingly, unhealthy behaviours are more likely among those who are poor and those subjected to chronic and institutionalized racism. These dynamics may be partially a consequence of a person's early life experiences, especially exposure to poverty, and increased stress. A clear example of this is the high levels of hypertension among African Americans that have been attributed to living under conditions of chronic racism and **social exclusion** (Krieger, 2005, 2009).

Health Inequities

Individualist explanations focus on individual choices and behaviours to explain poor health. Culturalist explanations similarly focus on individuals, often using individual's cultural affiliations as explanations for poor health. Materialist, neo-materialist, life course, and psychosocial explanations try to illuminate the pathways to poorer health by focusing on how social determinants of health impact health status. These explanations focus on the fundamental causes of diseases and how power dynamics in the distribution of societal resources shape constraints, opportunities, and access to resources necessary for health (Frohlich et al., 2006; Link & Phelan, 1995). It is the fundamental causes or social conditions that create "unequal chances in life" (Shaw, Dorling, Gordon, & Davey Smith, 1999). For example, HIV has been found to proliferate in risk environments such as impoverished neighbourhoods, where there is less information and fewer resources to reduce associated risks associated, with differential impacts along the lines of gender and ethnicity (Rhodes, 2002; Rhodes, Singer, Bourgois, Friedman, & Strathdee, 2005; Zierler & Krieger 1997). Attention to the role of power in the distribution of economic, social, and cultural resources and opportunities is fundamental to addressing the conditions in which vulnerability to poor health is created (Frohlich et al., 2006).

Health inequities are those differences in health that are unfair or unjust and are created by social conditions that are potentially remedial (Dahlgren and Whitehead, 2006). This unfairness and potential for remediation distinguishes **health equity** from **health inequalities**, which are differences in health that may be positive or negative. The term **health disparities** is sometimes used interchangeably with health inequities. However, health disparities usually refers to differences in health status among ethnic groups and as a consequence of racism. The existence of health inequities provides considerable evidence of vulnerability to social conditions in both developed and developing countries. As a consequence of historical abuses of power through colonial processes, health equities are particularly profound among indigenous populations throughout the world (Nettleton, Napolitano, & Stephens, 2007; Stephens, Nettleton, Porter, Willis, & Clark, 2005). For example, in Canada, the health of Aboriginal people, including First Nations, Inuit and Métis people, has been identified as poorer than that of the general population (Frohlich et al., 2006; Kendall, 2009; MacMillan et al., 2008; Waldram, Herring, & Young, 2006; Willows, Veugelers, Raine, & Kuhle, 2009), and this poor health is directly tied to racist treatment by the state and individuals (Frohlich et al., 2006; Veenstra, 2009).

Who Is Vulnerable to Poor Health?

One approach to understanding poor health has been to focus on identifying individuals or groups who are at greater risk for poor health because the conditions in which they live increases their exposure to risks for poor health. Such groups are often described as vulnerable, marginalized, or **disadvantaged populations**. **Vulnerable populations** may be understood as subpopulations that are likely to have poorer health than the general population because of the conditions in which they live (Frohlich & Potvin, 2008).

Limitations of Identification of Vulnerable Groups

Identification of vulnerable groups has significant limitations that are important to consider in the provision of nursing care. First, people may or may not identify with a certain group; therefore, assuming someone is vulnerable because he or she appear to be a member of a particular group can be quite wrong. For example, although some elderly persons may be more vulnerable than the general population, this varies greatly. There is a range of experiences within any group. For example, although low income is an overall feature on average for many Aboriginal groups, many other Aboriginal individuals and groups have higher incomes and would not see themselves as poor. Second, identification of certain people as vulnerable may lead to negative stereotyping and false classifications of groups. Third, the identification of vulnerable groups is often associated with disease-specific conditions such as those at risk of HIV and fails to recognize the determinants of vulnerability such as poverty, housing, and food insecurity. Thus, although some groups can be misidentified as vulnerable, other vulnerable groups may not identified. Lastly, when health-care providers consider certain individuals to belong to a vulnerable group solely on the basis of assumed group membership, such assumptions can contribute to stereotyping and inaccuracies in assessment and labeling (Corley & Goren, 1998). For example, people who are homeless are often assumed, incorrectly, to abuse drugs or alcohol and that substance use is the root of the problem rather than lack of housing and income.

Marginalization can be understood as a process in which people who are relatively different from the dominant norm are moved to the periphery of society because of their identities, associations, experiences, or environments (Hall, 1999; Hall, Stevens, & Meleis, 1994). According to Hall, marginalization is "seen as a socio-political process, producing both vulnerabilities (risks) and strengths (resilience)" (Hall, 1999, p. 89). Numerous authors have identified that those experiencing marginalization are most often differentiated from the rest of the population on the basis of income, ability, ethnicity, religion, class, and gender (Aday, 1993; Anderson, 2000; Anderson & Reimer Kirkham, 1998; Hall, 1999; Hall et al., 1994; Sherwin, 1992). Based on their research, Hall (1999) and Hall et al. (1994) propose that marginalization is associated with increased vulnerability and poorer health outcomes than the general population. The term *disadvantaged populations* suggests that certain groups have fewer opportunities than others in the population to access resources necessary for good health. Relationships of power prevent access to a fair share of social, cultural, or economic resources. For example, the health of Aboriginal people in Canada has been profoundly impacted by colonial laws and practices such as the 1870s Indian Act that created a social hierarchy and shaped access to resources such as education, employment, social and health-care facilities, and control and access to lands that provided subsistence (Frohlich et al., 2006).

Differences in health status follow a **social gradient** or hierarchy that affects all people (Marmot, 2003; World Health Organization [WHO], 2003). The lower one is on the socioeconomic gradient, the poorer the health. Marmot, a leading authority on health inequalities, notes that "wherever we are in the social hierarchy, our health is likely to be better than those below us and worse than those above us. The socially excluded are at the end of the health spectrum, it is the status syndrome that is the challenge" (Marmot, 2004, p. 4). As socioeconomic wealth increases, so does health such that people at each higher income level have better health than those below them. It is not just the absolute gap between the rich and the poor but differences across the socioeconomic gradient that are of concern.

In other words, those with lower incomes and education, inadequate housing, poor working conditions, detrimental health behaviours, limited access to health care, and who lack early childhood support and/or social supports are more likely to develop poorer physical and mental health outcomes than those living in better circumstances (Jones, 2008, p. 2). It is the gap between different groups along a continuum that highlights the way that health outcomes change across different groups rather than absolute differences in health between the highest and lowest income groups. As Coburn (2006) argues, the greater the gap between high and low incomes in a country, the poorer is the overall health of the population.

Looking Upstream and Working Downstream

It is essential for nurses to understand the sources of vulnerability to poor health, particularly the sources that arise as result of the conditions in which people live, especially for those who experience poor health in society. The social determinants focus on those factors that all of us need for health and well-being, whereas the **determinants of inequities** are those social processes that operate in the production of unfair or injustice differences in health (Graham, 2004). Although we can look at populations who are vulnerable and the challenges to health they experience as part of nursing care, it is crucial to look at the root causes of vulnerability (social determinants and determinants of inequities) that produce poor health.

Patricia Butterfield urges nurses to look "upstream" to the social, political, and economic factors that shape the health of society (Butterfield, 1990). Nurses need to focus on the upstream factors that contribute to vulnerability to poor health in order to (1) participate in health care and society in ways that will lessen inequities, (2) understand how we can provide care within the context of their lives, and (3) provide care that takes inequities and vulnerabilities of individuals and groups into account. Many nurses work downstream, meaning that they are addressing existing health issues rather than prevention of illness, injury or disease, and promotion of health. Working downstream in the turbulent waters of health-care delivery can limit our ability to look upstream to social influences or to see social action as part of our everyday work. However, we need to both respond to the consequences and realities of health inequities that manifest in poor health and disease and take action on the social factors that create vulnerability to poor health. It is not adequate to simply respond to health problems without looking upstream to address the root causes that exacerbate vulnerabilities and inequities and focus on prevention of ill health and promotion of health. This approach is particularly relevant because it helps nurses to resist a dominant tendency to "blame the victim" that is deeply embedded in societal structures and supported by a belief that poor health is solely a matter of personal responsibility. Looking upstream helps us recognize and address the broader determinants of poor health through public health activities of disease, illness and injury prevention, and health promotion.

Intersecting Factors and Poor Health

Multiple factors intersect to produce poorer health for some individuals and groups than for others. An intersectional approach describes the multiple social circumstances that shape the lives of individuals and thereby their chances to be healthy. "An intersectional approach recognizes the unique experience of the individual based on the intersection of all relevant grounds—gender, colour, ethnicity, class, immigrant status, and disability. This argument acknowledges that disadvantage arises from the way society treats particular individuals, rather than from any characteristic inherent in those individuals" (Reynoso, 2004, p. 63).

Using an intersectional approach can help nurses understand that multiple circumstances generate multiple vulnerabilities, possibilities of susceptibility, and risk to poor health. For example, a person who lives in poverty and belongs to a socially marginalized or stigmatized group is made more vulnerable by the intersections of those circumstances (e.g., poverty, gender, ethnicity). The combination of different oppressive conditions produces vulnerability to health that is cumulative and greater than one form of oppression alone (Eaton, 1994).

What Living Conditions Contribute to Vulnerability?

The social determinants of health and the conditions in which people live have a greater impact on life expectancy and the development of disease-related conditions such as cardiovascular problems, diabetes, respiratory disease, and cancer than biomedical or behaviour risk factors or access to health care (Raphael, 2009a). The social determinants of health have

been variously defined and often include a broad range of factors such as housing, income, education, employment and working conditions, physical environment, social support/inclusion as well as gender, age, and ethnicity considerations (Raphael, 2009b). Lack of access to resources to meet basic needs such as income, housing, food, and social support produces a high level of vulnerability. Although it is important to understand that there are many factors that impact vulnerability and that vulnerability to poor health increases for everyone as living conditions decline, our emphasis here is on situations of severe material and social deprivation that create high levels of vulnerability and health inequities among certain groups of people for whom nurses care.

Poverty

Income is a primary social determinant of vulnerability and health inequities (Wilkinson & Pickett, 2006). To date, a strong link has been found between vulnerability to poor health and socioeconomic factors that encompass issues related to income and poverty. In an analysis of 155 research papers, Wilkinson and Pickett found that 70% of the studies supported the finding that the greater disparities in income were accompanied by poorer health of the population. However, it is not always clear to what degree poverty perpetuates or follows poor health. As suggested earlier in this chapter, there are number of ways that health inequities associated with income come to be. Material deprivation entails living in poverty, which does not allow one to meet basic needs such as food, housing, and other essentials of daily living. Lack of income can impact resources needed to take up healthy behaviours. In societies where there are greater income differentials, people who are poor live and work in more stressful conditions. Further possibilities are that when there is greater income inequality, there is greater emphasis on lower taxes and reducing government spending at the expense of investment in health and social services to address poverty and more psychological stress related to social comparisons (Frohlich et al., 2006; Wilkinson & Pickett, 2010).

Poverty in Canada

In Canada, there is evidence that being lower on the social hierarchy is associated with poorer health, especially among those living in rural settings, low income seniors, street youth, people who are homeless, and lone-parent families (Butler-Jones, 2008). Aboriginal people and newcomers to Canada are disproportionately affected by poverty. Canada has a high rate of child poverty, which correlates to the large number of children living in families that have little access to income, most of which are single-parent families headed by women. Premature death and increased incidence of chronic diseases and ill health are a reality for many low-income Canadians today (Hwang et al., 2009).

Poverty in Canada has worsened in recent decades by the erosion of social safety nets through changes to eligibility for social assistance, employment and disability insurance, and low and declining rates of social assistance. Inadequate minimum wages make it difficult to impossible for people to sustain themselves (Eggleton & Segal, 2009). In spite of increases in the cost of living, social assistance rates across Canada have not risen in more than a decade (Eggleton & Keon, 2008; Eggleton & Segal, 2009). Likewise, minimum wages across the country are often lower than the cost of living, making adequate food and housing unattainable. For example, social assistance rates in British Columbia dropped the fastest in the country with changes to welfare policies effectively moving people into homelessness as well as into housing and food insecurity (Wallace, Klein, & Reitsma-Street, 2006). Throughout Canada, the number of people who are homeless has been growing, and in some cities, such as Vancouver, homelessness has doubled since 2002 with 22% increases in homelessness between 2005 and 2008 (Goldberg & Graves, 2005; Social Planning and Research Council of British Columbia et al., 2008). Similar trends have been reported in other Canadian cities including Calgary, Edmonton, Halifax, Toronto, and Ottawa. From an **intersectionality perspective**, these policy changes will impact differently those affected so the experience and nature of homelessness varies for women and men, youth, families, Aboriginal peoples, veterans, and those who have been incarcerated.

Policy and Poverty Trends

Some have observed that these trends in poverty, housing, and food insecurity are the result of policies that have systematically eroded our social safety net and the investment into social programs such as low-cost affordable housing (Shapcott, 2009). Thus, policy responses to these problems must necessarily focus on changing the structural determinants of inequities such as adequate income for living and affordable housing to counter this trend of deepening poverty. For example, the Canadian Senate recommended the introduction of guaranteed annual incomes for all (Eggleton & Segal, 2009). Guaranteed annual incomes have been found to result in lower use of health-care services and to positively impact health and wellbeing (Canadian Institutes of Health Research, 2009). These are important areas of policy work to reduce vulnerability to poor health. Nurses must understand the dynamics between poverty, policy, and health not only to better understand those for whom they provide care but also to counter victim blaming that suggests that individuals are responsible for their own poverty and to support antipoverty efforts.

Physical and Built Environment

Those most vulnerable to poor health often live in areas where poverty is concentrated. The neighbourhoods in which we live impact our opportunities for employment, social networks, and personal health behaviours (Jones, 2008). Access to nutritious food is often limited in low-income areas because of lack of grocery stores and availability of nutritious food items such as fruits and vegetables; these areas are known as food deserts. In some neighbourhoods,

there is a preponderance of convenience stores and fast-food outlets that provide poor-quality foods often at a higher cost; even when the cost of purchasing a fast-food meal is low, the long-term costs to the consumer are high. Opportunities for social interaction may be limited by the very nature of neighbourhoods such as a lack of parks and green spaces that encourage social and environmental interaction.

Housing

Housing is the nexus through which the other determinants of health operate (Dunn, Hayes, Hulchanski, Hwang, & Potvin, 2006). The ability to interact with others, prepare food, have time to oneself, rest, and sleep are all impacted by the availability of adequate housing. Housing affordability is the most common factor affecting housing insecurity (Canada Mortgage and Housing Corporation [CMHC], 2009). Housing insecurity is experienced when individuals and families are required to spend more than 30% of their income on rent. Many low-income people face housing insecurity because safe and affordable housing is simply unavailable. Housing is a particular problem in urban centres where housing costs are high and on Canadian reserves where the quality of housing is often poor and overcrowded.

In Canada, the definition of core housing need captures more explicitly the requirements for housing stability and safety. Core housing need refers to housing deficiencies, those not in adequate condition (e.g., requires major repairs or does not meet health and safety standards), that may not be suitable in size and are not affordable (CMHC, 2009). "A household is in core housing need if its housing does not meet one or more of the adequacy, suitability or affordability standards and it would have to spend 30 percent or more of its before-tax income to pay the median rent of alternative local market housing that meets all three standards" (CMHC, 2009, p. 1). In spite of improvements in Canada, Nunavut, Yukon, and Northwest Territories along with British Columbia, Ontario, Newfoundland, and Labrador have the highest levels of core housing need. For example, in 2006, 223,700 British Columbian households (15.8%) were estimated to be in core housing need. As well, almost 25% of British Columbia renter households were paying 50% or more of their income on housing (BC Housing, 2006). Many of these were lone-parent and Aboriginal families. In British Columbia, 28% of those people in core housing need are Aboriginal households (Housing Policy Branch, 2008). If housing expenditures are a relatively large proportion of an individual or family's income (greater than 30%), then there is less income for individuals and families to use in exercising control and discretion in lifestyle and living conditions.

How Housing Impacts Health

Housing impacts health through various means. Shaw (2004) describes both the hard and soft aspects of housing that impact health. Shaw states, "[housing is] a component of general wellbeing, ontological security, and the perception of social status, in both individual and community contexts; conversely, housing debt, poor housing, and deprived areas can be seen as potentially harmful" (Shaw, 2004, pp. 397–398). The hard aspects are those material conditions that both directly and indirectly impact health, such as the physical conditions of housing, the neighborhood in which one lives, and access to services and amenities. According to Shaw (2004), housing is a proxy indicator of wealth and socioeconomic status. In a summary of the evidence of housing and health, Shaw (2004) highlights key role that inadequate housing conditions, including overcrowding, have on the development of health conditions and injuries. For example, living in damp conditions and presence of mould is associated with increased respiratory problems, and overcrowding is associated with the transmission of communicable diseases such as tuberculosis (TB). Other problems include poisoning, such as that associated with lead paint or lead pipes in older homes, carbon monoxide, and radon. Lastly, increased injuries in the home can be associated with inadequate housing that disproportionately affects those who are disadvantaged on the socioeconomic gradient.

The soft aspects of housing focus on the meaning of home (Dunn, 2002; Shaw, 2004). Shaw observes that home can be a place of security that provides constancy, support for carrying out daily routines, exercising individual control and identity construction (Shaw, 2004). Owning a home can be a source of ontological security (a sense of order and continuity in regard to an individual's experiences), but it can also be a source of stress associated with psychological stress of mortgage payments, debt, and worry. The meaning of home is also associated with mental health, well-being, and sense of self. A home can be a site in which one can foster social contact and relationships, but homes can also be a site of social isolation, violence, and abuse that impact well-being and security. As Shaw (2004) and others have observed, notions of home are highly individualized constructions, and home is not always a refuge (Kidd & Davidson, 2007; Robinson, 2005; Taylor-Seehafer, Jacobvitz, & Steiker, 2008; Tomas & Dittmar, 1995).

Homelessness

Homelessness is an extreme example of the negative impacts that poverty and lack of adequate housing can have on health (Shaw, 2004). Canada has seen an unprecedented growth in homelessness since 1980s. Homelessness is often used as "catch all word" that is not always clearly defined (Hulchanski, Campsie, Chau, Hwang, & Paradis, 2009). The Canadian definition of homelessness describes a range of housing situations for individuals and families who do not have permanent stable housing and are unlikely to obtain it (Canadian Homelessness Research Network, 2012). The definition "describes a range of housing and shelter circumstances, with people being without any shelter at one end, and being insecurely housed at the other" (Canadian Homelessness Research Network, 2012, p. 1). There are

four categories of homelessness and housing vulnerability: (1) unsheltered, which refers to street homelessness including living outside or uninhabitable buildings; (2) emergency sheltered, living in homeless shelters, or shelters for women experiencing violence; (3) provisionally accommodated, which includes those who are in transitional housing and do not have permanent housing; and (4) at risk of homelessness, which includes those living in housing situations where their housing does not meet public health and safety standards or they are paying more than 30% of their income for housing.

This definition identifies both those who are homeless and those at risk for homelessness in relation to structural factors (e.g., housing situation) and provides for potential acknowledgement of broader social factors such as income policies, deinstitutionalization, housing affordability, and availability (e.g., rising costs and loss of social housing programs) that contribute to homelessness. However, homelessness is not necessarily a static state because people may move between different living situations including sleeping outdoors, with family and friends, shelters, and housing. Further, people experiencing homelessness are not a homogenous group, and there is a high degree of diversity on how policies that create homelessness impact those who experience homelessness.

Those who are homeless are more likely to die prematurely, often 20 to 25 years earlier than the rest of the population (Hwang, 2000, 2004; Nordentoft & Wandall-Holm, 2003; Wright & Tompkins, 2005). In Germany, the average age of death for people that are homeless was 44.5 years (Wright & Tompkins, 2005). In Canada, Spittal et al. (2006) found that women who were homeless and using drugs were 50 times more likely to die prematurely than other women in the population. Also, more recently in Canada, Hwang et al. (2009) found that mortality was increased for people who live in shelters, rooming houses, and hotels. These authors found that life expectancy at age 25 years for men living in such situations was approximately 42 years of age and 52 years of age for women. The mortality rate for people living in such housing conditions was significantly higher than others in the poorest fifth of the general population.

Homelessness is associated with poor health. People who have experienced or are experiencing homelessness suffer more frequently from conditions such as respiratory problems, problematic substance use, poor mental health and mental illness, suicide, violence, and accidents (Begin, Casavant, Chenier, & Dupuis, 1999; Eberle, Kraus, Pomeroy, & Hulchanski, 2001; Wright & Tompkins, 2005). In addition, people that are homeless experience difficulties associated with day-to-day living conditions including skin conditions such as scabies, foot problems, and dental decay (Eberle et al., 2001; Hwang, 2001). Living outdoors (rooflessness) is associated with exposure to the elements and may result in heat stroke, sunburn, frostbite, and increased incidence of accidents. Increased incidence of head injuries has been documented among those who are homeless (Hwang et al., 2008). There is a higher rate of chronic and communicable diseases associated with homelessness including TB, sexually transmitted diseases (STDs), HIV, AIDS, and hepatitis C (Begin et al., 1999; Eberle et al., 2001; Frankish, Hwang, & Quantz, 2005; Wright & Tompkins, 2005).

There is a wealth of literature on the prevalence of mental illness and substance use in the homeless population. For example, in Vancouver and Victoria, mental health problems, including substance use, have been identified in a significant proportion of those who are homeless (Social Planning and Research Council of British Columbia et al., 2009; Victoria Coolaid Society, 2007). Specific health concerns differ according to individual circumstances, age, gender, and ethnicity (Cheung & Hwang, 2004). For example, homeless women are at higher risk for depression, sexual abuse, HIV, and STDs than homeless men. Increased economic costs and use of more expensive emergency services have been associated with homelessness, mental illness, and substance use (Folsom et al., 2005). Conversely, obtaining housing with integrated supports has been shown to reduce costs associated with hospitalization, emergency department use, and the criminal justice system (City of Victoria, 2007; Larimer et al., 2009).

The pathways between poor health and homelessness are complex and run in both directions. According to the Institute of Medicine (1988), there is a complex relationship between homelessness and health in that poor health may precede homelessness, poor health may be a consequence of homelessness, and homelessness may exacerbate difficulties in addressing and managing health problems. However, as Shaw observes, "although debate exists about the extent to which health problems precede or result from homelessness, and evidence exists for both causal directions, this is not the key issue here, because either pathway confirms the close relationship between health problems and inadequate housing" (Shaw, 2004, p. 407). More to the point, Drew et al. state, " the most basic health problem of homeless people is lack of a home; to condemn someone to homelessness is to visit him or her with a host of other evils" (Drew et al., 1989, p. 1). An understanding of the causes and consequences of homelessness can assist nurses in providing relevant and empathetic care and contribute to efforts that seek to reduce or end homelessness by addressing root causes.

Food Insecurity

Access to healthy and nutritious food is a growing problem for many Canadian households including those who are homeless. Since the opening of the first food bank in Edmonton in 1981, the number of food banks has grown (Food Banks Canada, 2009). In 2007, there were 673 food banks and approximately 2,800 affiliated agencies. Today, there are at least 983 food banks and more than 2,900 affiliated agencies. In March 2012, more than 882,188 individual Canadians used a food bank (Food Banks Canada, 2012). According to Food Banks Canada, this is a 31% increase over 2008 and 2.4% higher than 2011. However, this does not capture the wide ranging problem of hunger and the establishment of food banks in settings such as universities, schools, and other institutions. For example, university students are often vulnerable to food insecurity because of limited income, but often, this is seen as a short-term rather than long-term situation.

According to the Hunger Count 2012 (Food Banks Canada, 2012), most households using food banks cited three primary sources of income including social assistance (including disability income) (65.8%), employment (11.4%), and pensions (6.85%). The use of food banks by those on social assistance and in the labor force and on pensions suggest these incomes are inadequate to make ends meet. Food is a disposable cost and may be a lower priority than paying one's rent which is a fixed cost. According to Food Banks Canada and the Hunger Count (2012), 38.4% of those helped are children and youth. The breakdown of Canadians using food banks by household type is as follows:

- 48.6% of assisted households are families with children
- 11.4% are couples without children
- 40% are single people

Among all of these households who use food banks, 48.4% are women, 11.3% are Aboriginal peoples, 11.1% are immigrants and refugees, 4.1% are seniors, and 3% are college students. Further, only 7.7% own their own home, and most (63.6%) live in rental accommodations or social housing (21.8%).

Food insecurity is a major concern for a diverse group of people with low incomes. In addition to food banks, many people may access other charitable organizations to meet needs for food through meal programs. Many charitable organizations across Canada are working to feed people as social and economic policies make it increasingly impossible for people to do so for themselves. However, food distribution is poorly regulated, is often of poor quality, insufficient in quantity, depends on fluctuating availability of contributions, and is sometimes hampered by food safety regulations (Bocskei & Ostry, 2010; Tarasuk, 2005). As a charity response to hungry, food banks and other agencies are an emergency response to inequitable social policies.

Despite such efforts, people routinely go hungry in Canada with significant consequences for health (Tarasuk, 2005). Children go to school hungry, affecting their ability to learn, and many people go without adequate nutrients for health and well-being. Family members often go hungry in Canada so that children can eat. For example, studies in Atlantic Canada have shown that women routinely go hungry to feed their children (McIntyre et al., 2002; McIntyre et al., 2003). People with precarious employment, such as men who work as casual day laborers, or seasonal farm workers, often have to work without eating until they are paid at the end of the day. This can put people at high risk for accidents (e.g., in construction where the use of such day laborers is common, or on farms), dehydration, electrolyte imbalances, dizziness, and so on.

Enhancing food security is part of a nurses' role that can be enacted in various settings. For example, nurses can work to ensure adequate nutrition for people while in hospital and upon discharge through referrals as well as connection to community services and resources. Some housing situations may have inadequate or nonexistent cooking facilities such as no fridge or only a hot plate. Public health nurses often participate in the development of food security initiatives such as community kitchens, community gardens, and food cooperatives. Understanding the living conditions that contribute to food insecurity is crucial in the development of programs that are relevant.

Social Exclusion

Living conditions impact health, and the impact is profound when people are living in impoverished social and economic conditions, characterized by income, housing, and food insecurity. Health is further compromised by the social exclusion that routinely accompanies and contributes to production of such conditions (Galabuzi, 2009):

> Social exclusion is an expression of unequal relations or power among groups in society, which then determine unequal access to economic, social, political and cultural resources. The assertion of certain forms of economic, political, social, and cultural privilege, or the normalization of certain ethnocultural norms by some groups, occurs at the expense of and ultimately, marginalization of others. (Galabuzi, 2009)

Social exclusion encompasses the structures and processes that shape inequality and access to resources that determine participation in society and shape health outcomes. Social exclusion may be based on many forms of discrimination along the lines of class, gender, sexual orientation, ability, age, religion, and ethnicity (Benoit & Shumka, 2009). For example, being unable to afford serviceable clothing and access washing facilities leads to people being made to feel unwelcome or being barred from public spaces, affecting well-being and access to resources, including employment.

Although Canada has embraced the social determinants of health as a basis for public policy since 1970s (Health and Welfare Canada, 1986; Health Disparities Task Group of the Federal/Provincial/Territorial Advisory Committee on Population Health and Health Security, 2005; Lalonde, 1974; WHO, 1986), the primary emphasis of health promotion efforts has been on lifestyle and individual behaviour modification. Yet, as we have previously discussed, health is profoundly impacted by the social conditions in which people live, and access to resources for health is increasingly scarce as living conditions decline. For example, barriers to employment are created by poverty (e.g., lack of access to transportation, lack of access to appropriate clothing and equipment for work), discrimination (e.g., gender discrimination and racism), and stigma (e.g., related to poverty and mental illness), with all of these influences intersecting.

Some of the same groups are repeatedly affected by income, housing, and food insecurity as well as unemployment and marginalization because of their social positioning on the basis of income in combination with age, gender, ethnicity, ability, sexual orientation, and so on. Thus, it is crucial for nurses to understand lifestyle and choices within the context of people's lives including the impact of the social determinants of health and to understand how social processes contribute to vulnerability to poor health.

What Social Processes Contribute to Vulnerability and Poor Health?

Although vulnerability is produced in certain living conditions, those living conditions and associated vulnerabilities are created and sustained by intersecting social, political, and economic factors. These dynamics are due in part to the fact that political systems, social structures, and economic arrangements determine who has power and control in decision-making about resources and who has access to those resources (Anderson et al., 2009; Young, 2001). These power differences are more evident if we consider problems such as stigmatization, racialization, marginalization, and discrimination associated with class, age, sexual orientation, ethnicity, gender, and ability.

Stigmatization, racialization, and discrimination are associated with psychosocial stress that can contribute to health problems including hypertension, poor mental health, and problematic substance use (Galabuzi, 2009). For example, people who are homeless frequently encounter stigmatizing attitudes that equate homelessness with drug use and lack of motivation to work. Discriminatory treatment can become part of everyday experiences. In spite of espoused Canadian values for diversity, people from nondominant cultures are frequently discriminated against in access to employment and educational opportunities. Gender is also important in discrimination on access to resources such as education and employment. This kind of stigmatization and discrimination negatively affects people's access to material resources, self-esteem and self-worth, and impact health and the development of health inequities (Hodgetts, Radley, Chamberlain, & Hodgetts, 2007; Krieger, 1999; Raphael, 2009a).

Stigmatization and discrimination are deeply embedded into both society and the health-care systems in which nurses live and work (Anderson & Reimer Kirkham, 1998). In part, this can be understood as a result of the fact that the more dominant groups in society (e.g., those with power, money, and resources) who are predominantly from certain social positions (e.g., male, white, and of European descent) have been key in the development of political, legal, educational, and social systems such as health care (Anderson & Reimer Kirkham, 1998). For example, historically women's health-care concerns have been more likely to be dismissed rather than taken seriously. Lack of understanding related to cultural differences in health care on the part of health-care providers can contribute to judgments and racial stereotyping that negatively impact **access to health care** (Browne, Johnson, Bottorf, Grewal, & Hilton, 2002). Browne (2005, 2007) and Browne and Fiske (2001) identified that perceived racism toward Aboriginal women affected their ability to access care, their health and well-being, and their future access to health care. Similarly, people who use illegal drugs often feel highly stigmatized and judged when they access health-care services (Butters & Erickson, 2003; Crockett & Gifford, 2004; Lloyd, 2010; McLaughlin, McKenna, Leslie, Moore, & Robinson, 2006). Fear of negative experiences and treatment that triggers past trauma and perpetuates feelings of low self-esteem and marginalization can result in delays in accessing care or even in avoidance of care. Multiple sources of stigma and discrimination impact access to health-care services and exacerbate vulnerability to poor health and health inequities.

Are People Merely Victims of Circumstance?

Individuals make choices and enact autonomous decision-making within the constraints of the social conditions that shape their lives (Sherwin, 1998). Another way of saying this is that individuals can make choices to the degree that their life circumstances permit. Thus, the health of individuals is affected by the interaction of individual and structural determinants.

Through the eyes of a patient

All of my disposable income goes toward food and rent. I have nothing left to pay for the fitness classes, and if I did, no way to pay for childcare and transportation to get there. I work all day and then have to prepare dinner, care for my children and help them with homework, then the only free time I have is once they are in bed. I don't even feel safe to walk or run in my neighbourhood. I feel like I have no choices to try to improve my health through fitness.

(*personal reflection of Adele S., single mother*)

Individuals do not have unlimited choice but make choices within as set of life circumstances that vary based on social positioning and accompanying resources and power. Understanding that we all make choices within different life circumstances can help us to understand that although individuals have autonomous choices, one's range of choices is limited by social conditions and living circumstances. Lifestyle changes involving fitness may not be a high priority. For nurses, understanding life circumstances can be a key to understanding both the behaviours and needs of people affected by various life circumstances. Teaching lifestyle modification must always be done with acute awareness of the circumstances of people's lives.

Think   Constrained Choices

You are walking with your friend downtown. As you are making your way to the nearest café for lunch, your friend points to someone pushing a shopping cart and says, "I don't understand why people choose to be homeless and sleep outside." You are quiet as you think how to respond to this comment. You reflect that if your house burned to the ground, you would have the option of staying in a hotel or renting a new apartment because you could pay for these options. However, if you did not have financial resources, your choices would be limited to living an emergency shelter, with friends, or outdoors. In an emergency shelter, you would be staying in a room with at least three other people whom you don't know, and you would have to leave your belongings outside. So your choices are to stay outside and keep your belongings or leave your belongings and sleep in the emergency shelter. Also, if you are in an emergency shelter, you would not necessarily have unlimited access to bathing facilities or the ability to rest during the day. Your sleep at night might be disrupted by the person in the next bed who is coughing throughout the night. You may lie awake worrying about your situation or fear being attacked by the person next to you. All of this would impact your ability to work and keep employment, assuming you are able to work.

How do poverty and homelessness impact available choices for people? Identify the stressors inherent with staying in an emergency shelter. Can any of these stressors be addressed or mitigated? How so?

Understanding behaviours as a product of social circumstances can assist us to understand different choices and move from blaming individuals for poor choices to contextualized knowledge (Pauly, MacKinnon, & Varcoe, 2009). For example, tobacco smoking, once considered a personal choice, is now more commonly viewed as a public health problem because of the active marketing of tobacco by cigarette companies through popular media. In fact, some groups such as young women have been actively targeted to increase cigarette sales (Mechanic & Tanner, 2007). Further, higher rates of tobacco use in low-income populations may not simply be a lifestyle choice but a response to coping with difficult living situations. For example, Bottorff et al. have shown how in Aboriginal communities, women, and children's exposure to tobacco is shaped by economic and rural conditions and the consequences of colonial policies currently still in effect (Bottorff et al., 2009).

Individuals also have different levels of capacity to make decisions. Self-determination or the ability to make choices assumes that one has the necessary skills and resources to make decisions. At a minimum level, to be self-determining, one must have the mental ability, have access to information, and be free of undue coercion. Beyond that, individuals may have different needs and wants for information. Further, individuals may have limited experience and ability in decision-making. Some have suggested that the stress of poverty in early childhood can negatively impact self-regulation and decision-making (Dunn, 2010). Individuals may have few positive experiences or skills in decision-making related to even basic life skills such as financial management and grocery shopping.

I'm a nurse working in a reproductive outpatient clinic. My first patient of the day is Melissa, a young woman seeking a therapeutic abortion. As I talk with Melissa about her decision, Melissa bursts into tears and says she doesn't know if she is making the right decision. She turns to me and says, "You seem like a smart woman, what would you do?" I comfort her and acknowledge that this must be a difficult decision. Melissa says that she is in a relationship with a man 20 years older than her who is physically violent at times and makes all of the decisions in their relationship. Melissa fears that she will be unable to provide a safe home for a child if she stays in this relationship and that if she leaves the relationship she will be unable to provide financially for her child. Prior to this relationship, she lived with her parents who made all of her decisions for her. She turns to me and says, "Please just tell me what to do, I don't know what to do." Her resources and experience with decision-making have been severely limited by her previous life experiences.

(personal reflection of a nurse)

To summarize, vulnerability is not merely a characteristic of individuals but the production of risk as a result of social conditions that impact the development of poor health and health inequities. Social positioning reflects socioeconomic status, age, ability, gender, and ethnicity (Graham, 2004). One's social position in society determines access and availability of resources for health. As a result of social, political, and economic conditions that impact social position, some individuals and groups are more vulnerable to poor health than others. Vulnerability to poor heath is made worse when social conditions and social processes interact with individual factors, contributing to the development of health inequities that negatively impact some groups more than others. Social positioning reflects an individual's place within society. Vulnerability is affected both by the social factors that determine health (the determinants of health) and the social processes that underlie the distribution of the resources for health (Bourgois, 2002; Graham, 2004; Marmot, 2007). It is within these varying social conditions that people make decisions about their lives.

Can Improving Access to Health Care Reduce Vulnerability?

The social determinants of health lay out the conditions necessary for good health. Access to health care is one but not necessarily the most powerful determinant of health (Marmot, 2003; WHO, 2003). The strong focus of acute health-care services on diagnosis and treatment of disease in part limits the impact of access to health care on health outcomes.

Barbara Starfield, a researcher and proponent of enhancing health equity, has found that the type of health care is important and that access to primary care can improve the health of people who are vulnerable to poor health because of the conditions in which they live (Starfield, Shi, & Macinko, 2005). Although access to hospitals and medical care seems to have little impact on vulnerability to poor health, access to primary care seems to make an important contribution to improving the health of vulnerable populations.

Primary care may be delivered by interdisciplinary teams that include nurses. For example, many urban inner city health-care centres employ both registered nurses and nurse practitioners as part of the health-care team. In the north, nurses often work in settings where they deliver both primary care and public health services as nurse practitioners and outreach nurses. Nurses in hospitals also have an important role to play in enhancing access to health care. There are at least two important aspects to this role. First, nurses in hospitals are often the first contact that people have as they access health services. Fear of stigma and discrimination can negatively affect people's ability to access health-care services and may result in them actually avoiding or delaying health care until they are very ill. The way that people are greeted and made to feel welcome is especially important for those who are vulnerable to poor health because of poverty and stigmatizing conditions (Pauly, 2008; Wen & Hudak, 2007). Respectful treatment and care can be a power antidote to the discrimination that individuals affected by disadvantage face daily. Secondly, in providing nursing care, nurses can shape their care to include the conditions that influence the ability of individuals to manage and care for themselves.

I am a registered nurse on a surgical unit and was preparing to discharge George home to recover following abdominal surgery. I know that while in hospital, George's roommate told him that he will have to find a new place to live. George is currently unemployed because of a chronic back injury and is going to apply for social assistance. Normally, my main focus in planning for discharge would be to describe the supplies that need to be purchased for dressing changes at home. In George's case I wondered if I should give George some extra dressing supplies and information on where to obtain the supplies without cost. Further, I was concerned that George might have difficulties keeping the wound clean as he mentioned he might just camp somewhere or stay in a shelter until he can get things sorted out and find a cheap place to rent. I have heard that some of the cheapest housing is in old hotels that are not in good repair and that living in single-room occupancy units or an emergency shelter would create difficulty in affording privacy for completing wound care, storage of supplies or even clean water necessary for wound care.

Also, I started to think about nutrition and the need for George to have sufficient calories for adequate wound healing, particularly good sources of protein. Living on a low income and in poverty often makes it difficult to obtain nutritionally adequate diets (Vozoris & Tarasuk, 2003). Being on a low income meant that George might obtain the needed calories, but these calories are often obtained from high-carbohydrate foods, not from the protein-rich foods needed for wound healing. Knowing all of this, I focused by discharge teaching on providing information and facilitating access to resources to assist George to implement discharge instructions, improve the conditions necessary for health, and prevent complications and readmissions.

(personal reflection of a nurse)

What Can Nurses Do to Reduce Vulnerability to Poor Health?

Reducing vulnerability to poor health requires policy to ensure that the structural determinants of health are in place and that where inequities exist additional resources are available to assist those vulnerable to poor health. Consistent with this, nurses can work with and strengthen community resources to reduce vulnerability to poor health. In the past, recommended strategies included empowerment and capacity building of individuals, families, and communities to counter vulnerability. Concepts such as community empowerment and capacity have been more recently replaced by strategies to promote social cohesion and social capital that are more focused on societal networks (Labonte, 2009). Labonte argues that such socially oriented concepts have an advantage over the earlier community-oriented empowerment concepts because they direct attention to the context in which communities operate (i.e., political systems and structures). However, he cautions that there are challenges associated with including people who have been systematically excluded without also making fundamental structural changes. He poses the question, "How does one go about including individuals and groups into a set of structured social relationships that were responsible for excluding them in the first place?" (Labonte, 2009, p. 271). He suggests that concern should be with the conditions that create exclusion and those who benefit rather than with excluded groups. Thus, our understanding of social inclusion should be built on understanding the power dynamics and social structures that have resulted in exclusion.

As registered nurses, we should be particularly concerned with understanding how social, political, and economic structures systematically exclude certain individuals and groups. For example, those experiencing homelessness are often excluded from the development of plans and strategies to reduce homelessness. The importance of including individuals in such discussions can help to provide insight into the very structures and processes that result in exclusion. The achievement of **social justice** requires that inequities in political structures and processes be addressed. Some, such as Young (1990, 2001), have suggested that fostering participatory processes of those systematically excluded is critical and that we ought to begin with understanding of differences between groups. In particular, this requires an understanding that individuals come with a unique perspective and capacity but few opportunities to express their perspectives and exercise decision-making and capacity. Nurses can play an important role in supporting development of existing capacity through provision of opportunities to participate in processes related to health and nursing services as well as in political and policy forums. Such participation can radically reform the delivery of nursing care and other services and policies. Understanding differences can illuminate aspects of programs and policies that exclude individuals.

What Is the Role of Nursing in Promoting Health Equity?

Nursing has long had a historical commitment to ameliorating conditions that produce vulnerability to poor health and the promotion of social justice. We can look back to Florence Nightingale, who cared for those wounded in the Crimean War and her efforts to not only care for them but also ensure the environment was conducive to healing and restoration of health. The Grey Nuns, who established hospitals for the poor first in Montreal and then Western Canada, are among early Canadian nurse leaders to promote social justice (Hardill, 2006). Lillian Wald, a public health nurse, provided care and sought to change the social conditions of people who were living in the impoverished Henry Street Settlements on the lower east side of New York City through the establishment of public health nursing services (Buhler-Wilkerson, 1993; Hardill, 2006). A Canadian nurse, Ethel Johns, worked in the early 1900s to foster racial equality particularly for black nurses in the United States (Grypma, 2003).

The commitment to promote health equity and social justice is written into the Canadian Nurses Association (CNA) Code of Ethics for Registered Nurses (Canadian Nurses Association [CNA], 2008) and in some cases provincial nursing practice standards. One of the seven values in the CNA Code of Ethics is to promote justice (see Box 4.3 in Chapter 4). Under the value of justice, nurses have ethical responsibilities not to discriminate in the provision of care, refrain from stigmatizing responses, do not engage or be complicit in demeaning or degrading treatment, and ensure fair allocation of resources (CNA, 2008). These values are consistent with the promotion of social justice. Part II of the CNA Code outlines the ethical endeavors of nurses highlighting their responsibilities to promote, advocate, and work toward equity and the reduction of social inequities.

These ethical endeavors include recognition of social, political, and economic factors that shape health and inequities, utilization of principles of **primary health care**; recognize and advocate for the social determinants of health in policies and programs; and work to improve the quality of life for disadvantaged and/or vulnerable populations.

What Is Nursing's Role in Addressing Systemic Health Inequities?

In their work, nurses can see firsthand the impact of living conditions on poor health and have a position of unique understanding and insight into the contextual factors that shape the health of people in various social circumstances. This kind of knowledge is essential for contextualizing nursing care and foregrounding understanding that all people are differentially impacted by social conditions and that living conditions vary dramatically between the rich and poor. It may be very difficult for someone who has always lived in a house with a lock on the door, clean running water, and electrical and plumbing systems in good working repair to imagine the health risks, difficulties, and fears associated with living in a house that does not have a working lock or a roof that keeps out the rain or to imagine being homeless with the only option being to sleep in an emergency shelter on a cot in a room with two, three, four, or more strangers.

Nurses may advocate for changes in health and social conditions through their employment settings by increasing awareness of the social determinants of health and inequities among the health-care team as well as managers and organizational leaders. Public health nurses have always included political action as an important strategy in doing their work and have been leaders in the development of actions that address poverty, homelessness, housing, food security, and so on (Community Health Nurses of Canada, 2009). Nurses may choose to work in settings that allow them to work directly with those vulnerable to poor health. For example, some nurses have taken up work in rural and remote communities, or in urban inner cities, or sought work internationally to address inequities associated with war, extreme poverty, and HIV in many countries around the world. Secondly, nurses may be involved outside of their employed role to work locally, nationally, or internationally with nursing professional groups or other groups and organizations committed to addressing the promotion of health equity. For example, nurses can join antipoverty groups, housing action groups, and others who are promoting policies and programs that reduce health inequities. Thirdly, and most importantly, nurses everywhere, in every work setting can counter stigma and discrimination, promote understanding of the context of peoples' lives, and advocate for equitable access and equitable policies at all levels.

Regardless of their work setting or professional involvements within and outside of nursing, addressing vulnerability to poor health and health inequities requires that nurses think politically every day. They can engage peers and leaders in discussions related to systemic problems that are exacerbating vulnerability to poor health and health inequities. They may choose to write letters to the editors or opinion editorials that bring greater public awareness to the issues facing people at risk of poor health. Students particularly may have opportunities to do this kind of thing as part of a course assignment and clinical experiences.

Now that Sasha has learned about the social, political, and economic conditions that shape health, it is much clearer to her what role she can play as both a student and as a registered nurse. She recognizes the importance of not judging behaviours without contextualizing the conditions that shape health behaviours and the role that income, housing, and food security play in shaping the actions of people and their ability to follow through on health education and lifestyle changes. During her placement, she joined forces with other nursing students and some fourth-year dentistry students to support the opening of a free dental and oral health clinic. The experience and knowledge she has gained from this placement are something that she will take with her regardless of where she works in nursing following graduation. At the end of her placement, she has decided to write an opinion editorial to her local newspaper to raise awareness of the broader conditions that shape the health of people at the centre where she is completing her placement. She recognizes that part of her professional and ethical responsibility is to advocate for changes in social conditions that will improve health and well-being of people most impacted by living conditions because of poverty and homelessness. She feels she has benefitted significantly by placing her clinical experience into context of the social determinants of health and the determinants of health inequities. This knowledge will help her to better assess and plan care for clients who are vulnerable to poor health whether she works in acute care or community settings.

Critical Thinking Case Scenarios

▶ As a student, your family and friends are curious about your current student placement at an agency serving homeless people. They wonder why a nurse would be placed in such a setting and ask, "Why aren't you learning about real nursing in hospitals?" They wonder why you are wasting your time with "those people" who are just too lazy to go out and get a job. Your family in particular is worried about your safety as they have heard there is a lot of drug use in that area and fear that you might be robbed or assaulted.

1. What images of homelessness are being presented in this scenario?
2. How have your attitudes, values, and beliefs been shaped by your own experiences and social positioning?
3. What are the causes of homelessness?

4. What are the health consequences associated with homelessness?
5. What is the role of nursing in advocating for better social conditions and how can nurses impact health by facilitating access to health care?

▶ In your clinical placement, you are faced with a request from a client for money. He tells you that he and his family are having difficulty paying their rent this month and that if they don't pay their rent, they will likely lose their housing. You know that the vacancy rate in the city is low and that if they lose their place they are at risk for homelessness.

1. What are some of the ethical issues nurses confront in working with vulnerable populations?
2. What might be sources of guidance related to professional boundaries in such situations (e.g., CNA Code of Ethics, provincial nursing practice standards)?

▶ A few of your friends have asked you to go out to a local club and on the way, you see someone you know who is panhandling. She asks you and your friends for money. She smiles at you but you quickly walk on, pretending that you do not know her.

1. How should nurses react to clients outside their work setting?
2. What might be sources of guidance related to your professional obligations in such situations?
3. What are the professional boundaries in such situations?
4. How do nurses navigate their professional role in their personal life?

▶ All of the nurses on the acute care unit where you are working dislike caring for people who come in with complications of drug or alcohol use. Recently, a man has been admitted because of chronic alcohol problems and complications of diabetes. It is likely he is going to lose his leg. One of your colleagues observes, "just another drunk." The man is often left unattended and left to lie in wet sheets for hours. When nurses go into the room, he is often angry and shouts at them to "get the hell out of here." Several of the nurses refer to him as a "difficult patient" and try to avoid caring for him.

1. What are the ethical issues and concerns raised in this scenario?
2. What standards of ethical practice are being violated?
3. As a student, what is your role in such situations?
4. What cultural norms have been created in this situation?
5. What societal stereotypes and norms are being reproduced in such situations?
6. What are the ethical responsibilities of nurses in such situations?

▶ A young woman with two children tells you that she has run out of money this month and will not be able to purchase any food until her next social assistance cheque arrives in a week. She tells you that she has enough cereal to last several days and that she doesn't need to eat. She has been to the food bank but has used up her allocated amount. She says don't worry, we will be okay as long as I can keep paying the rent.

1. What ethical issues are raised by this situation?
2. What actions might the nurse take in her professional role to assist this mother?
3. What actions might the nurse take to address underlying systemic issues embedded in this situation?

Multiple-Choice Questions

1. The use of food banks in Canada is primarily associated with:
   a. Low socioeconomic status
   b. Homelessness
   c. Female-headed households
   d. Urban settings
   e. Aboriginal peoples

2. The social determinants of health are:
   a. The same as the determinants of health inequities
   b. Living conditions that shape the health of the population
   c. More likely to impact very low–income earners
   d. Part of access to health-care services
   e. Less likely to impact the health of vulnerable populations than the rest of the population

3. Health inequities are:
   a. Differences in health status both positive and negative
   b. Amenable to change
   c. The same as health inequalities
   d. Associated primarily with vulnerable populations
   e. Not a concern in wealthy countries such as Canada

4. Actions to reduce health inequities include:
   a. Increasing privatization of health care
   b. Establishment of welfare limits and stricter eligibility criteria
   c. Guaranteed annual incomes
   d. Continued gentrification and for profit ownership in the housing market
   e. Increasing the establishment of food banks

5. The nursing role to reduce vulnerability to the conditions that contribute to poor health through action on health equity and social justice is:
   a. Part of every nursing role regardless of setting
   b. Not related to professional nursing responsibilities in acute care settings
   c. Assumed as a practice standard in all provinces
   d. Is an added responsibility beyond professional and ethical responsibilities
   e. Takes priority over clinical care

REFERENCES AND SUGGESTED READINGS

Aday, L. (1993). *At risk in America: The health and health care needs of vulnerable populations in the United States.* San Francisco, CA: Jossey-Bass.

Aday, L. (1997). Vulnerable populations: A community-oriented perspective. *Family and Community Health, 19*(4), 1.

Anderson, J. (2000). Gender, 'race' poverty, health and discourse of health reform in the context of globalization: A post-colonial feminist perspective in policy research. *Nursing Inquiry, 7*(4), 220.

Anderson, J., & Reimer Kirkham, S. (1998). Constructing nation: The gendering and racializing of the Canadian health care system. In V. Strong-Boag, S. Grace, A. Eisenberg, & J. Anderson (Eds.), *Painting the maple: Essays on race, gender and the construction of Canada* (p. 242). Vancouver, BC: UBC Press.

Anderson, J. M., Rodney, P., Reimer-Kirkham, S., Browne, A. J., Khan, K. B., & Lynam, M. J. (2009). Inequities in health and healthcare viewed through the ethical lens of critical social justice: Contextual knowledge for the global priorities ahead. *Advances in Nursing Science, 32*(4), 282–294.

BC Housing. (2006). *Housing matters BC.* Retrieved from http://www.bchousing.org/programs/Housing_Matters_BC

Begin, P., Casavant, L., Chenier, N., & Dupuis, J. (1999). *Homelessness.* Retrieved from http://www.parl.gc.ca/information/libaray/PRBpubs/prb991-e.htm

Benoit, C., & Shumka, L. (2009). Gendering the population health perspective: Fundamental determinants of women's health. Vancouver, BC: Women's Health Research Network.

Bocskei, E., & Ostry, A. (2010). Charitable food programs in Victoria, B.C. *Canadian Journal of Dietetic Practice and Research, 71*(1), 2–4.

Bottorff, J., Carey, J., Mowatt, R., Varcoe, C., Johnson, J. L., Hutchinson, P., . . . Wardman, D. (2009). Bingo halls and smoking: Perspectives of First Nations women. *Health and Place, 15*, 1014–1021.

Bourgois, P. (2002). Anthropology and epidemiology on drugs: The challenge of cross-methodological and theoretical dialogue. *International Journal of Drug Policy, 13*(4), 259–269.

Browne, A. J. (2005). Discourses influencing nurses' perceptions of First Nations patients. *Canadian Journal of Nursing Research, 37*(4), 62–87.

Browne, A. J. (2007). Clinical encounters between nurses and First Nations women in a Western Canadian hospital. *Social Science & Medicine, 64*(10), 2165–2176.

Browne, A. J., & Fiske, J. A. (2001). First Nations women's encounters with mainstream health care services. *Western Journal of Nursing Research, 23*(2), 126–147.

Browne, A. J., Johnson, J. L., Bottorff, J. L., Grewal, S., & Hilton, B. A. (2002). Recognizing discrimination in nursing practice. *Canadian Nurse, 98*(5), 24.

Browne, A. J., Smye, V. L., Rodney, P., Tang, S., Mussell, W., & O'Neil, J. (2011). Access to primary care from the perspective of Aboriginal patients at an urban emergency department. *Qualitative Health Research, 21*(3), 333–348.

Buhler-Wilkerson, K. (1993). Bringing care to the people: Lillian Wald's legacy to public health nursing. *American Journal of Nursing, 83*, 1778–1786.

Butler-Jones, D. (2008). *Report on the state of public health in Canada.* Retrieved from http://www.phac-aspc.gc.ca/publicat/2008/cphor-sphc-respcacsp/pdf/CPHO-Report-e.pdf

Butterfield, P. (1990). Thinking upstream: Nurturing a conceptual understanding of the societal context of health behavior. *Advances in Nursing Science, 12*(2), 1–8.

Butters, J., & Erickson, P. G. (2003). Meeting the health care needs of female crack users: A Canadian example. *Women and Health, 37*(3), 1.

Calderone, J. L. (1990). The influence of gender on the frequency of pain and sedative medication administered to postoperative patients. *Sex Roles, 23*, 713–725.

Canada Mortgage and Housing Corporation. (2009). *Canadian housing observer.* Ottawa, ON: Author. Retrieved from https://www03.cmhc-schl.gc.ca/catalog/productDetail.cfm?cat=122&itm=13&lang=en&fr=1385556242597

Canadian Homelessness Research Network. (2012). *Canadian definition of homelessness.* Toronto, ON: Author.

Canadian Institutes of Health Research. (2002). *Charting the course: Canadian population health initiative—A pan-Canadian consultation on population and public health priorities.* Ottawa, ON: Author.

Canadian Institutes of Health Research. (2009). *Research profile—Life in a town without poverty.* Retrieved from http://www.cihr-irsc.gc.ca/e/40308.html

Canadian Mortgage and Housing Corporation. (2009). *Research highlight: 2006 Census Housing Series: Issue 2—The Geography of Core Housing Need, 2001-2006.* Ottawa, ON: Author.

Canadian Nurses Association. (2008). *Code of ethics for registered nurses* (2008 centennial edition). Retrieved from http://www.cna-nurses.ca/CNA/practice/ethics/code/default_e.aspx

Cheung, A. M., & Hwang, S. W. (2004). Risk of death among homeless women: A cohort study and review of the literature. *Canadian Medical Association Journal, 170*(8), 1243–1247.

City of Victoria. (2007). *City of Victoria Mayor's Task Force on breaking the cycle of mental illness, addiction and homelessness: Report of the expert panel.* Victoria, BC: Author.

Cleeland, C. S., Gronin, R., Hatfield, A. K., Edmonson, J. H., Blum, R. H., Stewart, J. A., & Pandya, K. J. (1994). Pain and its treatment in outpatients with metastatic cancer. *New England Journal of Medicine, 330*, 592–596.

Coburn, D. (2006). Health and health care: A political economy perspective. In D. Raphael, T. Bryant, & M. Rioux (Eds.), *Critical perspectives on health, illness and health care: Staying alive* (pp. 59–84). Toronto, ON: Canadian Scholars' Press.

Community Health Nurses of Canada. (2009). *Public Health Nursing Discipline Specific Competencies Version 1.0.* Retrieved from http://www.chnc.ca/phn-nursing-competencies.cfm

Corley, M., & Goren, S. (1998). The dark side of nursing: Impact of stigmatizing responses on patients. *Scholarly Inquiry for Nursing Practice, 12*(2), 99.

Crockett, B., & Gifford, S. M. (2004). "Eyes wide shut": Narratives of women living with hepatitis C in Australia. *Women and Health, 39*(4), 117.

Dahlgren, G., & Whitehead, M. (2006). *European strategies for tackling social inequities in health: Levelling up part 2.* Copenhagen, Denmark: World Health Organization.

Drew, A., Bassuk, E., Breakey, W., Fischer, A., Halpern, C., Smith, G., . . . Wolfe, P. (1989). Health care for the homeless. *Society, 26*(4), 4–5.

Dunn, J. R. (2002). Housing and inequalities in health: A study of socioeconomic dimensions of housing and self reported health from a survey of Vancouver residents. *Journal of Epidemiological Community Health, 56*(9), 671–681.

Dunn, J. R. (2010). Health behavior vs the stress of low socioeconomic status and health outcomes. *Journal of American Medical Association, 303*(12), 1199–1200.

Dunn, J., Hayes, M., Hulchanski, J. D., Hwang, S., & Potvin, L. (2006). Housing as a socio-economic determinant of health: Findings of a national needs, gaps and opportunities assessment. *Canadian Journal of Public Health, 97*, S11–S15.

Eaton, M. (1994). Patently confused, complex inequality and Canada v. Mossop. *Review Constitutional Studies*, 203–209.

Eberle, M., Kraus, D., Pomeroy, S., & Hulchanski, D. (2001). *Homelessness—Causes & effects: A profile, policy review and analysis of homelessness in British Columbia.* Vancouver, BC: Government of British Columbia. Retrieved from http://www.homelesshub.ca/

(S(lp5jad55vccsf0uljvffhric))/Library/Homelessness---Causes-and-Effects-The-Costs-of-Homelessness-in-British-Columbia-47782.aspx

Eggleton, A., & Keon, W. (2008). *Poverty, housing and homelessness: Issues and options. First Report of the Subcommittee on Cities of the Standing Senate Committee on Social Affairs, Science and Technology.* Retrieved from http://www.parl.gc.ca

Eggleton, A., & Segal, H. (2009). *In from the margins: A call to action on poverty, housing and homelessness. Report of the subcommittee on Cities.* Retrieved from http://www.parl.gc.ca/Content/SEN/Committee/402/citi/subsite-dec09/Report_Home-e.htm

European Federation of National Association Working with the Homeless. (2007). ETHOS: European typology on homelessness and housing exclusion. Retrieved from http://www.feantsa.org

Folsom, D., Hawthorne, W., Lindamer, L., Gilmer, T., Bailey, A., Golshan, S., . . . Jeste, D. (2005). Prevalence and risk factors for homelessness and utilization of mental health services among 10,340 patients with serious mental illness in a large public mental health system. *American Journal of Psychiatry, 162*(2), 370–376.

Food Banks Canada. (2009). *Hunger count 2009: A comprehensive report on hunger and food bank use, and recommendations for change.* Toronto, ON: Author.

Food Banks Canada. (2012). *Hunger Count 2012: A comprehensive report on hunger and food bank use in Canada, and recommendations for change.* Toronto, ON: Author.

Frankish, C. J., Hwang, S. W., & Quantz, D. (2005). Homelessness and health in Canada: Research lessons and priorities. *Canadian Journal of Public Health, 96*(Suppl. 2), S23–S29.

Frohlich, K. L., & Potvin, L. (2008). The inequality paradox: The population approach and vulnerable populations. *American Journal of Public Health, 98*(2), 216–221.

Frohlich, K., Ross, N., & Richmond, C. (2006). Health disparities in Canada today: Some evidence and a theoretical framework. *Health Policy, 79,* 132–143.

Galabuzi, G. (2009). Social exclusion. In D. Raphael (Ed.), *Social determinants of health: Canadian perspectives* (2nd ed., pp. 252–268). Toronto, ON: Canadian Scholars' Press.

Goldberg, M., & Graves, J. (2005). *On our streets and in our shelters: Results of the 2005 Greater Vancouver Homeless Count.* Vancouver, BC: Social Planning and Research Council of British Columbia.

Graham, H. (2004). "Social determinants and their unequal distribution: Clarifying policy understandings." *The Milbank Quarterly, 82*(1), 101–124.

Green, A., Carney, D., Pallin, D., Ngo, L., Raymond, K., Iezzoni, L., & Banaji, M. (2007). Implicit bias among physicians and its prediction of thrombolysis decisions for black and white patients. *Journal of General Internal Medicine, 22*(9), 1231–1238.

Grypma, S. J. (2003). Profile of a leader: Unearthing Ethel John's "buried" commitment to racial equality, 1925. *Nursing Leadership, 16,* 439–447.

Hall, J. M. (1999). Marginalization revisited: Critical, postmodern, and liberation perspectives. *Advances in Nursing Science, 22*(2), 88.

Hall, J. M., Stevens, P., & Meleis, A. I. (1994). Marginalization: A guiding concept for valuing diversity in nursing knowledge development. *Advances in Nursing Science, 16*(4), 23.

Hardill, K. (2006). From the Grey Nuns to the streets: A critical history of outreach nursing in Canada. *Public Health Nursing, 24*(1), 91–97.

Health and Welfare Canada. (1986). *Achieving health for all: A framework for health promotion.* Ottawa, ON: Minister of Supply and Services. Retrieved from http://www.hc-sc.gc.ca/hcs-sss/pubs/system-regime/1986-frame-plan-promotion/index-eng.php

Health Disparities Task Group of the Federal/Provincial/Territorial Advisory Committee on Population Health and Health Security. (2005). *Reducing health disparities—Roles of the health sector: Recommended policy directions and activities.* Ottawa, ON: Minister of Health.

Hodgetts, D., Radley, A., Chamberlain, K., & Hodgetts, A. (2007). Health inequalities and homelessness: Considering material, spatial and relational dimensions. *Journal of Health Psychology, 12*(5), 709–725.

Housing Policy Branch. (2008). *Developing an off-reserve Aboriginal housing action plan for British Columbia: A discussion paper to support community engagement.* Retrieved from http://nationtalk.ca/story/developing-an-off-reserve-aboriginal-housing-action-plan-for-british-columbia/

Hulchanski, J. D., Campsie, P., Chau, S., Hwang, S., & Paradis, E. (2009). Introduction. Homelessness: What's in a word? In J. D. Hulchanski, P. Campsie, S. Chau, S. Hwang, E. Paradis (Eds.), *Finding home policy options for addressing homelessness in Canada.* Toronto, ON: Cities Centre Press, University of Toronto.

Hwang, S. (2000). Mortality among men using homeless shelters in Toronto, Ontario. *Journal of the American Medical Association, 283*(16), 2152–2157.

Hwang, S. W. (2001). Homelessness and health. *Canadian Medical Association Journal, 164*(2), 229–233.

Hwang, S. (2004). Risk of death among homeless women: A cohort study and review of the literature. *Canadian Medical Association Journal, 170*(8), 1243–1247.

Hwang, S., Colantonio, A., Chiu, S., Tolomiczenko, G., Kiss, A., Cowan, L., . . . Levinson, W. (2008). The effect of traumatic brain injury on the health of homeless people. *Canadian Medical Association Journal, 179*(8), 779–784.

Hwang, S., Wilkins, R., Tjepkema, M., O'Campo, P., & Dunn, J. (2009). Mortality among residents of shelters, rooming houses, and hotels in Canada: 11 year follow-up study. *British Medical Journal, 339.*

Institute of Medicine. (1988). *Homelessness, health and human needs.* Washington, DC: National Academy Press.

Kendall, P. (2009). *Pathways to health and healing: Second report on the health and well-being of Aboriginal People in British Columbia.* Victoria, BC: Ministry of Healthy Living and Sport.

Kidd, S. A., & Davidson, L. (2007). "You have to adapt because you have no other choice": Stories of strength and resilience of 208 homeless youth in New York City and Toronto. *Journal of Community Psychology, 35*(1), 219–238.

Krieger, N. (1999). Embodying inequality: A review of concepts, measures, and methods for studying health consequences of discrimination. *International Journal of Health Services, 29*(2), 295–352.

Krieger, N. (2005). Embodiment: A conceptual glossary for epidemiology. *Journal of Epidemiological Community Health, 59,* 350–355.

Krieger, N. (2009). Putting health inequities on the map: Social epidemiology meets medical/health geography—An ecosocial perspective. *GeoJournal, 74,* 74–89.

Labonte, R. (2009). Social inclusion/exclusion and health: Dancing the dialectic. In D. Raphael (Ed.), *Social determinants of health: Canadian perspectives* (2nd ed., pp. 269–279). Toronto, ON: Canadian Scholars' Press.

Lalonde, M. (1974). *A new perspective on the health of Canadians: A working document.* Ottawa, ON: Health Canada.

Larimer, M., Malone, D., Garner, M., Atkins, D., Burlingham, B., Lonczak, H., . . . Marlatt, G. A. (2009). Health care and public service use and costs before and after provision of housing for chronically homeless persons with severe alcohol problems. *Journal of American Medical Association, 301*(13), 1349–1357.

Link, B., & Phelan, J. (1995). Social conditions as fundamental causes of diseases. *Journal of Health and Social Behavior, 35,* 80–94.

Lloyd, C. (2010). *Sinning and sinned against: The stigmatization of problem drug users.* London, United Kingdom: Drug Policy Commission.

MacMillan, H. L., Jamieson, E., Walsh, C. A., Wong, M. Y. Y., Faries, E. J., McCue, H., . . . Offord, D. D. (2008). First Nations women's mental health: Results from an Ontario survey. *Archives of Women's Mental Health, 11,* 109–115.

Marmot, M. G. (2003). Understanding social inequalities in health. *Perspectives in Biology and Medicine, 43*(3), S9–S23.

Marmot, M. G. (2004). *The status syndrome: How social standing affects our health and longevity.* London, United Kingdom: Times Books.

Marmot, M. G. (2007). Achieving health equity: From root causes to fair outcomes. *Lancet, 370,* 1153–1163.

McDonald, D. D. (1994). Gender and ethnic stereotyping and analgesic administration. *Research in Nursing and Health, 17,* 5–49.

McIntyre, L., Glanville, N., Officer, S., Anderson, B., Raine, K., & Dayle, J. (2002). Food insecurity of low-income lone mothers and their children in Atlantic Canada. *Canadian Journal of Public Health, 93*(6), 411–415.

McIntyre, L., Glanville, N., Raine, K., Dayle, J., Anderson, B., & Battaglia, N. (2003). Do low-income lone mothers compromise their nutrition to feed their children? *Canadian Medical Association Journal, 168*(6), 686–691.

McLaughlin, D., McKenna, H., & Leslie, J. (2000). The perceptions and aspirations illicit drug users hold toward health care staff and the care they receive. *Journal of Psychiatric and Mental Health Nursing, 7,* 435.

McLaughlin, D., McKenna, H., Leslie, J., Moore, K., & Robinson, J. (2006). Illicit drug users in Northern Ireland: Perceptions and experiences of health and social care professionals [Research]. *Journal of Psychiatric and Mental Health Nursing, 13*(6), 682–686.

Mechanic, D., & Tanner, J. (2007). Vulnerable people, groups, and populations: Societal view. *Health Affairs, 26*(5), 1220–1230.

Napravnik, S., Royce, R., Walter, E., & Lim, W. (2000). HIV-1 infected women and prenatal care utilization: Barriers and facilitators. *AIDS Patient Care and STD's, 14*(8), 411.

Nettleton, C., Napolitano, D. A., & Stephens, C. (2007). *An overview of current knowledge of the social determinants of indigenous health.* Geneva, Switzerland: World Health Organization Commission on the Social Determinants of Health.

Nordentoft, M., & Wandall-Holm, M. (2003). 10 year follow up study of mortality among users of hostels for homeless people in Copenhagen. *British Medical Journal, 327,* 1–4.

Pauly, B. M. (2008). Shifting moral values to enhance access to health care: Harm reduction as a context for ethical nursing practice. *International Journal of Drug Policy, 19,* 195–204.

Pauly, B. M., MacKinnon, K., & Varcoe, C. (2009). Revisiting "Who gets care?" Health equity as an arena for nursing action. *Advances in Nursing Science, 32*(2), 118–127.

Peter, F. (2004). Health equity and social justice. In S. Anand, F. Peter, & A. Sen (Eds.), *Public health, ethics and equity* (pp. 93–106). New York, NY: Oxford University Press.

Phelan, J., Link, B., & Tehranifar, P. (2010). Social conditions as fundamental causes of health inequalities: Theory, evidence, and policy implications. *Journal of Health and Social Behavior, 51,* S28–S40.

Public Health Agency of Canada. (2007). Canada's response to WHO Commission on the Social Determinants of Health: Glossary. from http://www.phac-aspc.gc.ca/sdh-dss/glos-eng.php

Raphael, D. (2009a). *Social determinants of health: Canadian perspectives* (2nd ed.). Toronto, ON: Canadian Scholars' Press.

Raphael, D. (2009b). Social determinants of health: An overview of key issues and themes. In D. Raphael (Ed.), *Social determinants of health: Canadian perspectives* (2nd ed., pp. 2–19). Toronto, ON: Canadian Scholars' Press.

Raphael, D. (2009c). Social structure, living conditions and health. In D. Raphael (Ed.), *Social determinants of health: Canadian perspectives* (2nd ed., pp. 20–40). Toronto, ON: Canadian Scholars' Press.

Reynoso, J. (2004). Perspectives on intersections of race, ethnicity, gender, and other grounds: Latinas at the margins. *Harvard Latino Law Review, 7,* 63–73.

Rhodes, T. (2002). The 'risk environment': A framework for understanding and reducing drug-related harm. *International Journal of Drug Policy, 13*(2), 85–94.

Rhodes, T., Singer, M., Bourgois, P., Friedman, S. R., & Strathdee, S. A. (2005). The social structural production of HIV risk among injecting drug users. *Social Science and Medicine, 61,* 1026–1044.

Robinson, C. (2005). Grieving home. *Social and Cultural Geography, 6*(1), 47–60.

Shapcott, M. (2009). Housing. In D. Raphael (Ed.), *Social determinants of health: Canadian perspectives* (pp. 201–215). Toronto, ON: Canadian Scholars' Press.

Shaw, M. (2004). Housing and public health. *Annual Review of Public Health, 25,* 397–418.

Shaw, M., Dorling, D., Gordon, D., & Davey Smith, G. (1999). *The widening gap: Health inequalities and policy in Britain.* Bristol, United Kingdom: Bristol Policy Press.

Sherwin, S. (1992). *No longer patient: Feminist ethics & health care.* Philadelphia, PA: Temple University Press.

Sherwin, S. (1998). A relational approach to autonomy in health care. In S. Sherwin & The Feminist Health Care Ethics Research Network (Eds.), *The politics of women's health* (p. 19). Philadelphia, PA: Temple University Press.

Smedley, B. (2012). The lived experience of race and its health consequences. *American Journal of Public Health, 102,* 933–935.

Social Planning and Research Council of British Columbia, Eberle Planning and Research, Jim Wood and Associates, Grave, J., Hathala, K., Campbell, K., . . . Goldberg, M. (2008). *Still on our streets . . . Results of the 2008 Metro Vancouver homeless count.* Vancouver, BC: Greater Vancouver Regional Steering Committee on Homelessness.

Spittal, P., Hogg, R., Li, K., Craib, M., Recsky, C., Johnston, J., . . . Wood, E. (2006). Drastic elevations in mortality among female injection drug users in a Canadian setting. *AIDS Care, 18*(2), 101–108.

Starfield, B., Shi, L., & Macinko, J. (2005). Contribution of primary care to health systems and health. *The Milbank Quarterly, 83*(5), 457–502.

Stephens, C., Nettleton, C., Porter, J., Willis, R., & Clark, S. (2005). Indigenous peoples' health: Why are they behind everyone, everywhere? *The Lancet, 366*(9479), 10–13.

Stevens, P. (1992). Who gets care? Access to health care as an arena for nursing action. *Scholarly Inquiry for Nursing Practice, 6*(3), 185.

Tarasuk, V. (2005). Household food insecurity in Canada. *Topics in Clinical Nutrition, 20*(4), 299–312.

Taylor-Seehafer, M., Jacobvitz, D., & Steiker, L. H. (2008). Patterns of attachment organisation, social connectedness and substance use in a sample of older homeless adolescents. *Family Community Health, 31*(Suppl. 1), S81–S88.

Tomas, A., & Dittmar, H. (1995). The experience of homeless women: An exploration of housing histories and the meaning of home. *Housing Studies, 10*(4), 493–515.

Veenstra, G. (2009). Racialized identity and health in Canada: Results from a nationally representative survey. *Social Science & Medicine, 69*(4), 538–542. doi:10.1016/j.socscimed.2009.06.009

Victoria Coolaid Society. (2007). *Homeless needs survey: Housing first-plus support.* Victoria, BC: Author.

Vozoris, N. T., & Tarasuk, V. S. (2003). Household food insufficiency is associated with poorer health. *The Journal of Nutrition, 133*(1), 120–126.

Waldram, J. B., Herring, A., & Young, T. K. (2006). *Aboriginal health in Canada: Historical, cultural and epidemiological perspectives* (2nd ed.). Toronto, ON: University of Toronto Press.

Wallace, B., Klein, S., & Reitsma-Street, M. (2006). *Denied assistance: Closing the front door on welfare in BC.* Vancouver, BC: Canadian Centre for Policy Alternatives & Vancouver Island Public Interest Research Group.

Wen, C. K., & Hudak, P. L., & Hwang, S. H. (2007). Homeless people's perceptions of welcomeness and unwelcomeness in healthcare encounters. *Journal of General Internal Medicine,* 1011–1017.

Whitehead, M., & Dahlgren, G. (2006). *Concepts and principles for tackling social inequities in health: Levelling up part 1.* Copenhagen, Denmark: World Health Organization.

Wilkinson, R. G., & Pickett, K. (2006). Income inequality and population health: A review and explanation of the evidence. *Social Science & Medicine, 62,* 1768–1784.

Wilkinson, R. G., & Pickett, K. (2010). *The spirit level: Why equality is better for everyone.* Toronto, ON: Penguin Books.

Willows, N. D., Veugelers, P., Raine, K., & Kuhle, S. (2009). Prevalence and sociodemographic risk factors related to household food security in Aboriginal peoples in Canada. *Public Health Nutrition, 12,* 1150–1156.

World Health Organization. (1986). *Ottawa Charter for health promotion.* Retrieved from http://www.who.int/healthpromotion /conferences/previous/ottawa/en

World Health Organization. (2003). *Social determinants of health: The solid facts.* Geneva, Switzerland: Author.

World Health Organization, Commission on Social Determinants of Health. (2008). *Closing the gap in a generation: Health equity through action on the social determinants of health.* Geneva, Switzerland: Author. Retrieved from http://www.who.int/social_determinants /thecommission/finalreport/en/index.html

Wright, N., & Tompkins, C. (2005). *How can health care systems effectively deal with the major health care needs of homeless people?* Copenhagen, Denmark: World Health Organization Regional Office for Europe.

Young, I. M. (1990). *Justice and the politics of difference.* Princeton, NJ: Princeton University Press.

Young, I. M. (2001). Equality of whom? Social groups and judgments of injustice. *The Journal of Political Philosophy, 9*(1), 1–8.

Zierler, S., & Krieger, N. (1997). Reframing women's risk: Social inequalities and HIV infection. *Annual Reviews of Public Health, 18,* 401–436.

chapter 39

Aboriginal People and Nursing

FJOLA HART WASEKEESIKAW AND MICHÈLE PARENT

*S*andra is a first-year student in a baccalaureate nursing education program in Western Canada. During a simulated session for conducting health assessments, her learning scenario is to provide care to an Aboriginal woman. Like her classmates, she is looking forward to providing nursing care in various clinical settings. However, she has some trepidation about caring for Aboriginal people because she knows very little about this population. She asks, "Who are the Aboriginal people in Canada? What do I need to know about them as a nursing student?"

CHAPTER OBJECTIVES

By the end of this chapter, you will be able to:

1. Describe the diversity that exists among the Aboriginal Peoples of Canada.
2. Reflect on and discuss how the treaties and land claims signed between the Aboriginal people and the Government of Canada have established a unique relationship for First Nations, Inuit and Métis, peoples in Canada.
3. Describe the impact of historical Canadian government colonizing practices toward First Nations, Inuit and Métis, peoples and how they affect the contemporary lives of Aboriginal people.
4. Apply learning to improve cultural safety in nursing care to First Nations, Inuit, and Métis individuals, families, and communities.

KEY TERMS

Aboriginal People With a lower case *p* for *people*, refers to more than one Aboriginal person rather than a group; for example, Inuit people.

Aboriginal Peoples A collective name for all of the original peoples of Canada and their descendants. The Constitution Act of 1982 specifies that the Aboriginal Peoples in Canada are composed of three groups—Indian, Inuit, and Métis people.

Assimilation The social process of absorbing one cultural group into another. It is also the process by which language or culture comes to resemble that of another group. It is the cultural domination by another society.

Colonialism The practice where countries such as England ruled nations as colonies and developed trade for the benefit of the ruling country.

Colonization The outcome of a process of colonialism. This included attempts to assimilate Aboriginal Peoples into European lifestyles through force, if necessary. The Indian Act, residential schools, and land alienation processes were all designed to assimilate First Nations people.

Cultural Competence In nursing practice, refers to the development of skills, knowledge, and attitudes among health-care providers in learning about (1) themselves and (2) the contexts that shape experiences of their patients' cultures, health, and accessing health-care services.

Cultural Safety A notion that has arisen out of the history and legacy of colonialism. Nursing's response to this history is the promotion of cultural awareness and sensitivity that seeks to be familiar with respect and nurture the unique and dynamic cultural identities of all individuals and their families. Fundamentally, it is the creation of a safe environment in which the needs, expectations, and rights of individuals and their families are met within unique contexts.

First Nations A term that came into common usage in the 1970s to replace *Indian*, a word many found offensive. Despite its widespread use, there is no legal definition for the term *First Nations* in Canada. It refers to both Status and non-Status Indians. In addition, some have adopted the term *First Nations* to replace the word *band* or *reserve* when identifying their community.

Historical Trauma The cumulative emotional and psychological wounding over the lifespan and across generations emanating from massive group trauma.

Indian People belonging to one of the three groups identified as Aboriginal in the Constitution Act of 1982 in addition to the Inuit and Métis. Also, Indians in Canada may be further categorized as non-Status, Status, and/or Treaty Indians. The term *Indian* is a legal term, and its use in this chapter reflects this.

Indian Act Canadian federal legislation, first passed in 1876, that sets out certain federal government obligations and regulates the management of Indian reserve lands. The act has been amended several times. The Indian Act's most recent amendment was in 1985.

Indigenous Peoples Descendants of those who inhabited a country or a geographical region at the time when people of different cultures or ethnic origins arrived in their lands. The new arrivals became dominant through conquest, occupation, settlement, or other means. The indigenous people of Canada are the Aboriginal people.

Inuit In the Inuit language, *Inuktitut*, the word meaning "people" or "human beings." The Inuit are one of three groups recognized as Aboriginal in the Constitution Act of 1982, along with Indian and Métis.

Kitimakisowin A Cree word that refers to all kinds of poverty. If this is not addressed adequately, then there is risk for serious emotional, mental, physical, and spiritual problems and even death.

Land Claims Also known as *Aboriginal claims* in Canada. There are two types of land claims: comprehensive claims and specific claims. Comprehensive claims always involve land; they deal with the unfinished business of treaty making in Canada. These claims arise in areas of Canada where Aboriginal land rights have not been dealt with by past treaties or through other legal means. The Inuvialuit Final Agreement reached in 1984 is an example of a comprehensive claim. This Agreement is also known as a *modern treaty*. Specific claims, on the other hand, are not necessarily land-related. These claims deal with past grievances of First Nations related to Canada's obligations under historic treaties or the way it managed First Nations' funds or other assets.

Métis One of the three identified groups of Aboriginal Peoples recognized by the Constitution Act of 1982. Historically, the term *Métis* applied to the children of one of the following: French fur trading men and Prairie Cree women, English or Scottish trading men and Dene women, or British men and Inuit women of Newfoundland and Labrador.

Non-Status Indian People who consider themselves Indians or members of First Nations but are not entitled to be registered under the Indian Act. Their ancestors were never registered, or they lost their status under former provisions of the Indian Act. Non-Status Indian people are not entitled to the same rights and benefits available to the Status Indian person.

Status Indian People who are entitled to have their names included on the Indian Registry, an official list maintained by the federal government. Certain criteria determined by the federal government permits which individuals can be registered as a Status Indian. Only Status Indian people are recognized as Indian under the Indian Act and as such are entitled to certain rights and benefits under the law.

Traditional Culture Refers to the knowledge, attitudes, beliefs, customs, and values that are important historically and contemporarily among a particular group of people.

Traditional Territory The lands that have been used for traditional purposes such as hunting and fishing and, usually but not always, have an accompanying map to mark the boundaries.

Treaty Indian A person is also known as a Status Indian who belongs to First Nations that signed a treaty with the Crown. The Dakota people within Manitoba do not have treaties with the Crown; however, their land is considered reserve land under Canada's Indian Act.

Treaty Making Refers to the process that existed for thousands of years and served to build relationships between First Nations. First Nations people made treaties before western European settlements existed in the United States. Even though the ceremony and the items used within the First Nations' treaty-making process may differ from culture to culture, it generally followed the format of introductions, gift giving, time spent getting to know each other, negotiations, and the formalization of the treaty through ceremony such as smoking a pipe. After the ceremony, the treaty would then be seen as a tri-party agreement between the two parties with the Creator as a witness. In Canada, the Royal Proclamation of 1763 provided legal principles for treaty making between the Crown and First Nations. Western Europeans engaged in the treaty-making process in order to establish protocols between First Nations and non-First Nations parties.

Who Are the Aboriginal Peoples of Canada?

What do you think about when you hear the phrase, "Aboriginal Peoples of Canada"? An image of what an Aboriginal person may look like may come to mind. Or, possibly, an impression based on stories you may have read in the local newspapers or seen on television. There are many possible thoughts and images, and these are dependent on your past experiences and access to information.

The **Aboriginal Peoples** of Canada are diverse. The term *Aboriginal Peoples* is the collective name for all of the original people of Canada and their descendants. The Constitution Act of 1982 specifies that the Aboriginal Peoples in Canada are composed of three groups—Indian, Inuit, and Métis people. There are more than 50 Aboriginal languages, over 600 reserves, hundreds of Métis and Inuit communities, and thousands of Aboriginal people living in towns and cities in Canada. However, when all the people are lumped together under the term *Aboriginal*, how they see and interpret the world, the beliefs they hold, and their health and healing practices are homogenized; that is, the great diversity among people disappears, and the expectations and impressions of a people emerge.

This chapter introduces you to basic information that registered nurses require as they develop their competence in providing culturally safe care to Aboriginal individuals, families, and communities. Moreover, you are offered basic guidance to foster your development of respectful nursing practice when caring for Aboriginal patients. This basic information is foundational to the provision of competent care; however, this information does not constitute culturally safe care in of itself.

The Aboriginal Peoples of Canada

The Canadian Constitution Act of 1982 legally recognizes three distinct indigenous groups—the Indian people, Inuit, and Métis—as the Aboriginal Peoples of Canada. This Act also recognized and affirmed Aboriginal and treaty rights. Each of these groups will be briefly introduced to assist you in developing a basic understanding of the current demographics of Aboriginal people both regionally and nationally.

The First Nations of Canada

The **First Nations** are the descendants of the original inhabitants of Canada. First Nations people or **Indians** as noted in the Canadian Constitution Act of 1982 are generally registered under Canada's **Indian Act**. The term *Indian* is a legal term, and its usage is reflected accordingly in this chapter. The Indian Act is Canadian federal legislation, first passed in 1876, that sets out certain federal government obligations and regulates the management of Indian reserve lands. The act has been amended several times with its most recent amendment completed in 1985. The act has resulted in **status** (or **treaty Indians**) and **non-status** Indians. Indian people may live on-reserve or off-reserve in rural or urban areas. There are 615 reserves in Canada, and these are generally situated within the First Nations peoples' traditional territories. To get an idea about the number and location of First Nations in a specific province or territory, the Assembly of First Nations provides a listing of its organizations on their website. Internet links to each of the First Nations political organizations can provide access to listing of First Nations or communities within that region. In addition, some of these organizations provide maps of their traditional territories. For example, the Algonquin Nation of Ontario displays a map of their traditional territory on their website. It is important to note that many of their members reside in Ottawa and other cities in the area.

According to the 2011 Canadian Census, nearly one half (49.3%) of the First Nations total population resides on reserves and settlements (Statistics Canada, 2011). However, since some First Nations did not participate in the enumeration process, this information is considered an estimate. Over one half (55.5%) of the First Nations population in Canada reside in Ontario (23.6%), British Columbia (18.2%), and Alberta (13.7%). However, it is important to note that First Nations people living in these three provinces accounted for less than 4% of the population in each of these provinces. It is also important to notice that First Nations people represented the largest portion of the total population of the Northwest Territories, followed by Yukon, Manitoba, and Saskatchewan (Statistics Canada, 2011). First Nations people accounted for almost one third of the total population of the Northwest Territories, close to one fifth of the total population of Yukon and about 10% of the population of Manitoba and that of Saskatchewan.

The Inuit of Canada

For more than 4,000 years, the **Inuit**, a founding people of what is now Canada, have occupied the Arctic land and waters from the Mackenzie Delta in the west to the Labrador coast in the east and from the Hudson's Bay coast to the islands of the High Arctic. There are 59,000 Inuit in Canada, living mainly in 53 Inuit communities spread out over four Inuit regions: Inuvialuit Settlement Region (Northwest Territories), Nunavut, Nunavik (Northern Quebec), and Nunatsiavut (Northern Labrador). These four regions are collectively known as *Inuit Nunangat*. The term *Inuit Nunangat* is a Canadian Inuit term that includes land, water, and ice. Inuit consider the land, water, and ice of their homeland to be integral to their culture and way of life. In the language of the Inuit, Inuktitut, the word *Inuit* means the people or human beings. The Inuit are one of three groups recognized as Aboriginal in the Constitution Act of 1982, along with Indian and Métis.

Nunavut has the largest Inuit population in Nunangat with 43,460 residents (Statistics Canada, 2011). Nunavik has the second highest Inuit population with 10,750 Inuit people including those living in Chisasibi, a community located outside Nunavik territory. Inuvialuit Settlement Region has 3,310 Inuvialuit residents, and Nunatsiavut has 2,325 Inuit residents. The Inuit Tapiriit Kanatami is the national voice for the Inuit in these regions, providing links to each region's Inuit **land claim** organization offices.

The Métis of Canada

In 2002, the Métis National Council (MNC) developed the definition of **Métis** nation, meaning the Aboriginal people descended from the historic Métis nation, which is now composed of all Métis nation citizens and is one of the Aboriginal Peoples of Canada in the Constitution Act of 1982. Specifically, a Métis is a person who self-identifies as Métis, is of historic Métis nation ancestry, is distinct from other Aboriginal Peoples, and is accepted by the Métis nation. The Métis Nation's Homeland is based on the traditional territory on which the Métis people have historically lived in North America. This territory roughly includes the three prairie provinces—Manitoba, Alberta, and Saskatchewan; parts of Ontario, British Columbia, and the Northwest Territories; as well as parts of the northern United States (i.e., North Dakota, Montana).

According to Statistics Canada (2011), of those who stated that they were Métis (and note that this is different from the MNC definition of Métis), the majority (84.9%) live in the western provinces and Ontario. Another way of relating this same information is to rank the provinces—Alberta has the largest Métis population with 21.4%. This is followed by Ontario (19%), Manitoba (17.4%), British Columbia (15.4%), and Saskatchewan (11.6%). In addition, 9.1% of Métis live in Quebec, 5.1% in the Atlantic provinces, and 1% in the territories.

Twenty-five percent of Canadian Métis live in four western census metropolitan areas. Of these, Winnipeg has the highest Métis population in Canada, which is about 46,325. It is followed by Edmonton with 31,780, Vancouver with 18,485, and Calgary with 17,520. Also, 11,520 Métis live in Saskatoon. The rest reside in smaller urban centres with populations under 100,000. In addition, some of the Métis people reside on Métis settlements.

The MNC has a website that provides an Internet link to each of the Métis governments; the Métis Nation of Ontario, Manitoba Métis Federation, Métis Nation Saskatchewan, the Métis Nation of Alberta, and the Métis British Columbia Nation. Explore these websites for information about the regional locations of the Métis populations. For example, the Métis Nation of Alberta provides a listing of settlements. The Aboriginal Relations Government of Alberta has a website that shows the settlements on a map. Develop a basic understanding of current demographics of Aboriginal Peoples in the province or territory in which you are practicing nursing.

Language and Geographic Territories

The diversity of the Aboriginal Peoples of Canada originates with their ancestral language groups and traditional geographic territories. They are descendants from the original inhabitants of the land that is now known as *Canada*.

Traditional territory refers to the geographic area including land, water, and ice identified by a First Nations, Inuit, or Métis community on which they or their ancestors resided. The original residents were among the **indigenous peoples** of the United States who lived on this continent long before the Europeans arrived in the 1500s (Dickason, 2006). It has been estimated that there were flourishing indigenous communities dating from 14,000 years or more before our present day. Across North America, the indigenous peoples hunted, fished, produced tools and weapons, and gathered seasonally available food on land, water, and ice that would become known today as traditional territories. The geography of these traditional areas determined daily living customs, creating strong bonds between the tribal cultures and the lands. At the time when the Europeans arrived, there were thousands of tribes or bands of indigenous peoples residing in the United States. Estimates of the indigenous populations vary between 4,000,000 and 5,000,000 individuals in North America. The indigenous peoples were great travelers too. They travelled far and wide communicating and conversing in at least 50 to 60 distinct languages and dialects. Even though there was tremendous geographical distance between indigenous peoples' traditional territories, for the most part, their cultures, values and beliefs, and ways of living were very similar. Indeed, the diverse geographical locations favored an abundance of resources in one area, which could then be traded with other indigenous peoples who lacked or desired certain foods and natural resources. There were already well established transportation and communications routes in existence via the rivers and waterways, which would later be used by the European fur traders and explorers who came to the Canadian shores in the late 1500s and 1600s. The indigenous peoples' attitude about the land was to live in harmony with it—the land was there for the livelihood and sustenance of all human beings and animals (Box 39.1). This was in stark contrast to that of European attitudes where land ownership prevailed along with the expectation of exploitation of all the land's natural resources. The term *indigenous peoples* is used to describe the descendants of those who inhabited a country or a geographical region at the time when people of different cultures or ethnic origins arrived in their lands. The indigenous people of Canada are the Aboriginal people.

There are 11 ancestral language groups. Ten are First Nations and one is Inuit. These groups are Algonkian, Athapaskan, Inuit, Haidan, Iroquoian, Kutenaian, Salishan, Siouan, Tlingit, Tsimshian, and Wakashan. It is within these major groupings that about 59 ancestral languages are situated. In addition to the First Nations and Inuit languages, the Métis language is Michif. There are three dialects of

---

BOX 39.1 The People of Inuit Nunangat

The Inuit have a 5,000-year cultural heritage that has been sustained within Arctic territory marked by the eastern coast of present day Russia, across Alaska, and Canada to the east coast of Greenland. The Canadian territory known as Inuit Nunangat stretches about 2,800 km from west to east and crosses over four time zones. It extends roughly from the tree line in the south and about 3,000 km north.

Inuit Nunangat is large (i.e., approximately 6,000,000 km^2), and it is diverse with many different landscapes, seascapes, climatic zones, and ecological systems. It is important to the Inuit that it is understood that their territory encompasses the sea and the sea ice and fresh water lakes and rivers in addition to the land. The diversity of the land and sea has had and continues to have great influence on their cultural groups' heritage and language. The strength and vitality of Inuit culture in Canada is anchored to their capacity to use the environments and harvest the wildlife resources from the sea, land, and fresh water.

Source: Inuulitsivik Health Centre. (n.d.). *Northern life and Inuit culture.* Retrieved from http://www.inuulitsivik.ca/northern-life-and-inuit-culture

---

Michif in Canada. For example, Cree is most often spoken among the Métis in Canada who converse in an Aboriginal language. They also speak Dene, Ojibwa, and other Algonkian languages.

Become familiar with the traditional geographic territories and language groups of Aboriginal Peoples in the region in which you practice nursing. It is important that this understanding come from the perspective of the Aboriginal people. Consult individual First Nations and Inuit government offices' websites to obtain information about the languages spoken within a given region. For example, the first language of the people at Wasagamack First Nations in northern Manitoba Island Lake area is Oji-Cree. For another example, there are three dialects of Inuvialuktun spoken by the Inuvialuit: Uummarmiut, Siglit, and Kangiryuarmiut (Box 39.2).

BOX 39.2 Do You Speak Any of the Aboriginal Languages?

Actually you do! Here are a few of the adopted First Nations' place names for locations and regions across Canada:

Canada, adopted from the term *Kanata*, and means "settlement" or "village"

Etobicoke is the Ojibwa term designating "the place where the alders grow"

Ontario, a Huron term denotes "beautiful lake"

Manitoba, a Cree term means "the strait of the spirit or manitobau"

Nunavut is the Inuktitut term for "our land"

Quebec is an Algonkian word for "narrow passage"

Saskatchewan is the Cree term for "swift flowing river"

How might Sandra feel after having learned that her patient in the simulated session is from Berens River First Nations? What kind of information she might gather from the Internet knowing the patient's place of residence? Berens River First Nations is an Ojibway community in northern Manitoba that is accessible by winter road, boat, and airplane. How might she incorporate this information as she continues on with her patient assessment? Consider how Sandra might feel if her patient case scenario only stated that her patient was Aboriginal.

Relationship Between the Aboriginal People and the Government of Canada

Treaties were foundational to the indigenous people. They created mutually beneficial alliances with each other. These alliances established relationships among them, which included trade, safe passage through territories, peace and friendship, and other obligations and responsibilities. **Treaty making** was instrumental among the Aboriginal Peoples long before the Europeans arrived and was done to establish peace, regulate trade, share land and resources, and arrange mutual defense. Treaty making among the Europeans had a different meaning; it served to recognize independence, claim sovereignty, and formally marked mutual respect (Box 39.3).

The first treaties that indigenous people entered with the British Crown (in what is now known as Canada) were peaceful and relationship-building by design. The relationship between the Government of Canada and the Aboriginal Peoples of Canada is rooted in the historical treaties, which were based on mutual intent by the First Peoples and the newcomers (Royal Commission on Aboriginal Peoples [RCAP], 1996). The treaties reveal the relationship between the indigenous people and the newcomers.

The Royal Proclamation of 1763 was a significant document between the Aboriginal Peoples and non-Aboriginal people. This arrangement permitted Aboriginal and non-Aboriginal

BOX 39.3 Canadians Are Treaty People

Did you know that Canadians are also treaty people? There is a misconception that only First Nations peoples are part of the treaties. However, in reality, Canadians are also part of treaty. The treaties laid the foundation so that Canadians could enjoy the benefits of living in this country, such as owning a home. Consistent with all treaties, both First Nations peoples and Canadians have obligations in honouring these treaties. See the Office of the Treaty Commissioner short video at http://www.otc.ca/WE_ARE_ALL_TREATY_PEOPLE/. See also James Wilson, Commissioner of the Treaty Relations Commission of Manitoba at http://www.winnipegfreepress.com/opion/westview/in-canada-we-are-all-treaty-people-155890525.html

BOX 39.4 Treaty Making between Aboriginal Peoples and Canada

Treaty making between Aboriginal Peoples and Canada continues today. The James Bay and Northern Quebec Agreement, signed in 1975, was the first modern land claims agreement. Since then, 21 modern treaties have been signed. These include the Inuvialuit Final Agreement, June 1984; Nunavut Land Claims Agreement, May 1993; Sahtu Dene and Métis Comprehensive Land Agreement, September 1993; and the Tsawwassen First Nations Final Agreement, March 2009. The Land Claims Agreements Coalition has a website that provides a schedule of the modern land claim agreements and a map showing the geographic areas in Canada in which the modern treaties are in effect.

people to divide and share sovereignty rights to the lands of Canada. It was more than 100 years later, in 1867, when the first confederal agreement with the First Nations would allow for power sharing among diverse peoples and governments. Additional treaties, including those known as the *numbered treaties*, between the First Nations and the newcomers created mutually binding obligations between two or more nations of peoples. These historical treaties demonstrate the unique relationship between the Aboriginal Peoples of Canada and the Government of Canada (representative of the Queen of England). No other population in Canada has this status—historical or contemporary (Dickson & McNab, 2009). In addition to historical treaties, First Nations, Inuit and Métis, people continue to make treaties with Canada. These are called *contemporary treaties* (Box 39.4).

Assimilation and Colonization

In the 1800s, the treaties between Aboriginal and non-Aboriginal governments were undermined by policies and **colonization** practices intended to remove Aboriginal people from their lands, suppress Aboriginal nations and their governments, undermine Aboriginal cultures, and stifle Aboriginal identity (RCAP, 1996). The Indian Act, residential schools, relocation of communities, and reserve policy were specific strategies to assimilate. **Assimilation** is the social process of absorbing one cultural group into another. It also includes the process by which language or culture comes to resemble that of another group. It is the cultural domination by another society. Become familiar with the range of Canadian colonization processes used over the centuries because **colonialism** is one of the social determinants of Aboriginal Peoples' health (Loppie Reading & Wien, 2009).

Residential Schools

The first Indian residential schools were established in Canada in the 1620s. The federal government viewed residential schools as being essential for assimilating indigenous people. By 1874, the Canadian government began removing First Nations children from their families and communities and placing them in Indian residential schools (Frideres, 2011, p. 58). Children were forbidden to speak their first language and practice their cultural traditions. Many were emotionally, physically, and sexually abused by the clergy. The dramatic effect of Indian residential schools on children and their families included the following:

- Loss or disruption of language;
- Suppression of spiritual practices and beliefs;
- Suppression of culture through enforced changes in daily living routines including diet, play, contributions to family living (i.e., setting up trap lines), personal grooming, and clothing practices; and
- Disruption of families through placement in distant schools with no home visits allowed.

It was believed that by learning English and adopting Christianity and White settler customs, new non-Aboriginal lifestyles would be passed on to the next generation and after a generation or two would leave First Nations cultures in its wake. However, this was not the case. Rather, the legacy of Indian residential schools became one of pain and suffering for the survivors of residential schools and intergenerational trauma for indigenous people (Box 39.5).

The Legacy of Historical Trauma

As the result of colonization processes, many Aboriginal people are survivors of historic trauma, which include traumas within and beyond their lifespan. "**Historical trauma** is cumulative emotional and psychological wounding over the lifespan and across generations, emanating from massive group trauma" (Brave Heart, 2003, p. 7; Brave Heart, Chase, Elkins, & Altschul, 2011). Historical unresolved grief is the multifaceted response to loss that accompanies trauma. Aboriginal people have experienced many losses as result of massive group trauma because of colonial policies, including the following:

- Loss of culture,
- Loss of language,
- Loss of heritage,
- Loss of identity,
- Loss of parenting skills,
- Intergenerational family violence,
- Loss of land and livelihood, and
- Loss of autonomy and self-determination.

Wesley-Esquimaux and Smolewski (2004) describe historic trauma as "a cluster of traumatic events" and as "a causal factor operating in many different areas of impact" (p. 65). These traumatic events remain as hidden collective memories of trauma or a collective non-remembering that is passed from generation to generation. In addition, historic trauma disrupts adaptive social and cultural patterns and changes them into maladaptive ones that exhibit in symptoms. Similar to the hidden collective memories of trauma, symptoms may be passed from generation to generation. Symptoms that parents exhibit (e.g., family violence) act to traumatize and disrupt adaptive social adjustments in children. Children internalize symptoms, in turn taking on the behaviours of their parents, and the trauma continues onto the next generation. It is important to note that there is no single historical trauma response, yet equally important, not every First Nations, Inuit or Métis, person is overwhelmed by historic trauma.

BOX 39.5   The Removal of Aboriginal Children

The *Sixties Scoop* is a term coined by Patrick Johnston in his 1953 report, *Native Children and the Child Welfare System*, refers to the practice of fostering or adopting out Aboriginal children, usually into white families. During the 1960s and 1970s, as fewer Aboriginal children were being sent to residential school, the provincial and federal child welfare systems emerged as the new method of colonization. Child welfare workers removed Aboriginal children from their families and communities that were deemed unfit and placed them into non-Aboriginal homes located within the same or a different province, sometimes in other countries. In 1983, the Canadian Council on Social Development completed a statistical overview of Aboriginal children in the care of child welfare authorities across Canada. It found that Aboriginal children were highly overrepresented in the child welfare system as the result of the Sixties Scoop. Aboriginal children were 4.5 times more likely than non-Aboriginal children to be in the care of child welfare authorities.

Source: Aboriginal Justice Implementation Commission. (n.d.). *Justice System and Aboriginal People.* Retrieved from http://www.ajic.mb.ca /volume/shapter14.html

Kitimakisowin

Kitimakisowin is a Cree concept that aptly describes the devastating effects of colonization on First Nations, Inuit, and Métis peoples. **Kitimakisowin** refers to all kinds of poverty, and if these are not addressed adequately, there is risk for serious emotional, mental, physical, and spiritual problems and even death (Aboriginal Nurses Association of Canada, 2001; Dion Stout & Jodoin, 2006). Five areas of kitimakisowin include the following:

- The poverty of participation as result of marginalization
- The poverty of understanding as result of poor education
- The poverty of affection resulting from the lack of support and recognition
- The poverty of subsistence as result of inadequate resources
- The poverty of identity given the imposition of alien values, beliefs, and systems on local and regional cultures

Historical trauma, unresolved historical grief, and intergenerational posttraumatic stress disorder are also used to describe the effects of colonization on Aboriginal people (McCormick, 2009).

Is Colonization Over?

Is colonization over and now past history? Essentially no; however, many First Nations are working their way to overcome the effects of colonization. It is a challenge, if not impossible, to overcome the oppression that is the legacy of colonization because it continues well into 21st century Canada. Even though Prime Minister Harper offered an apology in the House of Commons on June 11, 2008, on behalf of Canadians for the Indian residential schools system, this does not mean that the government systemic prejudice toward Aboriginal people has changed. For example, one of the first acts of the Conservative Government when it took office in 2006 was to set aside the recently signed Kelowna Accord that sought to establish a new relationship between government and the First Nations (Frideres, 2011). Although Prime Minister Paul Martin endorsed the Kelowna Accord, it was not implemented because the liberal government was subsequently defeated in February 2006. Another example where the opportunity to change the relationship between government and First Nations people was the Royal Commission on Aboriginal Peoples. The commission spent 5 years conducting research and consulting with Aboriginal and non-Aboriginal Canadians and received recommendations on how the federal government might change its relationship with First Nations people. Unfortunately, nearly all of the recommendations were rejected or ignored.

Think   One of your nursing study group friends states, "I am tired of hearing about the woes of residential school. I wish they would just get over it. I was not even born when residential schools existed." Even though you quickly note that the last residential school closed in 1996, you do not say anything. Rather, you pause to consider your colleague's words. You reflect that colonizing practices are a part of Canadian history that has been essentially hidden, until recently, from the view of the general Canadian population.

Through the eyes of a student

I had no idea that there was so much to learn about First Nations, Inuit and Métis, people. For example, I did not know about the unique status that Aboriginal people have in Canada. When I was in school, the history we took was from the view of the non-Aboriginal historian. As result, I did not see that Aboriginal people were part of Canadian history; they were largely absent from my view. I am not certain though how knowing First Nations, Inuit and Métis, history will affect the nursing care I provide if I have an Aboriginal patient.

(personal reflection of a first-year nursing student)

Aboriginal Peoples of Canada in the Present Day

According to Canada's most recent census of 2011, over 1 million individuals have identified as an Aboriginal person (1,400,685), thus comprising 4.3% of Canada's total population. Figure 39.1 shows the trend in population who have indicated they are Aboriginal during the period from 1901 to 2006.

Aboriginal populations have increased by 20.1% between 2006 and 2011 compared to 5.2% for non-Aboriginal populations (Statistics Canada, 2011). Aboriginal children aged 14 years and younger represented over one quarter (28%) of all the Aboriginal population in Canada, and they comprised 7% of all children in Canada. Aboriginal youth from ages 15 years to 24 years comprised 18.2% of the total Aboriginal population and 5.9% of all youth in Canada. In comparison, non-Aboriginal youth comprised 12.9% of non-Aboriginal population. There are close to 4 million non-Aboriginal youth in Canada (Fig. 39.2).

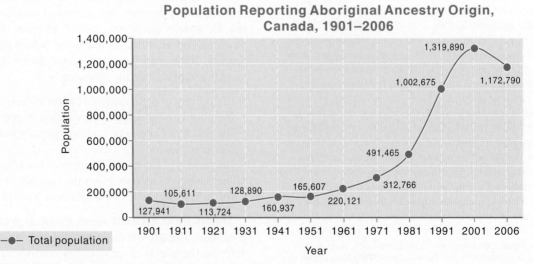

Figure 39.1 Trend in Aboriginal ancestry.

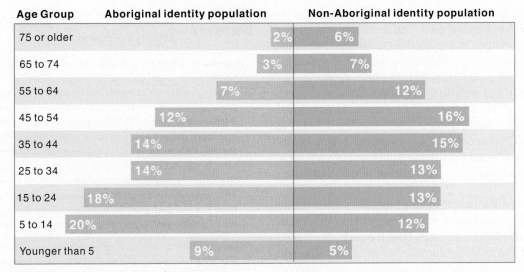

Age Group	Aboriginal identity population	Non-Aboriginal identity population
75 or older	2%	6%
65 to 74	3%	7%
55 to 64	7%	12%
45 to 54	12%	16%
35 to 44	14%	15%
25 to 34	14%	13%
15 to 24	18%	13%
5 to 14	20%	12%
Younger than 5	9%	5%

Figure 39.2 Aboriginal identity by age group.

Most significant is that Aboriginal populations are increasingly urban, with 54% of the population residing in urban centres. The city of Winnipeg (Manitoba) has the highest number of Aboriginal people followed by Edmonton (Alberta) and Vancouver (British Columbia). Other urban centres with large Aboriginal populations include Toronto (Ontario), Calgary (Alberta), Saskatoon (Saskatchewan), and Regina (Saskatchewan). There are also smaller urban centres with large Aboriginal populations such as Thompson (Manitoba), Prince Rupert (British Columbia), and Prince Albert (Saskatchewan).

Recent Trends

Why are there so many Aboriginal people now residing in urban centres? The 2011 Canadian census data indicates that almost one half of First Nations live off-reserve. There are various reasons for this current trend, especially among the First Nations peoples who are migrating to cities from their reserve or rural communities. This urban migration is the result of lack of opportunities for education and employment, an attempt to improve their overall living conditions and socioeconomic status, the need for better health-care services, and the need for better housing as a consequence of inadequate housing in their home communities. According to the Urban Aboriginal Peoples Study (Environics Institute, 2010), the leading life aspiration of urban Aboriginal people today is pursuing higher education. This is especially so for those who are younger and less affluent. Aboriginal people see higher education as a path to a good job or career for their own and future generations. Aboriginal women are more likely to migrate to larger municipalities seeking more opportunities for employment and education and after a marital breakdown and spousal abuse or violence. However, even though Aboriginal Peoples are migrating to urban centres with the hope of improving their lifestyle and thus their health, they are at risk for experiencing racism, prejudice, poverty, and marginalization. Young urban Aboriginal women are at extremely high risk for sexual exploitation and violence (Box 39.6).

Health disparities exist between the First Nations peoples who live off-reserve when compared to those who live on-reserve. There is more First Nations people on-reserve than off-reserve who report they have diabetes and high blood pressure and who are smokers. Overall, the data suggests that Aboriginal Peoples living off-reserve experience better health and a well-being than individuals living on-reserve. For more detailed information, read the national health survey of on-reserve communities, *First Nations Regional Health Survey (RHS) 2008/10 National Report on Adults, Youth and Children Living in First Nations Communities* at the First Nations Information Governance Centre website.

What Are the Determinants of Health for Aboriginal People?

Determinants of health are essentially factors that contribute to the health of a population. These factors are identified within several frameworks that offer differing approaches to health and well-being (Wilson & Rosenberg, 2002).

BOX 39.6 Missing and Murdered Aboriginal Women

According to the Native Women's Association of Canada, 582 occurrences of missing or murdered Aboriginal women and girls have occurred primarily within the last three decades. Racist and sexist stereotypes deny the dignity and worth of indigenous women, encouraging some men to feel they can get away with violent acts of hatred against them. At the 2013 National Forum on Community Safety and Ending Violence, the assembly called for a national inquiry and an action plan. Their recommendations, acknowledging these are important matters for all Canadians, included change through unity among indigenous peoples; improved focus on creating safe homes and communities through prevention and personal responsibility; engagement of men in actively preventing violence; and greater awareness throughout society.

Some of these factors include the physical and social environments, biologic endowment, and access to and quality of health care. Other factors include social and individual dimensions where social conditioning and the interrelationship dynamics of social status and class have significant impacts on health and well-being. The literature also explores determinants of health frameworks specific to Aboriginal people (Loppie Reading & Wien, 2009; Reading, Kmetic, & Gideon, 2007). Determinants of Aboriginal health frameworks tend to be used for striving equity and as such serve as a means to achieving equality in the health of the Aboriginal population.

Aboriginal people have lower life expectancy rates, higher infant mortality rates, lower incomes and educational levels, and higher unemployment rates. Health outcomes statistics are of concern to nursing education, practice, and research. However, when using these frameworks in their practice, nurses need to be mindful because there may be a tendency to view Aboriginal people as "disadvantaged, impoverished, and/or unemployed." According to the *First Nations Regional Health Survey (RHS) 2008/10: National report on adults, youth and children living in First Nations communities*, traditional culture affects the health and well-being of a population (First Nations Information Governance Centre, 2012).

Traditional Culture

In general, **traditional culture** refers to the knowledge, attitudes, beliefs, customs, and values that are important historically and contemporarily among a particular group of people. Traditional teachings or ways may be expressed, for example, through art, ceremonies, dances, fishing, hunting, preparation of (i.e., drying and smoking fish) and eating traditional foods, games, songs, and stories. Cultural traditions tend to be carried out by elders, traditional healers, and other persons designated by the community. There are some key points about First Nations people and traditional cultures. First, despite the negative effect of assimilation has had on First Nations people and their traditional cultures, many aspects of their traditional cultures continue to thrive. Second, First Nations people who participate in traditional culture can take many forms including attending community cultural events, visiting a traditional healer, speaking or understanding a First Nations language, or valuing traditional spirituality. Third, there is an association between First Nations people's participation in traditional culture with many benefits, including greater perceived control over one's life, greater spiritual balance, less substance use and abuse, and less depression. It is also noteworthy that urban Aboriginal people face challenges to their cultural identity, which include discrimination and racism, exclusion from opportunities for self-determination, and difficulty finding culturally appropriate health services. Subsequently, it is important for nurses to know that cultural traditions can influence the health of Aboriginal people in Canada. See Box 39.7 for two examples where traditional cultural practices have influenced children and young adults in making choices that affect their health.

BOX 39.7 How Can "Culture" Influence Healthy Lifestyle Choices?

Example #1: There is a high rate of smoking among Aboriginal youth, and it is well documented that individuals who begin smoking earlier are at higher risk for a range of mental and physical health issues across the lifespan. In a pilot study (McKennitt & Currie, 2012), there was significant reduction in intentions to smoke among Aboriginal children who received the culturally sensitive smoking prevention program. The small sample size did not allow a direct comparison of the efficacy of the culturally sensitive and standard programs. However, the findings suggested a smoking prevention program that has been culturally adapted for Aboriginal children might reduce future smoking intentions among Aboriginal grade 4 students.

Example #2: Illicit and prescription drug use disorders are two to four times more prevalent among Aboriginal people in North America than the general population (Currie, Wild, Schopflocher, Laing, & Veugelers, 2013). The results showed that cultural participation was a protective factor associated with reduced illicit and prescription drug problems. Increased self-esteem partially explained the effect of cultural participation by Aboriginal adults. As result of their findings, these authors advise the encouragement of programs and services that support Aboriginal people who strive to maintain their cultural traditions within cities.

Source: Currie, D. L., Wild, T. C., Schopflocher, D. P., Laing, L., & Veugelers, P. (2013). Illicit and prescription drug problems among urban Aboriginal adults in Canada: The role of traditional culture in protection and resilience. *Social Science and Medicine, 86*, 1–9; McKennitt, D. W., & Currie, C. L. (2012). Does a culturally sensitive smoking prevention program reduce smoking intentions among Aboriginal children? A pilot study. *American Indian and Alaska Native Mental Health Research, 19*(2). Retrieved from http://www.metiscentreresearch.ca/articles/does-culturally-sensitive-smoking-prevention-program-reduce-smoking-intentions-among-aborig

---

The Strength of Aboriginal People

It may be considered remarkable that Aboriginal people have maintained their identities despite government-imposed assimilative practices. Their strength came in the form of resistance to these practices, resilience against harsh conditions, and reclaiming of cultural traditions and language.

Resistance

Even though there was concerted effort by the Government of Canada to assimilate Aboriginal people into general society, First Nations, Inuit and Métis, people have and continue to resist assimilation. What forms has this resistance taken? According to the RCAP (1996), the relationship between First Nations and Canada shifted with the government's White Paper 1969. This document proposed to abolish the Indian Act and the special relationship that Canada had with the First Nations people. First Nations were unanimous in their rejection of this proposition because it would mean the end of their existence as distinct peoples. First Nations, Inuit and Métis, people studied their history and found that they have rights arising from the spirit and intent of their treaties and the Royal Proclamation of 1763 and took heart from decisions of the Canadian courts (most of which were from 1971), affirming their special relationship with the Crown and their unique interest in the traditional lands. First Nations, Inuit and Métis, set about beginning to rebuild their communities and their nations with newfound purpose.

The roots of resistance among Aboriginal people were present before 1969 when the White Paper was introduced. Dion Stout and Kipling (2003), in describing residential school survivor experiences, relate that acts of individual or collective resistance took many forms. Resistance served the purpose of giving a sense of control over one's surroundings and solidarity with others who were also resisting (p. 45). It provided children with a way of registering their opposition to an oppressive system, even if they realized they were not powerful enough to confront it directly. Dion Stout and Kipling (2003) describe food theft as one of the most frequently cited acts of resistance. The meals provided by school staff often left the children feeling hungry, so stealing foodstuffs such as fruit, bread, and meat from the kitchens and pantries was considered, by the children, a matter of necessity. These activities involved elaborate planning and provided students with an opportunity to work together in pursuit of a common cause. Equally interesting is that food stolen in this way was generally shared with smaller children who were too young to take part in the planned operation. The stealing of food was one of many forms of resistance used by residential schoolchildren. Among the coping strategies used by residential school survivors, resistance is cited as similar to the flexible, problem-solving behaviours and hallmarks of a resilient person (Box 39.8).

BOX 39.8 Three Generations of Resilience

Resilience is a digital story by Roberta Stout. A digital story is described on the Prairie Women's Health Centre of Excellence (PWHCE) website as a 2 to 5 minute video, a personal narrative coupled with a collection of still images, video, and music used to illustrate an individual's story. In her story, Stout talks about how resilience is being passed through three generations in her family—from her mother, a residential school survivor, to her own child. *Resilience* is one of six digital stories in the kiskino mâto tapanâsk (a Plains Cree phrase that means "the crying wagon/school bus") series, Intergenerational Effects on Professional First Nations Women Whose Mothers are Residential School Survivors. In this research project, six First Nations women share their stories, in their own words, of their understanding of how they had been impacted by the schools. Their stories speak of the emotional and healing journeys of mothers and daughters. To see the videos go to the PWHCE website under the section, "Digital Stories—First Nations Women Explore the Legacy of Residential Schools."

The impetus for the Idle No More movement is in centuries old resistance as indigenous nations and their lands suffered the impacts of exploration, invasion and colonization (Idle No More, 2012). The Idle No More events seek to assert indigenous inherent rights to sovereignty and reinstitute traditional indigenous laws and the treaties by protecting the lands and waters from corporate destruction.

Resilience

Resilience is a concept used to explain or understand positive adaptation to life despite harsh conditions (Fleming & Ledogar, 2008). Early models of resilience focused on individuals; however, there is ongoing research to find models that reflect resilience at multiple levels of the Aboriginal individual, family, community, and culture (Fast & Collin-Vézina, 2010). Resilience is passed from one generation to another.

Indigenous peoples' stories are intellectual traditions that can disrupt colonial narratives of history, recognize injustice, celebrate resistance, and envision the future. Researchers and communities are increasingly recognizing the healing properties of visual and narrative approaches (see Box 39.8). Reclaiming is one of the characteristics of resilience.

Reclaiming

First Nations, Inuit and Métis, people have experienced much loss through colonization; however, they have set about reclaiming their identity, language, and culture. Indigenous languages are the medium for the transmission and survival of indigenous consciousness, cultures literature, histories, religions, political institutions, and values. The reclaiming of indigenous language began in the early 1970s when First Nations people embarked on taking control of Indian education. "Indian control of Indian education" was based on parents wanting their children to participate fully in Canadian society while developing their personal and community potential through fully actualized linguistic and cultural identity from within their own indigenous contexts. This goal suggests the relationship between indigenous language usage and reclaiming identity as well as the relationship between indigenous language and relating knowledge within an indigenous cultural context. In the digital story *Resilience* (refer to Box 39.8), Roberta Stout talks about how she reclaimed her Cree language and identity. Some First Nations, Inuit and Métis, people have maintained their primary language, whereas others are striving to regain theirs. There are still other Aboriginal people whose primary language is English or French.

What Health Services Are Available to Aboriginal People in Canada?

There are various health services available to Aboriginal people in Canada, some of which are located on reserve land in rural and remote and isolated communities. Other services are provided in urban settings.

Health Canada

The Federal Indian Health Policy was developed in recognition of the federal government legal and traditional responsibilities to Indians (Box 39.9). Basic to this policy is the preservation and enhancement of First Nations' cultures and traditions. Health Canada through First Nations and Inuit Health provides nursing services in First Nations south of the 60th parallel in rural, remote, and isolated communities. Health Canada documents 76 nursing stations and more than 195 health centres serving more than 600 First Nations communities across Canada. Registered nurses working in these settings collaborate with a team of health-care professionals and health workers at the local community health service system. In about one half of the health facilities, nurses are employed by First Nations band councils, where First Nations have entered into agreements with Health Canada so they can administer their own health services.

Even though health centres and nursing stations are located on reserves, there are differences between them. Health centres are generally located in the rural parts of Canada, and nursing stations are located in remote, isolated, and semi-isolated Aboriginal communities. Nursing stations generally provide primary health care, public health, emergency, and treatment services; they attend to all medical emergencies and ready to patient for medical evacuation, if warranted. Nursing services at the nursing station is provided within an expanded scope of nursing practice on a 24-hour, 7 days a week basis. Because there are no physicians located at nursing stations, nurses can communicate via telephone with medical personnel located at larger tertiary centres.

Nursing Stations

Nursing stations are located in remote and isolated communities south of the 60th parallel. Registered nurses in this setting use the primary health-care model approach to common health problems across the lifespan. Health assessments, treatment, and emergency services are provided, and comprehensive health promotion/disease prevention programs are delivered. An example of services provided by the Webequie First Nations nursing station can be found in Box 39.10.

Health Centres

Health centres are located in First Nations communities in rural areas of Canada. Registered nurses in this setting work with community members to identify health priorities and plan programs to address these needs. Based on public health principles, nurses participate in the provision of a full range of community health programs with emphasis on health promotion, illness prevention, and health protection across the lifespan.

Health Services in First Nations Communities

Since 1989, support and processes were put into place for the transfer of Indian health services from Medical Services of

---

BOX 39.9 **Federal Indian Health Policy**

The goal of Federal Indian Health Policy is to achieve an increasing level of health in Indian communities, where the key is that Indian communities themselves fill an active and positive role in generating and maintaining physical, mental, and social well-being.

The Federal Indian Health Policy plan is built on three pillars.

1. Community development
   Through socioeconomic development and cultural and spiritual development, the goal is to minimize and remove conditions of poverty and apathy.
2. Traditional relationship of the Indian people to the federal government
   The federal government advocates for the interests of Indian communities within Canadian society and its institutions. Promoting the capacity of Indian communities to achieve their aspirations is contingent on open communication and encouraging greater Indian involvement in planning, budgeting and delivery of health programs.
3. The Canadian health system
   This complex and interdependent system of specialized and interrelated elements and participants includes federal, provincial, or municipal governments; Indian bands; and the private sector.

The most significant federal roles are public health activities on reserves, health promotion, and identification and mitigation of environmental hazards to health. Diagnosis and treatment of acute and chronic disease, and rehabilitating the sick are among the most important roles for provincial and private sectors. Indian communities play a significant role in health promotion as well as identifying the specific needs of their community health services.

Source: Health Canada. (n.d.). *About Health Canada. Indian Health Policy 1979.* Retrieved from http://hc-sc.gc.ca/ahc-asc/branch-dirgen/fnihb-dgspni/poli_1979-eng.php

---

BOX 39.10 **The Webequie First Nations Nursing Station**

The Webequie First Nations Nursing Station operates with three nurses, a community health representative (CHR), and two full-time counsellors. A doctor visits the community twice a month. Other health-care professionals such as dentists, optometrists, and mental health workers visit the station infrequently. Aboriginal staff serves as interpreters and assistants.

Nurse practitioners serving isolated northern communities are called on to assume some of the roles of doctors. Nurse practitioners are on call for 24 hours a day to handle emergencies and have 24-hour access to doctors for consultations support. Patients in critical condition are transported by air ambulance out of the community to receive treatment in a larger facility.

Source: Webequie First Nation. (n.d.). *Nursing station.* Retrieved from http://www.webequie.ca/article/nursing-station-137.asp

Health and Welfare Canada (now known as Health Canada) to First Nations and Inuit communities that wanted assume this responsibility. This was in keeping with the goal of the Indian Health Policy that was adopted by the federal government in 1979 "to achieve an increasing level of health in Indian communities, generated and maintained by the Indian communities themselves" (Health Canada, n.d., para. 1). Since then, many First Nations have gone through the health services transfer process that gradually moves control of resources and responsibility for community health services and programs into the hands of First Nations communities.

First Nations, through their chief and band council, enter into funding agreements with Health Canada in order to administer their health services and programs. The First Nations health administrator or health director oversees the day-to-day management of these health services and programs. The result of this transfer process is that communities manage and administer their health resources based on community needs and priorities. These may include a wide range of services such as prenatal classes, well-baby clinics, immunization programs, school health, oral health, home and community care, addictions and mental health, health education, and non-insured health benefits. The Non-Insured Health Benefits Program is Health Canada's national health benefit program that provides coverage for benefit claims for a specified medically necessary range of drugs, dental care, vision care, medical supplies and equipment, short-term crisis intervention, mental health counseling, and medical transportation for eligible First Nations people and Inuit. As a result of these various programs (Dobbelsteyn, 2006), the interdisciplinary health team in an Aboriginal community may include the following: registered nurses, licensed/registered practical nurses, community health representatives, dentist, dental hygienist, physician, psychologist, social workers, elders, traditional healers, mental health workers, and addiction workers. Many First Nations communities have developed vision and mission statements to guide the delivery of these programs. It is important to recognize that a local health-care system exists in Aboriginal communities.

Health Services in Urban Centres

In addition to using the health services that are available to the general Canadian public in cities and towns, there are health services that are specific to Aboriginal people. For example, the Wabano Centre is considered a "gateway to health" for Aboriginal people in Ottawa where health care is accessed and connections to support services are made. One of its programs makes available services incorporating Aboriginal beliefs, values, and traditions that promote holistic healing. The Wabano Centre has become a known authority on Aboriginal needs and issues in the Ottawa area and is part of the extensive network of health care, social services, youth engagement and support, and mental health services. The Wabano Centre works closely health networks, police, and first responders.

Nursing Care and First Nations, Inuit and Métis People

The nursing student's first task is to develop an understanding about the political climate and the general Canadian societal attitudes about Aboriginal people. A nurse can better examine his or her own beliefs and attitudes and determine whether anything needs to be reevaluated in light of this new knowledge when equipped with the understanding of how politicians, programs, schools, institutions, and media continue to perpetuate the stereotypes and negative attitudes (Foster, 2006). It may also be helpful to read the *United Nations Declaration on the Rights of Indigenous Peoples* (United Nations, 2008). Adopted by the United Nations General Assembly in 2007, this declaration lays down the individual and collective rights of indigenous peoples and their rights to culture, identity, language, employment, health, education, and other issues. It also prohibits discrimination against indigenous peoples and promotes their full and effective participation in all matters that concern them and their right to remain distinct and to pursue their own visions of economic and social development.

Nursing care is enhanced through learning more about First Nations, Inuit and Métis, history and culture. In addition to learning about Aboriginal people since settlers arrived on the shores of the United States, learn about indigenous societies in the United States prior to 1492 (Mann, 2005). Whenever the opportunity arises, take part in cultural awareness workshops (Box 39.11).

Intercultural Communication

Effective communication in health-care relationships has been linked to improved patient self-care (Marks & Shive, 2008) and outcomes (Charlton, Dearing, Berry, & Johnson, 2008; Kreps & Thornton, 1992, as cited in Quine, 2009). Lacking the ability to effectively communicate with Aboriginal patients is a patient safety issue because health professionals may avoid interactions and not provide appropriate care to patients (Quine, 2009, p. 104). Intercultural communication is important to understand and needs to be improved, especially with respect to non-Aboriginal nurses and

---

BOX 39.11 Remote Nursing Certified Practice

In 2010, Remote Nursing Certificate Practice (RNCP), a new category of registered nurse regulation was implemented in the province of British Columbia, Canada (Tarlier & Browne, 2011). It was created specifically to regulate the practice of registered nurses employed in remote communities. The RNCP initiative was preceded by the implementation of the nurse practitioner role in British Columbia following legislative and regulatory changes made in 2005. As of March 31, 2010, nurses employed in remote First Nations communities in British Columbia are required to be RNCP-certified.

Source: Tarlier, D. S., & Browne, A. J. (2011). Remote nursing certified practice: Viewing nursing and nurse practitioner practice through a social lens. *Canadian Journal of Nursing Research, 43*(2), 38–61.

Aboriginal patients (Quine, 2009). Research about nurse–patient communication is limited, and more is needed.

In a study conducted in Saskatchewan, the ability of nursing students to communicate with Aboriginal patients was explored (Quine, 2009). Using mixed methods, the researcher demonstrated that intercultural communication is anxiety provoking and a contributing factor to student stress. Intercultural anxiety decreases when nursing students reported having experiences with persons of Aboriginal ancestry. Experiences that typically improve self-efficacy in nursing students include exposure to high-quality education materials on the history of Aboriginal people and health issues; personal relationships with Aboriginal people; observation or participation in cultural events and traditions; and clinical rotations involving Aboriginal people, settings, and experiential projects (Parent, 2010; Quine, 2009). More than one type of experience is required over time; however, we do not know enough about these experiences and how they impact learning (Quine, 2009, p. 105).

Cultural Immersion

The idea that nursing students immerse themselves in Aboriginal culture and knowledge has not been researched in depth. In fact, there is controversy in the literature about cultural immersion in general and the impacts of these experiences on **cultural competence** among nursing students (Harrowing, Gregory, O'Sullivan, Lee, & Doolittle, 2012). The evidence is not clear on its specific impacts on nursing students' learning, and researchers have not examined students immersed over time in different settings (urban, rural, reserve) across Aboriginal contexts. However, Quine's study sheds light on the topic that students who have experiences with Aboriginal people and communities reported more effective intercultural communication knowledge and skills as compared to students who did not have such experiences (Quine, 2009). Quine also found that most nursing students reported not having much exposure or experience working with and for Aboriginal people and communities (Quine, 2009, p. 57). The opportunities to work with Aboriginal people should be actively sought out; that is, patient care assignments, placements in Aboriginal communities, and service learning with urban Aboriginal health and social services. In order to avoid racism and to promote equity in health care, it can serve nursing students and faculty well to receive education about working with and for Aboriginal people and communities, whether it be for education, practice, research, and policy endeavours. Beyond cultural competence, such experiences may assist students to understand the need for **cultural safety** when working with Aboriginal people. Canada has a history of "power over" Aboriginal people. And thus, it is important to think about how the current health care system, and the nursing care therein, can replicate power-over situations with Aboriginal patients, families, and communities.

Traditional Ways and a Changing Demographic

Aboriginal patients may make use of traditional practices or approaches to health and healing. Nurses are in a position to serve as advocates, within the health-care system, on behalf of their Aboriginal patients.

Significant demographic changes in the Aboriginal population influence the characteristics of the patient population and are of interest to nurses. "Improvements in life expectancy and declines in fertility rates [make it so] the Aboriginal population aged 65 years of age and older is projected to more than double from 2001 to 2017" (Wilson, Rosenberg, & Abonyi, 2011, p. 356). The use of health-care services by the older Aboriginal population is predicted to grow; there is then a greater need to facilitate the use of traditional approaches to care within Western models. The extent to which Aboriginal people turn to and use traditional practices to maintain and promote health is not known, but there seems to be differences according to age groups. "The effects of the residential school system including the loss of traditional approaches to healing might explain for example why older Aboriginal people are less likely to have had contact with a traditional healer than younger Aboriginal people" (Wilson et al., 2011, p. 361).

Traditional Healing

"Despite a complex colonial legacy . . . Aboriginal peoples . . . strive for equitable, effective, and culturally appropriate healthcare" (Jull & Giles, 2012, p. 70). Across regions and cultural groups within the Aboriginal population, there are variations in the traditional approaches preferred. Not all Aboriginal people practice and use traditional healing methods in the same way, some people may not practice any traditional ways. Sweetgrass smudging ceremonies, sweat and healing lodge ceremonies, healing circles, medicine teachings may be crucial in promoting health, depending on the patient. Ask the patient what is important to him or her in terms of health and healing. Another way to gain a better understanding of different approaches to health and healing is to consult and work with Aboriginal elders. The significant role of elders within nursing education has been identified in past research (Mahara, Duncan, Whyte, & Brown, 2011). Elders are promoted in the classroom for their ability to introduce cultural practices and to share knowledge of traditional foods and healing practices with nursing student (Mahara et al., 2011, p. 5). Please see the interactive resource at website called FourDirectionsTeachings.com to learn about indigenous knowledge and philosophy from five diverse First Nations in Canada. It is important to know that there are additional variations on these teachings.

*S*andra, although very busy with her nursing course work, has been able to spend some time during the past week retrieving information about Aboriginal people from the various Aboriginal Internet websites. She has learned more about the historical context (colonization, residential schools, treaties, and historical trauma) and its impact on the health of Aboriginal Peoples. She says, "At first, I was uncertain about how the information I was reading in first year on Aboriginal people would help me when it came time for me to provide nursing care. The information in this textbook is really just the beginning. It is giving me a point of reference as I move through my nursing studies.

Building Authentic Relationships

Building authentic and genuine relationships with Aboriginal people and communities will help nurses positively influence how people experience the health-care system. When health professionals build genuine relationships, open dialogue emerges and more responsive ways of serving the people ensue (Zeidler, 2011). Using qualitative methods, Zeidler (2011) explored how health professionals can build relationships with Aboriginal people. The researcher confirmed that health professionals have the opportunity in their role to significantly impact on the quality of the health-care relationships with Aboriginal people. For example, "when non-Aboriginal professionals encourage traditional language and make an effort to learn and use it, this shows respect for the culture and the people" (Zeidler, 2011, p. 142). Showing respect demonstrates professionalism, and in nursing, developing and maintaining therapeutic relationships with patients is key.

The following issues related to respect have been of concern to both nurses and patients.

- Disrespect, prejudice, and discrimination;
- Failure of the health-care personnel to consider the patient's perspective;
- Failure to provide sufficient privacy;
- Failure to provide adequate explanations for medical or nursing procedures and results;
- Use of a harsh or condescending tone with elders, patients, or family members;
- Leaving clients to feel misunderstood unaccepted and lessened as individuals through verbal and nonverbal behaviours of staff.

In order to promote positive respectful relationships with patients, nurses can support their work with best practice guidelines on establishing therapeutic relationships (Registered Nurses' Association of Ontario [RNAO], 2006). The recommendations of interest from Registered Nurses' Association of Ontario (RNAO) are (1) nurses need to acquire sufficient knowledge to participate effectively in relationships and (2) nurses are encouraged to engage in self-reflection. This type of self-reflection requires "nurses to reflect on their own cultural identity and to practice in a way that affirms the culture of clients" (Mahara et al., 2011, p. 3). Ziedler's research identified several themes that can guide health professionals in their quest to build

authentic relationships with Aboriginal people (Ziedler, 2011, p. 139):

(a) listen,
(b) be aware of the impact of the past,
(c) learn about the history and traditions,
(d) share who you are,
(e) learn from others who know about Aboriginal people,
(f) know the people and community before providing assessments,
(g) be community-focused, and
(h) support traditional culture and language as appropriate.

These themes were supported in other research in which a focus on understanding the local specific context of Aboriginal people was also recommended (Mahara et al., 2011). Fundamental to establishing relationships of respect and recognition, nurses are encouraged to develop genuine understanding and acceptance of all patient populations.

Through the eyes of a nurse

*I*t seems to me that the nursing students today are asking more questions about Aboriginal people. Some of their questions suggest a deeper awareness of the diversity among Aboriginal people. This presents a challenge to those of us who have not taken courses on the history of Aboriginal people as part of our basic nursing education. Thank goodness I have taken the Aboriginal cultural awareness course that this hospital provides as it has been beneficial in how I view the Aboriginal patients in my care. I believe nurse graduates who have taken this course will be in a better position to create effective communication with Aboriginal patients in their care as Aboriginal people's health are affected by unique determinants such as colonialism, racism, and the effects of residential schools.

(personal reflection of a nurse)

Through the eyes of a student

I am glad that information on Aboriginal Peoples was provided in our textbooks. I think, though, that talking with my Aboriginal patients was where I learned the most. Now that I am in the last year of the program, I have had the opportunity to work with some Aboriginal patients in my clinical practice. Many of my patients have been from the Métis settlements and Treaty Six First Nations. My patients taught me what was important to them and how I could provide good nursing care. I also listened a lot. I learned about the importance of respectful communication, and I did not make any assumptions about my patients. I had to get to know them to understand what was at stake for them and what mattered to them.

(personal reflection of a nursing student)

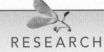

RESEARCH

THE EXPERIENCE OF ABORIGINAL NURSING STUDENTS

The experiences of undergraduate Aboriginal nursing students in two Canadian schools of nursing and how the contextual factors (i.e., historical, social, cultural, political, and ideological) shaped or influenced their experiences were examined. The purpose of this study was to provide nurse educators and educational administrators with more information about factors that enhanced or hampered the educational experiences of Aboriginal nursing students. This is in keeping with the need to improve recruitment and retention of Aboriginal Peoples in nursing.

Study

A critical ethnography was conducted using audiotaped interviews with Aboriginal nursing students, Aboriginal nurses, nursing faculty members, and individuals who were identified as knowledgeable about the context that might shape the experiences of nursing students. Other data sources included reflexive and descriptive field notes from fieldwork in the classroom and laboratory practice sessions, and texts from the participating schools. Nursing textbooks, course syllabi, policies, procedures, clinical evaluation forms, and websites were randomly selected and analyzed to explicate how texts shaped the Aboriginal nursing students' experiences.

Conclusions

Recommendations were developed to improve recruitment and retention of Aboriginal nursing students. The recommendations were as follows: Nurse educators collaborate with Aboriginal students, nurses, agencies, and communities to develop a contextual foundation in curriculum development and instructional design. More inclusive teaching strategies can be incorporated by using reflexivity. Second, formal mentorship programs may enhance Aboriginal nursing students' experiences. Third, educational administrators may consider establishing formal antiracist policies and resources to support and sustain urban and campus adjustment for Aboriginal nursing students. Fourth, conduct future research to identify how different explanatory models influence student–teacher relationships.

Martin, D. E., & Kipling, A. (2006). Factors shaping Aboriginal nursing students' experiences. Nurse Education in Practice, 6, 380–388. Retrieved from http://www.ncbi.nlm.nih.gov/pubmed/19040905

Critical Thinking Case Scenarios

▶ Mrs. Tucktoo is now 32 weeks pregnant according to the first ultrasound you did at 16 weeks. A repeat ultrasound at your next clinic when she was 29 weeks pregnant showed good growth. She presents at the nursing station at 11 PM complaining of slight bleeding and lower abdominal cramping. The latest weather report shows a major storm approaching, which could possibly shut down the area for the next few days. With windchill, the temperature on the runway is −60°C. The regular doctor is on holiday, and the replacement nurse (with some labour and delivery experience) has been there for a week. She phones you for your advice.

What additional information will you need from the nurse? What decisions need to be made first?

▶ Complete the following reflective exercise on communication:

I have some understanding of appropriate communication with the patient and taking into consideration the social, political, linguistic, economic, and spiritual realm of that patient.

I am comfortable that I am able to use plain language relevant to the patient or client in a way that makes the person feel engaged in the encounter.

I have some understanding of being able to respect the patient or client's culture, age, and beliefs.

I have an understanding that I bring my own life experiences and attitudes to the relationship.

▶ Additional discussion questions for learners:

To what extent are your patient's health concerns linked to social determinants of health as opposed to only the patient's biologic background?

How can you support patients who have cultural-based needs that are not being met?

Are you surprised by the outcomes, answers, or issues that were discussed today?

Has anyone encountered similar scenarios in their education or practice so far? If so, how did you manage them? How could you change your approach next time?

Would your decision, opinion, or perspective change if your patient was from another cultural background?

Multiple-Choice Questions

1. Approximately how many indigenous people are there living worldwide?
   a. 50 million
   b. 200 million
   c. 300 million
   d. 450 million

2. In Canada, how many groups are recognized as indigenous?
   a. 1
   b. 3
   c. 4
   d. 5

3. How many Aboriginal languages are spoken in Canada today?
   a. 11
   b. 23
   c. 50
   d. More than 60

4. On September 13, 2007, the United Nations General Assembly adopted the *Declaration on the Rights of Indigenous Peoples*. Which country or countries voted against the declaration?
   a. Australia
   b. Canada
   c. United States
   d. Australia, Canada, New Zealand, and United States

5. In what year was the Indian Act officially legislated in Canada?
   a. 1876
   b. 1891
   c. 1900
   d. 1922

6. In what year was the Indian Act amended to make residential school attendance compulsory for all First Nations children ages 7 to 15 years?
   a. 1886
   b. 1900
   c. 1920
   d. 1934

Suggested Lab Activities

● Select a local community for a First Nations, Métis or Inuit, patient and identify the range of healing and wellness practices available to this patient. Go to the community's website to obtain contact information.

Evaluation points

Understands the range of practices within local community

Demonstrates openness in interview style to other health practices

Is aware of two to three local healing resources and practices common in the population served (e.g., sweat lodge, fasts, smudging ceremony, elders, going into bush, attending ceremonies, sundance, potlatch, natural remedies, church)?

REFERENCES AND SUGGESTED READINGS

Aboriginal Nurses Association of Canada. (2001). *An aboriginal nursing specialty*. Ottawa, ON: Author.

Brave Heart, M. Y. (2003). The historical trauma response among Natives and its relationship with substance abuse: A Lakota illustration. *Journal of Psychoactive Drugs, 35*(1), 7–13.

Brave Heart, M. Y., Chase, J., Elkins, J., & Altschul, D. B. (2011). Historical trauma among indigenous peoples of the Americas: Concepts, research, and clinical considerations. *Journal of Psychoactive Drugs, 43*(4), 282–290.

Canadian Association of Schools of Nursing. (2013). *Integration of culture, society, history and context into nursing education*. Ottawa, ON: Author.

Charlton, C., Dearing, K., Berry, J., & Johnson, M. (2008). Nurse practitioners' communication styles and their impact on patient outcomes: An integrated literature review. *Journal of the American Academy of Nurse Practitioners, 20*(7), 382–388. doi:10.1111/j.1745-7599.2008.00336.x

Dickason, O. (2006). *A concise history of Canada's First Nations*. Oxford, England: Oxford University Press.

Dickason, O. P., & McNab, D. T. (2002). *Canada's First Nations. A history of founding peoples from earliest times* (3rd ed.). Oxford, England: Oxford University.

Dickason, O. P., & McNab, D. T. (2009). *Canada's First Nations: A history of founding peoples from earliest times* (4th ed.). Don Mills, ON: Oxford University Press.

Dion-Stout, M., & Jodoin, N. (2006). *MCH screening tool project: Final report*. Ottawa, ON: Maternal & Child Health Program, First Nations and Inuit Health Branch.

Dion Stout, M., & Kipling, G. (2003). *Aboriginal people, resilience and the residential school legacy*. Ottawa, ON: Aboriginal Healing Foundation. Retrieved from http://www.ahf.ca/downloads /resilience.pdf

Dobbelsteyn, J. L. (2006). Nursing in First Nations and Inuit communities in Atlantic Canada. *Canadian Nurse, 102*(4), 32–35.

Environics Institute. (2010). *Urban aboriginal peoples study*. Toronto, ON: Author. Retrieved from http://www.uaps.ca/wp -content/uploads/2010/03/UAPS-Main-Report_Dec.pdf

Fast, E., & Collin-Vézina, D. (2010). Historical trauma, race-based trauma and resilience of indigenous peoples: A literature review. *First Peoples Child and Family Review, 5*(1), 126–136.

First Nations Information Governance Centre. (2012). *First Nations Regional Health Survey (RHS) 2008/10: National report on adults, youth and children living in First Nations communities*. Ottawa, ON: Author. Retrieved from http://www.fnigc.ca/sites/default /files/First%20Nations%20Regional%20Health%20Survey%20 %28RHS%29%202008-10%20-%20National%20Report.pdf

Fleming, J., & Ledogar, R. J. (2008). Resilience, an evolving concept: A review of literature relevant to aboriginal research. *Pimatisiwin, 6*(2), 7–23.

Foster, C. H. (2006). What nurses should know when working with aboriginal communities. *Canadian Nurse, 102*(4), 28–31.

Frideres, J. S. (2011). *First Nations in the twenty-first century*. Don Mills, ON: Oxford.

Harrowing, J. N., Gregory, D. M., O'Sullivan, P. S., Lee, B., & Doolittle, L. (2012). A critical analysis of undergraduate students' cultural immersion experiences. *International Nursing Review, 59*(4), 494–501. doi:10.1111/j.1466-7657.2012.01012.x

Health Canada. (n.d.). *About Health Canada. Indian Health Policy 1979*. Retrieved from http://hc-sc.gc.ca/ahc-asc/branch-dirgen/ fnihb-dgspni/poli_1979-eng.php

Idle No More. (2012). *The story*. Retrieved from http://www .idlenomore.ca/story

Jull, J. E. G., & Giles, A. R. (2012). Health equity, aboriginal peoples and occupational therapy. *The Canadian Journal of Occupational Therapy, 79*(2), 70–76. Retrieved from http://search.proquest .com/docview/1001944094?accountid=13480

Loppie Reading, C., & Wien, F. (2009). *Health inequalities and social determinants of aboriginal peoples' health*. Prince George, BC: National Collaborating Centre for Aboriginal Health. Retrieved from http://www.nccah-ccnsa.ca/docs/social%20determinates/NCCAH-Loppie-Wien_Report.pdf

Magocsi, P. (2002). *Aboriginal peoples of Canada: A short introduction*. Toronto, ON: University of Toronto Press.

Mahara, M., Duncan, S. M., Whyte, N., & Brown, J. (2011). It takes a community to raise a nurse: Educating for culturally safe practice with Aboriginal peoples. *International Journal of Nursing Education Scholarship, 8*(1), 1–13. doi:10.2202/1548-923X.2208

Mann, C. (2005). *New revelations of the Americas before Columbus*. New York, NY: Knopf.

Marks, R., & Shive, S. E. (2008). Ethics and patient—Provider communication. *Health Promotion Practice, 9*(1), 29–33. doi:10.1177/1524839907312094

McCormick, R. (2009). Aboriginal approaches to counseling. In E. Kirmayer & V. Guthrie Valaskakis (Eds.), *Healing traditions: The mental health of aboriginal peoples in Canada* (pp. 337–354). Vancouver, BC: University of British Columbia Press.

McIntyre, M., & McDonald, C. (2010). *Realities of Canadian nursing: Professional, practice, and power issues* (3rd ed.). Philadelphia, PA: Lippincott Williams & Wilkins.

Morrison, B., & Wilson, C. (2004). *Native peoples: The Canadian experience* (3rd ed.). Oxford, England: Oxford University Press.

Parent, M. (2010). *A Delphi study on nursing education: A consensus on ideal programs for Aboriginal students* (Doctoral dissertation, Capella University). Retrieved from http://gradworks.umi.com/3398744.pdf

Quine, A. (2009). *Intercultural anxiety and cultural self-efficacy among Saskatchewan nursing students: Examination of experiences working with aboriginal persons with diabetes*. Regina, SK: University of Regina.

Reading, J. L., Kmetic, A., & Gideon, V. (2007). *First Nations wholistic policy and planning model. Discussion paper for the World Health Organization Commission on Social Determinants of Health*. Ottawa, ON: Assembly of First Nations. Retrieved from http://ahrnets.ca/files/2011/02/AFN_Paper_2007.pdf

Registered Nurses' Association of Ontario. (2006). *Establishing therapeutic relationships*. Retrieved from http://rnao.ca/sites/rnao-ca/files/Establishing_Therapeutic_Relationships.pdf

Royal Commission on Aboriginal Peoples. (1996). *The report of the Royal Commission on Aboriginal Peoples*. Retrieved from http://www.parl.gc.ca/content/lop/researchpublications/prb9924-e.htm

Statistics Canada. (2011). *Aboriginal peoples in Canada: First Nations, Métis and Inuit*. Retrieved from http://www12.statcan.gc.ca/nhs-enm/2011/as-sa/99-011-x/99-011-x2011001-eng.cfm

United Nations. (2008). *United Nations declaration on the rights of indigenous peoples*. Geneva, Switzerland: Author. Retrieved from http://www.un.org/esa/socdev/unpfii/documents/DRIPS_en.pdf

Waldram, J., Herring, A., & Young, T. K. (2007). *Aboriginal health in Canada. Historical, cultural, and epidemiological perspectives* (2nd ed.). Toronto, ON: University of Toronto Press.

Wesley-Esquimaux, S. S., & Smolewski, M. (2004). *Historic trauma and aboriginal healing*. Ottawa, ON: Aboriginal Health Foundation. Retrieved from http://www.ahf.ca/downloads/historic-trauma.pdf

Wilson, K., & Rosenberg, M. (2002). Exploring the determinants of health for First Nations peoples in Canada: Can existing frameworks accommodate traditional activities? *Social Science & Medicine, 55*, 2017–2031.

Wilson, K., Rosenberg, M., & Abonyi, S. (2011). Aboriginal peoples, health and healing approaches: The effects of age and place on health. *Social Science & Medicine, 72*(3), 355–364. doi:10.1016/j.socscimed.2010.09.022

Zeidler, D. (2011). Building a relationship: Perspectives from one First Nations community. *Canadian Journal of Speech-Language Pathology & Audiology, 35*(2), 136–143. Retrieved from http://www.caslpa.ca/english/resources/database/files/2011_CJSLPA_Vol_35/No_02_103-213/Zeidler_CJSLPA_2011.pdf

Spirituality and Nursing: Presence and Promise

chapter 40

KAREN SCOTT BARSS, VELNA CLARKE ARNAULT, AND MARIE SHERRY MCDONALD

Amira, Tommy, and Willa are first-year nursing students doing a clinical rotation in a long-term care facility. They have enjoyed caring for residents of varying ages, ethno-cultural backgrounds, and lengths of time living in the facility. At the end of their shift, their clinical teacher mentions they will be having a discussion the next day about addressing spirituality in their care. As they walk together to the locker room, they have the following conversation. These comments and questions come up:

"I get that being a nurse means caring for the whole person, but is it really necessary to talk so specifically about spirituality? Isn't that a little too personal?"
"We talked about it in class, but I still don't really know what it means."
"With so many different cultural backgrounds here, how are we supposed to know what the patient would even want?"

CHAPTER OBJECTIVES

By the end of this chapter, you will be able to:

1. Recognize characteristics of spirituality including its subjective and ever-evolving nature.
2. Discuss the role of spirituality in health and healing.
3. Describe the diversity of spiritual beliefs and worldviews among people in Canada.
4. Understand the impact of colonization on spirituality within Aboriginal populations and on spirituality within Canadian health care.
5. Identify spiritual needs and strengths to be addressed within holistic care.
6. Highlight inclusive language and guidelines that help you talk with patients in culturally safe, nonintrusive ways about their spirituality and its relevance to their health and healing.
7. Explain your responsibilities as a nurse on the interdisciplinary health-care team in relation to spiritual assessment and care.
8. Explore your own spirituality in preparation for helping patients mobilize their spirituality to promote optimum healing.
9. Express your fears and hopes in relation to addressing the spiritual dimension of holistic nursing care.
10. Tend your own spiritual needs and that of your colleagues to promote a healthy workplace environment.

KEY TERMS

Healing The process of moving toward wholeness in all dimensions of health, encompassing the mental, emotional, physical, relational, cultural, and spiritual; as such, it may or may not be associated with curing disease or disorder.

Inclusive Spiritual Care Relevant, nonintrusive care that tends to the spiritual dimension of health by addressing universal spiritual needs, honouring unique spiritual worldviews, and helping individuals to explore and mobilize factors that can help them gain/regain a sense of trust in order to promote optimum healing.

Religion An organized way of expressing and nurturing spirituality through affiliations, rites, and rituals based on creeds, codes of conduct, and communal practices.

Sacred Space A spiritually healing environment in which individuals are supported and nurtured, in which they feel spiritually calm, where they are connected to elements of nature, and in which health and well-being are promoted.

Spirit The essence of the individual being, expressed and experienced through multifaceted connections with oneself, others, the environment, and with a universal life force as it is understood by the individual.

(continued on page 1064)

Spiritual Dimension of Health   The dimension of health associated with "matters of the spirit," as ultimately defined by each individual.

Spirituality   A highly subjective and ineffable concept that defies standard definition and encompasses the individual's beliefs; expressions of these beliefs; perceptions of the meaning of life and death; and how the person relates to self, others, the world, and the possibility of a greater power.

Spiritual Practices   Processes of inner quieting to help attain a state of calm centeredness and receptive awareness, which nurtures the spirit and deepens insight, attention, and compassion for oneself and others.

Suffering   Distress, pain, or anguish, whether physical, mental, emotional, and/or spiritual, that can challenge the very trust we have in life.

Transcendence   An experience of moving to higher levels of self-awareness, consciousness, and spiritual well-being that offers individuals new possibilities and choices in their lives and in their relationships.

Unconditional Presence   A way of being with patients that involves a deeply authentic connectedness and produces an unconditional acceptance of each patient's essence or spirit, regardless of feelings, behaviours, challenges, or any part of their lived experience.

Worldview   A mental map containing a set of core beliefs and meanings that we use to explain the world around us and guide our way of being in the world.

The Nature of Spirituality

What comes to mind when you hear the word *spirituality*? What emotions come up when you hear this word? Understanding the nature of spirituality and your experiences of it are key aspects of preparing yourself to address spirituality in your nursing practice. Such preparation will help you to confirm your patients' understanding and empathize with their responses to spiritual exploration. It will also help you explore and nurture your own spirituality, an essential element in being able to help patients explore theirs (Kalish, 2012). As such, this chapter is intended not only to help you learn about spirituality in nursing but also to help nurture your spirit as you prepare for holistic nursing practice.

What Is Spirituality?

This is a vital question without a definitive answer. **Spirituality** remains a highly subjective, complex, and ineffable concept that defies development of a standard definition (Kalish, 2012; Pesut, 2008; Pike, 2011; Young & Koopsen, 2011). As such, a diverse range of definitions abound in the nursing and interdisciplinary literature. For purposes of introduction, spirituality can perhaps be best described as that which encompasses the individual's beliefs, expressions of these beliefs, perceptions of the meaning of life and death, and how the person relates to oneself, others, the world, and possibly a greater power (Kalish, 2012; Pesut, 2008; Pike, 2011; Young & Koopsen, 2011). Spirituality is the expression of one's **spirit**, which is the essence of our being, expressed and experienced through multifaceted connections with ourselves, others, the environment, and a universal life-force as understood by each of us (Pike, 2011; Seaward, 2012; Young & Koopsen, 2011). Spirituality is an integral part of the health, healing, and well-being of every individual. It is intertwined with every aspect of life and provides purpose, meaning, strength, and guidance in shaping the journey of life (Young & Koopsen, 2011, pp. 9, 114).

Given the highly personal nature of spirituality, the question, "What is spirituality?" is best answered by each patient for whom you provide care (Pesut, 2009). In the context of nursing practice, then, "the answer may be to understand its meaning for others, so that by recognizing the manifestations of spirituality, spiritual needs can be acknowledged as such" (Pike, 2011, p. 745). Your ability to focus on the patient's perspective will set the tone for truly patient-centered care.

What Is the Difference Between Spirituality and Religion?

Spirituality and *religion* are terms that are often used interchangeably even though they are quite different in many ways. **Religion** is an organized way of expressing and nurturing spirituality through affiliations, rites, and rituals based on creeds, codes of conduct, and communal practices (Pike, 2011; Young & Koopsen, 2011, pp. 90–91). Religion may or may not play a role in individual spirituality (Brewer, 2011; Pike, 2011; Young & Koopsen, 2011).

In 2009, Koenig found that 12.5% of Canadians described themselves as nonreligious and 1.9% as atheist. Bibby reported in 2011 that approximately 25% of Canadians embrace religion as a part of their spiritual lives. Meanwhile, Jedwab's 2010 Carlton University survey indicated that two in three Canadians qualified as following a religion or being spiritual. Jedwab concluded that "Canadians are split on the degree to which they follow a religion and around whether or not they are spiritual" (Jedwab, 2010, p. 4).

Whether or not an individual's spirit is nurtured by religion, or even expressed in spiritual terms, depends on the individual's worldview. A **worldview** is "a commitment, a fundamental orientation of the heart, that can be expressed as a story or a set of presuppositions (assumptions which may be true, partially true, or entirely false) that we hold (consciously or subconsciously, consistently or inconsistently) about the basic constitution of reality, and that provides the foundation on which we live and move and have our being" (Sire, 2004, as cited in Young & Koopsen, 2011, p. 26). In her seminal work, Canadian nurse scholar Barbara Pesut has defined *worldviews* as "the mental maps we use to explain the world around us," maps that contain a set of core beliefs and meanings that ultimately drive our behaviour (Pesut, 2003,

BOX 40.1 Perspectives From Various Worldviews: Spirituality and Related Concepts

- The word *spirituality* is derived from the Latin *spiritus*, meaning breath; it is also related to the Greek *pneuma* (or breath), which refers to the vital spirit or soul (Young & Koopsen, 2011, p. 9). It is the essence of who and how people are in the world and, like breathing, is essential to human existence (Young & Koopsen, 2011, p. 9).
- *Religion* is derived from the Latin word *re-ligare*, which means to reconnect or retie (Young & Koopsen, p. 90).
- *Theism* derives from the Greek *theos* meaning "god"; it is most often affiliated with a spiritual understanding wherein "God is infinite and personal, transcendent and immanent, omniscient, sovereign, and good" (Sire as cited in Young & Koopsen, 2011, p. 27).
- *Existentialism* comes from the ancient Greeks; it refers to a practical philosophy focusing on what can be learned from our lived experience. Existentialism "is a way of asking questions about life, rather than teaching a prescribed body of knowledge" (Adams, 2011, p. 8).
- In an Aboriginal worldview, the dimension of spirituality is difficult to discuss separately from the mental, emotional, physical, and sociocultural dimensions of health because there is such a focus on interconnection, relationships, and balance. "Humankind has not woven the web of life. We are but one thread within it. Whatever we do to the web, we do to ourselves. All things are bound together. All things connect." (Chief Seattle, 1855, as cited in Seaward, 2012, p. 178).
- Many Eastern spiritual traditions speak of the sacred as *chi* or universal energy that flows through everything and everyone (Seaward, 2012). Many healing modalities draw on this perspective.
- Feminist theology challenges spirituality and religion's traditionally male-oriented language (eg: God as *He*) and encourages language that fosters feminine, masculine, and non-gendered images of the sacred (Chittister, 2012).
- Aldous Huxley, a humanist author, described human spirituality as "a transcendent reality beyond cultures, religions, politics, and egos" (Seaward, 2012, p. 167).

p. 291). As a nurse, it is essential that you respect and seek to understand your patients' worldviews if you are to help them engage in life-giving, health-promoting behaviours. One important way you can do so is to avoid assumptions about whether or not religion (or spirituality) is integral to a patient's sense of self. Box 40.1 features perspectives on spirituality and related concepts from various worldviews.

Think Based on what you've read so far, write your own definition of spirituality that reflects your worldview. Include in that definition any related concepts that may be integral to your spirituality. Then, explore these reflective questions:

What implications does your personal definition of spirituality have for your nursing practice? How might it inform and/or challenge your role as a nurse?

The Relationship Between Spirituality and Health

A clear understanding of the relationship between spirituality and health will assist you and your patients in addressing the spiritual dimension of health as part of their holistic care. The **spiritual dimension of health** is defined as the dimension of health associated with matters of the spirit, as ultimately defined by each individual (Scott Barss, 2012a, p. 25). The spiritual dimension may or may not involve a sense of connection to a divine presence or to religious structures or traditions and is associated with universal spiritual needs such as those identified in the nursing literature and featured in Figure 40.1 (Kalish, 2012; Narayanasamy, 2011; Pike, 2011; Young & Koopsen, 2011). The spiritual dimension also relates to individuals' spiritual strengths, which are described in various ways across ethno-cultural groups, religious traditions, and professional disciplines (Clarke & Holtslander, 2010; Seaward, 2012; Young & Koopsen, 2011). See Figure 40.2 for examples of spiritual strengths. Later in the chapter, we explore how you can address such spiritual needs and strengths in your nursing practice.

For now, it is important for you to gain an understanding of how the spiritual dimension of health interrelates with the physical, mental, emotional, cultural, and relational dimensions of health. It is also important for you to become acquainted with what the interdisciplinary literature has to say about the role of spirituality in health promotion.

What Does Spirituality Have to Do With Health?

Literature across health-care disciplines has come to acknowledge spirituality as integral to holistic health promotion (Kalish, 2012; Koenig, 2011; Pike, 2011; Plante, 2010;

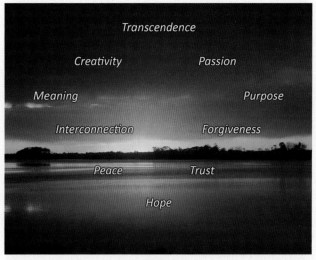

Figure 40.1 Universal spiritual needs. (Photo by Moira Theede BSN; Source: Saskatchewan Collaborative Bachelor of Science in Nursing [SCBScN] Program, CNUR 208 Spirituality & Health Course)

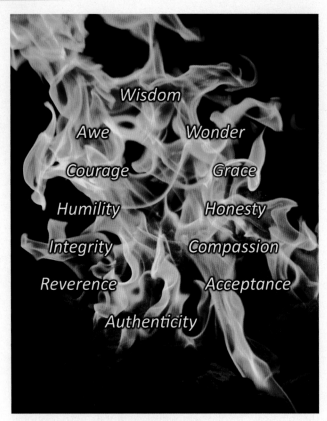

Figure 40.2 Examples of spiritual strengths.
(Photo by Moira Theede BSN; Source: Saskatchewan Collaborative Bachelor of Science in Nursing [SCBScN] Program, CNUR 208 Spirituality & Health Course)

toward wholeness in all dimensions of health, encompassing the mental, emotional, physical, relational, cultural, and spiritual; as such, it may or may not be associated with curing disease or disorder (Mariano, 2013; Puchalski & Ferrell, 2010; Rakel & Jonas, 2012; Scott Barss, 2012a). The healthcare literature, which integrates evidence-based care from all healing systems (i.e., biomedical and complementary), recognizes healing can be significantly enhanced when individuals experience a sense of trust in their healing process and relationships (Rakel & Jonas, 2012; Rakel & Weil, 2012; Scott Barss, 2012a). Such enhanced outcomes are mediated through activation of the healing response, a phenomenon increasingly validated by the field of psychoneuroimmunology (PNI) wherein fulfilled spiritual needs affiliated with trust are observed to promote enhanced overall physiological functioning and openness to mental, emotional, spiritual, and relational growth and well-being (Fortney, 2012; Parachini, 2011; Scott Barss, 2012a; Seaward, 2012; Wright & Bell, 2010).

The interconnection of spirituality with other dimensions of health can be understood in various ways, depending on one's worldview. For many, this interconnection is best understood through research. (See Table 40.1, which summarizes key findings to date on religion, spirituality, and specific health conditions.) For others, the integral relationship between spirituality and wellness is best understood through traditional teachings such as the medicine wheel (Fig. 40.3). Still others best understand this relationship through a philosophical lens such as existentialism (Table 40.2).

Remember Tommy, Amira, and Willa from the opening scenario? They could use information from the research in Table 40.1, the medicine wheel in Figure 40.3, and/or the existential embodied worldview in Table 40.2 to explore how spirituality relates to health promotion. Each student would likely choose different information to deepen his or her understanding of this interrelationship. Each could also use some of this information to better understand how each patient might view this interrelationship. For example, Tommy is caring for Margaret, who he knows follows traditional Aboriginal teachings, so he thinks about finding the right time to ask her about these teachings and how they affect her health and healing. Amira, who is caring for Matt, a young man who became quadriplegic following a car accident, wonders if he would be interested in some of the spirituality and health research because he is a part-time university student who has also struggled with depression. Meanwhile, Willa finds herself thinking about her patient, Annie, who has significant cognitive impairment, but who loves to sing old songs and receive hand massages. She thinks about how Annie experiences life through her body and through the images and memories she recalls—and realizes that these things are a form of spiritual care that promote Annie's well-being and quality of life.

Young & Koopsen, 2011). The World Health Organization cites spiritual well-being as critical to overall well-being (Seaward, 2012). Spiritual well-being may be considered the ability to develop our spiritual nature to its fullest potential. This would include our ability to discover and realize our own basic purpose in life; learn how to experience love, joy, peace, and fulfillment; and to help ourselves and others achieve their full potential (Young & Koopsen, 2011, p. 20). It makes sense that nurturing and realizing these positive states can significantly enhance our own and others' mental, emotional, and relational well-being, which, in turn, has the potential to also enhance our own and others' physical well-being in ways that we will now explore.

In ongoing research, spiritual well-being has been associated with decreased anxiety, depression, loneliness, and addictive behaviour. It has also been associated with enhanced coping, resilience, compassion, longevity, and an overall sense of trust in one's ability to navigate life's challenges, including those associated with the end of life (Armstrong, 2010; Balbuena, Baetz, & Bowen, 2013; Koenig, 2011; Luchetti, Luchetti, & Koenig, 2011). This overall sense may derive from trust in the deepest part of oneself, in life, in creation, or in a divine presence.

This sense of trust is pivotal in promoting optimal healing (Scott Barss, 2012a). **Healing** is the process of moving

| TABLE 40.1 | Summary of Findings on Religion, Spirituality, and Specific Health Conditions |

	All Studies			Best Studies		
	Negative % (n)	Positive % (n)	Total n	Negative % (n)	Positive % (n)	Total n
Positive Emotions						
Well-being	1 (3)	79 (256)	326	196 (1)	82 (98)	120
Hope	0 (0)	73 (29)	40	0 (0)	50 (3)	6
Optimism	0 (0)	81 (26)	32	0 (0)	73 (8)	11
Meaning and purpose	0 (0)	93 (42)	45	0 (0)	100 (10)	10
Self-esteem	3 (2)	61 (42)	69	8 (2)	68 (17)	25
Personal control	14 (3)	62 (13)	21	33 (3)	44 (4)	9
Negative Emotions/Disorders						
Depression	6 (28)	61 (272)	444	7 (13)	67 (119)	178
Suicide	3 (4)	75 (106)	141	4 (2)	80 (39)	49
Anxiety	11 (33)	49 (147)	299	10 (7)	55 (38)	67
Alcohol use/abuse	1 (4)	86 (240)	278	1 (1)	90 (131)	145
Drug use/abuse	1 (2)	84 (155)	185	1 (1)	86 (96)	112
Human Virtues						
Forgiveness	0 (0)	85 (34)	40	0 (0)	70 (7)	10
Altruism	11 (5)	70 (33)	47	10 (2)	75 (15)	20
Gratefulness	0 (0)	100 (5)	5	0 (0)	100 (3)	3
Social Connections						
Social support	0 (0)	82 (61)	74	0 (0)	93 (27)	29
Marital stability	0 (0)	86 (68)	79	0 (0)	92 (35)	38
Social capital	0 (0)	79 (11)	14	0 (0)	77 (10)	13
Delinquency/crime	3 (3)	79 (82)	104	2 (1)	82 (49)	60
Health Behaviours						
Exercise	16 (6)	68 (25)	37	10 (2)	76 (16)	21
Diet	5 (1)	62 (13)	21	0 (0)	70 (7)	10
Cholesterol	13 (3)	52 (12)	23	11 (1)	56 (5)	9
Weight	39 (14)	19 (7)	36	44 (11)	20 (5)	25
Risky sexual activity	1 (1)	86 (82)	95	0 (0)	84 (42)	50
Cigarette smoking	0 (0)	90 (123)	137	0 (0)	90 (75)	83
Disease Detection/Prevention						
Screening	18 (8)	64 (28)	44	22 (6)	52 (14)	27
Compliance	15 (4)	56 (15)	27	40 (2)	60 (3)	5
Physiological Functions						
Immune function	4 (1)	56 (14)	25	0 (0)	60 (6)	10
Endocrine function	0 (0)	74 (23)	31	0 (0)	69 (9)	13
Cardiovascular function	6 (1)	69 (11)	16	8 (1)	69 (9)	13
Medical Diseases and Mortality						
Coronary heart disease	5 (1)	63 (12)	19	8 (1)	69 (9)	13
Hypertension	11 (7)	57 (36)	63	13 (5)	62 (24)	39
Cerebrovascular disease	11 (1)	44 (4)	9	12 (1)	67 (4)	6
Dementia	14 (3)	48 (10)	21	21 (3)	57 (8)	14
Cancer	12 (3)	56 (14)	25	6 (1)	65 (11)	17
Mortality	6 (7)	68 (82)	121	4 (4)	66 (61)	92
				6 (1)	76 (13)*	17

"Negative" indicates worse health, "positive" indicates better health. Not included here are studies that found no association, mixed (positive and negative) findings, or complex results that were too hard to decipher; "total," however, includes all studies (negative, positive, no association, mixed, complex). "Best" studies were those studies whose research methodology rated a 7 or higher out of a possible 10 points maximum.

*Very best studies (i.e., quality ratings of 9 or 10 out of 10)

Source: Koenig, H. (2011). *Spirituality and health research: Methods, measurement statistics and resources.* West Conshohocken, PA: Templeton Press, pp. 19–20.

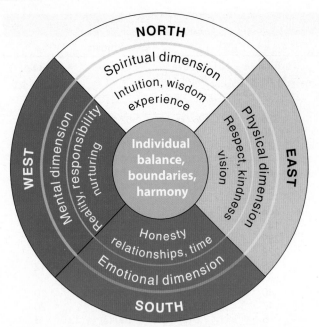

Figure 40.3 The medicine wheel. (Adapted from Clarke, V., & Holt-slander, L. [2010]. Finding a balanced approach: Incorporating teachings in the care of Aboriginal people at the end of life. *Journal of Palliative Care, 26*[1], 34–36. [Shared with the approval of the Elders].) Note: Medicine Wheels vary depending on each First Nation's teachings. The above Medicine Wheel reflects the Western Ojibwe Cree tradition.

Why Be Concerned About a Patient's Spirituality?

All health-care professionals need to be attuned to a patient's spirituality because of its well-documented potential to reduce suffering, promote optimum healing, and assist patients to cope with their health challenges (Young & Koopsen, 2011, p. 10). If health-care providers fail to address patients' spiritual needs, we not only miss significant opportunities to optimize their health outcomes but we also place patients at significant risk to experience greater suffering and a compromised ability to navigate the challenges they face (Koenig, 2011; Scott Barss, 2012a; Wright & Bell, 2010). In this respect, spiritual care is central to offering safe and ethical care.

Therefore, nurses need to be concerned with a patient's spirituality as an integral part of holistic practice (Jackson, 2011). Nursing has a long history of practicing and researching spiritual care (Kalish, 2012; O'Brien, 2011; Olson & Clark, 2010). Nurses are often the health-care team members who spend the most time with patients. They are likely to witness patients' spiritual strengths and needs, and through the nurse–patient relationship help patients explore how they might integrate their spirituality into their healing process (Johnston Taylor & Mamier, 2013). Although nursing is just one of many disciplines on the health-care team that address spirituality, nurses play a pivotal role in determining whether or not patients' spirituality is addressed and mobilized to promote health and healing (Carr, 2010; Johnston Taylor & Mamier, 2013).

Challenges in Addressing Spirituality in Nursing Practice

Although the importance of spirituality in health and healing is well documented in nursing theory and history, nurses continue to identify several challenges in integrating spirituality into their practice, such as fear and lack of

TABLE 40.2	An Existential Embodied Worldview				
Embodied refers to the way in which humans experience and interpret life through our bodies, not just our mind or our spirit; we feel, sense, move, and experience all living moments with, from, and through our bodies.					
A Human Being Is Thrust/Thrown/ Situated/Born in "a Priori World":	A Human Being Is Embodied Caring:	A Human Being Is Embodied Spirituality:	A Human Being Is Embodied Self-Interpreting:	A Human Being Is Embodied:	Is Embodied in Time:
Each person is situated in existing relationships, linguistic skills, traditions, embedded in the culture. (The world is beforehand.)	Each person has values (e.g., independence, ethical caring, social morality, commitment to self and others).	Each person has spiritual practices and processes that help to expand the authentic self, meet spiritual needs, and gain freedom from vulnerability.	Each person self-interprets one's own lived experience through metaphors, dreams, visions, and existential questions to resolve dilemmas of existence such as suffering.	Each person experiences (through the body) suffering around loss of some part of self.	Each person is in process over time, moment to moment, carrying the past is in one's body but influencing and remolding the present into the future.
What are the person's metaphors for being in his or her world?	*What matters to the person? What are his or her care practices?*	*What innate wisdom can the person access?*	*What possibilities and choices are available for person being in his or her world?*	*Where in the body does the person experience a potential "felt sense of life"?*	*What are the distressing life situations and strengths related to the now situation?*

Adapted from McDonald, M. (2012). *Nurses' experience of workplace violence before and after a focusing workshop* (Unpublished master's thesis). St. Stephen's College, Edmonton, AB.

support (Carr, 2010; Kalish, 2012). Acknowledgment of challenges you may face within yourself and in your professional environment is central to preparing yourself to address spirituality in your nursing practice (Carr, 2010; Kalish, 2012). This acknowledgment helps you know that you are not alone in these challenges and that any concerns you have about addressing spirituality are valid and important to explore.

What Challenges Do Nurses Face in Addressing Spirituality?

Tracy Carr's 2010 Atlantic Canadian study of barriers and challenges to spiritual nursing care reported that health-care culture often discourages interaction with patients at a spiritual level within an environment experienced by nurses as uncaring, time-pressured, and technologically focused in contrast to one that facilitates trust, compassion, and connection. Often, nurses receive mixed messages in their workplaces or educational preparation about the importance or relevance of spiritual nursing care (Carr, 2010; Kalish, 2012; Scott Barss, 2012b). As a result, nurses often feel uncomfortable addressing spirituality, fearing that such care is intrusive, irrelevant, or beyond their expertise, particularly when patients' belief systems are different than their own (Chan, 2009; Narayanasamy, 2011; Scott Barss, 2012b).

How Can Nurses Overcome Challenges in Addressing Spirituality?

In short, nurses can and do overcome internal and external barriers to spiritual exploration by

- Naming and exploring their fears and concerns
- Deepening their spiritual awareness and growth
- Finding supportive mentors who model and nurture holistic practice
- Gaining awareness about various spiritual beliefs and practices
- Knowing and following guidelines for spiritual assessment and care
- Receiving educational opportunities to learn the art and science of spiritual care and to demonstrate their competency in offering it.

The remainder of this chapter is intended to help you in each of these areas.

Think You have noticed when you are reviewing patients' charts that there is usually very little written by the nurses about the spiritual aspect of their care. Although you occasionally notice that staff from the spiritual care department come to the nursing station to find patients who have been referred to them, you rarely hear the nurses talk about their patients' spiritual needs. This lack of information and communication about spiritual care in nursing can make it really difficult to feel comfortable addressing this aspect of patient care.

Consider the following important self-reflective questions to help you begin to address the spiritual aspect of patient care:

- What are your fears and concerns about caring for the spiritual dimension of health?
- How/With whom can you explore these fears and concerns?
- Who do you know does a really good job of addressing spirituality within his or her nursing practice and/or healthcare discipline?
- What can you learn from these mentors?
- What can your patients teach you about offering spiritual care?

Responsibilities of the Nurse in Offering Spiritual Care

Standards of care from various professional bodies outline your responsibilities around spiritual care. Specific examples of such standards are those set by the Canadian Nurses Association (CNA, 2010), the International Council of Nurses (ICN, 2006), the Canadian Council on Health Services Accreditation (Accreditation Canada, 2013), and The Joint Commission on Accreditation of Healthcare Organizations (JCAHO, 2005; Pinto, March, Johnston Taylor, & Pravikoff, 2010). These standards are reflected in the following description of your nursing responsibilities in relation to spiritual care.

Offering Inclusive Spiritual Care

In order to maintain cultural safety (see Chapter 13), it is essential that spiritual care be offered in an inclusive manner (CNA, 2010; ICN, 2006; Pinto et al., 2010). **Inclusive spiritual care** is relevant, nonintrusive care that tends to the spiritual dimension of health by addressing universal spiritual needs, honouring unique spiritual worldviews, and helping individuals to explore and mobilize factors that can help them gain/regain a sense of trust in order to promote optimum healing (Scott Barss, 2012a).

Taking an inclusive approach to spiritual care is particularly vital in Canada's pluralistic society, wherein a multiplicity of religions and perspectives coexist (Stats Canada, 2013). Gaining understanding of the widely variant spiritual worldviews present among Canada's peoples will be a lifelong process for each of us. Each patient we care for will be our best teacher in this regard because each individual experiences and expresses his or her personal spirituality in a unique and ever-evolving manner. However, an introduction to relevant trends and worldviews in our country can be a helpful beginning in becoming attuned to culturally safe spiritual care. Box 40.2 highlights several Canadian trends of which you need to be aware.

Ensuring Ethical Inquiry and Follow-Up

All patients have the right to be offered spiritual care (JCAHO, 2005; Pinto et al., 2010). They also have the right to decline it; similarly, they have the right to have it offered at

BOX 40.2   Spiritual and Religious Trends in Canada

- The number of Canadians identifying themselves as having "No Religious Affiliation" is steadily increasing (Bibby, 2011; Statistics Canada, 2013).
- Native Canadian spirituality is recovering from the effects of colonization and oppression, as many Aboriginal people renew their interest in First Nations' traditional ceremonies that were once outlawed by the Canadian Government (Binda, 2011; First Nations Studies Program at University of British Columbia; Statistics Canada, 2013)
- Christians remain the largest religious group but are declining as a percentage of the population (figures vary, depending on the denomination). The latter trend is also evident in the Jewish community, indicating a trend across Western/European-based faiths (Bibby, 2011; Statistics Canada, 2013).
- Within Christianity, conservative groups are showing the greatest growth (Bibby, 2011; Statistics Canada, 2013).
- The number of Canadians self-identifying as Muslim, Hindu, Buddhist, and Sikh is steadily and significantly increasing, as are a number of other less predominant groups. (Statistics Canada, 2013).
- Materialism, constant change, and a rapid pace of life (associated with our predominant consumer culture) can serve as distractions from engagement in spiritual or religious practice (Armstrong, 2010; Bibby, 2011; Stukes, 2011).
- Many continue to resonate with or be influenced in some way by their natal religious tradition(s) (Armstrong, 2010; Bibby, 2011).
- Globalization and technological advances offer individuals unprecedented direct access to spiritual teachings from a wide variety of traditions and practices, prompting a growing "interspiritual movement," which also recognizes that many people tend to their spiritual needs outside of a specific tradition (Seaward, 2012; Teasdale, 1999).
- Spirituality continues to be self-identified as important to most people, particularly in times of illness or crisis (Bibby, 2011; Jedwab, 2010).

the depth and in ways they see as relevant to their health care (Pinto et al., 2010). It is essential for you to carefully discern whether the context of your therapeutic relationship with a given patient ethically affords deeper exploration, given the existing level of nurse–patient trust and the anticipated length of that relationship. In other words, it is unethical to open up this personal area for exploration unless supportive intervention is possible. Attentiveness to establishing and maintaining healthy therapeutic boundaries is essential in facilitating spiritual exploration at a level appropriate to the context and length of each nurse–patient relationship (see Chapter 26).

Throughout the process of spiritual exploration, it is essential to ensure patients' spiritual, psychological, and physical safety by providing appropriate referral and follow-through in relation to concerns shared as a result

of engaging in spiritual care (CNA, 2010; ICN, 2006). For example, a patient may have both counseling and spiritual care needs because psychological well-being and spiritual well-being, while interrelated, are different dimensions of health (Todres, 2011).

Clarifying the Role of Nursing on the Spiritual Care Team

Although nurses play a significant role in facilitating spiritual care, it is important that we do so within the scope of our practice. We may be able to help patients explore and tend their spiritual needs, but it is important to recognize that specialized skills and wisdom from a particular worldview or professional discipline may be necessary to effectively do so. In such instances, referral to specialized spiritual care providers is essential to safe practice. Conversely, it is important as nurses that we not underestimate our own ability to offer timely and safe spiritual care if we have a strong rapport with patients and are able to effectively help them address their spiritual concerns.

Providing Verbal and Nonverbal Care of the Spirit

Everyone on the health-care team can offer spiritual care in many ways, whether verbally or nonverbally. As nurses, we can do so by

- noticing cues in patients' environments and communication (verbal and nonverbal) that alert us to important aspects of their spirituality and then acknowledging and integrating them into their care (e.g., symbols, rituals, imagery—see "Traditions and Practices" on pp. 12–15 for how these might be integrated into care);
- listening attentively and empathetically to patients' stories and experiences;
- using appropriate touch, voice tone, and other compassionate actions that nurture the spirit in the course of all our nursing interventions; this is especially important for non-verbal and cognitively-impaired patients (Dossey, 2013; O'Brien, 2011; Wright, 2010; Young & Koopsen, 2011).

In nursing, we engage in both "doing" and "being" interventions (Dossey, 2013, p. 13). "Doing" interventions include active measures, such as medications, procedures, and treatments; "being" interventions do not employ such concrete measures but instead use "states of consciousness" and are viewed as having a transcendent quality (Dossey, 2013, p. 13). Examples are the various mind–body–spirit interventions that are in keeping with patients' needs and your practice scope and philosophy (see Chapter 3). Of particular relevance to spiritual care are the "being" interventions of imagery, quiet contemplation, and the presence and intention of the nurse (Dossey, 2013, p. 13). It is our responsibility as nurses to find creative ways of integrating "being" with "doing" so our actions and our words tend consistently to our patients' spirits during our daily interventions.

Developing Unconditional Presence

Our way of being is so essential to being able to offer safe, sensitive, timely spiritual care that it is important to explore ways to intentionally, actively, and continually deepen our ability to be unconditionally present to our patients. **Unconditional presence** is a way of being with patients that involves a deeply authentic connectedness that transcends day-to-day nursing and produces an unconditional acceptance of the patient's essence or spirit, regardless of feelings, behaviours, challenges, or any part of the patient's lived experience (Dossey, 2013; Koerner, 2011; Mariano, 2013; McDonald, 2012; Rogers, 1961). Drawing on the foundational interpersonal skills discussed in Chapter 26, unconditional presence involves deep levels of nonjudgmental curiosity, acknowledgment, attending, allowing, and openness in relation to every part of the patient (Koerner, 2011; McDonald, 2012).

As Koerner (2011) states, unconditional presence means that we engage fully with patients' issues, "gaining strength and wisdom ourselves from their unique moments of courage and brokenness as they gather up the broken fragments of their life. With compassionate nonjudgment, we support their movement toward a revised version of health or to a peaceful death" (p. 96).

Unconditional presence can lead to a spiritual experience and spiritual strength-building and development (Koerner, 2011; McDonald, 2012). For example, a patient living with addictions who experiences his nurse's unconditional presence may experience a deep sense of grace and acceptance, which inspires him to trust in his spiritual strengths and to feel safe enough to engage in spiritual exploration that enhances his resilience and promotes his recovery. Spiritual care begins with unconditional presence; "when we encounter another at the level of spirit, we open to the sacredness of the present moment" (Burkhardt & Nagai-Jacobson as cited in Young & Koopsen, 2011, p. 20).

Think Envision a patient–care situation in which you have had (or would anticipate) difficulty feeling unconditionally present to a patient and/or to the sacredness of the present moment. Using the following guidelines, visualize how you might practice developing the four qualities of unconditional presence: curiosity, acknowledging, attending/allowing, and openness.

Unconditional Curiosity

See yourself approaching the patient with a respectful curiosity and willingness to explore holistically this experience of being unconditionally present to the patient–nurse interaction.

Unconditional Acknowledging

Now become aware of, acknowledge, and name to the patient what you see/hear/sense/notice is happening for her in this moment, using empathetic statements to convey your unconditional acknowledging of the patient's experience (e.g., "I hear much despair within you right now"). Become aware of, acknowledge, and name to yourself what is happening to you as the nurse in this moment (e.g., "I am feeling fear, defensiveness, anxiety," etc.); explore within yourself whether any part of your current experience is relevant to the patient's exploration. If so, authentically acknowledge your experience to the patient through appropriate self-disclosure. If not, honestly acknowledge to yourself any need you have to further process your experience outside the therapeutic relationship. (See Chapter 26 for guidelines around appropriate use of therapeutic self-disclosure.)

Unconditional Attending and Allowing

Keep noticing what your mind, body, and spirit is experiencing in the moment; without rushing, allowing space for this experience.

Keep supporting the patient in observing and experiencing her thoughts, feelings, physical sensations and any other part of her experience. Envision how you would convey to the patient that there is time and space to honour her experience (e.g., "Take all the time you need to be with what you are experiencing." "No rush.").

Unconditional Openness

Now give yourself gentle permission to be more open to your felt bodily experience (i.e., what you feel in your "core" or your "gut"). In doing so, you also offer permission and support to your patient to be more open to her experience with no judgment, no fixing, no changing—to just be unconditionally present with what is in the now.

Guidelines for Spiritual Assessment and Care

Because unconditional presence is so much a part of spiritual care, it is inherent that spiritual assessment and care are inseparable. The moment we are unconditionally present to another's spiritual needs and strengths (whether through deep listening, careful observation, or gentle inquiry), we are, indeed, offering care at a spiritual level (O'Donohue & Quinn, 2011). The spirit is nurtured simply by attention being paid to it through respectful, compassionate assessment; relevant, ethical follow-up interventions that arise seamlessly out of this exploration will further tend to spiritual needs. As such, specific guidelines for spiritual assessment and care are addressed in an integral way (Plotnikoff & Dandurand, 2012).

Many spiritual assessment and care models appear in the nursing literature (Baldacchino, 2010; Kalish, 2012; Young & Koopsen, 2011). It will be important for you to explore various models as you develop your skills and adapt your holistic practice to different contexts. To help you begin, this chapter introduces you to a Canadian model particularly designed for use in a pluralistic health-care context, the T.R.U.S.T. Model for Inclusive Spiritual Care (Scott Barss, 2012a). This evidence-based model lends itself to use with other models that may be more culturally relevant in particular settings; for example, the medicine wheel with Aboriginal patients who follow First Nations traditional teachings; pastoral care-based models with patients who identify strongly with a religious tradition; humanistic models with patients who identify most with a secular context (Scott Barss, 2012a). This resource also lends itself to use with various indicator-based tools and scales for nurses and patients who identify with quantifying or measuring aspects of their spirituality (Baldacchino, 2010). In any case, the T.R.U.S.T. Model can facilitate early identification of how patients prefer to address their spiritual needs (Fig. 40.4.)

T.R.U.S.T. is an affirmation of inclusive spiritual care for those both offering and receiving care. Its imagery, symbolizing associated risk and potential during times of crisis, is a reminder of how essential it is to offer spiritual care at these pivotal times in the healing process. It is also intended to remind you and your patients to trust in your unique abilities, worldviews, and relationships in order to promote spiritual and overall well-being for self and others. T.R.U.S.T. offers a nonlinear outline for exploring the five domains illustrated in Figure 40.5. These domains are *traditions and practices*, *reconciliation*, *understandings*, *searching*, and *teachers*. These domains reflect recommended best practices and standards and cue assessment of all required areas. Spiritual exploration can begin on any one of these interconnected domains or stems, as determined through deep listening for the patient's uppermost concerns.

Some initial assessment questions and guidelines that can help you meet the minimum standards for spiritual care in nonintrusive, patient-centered ways are highlighted in Box 40.3. Sample questions that may be helpful for patients to explore at the appropriate time of readiness, determined by the spiritual needs and strengths they demonstrate and voice (Scott Barss, 2012a), are found in Box 40.4. For purposes of introduction and deeper understanding of related issues, we will explore the five domains of T.R.U.S.T. chronologically from left to right.

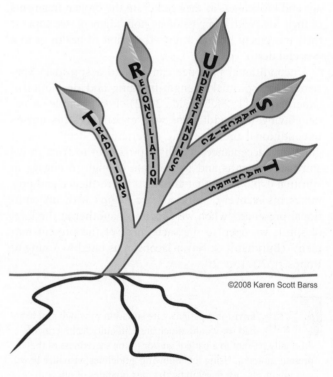

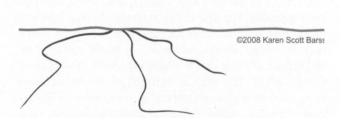

*Broken spirits
cracked open and exposed
remain ...*

*... until warmth and light,
the life-giving flow of
compassion
takes root, nurtures forth
new shoots of trust.*

©2008 Karen Scott Barss

Figure 40.4 T.R.U.S.T.—An affirmation for inclusive spiritual care. (Permission for use granted by Karen Scott Barss, 2014)

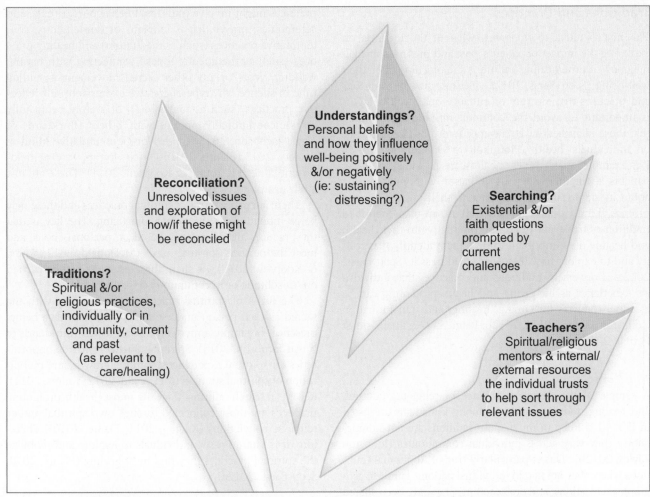

Understandings?
Personal beliefs
and how they influence
well-being positively
&/or negatively
(ie: sustaining?
distressing?)

Reconciliation?
Unresolved issues
and exploration of
how/if these might
be reconciled

Searching?
Existential &/or
faith questions
prompted by
current
challenges

Traditions?
Spiritual &/or
religious practices,
individually or in
community, current
and past
(as relevant to
care/healing)

Teachers?
Spiritual/religious
mentors & internal/
external resources
the individual trusts
to help sort through
relevant issues

TRUST Model for Spiritual Assessment and Care © Karen Scott Barss 2008

Figure 40.5 T.R.U.S.T.—Domains for spiritual exploration.
(Permission for use granted by Karen Scott Barss, 2014)

BOX 40.3   T.R.U.S.T. Initial Assessment Questions and Guidelines

Refer to Figure 40.5:

Initiating conversation about the very personal aspect of spirituality is most comfortable and effective when its relevance is clear. This relevance can be clarified by a statement like:

"As part of offering holistic care, we would like to be aware of anything you consider to be important in relation to the spiritual aspect of your care."

You may need to follow with some health teaching something like the following:

"The spiritual aspect of care has to do with things like finding ways to be hopeful and exploring how our beliefs might sustain us through difficult times like you're experiencing right now. More and more we are recognizing in health care how important these things are in promoting the best possible outcome."

Somewhere in the ensuing initial assessment conversation(s) the previous questions need to be addressed in a nonlinear, nonintrusive, patient-centered manner.

Note: Each of the questions themselves are closed-ended (i.e., answerable with a "yes" or a "no") in order to avoid assumption that the individual has/wishes to share related information.

During the conversation, explore how spiritual care can be integrated into the patient's holistic care in an individualized, nonintrusive manner. Specific expansion on the initial assessment questions will depend on patients' responses to each of the initial assessment questions. For example:

If the answer is "yes" . . . *"What are these? How can we help to integrate them into your health-care/healing process?"*

If the answer is "no" . . . *"Sometimes people become aware of and/or feel more comfortable sharing spiritual concerns as they become better acquainted with the health-care team. Please feel free to raise any such concerns that may come up at any time and to ask us to help seek out any resources you'd like."*

Permission for use granted by Karen Scott Barss, 2014.

Traditions and Practices

The first *T* refers to *traditions*, wherein the focus is on exploring the impact of patients' past and present spiritual/religious/cultural/healing traditions and practices upon their well-being (Scott Barss, 2012a). Because not all traditions and practices may nurture or enhance one's well-being, it is important to avoid the common mistake of assuming that those identified have relevance to or positive influence on individuals' health (Plotnikoff & Dandurand, 2012). For example, many times, health-care providers will ask patients about their religious affiliation without inquiring about its significance or relevance to their current healing process. If individuals experience all or part of an identified tradition as irrelevant or counterproductive to their health and healing, it is important to help them identify that reality and to explore how they wish to address it (Scott Barss, 2012a). Conversely, traditions and practices that individuals experience as life-giving and health-promoting can be essential catalysts for coping, healing, and transformation (Johnston Taylor, 2012a, 2012b; Plante, 2010; Puchalski & Ferrell, 2010).

Traditions

A sample of the trends and range of religious, cultural, and healing traditions present among Canadians are listed in Box 40.2. Keep in mind such traditions are not homogenous; they vary across individual communities (Johnston Taylor, 2012b). This is particularly true of Aboriginal traditions where they are tied to individual nations, families, geographical locations, and oral teachings that have been shared across generations (Clarke & Holtslander, 2010; Trudeau & Cherubini, 2010). Also, individuals within a tradition will fall along a continuum from liberal to conservative in their beliefs (Johnston Taylor, 2012b).

Remember, too, that individuals might follow more than one tradition, depending on their history and preferences. For example, many Aboriginal Canadians blend First Nations and Christian traditions, given their history with both (Clarke & Holtslander, 2010). Similarly, many Canadians draw on various religious and nonreligious traditions to nurture their spirituality. For example, an individual might belong to a Christian faith community, attend Buddhist meditation classes, and engage in readings from various religious and secular traditions such as Taoism and humanism (Young & Koopsen, 2011). Others would describe themselves as unaffiliated with any particular tradition (Stukes, 2011; Young & Koopsen, 2011).

Practices

Spiritual practices are defined as processes of inner quieting to help attain a state of calm centeredness and receptive awareness which nurtures the spirit and deepens insight, attention and compassion for oneself and others (The Centre for Contemplative Mind in Society, 2013; Puchalski & Ferrel, 2010; Scott Barss, 2012a). Spiritual practices might involve traditional behaviours, rituals, and ceremonies; prayer that is religious or nonreligious; contemplative practices (such as meditation) and healing practices (such as therapeutic touch) connecting with nature; walking, yoga, or any other sacred movement; spending time in silence; any type of creative expression; self-reflective practices (such as journaling); or simply being fully and unconditionally present with others (Burkhardt & Nagai-Jacobson, 2013; Centre for Contemplative Mind in Society, 2013; Plante, 2010; Ulrich, Evron, & Ostenfeld-Rosenthal, 2011; Young & Koopsen, 2011). These are just a few examples.

There are many forms of spiritual practices and these may be as individual as the person practicing. The key is that the practices are intentional, based on personal choice and meet the person's spiritual needs (McDonald, 2012; Young & Koopsen, 2011). As such, these practices can be carried out in solitude or in community (Fig. 40-6).

The focus of spiritual practices is to connect with the sacred as each person understands it—whether as a being, presence, or simply a mystery beyond words (Burkhardt & Nagai-Jacobson, 2013). Spiritual practices provide opportunities for spiritual experiences, spiritual growth, and mobilization of spiritual strength (McDonald, 2012; Todres, 2011). Recent research affirms that the most health-promoting practices are those connected to one's own spiritual and/or religious convictions (Koenig, 2011; Plante, 2010). Therefore, it is vital to assist individuals to explore and mobilize the spiritual practices they find most healing (Plante, 2010; Scott Barss, 2012a).

Through the eyes of a student

I felt very humbled today. I had decided I was going to teach my patient a relaxation exercise because I noticed how anxious he was yesterday. I sensed from the beginning that he was just doing it to be nice to a student. I think it made him more anxious—and maybe even a little annoyed by the time we finished. I finally got up the courage to check in with him, smiling and saying, "I'm not sure that was feeling right for you." He looked so relieved and said, "Actually, no, it wasn't. I just don't connect with 'relaxation' or 'meditation' or whatever pop culture calls it. It feels so . . . structured . . . and almost . . . empty . . . for me. I have a very strong Christian faith—and I've recently been learning about something called *centering prayer.* I find it so comforting . . . and restful. It's funny, though, I haven't thought to do it since I've been in the hospital, so this has been a helpful reminder." I realized I hadn't even asked him what he already finds calming—and that I had just chosen something that works for me. I am very lucky to have had this experience with someone who was so tolerant of the assumptions I made. I'll never forget it.

(personal reflection [clinical journal entry] of a first-year nursing student)

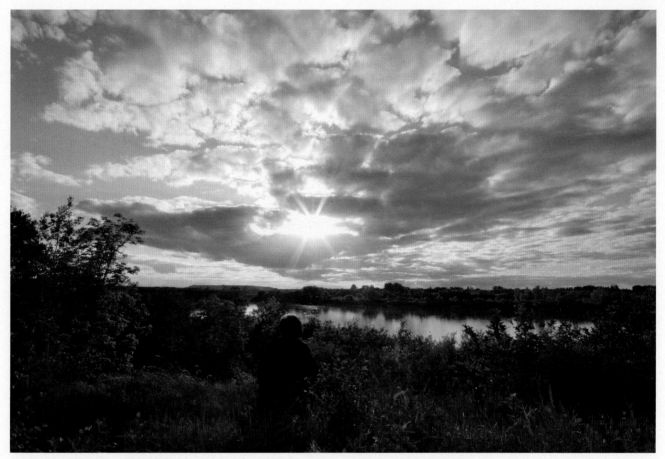

Figure 40.6 Meditation. Daily spiritual practices in keeping with each individual's worldview can be central to health promotion and restoration (Koenig, 2011; Plante, 2010). (Photo copyright Moira Theede, BSN)

Integrating Patient Traditions and Practices Into Health Care

Assisting patients to actively draw on their traditions and practices in the health-care context can be challenging, given the vast range of traditions and the need to maintain appropriate therapeutic boundaries in implementing interventions around this very personal aspect of care (Fowler, Reimer-Kirkham, Sawatzky, & Johnston Taylor, 2012). Knowledge of relevant resources and of your professional boundaries is essential, as is consultation with spiritual and cultural workers. (Further related guidance is offered in exploring the domain of "Teachers" on pp. 20–22.) Similarly, consultation with nursing colleagues and agency policies is vital to ensure that professional boundaries around spiritual care are not only maintained but are also clearly perceived to be maintained by all members of the health-care team. Such consultation helps ensure that the principles of patient-centeredness and cultural safety are being upheld, protecting both patients and nurses from any potential boundary violations that may arise from one individual's traditions or practices being imposed on another (Fowler et al., 2012; Young & Koopsen, 2011). The following general guidelines can help you safely assist patients to integrate their traditions and practices into their health care and healing.

Patient Choice

Engagement in the tradition or practice needs to be initiated by the patient. For example, it would be inappropriate for you to suggest to a patient that he or she engage in prayer, but if the patient self-identifies this practice as helpful, it would be important for you to offer encouragement and relevant resources (Young & Koopsen, 2011).

Mutual Comfort and Appropriate Consultation

If a patient asks you to share in a spiritual practice, you need not do so if it is incongruent with your own worldview (e.g., prayer; engagement in a ceremony from a particular tradition). However, it is your responsibility to help the patient connect with other sources of support. Should you feel comfortable meeting the patient's request to engage in the practice together, remember to consult with colleagues and supervisors to ensure your professional safety and clear communication about the appropriateness of this intervention (Olson & Clark, 2010; Pinto et al., 2008).

Health and Safety Considerations

You have a responsibility to encourage health-promoting traditions and practices. Although patients ultimately have a right to engage in whatever communities and activities they choose, it is our responsibility as nurses to help patients

BOX 40.4 T.R.U.S.T. Sample Reflective Questions

Traditions and Practices

- *Are there things about your spiritual, religious, cultural, and/or healing traditions/practices/experiences you would like the health-care team to be aware of? How might these affect how we work together?*
- What practices, activities, or issues are you inspired by/passionate about? How can these be integrated into your healing? What new practices, activities, or issues might you like to explore?
- Do you have affiliation with any particular spiritual, religious, cultural, and/or healing tradition(s)? If so, do you see it/them as a current source of strength? Of distress? How so? Are there aspects of/experiences with your tradition(s) that you feel contribute to your well-being? Compromise your well-being?
- What do/does your tradition(s) say about the nature of suffering? How do you feel about that?
- What gives you hope? How can we help you connect to your sources of hope?
- How are you creative in your daily life? Your coping? How can this creativity be applied to your current challenges? To your life in general?

Reconciliation

- *Are there any unresolved issues you would like support in exploring at this time?*
- Are there situations, choices, or actions of others in your life with whom you cannot currently make peace? How does this influence your sense of well-being? What do you wish to do with this awareness?
- Do you find yourself focusing on past choices or actions that you regret? How does this focus influence your sense of well-being? What do you wish to do with this awareness?
- What does "reconciliation" mean to you? What would reconciliation look/feel like to you? What might be the benefits of reconciliation?
- Do your current spiritual/religious/cultural traditions play a role in finding reconciliation? What do their teachings say about reconciliation/forgiveness/nonattachment/rebalancing? Do they assist/interfere? How so?
- Have you found anything positive arising from your painful experiences (e.g., development of inner strengths you didn't know you had; closer relationships; deeper trust; lessons learned; deeper appreciation for the good times; a sense of purpose or meaning, more creative coping)? If so, how does/can this enhance your daily life amidst the difficulties you face? If not, does it feel okay, for now, to grieve the losses associated with your difficulties?
- What/who can sustain you until you feel more hopeful/peaceful? Do you see yourself being able to feel more hopeful/peaceful?

Understandings

- *Are there particular personal beliefs or practices sustaining you/offering you comfort at this time? How can we help you draw on these for strength?*
- Are you aware of any beliefs or questions that are distressing/compromising your well-being? If so, how do you wish to address these? Do you see it as possible to eventually transform them into ones that promote wellness?
- Are there particular spiritual, religious, or cultural influences that influence or inform your understandings? How do you feel about these influences?
- What do you believe about the nature of suffering? How do you think these beliefs are influencing your current healing process?
- What gives your life meaning? Is there any meaning that you make in relation to your current difficulties? If so, what? How does this influence the way you navigate your circumstances?
- Has this experience prompted you to ponder your overall life's purpose(s)? If so, what is your sense about it/them? How does this influence your well-being/your approach to life/your healing process?

Searching

- *Are there spiritually oriented questions about your current difficulties that you would like an opportunity to explore?*
- How have your current difficulties influenced your beliefs? Are there any of your previously held beliefs that you are currently questioning? How do you feel about questioning these beliefs? Does this type of questioning feel safe/unsafe? What/who contributes to this sense of safety/risk?
- What answers about life/death/spirituality are you currently seeking? How difficult is this searching?
- What/who is a source of disillusionment for you? Have you had an opportunity to grieve associated losses? If not, how might you do so?
- Has the imposition of others' beliefs added to your distress? If so, how? How can you gain protection from these intrusions?

Teachers

- *Are there people/groups/resources you find helpful in exploring spiritual questions? How can they be involved in your healing process?*
- Who do you consider to be your spiritual teachers/mentors/leaders/companions?
- What readings and activities do you find personally inspiring or comforting? How might they contribute to your healing? How can you draw these resources into your regular routine?
- What new mentors, readings, activities, and events would you like to access?
- What resources within yourself can you name and draw upon? What new internal resources would you like to develop?

Note: Bold, italicized questions have been identified as suitable for initial assessment/trust-building.

Source: Scott Barss, K. (2012a). T.R.U.S.T.: An affirming model for inclusive spiritual care. *Journal of Holistic Nursing, 30*(1), 24–34. doi:10.1177/0898010111418118. Permission for use granted by Karen Scott Barss, 2014.

make informed choices about whether or not a tradition or practice is healthy in the context of their current health challenges. For example, if your sense was that a particular tradition or practice was compromising a patient's health by being disempowering or abusive, it would be important to help the patient explore how this might influence his or her healing, drawing on specialized spiritual care expertise as relevant to his or her worldview.

Day-to-Day Practices and Care

Be attentive to spiritual practices that may influence your day-to-day nursing care. For example, in many First Nations traditions, hair braids are sacred because they are an expression of one's relationship to the Creator. Similarly, various head coverings have deep religious significance to many Muslim, Sikh, and Hindu Canadians. These practices may be so much a part of individuals' way of being that they don't think to mention them when you inquire about their practices. However, if you are practicing unconditional presence, you will be guided by your careful observations and reverent inquiries about patient needs and preferences as you provide care. Doing so will not only allow you to assist patients with their activities of daily living (ADL) in a nonintrusive way but will also help you be attentive to openings to talk about how these practices influence patients' overall health and well-being (Johnston Taylor, 2012a, 2012b).

Conflicts With Traditions

Listen carefully for suffering that may have become associated with involvement in a religious or cultural tradition. Patients may have experienced marginalization and traumatization through related doctrine, interpretations, and even boundary violations (Aboriginal Healing Foundation, 2009, 2012; Stukes, 2010; Young & Koopsen, 2011). For example, many gay, lesbian, bisexual, and transgendered people have been rejected by (or have distanced themselves from) their religious communities (Stedman, 2012). Many others have been persecuted when their beliefs are at odds with a particular religious viewpoint. It is particularly important in these circumstances that our language is inclusive, so we don't inadvertently trigger emotions or reactions that could be a barrier to patients' trust in you.

Whether positive and/or negative, patients' experiences with spiritually related traditions can have significant implications for their health and healing, which need to be considered and sensitively addressed within the therapeutic relationship.

Reconciliation

The *R* in T.R.U.S.T. stands for *reconciliation*, a reminder to explore any unresolved issues the patient might wish to reconcile. Reconciliation is an often lengthy process of making peace with oneself, others, or losses and challenges in our lives (The Fetzer Institute, 2013). Reconciliation might mean finding acceptance of the immediate crisis or circumstances at hand so the patient can eventually move into a health-promoting state of trust (Scott Barss, 2012a). Reconciliation might also involve a self-identified need for healing within a community, a relationship, or oneself (Rindfleisch & Reed, 2012). Given enough time and support, reconciliation may assist individuals to make meaning of their painful experiences and move toward greater wholeness (The Fetzer Institute, 2013; Rindfleisch & Reed, 2012; Wright & Bell, 2010).

To this end, it is particularly important that exploration includes identification of the patient's personal meaning of reconciliation. For example, patients identifying with a Western worldview may equate it with such concepts as grace or forgiveness (Rindfleisch & Reed, 2013; Scott Barss, 2012a). Someone who identifies strongly with an Aboriginal worldview may use words describing the return to a natural state of balance and harmony (Binda, 2011; Calestani, White, Hendricks, & Scemons, 2012). Similarly, an individual who identifies most with an Eastern worldview may prefer to use language such as letting go of hurt or returning to the flow of life (Johnston Taylor, 2012b; O'Brien, 2011; Scott Barss, 2012a). Only through ongoing reflective dialogue will patients be able to find voice for and affirm the personal language that helps make meaning of their distress (McDonald 2012; Scott Barss, 2012a; Wright & Bell, 2010).

It is important to recognize that an absence of reconciliation can involve profound suffering. **Suffering** is any physical, emotional, and spiritual distress, pain, and anguish (Wright & Bell, 2010, p. 74). It may also involve a sense of chaos that can be overwhelming to the point of despair (Bridges, 2004; Gregory, 1994; Travelbee as cited in Meleis, 2012). Suffering is a spiritual phenomenon that can challenge the very trust we have in life or in our ability to heal (Johnston Taylor, 2012a; Scott Barss, 2012a). As pioneer nurse theorist Joyce Travelbee described it, "To suffer is to be immersed in a black ocean of pain" (Travelbee, 1966, p. 89).

Issues Relating to Reconciliation

Understanding common issues associated with reconciliation will help you listen for and address related spiritual needs. Unresolved loss, grief, and trauma are associated with profound spiritual pain that can significantly compromise health and healing (Wright & Bell, 2010; Young & Koopsen, 2011). As nurses, we witness daily the grief associated with a loss of health, independence, dreams, relationships, and even life itself. In particular, death often is not embraced easily; therefore, fear of death and avoidance of its reality can bring additional suffering (Puchalski & Ferrell, 2010; Young & Koopsen, 2011). So great is such loss and suffering that its reconciliation may prompt us (patients and nurses alike) to draw on or further develop what is deepest within us, our spirituality (Young & Koopsen, 2011).

Such losses are compounded when individuals experience trauma (Wright & Bell, 2010; Young & Koopsen, 2011). Trauma is an injury (which could be mental, emotional, physical, or spiritual) involving actual or feared death or serious injury, which triggers feelings of intense fear, helplessness, and loss of control (Levine, 2010; Rosenbloom, Williams, & Watkins, 2010). On a spiritual level, trauma often results in a "broken spirit" wherein the very will to heal is lost (Wilson, 2004, p. 109).

A broken spirit can, of course, have a ripple effect on an entire group of people. An important example is the far-reaching effect on the families and communities of countless refugees who have sought asylum in Canada from political oppression, war, torture, and other atrocities (Wilson, 2004). Another example is the brokenness experienced by generations of Aboriginal Canadians through the residential schools. This, too, is an essential example to highlight because this trauma was of such a magnitude that Aboriginal people are still in the process of reconciling related suffering across our country (Truth and Reconciliation Commission of Canada [TRC], 2012).

For approximately a century, beginning in the 1880s, Aboriginal children experienced mandatory attendance at government-run residential schools (Aboriginal Healing Foundation, 2012; Partridge, 2010). The resulting loss of traditional values and beliefs, language, and connections to family, elders, and societies meant that the cultural connections vanished from their lived experience and that of generations to follow. Such losses were often compounded by the trauma of verbal, physical, emotional, mental, spiritual, and sexual abuse. The resulting cycles of abuse, alcoholism, decreased self-esteem, and learned dependency are referred to as the 'intergenerational effects of residential school' (Getty, 2010).

Today, a resurgence of understanding Aboriginal worldviews, spirituality, and culture is part of the healing process for many survivors and their descendants as they seek reconciliation (Binda, 2011; Lavalle & Poole, 2010; Robbins & Dewar, 2011). Similarly, non-Aboriginal Canadians are seeking reconciliation related to regret and guilt associated with their involvement in the tragic policies and practices of the residential schools (TRC, 2012).

Along with that of other spiritual leaders and ethicists, the seminal work of Willie Ermine has validated the importance of sharing "ethical space" to promote healing between Aboriginal Canadians and other Canadians (Ermine, 2007, p. 193). The Truth and Reconciliation Commission of Canada (TRC) is among many initiatives aimed toward healing Canadians affected by our residential school legacy, with a necessary focus on how everyone can participate in healing the broken spirits and broken communities of Aboriginal Canadians (TRC, 2012). "The truth of our common experiences will help set our spirits free and pave the way to reconciliation" (TRC, 2012, p. 1). Such initiatives offer resources we can draw on when we encounter patients whose health has been affected by related suffering. For example, the TRC offers many web-based resources and face-to-face opportunities across the country to validate and support individuals in their progression toward healing. Such initiatives also can help us understand the lengthy process of healing and serve as strong examples of healthy reconciliation.

Margaret has just received a terminal diagnosis of breast cancer. She has declined any active treatment based on her poor prognosis and her wish to feel as well as she can during her remaining time. Because Tommy has taken the time to understand her views, Margaret is very comfortable talking with him. She voices that she is at peace with dying, but she is worried about her funeral plans. She tells Tommy she would like certain First Nations traditional ceremonies included, but that her children are uncomfortable with this because these ceremonies are not in keeping with the Christian traditions they follow. Margaret is torn because she sees the traditional ceremonies as vital for her peaceful transition to the Spirit World, but she also feels a great responsibility to help her children make peace with her passing.

Tommy initially feels overwhelmed by this challenging situation and by his own feelings of sadness. He talks with his clinical teacher who listens carefully, validates his feelings, and reminds him of the comfort he is already bringing to Margaret by creating a safe place to share her concerns. Tommy considers what a privilege it is to accompany Margaret on her journey and realizes there are many resources both he and Margaret can draw upon for support, such as the agency's Elder and other spiritual care staff Margaret wishes to involve. He also realizes that, in the process, he will learn much about making peace with what life brings.

Beginning the Process of Reconciliation

Compassionately acknowledging suffering and being willing to bear witness to suffering are the first steps toward reconciliation; doing so can initiate the healing response (Scott Barss, 2012a; Wright & Bell, 2010). Because the need for reconciliation is often associated with past or present grief, loss, and trauma, it is critical that the patient's interpretations, personal boundaries, and pacing be respected throughout any resulting exploration—and that sufficient personal and professional support is consistently available. Even if our time with patients is short, we can help them find freedom from blame and shame that is often felt around painful experiences. Specifically, nurses can

- offer patients reminders that they are not to blame for life circumstances beyond their control but do have a choice about how to respond to them (Rosenbloom et al., 2010).
- ensure our unconditional presence is shared when patients are seeking self-acceptance around past choices and mistakes (Rindfleisch & Reed, 2012).
- refrain from pressuring patients to engage in the difficult work of reconciliation. Any sense of judgment or rushing of the process has the potential not only to block healing but also to further traumatize the individual (Rindfleisch & Reed, 2012).
- arrange timely and relevant referral to any counselors and/or specialized spiritual mentors if patients identify a readiness to engage in reconciliation (Young & Koopsen, 2011).

- avoid the temptation to try to make meaning of patients' suffering (Wright & Bell, 2010; Young & Koopsen, 2011). Doing so can inadvertently trivialize their suffering and interfere with their ability to eventually make their own meaning of their experiences (Wright & Bell, 2010).
- help patients to identify sources of hope and meaning that can sustain them throughout the reconciliation process (Wright & Bell, 2010; Young & Koopsen, 2011).

The moments you share with patients along the way can be pivotal in helping them navigate their suffering. As Canadian nurse therapist Lorraine Wright says in her seminal work, "Softening suffering is the heart of nursing" (Wright, 2007, p. 394). Softening suffering does not rid the experience of suffering. However, when it is transformed, there is a spiritual strengthening for patients, families, and communities so they can move forward in their lives (Wright, 2007; Wright & Bell, 2010).

Think

One of your patients, Olive, a young Aboriginal woman, had surgery a couple of days ago in relation to injuries sustained through domestic violence. She has been very open about the incident in conversations with you. You acknowledge her spiritual strengths of honesty and acceptance and then gently inquire about what is helping her to cope so well after a relatively short time. She smiles shyly and tells you the following story:

I was sitting on the hospital bed after I was beaten up. I remember thinking, "Why did this happen to me?" Just as I had this thought, my sister walked in and took one look at me and cried. I joked with her . . . "Do I look that bad?" laughing a little to lighten the mood. After a while, my sister said to me, "I believe this happened to you for a reason. You are going through this so you can help others in the future." I thought to myself, "Others in the future? Are you crazy? I wouldn't wish this on anyone . . ." I calmed down and reflected on what she said. Many hours after she left, I prayed, "Creator, what message do I need to get out of this? Help me understand what I am supposed to learn." Not long after I finished praying, my elder walked into my room, and in his quiet manner said, "I was expecting to see you here today." At first, I was shocked but then . . . somehow . . . not surprised. Maybe there is something to what my sister said.

You know it is important to refrain from trying to make meaning on others' behalf. Therefore, you find it surprising that Olive's sister would share her interpretations with her so early in her healing process. Still, their interaction prompted important reflection for Olive about what this experience might mean. How do you respond to Olive?

(Since this is a particularly challenging scenario, an example of an appropriate response is provided below, based on guidelines provided in this chapter and with guidelines for sound therapeutic communication as outlined in Chapter 26.)

It sounds like your sister and your elder are both deeply connected to you. I also hear within you a strong sense of being guided. I admire how you are already considering the possibility that something good might come out of what you're going through. Are there any other ways we can support you and your spiritual exploration as you continue to sort through what all this means?

(This response honours Olive's experience without giving advice, imposing any differing beliefs you may have, or attempting to make meaning for her—all important pitfalls for you to avoid in your professional role.)

Understandings

Individuals' personal beliefs can be key sources of hope and meaning during the reconciliation process. However, personal beliefs can also block healing if they fail to be health-promoting. The *U* in T.R.U.S.T. addresses *understandings*, which refers to the individual worldview and associated personal beliefs that can significantly influence well-being (Scott Barss, 2012a). Given the substantial validation in scientific literature about the ability of our beliefs to influence health positively or negatively, it is essential for individuals and their caregivers to be aware of which beliefs are sustaining, inspiring, and health-promoting and which ones are distressing, disempowering, and health-compromising (Pinto et al., 2008; Wright & Bell, 2010). Identifying the former creates opportunity to mobilize such affirming beliefs, whereas identifying the latter offers invitation for individuals to challenge unhealthy beliefs and to eventually find related reconciliation (Rakel & Wiel, 2012; Rindfleisch & Reed, 2012; Wright & Bell, 2010).

Helping Patients Explore Their Beliefs

The beliefs and illness model developed by Canadian nurse therapists Wright and Bell (2010) is an important resource to help patients challenge beliefs that are blocking healing and draw on beliefs that can foster healing. Although you may draw more on Wright and Bell's specialized work later on in your career, the following guidelines based on their work will help you get started:

- Ask patients specifically about what beliefs are helping them cope with their current challenges, then provide validation and encouragement to draw on such convictions. Otherwise, patients may forget to fully tap into these.
- Listen carefully for any beliefs (distressing and/or sustaining) that are evident in patients' reflections. If your rapport with the patient feels strong enough, share your observations about what you heard; doing so may foster important awareness and ease suffering.
- Offer health-teaching and validation that challenging unhelpful beliefs and searching for helpful ones is a natural and healthy part of the healing process.
- Be intentional about not imposing your own beliefs on patients. Doing so may compromise cultural safety and intrude on the deeply personal process of forging beliefs that will foster healing.

Through the eyes of a nurse

*S*pirituality is part of my practice, but it is a very personal part. Sharing your faith is not seen as a professional thing to do, and in nursing, we are taught to be professional so I am hesitant to talk about it and admit to you that it is part of my care. To me, it can be the true essence of everything—of life, of death.

(continued on page 1080)

Through the eyes of a nurse (continued)

I do share my own beliefs if they [patients] are asking and they are feeling lost. I feel comfortable because I have my own beliefs together. People ask a lot of questions about the end, where they are going—especially if they haven't finished their business yet. Sometimes, I just pray to myself.

(personal reflection shared by Jane, an experienced oncology nurse who has been identified by her colleagues and patients as exemplary in research carried out by Canadian nurse-scholar, Beth Perry [Perry, 2009, p. 192])

Searching

The *S* in T.R.U.S.T. refers to *searching*, as in seeking understanding or searching for answers (Scott Barss, 2012a). Reconciliation and realization of health-promoting spiritual understandings is, of course, impossible without considerable exploration of existential and/or faith questions prompted by current suffering (Plotnikoff & Dandurand, 2012; Rindfleisch & Reed, 2012; Wright & Bell, 2010). Frequently, individuals' previously held beliefs are no longer serving them, creating a strong need for them to challenge old beliefs and seek new ones that can help make meaning of their current distress (Travelbee, 1966). Nurses can offer invaluable encouragement as patients explore the mystery of suffering (Wright & Bell, 2010). Rather than mainly focusing on fixing the body as the problem, nurses can support the patient to self-reflect and self-interpret their health challenges through their own worldview (Carr, 2010).

Common Spiritual/Existential Questions Prompted by Suffering

You can prepare to support patients' exploration by gaining understanding of the kinds of questions they may be pondering. This understanding will help you listen deeply for your patients' unspoken worries. Box 40.5 highlights common existential and faith questions prompted by illness.

Understanding and Supporting Spiritual Growth and Development

The nature of individuals' existential and faith questions and how they approach them is greatly influenced by where they are on their spiritual journey. For example, individuals in the early stages of spiritual development may need more support during health crises than those in later stages who are experienced at tapping into their spirituality to help navigate adversity (Young & Koopsen, 2011).

There are many ways of conceptualizing the spiritual journey (Fig. 40-7). A brief introduction to a few such ways may help you better understand where your patients are coming from spiritually. The classic works of Peck (1978) and Fowler (1981) conceptualized several stages of spiritual development. Their work raised awareness that our spiritual dimension undergoes various developmental phases akin to those described in other developmental theories you have studied.

BOX 40.5   Spiritual/Existential Questions Arising from Suffering

Common Existential or Faith Questions About Health Crises

Why is this happening to me?
Is this experience a test?
Am I being punished?
Am I to blame?
Is there something I can or am supposed to learn?
Is this experience in vain/meaningless?
Can I carry on? How?
What can/can't I control?

Common Existential or Faith Questions About Dying

Who will remember me?
What has my life meant?
How do I make peace with dying? With my past?
What will happen to me/my family after I die?

Based on O'Brien, M. (2011). *Spirituality in nursing: Standing on holy ground* (4th ed.). Mississauga, ON: Jones & Bartlett; Parachini, P. (2011). Attentiveness to the spiritual needs of the seriously ill. *Presence: An International Journal of Spiritual Direction, 17*(4), 51–58; Puchalski, C., & Ferrell, B. (2010). *Making healthcare whole: Integrating spirituality into patient care.* West Conshohocken, PA: Templeton Press; Wright, L., & Bell, J. (2010). *Beliefs and illness: A model for healing.* Calgary, AB: 4th Floor Press; Young, C., & Koopsen, C. (2011). *Spirituality, health and healing: An integrative approach* (2nd ed.). Toronto, ON: Jones & Bartlett.

Of course, people all develop at their own pace and may move back and forth through these stages, depending on their experiences and choices (O'Brien, 2011; Stukes, 2011). Dr. Brian Luc Seaward, a pioneer in mind–body–spirit healing, acknowledges this reality in his discussion of spiritual dormancy wherein one may choose not to recognize the importance of the spiritual dimension of life, individually or socially (Seaward, 2012, p. 168). He also describes what he calls a state of spiritual bankruptcy, a lack of spiritual direction, values, or less than desirable behaviours and choices. Many times, crisis or illness can prompt a sense of spiritual hunger which Seaward defines as "the quest for understanding life's bigger questions, the bigger picture, and how each of us fits into it" (Seaward, 2012, p. 168).

All cultural and religious traditions have related teachings and practices about such spiritual hunger and searching. For example, the Buddhist tradition speaks of awakening and experiencing enlightenment, whereas the Christian tradition speaks of having a revelation or experiencing salvation. Many Aboriginal traditions involve vision quests for individuals as they navigate rites of passage and gain spiritual wisdom at various times in the life cycle. (Anderson, Pakula, Smye, Peters, & Schroeder, 2011). Such quests involve an elder to guide the journey, interpret visions, and pass on wisdom (Binda, 2011; McAdam, 2009; Wilson & Restoole, 2010).

Mythologist Joseph Campbell drew on such teachings to develop his classic template of the human journey and the three stages of spiritual growth: departure, initiation, and return (Seaward, 2012). Whatever form it takes, spiritual searching invites the possibility of **transcendence**, the process of moving to higher levels of self-awareness and

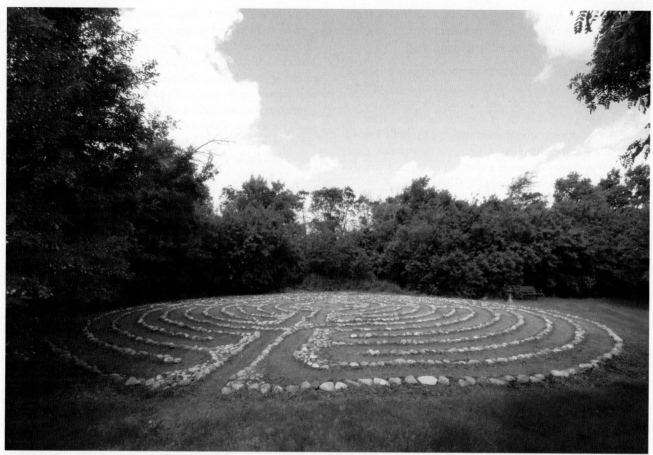

Figure 40.7 A labyrinth at Prairie View Chapel and Crematorium, Saskatoon, SK. The labyrinth is an ancient metaphor for the spiritual journey that has been found in various traditions. This form of walking meditation has reemerged today as a powerful tool for healing and transformation. (Source: http://labyrinthsociety.org; Photo copyright Moira Theede, BSN)

consciousness, which offers individuals new possibilities and choices in their lives and in their relationships (Sharpnack, Quinn Griffin, & Fitzpatrick, 2011; Young & Koopsen, 2011). Persons who go through transcending experiences spiritually grow into a "holistic human consciousness" and experience self-actualization (Conti-O'Hare, 2002, p. 88).

Such transcendence is not a necessary experience nor is it a goal that can be accomplished. At the same time, it is an opportunity that may unfold through the intentional and open spiritual searching often prompted by crises. Research on transcendence has shown that, when it does occur, its enhancement of a person's relationship with self, others, and the environment can increase hope, adaptation to illness, and spiritual well-being (Sharpnack et al., 2011; Thomas, Burton, Quinn Griffin, & Fitzpatrick, 2010).

As Tommy continues to care for Margaret, he realizes that he is learning more from her than she can learn from him at this point in his career. Prior to this experience, he had given little thought to the spiritual part of his life; Margaret, on the other hand, had spent years searching and finding answers as she made peace with the residential

school experiences and other hardships she has told Tommy about. Still, he realizes that he is offering an important gift to her by bearing witness to her stories, which are helping her prepare for her passing. As he reflects on this realization in postconference, Amira comments on how the conversations she has begun to have with Matt (the young man living with quadriplegia and depression) are like discovering new territory together, given their similar ages and inexperience with exploring spiritual questions. Further, she reflects that Matt has been more hopeful and more open lately as she has shared some of what she has been learning about the role of spirituality in healing.

Helping Patients Explore Their Questions

The safest and perhaps most powerful role you can play is simply to offer your unconditional presence as patients voice and explore their questions. You need not have the answers. In fact, it would be intrusive to try and provide the answers or attempt to draw conclusions on patients' behalf (Wright & Bell, 2010; Young & Koopsen, 2011). Some of the questions won't necessarily have answers, and each of us needs to find our own way to make peace with that reality (Scott Barss, 2012a). As they explore, patients may feel validated and encouraged to receive health teaching about

- the various ways of understanding the process of searching. Familiarizing yourself with and offering such information can help support patients' spiritual explorations.
- the nature and possibility of healing and transcendence. The timing of such information must be carefully considered; if it is too early in the process, the patient may experience it as false reassurance rather than a gentle sharing of hope (Carr, 2010; Wright & Bell, 2010).

Depending on your life experiences and comfort level, you may wish to leave such teaching to specialized spiritual care providers. However, do remember that you are one of many who can serve as supportive companions to patients during their process of searching.

Teachers

This brings us to the final *T* of T.R.U.S.T.: *teachers*, referring to the wide variety of spiritual/religious/personal mentors and internal/external resources that individuals might choose to help them sort through spiritual issues relevant to their healing process. These resources may include any of the patients' caregivers on the health-care team (volunteer or otherwise) with whom they have developed a strong sense of trust (Johnston Taylor & Mamier, 2013; Olson & Clark, 2010; Puchalski & Ferrell, 2010). They may also include trusted spiritual and/or religious leaders and healers, along with affiliated sacred texts and teachings (Johnston Taylor, 2012a, 2012b; Young & Koopsen, 2011). Others who might be deemed teachers may include any relationships, inspirational readings, educational events, retreats, or experiences individuals identify as helpful in meeting their spiritual needs (Young & Koopsen, 2011).

Through the eyes of a nurse

When my father was dying, it was not the nurses or chaplains or physicians who connected with him on a spiritual level. It was a volunteer who worked on the unit, passing out chocolate bars, juice, tea, and coffee. She and my father bonded immediately, and she had a profound impact on his spiritual sense, healing, and death. His face would light up when she walked into the room, and it was she who he entrusted with his final conversations. One day, I witnessed her quietly plucking dead flowers in a garden near the entrance of the hospital, and I thought about her gift of tending to the dying, and how my father found her accepting presence more helpful than anything else. Seems sometimes it's not about receiving spiritual "knowledge," but simply experiencing a human–spiritual connection—a kind of love—between a patient and another.

(personal reflection by a nurse, David, about professional learning gleaned from his personal observations as a family member)

As nurses, our most important quality in helping patients explore their potential spiritual teachers is our deep sense of humility. It allows us to be informed by colleagues; by patients and their self-identified, relevant traditional communities; and by the resources themselves. Such humility also allows us as caregivers to be deeply observant about internal resources evident within patients themselves and to share these observations with them to empower, inspire, and promote well-being (Plotnikoff & Dandurand, 2012; Scott Barss, 2012a; Young & Koopsen, 2011).

Helping Patients Discern and Integrate Internal Resources

As we share our unconditional presence with patients, we can listen and observe intentionally for their spiritual strengths (refer back to Fig. 40.2). You might hear patients and others refer to these strengths as, among other things, virtues, gifts of the spirit, or qualities (Koenig, 2011; Seaward, 2012; Young & Koopsen, 2011). Regardless of what the patient calls them, these strengths are spiritual in nature, as they are a part of the essence of the person. Often, we witness tremendous strength within patients in their most vulnerable moments. Vulnerability itself can be a strength if we can help patients feel safe enough to embrace it as a necessary part of the healing process (Parachini, 2011).

When we take the time to offer related observations, we can help patients remember their own sources of spiritual resilience and tap into them. It is also important to help patients learn to self-identify and draw on their inner resources. Helping them learn the relaxation and/or contemplative practices of their choice can assist them to recognize and listen to their inner wisdom (Plante, 2010; Young & Koopsen, 2011).

One such approach that is culturally safe and easy to learn is called *focusing* (Gendlin, 2007). Focusing is a skill for gaining awareness through listening quietly to our innate wisdom (Gendlin, 2007; McDonald, 2012; The Focusing Institute, 2012). Eugene Gendlin, the creator of *Focusing*, suggests that our bodies and brains know much more than we may realize (Gendlin, 2007). When we learn to do so, the experience of focusing can assist in shifting from experiencing the problem toward moving forward in life, putting us in touch with our interior strength (Gendlin, 2007, 2010; McDonald, 2012). This intervention is one that you may wish to integrate into your nursing practice as you gain experience and confidence (McDonald, 2012). The third suggested lab activity of this chapter offers you an opportunity to experience focusing. Each of us will have our own way of assisting patients to honour and draw on their internal resources. In doing so we have the opportunity to offer hope, solace, and sustenance when it is most needed.

Helping Patients Discern and Integrate External Resources

Assisting patients to connect with affirming and inspiring healing resources can be one of the most tangible and rewarding ways we can offer spiritual care. It can also be one of our most challenging tasks because relevant resources are so individual and potentially difficult to access. The following discussion will help you become familiar with resources to consider within the health-care system and broader community.

Spiritual, Cultural, and Pastoral Care Providers

Spiritual, cultural, and/or pastoral care providers (sometimes referred to as *chaplains* in some traditions) are required members of the interdisciplinary team in accredited health-care facilities (Young & Koopsen, 2011). They are professionally trained clergy, Elders or Knowledge keepers, clinical pastoral care workers, and cultural workers from various religious and cultural traditions (Canadian Association for Spiritual Care, 2014; Puchalski & Ferrell, 2010). Their role is to provide specialized spiritual care to any patients or staff requesting it and to assist them to connect with individualized spiritual care resources in the community. Some spiritual care departments include healing practitioners on their spiritual care team or in their referral options, so patients' spiritual care can be enhanced by healing modalities such as therapeutic touch and other energy modalities (Health Sciences Centre Winnipeg, 2012; Young & Koopsen, 2011).

Spiritual Leaders in the Community

Although it is unlikely that you will be familiar with all the varied spiritual leaders in the broader community, it is important for you to continually consider which ones individual patients might like to involve in their health care. Let patients be your teacher about proper terminology for their spiritual leaders. For example, Christian leaders may be known as ministers, pastors, or priests, depending on the denomination. Muslim leaders may be referred to as imams or mullahs, depending on the context. There are many types of Hindu leaders, such a Brahmins, swamis, and gurus (teachers). In some spiritual communities, there are no formal clergy, such as in earth-centered traditions like Wicca or pluralistic traditions such the Baha'i faith (Johnston Taylor, 2012b). Whatever their mentors' role or title, it is essential to ask patients whether or not the involvement of people from their spiritual community is relevant or helpful during the course of their health care.

Many Aboriginal patients who have chosen to follow First Nations traditional ways will want to make contact with an Elder or Knowledge Keeper during times of illness. The terms *Elder* and *Knowledge Keeper* are used interchangeably in some communities to acknowledge that chronological age is not the criteria for being chosen as a keeper of traditional knowledge. Communities recognize their Elders or Knowledge Keepers because they are respected and honoured for the sacred knowledge they hold. They play a vital role in sharing their wisdom, traditionally acquired over years of preparation (Binda, 2011; Brewer, 2011; Young & Koopsen, 2011). It is important to honour this part of the traditional knowledge system and encourage an understanding for both Aboriginal and non-Aboriginal people.

If you are assisting patients to make contact with an Elder/Knowledge Keeper it is important to follow protocol. (For clarity, the term *Elder* will be used in describing this protocol.) When approaching an Elder, it is important to offer a gift of tobacco, one of the sacred plants within First Nations teachings. In some circumstances, an honorarium is also appropriate. While meeting with the Elder, it is important to demonstrate reverence for the Elder's knowledge, refraining from asking explicit questions unless invited to, focusing more on hearing the teachings the Elder deems appropriate for the time, circumstances, and readiness of the individual seeking knowledge (Binda, 2011; Brewer, 2011; McAdam, 2009). Some of the teachings come from the stories told by the Elder, and it is up to the individual to discover their answers within the narrative (Mehl-Madrona, 2010). Often, a specialized spiritual or cultural worker can provide guidance during the process of connecting with an Elder (Young & Koopsen, 2011).

Spiritual Directors

Increasingly, individuals from various worldviews are seeking out spiritual directors or companions, those educated to engage in the process of accompanying people on the spiritual journey (Spiritual Directors International [SDI], 2013; Young & Koopsen, 2011). "Spiritual direction invites a deeper relationship with the spiritual aspect of being human," offering a place to explore spiritual practices and experiences and to address our growing desire for significance (SDI, 2013). In other words, spiritual directors help people discern their spiritual direction and how it can enhance their lives, well-being, and contributions to others. Spiritual directors can be found on the SDI website or by contacting local retreat centres that often offer spiritual direction and companioning.

Parish Nurses

Many nurses become specialized spiritual care providers either by becoming spiritual directors, engaging in clinical pastoral education (CPE), or entering into parish nursing. Parish nursing is a health ministry of faith communities that emphasizes the wholeness of body, mind, and spirit. Rooted in Christianity, this ministry grows out of the belief that all faith communities are places of health and healing and have a role in promoting wholeness through the integration of faith (Canadian Association of Parish Nursing Ministry [CAPNM], 2013). The roots of parish nursing are in early Christian communities where people attended to the sick (Carson & Koenig, 2011). Many hospitals developed from these religious communities (Carson & Koenig, 2011).

Parish nursing provides spiritual support and teaching for the patient, family, or community during times of illness (Carson & Koenig, 2011). The role of a parish nurse is to promote the integration of faith and health in various ways that reflect the context of the faith community; specific examples include health advocacy, counselling, and education, along with resource referral (CAPNM, 2013; Young & Koopsen, 2011).

Other Spiritual Resources and Mentors

It is important to keep in mind that many patients find their spiritual teachers outside of, or in addition to, a particular community; for example, healing practitioners or mentors and friends. Many people consider pets to be among their spiritual teachers, given the deep connection and healing associated with such relationships and animals' ability to embody spiritual strengths such as compassion, acceptance, and grace (Seaward, 2012; Young & Koopsen, 2011). Remember, any relationship that touches our spirit has the potential to teach us and contribute significantly to our well-being.

Connecting With Spiritual Care Resources

Once you explore with patients which spiritual care resources they find relevant and helpful, you can assist them to connect with those of their choice. It is essential to remember that specialized spiritual care providers on the interprofessional team can be consulted on a regular basis to enhance the quality of each patient's spiritual care, regardless of their denomination or worldview. Keep in mind that these specialized providers can assist you and your patients to identify readings, events, retreat centres, healing modalities, communities, and relationships that meet patients' spiritual needs and serve as teachers to both of you.

Through the eyes of a patient

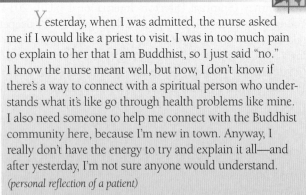

Yesterday, when I was admitted, the nurse asked me if I would like a priest to visit. I was in too much pain to explain to her that I am Buddhist, so I just said "no." I know the nurse meant well, but now, I don't know if there's a way to connect with a spiritual person who understands what it's like go through health problems like mine. I also need someone to help me connect with the Buddhist community here, because I'm new in town. Anyway, I really don't have the energy to try and explain it all—and after yesterday, I'm not sure anyone would understand.

(personal reflection of a patient)

Nursing Process in Spiritual Assessment and Care

There are various ways to conceptualize and organize information gathered during spiritual exploration with patients. The key is to identify which spiritual needs are currently unmet, what we can do to support each patient in meeting them, and what spiritual strengths can be supported and mobilized. From there, we can identify any nursing diagnoses necessary and proceed with planning, implementing, and evaluating spiritual care.

Identifying Spiritual Issues and Strengths

As you listen to patients, you will become attuned to which unmet spiritual needs are adding to their suffering and which fulfilled spiritual needs or strengths are fostering their healing. From there, you can document these issues and strengths in your care plans so they become an integral part of holistic care. Here is where familiarity with the nursing literature's information on universal spiritual needs and spiritual strengths can be particularly helpful (refer back to Figs. 40.1 and 40.2).

Nursing Diagnoses in Spiritual Care

Some nurses and agencies prefer to use formal North American Nursing Diagnosis Association (NANDA) nursing diagnoses such as Spiritual Distress (suffering associated with unmet spiritual needs) and Readiness for Enhanced Spiritual Well-Being (the ability to respond to adversity with spiritual strengths that meet spiritual needs; Ladwig & Ackley, 2014). Related diagnoses may be spiritual pain, alienation, anxiety, anger, loss, or despair (Ladwig & Ackley, 2014; O'Brien, 2011). See Box 40.6 for sample care plans.

Spiritual strengths and needs can also be integrated into related nursing diagnoses such as Risk for Ineffective Coping or Readiness for Enhanced Coping (Ladwig & Ackley, 2014). Other nurses and agencies simply identify the relevant spiritual need and/or strength rather than formulating a nursing diagnosis. In a traditional Aboriginal setting, the medicine wheel might be used to identify areas that are in and out of balance (Clarke & Holtslander, 2010).

Implementation

Once you have helped the patient to identify areas of need/strength and have identified any relevant nursing diagnoses, it is important then to implement the specific interventions co-identified with your patient as relevant and helpful in meeting unmet needs and enhancing existing strengths. Of course, communication with the rest of the interdisciplinary team is vital to facilitating safe, effective follow-up, as is documentation throughout the process (Young & Koopsen, 2011). See Box 40.7 for a sample of spiritual care documentation.

Evaluation of Spiritual Care

Evaluation of spiritual care can pose particular challenges because of its intangible, complex nature; many spiritual issues are immeasurable and won't be resolved during the time you care for the patient (Young & Koopsen, 2011). However, we can check to make sure that planned interventions have been carried out and take note of our patients' response to them (Ladwig & Ackley, 2014). "Perhaps the most effective way to measure the effectiveness of spiritual intervention is to ask the patient directly and carefully observe his or her physical, verbal, or non-verbal cues" (Young & Koopsen, 2011, p. 169). In this way, we can discern whether or not we have successfully "softened suffering" in the ways we would hope (Wright & Bell, 2010, p. 74).

Nurturing Spirituality in Ourselves and Our Workplaces

If we are to be unconditionally present enough to help soften or heal suffering within our patients, we need to continually find ways to maintain spiritual well-being within our workplaces and ourselves. Furthermore, our opportunities to enjoy life-giving environments and ways of being are as important as anyone else's. As your reading concludes, you are invited to focus specifically on how you can apply concepts from this chapter to enhance your own spiritual well-being and that of your colleagues and practice settings.

BOX 40.6 Sample Nursing Care Plans

Nursing Diagnosis: Spiritual Distress*

Related to:
Unmet spiritual needs arising from current health-care crisis

As evidenced by:
Voiced feelings of hopelessness
Voiced inability to make meaning of current circumstances

Goal:
The client will explore and name with the nursing student two unmet spiritual needs and one intervention to attend to each of them.

Interventions:

- Establish a trusting, culturally safe therapeutic relationship.
- Negotiate a time when the patient can express her distress and the nursing student can listen with unconditional presence.
- Use the T.R.U.S.T. Model to pose nonintrusive spiritual questions and facilitate a trust-based, culturally safe interaction.
- Provide patient teaching about spiritual needs.
- Assist patient to identify currently unmet spiritual needs.
- Assist patient to identify resources that can help address unmet spiritual needs.
- Make referral to specialized spiritual care providers and other resources if requested.
- Seek feedback from patient about her subjective experience of whether spiritual needs are met/not met by interventions implemented.
- Document spiritual needs identified, interventions implemented, and patient's self-reported outcomes.

Nursing Diagnosis: Readiness for Enhanced Spiritual Well-Being

Related to:
Health care currently incongruent with personal spiritual needs, strengths, beliefs, and practices

As evidenced by:
Desire expressed by patient to receive care that is in keeping with personal spiritual needs, strengths, beliefs, and practices

Goal:
Patient will share three examples with the nursing student regarding ways personal strengths, spiritual beliefs, and practices can be integrated into current health care to help address current spiritual needs.

Interventions:

- Establish a trusting, culturally safe therapeutic relationship.
- Negotiate a time when the patient can share spiritual needs/beliefs/resources and the nursing student can listen with unconditional presence.
- Use the T.R.U.S.T. Model to pose nonintrusive spiritual questions and facilitate a trust-based, culturally safe interaction.
- Assist patient to identify spiritual strengths and community resources that can be integrated into care.
- With permission from the patient, educate the staff on patient's cultural beliefs and practices as they relate to daily patient care.
- Advocate for spiritual ceremonies if requested.
- Make referral to specialized spiritual care providers if requested.
- Seek feedback from patient about impact of spiritual care on her subjective experience.
- Document spiritual needs/strengths/beliefs/resources identified, interventions implemented, and patient's self-reported outcomes.

* This, and all nursing diagnoses, may be adapted to reflect language in keeping with a particular worldview (eg: A nursing diagnosis from an Aboriginal perspective might be worded something like: 'Imbalance of the Spiritual Dimension')

(CNA, 2006; Ladwig & Ackley, 2014) (Note: publication date is 2014).

 Think Consider the following nursing diagnosis for a nursing practice setting/community:

Readiness for Enhanced Spiritual Well-Being in nursing practice settings

Related to: a strong desire by nurses to engage in advocacy that can promote spiritual well-being in the health-care workplace, within all on the interprofessional health-care team, and within those in their care.

As evidenced by: nurses creating "sacred space" in themselves and in their workplaces with the support of colleagues, mentors, and patients

Goal: Nursing fulfills its promise of "softening suffering" for all those giving and receiving care
(CNA, 2006; Ladwig & Ackley, 2014; Potter & Frisch, 2013; Wright & Bell, 2010)

How would you word your own nursing diagnosis or vision for nursing?

What mentors and colleagues share your vision?

How can you draw on their support and inspiration?

Addressing Spiritual Needs, Drawing on Spiritual Strengths

You can use any of the information in this chapter to support your own spiritual awareness and reflection. For example, exploration of some of the sample reflective questions affiliated with T.R.U.S.T. may bring helpful insights (see Box 40.4). Such resources may enrich or challenge spiritual exploration you already do elsewhere, or this information may introduce you to concepts you have not previously considered.

No matter where you are on your own journey, you can be sure that nursing will present you with many ongoing questions about the nature of suffering, life, and death. It is vital that you find safe places to meet your spiritual needs in whatever ways hold meaning for you. It is also vital to recognize and deepen the many spiritual strengths you bring to your work. Both you and your patients will benefit from your sharing of them.

When you take the time to have conversations with patients at a spiritual level, you receive privileged opportunities to

BOX 40.7   Sample Documentation of Spiritual Nursing Care

The following chart entry documents all aspects of the nursing process and describes how each of the domains of T.R.U.S.T. have been addressed.

Patient identifies her meditation community and practice as significant to her healing. Reports she requires no assistance to involve members of her community. Expressed appreciation in response to writer's invitation to put a sign on her door if she prefers not to be interrupted during her meditation times. States is having trouble making peace with her illness because she has led a very healthy lifestyle. States would be open to talking with someone from the spiritual care department if they can help her with this concern. Referral made via voice mail. States draws strength from a belief that something positive comes out of every experience. Also states she believes strongly that her meditation practice can help her heal. Voiced x 2 a sense that she must have "gone wrong somewhere, though" to have become ill in the first place. Noted to consider perspective offered that that there are many factors in health and illness beyond our control. Readily accepted positive feedback about her openness to making meaning of her experience. States she is open to ongoing related exploration with nursing and other disciplines as her energy allows. Facial expression and posture observed to be significantly more relaxed following above 1-1 interaction.

also witness and learn from their spiritual strengths. Although your focus is on promoting patients' well-being, such spirit-to-spirit conversations offer the possibility of a mutually beneficial experience for both the patient and you (Burkhardt & Nagai-Jacobson, 2013).

Questions for Personal Reflection

- What spiritual strengths do I bring to my nursing?
- How do I meet my spiritual needs?
- How does nursing challenge my ability to meet my spiritual needs?
- What spiritual wisdom have I already learned from my patients?
- What content from this chapter would I like to revisit to explore my own spirituality?

Creating Sacred Space Within Health Care

A **sacred space** is a "spiritually healing environment in which individuals are supported and nurtured, in which they feel spiritually calm, where they are connected to elements of nature, and in which health and well-being are promoted" (Young & Koopsen, 2011, p. 205).

When you compare this description to the noisy, rushed, stressful atmosphere of today's typical health-care setting,

you are likely to find sharp contrasts (Young & Koopsen, 2011). Barriers to spiritual care abound, as discussed earlier in the chapter. Furthermore, the CNA (2006) document, *Toward 2020: Visions for Nursing* suggests that the health-care system itself is experiencing despair related to workload, scheduling, minimal professional autonomy, and violence and abuse in the health-care setting. The World Health Organization has documented concerns about the level of distress and workplace violence in health-care settings (CNA, 2006; McDonald, 2012). Emotional, physical, and spiritual exhaustion have been associated with a lack of meaning, purpose, or sense of connection with colleagues (Wagner & Simington, 2011). Indeed, many workplace issues are contributing to unmet spiritual needs for nurses (Araujo & Sofield, 2011).

Although Willa, Tommy, and Amira experienced many affirming experiences with inspiring patients and supportive staff during their clinical rotation, they also experienced occurrences of nursing and other staff using inappropriate tone of voice, interaction, and body language toward residents, students, and one another. Each of the students in their clinical group expressed to their clinical teacher that they felt disrespected, unwanted, and helpless in such situations. They also voiced a strong desire to advocate for the residents, doing so through appropriate channels in consultation with their teacher. However, they recognized that as nursing students in the care facility for a short time, they could not accomplish long-standing changes. This led to a sense of discouragement by the end of their rotation. In final postconference, their clinical teacher asked the students to identify which of their spiritual needs were being compromised. Among those identified were the following:

- Meaning and purpose: "If I can't make my patients' lives better, what's the point?" (Willa)
- Interconnection: "I don't like feeling disconnected from people I work with; I also don't like ending the connection with my patients when I'm not sure they'll find that connection with someone else." (Tommy)
- Trust: "Sometimes, I feel quite disillusioned, like I'm losing my faith in nursing when I see some nurses so unhappy and uncaring." (Amira)

The clinical teacher led the students in a Focusing process that helped them to be unconditionally present to their experience. After a centering activity, the clinical teacher invited the students to simply be with the feelings and insights they had shared and then, after a few moments, to be aware of any new feelings or insights that surfaced. Students were encouraged to compassionately acknowledge all of their responses and experiences, without thinking that they needed to fix or problem-solve. Students were then gradually invited to reconnect with their surroundings and with one another.

Afterward, the clinical teacher invited students to consider, at their own pace, how their feelings and insights might influence their future nursing practice. Some students wanted some time to think about this, whereas others wanted to share. Among the responses was Willa's, who said, "I realized I don't ever want my behaviour to make a patient or coworker feel like I've felt. That's what I'm going to focus on now—in a way, maybe that's giving me a new sense of purpose."

Spirituality has the power to transcend adversity. There is hope to heal the despair many nurses feel. Individuals who have been able to integrate spirituality into their workplace have described their work as meaningful and purposeful and report a deep connection with others at work, in turn enhancing employee wellness, patient care, and organizational performance (Wagner & Simington, 2011).

As we integrate spirituality into our nursing practice by caring for our patients and each other at a spiritual level, we can help set the stage for broader systems change so that nursing practice settings can become safe, respectful, inclusive, compassionate, and ethical places for both the patient and the nurse (CNA, 2008). Creating a spiritually healthy workplace requires nurses to be conscious of how we engage in interactions with the patient, with the patient's family and community, with one another, and with other healthcare colleagues. In fact, the concept of sacred space applies to our inner state of being, not just the external environment (O'Donohue & Quinn, 2011; Wright & Sayre-Adams as cited in Young & Koopsen, 2011, p. 155). Therefore, it needs to begin with each of us. Ultimately, "we do not so much create sacred space, as become and be it. Who we are is sacred" (Wright & Sayre Adams as cited in Young & Koopsen, 2011, p.155.)

On the final day of the clinical rotation, Willa, Tommy, and Amira are walking to the locker room together for the last time. They talk about how much they've enjoyed their experience, despite the challenges they faced in their clinical setting. As they talk, they realize that this enjoyment was possible because of the depth of connection and trust they experienced with their patients, one another, and their clinical teacher. Willa, remembering their conversation at the beginning of the term about spirituality being too personal to talk about, says, "It's interesting that the more personal and spiritually oriented conversations were, the easier it was to deal with everything going on around us!" Tommy adds, "For sure, and without being personal, there's no way I would have ever been able to learn what I did about other people's beliefs and ways of looking at the world." Amira adds, "In the end, maybe the only way we could ever really 'get' what spirituality has to do with nursing was to experience it—person to person—or, maybe more accurately . . . spirit to spirit."

Critical Thinking Case Scenarios

▶ You are carrying out an initial spiritual assessment conversation with Jennifer, a third-year university student who has come to Addictions Services for her first appointment in relation to anxiety and habitual use of antianxiety medications and alcohol to cope. To help her see the relevance of this inquiry, you share with her a statement similar to that suggested in Table 40.1 about the increasing recognition of the role spirituality plays in enhancing health outcomes around chemical dependency. Jennifer expresses surprise, responding, "Really? I have a hard time seeing how religion has anything to do with my drinking." Consider what health teaching would be important to offer Jennifer. Write a possible response in your own words, keeping in mind that your time with Jennifer is limited.

▶ You have been engaged in a holistic assessment with Mohammed, a 48-year-old man who came to Canada 1 year ago as a refugee from Iraq. Mohammed was just admitted to the cardiac unit yesterday after experiencing a heart attack. He mentions he is not surprised this happened to him because he has had "nothing but trouble" for the last 10 years. He goes on to tell you about the various traumatic experiences he has had, which prompted him to flee his homeland. When you inquire about whether there are any spiritual or religious traditions or practices that have been helpful to him throughout his difficulties, he indicates he is a devout Muslim, but that he has been reluctant to attend any of the local mosques, given fears about his family's safety back in Iraq if it becomes known he is here. He also says, "Sometimes, I don't know what I believe anymore. I've seen people do terrible things in the name of religion, and I don't know who I can talk to." How would you go about helping Mohammed to connect with relevant and appropriate internal and external resources or "teachers"?

▶ Tim, a 35-year-old man living with schizophrenia, has been admitted to the inpatient psychiatry unit in relation to a psychotic episode. He also has been exhibiting symptoms of depression, which he openly acknowledges. He tells you that his belief in God is what keeps him going. He also shares with you his beliefs that he is a "messenger from God" and that he keeps hearing God's voice telling him he cannot sleep until he knows all in the hospital are willing to join his evangelical faith community. How do you respond?

Multiple-Choice Questions

1. Which of the following reflects current best practices for spiritual assessment and care?
   a. Asking standard questions in every interview to ensure patients are being treated equally
   b. Ensuring patients' psychological safety by leaving spiritual care to the specialists
   c. Refraining from assessment of the spiritual dimension if the patient doesn't raise the topic
   d. Ensuring patients' wishes, preferences, and worldviews are respected

2. The T.R.U.S.T. acronym for spiritual assessment and care cues you to explore:
   a. All the questions identified in the T.R.U.S.T. Model
   b. Spirituality in a linear, systematic fashion
   c. The individual's spiritual traditions, practices, beliefs, needs, and resources
   d. The associated plant imagery that is universally meaningful

3. As a nurse, you can safely help patients to integrate their spiritual traditions and practices into their health care by:
   a. Suggesting they pray about how to do so
   b. Providing encouragement and assisting them to find resources of their choice
   c. Offering to take them to the hospital chapel
   d. Participating in any tradition or practice they wish

4. Which of the following is true of spiritual practices? They are:
   a. Most effective when they draw on one's own convictions
   b. Religious behaviours and rituals
   c. Unrelated to spiritual needs
   d. Carried out in solitude

5. When making contact with a traditional Aboriginal Elder, it is important to:
   a. Understand that Elders are any of the old people within the community
   b. Come with tobacco and ask all the questions you want to ask
   c. Understand that Elders are those whom the community has recognized
   d. Come with tobacco and money to give the Elder

Suggested Lab Activities

During each of the following activities, it is important to practice sharing unconditional presence and creating sacred space. You can do so by sharing unconditional presence with your practice partner, maintaining confidentiality of any information shared, and trusting your intuition about what information is appropriate and safe to share in the context of your relationship with your practice partner.

● Review the sample introductory health teaching from the T.R.U.S.T. initial assessment questions and guidelines in Figure 40.5. How might you need to adapt such a statement to your own communication style and to the worldviews/needs of individual patients? (e.g., your patient may not relate to the word *spiritual*). Jot an alternate statement or two that feels natural for you and that maintains cultural safety. Discuss with a partner each of your responses and explore how they reflect your personal and professional style and the needs of individual patients.

For example, "Many times people find that illness stirs up a lot of difficult questions about life. As part of offering holistic care, we like to ask if there is anything you consider important for us to know about what you are going through and about your sources of strength during this difficult time. More and more, we are recognizing in health care how important it is to address these things so we can help promote the best possible outcome."

● Review the T.R.U.S.T. initial assessment questions and guidelines in Figure 40.5. Practice carrying out an initial spiritual assessment with a partner, taking turns as the nurse. One of you will use Scenario 1; the other will use Scenario 2. Afterward, debrief with your partner, focusing on how successful you were in either "leaving the door open" for future dialogue (if the answers were all "no") or providing appropriate referral and/or opportunity for deeper exploration (if any of the answers were "yes"). Identify any questions or issues you'd like to discuss with the rest of your lab group about this challenging but essential dimension of holistic assessment.

Scenario 1:

Nurse: You are completing an initial database/admission form with a patient who has just been admitted to your clinical area. This man/woman is scheduled tomorrow for major back surgery following a debilitating injury that has severely restricted his/her formerly active lifestyle. You come to the section of the form entitled "Spirituality." Using the T.R.U.S.T. guidelines for initial assessment, carry out an initial spiritual assessment in an inclusive, nonintrusive manner, providing clarification and validation as needed.

Patient: You are just being admitted as an inpatient in preparation for major back surgery, following a debilitating injury that has severely restricted your formerly active lifestyle. When inquiry is made about any spiritual needs you might have, you politely but consistently answer "no," as you consider this area of your life to be very private and do not see its relevance to your current health care. If your nurse offers you information that helps you see its relevance, you indicate that you will give it some thought and let the staff know if you have questions.

Scenario 2:

Nurse: You are completing an initial data base/admission form with a patient who has just been admitted to your clinical area. This man/woman has recently been diagnosed with a chronic illness. He/she has been admitted to hospital in hopes of stabilizing the currently unmanageable related symptoms.

You come to the section of the form entitled "Spirituality." Use the T.R.U.S.T. guidelines for initial assessment in Figure 40.5 to carry out an initial spiritual assessment in an inclusive, nonintrusive manner, providing clarification and validation as needed. Where appropriate, draw on relevant sample questions from Box 40.4 to continue patient-centered spiritual exploration.

Patient: You have recently been diagnosed with a chronic illness (pick one you are familiar with and/or that is relevant to your current clinical area; e.g., diabetes, depression, multiple sclerosis, schizophrenia). You are now being admitted to hospital in hopes of stabilizing the currently unmanageable accompanying symptoms.

When inquiry is made about any spiritual needs you might have, you indicate distress/confusion about why all this is happening to you and express interest in accessing supports available to help find reconciliation/make meaning in relation to your current experience. (Respond to the assessment questions according to your own spiritual beliefs/worldview or one with which you are familiar.) If you feel comfortable with your nurse, you may even begin to explore your spiritual questions with him/her.

● Invite a lab partner who you trust to share in this experience if it feels comfortable. Keep in mind that you can stop the experience at any point if you or your partner feel overwhelmed or wish to stop for any reason. Choose a comfortable setting and amount of space between one another. Take turns slowly reading the following Focusing experience to the other (who sits in a comfortable way with eyes either closed or gently gazing at the floor). Then, exchange roles.

A Focusing Experience:

I invite you to plant your feet on the floor and connect with the ground; perhaps wiggle your toes if that is okay. You may keep your eyes open or close them if you'd like. . . . I invite you now to move your mind inward and follow your breath. . . . Just notice your breathing—make no corrections in your breathing. . . . Rest your mind near your breathing and notice it. . . . Is it even? Shallow? Deep? Or do you notice any other breathing rhythms that you are becoming aware of? It's okay, however your breathing is in this moment.

Now if you can . . . I invite you to scan the rest of your body and do a gentle inventory of what is going on. If you can rest your mind at your feet and notice any sensations or feelings; gently progress to your ankles, shins, knees, legs, hips, pelvis, abdomen, now the chest, arms and hands, shoulders, neck, chin, ears, face, and finally your scalp. Take a gentle notice of your spine from your neck to your tail bone and back up again. . . . Just notice anything that may be going on that may be giving you some sort of bodily sensation, a feeling, or some kind of message. Perhaps there may be an image that pops up, or a phrase, or a saying, a poem or song, or a smell— these are all okay responses. I invite all of this, too, to be okay. Perhaps you are in pain, anxious, or concerned.

Again, I invite you to let all of this be okay. . . . These are human responses. If you can, just acknowledge unconditionally whatever comes to your awareness. I invite you to say a gentle, friendly, compassionate hello to all of your experiences, without thinking that you need to fix or problem solve.

Now take three nurturing breaths and gently come back to the outside world at your own pace, expressing gratefulness to your body and to your partner.

When both of you have completed the Focusing experience, debrief if you wish, focusing most on the process of your experience versus its content. Here are a few questions that may be helpful to explore either on your own or with your partner:

What was your experience of this process?

Were there any bodily felt sensations, feelings, or movements experienced?

Were there any images that bubbled up during the experience?

Were there any metaphors arising from your experience? (Gendlin, 2007, 2010; McDonald, 2012)

● Refer to Figure 40.3 and Table 40.2. Discuss the following questions with a lab partner:

What are the similarities and differences between these two worldviews? (See below points to consider in your discussion.)

With which of these worldviews do you identify most/least?

What other worldviews and traditions influence your perspectives on spirituality? On health?

If you were to create a drawing of your own worldview what would it look like?

How does your worldview influence your approach to spiritual assessment and care?

Some similarities and differences between the two worldviews:

A Priori World

From a Heideggerian existential perspective, the a priori world is the most important assessment that a nurse can do. This is because a person is already situated in an existing world with existing relationships, linguistic skills, practices, and traditions, embedded in the culture (the world is beforehand the birth of the human; McDonald, 2012). Please see Box 40.4 for assessment details.

Similar to existentialism, the Aboriginal holistic worldview has the philosophy of a good way of life and everyday practices, activities, language, and rituals are taken-for-granted knowledge (Clarke & Holtslander, 2010).

Both worldviews suggest that learning where persons come from, their history, their relationships, their traditions, etc., are important assessments (Clarke & Holtslander, 2010; McDonald, 2012).

Embodied Caring

The Aboriginal holistic worldview values interconnectedness and relationships, responsibility to others, connecting with their spirit to look from their worldview to understand their lived experience.

Similar to the Aboriginal holistic worldview, the existential worldview values interconnectedness and independence, ethical caring, social morality, commitment to self and others, and valuing others.

Embodied Spirituality

Existentialism will assess the person's spiritual practices and processes, expansion of the authentic self (transcendence), spiritual freedom from vulnerability, and spiritual needs (Barnett & Madison, 2012; Todres, 2011); whereas the holistic Aboriginal worldview supports a person's spiritual journey, accepts, and acts on his or her spirit, wisdom, and knowledge learned—sacred and general.

Embodied spirituality is a new facet in Heideggerian existentialism (McDonald, 2012); however, spirituality has been an embedded worldview for the Aboriginal peoples since the dawn of time (Clarke & Holtslander, 2010).

Embodied Self-Interpreting

The Aboriginal worldview uses the medicine wheel for self-reflecting and focusing on how the Aboriginal people self-interpret their experience of colonization and the "trauma effects of residential schools . . ." (Clarke & Holtslander, 2010, p. 34).

Existentialism views self-interpreting one's lived experience as not reflective or noncognitive and listens carefully for dilemmas of existence such as suffering and its various existentials (McDonald, 2012).

Being Is Embodied

Loss of some part of self through trauma and suffering is an existential worldview. We experience, live, respond, and move through our bodies (Madison, 2010).

Similarly, the Aboriginal worldview looks at historical loss of identity, culture, values, beliefs, colonization, residential schools, commonplace racism, "walking in my moccasins," and historical trauma. The Aboriginal people have experienced centuries of significant suffering and loss.

Embodied in Time

The Aboriginal worldview lives life through the past, present, and future, understanding how history affects the present, etc., when the time is right for doing, acting, reflecting, and learning.

The existential worldview sees the past in one's body influencing and remolding the present and the future (Heidegger, 1962; Madison, 2010).

REFERENCES AND SUGGESTED READINGS

Aboriginal Healing Foundation. (2009). *Response, responsibility, and renewal: Canada's truth and reconciliation journey.* Ottawa, ON: Aboriginal Healing Foundation Research Series.

Aboriginal Healing Foundation. (2012). *Helping Aboriginal people heal themselves.* Retrieved from http://www.ahf.ca.

Accreditation Canada. (2013). *Culture of care.* Retrieved from http://www.accreditation.ca/

Adams, M. (2011, October). Existential supervision. *Hermeneutic Circular: Newsletter of the Society for Existential Analysis,* 8–12.

Anderson, J., Pakula, B., Smye, V., Peters, V., & Schroeder, L. (2011). Strengthening aboriginal health through a place-based learning community. *Journal of Aboriginal Health,* 7(1), 42–53.

Araujo, S., & Sofield, L. (2011). Workplace violence in nursing today. In S. Prevost (Consulting Ed.) & S. Stark (Guest Ed.), *Victims of abuse: Nursing clinics of North America.* Philadelphia, PA: Saunders: Elsevier.

Armstrong, K. (2010). *Twelve steps to a compassionate life.* Toronto, ON: Knopf.

Balbuena, L., Baetz, M., & Bowen, R. (2013). Religious attendance, spirituality, and major depression in Canada: A 14-year follow-up study. *Canadian Journal of Psychiatry,* 58(4), 225–232.

Baldacchino, D. (2010). Indicator-based and value clarification tools. In W. McSherry & L. Ross (Eds.), *Spiritual assessment in healthcare practice* (pp. 95–118). Cumbria, England: M & K Publishing.

Barnett, L., & Madison, G. (Eds.) & Tudor, K. (Series Ed.). (2012). *Advancing theory in therapy. Existential therapy: Legacy, vibrancy and dialogue.* New York, NY: Routledge.

Bibby, R. (2011). *Beyond the gods and back: Religion's demise and rise and why it matters.* Lethbridge, AB: Project Canada Books.

Binda, J. (2011). *The renaissance of native spirituality: The journey of the spiritual seeker and traditional healing practices.* Bloomington, IN: iUniverse Books.

Bradford, K. (2013). *Authenticity and the play of unconditional presence in psychotherapy: From resolute searching to natural release forum.* Retrieved from http://www.daseinsanalyse.be /page14 .shtml

Brewer, L. (2011). Ancestors, elders, and the role of spirituality in late life. *The International Journal of Religion and Spirituality in Society,* 1(1), 37–43.

Bridges, W. (2004). *Transitions: Making sense of life's changes.* Boston, MA: Lifelong/DeCapo.

Brown, B. (2010). *The gifts of imperfection: Let go of who you think you're supposed to be and embrace who you are: Your guide to a wholehearted life.* Centre City, MN: Hazelden.

Burkhardt, M. A., & Nagai-Jacobson, M. G. (2013). Spirituality and health. In B. Dossey & L. Keegan (Eds.), *Holistic nursing: A handbook for practice* (6th ed., pp. 721–750). Boston, MA: Jones & Bartlett.

Calestani, M., White, N., Hendricks, J., & Scemons, D. (2012). Religion of native peoples and nursing. In M. Fowler, S. Reimer-Kirkham, R. Sawatzky, & E. Johnston Taylor (Eds.), *Religion, religious ethics, and nursing* (pp. 267–293). New York, NY: Springer Publishing.

Canadian Association for Spiritual Care. (2014). *About us.* Retrieved from http://www.spiritualcare.ca/page.asp?ID=2

Canadian Association of Parish Nursing Ministry. (2014). *Parish nursing ministry.* Retrieved from http://www.capnm.ca/

Canadian Nurses Association. (2006). *Toward 2020: Visions for nursing.* Retrieved from http://www.cna-ailc.ca

Canadian Nurses Association. (2008). *Code of ethics for registered nurses.* Ottawa, ON: Author.

Canadian Nurses Association. (2010). *Position statement: Spirituality, health and nursing practice.* Retrieved from http://www.cnaaiic.ca/ CNA/documents/pdf/publications/PS111 _Spirituality_2010_e.pdf

Carr, T. (2010). Facing existential realities: Exploring barriers and challenges in spiritual nursing care. *Qualitative Health Research,* 20(10), 1379–1392. doi:10.1177/1040732310372377

Carson, V., & Koenig, H. (2011). *Parish nursing: Stories of service and care.* Conshohocken, PA: Templeton Press.

Chan, M. (2009). Factors affecting nursing staff in practicing spiritual care. *Journal of Clinical Nursing,* 19(15–16), 2128–2136. doi:10.1111/j.1365-2702.2008.02690.x

Chittister, J. (2012). God our father, God our mother: In search of the Divine Feminine. In K. Schaaf, K. Lindahl, K. Hurty, & G. Cheen (Eds.), *Women, spirituality, & transformative leadership: Where grace meets power* (pp. 60–71). Woodstock, VT: Skylight Paths Publishing.

Clarke, V., & Holtslander, L. (2010). Finding a balanced approach: Incorporating medicine wheel teachings in the care of Aboriginal people at the end of life. *Journal of Palliative Care,* 26(1), 34–36.

Conti-O'Hare, M. (2002). *The nurse as wounded healer: From trauma to transcendence*. Sudbury, MA: Jones & Bartlett.

Dossey, B. (2013). Nursing: Integral, integrative, and holistic—Local to global. In B. Dossey & L. Keegan (Eds.), *Holistic nursing: A handbook for practice* (6th ed., pp. 3–58). Boston, MA: Jones & Bartlett.

Ermine, W. (2007). The ethical space of engagement. *Indigenous Law Journal, 6*(1), 193–203.

First Nations Studies Program at University of British Columbia. (2014). *The Indian act*. Retrieved from http://indigenous foundations.arts.ubc.ca/?id=1053#origins

Fortney, L. (2012). Recommending meditation. In D. Rakel (Ed.), *Integrative medicine* (3rd ed., pp. 873–881). Toronto, ON: Elsevier/Saunders.

Fowler, J. (1981). *Stages of faith: The psychology of human development and the quest for meaning*. New York, NY: Harper.

Fowler, M., Reimer-Kirkham, S., Sawatzky, R., & Johnston Taylor, E. (Eds.). (2012). *Religion, religious ethics, and nursing*. New York, NY: Springer Publishing.

Gendlin, E. T. (2007). *Focusing*. New York, NY: Bantam Dell.

Gendlin, E. T. (2010). *When you feel the body from the inside, there is a door*. Retrieved from http://www.focusing.org

Getty, G. (2010). The journey between western and indigenous research paradigms. *Journal of Transcultural Nursing, 21*(1), 5–14.

Gregory, D. (1994). The myth of control: Suffering in palliative care. *Journal of Palliative Care, 10*(2), 18–22.

Health Sciences Centre Winnipeg. (2012). *Spiritual health services*. Retrieved from http://www.hsc.mb.ca/placecard2.htm

Heidegger, M. (1962). *Being and time* (J. R. Macquarrie & E. Robinson, Trans.). Oxford, England: Blackwell.

Hessel, J. A. (2009). Presence in nursing practice: A concept analysis. *Holistic Nursing Practice, 23*(5), 276–281. doi:10.1097 /HNP.0b013e3181b66cb5

International Council of Nurses. (2006). *The ICN code of ethics for nurses*. Geneva, Switzerland: Author. Retrieved from http://www. icn.ch/images/stories/documents/about/icncode _english.pdf

Jackson, C. (2011). Addressing spirituality: A natural aspect of holistic care. *Holistic Nursing Practice, 25*(1), 3–7.

Jedwab, J. (2010). *To believe or not to believe, is that the question? Canadian views on religion.*. Association for Canadian Studies. Retrieved from http://cobourgatheist.ca/assets/downloads/ACS%20Survey%20 on%20Spirituality%20a20Religion%20in%20Canada.pdf

Johnston Taylor, E. (2012a). Religion and patient care. In M. Fowler, S. Reimer-Kirkham, R. Sawatzky, & E. Johnston Taylor (Eds.), *Religion, religious ethics, and nursing* (pp. 313–337). New York, NY: Springer Publishing.

Johnston Taylor, E. (Ed.). (2012b). *Religion: A clinical guide for nurses*. New York, NY: Springer Publishing.

Johnston Taylor, E., & Mamier, I. (2013). Nurse responses to patient expressions of spiritual distress. *Holistic Nursing Practice, 27*(4), 217–224.

Joint Commission on Accreditation of Healthcare Organizations. (2005). Evaluating your spiritual assessment process. *The Source, 3*(2), 6–7. Retrieved from http://www.ingentaconnect .com/content/jcaho/jcts

Kalish, N. (2012). Evidence-based spiritual care: A literature review. *Current Opinions & Support in Palliative Care, 6*(2), 242–246.

Kenney, C. (2011). *Transforming healthcare: Virginia Mason Medical Centre's Pursuit of the perfect patient experience*. New York, NY: CRC Press/Taylor & Francis.

Koenig, H. (2009). Research on religion, spirituality, and mental health: A review. *The Canadian Journal of Psychiatry, 54*(5), 283–291.

Koenig, H. (2011). *Spirituality and health research: Methods, measurement statistics and resources*. West Conshohocken, PA: Templeton.

Koerner, J. E. (2011). *Healing presence: The essence of nursing*. New York, NY: Springer Publishing.

Ladwig, G., & Ackley, B. (2014). *Mosby's guide to nursing diagnosis* (4th ed.). Maryland Heights, MI: Elsevier/Sanders.

Lavalle, L., & Poole, J. (2010). Beyond recovery: Colonization, health & healing for indigenous people in Canada. *International Journal Mental Health Addiction 8*, 271–281.

Levine, P. (2010). *An unspoken voice: How the body releases trauma and restores goodness*. Berkley, CA: North Atlantic Books.

Luchetti, G., Luchetti, A. L., & Koenig, H. G. (2011). Impact of spirituality/religiosity on mortality: Comparison with other health interventions. *Explore, 7*(4), 234–238.

Madison, G. (2010). Focusing on existence: Five facets of an experiential-existential model. *Person-Centered and Experiential Psychotherapies, 9*(3), 189–204.

Mariano, C. (2013). Holistic nursing: Scope and standards of practice. In B. Dossey & L. Keegan (Eds.), *Holistic nursing: A handbook for practice* (6th ed., pp. 59–84). Sudbury, MA: Jones & Bartlett.

McAdam, S. (2009). *Cultural teachings: First Nations protocols and methodologies*. Saskatoon, SK: Saskatchewan Indian Cultural Centre.

McDonald, S. (2012). *Nurses' experience of workplace violence before and after a focusing workshop* (Unpublished master's thesis). St. Stephen's College, Edmonton, AB.

Mehl-Madrona, L. (2010). *Healing the mind through the power of story: The promise of narrative psychiatry*. Rochester, VT: Bear & Co.

Meleis, A. (2012). *Theoretical nursing: Development and progress* (5th ed.). Philadelphia, PA: Lippincott Williams & Wilkins.

Narayanasamy, A. (2010). Recognising spiritual needs. In W. McSherry & L. Ross (Eds.), *Spiritual assessment in healthcare practice* (pp. 37–55). Cumbria, England: M & K Publishing.

Narayanasamy, A. (2011). Commentary on Chan M. F. (2009) Factors affecting nursing staff in practicing spiritual care. *Journal of Clinical Nursing, 20*(5–6), 915–916. doi:10.1111/j .1365-2702.2010.03653.x

O'Brien, M. (2011). *Spirituality in nursing: Standing on holy ground* (4th ed.). Mississauga, ON: Jones & Bartlett.

O'Donohue, H., & Quinn, S. (2011). Presence in a health care setting: Sacred time, sacred space, and sacred touch. *Presence: An International Journal of Spiritual Direction, 17*(4), 28–32.

Olson, J., & Clark, M. (2010). Spirituality. In A. J. Berman, S. Snyder, L. Yiu, L. Stamler, M. Buck, S. Bouchal, & S. Hirst (Eds.), *Kozier & Erb's Fundamentals of Nursing* (2nd Canadian ed., pp. 1471–1488). Toronto, ON: Pearson Education Canada.

Parachini, P. (2011). Attentiveness to the spiritual needs of the seriously ill. *Presence: An International Journal of Spiritual Direction, 17*(4), 51–58.

Partridge, C. (2010). Residential schools: The intergenerational impacts on aboriginal peoples. *Native Social Work Journal, 7*, p.33–62

Peck, S. (1978). *The road less travelled*. New York, NY: Simon and Schuster.

Perry, B. (2009). *More moments in time: Images of exemplary nursing*. Edmonton, AB: Athabasca University Press.

Pesut, B. (2003). Developing spirituality in the curriculum: Worldviews, intrapersonal connectedness, interpersonal connectedness. *Nursing Education Perspectives, 24*(6), 290–294.

Pesut, B. (2008). A conversation on diverse perspectives of spirituality in nursing literature. *Philosophy and Palliative Care, 9*, 98–109.

Pesut, B. (2009). Ontologies of nursing in an age of spiritual pluralism: Closed or open worldview? *Nursing Philosophy, 11*, 15–23.

Pike, J. (2011). Spirituality in nursing: A systematic review of the literature from 2006-10. *British Journal of Nursing, 20*(12), 743–749.

Pinto, S., March, P., Johnston Taylor, E., & Pravikoff, D. (2010). Spiritual needs of hospitalized patients: Evidence based care sheet. *Cinahl Information Systems, 50*, 2.

Plante, T. (Ed.). (2010). *Contemplative practices in action: Spirituality, meditation and health*. Santa Barbara, CA: Praeger.

Plotnikoff, G., & Dandurand, D. (2012). Integrating spiritual assessment and care. In D. Rakel (Ed.), *Integrative Medicine* (3rd ed., pp. 964–969). Toronto, ON: Saunders.

Potter, P. J., & Frisch, N. C. (2013). The holistic caring process. In B. M. Dossey & L. Keegan (Eds.), *Holistic nursing: A handbook for practice* (6th ed., pp. 145–160). Boston, MA: Jones & Bartlett.

Puchalski, C., & Ferrel, B. (2010). *Making healthcare whole: Integrating spirituality into patient care.* West Conshohocken, PA: Templeton Press.

Rakel, D., & Jonas, W. (2012). Creating optimal healing environments. In D. Rakel (Ed.), *Integrative medicine* (3rd ed., pp. 12–19). Toronto, ON: Saunders.

Rakel, D., & Weil, A. (2012). Philosophy of integrative medicine. In D. Rakel (Ed.), *Integrative medicine* (3rd ed., pp. 2–11). Toronto, ON: Saunders.

Rindfleisch, J., & Reed, G. (2013). Healing through forgiveness. In D. Rakel (Ed.), *Integrative Medicine* (3rd ed., pp. 867–872). Toronto, ON: Saunders.

Robbins, J., & Dewar, J. (2011). Traditional indigenous approaches to healing and the modern welfare of traditional knowledge, spirituality and lands: A critical reflection on practices and policies taken from the Canadian indigenous example. *The International Indigenous Policy Journal, 2* (4). Retrieved from: http://ir.lib.uwo.ca/iipj/vol2/iss4/2

Rogers, C. (1961). *On becoming a person: A therapist's view of psychotherapy.* New York, NY: Houghton Mifflin.

Rosenbloom, D., Williams, M., & Watkins, B. (2010). *Life after trauma: A workbook for healing* (2nd ed.). New York, NY: Guilford Press.

Scott Barss, K. (2012a). T.R.U.S.T.: An affirming model for inclusive spiritual care. *Journal of Holistic Nursing, 30*(1), 24–34. doi:10.1177/0898010111418118

Scott Barss, K. (2012b). Building bridges: An interpretive phenomenological analysis of nurse educators' clinical experience using the T.R.U.S.T. Model for inclusive spiritual care. *International Journal of Nursing Education Scholarship, 8*(1), 118.

Seaward, B. (2012). *Managing stress: Principles and strategies for health and well-being* (7th ed.). Mississauga, ON: Jones & Bartlett.

Sharpnack, P., Quinn Griffin, M., & Fitzpatrick, J. (2011). Self-transcendence and spiritual well-being in the Amish. *Journal of Holistic Nursing, 29*(2), 91–97.

Spiritual Directors International. (2013). *What is spiritual direction?* http://www.sdiworld.org/find-a-spiritual-director/what-is-spiritual-direction

Statistics Canada. (2013). *2011 national household survey data table: Religion, immigrant status, and period of immigration.* Retrieved from http://www12.statcan.gc.ca/nhs-enm/2011/dp-pd/dt-td/Rp-eng.cfm?LANG=E&APATH=3&DETAIL=0&DIM=0&FL=A&FREE=0&GC=0&GID=0&GK=0&GRP=1&PID=105399&PRID=0&PTYPE=105277&S=0&SHOWALL=0&SUB=0&Temporal=2013&THEME=95&VID=0&VNAMEE=&VNAMEF

Stedman, C. (2012). *Faithiest: How an atheist found common ground with the religious.* Boston, MA: Beacon Press.

Stukes, P. (2011). Healing the post-modern soul. *Presence: An International Journal of Spiritual Direction, 17*(4), 33–43.

Teasdale, W. (1999). *The mystic heart: Discovering a universal spirituality in the world's religions.* Novato, CA: New World Library.

The Centre for Contemplative Mind in Society. (2013). *Contemplative practices.* Retrieved from http://www.contemplativemind.org/practices

The Fetzer Institute. (2013). *Consider forgiveness: Forgiveness, love, reconciliation.* Retrieved from http://www.fetzer.org/resources/consider-forgiveness-forgiveness-love-reconciliation

The Focusing Institute. (2012). *Focusing.* Retrieved from http://www.focusing.org/

Thomas, J. C., Burton, M., Quinn Griffin, M. T., & Fitzpatrick, J. J. (2010). Self-transcendence, spiritual well-being and spiritual practices of women with breast cancer. *Journal of Holistic Nursing, 28,* 115–122.

Thornton, L., & Mariano, C. (2013). Evolving from therapeutic to holistic communication. In B. M. Dossey & L. Keegan (Eds.), *Holistic nursing: A handbook for practice* (6th ed., pp. 619–631). Boston, MA: Jones & Bartlett.

Todres, L. (2011). *Embodied enquiry: Phenomenological touchstones for research, psychotherapy and spirituality.* New York, NY: Palgrave MacMillan.

Travelbee, J. (1966). *Interpersonal aspects of nursing.* Philadelphia, PA: F. A. Davis.

Trudeau, L., & Cherubini, L. (2010). Speaking our truths in "a good way." *Canadian Journal of Native Education, 33*(1), 113–156.

Truth and Reconciliation Commission of Canada. (2012) *Our mandate.* Retrieved from http://www.trc.ca/websites/trcinstitution/index.php?p=7#Principles

Ulrich, A., Evron, L., & Ostenfeld-Rosenthal, A. (2011). Patients' views of CAM as spiritual practice. *Complementary Therapies in Clinical Practice, 17*(4), 221–225.

Wagner, J., & Simington, J. (2011). Spirit at work in long-term care. *Humane Healthcare, 10*(2). Retrieved from http://www.humanehealthcare.com/Article.asp?art_id=910

Wilson, D., & Restoole, J.-P. (2010). Tobacco ties: The relationship of the sacred to research. *Canadian Journal of Native Education, 33*(1), 29–45.

Wright, L. (2007). Softening suffering through spiritual care practices: One possibility for healing families. *Journal of Family Nursing, 14*(4), 394–411. doi:10.1177/1074840708326493

Wright, L., & Bell, J. (2010). *Beliefs and illness: A model for healing.* Calgary, AB: 4th Floor Press.

Young, C., & Koopsen, C. (2011). *Spirituality, health and healing: An integrative approach* (2nd ed.). Toronto, ON: Jones & Bartlett.

Nursing as Lifelong Learning

BETTY CRAGG

*S*amantha is a third-year nursing student doing a clinical rotation on a medical ward. During break time in the conference room, she sees a notice on the bulletin board announcing sessions to teach staff to use the new electronic record system. Samantha has used electronic records during other rotations and has found them easy to learn. She is surprised to hear one of the older nurses saying it would take at least three sessions to learn the charting system and she wasn't looking forward to having to learn something new. One of the other nurses then said, "We are constantly learning. Remember when we got the new monitors? They're computer-based and that was easy, but it is not always easy to learn new skills. I'll bet Samantha can help us learn how to use the new system because nursing students are used to using computers for school." Other nurses join the conversation commenting about the things they have learned in the past few months and how they have to keep learning to maintain the competencies required for registration every year.

CHAPTER OBJECTIVES

By the end of this chapter, you will be able to:

1. Explain the importance of continuous learning for maintaining a professional practice that is safe, ethical, and competent.
2. Describe how nursing knowledge is developed, modified, and disseminated.
3. Learn to identify your learning needs and effective strategies to fulfill them.
4. Identify strategies to maintain competence throughout your nursing career.
5. Describe methods to develop skills for interprofessional practice.
6. Plan the first steps in your nursing career.
7. Develop a plan for building and maintaining a personal professional portfolio.
8. Identify how a portfolio can be used in furthering your nursing career.

KEY TERMS

Career Planning A process of identifying a desired professional career path and the personal, educational, organizational, and social factors that need to be in place to accomplish that path.

Interprofessional Competence Ability of health-care providers from several health professions to communicate and work effectively together to enhance patient care.

Learning Contract A document that may be shared with others that specifies how learning will be accomplished, including outcomes, evidence of learning, and time lines for accomplishment.

Learning Plan A plan for meeting an identified learning need. It includes the outcomes desired and the means of achieving and evaluating the learning.

Lifelong Learning The continuous development of new knowledge, skills, and attitudes throughout a nurse's career.

Nursing Knowledge The unique knowledge based on which nurses build their practice. It is a combination of ideas, research evidence, and theories drawn from nursing and related fields.

Professional Competence Ability to demonstrate required competencies for various levels of professional practice or specialization.

Professional Portfolio An organized accumulation of evidence demonstrating competencies and achievements relevant to professional success.

Professional Socialization The process of assuming the knowledge base, attitudes, and values of a particular professional group.

Self-Directed Learning A process by which an individual takes responsibility for learning by identifying a learning need and developing a personal plan as well as implementation and evaluation strategies.

Nursing Knowledge

Nursing knowledge is the unique combination of theories, evidence, and experience that nurses apply to their practice. Nurses take information, research evidence, and theoretical perspectives from a broad range of academic disciplines, including social sciences, biologic sciences, medicine, and the humanities. They combine knowledge from these sources with understanding gained from experience in the practice of nursing, nurses' theoretical perspectives, and research unique to nursing to create a knowledge base they bring to their care of individuals, families, and communities. Nursing knowledge is applied in every interaction nurses have with patients or clients. Nursing knowledge expands through observations, identification of researchable questions, and application of new ideas to nursing practice.

Sources of Nursing Knowledge

As nurses, we have knowledge that has been handed down through nurses, midwives, wise women, and shamans who have practiced healing arts since the beginning of time. We have nursing knowledge developed through experience and the work of nurse scholars and researchers. We also use essential background knowledge from related fields such as the biomedical sciences (anatomy, physiology, pharmacology) and the social sciences (psychology, sociology, anthropology) and other health professions (medicine, nutrition, physiotherapy). In nursing school, in classes, labs, and clinical practice, we learn knowledge, skills, and attitudes necessary to practice as professional nurses. We develop more psychomotor, cognitive, and interpersonal skills as we start our careers as nurses and move into specialty areas. In our jobs, we learn what individuals and groups of patients and clients require for healing, health, and well-being. We learn theories in school that have been developed in nursing and related fields. Theories develop further, and applications change over time as research and experience inform our practice. We learn which theories are most useful to guide us as we practice our profession. Our practice is further shaped by evidence that includes research findings as well as through our professional and personal experience. Our interactions with patients lead to a deeper understanding of their conditions, their needs, and the nursing actions that are effective in providing good nursing care.

Development of Nursing Knowledge

Nursing knowledge develops in many ways; theory development and research are perhaps the most obvious ways in academic settings. Theories give us structure to organize our thinking about nursing and the health phenomena we encounter. We learn to frame questions and develop ideas and hypotheses to test through research. Research provides systematic study of particular questions. If the methods are sound and the situations are relevant to our practice, we can integrate the findings into our nursing care. Clinical guidelines provide a summary of research evidence, allowing us to use the best knowledge that exists. However, nurses working in direct contact with patients also develop knowledge. They modify their approaches based on what they find works, on the preferences of their patients, and what they learn from each other. They also ask questions about what the best nursing approach is or what is really going on with a particular population that can lead to formal research studies. The findings from that research can then inform nursing care internationally.

Through the eyes of a nurse

As nurses working in an environment of constant change, it is necessary for us to develop our knowledge and skills to cope with the demands of health care.
(personal reflection of Gurpreet, a surgical nurse)

How Is Nursing Knowledge Disseminated?

Nursing knowledge is disseminated in many ways, depending on the level of the student or nurse. Nursing schools base their programs and individual courses on the latest nursing knowledge. Researchers in universities and health-care institutions share their findings through local presentations, conferences, and publications. With more and more access to articles and other materials through the Internet, nurses in practice are able to identify the latest findings that are relevant to their specialty and can therefore modify their practice.

However, many nurses who have been practicing for years do not believe they have the skills and knowledge to access, review, and judge the quality and applicability of new findings. They may feel uncomfortable assessing the quality of research methods and findings. They may not have access to the latest literature or know how to find it. Going to conferences may be too expensive and time-consuming. If material is available but practicing nurses do not have the computer skills to find it or the critical appraisal skills to judge whether the findings of research should be integrated into their practice, the existence of knowledge will not lead to better patient care.

Evidence-Informed Practice

Health-care professions are increasingly emphasizing the need to base interventions on evidence. Getting new knowledge out to practitioners—what we think of as knowledge transfer—and encouraging them to use it has become a major field of study because although practitioners want to provide good care and may be aware of the push to use evidence as the basis for practice, they may not actually incorporate the latest findings into their care. Changing practice is difficult and involves persuading others to modify their approach. Persuasion takes time and energy that busy practitioners may not have, especially when the tried and true seems to be working just fine. To deal with some of these issues, there has been a move to summarize findings through clinical practice guidelines and provide sessions to teach frontline health workers to assess evidence. Institutional policies and procedures as well as interventions are expected to be informed by evidence. Similarly, this book uses published research findings to support the skills and procedures being taught.

Valuing Different Sources of Knowledge

In some circles, the systematic review of randomized controlled trials has been held up as the highest level of evidence (Centre for Evidence-based Medicine, 2010). All other forms of research, such as quasi-experimental designs, qualitative studies based on interviews with people who have lived through experiences, or practitioner experience, are given less value. This tendency to dismiss anything but the randomized controlled trial may be valid for drug trials and other interventions where it is ethically possible to try a new drug or treatment while using a placebo or usual approach with a control group. However, in many instances in nursing, we tend to be more inclusive in our acceptance of other forms of evidence (Registered Nurses Association of Ontario, 2010). It might be unethical to withhold a nursing approach or intervention in order to have a control group to demonstrate its efficacy. For example, how could we deliberately refuse to establish a therapeutic relationship with someone? Therefore, we have to rely on other forms of evidence and to value them as reflecting the realities of our practice. Experience is one source that also provides evidence allowing an expert nurse to choose one intervention over another.

Self-Directed Learning

Because knowledge is constantly evolving through research, theory, and experience, nurses cannot rely on what they learned in nursing school for the rest of their careers. They will have to continue to learn, and each nurse will have different learning needs. During your practice as a nurse, you will have to assume more and more control over what you learn and how you learn it. It begins as a student; as you make choices, you can develop skills as a self-directed learner that will be useful to you throughout your professional career. As a student, you decide which topic you will research for a paper or presentation. Which clinical area will you request for your integrative practicum experience? What electives will you choose? In an undergraduate nursing program, the curriculum determines much of the material you must learn to graduate. Your early focus is on the mastery of specific knowledge to succeed when you write the Canadian Registered Nurse Examination (CRNE) (Canadian Nurses Association [CNA], 2010a) or, as of 2015, the National

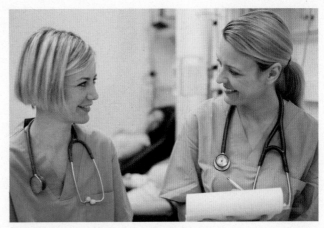

Figure 41.1 A senior nurse can be a good resource for a young or newly graduated nurse.

Council Licensure Examination (NCLEX) examinations and to practice safely as a nurse. Later, there may be educators where you work who have the responsibility for orientation and continuing education. With the wide variety of learning needs and experiences of working nurses, nurses have to assume personal responsibility for identifying their own learning needs and developing strategies to learn. The specialty area where you choose to practice, changes in equipment, medications, and approaches to practice will require you to continue to learn if you are to remain competent (Fig. 41.1).

In the case at the beginning of this chapter, Samantha knows how to learn new patient record systems. She is comfortable with computers and not afraid of experimenting. She knows the general principles of charting and can identify how they are incorporated in the electronic system. Nurses who are less comfortable with computer skills may turn to her as a nonthreatening expert to help them learn what they will need to know to meet the charting expectations of their jobs. However, Samantha herself recognizes that she does not know much about drugs prescribed for renal patients and their side effects. She decides that she must develop a plan to master the content she requires to give these medications safely and to assess her patients.

Identification of Knowledge Gaps

The first step in **self-directed learning** is identification of a learning need (Knowles, 1975). This need may be dictated externally by an employer or the arrival on the unit of a new piece of equipment. Internal driving forces may include discomfort with aspects of practice or a patient admitted with an unfamiliar condition, leading a nurse to seek to learn more. The identification of a learning need and a desire to fill a gap in knowledge are important first steps regardless of whether the need is to learn a psychomotor skill or an interpersonal skill. Adult learners learn best when

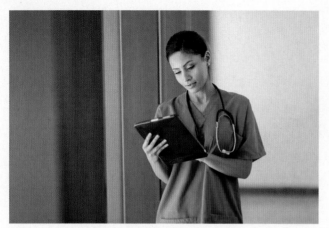

Figure 41.2 Learning new technology, such as use of a tablet device, can fill a knowledge gap.

they understand the need to develop further and have some control over the circumstances of their learning (Fig. 41.2).

Developing goals for your learning helps you to clarify exactly what you want to learn. If you express your goals vaguely, for example, "Know more about the aging process," it will be difficult to demonstrate to yourself or anyone else that you have learned what you wanted to. The clearer the goal, the more likely you are to achieve it. One approach to being sure your goal can be attained is to use the SMART acronym. This indicates the goal will be Specific, Measurable, Attainable, Relevant, and Time-framed (Brock University, n.d.; College of Nurses of Ontario, 2010). Therefore, instead of "Know more about the aging process," a SMART goal might include the following: "In the next month, use the Internet, library references, and information from elderly patients to identify five physiologic changes that occur after the menopause that have an impact on the musculoskeletal system of women and their impact on sense of well-being and physical activity."

Learning Style Preferences

People learn differently. Some prefer to read textbooks or articles or search the Internet, some like formal classes and lectures, others seek out experts for consultation or watch video recordings, whereas still others need to have hands-on experience to remember concepts and what to do in certain situations (Learning Styles Online, n.d.). We have all experienced various teaching–learning strategies in formal educational programs and informal situations and have learned from them, even if they do not completely meet our preferences. It is helpful to reflect on what learning strategies work best for you. For example, some people prefer to go from theory to practice, whereas others find it easier to learn theory after they have had a real-world experience to relate it to. Do you prefer to have clinical or simulation experience to which you can tie classroom learning or do you like to have a chance to master the theory before you are expected to deal with a problem in the real world? Reflecting on which

learning approaches work best for you and what alternatives may be satisfactory if you cannot completely match all your preferences is a good way to start directing your own learning. Many professors are upset because students do not come to class. In some cases, this is a reflection of poor priority setting and organization on the part of the students, but in others, students have recognized that lectures and group discussion are not the best way for them to master the material. They may feel that time spent reviewing the class notes online, researching on the Internet, and reading the textbook will be more effective for mastering the necessary content and to pass the exam. However, it is important for students to also consider the learning outcomes of the course or class. If developing group process skills is one of those outcomes, staying at home looking things up on the computer will not provide the interpersonal experience to build the necessary skills.

Through the eyes of a nurse

*L*earning is a lifelong process anyway; it happens in the conscious as well as the unconscious mind. However, **lifelong learning** conjures up images of an active learner. An active learner is one who keeps an open mind and a twinkle in the eye whether one is 20 or 70 years old. . . . The "lifelong learner" has the wisdom to know that active learning can go on for as long as one wishes to.

(personal reflection of Mari, a nurse educator)

Developing a Learning Plan/Contract

An organized plan for learning means you are more likely to achieve your goals. NurseOne (2010) has templates that help you reflect on learning needs and create a plan. Sometimes, a **learning plan** is framed as a **learning contract**, either with yourself or with someone else (University of Waterloo, n.d.). The contract may be with a teacher, a supervisor, a colleague, or a friend. Having someone else know about and support your desire to learn may provide an extra incentive to carry out your plan, particularly if it is for something you know you need to know but are not enthusiastic about. Establish a time frame for checking in on your progress. If it is a big task, identify interim points to check that you are making progress. It helps to measure success along the way, not only at the end. In self-directed learning, you usually don't receive a mark, so you have to develop ways of rewarding yourself for your successful mastery of the content you want to learn. If you realize you are not achieving your interim goals, you have an opportunity to revise your plan and renegotiate the contract. You may learn things you did not anticipate as you carry out your plan. Do not neglect this serendipitous learning. It may prove to be as valuable in the long run as the things you intended to learn (Table 41.1).

	Strategies to Achieve My Goal	Resources I Will Use for Learning	Evaluation Methods	Deadlines	If This Is a Learning Contract
TABLE 41.1 Learning Plan Template					
Learning Goal					
What do I want to learn?	What fits with my learning preferences and the resources (including time) available to me?	People, written and online resources, activities, formal learning activities, informal sources of information	How will I demonstrate to myself and others that I have achieved my goal? What are some interim steps that will show I am working toward my goal?	When do I hope to achieve my learning? When will I achieve my interim steps?	Who will I contract with to help me demonstrate my learning?

Using or modifying this table may help you develop learning plans for yourself. You may find you prefer a different way of organizing what you want to learn and how you want to learn it.

*S*amantha realizes she needs to learn more about renal medications. She has access to medication references on the unit, to a drug list on her, and to nurses who are experienced in giving medications to renal patients on the unit and assessing their effectiveness. There is also a consulting pharmacist who comes to the unit every morning.

Samantha decides to create a learning plan for herself. She consults her clinical instructor and agrees that a learning contract would help her to ensure she learns what she and her patients need her to know. Samantha has already identified that she is a visual learner. She likes to read material, follow diagrams, and map out the implications of material in her head before she applies her learning. However, she is also a relational learner, who likes to consult other people, including experts and fellow learners, and discuss her learning to confirm she is on the right track. Samantha draws up a learning contract and shares it with her clinical instructor. See Samantha's plan in Table 41.2.

In the course of implementing her plan, Samantha learns from the pharmacist how her profession can support nurses in dealing with problems with medications. One of the patients on the ward has real difficulty swallowing pills, and the pharmacist is helpful in providing alternatives. Samantha also learns that there is a clinical trial of a new medication occurring on the unit. She has the opportunity to review the research protocol, talk to the local leader of the study, administer the medication, talk to patients who have consented to join the study, and learn of some of their anxieties about whether they are on the medication or placebo and whether the medication is having any effect on their condition. Samantha did not plan to learn these things but realizes she has gained knowledge that she will use throughout her career.

Development of Critical Thinking Throughout Your Career

Developing clinical judgment through the exercise of critical thinking is a vital skill for every competent nurse to learn. We are able to deal with the unfamiliar and crises because of our thinking skills. We do not simply accept policies and procedures or blindly follow orders. We take into account the patient's condition, needs, and preferences; the context within which we are giving care; the norms and expectations of the profession and the institution; and our own values as we think through situations and reach decisions. While developing expertise and skills in a particular area of nursing, your critical thinking and problem-solving skills will also improve. Throughout this text, you have been presented with critical thinking exercises to help you develop these skills.

Through the eyes of a nurse

I consider my internal needs of striving for challenges and being the best you can be—not just in my personal life but also in my professional life. Lifelong learning to me satisfies these needs and allows the curiosity in me to thrive.
(personal reflection of Abha, a public health nurse)

Application/Adaptation of Knowledge to Unique Situations

It is in unique situations that thinking skills become most important when clinical judgment comes into play (Benner, Sutphen, Leonard, & Day, 2010). Rules, policies, and standards are needed because we literally have life and death in our hands and because nursing is a 24 hours–a-day/7 days–a-week activity where other nurses must be able to anticipate what their colleagues will do. Policies and procedures,

TABLE 41.2	**Samantha's Learning Plan**				
Learning Goal	**Strategies to Achieve My Goal**	**Resources I Will Use for Learning**	**Evaluation Methods**	**Deadlines**	**If This Is a Learning Contract**
List which meds are most frequently used.	Check out which renal meds are used most regularly on the floor.	Check the MARS for the renal meds in use this week.	List of common renal medications verified by teacher or experienced renal nurse	2 days	Clinical instructor will verify I achieved my interim and final goals.
Identify actions and side effects. Identify alternative medications.	Read about renal medications. Consult people who are knowledgeable about renal meds.	Use my pharmacology, pathophysiology, and adult nursing texts; PDA references; and reference manuals on the floor not only for the meds used this week but also for other common renal meds.	List of actions and side effects of each medication and nontraditional alternatives	First clinical day next week	
Identify how patients perceive being on renal meds.	Learn the patients' experience with renal meds.	Check out websites for meds and blogs of experiences of renal patients. Talk to nurses on the unit, MDs, and pharmacologist. Interview patients about their experiences.	Write a summary of patient perceptions.	By the end of the rotation	
Discharge— Teach one patient about medications.	Plan a teaching session.	Patient teaching theory from courses and texts	Carry out teaching: Patient will be able to explain the reasons for being on the medication and what side effects to look for.	By the end of the rotation	

MARS, Medication Administration Record.

Learning need: Increase understanding of renal medications.

practice guidelines, care maps, and other guides for practice are based on the usual, whereas it is the unusual situation that demands creativity. Some unusual circumstances might be the following: The patient is not responding as anticipated to the plan of care; there are no home supports to allow prompt discharge; and the patient's wife has been hospitalized herself for the same condition. The nurse works with the patient, the family, the community, other members of the nursing staff, and the entire interprofessional team to achieve the best care and outcomes for this particular person or group of people. Achieving the objective may require unorthodox approaches. If we allow ourselves to be too constrained by rules, we may not provide the best possible care. Rules may have to be broken or at least bent to provide optimal nursing care. In departing from usual practice, nurses must be able to justify their actions with clear rationales and communicate what has been done and why so that others can follow the train of thought and provide continuity of care. Justifying and communicating unusual decisions is as important as making them.

Developing Your Identity as a Nurse

Having a strong nursing identity creates comradeship and easy understanding among nurses. However, because nurses and members of other health-care professions are socialized into their own professional mindsets, communication among different professions may be difficult. Different professionals bring differing assumptions, concerns, and even vocabulary to a discussion. An interprofessional team working to plan patient care may be talking at cross-purposes at a risk to good patient care. For example, a nurse and physiotherapist are talking about transferring a patient. The nurse uses *transfer* in a plan to send the patient to long-term care; the physiotherapist is concerned about getting the patient from bed to chair. Until they realize they are using the same word for different things, they are not communicating.

It is important to reflect on the professional attitudes you are developing. Part of identifying your attitudes may come through sharing what you are learning about your profession. Take opportunities to share your experiences and your point of view with students from other health professions. You will learn to explain your views as a nurse and the things that concern nurses and will also help you to understand the perspective of other professionals. When health-care professionals can understand each other, patient care will be better and safer.

Professional Socialization

As you take nursing courses and learn to practice as a nurse, a process known as **professional socialization** is occurring. You are not only learning about nursing and how to practice but you are also becoming a nurse and forming an identity as a nurse. Nurses share values, attitudes, and beliefs with other members of the profession around the world. This socialization allows us to communicate better with each other, to understand the assumptions that are driving nurses' actions, and to work cooperatively with other members of our profession. Ask nurses how they became nurses, and you will get as many answers as people you ask. However, despite a unique path for each student, by the end of a nursing program, graduates have assumed a professional identity. The new graduate has become a nurse, and this professional identity will continue to change and develop with experience.

Novice to Expert

In a 1984 study, Benner used the Dreyfus model of expertise development to identify how nurses progress in their professional practice from being novices through advanced beginner, competent, and proficient stages to the level of expert. Whereas the novice is rule-bound and has difficulty putting things together, experts have developed intuitive knowledge that allows them to recognize patterns and anticipate problems earlier than any of the other groups. Nurses' comprehension of what it is to be a professional and how to exercise professional expertise also matures with continuing practice of the profession. However, being an expert in one field of nursing practice does not make a nurse an expert in all areas of nursing. Going back to school or changing jobs or specialties, a nurse reverts to an earlier phase of development.

Through the eyes of a nurse

Lifelong learning is a constant phenomenon within the field of nursing. As a nurse, I am constantly growing and learning through my experience with patients and families. Reflection on these interactions can reveal a wealth of knowledge and greater understanding of who I am and what I wish to become.
(personal reflection of Elisha, a medical nurse)

Maintaining Competence

When you graduate from your program, you will have attained entry-level **professional competence** as a registered nurse (RN). The CNA uses competencies to create the CRNE, and each provincial and territorial registering body has identified entry competencies for their new registrants. As a nurse works, the expectation is that additional competencies above and beyond those of the entering practitioner will be developed. The self-directed learning skills discussed at the beginning of the chapter are essential to develop and maintain your competence. Practicing nurses need to keep track of trends in their field and need to develop strategies for learning to accommodate change.

To protect the public, registering bodies expect practicing nurses to demonstrate each year that they have maintained their competence. Every provincial and territorial registering body has a continuing competency program that registrants must follow to renew their registration annually. There are some differences in requirements, but demonstrating self-reflection, development of learning plans, participation in continuing education, peer feedback, hours worked, and practice assessment are among ways required.

Through the eyes of a nurse

I think in terms of nursing, "lifelong learning" is a commitment that we all must make when becoming a nurse. There are always new ways of doing things or new knowledge being discovered or uncovered thus to provide the best care (which we as nurses strive to do). We must make a commitment to ourselves and to the public to be a continuous, lifelong learner.
(personal reflection of Nikki, nurse educator)

Many specialty groups have identified specific competencies required for skilled practice by nurses working within those specialties. The CNA (2010b) has developed a certification program to allow nurses to demonstrate that they have developed specialty knowledge and skills that exceed the expectations of a newly graduated nurse. The CNA certification process requires demonstration of learning through an examination and either examination or demonstration of continuous learning for renewal.

It remains the responsibility of each nurse to identify how the necessary knowledge and skills will be acquired to meet requirements of demonstrating that competence has been maintained. Learning may be through informal conversations, focused reading, going to continuing education sessions, or seeking a new credential. All are important ways of maintaining and increasing competence.

Nurse as Lifelong Learner

The nurse has many possible options to explore lifelong learning. From the informal learning that occurs on the unit to graduate-level education, learning opportunities abound. It is up to each nurse to create his or her own strategy to maintain learning throughout her professional life.

*S*amantha realizes that she will continue to learn throughout her career, but she may not yet be aware of all the options that will be available to her. Informal learning or formal courses and credit programs will be part of her further education. She can choose self-directed learning projects such as the one she used for renal medications. She may decide to attend in-service presentations within her workplace. She may even teach in-services in areas where she has expertise, for example, on electronic charting. Doing a good job of teaching others can be a valuable way to learn something thoroughly.

Informal Learning

Informal learning occurs every day, as we read online, watch the news, talk to colleagues, and interact with patients. Planned informal learning helps a nurse to focus what she wants to learn and helps her achieve her goals. The learning contract discussed on p. xx helps organize this kind of learning. There are also opportunities for gaining recognition or certification through demonstrating that informal learning has occurred. Some educational institutions have Prior Learning Assessment and Recognition programs that allow learners to receive credit when they demonstrate that they have met course objectives through work or other forms of informal learning.

Formal Learning

There are times when the best way to learn or to gain recognition for learning is to participate in formal learning activities. These can range from in-services that provide certification or recertification for skills such as advanced cardiac life support (ACLS) or hemodynamic monitoring to achieving a doctorate in nursing.

In-Services and Organization Meetings

In-services in the workplace may or may not provide certification, but they are frequently used as a way to reach a high proportion of nursing staff, spread new knowledge and techniques, reinforce correct approaches, or allow staff to share experiences and new knowledge they have acquired through attending conferences. Nursing organizations and specialty groups may have local meetings. These meetings usually include an educational component that allows nurses in the area to meet an expert or share new knowledge.

Conferences

Professional organizations, research groups, universities, and others hold local, national, or international conferences to allow those with similar interests to meet each other and share the latest findings. Going to conferences can be professionally rewarding because there are opportunities to network with practitioners from other locations, hear internationally recognized speakers, attend oral presentations reporting the latest findings that are not yet in the literature, and talk to poster presenters about their interests. Going to conferences can be expensive, so few nurses from any given area are able to attend. To spread the word, many local groups and employers ask attendees to share their experiences when they return.

Credit Courses—Certificates

To work in specialized areas, many employers require a formal course and/or certification. For example, many intensive care units (ICUs) require an ICU course before beginning nursing practice in that area. They may offer a program themselves, send new staff to a community college, or require the nurse have a certificate before hiring. One advantage of taking a specialty course from an educational institution is that recognition for the learning is more easily transferable to other settings. The in-house program at one hospital or employer may be recognized there, but you run the risk that other employers will not accept your formal learning as transferable to their organization.

The CNA certification program allows nurses to demonstrate their expertise in 19 specialized areas of nursing practice (CNA, 2010b). Because these nurses have taken a national examination, their knowledge is recognized across the country. Some post–RN baccalaureate programs give course recognition for certification. The learning methods nurses use to prepare for certificates vary. Some take formal courses, many join study groups or communicate with other learners online, and some choose to study alone.

Graduate Studies

Formal studies at the graduate level are also open to you as a bachelor's-degree–prepared nurse. Master's degrees in nursing, administration, education, epidemiology, and many other fields may be open to you. One factor to consider in taking graduate education is how the degree serves your goals, besides the intrinsic reward of learning more.

As a nurse committed to nursing, there are advantages to pursuing graduate studies in nursing. Whatever you choose, assess which career doors you are opening or closing with your choice of program. For example, if you want to become an academic, teaching nursing, a graduate degree in nursing is usually strongly preferred, if not required. If you enroll in a master's degree program in nursing, you can take electives in fields such as education or administration as you learn about nursing in more depth. Different universities emphasize different aspects of nursing. Some focus on advanced nursing practice in clinical specialty care or may include nurse practitioner credentials in areas such as primary health care, acute care, neonatal care, or nurse anesthesia. Other programs emphasize teaching, administration, or research. In each case, you will have a deeper understanding of the theory and practice of nursing and achieve greater sophistication in your knowledge of research.

Doctoral studies are generally focused on becoming a researcher in a specialized field of study, be it nursing or other fields. You will have several options open to you, and it is important to make a choice that suits your interests and abilities. Doctoral studies take a considerable amount of time and effort. There is also an expectation in the profession and society that a nurse who completes the doctorate in a field will provide leadership and pursue research in that field. Nurses with doctorates make up most faculties in university nursing schools and increasingly in colleges in Canada. They may take positions as nurse researchers in clinical agencies, and some work as administrators.

Learning as a Group Activity

Nursing is a group activity. Within health-care institutions, where approximately 85% of Canadian RNs work (CNA, 2009), one nurse cannot provide complete care to a patient. We have mechanisms to hand off our care to the next shift, to the nurse who is covering our lunch breaks, when we are leaving a primary nursing patient to the associate nurse, or when we share aspects of care with practical nurses or unregulated care providers. Just as we need to practice together, it helps if we learn together. Groups of nurses who have shared a learning experience are more likely to implement what they learned because they can reinforce each other in changing practice and together can explain to others what they gained from learning.

Learning with colleagues provides opportunities for greater depth because others may perceive things differently, ask questions that might never occur to us, and reinforce learning when we try to implement what we have learned. As a nursing student, you may have discovered that study groups help you to master difficult content. Nursing professors often assign group activities. These projects, presentations, and other group learning experiences allow you to learn the content and also learn group dynamics, how to deal with conflict, and how to optimize strengths within a group to accomplish more than any one person could manage. When group work is not required, it may still be useful to divide up what has to be learned so that each member of a group can master part of the content and then help the whole group get a sense of the bigger picture. Often, the best learning comes when you have to teach someone else. In the complex world of nursing practice, the more we can share our learning activities, the more likely we are to be able to join other nurses in providing the best possible nursing care.

Interprofessional Relationships

One skill that nurses and all health professionals must master is working with members of other health professions. Nurses need physicians for a medical diagnosis and treatment plan, physiotherapists to design an exercise and mobilization program for the patient, occupational therapists to assess needs for devices to support activities of daily living, social workers to mobilize community resources to support the family, and personal care workers to help maintain the patient at home. Nurses are often the co-coordinators of care for the patient, especially when planning discharge or long-term care. Knowing the particular expertise different professions may bring to your patient allows you to make appropriate consultations. Many professionals are confused about what nurses can do, so you also need to be able to explain the unique skills nurses add to a patient's care. Practice explaining to classmates and students in other professions what you are learning and share with them how your learning and scope of practice overlaps with, diverges from, or complements other professions. As your own nursing practice evolves, you will become more comfortable working with some individuals and professional groups than others. Your comfort level may partly lead to choosing one nursing specialty area over another. Even after years of practice, you cannot assume that you know all about the other professions you work with and how nursing relates to them. Just as nursing and nursing care evolve with theory development, more evidence, and lived experience, so other professions develop, and their evolution may not be parallel with that of nursing. Continuous learning with, from, and about students and practitioners from other professions will enrich your practice and help the whole team provide better care and promote patient safety.

Interprofessional Competencies

Interprofessional competence is another expectation of practicing nurses. National competencies have been developed for interprofessional practice (Canadian Interprofessional Health Collaborative, 2010). There are six competency domains that professionals must master to be effective members of interprofessional teams: role clarification, team functioning, patient/client/family/community-centred care, collaborative leadership, interprofessional communication, and interprofessional conflict resolution. Although these principles may seem fairly obvious, in reality, they may be difficult to achieve, given the differences in socialization, focus, and mind-set of different health professionals. Nurses have to learn to master interprofessional skills as well as those that lie specifically in the nursing domain. Increasingly, health-care education programs are requiring interprofessional learning experiences as part of the curriculum so that students have the opportunity to practice learning how to work together.

If there are no requirements for interprofessional learning experiences in your program, you can still seek out ways to learn more about other professions and how to work with them. There may be a chapter of the National Health Sciences Students' Association in your institution that sponsors interprofessional activities you can attend. During clinical placements, you can ask to attend patient care meetings where several professions provide input, especially if you can have an opportunity to present to the team the information about your assigned patient and nursing care. Seek opportunities to shadow members of other professions so that you can see how they approach patient care. Suggest to your clinical instructor that students from other professions who are assigned to your unit be invited to postconference to share their perceptions of patients on the unit and the care you can provide together.

Nursing Career Planning

The nursing profession has a wide range of career pathways open to you upon graduation. Your baccalaureate program is preparing you as a generalist who can function as a beginning practitioner in a wide variety of health-care settings. This means that after graduation, you can use your skills to specialize in a particular area of nursing practice. **Career planning** is important when you graduate and throughout your practice, but be aware that with a rapidly changing health-care system, there may be roles for nurses in the future that have not yet been envisioned. It is important to have a career plan, but remain open to unanticipated opportunities. You may become a critical care nurse or a community developer and work in a big city or a remote community overseas. You can pursue graduate studies or choose to develop expertise through remaining in one specialty area and learning as much as you can about it. You can be an educator, administrator, or researcher or combine any of those roles with being a practitioner. You may focus on your career or take time off while your children are young and return when they are older. You can choose to work part-time to maintain your nursing skills while you pursue other interests.

Challenges of an Abundance of Choices

Just as every student has a different path to becoming an RN, every RN will have a different career path. Some new graduates feel overwhelmed by the choices available to them. They may take the first job that comes along but not feel satisfied that they have made the best of the many choices available to them. It pays to make an inventory of what your best characteristics and skills are (Waddell, Donner, & Wheeler, 2009). What parts of nursing did you truly enjoy the most? Where do you want go with your career? What societal influences will affect your career? What are your particular values, skills, and interests? Your actions and decisions shape your career. Using your reflective and self-directed learning skills can help you to make the decisions that are best for you as a person and as a nurse.

Through the eyes of a nurse

*H*aving been a nurse for 28 years, I have learned things don't remain the same for very long. . . . Health problems change over time, and nurses always have to be aware of new illnesses, treatments, etc. Nursing is not a stagnant career choice. Change is constant, and you need to grow with the change.
(personal reflection of Maureen, a dialysis nurse)

Professional Portfolio Development

One way to demonstrate your knowledge and abilities is to maintain a **professional portfolio** (NurseOne, 2010). This process begins during your nursing education. The portfolio can begin informally; for example, if you have a box into which you throw all relevant documentation of what you have done, assignments you have completed, transcripts of marks, certificates for special training, letters of thanks or recognition you have received, or honors awarded to you. It can be electronic, paper-based, or mixed. At some point, order has to be imposed on the pile of documentation to make it tell a story about the skills you have developed and to help you persuade others that you have the background for opportunities you are interested in pursuing.

The professional portfolio can serve various functions. You may bring a short version of your portfolio to a job interview to demonstrate that you have already exhibited the skills required of the position. Although you may not have worked in a specific specialty area, your portfolio can show that you have transferable knowledge, skills, and attitudes that are relevant to a new position. You may put together a portfolio that demonstrates that you have already mastered the content of a formal program or course. This Prior Learning Assessment and Recognition (PLAR) process allows you to receive formal recognition of learning that you have gained in other ways.

A portfolio also allows you to review your own skills and talents to help you with the reflective practice requirements of many registering bodies. Some registering bodies require a portfolio to demonstrate participation in their continuing competence programs. If you are considering a career move, reviewing your portfolio can help you identify your professional strengths and any areas you would like to develop more fully by changing jobs. If you are seeking a promotion or other recognition, the portfolio is a way to show others what you have accomplished.

Although you may choose to keep everything that seems relevant to your career, when you are putting together a presentation for others, you should focus materials selectively to create a specific portfolio for your audience. Do you want to demonstrate that you coordinate things well? Then look through your previous experiences for times when you coordinated something. For example, you may have been the head lifeguard at a swimming pool when you were in university, making out the duty rosters and supervising the junior lifeguards. A cardiopulmonary resuscitation (CPR) certificate does not demonstrate coordination abilities, but advertisements for CPR recertification sessions you organized for your class and a schedule for the sessions do show these skills.

Nursing in the Future

Thinking about nursing in the future, we can predict that caring and health will remain the keystones of nursing and nursing practice. Where nurses practice, the tools and technologies they use, their scope of practice, and the challenges they face will probably be very different at the end of your career from what they are now. Nurses are pragmatic and flexible. When faced with new situations, problems, and opportunities, they seek the adventure that the future offers. Flexibility, curiosity, and a commitment to learning throughout your career will stand you in good stead as you face an uncertain future. Lifelong learning truly is a requirement for all practicing nurses. The CNA has done considerable work on what the future of nursing in Canada may be. Look at their reports and see if their predictions seem reasonable to you as you start your nursing career (CNA, 2006, 2010c). Many of the changes in nursing and health care that you experience will not be predictable, but that unpredictability can make your professional career more interesting and rewarding.

Samantha decides that she has enjoyed working with renal patients and thinks she may want to work with them when she graduates. She asks to have her integrative practicum placement on the renal unit of a different hospital. She also requests opportunities to go to the dialysis unit in that hospital and to spend time in the renal clinic so that she can have more opportunities to see the range of renal nursing. She learns there is an outreach program that offers the chance to make home visits as well. Samantha realizes that what she is taking in nursing school is just the beginning of professional learning that will continue for as long as she is a nurse.

Critical Thinking Case Scenarios

▶ You are an RN employed full-time in a long-term care setting where your responsibilities are primarily in management. Recently, you applied for a full-time position in an acute care setting and have been asked to come to an interview.

1. How will you go about identifying your learning needs to ensure that you provide safe care to the patients in this new setting and your new role?
2. Describe how a portfolio can be used to inform a future employer about the knowledge skills and experience that you possess.

▶ A patient is very persistent in asking you questions about her condition. Some of the information she is using seems to be very biased against the treatment her physician has been recommending. You realize she has been going online for additional information and is choosing websites that are selling unproven treatments and advocating actions that could lead to worsening of her symptoms.

1. How would you go about assessing online information on this condition and supporting this patient in her need for more knowledge?

▶ You are applying for a summer nursing internship position in a hospital in your hometown. You know there are three candidates for each job being offered.

1. How will you demonstrate that you are the best candidate for the position?
2. What documentation would you choose to bring with you to the interview?

▶ Recently, your unit manager announced that the hospital is investing in a different model of care delivery that will emphasize interprofessional teams.

1. How will you prepare to meet the six competency domains that professionals must master to contribute effectively to the team?
2. Conflict resolution is one of the six competency domains identified for interprofessional teams to master. What search strategies would you use to identify potential professional development opportunities for nurses seeking more information about conflict resolution?

Multiple-Choice Questions

1. A recently graduated nurse is taking action to ensure that nursing knowledge is the foundation of the care that she provides to patients and their families. The nurse should draw on which of the following potential sources of nursing knowledge? Select all that apply.
   a. The nurse's previous experiences in working with patients and families

b. Evidence from the fields of sociology and psychology

c. Reports from newspapers and magazines

d. Articles from academic journals

e. Theories relating to health and wellness

2. A nurse on a surgical unit admitted a patient who had a chest tube and needed to seek assistance from a colleague because of his unfamiliarity with the device. The nurse has resolved to embark on a process of self-directed learning and should begin by:

a. Finding a mentor who can guide him through the learning process

b. Conducting a detailed literature review, beginning with the relevant physiology

c. Admitting his lack of knowledge to the patient and the family

d. Identifying the specific learning needs that he requires in order to provide safe care

3. A patient has brought a medication to the hospital that he takes on a regular basis at home and which is not available from the hospital's pharmacy. The nurse knows that hospital policies preclude the use of medications that have been brought from home and not yet cleared by pharmacy. The nurse should:

a. Collaborate with other members of the care team to find a safe and workable solution.

b. Describe the policy to the patient and explain why it is unsafe for him to take the medication at this time.

c. Explain to the patient that he will need to sign a waiver and have it witnessed before taking the medication.

d. Withhold the drug and closely monitor the patient's health status.

4. A nurse has been working on a busy obstetrical unit for several years and has worked with a large number of patients with diverse health needs. What characteristic of the nurse's care would most clearly suggest that she has attained Benner's level of expertise?

a. The nurse is able to explain the rationale for her actions clearly.

b. The nurse never makes errors or has lapses in judgment when providing care.

c. The nurse's knowledge of medical diagnoses approximates that of the physicians'.

d. The nurse is able to reliably apply her intuition in order to guide her care.

5. An older adult patient will be returning home alone after hip replacement surgery. The nurse has met with the patient's physiotherapist and occupational therapist to address the patient's safety, mobility, and functional needs. This nurse has demonstrated:

a. Critical thinking

b. The principles of gerontology

c. Interprofessional competence

d. Advocacy for nursing

REFERENCES AND SUGGESTED READINGS

Benner, P. (1984). *From novice to expert: Excellence and power in clinical nursing practice*. Menlo Park, CA: Addison-Wesley.

Benner, P., Sutphen, M., Leonard, V., & Day, L. (2010). *Educating nurses: A call for radical transformation*. San Francisco, CA: Jossey-Bass.

Brock University. (n.d.). *How to write SMART goals*. Retrieved from http://www.brocku.ca/webfm_send/1394

Canadian Interprofessional Health Collaborative. (2010). *A national interprofessional competency framework*. Retrieved from http://www.cihc.ca/files/CIHC_IPCompetencies_Feb1210.pdf

Canadian Nurses Association. (2006). *Toward 2020: Visions for nursing*. Retrieved from http://www.cna-aiic.ca/CNA/documents/pdf/publications/Toward-2020-e.pdf

Canadian Nurses Association. (2009). *RN workforce profiles by area of responsibility 2007*. Retrieved from http://www.cna-aiic.ca/~/media/cna/page%20content/pdf%20en/2013/07/26/10/42/2007_rn_profiles_e.pdf

Canadian Nurses Association. (2010a). *Canadian Registered Nurse Examination June 2010–May 2015*. Retrieved from https://www.cna-aiic.ca/en/pages/blueprint-for-the-canadian-registered-nurse-examination-june-2010-may-2015

Canadian Nurses Association. (2010b). *CNA certification*. Retrieved from http://www.nurseone.ca/Default.aspx?portlet=StaticHtmlViewerPortlet&plang=1&ptdi=153

Canadian Nurses Association. (2010c). *The next decade: CNA's vision for nursing and health*. Retrieved from http://www.cna-aiic.ca/CNA/documents/pdf/publications/Next_Decade_2009_e.pdf

Centre for Evidence-based Medicine. (2010). *Oxford Centre for Evidence-based Medicine—Levels of evidence (March 2009)*. Retrieved from http://www.cebm.net/index.aspx?o=1025

College of Nurses of Ontario. (2010). *Developing SMART learning goals*. Retrieved from http://www.cno.org/Global/docs/qa/DevelopingSMARTGoals.pdf

Knowles, M. (1975). *Self-directed learning: A guide for learners and teachers*. New York, NY: The Adult Education Company.

Learning Styles Online. (n.d.). *Overview of learning styles*. Retrieved from http://www.learning-styles-online.com/overview/

NurseOne. (2010). *Homepage*. Retrieved from http://www.nurseone.ca/

Registered Nurses Association of Ontario. (2010). *Clinical practice guidelines and fact sheets*. Retrieved from http://www.rnao.org/Page.asp?PageID=1212&SiteNodeID=155&BL_ExpandID=

University of Waterloo. (n.d.). *Self-directed learning: Learning contracts*. Retrieved from https://uwaterloo.ca/centre-for-teaching-excellence/teaching-resources/teaching-tips/tips-students/self-directed-learning/self-directed-learning-learning-contracts

Waddell, J., Donner, G. J., & Wheeler, M. H. (2009). *Building your health care career: A guide for students*. Toronto, ON: Elsevier.

index

Note: Page numbers followed by *b*, *f*, *or t* indicate material in boxes, figures, or tables, respectively.